Wilbur McFadden, M.D.

S0-AHG-815

Wilbur McFadden, M.D.

GRIFFITH'S 5

MINUTE
CLINICAL
CONSULT

MARK R. DAMBRO, MD, FAAFP

Fort Worth, Texas
Formerly Assistant Professor of Medicine
and Director of Medical Computing
University of Arizona College of Medicine
Tucson, Arizona

JO A. GRIFFITH

Technical Editor

Previous editor:
H. Winter Griffith, MD
Editions 1993, 1994

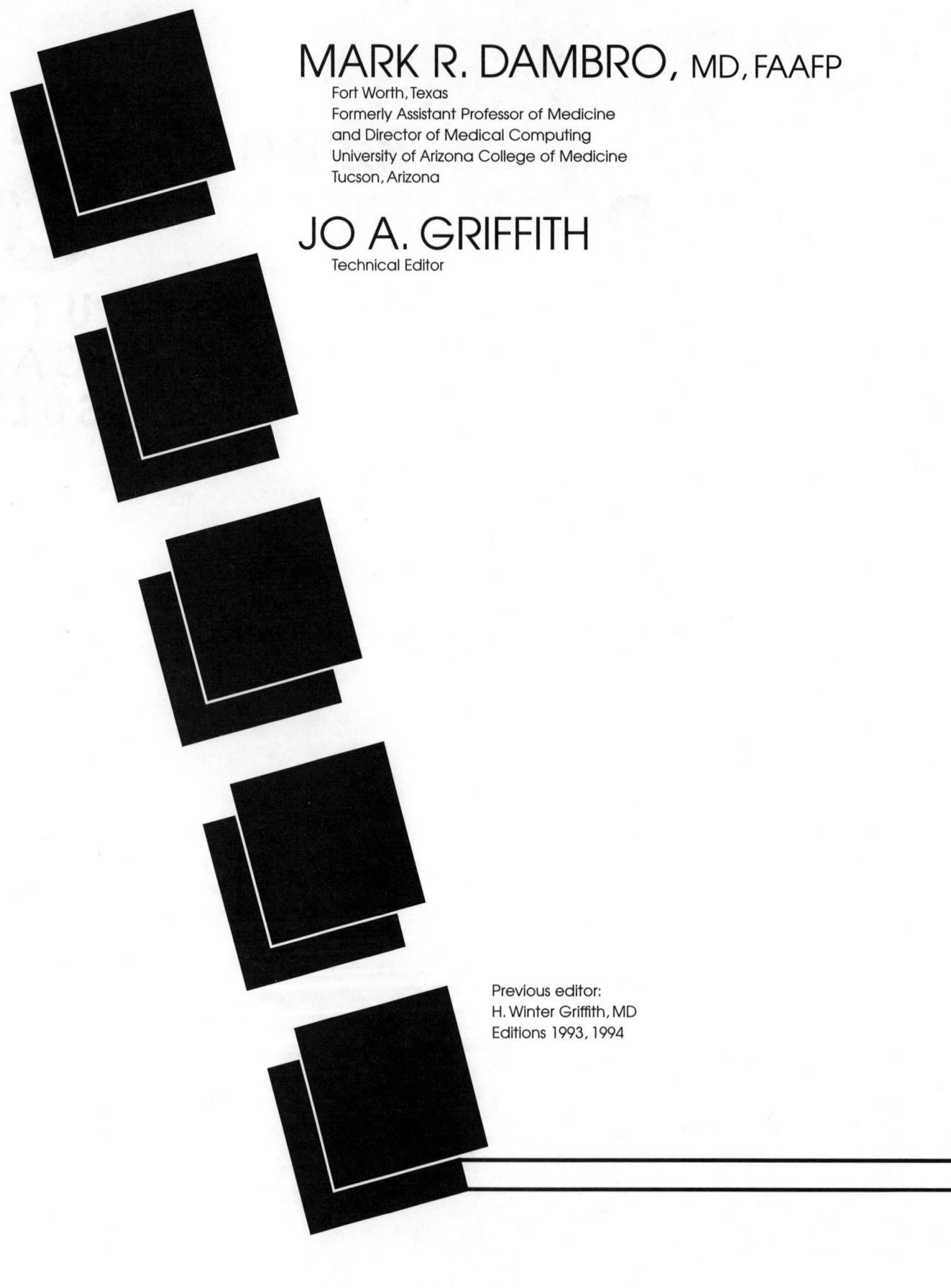

GRIFFITH'S 5
MINUTE
CLINICAL
CONSULT

Williams & Wilkins
A WAVERLY COMPANY

BALTIMORE • PHILADELPHIA • LONDON • PARIS • BANGKOK
BUENOS AIRES • HONG KONG • MUNICH • SYDNEY • TOKYO • WROCLAW

1998

Editor: Carroll C. Cann
Managing Editor: Joanne Husovsky
Marketing Manager: Daniell T. Griffin
Production Coordinator: Peter J. Carley
Project Editor: Robert D. Magee
Design Coordinator: Mario Fernandez
Typesetter: Maryland Composition Co., Inc.
Printer/Binder: RR Donnelley & Sons Company

Copyright © 1998 Williams & Wilkins

351 West Camden Street
Baltimore, Maryland 21201-2436 USA

Rose Tree Corporate Center
1400 North Providence Road
Building II, Suite 5025
Media, Pennsylvania 19063-2043 USA

All rights reserved. This book is protected by copyright. No part of this book may be reproduced in any form or by any means, including photocopying, or utilized by any information storage and retrieval system without written permission from the copyright owner.

Accurate indications, adverse reactions and dosage schedules for drugs are provided in this book, but it is possible that they may change. The reader is urged to review the package information data of the manufacturers of the medications mentioned.

Printed in the United States of America

ISBN 0-683-30578-6

The publishers have made every effort to trace the copyright holders for borrowed material. If they have inadvertently overlooked any, they will be pleased to make the necessary arrangements at the first opportunity.

To purchase additional copies of this book, call our customer service department at **(800) 638-0672** or fax orders to **(800) 447-8438.** For other book services, including chapter reprints and large quantity sales, ask for the Special Sales department.

Canadian customers should call **(800) 665-1148**, or fax **(800) 665-0103.** For all other calls originating outside of the United States, please call **(410) 528-4223** or fax us at **(410) 528-8550.**

Visit Williams & Wilkins on the Internet: **http://www.wwilkins.com** or contact our customer service department at **custserv@wwilkins.com**. Williams & Wilkins customer service representatives are available from 8:30 am to 6:00 pm, EST, Monday through Friday, for telephone access.

97 98 99 00
1 2 3 4 5 6 7 8 9 10

GRIFFITH'S *5 MINUTE CLINICAL CONSULT*—1998 represents the sixth annual edition of a quick medical reference for current medical diagnosis and treatment. These are the features:

SCOPE
One thousand topics arranged alphabetically and cross-indexed to synonyms of each. Approximately 585 **expanded** topics in a full format that contains enough detail to confirm the diagnosis and treat the problem. Approximately 414 **short** topics in a brief format.

CONTRIBUTING AUTHORS
Over 330 experienced clinicians writing on medical and surgical problems within their areas of interest and expertise.

CONSULTANTS
Thirty-eight authorities in fields of general and specialty practice. Review was for accuracy, currency, appropriateness, completeness, and safety. All medication entries and dosages were verified by a Doctor of Pharmacy and rechecked by the contributing authors prior to publication.

UPDATES
Annual. Assures inclusion of the most recent norms of practice and consensus of the majority of experts.

FORMAT
For the 585 major topics, a consistent, two-page, graphic, chart-like format, similar to the skeleton format discussed below. The six major divisions and 36 information blocks cover the major aspects of each disorder and are repeated for each topic.

BASICS	DIAGNOSIS	TREATMENT	MEDICATION	FOLLOW-UP	MISCELLANEOUS

- **BASICS**
  - Description
  - Genetics
  - Prevalence
  - Age
  - Signs and symptoms
  - Causes
  - Risk factors

- **DIAGNOSIS**
  - Differential
  - Laboratory
  - Pathological findings
  - Special tests
  - Imaging
  - Diagnostics

- **TREATMENT**
  - General measures
  - Surgical measures
  - Activity
  - Diet
  - Patient education

- **MEDICATION**
  - Drug(s) of choice
  - Contraindications
  - Precautions
  - Interactions
  - Alternate drugs

- **FOLLOW-UP**
  - Monitoring
  - Prevention
  - Complications
  - Prognosis

- **MISCELLANEOUS**
  - Associated conditions
  - Age-related factors
  - Pregnancy
  - Synonyms
  - ICD-9-CM
  - See also
  - Other notes
  - Abbreviations
  - References

PREFACE

A glance at the book's format will alert the reader to the fact that *Griffith's 5 Minute Clinical Consult* aptly lends itself to the realm of electronic media. Since its inception, the entire team has worked to make the data available in machine formats; CD-ROM, PC (PCMCIA) card, HTML (Internet), etc. It is my desire for the database to be easily accessible and to provide clinically relevant information to its readers. The database is available for several palmtop machines and is under development for several other popular platforms. Check the new web site (http://www.5mcc.com) for current information.

Toward this desire to make the data available and easily accessible, a web site is now available and is referenced in the chapters. That site, http://www.5mcc.com is certainly a work in progress, but today provides internet references that the author wants you to know about. In addition, all journal, textbook, and other "standard" references used in this book are available on this web site for your benefit.

This year, in addition to the web site, a new CD-ROM is available that includes the topic contents in a searchable format, with illustrations. Drs. Cowan and Miller have done an outstanding job of finding some excellent examples of many of the topics. I hope you'll find these illustrations helpful.

I wish to make this work continuously responsive to the needs of its readers and I thank those who have taken their time to write reviews and suggestions. I take your comments seriously and hope you will find many of them in this year's edition. This edition covers many new or newly expanded topics, and nearly 80% of the topics have new or edited material. This year a new Table of Contents sorts the topics by body system—I hope you find this valuable.

This book is a compilation of many people's efforts, including the contributing authors and the consultants who review the topics—each deserves a special thanks for their time. I'd especially like to also thank Mr. Carroll Cann, for his unending enthusiasm for this project; the staff at Williams & Wilkins who have done so much to keep the book and the concept of "The 5 Minute Clinical Consult" alive; my family for their patience and support; Drs. Gary Cowan and Scott Miller for their time in finding some really great photos and in helping me get them into a useful format; and finally, to Mrs. Jo Griffith whose persistent search for that elusive goal of perfection has so improved the book.

As before, I invite you to express your wishes regarding chapters for future editions. Send your comments and suggestions to:

Mark R. Dambro, MD
1650 W. Rosedale Street
Suite 307
Fort Worth, TX 76104

email: mrdambro@5mcc.com

BOARD OF CONSULTANTS

EDGAR ACHKAR, MD
Head, Section Gastrointestinal Diagnostic Laboratory
The Cleveland Clinic Foundation
Cleveland, OH

RODNEY D. ADAM, MD
Associate Professor of Medicine & Microbiology/Immunology
University of Arizona College of Medicine
Tucson, AZ

MICHAEL D. BAILIE, MD
Director and Senior Associate Dean
University of Illinois College of Medicine at Peoria
Peoria, IL

RUTH BECKER-SCHALLER, RN
School of Nursing
University of Arizona College of Medicine
Tucson, AZ

ROBERT C. BECKERMAN, MD
Professor of Pediatrics and Physiology
Chief, Pediatric Pulmonary Section
Tulane University School of Medicine
New Orleans, LA

JAMES B. BENJAMIN, MD
Associate Professor of Surgery
University of Arizona College of Medicine
Tucson, AZ

TIMOTHY L. BLACK, MD, FACS, FAAP
Medical Director of Trauma
Cook Children's Hospital
Fort Worth, TX

DENNIS W. BOULWARE, MD, FACP
Professor of Medicine
Division of Clinical Immunology & Rheumatology
The University of Alabama at Birmingham
Birmingham, AL

JAMES J. CORRIGAN, JR., MD
Dean
Professor of Pediatrics and Internal Medicine
Tulane University School of Medicine
New Orleans, LA

GARY COWAN, MD
Private Practice, Ophthalmology
Fort Worth, TX

STEVEN G. ECONOMOU, MD
Chairman, General Surgery
Presbyterian-St. Lukes Hospital
Chicago, IL

ATILLA ERTAN, MD
Professor of Medicine
Chief of Gastrointestinal Section, Methodist Hospital
Baylor College of Medicine
Houston, TX

JOHN L. EY, MD, MPH
Professor of Clinical Pediatrics
University of Arizona College of Medicine
Tucson, AZ

VINCENT A. FULGINITI, MD
Chancellor
Professor of Pediatrics
University of Colorado Health Sciences Center
Denver, CO

GALE GARDNER, MD, FACS
Clinical Professor
Department of Otolaryngology
University of Tennessee, Memphis
Memphis, TN

KAREN A. HARDY, MD
Chief, Pediatric Pulmonary & Cystic Fibrosis Center
California Pacific Medical Center
San Francisco, CA

WILLIAM E. HATHAWAY, MD
Professor Emeritus of Pediatrics
University of Colorado School of Medicine
Tucson, AZ

D. ROBERT HOWARD, MD
Professor of Family & Community Medicine
Mercer University School of Medicine
Ellenwood, GA

JOHN J. HUTTER, JR., MD
Professor of Pediatrics
Chief, Pediatric Hematology/Oncology
University of Arizona College of Medicine
Tucson, AZ

PHILIP E. JAFFE, MD
Associate Professor, Dept. of Medicine, Gastroenterology Section
University of Arizona College of Medicine
Medical Director, Gastrointestinal Endoscopy Lab,
University Medical Center
Tucson, AZ

DAVID G. JOHNSON, MD
Professor of Internal Medicine & Pharmacology
University of Arizona College of Medicine
Tucson, AZ

Board of Consultants

WILLIAM P. JOHNSON, MD
Clinical Assistant Professor of Medicine
Chief, Section of General Medicine
University of Arizona College of Medicine
Tucson, AZ

LISA KAUFMANN, MD
Clinical Assistant Professor
Department of Medicine
University of Arizona College of Medicine
Tucson, AZ

STEVEN R. KNOPER, MD
Research Assistant Professor
Respiratory Sciences Center
University of Arizona College of Medicine
Tucson, AZ

MARCIA G. KO, MD
University of Arizona College of Medicine
Tucson, AZ

JACQUES R. LECLERC, MD
Director, Division of Hematology
Montreal General Hospital
Montreal, Quebec CANADA

DANIEL O. LEVINSON, MD
Department of Family and Community Medicine
University of Arizona College of Medicine
Tucson, AZ

MIRIAM LEVINSON, PHARMD
Clinical Specialist, Drug Information
Meriter Hospital
Madison, WI

JOHN E. LEWY, MD
Professor and Chairman
Department of Pediatrics
Tulane University School of Medicine
New Orleans, LA

ELMER S. LIGHTNER, MD
Professor of Pediatrics
Department of Pediatrics
University of Arizona College of Medicine
Tucson, AZ

LEONARD S. LILLY, MD
Associate Professor of Medicine
Harvard Medical School
Brigham's and Women's Hospital
Boston, MA

ACHI LUDOMIRSKY, MD
Associate Professor of Pediatrics
University of Michigan
C.S. Mott Children's Hospital
Ann Arbor, MI

MARY ANNE MANGELSEN, MD, PHD, FACP
Chelsea, MI

EDWIN H. MCDOWELL, MD
Private Practice, Urology
Orlando, FL

SCOTT D. MILLER, MD
Private Practice, Dermatology
Fort Worth, TX

LARRY MILLIKAN, MD
Chairman, Department of Dermatology
Tulane University School of Medicine
New Orleans, LA

SAMUEL L. MOSCHELLA, MD, FACP
Clinical Professor Dermatology (Emeritus)
Harvard Medical School
Senior Consultant, Lahey Clinic
Burlington, MA

K. J. OOMMEN, MD
Associate Professor
Department of Neurology
University of Oklahoma College of Medicine
Oklahoma City, OK

CAROLYN RUBY, PHD
Health Education Program
American Academy of Family Physicians
Kansas City, MO

STEVEN M. SHAW, MD
Private Practice
Tucson, AZ

ROBERT W. SNYDER, MD, PHD
Department of Ophthalmology
University of Arizona College of Medicine
Tucson, AZ

CHARLES R. UNDERWOOD, MD
Private Practice - Retired
Marietta, GA

DANIEL K. WINSTEAD, MD
Department of Psychiatry & Neurology
Tulane University School of Medicine
New Orleans, LA

RALPH M. WYNN, MD
Professor of Obstetrics & Gynecology and Pathology
State University of New York Health Science Center at Brooklyn
Brooklyn, NY

STONEY A. ABERCROMBIE, MD
Professor, Family Medicine
Medical University of South Carolina
Greenwood, SC

ABDULRAZAK ABYAD, MD, MPH, AGSF
Director, ABYAD Medical Center
Tripoli, Lebanon

RODNEY D. ADAM, MD
Associate Professor of Medicine & Microbiology/Immunology
University of Arizona College of Medicine
Tucson, AZ

ALAN ADELMAN, MD, MS
Department of Family and Community Medicine
Milton S. Hershey Medical Center
Hershey, PA

AUGUSTO AGUIRRE, MD
Associate Clinical Professor of Pathology
Ohio State University
Grant-Riverside Hospitals
Columbus, OH

RICHARD W. ALLINSON, MD
Clinical Associate Professor
Department of Ophthalmology
University of Arizona, VA Medical Center
Phoenix, AZ

PATRICIA ANDERSON, MD
Mt. Auburn Associates
Cincinnati, OH

VICENTE J. ARANO, MD
Private Practice
Yucca Valley, CA

HENRY ARGUINCHONA, MD
Physicians Clinic of Spokane
Spokane, WA

WATSON C. ARNOLD, MD
Director, Pediatric Nephrology
Cook Children's Medical Center
Fort Worth, TX

JEHAD Y. ASFOURA, MD
Assistant Professor, Clinical Internal Medicine
Northeastern Ohio Universities College of Medicine
Canton, OH

ROBERT L. ATMAR, MD
Department of Medicine
Baylor College of Medicine
Houston, TX

COLIN R. BAMFORD, MD
Department of Neurology
University of Arizona College of Medicine
Tucson, AZ

MUSTAFA BARUDI, MD
Assistant Professor of Pediatrics
Northeastern Ohio Universities College of Medicine
Tod Children's Hospital
Youngstown, OH

ROBERT P. BAUGHMAN, MD
Professor of Medicine
Pulmonary and Critical Care Medicine
University of Cincinnati Medical Center
Cincinnati, OH

KAY A. BAUMAN, MD, MPH
Professor
Department of Family Practice & Community Health
University of Hawaii School of Medicine
Mililani, HI

KARIL BELLAH, MD
Private Practice, Cardiologist
Lawrence, KS

BRUCE G. BELLAMY, MD
Saint Luke's Medical
Clinton, MO

JAMES B. BENJAMIN, MD
Associate Professor of Surgery
University of Arizona College of Medicine
Tucson, AZ

PAUL J. BENKE, MD, PHD
University of Miami School of Medicine
Miami, FL

GEORGE R. BERGUS, MD
Associate Professor
Department of Family Practice
University of Iowa
Iowa City, IA

WILLIAM H. BILLICA, MD
Assistant Director
Family Practice Residency Program
Good Samaritan Medical Center
Phoenix, AZ

RICHARD B. BIRRER, MD
Vice President, Physician Services
Chief Medical Officer
Catholic Medical Center
Jamaica, NY

Contributing Authors

TIMOTHY L. BLACK, MD, FACS, FAAP
Medical Director of Trauma
Cook Children's Hospital
Fort Worth, TX

BRUCE BLOCK, MD
Family Practice Residency Program
Shadyside Hospital
Pittsburgh, PA

MICHAEL BOESPFLUG, MD
Santa Clara Medical Clinic
Eugene, OR

JESS G. BOND, MD, MPH
Assistant Professor of Internal Medicine
Northeastern Ohio Universities College of Medicine
Akron, OH

MARJORIE A. BOWMAN, MD, MPA
Department of Family Practice & Community Medicine
University of Pennsylvania Health System
Philadelphia, PA

W. PAUL BOWMAN, MD
Medical Director, Hematology-Oncology
Cook Children's Medical Center
Fort Worth, TX

JOHN T. BOYER, MD
Professor, Department of Medicine
University of Arizona College of Medicine
Tucson, AZ

GEORGE R. BRADBURY, MD
Section of Orthopedic Surgery
University of Arizona College of Medicine
Tucson, AZ

MARIE A. BRISTER, MD
Resident, Family Practice
St. Francis Hospital of Evanston
Evanston, IL

DAVID E. BURTNER, MD
Vice Chairman and Professor
Department of Family & Community Medicine
Mercer University School of Medicine
Macon, GA

ROGER CADY, MD
Director, Headache Care Center
Springfield, MO

JOANNA M. CAIN, MD
Professor, Department of Obstetrics & Gynecology
University of Washington Medical Center
Seattle, WA

CYNTHIA GAIL CARMICHAEL, MD
Staff Physician
Richmond Health Center
Berkeley, CA

KEVIN CARMICHAEL, MD
Unit Chief
El Rio Special Immunology Associates
Tucson, AZ

JOHN Z. CARTER, MD
Private Practice, Family Practice/Geriatrics
Tucson, AZ

L. PHILIP CARTER, MD
Western Neurological, Ltd.
Tucson, AZ

ROY R. CASIANO, MD
Associate Professor
Department of Otolaryngology-Center for Sinus & Voice Disorders
University of Miami School of Medicine
Miami, FL

FRANK "CHIP" CELESTINO, MD
Associate Professor
Department of Family & Community Medicine
Bowman Gray School of Medicine
Winston-Salem, NC

JASON CHAO, MD, MS
Associate Professor, Department of Family Medicine
Case Western Reserve University
Cleveland, OH

ROBERT A. CHENEY, MD
Associate Clinical Instructor, Orthopaedic Surgery
Albany Medical College
Albany, NY

ANTHONY W. CHOW, MD, FRCPC, FACP
Professor of Medicine, Division of Infectious Diseases
The University of British Columbia
Vancouver, British Columbia CANADA

THOMAS W. CLARK, MS, MD
Private Practice
Newport News, VA

WILLIAM W. CLEVELAND, MD
Professor of Pediatrics
Director, Division of Endocrinology
University of Miami
Miami, FL

RICHARD D. CLOVER, MD
Department of Family and Community Medicine
University of Louisville
Louisville, KY

RICHARD W. COHEN, MD
Georgia Orthopaedics and Sports Medicine
Marietta, GA

RUSSELL G. COHEN, MD
Department of Surgery/Orthopedics
Arizona Health Sciences Center
Tucson, AZ

JOHN J. COLEMAN, MD
Professor of Surgery
Director, Plastic Surgery
Indiana University Medical Center
Indianapolis, IN

JACK G. COPELAND, MD
Professor, Department of Surgery
Section of Cardiovascular and Thoracic Surgery
University of Arizona College of Medicine
Tucson, AZ

ANTHONY J. COSTA, MD
Professor of Clinical Family Medicine
Northeastern Ohio Universities College of Medicine
Director, Family Practice Residency Program
Barberton Citizens Hospital
Barberton, OH

ALAN J. CROPP, MD, FCCP
Associate Professor of Internal Medicine
Northeastern Ohio Universities College of Medicine
Youngstown, OH

PAUL T. CULLEN, MD
Director, Family Practice Residency Program
The Washington Hospital
Washington, PA

J. P. W. CUNNINGTON, MD, FRCPC
Associate Professor of Medicine
McMaster University
Hamilton, Ontario CANADA

M. BEATRIZ CURRIER, MD
Department of Psychiatry
University of Miami School of Medicine
Miami, FL

ROBERT B. DAIGNEAULT, MD, FAAP
Assistant Clinical Professor
University of California, San Diego
San Diego, CA

JAMES E. DALEN, MD, MPH
Vice President for Health Sciences
Dean, College of Medicine
The University of Arizona College of Medicine
Tucson, AZ

MARK R. DAMBRO, MD, FAAFP
Private Practice
Fort Worth, TX

NANCY N. DAMBRO, MD
Cook Children's Medical Center
Fort Worth, TX

JERYL DANSKY, MD
Private Practice
Tucson, AZ

MARC DARR, MD
Private Practice
Mercy Integrated Health
Phoenix, AZ

JANICE E. DAUGHERTY, MD
Associate Professor of Family Medicine
East Carolina University School of Medicine
Greenville, NC

ROBERT DEMARCO, MD
Associate Professor of Clinical Internal Medicine
Northeastern Ohio Universities College of Medicine
Youngstown, OH

C. VAN DEVERE, MD
Associate Professor of Psychiatry
Northeastern Ohio Universities College of Medicine
Director, Pediatric Psychiatry at Children's Hospital Medical Center
Akron, OH

EMIL S. DICKSTEIN, MD, FACP
Associate Professor of Medicine
Northeastern Ohio Universities College of Medicine
Youngstown, OH

J. HARLAN DIX, MD, FACP
Clinical Associate Professor
Northeastern Ohio Universities College of Medicine
Killbuck, OH

MICHEL J. DODARD, MD
Assistant Professor
Clinical Family Medicine & Community Health
Jackson Memorial Hospital
Miami, FL

ROBERT DOLIN, MD
Department of Medicine
Kaiser Permanente
La Palma, CA

S. SHEVAUN DUIKER, MD
Assistant Residency Director
Swedish Family Practice
Littleton, CO

BURRIS DUNCAN, MD
Professor
Department of Pediatrics
University of Arizona College of Medicine
Tucson, AZ

DONALD F. EIPPER, MD
Associate Professor, Internal Medicine
Northeastern Ohio Universities College of Medicine
Akron General Medical Center
Akron, OH

STEVEN EISENSTEIN, MD
Private Practice
The Family Doctors of Northbrook
Northbrook, IL

NANCY ELDER, MD, MSPH
Assistant Professor
Oregon Health Sciences University
Portland, OR

GREG ELDERS, MD
Family Practice
Mountain Home, AR

PAMELA I. ELLSWORTH, MD
Pediatric Urology
Darthmouth-Hitchcock Medical Center
Lebanon, NH

KURT ELWARD, MD, MPH
Family Medicine of Albemarle
Clinical Assistant Professor, Department of Family Medicine
University of Virginia
Charlottesville, VA

JOSEPH G. EWING, MD
Assistant Professor of Family Practice
Family Practice Residency Program at Conroe
University of Texas Medical Branch, Galveston
Conroe, TX

ROBERT G. FANTE, MD
Clinical Assistant Professor
Department of Ophthalmology
University of Michigan
Milan, MI

NANCY P. FAWCETT, MD
Professor of Pediatrics
Department of Pediatrics
University of Miami School of Medicine
Miami, FL

Contributing Authors

ANDREW H. FENTON, MD, FACS
Assistant Professor of Surgery
Northeastern Ohio Universities College of Medicine
Akron General Medical Center
Akron, OH

MICHAEL FERREBEE, MD
Assistant Professor
Department of Pediatrics, Critical Care Division
West Virginia University School of Medicine
Morgantown, WV

SCOTT A. FIELDS, MD
Associate Professor
Family Medicine
Oregon Health Sciences University
Portland, OR

DOUGLAS P. FINE, MD
Professor and Chairman of Medicine
University of Oklahoma Health Sciences Center
Oklahoma City, OK

STANLEY FINEMAN, MD
Clinical Assistant Professor
Department of Pediatrics
Emory University School of Medicine
Marietta, GA

GENE S. FISCH, PHD
Director of Research
Department of Psychiatry
Kings County Hospital
Brooklyn, NY

DANIEL B. FISHBEIN, MD
Coordinator, Scientific Studies International Branch
Epidemiology Program Office
Centers for Disease Control
Atlanta, GA

JOSEPH A. FLORENCE, MD
Director, East Kentucky Family Practice Residency Program
University of Kentucky
Hazard, KY

GRANT C. FOWLER, MD
Associate Professor and Director
Hermann/LBJ Family Practice Residency
The University of Texas-Houston Medical School
Houston, TX

DAVID J. FRAMM, MD, FACC
Mecklenburg Medical Group
Charlotte, NC

DAVID FRANK, MD
Department of Family and Community Medicine
Milton S. Hershey Medical Center
Hershey, PA

ELIZABETH A. FRANKEL, MD
Residency Training Program
Children's National Medical Center
Washington, DC

JOHN FREEMAN, MD
Private Practice
Fort Worth, TX

WESLEY FURSTE, MD, FACS
Clinical Professor, Emeritus
Department of Surgery
Ohio State University
Columbus, OH

GREGORY G. GAAR, MD, FAAP, FACEP
Co-Medical Director
Florida Poison Information and Toxicology Resource Center
Tampa General Hospital
Tampa, FL

ERIC P. GALL, MD
Professor and Chairman
Department of Medicine
Finch University of Health Sciences
The Chicago Medical School
North Chicago, IL

JAMES M. GALLOWAY, MD, FACP, FACC
Director, Center for Native American Health
Assistant Professor of Clinical Medicine
University of Arizona College of Medicine
Tucson, AZ

LEONARD GANZ, MD
Electrophysiology Section
Cardiology Division
Allegheny General Hospital
Pittsburgh, PA

GALE GARDNER, MD, FACS
Clinical Professor
Department of Otolaryngology
University of Tennessee, Memphis
Memphis, TN

WILLIAM G. GARDNER, MD
Chairman, Department of Medicine
Akron General Medical Center
Akron, OH

KENT R. GEBHARDT, DO, FAAFP
Associate Clinical Assistant Professor
Family Practice and Community Medicine
University of Hawaii
Mililani, HI

MARK GERSTBURGER, DO
Smoky Hill Family Practice Residency Program
Salina, KS

JOHN P. GEYMAN, MD
Professor Emeritus of Family Medicine
University of Washington
Seattle, WA

JEFF RAY GIBSON, JR., MD
Department of Anesthesiology
Scott and White Clinic
Temple, TX

BRUCE C. GILLILAND, MD
Professor of Medicine and Laboratory Medicine
School of Medicine
University of Washington
Seattle, WA

MARSHALL GODWIN, MD
Hotel Dieu Family Medicine Center
Queen's University
Kingston, Ontario CANADA

GARY A. GOFORTH, MD, MTMH
Associate Professor of Family Medicine
Medical University of South Carolina
Medical Director, Faculty
Montgomery Center for Family Medicine
Greenwood, SC

PAUL R. GORDON, MD
Department of Family & Community Medicine
University of Arizona College of Medicine
Tucson, AZ

R. SCOTT GORMAN, MD
Mayo Clinic
Scottsdale, AZ

MARK A. GRABER, MD
Assistant Professor
Department of Family Medicine & Surgery
The University of Iowa
Iowa City, IA

CARMELO GRAFFAGNINO, MD, FRCP
Department of Medicine
Division of Neurology
Duke University Medical Center
Durham, NC

DAVID S. GRAY, MD
Community Hospital
Family Practice Residency
Santa Rosa, CA

J. THOMAS GRAYSTON, MD
Professor, Department of Epidemiology
University of Washington
School of Public Health and Community Medicine
Seattle, WA

RONALD A. GREENFIELD, MD
Professor of Medicine & Chief, Infectious Diseases Section
University of Oklahoma Health Sciences Center
Oklahoma City, OK

DAVID A. GRIESEMER, MD
Division of Child Neurology
Department of Neurology and Pediatrics
Medical University of South Carolina
Charleston, SC

JOHN GUISTO, MD
Associate Professor of Clinical Surgery
Section of Emergency Medicine, Department of Surgery
University of Arizona College of Medicine
Tucson, AZ

VLADIMIR HACHINSKI, MD, DSC, FRCP
Department of Clinical Neurological Sciences
The University of Western Ontario
London, Ontario CANADA

SAMI K. W. HADEED, MD
Pulmonary Medicine
Cook Children's
Fort Worth, TX

JANET M. HAHN, MD
Resident, Family Practice
St. Francis Hospital of Evanston
Evanston, IL

HETTY B. HALL, MD
Iowa City, IA

R. BRUCE HALL, MD
Private Practice, Orthopedics
Southern Bone & Joint Specialists
Dothan, AL

LARRY W. HALVERSON, MD
Director, Cox Family Practice Residency Program
Cox Health Systems
Springfield, MO

DAVID HANSON, MD
Smoky Hill Family Practice Residency Program
Salina, KS

CLYDE L. HARRIS, MD
Private Practice
Franklin, NC

IRWIN E. HARRIS, MD, MBA, MSHA, FACS
Orthopedic Oncology, Pediatric Orthopedics
Lakewood, CO

FERN R. HAUCK, MD, MS
Associate Professor and Director of Research
Department of Family Medicine
Loyola University Chicago Stritch School of Medicine
Maywood, IL

STEVEN J. HAVENER, MD
Private Practice
Mission, TX

HARRY W. HAVERKOS, MD
Medical Director
National Institute on Drug Abuse
Baltimore, MD

CATHRYN HEATH, MD
Assistant Professor of Family Medicine
UMDNJ Robert Wood Johnson Medical School
New Brunswick, NJ

DARELL E. HEISELMAN, DO, FCCM, FACP, FACC, FCCP
Chief, Critical Care Medicine, Akron General Medical Center
Professor, Northeastern Ohio Universities College of Medicine
Akron, OH

THOMAS W. HEJKAL, MD, PHD
Assistant Professor
Department of Ophthalmology
University of Nebraska Medical Center
Omaha, NE

SCOTT T. HENDERSON, MD
Assistant Professor of Family Practice
Family Practice Residency Program, Cheyenne
University of Wyoming
Cheyenne, WY

ERIC HENLEY, MD, MPH
Assistant Professor
Department of Family & Community Medicine
University of Illinois College of Medicine at Rockford
Rockford, IL

KEVIN M. HEPLER, MD, MBA
Private Practice
Camp Hill, PA

BARTON L. HODES, MD
Professor
Department of Ophthalmology
University of Arizona College of Medicine
Tucson, AZ

Contributing Authors

MICHAEL P. HOPKINS, MD
Chairperson, Department of Obstetrics & Gynecology
Akron General Medical Center
Professor, Northeastern Ohio Universities College of Medicine
Akron, OH

MARK HORATTAS, MD, FACS
Associate Professor
Department of Surgery
Northeastern Ohio Universities College of Medicine
Akron, OH

LAURENE L. HOWELL, MD
Associate Professor
Department of Otolaryngology
Oregon Health Sciences University
Portland, OR

DOUGLAS M. HOY, MD
Associate Clinical Professor
Department of Family Medicine
Medical College of Ohio
Bellevue, OH

DENNIS E. HUGHES, DO
Associate Program Director
Cox Family Practice Residency Program
Cox Health Systems
Springfield, MO

JOHN J. HUTTER, JR., MD
Professor of Pediatrics
Chief, Pediatric Hematology/Oncology
University of Arizona College of Medicine
Tucson, AZ

FRANK L. IBER, MD
Department of Gastroenterology
Department of Veterans Affairs
Hines, IL

HERBERT L. ISSAC II, MD
Resident, Family Practice
St. Francis Hospital of Evanston
Evanston, IL

CHARLES N. JACOBS, MD
Nephrologist
Waterville, ME

PHILIP E. JAFFE, MD
Associate Professor, Dept of Medicine, Gastroenterology Section
University of Arizona College of Medicine
Medical Director, GI Endoscopy Lab, University Medical Center
Tucson, AZ

STEVEN L. JAFFE, MD
Associate Professor of Psychiatry
Director, Adolescent Programs
Emory University
Atlanta, GA

PAUL J. JASTER, MD
Associate Director, Assistant Professor
Smoky Hill Family Practice Residency Program
Salina, KS

E. R. JEANS, MD, BSC, FRCPC
Head, Microbiology
Hamilton Civic Hospitals
Hamilton, Ontario CANADA

ERIC L. JENISON, MD
Professor of Clinical Obstetrics & Gynecology
Northeastern Ohio Universities College of Medicine
Akron General Medical Center
Akron, OH

CHARLES JENNINGS, MD, FACS
Lima Urology, Inc.
Lima, OH

PAUL JOHNSON, MD
Emergency Department
St. Luke's Hospital
Phoenix, AZ

FURNIE W. JOHNSTON, MD
Private Practice
Dothan, AL

SMITH L. JOHNSTON, III, MD, MS
NASA Medical Officer/Flight Surgeon
Flight Medicine Clinic/SD26
NASA Johnson Space Center
Houston, TX

GRAHAM S. KAISER, DO
Resident, Family Practice
St. Francis Hospital of Evanston
Evanston, IL

K. SHASHI KANT, MD
Professor of Medicine, Division of Nephrology and Hypertension
University of Cincinnati Medical Center
Cincinnati, OH

PAUL E. KAPLAN, MD
Bert C. Wiley Professor and Chair
Physical Medicine and Rehabilitation
Ohio State University, Dodd Hall Rehabilitation Center
Columbus, OH

WAYNE J. KATON, MD
Professor of Psychiatry, Vice Chair
Department of Psychiatry, School of Medicine
University of Washington Medical School
Seattle, WA

RICK KELLERMAN, MD
Director
Smoky Hill Family Practice Residency Program
Salina, KS

MICHAEL W. KELLY, PHARMD, MS
Clinical Assistant Professor
College of Pharmacy
University of Iowa
Iowa City, IA

ROBERT M. KERSHNER, MD, FACS
Clinical Professor, University of Utah Medical Center
Director, Orange Grove Center for Corrective Eye Surgery
Tucson, AZ

GEORGE E. KIKANO, MD
Director of Clinical Affairs
Department of Family Medicine
Case Western Reserve University
Cleveland, OH

MICHELLE D. KIMMEL, MD
Private Practice
Cushing, OK

SCOTT A. KINCAID, MD
Assistant Clinical Professor of Family Medicine
Medical College of Virginia, Richmond, VA
Radford, VA

MITCHELL S. KING, MD
Family Practice Residency Director
St. Francis Hospital of Evanston
Northbrook, IL

JEFFERY T. KIRCHNER, DO, FAAFP
Associate Director
Family Practice Residency Program
Lancaster General Hospital
Lancaster, PA

JULIENNE K. KIRK, PHARMD
Assistant Professor
Department of Family & Community Medicine
Bowman Gray School of Medicine
Winston-Salem, NC

EVAN W. KLIGMAN, MD
Professor and Head, Department of Family Medicine
University of Iowa College of Medicine
Iowa City, IA

MARY E. KLINK, MD
Physicians Plus Medical Group
Medical Director, Sleep Disorders Program
Meriter Hospital
Madison, WI

AUBREY L. KNIGHT, MD
Associate Director of Family Practice Education
Carilion Health Systems
Roanoke, VA

ROBERT KOWAL, MD
Cardiology Fellow
Brigham's and Women's Physician Group
Boston, MA

PETER KOZISEK, MD
Family Practice Residency of Idaho
Boise, ID

BRADLEY KUNZ, MD
Grant Family Practice Residency
Grant/Riverside Methodist Hospital
Columbus, OH

ALVIN LANGER, MD
Professor and Chairperson of Obstetrics & Gynecology
Associate Dean for Clinical Education
Northeastern Ohio Universities College of Medicine
Canton, OH

LARS C. LARSEN, MD
Associate Professor
Department of Family Medicine
East Carolina University School of Medicine
Greenville, NC

RICHARD A. LARSON, MD
Professor of Medicine
Director, Leukemia Program
The University of Chicago Medical Center
Chicago, IL

MARC LEDUC, MD
Private Practice
Port Clinton, OH

YATES P. LEE, MD
Resident, Family Practice
St. Francis Hospital of Evanston
Evanston, IL

MARK C. LEESON, MD, FACS
Associate Professor
Northeastern Ohio Universities College of Medicine
Akron, OH

GARY LEVINE, MD
Associate Professor, Department of Family Medicine
East Carolina University School of Medicine
Greenville, NC

BARCEY T. LEVY, PHD, MD
Assistant Professor
Department of Family Practice
University of Iowa
Iowa City, IA

RICHARD P. LEVY, MD
Professor of Internal Medicine
Northeastern Ohio Universities College of Medicine
Akron, OH

JAMES H. LEWIS, MD, FACP, FACG
Associate Professor of Medicine
Division of Gastroenterology
Georgetown University Medical Center
Washington, DC

THOMAS LEWIS, DDS
Private Practice
Bayside, CA

LEONARD S. LILLY, MD
Associate Professor of Medicine
Harvard Medical School
Brigham's and Women's Hospital
Boston, MA

CAROL B. LINDSLEY, MD
Professor of Pediatrics
Director, Pediatric Rheumatology
University of Kansas School of Medicine
Kansas City, KS

JOHN M. LITTLE, MD
Chief Medical Officer and Medical Director, Companion Healthcare
Clinical Associate Professor
University of North Carolina and University of South Carolina
Columbia, SC

PHIL LOBSTEIN, MD
Private Practice
Fort Worth, TX

DOROTHY LOWDER, RN
Holmes County Hospice
Killbuck, OH

ELYSE E. LOWER, MD
Associate Professor of Medicine
Hematology/Oncology Division
University of Cincinnati Medical Center
Cincinnati, OH

D. W. MACPHERSON, MD, MSC (CTM), FRCPC
Assistant Professor
Director, Regional Parasitology Laboratory
McMaster University/St. Joseph's Hospital
Hamilton, Ontario CANADA

Contributing Authors

BARBARA A. MAJERONI, MD
Assistant Professor
Department of Family Medicine
State University of New York at Buffalo
Buffalo, NY

MOHAMMAD MALIK, MD
Resident, Family Practice
St. Francis Hospital of Evanston
Evanston, IL

SYLVIA A. MAMBY, MD
Consultant
Division of Cardiovascular Diseases
Mayo Clinic, Scottsdale
Scottsdale, AZ

RICHARD M. MANDEL, MD
Assistant Clinical Professor
Internal Medicine
University of Arizona College of Medicine
Tucson, AZ

DANNEN D. MANNSCHRECK, MD
Assistant Director, Family Practice Residency Program
University of Illinois College of Medicine at Rockford
L.P. Johnson Family Health Center
Rockford, IL

ROBERT A. MARLOW, MD, MA
Associate Dean/Program Director
Family Practice Residency Program at Cheyenne
University of Wyoming
Cheyenne, WY

BRADLEY R. MARTIN, MD
Akron City Hospital
Akron, OH

ANNA N. MAXEY, MD
Grant Family Practice Residency
Grant/Riverside Methodist Hospitals
Columbus, OH

SUSANA MAY, MD, MPH
Private Practice
Assistant Clinical Professor of Family Medicine
Department of Family Medicine
University of Miami School of Medicine
Tavernier, FL

SUMNER T. MCALLISTER, MD
Resident, Family Practice
Grant Family Practice Residency
Columbus, OH

PATRICK J. MCCARVILLE, MD
Private Practice
Valley, NE

ELIZABETH MCCORD, MD, MS
Assistant Professor, Johnson City Family Practice Residency
East Tennessee State University
James H. Quillen College of Medicine
Johnson City, TN

K. PATRICIA MCGANN, MD, MSPH
Palo Alto Medical Foundation
Associate Professor of Clinical Medicine
Stanford University School of Medicine
Palo Alto, CA

DON MCHARD, MD
Staff Physician
Department of Family Practice
Cigna Healthcare of Arizona
Glendale, AZ

SEAN O. MCMENOMEY, MD
Department of Otolaryngology
Oregon Health Sciences University
Portland, OR

LEO C. MERCER, MD
Chief Executive Officer
Capital Coast Health
Wellington SOUTH NEW ZEALAND

GARY M. MILLER, MD
Marietta Neurological Associates
Marietta, GA

JAMES P. MILLER, MD, FACS, FAAP
Pediatric Surgical Associates of Fort Worth
Fort Worth, TX

JOSEPH I. MILLER, MD
Professor of Cardiothoracic Surgery
Department of Surgery
Chief, General Thoracic Surgery
The Emory University Clinic
Atlanta, GA

KARL E. MILLER, MD
Associate Professor
Department of Family Medicine
University of Tennessee College of Medicine
Chattanooga Unit
Chattanooga, TN

SANDRA MILLER, MD
Assistant Director, Residency
Family Practice Center
Good Samaritan Regional Medical Center
Phoenix, AZ

SCOTT D. MILLER, MD
Private Practice
Fort Worth, TX

LARRY MILLIKAN, MD
Chairman, Department of Dermatology
Tulane University School of Medicine
New Orleans, LA

JEFFREY F. MINTEER, MD
Associate Director
Family Practice Residency Program
The Washington Hospital
Washington, PA

CHARLES D. MITCHELL, MD
Division of Immunology & Infectious Diseases
Department of Pediatrics
University of Miami School of Medicine
Miami, FL

REZA MOATTARI, MD
Associate Professor of Medicine and Head, Endocrinology Division
Northeastern Ohio Universities College of Medicine
Chief, Endocrinology Section, Akron General Hospital
Akron, OH

SUSAN LOUISA MONTAUK, MD
Associate Professor of Clinical Family Medicine
Department of Family Medicine
University of Cincinnati College of Medicine
Cincinnati, OH

T. GLENDON MOODY, MD
Clinical Lecturer
Department of Ophthalmology
University of Arizona College of Medicine
Phoenix, AZ

DONALD W. MOORMAN, MD
Department of Surgery Education
Iowa Methodist Medical Center
Des Moines, IA

BARBARA J. MORANT, MD
Resident, Family Practice
St. Francis Hospital of Evanston
Evanston, IL

JULIE GRAVES MOY, MD, MPH
Private Practice
Austin, TX

BRIAN J. MURRAY, MD
Director
Student Health Services
University of California at San Diego
La Jolla, CA

JAMES A. NARD, MD
Department of Pediatrics
Tod Children's Hospital
Youngstown, OH

DIANE NEDDENRIEP, MD
Pediatric Pulmonary Associates
Tucson, AZ

ANN NEFF, MD
Department of Internal Medicine
Northeastern Ohio Universities College of Medicine
Canton Affiliated Hospitals
Canton, OH

GUY W. NEFF, MD
Department of Medicine, Section of Gastroenterology
Louisiana State University Medical Center
Shreveport, LA

DONALD A. F. NELSON, MD
Family Health Center
Cedar Rapids Medical Education Program
Cedar Rapids, IA

MICHAEL M. VAN NESS, MD
Department of Internal Medicine
Aultman Hospital
Canton, OH

JAMES C. NIEDERMAN, MD
Clinical Professor of Medicine and Epidemiology
Yale University School of Medicine
New Haven, CT

PETER T. NIEH, MD
Senior Staff
Department of Urology
Lahey Hitchcock Medical Center
Burlington, MA

CARLO NIGUIDULA, MD
Resident, Family Practice
St. Francis Hospital of Evanston
Evanston, IL

CAROLYN NINE, MD
Private Practice
Grosse Pointe Woods, MI

ROBERT NOECKER, MD
Assistant Professor
Department of Ophthalmology
University of Arizona
Tucson, AZ

LAURA L. NOVAK, MD
Barberton Citizens Hospital
Barberton, OH

MICHAEL A. ODDI, MD
Department of Surgery
Akron General Medical Center
Akron, OH

EDWIN J. OLSEN, MD, MBA
Department of Psychiatry
University of Miami School of Medicine
Miami, FL

BENJAMIN PARAS, MD
Fellow, Section of Neurosurgery
University of Arizona College of Medicine
Tucson, AZ

TEJAL PARIKH, MD
Private Practice
Tucson, AZ

JOSE R. PARKER, MD
Thomas Davis Medical Center
Family Practice
Glendale, AZ

JOHN E. PERCHALSKI, MD, FAAFP
Department of Family Medicine
Rardin Family Practice Center
Ohio State University
Columbus, OH

JOHN R. PERSON, MD
Fallon Medical Center
Worcester, MA

CLAUDIA A. PETERS, MD
Queen's Student Health Service
Queen's University
Kingston, Ontario CANADA

DANA W. PETERSON, MD
Internal & Family Medicine Associates
Albuquerque, NM

ELSIRA M. PINA, DO
Fellow, Pulmonary and Critical Care Medicine
University of Cincinnati Medical Center
Cincinnati, OH

GREGORY A. POLAND, MD
Professor
Department of Internal Medicine, Mayo Vaccine Research Group
The Mayo Clinic and Foundation
Rochester, MN

Contributing Authors

DAVID A. POPE, MD
Private Practice
Janesville, MN

WILLIAM A. PRIMACK, MD
Associate Professor of Pediatrics
University of Massachusetts Medical Center
Fallon Clinic
Auburn, MA

JAMES K. RADIKE, MD
Infectious Disease Consultant
Stillwater, OK

LEE P. RALPH, MD
Department of Family Medicine
University of California, San Diego Medical Group
La Jolla, CA

RAGHU RAM, MD
Kenmore, NY

KATHRYN REILLY, MD, MPH
Family Practice Residency Program
University of Oklahoma
Oklahoma City, OK

ANNE C. REITZ, MD
Resident, Family Practice
St. Francis Hospital of Evanston
Evanston, IL

RICK RICER, MD
Department of Family Medicine
University of Cincinnati College of Medicine
Cincinnati, OH

J. RANDALL RICHARD, MD
Associate Professor of Clinical Family Medicine, Northeastern Ohio
    Universities College of Medicine
Associate Residency Director, Barberton Citizens Hospital
Barberton, OH

CHARLES W. RICKETSON, MD, FRCPC
Victoria General Hospital
Victoria, British Columbia CANADA

MICHEL E. RIVLIN, MD
Department of Obstetrics & Gynecology
University of Mississippi Medical Center
Jackson, MS

TIMOTHY ROBINSON, DO
Private Practice
Bayside, NY

VANCE D. RODGERS, MD
Director, Inflammatory Bowel Disease Center
Scripps Clinic & Research Foundation
La Jolla, CA

DUANE C. ROE, MD
Associate Professor of Medicine
Northeastern Ohio Universities College of Medicine
Akron, OH

BRUCE M. ROTHSCHILD, MD
Professor, Northeastern Ohio Universities College of Medicine
Director, Arthritis Center of Northeast Ohio
Youngstown, OH

JAMES H. RUDICK, MD, FACP
Assistant Professor of Internal Medicine
Northeastern Ohio Universities College of Medicine
Canton, OH

BARRY S. RUSSMAN, MD
Professor, Pediatrics and Neurology
University of Connecticut Medical School
CT Children's Medical Center
Hartford, CT

GREGORY W. RUTECKI, MD
Professor of Medicine & Master Teacher
Northeastern Ohio Universities College of Medicine
Columbia Mercy Medical Center
Canton, OH

ANDRES M. SALAZAR, MD
Professor of Neurology, USUHS
Director, Defense & Veterans Head Injury Program
Walter Reed Army Medical Center
Washington, DC

RICHARD E. SAMPLINER, MD
Professor of Medicine
Chief of Gastroenterology Section
University of Arizona College of Medicine
Tucson, AZ

DOUGLAS H. SANDBERG, MD
Professor of Pediatrics
Div of Gastroenterology and Nutrition
Dept of Pediatrics
University of Miami School of Medicine
Miami, FL

ARTHUR SANDERS, MD
Professor, Section of Emergency Medicine
Department of Surgery
University of Arizona College of Medicine
Tucson, AZ

WILLIAM D. SAWYER, MD
President
China Medical Board of New York
New York, NY

DANIEL T. SCHELBLE, MD, FACEP
Chairman, Department of Emergency Medicine
Akron General Medical Center
Akron, OH

ROBERT M. SCHULTZ, MD
Director
Pediatric Endocrinology
Scottish Rite Children's Medical Center
Atlanta, GA

WAYNE H. SCHWESINGER, MD
Head, Section of General Surgery
Department of Surgery
The University of Texas Health Science Center at San Antonio
San Antonio, TX

E. NAN SCOTT, PHD
Associate Professor
University of Oklahoma Health Sciences Center & Veterans
    Administration Medical Center
Oklahoma City, OK

ROBERT H. SCOTT, MD
Faculty
Family Practice Residency
Swedish Medical Center
Seattle, WA

DAVID P. SEALY, MD
Director, Sports Medicine
Associate Professor & Associate Director
Self Memorial Hospital Family Medicine Residency
Greenwood, SC

MARK E. SEXTON, MD
Clinical Associate Professor
University of AZ, Department of Family & Community Medicine
Medical Director, FHP Inc.
Paradise Valley, AZ

WILLIAM V. SHARP, MD
Private Practice - Retired
Vero Beach, FL

MARK M. SHELTON, MD
Director, Infectious Diseases
Cook Children's Medical Center
Fort Worth, TX

ALBERT T. SHIU, MD, FACOG
Associate Professor of Obstetrics and Gynecology
Michigan State University
College of Human Medicine
Lansing, MI

GARY J. SILKO, MD
Director, Family Practice Residency Program
Saint Vincent Health Center
Erie, PA

SAMUEL SIM, MD
Department of Internal Medicine
Northeastern Ohio Universities College of Medicine
Canton Affiliated Hospitals
Canton, OH

RICHARD J. SIMENSEN, PHD
Associate Professor
Family Medicine
Self Memorial Hospital
Greenwood, SC

LEONARD N. SLATER, MD
Professor of Medicine, Infectious Diseases Section
University of Oklahoma Health Sciences Center
    & Veterans Affairs Medical Center
Oklahoma City, OK

ARTHUR R. SLAUGHTER, MD
Associate Director, Family Practice Education
Carilion Family Practice Residency Program
Vinton, VA

ROBERT J. SLIMAN, MD
Associate Professor
Department of Internal Medicine
Northeastern Ohio Universities College of Medicine
Canton, OH

W. PAUL SLOMIANY, MD
Assistant Director
Family Practice Residency Program
Washington Hospital
Washington, PA

H. GRATIN SMITH, MD, FAAP
Director of Pediatric Education
Family Practice Residency Program
Self Memorial Hospital
Greenwood, SC

JAY W. SMITH, MD
Dean for Academic Affairs
University of Arizona College of Medicine
Tucson, AZ

MICHAEL J. SMITH, MD
Assistant Professor of Orthopedic Surgery
Northeastern Ohio Universities College of Medicine
Akron, OH

STAN G. SMITH, MA, MB, FCFPC
Professor, Department of Family Practice
University of Saskatchewan
Saskatchewan, Saskatoon CANADA

NANCY SNAPP, MD, MPH
Family Practice Faculty
Swedish Family Practice Residency
Swedish Hospital Medical Center
Seattle, WA

GREGORY SNYDER, MD
Department of Family Medicine
State University of New York at Buffalo
Buffalo, NY

VERA Y. SOONG, MD
Chairperson
Department of Dermatology
Lloyd Noland Hospital
Fairfield, AL

NICHOLAS J. SPIRTOS, DO
Associate Professor
Director, Northeastern Ohio Fertility Center
Northeastern Ohio Universities College of Medicine & Akron City
    Hospital
Akron, OH

JEFFREY A. STEARNS, MD
Associate Professor
Family Medicine
University of Illinois College of Medicine
Rockford, IL

MICHAEL STRANGE, MD
Private Practice
Fort Worth, TX

THOMAS R. STRIGLE, MD
Private Practice
Findlay Surgical Associates
Findlay, OH

DAVID H. STUBBS, MD, FACS
Department of Surgery Education
Iowa Methodist Medical Center
Des Moines, IA

GREGG W. SUITS, MD
Private Practice
Hillsboro, OR

JACK L. SUMMERS, MD, PHD
Professor, Urology
Northeastern Ohio Universities College of Medicine
Chairman, Urology, Summa Health Systems
Akron, OH

GEOFFREY R. SWAIN, MD
Assistant Professor
Department of Family and Community Medicine
Medical College of Wisconsin
Milwaukee, WI

Contributing Authors

JAMES S. TAN, MD, FACP
Professor of Medicine
Chairman, Infectious Disease Section
Northeastern Ohio Universities College of Medicine
Akron, OH

DAVID H. THOM, MD, PHD
Assistant Professor, Department of Medicine
Division of Family and Community Medicine
Stanford University School of Medicine
Palo Alto, CA

MARK D. THOMAS, MD
Private Practice
Albuquerque, NM

WILLIAM L. TOFFLER, MD
Professor
Department of Family Medicine
Oregon Health Sciences University
Portland, OR

MOSHE S. TOREM, MD, FAPA
Professor & Chairman, Department of Psychiatry
Northeastern Ohio Universities College of Medicine
Chairman, Department of Psychiatry & Behavioral Sciences
Akron General Medical Center
Akron, OH

SHELDON M. TRAEGER, MD
Head, Intensive Care Service, Department of Internal Medicine
Summa Hospital System
Northeastern Ohio Universities College of Medicine
Akron, OH

FRANCISCO G. VALENCIA, MD
Section of Orthopedic Surgery
University of Arizona College of Medicine
Tucson, AZ

BRUCE T. VANDERHOFF, MD
Associate Director
Grant Family Practice Residency
Grant/Riverside Methodist Hospitals
Columbus, OH

DINA K. VARON, DDS, MS
Adjunct Assistant Professor of Pediatrics
University of Miami College of Medicine
Miami, FL

V. VASUDEVIAH, BSC, MBBS
Consultant
Bangalore, INDIA

RICHARD VIKEN, MD
Chairman, Department of Family Practice
The University of Texas Health Center at Tyler
Tyler, TX

CHRIS VINCENT, MD
Faculty
Family Practice Residency
Swedish Family Medicine
Seattle, WA

KENTON VOORHEES, MD
Assistant Clinical Professor
Medical Director Swedish Family Medicine Residency
Littleton, CO

KIMBERLE VORE, MD
Clinical Instructor
Washington Hospital
Washington, PA

GENE W. VOSKUHL, MD
Infectious Disease Section
University of Oklahoma Health Sciences Center
Oklahoma City, OK

STANLEY WALLACH, MD
Department of Medicine
Endocrine Division and Osteoporosis Center
Hospital for Joint Diseases/Orthopedic Institute
New York, NY

BRIDGET T. WALSH, DO
Department of Rheumatology
University of Arizona College of Medicine
Tucson, AZ

CHATRCHAI WATANAKUNAKORN, MD, FACP, FCCP
Professor of Internal Medicine
Northeastern Ohio Universities College of Medicine
Director, Infectious Disease Section, St. Elizabeth Health Center
Youngstown, OH

JOHN R. WATERSON, MD, PHD
Associate Professor of Pediatrics
Northeastern Ohio Universities College of Medicine
Akron, OH

AMY W. WAUG, MD
Resident, Family Practice
St. Francis Hospital of Evanston
Evanston, IL

KURT J. WEGNER, MD
Professor of Pediatrics
Neonatologist, Geneticist and Pediatric Consultant
Northeastern Ohio Universities College of Medicine
Tod Children's Hospital
Youngstown, OH

MARTIN E. WEINAND, MD
Associate Professor of Surgery
Division of Neurosurgery
University of Arizona College of Medicine
Tucson, AZ

BARRY D. WEISS, MD
Professor and Chairman
Department of Family Practice
University of Texas Health Science Center at San Antonio
San Antonio, TX

JEFFREY R. WELKO, MD
Director, Hyperbaric Oxygen Unit
Akron General Medical Center
Akron, OH

ROBERT L. WESTON, MD
Medical Director, International SOS
International Healthcare Network
La Jolla, CA

BERNHARD L. WIEDERMANN, MD
Associate Professor of Pediatrics, George Washington University
Director, Pediatric Residency Training Program
Children's National Medical Center
Washington, DC

GARY B. WILLIAMS, MD
Associate Professor of Surgery
Northeastern Ohio Universities College of Medicine
Akron, OH

FREMONT P. WIRTH, MD, FACS
Neurological Institute of Savannah
Savannah, GA

CHRISTOPHER M. WISE, MD
W. Robert Irby Associate Professor Medicine
Division of Rheumatology, Allergy & Immunology
Medical College of Virginia/Virginia Commonwealth University
Richmond, VA

JEFFREY D. WOLFREY, MD
Program Director, Family Practice Residency Program
Good Samaritan Hospital
Phoenix, AZ

MARK ERIC WORSHTIL, MD
Assistant Director
Family Practice Residency Program
Washington Hospital
Washington, PA

FRANCES WU, MD
Assistant Director
Somerset Family Practice Residency Program
Somerville, NJ

ALAYNE YATES, MD
Director, Division of Child Adolescent Psychiatry
John A. Burns School of Medicine
Kapiolani Medical Center
Honolulu, HI

WILLIAM F. YOUNG, JR., MD
Associate Professor of Medicine, Division of Hypertension,
    Endocrinology & Metabolism
Mayo Clinic and Foundation
Rochester, MN

CHERYL ZAGOZESKI, MD, CCFP
Department of Family Medicine
Plains Health Centre
Regina, Saskatchewan CANADA

RICHARD KENT ZIMMERMAN, MD, MPH
Assistant Professor, Departments of Family Medicine & Clinical
    Epidemiology & Health Services Administration
University of Pittsburgh
Pittsburgh, PA

CONTENTS

EXPANDED TOPICS

Contents

Contents

SHORT TOPICS

Contents

Contents

Contents

CONTENTS BY SYSTEM

SKIN/EXOCRINE

Contents

■ NERVOUS

Contents

PULMONARY

Contents

■ CARDIOVASCULAR

Contents

Contents

ENDOCRINE/METABOLIC

RENAL/UROLOGIC

Contents

HEMIC/LYMPHATIC/IMMUNOLOGIC

GASTROINTESTINAL

Contents

MUSCULOSKELETAL

Contents

REPRODUCTIVE

OTHER

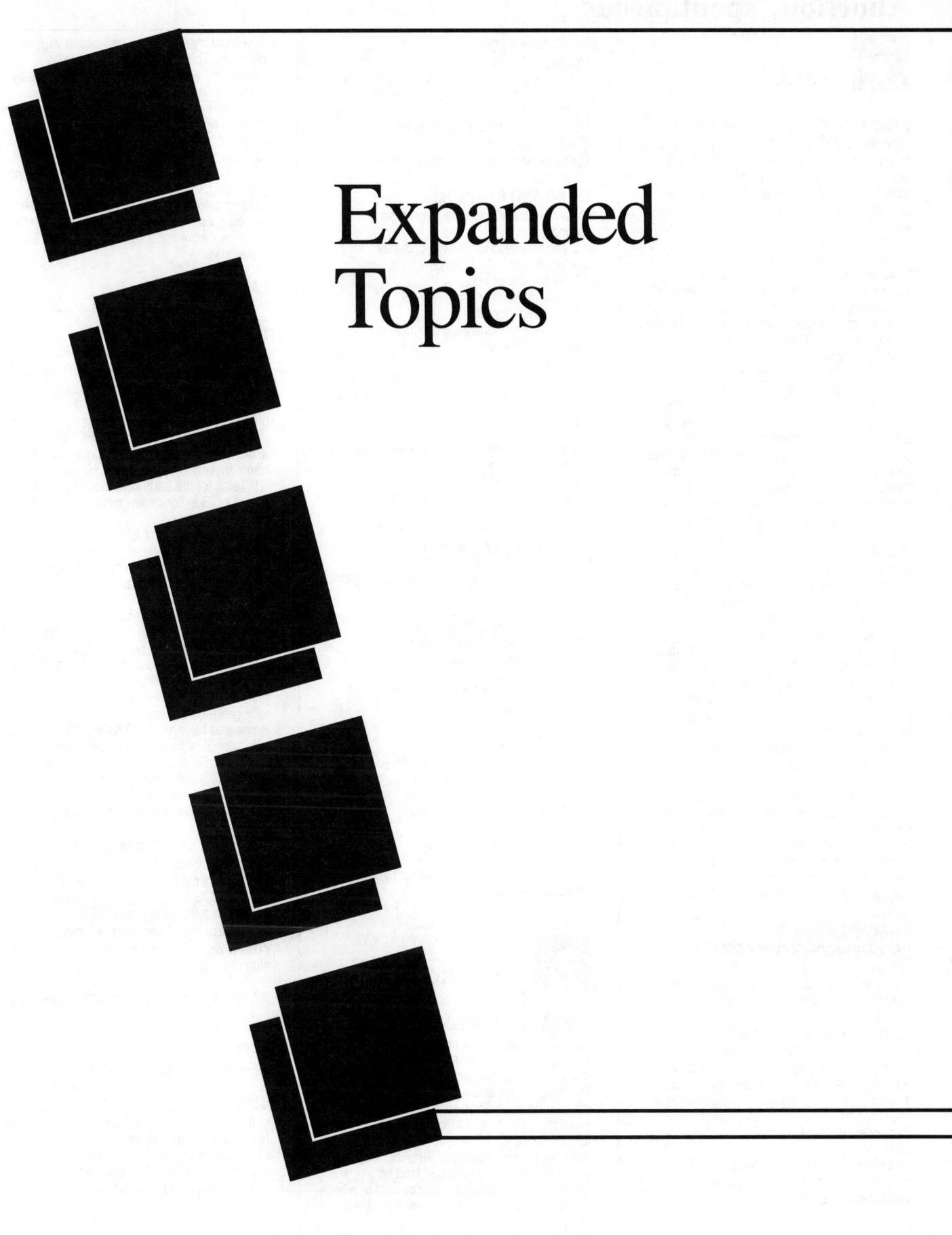

Expanded Topics

Abortion, spontaneous

BASICS

DESCRIPTION Abortion is the separation of products of conception from the uterus prior to the potential for fetal survival outside the uterus. Gestationally, the point at which potential fetal viability exists has been the subject of much legal and scientific debate, and definitions vary with locale and/or medical center; however, a "potentially viable" fetus generally weighs at least 500 grams and/or has a gestational age over 20 weeks.
• Spontaneous abortion: refers to expulsion of all (complete abortion) or part (incomplete abortion) of the products of conception from the uterus prior to the 20th completed week of gestation. Incomplete abortion tends to occur more often after the 10th gestational week, when the placenta and the fetus tend to be expelled separately. The placenta, either in whole or in part, can be retained and leads to continuing vaginal bleeding (sometimes profuse). Abortion is "threatened" when vaginal bleeding occurs early in pregnancy, with or without uterine contractions, but without dilatation of the cervix, rupture of the membranes, or expulsion of products of conception. Cervical dilation, rupture of membranes or expulsion of products in the presence of vaginal bleeding portends "inevitable abortion." Differentiation between threatened and inevitable abortion is desirable since management differs.
• Missed abortion: see Other Notes
• Induced abortion: refers to the evacuation of uterine contents/products of conception by either medical or surgical methodology
• Infected abortion: infection involving the products of conception and the maternal reproductive organs
• Septic abortion: dissemination of bacteria (and/or their toxins) into the maternal circulatory and organ system
• Habitual spontaneous abortion: three or more consecutive spontaneous abortions. Although repeated spontaneous abortions are often "chance" occurrences, many investigators recommend karyotyping of the parents and maternal evaluation for abnormalities (such as incompetent cervix) in cases of habitual abortion.
System(s) affected:
Reproductive,Endocrine/Metabolic
Genetics: Fetal (and to a much lesser extent maternal) chromosomal abnormalities greatly increase the incidence of spontaneous abortion
Incidence/Prevalence in USA:
• Estimated that 30-50% of all fertilized ova are spontaneously aborted. Most spontaneous abortions are clinically unrecognized because the fertilized/implanted ovum is expelled at or near the first missed period (i.e., prior to the traditional "hallmark" of potential pregnancy - amenorrhea).
• Approximately 10-15% of all recognized pregnancies end in clinically apparent spontaneous abortion

Predominant age:
• Young (< 15 years)
• Advancing age; women over 35 years of age have three times the risk of spontaneous abortion than women less than 30 years of age
• Incidence of induced abortion tends to decrease with age
Predominant sex: Female only

SIGNS AND SYMPTOMS
• In a previously diagnosed intrauterine pregnancy
  ◊ Vaginal bleeding (pink or brownish discharge)
  ◊ Uterine cramping
  ◊ Cervical dilation
  ◊ Ruptured membranes
  ◊ Passage of non-viable products of conception
  ◊ Fever
  ◊ Shock
  ◊ Soft, sub-involuted uterus

CAUSES
• The cause of most spontaneous abortions is unknown, however
  ◊ Chromosomal abnormalities (of the embryo/fetus) probably contribute to the majority
  ◊ Excessive caffeine consumption (over 2 cups of coffee/day) slightly increases the risk
• Improper implantation of fertilized ovum
• Abnormality of maternal reproductive organs
• Endocrine dysfunction
• Infectious systemic disease
• Poisons (including drugs and alcohol)
• Placental insufficiency abnormality
• Defective spermatozoa
• Trauma
• Therapeutic or criminal intervention
• Immunological factors

RISK FACTORS
• Fetal chromosomal abnormalities (100-fold increase in spontaneous abortion)
• Uterine abnormalities
• Maternal alcohol/drug ingestion
• Increasing maternal age
• Deteriorating health status (i.e., diabetes/thyroid disease)
• Infections with certain viruses or bacteria
• Previous abortions

DIAGNOSIS

DIFFERENTIAL DIAGNOSIS
• Ectopic pregnancy: a potentially life-threatening complication, difficult to distinguish from threatened abortion. Transvaginal ultrasonography can identify intrauterine gestational sacs at 32 days of gestation (at serum HCG levels of 1000-2000 IU). The absence of transvaginal ultrasound evidence of an intrauterine gestation with serum HCG over 1000 IU/L should be considered an ectopic pregnancy until proven otherwise. Culdocentesis may demonstrate free peritoneal blood.
• Cervical polyps, neoplasias, and/or

inflammatory conditions can cause vaginal bleeding. This bleeding is not usually associated with pain/cramping and is readily apparent on speculum exam.
• Hydatidiform mole pregnancy usually ends in abortion prior to the 20th week of pregnancy. Bloody discharge prior to abortion is common. An intrauterine grape-like appearing mass on the ultrasound is diagnostic. Human chorionic gonadotropin (HCG) is often positive.
• Membranous dysmenorrhea: characterized by bleeding, cramps and passage of endometrial casts can mimic spontaneous abortion. HCG is negative.

LABORATORY
• Cultures - for group B Streptococcus, gonorrhea and chlamydia
• Decreased hemoglobin
• Decreased hematocrit
• Vaginal cytology: karyopyknotic index near 20% indicates progesterone deficiency
• Human chorionic gonadotropin (HCG) - presumptive detection of pregnancy
  ◊ HCG (or its beta-subunit BHCG) can be assayed in urine and plasma, qualitatively and quantitatively
  ◊ Tests for the early detection of pregnancy detect HCG in concentrated urine within two weeks of ovulation
  ◊ Plasma assays of BHCG can provide presumptive evidence of pregnancy at implantation - one week after ovulation and one week prior to the first missed period
• Human chorionic gonadotropin (HCG) - assessment of fetal viability
  ◊ HCG concentration in maternal plasma rises rapidly from the second through the ninth gestational week. If plasma HCG is stable or declining, fetal viability and/or normal pregnancy is doubtful.
• Progesterone assay
Progesterone levels > 25 ng/mL are consistent with normal intrauterine pregnancy and are rarely seen in ectopic and/or non-viable pregnancy. A progesterone of < 5 ng/mL is ALWAYS an indicator of non-viable/non-intrauterine products of conception.
Drugs that may alter lab results:
• Heparin anticoagulants or ethylenediaminotetraacetic acid (EDTA) alter plasma HCG
• Phenothiazines alter urine HCG
Disorders that may alter lab results:
• Gross proteinuria, hematuria, elevated ESR alter urine HCG

PATHOLOGICAL FINDINGS Conceptual fragments

SPECIAL TESTS
• Progesterone estimation (RIA)

IMAGING
• Ultrasound examination for fetal viability and to rule out ectopic pregnancy
• Ultrasound imaging can be sensitive enough to confirm an intrauterine pregnancy in the fourth or fifth gestational week

DIAGNOSTIC PROCEDURES
• Two positive signs of early pregnancy are identification of fetal heart sounds (usually accomplished by Doppler instrumentation ≥ the ninth week of gestation) and identification of fetal parts/gestational sac by ultrasound
• Presumptive signs of pregnancy - increasing uterine size with corresponding increase in abdominal size, softening of the cervix, amenorrhea, breast soreness/swelling, presence of HCG in urine or blood
• Sterile speculum exam to determine bleeding source. Obtain cultures for group B Streptococcus, gonorrhea and chlamydia. Obtain catheterized urine for urinalysis/culture.
• A bimanual exam to assess uterine size and consistency/dilation of the cervix
• Careful assessment for adnexal mass/tenderness
• Consider a diagnosis of spontaneous abortion in a woman, of childbearing age, presenting with abnormal vaginal bleeding

TREATMENT

APPROPRIATE HEALTH CARE
Outpatient or inpatient, depending on severity of symptoms

GENERAL MEASURES
• Explore any first trimester vaginal bleeding
• Serial quantitative BHCG determination, progesterone assay, transvaginal/transabdominal ultrasonography
• Threatened abortion: bed rest (usually at home) and insert nothing per vagina. If bleeding is more severe (i.e., more than a heavy period), hospitalization and close observation are advisable.
• Type and screen for possible transfusion

SURGICAL MEASURES
• Inevitable or incomplete abortion: Dilatation and curettage (D&C) (usually suction)
• When completeness of an abortion is in doubt, a D&C for retained products should be performed
• Habitual abortion: Cerclage (cervical stitch) if cervical incompetence is suspected

ACTIVITY   If appropriate, bed rest

DIET   No special diet

PATIENT EDUCATION   American College of Obstetricians & Gynecologists, 409 12th St., SW, Washington, DC 20024-2188, (800)762-ACOG

MEDICATIONS

DRUG(S) OF CHOICE
• Bleeding following uncomplicated D&C or spontaneous abortion usually controlled by:

◊ Oxytocin (Pitocin) 3-10 units IM,or
◊ Methylergonovine (Methergine) 0.2 mg IM
• Analgesics if needed
• Rho(D) immune globulin if mother is Rh negative
• Beta-agonists (e.g. isoxsuprine) in threatened abortion
• Progesterone, if deficiency confirmed
Contraindications: None
Precautions: Do not give methylergonovine IV. Refer to manufacturer's literature.
Significant possible interactions: Refer to manufacturer's literature

ALTERNATIVE DRUGS   Perfusion of trophoblastic membrane vesicles reported to be 75% successful in selected patients

FOLLOWUP

PATIENT MONITORING
• Identification of products of conception within material expelled from the uterus confirms spontaneous abortion
• If abortion is complete, observe the patient for a period of time to check for further bleeding

PREVENTION/AVOIDANCE
• Any vaginal bleeding in a presumed or proven intrauterine pregnancy is abnormal and should be considered a "threatened" abortion until proven otherwise. In reality, vaginal bleeding in early pregnancy is common and often the bleeding source eludes diagnosis.
• In habitual abortion, the abortus should be sent for karyotyping. Explore other causes of habitual abortion with the couple to determine the best therapy.
• Special care and attention for the patient who has a subsequent pregnancy
• Surgical reinforcement of cervix for habitual abortion

POSSIBLE COMPLICATIONS
• Complications of D&C include uterine perforation, infection and bleeding
• Recurrent abortion
• Depression and feelings of guilt (patient may need counseling help)

EXPECTED COURSE/PROGNOSIS
• If bleeding ceases and pregnancy parameters continue normal progression, maternal prognosis is excellent. First trimester bleeding associated with preterm delivery, low birth weight infants (both preterm and term), and neonatal death.
• After D&C for incomplete or inevitable abortion and after complete abortion, prognosis is excellent
• Habitual abortion, prognosis for successful pregnancy is lower

MISCELLANEOUS

ASSOCIATED CONDITIONS
Hypothyroidism, diabetes mellitus

AGE-RELATED FACTORS
Pediatric: N/A
Geriatric: N/A
Others: N/A

PREGNANCY   Confined to pregnancy

SYNONYMS
• Miscarriage
• Habitual abortion
• Recurrent abortion

ICD-9-CM
• 634.9 Spontaneous abortion without mention of complications

SEE ALSO
• Ectopic pregnancy

OTHER NOTES   Missed abortion: Term abandoned in favor of more accurate descriptions (from better diagnostics) e.g., anembryonic gestation (molar pregnancy, empty sac) or first trimester intrauterine fetal demise. This term currently implies - retention of products of conception, embryonic, or fetal parts for eight weeks or more following embryonic or fetal demise.

ABBREVIATIONS   N/A

REFERENCES
• Cunningham FG, MacDonald PC, Gant NF, eds: Williams' Obstetrics. 19th Ed. Norwalk, CT, Appleton and Lange, 1993
• Wilcox AJ, et al: Incidence of early loss of pregnancy. New Engl J Med, 1988; 319:189-94
• Edmonds DK, et al: Early embryonic mortality in women. Fert Sterility. 1982;38:447-53
• Rempen A: Diagnosis and Viability of Early Pregnancy with Vaginal Sonography. J Ultras Med 1990; 9:711-716
• Daily CA, et al: The prognostic value of serum progesterone and quantitative B-Human Chorionic Gonadatropin in early human pregnancy. Am J Obstet Gynecol 1994;171:380-384
• Ohno M, et al: A Cytogenic study of spontaneous abortion with direct analysis of chorionic villi. Obstet Gynecol 1991;77(3):394-398
• Srisuphan W, et al: Caffeine consumption during pregnancy and association with late spontaneous abortion. Am J Obstet Gynecol 1986;154(1)
Illustrations: N/A
Internet references: http://www.5mcc.com

Author(s)
Kent R. Gebhardt, DO, FAAFP

Abruptio placentae

BASICS

DESCRIPTION Premature separation of otherwise normally implanted placenta. Sher's grades:
1: minimal or no bleeding; detected as retroplacental clot after delivery of viable fetus.
2: viable fetus with bleeding and tender irritable uterus.
3: type A with dead fetus and no coagulopathy; type B with dead fetus and coagulopathy (about 30% of grade 3's).
System(s) affected: Reproductive, Cardiovascular
Genetics: N/A
Incidence/Prevalence in USA:
• 1% of all deliveries
• 15% if one prior episode
• 20% if ≥ 2 prior episodes
Predominant age: All childbearing ages
Predominant sex: Female only

SIGNS AND SYMPTOMS
• Third trimester vaginal bleeding greater than one pad or tampon per hour
• Back pain, abdominal pain
• Uterine contractions, tenderness and/or hypertonia
• Blood loss may be concealed; clinical signs of shock may exceed estimated blood loss
• Since blood volumes increase in pregnancy, volume lost may exceed 30% before signs of shock or hypovolemia. Vital signs may be preserved even with significant loss.
• Narrowed pulse pressure, increased diastolic pressure, positive tilt test, orthostatic changes, or tachycardia may be soft signs of volume depletion
• Difficulty hearing fetal heart sounds or palpating fetus through a tender, tense, irritable uterus with bloody amniotic fluid
• Often constant pain with or without contractions
• In complete abruption, may find non-tender uterus

CAUSES
• Trauma of variable amounts; especially blunt abdominal trauma with anterior placental location in which external signs of trauma may be incongruent with fetal injury
• Sudden decompression of over-distended uterus as in hydramnios or twin gestation
• Cocaine use and abuse

RISK FACTORS
• Maternal smoking especially > 1 pack/day
• Multiparity
• Alcohol abuse
• Short umbilical cord
• Hypertension: pregnancy-induced and chronic
• Prior abruption
• Increased risk if hypertensive and parity > 3
• Preterm rupture of membranes, especially if bleeding occurs during observation interval - 5%
• Vaginal bleeding before spontaneous rupture of membranes - 25%

DIAGNOSIS

DIFFERENTIAL DIAGNOSIS Uterine rupture, placenta previa, vasa previa, marked bloody show, cervical and vaginal causes (e.g., chlamydia or gonorrhea with bloody, friable cervix), masses, other painful conditions (e.g., appendicitis, pyelonephritis), and labor.

LABORATORY
• Blood type, Rh, Coombs
• CBC with platelet count
• Prothrombin time (PT) , partial thromboplastin time (PTT), fibrinogen levels
• Cross match at least three units
Drugs that may alter lab results:
• Those affecting clotting parameters
• RhoD immune globulin less than 12 weeks prior may affect antibody test
Disorders that may alter lab results:
• Fibrinogen levels climb to 350-550 mg/dl (3.5-5.5 g/L) in third trimester and must fall to 100-150 mg/dl (1.0-1.5 g/L) before PTT will rise
• Fibrin split or degradation products are elevated in pregnancy so not very helpful in assessing disseminated intravascular coagulation (DIC)

PATHOLOGICAL FINDINGS
• Normocytic normochromic anemia with acute bleeding
• Elevated PT, PTT, fibrinogen levels below 100-150 mg/dl (1.0-1.5 g/L), platelets 20,000-50,000 if DIC active
• Positive Kleihauer-Betke reaction if fetal-maternal transfusion has occurred
• Positive antibody if RhoD isosensitization has occurred

SPECIAL TESTS
• Kleihauer-Betke for fetal-maternal transfusion
• Bedside clot test with red top tube of maternal blood with poor or non-clotting blood after 7-10 minutes indicating coagulopathy
• Apt test for fetal blood origin: mix vaginal blood with small amount tap water to cause hemolysis, centrifuge several minutes, mix pink hemoglobin containing supernatant with 1 cc 1% sodium hydroxide (NaOH) for each 5 cc supernatant, reading color in two minutes with fetal Hgb staying pink and adult turning yellow-brown
• Wright stain vaginal blood, observe for nucleated RBC's - usually of fetal origin
• Lecithin/sphingomyelin (L/S) ratio if delay of delivery is an option and length of pregnancy is preterm

IMAGING Although ultrasound may show sonolucent retroplacental clot, rounded placenta margin or thickened placenta, it is often not definitive - especially with posterior placement or mild abruption

DIAGNOSTIC PROCEDURES External uterine monitoring often shows elevated baseline pressure and frequent low amplitude contractions

TREATMENT

APPROPRIATE HEALTH CARE Hospitalize until stable

GENERAL MEASURES
• History and physical exam with past medical history, allergies, prior ultrasounds this gestation, and time of last meal
• In general, severe abruption best managed by delivery of fetus
• Sher's grade 1 - usual labor protocol
• Sher's grade 2 - varies with situation urgency
• Sher's grade 3 - vaginal delivery preferable if mother stable
• In trauma monitor inpatient at least 4 hours for evidence of fetal insult, abruption, fetal-maternal transfusion
• Early aggressive restoration of maternal physiology to protect fetus and maternal organs from hypoperfusion/DIC
• Stabilize vitals, keep Hct >30, urine output >30 cc/hr
• Bedrest with external fetal and labor monitoring, if fetus is viable
• Large bore 16-18 gauge IV crystalloid infusion, central line placement only after coagulation status has been assessed
• Attend to the basic ABC's with arterial blood gases (ABGs) if acidosis suspected
• Follow hemoglobin/hematocrit (H/H) and coagulation status every 1-2 hours
• Place intrauterine pressure catheter (IUC) since fetal risk climbs with elevated pressure
• Role of amniotomy to prevent amniotic fluid embolism is debatable but will speed delivery
• Positioning on left side may enhance venous return and cardiac output up to 30%
• Oxygen for all patients since oxygen consumption up 20% in pregnancy and fetus especially hypoxia sensitive
• If trauma without compromise after observation or small abruption and preterm may observe outpatient encouraging reduction of risk factors
• May need c/s after maternal stabilization if fetus viable and situation urgent

SURGICAL MEASURES N/A

ACTIVITY Bedrest until status defined

DIET NPO until status defined and cesarean section possibility ruled out

PATIENT EDUCATION In preterm mild abruption not necessitating delivery, teach about risks and causes

MEDICATIONS

DRUG(S) OF CHOICE
- Oxygen
- Saline or Ringer's lactate
- Whole blood and packed RBC's to keep hematocrit > 30
- May use oxytocin (Pitocin) augmentation to speed delivery
- Tocolytics like terbutaline, isoxsuprine or ritodrine may be used in mild non-compromising preterm abruption
- Rho(D) immune globulin for RhoD negative mother if undelivered or indicated after delivery
- 300 mcg RhoD immune globulin/15 cc fetal blood transfused, if Kleihauer-Betke test returns positive
- Fresh frozen plasma and platelet transfusions for coagulopathy with cryoprecipitate and fibrinogen given if indicated

Contraindications: Tocolytics should be withheld in preterm labor until abruption ruled out and fetal status defined

Precautions:
- Suffusion of blood into myometrium with weakening may increase risk of uterine rupture with oxytocin (Pitocin) augmentation
- Cryoprecipitate and fibrinogen may represent greater transfusion infection transmission risk

Significant possible interactions: Refer to manufacturer's profile of each drug

ALTERNATIVE DRUGS   N/A

FOLLOWUP

PATIENT MONITORING
- If not delivered, monitor for intrauterine growth retardation (IUGR)
- See regularly and assess for preterm labor

PREVENTION/AVOIDANCE   Eliminate risk factors when possible

POSSIBLE COMPLICATIONS
- Infection transfusion risks: Hepatitis, cytomegalovirus infection, HIV and others
- Sensitization from blood product transfusion

EXPECTED COURSE/PROGNOSIS
- 0.5% to 1% fetal mortality and 30-50% perinatal mortality
- With trauma and abruption 1% maternal and 30-70% fetal mortality
- Labor typically more rapid but hypotonus from blood suffusion may occur

MISCELLANEOUS

ASSOCIATED CONDITIONS
- Preeclampsia and other forms of hypertension in pregnancy
- Hypertension from collagen diseases such as lupus erythematosus
- Postpartum hemorrhage
- Maternal and fetal organ damage from hypoperfusion

AGE-RELATED FACTORS
Pediatric: N/A
Geriatric: N/A
Others: Multiparity, advanced maternal age - more at risk

PREGNANCY   This problem limited to pregnancy

SYNONYMS
- Placental abruption
- Premature separation of the placenta
- Couvelaire placenta

ICD-9-CM
641.2 Premature separation of placenta

SEE ALSO   Placenta previa

OTHER NOTES
- Increased pelvic blood flow of pregnancy may enhance blood loss
- Amniotic fluid embolism is rare but may present with DIC and severe respiratory distress
- Increased risk of fetal-maternal transfusion with trauma of anterior placenta location

ABBREVIATIONS   N/A

REFERENCES
- Scott CJ, et al: Emergencies in pregnancy. Patient Care 15,1991;132-150
- Lowe TW, et al: Placental abruption. Clinical OB Gyn 1990;33(3)
Illustrations: N/A
Internet references: http://www.5mcc.com

Author(s)
Mark E. Sexton, MD

Acetaminophen poisoning

BASICS

DESCRIPTION

• A disorder characterized by hepatic necrosis following large ingestions of acetaminophen. Symptoms may vary from initial nausea, vomiting, diaphoresis, and malaise to jaundice, confusion, somnolence, coma, and death. The clinical hallmark is the onset of symptoms within 24 hours of ingestion of acetaminophen-only or combination products.

• Acetaminophen poisoning is most often encountered following large single ingestions of acetaminophen-containing medications. However, poisoning also occurs following acute and chronic ingestions of lesser amounts in susceptible individuals including those who regularly abuse alcohol, are chronically malnourished, or take medications which affect hepatic metabolism of acetaminophen.

System(s) affected: Gastrointestinal, Renal/Urologic, Cardiovascular
Genetics: N/A
Incidence/Prevalence in USA:

• Over 105,000 ingestions of acetaminophen-containing medications reported by poison control centers in 1995
• 103 total deaths in 1995, one in children < 6

Predominant age:

• Occurs in children and adults at any age
• Approximately 48% of exposures are in children under 6 years

Predominant sex: No reported association

SIGNS AND SYMPTOMS

• Develop over the first 24 hours following large ingestions and may last as long as 8 days
• Severe symptoms indicate large ingestions or co-ingestants
• Fulminant hepatic failure occurs in less than 1% of adults and is very rare in children under 6 years
• Stage 1, first 24 hours
  ◊ Nausea
  ◊ Vomiting
  ◊ Diaphoresis
• Stage 2, 24-48 hours
  ◊ Right upper quadrant pain
  ◊ Typically less nausea, vomiting, diaphoresis, and malaise than in stage 1
• Stage 3, 72-96 hours
  ◊ Nausea, vomiting, malaise reappear
  ◊ Severe poisonings may result in jaundice, confusion, somnolence, and coma
• Stage 4, 7-8 days
  ◊ Resolution of clinical signs in survivors
• May develop gradually following long-term ingestion of smaller amounts of acetaminophen. Such patients may present in any stage 1-3 without a history of excessive acetaminophen ingestion.

CAUSES
Accidental or intentional ingestion of acetaminophen or combination medications containing acetaminophen

RISK FACTORS
• Age less than 6 years
• Concurrent oral poisoning with other substances
• Psychiatric illness
• History of previous toxic ingestions or suicide attempts
• Regular ingestion of large amounts of alcohol

DIAGNOSIS

DIFFERENTIAL DIAGNOSIS
• Consider presence of co-ingestants, especially alcohol
• Other ingested toxins which produce severe acute hepatic injury, including the mushroom Amanita phalloides and products containing yellow phosphorus or carbon tetrachloride

LABORATORY
• Plasma acetaminophen levels should be drawn on all patients 4 or more hours after ingestion (levels prior to 4 hours not helpful)
• A second acetaminophen level drawn 4-6 hours after the first level is recommended if the ingested acetaminophen is an extended release product (e.g., Tylenol Extended Relief) or is not known to be an immediate release product
  ◊ If the second level is higher than the first level or is close to the "possible risk" level on the Rumack-Matthew nomogram, it may be prudent to obtain additional acetaminophen levels every 2 hours until the levels stabilize or decline
• Screens for suspected co-ingestants (aspirin, iron, others) may be positive (especially when suicide is a possibility)
• With toxic ingestions, aspartate transaminase (AST; SGOT), alanine transaminase (ALT; SGPT), and bilirubin levels begin to rise in Stage 2 and peak in Stage 3. In severe poisonings, the PT will parallel these changes.
• AST levels over 1000 IU/L are consistent with the diagnosis and levels of 20,000 IU/L are not uncommon
• Laboratory abnormalities usually resolve by stage 4
• Renal function abnormalities are common in patients with hepatotoxicity
• Evidence of damage to the pancreas and heart may present following severe poisonings
Drugs that may alter lab results: None with clinically significant cross-reactivity with plasma acetaminophen assay
Disorders that may alter lab results: Diseases or toxic substances which damage the liver, particularly alcohol

PATHOLOGICAL FINDINGS
Centrilobular hepatic necrosis

SPECIAL TESTS N/A

IMAGING N/A

DIAGNOSTIC PROCEDURES None other than correlating plasma acetaminophen levels with the clinical presentation

TREATMENT

APPROPRIATE HEALTH CARE
• Contact a regional poison control center for management recommendations
• All patients should be evaluated at a health care facility
• Outpatient for non-toxic accidental ingestions
• Inpatient for toxic and intentional ingestions

GENERAL MEASURES
• The stomach of untreated patients should be emptied by ipecac or gastric lavage if within 4 hours of ingestion
• Patients may receive (especially if ingestion is 100-150 mg/kg) ipecac at home if alert and unable to be evaluated within 1 hour of ingestion
• Activated charcoal should be used, but preferably not within 1 hour of administration of the antidote N-acetylcysteine (NAC)
• NAC should be given when plasma acetaminophen concentrations measured 4 or more hours after ingestion are in the "possible risk" or higher levels on the Rumack-Matthew nomogram. This corresponds to acetaminophen levels greater than 150 µg/mL (993 µmol/L), 75 µg/mL (497 µmol/L), and 40 µg/mL (265 µmol/L) at 4 hours, 8 hours, and 12 hours after ingestion, respectively.
• NAC therapy may be effective up to 36 hours or more after ingestion

SURGICAL MEASURES N/A

ACTIVITY Restricted if significant hepatic damage has occurred

DIET No special diet except with severe hepatic damage

PATIENT EDUCATION
• Education of parents/caregivers during well child visits
• Anticipatory guidance for caregivers, family, and cohabitants of potentially suicidal patients
• Patient brochure: Child Safety: How to keep your home safe for your baby. American Academy of Family Physicians, 8880 Ward Parkway, Kansas City, MO 64114-2797
• Education of patients taking long-term acetaminophen therapy

Acetaminophen poisoning

MEDICATIONS

DRUG(S) OF CHOICE
• Three classes of medicine:
  ◊ Ipecac syrup
  ◊ Activated charcoal
  ◊ Acetylcysteine (N-acetylcysteine, NAC, Mucomyst)
• At home:
  ◊ Ipecac syrup may be given (especially if ingestion is 100-150 mg/kg) if the patient is alert and unable to be evaluated at a health care facility within 1 hour
  ◊ Ipecac syrup: Age 6 months-1 year 5 mL; age 1-12 years 15 mL; age > 12 years 30 mL. Give with 240 mL of water when possible; may repeat in 30 minutes if emesis has not occurred.
• Emergency facility/hospital:
  ◊ Patients evaluated within 4 hours of ingestion should have their stomachs evacuated. Gastric lavage is the preferred method.
  ◊ Activated charcoal: 1 g/kg for initial dose; preferably not within 1 hour of NAC administration. Additional concurrent use during NAC therapy is controversial.
  ◊ Acetylcysteine: oral loading dose of 140 mg/kg, followed by 70 mg/kg every 4 hours for 17 additional doses. Whenever possible, NAC therapy should be initiated within 8 hours following the toxic ingestion.

Contraindications:
• Ipecac should not be given to patients with decreased responsiveness
• Medication allergies

Precautions:
• Aggressive ipecac therapy may result in prolonged vomiting, thereby interfering with NAC administration
• To avoid risks of decreased effectiveness and aspiration, activated charcoal should be given at least 30 minutes to 1 hour after ipecac and never before ipecac
• NAC may cause significant nausea and vomiting due to it's sulfur content; consider administration by nasogastric tube. Nausea can be treated with metoclopramide (Reglan, 0.5-1 mg/kg IV) or ondansetron (Zofran) 0.15 mg/kg IV, for age > 4 years; usually 4 mg/dose

Significant possible interactions:
Activated charcoal given within 1 hour of NAC may adsorb the NAC, thereby limiting its effectiveness

ALTERNATIVE DRUGS
• IV NAC outside US; in approved trials within US
• Oral racemethionine (methionine)

FOLLOWUP

PATIENT MONITORING
Psychiatric follow-up after intentional ingestions

PREVENTION/AVOIDANCE
• Parent/caregiver education essential
  ◊ Education during well child exams regarding poisoning prevention
  ◊ Ipecac syrup at home
  ◊ Emergency telephone numbers

POSSIBLE COMPLICATIONS
Rare following recovery from acute poisoning

EXPECTED COURSE/PROGNOSIS
• Complete recovery with early therapy
• Fewer than 1% of adult patients develop hepatic failure
• Hepatic failure is very rare in children under 6 years

MISCELLANEOUS

ASSOCIATED CONDITIONS N/A

AGE-RELATED FACTORS
Pediatric: Hepatic damage at toxic acetaminophen levels is decreased in children less than 6 years
Geriatric: Hepatic damage may be increased if taking hepatotoxic medications chronically
Others: N/A

PREGNANCY
• Increased incidence of spontaneous abortion, especially with overdose at early gestational age
• Incidence of spontaneous abortion or fetal death appears increased when NAC treatment is delayed

SYNONYMS
• Paracetamol poisoning

ICD-9-CM
965.4 poisoning by aromatic analgesics (acetaminophen)

SEE ALSO N/A

OTHER NOTES N/A

ABBREVIATIONS
NAC = N-acetylcysteine

REFERENCES
• Anker AL, Smilkstein MJ: Acetaminophen - concepts and controversies. Emerg Med Clin N Amer 1994;12:335-49
• Lewis RK, Paloucek FP: Assessment and treatment of acetaminophen overdose. Clin Pharm 1991; l0:765-74
• Litovitz TL, Felberg L, White S, Klein-Schwartz W: 1995 Annual report of the American Association of Poison Control Centers Toxic Exposure Surveillance System. Am J Emerg Med 1996;14:487-537
Illustrations: N/A
Internet references: http://www.5mcc.com

Author(s)
Lars C. Larsen, MD

Acne rosacea

 BASICS

DESCRIPTION Chronic skin eruption with flushing and dilation of small blood vessels in the face, especially nose and cheeks. Sometimes associated with ocular symptoms (ocular rosacea).
System(s) affected: Skin/Exocrine
Genetics: People of Northern European and Celtic background commonly afflicted
Incidence/Prevalence in USA: Common
Predominant age: 30-50
Predominant sex: Female > Male

SIGNS AND SYMPTOMS
• Skin flush - prominent at onset
• Redness - lower half of nose, sometimes whole nose, forehead, cheeks, chin
• Conjunctivae red - (sometimes)
• Erythema, dusky - (in advanced cases)
• Blood vessels in involved area collapse under pressure
• Acne lesions form papules, pustules, and nodules; comedones are rare
• Telangiectasia
• Rhinophyma (sometimes) more common in males

CAUSES
• No proven cause. Possibilities include:
 ◊ Thyroid and gonadal disturbance
 ◊ Alcohol, coffee, tea, spiced food overindulgence (unproven)
 ◊ Demodex follicular parasite (suspected)
 ◊ Exposure to cold, heat, hot drinks
 ◊ Emotional stress
 ◊ Dysfunction of the gastrointestinal tract

RISK FACTORS N/A

 DIAGNOSIS

DIFFERENTIAL DIAGNOSIS
• Drug eruptions (iodides and bromides)
• Granulomas of the skin
• Cutaneous lupus erythematosus
• Carcinoid syndrome
• Deep fungal infection
• Acne vulgaris
• Seborrheic dermatitis

LABORATORY N/A
Drugs that may alter lab results: N/A
Disorders that may alter lab results: N/A

PATHOLOGICAL FINDINGS
• Inflammation around hypertrophied sebaceous glands, producing papules, pustules and cysts
• Absence of comedones and blocked ducts
• Vascular dilatation and dermal lymphocytic infiltrate

SPECIAL TESTS N/A

IMAGING N/A

DIAGNOSTIC PROCEDURES N/A

 TREATMENT

APPROPRIATE HEALTH CARE
Outpatient

GENERAL MEASURES
• Reassurance
• Treat psychological stress if present
• Avoid oil based cosmetics. Others are acceptable and may help women tolerate the symptoms.
• Electrodesiccation of permanently dilated blood vessels

SURGICAL MEASURES Surgical
treatment of rhinophyma

ACTIVITY No restrictions. Support physical fitness.

DIET Avoid any food or drink that causes facial flushing, e.g., hot drinks, spiced food, alcohol

PATIENT EDUCATION
• American Academy of Dermatology (708) 330-0230

MEDICATIONS

DRUG(S) OF CHOICE
• Low dose oral tetracycline 500-1000 mg/day
• Sulfur-containing local applications - alcohol-sulfur (Liquimat),sulfur (Fostril), resorcinol-sulfur (Rezamid), sulfacetamide-sulfur (Sulfacet-R)
• Topical steroids should not be used as they may aggravate rosacea
• Topical metronidazole 0.75% gel - apply each morning and at bedtime after cleansing skin; also available as a cream which may be better tolerated by some patients
• Topical erythromycin
• Topical clindamycin lotion preferred
Contraindications:
• Tetracycline: not for use in pregnancy or children < 8 years.
• Isotretinoin: teratogenic; not for use in pregnancy or in women or reproductive age who are not using a reliable birth control method.
Precautions:
• Tetracycline: may cause photosensitivity; sunscreen recommended.
Significant possible interactions:
• Tetracycline: avoid concurrent administration with antacids, dairy products, or iron.
• Broad-spectrum antibiotics: may reduce the effectiveness of oral contraceptives; barrier method recommended.

ALTERNATIVE DRUGS
• For severe cases, isotretinoin orally for 4 months.

FOLLOWUP

PATIENT MONITORING Occasional and as needed. Close followup for women using isotretinoin.

PREVENTION/AVOIDANCE No preventive measure known

POSSIBLE COMPLICATIONS
• Rhinophyma (dilated follicles and thickened bulbous skin on nose), especially in men
• Conjunctivitis
• Blepharitis
• Keratitis

EXPECTED COURSE/PROGNOSIS
• Slowly progressive
• Subsides spontaneously (sometimes)

MISCELLANEOUS

ASSOCIATED CONDITIONS
• Seborrheic dermatitis of scalp and eyelids
• Keratitis with photophobia, lacrimation, visual disturbance
• Corneal lesions
• Blepharitis
• Uveitis

AGE-RELATED FACTORS
Pediatric: Unlikely in this age group
Geriatric: Uncommon after age 60
Others: N/A

PREGNANCY Use of oral isotretinoin contraindicated

SYNONYMS Rosacea

ICD-9-CM 695.3 rosacea

SEE ALSO
• Blepharitis
• Dermatitis, seborrheic
• Uveitis
• Lupus erythematosus, discoid
• Acne vulgaris

OTHER NOTES N/A

ABBREVIATIONS N/A

REFERENCES
• Fitzpatrick TB, et al, eds: Dermatology In General Medicine. 4th Ed. New York, McGraw-Hill, 1993
• Habif T: Clinical Dermatology. 3rd Ed. St. Louis, CV Mosby, 1996
Illustrations: 8 available on CD-ROM
Internet references: http://www.5mcc.com

Author(s)
John M. Little, MD

Acne vulgaris

 BASICS

DESCRIPTION Acne is an androgenically stimulated, inflammatory disorder of the sebaceous glands, resulting in comedones, papules, inflammatory pustules and, occasionally, scarring
System(s) affected: Skin/Exocrine
Genetics: N/A
Incidence/Prevalence in USA: Virtually 100% of adolescents are affected to some degree. 15% will seek medical advice.
Predominant age: Early to late puberty, although some cases will persist into the third and fourth decade
Predominant sex: Male = Female (males tend to be more severely affected)

SIGNS AND SYMPTOMS
• Closed comedones (whiteheads)
• Open comedones (blackheads)
• Nodules or papules
• Pustules, with or without redness and edema ("cysts")
• Scars
• The lesions occur over the forehead, cheeks and nose, and may extend over the central chest and back

CAUSES Androgens stimulate the rate of keratin turnover in the sebaceous gland. The keratin plug, visible as a comedone, causes an accumulation of sebum in the gland. The presence of Propionibacterium acnes stimulates an inflammatory response to the sebum, which results in papule and pustule formation.

RISK FACTORS
• Adolescence
• Male sex
• Androgenic steroids, e.g., steroid abuse, some birth control pills
• Oily cosmetics, including cleansing creams, moisturizers, oil-based foundations
• Rubbing or occluding the skin surface, as may occur with sports equipment (helmets and shoulder pads), holding the telephone or hands against the skin
• Drugs - iodides or bromides, lithium, phenytoins
• Systemic corticosteroids
• Virilization disorders
• Hot, humid climate

 DIAGNOSIS

DIFFERENTIAL DIAGNOSIS
• Occupational exposure to tars, oils, grease
• Folliculitis
• Acne rosacea
• Steroid acne
• Perioral acne

LABORATORY N/A
Drugs that may alter lab results: N/A
Disorders that may alter lab results: N/A

PATHOLOGICAL FINDINGS
• Oiliness, thickening of the skin
• Hypertrophy of the sebaceous glands
• Perifolliculitis
• Scarring

SPECIAL TESTS Testosterone and its metabolites can be measured in those very rare cases when acne arises de novo in the previously unaffected adult

IMAGING N/A

DIAGNOSTIC PROCEDURES History and physical exam

 TREATMENT

APPROPRIATE HEALTH CARE
Outpatient

GENERAL MEASURES
• Comedone extraction: use a comedone extractor, after incising the thin layer of epithelium directly over the comedone
• Intralesional injection - of large cystic lesions with 0.5-1.0 mL of triamcinolone (Kenalog 20)
• Cleansing: gentle cleansing with a mild soap once or twice a day will control surface oiliness. More frequent washing will further irritate the skin and increase sebum production.
• Oil-free sun screens: although UV light results in some improvement in untreated acne, it will react adversely with the medications used to treat acne. Long-term UV exposure causes permanent skin damage.
• Stress management: may be helpful if acne flares with stress

SURGICAL MEASURES N/A

ACTIVITY Full activity. Physical conditioning important.

DIET
• Counsel regarding good nutrition
• No special diet has been shown to diminish acne. Chocolate and fatty foods do not aggravate acne.

PATIENT EDUCATION
• It is important for the patient to know that there is no cure for acne, that treatment only controls the lesions
• Any treatment measure takes a minimum of 4 weeks to show results
• The topical agents can cause redness and drying of the skin and most people need encouragement to persist with these useful agents
• For patient education materials favorably reviewed on this topic: American Academy of Dermatology, 930 N. Meacham Rd., P.O. Box 4014, Schaumburg, IL 60168-4014, (708)330-0230

MEDICATIONS

DRUG(S) OF CHOICE
• Topical medications, best for comedones and mild inflammatory acne
• Benzoyl peroxide starting at 5%, applied to dry skin at bedtime.
• Tretinoin (retinoic acid, Retin-A, Renova) starting with 0.025% cream, applied to dry skin at bedtime. Gel is available and is more drying; better for chest and back. Retinoic acid often causes an initial flare of lesions as it increases the turnover of previously formed keratin plugs.
• Topical erythromycin applied to cystic lesions, or
• Clindamycin, 2% solution in water or commercial formulation (Dalacin T), often helps cystic acne lesions
• Tetracycline 250 mg qid for 7-10 days, then tapering to the lowest effective dose
• Erythromycin 250 mg qid for 7-10 days, then tapering to the lowest effective dose
• Oral contraceptives, especially those with a very low androgenic activity
• Isotretinoin (Accutane), although associated with serious, dose-related side effects, can help patients who have severe pustular acne in spite of all the previous measures. Dosage is 0.5-1.0 mg/kg/day, in two doses, given for 12-16 weeks. A second course can be given after an 8-week interval. Common side effects include very dry skin, mucous membranes and cheilitis in effective doses, and lipid and liver function abnormalities.

Contraindications:
• Allergy
• Severe hepatic dysfunction - all oral agents
• Tetracycline: not for use in pregnancy or children < 8 years
• Isotretinoin: teratogenic; not for use in pregnancy or in women or reproductive age who are not using a reliable birth control method.

Precautions:
• Tetracycline: may cause photosensitivity; sunscreen recommended.

Significant possible interactions:
• Tetracycline: avoid concurrent administration with antacids, dairy products, or iron.
• Erythromycin: terfenadine (Seldane) and astemizole; ECG abnormalities
• Broad-spectrum antibiotics: may reduce the effectiveness of oral contraceptives; barrier method recommended.

ALTERNATIVE DRUGS   See previous discussion

FOLLOWUP

PATIENT MONITORING
• Monthly visits until adequate response is obtained
• Pre-treatment and monthly serum lipids, liver function tests, and pregnancy tests for patients on isotretinoin

PREVENTION/AVOIDANCE   N/A

POSSIBLE COMPLICATIONS
• Acne conglobata - a severe confluent inflammatory acne with systemic symptoms
• Facial scarring
• Psychological scarring

EXPECTED COURSE/PROGNOSIS
Gradual improvement over time

MISCELLANEOUS

ASSOCIATED CONDITIONS
• See risk factors
• Androgen-secreting tumors

AGE-RELATED FACTORS
Pediatric: Mild, self-limited acne can occur in the neonate
Geriatric: N/A
Others: N/A

PREGNANCY
• May result in a flare, or remission, of acne
• Isotretinoin: causes severe fetal malformations; effective contraception should be ensured one month prior to and one month following isotretinoin therapy.
• Erythromycin can be used during pregnancy, but would prefer topical agents whenever possible.

SYNONYMS   N/A

ICD-9-CM   706.1 Other acne

SEE ALSO   Acne rosacea

OTHER NOTES
• Acne is usually much more significant to the patient than it appears to the doctor
• Acne subsides with time
• Acne is often an "entry ticket"; frequently the adolescent also wants advice about life-style, contraception, physiology, etc.

ABBREVIATIONS   N/A

REFERENCES
• Fitzpatrick TB, et al: Color atlas and synopsis of clinical dermatology. 2nd Ed. New York, McGraw-Hill, 1992
• Fitzpatrick TB, et al, eds: Dermatology In General Medicine. 3rd Ed. New York, McGraw-Hill, 1987
• Pochi PE, Quan M: Acne Vulgaris. Amer Fam Phys Monograph, Spring, 1992
Illustrations: 12 available on CD-ROM
Internet references: http://www.5mcc.com

Author(s)
Gary Levine, MD

Addison's disease

BASICS

DESCRIPTION Adrenal hypofunction from primary disease (partial or complete destruction) of the adrenal gland with inadequate secretion of glucocorticoids and mineralocorticoids. An autoimmune process is the most common cause (80% of the cases) followed by tuberculosis. AIDS is becoming a more frequent cause.
• Addison's disease (primary adrenocortical insufficiency) is differentiated from secondary (pituitary failure) and tertiary (hypothalamic failure) causes of adrenocortical insufficiency (see Differential Diagnosis)
• Addisonian (adrenal) crisis - acute complication of adrenal insufficiency (circulatory collapse, dehydration, hypotension, nausea, vomiting, hypoglycemia); usually precipitated by acute physiologic stressor such as surgery, illness, exacerbation of co-morbid process, acute withdrawal of long term corticosteroid therapy
System(s) affected: Endocrine/Metabolic
Genetics: Autoimmune adrenal insufficiency shows some hereditary disposition. Familial glucocorticoid insufficiency may have recessive pattern; adrenoleukodystrophy may be X-linked. Frequent association with other autoimmune disorders.
Incidence/Prevalence: Approximately 4:100,000
Predominant age: All ages; usually 3rd to 5th decade
Predominant sex: Females > Males (slight)

SIGNS AND SYMPTOMS
• Weakness, fatigue
• Weight loss
• Dizziness; low blood pressure, orthostatic hypotension
• Increased pigmentation (extensor surfaces, hand creases, dental-gingival margins, buccal and vaginal mucosa, lips, areola, pressure points, scars; "tanning"; freckles; vitiligo)
• Anorexia; nausea; vomiting
• Chronic diarrhea
• Abdominal pain
• Decreased cold tolerance
• Salt craving
• Hair loss in females

CAUSES
• Autoimmune adrenal insufficiency (~80%)
• Tuberculosis (~20%)
• Waterhouse-Friderichsen syndrome (disseminated adrenal infection and subsequent infarction; meningococcemia most common; Pseudomonas aeruginosa common in children; atypical pathogens, CMV, Cryptococcus, MAC in immunosuppressed and AIDS)
• Fungal disease (histoplasmosis, blastomycosis, coccidioidomycosis)
• Bilateral adrenal hemorrhage and infarction (anticoagulants; 50% are in therapeutic range at time of hemorrhage)
• Metastatic (lung, breast, colon), lymphoma, Kaposi's sarcoma (tumor must destroy 90% of gland to produce hypofunction)

• Drugs (ketoconazole, etomidate)
• Surgical adrenalectomy
• Radiation therapy
• Sarcoidosis
• Hemochromatosis
• Amyloidosis
• Adrenoleukodystrophy
• Adrenomyelodystrophy
• Polyglandular endocrine syndromes
• Congenital (enzyme defects; hypoplasia; familial glucocortical deficiency)
• Idiopathic

RISK FACTORS
• Family history of autoimmune adrenal insufficiency. About 40% of patients have a first- or second-degree relative with one of the associated disorders.
• Taking steroids for prolonged periods, then experiencing severe infection, trauma or surgical procedures

DIAGNOSIS

DIFFERENTIAL DIAGNOSIS
• Secondary adrenocortical insufficiency
  ◊ Withdrawal of long-term corticosteroid use
  ◊ Sheehan's syndrome (postpartum necrosis of pituitary)
  ◊ Empty sella syndrome
  ◊ Surgical excision of pituitary
  ◊ Pituitary adenomas, carcinomas (rare), craniopharyngiomas
  ◊ Infiltrative disorders of pituitary (sarcoidosis, hemochromatosis, amyloidosis, histiocytosis X)
  ◊ Megestrol
• Tertiary adrenocortical insufficiency
  ◊ Pituitary stalk transection
  ◊ Trauma
  ◊ Disruption of production of corticotropic releasing factor (CRF)
• Myopathies
• Other causes of hypoglycemia
• Syndrome of inappropriate antidiuretic hormone (SIADH)
• Heavy metal ingestion
• Severe nutritional deficiencies
• Sprue syndrome
• Hyperparathyroidism
• Neurofibromatosis
• Peutz-Jeghers syndrome
• Porphyria cutanea tarda
• Salt-losing nephritis
• Bronchogenic carcinoma
• Anorexia nervosa
• Other causes of hypoglycemia

LABORATORY
• Low serum sodium
• Elevated serum potassium
• Elevated BUN
• Elevated serum calcium
• Hypoglycemia when fasted
• Metabolic acidosis
• Low cortisol level
• Elevated ACTH level
• Moderate neutropenia
• Eosinophilia
• Relative lymphocytosis
• Anemia
Drugs that may alter lab results: Digitalis
Disorders that may alter lab results: Diabetes mellitus

PATHOLOGICAL FINDINGS Atrophic adrenals in autoimmune adrenalitis. Infiltrative and hemorrhagic disorders produce enlargement with destruction of entire gland.

SPECIAL TESTS
• Rapid ACTH stimulation test: Cosyntropin 0.25 mg IV, measure pre-injection and 60 minute post-injection cortisol levels. Patients with Addison's disease have low to normal values that do not rise
• Metapyrone test
• Insulin-induced hypoglycemia test
• CRH may help distinguish secondary from tertiary adrenal insufficiency

IMAGING
• Abdominal CT scan
  ◊ Small adrenal glands in autoimmune adrenalitis
  ◊ Enlarged adrenal glands in infiltrative and hemorrhagic disorders
• Abdominal x-ray: may show adrenal calcifications
• Chest x-ray: may show adrenal calcifications, small heart size, calcification of cartilage

DIAGNOSTIC PROCEDURES A work-up to determine the cause of Addison's disease

TREATMENT

APPROPRIATE HEALTH CARE
• Outpatient
• Inpatient during adrenal crisis

GENERAL MEASURES
• Treatment for adrenal insufficiency is with glucocorticoid and mineralocorticoid replacement
  ◊ 5 S's of management of adrenal crisis: salt, sugar, steroids, support, search for precipitating illness
• Appropriate treatment for underlying cause (e.g., tuberculosis)

SURGICAL MEASURES N/A

ACTIVITY As tolerated

DIET Arrange for a diet that maintains sodium and potassium balances

PATIENT EDUCATION
• For patient education materials favorably reviewed on this topic, contact: National Addison's Disease Foundation, 505 Northern Blvd., Suite 200, Great Neck, NY 11021, (516)487-4992
• Patient should wear or carry medical identification with information about the disease and the need for hydrocortisone or other replacement therapy
• Instruct patient in self-administering of parenteral hydrocortisone for emergency situations (e.g., traveling in remote areas away from medical help)

MEDICATIONS

DRUG(S) OF CHOICE
• For chronic adrenal insufficiency:
  ◊ Hydrocortisone 15-20 mg orally each morning upon arising and 10 mg at 4-5 each afternoon is usual dosage (dosage may vary and is usually less in children's),PLUS,
  ◊ Fludrocortisone 0.05-0.2 mg orally once/day
• Acute adrenal insufficiency
  ◊ Hydrocortisone hemisuccinate 100 mg IV followed by 10 mg/hr infusion
  ◊ IV glucose, saline, plasma expanders
• For acute illnesses (fever, stress, minor trauma)
  ◊ Double the patient's ususal steroid dose
Contraindications: Refer to manufacturer's literature
Precautions:
• Patients with hepatic disease may need a reduced dose
• Elderly should have a slightly reduced dose
• Refer to manufacturer's literature for other precautions
Significant possible interactions: Refer to manufacturer's literature. Rifampin, phenytoin, and barbiturates may precipitate adrenal insufficiency in addisonian patients by inducing steroid-metabolizing liver enzymes

ALTERNATIVE DRUGS Prednisone 5 mg in AM and 2.5 mg at hs

FOLLOWUP

PATIENT MONITORING
• Verify adequacy of therapy - normal blood pressure, serum electrolytes normal, normal plasma renin, improvement of appetite and strength, increase in heart size to normal, normal blood glucose fasting level
• Lifelong medical supervision for signs of continued adequate therapy and avoidance of overdose

PREVENTION/AVOIDANCE
• No preventive measures known for Addison's disease
• Prevention of complications
  ◊ Anticipate adrenal crisis and treat before symptoms begin
  ◊ If nausea and vomiting preclude oral therapy, patient should seek medical help to start parenteral therapy
  ◊ Elective surgical procedures require adjustment in steroid dose
  ◊ Prevent exposure to infections

POSSIBLE COMPLICATIONS
• Hyperpyrexia
• Psychotic reactions
• Complications from underlying disease
• Over- or under-steroid treatment
• Hyperkalemic paralysis (rare)
• Addisonian crisis

EXPECTED COURSE/PROGNOSIS
• Good outlook with appropriate treatment. With adequate replacement therapy, life expectancy approximates normal
• Active tuberculosis or fungal disease responds to specific chemotherapy

MISCELLANEOUS

ASSOCIATED CONDITIONS
• Diabetes mellitus
• Grave's disease
• Hashimoto's thyroiditis
• Hypoparathyroidism
• Hypercalcemia
• Ovarian failure
• Pernicious anemia
• Myasthenia gravis
• Vitiligo
• Chronic moniliasis
• Sarcoidosis
• Sjogren's syndrome
• Chronic active hepatitis
• Schmidt's syndrome (multiple endocrine deficiency syndrome)
• Adrenoleukodystrophy

AGE-RELATED FACTORS
Pediatric:
• Hydrocortisone and fludrocortisone doses are lower than adults
• More difficult to diagnose
• Occurs in siblings
Geriatric: Acute adrenal crisis more likely
Others: N/A

PREGNANCY N/A

SYNONYMS
• Adrenocortical insufficiency
• Waterhouse-Friderichsen syndrome (adrenal crisis)
• Corticoadrenal insufficiency
• Primary adrenocortical insufficiency

ICD-9-CM
255.4 Corticoadrenal insufficiency

SEE ALSO N/A

OTHER NOTES N/A

ABBREVIATIONS N/A

REFERENCES
• Felig P, Baxter JD, Broadus AE, et al, eds: Endocrinology and Metabolism. 2nd Ed. New York, McGraw-Hill, 1987
• Hershman JM: Endocrine Pathophysiology: A Patient-Oriented Approach. 3rd Ed. Philadelphia, Lea & Febiger, 1988
• DeGroot LL, ed: Endocrinology. 2nd Ed. Philadelphia, WB Saunders Co, 1989
• Dale DC, Federman DD, eds: Scientific American Medicine. New York, Scientific American, Inc., 1997
Illustrations: N/A
Internet references: http://www.5mcc.com

Author(s)
Rick Kellerman, MD
Mark Gerstburger, DO

Adenovirus infections

BASICS

DESCRIPTION Usually self-limited febrile illnesses characterized by inflammation of conjunctivae and the respiratory tract. Adenovirus infections occur in epidemic and endemic situations.
• Common types
  ◊ Acute febrile respiratory illness (AFRI) affecting primarily children
  ◊ Acute respiratory disease (ARD) affecting adults
  ◊ Viral pneumonia affecting children and adults
  ◊ Acute pharyngoconjunctival fever (APC) affecting children, particularly after summer swimming
  ◊ Acute follicular conjunctivitis affecting all ages
  ◊ Epidemic keratoconjunctivitis (EKC) affecting adults
  ◊ Intestinal infections leading to enteritis, mesenteric adenitis and intussusception
System(s) affected: Pulmonary, Gastrointestinal, Renal/Urologic, Nervous, Hemic/Lymphatic/Immunologic, Musculoskeletal, Cardiovascular
Genetics: N/A
Incidence/Prevalence in USA: Very common infection, estimated at 2-5% of all respiratory infections. More common in infants and children.
Predominant age: All ages
Predominant sex: Male = Female

SIGNS AND SYMPTOMS
• Depends on type (see "Differential diagnosis")
In common with most respiratory forms:
• Headache
• Malaise
• Sore throat
• Cough
• Fever (moderate to high)
• Vomiting
• Diarrhea
• Mucosa exhibits patches of white exudate

CAUSES
• Adenovirus (DNA viruses 60-90 nm in size with 42 known serotypes)
• Different serotypes have different epidemiologies
• Most common known pathogens are:
  ◊ Types 1, 2, 3, 5, 7 cause respiratory illness
  ◊ Type 3 causes pharyngoconjunctival fever
  ◊ Types 4, 7, 21 cause acute respiratory disease
  ◊ Several other types may cause epidemic keratoconjunctivitis

RISK FACTORS
• Large number of people gathered in a small area (military recruits, college students at the beginning of the school year, daycare centers, community swimming pools, etc.)
• Immunocompromised at risk for severe disease

DIAGNOSIS

DIFFERENTIAL DIAGNOSIS
Early diagnosis depends on clinical evaluation. The following are the primary characteristics of the major adenovirus infections:
• Acute febrile respiratory illness:
  ◊ Nonspecific cold-like symptoms, similar to other viral respiratory illnesses (fever, pharyngitis, tracheitis, bronchitis, pneumonitis)
  ◊ Mostly in children
  ◊ Incubation period 2 to 5 days
  ◊ May be pertussis-like syndrome rarely
• Acute respiratory disease:
  ◊ Malaise, fever, chills, headache, pharyngitis, hoarseness and dry cough
  ◊ Fever lasts 2 to 4 days
  ◊ Illness subsides in 10 to 14 days
• Viral pneumonia
  ◊ Sudden onset of high fever, rapid infection of upper and lower respiratory tracts, skin rash, diarrhea
  ◊ Occurs in children aged a few days up to 3 years
  ◊ Common; severe illness occurs in subset
• Acute pharyngoconjunctival fever
  ◊ Spiking fever lasting several days, headache, pharyngitis, conjunctivitis, rhinitis, cervical adenitis
  ◊ Conjunctivitis is usually unilateral
  ◊ Subsides in about 1 week
• Epidemic keratoconjunctivitis
  ◊ Usually unilateral onset of ocular redness and edema, periorbital edema, periorbital swelling, local discomfort suggestive of foreign body
  ◊ Lasts 3 or 4 weeks

LABORATORY
• Viral cultures from respiratory, ocular or fecal sources can establish diagnosis
• Antigen detection in stool for enteric serotypes is available
• Serologic procedures such as complement fixation with a four fold rise in serum antibody titer identifies recent adenoviral infection
Drugs that may alter lab results: N/A
Disorders that may alter lab results: N/A

PATHOLOGICAL FINDINGS
• Varies with each virus, severe pneumonia may be reflected by extensive intranuclear inclusions
• Bronchiolitis obliterans may occur

SPECIAL TESTS Cultures and serologic studies if appropriate

IMAGING X-ray: bronchopneumonia in severe respiratory infections

DIAGNOSTIC PROCEDURES
• Biopsy (lung or other) may be needed in severe or unusual cases

TREATMENT

APPROPRIATE HEALTH CARE Ambulatory except for severely ill infants or those with epidemic keratoconjunctivitis or infants with severe pneumonia

GENERAL MEASURES Treatment is supportive and symptomatic. Infections are usually benign and of short duration.

SURGICAL MEASURES N/A

ACTIVITY Rest during febrile phases

DIET No special diet

PATIENT EDUCATION Avoid aspirin in children. Give instructions for nasal spray, cough preparations, frequent hand washing.

MEDICATIONS

DRUG(S) OF CHOICE
• Acetaminophen, 10-15 mg/kg/dose, for analgesia (avoid aspirin)
• Topical corticosteroids for conjunctivitis (after consulting an ophthalmologist)
• Cough suppressants and/or expectorants
Contraindications: Refer to manufacturer's literature
Precautions: Refer to manufacturer's literature
Significant possible interactions: Refer to manufacturer's literature

ALTERNATIVE DRUGS N/A

FOLLOWUP

PATIENT MONITORING For severe infantile pneumonia and conjunctivitis: daily physical exam until well

PREVENTION/AVOIDANCE
• Live types 4 and 7 adenovirus vaccine orally in enteric coated capsule reduces incidence of acute respiratory disease
• Frequent hand washing among office personnel and family members

POSSIBLE COMPLICATIONS
• Few if any recognizable long-term problems

EXPECTED COURSE/PROGNOSIS
• Self-limited, usually without sequelae
• Severe illness and death in very young and in immunocompromised hosts

MISCELLANEOUS

ASSOCIATED CONDITIONS
• Hemorrhagic cystitis (can be caused by adenovirus)
• Viral enteritis
• Intussusception and mesenteric adenitis

AGE-RELATED FACTORS
Pediatric: Viral pneumonia in infants may be fatal
Geriatric: Complications more likely
Others: N/A

PREGNANCY No special precautions

SYNONYMS N/A

ICD-9-CM
079.0 Adenovirus infection in condition classified elsewhere
462 Pharyngitis
480.0 Pneumonia due to adenovirus

SEE ALSO
• Conjunctivitis
• Intussusception
• Pneumonia, viral

OTHER NOTES Conjunctivitis sometimes called "pink eye"

ABBREVIATIONS N/A

REFERENCES
• Mandell GL, et al, eds: Principles and Practice of Infectious Diseases. 4th Ed. New York, Churchill Livingstone, 1995
• Fields BN, Knipe DM, eds: Virology. 2nd Ed. New York, Raven Press, 1989
Illustrations: N/A
Internet references: http://www.5mcc.com

Author(s)
Bernhard L. Wiedermann, MD

Alcoholism

BASICS

DESCRIPTION An illness characterized by significant physiologic, psychologic and/or social dysfunctions associated with persistent and excessive use of alcohol.
System(s) affected: Nervous, Gastrointestinal
Genetics: Twin and adoption studies support a genetic influence
Incidence/Prevalence in USA:
• 10% of men; 3.5% of women
• Lifetime prevalence for adults of 11.5-15.7%
Predominant age:
• All ages
• Highest prevalence of drinking problems is in the 18-29 age group. Subgroups of some age categories have higher prevalence rates.
Predominant sex: Males>Female (slightly)

SIGNS AND SYMPTOMS
• Behavioral
  ◊ Psychological and social dysfunction
  ◊ Marital problems (divorce or separation)
  ◊ Anxiety, depression, insomnia
  ◊ Social isolation or frequent moves
  ◊ Child or spouse abuse
  ◊ Alcohol-related arrests or legal problems (less likely in women)
  ◊ Preoccupation with recreational drinking
  ◊ Repeated attempts to stop or reduce drinking
  ◊ Loss of interest in non-drinking activities
  ◊ Employment problems (tardiness, absenteeism, decreased productivity, interpersonal problems at work, frequent job changes)
  ◊ Blackouts (not remembering what happened during drinking spells)
  ◊ Complaints by family members or friends about alcohol-related behavior
• Physical
  ◊ Gastrointestinal: anorexia, nausea, vomiting, abdominal pain, stigmata of chronic liver disease, peptic ulcer disease, pancreatitis, gastrointestinal malignancies
  ◊ Cardiovascular: modest hypertension, arrhythmias or palpitations (supraventricular), cardiomyopathy
  ◊ Respiratory: aspiration pneumonia, bronchitis and chronic pulmonary disease from associated cigarette smoking
  ◊ Genitourinary: impotence, menstrual irregularities, testicular atrophy
  ◊ Endocrine/metabolic: hypercholesterolemia, hypertriglyceridemia, cushingoid appearance, gynecomastia
  ◊ Dermatologic: signs of accidents and trauma, burns (esp. cigarette burns), bruises in various stages of healing, poor hygiene
  ◊ Musculoskeletal: old fractures and fractures in various stages of healing, myopathy
  ◊ Neurologic: cognitive deficits (e.g., mild impairment of recent memory), peripheral neuropathy, Wernicke-Korsakoff syndrome
  ◊ HEENT: plethoric facies, parotid hypertrophy, poor oral hygiene, head and neck malignancies

CAUSES
• Multifactorial including biological, psychological and sociocultural factors
• Possible biologic markers: brain neuro transmitters, cell membrane receptors, enzyme systems (monoamine oxidase and adenylate cyclase)
• No evidence for a characteristic personality predisposition

RISK FACTORS
• Alcohol use
• Use of other psychoactive drugs, including nicotine
• Family history of alcohol abuse
• Young, single male
• Heavy drinking - five or more drinks in one sitting, getting drunk at least once per week
• Peer group pressure
• Family or sociocultural background promoting intoxication; accepting it as a norm
• Increased accessibility of alcohol
• Adolescence (alcohol and drug use by peers or parents, delinquency, sociopathy in the parents, poor self-esteem, social non-conformity, and stressful life changes)

DIAGNOSIS

DIFFERENTIAL DIAGNOSIS
• Variety of medical and psychiatric disorders:
  ◊ Depression
  ◊ Anxiety states
  ◊ Bipolar or manic-depressive disease
  ◊ Essential hypertension
  ◊ Peptic ulcer disease
  ◊ Viral gastroenteritis
  ◊ Ischemic heart disease
  ◊ Cholelithiasis
  ◊ Viral hepatitis
  ◊ Diabetes
  ◊ Pancreatitis
  ◊ Hyperlipidemia
  ◊ Solar skin damage
  ◊ Breast tumor
  ◊ Primary endocrine disorder
  ◊ Primary seizure disorder

LABORATORY
• Three laboratory findings diagnostic of alcoholism, others are only suggestive, and when present, indicate advanced alcoholism
• Blood alcohol concentration:
  ◊ > 100 mg/dL (22 mmol/L) during an office visit
  ◊ > 150 mg/dL (33 mmol/L) without obvious signs of intoxication
  ◊ > 300 mg/dL (65 mmol/L) at any time
• Suggestive - if increased:
  ◊ Gamma-glutamyl transferase (GGT)
  ◊ Alanine aminotransferase (ALT)
  ◊ Aspartate aminotransferase (AST)
  ◊ Alkaline phosphatase
  ◊ Lactate dehydrogenase (LDH)
  ◊ Bilirubin (total)
  ◊ Amylase
  ◊ Uric acid
  ◊ Triglycerides
  ◊ Cholesterol (total and high density lipoprotein fraction)

  ◊ Mean corpuscular volume
  ◊ Prothrombin time
• Suggestive - if decreased:
  ◊ Calcium
  ◊ Phosphorus
  ◊ Magnesium
  ◊ Blood urea nitrogen
  ◊ White blood cell count
  ◊ Platelet count
  ◊ Hematocrit
  ◊ Serum protein
  ◊ Coagulopathy
Drugs that may alter lab results: See manufacturer's profile for each drug patient takes
Disorders that may alter lab results: Liver, heart, and kidney diseases

PATHOLOGICAL FINDINGS
• Liver: inflammation or fatty infiltration (alcoholic hepatitis), periportal fibrosis (alcoholic cirrhosis - occurs in only 20% of alcoholics)
• Gastric mucosa: inflammation, ulceration
• Pancreas: inflammation, liquefaction necrosis
• Intestine: flattening of villi, loss of enzymes
• Heart: interstitial fibrosis and myofibril atrophy (identical to other dilated cardiomyopathies)
• Immune system: depression of granulocyte production, lymphocyte proliferation response, and cell-mediated immunity
• Endocrine organs: elevated plasma cortisol levels, testicular atrophy, suppression of reproductive hormones in women
• Brain: cortical atrophy, enlarged ventricles

SPECIAL TESTS
• Psychological tests:
  ◊ Michigan Alcohol Screening Test (MAST): 25 item questionnaire, score > 5 indicates alcoholism, sensitivity 90%, specificity 74%
  ◊ Short MAST (SMAST): shortened version of the MAST, 13 questions, score > 3 indicates alcoholism, sensitivity 70%, specificity 74%
  ◊ CAGE: 4 questions, lower sensitivity and specificity, easily administered during a clinical interview, score > 2 suggests alcoholism
• Biologic tests:
  ◊ Mitochondrial AST-to-total AST ratio (investigational, limited availability, sensitivity 85-100%, specificity 81%)
  ◊ Acetate (investigational, limited availability, sensitivity 65%, specificity 92%)

IMAGING
• X-ray: multiple old rib fractures on chest x-ray suggests alcoholism
• CT scan, MRI of brain: cortical atrophy, structural lesions in the thalamic nucleus and basal forebrain

DIAGNOSTIC PROCEDURES Liver biopsy: for diagnosis of alcoholic hepatitis or cirrhosis

Alcoholism

TREATMENT

APPROPRIATE HEALTH CARE
• Inpatient or outpatient depending on:
◊ Severity of alcoholism
◊ Risk of major alcohol withdrawal (delirium tremens)
◊ Patient's health
◊ Social situation
◊ In some cases, detoxification is done as an inpatient, with the remainder of treatment done as an outpatient
• Indications for inpatient alcohol detoxification:
◊ Symptoms or complications of major withdrawal, history of delirium tremens
◊ Failure to complete prior outpatient detoxification
◊ Associated medical problem requiring hospitalization
◊ Significant psychiatric symptoms
◊ Depressive symptoms, particularly suicidal ideation
◊ Lack of physician or other care provider during withdrawal
◊ Lack of clear commitment to complete abstinence from alcohol
◊ Inadequate social support network (family/friends)

GENERAL MEASURES
• Supportive, non-judgmental attitude helpful
• Addiction specialist consult helpful

SURGICAL MEASURES N/A

ACTIVITY Fully active as tolerated

DIET
• Well balanced (malnutrition common)
• Alcohol interferes with the metabolism of most vitamins
• Patients with alcoholic hepatitis or ketoacidosis may have specific vitamin deficiencies, particularly thiamine
• Other deficiencies include magnesium, phosphate and zinc

PATIENT EDUCATION Information, literature and emotional support (crisis hot line) available from local Alcoholics Anonymous

MEDICATIONS

DRUG(S) OF CHOICE
• For detoxification and management of alcohol withdrawal syndrome:
(dose depends on patient's alcohol tolerance)
◊ Chlordiazepoxide (Librium)
◊ Diazepam (Valium)
◊ Lorazepam: in severe liver disease
◊ Phenobarbital: used less often
• Detoxification adjunct: used, as adjuncts to benzodiazepines, in doses adequate to control withdrawal symptoms, suppress seizures and

delirium tremens.
◊ Beta blockers (propranolol, atenolol): for persistent sinus tachycardia when other withdrawal signs are controlled
◊ Clonidine: relieves symptoms of autonomic hyperactivity (tremor, tachycardia, hypertension)
• To promote sobriety:
◊ Disulfiram: Contraindicated if patient in denial about alcoholism, is seeking a "quick fix", or if a serious medical condition or poor health status exists.
◊ Naltrexone: to reduce craving of alcohol
• Supplemental to all: thiamine
Contraindications: Patients who continue to drink while taking detox medications
Precautions:
• Use caution with severe liver disease, organic pain, organic brain syndromes
• Monitor for nystagmus, ataxia, excessive somnolence, slurred speech, other signs of intoxication
Significant Possible Interactions:
• Alcohol and benzodiazepines additive
• Other sedative hypnotics

ALTERNATIVE DRUGS N/A

FOLLOWUP

PATIENT MONITORING
• During detoxification: daily visits, if in-patient, frequent monitoring of vital signs
• Soon after patient completes treatment program: more frequent visits, e.g. weekly
• As patient more established in recovery: less frequent visits

PREVENTION/AVOIDANCE
• Preventive counseling of patients with a family history of alcoholism or other risk factors
• Anticipatory guidance for patients at increased risk due to life changes
• Public health and education measures

POSSIBLE COMPLICATIONS
• Relapse of drinking
• Wernicke-Korsakoff syndrome
• Neuropathy, dementia
• Increased susceptibility to infection
• Aseptic necrosis of the hip
• Malignancies (e.g., of gastrointestinal tract)
• Cirrhosis (women sooner than men)

EXPECTED COURSE/PROGNOSIS
• Chronic relapsing disease
• Untreated alcoholism is progressive and fatal

MISCELLANEOUS

ASSOCIATED CONDITIONS
• Nicotine addiction
• Depression, bipolar disorder and antisocial personality disorder
• Women have associated reproductive tract disorders, history of sexual abuse or incest; concurrent prescription drug dependence.

AGE-RELATED FACTORS
Pediatric:
• Substance abuse (often multiple) has negative impact on normal maturation and development, attainment of social, educational and occupational skills
• Watch for depression, suicide thought or attempts, family disruption, disorderly behavior, violence or destruction of property, poor school or work performance, sexual promiscuity, social immaturity, lack of hobbies or interests, isolation, moodiness
Geriatric:
• Alcoholism often missed; signs and symptoms may be different or attributed to chronic medical problem or dementia
• More hidden due to social unacceptability; self-reports of alcohol consumption inaccurate
• Elderly more sensitive to alcohol effects
• Assessment tools standardized on younger populations often inappropriate
Others: N/A

PREGNANCY
• Alcohol is a morphologic and behavioral teratogen. Greatest teratogenic effect occurs during the early weeks of fetal development.
• Women should abstain when planning conception and throughout pregnancy

SYNONYMS N/A

ICD-9-CM
• 303 Alcohol dependence syndrome
• 303.90 Other and unspecified alcohol dependence; unspecified drinking behavior

SEE ALSO N/A

OTHER NOTES N/A

REFERENCES
• National Institute on Alcohol Abuse and Alcoholism. Seventh Special Report to the US Congress on Alcohol and Health. DHHS: Rockville, MD, 1990
Illustrations: 4 available on CD-ROM
Internet references: http://www.5mcc.com

Author(s)
David Frank, MD

Aldosteronism, primary

BASICS

DESCRIPTION The clinical syndrome of hypertension, hypokalemia, low plasma renin activity, and increased aldosterone secretion.
• Unilateral aldosterone-producing adenoma (APA) - most common form (60%) and cured with unilateral adrenalectomy
• Idiopathic hyperaldosteronism (IHA) due to bilateral zona glomerulosa hyperplasia - second most common form (34%); not cured with surgery. Chronic medical therapy is treatment of choice.
System(s) affected: Endocrine/Metabolic
Genetics: Unknown
Incidence/Prevalence in USA:
• 0.5 to 2% of the hypertensive population
Predominant age: Usually diagnosed third to sixth decades
Predominant sex: APA more common in women

SIGNS AND SYMPTOMS
• Usually asymptomatic
• Marked hypokalemia may be associated with muscle weakness and cramping, headaches, palpitations, polydipsia, polyuria, or nocturia
• Mild to severe hypertension
• Funduscopy - benign or grade 1-2
• Edema (rare)
• Hypokalemia
• Metabolic alkalosis
• Relative "hypernatremia"
• Impaired glucose tolerance
• Increased incidence of renal cysts

CAUSES
• Unilateral aldosterone-producing adrenal adenoma (APA)
• Idiopathic hyperaldosteronism (IHA)
• Aldosterone-producing adrenocortical carcinoma
• Other rare subtypes

RISK FACTORS   N/A

DIAGNOSIS

DIFFERENTIAL DIAGNOSIS
• Diuretic use
• Renovascular hypertension
• Pheochromocytoma
• Renin-secreting tumor
• Malignant hypertension
• Congenital adrenal hyperplasia
• Deoxycorticosterone-producing tumor
• Exogenous mineralocorticoid
• High dose glucocorticoid therapy
• Apparent mineralocorticoid excess syndrome (congenital or acquired due to licorice ingestion)
• Liddle's syndrome

LABORATORY
• Hypokalemia with inappropriate kaliuresis
• Unsuppressible urine or plasma aldosterone levels
• Low ambulatory plasma renin activity
• High plasma aldosterone to renin ratio (> 20 in ng/dL [> 55 nmol/L] and ng/mL/h, respectively)
• Normal glucocorticoid excretion
Drugs that may alter lab results: The list of drugs and hormones capable of affecting the renin-angiotensin-aldosterone axis is extensive; examples include - spironolactone, estrogens, diuretics, ACE-inhibitors, vasodilators, calcium channel antagonists, and adrenergic inhibitors
Disorders that may alter lab results:
Malignant hypertension

PATHOLOGICAL FINDINGS Unilateral aldosterone-producing adrenal adenoma (APA), bilateral idiopathic adrenal hyperplasia (IHA), aldosterone-producing adrenocortical carcinoma

SPECIAL TESTS
• Aldosterone suppression test with either a high salt diet or saline infusion
• Posture study
• Spironolactone treatment trial
• Adrenal venous sampling (for aldosterone and cortisol)

IMAGING Adrenal computerized tomography (CT preferred over MRI). Use 3 mm cuts.

DIAGNOSTIC PROCEDURES Adrenal venous sampling

TREATMENT

APPROPRIATE HEALTH CARE
• Unilateral APA - unilateral adrenalectomy
• Bilateral IHA - chronic medical therapy

GENERAL MEASURES
• Unilateral APA - correct hypokalemia preoperatively with spironolactone
• Bilateral IHA - low sodium diet, regular isotonic exercise, maintenance of ideal body weight, tobacco avoidance, potassium-sparing agent, anti-hypertensive agent (e.g., calcium channel antagonist, ACE-inhibitor, low-dose thiazide diuretic)

SURGICAL MEASURES The treatment of choice for patients with an unilateral APA is adrenalectomy. Patients with bilateral IHA are treated medically.

ACTIVITY No limitations

DIET Low sodium

PATIENT EDUCATION N/A

MEDICATIONS

DRUG(S) OF CHOICE
• Potassium-sparing agent - spironolactone (Aldactone)or amiloride (Midamor)
• Antihypertensive agent - calcium channel antagonist, ACE-inhibitor, angiotensin-II receptor antagonist or low-dose thiazide diuretic
Contraindications: Potassium-sparing agent and ACE-inhibitors in renal failure, hyperkalemia, and pregnancy
Precautions: Monitor serum potassium closely after any adjustment in potassium replacement or potassium-sparing agent
Significant possible interactions: Lithium and diuretics, nonsteroidal anti-inflammatory agents with diuretics and ACE-inhibitors

ALTERNATIVE DRUGS
Peripheral alpha-1 antagonists (e.g., terazosin [Hytrin], doxazosin [Cardura]) or guanadrel (Hylorel) may be used to control hypertension during the diagnostic evaluation for primary aldosteronism

FOLLOWUP

PATIENT MONITORING
• Blood pressure checks
• Serum potassium check
• 24-hour urine aldosterone following surgery

PREVENTION/AVOIDANCE   N/A

POSSIBLE COMPLICATIONS   Cardiac arrhythmia associated with severe hypokalemia

EXPECTED COURSE/PROGNOSIS
Surgical removal of an APA results in cure of hypertension in approximately 70% of cases. Hypertension does not resolve immediately post operatively, but rather over 1 to 4 months.

MISCELLANEOUS

ASSOCIATED CONDITIONS   Cystic renal disease

AGE-RELATED FACTORS
Pediatric: Bilateral adrenal idiopathic hyperplasia is the most common form in children
Geriatric: N/A
Others: N/A

PREGNANCY   Treat hypertension with agents proven to be safe during pregnancy; avoid spironolactone and ACE-inhibitors

SYNONYMS
• Conn's syndrome
• Hyperaldosteronism

ICD-9-CM
255.1 hyperaldosteronism

SEE ALSO
• Hypertension
• Hypokalemia

OTHER NOTES
• Who should be screened for primary aldosteronism?
1)All patients with hypertension and spontaneous hypokalemia
2)All patients with treatment-resistant hypertension

ABBREVIATIONS
• APA = aldosterone-producing adenoma
• IHA = idiopathic hyperaldosteronism

REFERENCES
• Young WF Jr, Stanton AW, Grant CS, et al: Primary aldosteronism: adrenal venous sampling. Surgery 1996;120:913-920
• Young WF Jr, Hogan MJ: Renin-independent hypermineralocorticoidism. Trends Endocrinol Metab 1994;5:97
• Weinberger MH, Fineberg NS: The diagnosis of primary aldosteronism and separation of the two major subtypes. Arch Int Med 1993;153:2125-2129
Illustrations: N/A
Internet references: http://www.5mcc.com

Author(s)
William F. Young, Jr., MD

Alopecia

BASICS

DESCRIPTION Absence of the hair from skin areas where it normally is present
• Telogen effluvium - diffuse hair loss that results in decreased hair density but does not progress to complete baldness
• Anagen effluvium - diffuse shedding of hairs, including growing hairs, that may progress to complete baldness
• Cicatricial alopecia - also known as scarring alopecia and characterized by slick, smooth scalp without any evidence of follicular openings of hair
• Androgenic alopecia - hair loss occurring in either sex, caused by stimulation of the hair roots by male hormones
• Alopecia areata - patchy, non-scarring hair loss
• Traction alopecia - patchy, initially non-scarring hair loss
• Tinea capitis - patches of hair broken off close to the scalp, with or without associated inflammation, caused by fungus infection
System(s) affected: Skin/Exocrine
Genetics: In Caucasians, androgenic alopecia follows a dominant trait with incomplete penetrance. The hereditary incidence is notable not only in men but also in women with a strong family history of baldness.
Incidence/Prevalence in USA: 50% of Caucasian males by 50 years of age have noticeable male-pattern baldness. 37% of postmenopausal females show some evidence of hair loss.
Predominant age: The incidence of androgenic alopecia increases with increasing age. Tinea capitis and traction alopecia are more common in children.
Predominant sex: Male > Female

SIGNS AND SYMPTOMS
• Hair loss
• Pruritus (in tinea capitis)
• Scaling of the scalp (in tinea capitis)
• Broken hairs (in tinea capitis and traction alopecia)
• Tapered hair at the borders of the patch of alopecia (in alopecia areata)
• Easily removable hairs at the periphery of the patch of alopecia (in alopecia areata)
• Inflammation (in tinea capitis)

CAUSES
• Telogen effluvium
  ◊ Postpartum
  ◊ Drugs (oral contraceptives, anticoagulants, retinoids, beta blockers, chemotherapeutic agents, interferon)
  ◊ Stress (physical or psychological)
  ◊ Hormonal (hypo- or hyperthyroidism, hypopituitarism)
  ◊ Nutritional (malnutrition, iron deficiency, zinc deficiency)
  ◊ Diffuse alopecia areata

• Anagen effluvium
  ◊ Mycosis fungoides
  ◊ X-ray treatment
  ◊ Drugs (chemotherapeutic agents, allopurinol, levodopa, bromocriptine)
  ◊ Poisoning (bismuth, arsenic, gold, boric acid, thallium)
• Cicatricial alopecia
  ◊ Congenital and developmental defects
  ◊ Infection (leprosy, syphilis, varicella-zoster, cutaneous leishmaniasis)
  ◊ Basal cell carcinoma
  ◊ Epidermal nevi
  ◊ Physical agents (acids and alkali, burns, freezing, radiodermatitis)
  ◊ Cicatricial pemphigoid
  ◊ Lichen planus
  ◊ Sarcoidosis
• Androgenic alopecia
  ◊ Adrenal hyperplasia
  ◊ Polycystic ovaries
  ◊ Ovarian hyperplasia
  ◊ Carcinoid
  ◊ Pituitary hyperplasia
  ◊ Drugs (testosterone, danazol, ACTH, anabolic steroids, progesterones)
• Alopecia areata
  ◊ Unknown, but possibly autoimmune
• Traction alopecia
  ◊ Trichotillomania (direct self-pulling of the hair)
  ◊ Tight rollers or braids
• Tinea capitis
  ◊ Microsporum species
  ◊ Trichophyton species

RISK FACTORS
• Positive family history of baldness
• Physical or psychological stress
• Pregnancy
• Poor nutrition

DIAGNOSIS

DIFFERENTIAL DIAGNOSIS Search for type of alopecia and then for possible reversible causes

LABORATORY
• Thyroid function tests
• Complete blood count (may reflect an underlying immunologic disorder)
• Free testosterone and dehydroepiandrosterone sulfate (DHEA-S) in women with androgenic alopecia
• Serum ferritin
• VDRL or RPR for syphilis
• Lymphocyte T and B cell number (sometimes low in patients with alopecia areata)
Drugs that may alter lab results:
• Antifungal drugs may make KOH examination falsely negative
• Thyroid drugs and iodine preparations (including topicals) will alter thyroid function tests
Disorders that may alter lab results: N/A

PATHOLOGICAL FINDINGS Scalp biopsy with routine microscopy and direct immunofluorescence will aid in the diagnosis of tinea capitis, diffuse alopecia areata, and the scarring alopecias due to lupus erythematosus, lichen planus, and sarcoidosis

SPECIAL TESTS
• Light hair-pull test (positive in alopecia areata)
• Direct microscopic examination of the hair shaft
• Potassium hydroxide (KOH) examination of the scale, if present (positive in tinea capitis)
• Fungal culture of the scale, if present

IMAGING N/A

DIAGNOSTIC PROCEDURES Scalp biopsy (sometimes)

TREATMENT

APPROPRIATE HEALTH CARE
Outpatient

GENERAL MEASURES
• Telogen effluvium - maximum shedding 3 months after the inciting event (medication, stress, nutritional deficiency) and recovery following correction of the cause. Rarely permanent baldness.
• Anagen effluvium - shedding begins days to a few weeks after the inciting event with recovery following correction of the cause. Rarely permanent baldness.
• Cicatricial alopecia - hair follicles are permanently damaged. Only effective treatment is surgical (graft transplantation, flap transplantation, or excision of the scarred area).
• Androgenic alopecia - by 12 months of using topical minoxidil, 39% of subjects reported moderate to marked hair growth. Other treatments for androgenic alopecia are surgical (hair transplantation, scalp reduction, transposition flap, and soft tissue expansion).
• Alopecia areata - usually the disease resolves within three years without treatment. Recurrences are, however, common.
• Traction alopecia - only with discontinuation of the hair pulling will the disorder resolve. Psychologic or psychiatric intervention may be necessary. Successful therapeutic approaches have included medications, behavior modification, and hypnosis.
• Tinea capitis - six to eight weeks of therapy are often necessary. Careful handwashing and laundering of headwear and towels.

SURGICAL MEASURES N/A

ACTIVITY Fully active

DIET No special diet

PATIENT EDUCATION National Alopecia Areata Foundation, 714 C Street, San Rafael, CA 94901

MEDICATIONS

DRUG(S) OF CHOICE
• Androgenic alopecia - topical minoxidil (Rogaine) 2%
• Alopecia areata - high potency topical steroids
• Tinea capitis - griseofulvin [ultramicrosize] 250-375 mg/day in adults, 5.5-7.3 mg/kg/day in children. Alternatively, ketoconazole 200 mg once daily. Treatment for 6-8 weeks.
Contraindications:
• Griseofulvin - pregnancy, porphyria, hepatocellular failure
• Ketoconazole and cisapride (Propulsid) should not be used together
• Itraconazole and cisapride should not be used together
Precautions:
• Topical minoxidil
  ◊ Burning and irritation of the eyes
  ◊ Salt and water retention
  ◊ Tachycardia
  ◊ Angina (rare)
• Topical steroids
  ◊ Local burning and stinging
  ◊ Pruritus
  ◊ Skin atrophy
  ◊ Telangiectasias
  ◊ Hypothalamic-pituitary-adrenal (HPA) suppression if high-potency steroids used for prolonged duration
• Griseofulvin
  ◊ Photosensitivity reaction
  ◊ Lupus-like syndrome
  ◊ Oral thrush
  ◊ Granulocytopenia
• Ketoconazole
  ◊ Anaphylaxis
  ◊ Hepatotoxicity
  ◊ Oligospermia
  ◊ Neuropsychiatric disturbances
  ◊ Gynecomastia
• Itraconazole
  ◊ Hepatotoxicity
  ◊ Nausea, vomiting

Significant possible interactions:
• Topical minoxidil-guanethidine: may potentiate orthostatic hypotension (rare)
• Griseofulvin-warfarin: decreased activity of warfarin
• Griseofulvin-barbiturates: depressed activity of griseofulvin
• Ketoconazole-warfarin: may enhance the activity of warfarin
• Ketoconazole-isoniazid, rifampin: decreased activity of ketoconazole
• Ketoconazole-phenytoin: may alter the metabolism of either drug
• Itraconazole-terfenadine: prolonged QT and ventricular arrhythmias
• Itraconazole-astemizole: prolonged QT and ventricular arrhythmias
• Itraconazole-cisapride: contraindicated
• Itraconazole-digoxin: may result in elevated levels of digoxin
• H2 blockers or antacids-ketoconazole: decreased absorption of ketoconazole. If concomitant therapy needed, give H2 blocker or antacids at least 2 hours after ketoconazole dose. Avoid using the proton pump inhibitor omeprazole for the same reason.

ALTERNATIVE DRUGS N/A

FOLLOWUP

PATIENT MONITORING With ketoconazole, monitor liver enzymes

PREVENTION/AVOIDANCE N/A

POSSIBLE COMPLICATIONS N/A

EXPECTED COURSE/PROGNOSIS
• Telogen effluvium - rarely permanent baldness
• Anagen effluvium - rarely permanent baldness
• Cicatricial alopecia - the hair follicles are permanently damaged
• Androgenic alopecia - depends on treatment
• Alopecia areata - recurrences are common
• Traction alopecia - depends on behavior modification
• Tinea capitis - usually complete recovery

MISCELLANEOUS

ASSOCIATED CONDITIONS Alopecia areata - Down syndrome, vitiligo, diabetes

AGE-RELATED FACTORS
Pediatric: Tinea capitis only common form of alopecia
Geriatric: Androgenic alopecia more common after 50
Others: N/A

PREGNANCY Post partum hair loss is due to altered physiology during pregnancy

SYNONYMS
• Androgenic alopecia

ICD-9-CM
• 704.00 alopecia, unspecified
• 704.01 alopecia areata
• 704.09 other
• 110.0 dermatophytosis of the scalp and beard

SEE ALSO
• Lichen planus
• Tinea capitis
• Syphilis
• Cutaneous T cell lymphoma
• Acrodermatitis
• Werner's syndrome

OTHER NOTES N/A

ABBREVIATIONS
RPR = rapid plasma reagin
HPA = hypothalamic-pituitary axis

REFERENCES
• Bergfeld WF, Redmond GP: Androgenetic alopecia. Dermatologic Clinics 1987;5:491
• Mitchell AV, Krull EA, eds: Dermatologic Clinics 1987;5(3):483-603,
• Olsen EA: Primary Care 1989;16(3):768-787
• Burke KE: Hair loss. What causes it and what can be done about it. Postgrad Med 1989;85(6):52-77
Illustrations: 14 available on CD-ROM
Internet references: http://www.5mcc.com

Author(s)
Aubrey L. Knight, MD

Altitude illness

BASICS

DESCRIPTION Altitude illness is a spectrum of medical problems ranging from mild discomfort to fatal illness that may occur on ascent to higher altitude. It can affect anyone, including the most experienced and fit individual, who ascends to more than about 8,000 feet (2438 m). Several factors appear to be important in adaptation to altitude: How long the ascent takes, how high, and length of stay. There is a great deal of variation between people and an individual's response may vary from ascent to ascent.
• Acute mountain sickness (AMS): Begins within 4 to 6 hours after arrival at altitude, rare below 8,000 feet (2438 m), and affects most above 10,000 feet (3048 m)
• High altitude pulmonary edema (HAPE): Abnormal accumulation of fluid in the lungs. Begins 24 to 96 hours after arrival at altitude. Rare below 8,000 (2438 m) feet but affects more than 10% of individuals above 14,500 feet (4420 m).
• High altitude cerebral edema (HACE): Indicates swelling of the brain. It is the least common but most severe of the high altitude illnesses since it can result in permanent injury or death. Occurs 48 to 72 hours after arrival at altitude. Rare below 12,000 feet (3656 m).
System(s) affected: Pulmonary, Cardiovascular, Nervous
Genetics: N/A
Incidence/Prevalence: Unknown
Predominant age: Any age (young, well-conditioned climbers have a higher incidence of altitude illness, probably because they push themselves more)
Predominant sex: Male = Female

SIGNS AND SYMPTOMS
• AMS mild to moderately severe symptoms:
 ◊ Headache
 ◊ Lack of energy and appetite
 ◊ Mild nausea
 ◊ Dizziness
 ◊ Weakness
 ◊ Insomnia
• AMS severe symptoms:
 ◊ Increased headache
 ◊ Irritability
 ◊ Marked fatigue
 ◊ Shortness of breath with exercise
 ◊ Nausea and vomiting
 ◊ Irregular or periodic breathing at night (Cheyne-Stokes)
 ◊ Breathing apnea
• HAPE symptoms:
 ◊ Excessive shortness of breath on exertion
 ◊ Severe respiratory distress
 ◊ Shortness of breath at rest
 ◊ Dry cough and/or wheezing
 ◊ Heart rate and respiratory rate increased
 ◊ Marked periodic breathing present at night
 ◊ Gurgling breathing
 ◊ Frothy cough
 ◊ Wet crackling sounds in the lungs
 ◊ Confusion
 ◊ Coma

• HACE symptoms:
 ◊ Progressive headache that is unrelieved by mild pain relievers
 ◊ Lack of coordination (e.g., unable to perform a heel-to-toe walk)
 ◊ Confusion and bizarre behavior followed by unconsciousness
 ◊ Other symptoms of moderate AMS, such as dizziness, vomiting, and irritability, are usually present

CAUSES The physiology of altitude illness is still not completely understood. The fundamental problem results from the fact that with increasing altitude there is a progressive decrease in barometric pressure and a corresponding lower partial pressure of oxygen in inspired air, resulting in less oxygen delivery to the body.

RISK FACTORS
• In general, the faster the ascent and the higher, the more likely a person will experience symptoms of altitude illness
• Chronic illness
• Lack of conditioning

DIAGNOSIS

DIFFERENTIAL DIAGNOSIS
• Viral upper respiratory infection
• Gastroenteritis
• Pneumonia
• Other infections
• Cerebral vascular accident
• Ketoacidosis
• Pulmonary emboli
• Congestive heart failure

LABORATORY
• AMS: Laboratory studies are nonspecific and rarely required for diagnosis
• HAPE: WBC - often slightly elevated, erythrocyte sedimentation rate normal
• Arterial blood gas - may show hypoxia, hypocapnea, alkalosis
Drugs that may alter lab results: N/A
Disorders that may alter lab results: N/A

PATHOLOGICAL FINDINGS N/A

SPECIAL TESTS ECG may show only sinus tachycardia, possibly right heart strain

IMAGING Chest x-ray (in HAPE) shows Kerley's lines and a patchy distribution of edema

DIAGNOSTIC PROCEDURES N/A

TREATMENT

APPROPRIATE HEALTH CARE
Outpatient for mild cases, inpatient for severe cases

GENERAL MEASURES
• Therapy must be tailored to fit severity of disease and may be constrained by the environment
• Definitive treatment is to descend to a lower altitude. Dramatic improvement accompanies even modest reductions in altitude (as little as 1,000 feet [305 m]).
• Oxygen, given continuously at 1-2 liters per minute helps relieve symptoms. For severe symptoms, continuous oxygen should be administered and descent to a lower altitude is mandatory.
• AMS
 ◊ Descent rarely needed
 ◊ Fluids, light diet, curtailed activity
• HAPE and HACE
 ◊ Patient must be treated by immediate evacuation to a lower altitude. Occasionally, however, foul weather, lack of transportation or long distances prevent immediate evacuation. In these cases, supportive measures, such as bedrest and oxygen, will help.
 ◊ Hyperbaric therapy is another effective and practical alternative when descent is not possible. A portable hyperbaric chamber, the "Gamow Bag," made of fabric and weighing only 8 pounds (3.6 kg) can be inflated to 2 pounds per square inch (13.8 kPa) using a foot pump. This is equivalent to a drop in altitude of about 5,000 feet (1524 m). Improvement is usually immediate after being placed in the hyperbaric chamber.
 ◊ If patient is hospitalized, rule out any other pulmonary disease first, provide adequate oxygen (possibly by intubation or positive end-expiratory pressure [PEEP]), bed rest, diuresis if needed and postural drainage

SURGICAL MEASURES N/A

ACTIVITY Rest until symptoms clear

DIET Increased intake of fluids, a light diet, and avoidance of alcohol

PATIENT EDUCATION See guidelines in Prevention/Avoidance

MEDICATIONS

DRUG(S) OF CHOICE
• Aspirin or codeine can be used to relieve the headache. Antibiotics, if infection is present.
• Both dexamethasone and acetazolamide have been used to treat patients with severe symptoms of AMS. Dosage of dexamethasone is 8 mg initially, followed by 4 mg every six hours by mouth. Doses of acetazolamide of up to 1.0 g/day may be required for effective treatment.
• Dexamethasone may be effective in mild cases of HAPE, but this has not been proven
• Diuretics have not been useful
• Corticosteroids should be given even though their effectiveness is questionable
Contraindications: Refer to manufacturer's profile of each drug
Precautions: Refer to manufacturer's profile of each drug
Significant possible interactions: Refer to manufacturer's profile of each drug

ALTERNATIVE DRUGS N/A

FOLLOWUP

PATIENT MONITORING
• For mild cases, no followup needed
• For more severe cases, follow until symptoms subside
• If underlying cardiopulmonary or cardiovascular disease, follow as needed

PREVENTION/AVOIDANCE
• General guidelines
◊ Staged ascent: "Staging" is the process of remaining at an intermediate altitude (6600 to 9800 feet [2012 to 2988 m]) for a few days before attempting the ultimate altitude
◊ Conventional prescription for avoiding altitude illness is to allow one day to ascend and acclimatize each 1,000 feet (305 m) from elevations of 10,000 to 14,000 feet (3,048 to 4,267 m). Two days per 1,000 feet (305 m) at elevations above 14,000 feet (4267 m.
◊ Sleeping elevation - climber's maximum "climb high and sleep low" is a prudent practice for anyone going above 12,000 feet (3656 m)
◊ Adequate hydration - dehydration increases the likelihood of and worsens the symptoms of AMS
◊ Good physical conditioning
◊ Consider carrying a supply of oxygen
• Drug prophylaxis
◊ Acetazolamide (if patient has a history of problems at altitude and/or plans a rapid ascent to above 8,000 feet [2438 m] in a car or airplane). Dosage is usually 250 mg orally twice daily, starting 24 hours before ascent and continuing for two to three days while at altitude. Anyone with a known drug allergy to sulfa should avoid acetazolamide.
◊ Dexamethasone may significantly reduce the incidence and severity of acute mountain sickness. The dosage is 2 to 4 mg every six hours, begun the day of the ascent, continued for three days at the higher altitude, then tapered over five days. Adverse side effects are uncommon.

POSSIBLE COMPLICATIONS
• Without treatment, HACE can cause motor and sensory deficits, seizures and coma
• HAPE may progress to cyanosis and respiratory distress syndrome
• Patient may experience high altitude retinal hemorrhage (HARH) - can cause visual changes, but is usually asymptomatic

EXPECTED COURSE/PROGNOSIS
• Mild to moderate AMS resolves over 1-3 days. Patients may resume ascent once symptoms subside.
• HAPE and HACE patients can expect complete recovery, if there is no underlying disease. Should not resume ascent.
• Problems are more likely to recur in people who have had one or more attacks

MISCELLANEOUS

ASSOCIATED CONDITIONS N/A

AGE-RELATED FACTORS
Pediatric: Children under 6 are more susceptible than adults
Geriatric: Elderly more likely to have chronic conditions (coronary artery disease, congestive heart failure, chronic obstructive pulmonary disease) that may be exacerbated at altitudes of 6000-8000 feet (1829-2438 m)
Others: Women in premenstrual phase are more vulnerable

PREGNANCY N/A

SYNONYMS Mountain sickness

ICD-9-CM 289 mountain sickness acute

SEE ALSO N/A

OTHER NOTES N/A

ABBREVIATIONS
• AMS = acute mountain sickness
• HACE = high altitude cerebral edema
• HAPE = high altitude pulmonary edema

REFERENCES
• Zell SC, Goodman PH: Acetazolamide and dexamethasone in the prevention of acute mountain sickness. West J Med 1988;148:541
• Johnson TS, Rock PB: Current concepts, acute mountain sickness. New Engl J Med 1988;319:841
Illustrations: N/A
Internet references: http://www.5mcc.com

Author(s)
Tejal Parikh, MD
Kevin Carmichael, MD

Alzheimer's disease

BASICS

DESCRIPTION A degenerative organic mental disease characterized by progressive intellectual deterioration and dementia; usually occurring after age 65. The diagnosis is made on clinical grounds after ruling out treatable disorders with similar characteristics.
Long-term care cost to the nation is approximately $100 billion/year.
Usual course - progressive; chronic.
Genetics: Positive family history in 50% of cases. Markers on chromosomes: 1 and 14 (early onset disease); 12,19 (late onset); 21 (onset age 50-65).
System(s) affected: Nervous
Incidence/Prevalence in USA: 4 million cases/350 million people. 40% of those over age 85 are affected.
Predominant age: > 60
Predominant sex: Female > Male (slightly)

SIGNS AND SYMPTOMS
• Acalculia
• Agnosia
• Anhedonia
• Anxiety
• Apathy
• Aphasia
• Apraxia
• Confabulation
• Delusions
• Dementia
• Depression
• Impaired abstraction
• Intellectual decline
• Loss of interest
• Occupational dysfunction
• Personality change
• Progressive cognitive impairment
• Recent memory loss (key finding)
• Restlessness
• Sleep disturbances
• Social withdrawal
• Visuospatial distortion
• Weight loss
• Late signs – seizures, myoclonus, extrapyramidal dysfunction, incontinence

CAUSES
• Unknown, but toxic beta-amyloid deposits in neuritic plaques and arteriolar walls appear critical to pathogenesis. Beta-amyloid precursor gene localized to chromosome 21.
• Unsubstantiated possibilities - slow virus, herpes simplex type 1, metals (aluminum), accelerated aging, autoimmune attack

RISK FACTORS
• Aging
• Head trauma
• Low education level
• Down syndrome
• Positive family history
• Inheritance of the E4 allele of apolipoprotein E gene on chromosome 19

DIAGNOSIS

DIFFERENTIAL DIAGNOSIS
• Vascular dementia
• Multi-infarct dementia
• Dementia associated with Parkinson's
• Normal pressure hydrocephalus
• Creutzfeldt-Jakob disease
• End-stage multiple sclerosis
• Brain tumor – primary or metastatic
• Subdural hematoma
• Progressive multifocal leukoencephalopathy
• Metabolic dementia (hypothyroidism)
• Drug reactions
• Alcoholism and other addictions
• Dementia pugilistica
• Subcortical dementias
• Depression (persistent diminished interest and pleasure, insomnia or hyposomnia, psychomotor retardation, feelings of hopelessness and helplessness, thoughts of death, decreased ability to concentrate)
• Toxicity from liver or kidney failure
• Vitamin and other nutritional deficiencies
• Vasculitis
• Lewy body disease
• Neurosyphilis

LABORATORY
• To help rule out other causes of dementia:
  ◊ CBC
  ◊ Chemistry panel
  ◊ Thyroid function studies
  ◊ Folate and B-12 levels
  ◊ VDRL
  ◊ HIV antibody (selected cases)
Drugs that may alter lab results: N/A
Disorders that may alter lab results: N/A

PATHOLOGICAL FINDINGS
• Gross - diffuse cerebral atrophy in association areas, hippocampus, amygdala and some subcortical nuclei
• Micro - pyramidal cell loss
• Micro - decreased cholinergic innervation (other neurotransmitters variably decreased)
• Micro - neuritic senile plaques
• Micro - degeneration of locus ceruleus and basal forebrain nuclei of Meynert
• Neurofibrillary tangles
• Amyloid angiopathy common

SPECIAL TESTS
• Cerebrospinal fluid (depending on circumstances and clinical information)
• Extensive neuropsychological battery - only needed if clinical picture is confusing

IMAGING
• Head CT/MRI - moderate cortical atrophy, ventricular enlargement - to rule out infarcts, subdural hematomas, normal pressure hydrocephalus, neoplasm
• MRI-based hippocampal volumetry, positron emission tomography (PET) and single photon emission computed tomography (SPECT) are all rapidly approaching clinical usefulness as tools to distinguish early Alzheimer's disease from other dementias

DIAGNOSTIC PROCEDURES
• This is a clinical diagnosis - history, physical examination, tests (neurological and memory)
• More specific tests (CSF beta-amyloid, tau, AD7C levels; excessive pupillary dilatation to mydriatics) still investigational
• Testing for E4 allele of apolipoprotein E gene is available (but is not officially recommended) for assessing prognosis of early memory loss or predicting risk of dementia in patient's relatives

TREATMENT

APPROPRIATE HEALTH CARE
Outpatient, day care, nursing home (when necessary)

GENERAL MEASURES
• Supportive
• Optimize treatment of associated co-morbidities
• Exercises to reduce restlessness
• Occupational therapy
• Music therapy
• Continued cognitive challenge – shown to slow deterioration rate
• Analyze environment for safety and security
• Consider day care centers
• Assess needs of spouse/care giver
• Consider nursing home
• Referrals to:
  ◊ Visiting nurse
  ◊ Social worker
  ◊ Physical therapist
  ◊ Occupational therapist
  ◊ Lawyer
  ◊ Support groups

SURGICAL MEASURES N/A

ACTIVITY To whatever extent possible

DIET No special diet

PATIENT EDUCATION
• Printed patient and family information available from: Alzheimer's Association, 919 N. Michigan Ave., Suite 1000, Chicago, IL, (312)335-8700, (800)272-3900
• Help family understand the progressive nature of the disease
• Arrange durable power of attorney
• Advance directives planning as early as possible

MEDICATIONS

DRUG(S) OF CHOICE
• No specific drug therapy available for halting disease. Clinical studies are ongoing.
• Use as few drugs as possible. Alzheimer's patients tolerate them poorly.
• No drugs are helpful for – wandering, restlessness, fidgeting, uncooperativeness, hoarding, irritability. Use behavioral techniques.
• For depression (which occurs in 1/3 of patients), use selective serotonin reuptake inhibitors or trazodone (Desyrel). Start with half the usual adult dose.
• For insomnia – can try trazodone 25-100 mg qhs, zolpidem (Ambien) 5 mg qhs or temazepam (Restoril) 7.5-15 mg qhs
• For moderate anxiety/restlessness – can try low dose, short-acting benzodiazepines, but efficacy unproven
• For severe aggressive agitation, especially if psychotic features present (delusions, hallucinations), use low dose butyrophenones or phenothiazines. Resperidone (Resperidol) 0.5 -1.0 mg bid is newer antipsychotic agent useful in this setting due to excellent side effect profile. Remember to attempt periodic dose reductions or discontinuation, especially in nursing home patient (see OBRA [Omnibus Reconciliation Act] 1987).
• Carbamazepine (Tegretol) 100 mg bid-tid and propranolol (Inderal) 10-40 mg bid-tid also anecdotally reported in literature to help with severe aggressive agitation
• For memory enhancement – donepezil (Aricept) 5-10 mg qd has supplanted tacrine (Cognex) as the agent of choice. Indicated in mild to moderate disease (Folstein's MMSE scores 10-24). 30-50% of patients will respond - average response is moving patient back up the slope of decline by 12 months. Unlike tacrine, no liver toxicity seen. Most common side effects are gastrointestinal disturbances.
• A recent study supported efficacy of selegiline 5 mg bid and/or vitamin E, 1000 IU bid in slowing progression of disease
• NSAIDs and estrogen replacement therapy are consistently related to lesser incidence and slower progression of Alzheimer's disease. No standards for routine use exist.
• Also, randomized clinical trial exploring efficacy of corticosteroids is underway
Contraindications: Avoid anticholinergic drugs, such as tricyclic antidepressants (TCA) and antihistamines
Precautions:
• Tacrine (Cognex): Use with caution in persons with a history of neuromuscular disease, abnormal liver function tests, history of seizures or asthma
• Benzodiazepines may produce paradoxical excitation or daytime drowsiness
• Triazolam (Halcion) can produce confusion, memory loss and psychotic reactions in the elderly

Significant possible interactions:
• Antipsychotics: lithium may induce extrapyramidal symptoms and disorientation
• Benzodiazepines: increased serum phenytoin concentration. Cimetidine may increase the benzodiazepine concentration.
• Donepezil (Aricept) use with caution with anticholinergic medication or in patients with sick sinus syndrome or a history of peptic ulcers

ALTERNATIVE DRUGS N/A

FOLLOWUP

PATIENT MONITORING
• As often as necessary to treat poor nutrition, medical complications, monitor drug use, provide support for family, assess need for placement
• Serial mental status testing helpful
• Monitor caregiver burnout

EXPECTED COURSE/PROGNOSIS Poor; 8-10 year average survival

PREVENTION/AVOIDANCE
• None known for patient
• In near future, family members may seek genetic screening for presence of E4 allele of apolipoprotein E gene (kits already marketed)

POSSIBLE COMPLICATIONS
• Behavioral - hostility, agitation, wandering, uncooperativeness
• Metabolic - infection, dehydration, drug toxicity, malnutrition
• Others - falls, "sundowning"
• Family or caregiver burnout
• Depression occurs in third of patients
• Suicide – in early stages, especially if depression present

MISCELLANEOUS

ASSOCIATED CONDITIONS
• Down syndrome
• Depression
• Insomnia

AGE-RELATED FACTORS
Pediatric: N/A
Geriatric: A frequent and serious problem in this age group
Others: N/A

PREGNANCY N/A

SYNONYMS
• Presenile dementia
• Senile dementia of the Alzheimer's type (SDAT)
• Primary degenerative dementia

ICD-9-CM
290.0 Senile dementia, uncomplicated
290.10 Presenile dementia, uncomplicated
331.0 Alzheimer's disease

SEE ALSO
• Dementia
• Creutzfeldt-Jakob disease
• Hypothyroidism
• Alcoholism
• Depression
• Anemia, pernicious

OTHER NOTES N/A

ABBREVIATIONS
DAT = dementia of Alzheimer's type

REFERENCES
• Agency for Health and research: Recognition and initial assessment of Alzheimer's disease and related dementias: Clinical Practice Guidelines No. 19. Rockville, MD, US Dept of Health & Human Services, Nov 1996, AHCPR publication 97-0702
• Hyman BT: Apolipoprotein E genotype: utility in clinical practice in Alzheimer's disease. JAGS 1996;44:1469-1471
• Morrison-Bogorad M, Phelps C, Burkholtz N: Alzheimer's disease research comes of age -the pace accelerates. JAMA 1997;277:837-840
• National Institute on Aging. Progress report on Alzheimer's disease 1996. Washington, DC, NIA, HIH, US dept of Health & Human Services; 1996. NIH publication 96-4137
• Pendlebury W, Solomon PR: Alzheimer's disease. Ciba Clinical Symposia 1996;48(3):1-32
• Samo M, et al: A controlled trial of selegeline, alpha-tocopherol, or both as treatment for Alzheimer's disease. NEJM 1997;336:1216-1222
• Blass JP: Age-associated memory impairment and Alzheimer's disease. JAGS 1996;44:209
• Geldmacher DS, Whitehouse PJ: Evaluation of dementia. NEJM 1996;335:330-336
Illustrations: N/A
Internet references: http://www.5mcc.com

Author(s)
Frank "Chip" Celestino, MD

Amblyopia

BASICS

DESCRIPTION Amblyopia describes a reduction in visual acuity that cannot be corrected by eyeglasses or contact lenses in the absence of a structural or pathological abnormality of the eye.
System(s) affected: Nervous
Genetics: There is an increased incidence in children where one parent has a history of amblyopia
Incidence/Prevalence in USA: Approximately 2-2.5% in the general population
Predominant age: May be present from birth or may be detected at any age
Predominant sex: Male = Female

SIGNS AND SYMPTOMS Preschool vision screening is advisable to detect a decrease in visual acuity in one eye

CAUSES
• Strabismic amblyopia is a loss of visual acuity in an individual due to suppression of the images in eye which turns out or in
• Anisometropic amblyopia is present when one eye has a significantly different refractive error than the fellow eye and leads to visual blurring
• Refractive amblyopia is due to uncorrected high refractive error resulting in visual blurring in either or both eyes
• Deprivation amblyopia (amblyopia ex anopsia) is due to relative complete visual deprivation in one eye that can be caused by a congenital abnormality such as a corneal scar or cataract

RISK FACTORS None identified

DIAGNOSIS

DIFFERENTIAL DIAGNOSIS The diagnosis of amblyopia can be confused with an organic lesion causing decreased visual acuity and this must always be excluded before the diagnosis of amblyopia is considered

LABORATORY N/A
Drugs that may alter lab results: N/A
Disorders that may alter lab results: N/A

PATHOLOGICAL FINDINGS N/A

SPECIAL TESTS Examination by an ophthalmologist to screen for unequal refractive error, outward turning, or inward turning of the eye (strabismic amblyopia) and proper vision testing of the eye under monocular conditions. A complete slit lamp and dilated funduscopic examination is necessary to exclude an organic cause for the decreased visual acuity.

IMAGING N/A

DIAGNOSTIC PROCEDURES N/A

TREATMENT

APPROPRIATE HEALTH CARE All children should have complete visual examinations prior to starting school with each eye tested individually. Those children from families with a known history of amblyopia or strabismus should have special exams by an ophthalmologist.

GENERAL MEASURES
• Correction of the underlying disorder should be instituted at the earliest opportunity
• Full refractive correction and/or patching of the stronger eye to encourage visual development of the amblyopic eye is warranted
• Amblyopia never corrects itself spontaneously and will always require treatment. Children do not outgrow amblyopia.
• Surgical correction of an abnormal eye position may also be required

SURGICAL MEASURES N/A

ACTIVITY No restrictions

DIET No special diet

PATIENT EDUCATION All parents should be made aware of the need to have their children's eyes examined prior to starting school

MEDICATIONS

DRUG(S) OF CHOICE N/A
Contraindications: N/A
Precautions: N/A
Significant possible interactions: N/A

ALTERNATIVE DRUGS N/A

FOLLOWUP

PATIENT MONITORING Once the diagnosis of amblyopia is made, the patient needs to be seen frequently at the discretion of the ophthalmologist until complete resolution of the problem occurs

PREVENTION/AVOIDANCE None

POSSIBLE COMPLICATIONS If there is failure to institute proper therapy early, permanent and profound visual loss can be expected

EXPECTED COURSE/PROGNOSIS
Amblyopia is a treatable condition in most cases if the diagnosis is made early. Patching therapy, eyeglasses, and surgical correction of abnormal eye positions can result in near normalcy of vision when instituted early. Visual development occurs during the first several years of life and amblyopia therapy can be effective until approximately age 12.

MISCELLANEOUS

ASSOCIATED CONDITIONS Amblyopia is more common in families with a history of unequal refractive errors, high uncorrected refractive errors, and strabismus

AGE-RELATED FACTORS
Pediatric: More commonly seen in the pediatric age group early in life
Geriatric: When seen in the geriatric population, the diagnosis has usually been made early in childhood
Others: N/A

PREGNANCY N/A

SYNONYMS Lazy eye

ICD-9-CM
368.0

SEE ALSO
• Strabismus
• Refractive errors

OTHER NOTES
• Deficiency amblyopia: Also known as nutritional optic neuropathy or tobacco-alcohol amblyopia. Deficiencies of B1, B12, or riboflavine may be responsible. Treatment consists of balanced diet, vitamins, and avoidance of alcohol and tobacco.

ABBREVIATIONS N/A

REFERENCES
• Binocular Vision And Ocular Motility. In Ophthalmology Basic and Clinical Science Course. (American Academy of Ophthalmology)
• Harley RD: Pediatric Ophthalmology. Philadelphia, W.B. Saunders Co., 1983
Illustrations: N/A
Internet references: http://www.5mcc.com

Author(s)
Robert M. Kershner, MD, FACS

Amebiasis

 BASICS

DESCRIPTION Amebiasis is caused by the intestinal protozoan, Entamoeba histolytica. Infection results from ingestion of fecally contaminated food, such as garden vegetables or by direct fecal-oral transmission. Most persons are asymptomatic or have minimal diarrheal symptoms. In a few patients, invasive intestinal or extraintestinal (e.g., liver, and less commonly kidney, bladder, male or female genitalia, skin, lung, brain) infection results. Amebic abscess of the liver may develop during the acute attack or 1-3 months later; symptoms may be abrupt or insidious. Entamoeba histolytica has been divided into "pathogenic" and "nonpathogenic" strains. The pathogenic strains commonly cause invasive infection while the noninvasive strains cause only asymptomatic intestinal infection. More recently, the nonpathogenic strains have been assigned to a separate species, E. dispar. Unfortunately, the species cannot be distinguished in a routine clinical laboratory.

Incidence/Prevalence in USA: Probably < 1% overall, but much higher in some risk groups, such as areas with large immigrant populations

System(s) affected: Gastrointestinal, Renal/Urologic, Reproductive, Skin/Exocrine, Nervous

Genetics: N/A

Predominant age: All

Predominant sex: Male > Female; probably because of greater occupational exposure

SIGNS AND SYMPTOMS
- Noninvasive infection (up to 99%)
  ◊ Asymptomatic (90%)
  ◊ Mild diarrhea
  ◊ Abdominal discomfort
- Invasive intestinal infection
  ◊ Abdominal pain and tenderness
  ◊ Rectal pain
  ◊ Diarrhea
  ◊ Bloody stools
  ◊ Fever (30%)
  ◊ Systemic toxicity
- Extraintestinal infection
  ◊ Fever
  ◊ Systemic toxicity
  ◊ RUQ abdominal pain and tenderness
  ◊ Nausea and vomiting
  ◊ Diarrhea (50%)
  ◊ Hematuria, dysuria, urinary frequency and urgency

CAUSES Infection is transmitted through contaminated food or water, or through person-to-person contact

RISK FACTORS
- Low socioeconomic status
- Institutional living
- Male homosexuality
- Invasive disease is more common in certain geographic locations, including some parts of Mexico, South Africa, and India

 DIAGNOSIS

DIFFERENTIAL DIAGNOSIS
- Other infectious causes of colitis, including shigellosis, Campylobacter infection, pseudomembranous colitis, and occasionally salmonellosis or Yersinia infection
- Noninfectious causes of colitis include ulcerative colitis, Crohn's colitis and ischemic colitis
- Hepatic amebiasis must be distinguished from pyogenic liver abscess or superinfection of amebic abscess

LABORATORY
- Stool for ova and parasites (unfortunately, the sensitivity of this exam is poor). Diarrheal stool should be examined immediately for trophozoites in addition to fixed stool specimens (repeated as necessary). In invasive intestinal infection, stools are bloody, but fecal leukocytes are frequently absent.
- Serologic tests (especially indirect hemagglutination (IHA), positive in 85% of colitis patients and most patients with extraintestinal disease. Serologic tests should be done in patients with idiopathic inflammatory bowel disease to rule out amebiasis.
- In bladder infections – amoebae and/or cysts in urine

Drugs that may alter lab results: Many drugs interfere with stool exams

Disorders that may alter lab results: N/A

PATHOLOGICAL FINDINGS
- Colon biopsy
  ◊ Lysis of mucosal cells (flask ulcers)
  ◊ PAS-stained trophozoites
  ◊ Neutrophils at the periphery
- Liver biopsy
  ◊ Necrosis surrounded by a rim of trophozoites

SPECIAL TESTS N/A

IMAGING CT scan or ultrasound for hepatic infection

DIAGNOSTIC PROCEDURES
- Rectosigmoidoscopy with biopsy
- Needle aspirate of hepatic lesions may be needed to rule out pyogenic infection or superinfection

 TREATMENT

APPROPRIATE HEALTH CARE
Outpatient

GENERAL MEASURES
- Fluids and nutrition
- Electrolyte management

SURGICAL MEASURES With severe amebic colitis, surgery may be necessary

ACTIVITY In accordance with illness of patient

DIET As tolerated

PATIENT EDUCATION Avoid conditions of re-exposure

MEDICATIONS

DRUG(S) OF CHOICE
• Noninvasive infection
◊ Diiodohydroxyquin [also called iodoquinol] 650 mg tid for 20 days
• Invasive infection
◊ Metronidazole (Flagyl) 750 mg tid for 5-10 days, followed by a 20 day course of diiodohydroxyquin to eliminate intestinal carriage

Contraindications:
• Diiodohydroxyquin - use cautiously in patients with thyroid diseases. Contraindicated in hepatic or renal dysfunction. May cause optic neuritis or peripheral neuropathy.
• Known allergy to given medication

Precautions: None of the agents are proven safe in pregnancy, but pregnant women with invasive disease should still be treated

Significant possible interactions: Disulfiram reaction with ethanol

ALTERNATIVE DRUGS
• Noninvasive infection
◊ Diloxanide 500 mg tid for 10 days
◊ Paromomycin 500 mg tid for 10 days
• Invasive infection
◊ Dehydroemetine [as effective as metronidazole, but cardiotoxic] 1-1.5 mg/kg/day IM for 5 days
◊ Chloroquine [less effective] 600 mg base/day for 2 days, then 200 mg/day for 2-3 weeks. Children 10 mg/kg/day up to maximum of 300 mg/day.
◊ Tinidazole 600-800 mg tid for 5 days (not available in US)
◊ Secnidazole 2 gm single dose (not available in US)

FOLLOWUP

PATIENT MONITORING
Patient signs and symptoms, stool for ova and parasite

PREVENTION/AVOIDANCE
Avoid risk factors when possible

POSSIBLE COMPLICATIONS
• Toxic megacolon with rupture
• Rupture of hepatic abscess which may perforate into subphrenic space, right pleural cavity or other nearby organs
• Bladder perforation, urethral strictures, vesicointestinal fistula

EXPECTED COURSE/PROGNOSIS
Untreated invasive amebiasis is frequently fatal. With treatment, improvement usually occurs within a few days. Some patients with amebic colitis have irritable bowel symptoms for weeks after successful treatment. Relapses possible.

MISCELLANEOUS

ASSOCIATED CONDITIONS N/A

AGE-RELATED FACTORS
Pediatric: More severe in neonates
Geriatric: More severe in elderly
Others: More severe in patients on corticosteroids and other immunocompromised patients

PREGNANCY
More severe in pregnancy. Most agents are avoided in pregnancy (especially first trimester) because of concerns of teratogenicity, but invasive disease must still be treated. Paromomycin is sometimes recommended for noninvasive disease because it is not absorbed. Infectious disease consultation should be obtained.

SYNONYMS
• Amebic colitis
• Amebic dysentery

ICD-9-CM
006.0 Acute amebic dysentery without mention of abscess
006.3 Amebic liver abscess
006.5 Amebic brain abscess
006.8 Amebic infection of other sites
006.9 Amebiasis, unspecified

SEE ALSO
• Diarrhea, acute
• Diarrhea, chronic

OTHER NOTES N/A

ABBREVIATIONS N/A

REFERENCES
• Fedorak RN, Rubinoff MJ: Basic Investigation of a Patient with Diarrhea. In: Field M. ed. Diarrheal Diseases. Elsevier Science Publishing Co., Inc., New York, 1991:191-218
• Bruckner DA: Amebiasis. Clin Microbiol Rev 1992;5:356-369
• Ravdin JI, Petri WA Jr: Entamoeba histolytica (amebiasis). In: Mandell GL, Douglas RG, Bennett JE, eds. Principles and Practice of Infectious Diseases. 4th Ed. New York, Churchill Livingstone Inc., 1995:2395-2408
Illustrations: N/A
Internet references: http://www.5mcc.com

Author(s)
Rodney D. Adam, MD

Amenorrhea

BASICS

DESCRIPTION   The absence of menses.
• Primary amenorrhea - no menses by age 14 with absence of secondary sexual characteristics, or no menses by age 16 with normal secondary characteristics
• Secondary amenorrhea - the cessation of menses for three cycles
System(s) affected: Reproductive, Endocrine/Metabolic
Genetics: No known genetic pattern
Incidence/Prevalence in USA:
• Incidence of primary amenorrhea 0.3%
• Incidence of secondary amenorrhea 3.3%
Predominant age: Menarche to menopause
Predominant sex: Female only

SIGNS AND SYMPTOMS
• The absence of periods
• Galactorrhea
• Symptoms of hypothyroidism
• Symptoms of early pregnancy
• Signs of androgen excess
• Signs of estrogen deficiency

CAUSES
• Primary amenorrhea
  ◊ Imperforate hymen
  ◊ Agenesis of the uterus and upper 2/3 of the vagina (Mullerian agenesis)
  ◊ Turner's syndrome
  ◊ Constitutional delay
• Secondary amenorrhea
  ◊ Physiological - pregnancy, corpus luteal cyst, breast-feeding, menopause
  ◊ Suppression of the hypothalamic-pituitary axis - post pill amenorrhea, stress, intercurrent illness, weight loss, low body mass index
  ◊ Pituitary disease - ablation of the pituitary gland, Sheehan's syndrome, prolactinoma
  ◊ Uncontrolled endocrinopathies - diabetes, hypo- or hyperthyroidism
  ◊ Polycystic ovarian disease (POD), (Stein-Leventhal syndrome)
  ◊ Chemotherapy
  ◊ Pelvic irradiation
  ◊ Endometrial ablation (Asherman's syndrome)
  ◊ Drug therapy - systemic steroids, danazol, GRH-RH analogs, antipsychotics, OCP's
  ◊ Premature ovarian failure

RISK FACTORS
• Over-training (e.g., long-distance runner, ballet dancer)
• Eating disorders
• Psycho-social crisis

DIAGNOSIS

DIFFERENTIAL DIAGNOSIS   Includes all of the causes listed above. The most common cause of secondary amenorrhea is early pregnancy.

LABORATORY
• Pregnancy test if negative, obtain:
  ◊ Serum prolactin
  ◊ FSH
  ◊ LH
  ◊ TSH
  ◊ Blood sugar
Drugs that may alter lab results: N/A
Disorders that may alter lab results:
Pregnancy, menopause, hyperprolactinemia, ovarian suppression, endocrinopathy

PATHOLOGICAL FINDINGS   Due to underlying disease

SPECIAL TESTS
• Progesterone challenge test - 10 mg of medroxyprogesterone for 5 days orally.
  ◊ If withdrawal bleeding occurs, amenorrhea most likely due to anovulation
  ◊ If no bleeding, evaluate estrogen status (FSH, LH)

IMAGING
• Ultrasound may show cysts undetectable on pelvic examination
• Radiologic evaluation of the sella turcica if prolactinomas suspected (elevated serum prolactin)

DIAGNOSTIC PROCEDURES
• Laparoscopy - diagnosis of the streak ovaries of Turner's syndrome, or polycystic ovarian disease
• Hysterosalpingogram - to rule out Asherman's syndrome

TREATMENT

APPROPRIATE HEALTH CARE
Outpatient

GENERAL MEASURES   Definitive treatment depends on determining the cause of the amenorrhea. May not be necessary to treat all cases especially if just temporary amenorrhea.

SURGICAL MEASURES
• Hymenectomy, done as a day surgery, will be required for those whose primary amenorrhea is due to imperforate hymen
• Lysis at adhesions in Asherman's syndrome

ACTIVITY   No restrictions

DIET   Correct overweight or underweight by dietary management

PATIENT EDUCATION
• Consists of fully informing the patient of your findings, including the presence or absence of pregnancy, and of the underlying cause
• Specific educational resources can be utilized as necessary, e.g., prenatal classes, menopause support groups
• Specific information should be given about the expected duration of amenorrhea (temporary or permanent), effect on fertility, and the long-term sequelae of untreated amenorrhea (e.g., osteoporosis, vaginal dryness)
• Appropriate contraceptive advice should be given, as fertility returns before menses
• Additional support may be needed if the amenorrhea is associated with a reduction in, or loss of, fertility
• Society for Menstrual Cycle Research, 10559 N. 104th Place, Scottsdale, AZ 85258, (602)451-9731

MEDICATIONS

DRUG(S) OF CHOICE
• Progesterone replacement - medroxyprogesterone (Provera) 5 mg bid for 5 days, will result in a withdrawal bleed if the hypothalamo-pituitary-ovarian axis is intact and there is some endogenous estrogen production
• Estrogen replacement - estrogen, conjugated (Premarin) 0.625 mg for 25 days with progesterone added as above for the last 10 days will result in a withdrawal bleed if the uterus and lower genital tract are normal
• Use of hormonal therapies will not correct underlying problem. Other drugs might be required to treat specific conditions, e.g., bromocriptine for hyperprolactinemia.
• Use of hormonal replacement therapy is recommended after 6 months of amenorrhea (regardless of the primary cause) in order to reduce the risks of osteoporosis and hypercholesterolemia secondary to hypoestrogenism
• Calcium supplementation 1500 mg/day if cause is hypoestrogenism

Contraindications:
• Pregnancy
• Thromboembolic disease
• Previous myocardial infarct, cerebrovascular accident
• Estrogen-dependent malignancy
• Severe hepatic impairment or disease

Precautions:
• Diabetes
• Seizure disorder
• Migraine headache
• Smoker over 35

Significant possible interactions:
Barbiturates, phenytoin, rifampin, corticosteroids, theophyllines, tricyclics, oral anticoagulants (anticoagulant effect may be decreased)

ALTERNATIVE DRUGS
Use of oral contraceptives for hormonal replacement if patient has difficulty following above regimen

FOLLOWUP

PATIENT MONITORING
Depends on the cause, and the treatment chosen. If hormonal replacement is used, discontinuation after six months is advised, to assess spontaneous resumption of menses.

PREVENTION/AVOIDANCE
Maintenance of proper body mass index (BMI)

POSSIBLE COMPLICATIONS
• Estrogen deficiency symptoms, e.g., hot flushes, vaginal dryness
• Osteoporosis, in prolonged hypoestrogenic amenorrhea
• Increased risk of endometrial cancer in hyperestrogenism

EXPECTED COURSE/PROGNOSIS
Reflects the underlying cause. In secondary amenorrhea from hypothalamo-pituitary suppression, spontaneous resumption of menses with time (99% within 6 months) and correction of body mass index.

MISCELLANEOUS

ASSOCIATED CONDITIONS N/A

AGE-RELATED FACTORS
Pediatric: N/A
Geriatric: N/A
Others: N/A

PREGNANCY One of the primary causes

SYNONYMS N/A

ICD-9-CM
626.0 Absence of menstruation

SEE ALSO
• Polycystic ovarian disease
• Diabetes mellitus, insulin-dependent (IDDM or Type I)
• Diabetes mellitus, non-insulin dependent (NIDDM)
• Hypothyroidism, adult
• Hyperthyroidism

OTHER NOTES
• Use of hormonal replacement therapy is symptomatic and is discretionary if amenorrhea is temporary (e.g., hypothalamopituitary suppression)
• Patients who are amenorrheic and wish to become pregnant should not be given hormone replacement therapy, but should receive treatment for infertility based on specific cause
• Women less than age 30 with ovarian failure should have Karyotype analysis

ABBREVIATIONS N/A

REFERENCES
• Yen SSC, Jaffe RB, eds: Reproductive Endocrinology. 3rd Ed. Philadelphia, W.B. Saunders Co., 1991
• Speroff L, Glass R, Kase N, eds: Clinical Gynecology, Endocrinology and Infertility. 5th Ed. Baltimore, Williams & Wilkins, 1994
• Kiningham R, Apgar B, Schwenk T: Evaluation of amenorrhea, AM Fam Phys 1996;53:1185-1194
Illustrations: N/A
Internet references: http://www.5mcc.com

Author(s)
Barbara J. Morant, MD
Herbert L. Issac II, MD
Graham S. Kaiser, DO

Amyloidosis

BASICS

DESCRIPTION A disease characterized by increased deposition of amyloid fibrils in the tissues. Several different proteins may give rise to amyloid. These proteins are present due to their overproduction or decreased clearance. Their deposition may lead to compromise of vital organ function. The most common types of amyloidosis are:
• Primary amyloidosis: usually associated with the plasma cell disorders multiple myeloma and MGUS (monoclonal gammopathy of undetermined significance)
• Secondary amyloidosis: associated with several chronic inflammatory diseases such as rheumatoid arthritis, osteomyelitis, malaria, tuberculosis, and leprosy
• Familial (hereditary) amyloidosis: is sometimes associated with the genetic disease familial Mediterranean fever
• Hemodialysis amyloidosis: associated with renal hemodialysis

Incidence/Prevalence in USA: Not reported
System(s) affected: Endocrine/Metabolic, Cardiovascular, Pulmonary, Renal/Urologic, Musculoskeletal, Gastrointestinal, Nervous, Skin/Exocrine
Genetics: N/A
Predominant age: 60-70
Predominant sex: Male > Female (2:1)

SIGNS AND SYMPTOMS

May be highly variable depending upon which organ system is affected and to what degree:
• Fatigue, weight loss, gastroparesis, pseudo-obstruction, malabsorption, diarrhea, macroglossia
• Peripheral neuropathy, carpal tunnel syndrome
• Ascites, hepatomegaly
• Dyspnea, interstitial lung disease, congestive heart failure, arrhythmia, sudden death
• Hilar adenopathy, mediastinal adenopathy
• Symmetrical polyarthritis, rubbery peri-articular soft tissue swelling
• Translucent/waxy skin papules, purpura (especially peri-orbital purpura), edema
• Renal failure, nephrotic syndrome
• Dementia (may play a role in development of Alzheimer's disease)

CAUSES

• Primary amyloidosis: The amyloid consists of immunoglobulin light chains (AL) which are overproduced in plasma disorders.
• Secondary amyloidosis: The amyloid consists of amyloid fibrillary protein (AA), and its breakdown product, serum amyloid protein (SAA), which are overproduced in chronic inflammatory conditions
• Familial (hereditary) amyloidosis: The amyloid consists of transthyretin protein (ATTR) overproduced in the liver
• Hemodialysis Amyloidosis: The amyloid consists of beta-2-microglobulin which is normally cleared by the kidney, but cannot be cleared by hemodialysis

RISK FACTORS
• Underlying plasma cell dyscrasia
• Underlying chronic inflammatory disease
• Familial Mediterranean fever
• Hemodialysis

DIAGNOSIS

DIFFERENTIAL DIAGNOSIS
• Peripheral neuropathy - diabetes mellitus, alcoholism, vitamin deficiencies
• Carpal tunnel syndrome - hypothyroidism, trauma, rheumatoid arthritis, etc.
• Restrictive cardiomyopathy: acute viral myocarditis, endomyocardial fibrosis, sarcoidosis, hemochromatosis
• Nephrotic syndrome - glomerulonephritis, renal vein thrombosis
• Renal failure - glomerulonephritis, obstructive uropathy, toxin or drug-induced, acute tubular necrosis
• Symmetric polyarthritis - rheumatoid arthritis, psoriatic arthritis, SLE
• Interstitial lung disease - connective tissue diseases, infectious, sarcoidosis, drug-induced, pneumoconiosis
• Demential - Alzheimer's disease and multi-infarct dementia

LABORATORY
• Anemia may be present
• Hypothyroidism may be present due to amyloidosis of the thyroid
• Renal insufficiency will be present in almost 50% at presentation
• Proteinuria will be present in almost 80% at presentation
• In primary amyloidosis, an elevated monoclonal protein level will be found in the serum and/or urine
• In secondary amyloidosis, tests to assess the underlying inflammatory disease will be useful

Drugs that may alter lab results: N/A
Disorders that may alter lab results: N/A

PATHOLOGICAL FINDINGS
• Demonstration of amyloid deposits in tissues
• With Congo red staining, amyloid produces a green birefringence under polarized light
• Electron microscopy is the definitive diagnostic tool

SPECIAL TESTS N/A

IMAGING Echocardiography (if cardiac involvement is suspected)

DIAGNOSTIC PROCEDURES
• Rectal biopsy (70% positive)
• Bone marrow biopsy (20% positive)
• Abdominal fat pad biopsy
• Endomyocardial biopsy
• Renal biopsy

TREATMENT

APPROPRIATE HEALTH CARE
Outpatient except for serious complications (congestive heart failure, renal failure)

GENERAL MEASURES Change from hemodialysis to peritoneal dialysis, which clears beta-2-microglobulin, in those with hemodialysis amyloidosis

SURGICAL MEASURES
• Splenectomy may ameliorate this condition by decreasing the amount of amyloid produced
• Renal transplantation may improve the status of renal amyloidosis
• Liver transplantation may cure familial (hereditary) amyloidosis
• Other measures: Treatment of multiple myeloma with bone marrow translantation is an option for some patients

ACTIVITY Fully active as tolerated

DIET
• Low protein, low salt for renal failure patients
• Low salt for congestive heart failure patients

PATIENT EDUCATION
• For more information:
  ◊ National Organization for Rare Disorders (NORD), Box 8923, New Fairfield, CT 06812
  ◊ National Institute of Diabetes, Digestive and Kidney Disorders Information Clearinghouse, Bldg 31, Rm 9A04, Bethesda, MD 20892
• For genetic information and counseling referrals:
  ◊ March of Dimes Birth Defects Foundation, 1275 Mamaroneck Ave., White Plains, NY 10605
  ◊ National Center for Education in Maternal and Child Health

MEDICATIONS

DRUG(S) OF CHOICE
• Primary amyloidosis
◊ Treatment of the underlying plasma cell disorder may or may not affect the outcome
◊ Melphalan and prednisone are among the drugs of choice for plasma cell disorders. Colchicine may slow the progression of amyloid deposition.
• Secondary amyloidosis
◊ Treatment of the underlying inflammatory process with disease-specific medications usually improves the outcome (i.e., isoniazid and rifampin for M. Tuberculosis, methotrexate for rheumatoid arthritis)
◊ Tacrine and donepezil have been approved for mild to moderate dementia caused by Alzheimer's disease
• Familial amyloidosis
◊ Colchicine, 0.6 mg two or three times a day may decrease renal amyloidosis in this condition
• Hemodialysis amyloidosis
◊ None
Contraindications: Refer to manufacturer's literature
Precautions:
• Colchicine - bone marrow depression, including agranulocytosis, pancytopenia, thrombocytopenia, or aplastic anemia, may occur with prolonged administration. Monitor CBC periodically. Counsel patient to report symptoms/signs of infection promptly (headache, sore throat, fever).
• Tacrine - significant liver function abnormalities in up to one quarter of patients. Monitor LFT's closely.
Significant possible interactions: Refer to manufacturer's literature

ALTERNATIVE DRUGS   N/A

FOLLOWUP

PATIENT MONITORING
• Primary amyloidosis
◊ Regular testing of monoclonal protein levels to assess response to therapy
◊ Regular testing of renal function to assess response to therapy
• Secondary and hemodialysis amyloidosis
◊ Follow-up to assess control of the underlying disease process
◊ Regular testing of renal function to assess degree of impairment

PREVENTION/AVOIDANCE   N/A

POSSIBLE COMPLICATIONS   Despite intervention, worsening renal failure, heart failure, arthropathy, interstitial lung disease, and neuropathy are common

EXPECTED COURSE/PROGNOSIS
• Primary amyloidosis
◊ The prognosis is dependent upon the underlying disease
◊ Once renal failure has developed, the prognosis is usually less than one year
◊ Congestive heart failure has a four month prognosis
◊ Overall prognosis is 12-14 months. Women have better survival chances than men.
• Secondary amyloidosis
◊ The prognosis is much better, depending upon the ability to control the underlying inflammatory process
• Familial and hemodialysis amyloidosis
◊ Highly variable

MISCELLANEOUS

ASSOCIATED CONDITIONS
• Amyloid may bind Factor X leading to bleeding problems

AGE-RELATED FACTORS
Pediatric: N/A
Geriatric: In general, older individuals do less well
Others: N/A

PREGNANCY   No information available

SYNONYMS   N/A

ICD-9-CM
277.3 amyloidosis

SEE ALSO   N/A

OTHER NOTES   N/A

ABBREVIATIONS   N/A

REFERENCES
• Kelley WN, ed: Textbook of Internal Medicine, Philadelphia, J.B. Lippincott Co., 1989
• Kyle RA, et al: Primary Systemic Amyloidosis: multivariate analysis for prognostic factors in 168 cases. Blood 1986;68(1):220-4
• Cohen AS, et al: Survival of patients with primary (AL) amyloidosis. Colchicine-treated cases from 1976-1983 compared with cases seen in previous years (1961-1973). Am J Med 1987;82(6):1182-90
• Fiter J, et al: Methotrexate treatment of amyloidosis secondary to rheumatoid arthritis. Clinical Review of Spain 1995;195(6):390-392
Illustrations: 1 available on CD-ROM
Internet references: http://www.5mcc.com

Author(s)
R. Scott Gorman, MD

Amyotrophic lateral sclerosis

BASICS

DESCRIPTION A degenerative disease (or group of diseases) which affects the upper and lower motor neurons.
• Amyotrophic lateral sclerosis: the term applied to the sporadic and most common form of the disease. Includes a number of overlapping syndromes such as pseudobulbar palsy, progressive bulbar palsy, progressive muscular atrophy and primary lateral sclerosis.
• Familial ALS: an autosomal dominant or recessive disease which is clinically similar to sporadic ALS but probably represents a distinct entity pathologically and biochemically.
• ALS-Parkinson-dementia complex of Guam: an ALS like syndrome, often, but not always, associated with Parkinson's syndrome and dementia, which is prevalent amongst the Chamorro Indians of Guam (very rare in the USA).
Incidence/Prevalence in USA:
0.4-1.76/100,000 incidence; 5 in 100,000 prevalence
System(s) affected: Nervous
Genetics: N/A
Predominant age: Rare before age 40 years. Incidence increases with age.
Predominant sex: Male = Female

SIGNS AND SYMPTOMS
• Variable combinations of:
  ◊ Unexplained weight loss
  ◊ Focal wasting of muscle groups
  ◊ Limb weakness with variable symmetry and distribution
  ◊ Difficulty walking
  ◊ Difficulty swallowing
  ◊ Slurring of speech
  ◊ Inability to control affect (emotions)
  ◊ Atrophy of muscle groups, initially in a myotomal distribution
  ◊ Fasciculations (other than calves)
  ◊ Hyperactive deep tendon reflexes (including jaw jerk)
  ◊ Spares cognitive, oculomotor, sensory and autonomic functions

CAUSES
• Sporadic ALS - degeneration of the upper and lower motor neurons with their respective axons. Cause is unknown.
• Familial ALS - a genetically transmitted degenerative disease. Gene locus has been localized to the long arm of chromosome 21 and encodes the enzyme superoxide dismutase (SOD1). At this writing, although activity is reduced, levels of superoxide dismutase have not yet been proven to be low.
• ALS-Parkinson-dementia complex of Guam - possible relationship to ingestion of the cycad nut or to some other environmental toxin

RISK FACTORS
• Age over 40
• Family history of ALS

DIAGNOSIS

DIFFERENTIAL DIAGNOSIS
• Focal motor neuropathy
• Cervical spondylosis
• Lead intoxication
• Plasma cell dyscrasias
• Spinal muscular atrophy (adult form)
• Primary lateral sclerosis
• Familial spastic paraparesis
• Spinal multiple sclerosis
• Tropical spastic paraparesis

LABORATORY
• Anti GM1 autoantibodies in low titer commonly found
• Possibly reduced levels of nerve growth factor
• There is no simple reliable laboratory test available that confirms the diagnosis of ALS
Drugs that may alter lab results: N/A
Disorders that may alter lab results: N/A

PATHOLOGICAL FINDINGS
• Loss of Betz's cells in the motor cortex
• Atrophic or absent anterior horn cells of spinal cord
• Atrophic or absent neurons within the motor nuclei of the medulla and pons
• Degeneration of the lateral columns of the spinal cord
• Atrophy of the ventral roots
• Grouped atrophy of muscle (motor units)

SPECIAL TESTS N/A

IMAGING N/A

DIAGNOSTIC PROCEDURES
• Electromyography: denervation potentials (fibrillations, positive sharp waves) and often doublets are associated with prominent fasciculations (which suggest anterior horn cell dysfunction). Voluntary motor unit potentials have increased amplitude, long duration and/or polyphasia. The interference pattern is reduced for the force generated and individual motor units have a high rate of discharge.
• Muscle biopsy - will show groups of shrunken angulated muscle fibers (grouped atrophy) amid other groups of fibers with a uniform fiber type (fiber type grouping).

TREATMENT

APPROPRIATE HEALTH CARE
• Outpatient initially, may ultimately need nursing home placement and/or hospice
• Supportive care for complicating emergencies (aspiration, respiratory failure). Use of a respirator is a major ethical dilemma and is usually not suggested.

GENERAL MEASURES Prosthetic devices, e.g., wheelchair, etc.

SURGICAL MEASURES N/A

ACTIVITY As tolerated

DIET Modify as tolerated. May need tube feedings.

PATIENT EDUCATION Printed material for patients (and reference lists for physicians) available from The Muscular Dystrophy Association, (520)529-2000, (800)572-1717

MEDICATIONS

DRUG(S) OF CHOICE Riluzole produces a slight prolongation in life expectancy
Contraindications: N/A
Precautions: N/A
Significant possible interactions: N/A

ALTERNATIVE DRUGS Therapeutic trials of the efficacy of anti-oxidants (vitamins E, C, and beta-carotene), nerve growth factor and thyrotropin releasing hormone are being undertaken

FOLLOWUP

PATIENT MONITORING
• Initially every three months, frequency to be increased as need for symptomatic therapy develops

PREVENTION/AVOIDANCE N/A

POSSIBLE COMPLICATIONS
• Aspiration pneumonia
• Decubitus ulcers
• Pulmonary embolism

EXPECTED COURSE/PROGNOSIS
• ALS usually terminates in death within five years
• Patients predominantly manifesting progressive muscular atrophy have a better prognosis
• There have been reports of spontaneous arrest of the disease

MISCELLANEOUS

ASSOCIATED CONDITIONS None

AGE-RELATED FACTORS
Pediatric: Infantile and juvenile spinal muscular atrophies are conditions which are distinct from amyotrophic lateral sclerosis clinically and pathologically
Geriatric: Symptoms of ALS may inappropriately be attributed to age
Others: N/A

PREGNANCY Pregnancy is uncommon among affected individuals. Pregnancy would be unwise in any individual suffering from a disease with so poor a prognosis. If pregnancy did occur, the only foreseeable difficulties would be related to weakness.

SYNONYMS
• Motor neuron disease
• Lou Gehrig's disease
• ALS

ICD-9-CM
• 335.2 motor neuron disease
• 335.20 amyotrophic lateral sclerosis

SEE ALSO N/A

ABBREVIATIONS N/A

OTHER NOTES Also referred to as Mill's variant (unilateral involvement)

REFERENCES Rowland LP:
• Rowland LD, ed: Merritt's Textbook of Neurology. 9th Ed. Philadelphia, Williams & Wilkins, 1995
• Brown WF, Botton CF: Clinical Electromyography. 2nd Ed. Boston, Butterworth-Heinemann, 1993
Illustrations: N/A
Internet references: http://www.5mcc.com

Author(s)
Colin R. Bamford, MD

Anaerobic & necrotizing infections

BASICS

DESCRIPTION Gangrene is local death of soft tissues due to disease or injury and is associated with loss of blood supply. Anaerobic and necrotizing infections may be associated with gas.
System(s) affected: Skin/Exocrine, Cardiovascular
Genetics: N/A
Incidence/Prevalence in USA: Rare
Predominant age: Any
Predominant sex: Male = Female

SIGNS AND SYMPTOMS
• Local pain
• Foul odor
• Abnormally dark skin and tissues under skin (dark green to black)
• Crepitation (gas)
• Fever
• Rapid pulse
• Fulminant course leading to death without treatment

CAUSES
• Local injury
• Superimposed infection (surface or deep; local or distant)
• Pathologic conditions of large intestine
• Hematologic malignancies
• Severe neutropenia, related or not related to chemotherapy

RISK FACTORS
• Poor blood supply (arteriosclerosis)
• Old age
• Trauma
• Diabetes mellitus
• Malnutrition

DIAGNOSIS

DIFFERENTIAL DIAGNOSIS
Deep infections with muscle involvement
• Gas gangrene:
 ◊ Gas gangrene resulting from soft tissue trauma; clostridial myositis; clostridial myonecrosis
 ◊ Abdominal wall gas gangrene; postoperative clostridial sepsis of the abdominal wall; clostridial myonecrosis of the abdominal wall
 ◊ Nontraumatic, metastatic, clostridial myonecrosis; metastatic clostridial myositis; metastatic gas gangrene; gas gangrene without a visible wound
 ◊ Uterine clostridial infections
 ◊ Gas gangrene of the heart
 ◊ Gas gangrene of the brain
• Streptococcal myositis: anaerobic streptococcal myonecrosis; anaerobic streptococcal myositis
• Infected vascular gas gangrene; non-clostridial gas gangrene; non-clostridial myositis
• Synergistic necrotizing sepsis; synergistic necrotizing cellulitis
Superficial infections - with or without abscess
• Hemolytic streptococcal gangrene
• Acute, infectious staphylococcal gangrene
• Anaerobic cellulitis; crepitant phlegmon; clostridial cellulitis
• Necrotizing fasciitis; synergistic gangrene; non-clostridial anaerobic cellulitis; anaerobic cutaneous gangrene; perineal phlegmon; Fournier's gangrene. (Note: If there is extension to the tissues of the abdominal wall below the deep fascia, such as the anterior sheath of the rectus muscle, perineal phlegmon or Fournier's gangrene is a synergistic necrotizing sepsis rather than just a necrotizing fasciitis. These are similar infections but are in different locations.)
• Panophthalmitis
Simple clostridial contamination of wounds
Infiltration or injection or aspiration of gas into wounds
• Wounds with gas not produced by bacteria
• Injection of gas into wounds
 ◊ Therapy (e.g., hydrogen peroxide)
 ◊ Pranksters' jokes
 ◊ Malingerers
 ◊ Psychiatric problems
• Aspiration and dissemination of air into wounds by muscular activity
• Subcutaneous emphysema related to air leak syndrome or trauma
Gas in tissues after industrial accidents
• Magnesiogenous pneumagranuloma
Gas in tissues after injections of chemicals
• Injection of drugs
• Accidental injection of a foreign agent, such as benzene
Gas in tissues after laparoscopic examination and treatment

LABORATORY
• With severe gangrene, studies will reveal anemia and leukocytosis
• Gram smears for many possible organisms
• Daily serum creatine kinase determinations

Drugs that may alter lab results:
Antibiotics prior to culture
Disorders that may alter lab results: N/A

PATHOLOGICAL FINDINGS
• Necrosis of tissues with foul odor
• Sometimes, gas in tissues
• Microorganisms

SPECIAL TESTS
• Cultures and sensitivity tests for microorganisms reported to produce gas in human tissues:
 ◊ Gram-positive anaerobes: Cocci - Peptostreptococcus (anaerobic Streptococcus) (usually with group A Streptococcus [Streptococcus pyogenes, beta-hemolytic Streptococcus] or Staphylococcus aureus)
 ◊ Gram-positive anaerobes: Bacilli - Clostridium perfringens and other clostridia
 ◊ Gram-negative aerobes: Bacilli - Escherichia coli, Klebsiella pneumoniae, Enterobacter species, Proteus species (all usually in mixed infections)
 ◊ Gram-negative anaerobes: Bacilli - Bacteroides fragilis (usually with other gram-negative bacilli)

IMAGING Plain roentgenograms, gas in tissues; with MRI, edema

DIAGNOSTIC PROCEDURES
IMMEDIATE SURGICAL INTERVENTION with longitudinal incisions of skin, superficial fascia, deep fascia, and muscles to look for necrotic tissue and removal of necrotic tissues. Daily repetition if indicated

TREATMENT

APPROPRIATE HEALTH CARE
Hospital inpatient

GENERAL MEASURES
• Infectious disease consultation if possible
• Intravenous fluids with glucose, electrolytes, blood, vitamins
• Daily CBC and electrolytes in acute phase
• Prophylaxis for tetanus
• Hyperbaric oxygen: unclear therapeutic value; no delay of surgical intervention for hyperbaric oxygen therapy

SURGICAL MEASURES
• SURGICAL INTERVENTION FOR DIAGNOSIS AND DÉBRIDEMENT OF NECROTIC TISSUES; POSSIBLY DAILY
• Re-operation if possibility of spreading or unrecognized necrosis (with abnormal daily CK determination)
• Surgical repair for loss of skin and subcutaneous tissues

ACTIVITY Bedrest

DIET By mouth, as tolerated

PATIENT EDUCATION N/A

MEDICATIONS

DRUG(S) OF CHOICE
• Antibiotics: Determined by stained smears, cultures, and sensitivity tests (although anaerobic organisms are difficult to culture and identify). Dosage will vary according to clinical circumstances; refer to manufacturer's literature and suggestions of infectious disease consultant. Important: don't delay treatment if smear, cultures and tests negative.

```
-----------------------------
Gram stain  Presumed organism
-----------------------------
+ cocci     Streptococcus†
+ cocci     Staphylococcus
              aureus
+ bacilli   Clostridium spp
- bacilli   Bacteroides spp
- bacilli   Coliforms
-----------------------------
† anaerobic
```

◊ Gram-positive cocci: penicillin G, nafcillin (Unipen), clindamycin (Cleocin), metronidazole (Flagyl), or cephalosporins
◊ Gram-positive bacilli: penicillin G, clindamycin, metronidazole or cephalosporins
◊ Gram-negative bacilli (Bacteroides): clindamycin, metronidazole, cefoxitin (Mefoxin) [many B. frag. are resistant], ticarcillin (Ticar) or mezlocillin (Mezlin)
◊ Gram-negative bacilli (Coliforms): gentamicin (Garamycin), tobramycin (Nebcin), amikacin (Amikin), cephalosporins, ampicillin, mezlocillin, or ticarcillin
Contraindications: Sensitivity to drugs
Precautions:
• Recognize spreading gangrene when patient is receiving sedatives and analgesics
• Repeated gram smears, cultures and sensitivity tests for the best antibiotic(s) for the case being treated
Significant possible interactions: See manufacturer's profile of each drug.

ALTERNATIVE DRUGS   As above

FOLLOWUP

PATIENT MONITORING
• Diligence required to RECOGNIZE SPREADING GANGRENE
• Monitor effective blood levels of prescribed antibiotics
• Electrolytes
• Nutrition
• CK determinations daily for myonecrosis
• PROGRESS NOTES IN CHARTS DAILY OR AS OFTEN AS EVERY FEW HOURS

PREVENTION/AVOIDANCE
• Avoidance of trauma
• Good care of skin

POSSIBLE COMPLICATIONS
• Tissue and functional losses
• Amputation
• Death

EXPECTED COURSE/PROGNOSIS
• Good if early diagnosis and treatment, and if gangrene arrested at an early stage
• Fatal without treatment and possibly with treatment
• Fair if large intestine disease is recognized and removed

MISCELLANEOUS

ASSOCIATED CONDITIONS
• Diabetes mellitus with impaired blood flow
• Altered immunocompetence: Depressed immunocompetence may require an alteration of treatment, especially with tumor treatments

AGE-RELATED FACTORS
Pediatric: N/A
Geriatric: Diseases of the aged with debility and poor blood supply
Others: N/A

PREGNANCY   Treatment as for nonpregnant, but consider the pregnancy

SYNONYMS   N/A

ICD-9-CM
785.4 Gangrene
040.0 Gas gangrene
136.9 Unspecified infectious and parasitic diseases
682.9 Cellulitis and abscess at unspecified site (phlegmon)

SEE ALSO
• Tetanus

OTHER NOTES
• Group A Streptococcus: "flesh eating bacterium"

ABBREVIATIONS
CBC = complete blood cell count
MRI = magnetic resonance imaging

REFERENCES
• Barza, M: Myositis or fasciitis caused by Streptococcus pyogenes with the compartment and toxic shock syndromes. New Eng J Med 1995;333:113-119
• Associated Press: Court upholds $2.5 million malpractice award. J Am Med Assoc 1995;38:31
• Centers for Disease Control, Public Health Service, U.S. Department of Health and Human Services: ACIP. Use of vaccines and immune globulin in persons with altered immunocompetence. MMWR 42/RR-4: 1-18, 1993
• Fry DE: The importance of antibiotic pharmacokinetics in critical illness. AM J Surg 1996;172(suppl 6a):205-255
• Furste W, Lobe TE, Botros NM: Gangrenous soft tissue infections. Infections in Surgery 1985;4:837-878
• Furste W, Dolor MC, Rothstein LB, Vest CR: Carcinoma of the large intestine and nontraumatic metastatic clostridial myonecrosis. Diseases of Colon & Rectum 1986;29:899-904
• Furste W, Wheeler WL: Tetanus: a team disease. Curr Prob in Surg 1972;9:1-72
• Rice B: $15 million deep. Med Econ 1995;14:47-50
• Davies HD, McGeer A, Schwartz B, et al: Invasive group A streptococcal infections in Ontario, Canada. New Engl J Med 1996;335:547-554
• Golshani S, Simons AJ, Der R, et al: Necrotizing fasciitis following laparoscopic surgery. Surg Endosc 1996;10:751-754
• Holm SE: Invasive group A streptococcal infections. New Engl J Med 1996;335:590-591
• Shupak A, Shoshani O, Goldenberg I, et al: Necrotizing fasciitis: an indication for hyperbaric oxygenation therapy. Surg 1995;118:873-878
• Swartz MN: Use of antimicrobial agents and drug resistance. NEJM 1997;337:491-492
• Tibbles PM, Edelsberg JS: Hyperbaric-oxygen therapy. New Engl J Med 1996;334:1642-1648
Illustrations: N/A
Internet references: http://www.5mcc.com

Author(s)
Wesley Furste, MD, FACS
Augusto Aguirre, MD

Anaphylaxis

 BASICS

DESCRIPTION

• An acute, systemic reaction following antigen exposure in a sensitized person.
• A non-IgE mediated idiopathic anaphylactoid reaction also may occur. Anaphylactoid reactions are clinically indistinguishable from anaphylaxis and are treated in the same manner.
System(s) affected: Pulmonary, Cardiovascular, Skin/Exocrine, Gastrointestinal, Endocrine/Metabolic, Hemic/Lymphatic/Immunologic
Genetics: Genetic predisposition for sensitization to certain antigens
Incidence/Prevalence in USA:
• Incidence unknown
• Between 20,592 and 47,024 cases of idiopathic anaphylaxis occur per year
• Drug-induced anaphylaxis in 1/2,700 hospitalized patients
• 0.3-0.7/100,000/yr anaphylaxis deaths
Predominant age: All ages
Predominant sex: Male = Female

SIGNS AND SYMPTOMS

• Pruritus, flushing, urticaria, angioedema
• Dyspnea, cough, rhonchi
• Rhinorrhea, bronchorrhea, wheezing
• Difficulty swallowing
• Nausea, vomiting, diarrhea, cramps, bloating
• Tachycardia, hypotension, shock, syncope
• Malaise, shivering
• Mydriasis
• Central hypovolemia associated with peripheral hemostasis

CAUSES

• IgE mediated mast cell degranulation
• Complement activation (C3a, C4a, C5a) by antigen-antibody complexes that contain complement fixing antibodies
• Other non-IgE dependent anaphylaxis-like syndromes may be caused modulators of arachidonic acid metabolism, sulfiting agents, exercise induced anaphylaxis, and idiopathic recurrent anaphylaxis
• Some important causes of anaphylaxis are:
  ◊ Antimicrobials (e.g., penicillin)
  ◊ Blood products (especially in IgA deficient patients)
  ◊ Diagnostic chemicals (iodinated contrast media)
  ◊ Ethylene oxide gas (dialysis tubing, other sterilized products)
  ◊ Exercise
  ◊ Foods (e.g., peanuts, nuts, fish, crustaceans, mollusks, cow milk, eggs, soybean most common)
  ◊ Immunotherapy
  ◊ Insect stings (e.g., honeybees, wasps, kissing bugs, deer flies)
  ◊ Latex rubber (gloves, catheters)
  ◊ Macromolecules (e.g., chymopapain, insulin, dextran, glucocorticoid, protamine)
  ◊ Vaccines

RISK FACTORS Previous anaphylaxis; history of atopy or asthma

 DIAGNOSIS

DIFFERENTIAL DIAGNOSIS

• Anaphylactoid reactions: May occur after the first contact with substance, such as polymyxin, pentamidine, radiographic contrast media, aspirin
• Carcinoid syndrome
• Globus hystericus: may mimic pharyngeal edema.
• Hereditary angioedema: C1q esterase deficiency with painless, pruritus-free angioedema without urticaria, flushing or wheezing.
• Pheochromocytoma: Paradoxically, because of beta-2 stimulation, some patients have hypotensive attacks accompanied by tachycardia. Urticaria, angioedema, and wheezing absent.
• Pseudoanaphylactic reaction: After injection of procaine penicillin. Is a drug effect of procaine and not a penicillin allergy.
• Scombroid poisoning: From ingestion of dark meat fish (e.g., tuna, mackerel, mahi-mahi). Histamine-like mediator - symptoms include flushing, sweating, nausea, vomiting, diarrhea, headache, palpitations, dizziness, rash, swelling of face and tongue, respiratory distress, vasodilatory shock.
• Serum sickness: Occurs several days after exposure to inciting agent
• Systemic mastocytosis: Benign or malignant overgrowth of mast cells. Urticaria pigmentosa seen in benign form and the presence of reddish brown macular-papular cutaneous lesions which urticate after trauma - Darier's sign.
• Vasovagal reactions: Bradycardia and hypotension without tachycardia, flushing, urticaria, angioedema, pruritus, and wheezing
• Pulmonary embolism, foreign body aspiration, arrhythmia

LABORATORY

• Hypoxemia, hypercarbia, acidosis. Acidosis may cause apparent hyperkalemia by moving potassium extracellularly.
• Elevated serum and urine histamine (short-lived circulation)
• Elevated serum tryptase, a mast cell enzyme marker for allergic and anaphylactic reactions. Peak level: 30-90 minutes after reaction onset.
Drugs that may alter lab results:
Epinephrine and albuterol may cause apparent hypokalemia by shifting K+ intracellularly
Disorders that may alter lab results: N/A

PATHOLOGICAL FINDINGS N/A

SPECIAL TESTS N/A

IMAGING N/A

DIAGNOSTIC PROCEDURES N/A

 TREATMENT

APPROPRIATE HEALTH CARE

• Outpatient: Patients with cutaneous angioedema, urticaria, and minimal bronchospasm may be released when symptoms and signs have cleared. Continue antihistamines (diphenhydramine/cimetidine) and oral steroids for 72 hours.
• Moderate-severe anaphylaxis, admit observation; may need ventilatory support.
• Allergist referral, if anaphylaxis cause unclear
• Patients with anaphylaxis from insect stings benefit from desensitization immunotherapy

GENERAL MEASURES

• Treatment depends on severity
• Maintain a patent airway - endotracheal intubation and assisted ventilation may be necessary; possibly tracheostomy
• Oxygen
• Tourniquet placed proximal to injected or stung site if possible, to occlude lymphatic and venous drainage (but not arterial flow)
• IV fluids (normal saline/lactated ringers) restores intravascular volume; avoid precipitating CHF
• Monitor vital signs

SURGICAL MEASURES N/A

ACTIVITY Bedrest until anaphylaxis clears and patient hemodynamically stable

DIET Nothing until acute symptoms are controlled

PATIENT EDUCATION

• Printed patient information available from: Asthma & Allergy Foundation of America, 1717 Massachusetts Avenue, Suite 305, Washington, DC 20036,(800)7-Asthma or American Allergy Association, P.O. Box 7273, Menlo Park, CA 94026, (415)322-1663
• Medic-Alert type tags (Medic-Alert Foundation, Turlock, CA 95381-1009
• Avoid beta-blockers if possible
• Instruct patient in use of bee sting kit

 MEDICATIONS

DRUG(S) OF CHOICE
Immediate
• Epinephrine
  ◊ Less severe reaction: 0.3-0.5 mg (0.01 mg/kg in children)= (0.3-0.5 mL of a 1:1000 solution, 0.01 mL/kg in children), SQ q 20-30 minutes as needed up to 3 doses
  ◊ Life-threatening reactions: 0.5 mg (5 mL of a 1:10,000 solution)(for children: 0.05-0.1 mL/kg/dose) given IV slowly q 5-10 minutes as needed. If IV access not possible, endotracheal or intraosseous may be effective.
• Diphenhydramine, an H1 blocker 25-50 mg IV (IM or PO) immediately and then, q6h for 72 hours (children 1.25 mg/kg to 25 mg)

• Cimetidine, an H2 blocker, 300 mg IV over 3-5 minutes (children 5-10 mg/kg/dose) and then 400 mg PO bid is helpful and may be more effective than diphenhydramine.
• Corticosteroids: No immediate effect but should be administered in most cases to prevent prolonged or recurrent anaphylaxis
◊ Hydrocortisone sodium succinate 250-500 mg IV q 4-6 h (4-8 mg/kg for children), or
◊ Prednisone, 1 mg/kg in children, up to 60 mg, or
◊ Methylprednisolone 60-125 mg IV in adults. 1-2 mg/kg in children.
• Bronchodilator, if persistent bronchospasm
◊ Inhaled beta-2 agonists. Continuous nebulized albuterol of 10 mg/hr or 2.5 mg q 15-20 minutes is safe, effective and preferable to aminophylline as first line therapy.
◊ Aminophylline: many side effects, limited efficacy; no known good human studies
(1) 6 mg/kg IV bolus over 10-20 minute period in patients not on theophylline prior to admission
(2) 2.5 mg/kg IV bolus over 10-20 minutes in patients on theophylline prior to admission and without signs or symptoms of toxicity
(3) Follow bolus with infusion at 0.9 mg/kg/min
(4) Maintain blood level of 10-15 µg/mL
• Laryngeal edema:
◊ Epinephrine 5 mL 1:1000 by nebulizer. More effective than racemic epinephrine and usually available.
• Persistent hypotension
◊ Dopamine 200 mg in 500 mL of dextrose in water given by infusion pump. Titrate to blood pressure (3-20 mcg/kg/min)
◊ Glucagon: May be beneficial for resistant hypotension caused by concurrent beta-blockade therapy 50 mcg/kg IV bolus over 1 minute, or alternatively, because of short half-life, can give as continuous infusion at 5-15 mcg/min
• Normal saline or Ringer's lactate: As necessary to maintain tissue perfusion
• Oral antihistamines and steroids for 72 hours
Contraindications:
Refer to manufacturer's literature
Precautions:
Refer to manufacturer's literature
Significant possible interactions:
Theophylline levels will be increased by cimetidine

ALTERNATIVE DRUGS Several reports of tranexamic acid-1000 mg IV or sigma-aminocaproic acid for refractory anaphylaxis. Reserve for last resort in patient not responding to other therapy; these drugs not considered standard of care! Not to be used in pregnant women, or known vascular thrombosis.

FOLLOWUP

PATIENT MONITORING Follow vital signs closely during treatment and for several hours after anaphylaxis has resolved. Symptoms can recur for up to 72 hours.

PREVENTION/AVOIDANCE

• Avoid drugs, foods that cause the reaction
• Carry a pre-filled epinephrine syringe; avoid areas where insect exposure likely. Avoid wearing things that attract insects (e.g., perfumes, bright-colored clothing); avoid barefeet outdoors.
• Carry/wear medical alert ID about anaphylaxis-causing substance or event
• When radiologic contrast is unavoidable, use of low osmolar contrast agents (e.g., iothalamate) reduces risk of contrast reactions in those with previous contrast reaction to 3.1%; only 0.22% were considered severe. Stop beta-blockers before administering contrast materials; pre-treat with diphenhydramine (50 mg IV) and steroid (e.g., methylprednisolone 60 mg IV).
• Those with frequent (>6/year) episodes of idiopathic anaphylaxis should be treated prophylactically with prednisone 40-60 mg/day in a single a.m. dose, hydroxyzine-25 mg tid, and albuterol 2 mg po tid. The prednisone should be rapidly tapered to a qod regimen.
• Have latex-free kit (gloves, IVs, etc) available for treatment of latex allergic patients; some latex allergic patients will react to tropical fruits (e.g., kiwi, bananas)
• Avoid beta blockers

EXPECTED COURSE/PROGNOSIS

• Good prognosis if treated immediately; worse outcome with a delay of >30 minutes in administration of epinephrine
• Of those with idiopathic anaphylaxis - 60% are free of anaphylactic episodes at 2.5 years; most others were steroid free with a decrease in the number of episodes

POSSIBLE COMPLICATIONS

Hypoxemia; cardiac arrest; death

MISCELLANEOUS

ASSOCIATED CONDITIONS Asthma; atopy

AGE-RELATED FACTORS
Pediatric: N/A
Geriatric: Epinephrine may induce ischemia and myocardial infarction in those with cardiac disease; still the drug of choice. Be alert for anti-cholinergic and CNS side effects after giving diphenhydramine or cimetidine.
Others: N/A

PREGNANCY Epinephrine, other pressors may reduce placental blood flow; but may save life of mother and fetus

SYNONYMS
• Anaphylactoid reactions

ICD-9-CM
• 995.0 anaphylactic shock
• E947 other and unspecified drugs and medicinal substances
• E947.9 unspecified drug or medicinal substance

SEE ALSO
• Food allergy
• Insect bites & stings
• Urticaria

OTHER NOTES
• Allergy to one species of legume (e.g., peanuts) or one type of seafood (e.g., shrimp) doesn't mean allergy to all products in that category. Skin testing is prudent.
• MMR vaccine can be safely administered to those with a history of egg allergy since most egg allergies are related to the albumin.
• Penicillin allergic patients can generally tolerate second and third generation cephalosporins as well as monobactams (e.g., aztreonam); generally will be allergic to carbapenems (e.g., imipenem) and first generation cephalosporins
• IgA deficient patients should have washed RBCs for transfusion
• Those allergic to seafood are not allergic to iodine-based radiocontrast. Shellfish allergy is protein related.

ABBREVIATIONS N/A

REFERENCES
• Tintinalli JE, et al: Emergency Medicine, A Comprehensie Study Guide. 4th Ed. New York McGraw-Hill, 1995
• Patterson R, Hogan MB, Yarnold PR, Harris KE: Idiopathic anaphylaxis: An attempt to estimate the incidence in the United States. Archives of Internal Medicine 1995;155(8):869-871
Illustrations: N/A
Internet references: http://www.5mcc.com

Author(s)
Mark A. Graber, MD

Anemia, aplastic

BASICS

DESCRIPTION An anemia in which the bone marrow fails to produce adequate numbers of peripheral blood elements. Usual course - insidious. Pure red cell aplasia is a related syndrome that is caused by a selective failure of the production of erythroid elements. It can be associated with thymomas. Constitutional (Fanconi's) anemia is associated with congenital anomalies.
Genetics:
• Genetic pattern undetermined in acquired
• Autosomal recessive in constitutional
System(s) affected:
Hemic/Lymphatic/Immunologic
Incidence/Prevalence in USA: Not very common
Predominant age:
• Constitutional - children and young adults
• Acquired - all ages
Predominant sex: Male = Female

SIGNS AND SYMPTOMS
• Dyspnea
• Ecchymoses, petechiae
• Fatigue, fever
• Hemorrhage, menorrhagia, occult stool blood, melena, epistaxis
• Pallor
• Palpitations
• Progressive weakness
• Retinal flame hemorrhages
• Systolic ejection murmur
• Weight loss
• Constitutional:
  ◊ Short stature
  ◊ Microcephaly
  ◊ Radius and thumb anomalies
  ◊ Renal anomalies
  ◊ Hypospadias
  ◊ Hyperpigmentation

CAUSES
• Idiopathic (about 50% of the cases)
• Injury to pluripotential stem cells
• Destruction of pluripotential stem cells
• Immunologic injury
• Toxic exposure, e.g., benzene, inorganic arsenic
• Infectious hepatitis
• Radiation exposure
• Drugs - especially antibiotics, anticonvulsants, gold
• Pregnancy (rare)
• Inherited (constitutional anemia)

RISK FACTORS
• Viral illness
• Toxin exposure
• Tumors of thymus (red cell aplasia)

DIAGNOSIS

DIFFERENTIAL DIAGNOSIS
• Other causes of pancytopenia
• Myelodysplastic disorders
• Paroxysmal nocturnal hemoglobinuria
• Acute leukemia
• Hairy cell leukemia
• Systemic lupus erythematosus
• Disseminated infection
• Hypersplenism
• Transient erythroblastopenia of childhood

LABORATORY
• Pancytopenia
• Anemia
• Leukopenia
• Neutropenia
• Thrombocytopenia
• Increased bleeding time
• Decreased reticulocytes
• Increased serum iron secondary to transfusion
• Normal total iron binding capacity (TIBC)
• Borderline high mean corpuscular volume (MCV) > 104
• Hematuria
• Abnormal liver function tests (hepatitis)
• Increased fetal hemoglobin (Fanconi's)
• Increased chromosomal breaks under specialized conditions (constitutional anemia)
• Molecular determination of abnormal gene (Fanconi's)
Drugs that may alter lab results: N/A
Disorders that may alter lab results: N/A

PATHOLOGICAL FINDINGS
• Normochromic RBC
• Bone marrow:
  ◊ Increased iron stores
  ◊ Decreased cellularity (< 10%)
  ◊ Decreased megakaryocytes
  ◊ Decreased myelocytes
  ◊ Decreased erythroid precursors

SPECIAL TESTS
Chromosome breakage (constitutional anemia); fetal hemoglobin

IMAGING
• CT of thymus region if thymoma-associated RBC aplasia suspected
• Radiographs of radius and thumbs (constitutional anemia)
• Renal ultrasound (constitutional anemia)

DIAGNOSTIC PROCEDURES
Bone marrow biopsy

TREATMENT

APPROPRIATE HEALTH CARE
Inpatient. Referral to an institution that has experience in treating these patients is recommended.

GENERAL MEASURES
• Vigorous supportive measures
• Oxygen therapy
• Good oral hygiene
• Avoid causative agents
• Human leukocyte antigen (HLA) testing on all patients and their immediate families
• Transfusion support (judiciously prescribed)
• Immunosuppressive therapy (cyclosporine, corticosteroids, antithymocyte globulin [ATG]) if no suitable donor
• Androgen therapy if less severe

SURGICAL MEASURES
• Bone marrow transplantation for patients with severe aplastic anemia and an HLA-identical donor. Upper age restrictions on transplantations varies among institutions that perform them.
• Unrelated donor transplants, if other therapy fails
• Thymectomy for thymoma

ACTIVITY
Isolation procedures if neutropenic

DIET
No special diet, but nutritious diet important to improve resistance to infection

PATIENT EDUCATION
Printed patient information available from: Aplastic Anemia Foundation of America, P.O. Box 22689, Baltimore, MD 21203, (410)955-2803

MEDICATIONS

DRUG(S) OF CHOICE
• Antithymocyte globulin (ATG)
  ◊ It is a horse serum containing polyclonal antibodies against human T cells. Skin test patients to determine any hypersensitivity.
  ◊ Treatment for older patients and patients without a compatible donor
  ◊ Dosage is 10-20 mg/kg diluted in 500 mL saline, infused over 4-6 h for 8-14 consecutive days
  ◊ May be used as a single agent or in combination with corticosteroids
• Cyclosporine
  ◊ Dosage is 10 mg/kg initially, then taper to 5-10 mg/kg/day
  ◊ Monitor trough blood levels. Normal values for assays vary.
  ◊ 2-3 months trial may be necessary
• Androgens
  ◊ Clinical trials inconclusive
  ◊ Useful for some patients lacking other options and less severe patients
  ◊ Oxymetholone - 1-2 mg/kg/day orally
  ◊ 2-3 month trial usually necessary to assess response
• Prednisone for pure red cell anemia
Note: Relapses may occur after initial response to immunosuppressive therapy
Contraindications: Refer to manufacturer's literature
Precautions: Refer to manufacturer's literature
Significant possible interactions: Refer to manufacturer's literature

ALTERNATIVE DRUGS   Prednisone and cyclophosphamide

FOLLOWUP

PATIENT MONITORING   Close monitoring for all treatments. Drugs and other forms of treatment have numerous and severe side effects.

PREVENTION/AVOIDANCE
• Avoid possible toxic agents
• Use safety measures when working with radiation

POSSIBLE COMPLICATIONS
• Hemorrhage
• Infection
• Transfusion hemosiderosis
• Transfusion hepatitis
• Heart failure
• Complications of therapy
• Development of acute leukemia
• Neoplasm may complicate constitutional anemia

EXPECTED COURSE/PROGNOSIS
Depending on age and treatment available - guardedly favorable

MISCELLANEOUS

ASSOCIATED CONDITIONS   N/A

AGE-RELATED FACTORS
Pediatric:
• Pure red cell anemia (Diamond-Blackfan) and constitutional anemia are seen more often in children
• Idiopathic aplastic anemia is more common in adolescents
• Secondary aplastic anemia seen in children exposed to ionizing radiation or treated with cytotoxic chemotherapeutic agents
Geriatric: The elderly are more exposed to large numbers of drugs and therefore more susceptible to secondary aplastic anemia
Others: N/A

PREGNANCY   Pregnancy may be a cause of aplastic anemia (rare)

SYNONYMS
• Hypoplastic anemia
• Panmyelophthisis
• Refractory anemia
• Aleukia hemorrhagica
• Toxic paralytic anemia

ICD-9-CM
284 Aplastic anemia

SEE ALSO
• Myelodysplastic syndromes (MDS)
• Systemic lupus erythematosus (SLE)
• Leukemia, hairy cell
• Paroxysmal nocturnal hemoglobinuria

OTHER NOTES   N/A

ABBREVIATIONS   N/A

REFERENCES
• Williams WJ, et al: Hematology. 4th Ed. New York, McGraw-Hill, 1990
• Lee GR, et al: Wintrobe's Clinical Hematology. 9th Ed. Philadelphia, Lea & Febiger, 1993
Illustrations: N/A
Internet references: http://www.5mcc.com

Author(s)
John J. Hutter, Jr., MD

Anemia, autoimmune hemolytic

 BASICS

DESCRIPTION Acquired anemia induced by binding of autoantibodies and/or complement to the red cells
• Three main types
  ◊ Warm (37°C) antibody (80-90%)
  ◊ Cold reacting antibody (10%)
  ◊ Drug induced
System(s) affected:
Hemic/Lymphatic/Immunologic
Genetics: Unknown
Incidence/Prevalence in USA: 1/25,000 per year
Predominant age: < 50 years
Predominant sex: Female > Male

SIGNS AND SYMPTOMS
• Weakness
• Fatigue
• Exertional dyspnea
• Dizziness
• Palpitations
• Malaise
• Dyspnea
• Pallor
• Jaundice
• Splenomegaly
• Hepatomegaly
• Tachycardia
• Anemia (may be sudden and life threatening)

CAUSES
• Warm antibody
  ◊ Idiopathic (50%)
  ◊ Neoplasia (Leukemia, myeloma, lymphoma, thymoma)
  ◊ Collagen vascular disease
  ◊ Viral infection: e.g., hepatitis
• Cold antibody
  ◊ Idiopathic (50%)
  ◊ Infection (Mycoplasma, mononucleosis, viral)
  ◊ Neoplasia (lymphoma)
  ◊ Cold agglutinin disease
• Drug induced
  ◊ Methyldopa, quinidine, penicillin

RISK FACTORS Listed with Causes

 DIAGNOSIS

DIFFERENTIAL DIAGNOSIS Other hemolytic anemias

LABORATORY
• Direct Coombs' (antiglobulin test) - positive
• Anemia
• Increased mean corpuscular volume (MCV)
• Increased mean cell hemoglobin concentration (MCHC)
• Spherocytosis
• Poikilocytosis
• Anisocytosis
• Rouleaux
• Reticulocytosis
• Nucleated RBC
• Large polychromatophilic reticulocytes
• Hyperbilirubinemia
• Decreased haptoglobin
• Hemoglobinemia
Drugs that may alter lab results: N/A
Disorders that may alter lab results: N/A

PATHOLOGICAL FINDINGS
• Bone marrow hyperplasia
• Increased marrow hemosiderin

SPECIAL TESTS
• IgG antibody (warm)
• IgM antibody (cold)

IMAGING N/A

DIAGNOSTIC PROCEDURES N/A

 TREATMENT

APPROPRIATE HEALTH CARE
Inpatient

GENERAL MEASURES
• Warm antibody
  ◊ Mild - conservative therapy
  ◊ Moderate - prednisone
  ◊ Severe - high dose prednisone, immunosuppressant, packed red cell transfusion (which is difficult to crossmatch - need special blood bank techniques; in emergency, use most compatible crossmatch)
• Cold antibody
  ◊ Supportive
  ◊ Avoid cold
  ◊ Red cell transfusion (which is difficult to crossmatch - need special blood bank techniques; in emergency, use most compatible crossmatch)
  ◊ Consider high dose prednisone
• Drug induced
  ◊ Stop the offending drug
• Plasmapheresis/exchange transfusion for severe life-threatening cases

SURGICAL MEASURES Severe warm antibody - splenectomy

ACTIVITY Rest until asymptomatic

DIET No special diet

PATIENT EDUCATION Griffith, H.W.: Instructions for Patients; Philadelphia, 1994 W.B. Saunders Co

MEDICATIONS

DRUG(S) OF CHOICE Glucocorticoids - prednisone 1-2 mg/kg each day in divided doses. May need to be adjusted downward if needed for long-term treatment.
Contraindications: Refer to manufacturer's literature
Precautions: Refer to manufacturer's literature
Significant possible interactions: Refer to manufacturer's literature

ALTERNATIVE DRUGS
• Immunosuppressive drugs (if prednisone and splenectomy do not cure)
  ◊ Azathioprine (Imuran) 125 mg/day for up to 6 months
• Immune globulin, intravenous (IVIG)

FOLLOWUP

PATIENT MONITORING Monitor carefully if transfusion essential

PREVENTION/AVOIDANCE No preventive measures known

POSSIBLE COMPLICATIONS
• Shock (severe anemia)
• Thromboembolism
• Thrombocytopenic purpura (Evans's syndrome)

EXPECTED COURSE/PROGNOSIS
• Good with appropriate treatment
• If secondary to an underlying disorder, the prognosis is determined by the course of the primary disease

MISCELLANEOUS

ASSOCIATED CONDITIONS
• Systemic lupus erythematosus
• Chronic lymphocytic anemia
• Diffuse lymphomas

AGE-RELATED FACTORS
Pediatric: May occur in pediatric age group
Geriatric: Unusual in this age group; rule out neoplasia
Others: N/A

PREGNANCY N/A

SYNONYMS N/A

ICD-9-CM
283.0 Autoimmune hemolytic anemias

SEE ALSO N/A

OTHER NOTES N/A

ABBREVIATIONS N/A

REFERENCES
• Bennett JC, Plum FZ, eds: Cecil Textbook of Medicine. 20th Ed. Philadelphia, W.B. Saunders Co., 1996
• Rosenwasser LJ, Joseph BZ: Immunohematologic Disorders. JAMA 1992;268:2940-5
• Wheby MS, ed: Anemia. Medical Clinics of North America. Philadelphia, W.B. Saunders Co., 1992
Illustrations: N/A
Internet references: http://www.5mcc.com

Author(s)
Brian J. Murray, MD

Anemia, pernicious

BASICS

DESCRIPTION A disorder due to vitamin B12 deficiency. Pernicious anemia is invariably associated with atrophic gastritis and histamine-fast achlorhydria. Vitamin B12 cannot be absorbed in the terminal ileum without intrinsic factor (a secretion of the parietal cells of the gastric mucosa). Usual course - slowly progressive.
Genetics: HLA-DR2; HLA-DR4. Present in the rare form of pernicious anemia that is hereditary. Endemic areas - northern Europe, including Scandinavia.
System(s) affected:
Hemic/Lymphatic/Immunologic, Gastrointestinal, Nervous
Incidence/Prevalence: Unknown
Predominant age: Older adults (> 60 years)
Predominant sex: Male = Female

SIGNS AND SYMPTOMS
- Abnormal reflexes
- Anorexia; weight loss
- Ataxia
- Atrophic glossitis
- Babinski's sign - positive
- Confusion
- Congestive heart failure
- Dementia
- Depression
- Exertional dyspnea
- Extremity numbness
- Extremity paresthesias
- Hepatomegaly
- Pallor
- Palpitations
- Poor finger coordination
- Position sense - decreased
- Prematurely gray-haired
- Purpura
- Romberg's sign, positive
- Skin pigmentation increased
- Sore tongue
- Splenomegaly
- Tachycardia
- Tinnitus
- Vertigo
- Vibration sense - decreased
- Vitiligo
- Weakness

CAUSES
- Atrophic gastric mucosa
- Intrinsic factor deficiency
- Probable autoimmunity against gastric parietal cells
- Autoimmunity against intrinsic factor

RISK FACTORS
- Vegetarian diet, without B12 supplementation
- Gastrectomy
- Blind loop syndrome
- Fish-tapeworm infestation
- Malabsorption syndromes
- Drugs: oral calcium-chelating drugs, aminosalicylic acid, biguanides
- Chronic pancreatitis
- Alcoholism

DIAGNOSIS

DIFFERENTIAL DIAGNOSIS
- Folic acid deficiency
- Myelodysplasia
- Neurological disorders without B12 deficiency
- Liver dysfunction
- Hypothyroidism
- Hemolysis or bleeding
- Drug effects
- Alcoholism

LABORATORY
- Achlorhydria
- Anisocytosis
- Anti-intrinsic poikilocytosis factor antibody
- Anti-parietal cell antibody
- Direct hyperbilirubinemia
- Haptoglobin decreased
- Howell-Jolly bodies
- Hypergastrinemia
- Hypersegmented neutrophils
- LDH increased
- Leukopenia
- Macrocytic anemia
- Mean corpuscular volume - 110-140
- Pentagastrin stimulation - stomach pH > 6
- Peripheral blood smear - macro-ovalocytes
- Poikilocytes
- Serum ferritin increased
- Serum vitamin B12 level < 100 pg/mL (< 74 pmol/L)
- Thrombocytopenia

Drugs that may alter lab results: N/A
Disorders that may alter lab results:
- Falsely elevated MCV
  ◊ Cold agglutinins
  ◊ Hyperglycemia
  ◊ Marked hyperleukocytosis
- Falsely normal serum vitamin B12 level
  ◊ Myeloproliferative disorders
  ◊ Liver disease
- Falsely low serum B12 level
  ◊ Multiple myeloma
  ◊ Oral contraceptive intake
  ◊ Pregnancy
  ◊ Folate deficiency
  ◊ Transcobalamin I deficiency
  ◊ Recent isotope administration

PATHOLOGICAL FINDINGS
- Bone marrow - hypercellular, macrocytes, iron stores increased
- Nests of megaloblasts
- Giant metamyelocytes
- Macropolymorpholeukocytes
- Hypersegmented neutrophils
- Stomach - atrophic gastritis, goblet cells increased
- Parietal cell atrophy
- Chief cell atrophy
- Gastric cytology - cellular atypia
- Spinal cord - myelin degeneration of the dorsal and lateral tracts
- Peripheral nerve degeneration
- Degenerative changes of the posterior root ganglia

SPECIAL TESTS
- Schilling test plus intrinsic factor - normal vitamin B12 absorption
- Schilling test - decreased vitamin B12 absorption
- Gastric analysis - achlorhydria

IMAGING N/A:

DIAGNOSTIC PROCEDURES
- Bone marrow aspiration
- Detailed history and physical exam

TREATMENT

APPROPRIATE HEALTH CARE
Outpatient

GENERAL MEASURES
- Treatment must be continued for life
- Identification and treatment of the underlying disorder

SURGICAL MEASURES N/A

ACTIVITY Unlimited

DIET Emphasize meat, animal protein foods, legumes unless contraindicated

PATIENT EDUCATION Griffith, H.W.: Instructions for Patients, W.B. Saunders Co, Philadelphia (instructions to photocopy for patient)

MEDICATIONS

DRUG(S) OF CHOICE
• Parenteral Vitamin B12 (cyanocobalamin)
◊ 100 mcg subcutaneously for each dose
◊ Administer daily for the first week
◊ Administer weekly for one month
◊ Monthly injections for remainder of life
(patients may be taught to give self-injection)
Contraindications: None
Precautions: Do not give folic acid
supplements without vitamin B12 - may cause
fulminant neurological deficit
Significant possible interactions: N/A

ALTERNATIVE DRUGS   None

FOLLOWUP

PATIENT MONITORING
• Monthly injections of vitamin B12
• Endoscopy every 5 years to rule out gastric
carcinoma

PREVENTION/AVOIDANCE   Early
detection of anemia; workup of anemia

EXPECTED COURSE/PROGNOSIS
Anemia reversible with parenteral vitamin B12;
neurologic effects not reversible with parenteral
vitamin B12

POSSIBLE COMPLICATIONS
• Hypokalemia may complicate first week of
treatment
• Central nervous system symptoms may be
permanent if patient is not treated in less than
six months after symptoms begin
• Gastric polyps
• Stomach cancer

MISCELLANEOUS

ASSOCIATED CONDITIONS
• Autoimmune diseases including rheumatoid
arthritis, IgA deficiency
• Graves' disease
• Myxedema
• Iron deficiency
• Thyroiditis
• Vitiligo
• Idiopathic adrenocortical insufficiency
• Hypoparathyroidism
• Agammaglobulinemia
• Tropical sprue
• Celiac disease
• Crohn's disease
• Infiltrate disorders of the ileum and small
intestine

AGE-RELATED FACTORS
Pediatric:
• Juvenile pernicious anemia occurs in older
children and is the same in most respects as in
adults
• Congenital pernicious anemia - usually
evident before 3 years of age
Geriatric: More common in this age group and
often in association with other autoimmune
disorders, depression, and dementia
Others: N/A

PREGNANCY   N/A

SYNONYMS
• Addison's anemia
• Megaloblastic anemia due to B12 deficiency

ICD-9-CM
• 281.0 pernicious anemia
• 281.1 other vitamin B12 anemia

SEE ALSO   Tropical sprue

OTHER NOTES
• There is a 3-fold likelihood of developing
gastric carcinoma. Suggest endoscopy
approximately every 5 years even if
asymptomatic.
• Folic acid treatment in patients with
pernicious anemia is contraindicated

ABBREVIATIONS   N/A

REFERENCES
• Bennett JC, Plum F, eds: Cecil Textbook of
Medicine. 20th Ed. Philadelphia, W.B.
Saunders Co., 1996
• Williams WJ, Beutler E, Erslev AJ, et al, eds:
Hematology. 4th Ed. New York, McGraw-Hill,
1990
• Munseys W, ed: The Medical Clinic of North
America 1992;76(3)
Illustrations: 1 available on CD-ROM
Internet references: http://www.5mcc.com

Author(s)
Abdulrazak Abyad, MD, MPH, AGSF

Anemia, sickle cell

BASICS

DESCRIPTION
A chronic hemoglobinopathy transmitted genetically, marked by moderately severe chronic hemolytic anemia, periodic acute episodes of painful "crises," and increased susceptibility to intercurrent infections, especially S. pneumoniae. The heterozygous condition (Hb A/S) is called sickle cell trait and is usually asymptomatic, with no anemia.

System(s) affected:
Hemic/Lymphatic/Immunologic, Musculoskeletal

Genetics: Autosomal recessive, mostly in blacks. Homozygous presence of a variant hemoglobin, HbS or sickle hemoglobin. Heterozygous condition Hb A/S.

Incidence/Prevalence in USA:
Approximately 1 in 500 black Americans have sickle cell anemia; 8-10% black Americans have sickle trait

Predominant age: All ages
Predominant sex: Male = Female

SIGNS AND SYMPTOMS
- Often asymptomatic in early months of life
- After 6 months of age, earliest symptoms are pallor and symmetric, painful swelling of the hands and feet (hand-foot syndrome)
- Chronic hemolytic anemia
- Painful "crises" in bones, joints, abdomen, back, and viscera
- Mild scleral icterus
- Increased susceptibility to infections, especially pneumococcal sepsis and Salmonella osteomyelitis
- Functional asplenia
- Delayed physical/sexual maturation, especially boys
- Many multi-system complications, especially in later childhood and adolescence
- Acute chest syndrome (clinical picture consistent with pneumonia and/or infection)

CAUSES
- At molecular level: Hb S is produced by substitution of valine for glutamic acid in the sixth amino acid position of the beta chains of the hemoglobin molecule. When deoxygenated, Hb S polymerizes and forms long rods that change RBC from biconcave to sickle shape.
- At cellular level: Sickle RBCs are inflexible; odd shape and cell rigidity cause increased blood viscosity, stasis, and mechanical obstruction of small arterioles and capillaries, leading to distal ischemia. Sickle RBCs are also more fragile than normal, leading to hemolytic destruction in blood and reticuloendothelial system.
- At clinical level: Chronic anemia; a variety of "crises"; infections
  ◊ Vaso-occlusive crisis ("painful crisis"): Most common; pain results from tissue necrosis secondary to vascular occlusion and tissue hypoxia. Progressive organ failure and acute tissue damage results from repeated vaso-occlusive episodes.
  ◊ Aplastic crisis: Temporary suppression of RBC production in bone marrow by severe infection
  ◊ Hyperhemolytic crisis: Accelerated hemolysis; increased RBC fragility/shortened life span
  ◊ Sequestration crisis: Splenic sequestration of blood (only in infants/young children)
  ◊ Susceptibility to infection: Impaired/absent splenic function; defect in the alternate pathway of complement activation

RISK FACTORS
- Vaso-occlusive crisis
  ◊ Hypoxia
  ◊ Dehydration
  ◊ Infection
  ◊ Fever
  ◊ Acidosis
  ◊ Cold
  ◊ Anesthesia
  ◊ Strenuous physical exercise
- Aplastic crisis
  ◊ Severe infections
  ◊ Folic acid deficiency
- Hyperhemolytic crisis
  ◊ Acute bacterial infections
  ◊ Exposure to oxidant drugs

DIAGNOSIS

DIFFERENTIAL DIAGNOSIS
- Anemia: Other hemoglobinopathies, e.g., Hb SC disease, Hb C disease, Sickle cell-beta thalassemia
- Painful crisis: Other causes of acute pain in bones, joints, and abdomen. Seek infection and other precipitating causes.

LABORATORY
- Hb electrophoresis: Hb S predominates, variable amount Hb F, no Hb A. (In sickle cell trait, both Hb S and A are present).
- Screening tests: Sodium metabisulfite reduction-test; "Sickledex" test
- Anemia; hemoglobin approximately 8 g/dL (1.24 mmol/L); RBC indices usually normal but mean corpuscular volume (MCV) > 75 μm3 (> 75 fL)
- Reticulocytosis of 10-20%
- Leukocytosis; bands normal in absence of infection
- Thrombocytosis
- Peripheral smear: few sickled RBC's, polychromasia, nucleated RBC's
- Serum bilirubin mildly elevated (2-4 mg/dL [34-68 μmol/L]); fecal/urinary urobilinogen high
- ESR low
- Serum LDH elevated
- Haptoglobin absent

Drugs that may alter lab results: N/A
Disorders that may alter lab results:
- Infection
- Other anemias (e.g., iron deficiency)

PATHOLOGICAL FINDINGS
- Variable, dependent on tissue
- Hypoxia/infarction in multiple organs

SPECIAL TESTS   N/A

IMAGING.
- Bone scan (to rule out osteomyelitis)
- CT/MRI (to rule out CVA)
- Chest x-ray: often with enlarged heart

DIAGNOSTIC PROCEDURES   N/A

TREATMENT

APPROPRIATE HEALTH CARE
- General health care maintenance on outpatient basis should include assessment of growth/development, regular immunizations and Pneumovax, vision/hearing screening, and regular dental care
- Hospitalization required for most crises and complications

GENERAL MEASURES
- Infections/fever - prompt treatment with antibiotics
- Minimize factors that enhance sickling
- Painful crises - hydration (2 X maintenance fluids); analgesics (narcotic and non-narcotic)
- Transfusion needed with aplastic crises, severe complications (i.e., CVA), before surgery, and with recurrent debilitating painful crises

SURGICAL MEASURES   N/A

ACTIVITY
- Bedrest with crises. Otherwise, activity level as tolerated.
- Activity may be somewhat limited because of chronic anemia and poor muscular development

DIET
Well balanced diet with folic acid supplementation

PATIENT EDUCATION
- Guidelines for prompt management of fever, infections, pain, and specific complications should be reviewed at each visit
- Stress importance of keeping well-hydrated
- Teach early recognition of possible complications, especially education about priapism
- Genetic counseling

MEDICATIONS

DRUG(S) OF CHOICE
• Painful crises (mild, outpatient): non-narcotic analgesics (ibuprofen, acetaminophen)
• Painful crises (severe, hospitalized): parenteral narcotics, e.g., morphine, meperidine (Demerol) on fixed schedule; (PCA pump may be useful way of delivering narcotics) gradually lower dose and replace with oral medication as soon as possible (acetaminophen-codeine, ibuprofen). Correct dehydration and acidosis.
• Infections: prior to culture results, give antibiotic that covers S. pneumoniae and H. influenzae.
• Prophylactic penicillin controversial but often recommended
Contraindications: None
Precautions: Avoid high-dose estrogen oral contraceptives; consider Depo-Provera as alternate contraceptive
Significant possible interactions: None

ALTERNATIVE DRUGS
• Other NSAIDs
• Folic acid supplements

FOLLOWUP

PATIENT MONITORING
• Frequency determined by number/severity of crises and complications
• Early recognition/early treatment of infections. Parents/patient should be instructed that temperature of 101° F (38.3°C) or above requires immediate medical attention.
• All febrile patients require cultures (blood/urine), chest x-ray, CBC/reticulocytes
• For patients who receive chronic transfusions - monitor for hepatitis and hemosiderosis

PREVENTION/AVOIDANCE
Avoid conditions that precipitate sickling (hypoxia, dehydration, cold, infection, fever, acidosis, anesthesia).

POSSIBLE COMPLICATIONS
• Bone infarct
• Aseptic necrosis of femoral head
• Cerebrovascular accidents with neurologic sequelae
• Cardiac enlargement
• Cholelithiasis/abnormal liver function
• Chronic leg ulcers
• Priapism
• Hematuria/hyposthenuria
• Retinopathy
• Acute chest syndrome (infection/infarction), leading to chronic pulmonary disease
• Infections (pneumonia, osteomyelitis, meningitis, pyelonephritis). Increased risk of sepsis with each.
• Hemosiderosis (2° to multiple transfusions)

EXPECTED COURSE/PROGNOSIS
Anemia is lifelong. In second decade, number of crises diminish but complications more frequent. Some patients die in childhood, of CVA or sepsis. Most patients live to early-mid adulthood; few live > 50 years. Common causes of death are infections, thrombosis, pulmonary emboli, or renal failure.

MISCELLANEOUS

ASSOCIATED CONDITIONS
Psychosocial effects of chronic illness, especially low self-esteem, depression, and dependency. May need counseling, tutoring, and/or vocational training.

AGE-RELATED FACTORS
Pediatric:
• Sequestration crises and hand-foot syndrome seen only in infants/young children
• Functional asplenia in later childhood
• Adolescence/young adulthood:
◊ Frequency of complications and secondary organ/tissue damage increase with age
◊ Psychological complications, including body-image and sexual identity problems, interrupted schooling/career training, restriction of activities, stigma of chronic disease, low self-esteem, fear of future
Geriatric: N/A
Others: N/A

PREGNANCY
• Usually complicated and hazardous, especially 3rd trimester and delivery
• Complications include increased number/severity of crises, toxemia, infection, pulmonary infarction, phlebitis
• Fetal mortality 35-40%; abortions/stillbirths, prematurity
• Prophylactic partial exchange transfusion in 3rd trimester reduces maternal morbidity and fetal mortality

SYNONYMS
• Sickle cell disease
• Hb S disease
• S/S disease

ICD-9-CM
• 282.60 Sickle cell anemia, unspecified

SEE ALSO N/A

OTHER NOTES N/A

ABBREVIATIONS N/A

REFERENCES
• Serjeant GR: Sickle cell disease. 2 Ed. New York, Oxford University Press, 1992
• Radel E: Advances in the treatment of adolescents with sickle hemoglobinopathies. Adolescent Medicine State of the Art reviews: Chronic and Disability Disorders 1994;5(2):271-292
• Beutler E: The sickle cell diseases and related disorders. In: Williams Hematology. New York, McGraw-Hill, 1995:616-627
• Embury SH: Sickle Cell Disease-Basic Principles and Clinical Practice. New York, Raven Press, 1994
• Blum RW, ed: Chronic Illness and Disabilities in Childhood and Adolescence. Orlando, Grune and Statton, 1984:265-276
Illustrations: 1 available on CD-ROM
Internet references: http://www.5mcc.com

Author(s)
Mark R. Dambro, MD, FAAFP

Aneurysm of the aorta

BASICS

DESCRIPTION   A permanent, focal dilatation of the aorta. The clinical presentation relates to location, size, type, and comorbid factors. Some present with rupture, others with embolism or thrombosis. The management and indications for surgical repair is dictated by the natural history of the aneurysm, the type, the consequences of repair, and the general status of the patient. Types include:
◊ Infrarenal (90%)
◊ Thoracoabdominal which may extend from the chest to the abdomen, but always involve the suprarenal aorta.
◊ Dissection which may become aneurysmal (aneurysms do not dissect)
System(s) affected: Cardiovascular
Genetics: Familial propensity
Incidence/Prevalence in USA:
• 6% of males over age 65
• 4% of females over age 65
• 15,000 deaths per year related to aneurysms
Predominant age: Elderly
Predominant sex: Male > female (4:1)

SIGNS AND SYMPTOMS
• Asymptomatic; the majority
• Vague abdominal pain; may radiate to back or flank
• Pulsatile epigastric mass
• The triad of shock, pulsatile mass, and abdominal pain (perhaps with radiation to back, flank, or groin) suggests rupture of aneurysm
• Lower extremity ischemia
• Encroachment by aneurysm
◊ Vertebral body erosion
◊ Gastric outlet obstruction
◊ Ureteral obstruction
◊ Aortoenteric fistula, aortocaval fistula

CAUSES
• Atherosclerosis
• Dysfunctional connective tissue with diminished tensile strength (e.g., Marfan's)

RISK FACTORS
• Uncontrolled hypertension

DIAGNOSIS

DIFFERENTIAL DIAGNOSIS
• Abdominal masses transmitting aortic pulse
• Other causes of abdominal pain (e.g., peptic ulcer disease)
• Other causes of back pain (e.g., arthritis, metastatic disease)

LABORATORY
• Elevated ESR in inflammatory aneurysms
Drugs that may alter lab results: N/A
Disorders that may alter lab results: N/A

PATHOLOGICAL FINDINGS   N/A

SPECIAL TESTS   N/A

IMAGING
• Ultrasonography. Preferred study for initial diagnosis; but is not reliable for diagnosis of rupture
• CT scanning. Preferred preoperative study. Avoid contrast if patient has significant renal insufficiency. Diagnostic for inflammatory aneurysms
• MRI. Similar to CT and avoids contrast. MR angiography may replace arteriograms
• Aortography. Does not define outside dimensions of aneurysm
◊ Indications: associated renovascular hypertension; visceral angina; significant iliofemoral occlusive disease; suprarenal involvement; peripheral aneurysms; horseshoe or pelvic kidney; prior colectomy

DIAGNOSTIC PROCEDURES
• Coronary angiography may be warranted in some patients (33% have CAD), however, both angiography and bypass pose significant risks

TREATMENT

APPROPRIATE HEALTH CARE   Inpatient

GENERAL MEASURES
• Control hypertension carefully

SURGICAL MEASURES
• Repair when:
◊ Rupture occurs
◊ Size over 4.5cm (or > 6cm in poor surgical risk patients)
◊ Expansion > 0.5 cm/6 months
◊ Symptoms occur
• Poor surgical risk patients:
◊ Class III - IV angina; LVEF < 30 %; recent CHF or MI; severe valvular disease; unreconstructable CAD
◊ Serum creatinine > 3 mg/dL
◊ Home oxygen; PaO2 < 50 mmHg; FEV1<1L
◊ Cirrhosis with ascites
◊ Diffuse retroperitoneal fibrosis; hostile abdomen (e.g., irradiation, fistula, inflammatory bowel disease)
◊ Physiologic age > chronological age

ACTIVITY   Ad lib

DIET   Low fat

PATIENT EDUCATION   N/A

MEDICATIONS

DRUG(S) OF CHOICE
• Antihypertensives chronically
• For aneursym rupture, acute control of heart rate and blood pressure
  ◊ Propranolol in 0.5-1 mg IV doses every 5 minutes until the heart rate is 60-70 beats per minute plus
  ◊ Nitroprusside (Nipride) titrated to reduce systolic blood pressure to 100-110 mm Hg (13.3-14.6 kPa)

Contraindications:
• Propranolol - in bronchial asthma, diabetes mellitus, Raynaud's disease, sinus bradycardia, A-V heart block greater than first degree, in presence of MAO inhibitors, cardiogenic shock, CHF or right ventricular failure from pulmonary hypertension
• Nitroprusside - in treatment of compensatory hypertension, i.e., arteriovenous shunt, in patients with inadequate cerebral circulation, and for use during emergency surgery in moribund patients

Precautions:
• Use propranolol cautiously in patients with angina pectoris, cardiac failure, impaired renal or hepatic function, thyrotoxicosis, pre-excitation syndromes, diabetes, hypoglycemia or nonallergic bronchospasm. Propranolol may produce significant bradycardia, heart block or hypotension. Patients should not be suddenly withdrawn from beta blockers.
• Excessive nitroprusside or use in patients with renal or hepatic insufficiency may cause cyanide toxicity, through excessive production of serum thiocyanate.

Significant possible interactions:
• Propranolol interacts with may drugs
• Nitroprusside may have interactions with clonidine and other antihypertensives to enhance their hypotensive effects

ALTERNATIVE DRUGS N/A

FOLLOWUP

PATIENT MONITORING
• Hypertension control
• Lipid control
Elective repairs
• Peri-operative complications
  ◊ MI - 5%
  ◊ Renal failure - 6% chronic dialysis - 1%
  ◊ Pulmonary failure - 5-8%
  ◊ Ischemic colitis - 0.5-1%
  ◊ Wound infection - 2%
  ◊ Graft infection - < 0.5%
  ◊ Stroke - 0.5-1%
  ◊ Paraplegia - 0.2%
• Post-surgical monitoring
  ◊ Anastomotic aneurysms
  ◊ Graft infections
  ◊ Aortoenteric fistula
  ◊ Graft limb occlusion
  ◊ Additional aneurysms - thoracic, thoracoabdominal, femoral

PREVENTION/AVOIDANCE
• Screening not cost effective
• High risk groups & incidence
  ◊ Coronary disease: 5-9%
  ◊ Peripheral vascular disease: 10-15%
  ◊ First degree relative with AAA: 25%
  ◊ Obese patients > 65 yrs
  ◊ Presence of peripheral aneurysms

POSSIBLE COMPLICATIONS
• Rupture
• Associated dissection
• Thrombosis
• Embolization distally

EXPECTED COURSE/PROGNOSIS
• Usually expand over time (Laplace's Law: T=pr. Wall tension is directly related to blood pressure and the radius of the artery.) When wall tension exceeds wall tensile strength rupture occurs.
• 5 year rupture risk:

```
Diameter     Risk
---------------
  >7cm        75%
  6-7cm       35%
  5-6cm       25%
  0-5cm       low
---------------
```

• Mean expansion is 0.4cm/year
• Rupture risk is increased by
  ◊ Diastolic hypertension
  ◊ Tobacco use
  ◊ Diameter > 6 cm
  ◊ COPD
  ◊ Familial history
• Ruptured aneurysms
  ◊ 80% die before receiving definitive care and 50% of the remaining die during their treatment or hospitalization

MISCELLANEOUS

ASSOCIATED CONDITIONS
• Marfan's syndrome
• Ehlers-Danlos syndrome

AGE-RELATED FACTORS
Pediatric: Etiology more likely infectious or collagen disorders
Geriatric: More common in this age group and may present atypically
Others: N/A

PREGNANCY N/A

SYNONYMS
• Aortic aneurysms

ICD-9-CM
• 441.0 - 441.9 Aortic aneurysm and dissection

SEE ALSO
• Aortic dissection
• Marfan's syndrome
• Ehlers-Danlos syndrome
• Systemic lupus erythematosus (SLE)
• Takayasu syndrome
• Giant cell arteritis
• Polyarteritis nodosa
• Turner's syndrome

OTHER NOTES N/A

ABBREVIATIONS
CAD = coronary artery disease
CHF = congestive heart failure
COPD = chronic obstructive pulmonary disease
LVEF = left ventricular ejection fraction
MI = myocardial infarction

REFERENCES
• Irvin TT: Abdominal pain: A surgical audit of 1190 emergency admissions. Brit J Surg 1989;76:1121
• Johnston W, et al: Suggested standards for reporting on arterial aneurysms. J Vasc Surg 1991;13:452
• Mason JJ, et al: The role of coronary angiography and coronary revascularization before non cardiac vascular surgery. JAMA 1995;273:1919
• Porter JM, ed: The Year Book of Vascular Surgery. New York, Mosby - Year Book, Inc. 1997
• Rutherford B, ed: Vascular Surgery. 14th Ed. Philadelphia, WB Saunders Co., 1995
• Szilagyi DE, et al: Contribution of abdominal aortic aneurysmectomy to prolongation of life. Ann Surg 1966;164:678
Illustrations: N/A
Internet references: http://www.5mcc.com

Author(s)
David H. Stubbs, MD, FACS

Angina

BASICS

DESCRIPTION Symptom complex resulting from mismatch of myocardial oxygen demand and supply
• Classic angina - a sense of pressure or heaviness deep to the precordium, usually brought on by exertion or anxiety and relieved by rest.
• Anginal equivalent - exertional dyspnea or exertional fatigue which results from myocardial ischemia and is relieved by rest or nitroglycerin
• Variant angina - also referred to as Prinzmetal's angina describes angina occurring at rest of in atypical patterns such as after exercise or nocturnally. Prinzmetal's angina is caused by coronary artery spasm and is associated with ECG changes (usually ST elevation) during symptoms
• Unstable angina - pain which is new or which is changed in character to become more frequent, more severe or both. Unstable angina portends myocardial infarction in a certain percentage of patients.
System(s) affected: Cardiovascular
Genetics: Coronary artery disease has genetic implications.
Incidence/Prevalence in USA: The presenting symptom of coronary artery disease in 38% of men and 61% of women.
Predominant age: Most common in middle age and older men; postmenopausal women
Predominant sex: Male > Female

SIGNS AND SYMPTOMS
• Precordial pressure or heaviness, radiating to the back, neck or arms, brought on by exercise, emotional stress, meals, cold air or smoking, and relieved by rest or nitrates
• Discomfort may radiate to neck, lower jaw, teeth, shoulders, inner aspects of the arms or back
• Discomfort may be described with a clinched fist over the sternum (Levine's sign)
• Dyspnea on exertion may present as the only symptom

CAUSES
• Atherosclerosis of the coronary arteries
• Coronary artery spasm
• Thrombosis
• Aortic stenosis
• Hypertrophic cardiomyopathy
• Primary pulmonary hypertension
• Severe hypertension
• Aortic insufficiency

RISK FACTORS
• Family history of premature coronary artery disease (CAD)
• Hypercholesterolemia
• Hypertension
• Tobacco abuse
• Diabetes mellitus
• Male gender
• Advanced age

DIAGNOSIS

DIFFERENTIAL DIAGNOSIS
• Esophagitis
• Esophageal spasm
• Peptic ulcer
• Gastritis
• Cholecystitis
• Costochondritis
• Pericarditis
• Aortic dissection
• Pulmonary embolus
• Pulmonary hypertension
• Pneumothorax
• Radiculopathy
• Shoulder arthropathy
• Psychological - anxiety and panic disorders

LABORATORY
• Total cholesterol - frequently elevated
• HDL cholesterol - frequently reduced
• LDL cholesterol - frequently elevated
Drugs that may alter lab results: N/A
Disorders that may alter lab results: N/A

PATHOLOGICAL FINDINGS
Atherosclerosis of the coronary arteries

SPECIAL TESTS
• ECG - may show evidence of prior myocardial infarction. Other findings are nonspecific and tracings are frequently normal. Bundle branch block, Wolff-Parkinson-White syndrome or intraventricular conduction delay may make the ECG unreliable.
• Exercise stress testing

IMAGING
• Radionuclide scintigraphy
• Stress echocardiography
• Stress thallium
• Coronary angiography

DIAGNOSTIC PROCEDURES Rapid
sequence MRI may show coronary artery artery calcification and thereby identify coronary artery disease. It does not identify obstructive coronary lesions however.

TREATMENT

APPROPRIATE HEALTH CARE The patient's symptoms should be brought under control medically. If symptoms are unstable, hospitalization is warranted.

GENERAL MEASURES
• Treatment goal - involves reducing myocardial oxygen demand or to increase oxygen supply
• Noninvasive testing is often indicated as a means of stratifying the patient's risk for an event that might seriously compromise myocardial function
• Quit smoking
• Minimize emotional stress

SURGICAL MEASURES Coronary artery bypass graft surgery, angioplasty, stent placement, atherectomy in selected cases

ACTIVITY
• As tolerated after consulting physician
• Exercise program after physician's approval

DIET Low fat, low cholesterol diet

PATIENT EDUCATION American Heart Association, 7320 Greenville Avenue, Dallas, TX 75231, (214)373-6300

MEDICATIONS

DRUG(S) OF CHOICE
• Aspirin, 325 mg qd for all patients with coronary disease in whom this medication is not contraindicated (i.e., warfarin usage)
• Beta-blockers: atenolol 25-100 mg qd, metoprolol 25-100 mg bid or propranolol 30-100 mg bid-tid. Beta-blockers are effective in reducing the heart rate and thereby decreasing oxygen consumption and reducing angina. Adjust doses according to the clinical response. Aim to maintain resting heart rate of 50-60 beats per minute. Side effects are frequent and include fatigue, impotence, exacerbation of peripheral vascular and obstructive pulmonary disease, depression.
• Nitroglycerin 0.3-0.6 mg sublingually is the most effective therapy for acute anginal episodes. The dose may be repeated 2-3 times over a 10-15 minute time period; if the patient does not experience relief he/she should be instructed to seek medical attention immediately.
• Nitrates: long acting nitrates (mononitrates or transdermal nitrates) should be used with allowance for drug free interval of 10-14 hours to prevent tolerance. Tachyphylaxis occurs rapidly. Act through preload reduction and coronary vasodilatation. Side effects which include headaches and hypotension, tend to clear with continued usage. A beta-blocker or calcium channel blocker should be used in conjunction with the nitrates during the drug free interval.
• Calcium antagonist: long acting formulations of verapamil 160-480 mg qd or diltiazem 90-360 mg qd or nifedipine 30-120 mg qd or amlodipine 5-20 mg qd are available. The various agents have their own individual side effects (i.e., verapamil - constipation; nifedipine - peripheral edema). Neither verapamil nor diltiazem should be used in patient with compromised ventricular function (left ventricular ejection fraction < 40%). (Short-acting types should be avoided.)
• HMC CoA reductase inhibitors (e.g., pravastatin, lovastatin, and others) should be started for hypercholesterolemia. These drugs recently have been shown to decrease incidence of symptomatic CAD, and to reduce both myocardial infarction and death from MI. The new statin drug atorvastatin is particularly effective in lowering total cholesterol, LDL and triglycerides.
• Heparin: intravenously in therapeutic doses should be initiated in patients hospitalized with unstable angina
• Combination therapy: especially nitrates plus calcium antagonists may be used. Triple therapy with addition of beta-blockers may be necessary. Combination therapies should be used with care to avoid impairment of LV function.
Contraindications: Refer to manufacturer's literature
Precautions: Refer to manufacturer's literature

Significant possible interactions:
• Beta-blockers and calcium channel blockers
  ◊ May combine to produce symptomatic heart block although either class of drug may act alone in producing this side effect
  ◊ Care must also be taken when combining these classes of drugs (beta-blockers and calcium channel blockers) in patients with even moderately compromised ventricular function

ALTERNATIVE DRUGS
Lipid lowering drugs are often initiated in patients with unfavorable lipid profiles, whether symptomatic from CAD or not

FOLLOWUP

PATIENT MONITORING
• Depends on the frequency and severity of the complaints
• Hospitalization for initiation of intravenous heparin is indicated in patients diagnosed with unstable angina

PREVENTION/AVOIDANCE
• Discontinue tobacco, adherence to low fat/low cholesterol diet, regular aerobic exercise program
• Antilipidemics

POSSIBLE COMPLICATIONS
• Related to myocardial damage occurring during infarction
• Arrhythmia
• Cardiac arrest
• Congestive heart failure

EXPECTED COURSE/PROGNOSIS
• Variable and depending on the extent of coronary artery disease as well as left ventricular function
• Annual mortality is 3-4% overall

MISCELLANEOUS

ASSOCIATED CONDITIONS
• Hypercholesterolemia
• Claudication
• Mitral regurgitation
• Papillary muscle dysfunction
• Ventricular aneurysm
• Abdominal aortic aneurysm
• Hypertrophic subaortic stenosis
• Primary hyperthyroidism
• Pernicious anemia and other high output states

AGE-RELATED FACTORS
Pediatric: Suspect familial dyslipidemias in children presenting with manifestations of coronary artery disease
Geriatric: Patients may be very sensitive to the side effects of medications (i.e., beta-blockers - depression)
Others: N/A

PREGNANCY Other diagnosis should be excluded and the patient managed closely by an obstetrician and cardiologist as the metabolic demands of pregnancy will exacerbate symptoms and directly interfere with treatment

SYNONYMS
• Stenocardia
• Heberden's syndrome

ICD-9-CM
411.1 Angina, unstable
413 Angina pectoris
413.1 Prinzmetal's angina
413.9 Angina, unspecified

SEE ALSO N/A

OTHER NOTES N/A

ABBREVIATIONS N/A

REFERENCES
• Brandenburg RO, Fuster V, Giuliani ER, McGoon DC: Cardiology: Fundamentals and Practice, Chicago, Year Book Medical Publishers, 1987
• Braunwald E: Heart Disease: A Textbook of Cardiovascular Medicine. 4th Ed. Philadelphia, W.B. Saunders Co., 1992
Illustrations: N/A
Internet references: http://www.5mcc.com

Author(s)
Phil Lobstein, MD

Angioedema

BASICS

DESCRIPTION Rapid, localized edema of subcutaneous tissues up to several centimeters in diameter. Life threatening if larynx, pharynx is affected. Resolves in hours to days.
• Hereditary angioedema (HAE), type I: Recurrent episodes involving both skin and mucous membranes, without urticaria. 25% mortality. Many have abdominal pain from edema of intestinal mucosa. Due to hereditary deficiency of C1-esterase inhibitor (C1-INH).
• HAE, type II: Like type I, but has normal levels of non-functional C1-INH
• Acquired angioedema: Rare, in some patients with lymphoproliferative malignancies. Treatment of malignancy causes resolution of edema. Autoantibody inactivation or consumption of C1-INH.
• Vibratory angioedema: Rare. Local swelling in response to vibration. May be hereditary.
• Drug-induced angioedema:
  ◊ Immunologic hypersensitivity, as in penicillin reaction, or non-immunologic, as in aspirin or NSAID
  ◊ Angiotensin converting enzyme (ACE) inhibitor-induced angioedema has become the most common form of AE. non-immune; tendency to involve tongue, with life-threatening airway edema. Can't predict. May occur immediately, or many months after starting drug.
• Idiopathic angioedema: Acute or chronic
System(s) affected: Skin/Exocrine
Genetics: Hereditary angioedema is autosomal dominant
Incidence/Prevalence in USA:
Approximately 1 in 5,000. Accompanies urticaria 50% of time.
Predominant age: All ages (idiopathic).
Predominant sex: Male = Female (idiopathic)

SIGNS AND SYMPTOMS
• Occurs alone or with urticaria
• May occur as part of generalized anaphylactic reaction, potentially fatal
• May occur anywhere on body; usually face, extremities, genitalia; often asymmetric (e.g., half of upper lip, one earlobe)
• Rapid onset, usually resolves spontaneously in < 72 hours
• Very little itching in comparison to urticaria. May have stinging or burning sensation.

CAUSES Allergic or non-allergic, mediated by release of histamine from mast cells in subcutaneous tissues

RISK FACTORS Medications that cause allergic reactions, e.g., penicillin, aspirin. 0.2% of patients taking ACE inhibitors develop angioedema; some cases have proven fatal. Omeprazole and sertraline have also recently been implicated.

DIAGNOSIS

DIFFERENTIAL DIAGNOSIS
• Anaphylaxis
• Cellulitis
• Erysipelas
• Contact dermatitis
• Lymphedema
• Diffuse subcutaneous infiltrative process
• Localized edema

LABORATORY
• C4 assay (low in HAE). If C4 normal, do urticaria work-up.
• If C4 is low, do C1-INH assay (immunoreactive) for HAE type I, and C1-INH assay (functional) for HAE type II
• If not HAE, do neoplastic work-up to rule out acquired angioedema, vasculitis work-up (CBC, ANA, RA, ESR, skin biopsy) to rule out autoimmune disease
Drugs that may alter lab results:
Antihistamines, H2-blockers, tricyclic antidepressants
Disorders that may alter lab results: N/A

PATHOLOGICAL FINDINGS Edema, vasculitis and/or perivasculitis involving only subcutaneous tissues.

SPECIAL TESTS N/A

IMAGING N/A

DIAGNOSTIC PROCEDURES Skin biopsy (correlates poorly with clinical picture).

TREATMENT

APPROPRIATE HEALTH CARE Ensure airway patency first! Protect airway if mouth, tongue, throat are involved. CPR and transport to emergency facility if necessary.

GENERAL MEASURES Avoidance of known triggers. Cool, moist compresses to control itching.

SURGICAL MEASURES N/A

ACTIVITY As desired. HAE patients should avoid violent exercise, trauma.

DIET Avoidance of known trigger foods.

PATIENT EDUCATION Educate HAE patient to provide history of disease to health care workers.

Angioedema

MEDICATIONS

DRUG(S) OF CHOICE
• First generation antihistamines for acute angioedema
  ◊ Older children and adults: hydroxyzine (Vistaril) or diphenhydramine (Benadryl), 25-50 mg q6h
  ◊ Children under six: diphenhydramine 12.5 mg (elixir) q6-8h (5 mg/kg/day)
• Second generation H1 blockers are more expensive, about as effective as older antihistamines, but are less sedating (14% of patients, still less than 1st generation drugs), because they do not cross the blood-brain barrier.
  ◊ Terfenadine (Seldane) 60 mg bid or fexofenadine (Allegra) if Seldane not available
  ◊ Astemizole (Hismanal) 10 mg daily. Longest onset of action (3-4 days, so is not helpful for acute reactions), but has the longest duration of action (over 24 hours). This makes it good for chronic problems. Loading dose: 30 mg on day 1, 20 mg on day 2, then 10 mg daily.
  ◊ Loratadine (Claritin) 10 mg daily
  ◊ Acrivastine (Semprex) 8 mg TID
  ◊ Cetirizine (Zyrtec)10 mg daily. More sedating than others in this class.
• HAE therapy:
  ◊ Intubation if airway threatened
  ◊ Epinephrine 1:1000, 0.2-0.3 mL IV or subcutaneous
  ◊ Fresh frozen plasma (only works 1-12 days; no long-term benefit. May transmit hepatitis B).
  ◊ C1-INH, not yet available in USA
  ◊ Attenuated androgen - danazol. For prevention (increases amount of active C1-INH in both types I and II). Give 200-600 mg daily for 1 month, then 5 days on, 5 days off. Ineffective in other forms of C1-INH deficiency. Side effects: headaches, weight gain, hematuria.

Contraindications:
• Danazol not for use in childhood, pregnancy.

Precautions:
• Drowsiness with first generation drugs.
• Use caution when giving astemizole to patients in whom metabolism may be delayed.
• Second generation H1 blockers should be used with caution in pregnancy and the elderly.

Significant possible interactions: Do not give astemizole (Hismanal) or terfenadine (Seldane) to patients taking other inhibitors of the cytochrome P450 enzyme system (erythromycin, ketoconazole, cimetidine, etc) because of a potential for cardiac arrhythmia induction (torsades de pointes).

ALTERNATIVE DRUGS
Aminocaproic acid (epsilon-aminocaproic acid, EACA) was used before danazol available. Prevents activation of plasminogen and C1. Rarely can cause thrombophlebitis, embolism, myositis.

FOLLOWUP

PATIENT MONITORING
• Diagnostic work-up if symptoms severe, persistent or recurrent
• Protect airway if mouth, tongue, throat involved.

PREVENTION/AVOIDANCE
If etiology known, avoidance. Avoid ACE inhibitors in patients with history of angioedema.

POSSIBLE COMPLICATIONS
Anaphylaxis, respiratory compromise

EXPECTED COURSE/PROGNOSIS
Most with idiopathic do well. Chronic forms dependent on nature of defect.

MISCELLANEOUS

ASSOCIATED CONDITIONS Urticaria, anaphylaxis

AGE-RELATED FACTORS
Pediatric: N/A
Geriatric: N/A
Others: N/A

PREGNANCY

SYNONYMS
• Angioneurotic edema
• Quincke's edema

ICD-9-CM 995.1 (hereditary: 277.6)

SEE ALSO Urticaria

OTHER NOTES Same pathophysiology for urticaria and angioedema - localized anaphylaxis causes vasodilatation, vascular permeability of skin (urticaria) or subcutaneous tissue (angioedema)

ABBREVIATIONS
HAE = Hereditary angioedema

REFERENCES
• Cooper KD: Urticaria and angioedema: Diagnosis and evaluation. J Am Acad Dermatol 1991;25:166
• Greaves M, Lawlor F: Angioedema: Manifestations and management. J Am Acad Dermatol 1991;25:155
• Monroe EW: Nonsedating H1 antihistamines in chronic urticaria. Ann Allergy 1993;71:585-91
• Woosley R, Darrow WR: Analysis of potential adverse drug reactions - a case of mistaken identity. Amer J Cardiol 1994;74:208-209
Illustrations: N/A
Internet references: http://www.5mcc.com

Author(s)
John E. Perchalski, MD, FAAFP

Animal bites

BASICS

DESCRIPTION Bite wounds to humans from dogs, cats, other animals including humans
System(s) affected: Endocrine/Metabolic, Skin/Exocrine, Hemic/Lymphatic/Immunologic, Nervous
Genetics: N/A
Incidence/Prevalence in USA:
• Dog bites: 1200/100,000
• Cat bites: 160/100,000
• Snake bites: 15/100,000 non-venomous bites and 3/100,000 venomous bites per year. Lifetime prevalence for animal bite 50,000/100,000.
Predominant age: All ages, but children more likely to be affected
Predominant sex: Male > Female

SIGNS AND SYMPTOMS
• Bite wounds can be tears, punctures, scratches, avulsions or crush injuries
• Dog bites (80-90% of bites)
◊ Hands are most commonly affected with up to 68% of bites
◊ The face is the site of injury in up to 29% of cases, the lower extremities in 10%, and involvement of the trunk is uncommon
• Cat bites (10% of bites)
◊ Predominantly involve the hands, followed by lower extremities, face and trunk
◊ Are more likely to become infected because of puncture type of wounds

CAUSES
• Most bite wounds are from a domestic pet known to the victim. Large dogs are the most common source.
• Human bites are often the result of one person striking another in the mouth with a clenched fist

RISK FACTORS
• Dog bites are more common in the early afternoon, especially during warm weather. Male dogs more likely to bite.
• Clenched fist injuries are frequently associated with the use of alcohol

DIAGNOSIS:

DIFFERENTIAL DIAGNOSIS The diagnosis is straight forward. What is of concern is judging the risk to the patient from the injury and resulting infection.

LABORATORY
• 75% of bite wounds will yield a positive culture. Gram stain is sensitive but not specific for infecting organism. Wound culture is essential in directing therapy of infected wounds. Some pathogens are slow growing so cultures should be kept for 7-10 days.
• Dog bites - Pasteurella multocida is present in 25% of bites. Streptococcus viridans, Staphylococcus aureus, coagulase-negative Staphylococcus, Bacteroides, C. canimorsus, and Fusobacterium can also be found.
• Cat bites - Pasteurella multocida is present in 50% of bites. The wound is often contaminated by other mixed bacteria, including several species of both aerobic and anaerobic organisms.
• Human bites - Streptococcus species, Staphylococcus aureus, Eikenella corrodens and various anaerobic bacteria are common
• Other animal bites - scant information on the pathogens of these
Drugs that may alter lab results: Previous antibiotic therapy
Disorders that may alter lab results: N/A

PATHOLOGICAL FINDINGS N/A

SPECIAL TESTS N/A

IMAGING
• If bite wound is near a bone or joint, a plain radiograph is needed to check for bone injury and to use for comparison later if osteomyelitis is suspected
• In human bite wounds from clenched fist injuries, order plain film radiographs to check for metacarpal or phalanx fracture

DIAGNOSTIC PROCEDURES Surgical exploration might be needed to ascertain extent of injuries. Exploration should be performed on all serious hand wounds, especially clenched-fist injuries involving a joint.

TREATMENT

APPROPRIATE HEALTH CARE
Outpatient setting unless patient has fulminant infection requiring systemic antibiotics, close observation, or surgery

GENERAL MEASURES Elevation of the injured extremity to prevent swelling. Contact the local health department and consult about the prevalence of rabies in the species of animal involved.

SURGICAL MEASURES
• Copious irrigation of the wound with normal saline via a catheter tip is needed to reduce risk of infection
• Devitalized tissue needs débridement
• Débridement of puncture wounds not advised
• Consider surgical closure if the wound is clean after irrigation and bite is less than 12 hours old. Puncture wounds should be left open.
• Delayed primary closure in 3-5 days is an option for infected wounds
• Splint hand if it is injured
• Human bite wounds on the hands should not be primarily closed due to the high risk of infection. Large, gaping wounds should be reapproximated with widely space sutures or steristrips.

ACTIVITY No restriction

DIET No special diet

PATIENT EDUCATION Discussion with parents at "well child checks" should include education on how to avoid animal bites

Animal bites

MEDICATIONS

DRUG(S) OF CHOICE
• Consider anti-rabies therapy
• Use tetanus toxoid in those previously immunized, but more than 5 years since their last dose
• Consider tetanus immune globulin, human (TIG) in patients without a full primary series of immunizations
• Prophylactic therapy if wound seen in first 12 hours:
  ◊ Dog bite - penicillin V 500 mg po qid (child - 50 mg/kg/day po given qid) x 3 days
  ◊ Cat bite - amoxicillin-clavulanate 250-500 mg tid po; child 20-40 mg/kg/day po given tid
  ◊ Human bites - amoxicillin-clavulanate 250-500 mg tid po; child 20-40 mg/kg/day po given tid
  ◊ Snake bite - if venomous, the patient needs rapid transport to facility capable of definitive evaluation. If an envenomation has occurred, the patient will need to receive antivenin unless envenomation was only minimal. Be sure patient is stable for transport; consider measuring and or treating coagulation and renal status along with any anaphylactic reactions before transport.
  ◊ Others - amoxicillin-clavulanate (Augmentin) potassium - dosage - adult 250-500 mg po tid; child 20-40 mg/kg/day given tid
• Established infection
  ◊ Once patient has developed a clinical infection, amoxicillin-clavulanate potassium (Augmentin) can be used pending culture reports
Contraindications: Do not use penicillin-derived antibiotics in those with penicillin allergy
Precautions: Prescribe dosage of antibiotics by body weight and renal function
Significant possible interactions: Antibiotics may decrease efficacy of oral contraceptives

ALTERNATIVE DRUGS
• Alternative therapy for penicillin allergic patients: (for prophylaxis or empiric treatment):
  ◊ Approximately 10% cross reactivity with cephalosporins in penicillin allergic patients
  ◊ Dog bite - doxycycline if patient is older than 9 years, and in women only if they are not pregnant or breast feeding. Ceftriaxone or erythromycin can also be used. Avoid cephalexin due to resistant strains of P. Multocida.
  ◊ Cat bite - as for dog bite
  ◊ Human bite - cefoxitin 80-160 mg/kg/day (up to 12 grams), given in 3 or 4 equally divided doses. Usual dose is 1-2 grams q 6-8 hours; doxycycline can also be used.

FOLLOWUP:

PATIENT MONITORING
• Patient should be rechecked in 24-48 hours if not infected at time of first encounter
• Daily followup is warranted with active infections
• If antibiotics are used for an active infection, the duration of therapy should be 7-14 days depending on the severity of the infection and the clinical response

PREVENTION/AVOIDANCE   Instruct children and adults about animal hazards

POSSIBLE COMPLICATIONS
Complications from bites can include septic arthritis, osteomyelitis, extensive soft tissue injuries with scarring, sepsis, hemorrhage, death. Gas gangrene can take an exceedingly rapid course and should be treated very aggressively.

EXPECTED COURSE/PROGNOSIS
Wounds should steadily improve and close over by 7-10 days

MISCELLANEOUS

ASSOCIATED CONDITIONS   N/A

AGE-RELATED FACTORS
Pediatric: Young children are more likely to have severe bites
Geriatric:
• Serious injury from any bite wound is more common in persons greater than 50 years old, those with wounds in the upper extremities or those with puncture wounds
• Increased risk of infection in those greater than 50 years old
Others: N/A

PREGNANCY   No special precautions

SYNONYMS   N/A

ICD-9-CM
• 879.8 open wound(s) of unspecified site(s) without mention of complications
• 882.0 hand
• 873.40 face

SEE ALSO
• Rabies
• Snake Envenomations: Crotalidae
• Snake Envenomations: Elapidae
• Cellulitis
• Bartonella infections

OTHER NOTES   Rabies: Contact your local health department for information about the risk of rabies

ABBREVIATIONS   N/A

REFERENCES
• Wiggins ME, Akelman E, Weiss AC: The management of dog bite infections to the hand. Orthopedics 1994;17:617-623
• Griego RD, et al: Dog, cat and hume bites: A review. J AM Acad Dermatol 1995;33:1019-1029
• Cummings P: Antibiotics to prevent infection in patients with dog bite wounds: A meta-analysis. Ann Emerg Med 1994;23:535-540
• Lewis KT, Stilles M: Management of Cat and dog bites. Am Fam Phys 1995;52:479-485
Illustrations: N/A
Internet references: http://www.5mcc.com

Author(s)
George R. Bergus, MD

Ankylosing spondylitis

 BASICS

 DIAGNOSIS

 TREATMENT

DESCRIPTION
A chronic, usually progressive, condition in which inflammatory changes and new bone formation occurs at the attachment of tendons and ligaments to bone (enthesopathy)
• Sacroiliac joint involvement is the hallmark of ankylosing spondylitis with variable degrees of spinal involvement. However, 20-30% of patients also have larger peripheral joint involvement

System(s) affected: Musculoskeletal
Genetics: Familial clustering and higher than expected frequency of HLA-B27 tissue antigen
Incidence/Prevalence in USA:
• 0.5-5 per 1000 in white males
• Less common in women and Blacks
Predominant age:
• Usually symptoms begin in early twenties
• Onset of symptoms - rarely occurs after age 40
Predominant sex: Male > Female

SIGNS AND SYMPTOMS
• Subgluteal or low back pain and/or stiffness
• Insidious onset
• Onset usually in 3rd decade
• Duration greater than 3 months
• Morning stiffness
• Frequently awaken at night to "walk off" stiffness
• Improvement in stiffness with activity
• Increased symptoms with rest
• Pleuritic chest pain is often an early feature
• Thoracic and cervical spine complaints in advanced disease
• Hip, shoulder, or knee complaints
• Diminished range of motion in the lumbar spine in all three planes of motion
• Loss of lumbar lordosis
• Thoraco-cervical kyphosis (rarely occurs before ten years of symptoms)
• Aortic root dilatation (20%)
• Aortic regurgitation murmur (2%)
• Acute anterior uveitis (20-30%)
• Osteoporosis

CAUSES
Unknown

RISK FACTORS
• HLA-B27
• Positive family history
• 10% risk of developing AS (Ankylosing Spondylitis) for HLA-B27 positive child of spondylitic parent

DIFFERENTIAL DIAGNOSIS
• Reiter's syndrome
• Psoriatic arthritis
• Diffuse idiopathic skeletal hypertrophy (DISH)
• Spondylitis associated with inflammatory bowel disease
• Rheumatoid arthritis

LABORATORY
• HLA-B27 tissue antigen is present in 90% of patients compared to 5-8% incidence in general population
• Erythrocyte sedimentation rate (ESR) is elevated in 80% of cases, but correlates poorly with disease activity and prognosis
• Absent rheumatoid factor
Drugs that may alter lab results: N/A
Disorders that may alter lab results: N/A

PATHOLOGICAL FINDINGS
• Erosive changes coupled with new bone formation at attachment of tendons and ligaments to bone resulting in ossification of periarticular soft-tissues
• Synovial changes are indistinguishable from rheumatoid arthritis. Erosion of articular cartilage is less severe than in rheumatoid arthritis.

SPECIAL TESTS
• Synovial fluid - mild leukocytosis, decreased viscosity
• Cerebrospinal fluid - increased protein
• EKG - conduction defects
• Measurement of respiratory excursion of chest wall - less than 5 cm maximal respiratory excursion of chest wall measured at fourth intercostal space. Less than 2.5 cm is virtually diagnostic of ankylosing spondylitis.
• Wright-Schober test for lumbar spine flexion is abnormal

IMAGING
• Sacroiliac joint early - sclerosis on both sides of joint not extending more than 1 cm from articular surface
• Sacroiliac joint late - ankylosis of sacroiliac joint
• Spine - "squaring" of vertebral bodies and ossification of annulus fibrosis giving appearance of "bamboo spine". Ankylosis of facet joints.
• Peripheral joint - symmetric erosive changes in larger joints. Pericapsular ossification, sclerosis, loss of joint space.

DIAGNOSTIC PROCEDURES
• Physical examination
• Radiographs - sacroiliac joint films, lumbar spine series

APPROPRIATE HEALTH CARE
Outpatient

GENERAL MEASURES
• Posture training and range of motion exercises for spine are essential
• Firm bed
• Sleep in prone position or supine without a pillow
• Breathing exercises 2-3 times/day
• Swimming
• Physical therapy
• Stop smoking, if a smoker

SURGICAL MEASURES N/A

ACTIVITY
Encourage active lifestyle

DIET
No special diet

PATIENT EDUCATION
• For a listing of sources for patient education materials favorably reviewed on this topic, physicians may contact: American Academy of Family Physicians Foundation, P.O. Box 8418, Kansas City, MO 64114, (800)274-2237, ext. 4400

MEDICATIONS

DRUG(S) OF CHOICE
• Nonsteroidal anti-inflammatory drugs provide symptomatic relief
• Selection is empiric, but traditionally indomethacin, 50 mg tid or qid has been used
• Steroids and cytotoxic agents are not effective
Contraindications: See Precautions
Precautions:
• All patients on long term NSAID's should have renal function monitored
• NSAID's may aggravate peptic ulcer disease or cause gastritis
• Don't use NSAID's for patients with a bleeding diathesis or patients requiring anticoagulants
Significant possible interactions: Refer to manufacturer's profile of each drug

ALTERNATIVE DRUGS
Other NSAID's, such as sulindac, naproxen

FOLLOWUP

PATIENT MONITORING   Visits every six to twelve months to monitor posture and range of motion

PREVENTION/AVOIDANCE   N/A

POSSIBLE COMPLICATIONS
• Spine: Pseudarthrosis, cervical spine fracture (high mortality rate), C1-C2 subluxation, spondylodiscitis, cauda equina syndrome (rare)
• Peripheral joint ankylosis
• Pulmonary: Restrictive lung disease, diaphragmatic breathing, upper lobe fibrosis (rare)
• Cardiac: Conduction defects (20%), aortic insufficiency (2%)
• Uveitis

EXPECTED COURSE/PROGNOSIS
• Unpredictable course
• Prognosis good if mobility and upright posture maintained. Usually progressive disability.

MISCELLANEOUS

ASSOCIATED CONDITIONS
• Inflammatory bowel disease
• Uveitis
• Iritis

AGE-RELATED FACTORS
Pediatric: N/A
Geriatric: N/A
Others: N/A

PREGNANCY   N/A

SYNONYMS
• Rheumatoid spondylitis
• Marie-Strumpell disease

ICD-9-CM
720.0 ankylosing spondylitis

SEE ALSO
• Reiter's syndrome
• Crohn's disease of the colon
• Ulcerative colitis
• Arthritis, psoriatic
• Arthritis, rheumatoid (RA)

OTHER NOTES
Flexion contractures of the hip and ankylosis may be major contributors to poor posture. Hip arthroplasty should be strongly considered as it may restore upright posture. Heterotopic ossification may occur post operatively and appropriate prophylaxis should be considered.

ABBREVIATIONS   N/A

REFERENCES
• Calin A, ed: Spondyloarthropathies. New York, Grune & Stratton, 1983
• Calin A, Fries J: Ankylosing Spondylitis Discussions in Patient Management. Garden City, New York, Medical Examination Publishing Company, 1978
Illustrations: N/A
Internet references: http://www.5mcc.com

Author(s)
George R. Bradbury, MD
James B. Benjamin, MD

Anorectal abscess

 BASICS

DESCRIPTION Localized induration and fluctuance due to inflammation of the soft tissue near the rectum or anus. 80% are perianal, the remainder are intrasphincteric or supra-levator.
System(s) affected: Gastrointestinal, Skin/Exocrine
Genetics: No known genetic pattern
Incidence/Prevalence in USA: Common
Predominant age: All ages (most common in infants)
Predominant sex: Male > Female (4:1)

SIGNS AND SYMPTOMS
• Perirectal swelling for superficial abscesses
• Perirectal redness
• Perirectal tenderness
• Perirectal throbbing pain
• Fever and other toxic symptoms with deep abscesses
• If abscess is not accompanied by external swelling, digital exam will reveal a swollen tender mass
• Pain on defecation

CAUSES
• Bacterial invasion of the pararectal spaces, originating in an intersphincteric space which may begin with an abrasion or tear in lining of anal canal, rectum or perianal skin
• Organisms: usually mixed, E. coli, Proteus vulgaris, streptococci, staphylococci, bacteroides, pseudomonas aeruginosa

RISK FACTORS
• Inciting trauma
  ◊ Injections for internal hemorrhoids
  ◊ Enema tip abrasions
  ◊ Puncture wounds from eggshells or fish bones
  ◊ Foreign objects
  ◊ Prolapsed hemorrhoid
• Inflammatory bowel disease
• Chronic granulomatous disease
• Immunodeficiency disorders
• Hematologic malignancies (5-8% of these patients will have abscess at some time)

 DIAGNOSIS

DIFFERENTIAL DIAGNOSIS
• Carcinoma
• Retrorectal tumors
• Crohn's disease
• Primary lesions of syphilis
• Tuberculous ulceration

LABORATORY CBC - leukocytosis
Drugs that may alter lab results: N/A
Disorders that may alter lab results: N/A

PATHOLOGICAL FINDINGS
• Inflammation of anal mucosa
• Pus
• Inflammatory tissue

SPECIAL TESTS N/A

IMAGING Barium enema

DIAGNOSTIC PROCEDURES
Only indicated if diagnosis in doubt:
• Sigmoidoscopy - rule out unusual causes
• Proctoscopy - redness, induration of anus; tender mass

 TREATMENT

APPROPRIATE HEALTH CARE
• Outpatient surgery
• Inpatient surgery with IV antibiotics for supra-levator abscess or toxicity

GENERAL MEASURES N/A

SURGICAL MEASURES
• Perianal abscess
  ◊ Incise and drain abscess
  ◊ Local anesthetic frequently appropriate
  ◊ Pack wound with Iodoform gauze (24-48 hours)
• Ischiorectal abscess
  ◊ Incise and drain abscess
  ◊ General anesthetic usually required
  ◊ Pack wound with Iodoform gauze (removed after several days)
  ◊ Fistulectomy may be done at same time in selected cases
• After surgery:
  ◊ Sitz baths q 2-4 hours
  ◊ Heating pad, heat lamp or warm compress as needed for pain
  ◊ Encourage moving legs as soon as possible
  ◊ Prevent constipation

ACTIVITY Resume work and normal activity as soon as possible

DIET Increase fiber and fluid intake

PATIENT EDUCATION
• Sitz bath instruction
• Diet instructions
• Dressing change instructions
• Stress length of time to heal
• Stress physical cleanliness
• Possible development of fistula-in-ano
• Stress stool regularity

MEDICATIONS

DRUG(S) OF CHOICE
• Antibiotics - only for toxicity
• Stool softening laxatives
Contraindications: Refer to manufacturer's literature
Precautions: Refer to manufacturer's literature
Significant possible interactions: Refer to manufacturer's literature

ALTERNATIVE DRUGS   N/A

FOLLOWUP

PATIENT MONITORING   Routine postoperative care with attention to wound healing which should progress from the inside out

PREVENTION/AVOIDANCE
• Avoid constipation
• Don't use enemas
• Avoid rectal temperatures or medicines in immunocompromised patients

POSSIBLE COMPLICATIONS
• Possible anorectal fistula (in 25% of patients)
• Possible rectovaginal fistula
• Fecal incontinence due to rupture through sphincter muscle
• Recurrence of abscess if underlying cause not corrected

EXPECTED COURSE/PROGNOSIS
Slow healing depending on extent of disease, complete healing by 6 months if no complications (much faster in uncompromised patients)

MISCELLANEOUS

ASSOCIATED CONDITIONS
• Crohn's disease
• Other inflammatory disease such as appendicitis, salpingitis, diverticulitis
• Possibly perianal hidradenitis suppurativa, or HIV infection in patients with recurring perianal or ischiorectal abscesses

AGE-RELATED FACTORS
Pediatric: Common in first year of life
Geriatric: In elderly patients, a high pelvirectal abscess may cause no symptoms except lower abdominal pain and fever
Others: N/A

PREGNANCY   N/A

SYNONYMS   N/A

ICD-9-CM
566 Abscess of anal and rectal regions

SEE ALSO
• Anorectal fistula

OTHER NOTES   N/A

ABBREVIATIONS   N/A

REFERENCES
• Schwartz SI, Shires GT, Spences FC, Storer EH: Principles of Surgery. 4th Ed. New York, McGraw-Hill Book Co., 1984
• Ashcraft KW, Holder TM: Pediatric Surgery. 2nd Ed. Philadelphia, W.B. Saunders Co., 1993
• Fazio VW: Anorectal Disorders. In Gastroenterology Clinics of North America. Philadelphia, W.B. Saunders Co., 1987
• Schouten WR, van Vroonhoven TJ: Treatment of anorectal abscess with or without primary fistulectomy. Results of a prospective randomized trial. Dis Colon Rectum 1991;34:60-3
Illustrations: N/A
Internet references: http://www.5mcc.com

Author(s)
Timothy L. Black, MD, FACS, FAAP

Anorectal fistula

BASICS

DESCRIPTION Inflammatory track with one opening in the anal canal and another in perianal skin. Fistulas occur spontaneously or secondary to perirectal abscess. Most fistulas originate in the anal crypts at the anorectal juncture.
• Goodsall's rule
  ◊ If external opening is anterior to an imaginary line drawn horizontally through anal canal, fistula usually runs directly into anal canal
  ◊ If external opening is posterior to line, the fistula usually curves to posterior midline of anal canal
  ◊ In children, track is usually straight
• Classification
  ◊ Intersphincteric
  ◊ Transphincteric
  ◊ Suprasphincteric
  ◊ Extrasphincteric
System(s) affected: Gastrointestinal, Skin/Exocrine
Genetics: No known genetic pattern
Incidence/Prevalence in USA: Common
Predominant age: All ages
Predominant sex: Male = Female

SIGNS AND SYMPTOMS
• Constant or intermittent drainage or discharge
• Firm tender peri-anal lump
• External anal sphincter pain during and after defecation
• Spasm of external anal sphincter during and after defecation
• Anal bleeding
• Discoloration of skin surrounding the fistula
• Fistulous opening frequently granulose or scarred
• Possible fever

CAUSES
• Erosion of anal canal
• Extension from infection from a tear in lining in anal canal
• Infecting organism is commonly Escherichia coli

RISK FACTORS
• Injection of internal hemorrhoids, puncture wound from eggshells or fish bones, foreign objects, enema tip injuries
• Ruptured anal hematoma
• Prolapsed internal hemorrhoid
• Acute appendicitis, salpingitis, diverticulitis
• Inflammatory bowel disease (chronic ulcerative colitis, Crohn's disease)
• Previous perirectal abscess

DIAGNOSIS

DIFFERENTIAL DIAGNOSIS
• Pilonidal sinus
• Perianal abscess
• Urethroperineal fistulas
• Ischiorectal abscess
• Submucous or high muscular abscess
• Pelvirectal abscess (rare)
• Rule out: Crohn's disease; carcinoma; retrorectal tumors

LABORATORY CBC
Drugs that may alter lab results: N/A
Disorders that may alter lab results: N/A

PATHOLOGICAL FINDINGS
• Fistulous tract may be simple or multiple
• Fistulous tract has primary opening in anal crypt; secondary opening in anal skin, para-anal skin, perineal skin, or in rectal mucus membrane
• Anal sinus - opens in anal crypt
• Termination of sinus is blind and located in para-anal or pararectal tissue

SPECIAL TESTS N/A

IMAGING Lower GI series if inflammatory bowel disease suspected

DIAGNOSTIC PROCEDURES
• Proctoscopy
• Sigmoidoscopy
• Probe inserted into tract to determine its course (be careful not to create an artificial opening)

TREATMENT

APPROPRIATE HEALTH CARE
Outpatient surgery

GENERAL MEASURES Sitz baths 3-4 times per day until definitive surgery

SURGICAL MEASURES
• Fistulotomy - surgical incision of entire length of fistula (unroofing). Mucosal tract may be cauterized or curetted. Sphincterotomy.
• Fistulectomy - complete excision of tract is usually necessary. Sphincterotomy.
• General anesthesia or regional anesthesia usually required
• Postoperative - hot sitz baths
• Avoid constipation

ACTIVITY Resume work and normal activity as soon as possible

DIET Clear liquid diet until gastrointestinal function returns

PATIENT EDUCATION
• Stress peri-anal cleanliness
• Sitz baths

MEDICATIONS

DRUG(S) OF CHOICE
• Broad spectrum antibiotic if active infection
• Stool-softening laxative
Contraindications: Refer to manufacturer's literature
Precautions: Refer to manufacturer's literature
Significant possible interactions: Refer to manufacturer's literature

ALTERNATIVE DRUGS N/A

FOLLOWUP

PATIENT MONITORING Frequent followup examinations following surgery to ensure complete healing and assess continence

PREVENTION/AVOIDANCE N/A

POSSIBLE COMPLICATIONS
• Constipation (urge to defecate may be suppressed due to pain)
• Rectovaginal fistula
• Partial incontinence of fecal material if sphincter is divided
• Delayed wound healing
• Low grade carcinoma may develop in long-standing fistulas
• Recurrent anorectal fistula if fistula is incompletely opened or excised

EXPECTED COURSE/PROGNOSIS
• Surgical results usually excellent
• Postoperative healing requires 4-5 weeks for perianal fistulas; 12-16 weeks for deeper fistulas
• Postoperative healing may occur within 2-3 weeks in children

MISCELLANEOUS

ASSOCIATED CONDITIONS
• Possibly associated with penetrating injury, intestinal tuberculosis, ulcerative colitis
• Hidradenitis suppurativa
• Crohn's disease

AGE-RELATED FACTORS
Pediatric: Most common in infants. More frequent in males.
Geriatric: Constipation is a common complication
Others: N/A

PREGNANCY N/A

SYNONYMS
• Fistula-in-ano

ICD-9-CM
565.1 Anal fistula

SEE ALSO
• Anorectal abscess
• Crohn's disease

OTHER NOTES N/A

ABBREVIATIONS N/A

REFERENCES
• Kirsner JB, Shorter G, eds: Diseases of the Colon, Rectum and Anal Canal. Baltimore, Williams & Wilkins, 1989
• Sleisenger MH, Fordtran JS, eds: Gastrointestinal Disease: Pathophysiology, Diagnosis, Management. 5th Ed. Philadelphia, W.B. Saunders Co., 1994
• Schwartz SI, Shires GT, Spences FC, Storer EH: Principles of Surgery. 4th Ed. New York, McGraw-Hill Book Co., 1984
• Welch KJ, Randolph JG, Ravitcl MM, O'Neill JA, Rowe ML: Pediatric Surgery. 4th Ed. Chicago, Year Book Medical Publishers, 1986
Illustrations: N/A
Internet references: http://www.5mcc.com

Author(s)
Timothy L. Black, MD, FACS, FAAP

Anorexia nervosa

 BASICS

DESCRIPTION Body dissatisfaction; significant weight loss; amenorrhea (in females), not due to physical disease
Incidence/Prevalence in USA:
Approximately 1% of females; males comprise 5-10% of cases
System(s) affected: Nervous, Metabolic, Gastrointestinal, Cardiovascular, Reproductive
Genetics: N/A
Predominant age: Usually adolescents or young adults
Predominant sex: Female > Male

SIGNS AND SYMPTOMS
• Usually insidious in onset
• Onset may be stress related
• Pronounced weight loss (generally 15% below original or expectable weight)
• Deny that there is a problem
• Claim to feel fat even when emaciated
• Preoccupation with body size, weight control
• Reduction in total food intake, especially high calorie foods; food refusal
• Elaborate food preparation and eating rituals
• Extensive exercise, especially running or use of stair stepper
• Sexual disinterest
• Depression that may be secondary to inanition
• Cracked, dry skin, sparse scalp hair
• Fine, downy lanugo hair on extremities, face, and trunk
• Growth arrest
• Hypotension and bradycardia
• Hypothermia
• Peripheral edema
• Cognitive decline

CAUSES Unknown; thought to be largely emotional. Co-morbid major depression and/or dysthymia in 50-75% of patients. Obsessive-compulsive disorder in 10-13% of patients.

RISK FACTORS
• Perfectionistic personality
• Low self-esteem
• Achievement pressure; high self-expectations
• Acceptance of the culturally condoned ideal of slimness
• Ambivalence about dependence/independence
• Stress due to multiple responsibilities, tight schedules
• Unstable body image; perceptual distortions
• Early puberty

 DIAGNOSIS

DIFFERENTIAL DIAGNOSIS Inanition due to physical disorder; brain tumor; bulimia; depressive disorders with loss of appetite; food phobia; conversion disorder; schizophrenic disorder; body dysmorphic disorder

LABORATORY
• Findings are directly related to starvation, dehydration: no biological test is specific for anorexia
• Diminished plasma LH, FSH, T3
• Elevated growth hormone, cortisol, cholesterol, vasopressin
• Positive dexamethasone suppression test
• Diminished plasma tryptophan
• Diminished BUN, creatinine clearance
• Flat glucose tolerance curve, depressed fasting blood sugar
• Low resting metabolic rate
• Low CD4/CD8 ratio
• Prolonged QT interval
• Neutropenia with relative lymphocytosis
• Hypercarotenemia
• Low serum zinc
• Bone loss
• Abnormal CT, MRI
Drugs that may alter lab results: N/A
Disorders that may alter lab results: N/A

PATHOLOGICAL FINDINGS All are directly related to starvation
• Arrested maturation
• Pathological fractures
• Cognitive deficits
• Cracked, dry skin, sparse scalp hair
• Fine, downy lanugo hair on extremities, face, and trunk
• Hypotension and bradycardia
• Hypothermia
• Peripheral edema

SPECIAL TESTS Measure percent body fat

IMAGING Not indicated

DIAGNOSTIC PROCEDURES
• Psychological screening
• Eating Attitudes Test

 TREATMENT

APPROPRIATE HEALTH CARE
• Hospitalize if weight loss greater than 30% in 6 months; if patient is suicidal; if there is physiologic instability; or if there has been no response to outpatient therapy
• Initial goal should be weight restoration
• Partial hospitalization if patient more than 70% of ideal body weight, motivated and capable of interpersonal; relatedness

GENERAL MEASURES
• Inpatient:
  ◊ If possible admit to specialized eating disorders unit
  ◊ Bedrest with supervised meals until patient has gained 21 pounds (9.5 kg)
  ◊ 300 calorie (1.26 kJ) stepwise gradual increase in calories consumed
  ◊ Stepwise increase in activity as weight increases
  ◊ Assess psychological state and nutritional status
  ◊ Involve patient in establishing target weight
  ◊ Weigh daily at first, then 3 x per week
  ◊ Achieve 1-2 pound (0.45-0.91 kg) per week weight gain
  ◊ Supportive therapy within structured eating disorders program
  ◊ Tube feeding only as last resort
  ◊ Medicate for symptom relief
• Outpatient:
  ◊ Build trust, treatment alliance
  ◊ Assess psychological state and nutritional status
  ◊ Involve patient in establishing target weight
  ◊ Achieve gradual weight gain
  ◊ Weigh weekly at first, monthly when progress is evident
  ◊ Focus on overall indices of health, rather than weight gain alone
  ◊ Challenge fear of uncontrollable weight gain
  ◊ Consider cognitive-behavioral, educational-behavioral, individual, family, group or couples therapy
  ◊ Medicate for symptom relief

SURGICAL MEASURES N/A

ACTIVITY
• Stepwise increase as patient gains weight
• Monitor activity; gain patient's cooperation
• Focus on playful rather than goal oriented activities

DIET
• Goal is weight stabilization on a balanced diet with normal eating pattern
• Diminished ruminations about calories, weight

PATIENT EDUCATION
• Provide information on nutrition, metabolic balance
• Provide tools for self monitoring when appropriate
• Ask patient to keep a "food diary" listing feelings and foods eaten
• For patient education materials favorably reviewed on this topic, contact: Anorexia Nervosa & Related Eating Disorders, P.O. Box 5102, Eugene, OR 97405, (503)344-1144

MEDICATIONS

DRUG(S) OF CHOICE
• Fluoxetine (Prozac) 10-60 mg relieves symptoms and helps restore and maintain weight
• Short term anxiolytic therapy for starved inpatients (oxazepam 15 mg or alprazolam 0.25 mg before meals) to lessen anxiety about weight gain
Contraindications: Refer to manufacturer's literature
Precautions: Starved patients are more sensitive to medication, likely to suffer dangerous or lethal side effects due to compromised cardiac, liver and kidney function; caution is indicated
Significant possible interactions: Refer to manufacturer's literature

ALTERNATIVE DRUGS
• When patient is bulimic as well as anorexic and resistant to treatment, consider tricyclics - imipramine (Tofranil) 10 mg, gradual increase to 200 mg (higher doses in inpatient settings), or desipramine (Norpramin) 25 mg/day, increasing gradually to 150 mg/day. Monitor with EKG.
• Cyproheptadine (Periactin) 4 mg, increasing gradually if side effects permit, to 32 mg/day
• Cisapride (Propulsid) 10-20 mg before each meal and at bedtime for abdominal distension due to delayed gastric emptying
• Estrogen - estradiol 0.5-1 mg - does not enhance bone density in underweight patients, but may be used following weight gain
• Psyllium (Metamucil) preparations (1 tbs hs) to prevent constipation
• Therapeutic vitamin-mineral supplement

FOLLOWUP

PATIENT MONITORING
• Level of activity. Is the activity driven?
• Weigh weekly until stable, then monthly
• Depression, self-esteem, suicidal ideation
• Ruminations and rituals
• Repeat any abnormal lab values weekly or monthly

PREVENTION/AVOIDANCE
• Encourage rational attitude about weight
• Moderate overly high self-expectations
• Enhance self-esteem
• Diminish stress

POSSIBLE COMPLICATIONS
• Potassium depletion; cardiac arrhythmia; cardiac arrest
• Nitrogen depletion, exhaustion, collapse
• Cardiomyopathy, congestive heart failure
• Delayed gastric emptying
• Necrotizing colitis
• Convulsions, peripheral neuropathy
• Osteoporosis
• Too rapid initial weight gain can cause fluid retention and congestive heart failure

EXPECTED COURSE/PROGNOSIS
• Highly variable; relapse common
• Significant morbidity from cardiac arrest and eventual suicide
• Better outcome if patient hospitalized until weight in normal range
• Speed of weight gain does not predict treatment success
• Poor prognosis indicated by repeated hospitalization, failed treatment, initial low weight, vomiting, being married, poor maturation
• Patients often become depressed as (or after) they recover.
• Early age of onset indicates more favorable prognosis
• Many symptoms resolve spontaneously with weight gain
• Ruminations, rituals, social isolation, and abnormal attitudes toward food and the body often persist after weight gain

MISCELLANEOUS

ASSOCIATED CONDITIONS
• Major depression or dysthymia
• Social phobia
• Obsessive-compulsive disorder
• Other anxiety disorders
• Substance abuse disorder
• Borderline personality disorder

AGE-RELATED FACTORS
Pediatric: Growth can be compromised in preadolescence and early adolescence
Geriatric: Difficult to diagnose in elderly
Others:
• High risk
  ◊ Ballet dancers, models, cheerleaders
  ◊ Athletes, especially runners, gymnasts, weight lifters, body builders, jockeys, divers, wrestlers, figure skaters, field hockey players

PREGNANCY Unlikely due to amenorrhea

SYNONYMS N/A

ICD-9-CM
307.1 anorexia nervosa

SEE ALSO
• Amenorrhea
• Osteoporosis
• Idiopathic edema

OTHER NOTES N/A

ABBREVIATIONS N/A

REFERENCES
• Beaumont PJ, Russell JD, Touyz SW: Treatment of anorexia nervosa. Lancet 1993;341:1635-1640
• Yager J, et al: Practice Guidelines for the Eating Disorders. Am J Psychiatry 1993;150:207-228
• Salisbury JJ, Levine AS, Crow SJ, Mitchell JE: Refeeding, metabolic weight and weight gain in anorexia nervosa. Int J Eat Disord 1995;17:337-345
• Grinspoon S, Herzog DB, Kibanski A: Mechanisms and treatment options for bone loss in anorexia nervosa. In press: J of Clin Endocrin Metab
• Eckert ED, Halmi KA, Mardi P, et al: Ten year follow up of anorexia nervosa: clinical course and outcome. Psychol Med 1995;25:143-156
Illustrations: N/A
Internet references: http://www.5mcc.com

Author(s)
Alayne Yates, MD

Anxiety

BASICS

DESCRIPTION A common acute or chronic, fearful emotion with associated physical symptoms. DSM-IV-R recognizes the following sub types:
• Acute situational anxiety: Response to recent stressful event, usually transient symptoms
• Adjustment disorder with anxious mood: Persistent, maladaptive reaction following psychosocial stress and lasting up to six months
• Generalized anxiety disorder: Persistent underlying anxiety or adjustment disorder with anxious mood and significant symptoms of motor tension, autonomic hyperactivity and hypervigilance, lasting more than six months
• Panic disorder: Recurrent unexpected attacks with at least one attack (or more) associated with persistent concern about additional attacks, worries about implications of the attack (losing control, having a heart attack) or a significant change in behavior related to the attack; often leads to agoraphobia
• Post-traumatic stress disorder: Recurrent flashbacks or nightmares of catastrophic event by survivors, often associated with panic attacks and major depression
• Specific phobias: Intense recurrent fear of, and avoidance of, an object or situation
• Social phobia: Marked and persistent fear and avoidance of performance or social situations in which the person is exposed to unfamiliar people or scrutiny
• Obsessive-compulsive disorder: Persistent unwanted and disturbing thoughts and recurrent behavioral patterns (i.e., hand washing) which interfere with daily life
System(s) affected: Nervous
Genetics: Panic disorder - increased concordance in monozygotic versus dizygotic twins
Incidence/Prevalence in USA: 40 million (the most common psychiatric disorder in US)
• 12 month prevalence rate
   ◊ Panic disorder - female 3.2%, male 1.3%
   ◊ Obsessive compulsive disorder - female 2.6-3.1%, male 1.1-2.6%
   ◊ Agoraphobia - female 3.8%, male 1.7%
   ◊ Generalized anxiety disorder - female 4.3%, male 2.0%
Predominant Age: Mainly adults, highest prevalence in 20 to 45 year age group
Predominant Sex: Female > Male (social phobia female 5.27:male 3.87)

SIGNS AND SYMPTOMS Patterns vary with subtype of anxiety; not all present in each case
• Unrealistic or excessive anxiety or worry
• Sense of impending doom
• Nervousness
• Instability
• Tachycardia; palpitations
• Systolic click murmur
• Hyperventilation, choking sensation
• Labile hypertension
• Sighing respiration
• Nausea or abdominal distress
• Paresthesias
• Diaphoresis
• Dizziness or syncope
• Flushing
• Muscle tension
• Tremulousness
• Restlessness
• Chest tightness, pressure (pseudoangina)
• Headache, backaches, muscle spasm

CAUSES
• Panic disorder, social phobia and obsessive compulsive disorder are associated with genetic factors
• Psychosocial stressors commonly trigger anxiety disorders and may provoke a genetic diathesis
• Mediated by abnormalities of neurotransmitter systems (serotonin, norepinephrine and gamma-aminobutyric acid [GABA])

RISK FACTORS
• Social and financial problems
• Medical illness
• Family history
• Lack of social support

DIAGNOSIS

DIFFERENTIAL DIAGNOSIS
• Cardiovascular:
   ◊ Ischemic heart disease
   ◊ Valvular heart disease
   ◊ Cardiomyopathies
   ◊ Myocarditis
   ◊ Arrhythmias
   ◊ Mitral valve prolapse (most symptomatic cases are associated with panic disorder)
• Respiratory:
   ◊ Asthma
   ◊ Emphysema
   ◊ Pulmonary embolism
   ◊ Hamman-Rich syndrome
   ◊ Scleroderma
• CNS:
   ◊ Transient cerebral insufficiency
   ◊ Psychomotor epilepsy
   ◊ Essential tremor
• Metabolic and Hormonal:
   ◊ Hyperthyroidism
   ◊ Pheochromocytoma
   ◊ Adrenal insufficiency
   ◊ Cushing's syndrome
   ◊ Hypokalemia, hypoglycemia
   ◊ Hyperparathyroidism
   ◊ Myasthenia gravis
• Nutritional:
   ◊ Thiamine, pyridoxine, or folate deficiency
   ◊ Iron deficiency anemia
• Intoxication:
   ◊ Caffeine
   ◊ Alcohol
   ◊ Cocaine
   ◊ Sympathomimetics
   ◊ Amphetamines
• Withdrawal:
   ◊ Alcohol
   ◊ Sedative-hypnotics
• Other:
   ◊ Depression
   ◊ Panic disorder is associated with several physical disorders, including
(a) mitral valve prolapse (systolic click-murmur)
(b) labile hypertension
(c) migraine headaches
(d) irritable bowel syndrome

LABORATORY
• Selective use of laboratory tests, (with minimal to more extensive workup depending on clinical picture). Laboratory tests often normal in anxiety disorders.
• CBC and urinalysis
• Sequential serial multiple analysis (SMA-12 panel)
• Thyroid function studies
Drugs that may alter lab results: N/A
Disorders that may alter lab results: N/A

PATHOLOGICAL FINDINGS N/A

SPECIAL TESTS EEG, ECG, etc.

IMAGING Usually none; chest x-ray possibly

DIAGNOSTIC PROCEDURES
• Psychologic testing (e.g., Zung's anxiety self-assessment, Hamilton's anxiety scale)
• DSM-IV based interview

TREATMENT

APPROPRIATE HEALTH CARE
Outpatient

GENERAL MEASURES
• Should be based on careful workup and identification of etiology and subtype of anxiety disorders
• Adequate workup
• Identify co-existent substance abuse
• Counseling or psychotherapy along with medications
• Regular exercise program
• Biofeedback in selected cases
• Serial office visits
• Judicious reassurance after other medical disorders ruled out

SURGICAL MEASURES N/A

ACTIVITY Fully active

DIET No special diet

PATIENT EDUCATION
• For a listing of sources for patient education materials favorably reviewed on this topic, physicians may contact: American Academy of Family Physicians Foundation, P.O. Box 8418, Kansas City, MO 64114, (800)274-2237, ext. 4400
• National Institute of Mental Health (NIMH) - National Anxiety Awareness Program, 9000 Rockville Pike, Bethesda, MD 20892

MEDICATIONS

DRUG(S) OF CHOICE
• Acute situational anxiety:
◊ Short-term (up to 1 month) treatment with benzodiazepines; e.g., alprazolam (Xanax), clonazepam (Klonopin),lorazepam (Ativan), diazepam (Valium)
◊ Usual dose of alprazolam 0.25 mg 2-3 times daily, increase if needed in 0.25 mg increments
• Adjustment disorder with anxiety mood:
◊ Benzodiazepines as above
• Generalized anxiety disorder:
◊ Azapirones e.g., buspirone (BuSpar) begin 5 mg bid-tid; increase 5 mg q 2-3 days to maximum of 60 mg/day in divided doses
• Panic disorder and social phobia:
◊ TCAs, e.g., imipramine (Tofranil) begin with 10-25 mg qhs; increase by 10-25 mg/day q 2 weeks to maximum of 300 mg/day (100 mg/day maximum in geriatric and adolescent patients)
◊ SRIs - e.g., fluoxetine (Prozac) begin with 4 mg; increase by 4 mg q 5 days to maximum daily dosage of 20-40 mg; sertraline (Zoloft) begin with 25 mg; increase by 25 mg q 5 days; paroxetine (Paxil), begin with 10 mg; increase by 10 mg q 5 days
• Obsessive-compulsive disorder:
◊ Clomipramine (Anafranil), initially 25 mg bid; increase gradually to 250 mg/day if needed and as tolerated
◊ SRIs also effective - fluoxetine (Prozac) 40-100 mg/day or sertraline (Zoloft) 100-200 mg/day or paroxetine (Paxil) 20-50 mg/day
Contraindications:
• Benzodiazepines - 1st-trimester pregnancy, acute alcohol intoxication with depressed vital signs, acute angle-closure glaucoma, sleep apnea, history of personality disorder or substance abuse. Avoid long-term/prn use.
• Buspirone - concurrent MAO inhibitor use
• TCAs - acute myocardial infarction
Precautions:
• Benzodiazepines - advanced age, renal insufficiency, suicidal tendency, open-angle glaucoma. Sudden discontinuation increases risk of seizures, especially with alprazolam
• Benzodiazepines with short half-lives (e.g., alprazolam) increase potential for dependency and protracted withdrawal symptoms; extreme caution with severe panic disorder who are taking other CNS sedatives or who have a history of substance abuse/dependence
• Buspirone - hepatic and/or renal dysfunction. Buspirone will not protect against benzodiazepine withdrawal seizures; taper benzodiazepines.
• TCAs - advanced age, glaucoma, benign prostate hypertrophy, hyperthyroidism, cardiovascular disease, liver disease, urinary retention, MAO inhibitor treatment

Significant possible interactions:
• Benzodiazepines - cimetidine, ethanol, oral contraceptives, disulfiram, levodopa, rifampin
• Buspirone - MAO inhibitors
• TCAs - amphetamines, barbiturates, guanethidine, clonidine, epinephrine, ethanol, norepinephrine, MAO inhibitors, propoxyphene
• SRIs - MAO inhibitors (may cause fatal serotonin syndrome [confusion, hyperthermia, etc.])

ALTERNATIVE DRUGS
• Generalized anxiety disorder: Short-term use of benzodiazepine or TCA's
• Panic disorder: Although TCA's or serotonin reuptake inhibitors are the drugs of choice for panic disorder, they are slow in onset of action (2-3 weeks). Benzodiazepines may be helpful for initial control of symptoms until the TCA's are effective. Also, 10-20% of patients with panic do not tolerate side effects of TCA's. High potency benzodiazepines (alprazolam, clonazepam, lorazepam) or SRI's such as fluoxetine (Prozac), sertraline (Zoloft) or MAO inhibitors are effective alternatives.
• Obsessive-compulsive disorder: Fluoxetine (Prozac) initial dosage 20 mg, may increase by 20 mg each week to a dosage of 40-100 mg/day. Sertraline (Zoloft) also effective (initial dose 50 mg, increase by 50 mg every 2 weeks to maximum daily dosage of 150-200 mg). Paroxetine is also effective (initial dose 20 mg, increase by 10 mg every 2 weeks to a maximum dosage of 50 mg).
• Social phobia: Phenelzine - initial dose 15 mg bid, increase by 15 mg every week to a total dose of 45-90 mg. Benzodiazepines: Clonazepam 0.5 mg po tid, total dosage 1.5-4.5 mg.

FOLLOWUP

PATIENT MONITORING
• Followup by regular office visits
• Watch for and treat associated depression
• Monitor mental status on benzodiazepines and avoid drug dependence
• Monitor blood pressure, heart rate, anticholinergic side effects on TCA's
• Periodic serum levels, if indicated, for TCA's

PREVENTION/AVOIDANCE Management of stress, to extent possible, relaxation techniques, meditation

POSSIBLE COMPLICATIONS
• Impaired social/occupational functioning
• Drug dependence (benzodiazepines)
• Cardiac arrhythmias (TCA's)

EXPECTED COURSE/PROGNOSIS
• With active treatment, excellent results can often be obtained, especially with short-term anxiety disorders, including panic disorder
• Obsessive-compulsive disorder, and post-traumatic stress disorder are more difficult to treat, often requiring longer-term psychotherapy and medication (combination treatment)

MISCELLANEOUS

ASSOCIATED CONDITIONS
• Depression (commonly)
• Agoraphobia
• Alcohol or substance abuse
• Somatoform disorders

AGE-RELATED FACTORS
Pediatric: Reduced dosage of medications in adolescent
Geriatric: Reduced dosage of medications
Others: N/A

PREGNANCY
• Benzodiazepines - contraindicated in first-trimester of pregnancy, and with caution later in pregnancy and during lactation. May cause lethargy and weight loss in nursing infants; avoid breast feeding if mother taking benzodiazepines chronically or in high doses.
• TCAs - some evidence of fetal risk, especially in first trimester
• SRIs - taper and discontinue, if possible, in first trimester; may be used later in pregnancy

SYNONYMS
• Hyperventilation syndrome
• Panic disorder

ICD-9-CM
300.0 anxiety states

SEE ALSO N/A

OTHER NOTES N/A

ABBREVIATIONS
DSM-IV-R = Diagnostic and Statistical Manual of Mental Disorders. 4th edition
TCA = tricyclic antidepressant
SRI = serotonergic reuptake inhibitor

REFERENCES
• Katon W: Panic Disorder in the Medical Setting. Washington, D.C., American Psychiatric Press, 1991
• Roy-Byrne PP: Integrated Treatment of Panic Disorder. Am J Med. Suppl 1992;1A:495-545
• Landry MJ, Smith DE, et al: Benzodiazepine dependence and withdrawal: Identification and medical management. J Am Bd Fam Prac 1992;5:167-171
• Lydiard RB, Brawman-Mintzor O, et al: Recent developments in the psychopharmacology of anxiety disorders. J Consulting Clin Psychology. 1996;64:660-668
Illustrations: N/A
Internet references: http://www.5mcc.com

Author(s)
John P. Geyman, MD
Wayne J. Katon, MD

Aortic dissection

BASICS

DESCRIPTION Intimal tear in the aorta propagated via hematoma formation causing further dissection and separation producing a false lumen in the arterial wall.
• The Debakey classification:
  ◊ Type I: Involves the aortic root, aortic arch, and the descending aorta
  ◊ Type II: Involves only the ascending aorta
  ◊ Type III: Involves only the distal aorta beyond the origin of the left subclavian artery
System(s) affected: Cardiovascular
Genetics: Increased incidence among family members
Incidence/Prevalence in USA:
• 1 in 10,000 patients admitted to hospital; found 1 in 350 patients at autopsy
• 2000 new cases diagnosed annually
Predominant age: Dependent on etiology; Marfan's commonly present in the third and fourth decade; most common between the 6th and 8th decades
Predominant sex: Male > Female (3:1)

SIGNS AND SYMPTOMS
• Abrupt onset of tearing pain
• Shearing anterior chest pain which radiates to the interscapular region
• Back pain
• Syncope
• Symptoms of congestive heart failure
• Stroke
• Limb ischemia
• Abdominal pain
• Acute myocardial infarction
• Spinal cord syndromes/deficits
• Hypotension or hypertension
• Wide pulse pressure
• Murmur of aortic insufficiency
• Features of tamponade
• Dullness in left lung base (effusion)
• Pulse deficits or asymmetry
• Fever

CAUSES
• Cystic medionecrosis
• Iatrogenic during arterial catheterization

RISK FACTORS
• Hypertension
• Pregnancy
• Chest trauma
• Cocaine use
• Cardiovascular surgery

DIAGNOSIS

DIFFERENTIAL DIAGNOSIS
• Myocardial infarction
• Pulmonary embolism
• Pneumonia
• Pleurisy
• Pericarditis
• Pneumothorax
• Angina
• Acute pancreatitis
• Penetrating duodenal ulcer

LABORATORY No special studies required
Drugs that may alter lab results: N/A
Disorders that may alter lab results: N/A

PATHOLOGICAL FINDINGS
Approximately 60% of intimal tears occur in the proximal ascending aorta. The remainder are found between the origin of the left subclavian artery and ligamentum arteriosum, descending aorta (20%), aortic arch (10%), and the abdominal aorta. Although medionecrosis is found in normal aging aortas, it appears to be more extensive in patients who develop aortic dissection. Cystic medionecrosis is seen in patients with defects in elastin and connective tissue organization i.e., Marfan's, Ehlers-Danlos, etc. Death usually due to rupture and tamponade.

SPECIAL TESTS
• Electrocardiogram - LVH, nonspecific ST-T changes, electrical alternans with associated tamponade
• Echocardiogram - dilated aortic root, increased aortic posterior or anterior wall thickness, pericardial effusion, oscillating intimal flap

IMAGING Chest x-ray - widening of the superior mediastinum, left pleural effusion, haziness or enlargement of the aortic knob, double density of the descending aorta, irregular aortic contour, > 5 mm separation of intimal calcification from outer aortic contour, rightward displacement of the trachea, cardiomegaly.

DIAGNOSTIC PROCEDURES
• CT chest - demonstration of two lumens with hematoma formation, detection of intimal flap, differential flow between two lumens, compression of true lumen by false lumen
• Aortogram - demonstration of two lumens, detection of intimal flap, compression of true lumen, ulcer-like projections of contrast, arterial compromise, altered flow patterns, aortic insufficiency (not as sensitive as previous thought)
• Transesophageal echocardiography (TEE) - test of choice for hemodynamically unstable patients
• MRI - if available and patient hemodynamically stable, test of choice since same sensitivity as CT, but higher specificity

TREATMENT

APPROPRIATE HEALTH CARE
Admission to intensive care unit or transfer to operative suite

GENERAL MEASURES
• Treatment of choice - surgical for all ascending aortic dissections and medical for descending dissections without complications (Type III)
• Medical therapy is based on decreasing blood pressure and the "shearing" forces of myocardial contractility (dp/dt) to attempt to decrease intimal tear and hematoma propagation
• Arterial blood pressure monitoring is critical
• Careful observation for changes in mentation, neurological signs, or evidence of organ dysfunction
• A Foley catheter should be used to follow urine output
• Swan-Ganz catheterization may be very helpful to monitor cardiac performance and filling pressures during the use of vasoactive and cardiodepressive drugs
• Pain control may be difficult despite use of narcotics

SURGICAL MEASURES
• Surgical indications for Type III
  ◊ Increasing size of hematoma
  ◊ Impending rupture
  ◊ Inability to control pain
  ◊ Bleeding into pleural space

ACTIVITY Bedrest

DIET NPO until surgical evaluation is complete and patient classified as medical therapy only

PATIENT EDUCATION Depending on etiology, emphasis must be placed on risk factors and recurrence of symptoms

Aortic dissection

MEDICATIONS

DRUG(S) OF CHOICE Propranolol in 0.5-1 mg IV doses every 5 minutes until the heart rate is 60-70 beats per minute plus nitroprusside titrated to reduce systolic blood pressure to 100-110 mm Hg (13.3-14.6 kPa)

Contraindications:
• Propranolol - in bronchial asthma, diabetes mellitus, Raynaud's disease, sinus bradycardia, A-V heart block greater than first degree, in presence of monoamine oxidase inhibitors, cardiogenic shock, congestive heart failure or right ventricular failure from pulmonary hypertension
• Nitroprusside - in treatment of compensatory hypertension, i.e., arteriovenous shunt, in patients with inadequate cerebral circulation, and for use during emergency surgery in moribund patients

Precautions:
• Propranolol should be used cautiously in patients with angina pectoris, cardiac failure, impaired renal or hepatic function, thyrotoxicosis, pre-excitation syndromes, diabetes, hypoglycemia or nonallergic bronchospasm. Propranolol may produce significant bradycardia, heart block or hypotension. Patients should not be suddenly withdrawn from beta blockers.
• Nitroprusside may not lower blood pressure adequately in some patients, so another agent may be required. Excessive nitroprusside or use in patients with renal or hepatic insufficiency may cause cyanide toxicity, through excessive production of serum thiocyanate. Confusion and hyperreflexia are the early signs of thiocyanate toxicity. Because thiocyanate inhibits the uptake and binding of iodine, caution should be exercised in the presence of hypothyroidism. Thiocyanate blood levels should be followed after 48 hours of nitroprusside use. Because of the rapid onset and potency of nitroprusside, administration should be with the use of an infusion pump. Methemoglobinemia may be seen rarely.

Significant possible interactions:
• Propranolol may have interactions with adenosine, albuterol, alfentanil, amiodarone, barbiturates, bromazepam, chlorothiazide, chlorpromazine, chlorpropamide, chlorprothixene, cimetidine, clonidine, dextroamphetamine, diazoxide, dihydroergotamine, diltiazem, disopyramide, tricyclic antidepressants, encainide, epinephrine, flecainide, fluvoxamine, furosemide, glipizide, halofenate, haloperidol, heparin, ibuprofen, indomethacin, insulin, isoniazid, isoproterenol, lidocaine, lidoflazine, methacholine, methyldopa, metoclopramide, naproxen, nifedipine, phenylpropanolamine, procainamide, quinidine, reserpine, rifampin, ritodrine, sulfonylureas, theophylline, thioridazine, tocainide, tubocurarine, verapamil, warfarin.
• Nitroprusside may have interactions with clonidine and other antihypertensives to make their hypotensive effects cumulative

ALTERNATIVE DRUGS
• Labetalol, 10-20 mg IV bolus to a maximum of 300 mg total, then titrated to response with an infusion
• Trimethaphan, at an infusion rate of 1-2 mg/min
• Reserpine 0.5-2 mg intramuscularly every 4-8 hours. Onset of action is 1-3 hours.
• Methyldopa 250-500 mg every 6 hours. Unfortunately, it has a delayed onset of action of 4 to 6 hours and prolonged duration of 10 to 12 hours.

FOLLOWUP

PATIENT MONITORING
• Systolic blood pressure should be maintained at 120 mm Hg (16 kPa) or below as tolerated
• Routine chest x-rays and/or chest CT may be helpful in following the progress of any long-term medically treated patient
• Patients should have a one month follow-up visit, and then at three month intervals. During the follow-up, careful attention should be placed on signs and symptoms of aortic insufficiency, chest or back pain, and development of saccular aneurysms as displayed on chest roentgenogram.

PREVENTION/AVOIDANCE Long-term control of hypertension

POSSIBLE COMPLICATIONS
Redissection, localized saccular aneurysm, cardiac tamponade, aortic valvular insufficiency and progressive aortic enlargement

EXPECTED COURSE/PROGNOSIS
• Mortality of patients left untreated is: 20% in 24 hours, 60% in 2 weeks, approximately 90% in three months
• Hospital survival is estimated at approximately 70% in patients treated both medically and surgically
• Patients with ascending dissection treated early with surgery still have a mortality of 29-38%
• 10 year survival of all operated patients is 40%
• Redissection risk is 13% at 5 years; 23% at 10 years

MISCELLANEOUS

ASSOCIATED CONDITIONS
• Ehlers-Danlos syndrome
• Marfan's syndrome
• Aortic stenosis
• Coarctation of aorta
• Bicuspid valve
• Turner's syndrome
• Osteogenesis imperfecta
• Syphilis
• Relapsing polychondritis

AGE-RELATED FACTORS N/A
Pediatric: N/A
Geriatric: N/A
Others: N/A

PREGNANCY Aortic dissection may be associated with cystic medionecrosis of pregnancy and appears to have an increased associated risk with pregnancy. It is still unclear whether pregnancy itself is the originating factor or that it simply contributes to the worsening of an already pre-existing condition.

SYNONYMS
• Dissecting aneurysm

ICD-9-CM
441.0 Dissecting aneurysm (any part)

SEE ALSO N/A

OTHER NOTES N/A

ABBREVIATIONS N/A

REFERENCES
• Hirst AE Jr, Johns VJ Jr, Kim SW Jr: Dissecting aneurysm of the aorta: A review of 505 cases. Medicine 1958;37:217-219
• Cohn LH: Aortic dissection; new aspects of diagnosis and treatments. Hosp Practice1994;29(3):47-56, March 15
• DeSanctis RW, Doroghazi RM, Austen WG, Buckley MJ: Aortic dissection. N Engl J Med 1987;317:1060-1067
• Cigarroa JE, Isselbacher EM, et al: Diagnostic imaging in the evaluation of suspected aortic dissection. N Eng J Med 1993;328(1):35-43
• Summer T, Fehska W, et al: Aortic dissection: a comparative study of diagnosis with spiral CT, multiplanar transesophageal echocardiography, and MR imaging. Radiology 1996; 199(2): 347-52
Illustrations: N/A
Internet references: http://www.5mcc.com

Author(s)
Darell E. Heiselman, DO, FCCM, FACP, FACC, FCCP

- 67 -

Aortic valvular stenosis

BASICS

DESCRIPTION An acquired or congenital obstruction to systolic left ventricular outflow across the aortic valve
System(s) affected: Cardiovascular
Genetics: N/A
Incidence/Prevalence in USA:
• Except for mitral regurgitation due to myocardial disease, valvular aortic stenosis is the most common fatal cardiac valve lesion
• Bicuspid aortic valve has a frequency of 400 per 100,000 live births
Predominant age:
• Age < 30 years - predominantly congenital
• Age 30 to 70 years - most commonly congenital or rheumatic
• Age > 70 years - most commonly degenerative calcification of the aortic valve
Predominant sex:
• Congenital bicuspid valves: Male > Female (4:1)
• Congenital unicuspid valves: Male > Female (3:1)

SIGNS AND SYMPTOMS
• Angina pectoris (most frequent symptom, occurring in 50-70% of patients with severe aortic stenosis)
• Near syncope
• Syncope (often exertional, occurs in 15-30% of patients with severe aortic stenosis)
• Exertional dyspnea
• Orthopnea
• Paroxysmal nocturnal dyspnea
• Palpitations
• Fatigue
• Neurologic events (transient ischemic attack or cerebrovascular accident) due to embolization
• Systolic crescendo-decrescendo murmur, usually best heard at the second right sternal border (may have associated thrill) and may radiate into the carotid arteries
• Ejection (early systolic) click
• Prolonged ejection time
• Delayed, small carotid upstroke
• Delayed/decreased intensity of A2
• Paradoxical splitting of S2
• Left ventricular heave
• A high pitched diastolic blow may be present at the left sternal border (associated aortic regurgitation)

CAUSES
• Congenital etiologies
  ◊ Unicuspid valve
  ◊ Bicuspid valve (not inherently stenotic, but becomes so as a result of 'wear and tear' thickening and calcification; a calcified bicuspid valve is the most common cause of isolated aortic stenosis in adults)
  ◊ Three cusped valve with fusion of commissures
    ◊ Hypoplastic annulus
• Acquired etiologies
  ◊ Rheumatic (or, rarely, other inflammatory disease)
  ◊ Degenerative calcific aortic stenosis in the elderly

RISK FACTORS History of rheumatic fever

DIAGNOSIS

DIFFERENTIAL DIAGNOSIS
• Mitral regurgitation, either primary or secondary to underlying coronary artery disease or dilated cardiomyopathy. Mitral regurgitation, however, is usually an apical, high frequency, pansystolic murmur, often radiating to the axilla.
• Hypertrophic obstructive cardiomyopathy. This murmur is also a systolic crescendo-decrescendo murmur, but is best heard at the left sternal border and may radiate into the axilla. However, this murmur characteristically is intensified by moving from squatting to standing position and/or Valsalva's maneuver, and lessened by changing from standing to squatting.
• Aortic supravalvular stenosis
• Discrete subaortic stenosis

LABORATORY N/A
Drugs that may alter lab results: N/A
Disorders that may alter lab results: N/A

PATHOLOGICAL FINDINGS
• Left ventricular hypertrophy
• Myocardial interstitial fibrosis
• Aortic valvular calcification in older patients
• 50% incidence of concomitant coronary artery disease

SPECIAL TESTS ECG: Left ventricular hypertrophy, often with associated ST segment depression, conduction defects, left atrial enlargement, ventricular arrhythmias

IMAGING
• Chest x-ray
  ◊ May be normal in compensated, isolated valvular aortic stenosis
  ◊ Cardiac hypertrophy early, later cardiomegaly
  ◊ Post stenotic dilatation of the ascending aorta
  ◊ Calcification of aortic valve cusps (may require fluoroscopy to visualize)

DIAGNOSTIC PROCEDURES
• Echocardiography:
  ◊ Aortic valve morphology, thickening, calcifications
  ◊ Decreased aortic valve excursion
  ◊ Planimetry of aortic valve area
  ◊ Left ventricular hypertrophy
  ◊ Left ventricular ejection fraction
  ◊ Chamber dimensions
  ◊ Presence or absence of wall motion abnormalities suggestive of coronary artery disease
• With Doppler echocardiography:
  ◊ Transvalvular gradient
  ◊ Valve area
  ◊ Diastolic function
  ◊ Associated aortic regurgitation
• Cardiac catheterization:
  ◊ Transvalvular gradient
  ◊ Valve area

◊ Left ventricle ejection fraction
◊ Concomitant coronary artery disease

TREATMENT

APPROPRIATE HEALTH CARE
Outpatient except for surgical intervention

GENERAL MEASURES
• Aortic stenosis is a progressive disease. The asymptomatic patient with non-critical aortic stenosis can be closely followed with appropriate evaluation.
• All patients with valvular aortic stenosis should receive endocarditis prophylaxis, prior to dental work or invasive procedures regardless of age, etiology or severity of the stenosis (as recommended by the American Heart Association in Circulation, Vol 83, No 3, March, 1991)
• Patients with a rheumatic etiology should receive (in addition to endocarditis prophylaxis prior to dental work or invasive procedures) rheumatic fever prophylaxis, especially if less than 35 years of age, or continue to be in close contact with young children

SURGICAL MEASURES
• Prompt aortic valve replacement is clearly indicated in patients with symptomatic aortic stenosis
• Consider aortic valve replacement in asymptomatic patients with critical aortic stenosis (aortic valve area < 0.8 cm2 or gradient > 50 mm Hg [> 6.6 kPa]) particularly if there is left ventricular dysfunction, increasing cardiomegaly, and clinical symptoms
• Surgical valve replacement consists of the removal of the stenotic, native valve and placement of a prosthetic mechanical or tissue valve
• Balloon angioplasty of stenotic aortic valves may be of benefit in the pediatric patient with congenital disease. Also feasible (although one must expect suboptimal results) in the elderly, debilitated patient who may not tolerate valve replacement.

ACTIVITY In known or suspected severe aortic stenosis, vigorous physical activity is contraindicated

DIET No restrictions except sodium restriction in presence of congestive heart failure

PATIENT EDUCATION
• Educate the patient about the symptoms of symptomatic aortic stenosis and to report these promptly should they occur
• If moderate or severe aortic stenosis is known or suspected, instruct the patient to avoid vigorous physical activity
• Instruct the patient when prophylactic antibiotics are needed for medical or dental procedures

MEDICATIONS

DRUG(S) OF CHOICE
• None for treatment. Prophylactic antibiotics when needed.
• The use of vasodilators, nitrates, calcium channel blockers, beta blockers as well as diuretics are potentially hazardous in aortic stenosis and should be used very cautiously, if at all
Contraindications: N/A
Precautions: N/A
Significant possible interactions: N/A

ALTERNATIVE DRUGS N/A

FOLLOWUP

PATIENT MONITORING
• Asymptomatic patients without critical aortic stenosis should be followed with a history and physical examination every 3-6 months
• An echocardiogram should be performed every 6-12 months to assess progression
• Advise the patient to immediately report any symptoms referable to the aortic stenosis

PREVENTION/AVOIDANCE
• Bacterial endocarditis prophylaxis
• Rheumatic fever prophylaxis, where indicated
• Avoidance of vigorous physical activity

POSSIBLE COMPLICATIONS
• Progressive stenosis
• Sudden death
• Congestive heart failure
• Angina
• Syncope
• Hemolytic anemia
• Infective endocarditis

EXPECTED COURSE/PROGNOSIS
• Mean life expectancy in patients with aortic stenosis is 5 years after the onset of exertional chest discomfort, 3 years after the onset of syncope, 2 years after the development of heart failure
• Sudden death occurs in 15 to 20% of patients with symptomatic aortic stenosis

MISCELLANEOUS

ASSOCIATED CONDITIONS
• Coronary artery disease is present in 50% of patients with aortic stenosis
• Aortic regurgitation (particularly seen in calcified bicuspid valves and rheumatic disease)
• Mitral valve disease (primarily in rheumatic heart disease)

AGE-RELATED FACTORS
Pediatric: N/A
Geriatric: Increased incidence of degenerative calcific aortic stenosis
Others: N/A

PREGNANCY   Severe critical aortic stenosis tolerates poorly the hemodynamic changes in pregnancy, labor and delivery. Pregnancy should be avoided with critical aortic stenosis.

SYNONYMS N/A

ICD-9-CM
424.90 Endocarditis, valve unspecified, unspecified cause

SEE ALSO N/A

OTHER NOTES   As the left ventricle is relatively noncompliant in aortic stenosis, atrial contraction is an important component of diastolic filling. The loss of this component with the onset of atrial fibrillation can cause acute clinical and hemodynamic deterioration.

ABBREVIATIONS N/A

REFERENCES
• Brandenburg RO, et al: Cardiology: Fundamentals and Practice. New York, Year Book Publishers, 1987
• Dalen JE, Alpert JS: Valvular Heart Disease. 2nd Ed. New York, Little Brown & Co, 1987
• Hurst JW, et al: The Heart. 7th Ed. New York, McGraw-Hill, 1990
• Isselbacher KJ, et al, eds: Harrison's Principles of Internal Medicine. 13th Ed. New York, McGraw-Hill, 1994
Illustrations: N/A
Internet references: http://www.5mcc.com

Author(s)
James M. Galloway, MD, FACP, FACC

Appendicitis, acute

BASICS

DESCRIPTION Acute inflammation of the vermiform appendix
• First described by Fitz in 1886
• McBurney described the point of maximal tenderness
System(s) affected: Gastrointestinal
Genetics: Unknown.
Incidence/Prevalence in USA:
• 10/100,000
• Most common acute surgical condition of abdomen
• 1 in every 15 persons (7%) at some time in their life
Predominant age:
• Ages 10-30 - Male > Female (3:2)
• Over age 30 - Male = Female
Predominant sex: Slight male predominance

SIGNS AND SYMPTOMS
• Abdominal pain (100%) - periumbilical then right-lower-quadrant (RLQ). Pain lessened with flexion of thigh.
• Muscle guarding
• Anorexia (almost 100%)
• Nausea (90%)
• Vomiting (75%)-mild
• Obstipation
• Diarrhea-mild
• Sequence of symptom appearance (95%) - anorexia, then abdominal pain, then vomiting
• Slight temperature (one degree centigrade) elevation
• Slight tachycardia
• Patient frequently lies motionless with right thigh drawn up
• Maximal tenderness at "McBurney's point"
• Direct and referred RLQ tenderness
• Voluntary and involuntary guarding
• Cutaneous hyperesthesia at T10-12
• Rovsing's sign - RLQ pain with palpatory pressure in LLQ
• Psoas sign-pain with right thigh extension
• Obturator sign-pain with internal rotation of flexed right thigh
• Retrocecal appendix-flank tenderness in RLQ
• Pelvic appendix-local and suprapubic pain on rectal exam

CAUSES
• Obstruction of appendiceal lumen
  ◊ Fecaliths (most common)
  ◊ Lymphoid tissue hypertrophy
  ◊ Inspissated barium
  ◊ Vegetable, fruit seeds and other foreign bodies
  ◊ Intestinal worms (ascarids)
  ◊ Strictures

RISK FACTORS
• Adolescent males
• Familial tendency
• Intra-abdominal tumors

DIAGNOSIS

DIFFERENTIAL DIAGNOSIS
• Any cause of the "acute abdomen"
• 75% of erroneous diagnoses accounted for by acute mesenteric lymphadenitis, no organic pathologic condition, acute PID, twisted ovarian cyst, ruptured graafian follicle, acute gastroenteritis
• Also consider urologic causes, inflammatory bowel disease, colonic disorders, and other gynecologic diseases

LABORATORY
• Moderate leukocytosis - 10,000 to 18,000/mm3 in 75%
• Moderate polymorphonuclear predominance
• Urinalysis-elevated specific gravity, hematuria (sometimes), pyuria (sometimes), albuminuria (sometimes)
Drugs that may alter lab results:
• Antibiotics
• Steroids
Disorders that may alter lab results: N/A

PATHOLOGICAL FINDINGS
• Acute inflammation of the appendix
• Local vascular congestion
• Obstruction
• Gangrene
• Perforation with abscess (15-30%)

SPECIAL TESTS N/A

IMAGING (Used in differential diagnosis and to detect complications).
• KUB: gas-filled appendix; radiopaque fecalith; deformed cecum; fluid level; ileus; free air.
• Barium enema-non-filling appendix; RLQ mass effect
• Ultrasound-appendiceal inflammation; other pelvic pathology, such as inflammatory mass.
• CT scan for periappendiceal abscess

DIAGNOSTIC PROCEDURES
• Cornerstone of diagnosis is history and clinical findings
• Diagnostic laparoscopy - consider in young adult females
• Rectal and pelvic examinations
• Intensive in-hospital observation

TREATMENT

APPROPRIATE HEALTH CARE
• Inpatient surgery

GENERAL MEASURES
• Preoperative preparation
  ◊ Correction of fluid and electrolyte deficits
  ◊ Consider broad-spectrum antibiotic coverage

SURGICAL MEASURES
• Immediate appendectomy; open or laparoscopic
• Drainage of abscess, if present

ACTIVITY
• Early postoperative ambulation
• Return to full activity by 4 to 6 weeks postop

DIET Regular diet with return of bowel function, usually within 24 to 48 hours postop

PATIENT EDUCATION
• Restricted activity for 4 to 6 weeks postop
• Contact physician for development of postop anorexia, nausea, vomiting, abdominal pain, fever, or chills

Appendicitis, acute

MEDICATIONS

DRUG(S) OF CHOICE
• Uncomplicated acute appendicitis - one preoperative dose of broad spectrum antibiotic; cefoxitin (Mefoxin), cefotetan (Cefotan)
• Gangrenous or perforating appendicitis - broadened antibiotic coverage for aerobic and anaerobic enteric pathogens, dosage and choice of antibiotic should be adjusted based on intraoperative cultures. Continue antibiotics for 7 days postop or until patient becomes afebrile with normal white count. Pathogens usually sensitive to ampicillin, gentamicin, and clindamycin.
Contraindications: Documented allergy to specific antibiotic
Precautions: Adjust antibiotic dosages for elderly and renal failure patients
Significant possible interactions: Refer to manufacturer's literature for each drug

ALTERNATIVE DRUGS
• Metronidazole (Flagyl) - anaerobic coverage only
• Ampicillin-sulbactam (Unasyn)
• Ticarcillin-clavulanate (Timentin)

FOLLOWUP

PATIENT MONITORING Routine visits at 2 and 6 weeks postoperatively

PREVENTION/AVOIDANCE N/A

POSSIBLE COMPLICATIONS
• Wound infection
• Intra-abdominal abscess, sometimes diaphragmatic
• Fecal fistula
• Intestinal obstruction
• Incisional hernia
• Liver abscess (rare)
• Peritonitis with paralytic ileus

EXPECTED COURSE/PROGNOSIS
• Generally uncomplicated course in young adults with non-ruptured appendicitis.
• Factors increasing morbidity and mortality are extremes of age and appendiceal rupture.
• Morbidity rates:
  ◊ 3% with non-perforated appendicitis
  ◊ 47% with perforated appendicitis
• Mortality rates:
  ◊ 0.1% unruptured acute appendicitis
  ◊ 3% ruptured acute appendicitis
  ◊ 15% elderly patient with ruptured appendix

MISCELLANEOUS

ASSOCIATED CONDITIONS N/A

AGE-RELATED FACTORS
Pediatric:
• Rare in infancy
• Decreased diagnostic accuracy
• Higher fever, more vomiting
• Rupture earlier
• Rupture rate: 15 to 50%
• May return to full activities earlier
Geriatric:
• Decreased diagnostic accuracy
• Rupture rate: 67 to 90%
• Patients over 60 years of age account for 50% of deaths from acute appendicitis
Others: N/A

PREGNANCY
• Most common extra-uterine surgical emergency
• 1 in 2000 pregnancies
• Difficult diagnosis
• Appendix displaced superolaterally by gravid uterus
• Fetal mortality rate: 2 to 8.5%

SYNONYMS N/A

ICD-9-CM
540.0 appendicitis, with generalized peritonitis
540.9 appendicitis, without mention of peritonitis

SEE ALSO N/A

OTHER NOTES N/A

ABBREVIATIONS
KUB = kidney, ureter, bladder

REFERENCES
• Schwartz SI, ed: Principles of Surgery. 5th Ed. New York, McGraw-Hill, 1989
• Moody FG, ed: Surgical Treatment of Digestive Disease. 2nd Ed. Chicago, Year Book Medical Publishers, 1990
• Horattas MC, Guyton DP, Wu DA: Reappraisal of appendicitis in the elderly. American Journal of Surgery 1990;160:291-293
Illustrations: N/A
Internet references: http://www.5mcc.com

Author(s)
Andrew H. Fenton, MD, FACS
Thomas W. Clark, MS, MD
Donald W. Moorman, MD

Arterial embolus & thrombosis

 BASICS

DESCRIPTION The acute loss of perfusion distal to an occlusion of a major artery due to an embolus which migrates to the point of occlusion or a clot intrinsic to the point of occlusion (thrombosis). Both are true emergencies. Following obstruction of an artery, a soft coagulum forms both proximally and distally in the areas of stagnant flow. As the clot extends, collateral pathways are involved and the process becomes self-propagating. Ultimately, the venous circulation can be involved. The extent of vascular compromise is critical and determines the "golden" period of four to six hours. After this time, the profound ischemia leads to cellular death and is irreversible.

System(s) affected: Cardiovascular, Hemic/Lymphatic/Immunologic
Genetics: Can be associated with inheritable hypercoagulable and premature atherosclerotic syndromes
Incidence/Prevalence in USA: 50-100/100,000 hospital admissions. A leading cause of death and limb loss in the elderly.
Predominant age: Elderly
Predominant sex: Male > Female

SIGNS AND SYMPTOMS
• The five "P's": Pain, Pulselessness, Pallor, Paresthesias, and Paralysis. If any one is present, frequent re-evaluations indicated. Proximal occlusions lead to a more rapid progression of findings. Occlusion at the aortic bifurcation can produce bilateral findings.
  ◊ Pain: Diffuse in distal area. If persists, crescendo in nature. Predominates as first symptom in embolism. Not alleviated by change of position.
  ◊ Pulselessness: Mandatory for the diagnosis of embolism or thrombosis. Pedal pulses subject to observer error. Always compare to the opposite limb.
  ◊ Pallor: Skin color pale early, cyanotic later. Check extremity temperature left to right and top to bottom. Look for signs of chronic ischemia - skin atrophy, loss of hair, thick nails.
  ◊ Paresthesia: Numbness early with thrombosis. Light touch first to be lost. Not reliable in diabetics. Loss of pain and pressure indicate advanced ischemia.
  ◊ Paralysis: Motor defect occurs after sensory and indicates profound ischemia
• Distribution of emboli
  ◊ Femoral artery 30%
  ◊ Iliac artery 15%
  ◊ Aortic bifurcation 10%
  ◊ Popliteal artery 10%
  ◊ Brachial 10%
  ◊ Mesenteric arteries 5%
  ◊ Renal 5%
  ◊ Cerebral - estimated 15-20%
Level of occlusion
• Palpable pulses
  ◊ Absent below occlusion
  ◊ Accentuated above
• Symptoms typically start one joint below occlusion

CAUSES
• Emboli
  ◊ Cardiac
    - Atrial flutter/fibrillation
    - Valve disease
    - Myocardial infarction
    - Cardiomyopathy
    - Cardiac tumors
    - Endocarditis
  ◊ Aneurysms - cardiac, aortic, peripheral
  ◊ Paradoxical
• Thrombosis:
  ◊ Atherosclerotic occlusive disease
  ◊ Aortic and peripheral aneurysms - especially popliteal
  ◊ Hypercoagulable states
  ◊ Venous gangrene
  ◊ Drug abuse
  ◊ Heparin allergy
  ◊ Vascular bypass
• Trauma:
  ◊ Blunt
  ◊ Penetrating
  ◊ Vascular and cardiac interventional procedures

RISK FACTORS   See Causes

 DIAGNOSIS

DIFFERENTIAL DIAGNOSIS
Emboli vs thrombosis
• Emboli
  ◊ Myocardial diseases - myocardial infarction, arrhythmias - atrial fibrillation
  ◊ Aneurysms
  ◊ Pain as first symptom
• Thrombosis
  ◊ Absence of heart disease - arrhythmias/infarction
  ◊ Chronic vascular history
  ◊ Bilateral changes of chronic ischemia
  ◊ Numbness rather than pain as first symptom
  ◊ Vascular procedures - bypass/interventional
Acute aortic dissection
• Chest or back pain
Acute deep vein thrombosis
• Massive swelling and warm skin
Low flow states

LABORATORY
• Acute diagnosis is by history and exam: Laboratory data is for preoperative evaluation, elucidation of etiology, or documentation of severity of ischemia.
  ◊ EKG
  ◊ Myocardial/muscle isoenzymes
  ◊ Coagulation parameters
  ◊ Blood pH/bicarbonate
  ◊ Urine myoglobin
  ◊ Electrolytes
Drugs that may alter lab results: N/A
Disorders that may alter lab results: N/A

PATHOLOGICAL FINDINGS   N/A

SPECIAL TESTS
• Noninvasive - indirect:
  ◊ Doppler: presence or absence of flow
  ◊ A/ai (ankle/arm index): dorsal pedal/posterior tibial pressure divided by brachial pressure; a/ai > 0.30 favorable
• Noninvasive - direct
  ◊ Duplex imaging if time permits

IMAGING   N/A

DIAGNOSTIC PROCEDURES
• Arteriography
  ◊ Rarely indicated preoperatively in threatened limb
  ◊ May help differentiate thrombosis from embolus in non-threatened limb
  ◊ Useful with occluded grafts

 TREATMENT:

APPROPRIATE HEALTH CARE Based on detailed exam, history, and Doppler exam. Triage determines appropriate therapy.
• Viable
  ◊ Mild ischemic pain
  ◊ Normal neurologic exam
  ◊ Capillary refill present
  ◊ Arterial signals present by Doppler in distal extremity
  ◊ A/ai > 0.30
• Threatened
  ◊ Ischemic pain
  ◊ Mild neurologic deficit
    - Weakness of dorsiflexion
    - Minimal sensory loss - light touch and/or vibratory
  ◊ No pulsatile flow by Doppler
  ◊ Venous flow present
• Major ischemic changes - irreversible
  ◊ Profound sensory loss
  ◊ Muscle paralysis
  ◊ Absent capillary refill
  ◊ Skin marbling
  ◊ Muscle rigor
  ◊ No arterial or venous signals by Doppler

GENERAL MEASURES
• Time is of the essence
• In the threatened category nothing should delay appropriate therapy
• Unless contraindicated, systemic heparinization to decrease clot propagation and prophylaxis against further emboli
• Resuscitation and stabilization of patient to extent permitted by time

Viable - symptomatic
- Heparin (see Medications)
- Arteriography
- Embolism
  ◊ Surgical removal if acceptable operative risk, e.g., balloon embolectomy
  ◊ Anticoagulation vs intraarterial urokinase if prohibitive risk
- Thrombosis
  ◊ Trial of thrombolytics and correction of arterial defect if good risk
  ◊ Anticoagulation if poor risk or thrombolytics contraindicated

Threatened - salvageable
- Heparin (see Medications)
- Minimal delay to definitive therapy
- Arteriography
- Individualized thrombolysis and/or operative procedure (depending on extent of thrombosis and amenability for surgical removal)
- Thrombolysis to optimize alternatives
- Adjunctive operative therapy
  ◊ Intraoperative lytic therapy
  ◊ Bypass
  ◊ Patch angioplasty

Major ischemia - irreversible
- Arteriography usually not warranted
- Attempts at reperfusion contraindicated
- Anticoagulation
- Definitive amputation if possible

SURGICAL MEASURES See General Measures

ACTIVITY N/A

DIET N/A

PATIENT EDUCATION N/A

MEDICATIONS

DRUG(S) OF CHOICE
- Heparin
  ◊ 100 units/kg IV loading dose (approx 5,000-10,000 units)
  ◊ Continuous heparin infusion sufficient to double the PTT, generally 1000 to 1500 units/hour

Contraindications:
- Heparin:
  ◊ Allergy
  ◊ Bleeding diathesis
  ◊ Trauma (e.g., head injury)
  ◊ Hematuria/hemoptysis
  ◊ Acute aortic dissection
- Urokinase:
  ◊ Non-salvageable ischemia
  ◊ Recent MI
  ◊ Aneurysm
  ◊ Aortic dissection
  ◊ Stroke (CVA)
  ◊ Trauma
  ◊ Uncontrolled hypertension
  ◊ Recent operative procedure

Precautions: N/A
Significant possible interactions: N/A

ALTERNATIVE DRUGS
- Urokinase

FOLLOWUP

PATIENT MONITORING
Post operative monitoring:
- Anticoagulation
- Establish brisk diuresis
- Continued resuscitation and diagnosis
  ◊ Echocardiography
  ◊ See causes and risk factors
- Monitor perfusion stability
- Treat/eliminate causative factors

PREVENTION/AVOIDANCE
- Chronic anticogulation in atrial arrhythmia
- Reduction of risk factors for atherosclerosis

POSSIBLE COMPLICATIONS
- Acidosis
- Myoglobinuria
- Hyperkalemia
- Recurrent occlusion
- Failure to remove clot/obstruction

Compartment syndromes
- Reperfusion syndrome; delayed or instant
- Predisposing factors:
  ◊ Combined arterial injury
  ◊ Profound and prolonged ischemia
  ◊ Hypotension
- Occurs both in upper and lower extremities
- Clinical findings
  ◊ Severe pain
  ◊ Pain with passive muscle movement
  ◊ Hypesthesias of nerves in compartment
  ◊ Paralysis of nerves especially peroneal - foot drop
  ◊ Tender, tense edema
  ◊ Compartment pressure > 30-45 mm Hg
- Consequences of unrecognized compartment syndrome - acute
  ◊ Amputation
  ◊ Sepsis
  ◊ Myoglobin renal failure
  ◊ Shock
  ◊ Multiple organ failure
- Delayed
  ◊ Ischemic contracture
  ◊ Infection
  ◊ Causalgia
  ◊ Gangrene
- Treatment
  ◊ Vigilance
  ◊ Recognition
  ◊ Fasciotomy

EXPECTED COURSE/PROGNOSIS
- 90% good outcome with prompt treatment
- Delayed/untreated associated with high mortality and limb loss
- 20-30% hospital mortality associated with causative factors

MISCELLANEOUS

ASSOCIATED CONDITIONS
- Acute mesenteric ischemia
- Renal infarction
- Carotid/CVA
- Multiple emboli
- Digital microembolization

AGE-RELATED FACTORS
Pediatric: Rare in children
Geriatric: Most common age affected
Others: N/A

PREGNANCY Rare

SYNONYMS N/A

ICD-9-CM
- 444.0 Arterial embolism and thrombosis of abdominal aorta
- 444.21 Arterial embolism and thrombosis of upper extremity
- 444.22 Arterial embolism and thrombosis of lower extremity
- 444.81 Arterial embolism and thrombosis of iliac artery
- 444.9 Arterial embolism and thrombosis of unspecified artery

SEE ALSO N/A

OTHER NOTES N/A

ABBREVIATIONS
A/ai = Ankle/arm index

REFERENCES
- Rutherford RB, Flannigan DP, Gupta SK, et al: Suggested standards of reports dealing with lower extremity ischemia. J Vasc Surg 1986;64:80-94
- Brewster DC, Chin AK, Fogarty TJ: Arterial Thrombosis. In: Rutherford RB, ed. Vascular Surgery. 3rd Ed. Philadelphia, W.B. Saunders Co., 1989
- Miller DC., Roon AJ, eds: Diagnosis and Management of Peripheral Vascular Diseases. Menlo Park, CA., Addison-Wesley Co., 1982
Illustrations: N/A
Internet references: http://www.5mcc.com

Author(s)
David H. Stubbs, MD, FACS

Arterial gas embolism

BASICS

DESCRIPTION Air released from an over-pressurized alveolus enters the pulmonary capillaries then travels through the arterial circulation causing occlusion of the cerebral and/or coronary circulation.
• Arterial gas embolism is the most serious and rapidly fatal of all SCUBA diving injuries and is second only to drowning as the leading cause of death associated with sport diving.
• Arterial gas embolism occurs on ascent and the time from alveolar rupture to the manifestation of symptoms is nearly always less than ten minutes.
Incidence/Prevalence in USA: It is estimated (based on injury/mortality reports collected by Divers Alert Network) to occur in approximately 4 per 100,000 sport divers per year.
System(s) affected: Cardiovascular, Nervous, Musculoskeletal
Genetics: N/A
Predominant age: Young adult
Predominant sex: Male > Female

SIGNS AND SYMPTOMS
• Group 1: Neurologic symptoms only. Divers presenting with neurologic symptoms but without impairment of spontaneous respirations and cardiac function. May be impossible to clinically distinguish from severe decompression sickness.
  ◊ Asymmetrical multiplegia or paralysis
  ◊ Tingling or numbness
  ◊ Blindness or other visual disturbances
  ◊ Deafness
  ◊ Vertigo
  ◊ Dizziness
  ◊ Headache
  ◊ Confusion
  ◊ Convulsions
  ◊ Aphasia
  ◊ Personality change; from subtle changes to unconsciousness
• Group 2: Loss of consciousness, apnea, and cardiac arrest or dysrhythmia. Divers presenting with both neurologic and cardiac impairments. All of the above signs and symptoms plus those below are possible.
  ◊ Dysrhythmias
  ◊ Cardiac arrest

CAUSES
• Group 1: Localized obstruction of cerebral blood flow by an embolus of air. Local capillary endothelial damage with vasogenic edema leading to a rise in intracranial pressure and ischemia.
• Group 2: This is thought to be due to localized obstruction of both cerebral and coronary blood flow by an embolus of air

RISK FACTORS
• History of a rapid ascent
• History of panic during dive
• History of holding breath while diving
• History of loss of consciousness (or with other noted symptoms) within seconds to minutes after or during a dive

DIAGNOSIS

DIFFERENTIAL DIAGNOSIS
Decompression sickness

LABORATORY
• Hematocrit - increased indicating volume depletion
• Urinalysis - increased specific gravity indicating volume depletion
Drugs that may alter lab results: N/A
Disorders that may alter lab results: N/A

PATHOLOGICAL FINDINGS N/A

SPECIAL TESTS
• ECG

IMAGING
• Chest x-ray to rule out pneumothorax

DIAGNOSTIC PROCEDURES N/A

TREATMENT

APPROPRIATE HEALTH CARE
• Hospital based hyperbaric chamber capable of performing a U.S. Navy Table 6A recompression (165 fsw).

GENERAL MEASURES
• Immediate transport to a suitable hyperbaric chamber for recompression as soon as possible; do not delay with nonessential procedures.
• Transport by aircraft is justifiable if it will save a significant amount of time (aircraft must fly at low altitudes or be capable of maintaining cabin pressure at about one atmosphere)
• Life-saving measures (CPR) must take precedence to sustain life
• Administration of high flow maximum concentration oxygen therapy by a tight fitting mask or by intubation and mechanical ventilation during transport
• Keep patient in recumbent position while maintaining airway
• Maintain hydration with IV fluids
• For assistance and advice in locating the nearest treatment chamber in your area (world-wide) call DIVERS ALERT NETWORK (DAN) at any hour (919) 684-8111

SURGICAL MEASURES N/A

ACTIVITY None until after treatment

DIET None until after treatment

PATIENT EDUCATION DIVERS ALERT NETWORK (DAN) Non-Emergency Information Line (Mon-Fri 9-5 EST) (919)684-2948; membership line (800)446-2671

MEDICATIONS

DRUG(S) OF CHOICE None
Contraindications: N/A
Precautions: N/A
Significant possible interactions: N/A

ALTERNATIVE DRUGS None

FOLLOWUP

PATIENT MONITORING
• Frequent neurological checks in the acute pre-treatment and treatment phase
• Complete neurological assessment at one, three, six and twelve at months

PREVENTION/AVOIDANCE
• Strict adherence to diver safety protocols
• No diving after any dive injury or with any medical condition until evaluated and approved by a physician knowledgeable in diving medicine

POSSIBLE COMPLICATIONS
• Long term serious neurologic impairments
• Death

EXPECTED COURSE/PROGNOSIS
• Complete to partial resolution with adequate treatment

MISCELLANEOUS

ASSOCIATED CONDITIONS
• Pulmonary barotrauma leading to arterial gas embolism, can also cause pneumomediastinum, subcutaneous emphysema, pneumopericardium, pneumothorax, and pneumoperitoneum
• Always consider the possibility of decompression sickness in addition to arterial gas embolism in any SCUBA diver who has recently completed a dive

AGE-RELATED FACTORS
Pediatric: N/A
Geriatric: N/A
Others: N/A

PREGNANCY N/A

SYNONYMS
• Gas embolism
• Air embolism

ICD-9-CM
• 958.0 (any site)

SEE ALSO
• Decompression sickness

OTHER NOTES
• Any diver who has an onset of new symptom(s) or sign(s) after recently completing a SCUBA dive of any type, to any depth, for any period of time - serious consideration must be given as having sustained a dive related injury

ABBREVIATIONS
• DAN = Divers Alert Network
• AGE = arterial gas embolism

REFERENCES
• Shilling CW, ed: The Physicians Guide to Diving Medicine. New York, Plenum Press, 1984
• Strauss RH: Diving Medicine. Philadelphia, W.B. Saunders Co., 1976
Illustrations: N/A
Internet references: http://www.5mcc.com

Author(s)
Jess G. Bond, MD, MPH

Arteriosclerotic heart disease

BASICS

DESCRIPTION Arteriosclerosis means thickening of the arterial wall, along with loss of elasticity, that progressively blocks the coronary arteries and their main branches. The process is chronic, occurring over many years, and is the most common cause of cardiovascular disability and death. Elevated total serum cholesterol and low-density lipoproteins are involved in the development of arteriosclerosis as well as the process of aging and anatomic changes.
System(s) affected: Cardiovascular
Genetics: Tendency is inheritable
Incidence/Prevalence: Common. Causes 35% of deaths in men age 35-50. Death rate age 55-64 - 1:100.
Predominant age: Men 50-60, women 60-70, for peak clinical manifestations
Predominant sex: Male > Female

SIGNS AND SYMPTOMS
• May remain clinically silent, even in advanced stages, and in some instances of ischemia
• Clinical manifestations
  ◊ Substernal chest pain
  ◊ Exertional dyspnea
  ◊ Orthopnea
  ◊ Paroxysmal nocturnal dyspnea
  ◊ Extrasystoles
  ◊ Irregular rhythm
  ◊ Tachycardia
  ◊ Systolic murmur
  ◊ Cardiomegaly
  ◊ Pedal edema

CAUSES
• Atherosclerosis
• Narrowing of coronary arteries
• Embolism compromising coronary arteries at orifices
• Subintimal atheromas in large and medium vessels

RISK FACTORS
• Elevated low density lipoprotein (LDL)
• Decreased high density lipoprotein (HDL)
• Elevated triglycerides
• Smoking
• Family history of premature arteriosclerosis
• Obesity
• Hypertension
• Stress
• Sedentary life style
• Increasing age
• Male sex
• Female postmenopausal
• Diabetes mellitus

DIAGNOSIS

DIFFERENTIAL DIAGNOSIS N/A

LABORATORY
• Elevated triglycerides
• Elevated total cholesterol
• Elevated low density lipoproteins
• Decreased high density lipoproteins
Drugs that may alter lab results: N/A
Disorders that may alter lab results: N/A

PATHOLOGICAL FINDINGS
• Gross - narrowed coronary arteries
• Micro - cholesterol plaques on intima of coronary vessels
• Fibrotic subendothelial connective tissue of intima with plaque

SPECIAL TESTS
• ECG - ST segment depression, inverted T waves
• Exercise stress test - positive

IMAGING
• Stress thallium test - positive
• Angiography - narrowed coronary arteries
• Echocardiography
• Stress tests with and without contrast

DIAGNOSTIC PROCEDURES N/A

TREATMENT

APPROPRIATE HEALTH CARE
• Outpatient
• Inpatient for acute ischemic syndromes

GENERAL MEASURES
• Prevention of further progression of the disease
  ◊ Stop smoking (stop smoking programs, drugs)
  ◊ Treatment of hypercholesterolemia (diet, drugs)
  ◊ Increase high density lipoprotein (diet, exercise)
  ◊ Control of blood pressure
  ◊ Diabetes mellitus treated early and adequately
  ◊ Exercise
  ◊ Prophylactic aspirin
  ◊ Stress reduction
  ◊ Diet changes
  ◊ Weight loss
  ◊ Estrogen replacement therapy in postmenopausal women
• Treatment of complications
  ◊ Covered elsewhere under the individual topics (e.g., angina pectoris, myocardial infarction, heart failure, stroke, peripheral arterial occlusion, etc.)

SURGICAL MEASURES N/A

ACTIVITY Exercise may be helpful in preventing clinical coronary disease and useful for therapeutic measures

DIET
• Low-fat (20-30 grams of fat/day total intake)
• Weight-loss diet, if obesity a problem
• Increase soluble fiber

PATIENT EDUCATION For patient education materials favorably reviewed on this topic, contact: American Heart Association, 7320 Greenville Avenue, Dallas, TX 75231, (214)373-6300

MEDICATIONS

DRUG(S) OF CHOICE
• Aspirin, one 325 mg tablet/day unless contraindicated
• Cholesterol-lowering agents
  ◊ Cholestyramine or colestipol, (bile acid sequestrants) 12-32 gm orally BID-QID
  ◊ Nicotinic acid 2-6 gm daily in divided doses (may be helpful, but side effects restrict its use)
  ◊ Gemfibrozil 600 mg bid
  ◊ Probucol 500 mg bid
  ◊ HMG-CoA reductase inhibitors 20-80 mg daily; pravastatin (Pravachol), lovastatin (Mevacor), fluvastatin (Lescol)
Contraindications: Refer to manufacturer's literature
Precautions: SR form of niacin may be linked to hepatotoxicity. Refer to manufacturer's literature.
Significant possible interactions: Refer to manufacturer's literature

ALTERNATIVE DRUGS
• Ticlopidine - antiplatelet activity

FOLLOWUP

PATIENT MONITORING Monitor cholesterol, triglyceride levels, other preventive programs (weight loss, smoking cessation)

PREVENTION/AVOIDANCE See General measures

POSSIBLE COMPLICATIONS
• Myocardial infarction
• Ventricular fibrillation
• Congestive heart failure
• Angina pectoris
• Sudden cardiac death

EXPECTED COURSE/PROGNOSIS
Guardedly favorable. Many risk factors can be modified.

MISCELLANEOUS

ASSOCIATED CONDITIONS
• Obesity
• Hypertension
• Diabetes
• Hypercholesterolemia

AGE-RELATED FACTORS
Pediatric: Preventive measures can begin early (proper nutrition, exercise, weight control, smoking deterrent programs, etc.)
Geriatric: Greatest incidence in this age group
Others: N/A

PREGNANCY Practically non-existent in pregnant women

SYNONYMS
• Coronary artery disease (CAD)
• Coronary heart disease
• Coronary arteriosclerosis

ICD-9-CM 414.0 arteriosclerotic heart disease

SEE ALSO
• Angina
• Myocardial infarction

OTHER NOTES N/A

ABBREVIATIONS N/A

REFERENCES
• Hurst JW, et al: The Heart. 7th Ed. New York, McGraw-Hill, 1990
• Braunwald E. ed: Heart Disease: A Textbook of Cardiovascular Medicine. 4th Ed. Philadelphia, W.B. Saunders Co., 1992
Illustrations: N/A
Internet references: http://www.5mcc.com

Author(s)
Peter Kozisek, MD

Arthritis, infectious, bacterial

BASICS

DESCRIPTION Invasion of joints by live micro-organisms or their fragments. One of the few curable causes of arthritis. May allow early recognition of systemic infection/disease.

System(s) affected: Musculoskeletal
Genetics: N/A
Incidence/Prevalence in USA:
• Neisserial:
  ◊ Responsible for 50% of infectious arthritis
  ◊ Arthritis occurs in 0.6% of the 3% of women with gonorrhea
  ◊ Arthritis occurs in 0.1% of the 0.7% of men with gonorrhea
  ◊ Arthritis occurs in 7% of individuals with N. meningitidis
• Non-Neisserial:
  ◊ Perhaps half as frequent as Neisserial
Predominant age:
• Neisserial:
  ◊ Especially 15-40, can occur at any age
• Non-Neisserial:
  ◊ 50% Prior to age 2: 27% Staphylococcus, 20% Streptococcus, 33% Haemophilus, and 13% other gram negative rods
  ◊ 70% Age 2-14: 34% Staphylococcus, 29% Streptococcus, 13% Haemophilus, and 13% other gram negative rods
  ◊ Adult: 34% Staphylococcus, 38% Streptococcus, 2% Haemophilus, and 26% other gram negative rods
Predominant sex:
• Neisserial: Female > Male (4:1)
• Non-Neisserial: Male > Female (2:1)
• Subacute bacterial endocarditis-related: Male = Female

SIGNS AND SYMPTOMS
• Predominantly monoarticular (90%). (Haemophilus may be pauciarticular and Mycoplasma often presents as a migratory polyarthritis).
• Limited joint use/motion (especially in children)
• Joint effusion, tenderness
• Joint warmth - present in less than 50%
• Joint redness- present in less than 50%
• Loss of joint motion
• Tenosynovitis
• Sudden flare of one or two joints in a patient with underlying joint disease
• Fever - in 90% at some time during the course of the infection
• Chills, malaise
• Cutaneous lesions
• Peripheral neuropathy
• Back pain - especially in subacute bacterial endocarditis (SBE)
• Hypertrophic osteoarthropathy - rare, secondary to endocarditis
• Fretfulness - especially in children
• Dermato-arthritis - usually pustular skin lesions in gonorrhea - usually petechial rash in meningococcemia
• Bacteremic phase - migratory polyarthritis, tenosynovitis, high fever, chills, pustules
• Localized phase - usually monoarticular, low grade fever (80%)

CAUSES
• Hematogenous invasion by micro-organisms (80-90%)
• Contiguous spread (10-15%) from adjacent osteomyelitis in children
• Direct penetration of micro-organisms secondary to trauma or joint injection

RISK FACTORS
• Young patient with venereal exposure
• Concurrent extra-articular infection
• Prior arthritis in infected joint
• Rheumatoid arthritis
• Trauma
• Joint puncture or surgery
• Prosthetic joint
• Prior antibiotic, corticosteroid, or immunosuppressive therapy
• Serious chronic illness (e.g., diabetes, liver disease, malignancy, primary immunodeficiency)
• Defective phagocytic mechanisms (e.g., chronic granulomatous disease)
• Intravenous drug abuse
• Travel/habitat history
• Sickle cell anemia

DIAGNOSIS

DIFFERENTIAL DIAGNOSIS
• Gout
• Pseudogout (calcium pyrophosphate deposition disease)
• Spondyloarthropathy (Reiter's syndrome, psoriatic arthritis, ankylosing spondylitis, the arthritis of inflammatory bowel disease)
• Juvenile rheumatoid arthritis
• Type IIa hyperlipoproteinemia
• Foreign body synovitis
• Rheumatoid arthritis
• Rheumatic fever
• AIDS
• Cellulitis
• Palindromic rheumatism
• Neuropathic arthropathy
• Lyme arthritis
• Sarcoidosis
• Granulomatous arthritis

LABORATORY
• Synovial fluid usually cloudy with > 50,000 WBC/HPF, but may have fewer white blood cells present or over 100,000. (Caveat - cell count must be performed within 1 hour of obtaining specimen to be valid).
• Synovial fluid white count can be recognized as elevated (in presence of trauma) if RBC:WBC ratio significantly less than 700
• Polymorphonuclear leukocytes usually predominate in synovial fluid
• Synovial fluid glucose often more than 40 mg/dL (2.22 mmol/L) less than in a simultaneously obtained serum glucose value (in fasting patient). However, arthrocentesis should not be delayed simply to obtain fasting synovial fluid glucose level.
• Westergren erythrocyte sedimentation rate - often elevated, but normal in 20%

• Rheumatoid factor positive in 50% - if endocarditis present and in viral arthritis
• Anti-techoic acid antibodies - with Staphylococcus infection
• Elevated peripheral white blood cell count (in 50-90%)
• Cryoglobulins
• Immune complexes
• Febrile agglutinins (to include Brucella and rickettsial-related titers)
• Antistreptolysin O (ASO) titer is usually normal, exclusive of streptococcal infections
• Depressed synovial fluid and occasionally depressed serum levels of complement
• Microscopic hematuria in subacute bacterial endocarditis (SBE)
• Presence of crystals (e.g., urate or calcium pyrophosphate) does not exclude infectious arthritis
Drugs that may alter lab results:
Antibiotics
Disorders that may alter lab results: N/A

PATHOLOGICAL FINDINGS Synovial biopsy will reveal polymorphonuclear leukocytes and possibly the causative organism

SPECIAL TESTS
• Joint fluid - for gram stain (positive in 50%); culture (positive in 50-70%)
• Serum cidal level assessment of antibiotic adequacy is suggested with virulent organisms or therapeutic unresponsiveness (tenfold margin suggested)
• Blood, orifice, urine cultures. "Bedside culture" is recommended to enhance isolation of fastidious organisms.
• All cultures should be preserved and observed for at least 3 days and preferably 2 weeks. Observing synovial fluid cultures for at least 3 days allows isolation of fastidious organisms such as those of rat bite fever (Streptobacillus moniliformis and Spirillum minus).
• Neisserial infection generally requires use of special agars (e.g., chocolate or Thayer Martin) and relative anaerobic culturing conditions
• Countercurrent immunoelectrophoresis or complement fixation for specific bacterial antigens
• Polymerase chain reaction for specific bacterial DNA

IMAGING
• X-ray
  ◊ Soft tissue swelling
  ◊ Juxta-articular osteoporosis
  ◊ Radiolucent area (gas) in a joint space from gas forming organisms. (Caveat - may also occur normally as a "vacuum phenomenon").
  ◊ Effacement of the obturator fat pad (with hip involvement)
  ◊ X-ray changes are usually a late phenomenon
  ◊ Rarefaction of subchondral bone may occur as early as 2-7 days
  ◊ Joint space loss (secondary to cartilage destruction) may be seen as early as 4-10 days
  ◊ Erosions
  ◊ Joint destruction with ankylosis may occur as early as 2 weeks

• Other imaging techniques
◊ Technetium joint scans - reveal distribution of inflammation
◊ Gallium or Ceretec WBC scan-Indium scans - reveal inflammation as well as infection
◊ CT - to identify sequestration
◊ MRI - effusion, perhaps early cartilage damage, osteomyelitis

DIAGNOSTIC PROCEDURES
• Arthrocentesis with gram stain and culture - only positive in 50-70%. Must be done in all patients when possibility of infectious arthritis is considered. Arthrocentesis should probably be performed within 12 hours of suspicion.
• Arthrocentesis approach must avoid contaminated tissue (e.g., overlying cellulitis)

TREATMENT

APPROPRIATE HEALTH CARE
• Hospitalization for parenteral therapy
• Rarely an extremely compliant patient with a very sensitive organism might be treated as an outpatient

GENERAL MEASURES
• Repeat arthrocentesis to drain the joint, as fluid re-accumulates
• Avoid adding anti-inflammatory therapy so as not to compromise assessment of therapeutic response to antibiotic
• If a joint prosthesis is present in an infection, the infection is very difficult to eradicate, without removal of the prosthesis
• Treatment is continued for 1-2 weeks after total resolution of all signs of inflammation, 3-4 weeks for gram negative organisms, and 6-8 weeks if the joint was previously diseased (e.g., involved by arthritis)
• Intra-articular antibiotics are not required and may actually aggravate the arthritis

SURGICAL MEASURES Arthrotomy
indicated only if fluid accumulated is loculated and/or not amenable to needle drainage

ACTIVITY Limit activity or splint the joint
initially. Continuous passive motion may be used as an alternative approach.

DIET No special diet

PATIENT EDUCATION
• Rothschild, B.: Diagnosing and treating infectious arthritis. Geriatric Consultant. 5:14-15, 1986
• Arthritis Foundation pamphlet

MEDICATIONS

DRUG(S) OF CHOICE
• Neisserial
◊ Ceftriaxone 1 gm IM or IV every day for 14

days (but at least 7 days after symptoms resolve)
or
◊ Spectinomycin 2 gm IM every 12 hours for 10 days
• Non-Neisserial:
◊ Gram positive cocci in chains or clumps - nafcillin 150 mg/kg/day q 4-6 h IV/IM
◊ Gram positive diplococci - penicillin G 1.4 million units q6h
◊ Gram negative bacilli: In neonates - penicillin and gentamicin; in children age 6 months to 4 years - cefuroxime; in adult - penicillin or cephalosporin plus gentamicin, all at full dose. Add clindamycin, at full dose, in the presence of retroperitoneal or pelvic abscess.
◊ Gram negative pleomorphic organisms - clindamycin at full dose (clindamycin has gram negative activity only against anaerobes)
◊ No bacteria seen on smear - penicillin or cephalosporin plus gentamicin, all at full dose
Contraindications:
• Tetracycline: not for use in pregnancy or children < 8 years.
Precautions:
• Observe for allergic reactions/serum sickness
• Tetracycline: may cause photosensitivity; sunscreen recommended.
Significant possible interactions:
• Tetracycline: avoid concurrent administration with antacids, dairy products, or iron.
• Broad-spectrum antibiotics: may reduce the effectiveness of oral contraceptives; barrier method recommended.

ALTERNATIVE DRUGS
• Non-Neisserial
◊ In children age 6 months to 4 years - ampicillin [Chloramphenicol may be required to cover resistant Haemophilus]
◊ Infectious disease consult strongly advised to supplement rheumatologist input for Haemophilus infections
• Quinolones (e.g., ciprofloxacin)

FOLLOWUP

PATIENT MONITORING
• Recurrent arthrocentesis, as fluid re-accumulates - to verify sterilization of the joint and to verify reversion of inflammatory signs to normal
• If no definitive improvement within 48 hours, re-evaluate completely
• Complete blood count, liver and kidney function and urinalysis twice a week, while on antibiotics (perhaps with creatinine every other day when gentamicin used)
• Gentamycin levels
• It is essential to followup one week and a month after stopping antibiotics to detect any relapse

PREVENTION/AVOIDANCE
• Prophylaxis in presence of predisposing joint condition
• Condoms and discretion for STD protection

POSSIBLE COMPLICATIONS
• Death (9-33% in elderly, especially with gram negative organisms)
• Limited joint range of motion
• Flail or fused or dislocated joint
• Carpal tunnel syndrome
• Septic necrosis
• Sinus formation
• Ankylosis
• Osteomyelitis
• Postinfectious synovitis
• Shortening of the limb (in children)

EXPECTED COURSE/PROGNOSIS
• Early treatment should allow cure
• Delayed recognition/treatment complicated by morbidity and mortality

MISCELLANEOUS

ASSOCIATED CONDITIONS
• Systemic infection
• Infection elsewhere
• Immunodeficiency
• Immunosuppression

AGE-RELATED FACTORS
Pediatric: N/A
Geriatric: N/A
Others: N/A

PREGNANCY N/A

SYNONYMS
• Suppurative arthritis
• Septic arthritis

ICD-9-CM
711.9

SEE ALSO
• Reiter's syndrome
• Lyme disease

OTHER NOTES N/A

ABBREVIATIONS
HPF = high power field

REFERENCES
• Rothschild BM: Infectious Arthritis. Fairlawn, CT, Clinical AV, 1982
• Rothschild BM, Martin L: Paleopathology: Disease in the Fossil Record. London, CRC Press, 1993
• Kelly WW, Harris ED Jr, Rudd S, Sledge CB: Textbook of Rheumatology. Philadelphia, W.B. Saunders Co., 1993
• Gershwin ME, Robbins DL: Musculoskeletal Diseases of Children, New York, Grune & Stratton, 1983
Illustrations: N/A
Internet references: http://www.5mcc.com

Author(s)
Bruce M. Rothschild, MD

Arthritis, infectious, granulomatous

BASICS

DESCRIPTION Invasion of joints by live micro-organisms or their fragments. One of the few curable causes of arthritis. May allow early recognition of systemic infection/disease.
System(s) affected: Musculoskeletal
Genetics: N/A
Incidence/Prevalence in USA:
• One in three million
• Granulomatous arthritis occurs in 1-3% of patients with tuberculosis infections
Predominant age: Diffuse
Predominant sex:
• Male > Female (Brucella and mycobacterial)
• Female > Male (fungal)

SIGNS AND SYMPTOMS
• Predominantly monoarticular (90%). Fungal may present as a migratory polyarthritis.
• Joint tenderness
• Limited joint use/motion (especially in children)
• Joint effusion
• Joint warmth - present in less than 50%
• Joint redness - present in less than 50%
• Loss of joint motion
• Tenosynovitis
• Sudden flare of a single joint in a patient with underlying joint disease
• Fever - in 50% at some time during the course of the infection
• Chills
• Malaise
• Cutaneous lesions
• Peripheral neuropathy
• Back pain - especially in tuberculosis and brucellosis
• Hypertrophic osteoarthropathy
• Fretfulness - especially in children
• Doughy swelling, with minimal tenderness
• Dactylitis
• Diaphoresis
• Headache
• Hepatosplenomegaly
• Lymphadenopathy
• Erythema nodosum
• Iritis (with mycobacterial arthritis)

CAUSES
• Hematogenous invasion by microorganisms (80-90%)
• Contiguous spread (10-15%)
• Direct penetration of micro-organisms secondary to trauma

RISK FACTORS
• Concurrent acquired immunodeficiency disease
• Concurrent extra-articular infection
• Prior arthritis in infected joint
• Trauma
• Rheumatoid arthritis
• Joint puncture or surgery
• Prosthetic joint
• Prior antibiotic, corticosteroid, or immunosuppressive therapy
• Serious chronic illness (e.g., diabetes, liver disease, malignancy, primary immunodeficiency)
• Defective phagocytic mechanisms (e.g., chronic granulomatous disease)
• Intravenous drug abuse
• Exposure history (e.g., unpasteurized milk)
• Farmers, butchers, veterinarians
• Travel/habitat history
• Gardening, especially for sporotrichosis

DIAGNOSIS

DIFFERENTIAL DIAGNOSIS
• Gout
• Pseudogout (calcium pyrophosphate deposition disease)
• Spondyloarthropathy (Reiter's syndrome, psoriatic arthritis, ankylosing spondylitis, the arthritis of inflammatory bowel disease)
• Juvenile rheumatoid arthritis
• Type IIa hyperlipoproteinemia
• Foreign body synovitis
• Rheumatoid arthritis
• Rheumatic fever
• AIDS
• Cellulitis
• Palindromic rheumatism
• Neuropathic arthropathy
• Lyme arthritis
• Sarcoidosis
• Pyogenic arthritis

LABORATORY
• Synovial fluid usually cloudy with > 20,000 WBC/HPF, but may have fewer white blood cells present or over 100,000. (Caveat - cell count must be performed within 1 hour of obtaining specimen to be valid).
• Synovial fluid white count can be recognized as elevated (in presence of trauma) if RBC:WBC ratio significantly less than 700
• Polymorphonuclear leukocytes usually predominate in synovial fluid. (Granulomatous and viral arthritis may have a mononuclear cell predominance, but polymorphonuclear leukocytes usually predominate).
• Synovial fluid glucose often more than 40 mg/dL (2.22 mmol/L) less than in a simultaneously obtained serum glucose value (in fasting patient). However, arthrocentesis should not be delayed simply to obtain fasting synovial fluid glucose level.
• Synovial fluid eosinophilia may occasionally be seen in the healing phase of an infection, but parasitic (e.g., guinea-worm) infection must also be considered
• Westergren erythrocyte sedimentation - often elevated, but normal in 20%
• Rheumatoid factor positive in 50% - if endocarditis present
• Elevated peripheral white blood cell count
• Cryoglobulins
• Immune complexes
• Febrile agglutinins (to include Brucella and rickettsial related titers)
• Antistreptolysin O (ASO) titer is usually normal
• Depressed synovial fluid and occasionally serum levels of complement
• Presence of crystals in urine (e.g., urate or calcium pyrophosphate) does not exclude infectious arthritis
• Polymerase chain reaction for specific microorganisms
Drugs that may alter lab results: Insulin, antibiotics
Disorders that may alter lab results: Diabetes

PATHOLOGICAL FINDINGS Synovial biopsy may reveal granulomas and possibly the causative organism

SPECIAL TESTS
• Arthrocentesis - bacterial - for silver and acid fast stain and culture
• Arthrocentesis - mycobacterial - acid fast (positive in 20%); culture (positive in 80%)
• Drug sensitivity testing recommended
• Blood, urine cultures
• Sputum cultures
• Gastric lavage for acid fast - increases yield 7%
• Fungal blood cultures
• All cultures should be held for 3 days, preferably 2 weeks. (Observing synovial fluid cultures for at least 3 days allows isolation of fastidious organisms. Acid-fast cultures are held 6 weeks

IMAGING
• X-ray
  ◊ Soft tissue swelling
  ◊ Osteoporosis
  ◊ Effacement of the obturator fat pad (with hip involvement) or psoas shadow
  ◊ X-ray changes are usually a late phenomenon
  ◊ Rarefaction of subchondral bone
  ◊ Joint space loss
  ◊ Erosions
  ◊ Joint destruction with ankylosis
  ◊ Subchondral erosion with preservation of joint space is highly suggestive of granulomatous infection
• Other imaging techniques
  ◊ Technetium joint scans - reveal distribution of inflammation
  ◊ Gallium or Ceretec WBC scan-Indium scans - reveal inflammation as well as infection
  ◊ Computerized tomography - to identify sequestration
  ◊ Magnetic resonance imaging - perhaps early cartilage damage, osteomyelitis

DIAGNOSTIC PROCEDURES
• Arthrocentesis with gram, silver and acid fast stain, and culture. Must be done in all patients when possibility of infectious arthritis considered.
• Arthrocentesis approach must avoid contaminated tissue (e.g., overlying cellulitis)

TREATMENT

APPROPRIATE HEALTH CARE
• Fungal - initial hospitalization for parenteral therapy
• Mycobacterial - outpatient, once diagnosed
• Brucella - outpatient, once diagnosed

GENERAL MEASURES
• Repeat arthrocentesis to drain the joint, as fluid reaccumulates
• Avoid adding anti-inflammatory therapy so as not to compromise assessment of therapeutic response (to antibiotic)
• Infection associated with prosthetic joints may be difficult to eradicate without removal
• For Brucella or fungal infections, treatment is continued for 1-2 weeks after total resolution of all signs of inflammation, and 6-8 weeks if the joint was previously diseased (e.g., involved by arthritis)
• Anti-granulomatous therapy requires a long program (See Tuberculosis)
• Intra-articular antibiotics are not indicated
• Infectious disease consultation may be helpful

SURGICAL MEASURES
• Arthrotomy indicated only if fluid accumulated is loculated and/or not amenable to needle drainage

ACTIVITY
Limit/splint joint initially, while pursuing full passive range of motion. Continuous passive motion is an alternative approach.

DIET
As tolerated

PATIENT EDUCATION
• Rothschild, B.M.: Diagnosing and treating infectious arthritis. Geriatric Consultant, 5:14-15, 1986
• Arthritis Foundation
1314 Spring Street, NW
Atlanta, GA 30309
(404) 872-7100

MEDICATIONS

DRUG(S) OF CHOICE
• Medications based on sensitivity of organisms
• Mycobacterial: (use a combination of these three) isoniazid at 5 mg/kg, up to 300 mg po qd, rifampin at 10 mg/kg, up to 600 mg PO qd, and pyrazinamide at 15-30 mg/kg up to 2 gm/d. The latter is replaced after 2 months with ethambutol 15 mg/kg. Continue therapy for 9-24 months. Request infectious disease consultation.
• Brucella: tetracycline plus streptomycin or trimethoprim-sulfamethoxazole or rifampin (for dosage, see manufacturer's literature)
• Fungal infection: amphotericin B, ketoconazole, flucytosine (5-fluorocytosine) and even iodide, dependent upon organism
Contraindications:
• Tetracycline: not for use in pregnancy or children < 8 years.
Precautions:
• Observe for allergic reactions/serum sickness
• Tetracycline: may cause photosensitivity; sunscreen recommended.
Significant possible interactions:
• Tetracycline: avoid concurrent administration with antacids, dairy products, or iron.
• Ketaconazole - multiple drug intractions

ALTERNATIVE DRUGS
• See Tuberculosis

FOLLOWUP

PATIENT MONITORING
To verify sterilization of the joint and to verify reversion of inflammatory signs to normal
• Treatment of mycobacterial arthritis requires monthly complete blood count, liver and kidney function and urinalysis assessment
• It is essential to followup frequently after stopping antibiotics to detect relapse

PREVENTION/AVOIDANCE
Prophylaxis in presence of predisposing joint condition

POSSIBLE COMPLICATIONS
• Limited joint range of motion
• Flail or fused joint
• Carpal-tunnel syndrome
• Septic necrosis
• Sinus formation
• Ankylosis
• Joint dislocation
• Osteomyelitis
• Shortening of the limb (in children)

EXPECTED COURSE/PROGNOSIS
• Early initiation of treatment should allow cure
• Delayed recognition/treatment complicated by increased morbidity and mortality

MISCELLANEOUS

ASSOCIATED CONDITIONS
• Systemic infection
• Infection elsewhere
• Immunodeficiency - (medication)
• Immunosuppression

AGE-RELATED FACTORS
Pediatric: Infrequent
Geriatric:
• Grave in elderly
• Tuberculosis much more likely to occur
Others: N/A

PREGNANCY N/A

SYNONYMS
• Fungal arthritis

ICD-9-CM
• 031.8 Mycobacterial arthritis
• 023.9 Brucellosis, unspecified
• 115.99 Fungal arthritis

SEE ALSO
• Brucellosis
• Atypical mycobacterial infection

OTHER NOTES
Infectious arthritis may be caused by many other organisms including bacterial (particularly neisseria), rickettsial, parasitic, fungal, and viral agents. Much of the information contained in this profile applies to these other organisms as well as to granulomatous infections.

ABBREVIATIONS
HPF = high power field

REFERENCES
• Rothschild BM: Infectious Arthritis. Fairlawn, CT, Clinical AV, 1982
• Gershwin ME, Robbins DL: Musculoskeletal Diseases of Children. New York, Grune & Stratton, 1983
• Rothschild BM, Martin L: Paleopathology: Disease in the Fossil Record. London, CRC Press, 1993
• Kelly WW, Harris ED Jr, Ruddy S, Sledge CB: Textbook of Rheumatology. Philadelphia, W.B. Saunders Co., 1993
Illustrations: N/A
Internet references: http://www.5mcc.com

Author(s)
Bruce M. Rothschild, MD

Arthritis, juvenile rheumatoid (JRA)

BASICS

DESCRIPTION Juvenile rheumatoid arthritis (JRA) is the most common form of chronic arthritis in children and a major cause of musculoskeletal disability. There are three subtypes of the disease, determined by the clinical characteristics occurring within the first six months of illness.
• Systemic (sys) JRA: occurs in 10-20% of affected children; usually characterized by a febrile onset and evanescent rash with multiple physical and laboratory abnormalities
• Polyarticular (poly) JRA: occurs in 30-40% of affected children; characterized by multiple (> 4) joint involvement and minimal systemic features
• Pauciarticular (pauci) JRA: occurs in 40-50% of affected children; characterized by ≤ 4 joints involved, usually larger joints; a risk for chronic uveitis in young girls and axial skeletal involvement in older boys
System(s) affected: Musculoskeletal, Hemic/Lymphatic/Immunologic
Genetics: HLA-B27 histocompatibility antigen associated with risk of evolving spondyloarthropathy in older boys with pauci JRA. Weaker HLA associations exist for other subtypes (HLA-DR5; HLA-DR8; HLA-DR4).
Incidence/Prevalence in USA: Prevalence approximately 1/1000 children; incidence 1/10,000 children
Predominant age: 1-4 years and 9-14 years
Predominant sex: Female > Male

SIGNS AND SYMPTOMS
• Systemic
  ◊ Arthralgias/arthritis
  ◊ Chest pain, pericardial friction rub
  ◊ Dyspnea
  ◊ Fatigue
  ◊ Fever
  ◊ Hepatosplenomegaly
  ◊ Lymphadenopathy
  ◊ Myalgias
  ◊ Rash
  ◊ Weight loss
• Polyarticular
  ◊ Arthralgia/arthritis
  ◊ Cold intolerance
  ◊ Difficulty writing
  ◊ Fatigue
  ◊ Growth retardation
  ◊ Hand weakness
  ◊ Limitation of motion
  ◊ Malaise
  ◊ Morning stiffness
  ◊ Rheumatoid nodules
  ◊ Synovial cysts
  ◊ Synovial thickening
  ◊ Weight loss
• Pauciarticular
  ◊ Abnormal gait
  ◊ Eye pain, redness
  ◊ Joint swelling
  ◊ Leg length abnormality
  ◊ Morning stiffness
  ◊ Photophobia

CAUSES Multifactorial including abnormal immune response, genetic predisposition and environmental triggers, possibly infectious

RISK FACTORS
• HLA-B27 in pauci JRA increases risk for development of spondyloarthropathy
• Rheumatoid factor positivity increases risk for severe arthritis in poly JRA
• ANA positivity increases risk for uveitis in pauci and poly JRA

DIAGNOSIS

DIFFERENTIAL DIAGNOSIS Other rheumatic diseases, especially SLE and dermatomyositis; atypical bacterial or viral infections; hemoglobinopathies; malignancy; vasculitis; rheumatic fever; Lyme disease; post-infectious arthritis; musculoskeletal developmental abnormalities; sympathetic dystrophy

LABORATORY
• WBC normal or markedly elevated (sys)
• Hb normal or low (especially sys)
• Platelet count normal or elevated
• ANA positive, 40% (poly or pauci)
• RF positive, 10-15% (usually polys)
• HLA-B27 positive, 70% in pauci boys
• Sedimentation rate (ESR) elevated in most patients with active disease; > 100 mL/hr (Westergren) in active systemic disease
Drugs that may alter lab results: Anti-inflammatory therapy may alter CBC and ESR
Disorders that may alter lab results: Hemoglobinopathies (ESR)

PATHOLOGICAL FINDINGS Synovium shows hyperplasia of synovial cells, hyperemia and infiltration of small lymphocytes and mononuclear cells

SPECIAL TESTS
• Echocardiography (pericarditis)
• Radionuclide scans (infection, malignancy)

IMAGING
• Early radiographic changes - soft tissue swelling, periosteal reaction, juxta-articular demineralization; later changes include joint space loss, articular surface erosions, subchondral cyst formation, sclerosis and joint fusion
• CT and MRI very helpful in delineating early erosions

DIAGNOSTIC PROCEDURES
• Joint fluid aspiration and analysis helpful in excluding infection
• Synovial biopsy occasionally indicated in persistent, atypical monoarthritis

TREATMENT

APPROPRIATE HEALTH CARE
• Outpatient care except for initial diagnostic workup of systemic JRA disease and complications for all subtypes
• Patients require regular (every 4 months in patients with pauciarticular disease) ophthalmic exams to uncover asymptomatic eye disease .

GENERAL MEASURES Physical therapy including daily home exercise program required for joints with limited motion; moist heat, sleeping bag or electric blanket to relieve morning stiffness

SURGICAL MEASURES Total hip replacement for severe disease may be needed

ACTIVITY
• Full activity as tolerated
• Regular school. May need modified physical education program.

DIET Regular diet with special attention to adequate calcium, iron, protein and caloric intake

PATIENT EDUCATION
• Ongoing education of patients and families needed with special attention to psychosocial needs, behavioral strategies for dealing with pain and noncompliance, and utilization of health care resources
• Printed and audio-visual information available from local Arthritis Foundation

Arthritis, juvenile rheumatoid (JRA)

MEDICATIONS

DRUG(S) OF CHOICE
• First-line:
◊ Nonsteroidal anti-inflammatory medications (NSAID's) adequate in approximately 60% of patients. Average of 2-3 trials needed to determine most effective drug for an individual patient; adequate duration of trial for given NSAID 4-6 weeks (if no adverse reaction). Drugs for children include:
 - Aspirin 75-90 mg/kg/d
 - Ibuprofen (Motrin, Advil, Nuprin) 30-50 mg/kg/d (usual dose is 40 mg/kg/d)
 - Naproxen (Naprosyn, Aleve) 10-20 mg/kg/d
 - Tolmetin sodium 15-30 mg/kg/d
• Second-line:
◊ 30-40% of patients ultimately require addition of disease-modifying antirheumatic drug (DMARD) e.g., gold, antimalarials, penicillamine, methotrexate
◊ Other agents - corticosteroids for serious cardiac involvement or unresponsive uveitis; Immune globulin, intravenous (IVIG) or cyclosporine in selected patients
Contraindications: Known allergies
Precautions: All (except salicyl salicylate) affect platelet adhesiveness and may worsen a bleeding diathesis. Use caution with all NSAID's in renal insufficiency and hypovolemic states.
Significant possible interactions: NSAID's may lower serum levels of digitalis and anticonvulsants, and blunt the effect of loop diuretics. NSAID's may increase serum methotrexate levels.

ALTERNATIVE DRUGS
Other NSAID's; analgesics for pain control

FOLLOWUP

PATIENT MONITORING
• Patients on NSAID's - CBC, urinalysis, minimum every 3-4 months
• Patients on aspirin and/or other salicylates - transaminase and salicylate levels, weekly for first month, then every 3-4 months
• Patients on gold - monthly CBC, urinalysis
• Patient on methotrexate - monthly liver function tests, CBC
• Ophthalmologic monitoring for antimalarials

PREVENTION/AVOIDANCE
• Avoid salicylate therapy during serious viral illness or following varicella exposure due to possible risk for Reye's syndrome
• No known preventive measures for JRA

POSSIBLE COMPLICATIONS
• Blindness
• Band keratopathy
• Glaucoma
• Short stature
• Debilitating joint disease
• Patient on NSAID's
 ◊ Peptic ulcer
 ◊ Gastrointestinal hemorrhage
 ◊ Rashes
 ◊ CNS reactions
 ◊ Renal disease
 ◊ Leukopenia
• Patient on DMARD's
 ◊ Bone marrow suppression
 ◊ Hepatitis
 ◊ Renal disease
 ◊ Dermatitis
 ◊ Mouth ulcers
 ◊ Retinal toxicity (antimalarials)

EXPECTED COURSE/PROGNOSIS
• 70-80% ultimately remit, but functional ability depends on adequacy of long-term therapy (disease control and maintaining muscle and joint function)
• Poorest prognosis in polyarticular patients with positive rheumatoid factor (RF); and in systemic juvenile arthritis

MISCELLANEOUS

ASSOCIATED CONDITIONS Other autoimmune disorders

AGE-RELATED FACTORS
Pediatric: Behavioral and compliance problems frequent in toddlers and teenagers
Geriatric: N/A
Others: N/A

PREGNANCY Unpredictable effect on disease activity

SYNONYMS
• Juvenile chronic arthritis
• Juvenile arthritis
• Still's disease

ICD-9-CM
• 714 polyarticular juvenile rheumatoid arthritis, chronic
• 714.31 systemic onset JRA
• 714.32 pauciarticular onset
• 714.33 polyarticular onset JRA

SEE ALSO N/A

OTHER NOTES Treatment goal is to control active disease as well as extra-articular manifestations in order to maintain musculoskeletal function as normal as possible

ABBREVIATIONS
• JRA = juvenile rheumatoid arthritis
• RF = rheumatic factor
• DMARD = disease modifying antirheumatic drug

REFERENCES
• Schaller JG: Juvenile Rheumatoid Arthritis. Pediatrics in Review 1980;2(6), 163-174
• Cassidy JT, Petty RE: The Textbook of Pediatric Rheumatology. 3rd Ed. New York, Churchill Livingstone, 1995
Illustrations: 1 available on CD-ROM
Internet references: http://www.5mcc.com

Author(s)
Carol B. Lindsley, MD

Arthritis, osteo

BASICS

DESCRIPTION   Osteoarthritis (OA) is the most common form of joint disease. Involves progressive loss of articular cartilage and reactive changes at joint margins and in subchondral bone.
• Primary
  ◊ Idiopathic
  ◊ Divided into subsets depending on clinical features
• Secondary
  ◊ Childhood anatomic abnormalities (e.g., congenital hip dysplasia, slipped femoral epiphyses)
  ◊ Inheritable metabolic disorders (e.g., alkaptonuria, Wilson's disease, hemochromatosis)
  ◊ Neuropathic arthropathy (Charcot's joints)
  ◊ Hemophilic arthropathy
  ◊ Acromegalic arthropathy
  ◊ Paget's disease
  ◊ Hyperparathyroidism
  ◊ Noninfectious inflammatory arthritis (e.g., rheumatoid arthritis, spondyloarthropathies)
  ◊ Gout, calcium pyrophosphate deposition disease (pseudogout)
  ◊ Septic or tuberculous arthritis
  ◊ Post-traumatic
System(s) affected: Musculoskeletal
Genetics: Unknown
Incidence/Prevalence in USA:
• Estimates of radiographic evidence of OA - range from 33% to almost 90% in those people over the age of 65
• Approximately 60 million patients at any one time
Predominant age:
• Over age 40 (for symptomatic disease)
• Leading cause of disability in those over age 65
Predominant sex: Male = Female

SIGNS AND SYMPTOMS
• Slowly developing joint pain
• Pain that follows use of a joint
• Stiffness (especially morning and after sitting) of less than 15 minutes duration
• Joint enlargement (e.g., Heberden's nodes of distal interphalangeal joints)
• Decreased range of motion
• Tenderness usually absent; may be associated with synovitis, with tenderness along joint margin
• Crepitation as late sign
• Local pain and stiffness with osteoarthritis of spine, with radicular pain (if there is compression of nerve roots)

CAUSES   Biomechanical, biochemical, inflammatory, and immunological factors are all implicated in pathogenesis of osteoarthritis

RISK FACTORS
• Age over 50
• Obesity (weight bearing joints)
• Prolonged occupational or sports stress
• Injury to a joint

DIAGNOSIS

DIFFERENTIAL DIAGNOSIS
• Distinguish from other types of arthritis by absent systemic findings, minimal articular inflammation, and distribution of involved joints (e.g., distal and proximal interphalangeal joints, not wrist and metacarpophalangeal joints)
• In spine, distinguish from osteoporosis, metastatic disease, multiple myeloma, other bone disease

LABORATORY   Not helpful (sedimentation rate not increased)
Drugs that may alter lab results: N/A
Disorders that may alter lab results: In secondary OA, the underlying disorder may have abnormal lab results, e.g., hemochromatosis - abnormal iron studies

PATHOLOGICAL FINDINGS
• Synovial fluid may have a slightly increased white blood cell count, predominantly mononuclear
• Calcium pyrophosphate dihydrate and/or apatite crystals may occasionally be seen in effusions and require polarized light microscopy or special techniques to see
• Subchondral bone trabecular microfractures
• Degradation response produced by release of proteolytic enzymes, collagenolytic enzymes, prostaglandins, and immune responses

SPECIAL TESTS   N/A

IMAGING   X-rays usually normal early; later often show narrowed joint space, osteophyte formation, subchondral bony sclerosis, and cyst formation. Erosions may occur on surface of distal interphalangeal (DIP) and proximal interphalangeal (PIP) joints when OA is associated with inflammation (erosive osteoarthritis).

DIAGNOSTIC PROCEDURES
• Joint aspiration
  ◊ May be helpful to distinguish between OA and chronic inflammatory arthritides
  ◊ OA - cell count usually < 500 cells/mm3, predominantly mononuclear
  ◊ Inflammatory - cell count usually > 2000 cells/mm3, predominantly neutrophils

TREATMENT

APPROPRIATE HEALTH CARE
Outpatient

GENERAL MEASURES
• Reassurance of absence of generalized systemic disease, with recognition of potential disability from osteoarthritis
• Weight reduction if obese
• General fitness program
• Heat (local, tub baths, etc.)
• Physical therapy to maintain or regain joint motion and muscle strength. Quadriceps strengthening exercises can relive pain and disability of the knee.
• Protect joints from overuse (e.g., cane, crutches, walker, neck collar, elastic knee support)

SURGICAL MEASURES   Surgery may be indicated in advanced disease (e.g., osteotomy, debridement, removal of loose bodies, joint replacement)

ACTIVITY   As active as tolerated

DIET   No special diet

PATIENT EDUCATION
• For a listing of sources for patient education materials favorably reviewed on this topic, physicians may contact: American Academy of Family Physicians Foundation, P.O. Box 8418, Kansas City, MO 64114, (800)274-2237, ext. 4400

MEDICATIONS

DRUG(S) OF CHOICE
• Acetaminophen for relief of pain. If not effective, nonacetylated salicylates (e.g., salsalate, choline-magnesium salicylate), or low dose ibuprofen ≤ 1600 mg/d.
• Other NSAIDs can be used and have similar efficacy. Their prolonged use is associated with significant side effects, especially in the elderly. Since pain in osteoarthritis varies from day to day, brief course of a short acting NSAID are preferable.
• Opioid analgesics (e.g., codeine, oxycodone, propoxyphene) should be restricted for treatment of acute episodes of pain
Contraindications: NSAID's are contraindication if there is renal disease, congestive failure, hypertension, active peptic ulcer disease or previous hypersensitivity to a NSAID or aspirin (asthma, nasal polyps, urticaria/angioedema, hypotension)
Precautions:
• In patients with history of peptic ulcer disease, or risk factors for upper GI bleeding, acetaminophen is recommended. If a NSAID is necessary because of an inadequate response to acetaminophen, it should be given with misoprostol. Risk factors for upper GI bleeding are a previous history of bleeding or peptic ulcer, age 65, concomitant use of oral corticosteroids or anticoagulants.
• Oral or parenteral adrenal corticosteroids are contraindicated
• Combinations of 2 or more NSAIDs are contraindicated because of increased risk of adverse reactions without concomitant improved efficacy
Significant possible interactions:
• NSAID's reduce effectiveness of ACE inhibitors and diuretics
• Aspirin and NSAID's may increase effects of anticoagulants
• Increased hypoglycemic effects of oral hypoglycemics with aspirin
• Avoid concomitant use of aspirin with NSAID's
• Salicylates reduce effectiveness of spironolactone (Aldactone) and uricosurics
• Corticosteroids and some antacids increase salicylate excretion, while ascorbic acid and ammonium chloride reduce salicylate excretion and may cause toxicity

ALTERNATIVE DRUGS
• Tailor drug to patient, and switch if response is not adequate
• Judicious use of intra-articular injections of corticosteroids for selected acute flare-ups of joints. No more than 3-4/year intra-articular corticosteroid injections up to a maximal total of 12 injections per joint. Intra-articular corticosteroid injections, if excessive, can accelerate joint deterioration.
• Non-acetylate salicylates - salsalates, e.g., magnesium salicylate, choline salicylate, provide anti-inflammatory action without significant antiplatelet effects; also have less GI toxicity
• Capsaicin cream - local application relieves pain - most effective in small joints of the hand. May cause a local burning.

FOLLOWUP

PATIENT MONITORING
• Follow range of motion and functional status at regular intervals
• Watch for GI blood loss and follow cardiac, renal and mental status in older patients on NSAID's or ASA
• Periodic CBC, renal function tests, stool for occult blood

PREVENTION/AVOIDANCE Followup of secondary causes

POSSIBLE COMPLICATIONS
• Decompensated CHF, GI bleeding, decreased renal function on NSAID's or ASA
• Hypoglycemic reactions in diabetic patients taking aspirin (rare)
• Infection or accelerated cartilage loss with intra-articular corticosteroids

EXPECTED COURSE/PROGNOSIS
• Tends to be progressive
• Early in course, pain relieved by rest; later, pain may occur at rest and at night
• Joint effusions may occur, especially in knees
• Joint enlargement occurs later in course due to bony enlargement
• Osteophyte (spur) formation, especially at joint margins, as disease progresses
• Advanced stage with full thickness loss of cartilage down to bone

MISCELLANEOUS

ASSOCIATED CONDITIONS N/A

AGE-RELATED FACTORS
Pediatric: N/A
Geriatric:
• Prevalence increases with age
• Almost universal over 65 (by x-ray but not clinically)
Others: N/A

PREGNANCY ASA and NSAID's with some risk to fetus during pregnancy; compatible with breast feeding

SYNONYMS
• Osteoarthrosis
• Degenerative joint disease

ICD-9-CM 715.9 Osteoarthritis, unspecified whether generalized or localized

SEE ALSO N/A

OTHER NOTES Surgery may be indicated in advanced disease (for example joint replacement, fusion)

ABBREVIATIONS N/A

REFERENCES
• Kelly HE, Ruddy S, Sledge CB, eds: Textbook of Rheumatology. 4th Ed. Philadelphia, W.B. Saunders Co., 1993
• Schroeder SA, Krapp MA, Tierney LM, McPhee SI: Current Medical Diagnosis and Treatment. Norwalk, CT, Appleton and Lange, 1991:593-594
• Johnson GE: Essentials of Drug Therapy. Philadelphia, W.B. Saunders Co., 1991
• Ellsworth AJ, Bray RF, Bray BS, Geyman JP: The Family Practice Drug Handbook. Chicago, Mosby-Year Book, 1991:180, 186-187
Illustrations: N/A
Internet references: http://www.5mcc.com

Author(s)
John P. Geyman, MD
Bruce C. Gilliland, MD

Arthritis, psoriatic

 BASICS

DESCRIPTION Arthritis associated with psoriasis. Serologic tests for the rheumatoid factor are usually negative. Patients exhibit sausage-shaped digits and characteristic radiologic changes. Psoriatic arthropathy occurs in about 5% of individuals with psoriasis, especially those with psoriatic nail disease. There are several forms that have been described although the separation into these forms is not distinct. They are called by different descriptive terms by various authors.
• Forms of psoriatic arthropathy:
  ◊ Psoriatic nail disease and distal interphalangeal involvement (classic psoriatic arthritis). Characteristics - nail pitting, transverse depressions, subungual hyperkeratosis, distal interphalangeal arthritis.
  ◊ Arthritis mutilans - a destructive, resorptive arthropathy. Produces the so-called opera-glass hand.
  ◊ Symmetric polyarthropathy resembling rheumatoid arthritis - may be indistinguishable from RA and may represent coincidental rheumatoid arthritis in a patient who has psoriasis
  ◊ Asymmetric oligoarthropathy - little relationship between joint and skin activity; joints involved may be both large and small
  ◊ Psoriatic spondylitis - asymmetrical spondylitis and sacroiliitis
System(s) affected: Musculoskeletal, Skin/Exocrine
Genetics: HLA-B27 usually present in patients with spondylitis-type psoriatic arthropathy. Psoriasis itself is associated with HLA-B13, HLA-Bw17, HLA-Cw6, HLABw38, HLA-DR4 and HLA-DR7
Incidence/Prevalence in USA: Uncommon, approximately 5% of individuals have psoriatic skin disease
Predominant age: Onset age 30-35
Predominant sex: Female > Male (slightly)

SIGNS AND SYMPTOMS
• Joint swelling, tenderness, warmth, restricted movement
• Distribution of arthritis dependent upon form of psoriatic arthritis
• Nail changes - pitting, transverse ridging, onycholysis, keratosis, yellowing and destruction of the entire nail
• Fever
• Malaise
• Psoriasis - variable severity
• Other symptoms applying characteristically to the several types of psoriatic arthropathy. See description.

CAUSES
• Unknown
• Probably genetically related

RISK FACTORS
• Psoriasis
• Positive family history

 DIAGNOSIS

DIFFERENTIAL DIAGNOSIS
• Psoriasis
• Seropositive inflammatory polyarthritis
• Rheumatoid arthritis
• Osteoarthritis
• Gout
• Reiter's syndrome
• Ankylosing spondylitis

LABORATORY
• Serum rheumatoid factor - negative
• Elevated erythrocyte sedimentation rate
• Elevated uric acid
• Anemia
• HLA B27 - spondylitis
Drugs that may alter lab results: N/A
Disorders that may alter lab results: N/A

PATHOLOGICAL FINDINGS Synovitis (resembling rheumatoid arthritis)

SPECIAL TESTS N/A

IMAGING
• X-ray
  ◊ Gross destructive changes of isolated small joints
  ◊ Peripheral arthritis mutilans
  ◊ Erosions, ankylosis
  ◊ Extensive bone resorption to cause "opera-glass hand"
  ◊ Fluffy periostitis
  ◊ Atypical spondylitis with syndesmophyte formation
  ◊ Acro osteolysis, "pencil-in-cup" appearance
  ◊ Asymmetric sacroiliitis
  ◊ Absence of osteoporosis

DIAGNOSTIC PROCEDURES N/A

 TREATMENT

APPROPRIATE HEALTH CARE
Outpatient

GENERAL MEASURES
• Immobilizing splints
• Isometric exercises and swimming later
• Paraffin baths or other heat therapy
• Protect affected joints
• Regular, moderate exposure to sun
• Psoriatic skin care

SURGICAL MEASURES N/A

ACTIVITY Encourage exercise (particularly swimming) to maintain strength and flexibility

DIET No special diet

PATIENT EDUCATION
• Stress non-contagious
• Arthritis Foundation referral
• For a listing of sources for patient education materials favorably reviewed on this topic, physicians may contact: American Academy of Family Physicians Foundation, P.O. Box 8418, Kansas City, MO 64114, (800)274-2237, ext. 4400
• Arthritis Foundation, 1314 Spring Street N.W., Atlanta, GA 30309, (404)872-7100

MEDICATIONS

DRUG(S) OF CHOICE
• Several options available depending on involvement of skin and joints:
◊ Nonsteroidal anti-inflammatory drugs in usual doses. There is no evidence for superiority of any one NSAID in psoriatic arthritis.
◊ Low-dose systemic steroids, if necessary
◊ Topical therapy including steroids for skin
◊ PUVA therapy may be helpful for skin lesions
• Others sometimes useful:
◊ Methotrexate, used only specific guidelines and by someone experienced with its use.
◊ Gold salts
◊ Antimalarials (controversial)
◊ Sulfasalazine
◊ Immunosuppressives in resistant cases
◊ Cyclosporine in resistant cases

Contraindications:
• Antimalarials can provoke exfoliative dermatitis
• NSAID's may flare psoriasis
• Methotrexate contraindicated in HIV positive patients

Precautions: Phenylbutazone may cause bone marrow depression. NSAID's and ASA may cause gastritis and renal failure. Refer to manufacturer's literature.

Significant possible interactions:
NSAID's may impair methotrexate excretion and cause methotrexate toxicity. Refer to manufacturer's literature.

ALTERNATIVE DRUGS
Etretinate 0.5-1.0 mg/kg/day in 2 divided doses (severe side effects, avoid during pregnancy since it is highly teratogenic) may be helpful for psoriasis

FOLLOWUP

PATIENT MONITORING
Frequent for medication adjustment and encouragement

PREVENTION/AVOIDANCE N/A

POSSIBLE COMPLICATIONS
• Chronicity
• Severe deforming arthritis (arthritis mutilans)
• Spondylitic form of arthritis with sacroiliitis and spinal involvement

EXPECTED COURSE/PROGNOSIS
• Course - acute, intermittent
• More favorable than rheumatoid arthritis (except for arthritis mutilans)
• Treatment of skin lesions can sometime improve arthritic symptoms
• Joint surgery is at least as successful as for rheumatoid arthritis; (RA) infectious complications are more common than RA

MISCELLANEOUS

ASSOCIATED CONDITIONS Psoriasis

AGE-RELATED FACTORS
Pediatric: Not commonly seen in this age group
Geriatric: Arthritic symptoms worse
Others: N/A

PREGNANCY N/A

SYNONYMS Psoriasis, arthropathic

ICD-9-CM 696.0 Psoriatic arthropathy

SEE ALSO N/A

OTHER NOTES N/A

ABBREVIATIONS N/A

REFERENCES
• Kelley WN, Harris ED, Ruddy S, et al: Textbook of Rheumatology. 5th Ed. Philadelphia, W.B. Saunders, 1997
• Koopman WJ, eds: Arthritis and Allied Disorders. 13th Ed. Philadelphia, Lea & Febiger, 1997
• Kippel JH, Dippe PA, eds: Rheumatology. St. Louis, Mosby, 1994
Illustrations: N/A
Internet references: http://www.5mcc.com

Author(s)
John T. Boyer, MD

Arthritis, rheumatoid (RA)

BASICS

DESCRIPTION A chronic systemic inflammatory disease of unknown etiology with a predilection for joint involvement. Articular inflammation may be remitting, but if continued usually results in joint damage and disability. Certain extra-articular manifestations are characteristic, including rheumatoid nodules, arteritis, neuropathy, scleritis, pericarditis, and splenomegaly.
System(s) affected: Musculoskeletal, Hemic/Lymphatic/Immunologic, Pulmonary, Cardiovascular, Nervous
Genetics: Seropositive RA aggregates in families. Genetic factors versus their interaction with environmental facilitators is unclear. HLA-DR4 is found in 70% of Caucasian seropositive patients compared to 25% of controls. Increased relative risk of 4-5 times for the DR4 positive person, although a minority are affected. African Americans tend not to exhibit this predilection.
Incidence/Prevalence in USA:
• 0.3-1.5%; women affected twice as often, but men and women have equal prevalence of erosive disease
• Prevalence in Native Americans is 3.5-5.3%
Predominant age: Third to sixth decades
Predominant sex:
• Female > Male (overall incidence and prevalence of articular manifestations)
• Male > Female (exhibit more systemic disease)

SIGNS AND SYMPTOMS
• Joints: most often involved are wrists, knees, elbows, shoulders, ankles, metarsal-phalangeal and subtalar joints with swelling, joint heat, joint deformity,morning stiffness, pain on passive motion
• Systemic: fatigue, depression, malaise, anorexia, rheumatoid nodules, lymphadenopathy, splenomegaly, ocular disease, entrapment neuropathies

CAUSES Antibodies complexed with complement in the joint space result in inflammation.

RISK FACTORS
• HLA-DR4
• Family history
• Native American ethnicity
• Female gender, age 20-50 years

DIAGNOSIS

DIFFERENTIAL DIAGNOSIS
Sjögren's syndrome, sarcoidosis, poly-myositis, erosive osteoarthritis, seronegative polyarthritis, vasculitis, gout, pseudogout, inflammatory bowel disease, hypersensitivity reactions, Reiter's syndrome, Behçet's syndrome, psoriatic arthritis, systemic lupus erythematosus, Lyme disease, scleroderma, chronic infection, occult malignancy. Early clinical involvement of wrists speaks against osteoarthritis.

LABORATORY
• Hematocrit - mild anemia common
• Sedimentation rate: usually elevated; helpful adjunct to follow disease activity
• Rheumatoid factor: > 1:80 in 70-80% of patients with RA
• ANA: present in 20-30%.
• Electrolytes, creatinine, liver function, urinalysis to assess organ comorbid states, and provide a baseline to gauge potential adverse events
• Synovial fluid
  ◊ Yellowish - white, turbid, poor viscosity
  ◊ "Mucin clot" poor due to degradation of hyaluric acid by lysosomal enzymes
  ◊ WBC increased (3500-50,000)
  ◊ CH50 is lower than serum
  ◊ Protein: approximately 4.2 g/dL (42 g/L)
  ◊ Serum-synovial glucose difference ≥ 30 mg/dL (≥ 1.67 mmol/L)
Drugs that may alter lab results: Prior treatment with immunosuppressives may "normalize" results
Disorders that may alter lab results: N/A

PATHOLOGICAL FINDINGS
• Synovial infiltration by lymphocytes, plasma cells, and macrophages
• Hypertrophy and hyperplasia of synovial lining cells
• Local production of "self-associating" IgG

SPECIAL TESTS None; biopsy of nodules is not indicated in diagnosis

IMAGING
• X-rays rarely necessary in diagnosis, but useful in following the progression of disease
• Arthrography - to define joint abnormalities or injury to a supporting structure
• Bone scan - if aseptic necrosis is suspected
• CT/MRI - useful in specific situations such as cervical spine symptoms

DIAGNOSTIC PROCEDURES
• American College of Rheumatology criteria: (5 of the 7 must be present. Numbers 1-4 must be continuous > 6 weeks.)
1. Morning stiffness > 1 hour's duration
2. Arthritis of at least three joint groups with soft tissue swelling or fluid
3. Swelling involving at least one of the following joint groups: proximal interphalangeal, metacarpophalangeal, or wrists
4. Symmetrical joint swelling
5. Subcutaneous nodules
6. Positive rheumatoid factor test
7. Radiographic changes consistent with RA

TREATMENT

APPROPRIATE HEALTH CARE Primarily outpatient except for emergencies or orthopedic procedures. Key elements are ongoing evaluation of disease activity and extent of synovitis, structural damage, and psycho/social functional status.

GENERAL MEASURES
• Intervene before joint damage occurs
• Emphasis on exercise and mobility; reduction of joint stress; general health care; patient education

SURGICAL MEASURES Possibly surgery for severe mechanical symptoms (consider long-term outcomes, risk/benefits, and cumulative effects of medical therapies on surgical decisions)

ACTIVITY
• Encourage full activity, but avoid heavy work and vigorous exercise during active phases due to risk of intensifying joint inflammation
• Hydrotherapy or water exercise is effective

DIET No special diet

PATIENT EDUCATION American Rheumatism Association (800)282-7023

MEDICATIONS

DRUG(S) OF CHOICE
"Pyramid of therapy" (beginning with anti-inflammatories and moving to disease modifying regimens) controversial. Don't delay disease modifying agents (DMARDs) beyond 3 months, if patient has ongoing joint pain/morning stiffness, active synovitis, or persistent increase in ESR/CRP despite appropriate dose NSAIDs.
• Early disease or acute/chronic inflammation
  ◊ Aspirin or other NSAID
• Severe disease or to minimize disease activity while awaiting DMARDs to act, decrease activity for a short period of time, or control active disease when NSAIDs/DMARDs have failed.
  ◊ Prednisone: 5-15 mg q day
• Persistent disease activity (chronic synovitis, AM stiffness, increased ESR/CRP, extra-articular disease) - add DMARDs; HCQ or SSZ often chosen first.
  ◊ Intraarticular steroid - at times
  ◊ Antimalarials: hydroxychloroquine (HCQ, Plaquenil) 400 mg q hs for 2-3 months, then 200 mg/hs; 6 month trial usual
  ◊ Auranofin 6-10 mg/d po; reevaluate in 6 months or 1 gram total. Injectable gold: weekly for 22 weeks, then q 2-4 weeks

◊ Sulfasalazine (SSZ): 500 mg/d, increasing to 2 g/d over one month; max: 2-3 g/day; 6 month trial

◊ Penicillamine (d-penicillamine): 250 mg/d initially, increasing slowly to 750-1000 mg/day; 9 month trial with 8-12 weeks at maximum dosage

◊ Azathioprine

◊ Methotrexate: 5-15 mg/wk po; 3-6 month trial - for steroid dependent disease or after other measures unsuccessful. MTX is the DMARD with most predictable benefit. Role in earlier disease debated; many recommend MTX in early stage disease

Contraindications: N/A

Precautions:
• Consider 1)misoprostol for patients on NSAIDs chronically, 2) folic acid supplementation (1-2 mg/d) for patients on MTX
• Avoid NSAID combinations

Significant possible interactions:
• NSAIDs:
  ◊ Antacids: reduce absorption
  ◊ Anticoagulants: increase bleeding risk
  ◊ Oral hypoglycemic agents (OHA): Aspirin, phenylbutazone, and oxyphenbutazone may potentiate the activity of OHA's; others currently available do not
  ◊ Antihypertensive/diuretics: NSAID's may attenuate the effect of diuretics, beta-blockers, hydralazine, prazosin, and ACE inhibitors
  ◊ Lithium: Elevation of plasma lithium levels may occur, especially with indomethacin and diclofenac
  ◊ Methotrexate: Salicylate inhibits the renal clearance of methotrexate, and toxic levels may occur
  ◊ Phenytoin: Phenylbutazone inhibits metabolism of phenytoin. Salicylates increase the concentration of phenytoin.
  ◊ Probenecid: Inhibits renal clearance of several NSAID's

ALTERNATIVE DRUGS Combinations of DMARDs: MTX/HCQ, MTX/SSZ, and gold/HCQ. Most effective combinations unclear.

FOLLOWUP

PATIENT MONITORING
• Discuss prognosis, treatment options (time and cost), adverse effects, lab and PE monitoring , patient preferences
• Duration of morning stiffness
• Time of onset of fatigue
• NSAID need/day
• Grip strength
• Number of joints that are tender or painful on passive range-of-motion
• Degree of swelling of affected joints
• Functional status assessment
• Progress of established disease on x-ray
• ESR - often best test of disease activity
• Other lab testing, depend on medications and disease progression

PREVENTION/AVOIDANCE
• Possible association of oral contraceptive use with decreased risk of RA

POSSIBLE COMPLICATIONS
• Erosive arthritis and joint destruction
• Skin vasculitis
• Pericarditis
• Intracardiac rheumatoid nodules causing valvular, conduction abnormalities
• Pleural, subpleural disease; interstitial fibrosis
• Mononeuritis multiplex, median nerve entrapment
• Sjögren's syndrome, scleral rheumatoid nodules
• Felty's syndrome

EXPECTED COURSE/PROGNOSIS
• Progressive decline in function has been the usual course; this may be altered significantly with proper medical, surgical, and physiotherapeutic interventions.
• Poor prognosis: early age at onset, high RF titer, high ESR, swelling of > 20 joints, extra-articular disease
• Complete remission defined as absence of: 1) symptoms of active inflammatory joint pain. 2) morning stiffness, 3) fatigue, 4) synovitis on physical exam, 5) progression of x-ray damage, 6) elevation of ESR

MISCELLANEOUS

ASSOCIATED CONDITIONS Sjögren's; Felty's

AGE-RELATED FACTORS
Pediatric: See Juvenile RA
Geriatric:
• Onset uncommon (20% of persons over age 60 with the disease)
• Despite improved treatment, expect increased contribution/interaction of other age-related comorbidities. Pericarditis, septic arthritis, Sjögren's syndrome more common.
• Less tolerance to medications; increased incidence of hydroxychloroquine- associated-maculopathy, D-penicillamine rash, and sulfasalazine induced nausea and vomiting. Toxicity from parenteral gold not age-related.
Others: N/A

PREGNANCY
• Childbearing age women require effective contraception when DMARDs given. Modify regimen if pregnancy or breast-feeding desired.
• Labor/delivery pose no serious problems, unless severe mechanical joint disease
• > 75% of RA patients improve during pregnancy (in spite of discontinuing medications, e.g., gold and methotrexate). Occasionally, first episodes occur during pregnancy. Relapse occurs within 6 months after delivery.

• No increased number of fetal abnormalities. Presence of Sjögren's syndrome and anti-Ro antibody associated (especially in mother's with lupus) with congenital complete heart block.

SYNONYMS N/A

ICD-9-CM
714.0 Rheumatoid arthritis
714.1 Felty's syndrome

SEE ALSO
• Arthritis, juvenile rheumatoid (JRA)
• Arthritis, osteo

OTHER NOTES
• Functional ability - general classification
  ◊ Class I: No restriction of ability to perform normal activities
  ◊ Class II: Moderate restriction but adequate to perform normal activities
  ◊ Class III: Marked restriction, inability to perform most duties of the patient's usual occupation or self-care
  ◊ Class IV: Incapacitation or confinement to a bed or wheelchair
• Functional ability tasks (Pincus, et al): To dress self; To get in and out of bed; To eat and drink with utensils; To walk outside on flat ground; To wash and dry entire body; To bend down & pick up clothing from floor; To turn regular faucets on and off; To get in and out of car

ABBREVIATIONS
ARA = American Rheumatism Association

REFERENCES
• Schumacher HR, ed: Primer on Rheumatic Diseases. 9th Ed. Atlanta, Arthritis Foun, 1988
• American Rheumatism Association: A Uniform Database for Rheumatic Diseases, 1985 (obtainable from ARAMIS, Suite 3301, Welch Road, Palo Alto, CA 94304)
• Pincus T, Callahan LF, Brooks RH, et al: Self-report questionnaire scores in rheumatoid arthritis compared with traditional physical, radiographic, and laboratory measures. Ann Intern Med 1989;110:259
• ACR Ad Hoc Committee on Clinical Guidelines. Guidelines for the management of RA. Arthritis & Rheumatism. 1996; 39:713-722
• ACR Ad Hoc Committee on Clinical Guidelines. Guidelines for monitoring drug therapy. Arthritis & Rheumatism. 1996; 39:723-731
Illustrations: 5 available on CD-ROM
Internet references: http://www.5mcc.com

Author(s)
Kurt Elward, MD, MPH

Artificial insemination

BASICS

DESCRIPTION Artificial insemination is the placement of washed sperm into the female reproductive tract. Placement can be intracervical, intrauterine, intraperitoneal, or intrafollicular. Most common is intrauterine insemination (IUI). Sperm are washed to reduce antigenicity. Insemination can be with partner's sperm or therapeutic insemination with donor sperm (TID).
System(s) affected: Reproductive, Endocrine/Metabolic
Genetics: N/A
Incidence/Prevalence in USA: Varies, depending on etiology of infertility, i.e., male factor is responsible for approximately 35% of cases of infertility, and a cervical factor is responsible for approximately 10% of cases
Predominant age: Reproductive age women (18-45 years of age)
Predominant sex: Female only

SIGNS AND SYMPTOMS Inability to conceive

CAUSES
• Indications for IUI include:
  ◊ Male factor infertility
  - Oligospermia
  - Asthenospermia
  - Hypospadias
  - Retrograde ejaculation
  - Coital dysfunction
  ◊ Female factors
  - Cervical mucous abnormalities
  - Poor postcoital test
  ◊ Unexplained infertility

RISK FACTORS
• Male factor 35%
• Cervical factor 10%

DIAGNOSIS

DIFFERENTIAL DIAGNOSIS
• Primary female cervical factor?
• Primary male factor?

LABORATORY
• Semen analysis
• Postcoital test
• Sperm antibody testing
Drugs that may alter lab results:
Clomiphene citrate (Clomid)
Disorders that may alter lab results:
• Abnormal pH of vagina or cervical mucus
• Bacterial infection semen/mucus

PATHOLOGICAL FINDINGS
• Chronic cervicitis
• Chronic prostatitis

SPECIAL TESTS
• Zona free hamster sperm penetration assay
• Bovine cervical mucus sperm penetration test

IMAGING Hysterosalpingogram

DIAGNOSTIC PROCEDURES Postcoital test

TREATMENT

APPROPRIATE HEALTH CARE
Outpatient

GENERAL MEASURES
• Intrauterine insemination should be closely timed with ovulation. Ovulation prediction kits detect the luteinizing hormone (LH) surge which precedes ovulation by 12-36 hours. Intrauterine insemination is performed the day of or the day after the LH surge.
• The volume of inseminate that can be transferred into the uterus is 0.25 to 0.5 mL. Small amounts are used to avoid cramping and flushing the oocyte out of the tube. The volume is also limited by space within the uterus.
• Intrauterine insemination is an office procedure. First, the position of the uterus is determined. A speculum is placed in the vagina and the cervix is visualized. The sample of washed sperm is placed into the uppermost portion of the uterine cavity using an insemination catheter with a disposable tuberculin syringe. Occasionally a tenaculum is needed on the anterior lip of the cervix to straighten the endocervical canal. Cervical dilatation or paracervical block is rarely required. The sample is injected slowly over 30-60 seconds.

SURGICAL MEASURES N/A

ACTIVITY No restrictions

DIET No special diet

PATIENT EDUCATION No vaginal lubricants or douching

Artificial insemination

MEDICATIONS

DRUG(S) OF CHOICE
• Clomiphene citrate (Clomid) or human menopausal gonadotropins - menotropins (Pergonal) may be used for controlled ovarian hyperstimulation and ovulation may be initiated by the administration of human chorionic gonadotropin (HCG), an LH-like molecule. Intrauterine insemination is performed 24-36 hours after HCG administration. Clomid predisposes to poor cervical mucus, which can adversely alter sperm/mucus interaction.
• Dosages:
  ◊ Clomiphene: 50 mg daily x 5 days to induce ovulation
  ◊ Menotropins (Pergonal): 75 IU FSH/75 IU LH IM daily x 12 days; then a single dose of chorionic gonadotropin 10,000 IU/day after last dose of menotropins
Contraindications:
• Uncontrolled thyroid and adrenal dysfunction
• An intracranial lesion
• High follicle-stimulating hormone (FSH) level indicating primary ovarian failure
• Abnormal bleeding of undetermined etiology
• Ovarian cysts of unknown origin
• Hypersensitivity
• Pregnancy
Precautions:
• Multiple births - Clomid 8%, Pergonal 25%
• Severe ovarian hyperstimulation (ascites, pleural effusion, dehydration, electrolyte imbalance, pain)
• Ovarian torsion
Significant possible interactions: N/A

ALTERNATIVE DRUGS Estrogen in follicular phase of cycle to improve mucus

FOLLOWUP

PATIENT MONITORING
• Those patients on Clomid require a bimanual exam on a monthly basis
• Patients on Pergonal require serum estradiol measurements and pelvic sonography to monitor ovarian response

PREVENTION/AVOIDANCE N/A

POSSIBLE COMPLICATIONS
• Uterine cramping
• Mild vasomotor symptoms
• Infection
• Theoretical but unproven risk is development of antisperm antibodies in response to increase exposure of the immune system to sperm antigens

EXPECTED COURSE/PROGNOSIS
• Virtually all pregnancies that result, occur within the first six treatment cycles. A 6 month treatment interval usually represents an adequate therapeutic trial.
• There is a documented increase in efficacy with combination of intrauterine insemination and controlled ovarian hyperstimulation (Pergonal)
• The highest success rates are seen with idiopathic or cervical factor problems
• The poorest outcome is with male factor
• Monthly fecundities of 14% have occurred with therapeutic inseminations utilizing fresh semen

MISCELLANEOUS

ASSOCIATED CONDITIONS Causes of infertility

AGE-RELATED FACTORS
Pediatric: N/A
Geriatric: N/A
Others:
• Fecundity is inversely related to maternal age
• Contraindications to artificial insemination
  ◊ Infection (acute cervicitis, endometritis, acute prostatitis, epididymitis, salpingo-oophoritis)
    ◊ Pregnancy
    ◊ Unexplained uterine bleeding

PREGNANCY N/A

SYNONYMS
• Therapeutic Insemination
• Intrauterine Insemination

ICD-9-CM 628.4

SEE ALSO N/A

OTHER NOTES For donor insemination, only frozen semen is used and only after a 6 month period of "quarantine" to minimize danger of transmission of HIV

ABBREVIATIONS
• LH = luteinizing hormone
• HCG = human chorionic gonadotropin

REFERENCES
• Yen SSC, Jaffe RB, eds: Reproductive Endocrinology. 3rd Ed. Philadelphia, W.B. Saunders Co., 1991
• Berek JS, ed: Novak's Gynecology. 12th Ed. Williams & Wilkins, Baltimore, 1996
Illustrations: N/A
Internet references: http://www.5mcc.com

Author(s)
Barbara A. Majeroni, MD

Asbestosis

BASICS

DESCRIPTION A form of pneumoconiosis that can develop 15-20 or more years after regular exposure to asbestos (a heat-resistant and insulating material) has stopped. It is characterized by diffuse interstitial fibrosis. Causes pleural plaques and mesotheliomas of pleura and peritoneum. It increases the risk of tuberculosis and lung cancer in cigarette smokers. Usual course - chronic; progressive.
System(s) affected: Pulmonary
Genetics: No known genetic pattern
Incidence/Prevalence in USA: Less than 10 cases/100,000 people in the U.S. are diagnosed each year. More than a million people have been exposed to significant levels of asbestos.
Predominant age: Middle age (40-75 years)
Predominant sex: Male > Female

SIGNS AND SYMPTOMS
• Chest discomfort
• Clubbed fingers
• Crackles
• Cyanosis
• Exertional dyspnea
• Fatigue
• History of asbestos exposure at least 10 years previously
• Malaise
• Nonproductive cough
• Pleural effusion
• Pleuritic pain
• Pulmonary hypertension

CAUSES
• Occupational exposure to asbestos dust or asbestos fibers
• Secondary exposure in families of workers
• Inhalation of asbestos dust
• Macrophage-induced damage to lung parenchyma

RISK FACTORS
• Cigarette smoking - can enhance retention of asbestos fibers
• Asbestos workers
• Mine workers

DIAGNOSIS

DIFFERENTIAL DIAGNOSIS Other pneumoconioses (siderosis, stannosis,(due to inhalation of tin oxide), baritosis, coal worker's pneumoconiosis, silicosis, talcosis, shaver's disease)

LABORATORY
• Hypoxemia
• Bronchoalveolar lavage - macrophages, asbestos fibers
Drugs that may alter lab results: N/A
Disorders that may alter lab results: N/A

PATHOLOGICAL FINDINGS
• Lung:
  ◊ Parietal pleural thickening
  ◊ Parietal pleural calcification
  ◊ Interstitial inflammation
  ◊ Interstitial fibrosis
  ◊ Alveolar wall fibrosis
  ◊ Extensive pulmonary fibrosis
  ◊ Alveolar destruction
  ◊ Cystic changes

SPECIAL TESTS
• Pulmonary function test:
  ◊ Decreased vital capacity
  ◊ Decreased total lung capacity
  ◊ Normal FEV1/FVC ratio
  ◊ Decreased diffusing capacity

IMAGING
• Lung scan
  ◊ Alveolar capillary dysfunction
  ◊ Small airway narrowing
• Chest x-ray
  ◊ Calcified pleural plaques
  ◊ Irregular, linear opacities
  ◊ Bilateral pleural effusion
  ◊ Pleural thickening
  ◊ Interstitial fibrosis
  ◊ Honeycombed lung
  ◊ Round atelectasis

DIAGNOSTIC PROCEDURES
Bronchoscopy

TREATMENT

APPROPRIATE HEALTH CARE
Outpatient

GENERAL MEASURES
• There is no effective treatment once asbestosis has developed
• Malignancy surveillance
• Avoid tobacco smoking
• Relieve respiratory symptoms (chest physiotherapy)
• Manage hypoxia
• Manage cor pulmonale

SURGICAL MEASURES N/A

ACTIVITY As tolerated. Physical conditioning to the extent possible, conservation of energy when necessary.

DIET No special diet

PATIENT EDUCATION Printed patient information available from: Asbestos Victims of America, P.O. Box 559, Capitola, CA 95010, (408)476-3646 or American Lung Association, 1740 Broadway, New York, NY 10019, (212)315-8700

Asbestosis

MEDICATIONS

DRUG(S) OF CHOICE
• Supplemental oxygen for advanced disease
• Bronchodilators, if needed
Contraindications: N/A
Precautions: N/A
Significant possible interactions: N/A

ALTERNATIVE DRUGS
• Antibiotics for respiratory infections
• Diuretics
• Digitalis

FOLLOWUP

PATIENT MONITORING
• Chest x-ray
• Occasional pulmonary function tests
• Treat infections promptly

PREVENTION/AVOIDANCE
• Avoid asbestos
• If working with asbestos, strictly follow all safety guidelines
• Avoid tobacco smoke

EXPECTED COURSE/PROGNOSIS
• Severity depends on duration of exposure and on intensity of exposure
• Lung disease irreversible
• Further increased lung cancer risk with smoking
• Increased risk for mesotheliomas
• Increased risk for tuberculosis

POSSIBLE COMPLICATIONS
• Squamous cell lung carcinoma
• Pulmonary adenocarcinoma
• Pleural mesothelioma
• Peritoneal mesothelioma
• Diffuse interstitial pulmonary fibrosis
• Restrictive lung disease
• Asphyxiation

MISCELLANEOUS

ASSOCIATED CONDITIONS N/A

AGE-RELATED FACTORS
Pediatric: N/A
Geriatric: More likely to have terminal respiratory illness
Others: N/A

PREGNANCY N/A

SYNONYMS Asbestos pneumoconiosis

ICD-9-CM
501 asbestosis

SEE ALSO N/A

OTHER NOTES N/A

ABBREVIATIONS

REFERENCES
• LaDou J, ed: Occupational Medicine. Norwalk, CT, Appleton and Lange, 1990
• Rosenstock L, Cullen MR: Clinical Occupational Medicine. Philadelphia, W.B. Saunders Co., 1986
Illustrations: N/A
Internet references: http://www.5mcc.com

Author(s)
Nancy N. Dambro, MD

Ascites

BASICS

DESCRIPTION Effusion and accumulation of fluid in the abdominal cavity. Ascites may occur in any condition that causes generalized edema. In children, nephrotic syndrome and malignancy are the predominant causes. In adults, cirrhosis, heart failure, nephrotic syndrome and chronic peritonitis are most common.
System(s) affected:
Hemic/Lymphatic/Immunologic, Cardiovascular, Gastrointestinal, Renal/Urologic
Genetics: N/A
Incidence/Prevalence in USA:
Determined by etiology
Predominant age: Determined by etiology
Predominant sex: Determined by etiology

SIGNS AND SYMPTOMS
- Abdominal pain
- Abdominal discomfort
- Abdominal distention
- Tight clothing
- Shortness of breath
- Anorexia
- Nausea
- Early satiety
- Pyrosis; heartburn
- Flank pain
- Weight gain
- Orthopnea
- Abdominal fluid wave
- Shifting dullness
- Penile edema
- Scrotal edema
- Umbilical herniation
- Pleural effusion
- Pedal edema
- Rales
- Tachycardia

CAUSES
- Peritoneal infection and inflammation:
  ◊ Tuberculosis
  ◊ Fungus disease
  ◊ Chronic bacterial (foreign body, fistula)
  ◊ Ruptured viscus
  ◊ Granulomatous peritonitis
  ◊ Filariasis
- Metabolic diseases
  ◊ Hypothyroidism
  ◊ Cirrhosis
  ◊ Prehepatic and posthepatic portal hypertension
  ◊ Myxedema
  ◊ Nephrogenous
  ◊ Marked hypoalbuminemia (< 2 gm/dL)
- Heart and hepatic congestion
  ◊ Congestive heart failure
  ◊ Constrictive pericarditis
  ◊ Tricuspid stenosis or insufficiency
- Traumatic
  ◊ Pancreatic fistula
  ◊ Biliary fistula
  ◊ Lymphatic fistula (chylous)
  ◊ Hemoperitoneum (trauma, ectopic pregnancy, tumor)

- Malignancy
  ◊ Peritoneal seeding - ovarian, colon, pancreas and others
  ◊ Lymphatic obstruction - leukemia, lymphoma

RISK FACTORS Those associated with possible causes

DIAGNOSIS

DIFFERENTIAL DIAGNOSIS
- Obesity
- Air and liquid in distended intestine
- Fluid type:
- Transudate
  ◊ Likely causes include: Congestive heart failure, constrictive pericarditis, cirrhosis, nephrotic syndrome, hypoalbuminemia
- Exudate
  ◊ Likely causes include: Neoplasm, tuberculosis, pancreatitis, myxedema, biliary pathology, Budd-Chiari syndrome

LABORATORY
- Ascitic fluid (must be sampled in all new onset, or new to treatment cases; obtain in all:
  ◊ Culture through inoculating blood culture bottles
  ◊ Total cell count < 500 mm3
  ◊ PMN < 200 mm3
  ◊ Albumin in both serum and ascites calculate. Serum - ascites < 1.1 gm indicates inflammation or exudate, > 1.1 gm indicates portal hypertension. Protein > 2.0 gm (some would suggest 2.5 gm) indicates exudate.
- Of use in specific circumstances
  ◊ Lactate dehydrogenase < 200 IU/L
  ◊ Amylase
  ◊ Acid fast or fungal cultures
  ◊ Cytology
  ◊ Triglycerides (with a serum test)
- In blood
  ◊ Creatinine < 1.4 mg/dL
  ◊ Electrolytes
- In urine - sodium levels in a single sample:
  ◊ < 10 mEq/L diuretic response unlikely
  ◊ > 10-70 mEq/L diuretic response likely
  ◊ > 70 mEq/L diuretics unnecessary
Drugs that may alter lab results: Refer to laboratory test reference
Disorders that may alter lab results: Refer to laboratory test reference

PATHOLOGICAL FINDINGS N/A

SPECIAL TESTS Laparoscopy

IMAGING Sonography or CT scan

DIAGNOSTIC PROCEDURES
- Diagnostic paracentesis

TREATMENT

APPROPRIATE HEALTH CARE May be outpatient or inpatient depending on physical condition

GENERAL MEASURES
- For all patients
  ◊ Some sodium restriction required, must be most severe when urine sodium is very low
  ◊ Select a sodium restriction that patient can attain at home; treatment usually required 3-6 months
  ◊ Water restriction only necessary if sodium < 130 mEq/L
  ◊ Any persistent elevation of creatinine to > 2.5 mg/dL should lead to decreasing diuretic doses and therapeutic paracentesis
  ◊ Daily record of weight to monitor gains and losses
- For ascites with edema
  ◊ Salt restriction and diuretics usually effective
  ◊ Maximum weight loss of 5 lbs/day
  ◊ Weekly electrolytes on serum during rapid weight loss
- For ascites without edema
  ◊ Dietary restrictions and diuretics as above
  ◊ Maximum loss of 2 lbs/day
- For ascites failing to respond or rising creatinine
  ◊ Paracentesis up to 10 L. Replace albumin for all removals > 5 L at rate of 10 gm IV albumin for each liter beyond 5 removed.

SURGICAL MEASURES In chronic, refractory cases, consider peritoneovenous shunt or transjugular intrahepatic portal shunt (TIPS)

ACTIVITY Bedrest of benefit in heart failure and when leg edema is prominent, otherwise of limited value.

DIET Sodium restriction needed for several months; regulate on a diet that can be followed outside hospital

PATIENT EDUCATION Diet restrictions

MEDICATIONS

DRUG(S) OF CHOICE
• Diuretics are needed in nearly all patients
◊ Spironolactone 100-300 mg/day orally in one dose best for cirrhotic ascites; furosemide 40-120 mg/day orally best for all other etiologies. May use together.
◊ Dose should be sufficient to obtain net sodium loss in urine
◊ Spot sodium in mEq/L x estimated urine output (1 L if no information) should equal estimated dietary sodium. Increase diuretics daily until this is attained. Measure serum electrolytes before each dose change.
Contraindications: See manufacturer's literature
Precautions: In hospital, or when rapid diuresis, observe creatinine weekly. NSAIDs may worsen or initiate oliguria or azotemia. Potassium supplements are usually required when diuresis exceeds 1 lb/day.
Precautions: Observe patients closely for signs of volume depletion, encephalopathy and renal insufficiency. NSAIDs may worsen or initiate oliguria or azotemia.
Significant possible interactions: Avoid concomitant use of potassium supplements if spironolactone is used alone

ALTERNATIVE DRUGS   Other diuretics

FOLLOWUP

PATIENT MONITORING
• For ascites - changes in body weight and urinary sodium to measure response to therapy
• Monitoring as needed for other therapies

PREVENTION/AVOIDANCE   Dependent upon etiology

POSSIBLE COMPLICATIONS
• Overly aggressive diuresis may lead to hypokalemia, worsening hepatic encephalopathy, intravascular volume depletion, azotemia, and possibly to renal failure and death
• Sympathetic pleural effusion
• Other complications as may be associated with cause of ascites

EXPECTED COURSE/PROGNOSIS
• Ascites is rarely life-threatening. Conservative therapy usually successful.
• Prognosis variable depending upon the underlying cause

MISCELLANEOUS

ASSOCIATED CONDITIONS   Listed in Causes

AGE-RELATED FACTORS
Pediatric: N/A
Geriatric: N/A
Others: N/A

PREGNANCY   N/A

SYNONYMS   N/A

ICD-9-CM
789.5 ascites

SEE ALSO
• Congestive heart failure
• Nephrotic syndrome
• Cirrhosis of the liver

OTHER NOTES   N/A

ABBREVIATIONS
NSAID = Non-steroid anti-inflammatory drug

REFERENCES   Schiff L, Schiff EB, eds: Diseases of Liver. 7th Ed. Philadelphia, Lippincott, 1994
Illustrations: N/A
Internet references: http://www.5mcc.com

Author(s)
Frank L. Iber, MD

Aspergillosis

 BASICS

DESCRIPTION
Disease caused by a ubiquitous mold that primarily involves the lungs. Disease frequently lethal in neutropenic and bone marrow transplant (BMT) patients. Syndromes include:
• Allergic aspergillosis
  ◊ Extrinsic allergic alveolitis - hypersensitivity pneumonitis in individuals repeatedly exposed to the fungus.
  ◊ Allergic bronchopulmonary aspergillosis (ABPA) - pulmonary infiltrates, mucous plugging; secondary to allergic reaction to fungus.
• Aspergillomas: "fungus ball" saprophytic colonization within pre-existing pulmonary cavities.
• Invasive aspergillosis: most common and severe in BMT and neutropenic patients. Also occurs with increased frequency in other immunocompromised persons, such as those with solid organ transplant or high dose corticosteroids; commonly fatal.
System(s) affected: Pulmonary, Nervous, Gastrointestinal, Musculoskeletal, Cardiovascular
Genetics: No known genetic pattern
Incidence/Prevalence in USA: Rare
Predominant Age: None
Predominant Sex: Male = Female

SIGNS AND SYMPTOMS
• Allergic - cough, wheezing, constitutional symptoms, plug expectoration
• Aspergillomas - hemoptysis; manifestations of underlying disease
• Invasive - fever, cough, rales, rhonchi; toxicity; CNS signs; GI bleeding

CAUSES
Aspergillus species in decreasing order of frequency: fumigatus, flavus, niger

RISK FACTORS
• Allergic - exposure, asthma
• Aspergillomas - COPD, bronchiectasis, TB, malignancy
• Invasive - neutropenia, corticosteroid therapy

 DIAGNOSIS

DIFFERENTIAL DIAGNOSIS
• Allergic - other causes of asthma and hypersensitivity pneumonitis.
• Aspergillomas - neoplasm, TB
• Invasive - bacterial pneumonia, pulmonary hemorrhage, drug toxicity, malignancy; mucor (sinuses).

LABORATORY
• ABPA - eosinophilia, immediate skin reactivity to aspergillus antigen, precipitating–serum antibodies to aspergillus, elevated serum IgE concentrations.
• Invasive - sputum culture, cultures of bronchoalveolar lavage or bronchial washings; biopsy is definitive; blood cultures almost never positive
Drugs that may alter lab results: None
Disorders that may alter lab results: None

PATHOLOGICAL FINDINGS
Necrotizing pneumonia, hemorrhagic infarcts, blood vessel invasion; branching septate hyphae if organism seen microscopically

SPECIAL TESTS
• ABPA - immediate skin reactivity to aspergillus antigen, precipitating serum antibodies (precipitins) against aspergillus antigens, elevated serum IgE concentrations, elevated serum IgE and IgG antibodies specific to A. Fumigatus.
• Invasive - none

IMAGING
Chest x-ray - fleeting infiltrates (ABPA), round intracavity mass (aspergillomas); nodular or patchy infiltrates progressing to diffuse consolidation and cavitation (invasive)

DIAGNOSTIC PROCEDURES
Bronchoscopy, bronchial washings, bronchoalveolar lavage or transthoracic needle aspiration may be helpful in isolating organism in invasive disease; open lung biopsy is diagnostic but often not possible in severely ill, ventilated patients.

 TREATMENT

APPROPRIATE HEALTH CARE
• Allergic - outpatient usually
• Aspergillomas - outpatient usually
• Invasive - inpatient

GENERAL MEASURES
• Allergic
  ◊ Extrinsic allergic alveolitis - drug therapy, exposure avoidance.
  ◊ ABPA - corticosteroids
• Aspergillomas - individualized therapy ranging from no therapy to surgical resection of cavities in cases of severe hemoptysis; systemic antifungal therapy is seldom useful
• Invasive - (prognosis tends to be poor) high dose intravenous antifungal therapy; treatment of underlying disease; ?adjunctive cytokine therapy to reverse neutropenia

SURGICAL MEASURES N/A

ACTIVITY As tolerated

DIET No special diet

PATIENT EDUCATION To specifics of individual circumstances.

Aspergillosis

MEDICATIONS

DRUG(S) OF CHOICE
- Allergic
  ◊ Extrinsic allergic alveolitis - bronchodilators, cromolyn sodium, steroids
  ◊ ABPA - steroids
- Aspergillomas - none
- Invasive - high dose amphotericin B - up to 1 mg/kg/day. The lipid formulations of amphotericin may be useful if patients develop nephrotoxicity from amphotericin B.

Contraindications: Refer to manufacturers literature

Precautions: Amphotericin B can cause significant renal insufficiency and electrolyte abnormalities. Saline infusion at the time of amphotericin B administration may decrease the nephrotoxicity.

Significant possible interactions: Concomitant use of amphotericin B and other nephrotoxic drugs (aminoglycosides, cyclosporine, etc) can accelerate development of renal insufficiency; likewise, concomitant Amphotericin B and diuretics use can accelerate electrolyte depletion.

ALTERNATIVE DRUGS
Itraconazole is occasionally useful as an alternative agent

FOLLOWUP

PATIENT MONITORING
- Allergic
  ◊ Extrinsic allergic, alveolitis - spirometry
  ◊ ABPA - chest x-ray, IgE levels
- Aspergillomas - chest x-ray, symptoms
- Invasive - chest x-ray, CBC

PREVENTION/AVOIDANCE
- Allergic - avoid exposure
- Aspergillomas - treatment of underlying diseases, i.e., COPD, etc.

EXPECTED COURSE/PROGNOSIS
- Allergic - with treatment prognosis is good; untreated can progress to severe fibrosis, COPD
- Aspergillomas - prognosis more related to underlying disease
- Invasive - poor prognosis

POSSIBLE COMPLICATIONS
- Allergic - bronchiectasis, pulmonary fibrosis, obstructive lung disease
- Aspergillomas - hemoptyses
- Invasive - metastatic infection of CNS, GI tract and other organs; death

MISCELLANEOUS

ASSOCIATED CONDITIONS
- Allergic - asthma
- Aspergillomas - COPD, TB, pulmonary mycoses, silicosis, sarcoidosis, non-tuberculosis mycobacteria, ankylosing spondylitis, malignancy
- Invasive - neutropenia

AGE-RELATED FACTORS
Pediatric: N/A
Geriatric: N/A
Others:
- Allergic - Tends to occur in younger patients < 35.
- Aspergillomas - older patients with chronic lung disease
- Invasive - all ages

PREGNANCY N/A

SYNONYMS
- Hypersensitivity pneumonitis
- Fungus ball

ICD-9-CM 117.3 aspergillosis

SEE ALSO N/A

OTHER NOTES N/A

ABBREVIATIONS ABPA = allergic bronchopulmonary aspergillosis

REFERENCES
- Mandell GL, et al, eds: Principles and Practice of Infectious Diseases. 4th Ed. Churchill Livingstone, New York, 1995
- Levitz SM: Aspergillosis. Inf Dis Clin NA 1989;3:1:1-18
- Rosenberg M, Patterson R, Mintzer R, Cooper BJ, Roberts M, Harris KE: Clinical and immunologic criteria for the diagnosis of allergic bronchopulmonary aspergillosis. Ann Int Med 1977;86:405-414
- Denning DW, Stevens DA: Antifungal and surgical treatment of invasive aspergillosis: Review of 2,121 published cases. Rev Inf Dis 1990;12(6):1147-1201

Illustrations: 1 available on CD-ROM
Internet references: http://www.5mcc.com

Author(s)
Rodney D. Adam, MD

Asthma

BASICS

DESCRIPTION A disorder of the tracheobronchial tree characterized by mild to severe obstruction to airflow. Symptoms vary, generally episodic or paroxysmal, may be persistent. The clinical hallmark is wheezing, but cough may be the predominant symptom. Commonly misdiagnosed as recurrent pneumonia or chronic bronchitis.
• Acute symptoms are characterized by narrowing of large and small airways due to spasm of bronchial smooth muscle, edema and inflammation of the bronchial mucosa, and production of mucus
• Occurs in a setting in which asthma is likely and other, rarer conditions have been excluded
System(s) affected: Pulmonary
Genetics: Search for an asthma gene underway; there is a familial association of reactive airway disease (RAD), ectopic dermatitis, and allergic rhinitis
Incidence/Prevalence in USA:
• 10 million new cases each year, however, there is confusion due to lack of a uniform definition
• 7-19% of children
• A leading cause of missed school days - 7.5 million/year
Predominant age:
• 50% of cases are children under 10
• Young adult (16-40 years), but may occur at any age
Predominant sex:
• Children under 10: Male > Female
• Puberty: Male = Female
• Adult onset: Female > Male

SIGNS AND SYMPTOMS
Variation in pattern of symptoms; paroxysmal, constant, abnormal pulmonary function tests without symptoms
• Wheezing
• Cough
• Periodicity of symptoms
• Prolonged expiration
• Hyperresonance
• Decreased breath sounds
• Nocturnal attacks
• Pulsus paradoxus
• Cyanosis
• Tachycardia
• Accessory respiratory muscle use
• Flattened diaphragms
• Nasal polyp; seen in cystic fibrosis and aspirin sensitivity
• Clubbing is not seen in asthma
• Growth is usually normal

CAUSES
• Allergic factors
  ◊ Airborne pollens
  ◊ Molds
  ◊ House dust (mites)
  ◊ Animal dander
  ◊ Feather pillows
• Other factors
  ◊ Smoke and other pollutants
  ◊ Infections, especially viral
  ◊ Aspirin, tartrates
  ◊ Exercise

◊ Sinusitis
◊ Gastroesophageal reflux
◊ Sleep (peak expiratory flow rate [PEFR] lowest at 4 am)
• Current research focuses on inflammatory response (including abnormal release of chemical mediators, eosinophil chemotactic factor, neutrophil chemotactic factor, and others)

RISK FACTORS
• Positive family history
• Viral lower respiratory infection during infancy

DIAGNOSIS

DIFFERENTIAL DIAGNOSIS Foreign body aspiration - always consider; cystic fibrosis; viral respiratory infections (croup, bronchiolitis); epiglottitis; bronchopulmonary aspergillosis; tuberculosis; hyperventilation syndrome; mitral value prolapse; habit cough; recurrent pulmonary emboli; congestive heart failure; chronic obstructive pulmonary disease; hypersensitivity pneumonitis

LABORATORY
• CBC normal
• Nasal eosinophils
• Immunoglobulins
  ◊ Screen for immunodeficiency
  ◊ IgE elevated in allergic bronchopulmonary aspergillosis (ABPA)
• Sweat test in chronic childhood asthmatics
• Arterial blood gases in status asthmaticus
Drugs that may alter lab results: N/A
Disorders that may alter lab results: N/A

PATHOLOGICAL FINDINGS Smooth muscle hyperplasi; mucosal edema; thickened basement membrane; inflammatory response; hyperinflated lungs; mucus plugging; bronchiectasis is not seen except in association with ABPA; increased airway resistance; decreased airflow rates; ventilation-perfusion mismatching

SPECIAL TESTS
• Home monitoring of peak flow rates - report if drops below 70% of baseline
• Pulmonary function tests - reversible airway obstruction
• Allergy testing
• PPD yearly
• Exercise tolerance testing

IMAGING Chest x-ray (hyperinflation, atelectasis, airleak)

DIAGNOSTIC PROCEDURES
• Bronchoscopy: rarely indicated.
• Spirometry: decreased FEV1
• Chest x-ray: do at least one, but not necessary with each exacerbation

TREATMENT

APPROPRIATE HEALTH CARE
• Outpatient
• Inpatient for bronchospasm not relieved by beta-agonists and steroids

GENERAL MEASURES
• Eliminate irritants
• Education is essential
• Appropriate prophylactic management with anti-inflammatories such as cromolyn sodium, inhaled steroids
• Increase beta-agonists in response to symptoms
• Consider hyposensitization
• The following are NOT recommended: mist, large volumes of fluid, breathing exercises, IPPB

SURGICAL MEASURES N/A

ACTIVITY Early diagnosis and appropriate treatment facilitate unrestricted activity.

DIET No special diet

PATIENT EDUCATION
• Printed patient information available from:
  ◊ American Lung Association, 1740 Broadway, New York, NY 10019, (212)315-8700
  ◊ Asthma and Allergy Foundation of America, Suite 305, Washington, DC 20036, (800)7-ASTHMA, (800)727-8462

MEDICATIONS

DRUG(S) OF CHOICE
• Six major classes of drugs are used:
  ◊ Cromoglycate and nedocromil
  ◊ Steroids (beclomethasone, prednisone, etc)
  ◊ Beta-agonists (albuterol, bitolterol, salmeterol, etc)
  ◊ Methylxanthines (theophylline)
  ◊ Anticholinergics (atropine, ipratropium bromide)
  ◊ Leukotnene antagonists, a new class, introduced in 1997
• Mild intermittant asthma: brief wheezing once or twice a week:
  ◊ Intermittent use of beta-agonist (MDI or nebulizer)
  ◊ New longer-acting beta-agonists are for less frequent use (every 6-12 hours)
  ◊ Oral beta-agonist or theophylline may be considered, but have more side effects
• Mild persistant asthma: symptoms > 2 times a week, but < 1 time a day, affects activity. Once daily medication - choose from:
  ◊ Cromolyn sodium qid or nedocromil bid
  ◊ Inhaled steroids (low doses)
  ◊ Consider afirlukast or zileuton
  ◊ Consider oral theophylline; not preferred

- Moderate asthma: weekly symptoms interfering with sleep or exercise, occasional ER visits, PEFR 60-80% of predicted
  ◊ Regular maintenance schedule
  ◊ Inhaled steroids (beclomethasone diproprionate) 400 µg/day.
  ◊ Consider cromolyn sodium qid or nedocromil bid
  ◊ If not controlled with moderate dose inhaled steroid (600 µg/day), consider addition of oral slow-release xanthines or inhaled ipratropium bromide
  ◊ Consider zafirlukast or zileuton
- Moderate persistant asthma: daily symptoms, affecting activity, occasional ER visits; PEFR 60-80% predicted
  ◊ Regular maintenance schedule
  ◊ Inhaled steroids (beclomethasone diproprionate) 400 µg/day.
  ◊ Consider cromolyn sodium qid or nedocromil bid
  ◊ If not controlled with moderate dose inhaled steroid (600 µg/day), consider addition of oral slow-release xanthines or inhaled ipratropium bromide
  ◊ Consider zafirlukast or zileuton
- Severe persistant asthma: frequent symptoms affecting activity, nocturnal symptoms, frequent hospitalizations, PEFR <60% predicted, not interfering with growth or development
  ◊ Cromolyn sodium as above; also ipratropium
  ◊ High dose inhaled steroids; some patients may need alternate day oral steroids
  ◊ Theophylline often useful, particularly for nighttime symptoms; therapeutic level 10-20 µg/mL (56-111 µmol/L)
  ◊ Consider zafirlukast or zileuton
- Acute exacerbation - outpatient management
  ◊ Inhaled beta-agonist (albuterol) to reverse airflow obstruction
  ◊ Look for increased work of breathing, air leak syndromes, atelectasis, lowered PEFR
  ◊ Short course of steroids, 2mg/kg po qam for 5-7 days
  ◊ IV aminophylline adds toxicity only
  ◊ Observe at least one hour
- Delivery systems
  ◊ Children under 2 - nebulizer or MDI with valved spacer and mask
  ◊ Children 2-4 years - MDI and valved spacer
  ◊ Over 5 years - MDI or powder inhaler
- Hospital management
  ◊ Steroids IV: methylprednisolone (Solu-Medrol) 2 mg/kg once, then 1 mg/kg IV q6h
  ◊ Frequent beta-agonist aerosols
  ◊ Ipratropium neb and/or aminophylline IV drip if not responding well
  ◊ Rarely: isoproterenol or terbutaline IV; mechanical ventilation

Contraindications:
- Sedatives, mucolytics
- Antibiotics are usually not necessary
- Avoid beta-adrenergic blocking drugs

Precautions: Concern regarding deleterious effects of chronic use of beta agonists. Use only when symptomatic (chronic asthma may necessitate chronic use). If on chronic beta agonist, should also be on anti-inflammatory.

Significant possible interactions:
Erythromycin and ciprofloxacin slow theophylline clearance and can increase levels 15-20%.

ALTERNATIVE DRUGS
- Ketotifen
- H1-antagonists
- Troleandomycin (TAO)
- methotrexate
- Immune globulin, intravenous (IVIG)
- Furosemide (Lasix)

FOLLOWUP

PATIENT MONITORING
- PEFR meter at home - record for trend; call if < 70% baseliine, ER if < 50% baseline
- pH and arterial blood gases
- Oximetry
- Electrolytes

PREVENTION/AVOIDANCE
- Co-management is essential
  ◊ Understand medication, inhalers, nebulizers, peak flow meters
  ◊ Monitor symptoms, peak flows
  ◊ Pre-arranged action plan for exacerbations
  ◊ Written guidelines
- Investigate and control triggering factors (pollutants, exercise, house-dust mite, molds, animal dander) if severe
- Annual influenza immunization
- Avoid aspirin
- Avoid sulfites and tartrazine (food additives)

POSSIBLE COMPLICATIONS
- Respiratory failure; mechanical ventilation
- Atelectasis in 25% of hospitalized patients
- Flaccid paralysis after exacerbation (self-limited)
- Death
- Air leak syndromes (pneumothorax, etc.)
- SIADH
- Altered theophylline metabolism

EXPECTED COURSE/PROGNOSIS
- Excellent, with attention to general health and use of medications to control symptoms
- Less than 50% of children with asthma "outgrow it"
- Mortality risk increases with:
  ◊ Greater than 3 emergency room visits/year
  ◊ Nocturnal symptoms
  ◊ History of ICU admission
  ◊ Mechanical ventilation
  ◊ Greater than 2 hospitalizations/year
  ◊ Steroid dependence (systemic use)
  ◊ History of syncope with asthma
- Mortality rates are increasing
- If responsive to treatment is poor, review diagnosis and compliance prior to adding more potent therapy

MISCELLANEOUS

ASSOCIATED CONDITIONS
- Reflux esophagitis
- Sinusitis

AGE-RELATED FACTORS
Pediatric: 50% of new cases of asthma occur in children below 10 years
Geriatric: Unusual for initial episode to occur
Others: N/A

PREGNANCY
- About 50% of asthma patients have no changes, 25% seem to improve and 25% have worse symptoms
- Stress prevention
- Avoid medications with contraindications

SYNONYMS
- Bronchial asthma
- Reactive airway disease

ICD-9-CM
- 493.0 extrinsic asthma
- 493.1 intrinsic asthma
- 493.9 asthma, unspecified

SEE ALSO
- Cystic fibrosis
- Bronchitis
- Immunodeficiency diseases
- Bronchiolitis
- Laryngotracheobronchitis
- Epiglottitis
- Congestive heart failure
- Chronic obstructive pulmonary disease & emphysema
- Hypersensitivity pneumonitis
- Tuberculosis

OTHER NOTES Antihistamines are not contraindicated in asthma

ABBREVIATIONS
- ABPA = allergic bronchopulmonary aspergillosis
- PFT = pulmonary function test
- RAD = reactive airway disease
- TAO = toleandromycin
- PEFR = peak expiratory flow

REFERENCES
- Murray JF, Nadel JA, eds: Textbook of Respiratory Medicine. Philadelphia, W.B. Saunders Co., 1988
- Barnes PJ: A new approach to the treatment of asthma. New Engl J Med 1989;321:1517
- NHLBI Guidelines, 1997
- Rachelefsky G, Warner J: International Consensus on the Management of Pediatric Asthma. Ped Pulmon 1993;15:125-127
Illustrations: N/A
Internet references: http://www.5mcc.com

Author(s)
Nancy N. Dambro, MD

Atelectasis

 BASICS

DESCRIPTION Atelectasis (lung collapse) is a portion of lung which is non-aerated, but otherwise normal. May be an asymptomatic finding on chest roentgenogram or associated with symptoms. Pulmonary blood flow to area of atelectasis is usually reduced, thereby limiting shunting and hypoxia. Diagnosis and therapy are directed at basic cause.
System(s) affected: Pulmonary, Cardiovascular
Genetics: Depends on basic condition e.g., cystic fibrosis, asthma, congenital heart disease, etc.
Incidence/Prevalence in USA: Common in general anesthesia and in intensive care with high inspired oxygen concentrations
Predominant age: All ages
Predominant sex: Male = Female

SIGNS AND SYMPTOMS
• Small atelectasis
  ◊ Commonly asymptomatic
  ◊ Produces no change in the overall clinical presentation
• Large atelectasis:
  ◊ Tachypnea
  ◊ Cough
  ◊ Hypoxia which resolves in some cases over 24-48 hours
  ◊ Dullness to percussion
  ◊ Absent breath sounds if airway is occluded
  ◊ Bronchial breathing if airway is patent
  ◊ Diminished chest expansion
  ◊ Tracheal or precordial impulse displacement
  ◊ Wheezing may be heard with focal obstruction

CAUSES
• Increased alveolar surface tension due to cardiogenic or non-cardiogenic pulmonary edema, primary surfactant deficiency, or infection
• Resorptive atelectasis due to airway obstruction from lumenal blockage (mucus, tumor, foreign body), airway wall abnormality (edema, tumor, bronchomalacia, deformation), or extrinsic airway compression (cardiac, vascular, tumor, adenopathy)
• Compression of the lung (lobar emphysema, cardiomegaly, tumor)
• Increased pleural pressure due to fluid or air in the pleural space (pneumothorax, effusion, empyema, hemothorax, chylothorax)
• Chest wall restriction due to skeletal deformity and/or muscular weakness (scoliosis, neuromuscular disease, phrenic nerve paralysis, anesthesia)

RISK FACTORS
• Varies with condition producing atelectasis
• Atelectasis following anesthesia is increased in smokers, obese individuals, and individuals with short, wide thoraces
• Asthma

 DIAGNOSIS

DIFFERENTIAL DIAGNOSIS
• Atelectasis is not a specific diagnosis, but rather a result of disease or distorted anatomy. The differential is thus found under Causes.
• The roentgenographic differential includes pneumonia, fluid accumulation, lung hypoplasia, or tumor

LABORATORY N/A
Drugs that may alter lab results: N/A
Disorders that may alter lab results: N/A

PATHOLOGICAL FINDINGS
• Pathology varies with cause
• Obstructive atelectasis - non-aerated lung without inflammation or infiltration

SPECIAL TESTS N/A

IMAGING
• Chest roentgenography
  ◊ May demonstrate linear, round, or wedge shaped densities
  ◊ Right middle lobe and lingular atelectasis will obscure the ipsilateral heart border
  ◊ Lower lobe atelectasis will obscure the diaphragm
  ◊ Air bronchograms are usually absent in obstructive atelectasis
  ◊ Evidence of possible airway compression, pleural fluid or air should be sought
  ◊ Diffuse microatelectasis in surfactant deficiency may lead to a ground-glass appearance with striking air bronchograms
  ◊ Mediastinal structures and the diaphragm move toward the atelectatic region
  ◊ Adjacent lung may show compensatory hyperinflation

DIAGNOSTIC PROCEDURES
• Bronchoscopy to assess airway patency. (Bronchoscopy as therapy is controversial with the exception of foreign body or other structural causes).
• Echocardiography to assess cardiac status in cardiomegaly
• Chest CT or MRI to visualize airway and mediastinal structures
• Barium swallow to assess mediastinal vascular compression
• Other procedures vary with potential cause

 TREATMENT

APPROPRIATE HEALTH CARE Varies with severity

GENERAL MEASURES
• Varies with severity and cause of atelectasis
• Ensure adequate oxygenation and humidification
• Chest physiotherapy with percussion and postural drainage. Consider adding treatments using new airway clearance techniques such as Positive Expiratory Pressure (PEP) mask.
• Incentive spirometry
• Positive pressure ventilation or continuous positive airway pressure in subjects with neuromuscular weakness

SURGICAL MEASURES N/A

ACTIVITY Encourage activity, mobilization as tolerated

DIET No special diet

PATIENT EDUCATION Encourage activity as appropriate. Instruct in basic cause and its therapy.

Atelectasis

MEDICATIONS

DRUG(S) OF CHOICE
• Bronchodilator therapy (beta-agonist aerosol)
• Other therapies directed at basic cause - antibiotics, foreign body removal, tumor therapy, cardiac medication, steroids in asthma
Contraindications: Refer to manufacturer's literature
Precautions: Refer to manufacturer's literature
Significant possible interactions: Refer to manufacturer's literature

ALTERNATIVE DRUGS N/A

FOLLOWUP

PATIENT MONITORING
• Varies with cause and patient status
• In simple atelectasis associated with asthma or infection, monthly visits are adequate

PREVENTION/AVOIDANCE
• Avoidance of 100% inspired oxygen (which can rapidly absorb causing atelectasis)
• Foreign body/aspiration precautions
• Postoperative mobilization and/or rotation
• Institute therapies such as chest physiotherapy and incentive spirometry as preventive maneuvers in at-risk patients

POSSIBLE COMPLICATIONS
• Infection with chronic lung damage is an unlikely, but unfortunate complication
• Atelectasis is rarely life-threatening and usually spontaneously resolves

EXPECTED COURSE/PROGNOSIS
• Resolution with medical therapy
• Surgical therapy needed only for certain causes, or if chronic infection and bronchiectasis supervene

MISCELLANEOUS

ASSOCIATED CONDITIONS N/A

AGE-RELATED FACTORS Very young and very old patients with limited mobility at greater risk
Pediatric: Congenital airway obstruction due to mediastinal cysts, tumor, or vascular rings; foreign body aspiration
Geriatric: Primary and secondary lung tumors sometimes associated
Others: Asthma

PREGNANCY Management is similar to non-pregnant and varies with cause

SYNONYMS Lung collapse

ICD-9-CM 518.0

SEE ALSO
• Asthma
• Pneumonia, viral
• Pneumonia, bacterial
• Pneumonia, mycoplasma

OTHER NOTES
• Round atelectasis:
    ◊ A pleural based round density on chest roentgenogram with a comet tail of vessel and airway
    ◊ More common in patients with asbestos exposure
    ◊ May mimic tumor, but can usually be definitively diagnosed with imaging studies thereby avoiding surgery

ABBREVIATIONS N/A

REFERENCES
• Hazinski TH: Atelectasis. In: Chernick V, ed. Kendig's Disorders of the Respiratory Tract in Children. 5th Ed. Philadelphia, W.B. Saunders Co., 1990
• Marini JJ, Pierson DJ, Hudson LD: Acute lobar atelectasis: a prospective comparison of fiberoptic bronchoscopy and respiratory therapy. Am Rev Respir Dis 1971;119:971
• Rickstenste, Sventrik, et al: Effects of peiodic positive airway pressure by mask on postoperative pulmonary function. Chest 1986;6:774-781
Illustrations: N/A
Internet references: http://www.5mcc.com

Author(s)
Nancy N. Dambro, MD

Atherosclerosis

BASICS

DESCRIPTION The common form of arteriosclerosis in which deposits of yellowish plaques (atheromas) containing cholesterol, lipoid material, and lipophages are formed within the intima and inner media of large and medium sized arteries.
System(s) affected: Cardiovascular
Genetics: Probable genetic link; many risk factors for atherosclerosis (lipid metabolism, hypertension, and diabetes) are clearly inheritable
Incidence/Prevalence in USA:
• Common, but declining steadily. The effects upon the brain, heart, kidneys, extremities and other vital organs form the leading cause of morbidity and mortality in the USA and most Western countries.
• Complications of atherosclerosis account for 1/2 of all deaths, and 1/3 of deaths in persons between ages 35-65
Predominant age: 35 and older
Predominant sex: Male > Female

SIGNS AND SYMPTOMS
• Characteristically silent until atheromas produce:
    ◊ Stenosis
    ◊ Thrombosis
    ◊ Aneurysm
    ◊ Embolus
• For lists of possible symptoms see the following titles elsewhere in this book:
    ◊ Essential hypertension
    ◊ Coronary arteriosclerosis
    ◊ Congestive heart failure
    ◊ Cerebrovascular accident
    ◊ Atrial arrhythmias
    ◊ Ventricular arrhythmias
    ◊ Renal failure, chronic
    ◊ Dissecting aneurysm
    ◊ Thrombosis and embolism, arterial

CAUSES
• Biochemical, physiologic, environmental factors that lead to thickening and occlusion of the lumen of arteries
• Aging (some degree of atherosclerosis is universal)
• One or more of the risk factors listed below

RISK FACTORS
• Hypertension
• Tobacco smoking
• Diabetes mellitus
• Obesity
• Male gender
• Physical inactivity
• Increasing age
• Family history of premature atherosclerosis
• Decreased high-density lipoprotein (HDL) cholesterol
• Increased low-density lipoprotein (LDL) cholesterol

DIAGNOSIS

DIFFERENTIAL DIAGNOSIS N/A

LABORATORY Associated with elevated serum cholesterol; elevated LDL and low HDL
Drugs that may alter lab results: N/A
Disorders that may alter lab results: N/A

PATHOLOGICAL FINDINGS
• Early changes (simple) potentially reversible
    ◊ Accumulation of lipid-laden cells in the intimal layer of the artery (usually monocytes/macrophages from circulating blood)
    ◊ Lipid streaks in aortas and coronary arteries
• Late changes (complicated) usually reversible
    ◊ Atheromatous plaques with necrosis, fibrosis, calcification
        ◊ Weakening of elastic lamellae
        ◊ Neovascularization
        ◊ Arterial obstruction
        ◊ Thrombosis

SPECIAL TESTS N/A

IMAGING Extensively calcified atherosclerotic plaques may be identified in major blood vessels on x-ray

DIAGNOSTIC PROCEDURES
• X-ray (often incidental finding)
• Associated with hypercholesterolemia; elevated LDL and low HDL

TREATMENT

APPROPRIATE HEALTH CARE
Outpatient until complications occur; emphasis on prevention

GENERAL MEASURES
• For details see the following titles:
    ◊ Essential hypertension
    ◊ Congestive heart failure
    ◊ Cerebrovascular accident
    ◊ Renal failure, chronic
    ◊ Dissecting aneurysm
    ◊ Thrombosis & embolism, arterial

SURGICAL MEASURES N/A

ACTIVITY Encourage physical fitness

DIET
Recommended daily intake
• Initial diet; Step 1
    ◊ Total fat - < 30% of total calories; saturated fat < 10%
    ◊ Carbohydrates - 50-60% of total calories
    ◊ Protein - 10-20% of total calories
    ◊ Cholesterol - < 300 mg a day
    ◊ Total calories - amount required to achieve and maintain desirable weight
    ◊ Sodium - 1650-2400 mg
    ◊ Alcohol - < 30 g
• Initial diet; Step 2
    ◊ Total fat - < 30% of total calories; saturated fat < 7%
    ◊ Carbohydrates - 50-60% of total calories
    ◊ Protein - 10-20% of total calories
    ◊ Cholesterol - < 200 mg a day
    ◊ Total calories - amount required to achieve and maintain desirable weight
    ◊ Sodium - 1650-2400 mg
    ◊ Alcohol - < 30 g

PATIENT EDUCATION
• Crucial parts of preventing and treating atheroscleroses involve nutrition, fitness, and smoking cessation
• Extensive educational materials available from many agencies (e.g., American Heart Association, U.S. Government Printing Office, National Cholesterol Education Program). Use these to help teach patients how to avoid or eliminate risk factors.

MEDICATIONS

DRUG(S) OF CHOICE
- For details see the following titles:
  ◊ Essential hypertension
  ◊ Coronary arteriosclerosis
  ◊ Congestive heart failure
  ◊ Stroke
  ◊ Atrial arrhythmias
  ◊ Ventricular arrhythmias
  ◊ Renal failure, chronic
  ◊ Dissecting aneurysm
  ◊ Thrombosis and embolism, arterial
  ◊ Angina
  ◊ Myocardial infarction
  ◊ Arteriosclerotic heart disease

Contraindications: Refer to manufacturer's literature

Precautions: Refer to manufacturer's literature

Significant possible interactions: Refer to manufacturer's literature

ALTERNATIVE DRUGS See specific titles

FOLLOWUP

PATIENT MONITORING See specific titles

PREVENTION/AVOIDANCE Eliminate risk factors - all or as many as possible

POSSIBLE COMPLICATIONS
- Coronary artery disease
- Renal failure
- Cerebrovascular accidents
- Dissecting or ruptured aneurysms
- Congestive heart failure
- Cardiac arrhythmias
- Sudden death

EXPECTED COURSE/PROGNOSIS
Avoiding risk factors has greatly decreased mortality rates in the past decade

MISCELLANEOUS

ASSOCIATED CONDITIONS
- Essential hypertension
- Coronary arteriosclerosis
- Congestive heart failure
- Cerebrovascular accident
- Atrial arrhythmias
- Ventricular arrhythmias
- Renal failure, chronic
- Aortic dissection
- Thrombosis and embolism, arterial

AGE-RELATED FACTORS
Pediatric: Fatty streaks and deposits in the intima of the aortas of all children begin as early as age 3 years
Geriatric: Atherosclerosis happens to all who live long enough. Its effects and complications can be minimized and/or delayed by avoiding all risk factors possible.
Others: N/A

PREGNANCY N/A

SYNONYMS N/A

ICD-9-CM
414.0

SEE ALSO
- Hypertension, essential
- Congestive heart failure
- Stroke (Brain attack)
- Renal failure, chronic
- Aortic dissection
- Arterial embolus & thrombosis

OTHER NOTES N/A

ABBREVIATIONS N/A

REFERENCES
- Hurst JW, et.al: The Heart. 7th Ed. New York, McGraw-Hill, 1990
- Hunninghake D, ed: Lipid disorders. Medical Clinics of North America. Vol. 78, No. 1, Jan., 1994
- Guidelines for cardiopulmonary resuscitation and emergency cardiac care. JAMA 1992;268(16)28
Illustrations: 4 available on CD-ROM
Internet references: http://www.5mcc.com

Author(s)
Joseph A. Florence, MD

Atherosclerotic occlusive disease

 BASICS

DESCRIPTION A peripheral arterial disease can be acute or chronic. There is obstruction or narrowing of the lumen of the aorta and its major branches causing interruption of blood flow, usually to feet and legs. Involved arteries may include mesenteric and celiac arteries. Occlusions cause ischemia, discomfort, skin ulceration and gangrene.
System(s) affected: Cardiovascular
Genetics: Family history of early complications of atherosclerosis
Incidence/Prevalence in USA: Increases with age (parallels atherosclerosis)
Predominant age: Older adults
Predominant sex: Male > Female (2:1)

SIGNS AND SYMPTOMS
• Intermittent claudication - exercise induced pain that is relieved by rest is pathognomonic
• Site of occlusion determines site of pain
• Occlusion of abdominal aorta and/or iliac vessels produce claudication in the back, buttocks and hips
• Femoral obstruction causes pain in the calf
• The degree of occlusion determines the exercise tolerance and if severe enough produces pain at rest
• Pulses are diminished or absent
• The limb is cold and pale and typically develops dependent rubor
• Atrophic skin changes often result in shiny hairless skin

CAUSES
• Almost always a complication of atherosclerosis
• Mechanism of occlusion - embolus, thrombosis, fracture, or trauma

RISK FACTORS
• Smoking
• Hyperlipidemia
• Diabetes
• Hypertension
• Physical stress

 DIAGNOSIS

DIFFERENTIAL DIAGNOSIS
• Thromboangiitis obliterans (inflammatory disease primarily affecting young male smokers)
• Fibromuscular dysplasia of the peripheral vessels (rare)

LABORATORY N/A
Drugs that may alter lab results: N/A
Disorders that may alter lab results: N/A

PATHOLOGICAL FINDINGS
• Occluding mass in lumen of thrombosed artery
• Calcareous deposits in occluded vessel in medial coat with atheromas

SPECIAL TESTS Doppler ultrasound to compare systolic pressure in upper and lower limbs (ankle: brachial ratio should be higher than 0.95 at rest)

IMAGING Angiography for an individual who may be a candidate for surgery

DIAGNOSTIC PROCEDURES History and physical

 TREATMENT

APPROPRIATE HEALTH CARE
Outpatient for conservative management. Inpatient for surgery or more severe cases.

GENERAL MEASURES
• Smoking cessation
• Foot and limb care
• Graduated exercise program
• Weight control
• Pain management
• Cholesterol management
• Appropriate treatment of coexisting disease, i.e., diabetes
• Infection control
• Lifestyle modification

SURGICAL MEASURES
• Indications for surgery are ischemic pain at rest, or changes likely to lead to amputation, or intolerable symptoms
• The procedure depends upon site of lesion. Includes endarterectomy, bypass procedures, transluminal angioplasty, and amputation.
• Patients with aorto-iliac disease tend to have good surgical results to a disabling disorder
• Surgery should not be performed for femoral popliteal disease unless symptoms are very severe or disabling
• Bypass surgery for vessels distal to popliteal artery has little success
• Patch grafting
• Atherectomy
• Laser angioplasty
• Stents (wire plastic mesh to stretch and mold to the arterial wall to prevent re-occlusion)
• Amputation with failure of arterial reconstructive surgery or with development of gangrene, persistent infection, or intractable pain

ACTIVITY To the degree that symptoms permit

DIET
• Good diet control
• Lose weight, if overweight

PATIENT EDUCATION
• Educate patient regarding symptoms or signs that require early assessment by physician
• Teach careful foot care
• Avoid elevating or applying heat to affected parts
• Urge early ambulation after surgery
• Assist patient with a stop smoking program

MEDICATIONS

DRUG(S) OF CHOICE
• Vasodilator drugs are ineffective
• Pentoxifylline (Trental) for reducing blood viscosity and increasing red cell flexibility may help. Usual dose 400 mg tid.
• Aspirin to decrease platelet aggregation
Contraindications: In patients sensitive to xanthines
Precautions: Most adverse effects are gastrointestinal. Dizziness and headache are also common.
Significant possible interactions: Use cautiously in patients on oral coagulants. Monitor closely for bleeding complications.

ALTERNATIVE DRUGS   Anticoagulants

FOLLOWUP

PATIENT MONITORING
• For acute phase with surgery, closely follow all aspects of postoperative recovery
• For mild chronic cases, follow patient at regular intervals, frequency dependent upon severity of symptoms
• Management/modification of risk factors

PREVENTION/AVOIDANCE
• Periodic health maintenance measures
• Healthy lifestyle including appropriate diet and adequate exercise
• Avoidance of smoking

POSSIBLE COMPLICATIONS
• Necrosis
• Gangrene
• Limb amputation

EXPECTED COURSE/PROGNOSIS
Course varies from slow progression with easily controlled symptoms to rapid deterioration with severe symptoms requiring surgical intervention

MISCELLANEOUS

ASSOCIATED CONDITIONS
• Atherosclerosis
• Arteriosclerosis obliterans
• Fibromuscular dysplasia
• Thromboangiitis obliterans
• Takayasu's arteritis
• Abdominal aortic coarctation
• Radiation injury
• Popliteal artery entrapment syndrome
• Popliteal cystic degeneration
• Arteritis

AGE-RELATED FACTORS
Pediatric: N/A
Geriatric: N/A
Others: N/A

PREGNANCY   N/A

SYNONYMS
• Peripheral arterial disease
• Occlusive arterial disease

ICD-9-CM
• 444.22 Occlusion, arteries of extremities, lower
• 444.21 Occlusion, arteries of extremities, upper

SEE ALSO
• Arteriosclerosis obliterans

OTHER NOTES   N/A

ABBREVIATIONS   N/A

REFERENCES
• Marcus ML: The Coronary Circulation in Health and Disease. New York, McGraw-Hill, 1983
• Hurst JW, et al: The Heart. 7th Ed. New York, McGraw-Hill, 1990
• Braunwald E, ed: Heart Disease: A Textbook of Cardiovascular Medicine. 4th Ed. Philadelphia, W.B. Saunders Co., 1992
Illustrations: N/A
Internet references: http://www.5mcc.com

Author(s)
Stan G. Smith, MA, MB, FCFPC

Atrial fibrillation

BASICS

DESCRIPTION Atrial fibrillation (AF) is a chronic or paroxysmal arrhythmia characterized by chaotic electrical activity. The electrophysiologic mechanism is most likely multiple reentrant wavelets within the atria. Because the AV node is bombarded with nearly continuous atrial electrical impulses, the ventricular response is irregular and usually rapid (up to or exceeding 180 beats per minute). Symptoms vary from none to mild (palpitations, lightheadedness, fatigue, poor exercise capacity) to severe (angina, dyspnea, syncope), and are frequently more serious in patients with significant structural heart disease. In some patients with Wolff-Parkinson-White syndrome, AF may be extremely rapid and degenerate into ventricular fibrillation.

System(s) affected: Cardiovascular, Nervous
Genetics: No specific genetic pattern in most patients
Incidence/Prevalence in USA: Estimated at 1 per 1000 adults per year; estimated at 2-4% of adult population
Predominant age: Prevalence increases with age:

Age	AF cases/1000
25-35	2-3
55-64	30-40
62-90	50-90

Predominant sex: Male > Female

SIGNS AND SYMPTOMS
• Irregular pulse
• Tachycardia
• Heart failure
• Hypotension
• Palpitations
• Lightheadedness
• Poor exercise capacity
• Fatigue
• Dyspnea
• Angina
• Near syncope/syncope
• Stroke
• Arterial embolization

CAUSES
• Hypertensive heart disease
• Valvular/rheumatic heart disease
• Coronary artery disease
• Acute myocardial infarction
• Pulmonary embolus
• Cardiomyopathy
• Congestive heart failure
• Infiltrative heart disease
• Pericarditis
• Intoxication/ingestion (e.g., ethanol in "Holiday Heart")
• Hyperthyroidism
• Postoperative state (especially cardiothoracic surgery)
• Sick sinus syndrome (tachycardia-bradycardia syndrome)
• Idiopathic (including "lone" atrial fibrillation)

RISK FACTORS
• Hypertension
• Diabetes mellitus
• Left ventricular hypertrophy
• Coronary artery disease
• Congestive heart failure
• Rheumatic heart disease

DIAGNOSIS

DIFFERENTIAL DIAGNOSIS
• Multifocal atrial tachycardia (MAT)
• Sinus tachycardia with frequent atrial premature beats
• Atrial flutter (see below)

LABORATORY
• ECG is diagnostic; low amplitude fibrillatory waves without clear P waves; irregularly irregular pattern of QRS complexes
• Holter monitor and event monitor helpful in diagnosing paroxysmal atrial fibrillation (PAF)
• Echocardiogram to assess for structural heart disease
• Thyroid function tests
Drugs that may alter lab results: N/A
Disorders that may alter lab results: N/A

PATHOLOGICAL FINDINGS
• Atrial dilatation
• Atrial injury (chronic or acute)
• Atrial thrombus, especially in atrial appendage
• Sclerosis/fibrosis of SA node
• Coronary artery disease, valvular/rheumatic disease, cardiomyopathy, pulmonary embolus, etc.

SPECIAL TESTS
• Ventilation-perfusion scan or pulmonary angiography if pulmonary embolus suspected
• Transesophageal echocardiography may be useful in detecting left atrial appendage thrombus and therefore risk of stroke with cardioversion; controversial at present

IMAGING
• Chest x-ray to screen for cardiopulmonary abnormalities
• Echocardiogram to assess for structural heart disease

DIAGNOSTIC PROCEDURES As above

TREATMENT

APPROPRIATE HEALTH CARE
• Inpatient if significant symptoms, extremely rapid ventricular rate, initiating antiarrhythmic therapy, if AF triggered by acute process (acute myocardial infarction, congestive heart failure, pulmonary embolus, etc.)
• Outpatient management appropriate for many patients

GENERAL MEASURES
• Avoidance of potential risks
  ◊ Avoid ethanol, caffeine, nicotine
  ◊ Management of underlying structural heart disease
• Prevention of complications
  ◊ Anticoagulation to reduce the risk of embolic complications
  ◊ Antibiotic prophylaxis if AF is due to valvular heart disease
• Therapy strategies (ongoing trials compare these two strategies)
  ◊ Ventricular rate control with AV nodal blocking agents
  ◊ Restore and maintain sinus rhythm with antiarrhythmic drugs

SURGICAL MEASURES
Nonpharmacological therapies
• Cardiac surgery (e.g., the "maze procedure") may be considered in severely symptomatic, medically refractory patients
• Permanent dual chamber pacing may reduce incidence of AF in patients with sick sinus syndrome
• Radiofrequency catheter ablation of AV node with permanent pacemaker implantation is a reasonable alternative in symptomatic medically refractory patients
• Radiofrequency catheter ablation procedures to approximate the "maze" or other surgical approaches to prevent AF recurrence are investigational at present
• Implantable atrial defibrillators to detect and cardiovert paroxysms of AF are investigational at present

ACTIVITY
• As tolerated
• With medical management, minimal functional impairment in many patients

DIET As appropriate for underlying heart disease and other comorbidities

PATIENT EDUCATION
Printed material available from:
• Du Pont Pharmaceuticals, Wilmington, DE 19880-0026, (800)341-4004
• Marion Merrell Dow Inc., Customer Service Dept., Box 8480, Kansas City, MO 64114, (800)362-7466

MEDICATIONS

DRUG(S) OF CHOICE
Note: Clinical risk factors for stroke include age > 65, diabetes, hypertension, history of prior stroke or transient ischemic attack (TIA), and prior history of congestive heart failure. Echocardiographic risk factors for stroke include left atrial enlargement, mitral regurgitation, and left ventricular dysfunction.
• Anticoagulation:
  ◊ Unless contraindications to anticoagulants exist, patients with chronic AF with any of these risk factors should receive warfarin to maintain an international normalized ratio (INR) of 2.0-3.0

◊ Patients in whom warfarin is contraindicated should receive aspirin 325 mg/day. Aspirin 325 mg/day, is appropriate in low risk patients (e.g., age < 65 years with no risk factors for stroke). Data are fewer with paroxysmal AF, though treatment guidelines are the same for chronic AF.

• Debate exists as to whether controls of the ventricular rate during AF or maintenance of sinus rhythm should be objective of medical therapy. This is being evaluated in an ongoing multicenter clinical trial called AFFIRM.

• Control of ventricular rate
◊ Beta-blockers (propranolol, metoprolol, atenolol, nadolol, etc.)
◊ Non-dihydropyridine calcium channel blockers (diltiazem and verapamil)
◊ Cardiac glycosides (digoxin). Frequently less effective than other agents in controlling the ventricular response.

• Conversion to/maintenance of sinus rhythm:
◊ Direct current (DC) cardioversion. Antiarrhythmic therapy for chemical cardioversion and maintenance of sinus rhythm following cardioversion is controversial due to the risk of pro-arrhythmia.
◊ Ibutilide, an intravenous type III agent, has recently been approved for chemical cardioversion of atrial fibrillation and flutter of short duration (less than 90 days)
◊ If the duration of AF is more tha 24-48 hours or is unknown, patients should be treated with warfarin for at least 3 weeks before and after cardioversion. Transesophageal echocardiography to visualize left atrial thrombus has been proposed to expedite cardioversion.
◊ Chronic oral antiarrhythmic therapy initiated with continuous cardiac monitoring to suppress AF recurrences
   - Type IA (procainamide, disopyramide, quinidine)
   - Type IC (flecainide, propafenone) only in patients with structurally normal hearts
   - Type III (sotalol, amiodarone)
• Acute therapy for hemodynamically compromised patients:
◊ Heparin for anticoagulation
◊ IV beta or calcium channel blocker for control of ventricular rate
◊ IV procainamide and/or DC cardioversion

Contraindications:
• Active bleeding precludes anticoagulation; risk of bleeding is a relative contraindication to long-term anticoagulation
• Warfarin is contraindicated in patients with prior history of warfarin skin necrosis
• Type IC drugs are contraindicated in patients with coronary artery disease and other forms of structural heart disease
• Type IA drugs and sotalol should not be used in patients with torsade de pointes history

Precautions:
• With type IA drugs, ibutilide and sotalol, the risk of torsade de pointes increases with the extent of QT interval prolongation (i.e., the QTc). In these patients, avoid other drugs that prolong the QT interval (phenothiazines, tricyclic antidepressants, terfenadine, astemizole, erythromycin, etc.). Avoid hypokalemia and hypomagnesemia. Torsade de pointes due to drug induced long QT syndrome is said to be "pause dependent" as

the risk increases with bradycardia, heart block, and sinus pauses.
• In many patients, adequate medical therapy of AF will cause bradycardia necessitating a permanent pacemaker.
Significant possible interactions:
• Quinidine increases digoxin levels
• Amiodarone increases digoxin levels and enhances effects of warfarin

ALTERNATIVE DRUGS N/A

FOLLOWUP

PATIENT MONITORING
• ECG/Holter monitor to assess maintenance of sinus rhythm, control of ventricular rate during AF
• Frequent PT to maintain INR at 2.0-3.0
• ECG to monitor QTc interval in patients on antiarrhythmic therapy

PREVENTION/AVOIDANCE
• Ethanol may trigger AF in some patients
• In cardiomyopathy/heart failure, hemodynamic decompensation may trigger AF

POSSIBLE COMPLICATIONS
• Embolic stroke
• Peripheral arterial embolization
• Significant complications of pharmacologic therapy (bradyarrhythmias and torsade de pointes)
• Bleeding with anticoagulation

EXPECTED COURSE/PROGNOSIS
• Stroke risk low with long-term anticoagulation
• AF increases the risk of cardiovascular morbidity and mortality, but long-term prognosis may be a function of underlying structural heart disease

MISCELLANEOUS

ASSOCIATED CONDITIONS
• Wolff-Parkinson-White syndrome
• Sick sinus syndrome
• Atrial flutter:
◊ A related arrhythmia with regular atrial electrical activity, typically at a rate of 250-350, manifested as sawtooth "flutter" waves on the ECG. 2:1 or 4:1 conduction through the AV node to the ventricle is usual, so the pulse is frequently regular.
◊ Many patients have both AF and atrial flutter
◊ Management for these closely related arrhythmias is similar, though atrial flutter is more difficult to control pharmacologically but more easily electrically cardioverted than AF
◊ Although atrial flutter alone may pose less of a risk of thromboembolism than AF, guidelines for anticoagulation of atrial flutter and AF are similar

◊ Radiofrequency catheter ablation to cure atrial flutter is becoming more widely applied in patients without AF

AGE-RELATED FACTORS
Pediatric: Though extremely uncommon in children with structurally normal hearts, AF may be seen in the setting of congenital heart disease and following surgical repair
Geriatric: Both the incidence of AF and the risk of stroke increase with age
Others: Young patients at lower risk for stroke. The risk of stroke is extremely low in young patients without structural heart disease, so called "lone atrial fibrillation."

PREGNANCY
• AF is unusual during pregnancy in the absence of structural heart disease (e.g., rheumatic mitral stenosis)
• Digoxin is safe during pregnancy; beta-blockers, procainamide, and quinidine are probably safe. There is limited information regarding calcium blockers.
• Risk of fetal hemorrhage makes anticoagulation problematic; moreover, warfarin causes fetal anomalies. SC heparin is probably the best choice if long-term anticoagulation is necessary.
• DC cardioversion does not seem to adversely affect the fetus

SYNONYMS
• AF; A Fib = atrial fibrillation

ICD-9-CM
427.3 Atrial fibrillation and flutter
427.31 Atrial fibrillation
427.32 Atrial flutter

SEE ALSO
• Atrial flutter
• Wolff-Parkinson-White syndrome

OTHER NOTES N/A

ABBREVIATIONS
• AF = atrial fibrillation
• CAF = chronic atrial fibrillation
• PAF = paroxysmal atrial fibrillation
• PT = prothrombin time
• INR = international normalized ratio

REFERENCES
• Pritchett ELC: Management of atrial fibrillation. N Engl J Med 1992;326:1264-71
• Prystowsky EN, Benson DW, Fuster V, et al: Management of patients with atrial fibrillation. Circulation 1996;93:1262-77
• The National Heart, Lung, and Blood Institute Working Group on Atrial Fibrillation. Atrial Fibrillation: Current Understandings and Research Imperatives. J Am Coll Cardiol 1993;22:1830-4
Illustrations: 1 available on CD-ROM
Internet references: http://www.5mcc.com

Author(s)
Leonard Ganz, MD
Leonard S. Lilly, MD

Atrial septal defect (ASD)

BASICS

DESCRIPTION A defect or opening in the atrial septum allowing flow of blood between the two chambers. Shunting is typically left to right and occurs late in ventricular systole and early diastole. The degree of shunting depends on 1) the size of the defect, and 2) the relative compliance of the two ventricles. There can be minimal right to left shunting in early ventricular systole, especially during inspiration. Symptoms typically occur due to right ventricular and pulmonary vascular volume overload sometimes with resultant pulmonary hypertension.
Types:
• Ostium secundum - occurs in the region of the fossa ovalis (most common)
• Sinus venosus - occurs in the superior-posterior septum
• Ostium primum - occurs in the inferior portion of the septum
System(s) affected: Cardiovascular and Pulmonary
Genetics: Congenital, associated with multiple syndromes. rarely familial.
Incidence/Prevalence in USA: Accounts for 10% of congenital heart defects
Predominant age: Newborn, but may be diagnosed at any age
Predominant sex: Female > Male (2:1)

SIGNS AND SYMPTOMS
• Childhood symptoms - usually minimal. Can include failure to thrive and frequent pulmonary infections
• Adult symptoms - easy fatigability, dyspnea on exertion, heart failure (late)
• Signs vary according to extent of shunting and include:
• Right ventricular lift
• Palpable pulmonary artery pulse
• Fixed, widely-split S2
• Pulmonic flow murmur
• Low pitched diastolic murmur at left upper sternal border
• Cyanosis and clubbing

CAUSES Unknown

RISK FACTORS Congenital heart disease family history

DIAGNOSIS

DIFFERENTIAL DIAGNOSIS Other congenital heart disease

LABORATORY N/A
Drugs that may alter lab results: N/A
Disorders that may alter lab results: N/A

PATHOLOGICAL FINDINGS
• Gross defect in atrial septum
• Dilated right atrium
• Enlarged pulmonary artery

SPECIAL TESTS
• ECG findings:
  ◊ Ostium secundum - rightward axis, right ventricular hypertrophy, rSR' pattern
  ◊ Sinus venosus - leftward axis, inverted P wave in lead III
  ◊ Ostium primum - leftward axis
Note: All may be associated with PR prolongation

IMAGING
• X-ray - varying degrees of cardiac enlargement
• Cardiac catheterization (indicated in select patients) demonstrates right ventricle enlargement and location of the shunt
• Echocardiography

DIAGNOSTIC PROCEDURES
• Cardiac angiography
• Echo and Doppler
• Transesophageal echo in adults

TREATMENT

APPROPRIATE HEALTH CARE Inpatient for work-up and when surgery is indicated

GENERAL MEASURES N/A

SURGICAL MEASURES
• Surgical repair (particularly when the pulmonary systemic flow ratio is ≥ 2:1)
• Surgical repair delayed until preschool age (3-4) except for large defects to be repaired earlier
• Small atrial septal defect - primary closure with umbrella-like patch via cardiac catheter is an alternative to open heart surgery

ACTIVITY As tolerated

DIET No special diet

PATIENT EDUCATION For patient education materials on this topic, contact: American Heart Association, 7320 Greenville Avenue, Dallas, TX 75231, (214)373-6300

Atrial septal defect (ASD)

 MEDICATIONS

DRUG(S) OF CHOICE N/A
Contraindications: N/A
Precautions: N/A
Significant possible interactions: N/A

ALTERNATIVE DRUGS N/A

 FOLLOWUP

PATIENT MONITORING Until defect has closed

PREVENTION/AVOIDANCE N/A

POSSIBLE COMPLICATIONS
• Congestive heart failure
• Cyanosis
• Late-onset arrhythmias 10-20 years after surgery (5%)
• Stroke

EXPECTED COURSE/PROGNOSIS
• Course - chronic
• 50% mortality by age 50 in untreated patients
• Favorable in surgically treated symptomatic patients

 MISCELLANEOUS

ASSOCIATED CONDITIONS
• Mitral stenosis
• Anomalous pulmonary venous return
• Multiple congenital syndromes

AGE-RELATED FACTORS
Pediatric: Most frequently appears in this age group
Geriatric: Defects in older persons may still be closed surgically
Others: N/A

PREGNANCY N/A

SYNONYMS N/A

ICD-9-CM 429.71 Atrial septal acquired

SEE ALSO
• Ventricular septal defect
• Patent ductus arteriosus
• Tetralogy of Fallot
• Pulmonic valvular stenosis
• Aortic valvular stenosis
• Coarctation of the aorta
• Transposition of the great vessels
• Complete atrioventricular (AV) canal
• Tricuspid atresia
• Truncus arteriosus

OTHER NOTES N/A

ABBREVIATIONS N/A

REFERENCES
• Friedman WF, Perloff JK: Congenital heart disease in infancy and childhood. In: Braunwald E, ed. Heart Disease. 4th Ed. Philadelphia, W.B. Saunders Co., 1992
• Hillis DL, Lange RA, Winniford MD, Page RL: Manual of Clinical Problems in Cardiology. New York, Little, Brown and Co., 1995
Illustrations: N/A
Internet references: http://www.5mcc.com

Author(s)
Robert Kowal, MD

Attention deficit hyperactivity disorder

 BASICS

DESCRIPTION A behavior problem characterized by a short attention span, low frustration tolerance, impulsivity, distractibility, and usually, hyperactivity. This can result in poor school performance, difficulty in peer relationships, and parent/child conflict.
System(s) affected: Nervous
Genetics: Familial pattern
Incidence/Prevalence in USA: 5% of school aged children
Predominant age:
• Onset < 7 years old
• Lasts into adolescence and adulthood
• 50% meet diagnostic criteria by age 4
Predominant sex: Males > Females (4-6:1)

SIGNS AND SYMPTOMS
DSM-IV-R Criteria - either 6 or more inattention criteria or 6 or more hyperactivity/impulsivity criteria
• Inattention
◊ Careless mistakes in tasks
◊ Difficulty sustaining attention
◊ Doesn't seem to listen
◊ Doesn't follow through or finish
◊ Difficulty organizing tasks
◊ Avoids tasks which require sustained mental effort
◊ Loses things
◊ Easily distracted
◊ Forgetful
• Hyperactivity/impulsivity
◊ Fidgets
◊ Difficulty remaining seated
◊ Runs or climbs excessively
◊ Difficulty playing quietly
◊ Acts as if "driven by a motor"
◊ Talks excessively
◊ Blurts out answers before question is complete
◊ Has difficulty awaiting turn
◊ Interrupts others

CAUSES Polyfactorial

RISK FACTORS
• Association with poor prenatal health (preeclampsia, drug and alcohol use, smoking)
• Co-morbid conditions (associated with, but not caused by)
◊ Learning disabilities
◊ Tourette's
◊ Mood disorders
◊ Oppositional defiant disorder
◊ Conduct disorder

 DIAGNOSIS

DIFFERENTIAL DIAGNOSIS
• Refer to DSM IV-R (see References)
• Activity level appropriate for age
• Dysfunctional family situation
• Learning disability (dyslexia, etc.))
• Hearing/vision disorder
• Oppositional/defiant disorder (see DSM IV-R)
• Conduct disorder (see DSM IV-R)
• Lead poisoning
• Medication reaction (decongestant, antihistamine, theophylline, phenobarbital)
• Tourette's
• Pervasive developmental delay
• Hyperthyroidism (rare)
• Absence seizures (attention deficit only)

LABORATORY Rarely needed, can check lead level
Drugs that may alter lab results: N/A
Disorders that may alter lab results: N/A

PATHOLOGICAL FINDINGS
• "Soft" neurological signs - nonspecific (Romberg, mixed hand preference, etc.)
• Motor tics can be present (cough, noise, scratching)

SPECIAL TESTS
• Learning disability evaluation (mismatch of IQ and achievement) - usually by school
• Behavior rating scales to be completed by parents and teachers. Often repeated after therapy is started to gauge differences - Conner's scale, AcTERs scale.
• Good psychosocial evaluation of home environment
• Continuous Performance Tests - rapid fire computer test - high false negative
• See References

IMAGING Not needed

DIAGNOSTIC PROCEDURES Diagnosis is by DSM-IV criteria. (Do not need EEG unless symptoms highly suggestive of seizure disorder [e.g., absence seizures]).

 TREATMENT

APPROPRIATE HEALTH CARE
Outpatient

GENERAL MEASURES
• Parent/school/patient education
• Work closely with teacher
• Avoid unproved therapies

SURGICAL MEASURES N/A

ACTIVITY
• Allow for increased activity in safe environment
• Often respond well to water play/bathtubs

DIET No dietary changes have been proven to help ADHD. Parents can experiment with non-harmful diets by eliminating:
• Sugar
• Dyes
• Additives

PATIENT EDUCATION
• Key points for parents:
◊ Reinforce good behavior (with rewards and attention)
◊ Make eye contact with each request
◊ One task at a time
◊ Time out (brief) for problems
◊ Stop behavior before it escalates
◊ Find things child is good at and emphasize these
◊ Some families benefit from "anger training," "social training" and family therapy
◊ Educate parents to realistic expectations
◊ Awareness of child advocate groups and support groups
◊ Help to deal with negative feelings
• Key points for teachers:
◊ Short work sessions
◊ Clear rules
◊ Immediate consequences
◊ Reinforce good behavior
◊ Coordinate homework with parent (child may not bring home messages)
◊ See References

Attention deficit hyperactivity disorder

MEDICATIONS

DRUG(S) OF CHOICE
• Methylphenidate (Ritalin): 0.3-0.7 mg/kg/day up to 60 mg/day, lasts 3-4 hours, given am, noon, and ±4 pm, alter dose every week until effective, also comes in sustained release (SR) form
• Pemoline (Cylert): 18.75 mg-112.5 mg/day, long acting, alter dose q 2 weeks, may need to monitor liver function, chewable tablets available
• Additional information:
◊ Many children need 4pm dose for homework and peer interactions
◊ Long acting drugs may be less effective, and should not be discontinued on weekends and short holidays
◊ Therapy should be started low and adjusted
◊ End point is - improved grades, improved rating scales, and improved peer interactions
◊ If not responding, check compliance and consider another diagnosis
◊ The government limits methylphenidate production each year, and pharmacies may run out in November
◊ Some physicians give "holidays" off drugs in the summer and a few patients can have weekend "holidays"
◊ Methylphenidate has become a drug of abuse and should be monitored carefully
◊ Some children experience withdrawal (tearfulness, agitation) after a missed dose
Contraindications: N/A
Precautions: The manufacturer recommends:
• Don't crush sustained-release tablets
• Monitoring LFTs in pemoline every 3-6 months
• In coexisting Tourette's syndrome, methylphenidate may unmask tics
Significant possible interactions: N/A

ALTERNATIVE DRUGS
• Dextroamphetamine (Dexedrine) - 0.1-0.5 mg/kg/day, rarely used, indicated in age 3 and up, comes in elixir form
• Clonidine - helpful for motor tics - 4-5 µg/kg/day
• Tricyclics - useful if stimulants not working, or there is an accompanying mood disorder; not officially indicated, consider EKG to rule out conduction abnormalities (sudden death has been reported). Useful in older children when methylphenidate is less effective.
• Selective serotonin reuptake inhibitors (SSRIs) have not shown any clear benefit

FOLLOWUP

PATIENT MONITORING
• Parent/teacher rating scales (i.e., Conner's scale) initially, in 2 weeks, and regularly
• At least quarterly office visits to monitor side effects and efficacy:
◊ Increased blood pressure
◊ Insomnia
◊ Headache
◊ Abdominal pain
◊ Poor growth
• Some physicians obtain look-alike placebo Ritalin from CIBA for blinded trials

PREVENTION/AVOIDANCE
• Children are at risk for: abuse, depression, social isolation
• Parents need regular support and advice
• Establish contact with teacher each school year

POSSIBLE COMPLICATIONS
• Medications can cause headaches, abdominal pain (take with meals), growth delay
• Untreated ADHD can lead to: failing school, parental abuse, social isolation, poor self esteem

EXPECTED COURSE/PROGNOSIS
• Lasts through school years and into adulthood
• It becomes easier to control with increasing age
• Encourage career choices which allow patient autonomy and mobility
• No increased incidence of delinquency unless other co-morbid features exist (e.g., conduct disorder)

MISCELLANEOUS

ASSOCIATED CONDITIONS See Risk Factors

AGE-RELATED FACTORS
Pediatric: N/A
Geriatric: N/A
Others: N/A

PREGNANCY Avoid stimulant medications in pregnancy

SYNONYMS
• Attention deficit disorder
• Hyperactivity
• Hyperkinesis
• Minimal brain disorder

ICD-9-CM
• 314.00 Attention deficit disorder
• 314.01 With hyperactivity

SEE ALSO N/A

OTHER NOTES N/A

ABBREVIATIONS
ADD = Attention Deficit Disorder
LFT = liver function test

REFERENCES
• Behrman RE, Kliegman M, eds: Nelson Textbook of Pediatrics, Philadelphia, W.B. Saunders Co., 1994
• American Psychiatric Association: Diagnostic and Statistical Manual of Mental Disorders. 4th Ed, Revised. Washington, DC, American Psychiatric Association, 1994
• Barkley RA: ADHD - A Handbook for Diagnosis and Treatment, New York, Guilford Press, 1990
• Connors Rating Scale, Multihealth Systems Inc., 1-800-456-3003
• AcTERs Scale: Institute for Child Behavior and Development, 51 Gerty Dr., Champaign, IL 61820
• Children with ADD (The ADD Warehouse), 499 NW 70th Ave., Suite 109, Plantation, Florida 33317, 1-305-587-3700
• ADDA, 430 West Park Blvd., Plano Texas 75093
• Local Board of Mental Retardation/Developmental Disabilities
• The Parents Guide to Attention Deficit Disorders, Hawthorne Education Services, Columbia, Missouri 65205, 1-314-874-1710
Illustrations: N/A
Internet references: http://www.5mcc.com

Author(s)
Laura L. Novak, MD

Autism

BASICS

DESCRIPTION Autism is a pervasive developmental disorder of early childhood characterized by severe impairment in:
• Effective social skills
• Absent or impaired language development
• Repetitive and/or stereotyped activities and interests, especially inanimate objects
System(s) affected: Nervous
Genetics: High concordance in monozygotic twins, increased prevalence in siblings
Incidence/Prevalence in USA: 3-5 per 10,000 school age children
Predominant age: Onset prior to age 3, but generally abnormal development is apparent well before
Predominant sex: Male > Female (5:1)

SIGNS AND SYMPTOMS
• Impairment in social interaction:
   ◊ Inadequate or lack of use of multiple non-verbal behaviors, such as postures and facial expression
   ◊ Failure to develop appropriate peer relationships
   ◊ Lack of sharing interests and achievements
   ◊ Lack of social and/or emotional reciprocity
• Communication impairment:
   ◊ Delay or lack of development of spoken language without accompanying alternative modes of communication
   ◊ Impairment in initiating and sustaining conversation
   ◊ Idiosyncratic language with stereotyped or repetitive usage
   ◊ Lack of developmentally appropriate play, especially imitative
• Repetitive and stereotyped patterns of behavior:
   ◊ Abnormal preoccupations either in intensity or focus
   ◊ Inflexibility to non-functional activities
   ◊ Stereotyped or repetitive motor mannerisms
   ◊ Preoccupation with inanimate objects and their parts

CAUSES Unknown

RISK FACTORS Associated with increased risks during pregnancy, labor and delivery. Maternal rubella.

DIAGNOSIS

DIFFERENTIAL DIAGNOSIS
• Other mental and CNS disorders including:
   ◊ Schizophrenia
   ◊ Elective mutism
   ◊ Language disorder
   ◊ Mental retardation
   ◊ Stereotyped movement disorder
• Other pervasive developmental disorders including:
   ◊ Rett's disorder
   ◊ Childhood disintegrative disorder
   ◊ Asperger's disorder

LABORATORY N/A (other than to rule-out associated conditions)
Drugs that may alter lab results: N/A
Disorders that may alter lab results: N/A

PATHOLOGICAL FINDINGS N/A

SPECIAL TESTS
• Psychological testing using early childhood instruments, such as the Bailey or using non-verbal instruments, such as the Leiter
• Intellectual level needs to be established and monitored, as it is one of the best measures of prognosis
• EEG to rule-out brain damage and associated conditions. Autistic children have a markedly higher incidence of epilepsy which increases with age.

IMAGING Could be useful in ruling out associated conditions

DIAGNOSTIC PROCEDURES
• Developmental history
• Psychiatric examination
• Psychological testing
• Comprehensive language assessment

TREATMENT

APPROPRIATE HEALTH CARE
Comprehensive structured educational programming of a sustained and intensive design

GENERAL MEASURES Parent support groups and respite programs

SURGICAL MEASURES N/A

ACTIVITY As tolerated by the child

DIET No special diet

PATIENT EDUCATION The Autism Society of America, 8601 Georgia Ave., Suite 503, Silver Spring, MD 20910; 301-565-0433

MEDICATIONS

DRUG(S) OF CHOICE None
Contraindications: N/A
Precautions: N/A
Significant possible interactions: N/A

ALTERNATIVE DRUGS
• Stimulant medications may be used to address concomitant symptoms of attention deficit disorder, such as impulsiveness, hyperactivity and inattention
• Fenfluramine, probably effects attentional symptoms as does other stimulants
• SSRI antidepressants, such as fluoxetine and sertraline have shown some help in reducing ritualistic behavior and improving moods
• Clomipramine (Anafranil), a tricyclic antidepressant, has been reported to decrease some forms of self-injurious behavior, obsessive/compulsive symptoms and compulsive, aggressive behavior
• Buspirone (BuSpar) has in some individuals reduced hyperactivity and stereotyped behavior
• Neuroleptics have been used with limited effectiveness
• Risperidone (Risperdal) in low doses has helped in some case reports

FOLLOWUP

PATIENT MONITORING
• Constant by caregivers. As indicated by physician, prescribed medical management.
• Intellectual and language testing every two years in childhood.

PREVENTION/AVOIDANCE None known

POSSIBLE COMPLICATIONS Increasing incidents of seizure disorders

EXPECTED COURSE/PROGNOSIS
• Prognosis is closely related to initial intellectual abilities with only 20% functioning above the mentally retarded level
• Communicative language development before age five is also associated with a better outcome
• The general expected course is for a life-long need of supervised structured care. Only 1-2% become independent.

MISCELLANEOUS

ASSOCIATED CONDITIONS
• Mental retardation
• Attention deficit/hyperactivity disorder
• Phenylketonuria, tuberous sclerosis, and fragile X syndrome

AGE-RELATED FACTORS
Pediatric: Onset seen only in children under three
Geriatric: N/A
Others: N/A

PREGNANCY Increased risk of autism in complications of pregnancy, labor and delivery

SYNONYMS
• Early infantile autism
• Childhood autism
• Kanner's autism

ICD-9-CM
299.00 Infantile autism

SEE ALSO N/A

OTHER NOTES N/A

ABBREVIATIONS N/A

REFERENCES
• Volkmar FR, Cohen DJ: Autism: Current Concepts In: Volkmar FR, ed. Child and Adolescent Psychiatric Clinics of North American. Philadelphia, W.B. Saunders Co., 3;1:43-52, January, 1994
• Volkmar FR: Autism and the Pervasive Developmental Disorders. In: Lewis M, ed. Child and Adolescent Psychiatry; A Comprehensive Textbook. Baltimore, Williams and Wilkins, 1991
• Diagnostic and Statistical Manual of Mental Disorders. 4th Ed. American Psychiatric Association, Washington, D.C., 1994
Illustrations: N/A
Internet references: http://www.5mcc.com

Author(s)
C. Van Devere, MD

Balanitis

BASICS

DESCRIPTION
Balanitis: inflammation of glans penis
Posthitis: inflammation of the foreskin
System(s) affected:
Skin/Exocrine, Renal/Urologic
Genetics: N/A
Incidence/Prevalence in USA: N/A
Predominant age: Adult
Predominant sex: Male only

SIGNS AND SYMPTOMS
• Pain, penile
• Dysuria
• Drainage, site of infection
• Erythema
• Prepuce swelling
• Ulceration
• Plaques

CAUSES
• Allergic reaction (condom latex, contraceptive jelly)
• Fungal (Candida albicans) and bacterial infections (Borrelia vincentii, streptococci)
• Fixed drug eruption (sulfa, tetracycline, barbital)
• Plasma cell infiltration (Zoon's balanitis)
• Autodigestion by activated transplant exocrine enzymes

RISK FACTORS
• Presence of foreskin
• Oral antibiotics in male infants can predispose to Candida balanitis

DIAGNOSIS

DIFFERENTIAL DIAGNOSIS
• Leukoplakia
• Lichen planus
• Psoriasis
• Reiter's syndrome
• Lichen sclerosus et atrophicus
• Erythroplasia of Queyrat
• Balanitis Xerotica obliterans

LABORATORY
• Microbiology culture
• Wet mount
• Serology for syphilis
• Serum glucose
Drugs that may alter lab results: None
Disorders that may alter lab results: None

PATHOLOGICAL FINDINGS   Plasma cells infiltration with Zoon's balanitis

SPECIAL TESTS   Biopsy, if balanitis persistent

IMAGING   N/A

DIAGNOSTIC PROCEDURES   Biopsy, if persistent

TREATMENT

APPROPRIATE HEALTH CARE
Outpatient

GENERAL MEASURES
• Warm compresses or sitz baths
• Local hygiene

SURGICAL MEASURES   Consider circumcision as preventative measure

ACTIVITY   No limitations

DIET   No special diet

PATIENT EDUCATION
• Need for appropriate hygiene
• Avoidance of known allergens

MEDICATIONS

DRUG(S) OF CHOICE
• Fungal - clotrimazole (Lotrimin) 1% bid to affected area or nystatin (Mycostatin) bid to qid to affected area
• Bacterial - bacitracin qid to affected area or neomycin-polymyxin B-bacitracin (Neosporin) qid to affected area. If infection, cephalosporin or sulfa drug by mouth or injection.
• Dermatitis - topical steroids qid to affected area
• Zoon's balanitis - topical steroids qid
Contraindications: Refer to manufacturer's profile of each drug
Precautions: Refer to manufacturer's profile of each drug
Significant possible interactions: Refer to manufacturer's profile of each drug

ALTERNATIVE DRUGS N/A

FOLLOWUP

PATIENT MONITORING Every 1-2 weeks until etiology has been established. Persistent balanitis may require biopsy to rule out malignancy.

PREVENTION/AVOIDANCE
• Proper hygiene and avoidance of allergens
• Circumcision

POSSIBLE COMPLICATIONS
• Meatal stenosis
• Premalignant changes from chronic irritations
• Urinary tract infections

EXPECTED COURSE/PROGNOSIS With appropriate treatment it should resolve

MISCELLANEOUS

ASSOCIATED CONDITIONS Diabetes mellitus

AGE-RELATED FACTORS
Pediatric: Oral antibiotics predispose infants to candida balanitis
Geriatric: Condom catheters can predispose to balanitis
Others: N/A

PREGNANCY N/A

SYNONYMS N/A

ICD-9-CM
607.1 balanitis
112.2 candida
099.8 venereal

SEE ALSO N/A

OTHER NOTES N/A

ABBREVIATIONS N/A

REFERENCES
• Gillenwater JY, Grayhack JT, Howard SS, Duckett JW: Adult and Pediatric Urology. 2nd Ed. Mosby Year Book, Philadelphia, 1991
• Zoon JJ: Balanoposthite chronique cireonscrite benigne à plasmacytes (contra èrythroplasie de Queyrat). Dermatologica 1952;105:1
• Tom WW, Munda R, First MR, et al: Autodigestion of the glans, penis and urethra by activated transplant pancreatic exocrine enzymes. Surgery 1987;102:99-101
Illustrations: 2 available on CD-ROM
Internet references: http://www.5mcc.com

Author(s)
James P. Miller, MD, FACS, FAAP
Timothy L. Black, MD, FACS, FAAP

Barotitis media

BASICS

DESCRIPTION Acute or chronic traumatic inflammation of the middle ear space secondary to the rapid development of a negative (or less commonly a positive) pressure differential between the surrounding atmosphere of the external canal and the middle ear compartments (tympanic cavity, eustachian tube, and mastoid air cells) This situation is brought about by the inability of the eustachian tube to adequately equilibrate the middle ear air pressure with the moment-to-moment changes in the environmental atmospheric pressures while descending or ascending in air (flight) and/or especially in water (diving). This causes the retraction or protraction of the tympanic membrane with subsequent inflammation and/or rupture. This also may cause asymmetric pressure stimulation of the inner ear and vestibular end-organ.
System(s) affected: Nervous
Genetics: N/A
Incidence/Prevalence in USA: The most common medical disorder experienced by SCUBA divers. Also highly prevalent among aircraft flight personnel (especially high-performance jet aircraft), passengers, and sky divers.
Predominant age: All ages
Predominant sex: Male = Female

SIGNS AND SYMPTOMS
• Abrupt in onset
• Otalgia (ear pain)
• Feeling of fullness in ear
• Conductive hearing loss
• Dizziness
• Tinnitus
• Vertigo
• Nausea and vomiting
• Transient facial paralysis
• With tympanic membrane rupture the ability to blow air and/or fluid out one's ear while performing a Valsalva maneuver or when sneezing
• Crying in children (which is their only means of autoinflation)

CAUSES
• Rapid descent or ascent with eustachian tube obstruction
  ◊ Eustachian tube lock
  ◊ Upper respiratory infections - sinusitis, rhinitis, tonsillitis, and adenoiditis
  ◊ Overzealous forceful Valsalva maneuver (in ascent with vestibular stimulation)
  ◊ Allergic rhinitis
  ◊ Non-allergic rhinitis with eosinophilia
  ◊ Obstructing nasal polyps
  ◊ Deviated nasal septum
  ◊ Congenital abnormalities of inner/middle ear (cleft palate)
  ◊ Nasopharyngeal tumors
• Rapid descent or ascent with external ear canal occlusion
  ◊ Otitis externa (swimmer's ear)
  ◊ Impacted cerumen
  ◊ Ear plugs

• Trauma to external and middle ear
  ◊ Activities involving external ear trauma - boxing, soccer, water skiing, accidents, etc.
  ◊ Overzealous use of cotton swab in cleaning ear canals

RISK FACTORS
• Participating in high risk activities without adequate eustachian tube autoinflation (Valsalva maneuver, swallowing) and/or with any of the listed causes of eustachian tube and external ear canal dysfunction:
• SCUBA diving
• Airplane flight
• Sky diving
• High altitude mountain travelers
• High altitude elevator rides
• Hyperbaric oxygen chamber therapy
• High impact sports
• Infants and young otologically healthy children have difficulty in dilating the eustachian tube (by swallowing) even at small pressure changes and therefore are at higher risk (especially with upper respiratory infection)

DIAGNOSIS

DIFFERENTIAL DIAGNOSIS
• Serous otitis media
• Acute and chronic otitis media
• External otitis
• Myringitis bullosa

LABORATORY N/A
Drugs that may alter lab results: N/A
Disorders that may alter lab results: N/A

PATHOLOGICAL FINDINGS
• Tympanic membrane retraction or protraction with hemotympanum or rupture
• Edema of mucosal lining and capillary engorgement with transudation of middle ear effusion
• Inner ear involvement with rupture of the round or oval windows and leakage of perilymph into the middle ear and perilymphatic fistula development

SPECIAL TESTS N/A

IMAGING Only to rule out suspected nasopharyngeal tumor or sinusitis

DIAGNOSTIC PROCEDURES
• Otoscopic exam
• Audiogram - conductive (middle ear) versus mixed (inner ear) loss
• Surgical exploration to rule out inner ear involvement if suspected

TREATMENT

APPROPRIATE HEALTH CARE
• Outpatient generally
• Inpatient for complicating emergencies, e.g., incapacitating pain requiring myringotomy, large tympanic perforation requiring tympanoplasty

GENERAL MEASURES
• Perform Valsalva method of eustachian tube autoinflation (patient inhales then closes nose with thumb and index finger on nasal alae, then exhales with mouth closed). This will equalize pressures, relieve pain, and restore hearing. This usually needs to be repeated several times during descent or ascent.
• Nasal decongestant spray with repeated applications
• Antihistamines
• If the suggested maneuvers are unsuccessful return to higher altitude if possible and repeat Valsalva
• If ear block occurs, then outpatient politzerization must be performed followed by systemic and oral decongestants
• If associated infection, treat with appropriate antibiotics

SURGICAL MEASURES N/A

ACTIVITY
• No flying or diving until complete resolution of all signs and symptoms and Valsalva maneuver can be performed
• In severe cases, bedrest

DIET Avoid food allergens that cause rhinitis

PATIENT EDUCATION
• Teach Valsalva maneuver
• Educate on how to create allergy-free environment
• Divers Alert Network of Duke University Medical Center, information line, (919) 684-2948

MEDICATIONS

DRUG(S) OF CHOICE
• Decongestants:
  ◊ 0.05% oxymetazoline (Afrin, Afrin 12-Hour) two initial sprays 5 minutes apart then q12h
  ◊ 0.05% phenylephrine (Neo-Synephrine) two initial sprays 5 minutes apart then q12h
  ◊ Pseudoephedrine (Sudafed 12-hour, Afrinol) 120 mg q12h po
  ◊ Phenylpropanolamine (Propagest) 25 mg q12h po
• Antihistamines for allergic component:
  ◊ Diphenhydramine (Benadryl) 25-50 mg q6h
  ◊ Loratadine (Claritin) 10 mg qday
  ◊ Fexofenadine (Allegra) 60 mg qday (60 mg qday in patients with decreased renal function)

Contraindications:
• Previous allergic reactions
• Hypertension
• Drowsiness
• Erythromycin and terfenadine or astemizole; cardiac toxicity.

Precautions:
• All medications must be used on the ground to rule out idiosyncratic reactions that could incapacitate in an airplane or underwater environment
• Elderly are more susceptible to drug side effects, especially with diphenhydramine

Significant possible interactions: Refer to manufacturer's profile of each drug. Terfenadine and astemizole have many possible intractions. Avoid with macrolide antibiotics, ketoconazole.

ALTERNATIVE DRUGS Loratadine

FOLLOWUP

PATIENT MONITORING
• Otoscopic until symptoms clear
• In severe cases, audiograms

PREVENTION/AVOIDANCE
• Avoid altitude changes with any risk factors for eustachian tube dysfunction
• Chewing gum while flying especially for children
• Use of recommended medications before the activity

POSSIBLE COMPLICATIONS
• Permanent hearing loss
• Ruptured tympanic membranes
• Serous otitis media

EXPECTED COURSE/PROGNOSIS
• Ear block - hours to days with complete resolution and return to flight or diving in days to weeks
• Tympanic rupture - weeks to months

MISCELLANEOUS

ASSOCIATED CONDITIONS
• Aerosinusitis
• Aerodontalgia
• Face mask squeeze
• Epistaxis
• Alternobaric vertigo
• Unequal caloric stimulation vertigo
• Anxiety - leading to panic attack
• Temporomandibular joint syndrome
• Inner ear cochlear damage and/or perilymph fistula

AGE-RELATED FACTORS
Pediatric: Healthy children have difficulty in dilating the eustachian tube (by swallowing) even at small pressure changes and therefore are at higher risk (especially with upper respiratory infection)
Geriatric: Drug side effects
Others: N/A

PREGNANCY   Increased nasal congestion

SYNONYMS
• Aerotitis
• Otitic barotrauma
• Middle ear barotrauma
• Middle ear squeeze

ICD-9-CM
• 993.0 barotrauma, otic
• 993.1 barotrauma, sinus

SEE ALSO   N/A

OTHER NOTES   N/A

ABBREVIATIONS
SCUBA = self-contained underwater breathing apparatus

REFERENCES
• Paparella MM, Shumrick DA, et al, eds: Otolaryngology. 4th Ed. Philadelphia, W.B. Saunders Co., 1991
• Dehart R, ed: Fundamentals of Aerospace Medicine. Philadelphia, Lea & Febiger, 1985
Illustrations: N/A
Internet references: http://www.5mcc.com

Author(s)
Smith L. Johnston, III, MD, MS

Bartonella infections

BASICS

DESCRIPTION Bartonella infections cause manifestations in two broad categories:
• Localized skin lesions and prominent regional lymphadenitis, i.e., typical cat scratch disease (CSD). Atypical CSD manifestations often represent disseminated infection.
• Primary bacteremia, potential for persistent disseminated infection with localized inflammatory (and neovascular) lesions in a variety of organ systems and/or ongoing bacteremia.
System(s) affected: Nervous, Cardiovascular, Musculoskeletal, Pulmonary, Gastrointestinal, Skin/Exocrine, Hemic/Lymphatic/Immunologic
Genetics: No defined genetic predisposition
Incidence/Prevalence in USA:
• Non-B. bacilliformis infections:
◊ CSD: estimated 9.3/100,000 people (approximately 25,000 cases annually)
• Others, no incidence estimates
Predominant age:
• B. henselae infections:
◊ CSD: 55% in persons < 18 years old
◊ BA/BP, bacteremia, endocarditis, other syndromes: predominantly adults
Predominant sex: Non-B. bacilliformis infections: Male > Female

SIGNS AND SYMPTOMS
• Carrión's disease (the spectrum of B. bacilliformis infection)
◊ Oroya fever (acute bacteremia): abrupt onset 3 weeks after inoculation, morbid course; severe anemia due to bacterial invasion of erythrocytes, many complications
◊ Asymptomatic persistent bacteremia: <15% of Oroya fever survivors not treated with antibiotics
◊ Verruga peruana: crops of nodular angiomatous skin lesions months after Oroya fever; mucosal and internal lesions also; involute in months to years
• Typical CSD (89% of cases)
◊ 4-6 days after inoculation: 50-75% develop 2-3 mm macule at the trauma site; progresses to a papule or pustule
◊ Regional adenopathy 1-8 weeks post-inoculation; sole manifestation in up to 50%
◊ Nodes involved: 80% upper extremities, neck, head
◊ Suppuration of involved nodes: 15%.
◊ Malaise and/or fever: 30% of patients
◊ Spontaneous resolution: 2-4 months for majority
• Atypical CSD (11% of cases)
◊ Parinaud's oculoglandular syndrome: granulomatous conjunctivitis and ipsilateral preauricular lymphadenitis
◊ Neuroretinitis: usually unilateral; macular star exudate, papilledema, retinal nodules, angiomatous subretinal changes; self-limited, with return of visual acuity to near-baseline; concurrent B. henselae bacteremia found in some

◊ Encephalopathy: mild-profound changes of higher cortical functions; seizures; neurologic sequelae rare
◊ Other manifestations self-limited, sequelae rare: granulomatous hepatitis/splenitis, osteolysis, atypical pneumonitis, others
• Bacteremia due to non-B. bacilliformis species: short-term fatality uncommon
◊ B. quintana: (Eponyms: Trench fever, Wolhynia fever, shin-bone fever, quintan fever) Incubation days-weeks; sudden onset of fever, non-specific symptoms/signs; self-limited illness may be brief (4-5 days), prolonged (2-6 weeks), most commonly paroxysmal (3-5 episodes of 5 days duration).
◊ B. henselae: HIV-infected: insidious onset of fatigue, malaise, aches, weight loss, recurring fevers, headache; localizing findings uncommon. HIV-uninfected: abrupt onset of fever, may persist or become relapsing; myalgias, arthralgias, headache; localizing findings unusual; asymptomatic persistence can evolve.
• Endocarditis: fever, new or changed heart murmur
• Bacillary angiomatosis/peliosis (BA/BP): neovascular proliferation disorders
◊ BA: mostly immunocompromised hosts, e.g., HIV-infected; involves skin (crops of subcutaneous or dermal nodules, and/or skin-colored to purple papules; may ulcerate with serous or bloody drainage, and crusting), regional lymph nodes, internal organs; B. henselae and B. quintana both inculpated
◊ BP involves liver and spleen in HIV-infected and other immunosuppressed persons; can involve lymph nodes as well; nonspecific clinical manifestations
• Neurologic in HIV-infected: cognitive dysfunction, behavioral disturbances; may be mistaken for HIV-related or other dementia, psychiatric disease

CAUSES
• B. bacilliformis: Carrión's disease (limited to the Andes mountains)
• B. quintana: Trench fever, BA/BP, endocarditis
• B. henselae: Acute and persistent bacteremia, BA/BP complex, non-neovascular inflammation including endocarditis and CSD, neurologic manifestations
• B. elizabethae: Bacteremia with endocarditis (1 reported case)
• B. claridgeae: CSD (1 reported case)

RISK FACTORS
• Vector exposure with cutaneous inoculation
◊ B. bacilliformis: Sandflies of the genus Lutzomyia (formerly Phlebotomus)
◊ B. quintana: Human body louse, possibly others as yet unidentified
◊ B. henselae: Domestic cat (especially scratch/bite from kitten < 1 year old), possibly cat fleas, possibly ticks
◊ B. elizabethae: unknown
• Cell-mediated immune dysfunction (a role in BA/BP, possibly endocarditis)
◊ HIV infection, especially with CD4+ lymphocyte count < 100/µL
◊ Chronic corticosteroid, azathioprine, cyclophosphamide, cyclosporine, ethanol

DIAGNOSIS

DIFFERENTIAL DIAGNOSIS
• Typical CSD: other causes of unilateral lymphadenopathy: Sporothrix schenckii, Pasturella species, Yersinia pestis, Francisella tularensis, mycobacteria, Erysipelothrix rhusiopathiae, staphylococci, streptococci, other agents associated injection drug use, lymphoma, metastatic malignancy
• Atypical CSD: other agents causing similar syndromes
• Non-bacilliformis Bartonella species bacteremia syndromes
◊ In immunocompromised, especially HIV-infected: Cryptococcus neoformans, Histoplasma capsulatum, Coccidioides immitis, Mycobacterium avium-complex
◊ After recent arthropod exposure: rickettsial infections, tularemia, plague, babesiosis, borreliosis (location-dependent).
◊ After cat/dog scratch/bite: Pasturella species infection
◊ Viral illnesses: influenza, infectious mononucleosis, acute hepatitis, etc.
• Endocarditis: other fastidious/slow-growing bacteria associated with endocarditis, e.g. species of Haemophilus, Actinobacillus, Cardiobacterium, Eikenella, Kingella, Coxiella
• BA/BP: Kaposi's sarcoma; pyogenic granuloma
• Neurologic in HIV-infected: other causes of encephalopathy, e.g., primary HIV-related, tertiary syphilis, cryptococcal meningitis, toxoplasmosis of brain, progressive multifocal leukoencephalopathy, alcohol or drug abuse

LABORATORY
• Non-bacilliformis Bartonella spp
◊ Blood cultures: lysis-centrifugation (Isolator) cultures plated on blood or chocolate agar, incubated at 35-37°C in 5% CO2 > 2 weeks; enriched broth media, e.g. Bactec, incubated at 35-37°C in 5% CO2 >2 weeks and subculture to agar if bacilli detected by periodic acridine orange staining.
◊ Tissue cultures: recovery from tissue homogenate plated on blood or chocolate agar may require >4 weeks
◊ 1st generation serologic tests available in reference labs
Drugs that may alter lab results: Antibiotics: cultures falsely negative
Disorders that may alter lab results: N/A

PATHOLOGICAL FINDINGS
• Verruga peruana: neovascular proliferation, bacteria uncommonly identified
• CSD: stellate abscesses, mixed inflammatory infiltrates, granulomata, follicular hyperplasia of lymph nodes; bacilli in tissue demonstrable by silver impregnation stains (Warthin-Starry or Steiner) in about 1/3 cases
• Endocarditis: Warthin-Starry stained bacilli may be seen in vegetations

- BA/BP
  ◊ BA lesions: lobular proliferations of small blood vessels containing cuboidal endothelial cells interspersed with inflammatory cells, mostly neutrophils. Fibrillar- or granular-appearing amphophilic material often seen in interstitium hematoxylin and eosin stain. Warthin-Starry stain or electron microscopy demonstrate these to be clusters of bacilli.
  ◊ BP: involved organs contain blood-filled, partially endothelial cell-lined cystic structures and surrounding clumps of bacilli (identified by Warthin-Starry stain) in the midst of inflammatory cells.
- Neurologic in HIV-infected: little information

SPECIAL TESTS
- Skin testing reagents: not commercially available or standardized
- Co-incubation of tissue homogenates with cell culture lines to enhance culture recovery; PCR and immunohistochemical labeling for non-culture detection in tissue: currently remain research tools

IMAGING
Ultrasonography or CT as indicated

DIAGNOSTIC PROCEDURES
- Biopsies for histology/culture of cutaneous nodules, lymph nodes, or internal organs as necessary
- Typical CSD; traditionally, diagnosis required 3 of 4 criteria fulfilled:
(1) Animal contact (usually cat or dog) resulting in a scratch, abrasion or ocular lesion
(2) Positive skin test with cat scratch antigen (not available commercially)
(3) Characteristic lymph node pathology
(4) Absence of evidence of other causes of lymphadenopathy
- Serologic testing preferable alternative to skin testing
- Atypical CSD: compatible syndrome, absence of other evident cause; positive skin or serologic testing
- Bacteremia: clinical suspicion; use of appropriate culture methods
- Endocarditis: compatible clinical syndrome, evidence of valve lesion (ultrasonographic or tissue), positive culture of blood or valve (or non-culture demonstration, e.g., immunohistochemistry, polymerase chain reaction [PCR])
- BA/BP: biopsy for definitive diagnosis; presumptive diagnosis by response to appropriate antibiotics
- Neurologic in HIV-infected:
(1) compatible clinical syndrome plus elevated antibodies in CSF or detection in CSF by culture or PCR
(2) no other cause

TREATMENT

APPROPRIATE HEALTH CARE
- Outpatient for uncomplicated infection
- Initial hospitalization may be necessary for complications

GENERAL MEASURES
- CSD: symptom-specific supportive therapy, e.g., aspiration of suppurative lymph nodes to alleviate pain
- Other syndromes (perhaps including CSD-associated neuroretinitis and encephalopathy): antibiotic therapy

SURGICAL MEASURES N/A

ACTIVITY Fully active for uncomplicated disease

DIET No special diet

PATIENT EDUCATION N/A

MEDICATIONS

DRUG(S) OF CHOICE
- B. bacilliformis infection: chloramphenicol 500 mg po qid for 1 week
- Non-bacilliformis Bartonella infections including bacteremia without endocarditis, cutaneous BA + local lymph node involvement, CSD-associated neuroretinitis and encephalopathy, B. henselae-related neuro-psychiatric disorders in HIV-infected:
  ◊ Erythromycin 500-1000 mg po qid or doxycycline 100 mg po qid for 4 weeks in immunocompetent; 8-12 weeks in immunocompromised (rifampin may play adjunctive role)
- Endocarditis, visceral or bony involvement with BA/BP: Erythromycin 500-1000 mg qid or doxycycline 100 mg bid x 2-4 weeks parenteral; complete 8-12 weeks po
Contraindications: N/A
Precautions: N/A
Significant possible interactions: N/A

ALTERNATIVE DRUGS
- B. bacilliformis infection: tetracyclines
- Non-bacilliformis Bartonella infections: other tetracyclines, azithromycin, clarithromycin, chloramphenicol, ofloxacin, ciprofloxacin
- Antibiotics for typical CSD: no proven response to many agents including erythromycin, doxycycline, penicillin, cephalosporins, but there are anecdotal reports of efficacy of rifampin > ciprofloxacin > gentamicin > trimethoprim-sulfamethoxazole

FOLLOWUP

PATIENT MONITORING Relapse may occur in non-CSD syndromes if therapy is too brief, close follow-up after completion of antibiotics is warranted

PREVENTION/AVOIDANCE Avoid contact with potential vectors, especially young cats. If cat scratch or bite occurs, wash the wound promptly and thoroughly.

POSSIBLE COMPLICATIONS Relapse, especially in HIV infection

EXPECTED COURSE/PROGNOSIS
- CSD - spontaneous resolution usually in 2-4 months without specific therapy
- Other syndromes - with proper treatment, full resolution; if relapse, consider long-term suppressive antibiotics after retreatment

MISCELLANEOUS

ASSOCIATED CONDITIONS In advanced HIV infection, other opportunistic infections may be present

AGE-RELATED FACTORS
Pediatric: N/A
Geriatric: N/A
Others: N/A

PREGNANCY N/A

SYNONYMS N/A

ICD-9-CM
- 078.3 Cat scratch disease
- 083.1 Trench fever (B. quintana bacteremia)
- 083.8 Other Bartonella-related diagnoses, including BA/BP
- 088.0 B. bacilliformis infections (Oroya fever, verruga peruana)

SEE ALSO N/A

OTHER NOTES N/A

ABBREVIATIONS
CSD = Cat Scratch Disease
BA = Bacillary angiomatosis
BP = Bacillary peliosis
HIV = Human immunodeficiency virus

REFERENCES
- Margileth AM. Cat scratch disease. Adv Pediatr Infect Dis 1993;8:1-21
- Regnery RL, Childs JE, Koehler JE: Infections associated with Bartonella species in persons infected with the human immunodeficiency virus. Clin Infect Dis 1995;21(S1):S94-S98
- Slater LN, Welch DF: Rochalimaea species (recently renamed Bartonella). In: Mandell GL, Bennett JE, Dolin R, eds. Principles and Practice of Infectious Diseases, 4th edition. New York, Churchill Livingstone, 1995:429-435
Illustrations: 2 available on CD-ROM
Internet references: http://www.5mcc.com

Author(s)
Leonard N. Slater, MD

Basal cell carcinoma

BASICS

DESCRIPTION Malignant tumor of the skin originating from the basal cells of the epidermis and its appendages. Rarely metastasizes but capable of local tissue destruction.
System(s) affected: Skin/Exocrine
Genetics: More common in fair-skin blondes and redheads
Incidence/Prevalence in USA:
Approximately 400,000 cases/year
Predominant age: Generally > 40 but incidence is increasing in younger populations
Predominant sex: Males > Female (although incidence is increasing in females)

SIGNS AND SYMPTOMS
• Begins as a small, smooth surfaced, well defined nodule
• Color pink to red
• "Pearly" translucent border
• Telangiectatic vessels overlying
• May have varying degrees of melanin pigment
• As nodule enlarges, central ulceration and crusting occurs

CAUSES
• Sun exposure
• Inorganic arsenic exposure

RISK FACTORS
• Chronic sun exposure
• Light complexion
• Tendency to sunburn
• Male sex although increasing risk in women due to lifestyle changes e.g., suntan parlors, etc.

DIAGNOSIS

DIFFERENTIAL DIAGNOSIS Sebaceous hyperplasia, intradermal nevi (pigmented and non-pigmented), molluscum contagiosum

LABORATORY Pathologic examination required to confirm diagnosis
Drugs that may alter lab results: N/A
Disorders that may alter lab results: N/A

PATHOLOGICAL FINDINGS Nidus of basal cells extending into dermis. Characteristic cells resemble normal basal cells with large basophilic, oval nuclei. Rare mitoses. Tumor cells arranged in palisades at periphery.

SPECIAL TESTS N/A

IMAGING N/A

DIAGNOSTIC PROCEDURES Biopsy mandatory to confirm diagnosis

TREATMENT

APPROPRIATE HEALTH CARE
Outpatient unless extensive lesion

GENERAL MEASURES N/A

SURGICAL MEASURES
• Treatment selection varies with extent and location of lesion, tumor border distinctiveness
• High risk areas - inner canthus, nasolabial sulcus, philtrum, preauricular area, retroauricular sulcus, lip, temple
• Curettage and electrodesiccation - nodular lesion < l cm, in low risk area, if not deeply invasive. Requires specialized training and experience in surgical technique.
• Excision - useful for lesions in high risk areas, not as dependent on lesion size. Poor choice if multiple lesions. Requires appropriate training.
• Cryosurgery - reserved for small lesions in low risk area. Requires specialized training and equipment. May want pre- and post-treatment biopsies.
• Moh's surgery - the preferred microsurgically-controlled surgical treatment for lesions in high risk area, for recurrent lesion, if there is an aggressive growth pattern. Requires referral to appropriately trained dermatologic surgeon.
• Radiation - useful for patients who could not tolerate minor surgical procedures (e.g., elderly patients). Also may be used when preservation of local tissue important such as near lips and eyelids.

ACTIVITY No restrictions except to avoid overexposure to sun

DIET No special diet

PATIENT EDUCATION
• Teach patient appropriate sun avoidance techniques, sunscreens, etc.
• Skin self exam

MEDICATIONS

DRUG(S) OF CHOICE Topical antibiotics after excision for 24 to 48 hours (optional)
Contraindications: N/A
Precautions: N/A
Significant possible interactions: N/A

ALTERNATIVE DRUGS N/A

FOLLOWUP

PATIENT MONITORING Every month for 3 months, then twice yearly for 5 years, yearly thereafter

PREVENTION/AVOIDANCE
• Sunscreens
• Hats, long-sleeve shirts
• Avoid excessive tanning

POSSIBLE COMPLICATIONS
• Local recurrence and spread. Usually recurrences will appear within 5 years.
• Metastasis (rare)

EXPECTED COURSE/PROGNOSIS
• Proper treatment yields 90-95% cure
• Most recurrences happen within 5 years
• Development of new basal cell carcinomas. 36% of patients will develop a new lesion within 5 years.

MISCELLANEOUS

ASSOCIATED CONDITIONS
• Xeroderma pigmentosum
• Basal cell nevus syndrome

AGE-RELATED FACTORS
Pediatric: Rare in children
Geriatric: Greater frequency in geriatric patients
Others: N/A

PREGNANCY N/A

SYNONYMS
• Basal cell epithelioma
• Rodent ulcer

ICD-9-CM
• 173.3 (face)
• 173.4 (scalp, neck)
• 173.5 (trunk)
• 173.6 (upper limb)
• 173.7 (lower limb)
• 173.9 (site unspecified)

SEE ALSO N/A

OTHER NOTES N/A

ABBREVIATIONS N/A

REFERENCES
• Fitzpatrick TN, et al: Dermatology in General Medicine. New York, McGraw-Hill, 1987
• Friedman RJ, et al: Cancer of the Skin. Philadelphia, W.B. Saunders Co., 1991
Illustrations: 10 available on CD-ROM
Internet references: http://www.5mcc.com

Author(s)
John M. Little, MD

Behçet's syndrome

BASICS

DESCRIPTION Rare multisystem, chronic disease characterized by oral and genital mucocutaneous ulcerations, skin rashes, arthritis, thrombophlebitis, uveitis, colitis, and neurologic symptoms.
• Endemic in Japan and Northeastern Mediterranean region.
System(s) affected: Skin/Exocrine, Reproductive, Nervous, Renal/Urologic, Musculoskeletal
Genetics: One report in a mother and newborn (A. Fam, Ann Rheumatic Dis 1981;40:509-512). Very rarely familial.
Incidence/Prevalence in USA:
• 1/100, 000 prevalence
• 670/100,000 in Japan
Predominant age: 3rd to 4th decades
Predominant sex: Male > Female; as frequently to twice as often. Some studies suggest equal frequency.

SIGNS AND SYMPTOMS
• Aphthous stomatitis
• Genital ulcers - painful in the male, painless in the female
• Dermal - papulovesicular, erythema nodosum, pathergy, erythema multiforme, vasculitis, pyoderma
• Ocular - iritis, iridocyclitis, chorioretinitis, hypopyon, hemorrhage, papilledema, optic atrophy
• Morning stiffness - in 1/3
• Polyarthritis - self-limited and predominantly affecting lower extremities
• Thrombophlebitis - peripheral, pulmonary, cerebral, Budd Chiari syndrome
• Neurologic - cranial nerve palsy, hemiplegia, intracranial hypertension, meningomyelitis and recurrent meningitis, confusional state
• GI - aphthous ulcers, colitis, melena
• Pulmonary infiltrates - possibly related to thrombosis
• Myopathy/myositis - rare
• Peripheral gangrene - rare
• Epididymitis
• Glomerulonephritis - rare

CAUSES
• Unknown
  ◊ Classified as vasculopathy or autoimmune
  ◊ HLA-B5 alloantigen relationship
  ◊ Possible environmental toxin - heavy metals, pesticides
  ◊ Possibly English walnuts or Ginko nuts
  ◊ Fibrinolysis abnormality
  ◊ One report associated with HIV infection
(C. Stein, J Rheumatol 1991;18,1427-8)

RISK FACTORS See Causes

DIAGNOSIS

DIFFERENTIAL DIAGNOSIS
• Reiter's syndrome and other forms of spondyloarthropathy
• Inflammatory bowel disease (Crohn's disease and ulcerative colitis)
• Syphilis
• Erythema nodosum
• Aphthous stomatitis
• Herpes simplex
• Stevens-Johnson syndrome
• Vasculitis
• Multisystem disease
• Thrombophlebitis related to coagulation factor deficiency
• Mollaret's meningitis

LABORATORY
• Erythrocyte sedimentation rate elevation, but can be normal
• Immune complexes detected by Raji cell and C1q solid phase assays
• Cryoglobulin
• Hypergammaglobulinemia
• Circulating anticoagulation (rare)
• Anti-cardiolipin antibody (rare)
Drugs that may alter lab results: N/A
Disorders that may alter lab results: N/A

PATHOLOGICAL FINDINGS
• May be no recognizable changes
• Mononuclear perivascular infiltration
• Mononuclear infiltrate in synovium
• Endothelial cell swelling
• Partial obliteration of vascular lumen
• Neutrophilic dermatitis (Sweet syndrome) rarely

SPECIAL TESTS
• None specific for Behçet's, but helpful in following disease course:
  ◊ Depression of plasma antithrombin III levels with active disease
  ◊ Increased fibrinolytic activity during attacks
  ◊ Anti-neutrophil cytoplasmic antigen antibodies, perinuclear variety
  ◊ Demyelinating antibodies in neuro-Behçet's syndrome
  ◊ Anti-cardiolipin antibodies, lupus anticoagulants
  ◊ Anti-endothelial antibodies

IMAGING N/A

DIAGNOSTIC PROCEDURES
• Careful history and physical and frequent reevaluation
• Synovial fluid - inflammatory effusion
• Arteriography - for aneurysms or thrombosis

TREATMENT

APPROPRIATE HEALTH CARE Usually outpatient. Inpatient usually required for neurologic complications

GENERAL MEASURES According to body system involved

SURGICAL MEASURES N/A

ACTIVITY As tolerated

DIET No special diet

PATIENT EDUCATION
• American Behçet's Association, 421 21st Avenue SW, Rochester, MN 55902, (507)281-3059

MEDICATIONS

DRUG(S) OF CHOICE
- Colchicine: 0.6 mg bid
- Topical ocular steroids
- Prednisone: 1 mg/kg for severe involvement, especially CNS
- Azathioprine: 2-3 mg/kg/day po
- Methotrexate: Use the lowest possible dose; perhaps 7.5 mg/week

Contraindications:
- Thalidomide contraindicated in pregnancy
- Refer to manufacturer's literature

Precautions:
- Refer to manufacturer's literature
- Absorption of drugs such as amitriptyline, diazepam, carbamazepine, phenytoin, and acetaminophen may be reduced

Significant possible interactions: Refer to manufacturer's literature

ALTERNATIVE DRUGS
- Cyclosporine
- Levamisole - 100-150 mg two days per week
- Chlorambucil - but concern with respect to toxicity, especially its malignant potential
- Thalidomide
- Cyclophosphamide: 50-100 mg/day q am. Patient should drink 8-10 glasses of water/day and report any blood in the urine.

FOLLOWUP

PATIENT MONITORING Dependent on severity of system involvement and medication monitoring

PREVENTION/AVOIDANCE Avoid English walnuts

POSSIBLE COMPLICATIONS
- Death
- Blindness
- Paralysis
- Embolism/thrombosis - pulmonary, vena cava, peripheral
- Aneurysms
- Amyloidosis
- Thrombotic events, especially when anticardiolipin antibodies present

EXPECTED COURSE/PROGNOSIS
- Normal life expectancy, except with neurologic involvement
- Possible vision impairment

MISCELLANEOUS

ASSOCIATED CONDITIONS
- Amyloid
- Sweet syndrome

AGE-RELATED FACTORS
Pediatric: Rare
Geriatric: Rare
Others: N/A

PREGNANCY
- Thalidomide contraindicated in pregnancy
- Possible increase in thrombosis and fetal demise

SYNONYMS
- Mucocutaneous ocular syndrome
- Franceschetti-Valerio syndrome

ICD-9-CM 136.1 Behçet's syndrome

SEE ALSO N/A

OTHER NOTES N/A

ABBREVIATIONS N/A

REFERENCES
- International diagnostic study group for Behçet's disease. Evaluation of ('classification') criteria in Behçet's disease - Towards internationally agreed criteria. Brit J Rheumatol 1992;31:299-308
- Mizushima Y: Behçet's disease. Curr Opin Rheumatol 1991;3:32-35
- Hashimoto T, Takeuchi A: Treatment of Behçet's disease. Curr Opin Rheumatol 1992;4:31-34
- Shimizu T, et al: Behcet disease. Semin Arthritis Rheum 1979; 8:223-260
- Chaleby K: Clin Chem 1987;33:1679-1681
- O'Duffy JD: Behcet's disease. Curr Opin Rheumatol 1994;6:39-43 (note: this is better than the more recent Curr Opin Rheumatol reviews)
- Hamuryudan V, et al: Systemic interferon alpha-2b treatment in Behcet syndrome. J Rheumatol 1994;21:1098-1100
- Pacor ML, et al: Cyclosporin in Behcet's disease. J Rheumatol 1994;13:224-227
- Huong DL, et al: Arterial lesions in Behcet's disease. J Rheumatol 1995;22:2103-2113
- Akman-Demir G, et al: Seven year follow-up of neurologic involvment in Behcet syndrome. Arch Neurol 1996;53:691-768
- Gerber S, et al: Long-term MR follow-up of cerebral lesions in neuro-Behcet's disease. Neuroradiol 1996;38:761-768

Illustrations: 1 available on CD-ROM
Internet references: http://www.5mcc.com

Author(s)
Bruce M. Rothschild, MD

Bell's palsy

BASICS

DESCRIPTION Paralysis or weakness of the muscles supplied by the facial nerve, typically unilaterally, due to inflammation and swelling of the facial nerve within the facial canal
• Bell's palsy: Idiopathic
• Ramsay Hunt syndrome: Bell's palsy associated with vesicles within the outer ear canal or behind the ear, due to herpes zoster infection
• Facial diplegia: The simultaneous development of bilateral Bell's palsy is highly unusual and conditions such as Guillain-Barré syndrome and chronic meningitis should be considered as possible explanations.
System(s) affected: Nervous
Genetics: There is a familial tendency toward Bell's palsy
Incidence/Prevalence in USA: 25 in 100,000
Predominant age: Affects all ages. Most common in individuals over 30 years of age.
Predominant sex: Male = Female

SIGNS AND SYMPTOMS
• Sudden onset or onset over days
• Unilateral total or partial paralysis of the facial muscles
• Mild "numbness" on the affected side
• Ipsilateral inadequate tear production; ipsilateral tearing
• Ipsilateral loss of taste
• Ipsilateral ear ache

CAUSES
• Bell's palsy
  ◊ Inflammation of the facial nerve within the facial canal
  ◊ Exposure to cold
  ◊ Probably viral
• Ramsay-Hunt syndrome
  ◊ Herpes zoster
  ◊ Rarely herpes simplex

RISK FACTORS
• Age over 30
• Exposure to cold

DIAGNOSIS

DIFFERENTIAL DIAGNOSIS
• Neoplastic
  ◊ Carcinomatous meningitis
  ◊ Leukemic meningitis
  ◊ Tumors of the parotid gland
  ◊ Tumors of the base of the skull
• Infectious
  ◊ Chronic meningitis
  ◊ Bacterial meningitis
  ◊ Osteomyelitis of the base of the skull
  ◊ Otitis media
  ◊ Leprosy
• Other
  ◊ Sarcoidosis
  ◊ Melkersson-Rosenthal syndrome (facial paralysis with scrotal tongue)
  ◊ Head injury with fracture of the temporal bone
  ◊ Brainstem stroke (anterior-inferior cerebellar artery)
  ◊ Multiple sclerosis
  ◊ Guillain-Barré syndrome (can initially present as a very typical Bell's palsy)

LABORATORY
• CSF protein - mildly elevated in 1/3 of cases
• CSF cells - mildly elevated in 10% of cases, with a mononuclear cell predominance
Drugs that may alter lab results: N/A
Disorders that may alter lab results: N/A

PATHOLOGICAL FINDINGS
• Edema of the facial nerve
• Occasional hemorrhagic streaks
• Dilatation of the vasa nervorum
• Infiltration of mononuclear cells in some cases
• Atrophy of the facial nerve

SPECIAL TESTS
• Electromyography in the first three weeks after onset of the condition manifests a decreased or absent interference pattern on the affected side, which reflects a reduction or absence of function of the facial motor units. After three weeks, denervation potentials (fibrillations) are typically seen. Eventually, with recovery, low-amplitude, short-duration, polyphasic (nascent) motor units may appear in previously denervated areas. Recovery may be incomplete.
• Nerve conduction velocities may reveal absence or attenuation of the evoked potential, slowing of the conduction velocity or a normal conduction velocity and amplitude
• Blink reflex - the electrophysiological equivalent of the corneal reflex, should be abnormal in all cases

IMAGING
MRI to rule out posterior fossa lesions and intracanalicular 8th nerve tumors if clinical suspicion is high

DIAGNOSTIC PROCEDURES
Spinal tap may reveal an elevated protein or cell count, however, it is usually not necessary

TREATMENT

APPROPRIATE HEALTH CARE
Outpatient except for surgical decompression (very controversial and largely abandoned)

GENERAL MEASURES
• Close and patch ipsilateral eye
• Methylcellulose eye drops

SURGICAL MEASURES N/A

ACTIVITY
Fully active. Use caution in activities requiring keen depth perception.

DIET No special diet

PATIENT EDUCATION
Explanation and reassurance when appropriate

MEDICATIONS

DRUG(S) OF CHOICE
• Corticosteroids: Prednisone 80 mg po qd for three days, then 60 mg po qd for three days, then 40 mg po qd for three days, then 20 mg po qd for three days, then discontinue use. Course of treatment to begin immediately after onset of Bell's palsy. There is little benefit in starting steroids after four days.
• Antiviral agents with activity against herpes group of viruses in Ramsay-Hunt syndrome and idiopathic Bell's palsy
Contraindications: Pre-existing infections including tuberculosis and systemic mycosis
Precautions: Use with discretion in pregnancy, peptic ulcer disease, and diabetes
Significant possible interactions: MMR, OPV, and other live vaccines

ALTERNATIVE DRUGS N/A

FOLLOWUP

PATIENT MONITORING
• Recheck monthly for six to twelve months
• Look for evidence of corneal abrasions. Expect early recovery.

PREVENTION/AVOIDANCE N/A

POSSIBLE COMPLICATIONS
• Unmasking of subclinical infection (such as tuberculosis) by steroid usage
• Steroid induced psychological disturbances
• Corneal abrasion and ulceration

EXPECTED COURSE/PROGNOSIS
Complete, partial or no recovery of function. Patients with partial denervation typically fully recover. Patients with total denervation usually partially recover, but may exhibit aberrant regeneration (e.g., crocodile tears) or hemifacial spasm as long term complications.

MISCELLANEOUS

ASSOCIATED CONDITIONS N/A

AGE-RELATED FACTORS
Pediatric: N/A
Geriatric: N/A
Others: N/A

PREGNANCY Use steroids cautiously in pregnancy. Consult with obstetrician.

SYNONYMS
• Idiopathic facial paralysis

ICD-9-CM 351.0 Bell's palsy

SEE ALSO
• Herpes simplex
• Herpes zoster

OTHER NOTES N/A

ABBREVIATIONS N/A

REFERENCES Dyck PJ, Thomas PK, et al, eds: Peripheral Neuropathy. 3rd Ed. Philadelphia, W.B. Saunders Co., 1993
Illustrations: N/A
Internet references: http://www.5mcc.com

Author(s)
Colin R. Bamford, MD

Bladder injury

BASICS

DESCRIPTION Due to its well protected location, bladder rupture is unusual. Injury most often secondary to penetrating or blunt trauma and classified as contusion, intraperitoneal or extraperitoneal rupture.
System(s) affected: Renal/Urologic
Genetics: N/A
Incidence/Prevalence in USA: N/A
Predominant Age: N/A
Predominant Sex: N/A

SIGNS AND SYMPTOMS
• Suprapubic pain
• Urinary retention
• Hematuria (94%)
• Muscle rigidity over lower abdomen
• No peritonitis

CAUSES
• Forceful blunt or penetrating blow to lower abdomen

RISK FACTORS
• Distended bladder at the time of trauma
• Congenital malformation of bladder
• Prior pelvic or bladder surgery
• Frequently associated with pelvic fractures

DIAGNOSIS

DIFFERENTIAL DIAGNOSIS
• Rupture of the urethra
• Rupture of abdominal viscus
• Pelvic fracture with hematoma

LABORATORY Hematuria on urinalysis
Drugs that may alter lab results: None
Disorders that may alter lab results: None

PATHOLOGICAL FINDINGS
• Jagged irregular tear in the bladder
• Perforation at the dome of bladder near urachus (blunt trauma)
• Extensive perivesicle hematoma

SPECIAL TESTS None

IMAGING
• Cystogram with drain out film
• Urethrogram

DIAGNOSTIC PROCEDURES
• Rarely is cystoscopy indicated

TREATMENT

APPROPRIATE HEALTH CARE Inpatient

GENERAL MEASURES
• Extraperitoneal rupture, insert foley, admit, comfort care
• Antibacterial coverage, broad spectrum
• Anticholinergics for spasm
• Pain medication as required

SURGICAL MEASURES
• Intraperitoneal rupture, immediate surgical repair
• Blunt trauma, contusion, comfort care
• Penetrating injury, exploration, surgical repair

ACTIVITY Full activity when associated injuries permit

DIET No special diet

PATIENT EDUCATION Printed material available from multiple sources

MEDICATIONS

DRUG(S) OF CHOICE
• Broad spectrum coverage, ciprofloxacin (Cipro) 500 mg bid
• Opium and belladonna suppositories q 6-8 hr prn spasms
• Oxybutynin (Ditropan) 5-10 mg tid for spasms
• Adequate pain control as required
Contraindications: Refer to manufacturer's profile of each drug
Precautions: Avoid quinolones (e.g., ciprofloxacin) in children
Significant possible interactions: Refer to manufacturer's profile of each drug

ALTERNATIVE DRUGS
• Other quinolones
• Other antispasmodics; e.g., flavoxate

FOLLOWUP

PATIENT MONITORING
• Cystogram repeat in 7-10 days
• Remove catheter when bladder sealed
• Periodic check for infection and stricture formation

PREVENTION/AVOIDANCE
• Use seat belts
• Auto air bag

POSSIBLE COMPLICATIONS
• Infection
• Fistula formation (rare)
• Peritonitis (rare)

EXPECTED COURSE/PROGNOSIS
• Complete recovery
• Stricture (uncommon) - only long term complication

MISCELLANEOUS

ASSOCIATED CONDITIONS
• Frequently associated with pelvic fractures

AGE-RELATED FACTORS
Pediatric: Position of bladder makes intraperitoneal rupture more common
Geriatric: N/A
Others: N/A

PREGNANCY N/A

SYNONYMS N/A

ICD-9-CM
596.9 Unspecified disorder of bladder

SEE ALSO N/A

OTHER NOTES N/A

ABBREVIATIONS N/A

REFERENCES Walsh PC, Gittes RF, Perlmutter AD: 6th Ed. Campbell's Urology. Philadelphia, W.B. Saunders Co., 1992
Illustrations: N/A
Internet references: http://www.5mcc.com

Author(s)
Jack L. Summers, MD, PhD

Blastomycosis

 BASICS

DESCRIPTION An uncommon, systemic, fungal infection with a broad range of manifestations including pulmonary, skin, bone and genitourinary involvement
System(s) affected: Skin/Exocrine, Pulmonary, Musculoskeletal, Renal/Urologic, Endocrine/Metabolic
Genetics: N/A
Incidence/Prevalence in USA: Ranges from 0.4-4 cases per 100,000 population per year. Higher prevalence in states bordering the Mississippi and Ohio Rivers. Sporadic cases occurring in other areas.
Predominant age: Adults, but 10-20% of cases occur in children
Predominant sex: Male > Female

SIGNS AND SYMPTOMS
• Acute infection
  ◊ Onset may be abrupt or insidious
  ◊ May be asymptomatic and self-limiting
  ◊ Incubation period 30-45 days
  ◊ Fever, chills, myalgias, arthralgias
  ◊ Cough initially nonproductive, then productive
  ◊ Hemoptysis (common)
  ◊ Erythema nodosum
• Pulmonary blastomycosis
  ◊ 60-90% of cases
  ◊ Three forms - acute, chronic, asymptomatic
  ◊ Cough - nonproductive to productive
  ◊ Hemoptysis
  ◊ Weight loss
  ◊ Pleuritic chest pain
  ◊ Pleural effusions - 10%
  ◊ Respiratory failure in small percentage
  ◊ Upper lobe fibronodular infiltrates - 50%
  ◊ Mass lesion - 30%
  ◊ Diffuse pulmonary infiltrates; cavitation (uncommon)
  ◊ Pleural thickening
• Cutaneous blastomycosis
  ◊ Most common extrapulmonary manifestation - 40-80%
  ◊ May occur with or without pulmonary disease
  ◊ Two types of lesions
  ◊ Verrucous lesions begin as small papulopustular lesions, slowly spread, become crusted, have sharp borders; central clearing with scar formation and depigmentation; microabscesses noted at periphery of lesion
  ◊ Ulcerative lesions (initially pustules) form shallow ulcers with raised edges and granulating base
  ◊ Mucosal lesions may occur
  ◊ Regional adenopathy (uncommon)
  ◊ Subcutaneous nodules - cold abscesses

• Skeletal blastomycosis
  ◊ Occurs 25-50% of extrapulmonary cases
  ◊ Long bones, vertebrae, ribs most commonly involved
  ◊ Well circumscribed osteolytic lesions
  ◊ May present with contiguous soft tissue abscesses and/or sinus tracts
  ◊ Paraspinous abscess may occur in vertebral disease
  ◊ Acute or chronic arthritis may result from extension of contiguous osteomyelitis
• Genitourinary blastomycosis
  ◊ Occurs in 10-30% of cases
  ◊ Involves prostate most commonly but also epididymis and testes
  ◊ Outflow obstruction
  ◊ Enlarged tender prostate
  ◊ Involvement of female genitalia uncommon and usually acquired through sexual contact
• Other
  ◊ Central nervous system involvement with acute or chronic meningitis, epidural or cerebral abscesses
  ◊ Liver, spleen, pericardium, thyroid, gastrointestinal tract, adrenal gland may each be involved

CAUSES
• Inhalation of spores of Blastomyces dermatitidis into lung with spread to other organ systems by lympho-hematogenous dissemination
• Primary inoculation of skin may rarely occur
• Female genital infection may result from sexual transmission
• Reactivation of previous infection may occur in immunocompromised patients including those with AIDS

RISK FACTORS
• Occupational or recreational exposure to soil containing spores of B. dermatitidis
• Residence in areas of increased disease prevalence
• Rarely associated with AIDS

DIAGNOSIS

DIFFERENTIAL DIAGNOSIS
• Pulmonary - acute bacterial pneumonia, tuberculosis, other fungal diseases, bacterial lung abscess, empyema, bronchogenic carcinoma
• Cutaneous - bacterial pyoderma, cutaneous mycobacterial infection, other cutaneous fungal infections (sporotrichosis, histoplasmosis, cryptococcosis), squamous cell carcinoma
• Bone - bacterial osteomyelitis, tuberculosis, neoplastic disease
• Genitourinary - bacterial prostatitis, prostate cancer, other fungal infections, tuberculosis

LABORATORY
• Culture of B. dermatitidis from tissue or body secretions on Sabouraud's or other enriched media
• Demonstration of yeast forms (5-15 micrometers in diameter, with refractile cell wall, broad-based budding and no capsule) in tissue or body secretions by wet mount or special stains
• Serologic tests include complement fixation, enzyme-linked immunoassay, immunodiffusion precipitin antibody tests. All have variable sensitivity and low specificity and are not helpful in diagnosis.
• Delayed hypersensitivity skin testing with blastomycin also has low sensitivity and specificity and not useful in diagnosis
Drugs that may alter lab results: N/A
Disorders that may alter lab results: Histoplasma cross-reacts with serologic tests for blastomycosis

PATHOLOGICAL FINDINGS
• Early inflammatory response with polymorphonuclear leukocytes followed by granuloma formation with lymphocytes and macrophages
• Granulomas do not show caseation necrosis
• Yeast is often found attached to or inside monocytes, macrophages and giant cells

SPECIAL TESTS
• Special staining of tissue with Gomori methenamine silver stain
• Periodic acid-Schiff's stain colors cell wall pink or red
• Mucicarmine stain helps differentiate from encapsulated Cryptococcus

IMAGING
• CT scan of head for CNS lesions
• CT scan of spine for vertebral lesions
• Bone scan for skeletal lesions
• Chest x-ray may show upper lobe fibronodular infiltrates, consolidation, diffuse alveolar infiltrates, mass lesions or pleural thickening

DIAGNOSTIC PROCEDURES
• Aspiration of abscess contents for wet mount and culture
• Needle or surgical biopsy of involved tissue

Blastomycosis

TREATMENT

APPROPRIATE HEALTH CARE
• Acute pulmonary blastomycosis may be treated with oral itraconazole as an outpatient
• Chronic blastomycosis, overwhelming pneumonia, or extrapulmonary disease should be treated initially with intravenous amphotericin B as a hospital patient

GENERAL MEASURES
• Systemic antifungal therapy is indicated for all cases of extrapulmonary blastomycosis
• Systemic antifungal therapy is indicated for all but the very mild or asymptomatic pulmonary cases in which a trial of observation may be appropriate

SURGICAL MEASURES
• Surgical débridement of bone lesions if there are areas of devitalized bone
• Surgical drainage of large cutaneous abscesses or pleural empyemas

ACTIVITY No restrictions, once patient is released from hospital

DIET No special dietary requirement

PATIENT EDUCATION Counsel patient and family on potential adverse effects associated with antifungal therapy, duration of therapy required and potential for relapse or chronic infection

MEDICATIONS

DRUG(S) OF CHOICE
• Milder forms
  ◊ Itraconazole (Sporanox) 200 mg po twice daily for at least 6 months
• Severe forms
  ◊ Amphotericin B (Fungizone): 0.5-0.8 mg/kg IV over 4-6 hours daily for a cumulative dose of 1.5-2 gm
   - First dose of amphotericin B is given as a test dose of 1 mg in 200 mL dextrose 5% in sterile water intravenously over 2-4 hours
   - Dose is increased by 10 mg daily until a maintenance dose of 0.5 mg-0.8 mg per kg per day is reached. Slow escalation is not appropriate for severe blastomycosis. Full dose can be given on 1st or 2nd day of treatment.
   - Rigors can be prevented by pre-infusion dose of meperidine 50 mg
   - To reduce infusion-related fever, pre-infusion acetaminophen and diphenhydramine
Contraindications: Life threatening intolerance to amphotericin such as anaphylaxis

Precautions:
• Monitor for hypotension during the infusion
• Monitor renal function, serum sodium, potassium and magnesium, and CBC twice weekly during therapy
• Replace potassium and magnesium as indicated
• When serum creatinine rises to 1.6 mg/dL (141 μmol/L) or greater, dosage interval should be changed to 48 hours
• Watch for phlebitis at infusion site
Significant possible interactions: Avoid use of potentially nephrotoxic drugs such as aminoglycosides which may potentiate nephrotoxicity of amphotericin B

ALTERNATIVE DRUGS
Efficacy of alternate regimens not well established by controlled studies
• Ketoconazole (Nizoral): 400-800 mg po daily for 6 months
• Hydroxystilbamidine isethionate useful in some patients

FOLLOWUP

PATIENT MONITORING
• Monitor closely during early therapy
• Frequency of followup depends on severity of disease
• Monitor serum electrolytes, creatinine and CBC twice weekly during amphotericin B therapy
• Post-therapy followup every 3 months for 2 years then twice yearly

PREVENTION/AVOIDANCE
• Unknown
• Condoms for sexual encounters

POSSIBLE COMPLICATIONS
Treatment-induced nephrotoxicity, electrolyte imbalance, anemia

EXPECTED COURSE/PROGNOSIS
• Cure in over 90% with appropriate therapy
• Relapse in less than 10% of cases
• Relapse rate higher with ketoconazole therapy
• Adverse reactions with amphotericin B are frequent and significant

MISCELLANEOUS

ASSOCIATED CONDITIONS N/A

AGE-RELATED FACTORS
Pediatric: Uncommon in children
Geriatric: Prognosis is worse in elderly patients with significant underlying pulmonary or renal disease
Others: N/A

PREGNANCY Safety of amphotericin B and ketoconazole in pregnancy has not been established

SYNONYMS North American blastomycosis

ICD-9-CM 116.0

SEE ALSO N/A

OTHER NOTES N/A

ABBREVIATIONS N/A

REFERENCES
• Mandell GL, ed: Principles and Practice of Infectious Diseases. 4th Ed. New York, Churchill Livingstone, 1995
• Bradsher RW: Blastomycosis. Infectious Disease Clinics of North America 1988:877
• Brown LR, et al: Mayo Clin Proc 1991;66:29-38
Illustrations: N/A
Internet references: http://www.5mcc.com

Author(s)
William G. Gardner, MD

Blepharitis

BASICS

DESCRIPTION An inflammatory reaction of the eyelid margin. It usually occurs as seborrheic (nonulcerative) or as staphylococcal (ulcerative) blepharitis. Both types may coexist.
System(s) affected: Skin/Exocrine
Genetics: N/A
Incidence/Prevalence in USA: Common (the most frequent ocular disease)
Predominant age: Adult
Predominant sex: Male = Female

SIGNS AND SYMPTOMS
• Staphylococcus aureus blepharitis
  ◊ Itching
  ◊ Lacrimation; tearing
  ◊ Burning
  ◊ Photophobia (light sensitivity)
  ◊ Usually worse in morning
  ◊ Recurrent stye (external hordeolum, or internal hordeolum)
  ◊ Recurrent chalazia (chronic inflammation of meibomian glands)
  ◊ Fine, epithelial keratitis, lower half of cornea
  ◊ Ulcerations at base of eyelashes
  ◊ Broken, sparse, misdirected eyelashes(trichiasis)
• Seborrheic blepharitis
  ◊ Lid margin erythema
  ◊ Dry flakes, oily secretions on lid margins and/or lashes
  ◊ Associated dandruff of scalp, eyebrows
  ◊ Sometimes nasolabial erythema, scaling
• Mixed blepharitis (seborrheic with associated Staph aureus)
  ◊ Most common type of blepharitis
  ◊ Symptoms and signs of both staph and seborrheic present

CAUSES
• Seborrheic
  ◊ Accelerated shedding of skin cells with associated sebaceous gland dysfunction
  ◊ P. ovale and P. orbiculare yeasts often colonize
  ◊ Oil and skin cells foster staph growth
• Staphylococcus
  ◊ Usually part of mixed blepharitis
  ◊ Colonization of Zeis glands of lid margin and meibomian glands posterior to lashes, with Staphylococcus aureus
  ◊ Impetigo contagiosa-staph
  ◊ Infectious eczematoid dermatitis-Staphylococcus is the hapten
  ◊ Staphylococcus scalded skin syndrome - entire body involved (in young children)
  ◊ Angular blepharitis-staph - most frequent bacteria involved
• Other types of blepharitis
  ◊ Contact dermatitis with or without secondary Staphylococcus infection
  ◊ Meibomian gland dysfunction

RISK FACTORS
• Candida
• Seborrheic dermatitis
• Acne rosacea
• Diabetes mellitus
• Immunocompromised state (AIDS, chemotherapy, etc.)

DIAGNOSIS

DIFFERENTIAL DIAGNOSIS
• Masquerade syndrome:
  ◊ Persistent inflammation and thickening of eyelid margin may indicate squamous cell, basal cell, or sebaceous cell carcinoma masquerading as "blepharitis"
  ◊ These carcinomas may also mimic styes or chalazions
  ◊ Sebaceous cell carcinoma has a 23% fatality rate (found in one study of eyelid sebaceous cell carcinomas). Up to one half of potentially fatal sebaceous cell carcinoma may resemble benign inflammatory diseases, particularly chalazions and chronic blepharoconjunctivitis.
  ◊ Any swelling or inflammation of eyelid which does not resolve promptly (within one month) with treatment, is suspect as a possible underlying carcinoma

LABORATORY N/A
Drugs that may alter lab results: N/A
Disorders that may alter lab results: N/A

PATHOLOGICAL FINDINGS Acute or chronic inflammatory cell types

SPECIAL TESTS
• Cultures in atypical blepharitis
• Biopsy in atypical cases that are suspect for carcinoma

IMAGING N/A

DIAGNOSTIC PROCEDURES See Special Tests

TREATMENT

APPROPRIATE HEALTH CARE
Outpatient

GENERAL MEASURES
• Mild seborrheic blepharitis (dry flakes, minimal inflammation) - apply eyelid margin scrubs with eyelid cleanser at least once daily
• If Staphylococcus likely, follow lid scrubs with application of bacitracin, or (second choice), erythromycin ophthalmic ointment, to eyelid margins, using cotton tipped applicator
• Clean lids and apply ointment nightly in mild cases, up to four times daily in severe cases
• Discontinue soft contact lenses until condition cleared
• Chronic recurrent blepharitis requires referral to ophthalmologist for evaluation as to whether patient should continue in lenses

SURGICAL MEASURES N/A

ACTIVITY No restrictions

DIET No restrictions

PATIENT EDUCATION
• Blepharitis "Fact Sheet" from American Academy of Ophthalmology (see References for ordering information)
• Advise patient that blepharitis is a chronic condition, prone to recurrence if hygiene (lid scrubs) are not maintained after antibiotic treatment is discontinued

MEDICATIONS

DRUG(S) OF CHOICE
• Topical treatment, if Staphylococcus likely, application of bacitracin, or (second choice), erythromycin ophthalmic ointment
• In some cases of Staphylococcus blepharitis (e.g., rosacea), systemic tetracycline 250 mg qid x several weeks, tapering to 250 mg daily for one to three months, or doxycycline 100 mg bid po. Alternative is oxacillin 250 mg qid for 1-2 weeks. Used for persistent (despite topical treatment) lid inflammation or recurrent meibomian styes.

Contraindications:
• Allergy to medication
• Tetracycline: not for use in pregnancy or children < 8 years

Precautions:
• Avoid medication containing neomycin, as it is sensitizing
• Tetracycline: may cause photosensitivity; sunscreen recommended

Significant possible interactions:
• Tetracycline: avoid concurrent administration with antacids, dairy products, or iron
• Broad-spectrum antibiotics: may reduce the effectiveness of oral contraceptives; barrier method recommended

ALTERNATIVE DRUGS
Quinolones may be helpful for persistent or recurrent Staphylococcal blepharitis

FOLLOWUP

PATIENT MONITORING   Every 2 months

PREVENTION/AVOIDANCE   Follow treatment guidelines

POSSIBLE COMPLICATIONS
• Hordeolum (stye)
• Scarring of eyelid margin
• Misdirection of eyelashes (trichiasis)
• Corneal infection

EXPECTED COURSE/PROGNOSIS
Long-term eyelid hygiene required to control

MISCELLANEOUS

ASSOCIATED CONDITIONS   See
diagnosis section above regarding blepharitis masquerade syndromes

AGE-RELATED FACTORS
Pediatric: N/A
Geriatric: N/A
Others: N/A

PREGNANCY   N/A

SYNONYMS   N/A

ICD-9-CM
373.00 Blepharitis

SEE ALSO   N/A

OTHER NOTES   N/A

ABBREVIATIONS   N/A

REFERENCES
• Tasman W, ed: Duane's Clinical Ophthalmology. Philadelphia, J.B. Lippincott Co., 1997
• Boniuk M, Zimmerman LE: Sebaceous carcinoma of the eyelid, eyebrow, caruncle, and orbit. Trans Am Acad Ophthalmol Otolaryngol 1968;72:619
• Rao NA, McLean IW, Zimmerman LE: Sebaceous carcinoma of the eyelids and caruncles: Correlation of clinicopathological features of prognosis. In: Jakobic FA, ed. Ocular and Adnexal Tumors. Birmingham, Aesculapius 1978:461
• American Academy of Ophthalmology, Department of Patient Education: Blepharitis Fact Sheet. San Francisco, American Academy of Ophthalmology. Available for order as tear-off pads, phone (415)-561-8500 to order or write AAO, P.O. Box 7424, San Francisco, CA 94120-7424
Illustrations: N/A
Internet references: http://www.5mcc.com

Author(s)
T. Glendon Moody, MD

Bone tumor, primary malignant

BASICS

DESCRIPTION Primary malignant bone tumors are rare. Four types make up the majority.
• Malignant fibrous histiocytoma (MFH) - a pleomorphic sarcoma of storiform pattern without differentiation
• Osteosarcoma - similar to malignant fibrous histiocytoma with differentiation to osteoid production
• Chondrosarcoma - cellular cartilaginous lesion with abundant binucleate cells, myxoid areas, and pushing borders
• Ewing's sarcoma - small, blue-round cell neoplasm
System(s) affected: Musculoskeletal
Genetics:
• Ewing's sarcoma has 11/22 chromosomal translocation and EW5-FLI-1 fusion protein
• Osteosarcomas shows loss of retinoblastoma and p53 suppressor genes and amplification of the genes C-myc, mdm-2, SAS, and cyclin-dependent kinase
Incidence/Prevalence in USA:
Rare: 5000 bone and soft tissue sarcomas per year, a practicing orthopedic surgeon may see one primary malignant tumor of bone in every five years of practice. Ewing's sarcoma is less common in blacks.
Predominant age:
• MFH - teens and elderly
• Osteogenic sarcoma - teens and early twenties
• Chondrosarcoma - very young and very old
• Ewing's sarcoma - children, teens, and early twenties
Predominant sex: Male = Female

SIGNS AND SYMPTOMS
• Pain with weight bearing, at rest and at night
• Swelling
• Tenderness
• Fracture with minor trauma
• Minor injury may bring attention to lesion

CAUSES
• Generally unknown
• MFH often follows irradiation or arises in old bone infarct
• Osteosarcoma has association with loss of suppressor retinoblastoma and p53 genes
• Chondrosarcoma may arise in pre-existing enchondroma or exostosis

RISK FACTORS
• Multiple enchondromatosis (Ollier's disease)–chondrosarcoma
• Multiple hereditary exostosis–chondrosarcoma
• Previous irradiation, risk factor for MFH
• Previous history of bilateral retinoblastoma–osteosarcoma

DIAGNOSIS

DIFFERENTIAL DIAGNOSIS
• Solitary metastatic lesion or myeloma especially in the patient over age 40
• Lymphoma at any age
• Benign bone tumors and benign bone tumors that look aggressive (aneurysmal bone cyst, giant cell tumor, eosinophilic granuloma)
• Infection (osteomyelitis)
• Metabolic bone disease (osteopenia, Paget's, hyperparathyroidism)
• Synovial diseases (pigmented villonodular synovitis, synovial chondromatosis, degenerative or inflammatory synovitis)
• Myositis ossificans and repair reaction to trauma
• Avascular necrosis

LABORATORY
• Generally unhelpful
• 50% of osteosarcomas have an elevated alkaline phosphatase
• Ewing's sarcoma may be associated with an elevated ESR and LDH
• Acid phosphatase, prostatic specific antigen to exclude prostatic carcinoma
• Calcium, P04, alkaline phosphatase
• Thyroid function tests to exclude thyroid carcinoma
• Elevated ESR and WBC in osteomyelitis
• Serum protein electrophoresis and urine electrophoresis to exclude myeloma
Drugs that may alter lab results: N/A
Disorders that may alter lab results: N/A

PATHOLOGICAL FINDINGS
• Histology and special studies in combination with radiographic findings confirms the diagnosis
• PAS staining before and after glycogen digestion with diastase is useful in confirming the diagnosis in 80% of Ewing's sarcomas
• Electron microscopy: glycogen granules in Ewing's sarcoma; neurosecretory granules in neuroectodermal tumors; Birbeck bodies in histiocytosis-X

SPECIAL TESTS
• Open biopsy or needle biopsy. Needle biopsies may not provide enough tissue for frozen section, touch prep, permanent section, snap freezing, electron microscopy, cytogenetic and molecular studies, DNA indices, immunoperoxidase staining and immunophenotyping (lymphoma).
• Biopsy of associated soft tissue mass may lessen the risk of pathologic fracture
• Biopsy tract should to be excised in continuity with the tumor at the time of resection.

IMAGING
• Plain films provide the most important information regarding the nature of the lesion and guide further testing
• Bone scan - prior to biopsy, looking for other lesions
• CT scan for cortical destruction and internal calcification or ossification. Abdominal CT, MRI or renal ultrasound to exclude hypernephroma.
• MRI scan determines the extent of marrow involvement and associated soft tissue mass
• Chest x-ray and chest CT for metastatic disease.
• Mammogram to exclude breast carcinoma

DIAGNOSTIC PROCEDURES
• Rectal exam for prostatic nodules
• Laboratory studies for metabolic bone disease

TREATMENT

APPROPRIATE HEALTH CARE Inpatient surgery

GENERAL MEASURES N/A

SURGICAL MEASURES
• Resection with adequate margin is required to minimize risk of local persistence
• For MFH and osteosarcoma, pre-resection neo-adjuvant chemotherapy treats micrometastatic disease immediately, allows time for ordering replacement prosthesis and bone graft, allows for an in vivo assessment of the chemotherapy responsiveness of the tumor, and may facilitate limb salvage by allowing a "safer" close margin
• Chondrosarcoma in the extremities should be treated exclusively by surgery unless it is of the mesenchymal or de-differentiated high grade variety
• Ewing's sarcoma was traditionally treated with chemotherapy and surgery was limited to those lesions that were extremely large, associated with pathologic fracture, or involved an expendable bone. Most Ewing's sarcoma lesions were irradiated. However, despite irradiation, local recurrence is common up to 25% in pelvic lesions. Therefore, surgery with limb salvage is increasingly accepted. A dramatic decrease in size in Ewing's sarcoma occurs after initial chemotherapy and a decision can then be made after restaging as to whether to irradiate or to resect the primary lesion.
• The treatment goal is to minimize local recurrence while preserving function. Limb salvage is employed whenever a safe margin can be obtained.

ACTIVITY Varies with stage of disease and treatment

DIET No special diet

PATIENT EDUCATION Refer to local branch of American Cancer Society for information and support groups

Bone tumor, primary malignant

MEDICATIONS

DRUG(S) OF CHOICE
These drugs are administered according to specific protocols. Other protocols may be appropriate.
- MFH and osteosarcoma:
  ◊ Doxorubicin (Adriamycin)
  ◊ Intra-arterial and intravenous cisplatin
  ◊ High dose methotrexate with leucovorin rescue
  ◊ Ifosfamide [with mesna to protect against hemorrhagic cystitis]
  ◊ Cyclophosphamide (Cytoxan)
  ◊ Dactinomycin (actinomycin-D)
  ◊ Bleomycin
- Liposome-encapsulated muramyl tripeptide phosphatidylethanolamine (liposomal MTP-PE) immune modulating agent for osteosarcoma (under trial in CCSG and POG)
- Ewing's sarcoma:
  ◊ Cyclophosphamide
  ◊ Vincristine
  ◊ Actinomycin D
  ◊ Doxorubicin (Adriamycin)
  ◊ Ifosfamide
  ◊ Etoposide

Contraindications: Refer to manufacturer's literature
Precautions:
- Left ventricular dysfunction with Adriamycin. Cumulative dose > 450 mg/m2 increases risk. Follow with serial echocardiograms and/or MUGA scans when cumulative dose > 250 mg/m2.
- With high dose methotrexate, hydration, alkalinization of the urine, and close monitoring of plasma levels are needed
Significant possible interactions:
- Myelosuppression
- Renal tubular dysfunction with ifosfamide
- Renal and hepatic dysfunction and GI mucositis with methotrexate
- Nephrotoxicity and ototoxicity with cisplatin

ALTERNATIVE DRUGS
- Ondansetron (Zofran), dronabinol (Marinol), metoclopramide (Reglan), and others for nausea control
- Cyclosporin-A is used in clinical trials to reverse effect of multiple drug resistance gene (MDR-1) expression of P-glycoprotein in metastatic osteosarcomas (verapamil has toxicity)

FOLLOWUP

PATIENT MONITORING
- Patients who require adjuvant chemotherapy are treated after resection of the tumor with maintenance chemotherapy
- Blood counts for myelosuppression
- Serial echocardiograms when Adriamycin is being used. G-CSF often used to minimize neutropenia.

- Chest x-rays obtained every two months for the first year, every three months for the second year, and every four months in the third year
- CT scans of the lungs are initially repeated every six months during first two years
- Ewing's sarcoma may recur > 5 years after diagnosis

PREVENTION/AVOIDANCE None identified

POSSIBLE COMPLICATIONS
- Limb salvage with any primary malignant bone tumor is fraught with potential complications
- Micrometastatic disease may have occurred at the time of presentation and can appear at any time during the course of treatment or followup
- Local recurrence risk for osteosarcoma with limb salvage is about 10%
- There can be leg length discrepancy, infection, wound dehiscence, skin coverage problems, arterial and nerve injury, non-union of bone grafts, and mechanical loosening of prosthetic implants
- Thoracotomy and continued chemotherapy is often recommended for metastatic disease to the lung
- Ewing's sarcoma, metastatic to the lung, is quite diffuse and is less amenable to thoracotomy

EXPECTED COURSE/PROGNOSIS
- With amputation alone, 80% of patients with osteosarcoma had pulmonary metastatic disease by two years. With chemotherapy, the five year disease-free survival rate is 50-85%.
- Favorable prognostic factors for MFH and osteosarcoma include responsiveness to chemotherapy, distal portions of the extremities, small size, age over ten
- Most chondrosarcomas are of lower grade and have a low risk of metastatic spread and low incidence of local recurrence after adequate surgery
- MFH, osteosarcoma, and Ewing's sarcoma have an overall 50% survival with combined treatment modalities

MISCELLANEOUS

ASSOCIATED CONDITIONS
- A higher incidence of chondrosarcoma is seen in patients with multiple hereditary exostosis, multiple enchondromatosis (Ollier's disease) and patients with enchondromatosis and hemangiomatosis (Maffucci's syndrome)
- Patients with enchondromatosis more often die of GI malignancies than metastatic chondrosarcoma

AGE-RELATED FACTORS
Pediatric: N/A
Geriatric: N/A
Others: N/A

PREGNANCY
- Increased growth of musculoskeletal malignancies during pregnancy
- Soft tissue desmoid tumors have estrogen and progesterone receptors

SYNONYMS N/A

ICD-9-CM
170.9 (unless otherwise specified)

SEE ALSO
- Osteitis deformans

OTHER NOTES
- Osteosarcoma variants like parosteal, periosteal, and intraosseous osteosarcoma are lower grade lesions with a more favorable prognosis, often not requiring chemotherapy. Other variants, post irradiation, and post-Paget's osteosarcoma metastasize early.
- Chordoma - rare malignant bone tumor that develops from the remnants of the primitive notochord. May be located in the sacrum or near the base of the skull. Usual course - slowly progressive; recurrent; cure possible.

ABBREVIATIONS
ESR = erythrocyte sedimentation rate
MUGA = nuclear multiple gated acquisition ventriculogram

REFERENCES
- Enneking WF: Musculoskeletal Tumor Surgery, Volumes I and II. New York, Churchill Livingstone, 1983
- Schajowicz F, McGuire MH: Diagnostic difficulties in skeletal pathology. Clinical orthopedics and Related Research 1991;240:281-310
- Womer RB: The cellular biology of bone tumors. Clinical orthopedics and Related Research 1991;262:12-21
- Simon MA: Limb salvage for osteosarcoma in the 1980's. Clinical orthopedics and Related Research 1991;270:264-270
- Velez-Yanguas, Warrier RP: The evolution of chemotherapeutic agents for the treatment of pediatric musculoskeletal malignancies, Orthopedic Clin NA 1996;27:545-549
Illustrations: N/A
Internet references: http://www.5mcc.com

Author(s)
Irwin E. Harris, MD, MBA, MSHA, FACS

- 133 -

Botulism

BASICS

DESCRIPTION An intoxication producing paralytic disease, caused by neurotoxins of Clostridium botulinum. The toxin prevents acetylcholine release at presynaptic membranes.
• Three forms exist:
 ◊ Foodborne botulism
 ◊ Infantile botulism
 ◊ Wound botulism
System(s) affected: Endocrine/Metabolic, Gastrointestinal, Nervous
Genetics: N/A
Incidence in the USA/Prevalence in USA:
• 0.034/100,000 with 75% the infantile form.
• Foodborne - 20 to 50 cases per year
• Infantile - 50 to 100 cases per year
• Wound botulism is rare
Predominant age:
• Foodborne - all ages
• Infantile mean age - 3 months
• Wound - usually young adult
Predominant sex:
• Foodborne and infantile - Male = Female
• Wound - Male > Female

SIGNS AND SYMPTOMS
• Foodborne
 ◊ Nonspecific findings early (nausea, vomiting, malaise, dizziness)
 ◊ Dry mouth
 ◊ Constipation, urinary retention
 ◊ Symmetric descending weakness or paralysis
 ◊ Cranial nerve paralysis (ptosis; extraocular muscle paresis; fixed, dilated pupils; dysphagia)
 ◊ Postural hypotension
 ◊ Muscle weakness, respiratory paralysis
 ◊ Variable deep tendon reflexes
 ◊ Afebrile
 ◊ Progression over few days
• Infantile
 ◊ Constipation - early sign
 ◊ Loss of head control
 ◊ Loss of suck
 ◊ Loss of facial expression and verbalization
 ◊ Symmetric descending weakness and cranial nerve paresis similar to foodborne form
 ◊ Diminished or absent deep tendon reflexes
 ◊ Autonomic dysfunction
 ◊ Afebrile
 ◊ Usual progression over 2-5 days, can be as short as few hours
• Wound
 ◊ Onset 4-14 days post injury
 ◊ Findings similar to foodborne botulism
 ◊ May be febrile

CAUSES
• Ingestion of C. botulinum neurotoxins (A, B, and E most common)
• Foodborne usually from home-canned vegetables or prepared foods
• Infantile from ingestion of spores in environment or occasionally in honey
• Wound due to contamination with toxin-producing C. botulinum

RISK FACTORS
• Foodborne - ingestion of home-canned or prepared foods
• Infantile - ingestion of honey. Breast feeding (controversial).

DIAGNOSIS

DIFFERENTIAL DIAGNOSIS
• Guillain-Barré syndrome
• Encephalitis
• Tick paralysis
• Myasthenia gravis
• Basilar artery stroke
• Congenital neuropathy or myopathy
• Sepsis
• Other poisonings (organophosphate, shellfish, Amanita mushrooms, atropine, aminoglycoside)

LABORATORY Routine tests including CSF exam normal
Drugs that may alter lab results: N/A
Disorders that may alter lab results: Underlying myoneural disease

PATHOLOGICAL FINDINGS Nonspecific

SPECIAL TESTS
• Stool contains organism and toxin
• Serum toxin present in foodborne form

IMAGING N/A

DIAGNOSTIC PROCEDURES
Electromyogram (EMG) shows characteristic brief, low voltage compound motor-unit, small amplitude, overly abundant action potentials (BSAPs), incremental response to repetitive stimulation

TREATMENT

APPROPRIATE HEALTH CARE Inpatient, with maximal monitoring capabilities, especially for respiratory failure

GENERAL MEASURES
• Meticulous airway management
• Physical therapy with range of motion exercise and assisted ambulation as tolerated
• Prevention of decubiti

SURGICAL MEASURES Wound excision débridement

ACTIVITY Bedrest initially

DIET
• Nasogastric feedings if needed
• Fluid restriction if inappropriate antidiuretic hormone (ADH) syndrome

PATIENT EDUCATION
• When preserving food at home, kill Clostridium botulinum spores by pressure cooking at 250°F (120°C) for 30 minutes
• Toxin can be destroyed by boiling for 10 minutes or cooking at 175°F (80°C) for 30 minutes
• Avoid honey in first year of life

Botulism

 ## MEDICATIONS

DRUG(S) OF CHOICE
• Foodborne
  ◊ Antitoxin therapy with trivalent A-B-E antitoxin [available at CDC (404) 639-3670 or 639-2888], one vial IV and one vial IM, repeat IV in 2-4 hours if symptoms persist
  ◊ Penicillin therapy of unclear value
• Infantile
  ◊ Antitoxin therapy not needed
  ◊ Penicillin therapy of unclear value
  ◊ Enemas may assist in removal of toxin
• Wound
  ◊ Antitoxin therapy with trivalent A-B-E antitoxin (available at CDC (404) 639-3753 or 639-2888), one vial IV and one vial IM, repeat in 2-4 hours if persistent symptoms
Contraindications: Aminoglycosides - may potentiate paralysis
Precautions: Serum sickness or hypersensitivity reactions in 20% of antitoxin recipients
Significant possible interactions: N/A

ALTERNATIVE DRUGS N/A

 ## FOLLOWUP

PATIENT MONITORING Cardiorespiratory monitoring during illness

PREVENTION/AVOIDANCE
• Avoid giving honey to infants
• Do not eat or taste food from bulging cans, or if food is off-smelling, discard it

POSSIBLE COMPLICATIONS
• Aspiration pneumonia
• Nosocomial infection
• Hypoxic tissue damage
• Death

EXPECTED COURSE/PROGNOSIS
• Foodborne and wound
  ◊ Mortality 25% (< 10% under 20 years of age), usually due to delayed diagnosis and respiratory failure
  ◊ Full recovery may require months
  ◊ Sequelae due to hypoxic insults
• Infantile
  ◊ Mortality < 1%
  ◊ Extended recovery period and sequelae as above

 ## MISCELLANEOUS

ASSOCIATED CONDITIONS N/A

AGE-RELATED FACTORS
Pediatric: Avoid honey for first year
Geriatric: N/A
Others: N/A

PREGNANCY N/A

SYNONYMS
• Sausage poisoning
• Kerner's disease

ICD-9-CM
005.1 Botulism

SEE ALSO Food poisoning, bacterial

OTHER NOTES Organism present in stools of 1-2% of healthy individuals

ABBREVIATIONS N/A

REFERENCES
• Mandell G, Douglas R, Bennett J: Principles and Practice of Infectious Diseases. 4th Ed. New York, Churchill Livingstone, 1995
• Oski F, DeAngelis C, Feigin R, Warshaw J: Principles and Practice of Pediatrics. Philadelphia, J.B. Lippincott, 1990
Illustrations: N/A
Internet references: http://www.5mcc.com

Author(s)
Bernhard L. Wiedermann, MD

Brain abscess

BASICS

DESCRIPTION Single or multiple abscesses within the brain, usually occurring secondary to a focus of infection outside the central nervous system. May mimic brain tumor but evolves more rapidly (days to a few weeks). It starts as a cerebritis, becomes necrotic, and subsequently becomes encapsulated.
System(s) affected: Nervous
Genetics: No known genetic pattern
Incidence/Prevalence in USA: Infrequent
Predominant age: Median age 30-40
Predominant sex: Male > Female (2:1)

SIGNS AND SYMPTOMS
• Recent onset of headache becoming severe
• Nausea and vomiting
• Mental changes progressing to stupor and coma
• Afebrile or low-grade fever
• Neck stiffness
• Seizures
• Papilledema
• Focal neurological signs depending on location

CAUSES
• Direct extension from otitis, mastoiditis, sinusitis or dental infection
• Cranial osteomyelitis
• Penetrating skull trauma
• Prior craniotomy
• Bacteremia from lung abscess, pneumonia
• Bacterial endocarditis
• Fungal infection of the nasopharynx
• Toxoplasma gondii (in AIDS patients)
• Cyanotic congenital heart disease
• Intravenous drug use
• No source found in 20%
• Most common infective organisms - streptococci, staphylococci, enteric gram-negative bacilli and anaerobes (usually same as source of infection), Nocardia

RISK FACTORS
• AIDS
• Immunocompromised
• IV drug abuse

DIAGNOSIS

DIFFERENTIAL DIAGNOSIS
• Brain tumors
• Stroke
• Resolving intracranial hemorrhage
• Subdural empyema
• Extradural abscess
• Encephalitis

LABORATORY
• WBC may be normal or mildly elevated
• Culture of abscess contents, predominant organisms include Toxoplasma (AIDS), Staphylococcus (trauma), aerobic or anaerobic bacteria, fungi (rare)
• Blood studies - mild polymorphonuclear leukocytosis, elevated sedimentation rate
Drugs that may alter lab results: Prior administration of antibiotics
Disorders that may alter lab results: N/A

PATHOLOGICAL FINDINGS
• Suppuration, liquification, encapsulation, depending on stage of evolution
• Fibrosis

SPECIAL TESTS Surgical burr hole with aspiration to make a specific bacteriologic diagnosis

IMAGING
• CT or MRI are diagnostic methods of choice - findings are dependent on stages of the abscess
• Radionuclide 117 IN-labeled leukocytes may distinguish abscess from neoplasm

DIAGNOSTIC PROCEDURES
• History, physical exam
• Lumbar puncture often contraindicated
• Search for primary source of infection (chest x-ray, skull film for fracture, sinus films, etc.)

TREATMENT

APPROPRIATE HEALTH CARE Inpatient for close observation, diagnostic evaluation, and specialty consultation (neurology, neurosurgery, infectious disease)

GENERAL MEASURES
• Palliative and supportive
• Medical therapy
  ◊ For surgical inaccessible, multiple abscesses
  ◊ For abscesses in early cerebritis stage
  ◊ Therapy directed toward most likely organism
  ◊ Small (< 2.5 cm) abscess

SURGICAL MEASURES
• Surgical therapy
  ◊ Mandatory when neurologic deficits are severe or progressive
  ◊ Used when the abscess is in the posterior fossa
  ◊ Abscess drainage - (via needle) under stereotactic CT guidance through a burr hole under local anesthesia, is most rapid and effective method. May be repeated if needed.
  ◊ Craniotomy - if abscess is large or multilocular
  ◊ Abscess resulting from trauma

ACTIVITY Bedrest until infection controlled and abscess evacuated or resolving, then up as tolerated

DIET IV fluids if nausea and vomiting present

PATIENT EDUCATION For patient education materials favorably reviewed on this topic, contact: Brain Research Foundation, 208 S. LaSalle Street, Suite 1426, Chicago, IL 60604, (312)782-4311

MEDICATIONS

DRUG(S) OF CHOICE
• Antibiotics according to organism if known
• If organism unknown, begin with penicillin G and metronidazole, or chloramphenicol (Chloromycetin), if metronidazole cannot be used
• Add oxacillin or nafcillin if trauma or IV drug user (use vancomycin in penicillin-sensitive patients)
• If gram-negative organism suspected (otic, GI, GU organ) add third-generation cephalosporin
• Abscess associated with HIV infection assumed to be due to Toxoplasma gondii - daily doses of sulfadiazine and pyrimethamine. (Therapy will be life-long in AIDS patients.)
• Anticonvulsants - phenytoin until abscess resolved or perhaps longer. Obtain anticonvulsant levels.
• Following surgical procedure - corticosteroids to reduce edema. Dexamethasone. Taper rapidly. Use usually limited to 1 week. Continue antibiotics for 6-8 weeks.
Contraindications: Sensitivity or allergy to any prescribed medications
Precautions:
• Sulfadiazine poorly water soluble. Patients must maintain adequate hydration or risk developing crystalluria.
• Decrease dosage of penicillins in patients with renal dysfunction
• Monitor serum levels of anticonvulsants
• Dose of pyrimethamine require for treatment of toxoplasmosis may approach toxic levels. Should observe for folic acid deficiency and treat with folinic acid (leucovorin) 5-15 mg (orally, IM, IV) if necessary
Significant possible interactions: Refer to manufacturer's literature

ALTERNATIVE DRUGS N/A

FOLLOWUP

PATIENT MONITORING
• Postsurgical monitoring as needed
• Serial CT or MRI - to confirm progressive resolution, early detection and management of complications

PREVENTION/AVOIDANCE
• Adequate treatment of otitis media, mastoiditis, dental abscess, other predisposing factors
• Prophylactic antibiotics after compound skull fracture or penetrating head wound

POSSIBLE COMPLICATIONS
• Permanent neurological deficits
• Surgical complications
• Recurrent abscess
• Seizures

EXPECTED COURSE/PROGNOSIS
Survival > 80% with early diagnosis and treatment

MISCELLANEOUS

ASSOCIATED CONDITIONS
• AIDS
• Congenital heart disease

AGE-RELATED FACTORS
Pediatric:
• About one third of cases in pediatric age group. Rarely found in infants under 1 year of age.
• Cyanotic congenital heart disease frequently associated
Geriatric: Age does not affect outcome as much as abscess size and state of neurological dysfunction at presentation
Others: N/A

PREGNANCY N/A

SYNONYMS Cerebral abscess

ICD-9-CM 324.0 Intracranial abscess

SEE ALSO N/A

OTHER NOTES N/A

ABBREVIATIONS N/A

REFERENCES
• Patel KS, Marks PV: Management of focal intracranial infections: Is medical treatment better than surgery? J Neuro Neurosurg Psychiatry 1990;53:472
• Maniglia AJ, Goodwin WJ, Arnold JE, et al: Intracranial abscesses secondary to nasal, sinus, and orbital infections in adults and children. Arch Otolaryngol Head Neck Surg 1989;115:1424
• Osenbach RK, Loftus CM: Diagnosis and Management of Brain Abscess. Neurosurgery Clinics of North America 1992;3:403-420
• Twomey CR: Brain diseases: An update. J Neuroscience Nursing 1992;24:34-39
• Adams RD, Victor M: Principles of Neurology. 5th Ed. New York, McGraw-Hill, 1993
• Rowland LD, ed: Merritt's Textbook of Neurology. 9th Ed. Baltimore, Williams & Wilkins, 1995
• Rakel RE, ed: Conn's Current Therapy. Philadelphia, W.B. Saunders Co., 1995
Illustrations: N/A
Internet references: http://www.5mcc.com

Author(s)
Mark R. Dambro, MD, FAAFP

Brain injury, traumatic

 BASICS

 DIAGNOSIS

 TREATMENT

DESCRIPTION
Traumatic brain injury (TBI) is a principal cause of death and disability in young adults, at an estimated cost of $39 billion per year in the USA
- Several themes underlie discussions of TBI:
  ◊ TBI comprises a spectrum of disorders in terms of severity and agent of injury
  ◊ The most common, closed head injury, is most often related to a rapid deceleration of the head, with or without impact, and results in relatively reproducible pathology
  ◊ TBI is a dynamic process. Not only does the pathologic picture evolve over the first few hours and days after trauma (often with devastating secondary injury), but the physiologic and clinical aspects of recovery continues for years.
  ◊ The prognosis often requires frequent revision because of the long period of recovery and the multiple, poorly understood variables involved
  ◊ The outcome from TBI is a composite of neurologic, cognitive, behavioral and psychosocial variables, where the last two variables are probably most important.
  ◊ The young adult brain has a remarkable ability to compensate for injury; a factor to consider in predicting long-term outcome and in evaluating the value of specific rehabilitation strategies
  ◊ The TBI patient often manifests a multitude of systemic abnormalities, as a consequence of both brain injury and concomitant trauma outside the brain. Changes in nutrition, cardiopulmonary status, circulating catecholamines, and coagulation are all important.

System(s) affected: Nervous, Cardiovascular, Endocrine/Metabolic
Genetics: N/A
Incidence/Prevalence in USA:
Incidence: 200/100,000; 500,000 hospitalizations and 75,000 deaths per year
Predominant age: 15-24
Predominant sex: Male > Female

SIGNS AND SYMPTOMS
- Loss of consciousness
- External signs of head injury
- Labored breathing
- Focal neurologic signs
- Decorticate or decerebrate rigidity
- Bloody cerebrospinal fluid
- Pupils unequal
- Rising blood pressure with increased intracranial pressure
- Posttraumatic amnesia

CAUSES
- Motor vehicle accident (50%)
- Falls
- Assault

RISK FACTORS
- Alcohol
- Prior head injury
- Contact sports

DIFFERENTIAL DIAGNOSIS
Without external evidence or history of head injury other causes of coma should be considered (e.g., drug overdose, infection, metabolic, vascular causes)

LABORATORY
N/A
Drugs that may alter lab results: N/A
Disorders that may alter lab results: N/A

PATHOLOGICAL FINDINGS
- Focal injury, including hematoma or contusion, most commonly seen in the orbito-frontal and anterior temporal lobes
- Diffuse axonal injury, which evolves over 12-24 hours and may occur even in mild head injury. A principal cause of long-term disability.
- Superimposed hypoxia/ischemia involving mainly the hippocampus and cortical vascular border zones
- Microvascular injury, also evolves over 6-12 hours and may persist for days. Is probably a major contributor to secondary brain swelling.
- Selective excitotoxic injury to reticular thalamus and hippocampal neurons, even after relatively mild injury. This may relate to chronic attentional and memory problems.
- Delayed secondary injury is one of the major determinants of ultimate tissue loss and of mortality. A cascade of biochemical events is set in motion by the trauma, including the generation of oxygen free radicals and the process of lipid peroxidation, release of kinins, excitotoxins, peptides, changes in calcium and magnesium metabolism and activation of the arachidonic acid chain. Acute management is aimed at minimizing this chain of events and protecting the brain from further injury.

SPECIAL TESTS
Drug and alcohol screen, diffuse intravascular coagulation panel in severe TBI

IMAGING
- CT scan acutely in all patients with coma, skull fracture, lateralized neurologic signs, or progressive deterioration of Glasgow Coma Scores (GCS)
- Cervical x-ray (associated cervical fracture seen in 5% of severe TBI)
- MRI scan may be useful in post-acute and chronic followup

DIAGNOSTIC PROCEDURES
- Sequential GCS and checks for lateralized neurologic deficit and/or pupillary paralysis
- Intracranial pressure monitoring in comatose patients

APPROPRIATE HEALTH CARE
Inpatient in intensive care unit for comatose patients

GENERAL MEASURES
- Acute management:
  ◊ Immediate cardiopulmonary resuscitation, avoid hypotension or hypoxia, since the traumatized brain is exquisitely sensitive to hypoxia/ischemia
  ◊ Intubate the deeply comatose patient, sedate and/or paralyze if necessary
  ◊ Frequent monitoring with sequential GCS. Beware of the "talk and die" patient, who initially appears well, but deteriorates quickly.
  ◊ Consider evacuation of intracranial hematomas within 4 hours of injury
  ◊ Emphasize a "team approach"
  ◊ Management of systemic metabolic abnormalities. Avoid excessive use of glucose, since hyperglycemia may be detrimental in acute TBI.
- Post-acute rehabilitation:
  ◊ Outcome from TBI is a composite of pre-injury status (intelligence, education) and neurologic, cognitive, behavioral and psycho-social deficits
  ◊ The most troublesome of these are often the behavioral and psycho-social
  ◊ The goal of rehabilitation is to aid the natural process of improvement and help the patient return to independent living
  ◊ While most TBI patients would probably benefit from some level of TBI-specific rehabilitation, the exact type and intensity of treatment for a given patient is debated
  ◊ Few, if any, rehabilitation strategies have been subjected to the level of scientific scrutiny applied to most other medical therapies
  ◊ Some over-zealous institutional programs could even be detrimental, particularly if they inadvertently foster continued dependence
  ◊ Rehabilitation should begin as soon as possible after injury
  ◊ Essential elements of treatment include proper counseling and support of patient and family, emphasis on training in decision making, behavioral modification, and return to independence

SURGICAL MEASURES
Dependent on injury and risk of complications

ACTIVITY
As tolerated

DIET
As tolerated

PATIENT EDUCATION
- Brain Injury Association help-line: 1-800-444-6443
- Printed patient information available from: A Chance to Grow, 5034 Oliver Avenue North, Minneapolis, MN 55430, (612)521-2266

MEDICATIONS

DRUG(S) OF CHOICE
• Acute management:
◊ Morphine 4-12 mg q 2-4 hours for sedation (if needed)
◊ Paralysis with pancuronium bromide 4 mg q 2-4 hours prn (if needed)
◊ Mannitol, 1 gm/kg/8 hours for increased intracranial pressure
◊ Barbiturate coma for persistent elevation of intracranial pressure
◊ Phenytoin seizure prophylaxis for 2 weeks after severe head injury (GCS < 8 , contusions or hematoma on CT scan)
◊ If seizures occur, then carbamazepine to maintain therapeutic blood level
◊ Use of mega-dose corticosteroids to control acute brain swelling remains very controversial and is generally not recommended. Oxygen Free Radical Scavengers appear promising, but remain experimental.
• Chronic management:
◊ Medical control of agitation and aggression remains largely empiric and highly individualized
◊ Avoid neuroleptics such as haloperidol
◊ Consider carbamazepine, lithium, tricyclic antidepressants, beta-adrenergic blockers such as propranolol, or buspirone
◊ "Activating" antidepressants such as amantadine, bromocriptine, desipramine, sertraline or methylphenidate may be useful in patients who are generally under-aroused with only occasional episodes of agitation
Contraindications: Refer to manufacturer's literature
Precautions: Refer to manufacturer's literature
Significant possible interactions: Refer to manufacturer's literature

ALTERNATIVE DRUGS
Diuretics, beta-blockers, and ACE inhibitors for maintaining the mean blood pressure between 110-120 mmHg. Higher pressures may increase cerebral edema. Calcium channel blockers may increase ICP.

FOLLOWUP

PATIENT MONITORING
• Schedule regular followup over the first 6-12 months post-injury, but especially over the first month
• Recommend a gradual return to work or school, even after mild to moderate head injury
• The post-concussion syndrome can follow even mild head injury without loss of consciousness and includes headaches, dizziness, fatigue and subtle cognitive or affective changes. Most of these improve markedly over the first 3 months.
• The most important element of mild TBI management, however, is the recognition that initially there is a genuine organic basis for all of these symptoms
• Proper counselling, symptomatic management and gradual return to normal activities is essential to prevent a post-traumatic neurosis which can become refractory to treatment

PREVENTION/AVOIDANCE
• Safety education
• Seat belts, bicycle and motorcycle helmets
• Protective headgear for contact sports

POSSIBLE COMPLICATIONS
• Delayed hematomas
• Maintain high levels of suspicion for chronic subdural hematoma, which may follow even "mild" head injury, especially in the elderly. Often present with headache, decreased mentation.
• Delayed hydrocephalus
• Emotional disturbances and psychiatric disorders resulting from head injury may be refractory to treatment
• Seizure disorders - in about 50% of penetrating head injuries, in about 20% of severe closed head injuries, and in < 5% of head injuries overall. Hematomas significantly increase risk of epilepsy.

EXPECTED COURSE/PROGNOSIS
• Gradual improvement for many
• 30-50% of severe head injuries may be fatal
• Prolonged coma may be followed by satisfactory outcome

MISCELLANEOUS

ASSOCIATED CONDITIONS
Alcohol and drug abuse

AGE-RELATED FACTORS
Pediatric: Outcome for children more positive, except in severe TBI
Geriatric:
• Poorer prognosis with increasing age
• Subdural hematomas are common after fall or blow; symptoms may be subtle
Others: None

PREGNANCY N/A

SYNONYMS
• Head injury
• Closed head injury

ICD-9-CM
800-804 Skull and facial fractures
850 Concussion
851 Cerebral laceration or contusion
852 Hematoma
854 Other cerebral injury

SEE ALSO
• Seizure disorders

OTHER NOTES N/A

ABBREVIATIONS
GCS = Glasgow Coma Score
ICP = intracranial pressure

REFERENCES
• Jennett B, Teasdale G: Management of Head Injury. Philadelphia, F.A. Davis Co., 1981
• Becker S, Gudeman D: Textbook of Head Injury. Philadelphia, W.B. Saunders Co., 1989
Illustrations: N/A
Internet references: http://www.5mcc.com

Author(s)
Andres M. Salazar, MD

Branchial cleft fistula

BASICS

DESCRIPTION A congenital, abnormal tract connecting the skin of neck with an internal structure, resulting from failure of closure of a branchial cleft.
• May involve branchial clefts I-IV
Genetics: 10% have family history
System(s) affected: head and neck
Incidence/Prevalence in USA: Unknown
Predominant age: By definition are all present at birth although may remain unnoticed for some time. (Branchial cleft cysts may not present until later childhood.)
Predominant sex: Unknown

SIGNS AND SYMPTOMS
• Presence of tiny external opening usually on neck
• Spontaneous mucoid drainage
• External openings may also be marked by a skin tag or cartilage
• Infection may rarely be the presenting sign with erythema, swelling, pain, fever
• 10% are bilateral

CAUSES
• The 1st branchial cleft contributes to the tympanic cavity and eustachian tube. Related fistulae are very rare and tend to be infra- or retroauricular. (Preauricular cysts and sinuses are not thought to be of branchial cleft origin.)
• The 2nd branchial cleft forms the hyoid bone and tonsillar fossa. Related fistulae (most common variant) course between the internal and external carotid arteries. Internal opening usually at level of tonsillar fossa. External opening along anterior border of sternocleidomastoid muscle.
• 3rd and 4th branchial clefts form parathyroid glands, thymus and portions of thyroid (parafollicular cells). Fistulae are rare, those from 3rd cleft course lateral to carotid artery, both should have external ostia on lower anterior neck.

RISK FACTORS Positive family history

DIAGNOSIS

DIFFERENTIAL DIAGNOSIS
• External sinuses
• Branchial cysts must be differentiated from cystic hygroma, dermoid cysts, lymphadenopathy

LABORATORY Culture if signs of infection
Drugs that may alter lab results: N/A
Disorders that may alter lab results: N/A

PATHOLOGICAL FINDINGS Lined by stratified squamous epithelium, may contain hair follicles, sweat glands, sebaceous glands, cartilage. Some are lined by ciliated columnar epithelium.

SPECIAL TESTS N/A

IMAGING N/A

DIAGNOSTIC PROCEDURES Sinogram or fistulogram may be done but is of little value

TREATMENT

APPROPRIATE HEALTH CARE
• Surgical excision
• Outpatient status usually appropriate

GENERAL MEASURES N/A

SURGICAL MEASURES
• Small transverse incision at external ostium with careful dissection of fistula
• Stepladder incisions may be needed
• End of fistula ligated flush with pharyngeal mucosa
• Drains are not used
• Antibiotics only for infection

ACTIVITY N/A

DIET N/A

PATIENT EDUCATION

MEDICATIONS

DRUG(S) OF CHOICE N/A
Contraindications: N/A
Precautions: N/A
Significant possible interactions: N/A

ALTERNATIVE DRUGS N/A

FOLLOWUP

PATIENT MONITORING
• Follow at weekly intervals, if infected, until resolution, than excision
• Postoperative visit at 2 weeks

PREVENTION/AVOIDANCE N/A

EXPECTED COURSE/PROGNOSIS
Good

POSSIBLE COMPLICATIONS
• Facial nerve injury
• Infection
• Carotid artery injury
• Possible recurrence if any epithelium remains
• Neoplastic degeneration of branchial remnants (about 250 reported cases) if not resected

MISCELLANEOUS

ASSOCIATED CONDITIONS Microtia and aural atresia occur with failure of development of 1st branchial cleft.

AGE-RELATED FACTORS
Pediatric: N/A
Geriatric: N/A
Others: N/A

PREGNANCY N/A

SYNONYMS N/A

ICD-9-CM
744.41 branchial cleft sinus or fistula

SEE ALSO N/A

OTHER NOTES Branchial cleft remnants, sinuses, cysts are also the result of failure of branchial cleft to complete its normal development

ABBREVIATIONS N/A

REFERENCES
• Ashcraft KW, Holder TM: Pediatric Surgery. 2nd Ed. Philadelphia, W.B. Saunders Co., 1993
• Welch KJ, Randolph JG, Ravitch MM, O'Neill JA, Rowe MI: Pediatric Surgery. 4th Ed. Chicago, Year Book Medical Publishers, Inc., 1986
Illustrations: N/A
Internet references: http://www.5mcc.com

Author(s)
Timothy L. Black, MD, FACS, FAAP

Breast abscess

BASICS

DESCRIPTION Collection of pus usually localized. Can be associated with lactation or fistulous tracts secondary to squamous epithelial neoplasm or duct occlusion.
System(s) affected: Skin/Exocrine
Genetics: N/A
Incidence/Prevalence in USA: Common
Predominant age:
• Subareolar abscess - postmenopausal
• Puerperal abscess - premenopausal
Predominant sex: Female

SIGNS AND SYMPTOMS
• Tender breast lump, fluctuant, usually unilateral
• Erythema
• Draining pus
• Local edema
• Systemic malaise
• Fever
• Nipple and skin retraction
• Proximal lymphadenopathy

CAUSES
• Puerperal abscesses - blocked lactiferous duct
• Subareolar abscess - squamous epithelial neoplasm with keratin plugs or ductal extension with associated inflammation
• Peripheral abscess - stasis of the duct

RISK FACTORS
• Puerperal mastitis 5-11% go on to abscess
• Diabetes
• Rheumatoid arthritis
• Steroids
• Silicone/paraffin implants
• Lumpectomy with radiation
• Heavy cigarette smoking
• Nipple retraction

DIAGNOSIS

DIFFERENTIAL DIAGNOSIS
• Carcinoma (inflammatory)
• Tuberculosis (may be associated with HIV infection)
• Actinomycosis
• Typhoid
• Sarcoid
• Syphilis
• Hydatid cyst
• Sebaceous cyst

LABORATORY
• Leukocytosis
• Elevated sedimentation rate
• Culture and sensitivity of drainage to identify pathogen, usually staphylococci or streptococcus. Non-lactational abscess associated with anaerobic bacteria.
Drugs that may alter lab results: None
Disorders that may alter lab results: None

PATHOLOGICAL FINDINGS
• Squamous metaplasia of the ducts
• Intraductal hyperplasia
• Epithelial overgrowth
• Fat necrosis
• Duct ectasia

SPECIAL TESTS None

IMAGING
• Ultrasound
• Mammogram - cannot exclude carcinoma

DIAGNOSTIC PROCEDURES
• Aspiration for culture
• Fine needle aspiration (FNA) not accurate to exclude carcinoma

TREATMENT

APPROPRIATE HEALTH CARE
Outpatient, unless systemically immunocompromised

GENERAL MEASURES
• Cold compresses
• Expression of milk

SURGICAL MEASURES
• Aspiration possibly under ultrasound guidance
• Incision and drainage with removal of loculations and biopsy of all non-puerperal abscesses to rule out carcinoma
• Open all fistulous tracts, especially in nonlactating abscesses

ACTIVITY No restrictions

DIET No restrictions

PATIENT EDUCATION
• Care of wound
• Breast feeding precautions

Breast abscess

MEDICATIONS

DRUG(S) OF CHOICE
• Nonsteroidal anti-inflammatory agents
• Erythromycin 250-500 mg qid
• First generation, oral cephalosporin
  ◊ Cephalexin 500 mg bid
  ◊ Cefaclor 250 mg tid
• Amoxicillin-clavulanate (Augmentin) 250 mg tid
• Clindamycin 300 mg tid if anaerobes suspected
Contraindications: Allergy to antibiotic
Precautions: Refer to manufacturer's profile of each drug
Significant possible interactions: Refer to manufacturer's profile of each drug

ALTERNATIVE DRUGS N/A

FOLLOWUP

PATIENT MONITORING Assure resolution to exclude carcinoma

PREVENTION/AVOIDANCE
• Early treatment of mastitis with milk expression and cold compresses
• Early treatment with antibiotics

POSSIBLE COMPLICATIONS Fistula

EXPECTED COURSE/PROGNOSIS
Good. Complete healing expected in 8 to 10 days, particularly if abscess can be incised and drained.

MISCELLANEOUS

ASSOCIATED CONDITIONS N/A

AGE-RELATED FACTORS
Pediatric: N/A
Geriatric: N/A
Others: N/A

PREGNANCY Most commonly associated with postpartum lactation

SYNONYMS
• Mammary abscess
• Peripheral breast abscess
• Subareolar abscess
• Puerperal abscess

ICD-9-CM
611.0 Acute, chronic, nonpuerperal
675.1 Puerperal, postpartum

SEE ALSO N/A

OTHER NOTES N/A

ABBREVIATIONS N/A

REFERENCES
• Benson EA: Management of breast abscesses. World J Surg 1989;13:753-756
• Dixon JM: Periductal mastitis/duct ectasia. World J Surg 1989;13:715-720
• Ferrara JJ, et al: Non surgical management of breast infections in non-lactating women. Am Surg 1990;56:668-671
• Olsen CG, Gordon RE: Breast disorders in nursing mothers. Am Fam Physician 1990;41:1509-1515
• Smallwood JA: Benign breast disease. Baltimore, Urban & Schwarzenberg, 1990
• Maier WP, et al: Nonlactational breast infection. Amer Surg 1994;60:247-250
• Bundred NJ, Dover MS, et al: Breast abscess and cigarette smoking. Br Jour Surg 1992;79(1):58-59
• Karstoup S, et al: Acute puerperal breast abscess: US-guided drainage. Radiology 1993;188(3):807-809
Illustrations: N/A
Internet references: http://www.5mcc.com

Author(s)
Thomas R. Strigle, MD
Donald W. Moorman, MD

Breast cancer

BASICS

DESCRIPTION Malignant neoplasm in the breast. Breast cancers are classified as noninvasive (in situ) or invasive (infiltrating) with approximately 70% of all breast cancers possessing a component of invasion.

System(s) affected: Skin/Exocrine, Pulmonary, Gastrointestinal, Musculoskeletal, Nervous

Genetics:
• Only 20% of patients have a significant family history of breast cancer. This predisposition tends to be autosomal dominant with maternal lineage.
• Recent studies have revealed families with breast cancer susceptibility genes including BRCA1 and BRCA2. Family history suggestive of breast cancer susceptibility genes include multiple first and second degree relatives with early breast cancer diagnosis and the presence of ovarian cancer. Approximately 1 in 400 U.S. women will carry a germ-line mutation for BRCA1. BRCA1 carriers have approximately an 85% chance of developing breast cancer in a lifetime. BRCA2 carriers have a higher risk of male breast cancer.

Incidence/Prevalence in USA:
• 1 in 8 women will develop breast cancer within a lifetime
• 150,000 new cases are diagnosed annually, and 50,000 women die annually

Predominant age: 30-80 with peak age 45-65

Predominant sex: Female > Male (1% occurs in male)

SIGNS AND SYMPTOMS
• Palpable mass (55%)
• Abnormal mammogram without a palpable mass (35%)
• Color change (peau d'orange)
• Dimpling
• Nipple retraction
• Breast enlargement
• Axillary mass
• Bone pain (rare)

CAUSES Unknown

RISK FACTORS
• Increased breast cancer risk occurs in first degree relatives (relative risk [RR] = 2.3), with bilateral disease in premenopausal relatives (RR = 10.5), or bilateral disease in postmenopausal relatives (RR = 5.0)
• Increased hormone risks include early menarche, late menopause, nulliparity or first full term pregnancy after age 30
• Women with a prior history of breast cancer or previous breast biopsies revealing atypical changes are at increased risk (5-10 times) for subsequent cancer
• Inconclusive risk factors include exogenous estrogen use, high dietary fat, or high alcohol use

DIAGNOSIS

DIFFERENTIAL DIAGNOSIS
• Differential diagnosis is extensive
• Benign breast disorders such as abscesses, hematomas, or fibroadenomas
• Proliferative breast diseases such as fibrocystic changes, ductal and lobular hyperplasia, or sclerosing adenosis
• Malignant breast diseases including sarcomas, lymphomas, or metastatic disease to breast

LABORATORY Complete blood counts and blood tests of liver and bone function are routinely performed at time of definitive diagnosis

Drugs that may alter lab results: None
Disorders that may alter lab results: None

PATHOLOGICAL FINDINGS
• Noninvasive cancers
◊ The percentage of non-invasive cancers diagnosed is increasing due to increased mammography screening
◊ Usually detected by abnormal mammogram
◊ Noninvasive cancers are of two types: Intraductal or intralobular. Intraductal cancers are subdivided by growth patterns: Micropapillary, cribriform, solid, or comedo. The comedo growth pattern is considered more aggressive.
• Invasive cancers
◊ Tend to present with a breast lump
◊ Subdivided into - not-otherwise-specified (50%), lobular (5%), Paget's disease (2%), and miscellaneous (metaplastic, neuroendocrine, or squamous cell carcinomas [1%])
◊ Patients with invasive histologies with medullary 6%, colloid 7%, tubular, papillary, and adenoid cystic carcinomas 2%, have improved survival

SPECIAL TESTS
• Assessment of estrogen receptor (ER) and progesterone receptor (PgR) activity on breast cancer tissue has diagnostic and prognostic significance
• Evaluation of HER-2/neu expression, epidermal growth factor receptor (EGF-R), cathepsin D, ploidy analysis, and S phase activity remains investigational
• CA 15-3 and carcinoembryonic antigen (CEA) are investigational blood tests

IMAGING
• Mammography, which detects 80% of breast cancers, is the best technique for the detection of minimal (< 0.5 cm) breast cancer. The most common abnormality representing cancer is an irregular mass. Microcalcifications can occur as the only sign of malignancy in 35% of breast cancers.
• Ultrasound may confirm whether a suspicious lump is solid or cystic
• After diagnosis, baseline bone scan, chest x-ray, and liver imaging (nuclear medicine scan or CT scan) are often performed

DIAGNOSTIC PROCEDURES
• Tissue confirmation of the suspicious mass or abnormal mammogram is essential. Biopsy may be excisional or incisional depending upon the size and location of the abnormality.
• Biopsy of non-palpable lesions is achieved with needle localization
• Cytologic confirmation of a palpable abnormality may be obtained by fine needle aspiration

TREATMENT

APPROPRIATE HEALTH CARE Patients are usually treated by a team consisting of a medical oncologist, a surgeon, and a radiation oncologist

GENERAL MEASURES
• The decision to treat with hormone or chemotherapy is very complex. Premenopausal women tend to respond more to cytotoxic chemotherapy, and postmenopausal women tend to obtain greater benefit with hormone therapy. Other important factors in the treatment decision include ER and PgR status, nuclear grade, site of metastasis, etc.
• Breast cancer treatment for early stage disease (Stage I or II)
◊ Consists of local control measures and treatment of micrometastatic disease
◊ Either modified radical mastectomy or lumpectomy followed by radiation
◊ Axillary nodal sampling should be performed with both procedures to assess probability of disease recurrence
◊ Disease-free and overall survival is similar with either procedure
◊ The optimal treatment for noninvasive or minimally invasive breast cancer is unclear
• Treatment of locally advanced breast cancer (Stage III)
◊ Is multidisciplinary with most patients receiving combination cytotoxic chemotherapy and radiation therapy prior to mastectomy
• Treatment of metastatic (Stage IV) disease
◊ Measures to provide symptom improvement
◊ Combinations of chemotherapy, hormone therapy, or radiation therapy

SURGICAL MEASURES See General Measures

ACTIVITY Minimal activity restrictions exist during treatment

DIET No proven relationship exists between breast cancer and diet

PATIENT EDUCATION
• Instruct patients in monthly breast self-examination to detect lumps, skin or nipple changes and the importance of mammography
• For a listing of sources for patient education materials, physicians may contact: American Cancer Society and the National Cancer Institute

MEDICATIONS

DRUG(S) OF CHOICE
• Adjuvant cytotoxic chemotherapy or hormone therapy is administered to many patients with Stage I or Stage II invasive disease to prevent cancer recurrence
• Therapeutic cytotoxic chemotherapy or hormone therapy is administered to patients with advanced or metastatic disease
• Metastatic disease is considered incurable, but treatable with remissions occurring in 30-40% of patients
• Combination chemotherapy with cyclophosphamide, methotrexate, fluorouracil, anthracyclines or taxanes are often used
• Tamoxifen is the most commonly used hormone agent in breast cancer; however, medroxyprogesterone and aminoglutethimide are also active agents
Contraindications: Strict hematologic, renal, hepatic, and cardiac guidelines need to be followed for the administration of cytotoxic chemotherapy
Precautions: Monitoring for infection is important for patients receiving chemotherapy
Significant possible interactions: Drug interactions are common and depend on combinations used. Refer to manufacturer's literature.

ALTERNATIVE DRUGS
• Additional efficacious chemotherapy drugs include vinblastine, cisplatin, thiotepa, mitomycin, etoposide and paclitaxel (Taxol)
• Ondansetron (Zofran), dronabinol (Marinol), metoclopramide (Reglan), and others for nausea control

FOLLOWUP

PATIENT MONITORING
• Up to 60% of patients with invasive disease will relapse within five years despite initial therapy
• The status of the axillary lymph nodes is the most important indicator for disease relapse
• Clinical evaluation and physical examination are most important to detect relapses
• The role of followup blood testing and roentgenographic studies (except mammography) is poorly established

PREVENTION/AVOIDANCE
• Decreasing dietary fat or alcohol has not been shown to alter breast cancer risk
• The synthetic anti-estrogen, tamoxifen, may be a useful prophylactic agent in high risk women
• Mammography
◊ In women over 50, mammography screening can reduce mortality by 30%
◊ All women over 35 should have baseline screening mammogram, and it should be repeated every 1-2 years between the ages of 40-49 and annually after 50
◊ Diagnostic mammography should be performed at the advice of the patient's physician

POSSIBLE COMPLICATIONS
• Post-operative: lymphedema (< 5% in modified radical mastectomy), seromas, wound infection, and limited shoulder motion
• Chemotherapy: nausea, vomiting, alopecia, leukopenia, bladder irritation, stomatitis, fatigue, and menstrual abnormalities
• Tamoxifen: hot flushes, menstrual irregularities including menopause, vaginal discharge, hypercalcemia, skin rashes, and possible endometrial carcinoma
• Irradiation: skin reaction, fibrosis (1%), brachial plexopathy (1%), rib fracture (1%), arm edema, pulmonary fibrosis (1%), and rarely second breast malignancy.

EXPECTED COURSE/PROGNOSIS
• 10 year Survival
◊ Noninvasive - 95%: Stage I occult: tumors < 1 cm with no axillary node involvement
◊ I occult - 90%: Stage I overt: tumors > 1 cm with no axillary node involvement
◊ II - 40%: Stage II: tumors < 5 cm or axillary node involvement
◊ III - 15%: Stage III: tumors > 5 cm or with chest wall or skin extension, inflammatory changes, or supraclavicular involvement
◊ IV - 0%: Stage IV: metastatic

MISCELLANEOUS

ASSOCIATED CONDITIONS Organ disease at metastatic sites

AGE-RELATED FACTORS Age-specific incidence of breast cancer increases sharply until menopause and continues to increase at a slower rate in the geriatric population
Pediatric: Breast cancer occurs rarely in children with the most common pathology being secretory carcinoma
Geriatric: There is a higher percentage of ER positive tumors (80%) in the geriatric population. This correlates with improved disease-free survival.
Others: N/A

PREGNANCY Breast cancer occurs infrequently during pregnancy (2.8%). Delay in diagnosis is common, and most series report poorer survival related to advanced stage at diagnosis.

SYNONYMS N/A

ICD-9-CM
174 Malignant neoplasm of female breast
175 Malignant neoplasm of male breast

SEE ALSO N/A

OTHER NOTES N/A

ABBREVIATIONS
• ER = estrogen receptor
• PgR = progesterone receptor

REFERENCES
• Fisher B, Redmond C, Poisson R, et al: Eight year results of the NSABP randomized clinical trial comparing total mastectomy and lumpectomy with or without radiation in the treatment of breast cancer. N Engl J Med 1989;320(13):822-828
• Harris JR, Lippman ME, Veronesi U, Willett W: Breast cancer (first of three parts). New Engl J Med 1992;327(5):319-328
• Harris JR, Lippman ME, Veronesi U, Willett W: Breast cancer (second of three parts). New Engl J Med 1992;327(6):390-398
• Harris JR, Lippman ME, Veronesi U, Willett W: Breast cancer (third of three parts). New Engl J Med 1992;327(7):473-480
• Jaiyesimi IA, Buzdar AU, Decker DA, Hortobagyi GN: Use of tamoxifen for breast cancer; twenty-eight years later. J Clin Oncol 1995;13:513-529
Illustrations: 1 available on CD-ROM
Internet references: http://www.5mcc.com

Author(s)
Elyse E. Lower, MD

Breast-feeding

BASICS

DESCRIPTION
• Advantages
◊ Fewer respiratory, gastrointestinal and otitis media infections
◊ Ideal food - easily digestible, nutrients well absorbed, less constipation
◊ Increased contact between mother and baby and, perhaps, added self-esteem for mother
◊ Economical, portable, easy to meet needs quickly
◊ Breast-feeding may decrease incidence of allergies in childhood
◊ Mothers often like it more than bottle feeding
◊ More rapid and complete reversion of mother's pelvis and uterus to pre-puerperal state
• Contraindications
◊ HIV infection; active TB
◊ Hepatitis is not a contraindication
◊ Substances of abuse will pass into human milk; please see Reference on drugs in lactation
• Physiology
◊ Stimulation of areola causes secretion of oxytocin
◊ Oxytocin is responsible for let-down reflex when milk is ejected from cells into milk ducts
◊ Sucking stimulates secretion of prolactin which triggers milk production. Thus milk is made in response to nursing and increases supply.
• Technique
◊ Get in comfortable position, usually sitting or reclining with baby's head in crook of mother's arm (side-lying position often useful following C-section delivery)
◊ Bring baby to mother to decrease stress on back
◊ Baby's belly and mother's belly should face each other or touch (belly-to-belly)
◊ Initiate the rooting reflex by tickling baby's lips with nipple or finger. As baby's mouth opens wide, mother guides her nipple to back of her baby's mouth while pulling the baby closer. This will ensure that the baby's gums are sucking on the areola, not the nipple.
System(s) affected: Endocrine/Metabolic, Skin/Exocrine
Genetics: N/A
Incidence/Prevalence in USA: According to 1995 Healthy People 2000 Update, 60% of new mothers breastfed in the early postpartum period (highest % since 1984).
Predominant age: 16-45
Predominant sex: Female only

SIGNS AND SYMPTOMS N/A

CAUSES N/A

RISK FACTORS N/A

DIAGNOSIS

DIFFERENTIAL DIAGNOSIS N/A

LABORATORY N/A
Drugs that may alter lab results: N/A
Disorders that may alter lab results: N/A

PATHOLOGICAL FINDINGS N/A

SPECIAL TESTS N/A

IMAGING N/A

DIAGNOSTIC PROCEDURES N/A

TREATMENT

APPROPRIATE HEALTH CARE
Outpatient

GENERAL MEASURES See Patient Education

SURGICAL MEASURES N/A

ACTIVITY No restrictions

DIET
• Adequate calorie and protein intake while nursing
• Drink plenty of fluids
• Continue prenatal vitamins
• Fluoride supplement unnecessary

PATIENT EDUCATION
• Antepartum
◊ Regular promotion of advantages of breast-feeding
◊ Discuss woman's postpartum plans, i.e., if going to work. Emphasize possibility of nursing part-time after returning to work or nursing until weaning the week before returning to work
◊ For some mothers, you need to explain that an occasional supplemental bottle can be used to give them time away from their baby
◊ Counsel women on technique
• Natural history
◊ Colostrum present in breast at birth but may not be seen
◊ Milk will not come in before 3rd day postpartum
◊ Frequent nursing (at least 9 or more times/24 hours) will lead to milk coming in sooner and in greater quantities
◊ Allow baby to determine duration of each nursing; baby will lose weight the first few days and may not get back to birth weight until day 10
• Postpartum
◊ Immediate breast-feeding after the birth
◊ Rooming-in to encourage on-demand feeding
◊ Observation of a nursing session by experienced physician, nurse or lactation consultant
◊ Avoid formula or water supplementation
◊ Review expectations, techniques. Be very encouraging.
◊ See in office within a few days of discharge, especially if first-time nursing
• Signs of adequate nursing
◊ Breasts become hard before and soft after feeding
◊ 6 or more wet diapers in 24 hours
◊ Baby satisfied; appropriate weight gain (average one ounce/day in first few months)
◊ Growth spurts - anticipate these around 10 days, 6 weeks, 3 months, and 4-6 months. Baby will nurse more often at these times for several days. This will increase milk production to allow for further adequate growth.
◊ Supplemental baby vitamins are unnecessary unless the baby has very limited exposure to sun (then needs vitamin D)
• Weaning
◊ Breast milk alone is adequate food for first 6 months
◊ Solids may be introduced at 4-6 months
◊ For mothers going to work, start switching the baby to bottle feeding during the hours mother will be gone about a week ahead of time. Do this by dropping a breast-feed every few days and substituting pumped breast milk or formula, preferably given by another caregiver.
◊ To increase the likelihood that baby will take a bottle occasionally, introduce it at 3-4 weeks and give once or twice a week

MEDICATIONS

DRUG(S) OF CHOICE N/A
Contraindications: N/A
Precautions: N/A
Significant possible interactions: N/A

ALTERNATIVE DRUGS N/A

FOLLOWUP

PATIENT MONITORING See mother and baby within a few days of hospital discharge if she is a first-time breast-feeder

PREVENTION/AVOIDANCE N/A

POSSIBLE COMPLICATIONS
• Plugged ducts (mother is well except for)
  ◊ Sore lump in one or both breasts without fever
  ◊ Use moist hot packs on lump prior to and during nursing; more frequent nursing on affected side; ensure good technique
• Mastitis
  ◊ Sore lump in one or both breasts plus fever and/or redness on skin overlying lump
  ◊ Use moist hot packs on lump prior to and during nursing; more frequent nursing on affected side; antibiotics covering for Staph. aureus (the most common organism) for at least 7 days
    ◊ Patients can be quite ill with mastitis
    ◊ Other possible sources of fever should be ruled out - endometritis, pyelonephritis in particular. Mother should get increased rest, use acetaminophen (Tylenol) as necessary. Fever should resolve within 48 hours or consider changing antibiotics. Lump should also resolve. If it continues, an abscess may be present requiring surgical drainage.
• Milk supply inadequate
  ◊ Check weight gain
  ◊ Review signs of adequate supply; review technique, frequency and duration of nursing
  ◊ Check to see if mother has been supplementing, thereby decreasing her own milk production
• Sore nipples
  ◊ Check technique
  ◊ Baby should be taken off the breast by breaking the suction with a finger in the mouth
  ◊ Air-dry nipples after each nursing; no breast creams and do not wash nipples with soap and water; check for signs of thrush in baby and mother
• Engorgement
  ◊ Usually develops after milk first comes in (day 3 or 4)
  ◊ Signs are warm, hard, sore breasts
  ◊ To resolve, offer baby more frequent nursing; may have to hand express a little milk to soften areola enough to let baby latch on; nurse long enough to empty breasts; generally resolves within a day or two
• Flat or inverted nipples
  ◊ When stimulated, inverted nipples will retract inward, flat nipples remain flat; should check for this on initial prenatal physical
  ◊ Nipple shells, a doughnut-shaped insert, can be worn inside the bra during the last month of pregnancy to gently force the nipple through the center opening of the shell
  ◊ Babies can nurse successfully even if the shell does not correct the problem before birth. A lactation consultant or La Leche League member may be a good resource in this situation. Another source: J Human Lactation. 9(1):27-29, 1993.

EXPECTED COURSE/PROGNOSIS
Healthy baby

MISCELLANEOUS

ASSOCIATED CONDITIONS N/A

AGE-RELATED FACTORS N/A
Pediatric: N/A
Geriatric: N/A
Others: N/A

PREGNANCY N/A

SYNONYMS N/A

ICD-9-CM N/A

SEE ALSO N/A

OTHER NOTES N/A

ABBREVIATIONS N/A

REFERENCES
• Briggs GG, et al: Drugs in Pregnancy and lactation. 4th Ed. Baltimore, Williams & Wilkins, 1994
• Riordan J, Auerback K: Pocket Guide to Breast-feeding and Human Lactation. Jones and Bartlett, 1997
• Walker M: Hospital Breastfeeding Policies & Protocols: A Model for the Short Stay. Lactation Associates, 1995
Illustrations: N/A
Internet references: http://www.5mcc.com

Author(s)
Eric Henley, MD, MPH

Breech birth

BASICS

DESCRIPTION At the time of delivery the fetal buttocks are the presenting part in the maternal pelvis
• Frank breech presentation - the fetal hips are flexed and the knees extended with the feet near the shoulders, accounting for 60-65% of breech presentations at term
• Incomplete breech presentation - one or both of the fetal hips are incompletely flexed, resulting in some part of the fetal lower extremity as the presenting part. Thus the terms single footling, double footling, knee presentation. Accounts for 25-35% of breech presentations.
• Complete breech - similar to frank breech except one or both knees are flexed rather than extended. Accounts for 5% of breech presentations.
System(s) affected: Reproductive
Genetics: Fetal anomalies including anencephaly, hydrocephalus, trisomy 21
Incidence/Prevalence in USA: 3-4% of singleton term deliveries and up to 15-30% of low birth weight infants (< 2500 grams)
Predominant age: N/A
Predominant sex: Female only

SIGNS AND SYMPTOMS
• Anus palpable on digital vaginal exam
• Leopold's maneuver reveals ballottable head in fundal region

CAUSES Probably a combination of one or more of the risk factors listed below

RISK FACTORS
• Fetal anomalies including anencephaly, hydrocephalus, trisomy 21
• Uterine anomalies
• Uterine relaxation associated with great parity
• Uterine overdistension as in polyhydramnios or multiple gestation
• Placenta previa
• Placental implantation in cornual-fundal region
• Low birth weight or premature infant

DIAGNOSIS

DIFFERENTIAL DIAGNOSIS Diagnosis is made by vaginal exam and confirmed by ultrasound. Can be confused with face presentation on digital vaginal exam.

LABORATORY None
Drugs that may alter lab results: N/A
Disorders that may alter lab results: N/A

PATHOLOGICAL FINDINGS Congenital malformation among term breech infants: Overall incidence 9.0%

SPECIAL TESTS N/A

IMAGING
• Ultrasound - confirms presenting part
• X-ray - flat plate of abdomen and pelvimetry to determine extent of head flexion and pelvic measurements

DIAGNOSTIC PROCEDURES N/A

TREATMENT

APPROPRIATE HEALTH CARE Inpatient for labor and delivery

GENERAL MEASURES N/A

SURGICAL MEASURES
• Breech delivery is accomplished either vaginally or by cesarean section
• When a patient presents in labor with the fetus in breech position, a decision about a trial of labor or immediate cesarean section must be made
• Obtain a flat plate of abdomen with pelvimetry and/or ultrasound to document fetal presentation, to check for fetal abnormalities, and to estimate fetal weight in deciding candidacy for vaginal delivery
• The selection criteria for vaginal delivery are fairly strict to reduce morbidity and mortality for both mother and infant
• Cesarean section is recommended in the following circumstances unless the fetus is too immature to survive:
  ◊ Large (> 3500 grams) or small (< 1500 grams) fetus, estimated by ultrasound or skilled observer
  ◊ Pelvic contraction or unfavorable pelvic shape (platypelloid and android)
  ◊ Hyperextended head
  ◊ Significant fetal heart rate abnormality
  ◊ Footling breech
  ◊ Severe fetal growth retardation
  ◊ Premature fetus greater than 26 weeks with mother in active labor
  ◊ Previous cesarean section
  ◊ Abnormal labor including failure to dilate, prolonged second stage, and failure of descent

• Cesarean section procedure:
  ◊ Prepare for cesarean section by starting IV fluids and obtaining blood type and screen, in all patients, in case needed for emergency
  ◊ A low transverse cesarean section may need to be extended vertically if there is difficulty with head entrapment
  ◊ General anesthesia with isoflurane can rapidly relax the uterus and allow delivery of an entrapped after-coming head
  ◊ Cord blood gases should be obtained following delivery
• Vaginal delivery procedures:
  ◊ The candidate for vaginal delivery needs to be attended by a birth attendant skilled in breech delivery, a scrubbed assistant, an anesthesiologist capable of rapid induction of general anesthesia, and an individual skilled in neonatal resuscitation
  ◊ Leave membranes intact as long as possible to prevent possible cord prolapse
  ◊ The patient should not push until fully dilated
  ◊ Cut large episiotomy to allow sufficient room for delivery
  ◊ The infant should not be touched before the umbilicus crosses the maternal perineum
  ◊ Traction prior to this point constitutes a complete breech extraction and is associated with higher risk of perinatal morbidity and mortality
  ◊ With the fetal back anterior, maintain downward traction while grasping the fetal hips until the scapula becomes visible
  ◊ Check for nuchal arm
  ◊ As one axilla becomes visible rotate the infant until the shoulders are oriented anteriorly and posteriorly allowing their delivery
  ◊ The fetal head is delivered in a face down position with either piper forceps or manual flexion of the head
  ◊ Cord blood gases should be obtained following delivery

ACTIVITY Bedrest during labor

DIET Nothing by mouth until delivery accomplished

PATIENT EDUCATION Come to the hospital at the first sign of labor

MEDICATIONS

DRUG(S) OF CHOICE None
Contraindications: N/A
Precautions: N/A
Significant possible interactions: N/A

ALTERNATIVE DRUGS N/A

FOLLOWUP

PATIENT MONITORING
• Continuous fetal heart rate monitoring should be done during labor and delivery
• Six weeks postpartum care is done as with other deliveries

PREVENTION/AVOIDANCE
• External version
  ◊ Conversion to vertex presentation can be attempted from 30-36 weeks gestation
  ◊ External version can cause abruption, premature rupture of membranes, and feto-maternal hemorrhage
  ◊ Should only be attempted with continuous fetal heart monitoring in the delivery suite where immediate cesarean section can be done
  ◊ Contraindications to external version include pelvic engagement of presenting part, placenta previa, previous uterine surgery, premature rupture of the membranes, or marked oligohydramnios

POSSIBLE COMPLICATIONS
• Trauma to head, soft tissue, brachial plexus and spinal cord - not always prevented by cesarean
• Asphyxia secondary to cord compression or prolapse

EXPECTED COURSE/PROGNOSIS
• Perinatal morbidity and mortality are much higher in breech births. A large proportion of the deaths are related to congenital abnormalities.
• In patients properly selected for vaginal delivery, potentially perinatal morbidity and mortality, and maternal morbidity are reduced
• For infants less than 1500 grams, there is a much higher rate of cerebral hemorrhage and perinatal death associated with vaginal compared to cesarean delivery

MISCELLANEOUS

ASSOCIATED CONDITIONS See Risk Factors

AGE-RELATED FACTORS
Pediatric: N/A
Geriatric: N/A
Others: N/A

PREGNANCY A problem of pregnancy

SYNONYMS N/A

ICD-9-CM
• Breech extraction (assisted) 72.52
• Above with forceps to after-coming head 72.51
• Total breech extraction 72.54
• Above with forceps to after-coming head 72.53
• Cesarean section lower uterine segment 74.1

SEE ALSO
• Placenta previa
• Premature labor

OTHER NOTES Maneuvers of cesarean breech delivery are similar to vaginal breech extraction and can be associated with severe trauma to the infant

ABBREVIATIONS N/A

REFERENCES Cunningham FG, MacDonald PC, Gant NF, eds: Williams' Obstetrics. 19th Ed. Norwalk, CT, Appleton and Lange, 1993
Illustrations: N/A
Internet references: http://www.5mcc.com

Author(s)
Kimberle Vore, MD

Bronchiectasis

BASICS

DESCRIPTION Chronic irreversible, abnormal dilatation of the bronchi, usually accompanied by infection and productive cough
System(s) affected: Pulmonary
Genetics: Associated with many conditions including some that are congenital or hereditary
Incidence/Prevalence in USA:
• No reliable figures available
• Less common than it once was, probably due to more effective treatment of childhood respiratory infections
Predominant age: Begins most often in early childhood, but symptoms may not appear until later in life
Predominant sex: Male = Female

SIGNS AND SYMPTOMS
• Cough
• Sputum - copious and purulent
• Hemoptysis
• Wheezing
• Coarse or moist crackles
• Cyanosis
• Digital clubbing
• Dyspnea
• Barrel chest
• Emaciation
• Fatigue
• Fever
• Recurrent pneumonia
• Tachycardia
• Tachypnea

CAUSES
• Alpha-1-antitrypsin deficiency
• Allergic bronchopulmonary aspergillosis
• Bronchial obstruction
• Cystic fibrosis
• Dyskinetic cilia syndromes
• Hypogammaglobulinemia
• Inhaling noxious chemicals
• Kartagener's syndrome (situs inversus, sinusitis, immotile spermatozoa, bronchiectasis)
• Necrotizing pulmonary infections
• Pulmonary abscess
• Severe lung infection in childhood (measles, adenovirus, influenza, pertussis, or bronchiolitis)
• Tuberculosis
• Congenital immunodeficiency syndromes
• Chronic aspiration

RISK FACTORS
• Repeated bouts of pneumonia
• Any chronic respiratory illness
• Retained foreign body

DIAGNOSIS

DIFFERENTIAL DIAGNOSIS
• Chronic bronchitis
• Chronic obstructive pulmonary disease
• Cystic fibrosis
• Pulmonary tuberculosis
• Allergic bronchopulmonary aspergillosis

LABORATORY
• Positive sputum culture (yields H. influenzae, Streptococcus pneumoniae, staphylococcal, klebsiella, pseudomonas, or anaerobes)
• Hypoxemia
• Leukocytosis, usually
• Serum immunoglobulins - check for hypogammaglobulinemia, IgE level helpful
Drugs that may alter lab results: N/A
Disorders that may alter lab results: N/A

PATHOLOGICAL FINDINGS
• Bronchial dilation
• Inflamed bronchi
• Purulent bronchorrhea
• Necrosis of bronchial mucosa
• Peribronchial scarring

SPECIAL TESTS
• Sweat test
• Skin test for aspergillus
• Bronchoscopy useful in locating bleeding site and to exclude adenoma or foreign body
• Ciliary biopsy with electron microscopy (EM)
• Pulmonary function tests
• Sputum culture/sensitivity, AFB, fungus

IMAGING
• Bronchography
  ◊ For definitive diagnosis, to help determine extent, and if surgery contemplated
  ◊ Bronchial dilation, truncated
• Chest x-ray
  ◊ Can be normal
  ◊ Coarse lung markings - honeycomb/tram tracks
  ◊ Air-fluid level
  ◊ Cystic lesions
  ◊ Atelectasis
• CT scan
  ◊ Shows dilation of airways with signet rings
  ◊ High resolution scans best

DIAGNOSTIC PROCEDURES
• Fiberoptic bronchoscopy
  ◊ Recommended when disease is of recent onset or is unilateral
  ◊ May be combined with bronchography
  ◊ Obtain culture

TREATMENT

APPROPRIATE HEALTH CARE
Outpatient except for possible surgery

GENERAL MEASURES
• Airway clearance techniques
  ◊ Chest physical therapy
  ◊ Percussion
• Postural drainage
• Hydration
• Bronchial artery embolization may be lifesaving for massive pulmonary hemorrhage
• Avoid cigarette smoking
• Bronchoscopy may be required for extraction of mucus or mycelial plugs, or if physiotherapy has failed

SURGICAL MEASURES
Segmental pulmonary resection for localized disease or refractory hemoptysis

ACTIVITY
As fully active as possible

DIET
No restrictions

PATIENT EDUCATION
Printed patient information available from: American Lung Association, 1740 Broadway, New York, NY 10019, (212)315-8700

MEDICATIONS

DRUG(S) OF CHOICE
• Bronchodilators
 ◊ Dependent on pulmonary function tests
 ◊ May be helpful for patients with associated asthma or aspergillosis
 ◊ Beta-adrenergic agonists (e.g., albuterol) given by metered dose inhaler with use of a spacer (reservoir device)
• Antibiotics
 ◊ Dependent on culture results, use at exacerbations
 ◊ Ampicillin: 250-500 mg orally q 6 hours (50 mg/kg/day in divided doses q 6-8 hours in children less than 20 kg)
or
 ◊ Trimethoprim-sulfamethoxazole: DS q12h
 ◊ Tetracycline: 250-500 mg orally q 6 hours
• Steroids
 ◊ Consider for patients with bronchopulmonary aspergillosis. IgE level guides steroid dosing.
Contraindications:
• Tetracycline: not for use in pregnancy or children < 8 years.
Precautions:
• Tetracycline: may cause photosensitivity; sunscreen recommended.
Significant possible interactions:
• Tetracycline: avoid concurrent administration with antacids, dairy products, or iron.
• Broad-spectrum antibiotics: may reduce the effectiveness of oral contraceptives; barrier method recommended.

ALTERNATIVE DRUGS
• For chronic persistent infection, long-term high dose of amoxicillin 3 g every 12 hours may be useful. It does not provide relief for everyone and has more side effects.
• Other broad-spectrum antimicrobials including anti-pseudomonals if required. Choice would depend on pathogen and susceptibility.
• Inhaled corticosteroids if reversible obstruction present
• Oxygen - if PO2 < 60 mm HG
• Nicotine replacement, consider to aid smoking cessation

FOLLOWUP

PATIENT MONITORING
• Frequent followup for progress of illness, prevention of infection, smoking cessation, and to check on physiotherapy
• At some point in followup, need to discuss with patient the possibility of mechanical ventilation and cardiopulmonary resuscitation in the future. The patient, family and provider should determine if this type of treatment is appropriate.

PREVENTION/AVOIDANCE
• Treat all pneumonias adequately
• Immunizations for viral illnesses (i.e., influenza)
• Immunization for pneumococcal pneumonia
• Routine childhood immunizations, e.g., pertussis, measles, Hib
• Genetic counselling if inherited etiology

EXPECTED COURSE/PROGNOSIS
• Chronic. Surgery may be curative if disease localized.
• Average life expectancy - 55 years

POSSIBLE COMPLICATIONS
• Recurrent pulmonary infections
• Pulmonary hypertension
• Secondary amyloidosis
• Cor pulmonale
• Brain abscess
• Massive hemoptysis
• Atelectasis
• Lung abscess

MISCELLANEOUS

ASSOCIATED CONDITIONS
• Sinusitis
• Cor pulmonale
• Kartagener syndrome
• Cystic fibrosis

AGE-RELATED FACTORS
Pediatric: Cystic fibrosis and other congenital disorders
Geriatric: Elderly more likely to need hospitalization for treatment
Others: N/A

PREGNANCY N/A

SYNONYMS N/A

ICD-9-CM
494 bronchiectasis

SEE ALSO N/A

OTHER NOTES
Conditions that may lead to bronchiectasis include severe pneumonia (especially measles, pertussis, adenoviral infections in children), necrotizing infections due to Klebsiella, staphylococci, influenza virus, fungi, mycobacteria, mycoplasma, bronchial obstruction from any cause (foreign body, carcinoma, enlarged mediastinal lymph nodes

ABBREVIATIONS N/A

REFERENCES
• Hardy KA: A review of airway clearance: New techniques, indications and recommendations. Respir Care 1994;39(5):440-445
• Lewiston NJ: Bronchiectasis in childhood. Pediatr Clin North Am 1984;31(4):865-878
• Marwah OS: Bronchiectasis: How to identify, treat and prevent. Postgrad Med 1995;97:149-159
Illustrations: N/A
Internet references: http://www.5mcc.com

Author(s)
Gregory Snyder, MD

Bronchiolitis

BASICS

DESCRIPTION Inflammation of the bronchioles, usually seen in young children, occasionally in high-risk adults. May be seasonal (winter and spring) and often occurs in epidemics. Usual course: insidious; acute; progressive.
Genetics: N/A
System(s) affected: Pulmonary
Incidence/Prevalence in USA: Medical care provided to 1000-1500/100,000 annually. Estimated incidence is higher.
Predominant age: newborn-2 years (peak age 2-6 months)
Predominant sex: Male > Female

SIGNS AND SYMPTOMS
• Anorexia
• Cough
• Cyanosis
• Expiratory wheezing
• Apnea
• Fever
• Grunting
• Inspiratory crackles
• Intercostal retractions
• Irritability
• Noisy breathing
• Otitis media
• Pharyngitis
• Tachycardia
• Tachypnea
• Vomiting

CAUSES
• Respiratory syncytial virus
• Parainfluenza
• Adenovirus
• Rhinovirus
• Influenza virus
• Chlamydia
• Eye, nose, mouth inoculation
• Exposure to adult with URI
• Day care exposure (significant)
• Idiopathic (many adult cases)

RISK FACTORS
• Contact with infected person
• Children in day care environment
• Heart-lung transplantation patient
• Adults - exposure to toxic fumes, connective tissue disease

DIAGNOSIS

DIFFERENTIAL DIAGNOSIS
• Asthma
• Vascular ring
• Lobar emphysema
• Foreign body
• Heart disease
• Pneumonia
• Reflux
• Aspiration
• Cystic fibrosis

LABORATORY
• Arterial blood gas - hypoxemia, hypercarbia, acidemia
• Respiratory viral culture - positive
• Respiratory viral antigens - positive
Drugs that may alter lab results: N/A
Disorders that may alter lab results: N/A

PATHOLOGICAL FINDINGS
• Abundant mucous exudate
• Mucosal - hyperemia, edema
• Submucosal lymphocytic infiltrate, monocytic infiltrate, plasmacytic infiltrate
• Small airway debris, fibrin, inflammatory exudate, fibrosis
• Peribronchiolar mononuclear infiltrate

SPECIAL TESTS
Infant pulmonary function studies

IMAGING
• Chest x-ray
   ◊ Focal atelectasis
   ◊ Air trapping
   ◊ Flattened diaphragm
   ◊ Increased anteroposterior diameter
   ◊ Peribronchial cuffing

DIAGNOSTIC PROCEDURES   N/A

TREATMENT

APPROPRIATE HEALTH CARE
• Most patients can be treated at home
• Inpatient indicated for patient with increased respiratory distress, cyanosis, and dehydration

GENERAL MEASURES
• Most critical phase is first 48-72 hours after onset. Treatment is usually symptomatic.
• Fluid at maintenance
• Mechanical ventilation in respiratory failure
• Isolation: contact; handwashing most important
• Antiviral agents for selected high-risk patients
• Cardio-respiratory monitoring
• Bronchodilators, especially inhaled
• Steroids may not change course - except in patients with reactive airway disease

SURGICAL MEASURES   N/A

ACTIVITY
• Avoid exposure to crowds, viral illness for 2 months
• Avoid smoke

DIET
• Frequent small feedings of clear liquids
• If hospitalized, may require intravenous fluids

PATIENT EDUCATION Griffith: Instructions for Patients; Philadelphia, W.B. Saunders Co.

MEDICATIONS

DRUG(S) OF CHOICE
• Oxygen
• Bronchodilators may be effective for acute symptoms. Corticosteroids do not change course, unless infant has reactive airway disease.
• Epinephrine aerosols may be of benefit
• For infants and children - ribavirin - inhaled antiviral agent active against RSV may be indicated in patients with underlying cardio-pulmonary disease, young age (< 6 weeks), or with severe RSV (elevated pCO2; require mechanical ventilation - use with caution via ventilator). Nebulize via small particle aerosol generator (SPAG).
• For adults - corticosteroids and bronchodilators may be effective in some patients
• Antibiotics only if secondary bacterial infection present (rare)
Contraindications: Refer to manufacturer's literature
Precautions: None
Significant possible interactions: None

ALTERNATIVE DRUGS N/A

FOLLOWUP

PATIENT MONITORING
• If patient is receiving home care, follow daily by telephone for 2-4 days
• For hospitalized patient, monitor as needed depending on severity of infection
• Bronchiolitis is associated with apnea.

PREVENTION/AVOIDANCE
• Hand washing
• Contact isolation of infected babies
• Persons with colds should keep contacts with infants to a minimum

EXPECTED COURSE/PROGNOSIS
• In most cases, recovery is complete within 7-10 days
• Mortality statistics differ, but probably under 1%
• High-risk infants (BPD, CHD) may have prolonged course

POSSIBLE COMPLICATIONS
• Bacterial superinfection
• Viral obliterative bronchiolitis
• Apnea
• Respiratory failure
• Death
• Increased incidence of RAD

MISCELLANEOUS

ASSOCIATED CONDITIONS
• Common cold
• Conjunctivitis
• Pharyngitis
• Otitis media
• Diarrhea

AGE-RELATED FACTORS
Pediatric: Most common in infants
Geriatric: N/A
Others: N/A

PREGNANCY N/A

SYNONYMS N/A

ICD-9-CM
466.1 acute bronchiolitis

SEE ALSO N/A

OTHER NOTES N/A

ABBREVIATIONS
• BPD = bronchopulmonary dysplasia
• CHD = congenital heart disease
• RAD = reactive airway disease
• SPAG = small particle aerosol generator

REFERENCES
• Mandell GL, ed: Principles and Practice of Infectious Diseases. 4th Ed. New York, Churchill Livingstone, 1995
• Fields BN, et al, eds: Virology. 2nd Ed. New York, Raven Press, 1990
Illustrations: N/A
Internet references: http://www.5mcc.com

Author(s)
Nancy N. Dambro, MD

Bronchiolitis obliterans & organizing pneumonia

 BASICS

DESCRIPTION   This is a specific reaction of lung tissue to a variety of injuries. The lungs show a pattern of multiple patchy pneumonia. These are seen on chest x-ray as patchy alveolar or ground glass opacifications with or without interstitial infiltrates and may have air bronchograms as well.
System(s) affected: Pulmonary
Genetics: N/A
Incidence/Prevalence in USA:
Uncommon
Predominant age: Reported cases range age 0-70, mean age 50's
Predominant sex: N/A

SIGNS AND SYMPTOMS
• Most cases present with a flu-like illness that lasts 4-10 weeks or longer. Most have been treated with antibiotics without success.
• Fever
• Dry cough
• Weight loss
• Dyspnea may be severe
• Crackles and perhaps squeaks over involved area
• Fatigue

CAUSES   Idiopathic. A complex response to a variety of injuries, such as toxic inhalation; post mycoplasma, viral and bacterial infection; aspiration; immunologic factors.

RISK FACTORS
• AIDS
• Immunocompromised patients, including transplant patients

 DIAGNOSIS

DIFFERENTIAL DIAGNOSIS
• Usual interstitial pneumonitis (UIP)
• Noninfectious diseases
• Tuberculosis
• Sarcoidosis
• Histoplasmosis
• Berylliosis
• Goodpasture's syndrome
• Neoplasm
• Polyarteritis nodosa
• Systemic lupus erythematosus
• Wegener's granulomatosis
• Sjögren's syndrome
• Chronic eosinophilic pneumonia
• Cryptogenic bronchiolitis

LABORATORY
• Leukocytosis with a normal differential
• Elevated ESR, usually quite elevated
• Negative cultures
• Negative serology for mycoplasma, Coxiella, Legionella, psittacosis, and fungus
• Negative viral studies
Drugs that may alter lab results: N/A
Disorders that may alter lab results: N/A

PATHOLOGICAL FINDINGS
• Intraluminal fibrosis of distal airspaces is the major pathologic feature
• Fibroblasts and plugs of inflammatory cells and loose connective tissue fill these distal airways
• The inflammatory cells are mainly lymphocytes and plasma cells
• Interstitial fibrosis is present
• The plugs of edematous granulation tissue in the terminal and respiratory bronchioles and alveolar ducts do not cause permanent damage

SPECIAL TESTS
• Pulmonary function shows a restrictive/obstructive pattern
• Flow-volume loop shows terminal airway obstruction
• Chest x-ray may show patchy alveolar opacities often in the mid or upper lung area. A ground glass pattern that may have air bronchograms.
• V/Q scan: matched patchy defects

IMAGING
• Chest x-ray - often appears more normal than the physical examination
• CT scans more accurately define the distribution and extent of the patchy alveolar opacities with areas of hyperlucency

DIAGNOSTIC PROCEDURES
• Open lung biopsy
• Transbronchial biopsy
• It may be well to use a trial of steroids as a diagnostic trial, though not all would agree
• If a diagnostic trial is successful, be prepared to treat the patient for at least a year

 TREATMENT

APPROPRIATE HEALTH CARE   Inpatient

GENERAL MEASURES
• Monitor blood gases or pulse oximetry
• Oxygen as necessary

SURGICAL MEASURES   N/A

ACTIVITY   As tolerated

DIET   No special diet

PATIENT EDUCATION   Followup is especially important. Relapse is common. Treatment is prolonged. If medication tapered too rapidly, relapse may well occur.

MEDICATIONS

DRUG(S) OF CHOICE
- Prednisone
  - ◊ 60 mg daily for 1-3 months
  - ◊ Then tapered over a few weeks to 20 mg (this dose may later be given as alternate day therapy). Increase length of taper for patients on long-term therapy to avoid precipitating Addisonian crisis.
  - ◊ Treatment may be needed for one year or more

Contraindications: Refer to manufacturer's literature

Precautions: Be aware of the patient's Mantoux status and history of peptic ulcer disease. Long-term steroid associated with significant adverse effects including Cushing's syndrome, fluid retention, osteoporosis, hyperkalemia, poor wound healing.

Significant possible interactions: Refer to manufacturer's literature

ALTERNATIVE DRUGS
- Steroids other than prednisone may be used
- One paper reported the use of erythromycin 600 mg/day for 3-4 months after initial control with prednisone
- Antimicrobials if original infection is persistent. Choice depends on the pathogen.

FOLLOWUP

PATIENT MONITORING
- Frequent visits, weekly initially
- Emphasize the need to continue the prednisone because of the chance of relapse
- Monitor the lung disease and the side effects of prednisone therapy (Mantoux, monthly CBC, funduscopic exam every 3-6 months)

PREVENTION/AVOIDANCE Except for prevention of relapse, none known

POSSIBLE COMPLICATIONS
- Bronchiectasis
- Death, but with proper treatment, recovery is usually complete without permanent sequelae

EXPECTED COURSE/PROGNOSIS
Complete recovery but individual case management is mandatory

MISCELLANEOUS

ASSOCIATED CONDITIONS
- Drug-induced pneumonitis
  - ◊ Paraquat poisoning
  - ◊ Amiodarone toxicity
  - ◊ Acebutolol toxicity
  - ◊ Freebase cocaine pulmonary toxicity
  - ◊ Overdose of L-tryptophan
  - ◊ Though most were treated with antibiotics only penicillamine and sulfasalazine have been implicated
- Infections
  - ◊ Chronic infectious pneumonia
  - ◊ Malaria
- Immuno-compromise
  - ◊ Bone marrow transplantation
- Connective tissue diseases
  - ◊ Rheumatic lung
  - ◊ Sjogren's syndrome
  - ◊ Polymyositis
  - ◊ Scleroderma
  - ◊ Essential mixed cryoglobulinemia
- Miscellaneous
  - ◊ Cystic fibrosis
  - ◊ Bronchopulmonary dysplasia
  - ◊ Renal failure
  - ◊ Congestive heart failure
  - ◊ Adult respiratory distress syndrome
  - ◊ Chronic eosinophilic pneumonia
  - ◊ Hypersensitivity pneumonitis
  - ◊ Histiocytosis X
  - ◊ Sarcoidosis
  - ◊ Pneumoconioses
  - ◊ Radiation pneumonitis

AGE-RELATED FACTORS
Pediatric: Rare, but has been reported after viral pneumonia (adenovirus influenza). Characteristics include delayed recovery, persistent cough, crackles or wheezing after pneumonia. The laboratory findings are generally not helpful. Imaging shows: V/Qm matched defects; HRCT, bronchiectasis, bronchogram, pruned tree appearance. Diagnosis confirmed by biopsy. Treatment includes steroids - 1 mg/kg/24 hrs for one month, followed by weaning over several months.
Geriatric: Not common
Others: Apparently only seen in adults

PREGNANCY N/A

SYNONYMS
- Intraluminal fibrosis of distal airways
- Idiopathic BOOP
- Cryptogenic organizing pneumonia (COP)
- Obliterative bronchiolitis

ICD-9-CM
491.8 Other chronic bronchitis

SEE ALSO N/A

OTHER NOTES This disease behaves differently than bronchiolitis obliterans (BO). BOOP is a restrictive problem, BO is an obstructive problem. BO causes permanent lung damage and BOOP is completely reversible.

ABBREVIATIONS
V/Q = ventilation-perfusion ratio
HRCT = high resolution computed tomography

REFERENCES
- Cordier JF, Loire R, Brune J: Idiopathic Bronchiolitis Obliterans Organizing Pneumonia. Chest 1989;96:999-1004
- Mueller NL, Staples CA, Miller RR: Bronchiolitis Obliterans Organizing Pneumonia: CT features in 14 patients. AJR 1990;154:983-987
- Epler GR, Colby TV, et al: Bronchiolitis Obliterans Organizing Pneumonia. N Eng J Med 1985;312:152-158
- Hardy KA, Schidlow D, Zaeri N: Obliterative Bronchiolitis in Children. CHEST 1988;93:460-466
- St John RC, Dorinsky PM: Cryptogenic broncolitis. Clin Chest Med 1993;14(4): 667-75
- Lynch DA: Imaging of small airways diseases. Clin Chest Med 1993;14(4):623-34
Illustrations: N/A
Internet references: http://www.5mcc.com

Author(s)
David A. Pope, MD

Bronchitis, acute

 BASICS

DESCRIPTION Inflammation of trachea, bronchi and bronchioles resulting from a respiratory tract infection. Generally self-limited with complete healing and full return of function.
System(s) affected: Pulmonary
Genetics: No known genetic pattern
Incidence/Prevalence in USA: Common
Predominant age: All ages
Predominant sex: Male = Female

SIGNS AND SYMPTOMS
• Preceding respiratory tract infection, such as a common cold with coryza, malaise, chills, slight fever, sore throat, back and muscle pain
• Cough, initially dry and unproductive, then productive. Later, mucopurulent sputum.
• Fever
• Fatigue, aching
• Hemoptysis
• Chest burning
• Dyspnea (sometimes)
• Rales, rhonchi, wheezing
• No evidence of pulmonary consolidation
• Pharynx injected

CAUSES
• Adenovirus
• Influenza
• Parainfluenza
• Chlamydia pneumoniae (TWAR agent)
• Bordetella pertussis
• Respiratory syncytial virus
• Coxsackievirus
• Herpes simplex
• Haemophilus influenzae
• Possibly fungi
• Mycoplasma
• Secondary bacterial infection as part of an acute upper respiratory infection
• Streptococcus pneumoniae
• Moraxella catarrhalis
• Mycobacterium tuberculosis
• Rhinovirus

RISK FACTORS
• Chronic bronchopulmonary diseases
• Chronic sinusitis
• Bronchopulmonary allergy
• Hypertrophied tonsils and adenoids in children
• Immunosuppression
• Air pollutants
• Elderly
• Infants
• Smoking
• Second-hand smoke
• Alcoholism
• Gastroesophageal reflux disease (GERD)
• Tracheostomy
• IgA deficiency
• Environmental changes

 DIAGNOSIS

DIFFERENTIAL DIAGNOSIS
• Influenza
• Bronchopneumonia
• Bronchiectasis
• Acute sinusitis
• Aspiration
• Cystic fibrosis
• Reactive airways disease
• Bacterial tracheitis
• Retained foreign body

LABORATORY
• Arterial blood gases - hypoxemia (rarely)
• Leukocytosis
• Sputum culture/gram stain
• Viral titers
• Mycoplasma titers
Drugs that may alter lab results: N/A
Disorders that may alter lab results: N/A

PATHOLOGICAL FINDINGS
• Mucosal hyperemia and inflammation
• Desquamation of columnar epithelium
• Mucopurulent exudate

SPECIAL TESTS Pulmonary function tests (seldom needed during acute stages) - increased residual volume, decreased maximal expiratory rate

IMAGING Chest x-ray - lungs normal if uncomplicated. Helps rule out other diseases or complications.

DIAGNOSTIC PROCEDURES Symptoms and signs

 TREATMENT

APPROPRIATE HEALTH CARE
Outpatient unless elderly or complicated by severe underlying disease

GENERAL MEASURES
• Rest
• Steam inhalations
• Vaporizers
• Antibiotics if bacterial etiology suspected
• Adequate hydration
• Stop smoking
• Treat associated illnesses (e.g., GERD)

SURGICAL MEASURES N/A

ACTIVITY Rest until fever subsides

DIET Increased fluids (up to 3-4 L/day) while febrile

PATIENT EDUCATION For patient education materials favorably reviewed on this topic, contact: American Lung Association, 1740 Broadway, New York, NY 10019, (212)315-8700

Bronchitis, acute

MEDICATIONS

DRUG(S) OF CHOICE
• Amantadine therapy if influenza A suspected; most effective if started within 24-48 hours of development of symptoms
• Decongestants if accompanied by sinus condition
• Antipyretic analgesic such as aspirin, in adults, 650 mg q 4-6 hours
• Antibiotics - for more severe symptoms (high fever persists, concomitant COPD, purulent discharge).
◊ amoxicillin 500 mg q8hrs or trimethoprim-sulfamethoxazole azole DS q12hrs for routine infection
◊ Macrolide - clarithromycin (Biaxin) 500 mg q12hr or azithromycin (Zithromax) Z-pack for PCN or sulfa allergy or mycoplasma infection
◊ Doxycycline 100 mg qd for 10 days if moraxcella, chlamydia or mycoplasma suspected
◊ Quinalone - ciprofloxacin (Cipro) 500 mg q12hr; ofloxacin (Floxin) 300-400 mg q12hr or levofloxacin (Levaquin) 500 mg qd for more serious infection or other antibiotic failure
• Cough suppressant for troublesome cough (not with COPD)
• Bronchodilators (aerosols/steroids)
Contraindications:
• Doxycycline should not be used during pregnancy
Precautions: Refer to manufacturer's literature. Watch for theophylline toxicity with macrolides and quinalones.
Significant possible interactions: Refer to manufacturer's literature

ALTERNATIVE DRUGS
• Other antibiotics if indicated by sputum culture (Moraxella needs different set of antibiotics)
• Antivirals
• Other macrolides or quinolones according to pathogen and sensitivity

FOLLOWUP

PATIENT MONITORING
• Oximetry until no longer hypoxemic
• Recheck for chronicity

PREVENTION/AVOIDANCE
• Avoid smoking
• Control underlying risk factors (asthma, sinusitis, reflux)
• Avoid exposure

POSSIBLE COMPLICATIONS
• Bronchopneumonia
• Acute respiratory failure

EXPECTED COURSE/PROGNOSIS
• Usual - complete healing with good return of function
• Can be serious in elderly or debilitated patients
• Cough may persist for several weeks after initial improvement
• Post-bronchitic reactive airways disease (rare)
• Bronchiolitis obliterans and organizing pneumonia (BOOP) (rare)

MISCELLANEOUS

ASSOCIATED CONDITIONS
• Asthma
• Epiglottitis
• Coryza
• Pharyngitis
• Croup
• Influenza
• Smoking
• Pneumonia
• Emphysema
• Sinusitis
• Bronchial obstruction
• Gastroesophageal reflux disease

AGE-RELATED FACTORS
Pediatric:
• Occurrence in this age group usually is in association with other conditions of upper and lower respiratory tract (trachea usually involved)
• Some children seem to be more susceptible than others (if repeated attacks, child should be evaluated for anomalies of the respiratory tract including immune deficiencies)
• If acute bronchitis is caused by respiratory syncytial virus, may be fatal
Geriatric: Can be a serious illness in this age group, particularly if part of influenza
Others: N/A

PREGNANCY N/A

SYNONYMS N/A

ICD-9-CM 466.0 acute bronchitis

SEE ALSO
• Asthma
• Chronic obstructive pulmonary disease & emphysema

OTHER NOTES N/A

ABBREVIATIONS
GERD = gastroesophageal reflux disease

REFERENCES
• Baum GL, Wolinsky E, eds: Textbook of Pulmonary Diseases. 4th Ed. Boston, Little, Brown & Co., 1989
• Murray JF, Nadel JA, eds: Textbook of Respiratory Medicine. Philadelphia, W.B. Saunders Co., 1988
• Seaton A, Seaton D, Leitch AG: Crofton and Douglas's Respiratory Diseases. Boston, Blackwell Scientific Publications, 1989
Illustrations: N/A
Internet references: http://www.5mcc.com

Author(s)
Alan J. Cropp, MD, FCCP

Brucellosis

BASICS

DESCRIPTION Systemic bacterial infection caused by Brucella species in infected animal products, or vaccine. Incubation period usually 5-60 days, but highly variable and may be several months. Characterized by intermittent or irregular fevers, with symptoms ranging from subclinical disease to infection of almost any organ system. Bone and joint involvement common. May be chronic or recurrent. Case fatality untreated less than 2%.
System(s) affected: Endocrine/Metabolic, Gastrointestinal, Renal/Urologic, Pulmonary, Nervous, Skin/Exocrine
Genetics: None; some evidence for intrauterine transmission
Incidence/Prevalence in USA: About 100/year (105 cases in 1992; 0.34/100,000), but probably underreported; common in developing countries. Recent cases reported from exposure to dairy products from Mexico. Reportable in all states except Nevada.
Predominant age: All ages, but especially 20-60 (occupational exposure), sometimes children (milk-related outbreaks)
Predominant sex:
• Male > Female (occupational exposure)
• Female ≥ Male (milk exposure)

SIGNS AND SYMPTOMS
• Fever (may be undulant, increased in afternoon and evening, maximum 101-104° daily); weakness; headache; sweating; chills; generalized aching; arthralgia (90%)
• Also common - weight loss, depression, irritability, hepatosplenomegaly (20-30%)
• Hepatic dysfunction (abnormal liver function test) 30-60%
• Gastrointestinal symptoms (unusual)
• Lymphadenopathy, especially cervical, inguinal (12-21%)
• Orchitis, epididymitis (normal urinalysis) (2-40%)
• Nephritis, prostatitis (rare)
• Cystitis
• Pulmonary - cough or other pulmonary symptoms, x-ray may be normal (15-25%)
• Cutaneous - many transient, non-specific rashes have been described; also, purpura from thrombopenia (5%)
• Visual disturbances, eye pain
• Chronic fatigue syndrome and various neuro-psychiatric symptoms described. Unclear relationship.
• Also localized suppurative infections (see Complications)

CAUSES
• Brucella ingestion from tissue or milk
• Worst disease: B. melitensis, B. suis; also B. canis, B. abortus. Enter through mucous membrane, broken skin, occasionally inhaled. Facultative intracellular parasite, releases endotoxin when destroyed.
• Person-to-person transmission rare

RISK FACTORS
• In US, from occupational exposure to infected animals (especially cattle, sheep). Veterinarians, meat processors, farm workers; who may experience accidental exposure to vaccine. 18 case outbreak in pork processing plant, 1992.
• Consumer exposure to unpasteurized milk products, cheese
• Exposure while traveling in countries where endemic (Mediterranean, N. and E. Africa, central Asia, India, Mexico, Central and South America)
• Worse in chronically ill, immunosuppressed, malnourished
• Iron deficiency increases susceptibility

DIAGNOSIS

DIFFERENTIAL DIAGNOSIS
• Many non-specific systemic febrile illnesses; a great mimic
• Tularemia
• Psittacosis
• Rickettsial disease
• Tuberculosis
• Visceral leishmaniasis
• Other disease of infected organs
• HIV infection

LABORATORY
• Isolation of organism from blood, discharge, bone or other tissue. Fastidious and slow-growing. Watch 3-4 weeks, with periodic subcultures. Automated systems shorten time, but not all recognize brucellosis. PCR exists, but not available in most clinical labs. Skin tests not standardized, not recommended for diagnosis.
• Acute illness: Blood culture is positive 70%, bone 90%
• May have thrombopenia, disseminated intravascular coagulation; granulopenia, lymphopenia, lymphocytosis. 30-60% with abnormal liver function test
• Serology: Brucella standard tube agglutination (STA) paired sera, > 1:160 or 4 x rise
• Recent development of more effective ELISA tests. With ELISA, IgM, IgG or IGA may be present at low levels > 1 year even if treated.
• IgM increased initially for several weeks, declines by 3 months
• IgG begins rise 2 weeks, may stay up (low levels) > 1 yr if treated or not treated (though IgM increase may be lower or gone by 6 months if treated, but can also persist > 1 year at low levels). IgG titer rises again with reinfection or reactivation. IgG titer > 1:160 at 1 year implies ongoing infection.

Drugs that may alter lab results: None
Disorders that may alter lab results: Serologic cross-reaction with F. tularensis, Yersinia enterocolitica, V. cholerae, or vaccinated patients. It has been misdiagnosed in culture as Moraxella phenylpyruvica.

PATHOLOGICAL FINDINGS
• Facultative intracellular; can survive inside phagocytic cells, circulate to regional lymph nodes, and into circulation. (Cell-mediated immunity necessary to kill intracellular organism.)
• Macrophages kill, releasing endotoxin that may cause symptoms of acute disease
• Variable tissue reaction depending on site, organisms. Causes local microabscesses; possibly some immune reaction in arthritis, including elevated C3, C4; ANA, RF

SPECIAL TESTS Echocardiogram depending on location

IMAGING
• Bone scan, CT, depending on location
• Chest x-ray - pleural effusion, lung cavitation
• Joint x-rays frequently normal, requiring scan or MRI

DIAGNOSTIC PROCEDURES Biopsy, aspiration depending on location

TREATMENT

APPROPRIATE HEALTH CARE
Outpatient in mild cases, hospitalization in severe illness. Cardiac care unit in patients with complicating cardiac disease.

GENERAL MEASURES
• Supportive care
• In milk-related outbreak, look for other cases

SURGICAL MEASURES Specific complications may require surgical drainage, or valve replacement in endocarditis

ACTIVITY Bedrest during febrile periods and restricted activity in acute cases

DIET No special diet. May need to provide supplemental foods, e.g., milk shakes, to counter weight loss.

PATIENT EDUCATION Food Safety and Inspection Service, Office of Public Awareness, Dept. of Agriculture, Room 1165-S, Washington, DC 20205, (202)447-9351

MEDICATIONS

DRUG(S) OF CHOICE
• Optimal therapy includes two drugs, at least one with good intracellular penetration
• Rifampin 600-900 mg and doxycycline 200 mg given together every day for at least 6 weeks (possible for several months with severe complications). 5% relapse rate, not related to drug resistance - use same drugs for relapse. Usual cause is localized sequestration of organisms, or noncompliance with medication.
• Steroids in Herxheimer's reaction, severe illness, pancytopenia
Contraindications: Avoid doxycycline in children, pregnant women
Precautions: May get Herxheimer's reaction when therapy initiated
Significant possible interactions:
• Rifampin is a potent inducer for the hepatic P450 enzyme system, and may increase metabolism of many drugs metabolized by the liver including: Acetaminophen, anticoagulants, barbiturates, benzodiazepines, beta-blockers, chloramphenicol, clofibrate, oral contraceptives, corticosteroids, cyclosporine, digoxin, disopyramide, estrogens, hydantoins, methadone, mexiletine, quinidine, sulfones sulfonylureas, theophyllines, tocainide, verapamil, enalapril, ketoconazole, halothane
• Doxycycline: Antacids, anticoagulants, barbiturates, carbamazepine, hydantoins, cimetidine, digoxin insulin, iron salts, lithium, methoxyflurane, oral contraceptives, penicillins, sodium bicarbonate

ALTERNATIVE DRUGS
• Doxycycline orally bid and streptomycin by injection - very effective. (Streptomycin currently not available in the USA except by special request from CDC in Atlanta.) Slightly more effective than doxycycline/rifampin, especially with spondylitis, but more toxic and less convenient.
• Trimethoprim-sulfamethoxazole (Co-trimoxazole) plus rifampin 15 mg/kg in children (don't use alone) - higher relapse rate. Use in children.
• Neither ceftriaxone nor ofloxacin nor ciprofloxacin alone is as effective in acute therapy or preventing relapses; recent study shows ofloxacin plus rifampin effective

FOLLOWUP

PATIENT MONITORING
Check serology at 6 months and 1 year for chronic disease (difficult to evaluate if continuing exposure). Investigate any evidence of complication, recurrence.

PREVENTION/AVOIDANCE
• Avoid infected milk
• For occupational exposure - caution, possibly vaccination, use of protective goggles, protective gloves

POSSIBLE COMPLICATIONS
• Relapse (5% overall)
• Localized suppurative infections - osteo-articular (20-85%). Includes arthritis (possibly also immune effect), bursitis, tenosynovitis, osteomyelitis, sacroiliitis, vertebral or paraspinous abscess.
• Endocarditis - rare, but main cause of death in brucellosis
• Thrombophlebitis
• Neuro-brucellosis - most are meningeal. Also peripheral neuritis (usually single, bilateral is possible), encephalitis, myelitis, radiculopathy. Possibly neuro-psychiatric symptoms; a chronic fatigue type syndrome may exist which may or may not represent organic disease.
• Intrinsic ocular lesions - uveitis, retinal thrombophlebitis, nummular keratitis
• Pneumonitis with pleural effusion
• Hepatitis
• Cholecystitis

EXPECTED COURSE/PROGNOSIS
• Untreated case fatality < 2%
• Most cases resolve with treatment. 2-3 weeks for acute uncomplicated cases, but at least 6 weeks treatment recommended
• Relapse rate overall, 5%

MISCELLANEOUS

ASSOCIATED CONDITIONS N/A

AGE-RELATED FACTORS
Pediatric: May be mild, subclinical
Geriatric: N/A
Others: Worse in chronically ill, immunosuppressed

PREGNANCY
May cause miscarriage or abortion, even in subclinical cases

SYNONYMS
• Undulant fever
• Malta fever

ICD-9-CM 023.9 Brucellosis, unspecified

SEE ALSO N/A

OTHER NOTES N/A

ABBREVIATIONS N/A

REFERENCES
• Berenson AS, ed: Control of Communicable Diseases Manual. 16th Ed. Washington, DC, American Public Health Association, 1995
• Mandell GL, ed: Principles and Practice of Infectious Diseases. 4th Ed. New York, Churchill Livingstone, 1995
• Radolph JD: Brucellosis, don't let it get your goat. Amer J of Med 1994;307(1):64-75
• Montejo JM, et al: Open randomized therapeutic trial of six antimicrobial regimens in brucellosis. Clinical Infectious Diseases 1993;16;671-676
• Trujillo IZ, Zavala AN, Caceres JG, Miranda CQ: Brucellosis. Infectious Dis Clin of NA 1994;8(1)
• Young E: An overview of human brucellosis. Clinical Inf Dis 1995;21:283-290
Illustrations: N/A
Internet references: http://www.5mcc.com

Author(s)
Nancy Snapp, MD, MPH

Bulimia nervosa

BASICS

DESCRIPTION Body dissatisfaction; recurrent binge eating, with or without purging by self-induced vomiting, laxatives, diuretics. Alternative pattern - binges followed by sharply restricted diet and/or vigorous exercise.
Incidence/Prevalence in USA: Approximately 2% of females; higher among university women. True incidence is not known as this is a secretive disease.
System(s) affected: Endocrine/Metabolic, Nervous, Gastrointestinal, Cardiovascular
Genetics: N/A
Predominant age: Adolescents and young adults
Predominant sex: Female > Male

SIGNS AND SYMPTOMS
• Patients may switch back and forth between anorexia and bulimia
• Onset may be stress related
• May be average weight or even somewhat obese; most are slightly below average weight but have frequent fluctuations in weight
• Deny that there is a problem
• Gobble high calorie foods during binge
• Claim to feel fat even when thin
• Preoccupation with weight control
• Food collection and hoarding
• Diet pill, diuretic, laxative, ipecac and thyroid medication abuse
• Calories expended through vigorous exercise, especially running, aerobics
• Diabetic patients often withhold insulin
• Depressed mood and self-depreciation following the binges
• Relief and increased ability to concentrate following the binges
• Vomiting (may be effortless)
• Abdominal pain
• Parotid swelling
• Eroded teeth
• Scarred hands
• Conflicted relationships
• Cardiomyopathy and muscle weakness due to ipecac abuse

CAUSES Unknown; thought to be largely emotional

RISK FACTORS
• Impulsive character traits
• Low self-esteem
• Achievement pressure; high self-expectations
• Acceptance of the culturally condoned ideal of slimness
• Ambivalence about dependence/independence
• Stress due to multiple responsibilities, tight schedules, competition
• Unstable body image; perceptual distortions

DIAGNOSIS

DIFFERENTIAL DIAGNOSIS
• Gastrointestinal disorder
• Anorexia
• Psychogenic vomiting
• Hypothalamic brain tumor
• Epileptic equivalent seizures
• Kluver-Bucy-like syndromes
• Kleine-Levin syndrome
• Body dysmorphic disorder

LABORATORY
• Elevated BUN
• Hypokalemia
• Hypomagnesemia
• Hypochloremia
• Elevated basal serum prolactin
• Positive dexamethasone suppression test
• Low CD4/CD8 ratio
Drugs that may alter lab results: N/A
Disorders that may alter lab results: N/A

PATHOLOGICAL FINDINGS
• Eroded tooth enamel
• Esophagitis, Mallory-Weiss tears
• Asymptomatic, non-inflammatory parotid enlargement
• Gastric dilatation
• Infarction and perforation of the stomach

SPECIAL TESTS
• ECG
• Gastric motility
• Thyroid, liver, renal function
• Drug screen

IMAGING Not indicated

DIAGNOSTIC PROCEDURES
Psychological screening: Eating Attitudes Test

TREATMENT

APPROPRIATE HEALTH CARE
• Most patients can be treated as outpatients
• Hospitalize if patient is suicidal; if there is lab or ECG evidence of marked electrolyte imbalance; marked dehydration; or if there has been no response to outpatient therapy

GENERAL MEASURES
• Inpatient:
  ◊ If possible, admit to eating disorders unit or unit with structured eating disorders program
  ◊ Supervised meals and bathroom privileges
  ◊ No access to the bathroom for 2 hours after meals
  ◊ Monitor weight and physical activity
  ◊ Assess psychological state and nutritional status
  ◊ Identify precipitants to bingeing
  ◊ Develop alternatives to purging
  ◊ Monitor electrolytes
  ◊ Focal individual and cognitive behavioral therapy. Frequent visits by physician.
  ◊ Gradually shift control to patient as she demonstrates responsibility
• Outpatient:
  ◊ Build trust, treatment alliance
  ◊ Assess psychological state and nutritional status
  ◊ Involve patient in establishing target goals
  ◊ Use self-monitoring techniques such as food diary
  ◊ Identify prodromal states, precipitants
  ◊ Focus on overall well-being, developing gratifying relationships
  ◊ Challenge fear of loss of control
  ◊ Cognitive-behavioral therapy is of established efficacy in individual or group formats. Individual and family therapy, nutritional education, relaxation techniques, couples therapy, self-help group may also be helpful.

SURGICAL MEASURES N/A

ACTIVITY
• Monitor excess activity
• Stress importance of playful, pleasurable activities

DIET
• Goal is a balanced diet with adequate calories and a normal eating pattern
• Diminished ruminations about calories, weight, purging
• Reintroduce feared foods

PATIENT EDUCATION
• Seriousness and consequences of bulimic behavior
• Information on nutrition, metabolic balance
• Tools for self monitoring when appropriate

Bulimia nervosa

MEDICATIONS

DRUG(S) OF CHOICE
- Fluoxetine (Prozac) 10-80 mg is the only FDA approved medication for bulimia
- Other commonly used medications are the tricyclic antidepressants (TCA's), monoamine oxidase inhibitors (MAO's), and serotonin reuptake inhibitors (SRI's). When patients do not respond to a drug in one class (or experiences side effects), try a drug of a different class. To prevent relapse, maintain antidepressant medication at full therapeutic dose for at least one year.
- TCA's - imipramine (Tofranil), 10 mg, gradual increase to 250 mg if needed (monitor with ECG) (maximum dosage for adolescents 100 mg) or desipramine, (Norpramin) 25 mg/day, increasing gradually to 150 mg/day if needed (monitor with ECG). Improvement is not necessarily related to blood level.
- SRI's - fluoxetine (Prozac) often in higher doses than used for depression, 40-80 mg/day, are usually necessary; sertraline (Zoloft), 50-200 mg/day; paroxetine (Paxil), 20-60 mg/day; fluvoxamine (Luvox), 50-200 mg/day may be used also
- MAO inhibitors - phenelzine (Nardil) 60-90 mg/day. Patients with atypical depression may respond to MAO inhibitors.

Contraindications: Refer to manufacturer's literature

Precautions: Serious toxicity following overdose is common

Significant possible interactions:
- Lithium and tricyclic medication can be lethal when administered to hypokalemic patients
- Fluoxetine may increase tricyclic levels; monitor levels of TCA's if started after fluoxetine (remember fluoxetine's long half-life)
- Because of danger of food related hypertensive crises, use irreversible MAO inhibitors only with fully cooperative patients
- To avoid the serotonin syndrome, allow 5 weeks between fluoxetine and beginning of MAO inhibitor

ALTERNATIVE DRUGS
- If there is an underlying bipolar disorder, patients may benefit from lithium (Eskalith), 300 mg bid, increase gradually to therapeutic blood level of 0.6-1.2 mEq/L (0.6-1.2 mmol/L)
- Ondansetron (Zofran) 4-8 mg tid between meals can help prevent vomiting
- Cisapride (Propulsid), 10-20 mg before each meal and at bedtime for post-prandial abdominal discomfort
- Note: Dishonesty and noncompliance are common
- Psyllium (Metamucil) preparations 1tbs hs with glass of water, can prevent constipation during laxative withdrawal

FOLLOWUP

PATIENT MONITORING
- Binge-purge activity
- Level of exercise activity
- Self-esteem, comfort with body and self
- Ruminations and depression
- Repeat any abnormal lab values weekly or monthly until stable

PREVENTION/AVOIDANCE
- Encourage rational attitude about weight
- Moderate overly high self-expectations
- Enhance self-esteem
- Diminish stress

POSSIBLE COMPLICATIONS
- Suicide
- Drug and alcohol abuse
- Potassium depletion; cardiac arrhythmia; cardiac arrest

EXPECTED COURSE/PROGNOSIS
- Highly variable, tends to wax and wane
- May spontaneously remit
- Most patients continue to binge/purge, but do so less often
- Patients who do not establish trust likely to drop out of therapy, be lost to follow-up
- Those who stay in therapy tend to improve
- Patients with personality disorders have a generally poor prognosis

MISCELLANEOUS

ASSOCIATED CONDITIONS
- Major depression and dysthymia
- Bipolar disorder
- Obsessive-compulsive disorder
- Social phobia and other anxiety disorders
- Schizophrenic disorder
- Substance abuse disorder
- Borderline personality disorder
- Compulsive shoplifting

AGE-RELATED FACTORS
Pediatric: N/A
Geriatric: N/A
Others: Infrequently diagnosed in men or in older women

PREGNANCY
- Poor nutritional status may affect fetus
- Binge-purge may increase or decrease during pregnancy

SYNONYMS N/A

ICD-9-CM
- 783.6 Bulimia
- 307.51 Bulimia overeating of nonorganic origin

SEE ALSO
- Hyperkalemia
- Laxative abuse
- Salivary gland tumors

OTHER NOTES
- Anorexic patients may deal with the frustration of chronic food deprivation by converting to bulimia
- High risk
  ◊ Ballet dancers, models, cheerleaders
  ◊ Athletes, especially runners, gymnasts, weight lifters, body builders, jockeys, divers, wrestlers, figure skaters, field hockey players
- Sub-clinical eating disorders are common in university populations
- Sexual abuse is not causally related to bulimia
- Chronic, extreme hypokalemia can occur without physical symptoms

ABBREVIATIONS
- MAO = monoamine oxidase
- SRI = serotonin reuptake inhibitors
- TCA = tricyclic antidepressant

REFERENCES
- Crow SJ, Mitchell JE: Rational therapy in eating disorders. Drugs 1994;48(3):372-379
- Goldstein DJ, et al: Long term fluoxetine treatment of bulimia nervosa. Br J Psychiatry 1995;166:660-666
- Yager J, et al: Practice Guidelines for the Eating Disorders. Am J Psychiatry 1993;150:207-228
- Beumont PJV, et al: Excessive physical activity in dieting disorder patients. Int J Eating Disorders 1994;15:21-36

Illustrations: N/A
Internet references: http://www.5mcc.com

Author(s)
Alayne Yates, MD

Burns

BASICS

DESCRIPTION Burns are tissue injuries caused by application of heat, chemicals, electricity, or irradiation to the tissue. Extent of injury (depth of burn) is result of intensity of heat (or other exposure) and the duration of exposure.
• Partial thickness: First degree involves superficial layers of epidermis. Second degree involves varying degrees of epidermis (with blister formation) and part of the dermis.
• Full thickness: Third degree involves destruction of all skin elements with coagulation of subdermal plexus
System(s) affected: Skin/Exocrine, Endocrine/Metabolic
Genetics: N/A
Incidence/Prevalence in USA:
• 2 to 5 million burns/year in USA require assistance, 1,000,000/year require hospitalization, 12,000/year die
• Burns are leading cause of accidental death in children
Predominant age: All ages
Predominant sex: Male = Female

SIGNS AND SYMPTOMS
• First degree
 ◊ Erythema of involved tissue
 ◊ Skin blanches with pressure
 ◊ Skin may be tender
• Second degree
 ◊ Skin is red and blistered
 ◊ Skin is very tender
• Third degree
 ◊ Burned skin is tough and leathery
 ◊ Skin is not tender

CAUSES
• Open flame and hot liquid are most common (heat usually 15-45°C or greater)
• Caustic chemicals or acids (may show little signs or symptoms for the first few days)
• Electricity (may have significant injury with very little damage to overlying skin)
• Excess sun exposure

RISK FACTORS
• Hot water heaters set too high
• Work place exposure to chemicals, electricity or irradiation
• Young children and elderly adults with thin skin are more susceptible to injury
• Carelessness with burning cigarettes
• Inadequate or faulty electrical wiring

DIAGNOSIS

DIFFERENTIAL DIAGNOSIS
• Toxic epidermal necrolysis
• Scalded skin syndrome

LABORATORY
• Hematocrit
• Type and cross
• Electrolytes
• Blood urea nitrogen
• Urinalysis
Drugs that may alter lab results: N/A
Disorders that may alter lab results:
Pre-existing cardiac disease

PATHOLOGICAL FINDINGS
• First degree: devitalization of superficial layers of epidermis, congestion of intradermal vessels
• Second degree: coagulation necrosis of varying depths of epidermis, clefting of epidermis (blister), coagulation of subdermal plexus, skin appendages intact
• Third degree: necrosis of all skin elements, coagulation of subdermal plexus

SPECIAL TESTS
• Children - glucose (hypoglycemia may occur in children because of limited glycogen storage)
• Smoke inhalation - arterial blood gas, carboxyhemoglobin
• Electric burns - electrocardiogram, urine myoglobin, creatine kinase (CK) isoenzymes

IMAGING
• Chest x-ray
• Xenon scan may be useful in suspected smoke inhalation

DIAGNOSTIC PROCEDURES
Bronchoscopy may be necessary in smoke inhalation to evaluate lower respiratory tract

TREATMENT

APPROPRIATE HEALTH CARE
• Hospitalization for all serious burns
 ◊ Second degree burns over 10% body surface area (BSA), any 3rd degree burn
 ◊ Burns of hands, feet, face or perineum
 ◊ Electrical/lightning burns
 ◊ Inhalation injury
 ◊ Chemical burns
 ◊ Circumferential burn
• Transfer to burn center for:
 ◊ 2nd and 3rd degree burns over 10% BSA in patients under 10 years and over 50 years of age
 ◊ 2nd and 3rd degree burns over 20% BSA in any age range
 ◊ Burns of hands, feet, face or perineum
 ◊ Electrical/lightning burns
 ◊ Inhalation injury
 ◊ Chemical burns
 ◊ Circumferential burn
 ◊ Chemical burns with threat of functional impairment

GENERAL MEASURES
Based on depth of burns and accurate estimate of total body surface area (BSA) involved (Rule of nines)
• Rule of nines
 ◊ Each upper extremity - adult and child 9%
 ◊ Each lower extremity - adult 18%; child 14%
 ◊ Anterior trunk - adult and child 18%
 ◊ Posterior trunk - adult and child 18%
 ◊ Head and neck - adult 10%; child 18%
• Quick estimate (for smaller burns)
 ◊ The surface area of the patient's hand is approximately 1% of their BSA.
• Tetanus prophylaxis
• Remove all rings, watches, etc., from injured extremities to avoid tourniquet effect
• Remove clothing and cover all burned areas with dry sheet
• Flush area of chemical burn (for approximately 2 hours)
• 100% oxygen administration in all major burns, consider early intubation
• Do not apply ice to burn site
• Nasogastric tube (high risk of paralytic ileus)
• Foley catheter
• Pain relief with narcotics-should only be given IV
• ECG monitoring in first 24 hours following electrical burn
• Whirlpool hydrotherapy followed by silver sulfadiazine (Silvadene) occlusive dressings in severe burns
• Once or twice a day cleansing with dressing changes
• Epilock may be used as dressing in selected patients (especially useful for outpatient treatment of minor burns)

• Burn fluid resuscitation
Calculate fluid resuscitation from time of burn, not from time treatment begins.
◊ 2-4 mL Ringer's lactate x body weight (kg) x % BSA burn (1/2 given in first eight hours, 1/4 in second eight hours and 1/4 in third eight hours). In children, this is given in addition to maintenance fluids and is adjusted according to urine output and vital signs.
◊ Colloid solutions are not recommended during the first 12-24 hours of resuscitation
• Surgical procedures
◊ Escharotomy may be necessary in constricting circumferential burns of extremities or chest
◊ Tangential excision with split thickness skin grafts
• Other
◊ Use of biological membranes or skin substitutes may be indicated for burn coverage

SURGICAL MEASURES See General Measures

ACTIVITY Early mobilization is the goal

DIET High protein, high calorie diet when bowel function resumes; nasogastric tube feedings may be required in early post-burn period. TPN if NPO expected for > 5 days.

PATIENT EDUCATION
• Use of sunscreen
• Access to electrical cords/outlets
• Isolate household chemicals
• Use low temperature setting for hot water heater
• Household smoke detectors with special emphasis on maintenance
• Family/household evacuation plan
• Proper storage and use of flammable substances

MEDICATIONS

DRUG(S) OF CHOICE
• Morphine small frequent IV doses (0.1 mg/kg/dose in children)
• Silver sulfadiazine (Silvadene) topically to burn site (can cause leukopenia)
• Electrical burn with myoglobinuria will require alkalinization of urine and mannitol
• No indication for prophylactic antibiotics
• Consider H2 blockers: cimetidine, ranitidine, famotidine, or nizatidine for stress ulcer prophylaxis in severely burned patients
Contraindications: Specific drug allergies
Precautions: Be alert for respiratory depression with narcotics
Significant possible interactions: Refer to manufacturer's profile of each drug

ALTERNATIVE DRUGS
• Mafenide (Sulfamylon) - full thickness burn (caution: metabolic acidosis)
• Silver nitrate 0.5% (messy, leaches electrolytes from burn and causes water toxicity)
• Povidone-iodine (Betadine) may result in Iodine absorption from burn, "tan eschar". Makes débridement more difficult.
• Travase-enzymatic débridement

FOLLOWUP

PATIENT MONITORING According to extent of burn and treatment

PREVENTION/AVOIDANCE Skin grafts or newly epithelialized skin is highly sensitive to sun exposure and thermal extremes

POSSIBLE COMPLICATIONS
• Gastroduodenal ulceration (Curling's ulcer)
• Marjolin's ulcer - squamous cell carcinoma developing in old burn site
• Burn wound sepsis-usually gram negative organisms
• Pneumonia
• Decreased mobility with possibility of future flexion contractures

EXPECTED COURSE/PROGNOSIS
• First degree burn: complete resolution
• Second degree burn: epithelialization in 10-14 days (deep second degree burns will probably require skin graft)
• Third degree burn: no potential for re-epithelialization, skin graft required
• Length of hospital stay and need for ICU care depends on extent of burn, smoke inhalation and age
• A 50% survival can be expected with a 62% burn in ages 0-14 years, 63% burn in ages 15-40 years, 38% burn in age 40-65 years, 25% burn in patients over 65 years
• 90% of survivors can be expected to return to an occupation as remunerative as their pre-burn employment

MISCELLANEOUS

ASSOCIATED CONDITIONS
• Smoke inhalation syndrome
◊ Occurs within 72 hours of burn
◊ Suspected in burns occurring in an enclosed space
◊ Intubation, ventilation with positive end-expiratory pressure (PEEP) assistance

AGE-RELATED FACTORS
Pediatric:
• Consider child abuse when dealing with hot water burns in children
◊ Observe distribution of burns
◊ Pay attention to straight lines, especially if bilateral
Geriatric: Prognosis poorer for severe burns
Others: N/A

PREGNANCY N/A

SYNONYMS N/A

ICD-9-CM
940 Burn confined to eye and adnexa
941 Burn of face, head, and neck
942 Burn of trunk
948.0 Burn, any degree <10% of BSA (fifth digit can indicate BSA involved in 3rd degree burn)
949.0 Burn, unspecified degree
949.1 Burn, first degree
949.2 Burn, second degree
949.3 Burn, third degree

SEE ALSO N/A

OTHER NOTES N/A

ABBREVIATIONS
BSA = body surface area

REFERENCES
• Gillespie RW, Dimik AR, Hallberg PW: Advanced Burn Life Support Course Provider's Manual. Lincoln, Nebraska Burn Institute, 1990
• Schwartz SI, Shires GT, Spencer FC, et al: Principles of Surgery. 4th Ed. New York, McGraw-Hill Book Co., 1984
• Touloukian RJ: Pediatric Trauma. 2nd Ed. St. Louis, Mosby Year Book, 1990
Illustrations: 3 available on CD-ROM
Internet references: http://www.5mcc.com

Author(s)
Timothy L. Black, MD, FACS, FAAP
James P. Miller, MD, FACS, FAAP

Bursitis

BASICS

DESCRIPTION A bursa is a sac that is formed or found in areas subject to friction, such as locations where tendons pass over bony landmarks. Most common sites are subdeltoid, olecranon, prepatellar, trochanteric, radiohumeral. They essentially lubricate the region with synovial fluid. Large bursae usually communicate with joints and are responsible for retaining the synovial fluid in place. Bursae are fluid-filled sacs that serve as a cushion between tendons and bones. Bywaters, an English rheumatologist, found at least 78 bursae symmetrically placed on each side of the body.
System(s) affected: Musculoskeletal
Genetics: N/A
Incidence/Prevalence in USA: Common. Traumatic bursitis more likely in patients less than 35 years of age.
Predominant age: 15-50 years (most common in skeletally mature)
Predominant sex: Males > Females

SIGNS AND SYMPTOMS
• Include pain/tenderness/decreased range of motion of affected region
• Erythema
• Swelling
• Crepitus sometimes found

CAUSES
• Bursitis may be acute or chronic, and its etiology is often unknown
• There are many types of bursitis, including infectious, traumatic, inflammatory or gouty
• Less often rheumatoid disease or TB as well as gout and pseudogout

RISK FACTORS Individuals who engage in repetitive and vigorous training or others who suddenly increase their level of activity (e.g., "weekend warriors"). Also, improper or over-zealous stretching may lead to injury.

DIAGNOSIS

DIFFERENTIAL DIAGNOSIS
• Tendinitis, strains and sprains
• Joint pains may be caused by gout, pseudogout, rheumatoid arthritis, osteoarthritis
• Arthritis. Many elderly patients think it is the cause of their pain. (Lars Goran-Larsson, a rheumatologist from Sweden, and John Barn, M.D., reviewed their referrals for a 26-month period and found that 108 of 600 (18%) patients had some form of soft tissue problem rather than arthritis).

LABORATORY
Following will all help in differentiating soft tissue disease from rheumatic and connective tissue disease:
• CBC
• ESR
• Serum protein electrophoresis
• Rheumatoid factor (RF)
• Serum uric acid
• Calcium
• Phosphorus
• Alkaline phosphatase
• VDRL
• Joint fluid analysis (when available)
Drugs that may alter lab results:
• ESR may be increased with coexistent use of dextran, methyldopa, methysergide, penicillamine, theophylline, vitamin A
• ESR may be decreased with coexistent use of quinine, salicylates, and drugs which cause a high glucose level
Disorders that may alter lab results: N/A

PATHOLOGICAL FINDINGS
• Acute - with early inflammation, bursa is distended with watery or mucoid fluid
• Chronic - bursal wall is thickened and inner surface is shaggy and trabeculated. The space is filled with granular, brown, inspissated blood admixed with gritty, calcific precipitations. Upper extremity tendonitis and bursitis are usually the result of repetitive microtrauma, probably resulting in disruption of fibers leading to pain, spasm and disability.

SPECIAL TESTS
ECG (if pain mimics cardiac pain)

IMAGING
• CT or MRI
• Calcific deposits may be seen on plain x-ray

DIAGNOSTIC PROCEDURES
• Aspiration of swollen bursa and evaluation of synovial fluid
• The clinician must differentiate infected from inflammatory bursitis. Fluid analysis and culture help make the diagnosis. If the gram stain and culture yield an infective cause, treat with appropriate antibiotics. If the etiology is inflammatory, give local care.

TREATMENT

APPROPRIATE HEALTH CARE
Outpatient; refer only difficult cases

GENERAL MEASURES
• Conservative therapy consists of rest, ice and local care, elevation, gentle compression (often referred to as RICE therapy [rest-ice-compression-elevation])
• Physical therapy/hydrocollator treatments
• Invasive therapy would include aspiration of the bursa, injection of steroids
• Have patient wear a triangular sling to protect arm and support shoulder
• Treatment of any underlying infection

SURGICAL MEASURES
In severe cases, possibly surgical excision

ACTIVITY
Rest and elevation of affected extremity

DIET
Consider changes if bursitis directly related to obesity/crystalline deposition

PATIENT EDUCATION
• Advice concerning prevention via appropriate warm-up and stretching and avoidance of repetitive injury
• Possible life-style changes to prevent recurrent joint irritation

MEDICATIONS

DRUG(S) OF CHOICE
• Nonsteroidal anti-inflammatories (NSAID's) or aspirin. Injectable steroids and stronger analgesics if needed.
• Antibiotic therapy if infection present
Contraindications: Refer to manufacturer's profile of each drug
Precautions: Refer to manufacturer's profile of each drug
Significant possible interactions: Refer to manufacturer's profile of each drug

ALTERNATIVE DRUGS
• Application of local analgesic balms, capsaicin cream, injection of a corticosteroid along with lidocaine
• Systemic steroids (if not contraindicated)

FOLLOWUP

PATIENT MONITORING
• Discontinue NSAID's as soon as possible to avoid side effects
• Some patients may require repeated injections (usually no more than three) of a corticosteroid and xylocaine

PREVENTION/AVOIDANCE
• Appropriate warm-up and cool-down maneuvers, avoidance of overuse or inadequate rest between workouts
• Range of motion exercises
• Maintain high level of fitness and general good health

POSSIBLE COMPLICATIONS
• Acute bursitis may progress to chronic
• Severe long-range limitation of motion

EXPECTED COURSE/PROGNOSIS
• Most bouts of bursitis heal without sequelae
• Repetitive acute bouts may lead to chronic bursitis necessitating repeated joint/bursal aspirations or eventually surgical excision of involved bursa

MISCELLANEOUS

ASSOCIATED CONDITIONS
• Tendinitis
• Sprains, strains
• Associated stress fractures

AGE-RELATED FACTORS
Pediatric: Look for other causes
Geriatric: More common
Others: N/A

PREGNANCY N/A

SYNONYMS N/A

ICD-9-CM
727.3 Other bursitis

SEE ALSO Tendinitis

OTHER NOTES N/A

ABBREVIATIONS N/A

REFERENCES
• Robbins SL, Cotran RS: Pathological Basis of Disease. 2nd Ed. Philadelphia, W.B. Saunders Co., 1989
• Rotstein BR: Soft tissue rheumatism of the upper extremities: diagnosis and management. Medline Professional, Sept, 1991
Illustrations: N/A
Internet references: http://www.5mcc.com

Author(s)
Timothy Robinson, DO
Richard B. Birrer, MD

Candidiasis

BASICS

DESCRIPTION Candida albicans and related species cause a variety of infections. Cutaneous candidiasis syndromes include erosio interdigitalis blastomycetica, folliculitis, balanitis, intertrigo, paronychia, onychomycosis, diaper rash, perianal candidiasis, and the syndromes of chronic mucocutaneous candidiasis. Mucous membrane infections include oral candidiasis (thrush), esophagitis, and vaginitis. The most serious manifestation of candidiasis is hematogenously disseminated candidiasis (sometimes referred to as acute systemic candidiasis).
System(s) affected: Skin/Exocrine, Gastrointestinal, Reproductive, Pulmonary, Renal/Urologic
Genetics: N/A
Incidence/Prevalence in USA:
Approximately 50/100,000. Hematogenously disseminated candidiasis affects at least 120,000 patients annually in the USA.
Predominant age: All ages are susceptible to hematogenously disseminated candidiasis. Premature neonates are at particularly high risk.
Predominant sex: Male = Female (hematogenously disseminated candidiasis)

SIGNS AND SYMPTOMS
• Fever
• Malaise
• Tachycardia
• Hypotension
• Altered mental status
• Hepatosplenomegaly
• Maculopapular or nodular skin rash

CAUSES
• Most Candida infections are due to Candida albicans. However, other important human pathogens include C. tropicalis, C. krusei, C. stellatoidea, C. pseudotropicalis, C. guilliermondi, C. parapsilosis, C. lusitaniae, C. lambica, and C. glabrata.
• Candida species colonize human mucocutaneous surfaces, and most infections are endogenously acquired from this reservoir
• Human-to-human transmission of Candida occurs in some settings

RISK FACTORS
• For hematogenously disseminated candidiasis:
  ◊ Neutropenia
  ◊ Antibacterial chemotherapy
  ◊ Indwelling intravascular access devices
  ◊ Prior hemodialysis
  ◊ Mucocutaneous candidiasis

DIAGNOSIS

DIFFERENTIAL DIAGNOSIS Includes a variety of cryptic bacterial infections and, in the neutropenic host, multiple opportunistic infections

LABORATORY N/A
Drugs that may alter lab results: N/A
Disorders that may alter lab results: N/A

PATHOLOGICAL FINDINGS The characteristic histopathology of lesions of Candida invasion of visceral organs is microabscess formation

SPECIAL TESTS
• The diagnosis is established by isolating the causative organism from blood cultures (lysis/centrifugation blood cultures are superior to broth culture techniques for this purpose) or other normally sterile body sites, or by demonstration of organisms in histopathologic specimens of normally sterile tissues
• Isolation of Candida from multiple sites should raise the diagnostic suspicion of hematogenously disseminated candidiasis

IMAGING Imaging techniques are generally not specifically useful in the diagnosis of hematogenously disseminated candidiasis. However, in the syndrome of hepatosplenic candidiasis (chronic systemic candidiasis) imaging of the liver and spleen by liver scan, ultrasound, or CT (the most sensitive) may be useful in suggesting this syndrome as the cause of persistent fever and liver dysfunction.

DIAGNOSTIC PROCEDURES If blood cultures remain consistently negative, excisional biopsy may be useful in diagnosis. Aspiration and biopsy of skin lesions occasionally seen with hematogenously disseminated candidiasis is also useful.

TREATMENT

APPROPRIATE HEALTH CARE Inpatient for hematogenously disseminated candidiasis

GENERAL MEASURES
• Fluid and electrolyte therapy is often required
• Hemodynamic and respiratory support may be required in seriously ill patients
• Removal of potentially infected intravascular access devices is imperative

SURGICAL MEASURES N/A

ACTIVITY As tolerated

DIET No special diet

PATIENT EDUCATION Patients should be advised of the nature of the infection and the toxicities associated with therapy

Candidiasis

MEDICATIONS

DRUG(S) OF CHOICE
• Fluconazole
◊ 400 mg IV daily for first week, followed by additional IV or oral therapy at the same dose for at least 2 weeks after last positive blood culture or last evidence of infection
◊ Has been shown to be as effective as amphotericin B therapy and less toxic for treatment of candidemia in patients who are not neutropenic, do not have AIDS, and are not severely immunosuppressed by therapy after organ transplantation
• Amphotericin B
◊ Is alternative therapy for any patient with candidemia and the preferred therapy for patients with neutropenia or severe immune compromise
◊ Administer first in a test dose of 1 mg and then in incrementally increasing doses to 0.3-0.7 mg/kg/day. (Some authorities administer full dose after the test dose. In a critically ill patient, slow increase in dose is not warranted). Depending on host status and form of hematogenously disseminated candidiasis, total dose requirement ranges from 200 mg to 2.0 gm over a therapeutic duration of 2-10 weeks.
Contraindications: The safety of amphotericin B therapy in pregnant patients has not been established
Precautions:
• Amphotericin B
◊ Toxicity is formidable. Acute reactions occur commonly during initiation of therapy, including fever, rigors, and hypotension. These can be ameliorated or eliminated by premedication with acetaminophen, ibuprofen or hydrocortisone, and tend to decline over time with continuing daily therapy. Use meperidine if needed to abort rigors.
◊ Azotemia is a common complication and may be an indication for reducing therapy in some patients (to reduce toxicity, not because of renal elimination of drug). Generally recommended to hold drug if BUN > 40 mg/dL (14.3 mmol/L) or creatinine > 3.0 mg/dL (266 μmol). Hold until above levels decline, then administer drug every other day. Maintenance of optimal fluid status and prevention of dehydration help minimize risk of azotemia. "Sodium loading" with 77 mEq (77 mmol) sodium daily (= 1 L 1/2 normal saline) has been suggested by some authorities to decrease renal toxicity.
◊ Significant hypokalemia (often requires therapy) and renal tubular acidosis (rarely requires therapy) may develop. Significant hypomagnesemia may worsen hypokalemia.
◊ Anemia commonly develops in patients on protracted therapy but is almost always reversible
◊ Headache and phlebitis are common
◊ Leukopenia, thrombocytopenia, and liver function abnormalities are rarely encountered

Significant possible interactions:
• Amphotericin B - concomitant therapy with cyclosporine or other nephrotoxic agents such as aminoglycoside or vancomycin may increase risk of amphotericin-induced nephrotoxicity
• Fluconazole - potentially important drug interactions may occur in patients receiving oral hypoglycemics, coumarin-type anticoagulants, phenytoin, cyclosporine, rifampin, theophylline or terfenadine or astemizole

ALTERNATIVE DRUGS
• Fluconazole therapy may be preferred for infections with C. lusitaniae, which may be resistant to amphotericin B
• Amphotericin B is preferred for infections with C. krusei which is likely resistant to fluconazole
• Other azole antifungals depending on activity and safety.

FOLLOWUP

PATIENT MONITORING Complete blood count, serum electrolytes, and serum creatinine should be measured at least twice weekly in patients on daily amphotericin B therapy. If blood cultures are positive, they should be repeated until negative.

PREVENTION/AVOIDANCE Fluconazole 400 mg/day reduces the incidence of candidiasis in patients undergoing induction therapy for acute leukemia or bone marrow transplantation

POSSIBLE COMPLICATIONS
• Of hematogenously disseminated candidiasis
◊ Pyelonephritis
◊ Endophthalmitis
◊ Endocarditis, myocarditis, pericarditis
◊ Arthritis, chondritis, osteomyelitis
◊ Pneumonitis
◊ Central nervous system infection

EXPECTED COURSE/PROGNOSIS
Overall mortality for patients with hematogenously disseminated candidiasis is 40-75%, with mortality attributable to candidemia being 15-37%

MISCELLANEOUS

ASSOCIATED CONDITIONS See Risk Factors

AGE-RELATED FACTORS
Pediatric: N/A
Geriatric: N/A
Others: N/A

PREGNANCY N/A

SYNONYMS N/A

ICD-9-CM
112.5 Candidiasis, disseminated
112.9 Candidiasis, unspecified site

SEE ALSO
• Candidiasis, mucocutaneous
• Vulvovaginitis, candidal

OTHER NOTES Other candidal infections: Intraperitoneal infection in patients with major abdominal surgery, biliary tract candidiasis, isolated lower urinary tract infection

ABBREVIATIONS N/A

REFERENCES
• Crislip MA, Edwards JE Jr: Candidiasis. Infect Dis Clinics North America 1989;3:103-133
• Fraser VJ, Jones M, Dunkel J, Sorfer S, Medoff G, Dunagan WC: Candidemia in a tertiary care hospital: Epidemiology, risk factors, and predictors of mortality. Clin Infect Dis 1992;15:414-21
• Rex JH, Bennett JE, Sugar AM, et al (for the Candidemia Study Group and the National Institute of Allergy and Infectious Diseases Mycoses Study Group): A randomized trial comparing fluconazole with amphotericin B for the treatment of candidemia in patients without neutropenia. N Engl J Med 1994;331:1325-1330
• Uzua O, Anaissie EJ: Problems and Controversies in the Management of Hematogenous Candidiasis. Clin Infect Dis 1996;22(Suppl 2):S95
Illustrations: 8 available on CD-ROM
Internet references: http://www.5mcc.com

Author(s)
Ronald A. Greenfield, MD
Douglas P. Fine, MD

Candidiasis, mucocutaneous

BASICS

DESCRIPTION A mucocutaneous disorder caused by infection with, most commonly, species of Candida. Candida is normally present, in very small amounts, in the oral cavity, gastrointestinal tract, and female genital tract.
• Candida vulvovaginitis - this common form of mucocutaneous candidiasis consists of infections located on the vaginal mucosa, often associated with cutaneous vulvar involvement as well
• Oropharyngeal candidiasis - a candida infection of the oral cavity ("thrush") and/or pharynx.
• Candida esophagitis - usually associated with an immunosuppressed host
• Gastrointestinal candidiasis - gastritis, sometimes with ulcers, usually associated with thrush. The small and large bowel can also be affected.
• Angular cheilitis - fissures formed by candida infection at the corners of the mouth.
System(s) affected: Skin/Exocrine, Gastrointestinal
Genetics: None known
Incidence/Prevalence in USA: Very common, particularly vaginal. Very common in persons with immunodeficiency
Predominant age:
• Infants and older geriatrics predominate for thrush and cutaneous infections
• Women during their child bearing years predominate for vaginitis
Predominant sex: Female > Male (due to the entity of Candida vaginitis)

SIGNS AND SYMPTOMS
• In pediatrics
  ◊ Oral lesions - white, raised, painless, distinct patches
  ◊ Perineal - erythematous maculopapular rash with white "satellite" pustules
• In adults (whether or not immunocompromised)
  ◊ Vulvovaginal lesions - thin to thick whitish, "cottage cheese" like discharge; erythematous patches in vagina, on labia, on vulva, or other areas of perineum. Range from asymptomatic to intense pruritus with "burning" irritation
• In immunocompromised hosts
  ◊ Oral lesions - white, raised, painless, distinct patches; erythematous slightly raised patches; thick dark brownish coating; deep fissures
  ◊ Esophagitis - dysphagia, odynophagia, retrosternal pain. Usually associated with thrush.
  ◊ Gastrointestinal - ulcerations, pain
  ◊ Balanitis - erythema, linear erosions and scaling

CAUSES Species of Candida albicans, and less frequently, Candida tropicalis

RISK FACTORS
• Immunosuppression
• Antibacterial therapy
• Douching, chemical irritants, other vaginitides predispose some women to yeast vaginitis
• Dentures
• Chronic steroids (oral or inhaled)
• Birth control pills
• Hyperglycemia

DIAGNOSIS

DIFFERENTIAL DIAGNOSIS
• Baby formula can mimic thrush
• Hairy leukoplakia can mimic thrush but does not rub off to an erythematous base, is KOH negative, and is usually on the lateral sides of the tongue.
• Other yeasts may present like candida

LABORATORY
• Potassium hydroxide 10% microscopic slide preparation ("KOH prep"). Breaks down epithelial cell walls allowing yeast forms to be more easily identified. Best if heated. Lack of slide identification does not rule out and, conversely, one may identify a scant number of fungal forms without symptoms or pathogenesis.
• Gram stain reveals gram positive yeast forms
• Culture - blood or Sabouraud's agar. A positive may be result of normal flora.
Drugs that may alter lab results:
• Douches and spermicides (intravaginal infection)
• Inadequately dosed antifungal medication
Disorders that may alter lab results: Other vaginitides (may obscure vaginal slide findings)

PATHOLOGICAL FINDINGS Slide prep - Mycelia (hyphae) or pseudomycelia (pseudohyphae) yeast forms. A polymorphonuclear leukocyte response is not usually seen.

SPECIAL TESTS N/A

IMAGING Esophageal candidiasis will sometimes reveal a "cobblestone" appearance with a barium swallow and, less commonly, fistulas or esophageal dilatation (from denervation)

DIAGNOSTIC PROCEDURES
• For KOH prep, will need sample of discharge or "coating" of infected area or ulcer
• Esophagitis may need endoscopic biopsy
• If a person who is HIV seropositive has thrush plus dysphagia, and dysphagia is relieved with Candida therapy, a diagnosis of "Candida esophagitis" can be assumed.

TREATMENT

APPROPRIATE HEALTH CARE
Outpatient

GENERAL MEASURES Screen both well infants and patients with severe immunodeficiency using appropriate history and physical at all routine visits

SURGICAL MEASURES N/A

ACTIVITY N/A

DIET A few authorities say rectal colonization may be decreased with active culture yogurt or other live lactobacillus, but no clear correlation

PATIENT EDUCATION
• Advise patients at risk for recurrence about antibacterial therapy overgrowth
• Inform appropriate patients of over-the-counter vaginitis medications
• Cotton underwear may allow for better perineal ventilation and, thus, a less suitable environment for yeast

MEDICATIONS

DRUG(S) OF CHOICE
• Vaginal (choose one):
  ◊ Miconazole (Monistat) 2% cream - one applicator or 100 mg suppositories, intravaginally q hs x 7 days
  ◊ Clotrimazole (Gyne-Lotrimin, Mycelex) - intravaginal suppositories 100 mg q hs x 6-7 days or 200 mg q hs x 3 days. 1% cream one applicator intravaginally q hs x 6-7 days.
  ◊ Nystatin (Mycostatin, Nilstat) 100,000 U/gram cream (one applicator) or 100,000 U tablets (one) intravaginally bid x 7 days
  ◊ Fluconazole (Diflucan) 150 mg tablet once
• Oropharyngeal:
  ◊ Clotrimazole (Mycelex) 10 mg troche, slowly dissolve in mouth 5 times per day, preferably over 20 minutes for 7-14 days (48 hours after disappearance of thrush) (first choice in most literature)
  ◊ Nystatin pastilles - 1 or 2, 4-5 times daily for 7-14 days (48 hours after disappearance of thrush)
  ◊ Nystatin oral suspension (100,000 units/ml) - Children apply 5-10ml QID for 10 days directly to oral lesions. Adults swish and swallow 5-10 mL over 20 minutes 4-5 times per day x 14 days. Prophylaxis for relapses consists of above dosages 2-5 times per day.
  ◊ Fluconazole (Diflucan) although a majority of fungal strains found in the oropharynx are likely to be resistant

- Esophagitis:
  ◊ Ketoconazole (Nizoral) 200-400 mg tablets - one po qd x 14-21 days
  or
  ◊ Fluconazole (Diflucan) 200 mg tablet one time, then 100 mg po qd x 10-21 days
- Gastrointestinal (therapy not well defined)
  ◊ Fluconazole 200 mg tablets - one po qd x 14-21 days
  or
  ◊ Amphotericin B (Fungizone) IV solution - variable dosing, see pharmacology texts for full appropriate administration information
- Note: Resistant candidiasis is common in severely immunocompromised hosts. Some patients with otherwise resistant oropharyngeal and/or esophageal infection benefit from amphotericin B, 50 mg 3 times a week.

Contraindications:
- Any drug is contraindicated if it causes severe allergic response or a severe adverse reaction
- Ketoconazole or nystatin (if swallowed) - severe hepatotoxicity
- Amphotericin B - renal failure

Precautions:
- Vaginal - miconazole is usually drug of choice in pregnancy
- Ketoconazole - rarely, men may have difficulty achieving erections secondary to this drug. May cause light sensitivity. Teratogen in pregnancy and probably excreted in milk. Not well studied in children. Anaphylaxis is reported. Hepatic toxicity has been noted, predominantly with long-term therapy.
- Fluconazole - adjust dose with renal compromise. Hepatotoxicity is rare but reported. Very expensive relative to other oral agents. Resistance has often been noted.
- Amphotericin B - renal toxicity and hypokalemia are common. Careful patient monitoring is mandatory. Ketotic diabetics should have well controlled blood sugars prior to administration. Safety during pregnancy is not established.

Significant possible interactions:
- Rarely seen with creams, lotions or suppositories
- Ketoconazole
  ◊ Antacids, H2 blockers (achlorhydria) - reduce ketoconazole concentration
  ◊ Amphotericin - drug antagonism; do not give together
  ◊ Antiretrovirals - many have problematic interactions with ketoconazole; check drug reference
  ◊ Coumadin - potentiates anticoagulation
  ◊ Hypoglycemics - enhanced hypoglycemia
  ◊ INH/rifampin - reduce ketoconazole concentration
  ◊ Cyclosporine - increased cyclosporine concentration
  ◊ Phenytoin - metabolism altered; check levels
  ◊ Terfenadine (Seldane), astemizole - ECG QT abnormalities
  ◊ Alcohol - disulfiram reaction possible
  ◊ Others - check drug interaction reference
- Amphotericin
  ◊ Nephrotoxic drugs - enhanced toxicity
  ◊ Corticosteroids - potentiates hypokalemia
  ◊ Ketoconazole - drug antagonism; do not give together
- Fluconazole

  ◊ Rifampin - decreased fluconazole concentrations
  ◊ Tolbutamide - decreased tolbutamide concentrations
  ◊ Warfarin, phenytoin, cyclosporine - metabolism altered; check levels

ALTERNATIVE DRUGS
- Vaginal
  ◊ Terconazole (Terazol) particularly for recurrent cases that may involve imidazole resistance. 0.4% cream - one applicator intravaginally q hs x 7 days; 0.8% cream/80 mg suppositories - one applicator or one suppository intravaginally q hs x 3 days
  ◊ Any of the antifungal creams or suppositories can be tried every month for a few days near menses to help curb recurrent infections
- Oropharyngeal
  ◊ Ketoconazole 200-400 mg po qd x 14-21 days
  ◊ Fluconazole 50-200 mg tablets - one po qd x 14-21 days
- Esophagitis
  ◊ Amphotericin B (variable dosing)

FOLLOWUP

PATIENT MONITORING
Immunocompromised persons may need to monitor themselves regularly. Use symptoms to monitor as well as "routine" KOH preps and or visual investigations during vaginal or oral exams.

PREVENTION/AVOIDANCE
- Antibiotics can potentiate candidiasis
- Candida overgrowth is more likely with pH changes from douching, chemicals (such as spermicides) or other vaginitises
- Moist environments are conducive to overgrowth of Candida. Cotton underwear may help deter some Candida infections.

POSSIBLE COMPLICATIONS
- Rarely develops major complications in immunocompetent persons
- With immunocompromised, generally depends on severity of immune status (CD4 count is the most common marker). Moderate immunodepression (CD4 200-500) may be associated with chronic candidiasis. With severe immunodepression (CD4 < 100) thrush can lead to esophagitis and, later, a full systemic infection can involve every organ system, particularly the kidney (candiduria).

EXPECTED COURSE/PROGNOSIS
- For immunocompetent individuals, a benign course and excellent prognosis is the norm. Recurrent vulvovaginitis may be associated with a colonized partner, but specifics have not yet been well documented.
- For severely immunosuppressed persons, candida may become an "AIDS defining illness" by CDC criteria and chronicity can cause much morbidity and, less commonly, mortality

MISCELLANEOUS

ASSOCIATED CONDITIONS
- Human immunodeficiency virus
- Other leukopenias
- Diabetes mellitus
- Cancer
- Other immunosuppressive disorders

AGE-RELATED FACTORS
Pediatric: Newborn thrush may be acquired in the birth canal
Geriatric: A common geriatric infection
Others: Vaginitis is common in women of childbearing age. Uncommon to see prepubertal or postmenopausal yeast vaginitis due to hormonal induced changes in the vaginal wall.

PREGNANCY
- No known fetal complications of maternal candida
- See specific "medication precautions" above
- Miconazole is usually drug of choice in pregnancy

SYNONYMS
- Monilia
- Thrush

ICD-9-CM
112.0 Candidiasis of mouth
112.1 Candidiasis of vulva and vagina
112.9 Candidiasis of unspecified site

SEE ALSO
- Candidiasis
- HIV infection & AIDS
- Vulvovaginitis, candidal

OTHER NOTES
- Most Candida infections are associated with endogenous flora
- Transmission from person to person is rare
- Occasionally Candida vaginitis may be sexually transmitted
- Rarely, oral Candida leukoplakia can be precancerous
- Esophageal candidiasis may occur concurrently with another infectious (e.g., herpes simplex virus, cytomegalovirus) esophagitis in severely immunocompromised persons
- Skin testing, often used to diagnose or exclude anergy, is positive in 70-85% of individuals randomly checked in studies

ABBREVIATIONS N/A

REFERENCES Reese RE, Betts RF, eds: A Practical Approach to Infectious Diseases. 3rd Ed. Boston, Little, Brown and Co., 1991
Illustrations: N/A
Internet references: http://www.5mcc.com

Author(s)
Susan Louisa Montauk, MD

Carbon monoxide poisoning

 BASICS

DESCRIPTION Carbon monoxide (CO) is produced by incomplete combustion of carbon containing compounds such as wood. Inhalation of CO leads to displacement of oxygen from binding sites on hemoglobin. CO has about 250 times the affinity for hemoglobin than oxygen.
Detrimental effects are related to tissue hypoxia from decreased oxygen content and a shift of the oxyhemoglobin dissociation curve to the left. CO also binds to cytochrome oxidase impairing mitochondrial function. Muscle activity is affected by CO by binding to myoglobin.
System(s) affected: Cardiovascular, Musculoskeletal, Nervous
Genetics: N/A
Incidence/Prevalence in USA:
Approximately 3800 deaths annually
Additional 10,000 individuals miss one or more days of work
Predominant age: N/A
Predominant sex: N/A

SIGNS AND SYMPTOMS
• Headaches
• Tinnitus
• Nausea
• Dizziness
• Weakness
• Confusion
• CNS depression
• Syncope
• Angina
• Tachycardia
• Cardiac dysrhythmias
• Nystagmus
• Ataxia
• Seizures
• Coma
• Cardiopulmonary arrest

CAUSES Carbon monoxide inhalation

RISK FACTORS
• Cigarette smokers
• Smoke inhalation
• Closed space with faulty furnaces or stoves
• Coal miners
• Mechanics (inhalation of car exhaust)
• Paint strippers
• Solvent manufacturing

 DIAGNOSIS

DIFFERENTIAL DIAGNOSIS Cyanide toxicity

LABORATORY Measurement of carboxyhemoglobin
Drugs that may alter lab results: N/A
Disorders that may alter lab results: N/A

PATHOLOGICAL FINDINGS N/A

SPECIAL TESTS N/A

IMAGING N/A

DIAGNOSTIC PROCEDURES N/A

 TREATMENT

APPROPRIATE HEALTH CARE
• Emergency room for mild poisoning
• Inpatient for moderate or severe poisoning

GENERAL MEASURES
• Removal from offending source
• Rapid reduction in tissue hypoxia with supplemental oxygen
• Supportive care as necessary
• Intubation and mechanical ventilation
• Volume resuscitation

SURGICAL MEASURES N/A

ACTIVITY Rest until COHgb reduced and symptoms abate

DIET N/A

PATIENT EDUCATION N/A

Carbon monoxide poisoning

MEDICATIONS

DRUG(S) OF CHOICE
• 100% Oxygen by tight fitting nonrebreather mask
• Hyperbaric oxygen for severe poisoning
• Mild poisoning: COHgb levels < 30%
  ◊ No signs or symptoms of cardiovascular or neurologic dysfunction
  ◊ Treatment - admission if COHgb > 25%
  ◊ Symptomatic medication - acetaminophen for headache etc.
  ◊ 100% Oxygen by nonrebreather until COHgb < 5%
  ◊ Patients with underlying heart disease should be admitted regardless of level of COHgb
• Moderate poisoning: COHgb 30-40%
  ◊ No signs or symptoms of cardiovascular or neurologic dysfunction
  ◊ Treatment - admission
  ◊ Cardiovascular status should be followed closely even in the absence of clear cardiac effects
  ◊ Determination of acid-base status - corrected by oxygen
  ◊ 100% Oxygen by nonrebreather until COHgb < 5%
• Severe poisoning: COHgb > 40%
  ◊ Cardiovascular or neurologic functional impairment at any COHgb
  ◊ Treatment - admission
  ◊ Cardiovascular function monitoring
  ◊ Acid-base status monitoring
  ◊ 100% Oxygen by nonrebreather until COHgb < 5%
  ◊ Hyperbaric oxygen immediately if available, if unavailable then treat as in moderate poisoning
  ◊ No improvement in cardiovascular or neurologic function within 4 hours - transport to nearest facility with hyperbaric oxygen, regardless of distance
Contraindications: N/A
Precautions: N/A
Significant possible interactions: N/A

ALTERNATIVE DRUGS   N/A

FOLLOWUP

PATIENT MONITORING
• Measurement of COHgb levels
• Arterial blood gases

PREVENTION/AVOIDANCE
• Maintenance of furnaces and stoves to avoid faulty combustion
• Adequate ventilation in high risk occupations

POSSIBLE COMPLICATIONS
• Myocardial infarction
• Long term neuropsychiatric complications
  ◊ Intellectual deterioration
  ◊ Memory impairment
• Personality changes
  ◊ Irritability
  ◊ Aggressiveness
  ◊ Violence
  ◊ Moodiness

EXPECTED COURSE/PROGNOSIS   Most survivors recover completely with only a minority developing chronic neuropsychiatric impairment

MISCELLANEOUS

ASSOCIATED CONDITIONS N/A

AGE-RELATED FACTORS
Pediatric: N/A
Geriatric: Higher incidence of cardiovascular and neurologic disease increasing complications
Others: N/A

PREGNANCY   Tissue hypoxia includes the fetus. Can cause significant fetal abnormalities depending on the developmental stage.

SYNONYMS N/A

ICD-9-CM
986 Toxic effect of carbon monoxide

SEE ALSO N/A

OTHER NOTES N/A

ABBREVIATIONS
• CO = Carbon monoxide
• COHgb = Carboxyhemoglobin
• CNS = Central nervous system

REFERENCES
• Murray JF, Nadel JA, eds: Textbook of Respiratory Medicine. Philadelphia, W.B. Saunders Co., 1988
• Ingbar DH, ed: Clinics in Chest Medicine: Respiratory Emergencies I. Philadelphia, W.B. Saunders Co., March, 1994
• Shoemaker WC, Ayers S, et al, eds: Textbook of Critical Care. Philadelphia, W.B. Saunders Co., 1989
• Ilano AL, Raffin TA: Management of Carbon Monoxide Poisoning. Chest 1990;91:165-169
Illustrations: N/A
Internet references: http://www.5mcc.com

Author(s)
Robert DeMarco, MD

Cardiac arrest

BASICS

DESCRIPTION Absence of effective mechanical cardiac activity.
This section is not a substitute for an American Heart Association approved ACLS course and is intended only as a quick reference.
System(s) affected: Cardiovascular
Genetics: N/A
Incidence/Prevalence in USA: 2:1000
Predominant Age: Increases with age
Predominant sex: Male > Female

SIGNS AND SYMPTOMS
• Unconscious secondary to CNS hypoperfusion
• No pulses in large arteries
• Apnea or agonal breathing
• Cyanosis or pallor

CAUSES
• Asystole (confirm in 2 leads; 11% actually fine V-fib)
• Ventricular fibrillation (V-fib)
• Pulseless ventricular tachycardia (V-tach)
• Pulseless electrical activity (PEA, previously known as electrical mechanical dissociation [EMD])

RISK FACTORS
• Male
• Increasing age
• Hypercholesterolemia
• Hypertension
• Cigarette smoking
• Positive family history of atherosclerosis

DIAGNOSIS

DIFFERENTIAL DIAGNOSIS
• Drugs: barbiturates, narcotics, calcium channel blockers, beta blockers, tricyclics
• Shock: septic or blood loss induced
• Hypothermia
• Pulmonary embolism
• Cardiac tamponade
• Pneumothorax

LABORATORY
• Arterial blood gas
• Electrolytes
• CBC
• Drug levels
• PT (international normalized ratio [INR]), PTT, type and cross, if indicated
Drugs that may alter lab results: Digoxin toxicity may cause hyperkalemia
Disorders that may alter lab results:
• Hypo- or hyperventilation will change pO_2 and pCO_2
• Acidosis increases serum potassium

PATHOLOGICAL FINDINGS Based on underlying cause

SPECIAL TESTS ECG

IMAGING Chest x-ray for endotracheal (ET) tube placement, pneumothorax. Consider echocardiogram for pericardial effusion.

DIAGNOSTIC PROCEDURES N/A

TREATMENT

APPROPRIATE HEALTH CARE
Prehospital emergency medical service (EMS) personnel, emergency department, "cardiac arrest team", intensive care setting

GENERAL MEASURES
• Defibrillation first
  ◊ Adult: 200, 300, or 360J
  ◊ Children: Use largest paddles that will fit on child even adult size if can get good contact. Defibrillate at 2J/kg once. Increase to 4J/kg twice.
• 100% oxygen by bag-valve-mask or endotracheal tube (preferred)
• Start 2 IV's as close to the heart as possible (central line OK but don't waste time). Large bore peripheral lines can deliver fluid more quickly than a central line. This is especially important in PEA secondary to hypovolemia.
• Perform CPR including closed chest compression. Intermittent abdominal compression and active compression /decompression show no survival advantage.
• Keep patient warm if possible, especially in children
• Monitor:
  ◊ Pulse after three initial defibrillations
  ◊ Check monitor between each defibrillation and after any intervention
  ◊ Use end-tidal CO2 monitor to assess gas exchange, if available. Esophageal intubation will produce a very low end-tidal CO2.

SURGICAL MEASURES
If indicated:
• Pericardiocentesis to treat cardiac tamponade
• Needle decompression (second intercoastal space mid clavicular line), then chest tube insertion to treat tension pneumothorax

ACTIVITY N/A

DIET N/A

PATIENT EDUCATION Suggest basic life support (BLS) training to all patients in your practice, especially those who have family members at risk for cardiac arrest

MEDICATIONS

DRUG(S) OF CHOICE
• Lidocaine, atropine, naloxone, and epinephrine [LANE] can all be given by endotracheal tube. Follow by 10 cc of NS or sterile water followed by bagging.
• Epinephrine:
  ◊ 1 mL = 1 mg (1:1000)
  ◊ 1 mL = 0.1 mg (1:10,000)
ADULT:
For ventricular tachycardia and pulseless ventricular tachycardia.
Use in order listed below:
• Defibrillate x3 at 200J, 300J, 360J
  ◊ Check monitor rhythm
  ◊ Follow each drug administration by repeated defibrillation at 360J
  ◊ Check monitor and pulses after each subsequent intervention
• Epinephrine: 1 mg IV and repeated every 3-5 minutes
  ◊ If 1 mg fails may use intermediate dose 2-5 mg IV every 3-5 minutes or high dose epinephrine 0.1 mg/kg every 3-5 minutes. No good evidence that high dose epinephrine increases survival.
• Lidocaine: 1.5 mg/kg IV, repeat in 5 minutes to total dose of 3 mg/kg
• Bretylium: 5 mg/kg IV push. Repeat in 5 minutes at dose of 10 mg/kg.
• Magnesium sulfate: 1-2 mg IV in suspected Torsades de pointes or refractory V-fib/V-tach. Some authors would use this before bretylium
• Procainamide 30 mg/min IV in refractory V-fib/V-tach (maximum dose of 17 mg/kg)
• Bicarbonate: 1 mEq/kg IV only in known preexisting bicarbonate responsive acidosis, tricyclic overdose, to alkalinize the urine in known overdose
For asystole
• CPR
• Confirm in 2 leads
• Consider possible causes including hypoxia, hyperkalemia, hypokalemia, preexisting acidosis, drug overdose, hypothermia
• Consider immediate transcutaneous pacing
• Epinephrine: 1 mg IV push repeated every 3-5 minutes
  ◊ May use intermediate dose or high dose epinephrine (2-5 mg IV or 0.1 mg/kg IV) every 3-5 minutes
• Atropine: 1 mg IV push every 3-5 minutes to total dose of 0.04 mg/kg
  ◊ Shorter atropine dosing intervals are acceptable (every 1-2 minutes)
• Consider termination of efforts if no reversible underlying cause is found

For pulseless electrical activity (PEA)
• Includes EMD, idioventricular rhythms, ventricular escape rhythms, bradyasystole rhythms, postdefibrillation idioventricular rhythms
• Assess blood flow by Doppler ultrasound if available
• Consider possible reversible causes: cardiogenic shock (weak pump), cardiac tamponade, tension pneumothorax, severe hypovolemia, pulmonary embolism (consider thrombolytics), hypothermia, hypoxia, acidosis, hyperkalemia, drug overdose such as beta-blockers, calcium channel blockers, tricyclics, digoxin, hyperkalemia
• Epinephrine: 1 mg IV push. Repeat every 3-5 minutes. Can use intermediate or high dose epinephrine (2-5 mg IV or 0.1 mg/kg IV respectively) every 3-5 minutes.
• Atropine: 1 mg IV every 3-5 minutes to total dose of 0.04 mg/kg: if absolute bradycardia (< 60 beats per minute) or relative bradycardia. May decrease interval to 1-2 minutes if desired.
CHILDREN:
(in alphabetical order)
• Atropine 0.01-0.02 mg/kg/dose; minimum dose is 0.1 mg, maximum single dose is 0.5 mg in child, 1.0 mg in adolescent
• Bretylium sulfate 5-10 mg/kg
• Epinephrine
 ◊ Bradycardia: 0.01 mg/kg IV/IO or 0.1 mg/kg ET (1:1000)
 ◊ Asystolic or pulseless arrest: First dose is 0.01-0.03 mg/kg IV/IO. Doses as high as 0.2 mg/kg may be effective.
 ◊ Infusion: 0.1 µg/kg/min. Titrate to desired effect (0.1 µg/kg/min-1.0 µg/kg/min)
• Lidocaine
 ◊ Bolus: 1 mg/kg/dose (maximum 3 mg/kg)
 ◊ Infusion: 20-50 µg/kg/min
• Sodium bicarbonate 1 mEq/kg/dose or 0.3 x kg x base deficit. Infuse slowly and only if ventilation adequate.
Contraindications: None during an arrest
Precautions:
• Bretylium will cause hypotension 15-20 minutes after injection
• Calcium can be use if known (pre-existing) hyperkalemia precipitated arrhythmia
• Magnesium is relatively contraindicated in renal failure but given consequences of not terminating rhythm, this is only a relative contraindication in this setting
Significant possible interactions: N/A

ALTERNATIVE DRUGS
• Asystole: Aminophylline 250 mg IV bolus has been effective in uncontrolled trials, but should be used only when conventional therapy has failed
• V-tach/V-fib: Amiodarone 150 mg IV over 10 minutes followed by 360 mg over next 6 hours. Now FDA approved for V-tach/V-fib unresponsive to other therapy. Initial 150 mg can be accelerated in code situation.

FOLLOWUP

PATIENT MONITORING Intensive care setting on continuous monitor, look for precipitating cause including serial EKG's and enzymes to rule out myocardial infarction

PREVENTION/AVOIDANCE Treat underlying disease

POSSIBLE COMPLICATIONS
• Can have significant neurologic, hepatic, renal, and cardiac ischemic injury
• May have rib fractures or pneumothorax from CPR

EXPECTED COURSE/PROGNOSIS
• Outcome related to underlying disease, age, duration of arrest, etc.
• Outcome poor if
 ◊ > 4 minutes to CPR or > 8 minutes to ACLS
 ◊ Arrest in field
 ◊ Resuscitation effort > 30 minutes
• About 14% survive in-hospital arrest; fewer after field arrest.

MISCELLANEOUS

ASSOCIATED CONDITIONS
• Coronary artery disease (cardiac arrest may be first presenting symptom)
• Valvular heart disease
• Hypertension

AGE-RELATED FACTORS
Pediatric: Bradycardia is most common initial form of cardiac arrest. Most frequently is primarily a response to underlying pulmonary disease and hypoxia. Adequate oxygenation and ventilation is especially important.
Geriatric: Poor risk for survival and long-term outcome
Others: N/A

PREGNANCY
• Displace uterus either manually or by placing a rolled towel or pad under right hip. If not able to resuscitate within 5-15 minutes, consider emergency C-section to relieve uterine obstruction and increase blood return to the heart. This may also be done to save the fetus if at a viable age.
• Consider amniotic fluid embolism or eclampsia related seizures as precipitating factors

SYNONYMS
• Code Blue

ICD-9-CM
427.5 Cardiac arrest

SEE ALSO N/A

OTHER NOTES N/A

ABBREVIATIONS
• ACLS = Advanced Cardiac Life Support
• EMD = electro-mechanical dissociation
• ET = endotracheal
• IO = intraosseous
• PEA = pulseless electrical activity

REFERENCES
• Emergency Cardiac Care Committee and Subcommittees: American Heart Association: Guidelines for Cardiopulmonary Resuscitation and Emergency Cardiac Care. JAMA 1992;268:16
• Graber MD: Emergency Medicine. In: Graber MD, et al, eds. The Family Practice Handbook. St. Louis, Mosby-Yearbook, 1994
Illustrations: N/A
Internet references: http://www.5mcc.com

Author(s)
Mark A. Graber, MD

Cardiac tamponade

BASICS

DESCRIPTION
Compression of cardiac chambers by acute pressure on the heart from increased volume and pressure of the pericardial fluid
• As fluid accumulates, pressure primarily affects the compliant cardiac wall and transmits the pressure transmurally, resulting in increased ventricular pressure. This decreases ventricular filling and reduces cardiac output by reducing stroke volume. Contraction is preserved until ventricular diastolic pressures rise enough to limit coronary perfusion.
• The compensatory mechanisms for tamponade are: Increased peripheral resistance, increased CVP and increased heart rate. All three increase myocardial oxygen denied the heart at a time when perfusion is limited.
• In some patients, pulsus paradoxus and equalization of pressures may not occur
• In patients with elevated left ventricular diastolic pressures (as with chronic hypertension), resistance to left ventricle (LV) filling is constant. Throughout the cardiac cycle, equalization of pressures in these patients may only be noted in the right heart chambers with LV pressures being higher than right ventricle (RV) pressures.
• The absence of pulsus paradoxus and classic hemodynamic finding does not rule out tamponade
System(s) affected: Cardiovascular
Genetics: N/A
Incidence/Prevalence in USA: N/A
Predominant age: N/A
Predominant sex: N/A

SIGNS AND SYMPTOMS
• Beck's triad - distant heart sounds, hypotension, distended neck veins
• Most common complaints are of intolerance to minimal activity and dyspnea. Later may develop agitation, CNS depression, coma and cardiac arrest.
• Decreased systolic blood pressure
• Narrow pulse pressure
• Pulsus paradoxus - greater than 15 mm Hg drop in systolic blood pressure between inspiration and expiration
• Neck veins may be distended and reveal a rapid systolic (X) descent and attenuated or absent diastolic (Y) descent
• Tachycardia - a compensatory mechanism to maintain output
• Right upper quadrant tenderness due to hepatic engorgement
• Increased area of cardiac dullness outside the apical point of maximum impulse

CAUSES
• Physiology of tamponade depends on size and rapidity of development
• Uremia
• Neoplasm - breast, lung, lymphoma, leukemia
• Postmyocardial infarction (Dressler's)
• Postoperative - as high as 30% post pericardiotomy
• Viral Infection - Coxsackie group B, influenza, echo, herpes
• Bacterial infection - S. aureus, M. tuberculosis, S. pneumoniae (rare)
• Fungal infection - M. capsulatum
• Lupus and rheumatologic disease
• Trauma
• Placement of central venous catheter, pacer wires
• Myxedema
• Drug induced

RISK FACTORS
• Cardiac tamponade should be suspected in the hemodynamically unstable patient:
  ◊ With known pericarditis
  ◊ Following blunt or penetrating chest trauma
  ◊ Following open heart surgery or cardiac catheterization
  ◊ With known or suspected intrathoracic neoplasm
  ◊ With suspected dissecting aortic aneurysm
  ◊ Renal failure on dialysis

DIAGNOSIS

DIFFERENTIAL DIAGNOSIS
• Tension pneumothorax
• Acute RV failure
• Chronic obstructive pulmonary disease
• Constrictive pericarditis
• Acute acceleration of chronic bronchitis
• Acute pulmonary emboli
• Fat emboli
• Excessive or rapid administration of fluids
• Abdominal distention from ascites or ileus
• Increased intrathoracic pressure from pneumothorax, hemothorax, airway obstruction, or mechanical ventilation
• Administration of vasopressors

LABORATORY
• CBC
• Sed rate
• Cardiac enzymes to rule out acute myocardial infarction
• Antinuclear antibodies (ANA)
• Rheumatoid factor
• BUN/creatinine
• Pericardial fluid for - culture of bacteria, fungus, mycobacteria, Gram stain, hematocrit, cell count, cytology, glucose, protein, rheumatoid factors, complement levels
Drugs that may alter lab results: N/A
Disorders that may alter lab results: N/A

PATHOLOGICAL FINDINGS
Pericardial blood usually does not clot, but occasionally will

SPECIAL TESTS
• ECG
  ◊ May show low voltage QRS complexes, ST segment elevation and PR segment depression of pericarditis
  ◊ Electrical alternans (R wave variation from beat to beat)
  ◊ Electrical alternans is seen in 10-20% of cases of tamponade and 50-60% of these are neoplastic in origin
• Right heart catheterization
  ◊ Equalization (within 2-3 mm) of right atrial, pulmonary artery, pulmonary capillary wedge pressure, left atrial and left ventricular diastolic pressure
  ◊ The intracardiac diastolic pressure will approximate the intrapericardial pressure
  ◊ The dip and plateau pattern of constriction or restriction pericardial disease is absent
  ◊ Loss of Y descent on atrial wave form

IMAGING
• Chest x-ray:
  ◊ May or may not show enlargement of cardiac shadow (if > 250 cc fluid present)
• Echocardiography:
  ◊ Diagnostic cardiac compression
  ◊ Doppler - right sided transvalvular flow greatly exaggerated; left sided flows greatly reduced with inspiration

DIAGNOSTIC PROCEDURES
N/A

TREATMENT

APPROPRIATE HEALTH CARE Inpatient

GENERAL MEASURES
• Maintain hemodynamic stability until definitive correction of the pericardial tamponade
• All patients should have q 15 minute blood pressures, heart rate and at a minimum CVP measurement. Strong consideration should be given to placement of a Swan-Ganz catheter if time allows.
• Fluids may be of temporary benefit, but rising filling pressures may further compromise coronary perfusion

SURGICAL MEASURES
• Pericardiocentesis surgical treatment:
◊ Indications - when there is rapid deterioration of hemodynamic function, when there is delay in operation for traumatic effusion and for diagnostic reasons
◊ If rapid re-accumulation is anticipated (as in malignancy) it may be helpful to insert a long term drainage catheter. Also consider instillation of sclerosing agents.
◊ Surgery should be performed under the most optimal circumstances available to the operation as the patient's condition allows
◊ Blind pericardiocentesis should be performed only in life threatening emergencies
◊ Ideally echocardiography can be brought to the bedside to assist in needle placement and progress of fluid removal
◊ Invasive monitoring is also helpful to follow decrease in pericardial pressures
◊ Fluoroscopy can also be used
◊ EKG guidance using the "V" lead to avoid contact with the epicardium may be useful
◊ 20% of patients with tamponade will have a negative tap because the pericardial sac contains coagulated material. Hemorrhagic pericardial effusions usually do not clot.

ACTIVITY Bedrest

DIET As tolerated

PATIENT EDUCATION N/A

MEDICATIONS

DRUG(S) OF CHOICE Isoproterenol may temporarily increase cardiac output
Contraindications: Refer to manufacturer's literature
Precautions: Refer to manufacturer's literature
Significant possible interactions: Refer to manufacturer's literature

ALTERNATIVE DRUGS N/A

FOLLOWUP

PATIENT MONITORING Close monitoring until stable

PREVENTION/AVOIDANCE None

POSSIBLE COMPLICATIONS
• Cardiac perforation and/or laceration at time of pericardiocentesis
• Pneumothorax at time of pericardiocentesis
• Constriction of pericardium

EXPECTED COURSE/PROGNOSIS
Good results expected with appropriate treatment

MISCELLANEOUS

ASSOCIATED CONDITIONS
• Myocardial infarction
• Aortic aneurysm

AGE-RELATED FACTORS
Pediatric: N/A
Geriatric: N/A
Others: N/A

PREGNANCY N/A

SYNONYMS N/A

ICD-9-CM 423.9 Unspecified disease of pericardium

SEE ALSO N/A

OTHER NOTES N/A

ABBREVIATIONS N/A

REFERENCES
• Heger JW, et al: Cardiology for the House Officer. Baltimore, Williams & Wilkins, 1982
• Civettee JM, Taylor RW, Kirby RR: Critical Care. Philadelphia, J.B. Lippincott, 1988
• Rippie JM, et al: Intensive Care Medicine. Boston, Little, Brown and Company, 1991
• Shoemaker WC, et al: Textbook of Critical Care. Philadelphia, W.B. Saunders Co., 1989
Illustrations: N/A
Internet references: http://www.5mcc.com

Author(s)
Bradley R. Martin, MD

Cardiomyopathy, end stage

BASICS

DESCRIPTION Congestive heart failure causing symptoms with less than normal activity or at rest and requiring "maximal medical therapy."
Ischemic cardiomyopathy is the product of long standing, severe coronary artery disease, usually associated with multiple myocardial infarctions, often also following multiple coronary bypass operations.
This myopathy and the majority of others share in common enlargement of the heart, increased wall tension, and wall stress of the left and right ventricles, decreased mechanical efficiency of cardiac function. The tendency to have sub-endocardial ischemia, because of increased wall stress, and increased end diastolic pressures. Markedly decreased ejection fraction of usually in the range of 20% (normal 65%). Because of the abnormal mechanics there is a tendency for these hearts to progressively enlarge with time.
System(s) affected: Cardiovascular
Genetics: Idiopathic hypertrophic subaortic stenosis well known to have a familial distribution
Incidence/Prevalence in USA:
• The number of patients dying from end stage heart disease, per year, under the age of 65, in the US today is approximately 60,000
• 35,000 to 70,000 of the population might benefit from cardiac replacement or chronic support
• Heart failure is the most rapidly growing form of heart disease
Predominant age:
• Ischemic cardiomyopathy is seen predominately in patients from the 5th decade of life and beyond
• Idiopathic and familial cardiomyopathies are seen at an earlier age, as are those related to congenital heart disease, viral cardiomyopathy, alcoholic cardiomyopathy and post partum cardiomyopathy
Predominant Sex: Male > Female (ischemic cardiomyopathy)

SIGNS AND SYMPTOMS
• Shortness of breath at rest
• Dyspnea on minimal exertion
• Paroxysmal nocturnal dyspnea
• Postprandial dyspnea
• Fatigue
• Syncope
• Tachypnea
• Cyanosis, pallor
• Cool vasoconstricted extremities
• Diaphoresis
• Jugular venous distention
• Bi-basilar inspiratory rales
• S3 cardiac gallop
• Liver and spleen enlargement
• Ascites, edema
• Chest pain

CAUSES
• Infectious
  ◊ Viral (e.g., Coxsackie virus)
  ◊ Poliomyelitis
  ◊ Diphtheria
  ◊ Toxoplasmosis
  ◊ Trichinosis
  ◊ Trypanosomiasis
  ◊ Acute rheumatic fever
• Congenital
  ◊ Congenital heart disease
  ◊ Glycogen storage disease
  ◊ Pompe's disease
  ◊ Hurler's syndrome
  ◊ Hunter's syndrome
  ◊ Fabry's disease
  ◊ Duchenne's muscular dystrophy
  ◊ Friedreich's ataxia
  ◊ Familial cardiomyopathies, such as "asymmetric septal hypertrophy"
• Toxic/metabolic
  ◊ Alcoholism
  ◊ Radiation
  ◊ Beriberi
  ◊ Kwashiorkor
  ◊ Potassium deficiency
  ◊ Cobalt
  ◊ Hemosiderosis
• Drugs
  ◊ Adriamycin
• Inflammatory
  ◊ Giant cell myocarditis
  ◊ Loeffler's eosinophilia
  ◊ Sarcoidosis
• Idiopathic
• Others
  ◊ Coronary artery disease
  ◊ Peripartum and postpartum
  ◊ Amyloidosis
  ◊ Idiopathic hypertrophic subaortic stenosis
  ◊ Endomyocardial fibrosis

RISK FACTORS
• Hypertension
• Hyperlipidemia
• Obesity
• Diabetes mellitus
• Smoking
• Stress
• Sedentary lifestyle
• Cardiac surgery

DIAGNOSIS

DIFFERENTIAL DIAGNOSIS
• Severe pulmonary disease
• Primary pulmonary hypertension
• Recurrent pulmonary embolism
• Hypothyroidism
• Some advanced forms of malignancy

LABORATORY
• Hyponatremia
• Pre-renal azotemia
• Mild hyperbilirubinemia
• ECG: left ventricular hypertrophy, ventricular strain pattern, left and right atrial enlargement are often seen. In ischemic cardiomyopathies evidence of previous myocardial infarctions indicated by Q-waves and poor R-wave progression in the precordial leads.
Drugs that may alter lab results:
Digoxin, Furosemide, ACE inhibitors (by improving cardiac function)
Disorders that may alter lab results: N/A

PATHOLOGICAL FINDINGS N/A

SPECIAL TESTS
• Cardiac catheterization may help differentiate between ischemic and other types of cardiomyopathy, elucidate intracavitary pressures, cardiac output, left ventricular function and coronary anatomy. In addition, cardiac catheterization provides an opportunity for assessment for pulmonary artery pressures and pulmonary vascular resistance (mean pulmonary artery pressure minus the mean left atrial [wedge] pressure divided by the cardiac output [normal 1.2])
• For transplant candidates, the following additional tests are recommended to rule out significant non-cardiac disease: Computed tomographic (CT) scans of the chest and abdomen; 24 hour creatinine clearance; routine pulmonary function studies (including blood gas determination); serologies for hepatitis A, B, C, HIV, Toxoplasma, CMV and EB virus; full panels of renal and liver function; a complete blood count with differential; and a Panorex dental x-ray. Additional diagnostic studies may be indicated if any findings are suspicious for disease which would be a contraindication to transplantation. For instance, any undiagnosed roentgenographic abnormality of the lungs is a contraindication to transplantation.

IMAGING
• Chest x-ray
  ◊ Cardiac enlargement is found in the majority of cardiomyopathies, which are termed dilated cardiomyopathies
  ◊ Generally, four chamber enlargement is seen and the cardiac silhouette on a posterior-anterior film occupies more than 50% of the transverse diameter
  ◊ Increased vascular markings to the upper lobes, indicating elevated pulmonary venous pressure
  ◊ Hazy diffuse densities in the hilar areas, indicating pulmonary edema
  ◊ Pleural effusions and curly B-lines in the periphery of the lung, indicating engorged pulmonary lymphatics
  ◊ In hypertrophic cardiomyopathies and cardiomyopathies characterized by normal cardiac size, chest x-ray generally demonstrates pulmonary signs of cardiac failure with a cardiac silhouette which is normal to upper limits in size

• Echocardiogram:
◊ In the dilated cardiomyopathies, demonstrates four chamber enlargement and global hypokinesias
◊ In hypertrophic cardiomyopathies, severe left ventricular hypertrophy
◊ In ischemic cardiomyopathy, the heart may be normal or enlarged
◊ Usually segmental abnormalities in contraction of the left ventricle can be detected, indicative of previous localized myocardial infarction
• Nuclear multiple gaited acquisition ventriculogram (MUGA):
◊ The best study to quantitate ejection fraction, which is often 25% or less

DIAGNOSTIC PROCEDURES N/A

TREATMENT

APPROPRIATE HEALTH CARE
Outpatient until time for myocardial transplant or for treatment of severe heart failure

GENERAL MEASURES
• Treatment of heart failure
• Treatment of electrolyte disturbances

SURGICAL MEASURES Myocardial transplant

ACTIVITY Limited by varying degrees. Bedrest may be necessary.

DIET Low fat, low salt, fluid restriction

PATIENT EDUCATION Careful instructions and precautions for all medications

MEDICATIONS

DRUG(S) OF CHOICE
• Dilated cardiomyopathies, in the usual recommended adult dosage include the following:
◊ Digoxin, 0.125-0.25 mg/day
◊ Furosemide 40-120 mg two to four times/day
◊ Potassium chloride 20 mEq for each 40 mg of furosemide
◊ ACE inhibitors - captopril 6.25-50 mg three times/day or enalapril 2.5-25 mg/day
◊ Isosorbide dinitrate 20-100 mg four times/day
◊ Hydralazine 5-25 mg four times/day (maximum of 300 mg/day divided)
◊ Oxygen 2-4 liters/minute by nasal cannula at bedtime

Contraindications:
• Digoxin - 1st or 2nd degree heart block
• Furosemide - oliguria, anuria, renal dysfunction

Precautions:
• Digoxin - in patients with renal dysfunction requiring quinidine therapy, the digoxin dosage should be lowered to 0.125 mg/day and level determined 4 or 5 days later. The potassium level must also be carefully monitored.
• Furosemide - a careful titration of patients with end stage heart disease is necessary when furosemide therapy is employed. Over diuresis may result in dehydration and severe hyponatremia. Potassium therapy is necessary accompaniment to furosemide therapy in order to prevent hypokalemia and hypochloremic alkalosis. A combination of high dose furosemide plus aminoglycoside antibiotics may cause nephrotoxicity or ototoxicity.
• ACE inhibitors - must be used with extreme care. If the patient's blood pressure is already low, it's safest to begin with captopril at a very low dose such as 6.25 mg 3 times/day. The after load reduction or drop in systolic blood pressure, experienced by patients on these drugs may lead to reduction in cardiac size and improved efficiency. Patients survive longer when on ACE inhibitors.

Significant possible interactions:
Digoxin - has many potentially significant interactions including antibiotics, amiodarone, verapamil, cholestyramine. Digoxin levels increase in patients on quinidine. Toxicity is more common in this setting.

ALTERNATIVE DRUGS
• IV continuous infusion of dobutamine. It may be applicable in an outpatient setting.
• Other ACE inhibitors at appropriate doses
• IV infusion of amrinone or milrinone

FOLLOWUP

PATIENT MONITORING Once a month followup is usually adequate

PREVENTION/AVOIDANCE Dietary control of salt and water intake, home blood pressure measurement, daily weight check by the patient are helpful in preventing problems

POSSIBLE COMPLICATIONS Worsening congestive heart failure, syncope, arrhythmias, sudden death

EXPECTED COURSE/PROGNOSIS
20-40% of the patients in New York functional class IV are expected to die within one year. With transplant, one year survival may be as high as 94%.

MISCELLANEOUS

ASSOCIATED CONDITIONS N/A

AGE-RELATED FACTORS
Pediatric: Idiopathic and familial cardiomyopathies are seen at an earlier age, as are those related to congenital heart disease, viral cardiomyopathy, alcoholic cardiomyopathy and postpartum cardiomyopathy
Geriatric: N/A
Others: N/A

PREGNANCY May occur postpartum

SYNONYMS N/A

ICD-9-CM
• 425.4 other primary cardiomyopathies
• 425.5 alcoholic cardiomyopathy

SEE ALSO
• Alcoholism
• Amyloidosis
• Diabetes mellitus, insulin-dependent (IDDM or Type I)
• Diabetes mellitus, non-insulin dependent (NIDDM)
• Diphtheria
• Hypertension, essential
• Hypothyroidism, adult
• Idiopathic hypertrophic subaortic stenosis (IHSS)
• Malnutrition, protein-calorie
• Poliomyelitis
• Rheumatic fever
• Sarcoidosis
• Toxoplasmosis
• Trichinosis
• Trypanosomiasis, East African
• Trypanosomiasis, West African

OTHER NOTES N/A

ABBREVIATIONS
CMV = cytomegalic inclusion virus
EBV = Epstein-Barr virus

REFERENCES
• Copeland JG: Cardiac Transplantation. Curr Probl Surg 1988;25(9):607-72
• Emery RW, et al: The cardiac donor: A six-year experience. Ann Thorac Surg 1986;41:356-362
• Wahlers T, et al: Donor heart related variables and early mortality after heart transplantation. J. Heart Transplant 1991;10:22-27
• Pickering JG, et al: Fibrosis in the transplanted heart and its relation to donor ischemic time. Circulation 1990;81:949-958
• Hosenpud JO, et al: Relation between recipient: Donor body size match and hemodynamics three months after heart transplantation. J. Heart Transplant 1989;8:241-243
Illustrations: N/A
Internet references: http://www.5mcc.com

Author(s)
Jack G. Copeland, MD

Carotid sinus syndrome

BASICS

DESCRIPTION   In carotid sinus syndrome (CSS), stimulation of one or both of the hypersensitive carotid sinuses at the bifurcation of the common carotid arteries produces brief episodes of faintness or loss of consciousness. Four types are described:
• Cardioinhibitory - is vagally mediated, causes bradycardia, sinus arrest or atrioventricular block
• Vasodepressor: a sudden drop of peripheral vascular resistance leads to hypotension without associated cardiac slowing
• Mixed - combined cardioinhibitory and vasodepressor changes
• Cerebral - extremely rare, carotid sinus hypersensitivity occurs without bradycardia or hypotension
System(s) affected: Cardiovascular, Nervous
Genetics: N/A
Incidence/Prevalence in USA: 64 out of 132 consecutive patients (48.5%) older than 65, evaluated for dizziness, falls or syncope were found to have carotid sinus type sensitivity
Predominant age: Elderly
Predominant sex: Male > Female

SIGNS AND SYMPTOMS
• Dizziness
• Syncope
• Falls
• Blurred vision
• Vertigo
• Tinnitus
• Bradycardia
• Hypotension
• Pallor
• Sweating
• Tachypnea
• No postictal symptoms

CAUSES
• Stimulation of the hypersensitive baroreceptors in the carotid sinus affects vagus and sympathetic nerve outflow
• Carotid body tumors
• Inflammatory and malignant lymph nodes in the neck
• Metastatic cancer

RISK FACTORS
• Organic heart disease
• Diffuse atherosclerosis
• Wearing tight collars
• Shaving over region of sinus
• Emotional upheaval
• Head movement

DIAGNOSIS

DIFFERENTIAL DIAGNOSIS
• Vasovagal syncope
• Postural hypotension
• Primary autonomic insufficiency
• Hypovolemia
• Arrhythmias
• Sick sinus syndrome
• Syncope secondary to reduced cardiac output
• Cerebrovascular insufficiency
• Emotional disturbances
• Other causes of syncope.

LABORATORY   N/A
Drugs that may alter lab results: N/A
Disorders that may alter lab results: N/A

PATHOLOGICAL FINDINGS   N/A

SPECIAL TESTS   With the patient in the supine position and while the ECG is monitored, manual massage of the carotid sinus causes asystole of more than 3 seconds (cardioinhibitory) and/or a drop in systolic BP of more than 50 mm Hg without decrease in heart rate (vasodepressor).

IMAGING   N/A

DIAGNOSTIC PROCEDURES
• Carotid sinus massage (check for potential contraindications before performing massage)
• Electrophysiologic studies such as tilt table test
• Electrocardiogram
• Carotid duplex scan

TREATMENT

APPROPRIATE HEALTH CARE
Outpatient

GENERAL MEASURES   Cardiac pacing (dual chamber) is the treatment of choice

SURGICAL MEASURES
• Denervation of the carotid sinus by surgery or radiation therapy for selected patients
• Implantation of a permanent pacemaker helps in preventing recurrent symptoms in patients with cardioinhibitory component
• Surgery for selected patients with atheromata

ACTIVITY   No restrictions

DIET   No special diet

PATIENT EDUCATION   Avoidance of exacerbating factors that might stimulate the carotid sinus - tight neck collar, shaving, turning of the head to one side, straining at stool

Carotid sinus syndrome

 MEDICATIONS

DRUG(S) OF CHOICE
• Anticholinergics - atropine for the cardioinhibitory type
• Sympathomimetics - ephedrine
• Theophylline
Contraindications: Refer to manufacturer's instructions
Precautions: Concomitant usage of digitalis, beta-blockers and alpha-methyldopa may accentuate response to carotid sinus massage
Significant possible interactions: Refer to manufacturer's instructions

ALTERNATIVE DRUGS
Fludrocortisone has been used in clinical trials for patients with vasopressor CSS

 FOLLOWUP

PATIENT MONITORING
Follow as an outpatient

PREVENTION/AVOIDANCE
Avoidance of pressure on the neck

POSSIBLE COMPLICATIONS
• Prolonged confusion
• Frequent falls leading to injuries and fractures

EXPECTED COURSE/PROGNOSIS
Serious if syncope associated with atheromatous narrowing of sinus artery or basilar artery

 MISCELLANEOUS

ASSOCIATED CONDITIONS
• Sick sinus syndrome
• Atrioventricular block

AGE-RELATED FACTORS
Pediatric: N/A
Geriatric: More likely to occur in elderly. Associated with atheromata.
Others: N/A

PREGNANCY
N/A

SYNONYMS
• CSS
• Carotid sinus syncope
• Carotid sinus hypersensitivity

ICD-9-CM
337.0

SEE ALSO
Atherosclerosis

OTHER NOTES
It is clinically important to distinguish CSS from sick sinus syndrome

ABBREVIATIONS
CSS = carotid sinus syndrome

REFERENCES
• McIntoch SJ, Lawson J, Kenny RA: Clinical characteristics of vasopressor, cardioinhibitory, and mixed carotid sinus syndrome in the elderly. Amer J of Med 1993;95(2):203-208
• Isselbacher KJ, et al, eds: Harrison's Principles of Internal Medicine. 13th Ed. New York, McGraw-Hill, 1994
• Braunwald E, ed: Heart Disease: A Textbook of Cardiovascular Medicine. 4th Ed. Philadelphia, W.B. Saunders Co., 1992
• Blane JJ, et al: Carotid sinus syndrome: acute hemodynamic evaluation of a dual chamber pacing mode. Pacing & Clin Electrophysiology 1995;18(10):1902-1908
Illustrations: N/A
Internet references: http://www.5mcc.com

Author(s)
George E. Kikano, MD

Carpal tunnel syndrome

 BASICS

 DIAGNOSIS

 TREATMENT

DESCRIPTION
This is the most common cause of peripheral nerve compression. The median nerve is compressed as it traverses the carpal tunnel in the wrist and hand. The tunnel is composed of the carpal bones dorsally and the transverse carpal ligament ventrally. It contains flexor tendons and the median nerve. Symptoms tend to affect the dominant hand but over half the patients experience bilateral symptoms.
System(s) affected: Musculoskeletal, Nervous
Genetics: Unknown, however a familial type has been reported
Incidence/Prevalence in USA: Most common entrapment neuropathy
Predominant age: 40 to 60
Predominant sex: Female > Male (3-6:1)

SIGNS AND SYMPTOMS
• Tingling or prickling sensations in the fingers
• Burning pain in the fingers particularly at night (acroparesthesias)
• The symptoms characteristically are relieved by shaking or rubbing the hands
• Arm pain
• Finger sensory loss
• Tinel's sign
• Phalen's sign
• During waking hours symptoms occur when driving the car, reading the newspaper and occasionally when using the hands for repetitive maneuvers
• Symptoms characteristically are confined to the thumb, index and middle finger but many patients do not distinguish this localization and feel the entire hand is affected
• Wasting of the thenar muscles is a late sign
• Weakness of the hand, however, for such tasks as opening jars is often noted by the patient early on in the disorder

CAUSES
• Causes include disorders which affect the musculoskeletal system in the region of the wrist including trauma or Colles' fracture, degenerative joint disease, rheumatoid arthritis, ganglion cyst, scleroderma
• Hypothyroidism and diabetes are frequently associated with this condition which also occurs with increased frequency during pregnancy
• Other miscellaneous causes include acromegaly, lupus erythematosus, leukemia, pyogenic infections, sarcoidosis, primary amyloidosis and Paget's disease
• Hyperparathyroidism, hypocalcemia

RISK FACTORS
Jobs which involve repetitive flexion and extension of the wrist may influence the development of carpal tunnel syndrome. Occupation as a seamstress, and more recently, that of computer operator may aggravate carpal tunnel syndrome. There is, however, no universal agreement that carpal tunnel syndrome is job related.

DIFFERENTIAL DIAGNOSIS
• Cervical spondylosis
• Generalized peripheral neuropathy
• Brachial plexus lesion

LABORATORY
• No one laboratory test is diagnostic
• Normal thyroid function studies and normal glucose metabolism studies may be helpful in excluding these conditions which may be associated with CTS
Drugs that may alter lab results: N/A
Disorders that may alter lab results: N/A

PATHOLOGICAL FINDINGS N/A

SPECIAL TESTS
• Electromyography will be abnormal in more than 85% of cases; prolonged distal latency of the median motor nerves; the most sensitive indicator is the median sensory distal latency which is prolonged. Furthermore the sensory nerve action potential may be reduced or unobtainable.
• Stimulation of the ulnar nerve should be done as well to exclude generalized polyneuropathy

IMAGING
Special x-ray views of the carpal tunnel may be obtained. These are of limited usefulness unless heterotopic calcification can be identified.

DIAGNOSTIC PROCEDURES
• Tinel's sign - tapping of the wrist proximal to the carpal tunnel may produce electric sensation perceived by the patient, a sign of nerve compression
• Phalen's sign - holding the wrist flexed may precipitate the paresthesias experienced by the patient within a few seconds
• A blood pressure tourniquet to cut off circulation to the arm may precipitate symptoms promptly

APPROPRIATE HEALTH CARE
• Outpatient
• Outpatient surgery

GENERAL MEASURES
• Splinting of the wrist in extension may provide significant relief of symptoms. Prolonged use of splinting if possible may allow some symptoms to resolve.
• Injection of the carpal tunnel with hydrocortisone (Medrol 40 mg/mL). 1 mL + 1% lidocaine (1 mL) may provide significant temporary relief. This is particularly useful during pregnancy.

SURGICAL MEASURES
• With few exceptions surgical decompression of the carpal tunnel by dividing the transverse carpal ligament completely provides almost complete relief of symptoms in the overwhelming majority of patients (greater than 95%)
• The procedure may be done as an outpatient under local anesthesia in the majority of cases
• Healing of the incision generally takes two weeks; an additional two weeks of recuperation may be required before the hand can be fully utilized for tasks requiring strength

ACTIVITY As tolerated

DIET No special diet

PATIENT EDUCATION
Carpal Tunnel Syndrome Foundation. For patient education materials favorably reviewed on this topic, contact: American Academy of Family Physicians Foundation, P.O. Box 8418, Kansas City, MO 64114, (800)274-2237, ext.4400

MEDICATIONS

DRUG(S) OF CHOICE Nonsteroidal anti-inflammatory agents such as ibuprofen 400 mg three or four times a day or naproxen sodium 500 mg twice a day will provide significant relief of symptoms in many patients
Contraindications: Gastrointestinal intolerance
Precautions: Gastrointestinal side effects of NSAID's may preclude their use in selected patients
Significant possible interactions: Refer to manufacturer's literature

ALTERNATIVE DRUGS Other NSAID's

FOLLOWUP

PATIENT MONITORING
• Patients treated with wrist splints or other palliative measures such as cortisone injections will require followup in the ensuing 4 to 12 weeks to assess the success of treatment modalities
• Patients treated surgically rarely experience recurrence of the disorder. Routine followup once healing of the incision has occurred is not necessary.

PREVENTION/AVOIDANCE Take a break once an hour when doing repetitive work involving hands

POSSIBLE COMPLICATIONS
• Post-op infection (rare)
• Injury to recurrent branch of the nerve

EXPECTED COURSE/PROGNOSIS
Untreated the condition can be expected to lead to numbness and weakness in the hand with atrophy of hand muscles and permanent loss function of the extremity

MISCELLANEOUS

ASSOCIATED CONDITIONS See Causes

AGE-RELATED FACTORS
Pediatric: N/A
Geriatric: N/A
Others: N/A

PREGNANCY May occur in pregnancy

SYNONYMS N/A

ICD-9-CM 354.0 Carpal tunnel syndrome

SEE ALSO N/A

OTHER NOTES N/A

ABBREVIATIONS N/A

REFERENCES
• Joynt RJ, ed: Clinical Neurology. Vol. 4. Philadelphia, J.B. Lippincott Co, 1990
• Seddon H: Surgical Disorders of the Peripheral Nerves. Baltimore, Williams and Wilkins Co., 1972
Illustrations: N/A
Internet references: http://www.5mcc.com

Author(s)
Fremont P. Wirth, MD, FACS

Cataract

BASICS

DESCRIPTION Any opacity of the lens, either localized or generalized. Single largest cause of blindness in the world, blinding an estimated 17 million people.
- Types include:
  ◊ Age-related ("senile") - over 90%
  ◊ Congenital - 1/250 newborns, 10-38% of childhood blindness
  ◊ Toxic/nutritional
  ◊ Systemic disease associated e.g., myotonic dystrophy, atopic dermatitis
  ◊ Metabolic - diabetes (accelerated sorbitol pathway), hypocalcemia, Wilson's disease
  ◊ "Complicated" - secondary to associated eye disease, e.g., uveitis (juvenile rheumatoid arthritis, sarcoid, etc.). Also secondary to occult tumor (melanoma, retinoblastoma).
  ◊ Trauma - heat (infrared), electrical shock, radiation, concussion, perforating eye injuries, intraocular foreign body

System(s) affected: Nervous
Genetics:
- Age related cataract has no clear pattern
- Congenital sometimes associated, e.g., heredofamilial systemic disorders (Laurence-Moon-Biedl syndrome), chromosomal disorders (Down syndrome)

Incidence/Prevalence in USA:
- 5% of age 52-62
- 46% of age 75-85 have significant vision loss (20/30 or worse)
- 92% of age 75-85 have some cataract changes

Predominant Age: Depends on type of cataract
Predominant Sex: Male = Female

SIGNS AND SYMPTOMS
- Age-related cataract:
  ◊ Blurred vision, distortion or "ghosting" of images
  ◊ Problems with visual acuity in bright light or night driving (glare)
  ◊ Falls or accidents
  ◊ Injuries (e.g., hip fracture)
  ◊ Signs on eye examination: A lens opacity consistent with the symptoms
- Congenital:
  ◊ Lens opacity present at birth or within three months after birth
- Often asymptomatic or parents notice child's visual inattention or strabismus (lazy eye)
  ◊ Leukocoria (white pupil reflex), strabismus, nystagmus, associated syndrome signs (as in Down or rubella syndromes)
  ◊ Visual acuity tests abnormal for one or both eyes
  ◊ Note: Must always rule out ocular tumor. Early diagnosis and treatment of retinoblastoma may be lifesaving.
- Other types of cataract:
  ◊ May present with decreased visual acuity complaint
  ◊ Appropriate history or signs to help in diagnosis

CAUSES
- Age-related cataract:
  ◊ Continual addition of layers of lens fibers throughout life creates hard, dehydrated lens nucleus which impairs vision (nuclear cataract)
  ◊ Aging alters biochemical and osmotic balance required for lens clarity, outer lens layers hydrate and become opaque, affecting vision
- Congenital:
  ◊ Usually obscure
  ◊ Drugs (corticosteroids in first trimester, sulfonamides, etc.)
  ◊ Metabolic - diabetes in mother, galactosemia in fetus
  ◊ Intrauterine infection - first trimester (rubella, herpes, mumps)
  ◊ Maternal malnutrition
- Other cataract types:
  ◊ Have in common that a biochemical/osmotic imbalance disrupts lens clarity
  ◊ Local changes in lens protein distribution lead to light scattering manifest as lens opacity

RISK FACTORS
- Aging
- Patient with one of the predisposing diseases

DIAGNOSIS

DIFFERENTIAL DIAGNOSIS
- An opaque appearing eye may be due to surface opacities of the cornea (scarring), lens opacities, tumor, retinal detachment, gliotic retinal scar. Biomicroscopic examination (slit lamp) or careful ophthalmoscopic exam should provide diagnosis. A visual acuity worse than 20/30, not easily correctable by glasses, and explainable by the degree of cataract noted on examination makes the diagnosis.
- In the elderly, visual impairment often due to multiple factors, e.g., cataract and macular degeneration both contributing to visual loss
- Age-related cataract - significant if symptoms and ophthalmic exam support cataract as major cause of vision impairment
- Congenital - lens opacity in absence of other ocular pathology such as tumor, nerve glioma, retinopathy of prematurity may be consistent with the visual loss. May cause severe amblyopia.
- Note: No cataract produces an afferent pupillary reaction defect (Marcus Gunn pupil). Abnormal pupillary reactions mandate further evaluation for other pathology.

LABORATORY N/A
Drugs that may alter lab results: N/A
Disorders that may alter lab results: N/A

PATHOLOGICAL FINDINGS Consistent with lens changes found in the type of cataract

SPECIAL TESTS
- Visual quality assessment: Glare testing, contrast sensitivity are sometimes indicated. (Hyperglycemic state as in poor diabetic control creates osmotic change within lens and may alter measurement of visual acuity and refractive state.)
- Retinal/macular function assessment: Potential acuity meter testing, fluorescein retinal angiography sometimes required

IMAGING N/A

DIAGNOSTIC PROCEDURES Noted above in special testing

TREATMENT

APPROPRIATE HEALTH CARE
Outpatient or inpatient surgery

GENERAL MEASURES
- Age-related cataract
  ◊ Since significant cataract may develop gradually, patient may not be aware of how it has changed his/her lifestyle. Physician may note a significant cataract and patient reports "no problems." Thus the evaluation requires physician/patient exchange of information.
  ◊ Pre-surgical evaluation - by the primary care physician includes physical exam, lab work (CBC, electrolytes, ECG). Patients on anticoagulants may need to temporarily discontinue one week before surgery if possible. Not always necessary, so need to discuss with ophthalmologist.

Cataract

SURGICAL MEASURES
• Age-related cataract
◊ Surgical removal of the cataract - indicated if visual impairment producing symptoms distressing to the patient, or interfering with lifestyle or occupation, or posing risk of fall or injury
◊ Since significant cataract may develop gradually, patient may not be aware of how it has changed his/her lifestyle. Physician may note a significant cataract and patient reports "no problems." Thus the evaluation requires physician/patient exchange of information.
◊ Surgical technique - cataracts are not removed by laser. Most surgical techniques include implantation of a plastic intraocular lens immediately following cataract extraction.
◊ Anesthesia - usually local, with anesthesiologist monitoring vital signs
◊ Pre-surgical evaluation - by the primary care physician includes physical exam, lab work (CBC, electrolytes, ECG). Patients on anticoagulants may need to temporarily discontinue one week before surgery if possible. Not always necessary, so need to discuss with ophthalmologist.
◊ Postoperative care - usually protective eye shield as directed, topical antibiotic and steroid ophthalmic medications. Avoid lifting, bending over for a few weeks.
• Congenital cataract
◊ Treatment is surgical removal of cataract. Newborn may need surgery within days to reduce risk of severe amblyopia. Use of implant lenses controversial.
◊ Postoperative care - long-term patching program for good eye to combat amblyopia. Refractive correction of operative eye, with multiple repeat examinations. Very difficult challenge for physician and parents.

ACTIVITY See above

DIET N/A

PATIENT EDUCATION See above

MEDICATIONS

DRUG(S) OF CHOICE There is no medication at present to prevent or slow the progression of cataracts
Contraindications: N/A
Precautions: N/A
Significant possible interactions: N/A

ALTERNATIVE DRUGS N/A

FOLLOWUP

PATIENT MONITORING
• As cataract progresses, the ophthalmologist may change spectacle correction to maintain vision. When this is no longer practical or successful, surgery is recommended.
• Following surgery, spectacle correction may be required to maximize visual acuity for the patient's need. Usually measured several weeks after surgery.

PREVENTION/AVOIDANCE
• Use of ultraviolet protecting glasses in sunny climates may slow progression of cataract, but this is not proven by controlled studies to date
• Antioxidants (vitamins C, E, etc.) theoretically beneficial, but not proven

POSSIBLE COMPLICATIONS Blindness

EXPECTED COURSE/PROGNOSIS
• Ocular prognosis good after cataract removal if no prior ocular disease.
• In congenital cataracts prognosis is often poor because of the high risk of amblyopia.

MISCELLANEOUS

ASSOCIATED CONDITIONS
• Diabetes
• Ocular diseases

AGE-RELATED FACTORS
Pediatric: See information on congenital cataracts
Geriatric: 92% of people over age 75 have cataracts
Others: N/A

PREGNANCY See information on congenital cataracts (e.g., rubella syndrome)

SYNONYMS N/A

ICD-9-CM
366.19 Age-related cataract
743.30 Congenital cataract

SEE ALSO N/A

OTHER NOTES If patient has cataract and symptoms do not seem to support recommended surgery, a second opinion by another ophthalmologist may be indicated

ABBREVIATIONS N/A

REFERENCES Tasman W, ed: Duane's Ophthalmology. Philadelphia, J.B. Lippincott Co., 1997
Illustrations: N/A
Internet references: http://www.5mcc.com

Author(s)
T. Glendon Moody, MD

Causalgia syndrome

BASICS

DESCRIPTION Pain syndrome following injury to bone and soft tissue. Pathogenesis is obscure.
System(s) affected: Nervous
Genetics: No known genetic pattern
Incidence/Prevalence in USA: Unknown
Predominant age: No predominant age
Predominant sex: Male > Female

SIGNS AND SYMPTOMS
• Deep aching pain
• Burning pain with superimposed lancinating pain
• Hyperesthesia
• Hyperalgesia
• Pain from a non-noxious stimulus
• Pain most likely in palm or sole, aggravated by minimal physical stimulus such as friction or heat
• Skin - discolored, edematous, cold, hyperesthetic, smooth, glossy
• Stiff joints
• Nails curved and brittle
• Hyperhidrosis

CAUSES
• Partial interruption of nerve conduction by injury, such as gunshot wounds
• Possible shunting of efferent sympathetic impulses into sensory fibers at site of injury in a mixed nerve
• Reflex sympathetic dystrophy

RISK FACTORS Trauma

DIAGNOSIS

DIFFERENTIAL DIAGNOSIS Rule out infection, hypertrophic scar, bone fragments, neuroma, central nervous system tumor or syrinx

LABORATORY N/A
Drugs that may alter lab results: N/A
Disorders that may alter lab results: N/A

PATHOLOGICAL FINDINGS
• Partial or complete damage to afferent nerve pathways and probably reorganized central pain pathways
• Most common nerves involved are median and sciatic
• Atrophy in affected muscles
• Incomplete nerve plexus lesion

SPECIAL TESTS N/A

IMAGING Bone scan

DIAGNOSTIC PROCEDURES
Intravenous regional sympathetic block with guanethidine or reserpine (this is a specialized anesthetic technique that may also be therapeutic)

TREATMENT

APPROPRIATE HEALTH CARE
Outpatient, except for operative procedures or intravenous sympathetic nerve blockade

GENERAL MEASURES
• Treatment is empirical
• Anesthetic blockade (chemical or surgical) of sympathetic nerve function (transient relief suggests that chemical or surgical sympathectomy will be helpful)
• Intravenous regional sympathetic block with guanethidine or reserpine by pain specialist or anesthetist
• Physical therapy (essential during all phases of treatment)
• Transcutaneous electric nerve stimulation (controversial)
• Inject myofacial painful trigger points
• Briskly rub the affected part several times per day
• Acupuncture can be tried
• Hypnosis
• Relaxation training (alternate muscle relaxing and contracting)
• Biofeedback
• Discourage maladaptive behaviors
• Refer the patient to a specialty pain clinic in difficult cases

SURGICAL MEASURES Sympathectomy sometimes necessary

ACTIVITY Maintain as high a level of physical and intellectual activity as possible

DIET No special diet

PATIENT EDUCATION
• Stress staying active physically
• Careful instructions about any prescribed medications

MEDICATIONS

DRUG(S) OF CHOICE
• Following agents reported to be of benefit in some cases:
  ◊ Prazosin, 1-8 mg orally in divided doses
  ◊ Phenoxybenzamine 40-120 mg daily, orally in divided doses. The initial dose should not exceed 10 mg.
  ◊ Nifedipine 10-30 mg tid
  ◊ Prednisone 60-80 mg/day orally, tapered over 2-4 weeks
  ◊ Tricyclic antidepressants (see manufacturers recommended dose)
• Anticonvulsants. (Require serum drug level monitoring, except for clonazepam. Doses must be individualized.):
  ◊ Carbamazepine 200-1000 mg/day orally
  ◊ Phenytoin 100-300 mg/day orally
  ◊ Clonazepam 1-10 mg/day orally
  ◊ Valproic acid 750-2250 mg/day orally, maximum of 60 mg/kg
• Skeletal muscle relaxant:
  ◊ Baclofen 10-40 mg/day orally - may act synergistically with carbamazepine and phenytoin
Contraindications: Refer to manufacturer's literature
Precautions: Refer to manufacturer's literature
Significant possible interactions: There are many with this group of drugs. Refer to manufacturer's literature.

ALTERNATIVE DRUGS
• Narcotics - only after all non-opioid therapies are exhausted
• Other alpha-adrenergic blockers or dihydropyridine calcium channel blockers may be tried though experience with them is limited

FOLLOWUP

PATIENT MONITORING
• Watch carefully for adverse reactions to medications
• Several different forms of therapy may need to be tried

PREVENTION/AVOIDANCE
• Mobilization following injury
• Avoidance of nerve damage during surgical procedures
• Splinting of an injured extremity for adequate period of time
• Adequate analgesics during recovery from injuries

POSSIBLE COMPLICATIONS
• Drug mishaps
• Joint contractures
• Contralateral spread of symptoms

EXPECTED COURSE/PROGNOSIS
• Course - variable; chronic; remitting
• Outlook only satisfactory, may need attempts at several treatment modalities. No one form of therapy is superior to others. Failure to respond to one form does not mitigate against success with another.
• Those patients receiving work compensation for an injury or secondary gain from family or friends are in a separate category and may never get well

MISCELLANEOUS

ASSOCIATED CONDITIONS
• Serious injury to bone and soft tissue
• Herpes zoster

AGE-RELATED FACTORS
Pediatric: N/A
Geriatric: Painful perception is frequently worse in older patients. Start with smaller than usual doses of drugs.
Others:
• Postherpetic neuralgia is a result of partial or complete damage to afferent nerve pathways
• Pain occurring in dermatomes as a sequela of herpes zoster

PREGNANCY   Many of the useful drugs are contraindicated in pregnancy

SYNONYMS
• Erythromelalgia, traumatic
• Weir Mitchell causalgia
• Minor causalgia
• Reflex sympathetic dystrophy
• Posttraumatic neuralgia
• Sympathetically maintained pain

ICD-9-CM
354.4 Causalgia of upper limb
355.71 Causalgia of lower limb
355.9 Causalgia, NOS

SEE ALSO   Herpes zoster

OTHER NOTES   N/A

ABBREVIATIONS   N/A

REFERENCES   Adams RD, et al, eds: Prinicipals of Neurology. 6th Ed. New York, McGraw-Hill, 1997
Illustrations: N/A
Internet references: http://www.5mcc.com

Author(s)
Dennis E. Hughes, DO

Celiac disease

BASICS

DESCRIPTION A chronic diarrheal disease characterized by intestinal malabsorption of virtually all nutrients and precipitated by eating gluten-containing foods.
System(s) affected: Gastrointestinal
Genetics: See Risk factors
Incidence/Prevalence in USA: 50-75 in 100,000
Predominant age: Two incidence peaks, age 1 and 60's
Predominant sex: Female > Male (3:2)

SIGNS AND SYMPTOMS
• Diarrhea
• Steatorrhea
• Muscle cramps
• Vertigo
• Nervousness
• Weight loss
• Failure to thrive
• Weakness
• Lassitude
• Fatigue
• Large appetite
• Abdominal distention
• Explosive flatulence
• Abdominal pain, nausea, vomiting are rare

CAUSES Sensitivity to gluten, specifically gliadin fraction

RISK FACTORS
• First order relatives - 10% incidence
• 71% in monozygotic twins

DIAGNOSIS

DIFFERENTIAL DIAGNOSIS Rule out short bowel syndrome, pancreatic insufficiency, Crohn's disease, Whipple's disease, hypogammaglobulinemia, tropical sprue, lymphoma, acquired immune deficiency syndrome, acute enteritis, giardiasis, eosinophilic gastroenteritis

LABORATORY
• Positive anti-gliadin IgA and IgG
• Positive anti-reticulum and anti-endomycial antibodies
• 72 hour fecal fat showing greater than 7% fat malabsorption
• D-xylose test showing malabsorption of this sugar
• Decreased calcium
• Decreased prothrombin time
• Decreased neutral fats
• Decreased cholesterol
• Decreased vitamin A
• Decreased vitamin B12
• Decreased vitamin C
• Decreased folic acid
• Decreased iron
• Decreased total protein
• Anemia
Drugs that may alter lab results: N/A
Disorders that may alter lab results: N/A

PATHOLOGICAL FINDINGS Small bowel biopsy - flattened villi, hyperplasia and lengthening of crypts, infiltration of plasma cells and lymphocytes in lamina propria

SPECIAL TESTS Endoscopy

IMAGING Upper GI series showing flocculation of barium, edema and flattening of mucosal folds

DIAGNOSTIC PROCEDURES Biopsy of the duodenal mucosa with repeat endoscopy and normal biopsy on a gluten-free diet is necessary before a firm diagnosis can be made.

TREATMENT

APPROPRIATE HEALTH CARE
Outpatient

GENERAL MEASURES Removal of gluten from the diet. Rice, corn and soybean flour are safe, palatable substitutes.

SURGICAL MEASURES N/A

ACTIVITY No restrictions

DIET Removal of gluten - wheat, rye, barley and those with gluten additives

PATIENT EDUCATION
• Clinical dietician
• Copy of gluten-free diet
• Possible lay self-help group
• American Celiac Society, 45 Gifford Avenue, Jersey City, NJ 07304, (201)432-1207.
• Gluten Intolerance Group (206) 325-6980

MEDICATIONS

DRUG(S) OF CHOICE
• Usually none
• Prednisone, 40-60 mg/day po in cases of refractory sprue

Contraindications: History of tuberculosis, fungus or herpes infections

Precautions: Use with caution in congestive heart failure, diabetes, peptic ulcer, myasthenia gravis

Significant possible interactions: Diuretics taken concomitantly may lead to potassium depletion

ALTERNATIVE DRUGS
May require supplemental calcium, calcium carbonate, 500 mg po bid, and vitamin D (ergocalciferol) 10-100 mcg/day; in severe malabsorption, up to 2.5 mg/day may be required

FOLLOWUP

PATIENT MONITORING
Repeat endoscopy after 6-8 weeks on a gluten-free diet (in selected cases)

PREVENTION/AVOIDANCE
Avoid all gluten containing products

POSSIBLE COMPLICATIONS
• Malignancy - less than 10% of patients (50% of which are small bowel lymphoma)
• Refractory sprue - may respond to prednisone 40-60 mg/day po
• Chronic ulcerative jejunoileitis - associated with multiple ulcers, intestinal bleeding, strictures, perforation, obstruction, peritonitis - 7% mortality
• Osteoporosis secondary to decreased vitamin D and calcium absorption
• Dehydration
• Electrolyte depletion
• Death (rare)

EXPECTED COURSE/PROGNOSIS
Good with correct diagnosis and adherence to gluten free diet. Feel better in seven days. All symptoms usually disappear in four to six weeks. It is unknown whether strict dietary adherence decreases cancer risk.

MISCELLANEOUS

ASSOCIATED CONDITIONS
• May have secondary lactase deficiency
• Extraintestinal manifestation may include marked decrease in bone density
• Dermatitis herpetiformis

AGE-RELATED FACTORS
Pediatric: Children reaching adolescence may outgrow intolerance to wheat but should be cautioned to watch for signs of recurrence in middle age
Geriatric: N/A
Others: N/A

PREGNANCY
No significant effect

SYNONYMS
• Sprue
• Gluten enteropathy
• Celiac sprue

ICD-9-CM
579.0 Celiac disease

SEE ALSO
N/A

OTHER NOTES
N/A

ABBREVIATIONS
N/A

REFERENCES
• McClave S: Celiac and Tropical Sprue. In: Chobanian SJ, Van Ness MM, eds. A Manual of Clinical Problems in Gastroenterology. 2nd Ed. Boston, Little-Brown, 1993
• Stenson WF: Gastrointestinal Diseases. In: Orland MJ, Saltman RJ, eds. A Manual of Medical Therapeutics. 25th Ed. Boston, Little-Brown,1986
• Trier JS: Celiac Sprue. In: Sleisenger MH, Fordtran JS, eds. Gastrointestinal Disease. 4th Ed. Philadelphia, W.B. Saunders Co., 1988
Illustrations: N/A
Internet references: http://www.5mcc.com

Author(s)
Michael M. Van Ness, MD

Cellulitis

BASICS

DESCRIPTION An acute, spreading infection of the dermis and subcutaneous tissue. Several entities are recognized:
• Cellulitis of the extremities - characterized by an expanding, red, swollen, tender or painful plaque with an indefinite border that may cover a wide area
• Recurrent cellulitis of the leg after saphenous venectomy - patients have an acute onset of swelling, erythema of the legs arising months to years after coronary artery bypass. (Surgery using lower extremity veins for by-pass grafts.)
• Dissecting cellulitis of the scalp - recurrent painful, fluctuant dermal and subcutaneous nodules
• Facial cellulitis in adults - a rare event. Patients usually develop pharyngitis, followed by high fever, rapidly progressive anterior neck swelling, tenderness and erythema associated with dysphagia
• Facial cellulitis in children - potentially serious. Swelling and erythema of the cheek develop rapidly, usually unilateral.
• Perianal cellulitis - bright perianal erythema extending from the anal verge approximately 2 to 3 cm onto the surrounding perianal skin
• Pseudomonas cellulitis - may be a localized phenomenon or it may occur during pseudomonas septicemia
System(s) affected: Skin/Exocrine
Genetics: No known genetic pattern
Incidence/Prevalence in USA: Unknown
Predominant age:
• Perianal cellulitis - principally in children
• Facial cellulitis - in adults, usually older than 50 years. In children, between 6 months and three years.
Predominant sex: Male = Female (perianal cellulitis more common in boys)

SIGNS AND SYMPTOMS
• General
  ◊ Local tenderness
  ◊ Pain
  ◊ Erythema
  ◊ Malaise
  ◊ Fever, chills
  ◊ Involved area is red, hot, and swollen
  ◊ Borders of the area are not elevated and not demarcated
  ◊ Regional lymphadenopathy is common
• Recurrent cellulitis
  ◊ Same as above
  ◊ Edema
  ◊ High fever, chills and toxicity
• Dissecting cellulitis of the scalp
  ◊ Purulent drainage from burrowing interconnecting abscesses
• Facial cellulitis in adults
  ◊ Malaise
  ◊ Anorexia
  ◊ Vomiting
  ◊ Itching
  ◊ Burning
  ◊ Dysplasia
  ◊ Anterior neck swelling
• Facial cellulitis in children
  ◊ Irritability
  ◊ Upper respiratory tract infection symptoms

• Perianal cellulitis
  ◊ Intense perianal erythema
  ◊ Pain on defecation
  ◊ Blood streaked stools
  ◊ Perianal pruritis

CAUSES
• By site
  ◊ Cellulitis of the extremities: Group A streptococcus, Staphylococcus aureus
  ◊ Recurrent cellulitis of the leg: Non-group A beta hemolytic Streptococci (group C,G,B)
  ◊ Dissecting cellulitis of the scalp: Staphylococcus aureus
  ◊ Facial cellulitis in adults: H. influenzae type B
  ◊ Facial cellulitis in children: H. influenzae type B, over 3 years with portal of entry: staphylococcal and streptococcal
  ◊ Synergetic necrotizing cellulitis: Mixed aerobic-anaerobic flora
  ◊ Intravenous drug use: Staphylococcus aureus, Streptococci, Enterobacteriaceae, Pseudomonas, Fungi
  ◊ Synergetic necrotizing cellulitis: Mixed aerobic-anaerobic flora
• Specific diseases
  ◊ Diabetes mellitus: Staphylococcus aureus, Streptococci, Enterobacteriaceae, Anaerobes
  ◊ Human bites: Eikenella corrodens
  ◊ Animal bites (cat and dog): Staphylococci, Pasteurella multocida
• Patient groups
  ◊ Neonates: Group B streptococcus
  ◊ Immunocompromised
    - Bacteria (Serratia, Proteus and other Enterobacteriaceae)
    - Fungi (Cryptococcus neoformans)
    - Atypical mycobacterium
  ◊ Children with nephrotic syndrome: E. coli
  ◊ Environmental and occupational exposures
    - Erysipelothrix rhusiopathiae
    - Vibrio species
    - Aeromonas hydrophilia
• Rare causes
  ◊ Anaerobic
  ◊ Clostridium perfringens (gas forming cellulitis)
  ◊ Tuberculosis
  ◊ Syphilitic gumma
  ◊ Fungal: Mucormycosis, Aspergillosis

RISK FACTORS
• General
  ◊ Previous trauma (laceration, puncture, human or animal bite)
  ◊ Underlying skin lesion (furuncle, ulcer)
  ◊ Surgical wound
  ◊ Recurrent cellulitis
  ◊ Post coronary artery bypass in patients whose saphenous veins have been removed
  ◊ Lower extremity lymphedema secondary to a) radical pelvic surgery b) radiation therapy c) neoplastic involvement of pelvic lymph nodes
  ◊ Mastectomy
  ◊ Diabetes mellitus
  ◊ Intravenous drug use
  ◊ Immunocompromised host
  ◊ Burns
  ◊ Environmental and occupational factors

DIAGNOSIS

DIFFERENTIAL DIAGNOSIS
• Perianal cellulitis
  ◊ Candida intertrigo
  ◊ Psoriasis
  ◊ Pin worm infection
  ◊ Inflammatory bowel disease
  ◊ Behavioral problem
  ◊ Child abuse
• Others
  ◊ Acute gout
  ◊ Fasciitis/myositis
  ◊ Mycotic aneurysm
  ◊ Ruptured Baker's cyst
  ◊ Thrombophlebitis
  ◊ Osteomyelitis
  ◊ Herpetic whitlow
  ◊ Cutaneous diphtheria
  ◊ Pseudogout

LABORATORY
• Aspirates from the point of maximum inflammation. Yield a 45% positive culture rate as compared to a 5% from leading edge culture.
• Blood cultures - potential pathogens isolated in 25% of patients
• Mild leucocytosis with a left shift
• A mildly elevated sedimentation rate
• CBC
Drugs that may alter lab results: Previous antibiotic therapy may alter the results
Disorders that may alter lab results: N/A

PATHOLOGICAL FINDINGS Biopsy of skin shows marked infiltration of the dermis with eosinophils and inflammatory changes

SPECIAL TESTS
• Serial serological testing with antistreptolysin O, anti-deoxyribonuclease B, and anti hyaluronidase tests may be successful in diagnosing cellulitis caused by group A, C, or G hemolytic streptococci
• Sinus drainage and culture of aspirate

IMAGING
• Gas forming cellulitis
  ◊ Plain x-rays show gas bubbles in the soft tissue
  ◊ CT shows gas and myonecrosis

DIAGNOSTIC PROCEDURES
• Skin biopsy
• Lumbar puncture should be considered for all children with H. influenzae type B cellulitis

Cellulitis

TREATMENT

APPROPRIATE HEALTH CARE
Outpatient for mild cases, inpatient for severe infections

GENERAL MEASURES
• Immobilization and elevation of the involved limb to reduce swelling may be needed in H. influenzae type B
• Sterile saline dressings to decrease local pain
• Moist heat to localize the infection
• Cool Burrow's compresses for pain relief

SURGICAL MEASURES
• Debridement for gas/purulent collections
• Intubation or tracheotomy may be needed for cellulitis of the head or neck
• Wide filleting incision in necrotizing cellulitis

ACTIVITY Ambulatory in mild infection; bedrest in severe infection

DIET Regular diet

PATIENT EDUCATION
• Good skin hygiene
• Avoid skin traumas
• Report early skin changes to physician

MEDICATIONS

DRUG(S) OF CHOICE
Treatment 10-30 days. Guided by culture results whenever possible.
• Mild early suspected streptococcal etiology: Aqueous penicillin G, 600,000 U, then IM procaine penicillin at 600,000 U q8-12 hrs
• Staphylococcal infection or no clues to etiology: penicillinase-resistant penicillin (e.g., oxacillin 0.5-1.0 g po q6 hrs)
• Severe infection: penicillinase-resistant penicillin (e.g., nafcillin 1.0-1.5 g IV q4 hrs)
• Gram negative bacillus as possible etiology: aminoglycoside (gentamicin) plus a semisynthetic penicillin
• Rapidly progressive cellulitis after a fresh water injury: penicillinase-resistant penicillin plus gentamicin or chloramphenicol
• Human bites: amoxicillin-clavulanate (Augmentin)
• Animal bites (cellulitis at the saphenous site): penicillin or nafcillin, in high dosage, IV for 7 days before switching to oral therapy
• Facial cellulitis in adults and children: (H. influenza B) cefotaxime IV
• Gas forming cellulitis: Aqueous penicillin G 10-20 million U/day IV
• Diabetes mellitus: Cefoxitin or if toxic, clindamycin and gentamicin
• Intravenous drug abuse: Vancomycin and gentamicin
• Compromised hosts: clindamycin and gentamicin
• Burn patients: vancomycin and gentamicin

Contraindications:
• Allergies to the antibiotic
Precautions: Renal failure, other organ failure
Significant possible interactions: Refer to manufacturer's literature

ALTERNATIVE DRUGS
• Mild infection
  ◊ Penicillin allergy: erythromycin, 500 mg po q6 hrs
• Severe infection
  ◊ Vancomycin 1.0-1.5 g/day IV
  ◊ Human bite and animal bites: IV cefoxitin
• Gas forming cellulitis
  ◊ Metronidazole 500 mg IV q6h
  ◊ Clindamycin 600 mg IV q8h

FOLLOWUP

PATIENT MONITORING
• A blood culture at the end of treatment to ensure cure
• Repeat needle aspirate culture
• Repeat blood count if patient was toxic
• Repeat lumbar puncture in case of meningitis

PREVENTION/AVOIDANCE
• Treatment of tinea pedis with antifungal (such as clotrimazole) will prevent recurrent cellulitis of the legs in patients who have had coronary bypass
• Avoid trauma
• Avoid swimming in fresh water or salt water in the presence of skin abrasion
• Avoid human or animal bite
• Use of support stocking with peripheral edema
• Good skin hygiene
• For recurrent cellulitis - prophylactic penicillin G (250-500 mg po bid)
• In H. influenzae cellulitis - rifampin prophylaxis for the entire family of an index case. Rifampin prophylaxis in day-care classroom in which one or two children exposed. Dosage: 20 mg/kg/day (maximum: 600 mg/day) for 4 days.

POSSIBLE COMPLICATIONS
• Bacteremia
• Local abscesses
• Super infection with gram negative organisms
• Lymphangitis especially in recurrent cellulitis
• Thrombophlebitis of lower extremities in older patients
• Dissecting cellulitis of the scalp - scarring; alopecia
• Facial cellulitis in children - meningitis in 8% of patients
• Gas forming cellulitis - gangrene; amputation; 25% mortality

EXPECTED COURSE/PROGNOSIS With adequate antibiotic treatment, outlook is good

MISCELLANEOUS

ASSOCIATED CONDITIONS
• Facial cellulitis in children
  ◊ Upper respiratory tract infection
  ◊ Unilateral or bilateral otitis media in 68% of patients
  ◊ Meningitis in 8% of patients
• Perianal cellulitis
  ◊ Pharyngitis may precede the infection
• Frontal sinus in adult
  ◊ Subacute bacterial endocarditis
  ◊ Scarlet fever
  ◊ Vaccinia
  ◊ Herpes simplex
  ◊ Herpes zoster

AGE-RELATED FACTORS
Pediatric: N/A
Geriatric: In cellulitis of lower extremities, patients are more prone to develop thrombophlebitis
Others: N/A

PREGNANCY N/A

SYNONYMS N/A

ICD-9-CM
682.9 Cellulitis

SEE ALSO
• Cellulitis, periorbital & orbital
• Erysipelas
• Animal bites
• Thrombophlebitis, superficial

OTHER NOTES N/A

ABBREVIATIONS N/A

REFERENCES
• Habif T: Clinical Dermatology. 3rd Ed. St. Louis, CV Mosby, 1996
• Mandell GL, ed: Principles and Practice of Infectious Diseases. 4th Ed. New York, Churchill Livingstone, 1995
Illustrations: 18 available on CD-ROM
Internet references: http://www.5mcc.com

Author(s)
Abdulrazak Abyad, MD, MPH, AGSF

Cellulitis, periorbital & orbital

BASICS

DESCRIPTION An acute, spreading infection of the dermis and subcutaneous tissue. Several entities are recognized. Cellulitis around the eyes is a potentially dangerous periorbital and orbital infection.
System(s) affected: Skin/Exocrine, Nervous
Genetics: No known genetic pattern
Incidence/Prevalence in USA: Unknown
Predominant age: N/A
Predominant sex: Male = Female

SIGNS AND SYMPTOMS
• Lid edema
• Rhinorrhea
• Orbital pain, tenderness
• Headache
• Conjunctival hyperemia
• Chemosis
• Ptosis
• Limitation to occular motion
• Increase intraocular pressure
• Disease in corneal sensation
• Congestion of retinal veins
• Chorioretinal stria
• Gangrene and sloughing of lids

CAUSES
• Cellulitis around the eye in adult
  ◊ Staphylococcus aureus most common
  ◊ Streptococcus pyogenes
  ◊ Streptococcus pneumonia
  ◊ Mixed infection
• Cellulitis around the eye in children less than five years
  ◊ H. influenzae most common

RISK FACTORS
• Trauma
• Chronic sinusitis (anaerobic)
• Acute sinusitis (aerobic)
• Retained orbital foreign bodies
• Puncture wound
• Surgical procedure: Exploration of orbital tumor, retinal detachment procedure, strabismus operation
• Acute dacryocystitis
• Dental or intracranial infection
• Bacteremia

DIAGNOSIS

DIFFERENTIAL DIAGNOSIS
• Retro-orbital cellulitis/abscess

LABORATORY
• Aspiration of fluid from the orbit is contraindicated
• Blood culture more likely to be positive in children < 5 years
• Culture of discharge from nasal mucosa, nasopharynx and conjunctiva
Drugs that may alter lab results:
Previous antibiotic therapy
Disorders that may alter lab results: N/A

PATHOLOGICAL FINDINGS N/A

SPECIAL TESTS Serial serological testing with antistreptolysin O, anti-deoxyribonuclease B, and anti hyaluronidase tests may be successful in diagnosing cellulitis caused by group A, C, or G hemolytic streptococci

IMAGING
• B-scan ultrasound
• Plain orbital and sinus films
• Computed tomography (CT) is the most accurate and provides the most important information
• Magnetic resonance imaging is the imaging modality of choice in diagnosing suspected cases of cavernous sinus thrombosis

DIAGNOSTIC PROCEDURES
• Skin biopsy
• Lumbar puncture should be considered for all children with H. influenzae type B cellulitis

TREATMENT

APPROPRIATE HEALTH CARE
Outpatient for mild cases, inpatient for severe infections

GENERAL MEASURES N/A

SURGICAL MEASURES
• Surgical debridement and/or drainage is needed if abscess develops or if clinical situation deteriorates despite adequate therapy in 24-48 hours or if visual acuity decreases
• In orbital mucormycosis, surgical debridement of devitalized tissue is extremely important

ACTIVITY
• Ambulatory in mild infection
• Bedrest in severe infection

DIET Regular diet

PATIENT EDUCATION
• Good skin hygiene
• Avoid skin traumas
• Report early skin changes to health professional

MEDICATIONS

DRUG(S) OF CHOICE
• In adults, nafcillin or oxacillin 1.5 g every 4 hours
• In children, ampicillin 200 mg/kg/day in divided doses intravenously plus nafcillin or oxacillin (100 mg/kg/day)
• Sinus decongestion - nasal sprays, oral decongestants, oral antihistamines

Contraindications:
• Allergies to the antibiotic
• Previous history of allergy to the drug

Precautions: Renal failure, other organ failure

Significant possible interactions: Refer to manufacturer's literature

ALTERNATIVE DRUGS
• In adults, cefotaxime or clindamycin or chloramphenicol or vancomycin
• In children, if H. influenzae resistant to ampicillin - third generation cephalosporin, cefotaxime or chloramphenicol
• In immunocompromised - piperacillin and gentamicin

FOLLOWUP

PATIENT MONITORING
Repeat imaging in patients with orbital cellulitis

PREVENTION/AVOIDANCE
• Avoid trauma
• Avoid swimming in fresh water or salt water in the presence of skin abrasion
• In H. influenzae cellulitis - rifampin prophylaxis for the entire family of an index case. Rifampin prophylaxis in day-care classroom in which one or two children exposed. Dosage - 20 mg/kg/24 h (maximum of 600 mg a day) for 4 days.

POSSIBLE COMPLICATIONS
• Osteomyelitis
• Strabismus
• Afferent pupillary defect
• Chronic draining sinus
• Scarred upper eyelid
• Profound visual loss
• Blindness
• Ophthalmoplegia
• Cavernous sinus thrombosis
• Meningitis
• Intracranial abscess
• Acute infarction of retina and choroid

EXPECTED COURSE/PROGNOSIS
With adequate antibiotic treatment, outlook is good

MISCELLANEOUS

ASSOCIATED CONDITIONS
Sinusitis ethmoiditis in children in 84% of patients

AGE-RELATED FACTORS
Pediatric: Newborn may acquire orbital cellulitis secondary to intrauterine infection
Geriatric: N/A
Others: N/A

PREGNANCY N/A

SYNONYMS N/A

ICD-9-CM
376.01 Orbital cellulitis

SEE ALSO
• Cellulitis
• Erysipelas
• Animal bites
• Thrombophlebitis, superficial

OTHER NOTES N/A

ABBREVIATIONS N/A

REFERENCES
• Habif T: Clinical Dermatology. 3rd Ed. St. Louis, CV Mosby, 1996
• Mandell GL, ed: Principles and Practice of Infectious Diseases. 4th Ed. New York, Churchill Livingstone, 1995
Illustrations: N/A
Internet references: http://www.5mcc.com

Author(s)
Abdulrazak Abyad, MD, MPH, AGSF

Cerebral palsy

 BASICS

DESCRIPTION A term used to describe a group of patients with a non-progressive disorder of movement or posture that is a result of a central nervous system abnormality that occurred prenatally, perinatally, or during the first three years of life
System(s) affected: Nervous
Genetics: Although familial cases have been described, this is not considered a genetic disease
Incidence/Prevalence in USA: 2.1 per 1,000 live births
Predominant age: Because of the definition, this problem is restricted to life. The disease is lifelong, although changes occur as the patient matures.
Predominant sex: Male = Female

SIGNS AND SYMPTOMS
Subtypes
• Spastic
  ◊ Associated and significant spasticity
  ◊ Contractures
  ◊ Mental retardation
  ◊ Aphonia
  ◊ Seizures
• Athetotic
  ◊ Usually normal intelligence
  ◊ Choreiform movements
  ◊ Muscular hypertrophy
• Ataxic
  ◊ Clumsy disposition
  ◊ Normal intelligence
  ◊ Some are highly talkative (cocktail party syndrome)
• Spastic diplegia
  ◊ Spares upper extremities
  ◊ Spastic (scissor gait)
  ◊ Normal intelligence

CAUSES
• 70% of the time, neither causes nor risk factors can be identified
• In utero infections, malformations, chromosomal abnormalities and strokes are causes

RISK FACTORS
• Prematurity
• Hypoxic ischemia
• Encephalopathy in the perinatal period
• Seizures in the perinatal period
• Interventricular hemorrhage in the perinatal period
• In utero infections
• Meningitis/encephalitis postnatally
• Child abuse

 DIAGNOSIS

DIFFERENTIAL DIAGNOSIS Children with muscle disease will appear floppy; however, the most common cause of the floppy baby syndrome is cerebral palsy

LABORATORY
• Laboratory data is not required to make the diagnosis.
• Other tests may help exclude Tay-Sachs metachromatic leukodystrophy, mucopolysaccharidosis
Drugs that may alter lab results: None
Disorders that may alter lab results: None

PATHOLOGICAL FINDINGS Central nervous system abnormalities: CT and MRI might show abnormalities of the brain including cysts, cerebral atrophy, calcification, tumors, malformation, strokes, etc.

SPECIAL TESTS Urine amino acid screening

IMAGING N/A

DIAGNOSTIC PROCEDURES
• History and careful physical exam
• EEG

 TREATMENT

APPROPRIATE HEALTH CARE
Outpatient

GENERAL MEASURES
• Physical therapy, occupational therapy, orthosis, adaptive equipment
• Medications by mouth usually not very successful; side effects occur before beneficial effects are present
• Alter muscle tone, assuming that the abnormal tone is adversely affecting function, by:
  ◊ Injection of botulinum toxin into the abnormal muscles
  ◊ Rhizotomy
  ◊ Continuous infusion of intrathecal baclofen

SURGICAL MEASURES Tendon transfers, release of contractures, rhizotomy to decrease spasticity

ACTIVITY Full activity depending upon the patient's dysfunction

DIET Normal diet, although constipation is frequent and stool softeners might be considered

PATIENT EDUCATION
• It is very important to educate the patient and parents about the child's disabilities as well as prognosis; mental retardation seen in 20-25% of patients with cerebral palsy.
• United Cerebral Palsy Associations, 7 Penn Plaza, Suite 804, New York, NY 10001, (800)USA-1UCP

MEDICATIONS

DRUG(S) OF CHOICE
• Medications to decrease spasticity (e.g., diazepam, dantrolene sodium and baclofen)
• Botulinum toxin (Botox) type A also to decrease spasticity
• Baclofen delivered intrathecally is of value
• Medications for epilepsy might have to be used
Contraindications: Refer to manufacturer's literature
Precautions: Refer to manufacturer's literature
Significant possible interactions: Refer to manufacturer's literature

ALTERNATIVE DRUGS
Other centrally acting muscle relaxants

FOLLOWUP

PATIENT MONITORING Followup visits are important - to determine the development of contractures and to determine the presence of associated problems including epilepsy, learning disabilities, strabismus, hearing loss and mental retardation.

PREVENTION/AVOIDANCE N/A

POSSIBLE COMPLICATIONS Chronicity with permanent disability

EXPECTED COURSE/PROGNOSIS
• The patient should improve in function with time
• Muscle tone may change for the worse during adolescence (does not mean that the disease is progressive)

MISCELLANEOUS

ASSOCIATED CONDITIONS
• Epilepsy
• Learning disabilities
• Mental retardation
• Behavioral problems
• Strabismus
• Hearing loss

AGE-RELATED FACTORS
Pediatric: Contractures will increase as a result of growth associated with asymmetrical muscle tone and strength. Scoliosis may develop as a result.
Geriatric: N/A
Others: N/A

PREGNANCY N/A

SYNONYMS
• Little disease
• Cerebral diplegia
• Infantile cerebral paralysis

ICD-9-CM
343.9 Infantile cerebral palsy, unspecified

SEE ALSO N/A

OTHER NOTES N/A

ABBREVIATIONS N/A

REFERENCES Russman BS, Gage JR: Cerebral Palsy. Current Problems in Pediatrics 1989;19(2):65-111
Illustrations: N/A
Internet references: http://www.5mcc.com

Author(s)
Barry S. Russman, MD

Cervical dysplasia

BASICS

DESCRIPTION Pre-invasive neoplastic epithelial changes in the transformation zone of the uterine cervix often associate with human papillomavirus infections
• Mild dysplasia (CIN I or SIL low grade) - cellular changes are limited to the lower one-third of the squamous epithelium
• Moderate dysplasia (CIN II or SIL high grade) - cellular changes are limited to the lower two-thirds of the squamous epithelium
• Severe dysplasia (CIN III or SIL high grade or carcinoma in situ) - cellular changes involves the full thickness of the squamous epithelium
System(s) affected: Reproductive
Genetics: N/A
Incidence/Prevalence in USA: Difficult to assess due to wide variability in false negative Pap smear reporting and uneven distribution of qualified colposcopists. Prevalence 3,600/100,000 at age 27-28.
Predominant age: The median age for carcinoma in situ is 28 years. Earlier lesions can be expected at younger ages
Predominant sex: Female only

SIGNS AND SYMPTOMS
• Frequently none
• Occasionally there is association with condyloma acuminatum in the vulva, vagina, or anus
• Occasionally there are co-existing sexually transmitted diseases in the lower reproductive tract, e.g., chlamydia, gonorrhea

CAUSES Strong linkage with infections by human papilloma viruses types 6, 11, 16, 18, 31, 33, and 35. Other types of the same virus have also been implicated.

RISK FACTORS
• Multiparity and pregnancy before age 20 years
• Multiple sexual partners
• Early age in first sexual intercourse
• Condyloma acuminatum infection elsewhere in the body
• Cigarette smoking
• Prostitution
• Lower socio-economic status

DIAGNOSIS

DIFFERENTIAL DIAGNOSIS
• Invasive carcinoma of the cervix
• Condyloma acuminatum

LABORATORY
• Pap smear
Drugs that may alter lab results:
• Surgical lubricants e.g., K-Y Jelly
Disorders that may alter lab results: N/A

PATHOLOGICAL FINDINGS
• Clumping of the nuclear chromatin material
• Reversal of the nuclear/cytoplasmic ratio
• Koilocytosis
• Hyperchromasia

SPECIAL TESTS
• Viral DNA hybridization (Virapap) and others
• Colposcopy
• PAPNET system to review negative Pap smears
• CYTYC 2000 thin prep Pap test (replacement of current Pap preparations)

IMAGING N/A

DIAGNOSTIC PROCEDURES
• Papanicolaou smear
• Colposcopy and directed cervical biopsies
• Cone biopsy (by cold knife, laser, or loop excision)
• Endocervical curettage
• Loop electrosurgical excision procedure (LEEP)
• Cervicography
• Speculoscopy
• Use of HPV DNA typing to select certain cases with borderline abnormalities, e.g., atypical squamous cells of undetermined significance (ASCUS), for closer followup and colposcopy

TREATMENT

APPROPRIATE HEALTH CARE
Outpatient

GENERAL MEASURES Office evaluation and observation

SURGICAL MEASURES Outpatient surgery - cryotherapy, laser ablative or excisional cone, cold knife cone, electro-surgical loop excision of transformation zone

ACTIVITY Four weeks of pelvic rest after cone biopsy

DIET No restriction

PATIENT EDUCATION See Followup section

Cervical dysplasia

MEDICATIONS

DRUG(S) OF CHOICE
• Treatment is primarily surgical
• Fluorouracil (Efudex) once or twice daily as 5% vaginal cream supplemental therapy
Contraindications: Hypersensitivity to 5-fluorouracil
Precautions:
• If hand is used in application of 5-fluorouracil, wash hand immediately afterwards
• Avoid contact of 5-fluorouracil with eyes, nose, or mouth
Significant possible interactions: N/A

ALTERNATIVE DRUGS   N/A

FOLLOWUP

PATIENT MONITORING Repeat Pap smears every 4 months during the first year after cone excision for severe dysplasia, every 6 months thereafter. For lesser lesions, repeat Pap smear yearly. Probe endocervical canal to assure patency.

PREVENTION/AVOIDANCE
• Monogamy of both sexual partners
• Use of condom during coitus if unable to practice monogamy
• Abstain from smoking
• Emphasize importance of yearly Pap smears for patients
• Ability to obtain skilled colposcopy service as needed
• Patient education (individually or by community services) to emphasize the need for Pap smear
• Educate medical care providers to make patient referrals for the screening service unless they provide it themselves

POSSIBLE COMPLICATIONS
• Some severe dysplasia will progress to invasive carcinoma of the cervix
• Possible complications following cone biopsy of the cervix:
  ◊ Hemorrhage
  ◊ Infection
  ◊ Cervical stenosis
  ◊ Cervical incompetence
  ◊ Infertility
  ◊ Incomplete excision of dysplastic tissue
  ◊ Recurrence

EXPECTED COURSE/PROGNOSIS
• Generally excellent
• Persistence of dysplasia can occur due to incomplete excision
• Recurrence of dysplasia can occur due to inability to eradicate the human papilloma virus in the patient's body or prevent new infections

MISCELLANEOUS

ASSOCIATED CONDITIONS
• Condyloma acuminatum
• Carcinoma of the cervix

AGE-RELATED FACTORS
Pediatric: Very rare
Geriatric: Less frequent
Others: This is usually a problem for the women in the reproductive age group. The median age is 28 years for severe dysplasia. For lesser lesions, the median ages tend to be much lower.

PREGNANCY
• Dysplasia may progress during pregnancy
• It is important to determine the severity of dysplasia and to exclude the presence of invasive carcinoma during pregnancy
• Dysplasia does not require definitive treatment during pregnancy
• Dysplasia by itself is not an indication for cesarean section

SYNONYMS   N/A

ICD-9-CM   622.1 Dysplasia of cervix (uteri)

SEE ALSO
• Condyloma acuminata
• Cervical malignancy

OTHER NOTES Squamous intraepithelial lesion (SIL) is in reference to Pap smear only

ABBREVIATIONS
• CIN = cervical intraepithelial neoplasia (CIN)
• SIL = squamous intraepithelial lesion (SIL)

REFERENCES
• Koss LG: Reducing the error rate in Papanicolaou smears. The Female Patient 1994;19:6
• Sherman ME, et al: PAPNET analysis of reportedly negative smears preceding the diagnosis of high grade intraepithelial lesion or carcinoma. Modern Pathol 19947(5):578-581
• Disaia PJ, Creasman WT: Clinical Gynecologic Oncology. 4th Ed. St. Louis, The C.V. Mosby Co., 1993
• Wright TC, Richart RM, Ferencz A: Electrosurgery for HPV-related diseases of the lower genital tract. New York, Arthur Vision, Inc. & Biovision, Inc., 1992
• Kurman RJ, ed: Blaustein's Pathology Of The Female Genital Tract. 3rd Ed. New York, Springer-Verlag, 1987
• Novak ER, Woodruff JD: Novak's Gynecologic and Obstetric Pathology With Clinical and Endocrine Relations. 8th Ed. Philadelphia, W.B. Saunders Company, 1979
• Herbst AL, Mishel DR, Stenchever MA, Drogemueller W: Comprehensive Gynecology. 2nd Ed. St. Louis, C.V. Mosby Co., 1992
• Richart R, Jones HW III, Reid R: Classification and Interpretation of Pap smears. ACOG Update 1993;18;10:1-10
Illustrations: N/A
Internet references: http://www.5mcc.com

Author(s)
Albert T. Shiu, MD, FACOG

Cervical hyperextension injuries

BASICS

DESCRIPTION Result from upward or backward injury to frontal head, jaw, and face. May involve:
• Soft tissues of neck - "whiplash"
• Vertebral structures - fractures, dislocations, ligamentous tears, and disc disruption
• Spinal cord - acute central cord syndrome (CCS) secondary to cord compression or vascular insult

System(s) affected: Musculoskeletal, Nervous

Genetics: Related to predisposing factors like ankylosing spondylitis associated with HLA-B27

Incidence/prevalence: About 1/4 of spinal injuries caused by hyperextension

Predominant age: Trauma and sports injuries most common in young adults, average age 29.4 years; CCS most common among elderly, average age 53 years

Predominant sex: Male > Female

SIGNS AND SYMPTOMS
• Neck pain, stiffness and tenderness
• Headaches
• Paresthesia
• Numbness
• Shoulder pain, spasms and tenderness; range of motion limitation; radicular signs
• Classically, with forehead, face, or jaw abrasion, laceration, or contusion
• CCS
  ◊ Typically distal upper extremity (UE) weakness or paralysis worse than proximal UE, worse than lower extremity
  ◊ Variable sensory changes and sphincter disturbances
  ◊ Horner's syndrome if C8-T11 involved

CAUSES
• Trauma
  ◊ Mostly vehicular accidents
  ◊ Sports injuries
  ◊ Falls
  ◊ Assaults

RISK FACTORS
Present in 65% of CCS
• Spinal stenosis
  ◊ Congenital
  ◊ Acquired - prior trauma, spondylosis
• Spinal rigidity
  ◊ Klippel-Feil syndrome
  ◊ Ankylosing spondylitis

DIAGNOSIS

DIFFERENTIAL DIAGNOSIS
• Herniated discs
• Arthritis
• Radiculopathy
• Myelopathy
• For CCS
  ◊ Bell's cruciate palsy
  ◊ Bilateral brachial plexus injuries

LABORATORY N/A
Drugs that may alter lab results: N/A
Disorders that may alter lab results: N/A

PATHOLOGICAL FINDINGS
• Whiplash - based on animal experiments
  ◊ Muscle tears of the longus colli and sternocleidomastoid
  ◊ Injuries to anterior longitudinal ligament
  ◊ Intervertebral discs and vertebral body endplates
  ◊ Retropharyngeal hematoma, rarely
• CCS
  ◊ Traditionally reported as central gray matter injury with hemorrhage
  ◊ Recent reports show predominantly white matter injury with involvement of the lateral column, particularly, corticospinal tracts ◊ Pathologic hallmark - diffuse axonal disruption
  ◊ With more severe injuries, central hemorrhage is seen

SPECIAL TESTS See Imaging

IMAGING
• Plain c-spine films still main initial diagnostic tool
  ◊ Static - c-spine series; findings of slight extension, prevertebral swelling from anterior longitudinal ligament disruption
  ◊ Dynamic - flexion/extension, only if asymptomatic neck and no neurologic deficits or change in level of consciousness
• CT scan or tomograms - better delineation of fractures, spinal canal status
• CT myelogram - alternative to MRI, show cutoffs of thecal sac and nerve sleeve
• MRI - diagnostic procedure of choice in CCS; show ligament and disc injuries, vertebral body endplate fractures, disc-endplate disruption

DIAGNOSTIC PROCEDURES Discussed in other sections; care needs to be taken to avoid overlooking subtle hyperextension injuries

TREATMENT:

APPROPRIATE HEALTH CARE
Outpatient or inpatients as required by injury

GENERAL MEASURES
Whiplash
• Depending on severity
  ◊ Activity restriction
  ◊ Soft to rigid collar
  ◊ Medicines - analgesics, muscle relaxants, anti-inflammatory
  ◊ Post resolution of spasms, repeat flexion/extension lateral c-spine to confirm stability
CCS
• See Medications
• If no instability, bed rest with soft collar for 4-6 weeks followed by mobilization with collar for another 4-6 weeks
Fractures
• Stability determined by usual radiologic criteria; surgical decompression and stabilization is indicated:
  ◊ In patients with incomplete spinal cord injuries and spinal canal compromise from bone, disc, subluxation, or hematoma
  ◊ In those who deteriorate or do not improve on conservative therapy
• Hangman's fracture - traumatic spondylolisthesis of the axis is a fracture through the C2 pedicles, often with subluxation of C2 over C3
  ◊ Usually stable, managed with orthosis, SOMI (sternal-occipital-mental orthosis)
  ◊ Unstable if C2 subluxation over C3 is over 50% of C3
  ◊ If excessive angulation of C2 over C3
  ◊ Treated with halo vest immobilization for 8-14 weeks when lateral films in flexion and extension again done
  ◊ If stable, rigid collar for additional 8-12 weeks
• Odontoid fracture - treated according to type
  ◊ I - through apex, may be unstable and require surgical fusion
  ◊ II - at base of neck, usually unstable; nonunion rates up to 30% on immobilization alone, especially if displacement more than 5 mm in patients more than 7 years old
  ◊ III - through C2 body, usually stable; immobilized in halo for 8-14 weeks, rigid collar for 8-14 weeks, then mobilization
• C3-C7 hyperextension fractures
  ◊ If stable, rigid collar for 8-14 weeks then mobilization
  ◊ If unstable, halo brace; serial lat c-spine films from supine to upright; if still unstable, surgical stabilization
  ◊ Post-op, followup x-rays until trabeculation across fracture site or interbody fusion achieved

Cervical hyperextension injuries

SURGICAL MEASURES
CCS
• In acute cases, surgery is associated with deterioration and increased complications, and therefore contraindicated
• Surgery may be indicated in patient who is improving and then deteriorates
• Otherwise, surgical decompression and stabilization performed only when neurologic function has reached a plateau or maximum recovery
• Fractures: See General Measures

ACTIVITY Rest and immobilization until pain is controlled; followed by gradual mobilization, and rehabilitation exercises if needed

DIET No special diet

PATIENT EDUCATION For patient instruction on prevention: THINK FIRST Foundation, 22 S. Washington St., Park Ridge, IL 60068, (708)692-2740

MEDICATIONS

DRUG(S) OF CHOICE CCS - methylprednisolone 30 mg/kg IV over 1 hour followed by 5.4 mg/kg IV per hour for 23 hours should be started within 8 hours of injury. It has been proven to improve neurologic outcome, motor and sensory function at 6 months and 1 year after incomplete spinal cord injury.
Contraindications: N/A
Precautions: N/A
Significant possible interactions: N/A

ALTERNATIVE DRUGS N/A

FOLLOWUP

PATIENT MONITORING
• Patients seen and checked with x-rays every 3-4 weeks for about 3 months, when bone healing is usually adequate
• Halo then replaced with rigid collar for next 3 months or rigid collar replaced with soft collar for comfort

PREVENTION/AVOIDANCE Wearing seat belts; using proper equipment when participating in sports activities

POSSIBLE COMPLICATIONS
• Persistent symptoms
• Nonunion of fractures
• Persistent instability requiring another procedure
• Reactions and infection related to orthosis

EXPECTED COURSE/PROGNOSIS
Most important prognostic factor is the initial neurologic status
• Whiplash - most patients recover well, mild symptoms resolving within 6 months
  ◊ On the average, more severe injuries without disc involvement resolve in 21 months
  ◊ 30 months for those with degenerative changes
  ◊ At 2 years, 42% complete recovery, 15% mild discomfort, 43% significant discomfort affecting work
• CCS
  ◊ Most patients recover motor strength within 2 weeks
  ◊ Younger patients have better prognosis
  ◊ Leg, bowel, and bladder function return first
  ◊ Return of arm strength follows, then that of hand
  ◊ However, upper extremities recover less well, and fine finger movements is usually not regained completely
  ◊ With cord contusion but no hematomyelia, 50% recover enough strength and sensation to ambulate independently although usually with spasticity
• Fracture-dislocation
  ◊ Hangman's fracture - 93-100% fusion rate after 8-14 weeks external immobilization
  ◊ Odontoid fracture - type III, 90% fusion with immobilization

MISCELLANEOUS

ASSOCIATED CONDITIONS N/A

AGE-RELATED FACTORS
Pediatric: N/A
Geriatric: N/A
Others: N/A

PREGNANCY N/A

SYNONYMS N/A

ICD-9-CM
952.0 Spinal cord injury without evidence of spinal bone injury, cervical

SEE ALSO N/A

OTHER NOTES N/A

ABBREVIATIONS N/A

REFERENCES
• Greenberg MS: Handbook of Neurosurgery. Florida, Greenberg Graphics, Inc., 1994
• Larson SJ: Hyperextension, hyperflexion, and torsion injuries of the spine. In Youman's Neurological Surgery. 3rd Ed, Philadelphia, W.B. Saunders Co., 1990:2392-2402
• McSwain NE, Martinez JA, Timberlake GA: Cervical Spine Trauma: Evaluation and Acute Management. New York, Thieme Medical Publishers, Inc.,1989
• Pitts LH, Wagner FC Jr: Craniospinal Trauma, New York, Thieme Medical Publishers, Inc., 1990
• Sonntag VKH, Francis PM: Controversies in spinal cord syndromes. In: Grafin SR, Northru BE, eds. Surgery For Spinal Cord Injuries. New York, Raven Press, 1993:15-30
• Wagner FC: Injuries to the cervical spine and spinal cord. In Youman's Neurological Surgery. 3rd Ed. Philadelphia, W.B. Saunders Co., 1990:2378-2391
Illustrations: N/A
Internet references: http://www.5mcc.com

Author(s)
Benjamin Paras, MD
Martin E. Weinand, MD

Cervical malignancy

BASICS

DESCRIPTION An invasive process initiated usually at the squamocolumnar junction either by the squamous or adenomatous (glandular) components of the cervical epithelium
System(s) affected: Reproductive
Genetics: Not known to be an inherited tendency
Incidence/Prevalence in USA: 17,000 new cases/year; majority of cases confined to cervix (Stage I)
Predominant age: 53 year old women, but possible increasing frequency in younger women
Predominant sex: Female only

SIGNS AND SYMPTOMS
• Irregular vaginal bleeding
• Post-coital vaginal bleeding
• Unusually foul-smelling discharge
• Dyspareunia
• Pelvic pain
• Hematuria
• Rectal bleeding
• Enlarged cervix

CAUSES Probably related to viral infections, including human papilloma virus

RISK FACTORS
• Human papilloma virus infection
• Human immunodeficiency virus infection
• Smoking
• High number of sexual partners
• Early age at first intercourse
• DES daughters
• Immunosuppression

DIAGNOSIS

DIFFERENTIAL DIAGNOSIS
• Cervicitis, severe
• Cervical polyp
• Carcinoma of endometrium with cervical extension
• Metastatic carcinoma, including choriocarcinoma

LABORATORY
• CBC (question of anemia secondary to chronic blood loss)
• Creatinine (question of ureteral obstruction)
• Liver function tests (question of metastases)
• Papanicolaou smear
Drugs that may alter lab results: N/A
Disorders that may alter lab results: Bleeding or inflammation may obscure presence of cancer cells

PATHOLOGICAL FINDINGS
• Invasive squamous carcinoma most common (80-85%)
• Invasive adenocarcinoma is second most common (15-20%)

SPECIAL TESTS
• Papanicolaou smear (Pap smear) for screening
• Colposcopy and endocervical sampling
• Diagnosis requires cervical tissue biopsy. Needs biopsy large enough to show cervical stroma to diagnose invasive nature.

IMAGING
• For advanced disease
◊ CT abdomen and pelvis for radiation planning and detection of lymph node metastases
◊ Lymphangiogram occasionally for diagnosis of lymph node metastases

DIAGNOSTIC PROCEDURES Cervical cone biopsy if early invasion or if question of invasion to determine depth of invasion

TREATMENT

APPROPRIATE HEALTH CARE
Dependent on depth of invasion

GENERAL MEASURES N/A

SURGICAL MEASURES
• Initial disease
◊ For lesions with less than 3 mm invasion from basement membrane, no lymphatic or vascular invasion and no confluent tongues
◊ Total abdominal hysterectomy
◊ Cone biopsy - later hysterectomy
◊ Vaginal hysterectomy
◊ For cancer confined to the cervix (Stage I) with invasion greater than 3 mm
◊ Radical hysterectomy with lymph node dissection
◊ Or primary radiation therapy
◊ For most lesions greater than Stage I, radiation with or without adjuvant chemotherapy is appropriate
• For recurrent disease
◊ Radiation or pelvic exenteration, if localized
◊ Chemotherapy, if metastatic
◊ Possible intraoperative radiation therapy

ACTIVITY As tolerated

DIET If radiation used, may need a lactose restricted diet

PATIENT EDUCATION
• "Sexuality and Cancer" pamphlet. American Cancer Society, 1599 Clifton Rd., Atlanta, GA 30329, (404)320-3333
• "What You Need to Know About Cancer of the Cervix" and "Cancer Treatments: Consider the Possibilities." National Institutes of Health, Building 31, Room 41-21, 9000 Rockville Pike, Bethesda, MD 20892, (301)496-4236.

MEDICATIONS

DRUG(S) OF CHOICE
• For adjuvant radiation therapy sensitization
  ◊ Fluorouracil
  ◊ Hydroxyurea
  ◊ Cisplatin
• For recurrent, metastatic disease
  ◊ Bleomycin
  ◊ Etoposide (VP-16)
  ◊ Cisplatin or carboplatin
  ◊ Ifosfamide [with mesna to protect against hemorrhagic cystitis]
Contraindications: Each drug has different contraindications and side effects. Refer to manufacturer's profile of each drug.
Precautions: Neutropenia and renal failure can occur with some combinations
Significant possible interactions: Refer to manufacturer's profile of each drug

ALTERNATIVE DRUGS
• Ondansetron (Zofran), dronabinol (Marinol), metoclopramide (Reglan), and others for nausea control

FOLLOWUP

PATIENT MONITORING
• Following initial therapy, evaluation with physical exam and pap smear
  ◊ Every three months for 1-2 years
  ◊ Every six months until five years
  ◊ After five years, yearly evaluations

PREVENTION/AVOIDANCE
• Pap smear may decrease incidence of invasive disease
• Stop smoking
• Decrease exposure to sexually transmitted diseases

POSSIBLE COMPLICATIONS
• Ureteral fistula (less than 2% with treatment)
• Hydronephrosis
• Uremia

EXPECTED COURSE/PROGNOSIS
• Stage I and II (60% of patients) 50-70% 5 year survival dependent upon risk factors
• Stage III 40% 5 year survival

MISCELLANEOUS

ASSOCIATED CONDITIONS
• Vaginal carcinoma in situ and invasive cancer
• Vulvar carcinoma in situ and invasive cancer
• Warts

AGE-RELATED FACTORS
Pediatric: N/A
Geriatric: May replace estrogen if ovaries removed
Others: Choice of initial therapy between radiation and radical surgery dependent on activity and general health of individual

PREGNANCY Can occur in pregnant patients. Choice of therapy and need for therapeutic abortion dependent on stage cell type and gestational age.

SYNONYMS
• Cancer of the uterine cervix
• Cervical cancer
• Cervical carcinoma

ICD-9-CM
180.0 Malignant neoplasm of cervix uteri

SEE ALSO N/A

OTHER NOTES N/A

ABBREVIATIONS
DES = diethylstilbestrol

REFERENCES
• Cain J: Cancer of the Uterine Cervix. In: Rakel R, ed. Conn's Current Therapy. Philadelphia, W.B. Saunders Co., 1991
• ACOG: Classification and Staging of Gynecologic Malignancies. No. 155, May, 1991
• Goodman J, Bowling M, Nelson J: Cervical Malignancies. Gynecologic Oncology. New York, Knapp/Berkowitz, 1986
Illustrations: N/A
Internet references: http://www.5mcc.com

Author(s)
Joanna M. Cain, MD

Cervical polyps

 BASICS

DESCRIPTION Pedunculated masses, usually single, which vary in size from a few millimeters to 3 centimeters and protrude from the cervix; may bleed
System(s) affected: Reproductive
Genetics: N/A
Incidence/Prevalence in USA: Common
Predominant age: Most often ages 30-50
Predominant sex: Female only

SIGNS AND SYMPTOMS
• Painless
• Intermenstrual bleeding (slight)
• May cause post-coital spotting

CAUSES
• Unknown for most
• Secondary reaction to cervical infection, erosion, or ulceration

RISK FACTORS None known

 DIAGNOSIS

DIFFERENTIAL DIAGNOSIS
• Prolapsed submucous myoma
• Other causes of intermenstrual bleeding

LABORATORY N/A
Drugs that may alter lab results: N/A
Disorders that may alter lab results: N/A

PATHOLOGICAL FINDINGS
• Benign hyperplastic endocervical epithelium often with large number of blood vessels
• Size may be increased by edema and inflammation

SPECIAL TESTS
• Diagnosis usually made by pelvic examination
• Perform Pap smear prior to treatment

IMAGING N/A

DIAGNOSTIC PROCEDURES
Characteristic appearance noted at time of pelvic examination

 TREATMENT

APPROPRIATE HEALTH CARE
Outpatient usually. Very large polyps may require removal in operating room.

GENERAL MEASURES N/A

SURGICAL MEASURES
• Simple surgical excision in office with snare, electrocautery, or liquid nitrogen, control bleeding with silver nitrate
• No douching following excision

ACTIVITY Avoid sexual intercourse until postoperative followup

DIET General diet

PATIENT EDUCATION Routine care instructions

MEDICATIONS

DRUG(S) OF CHOICE None
Contraindications: N/A
Precautions: N/A
Significant possible interactions: N/A

ALTERNATIVE DRUGS N/A

FOLLOWUP

PATIENT MONITORING Recheck at routine appointments, 1 and 6 weeks following surgical excision

PREVENTION/AVOIDANCE None known

POSSIBLE COMPLICATIONS
• Bleeding and mild pain with removal
• Spotting for 1 or 2 days

EXPECTED COURSE/PROGNOSIS
Almost always benign. Very rare incidence of dysplasia in polyp. Very rare possibility of malignancy arising.

MISCELLANEOUS

ASSOCIATED CONDITIONS None

AGE-RELATED FACTORS
Pediatric: Very rare
Geriatric: Rare
Others: N/A

PREGNANCY Delay removal until postpartum

SYNONYMS N/A

ICD-9-CM 622.7

SEE ALSO N/A

OTHER NOTES N/A

ABBREVIATIONS N/A

REFERENCES
• Danforth DM, Scott JR, et al, eds: Obstetric and Gynecology. 6th Ed. Philadelphia, J.B. Lippincott, 1990
• Novak ER, et al, eds: Novak's, Textbook of Gynecology. 11th Ed. Baltimore, Williams & Wilkins, 1988
Illustrations: N/A
Internet references: http://www.5mcc.com

Author(s)
Mark Eric Worshtil, MD

Cervical spine injury

BASICS

DESCRIPTION Though an over-simplification, it is best to classify injuries as flexion, extension, compression, or unknown
• Flexion injuries
  ◊ Anterior subluxation - best seen on lateral view of cervical spine as a kyphotic angulation at the point of ligamentous injury. Widening of spinous process at the point of injury may occur.
  ◊ Facet dislocation - unstable injury, especially when bilateral. Anterior displacement of vertebra (50% of its width) usually indicates bilateral facet dislocation.
  ◊ Compression fractures - usually associated with disruption of the posterior ligament complex and therefore unstable
  ◊ Clay-shovelers fracture - avulsion fracture of C7-C6 or T1 spinous process with intact posterior ligaments and therefore stable
• Extension injuries
  ◊ Hangman's fracture - fracture of the pars interarticularis of the axis. It accounts for 10-15% of fractures.
  ◊ Laminar fracture - difficult to see. Usually in older people who have spondylosis.
  ◊ Fracture posterior arch atlas - usually stable when an isolated injury
  ◊ Fracture dislocations - may resemble a flexion injury since the vertebral body is propelled forward and therefore appears as a flexion subluxation
• Compression
  ◊ Jefferson's fracture - a fracture of the arches of C1, best seen on the open mouth view as displacement of C1 lateral masses
  ◊ Burst fracture - seen on the AP radiograph as a vertical fracture of the body and on the lateral as a commutation of the body with varying degrees of retropulsion of the body
• Unknown mechanisms
  ◊ Odontoid fractures - best seen on the AP view, but lateral views may show a tilt or displacement
System(s) affected: Musculoskeletal, Nervous
Genetics: N/A
Incidence/Prevalence in USA: Cervical injuries account for twelve thousand deaths in the U.S. each year. One-half of these are from motor vehicular accidents.
Predominant age: Most common in ages 16-25
Predominant sex: Male > Female

SIGNS AND SYMPTOMS
• Pain, stiffness, and/or tenderness in an alert patient. If none of these are present the incidence of cervical spine injury is only 1-2%, provided the patient is alert and without alcohol or drug intake. (A lateral cervical spine x-ray should be taken routinely in all severe trauma).
• Head and/or facial trauma/lacerations in patients with altered consciousness

CAUSES Trauma

RISK FACTORS
• Motor vehicle accidents
• Diving accidents

DIAGNOSIS

DIFFERENTIAL DIAGNOSIS
• Joint, muscle or ligament inflammation
• Paresthesias
• Arthritis
• Cervical disk protrusion
• Cervical spondylosis

LABORATORY N/A
Drugs that may alter lab results: N/A
Disorders that may alter lab results: N/A

PATHOLOGICAL FINDINGS N/A

SPECIAL TESTS Tomograms may be obtained to visualize otherwise obscure fractures, but even these are usually inferior to imaging by CT. MRI is superior in evaluating soft tissue injury.

IMAGING
• The use of CT and MRI scanning has greatly facilitated diagnosis of obscure cervical injuries. The CT may be a little better in some bone injuries, especially in the foramen, while the MRI has the edge with soft tissue evaluation. Both are superior to any previous method.
• X-ray - a lateral view of the cervical spine is only 80-85% accurate in picking up abnormalities. Adding an AP and open mouth odontoid view will increase the accuracy of screening to 90-95%. However, in the presence of pain, tenderness, and/or stiffness, the use of a CT or MRI scan should be considered since 5-10% of cases will have normal radiographs even with a significant cervical injury.
• X-rays vary with the type of injury, but a few salient features to be observed are:
  ◊ Soft-tissue swelling on the lateral view of greater than 5 mm when measured from the inferior border of C3 to the trachea indicates a severe injury (except children)
  ◊ Widely divergent spinous processes on the lateral view indicates rupture of ligaments
  ◊ Abnormal widening of either a complete interspace or a portion of the anterior or posterior interspace on lateral view (compare with interspaces above and below)
  ◊ Malrotation of the spinous processes on the AP view (they should form a straight line)
  ◊ Inequality of the space on either side of the odontoid on open mouth views

DIAGNOSTIC PROCEDURES N/A

TREATMENT

APPROPRIATE HEALTH CARE
• Transportation
  ◊ A carefully applied rigid collar supplemented by sand bags on either side of the head on a rigid backboard is probably the safest method
  ◊ Oxygen should be given to all patients with injury to the spinal cord. (Patients with high cord lesions die of asphyxiation so assisted ventilation may be needed).
  ◊ 50% of serious cervical injuries will have associated head, chest, abdominal or major extremity injuries in association. Give first aid to these patients maintaining the "ABC" principle of airway, breathing, and circulation.
  ◊ Military antishock garment (MASG) can be used in cases of shock
  ◊ Start an intravenous line if it can be done rapidly. Otherwise, this should not be done as valuable time may be wasted. The principle of "load and go" in cases of ambulance or "swoop and scoop" in the case of helicopters is a good one if an acute care center is close at hand.
• Hospital
  ◊ Prior to dealing with the cervical injury, attention should be directed towards the ABC's (airway, breathing, circulation)
  ◊ Arterial oxygen should be measured immediately since oxygenation of an injured spinal cord helps prevent further damage and aids in recovery. If the oxygen partial pressure (pO2) is less than 70 mm of mercury, or the cervical lesion is above C5, intubation is indicated. If the patient is breathing, blind nasal intubation can be tried; otherwise the oral approach with a laryngoscope is necessary. Both require careful technique with avoidance of neck extension. If this cannot be done with ease or if there are severe facial injuries, a cricothyroidotomy should be done.
  ◊ A nasogastric (NG) tube should always be inserted to prevent vomiting, aspiration. It also prevents gastric dilatation with lung compression and difficult breathing.
  ◊ In most cases, volume replacement is best accomplished through the femoral route. The subclavian approach risks pneumothorax and further oxygenation problems.
  ◊ If a pneumothorax is present, a chest tube should always be inserted (first confirmed by x-ray). Needle aspiration is indicated only as a temporary measure to relieve symptoms in a tension pneumothorax prior to insertion of the tube.
  ◊ In all cord injuries, abdominal and chest CT scan should be done to rule out a severe intra-abdominal injury. This procedure is highly accurate while all physical findings and symptoms are unreliable. (The NG tube and an indwelling Foley catheter should be done prior to the scans.)

GENERAL MEASURES
• Spinal shock occurs in 25-40% of spinal cord injuries. It is characterized by systolic hypotension and bradycardia. The cause is loss of distal sympathetic tone.
• Head injuries alone do not cause hypotension but can cause hypertension
• Because patients with cervical trauma may sustain other significant injuries, systolic hypotension may be from blood loss and/or spinal shock. Remember that several liters of blood can be lost from a head or perineal wound.
• Shock other than from volume loss or spinal shock can come from pericardial tamponade, tension pneumothorax, or cardiac contusion

SURGICAL MEASURES Surgical management as needed for type of injury

ACTIVITY N/A

DIET N/A

PATIENT EDUCATION N/A

 ## MEDICATIONS

DRUG(S) OF CHOICE
• Methylprednisolone
◊ If given within 8 hours after the injury, has been shown to not only minimize further injury, but to improve both motor function and sensation for up to six months. This steroid apparently prevents lipid hydrolysis and subsequent destruction of the cell membrane.
◊ Initial dose: 30 mg/kg over a 15 minute period. Then 45 minutes later, 5.4 mg/kg/hr for the next 23 hours. See Bracken 1990, N Engl J Med 322:1405-1411.
Contraindications: None
Precautions: Intravenous cimetidine (Tagamet) 300 mg q6h or ranitidine (Zantac) 50 mg q8h can be given if a history of ulcer is present. In cases of multiple injuries this is a good way to prevent stress ulcer.
Significant possible interactions: None

ALTERNATIVE DRUGS
• Naloxone, nimodipine and thyrotropin releasing hormones have been tried with equivocal results. Tests are underway using chemotherapeutic drugs, but these await the outcome of several studies.
• Other H2 receptor antagonists

 ## FOLLOWUP

PATIENT MONITORING Critical care facilities must be available initially and later physical and occupational therapy units with special skills in spinal cord injuries

PREVENTION/AVOIDANCE N/A

POSSIBLE COMPLICATIONS
• Paresthesia
• Muscle weakness
• Reflex loss
• Sensory loss
• Radiculopathy

EXPECTED COURSE/PROGNOSIS In cases of significant cord injuries, the prognosis is guarded. Development of newer orthopedic devices can stabilize the spine and allow early mobilization, but do not help to reverse neurological damage if present.

 ## MISCELLANEOUS

ASSOCIATED CONDITIONS N/A

AGE-RELATED FACTORS
Pediatric: N/A
Geriatric: N/A
Others: N/A

PREGNANCY N/A

SYNONYMS Cervical fracture, dislocation

ICD-9-CM 952.0 Cervical spinal cord injury

SEE ALSO N/A

OTHER NOTES N/A

ABBREVIATIONS N/A

REFERENCES
• Torg JS, Sennett B, et al: Axial loading injuries to middle cervical spine segment. An analysis and classification of 25 cases. American Journal of Sports Medicine 1991:19(1):6-20
• Soderstrom CA, Brumback RJ: Orthopedic Clinics of North America 1986;17(1):3-13
• Bracken MB, et al: Efficacy of methylprednisolone in acute spinal cord Injury; JAMA 1984;251:45-52
• Bracken MB, et al: A randomized control trial of methylprednisolone or naloxone in the treatment of acute spinal cord injury. Results of the second acute spinal cord Injury study. N Engl J Med 1990;322:1405-1411
• Jacobs B: Cervical Fractures and Dislocations, Clinical Orthopedics 1975;109:18
Illustrations: N/A
Internet references: http://www.5mcc.com

Author(s)
Furnie W. Johnston, MD
R. Bruce Hall, MD

Cervical spondylosis

BASICS

DESCRIPTION Degenerative changes in the cervical vertebra and/or disk with spur formation and subsequent impingement of neural elements in a narrow cervical canal
System(s) affected: Musculoskeletal
Genetics: N/A
Incidence/Prevalence in USA: 30-40% of the population above age 40 years
Predominant age: Above 40 the incidence increases with each passing decade
Predominant sex: Male > Female (3:2)

SIGNS AND SYMPTOMS
• Pain in the posterior neck often associated with radiation into the arms
• Scapular pain
• Pain in the arms is almost always on the outer aspect of the arm at least to elbow level (coronary heart pain is almost always on the inner aspect of the arm)
• Radicular pain into the arms or scapular area may be present without neck pain
• Dysphagia may develop with large anterior osteophytes
• Weakness of extremities - upper and/or lower
• Bladder or bowel incontinence in severe cases
• If an osteophyte develops on a neurocentral joint and extends laterally, it can encroach on the vertebral artery and may cause dizziness, vertigo, tinnitus or interorbital blurring of vision. Symptoms are exacerbated by extremes of movement and even minor neck trauma.
• Loss of neck extension (common)
• Lateral flexion of the cervical spine is limited in the erect position, but greatly increased on lying down. (Functional disorders are not improved by lying down.)
• Long tract signs may develop in severe cases with positive Babinski
• Tenderness of biceps and pectoralis major in C5-6 segment disease
• Triceps tenderness in C6-7 segment disease

CAUSES Degenerative changes with osteophytes and disk space narrowing

RISK FACTORS N/A

DIAGNOSIS

DIFFERENTIAL DIAGNOSIS
• Cervical disk disease (the two often co-exist)
• Pancoast tumor of lung
• Rheumatoid arthritis
• Neurological disorders such as multiple sclerosis

LABORATORY N/A
Drugs that may alter lab results: N/A
Disorders that may alter lab results: N/A

PATHOLOGICAL FINDINGS N/A

SPECIAL TESTS N/A

IMAGING
• X-rays of cervical spine, AP, lateral open mouth odontoid and both oblique views should be obtained. Osteophytes and/or joint space narrowing will be evident.
• CT or MRI scans are quite valuable in cases where surgery is contemplated or the diagnosis is in doubt. It is not indicated in the great majority of cases as a careful history and physical examination coupled with routine cervical spine x-rays will make the diagnosis. The decision as to which is better, the CT scan or MRI, is controversial. The MRI depicts cord changes, enlargement, compression, or atrophy better. While the CT, especially in conjunction with myelography, shows the bony changes, especially in foramina involvement. MRI has the obvious advantage of not requiring a myelogram. Postoperatively, the MRI is excellent in evaluation of patients who have failed to obtain relief from surgery or have developed new symptoms. If this does not demonstrate a cause, then a CT scan with contrast can be obtained.

DIAGNOSTIC PROCEDURES N/A

TREATMENT

APPROPRIATE HEALTH CARE
Outpatient for conservative treatment, inpatient if surgery indicated

GENERAL MEASURES
• Acute phase - moist heat, gentle massage and temporary immobilization with a cervical collar that holds the neck in slight flexion. Intermittent cervical traction may be helpful, but the line of pull should be such that the neck is slightly flexed. Ultrasonic treatments, especially combined with gentle muscle stimulation (US-MS) for 15-20 minutes daily or bid may be helpful in the acute phase.
• Chronic - no treatment necessary except for non-narcotic analgesics for symptoms. Any type of activity or work which causes strain of the neck should be avoided.

SURGICAL MEASURES
• Indications: Severe pain unresponsive to conservative measures, significant or progression of neurologic deficits, long tract signs, vertebral artery syndrome
• Most common surgery is anterior interbody fusion with excision of disk and any accessible osteophytes

ACTIVITY Any activity which does not cause symptoms should be encouraged as the disease is chronic. Needless restrictions can make the patient a medical invalid.

DIET No special diet

PATIENT EDUCATION
• Personally instruct (or have a therapist instruct) in the proper use of orthopedic appliances. Cervical collars should produce a slight flexion of the neck as should traction. Avoid extension in all situations.
• Instruct patient in home traction to relieve symptoms; instruct patient in home exercise routine to relieve spasm and discomfort
• Instruct patients to report any weaknesses, eye symptoms, bladder or bowel incontinence immediately

Cervical spondylosis

MEDICATIONS

DRUG(S) OF CHOICE
• Acetaminophen (Tylenol) 500 mg qid is the safest regimen. Studies have shown it to be at least as effective as NSAID's.
• NSAID's - aspirin 1.0 gm qid is effective in many cases. If this fails, any of the other NSAID's are used with all having about the same success rate. Piroxicam 10 mg daily, tolmetin 600 mg tid are some examples. If aspirin therapy is used, salicylate levels should be obtained; therapeutic range is 10-30 mg/dL (0.724-2.17 mmol/L). Enteric-coated aspirin may be helpful to minimize GI upset.
• Cortisone should not be used in long term management. Occasional injections of trigger zones with 40 mg methylprednisolone (Depo-Medrol) may be used, but this should be saved for severe exacerbations.
• Trigger point injection of lidocaine 1%, injected into the "hot areas", especially in the scapular area. Often as effective in relieving symptoms alone as when combined with methylprednisolone
Contraindications: NSAID's, except aspirin, should not be used in patients with chronic liver disease. Use with caution in cases of ulcers. If NSAID's are used, misoprostol (Cytotec) 200 µg qid should be given concomitantly.
Precautions: Patients on long term NSAID's should be monitored with liver studies 6-8 weeks after initial treatment and then every 3-4 months
Significant possible interactions: Refer to manufacturer's profile of each drug

ALTERNATIVE DRUGS   Listed in Drug(s) of Choice

FOLLOWUP

PATIENT MONITORING   Patients should be seen in 3-4 weeks for evaluation of neurologic status. If this has not changed follow at intervals of 3-6 months, depending on severity of symptoms.

PREVENTION/AVOIDANCE   The midcervical spine is the area usually involved in spondylosis. This portion will develop a flexion deformity causing extension of the upper spine as the body tries to keep the head erect. Avoid any extension strain such as a "spinal manipulation," extension during intubation for a general anesthesia, or cervical strain from auto accidents, especially rear-end collisions. These can cause a basilar artery thrombosis or thrombosis of the posterior inferior cerebellar artery with a subsequent Wallenberg's syndrome. Dysphagia, pain and temperature loss to the same side of the face and opposite side of the body, nystagmus and Horner's syndrome are present in Wallenberg's syndrome.

POSSIBLE COMPLICATIONS   Loss of motion, especially extension, may require adjustments to certain occupations to prevent uncommonly significant muscle loss and instability of gait, bladder or bowel function

EXPECTED COURSE/PROGNOSIS
Fortunately, the prognosis is for a benign course in the overwhelming majority of cases, though for most of their lives patients will be plagued by pain which exacerbates often with no known cause

MISCELLANEOUS

ASSOCIATED CONDITIONS   Cervical disk disease

AGE-RELATED FACTORS
Pediatric: N/A
Geriatric: N/A
Others: N/A

PREGNANCY   As in the case of rheumatoid arthritis, the symptoms often improve but occasionally are made worse

SYNONYMS
• Cervical arthritis
• Cervical myelopathy
• Cervical osteophyte

ICD-9-CM   756.19 cervical spondylosis

SEE ALSO   N/A

OTHER NOTES   N/A

ABBREVIATIONS
US-MS = ultrasonic treatment with muscle stimulation

REFERENCES
• McNab I: Cervical Spondylosis: Clinical Orthopedics 1975;109:69-77
• Clifton AG, et al: Identifiable causes for poor outcome in surgery for cervical spondylosis. Neuroradiology 1990;177(2):313-325
• Karnaze MG, et al: Comparison of MR and CT myelography in imaging the cervical and thoracic spine. American Journal of Roentgenography 1988;150(2);397-403
Illustrations: N/A
Internet references: http://www.5mcc.com

Author(s)
Furnie W. Johnston, MD
R. Bruce Hall, MD

Cervicitis

BASICS

DESCRIPTION An inflammation of the uterine cervix. Infectious cervicitis may be caused by Chlamydia trachomatis, Neisseria gonorrhoeae, herpes simplex or Trichomonas vaginalis.
• Chronic cervicitis is characterized by inflammation of the cervix without an identified pathogen
System(s) affected: Reproductive
Genetics: N/A
Incidence/Prevalence in USA:
• Gonorrhea 166/100,000
• Chlamydia 290/100,000 women
• Trichomonas 1200/100,000
• Gonorrhea 2% of sexually active women under age 30
• Chlamydia 5-35% of women
• Trichomonas 5-25%
Predominant age: Infectious cervicitis is most common in adolescents, but can be seen in women of any age
Predominant sex: Female only

SIGNS AND SYMPTOMS
• Mucopurulent (yellow) discharge from the cervix
• Cervical erosion or erythema
• Easily induced endocervical mucosal bleeding
• Tenderness of cervix
• Postcoital bleeding
• Frequently asymptomatic

CAUSES
• Chlamydia trachomatis
• Neisseria gonorrhoeae
• Herpes simplex virus
• Trichomonas vaginalis
• Cause of chronic cervicitis unknown

RISK FACTORS
• Multiple sexual partners
• History of sexually transmitted disease
• Postpartum period

DIAGNOSIS

DIFFERENTIAL DIAGNOSIS
• Vaginal infections with Candida albicans or Trichomonas vaginalis extending onto the cervix
• Carcinoma of the cervix

LABORATORY
• Endocervical gram stain, more than 10 WBC's per high power field (hpf) suggests cervicitis
• Cervical cultures for C. trachomatis, N. gonorrhoeae
• Enzyme assays (Chlamydiazyme and others) sometimes used to screen for chlamydia
• Polymerase chain reaction (PCR) and ligase chain reaction (LCR) more sensitive than cultures for Chlamydia. LCR can be used with urine.
• Wet mount for Trichomonas vaginalis
• If ulcerations present, culture for herpes simplex virus
• Venereal Disease Research Laboratory (VDRL) or rapid plasma reagin (RPR) to rule out concurrent syphilis
Drugs that may alter lab results: Recent antibiotic treatment
Disorders that may alter lab results: N/A

PATHOLOGICAL FINDINGS Inflammatory changes on Pap smear

SPECIAL TESTS N/A

IMAGING N/A

DIAGNOSTIC PROCEDURES
Colposcopy is indicated in chronic inflammation, with biopsy of suspicious areas

TREATMENT

APPROPRIATE HEALTH CARE
Outpatient treatment

GENERAL MEASURES Chronic cervicitis with negative cultures and biopsies may be treated with cryosurgery

SURGICAL MEASURES N/A

ACTIVITY Full activity

DIET No special diet

PATIENT EDUCATION
• Advise patient to use condoms consistently
• If infectious etiology, advise patient to inform her partners

MEDICATIONS

DRUG(S) OF CHOICE
• If infectious cervicitis suspected, treat without awaiting culture results. Ceftriaxone (Rocephin) 125 mg IM single dose; followed by either doxycycline (Vibramycin) 100 mg po bid for 7 days or azithromycin (Zithromax) 1 g single dose
• For Trichomonas, metronidazole (Flagyl) 2 g single dose
• For herpes, acyclovir (Zovirax) 200 mg po 5 times daily (or 400 mg tid) for 7 days
• Chronic cervicitis associated with postmenopausal vaginal atrophic changes may respond to topical estrogen creams
Contraindications:
• Doxycycline should not be used in pregnant or nursing mothers
• Metronidazole contraindicated in first trimester of pregnancy
Precautions: Doxycycline should not be taken with milk, antacids, or iron containing preparations
Significant possible interactions:
Doxycycline - warfarin (Coumadin) and oral contraceptives may have their effectiveness reduced

ALTERNATIVE DRUGS
• Any of the following can be substituted for ceftriaxone:
  ◊ Cefixime 400 mg po once
  ◊ Ofloxacin 400 mg po once
  ◊ Spectinomycin 2 g IM once
• Erythromycin base or stearate 500 mg po qid, or erythromycin ethylsuccinate 800 mg po qid can be substituted for doxycycline
• Ofloxacin (Floxin) 300 mg po bid x 7 days

FOLLOWUP

PATIENT MONITORING
• Repeat cultures after treatment for chlamydia or gonorrhea are indicated in pregnant or high risk patients
• Annual Pap smears in sexually active patients screen for chronic cervicitis

PREVENTION/AVOIDANCE Patients with more than one sexual partner should be advised to use condoms at every encounter

POSSIBLE COMPLICATIONS
• Cervicitis with C. trachomatis or N. gonorrhoeae is associated with an 8-10% risk of subsequent pelvic inflammatory disease
• Moderate to severe inflammation is associated with condyloma acuminatum and cervical carcinoma

EXPECTED COURSE/PROGNOSIS
• Infectious cervicitis usually responds to systemic antibiotics
• Chronic cervicitis may be resistant to treatment, and should be monitored closely for cervical dysplasia

MISCELLANEOUS

ASSOCIATED CONDITIONS Patients with infectious cervicitis should be screened for other sexually transmitted diseases, syphilis, trichomonas, and possibly human immunodeficiency virus (HIV)

AGE-RELATED FACTORS
Pediatric: Infectious cervicitis in children should lead to investigation for possible sexual abuse
Geriatric:
• Chronic cervicitis in postmenopausal women may be related to lack of estrogen
• The possibility of infectious cervicitis should not be overlooked, as many geriatric patients remain sexually active
Others: Adolescents remain a high-risk group for sexually transmitted diseases

PREGNANCY Screen all pregnant women for infectious cervicitis because of the risk of transmission to the fetus

SYNONYMS Mucopurulent cervicitis

ICD-9-CM
• 616.0 cervicitis
• 098.15 acute gonococcal cervicitis
• 079.8 chlamydia infection

SEE ALSO
• Chlamydial sexually transmitted diseases
• Gonococcal infections
• Trichomoniasis
• Cervicitis, ectropion & true erosion
• Cervical dysplasia

OTHER NOTES The presence of Trichomonas does not rule out other concurrent infection

ABBREVIATIONS N/A

REFERENCES
• MMWR 1997;46:193-198
• Clinical Chemistry 1996;42:809-812
• Danforth DN, Scott JR, eds: Obstetrics and Gynecology. 7th Ed. Philadelphia, Lippincott, 1994
• The Medical Letter, 1995;37:117-122
• Obstet Gynecol 1997;89:556-560
• Med Clin N Am 1995;79:1277-1280
Illustrations: N/A
Internet references: http://www.5mcc.com

Author(s)
Barbara A. Majeroni, MD

Cervicitis, ectropion & true erosion

BASICS

DESCRIPTION
• Cervicitis - inflammatory changes due to infections
• Ectropion - eversion of the cervix in pregnancy
• True erosion - abrupt loss of overlying vaginal epithelium due to trauma, e.g., forceful insertion of vaginal speculum in patient with atrophic mucosa
System(s) affected: Reproductive
Genetics: N/A
Incidence/Prevalence in USA:
• Cervicitis - very common in sexually active women
• Ectropion - with oral contraceptive use; very common in pregnant women
• True erosion - occasionally seen in postmenopausal women
Predominant Age: Sexually active women
Predominant Sex: Female only

SIGNS AND SYMPTOMS
• Cervicitis - metrorrhagia, post-coital bleeding, vaginal discharge
• Ectropion - red cervix due to color of the columnar epithelium
• True erosion - vaginal bleeding, sharply defined ulcers of cervix

CAUSES
• Cervicitis - Chlamydia trachomatis, Trichomonas vaginalis
• Ectropion - hormonal changes with oral contraceptive use (especially with progesterone) or during pregnancy,
• True erosion - injury to atrophic epithelium due to estrogen deficiency in menopause

RISK FACTORS
• Cervicitis - sexual contact with infected partner(s), recurrence due to inadequate therapy
• Ectropion - pregnancy
• True erosion - estrogen deficiency, trauma

DIAGNOSIS

DIFFERENTIAL DIAGNOSIS
• Cervical dysplasia
• Carcinoma of the cervix

LABORATORY
• Saline and potassium hydroxide preparation of cervical/vaginal smears
• Chlamydiazyme or chlamydia cell culture, gonorrhea culture
• Papanicolaou (Pap) smear of the cervix
• Chlamydia DNA probe
Drugs that may alter lab results: N/A
Disorders that may alter lab results: N/A

PATHOLOGICAL FINDINGS
• Cervicitis - acute and chronic inflammatory changes, presence of infective organisms
• Ectropion - none/squamous metaplasia
• True erosion - sharply defined ulcer borders, loss of epithelium

SPECIAL TESTS   None

IMAGING   None

DIAGNOSTIC PROCEDURES
Colposcopy

TREATMENT

APPROPRIATE HEALTH CARE
Outpatient

GENERAL MEASURES   N/A

SURGICAL MEASURES   N/A

ACTIVITY   No restrictions

DIET   No special diet

PATIENT EDUCATION   Provide printed material about sexually transmitted diseases and about estrogen deficiency and estrogen replacement therapy

Cervicitis, ectropion & true erosion

MEDICATIONS

DRUG(S) OF CHOICE
• Trichomoniasis - metronidazole 500 mg bid for 7 days or 2 g once or 1 g bid for 2 doses
• Chlamydial infection - for non-pregnant women, doxycycline 100 mg bid po for 7 days; for pregnant women, erythromycin base 500 mg qid po for 7 days, or erythromycin ethylsuccinate 800 mg qid for 7 days
• Ectropion - none
• True erosion - estrogen, conjugated vaginal cream daily for 2 weeks, follow by estrogen replacement therapy

Contraindications:
• Metronidazole - first trimester of pregnancy
• Doxycycline - pregnancy or lactation
• Estrogen - see extended list of contraindications to estrogen use in standard texts

Precautions:
• Metronidazole - possible fetal harm if used in first trimester of pregnancy, disulfiram reaction with alcohol
• Doxycycline - possible fetal harm if used during pregnancy, staining of the infant's teeth if used during breast-feeding, allergy, photosensitization
• Erythromycin - nausea or vomiting
• Estrogens - history of estrogen dependent neoplasms, history of thromboembolic diseases, see extended list of contraindications to estrogen therapy in standard texts

Significant possible interactions:
• Metronidazole and alcohol
• Doxycycline and dairy products, iron preparations, warfarin, and oral contraceptives (use backup contraceptive method)
• Erythromycin with terfenadine (Seldane) or astemizole - may increase latter's levels with subsequent ECG changes
• Erythromycin and theophylline (elevated theophylline level)
• Estrogen - N/A

ALTERNATIVE DRUGS
• Metronidazole - sulfanilamide-aminacrine-allantoin cream (AVC cream)
• Doxycycline - erythromycin or azithromycin
• Erythromycin - clindamycin
• Estrogen - lubricant, same as that used for vaginal speculum
• Azithromycin 1 g for one dose only (pregnancy category B)
• Ofloxacin 300 mg bid x 7 days
• Amoxicillin-clavulanate (Augmentin) 250 mg po q8h for 7 days

FOLLOWUP

PATIENT MONITORING
• Trichomoniasis - repeat vaginal smear until infection is cleared
• Chlamydial infection - repeat chlamydial culture post antibiotic therapy
• Estrogen deficiency - re-examine in one month to confirm healing

PREVENTION/AVOIDANCE
• Trichomoniasis or chlamydial infection - treatment of sexual partners and use of condom during coitus
• Estrogen deficiency - estrogen replacement therapy

POSSIBLE COMPLICATIONS N/A

EXPECTED COURSE/PROGNOSIS
• Cervicitis - excellent healing once infection is eradicated
• Ectropion - spontaneous regression postpartum, cessation or oral contraceptive use
• True erosion - spontaneous healing

MISCELLANEOUS

ASSOCIATED CONDITIONS
• Gonorrhea
• Bacterial vaginosis

AGE-RELATED FACTORS
Pediatric: N/A
Geriatric: Menopause
Others: N/A

PREGNANCY
• Ectropion
• Azithromycin should be used with caution
• Doxycycline should not be used in pregnancy

SYNONYMS N/A

ICD-9-CM 616.0

SEE ALSO N/A

OTHER NOTES N/A

ABBREVIATIONS N/A

REFERENCES
• Disaia PJ, Creasman WT: Clinical Gynecologic Oncology. 3rd Ed. St. Louis, The C.V. Mosby Company, 1989
• Herbst AL, Mishell DR, Stenchever MA, Droegemueller W: Comprehensive Gynecology. 2nd Ed. St. Louis, The C.V. Mosby Co., 1992
• Kurman RJ, ed: Blaustein's Pathology Of The Female Genital Tract. 3rd Ed. New York, Springer-Verlag, 1987
• Novak ER, Woodruff JD: Novak's Gynocologic and Obstetric Pathology With Clinical and Endocrine Relations. 8th Ed. Philadelphia, W.B. Saunders Company, 1979
• Lebhere TB: In: Hacker NF, Moore JG, eds. Essentials Obstetrics and Gynecology. 2nd Ed. Philadelphia, W.B. Saunders Co., 1992
Illustrations: N/A
Internet references: http://www.5mcc.com

Author(s)
Albert T. Shiu, MD, FACOG

Chancroid

 BASICS

DESCRIPTION A sexually transmitted disease characterized by painful genital ulcerations and inflammatory inguinal adenopathy. It is uncommon in the United States but found worldwide. Chancroid is endemic in developing countries.
System(s) affected: Reproductive, Skin/Exocrine
Genetics: N/A
Incidence/Prevalence in USA:
Approximately 1,000 cases annually (1993, 1994, 1995 - CDC data). Actual numbers felt to be greater due to underreporting of cases.
Predominant age: Teenagers and adults
Predominant sex: Male > Female

SIGNS AND SYMPTOMS
• Tender genital papule that ulcerates after 24 hours
• Irregular edged, painful ulcer(s)
• Ulcers may be 1 mm to 5 cm in size
• Ulcers may occur on the shaft of the penis, glans and meatus in men
• Ulcers in women most commonly occur in labia majora but also seen in labia minora, perineum, thigh, and cervix
• Painful inguinal adenopathy with abscess (bubo) formation in 30% of patients
• Atypical presentations include folliculitis and foreskin abscess

CAUSES Haemophilus ducreyi (gram negative bacterium)

RISK FACTORS
• Multiple sexual partners
• Uncircumcised males
• Prostitutes often are carriers

 DIAGNOSIS

DIFFERENTIAL DIAGNOSIS
• Syphilis
• Herpes Simplex Virus (HSV 1 and 2)
• Lymphogranuloma venereum (LGV)
• Granuloma inguinale

LABORATORY Serologic testing for antibody with ELISA technique. Gram stain; culture of organism on Mueller-Hinton agar with incorporated vancomycin. Polymerase chain reaction (PCR) where available.
Drugs that may alter lab results:
Previous antibiotics
Disorders that may alter lab results:
None expected

PATHOLOGICAL FINDINGS "School of fish" pattern on gram stain

SPECIAL TESTS N/A

IMAGING N/A

DIAGNOSTIC PROCEDURES
• Gram stain and culture of ulcer exudate
• Aspiration of inguinal bubo (lymph node)
• Dark-field examinations of exudate to rule out Treponema pallidum

 TREATMENT

APPROPRIATE HEALTH CARE
Outpatient treatment

GENERAL MEASURES
• Saline or Burow's solution soaks to ulcers
• Aspiration of buboes if greater than 5 cm

SURGICAL MEASURES N/A

ACTIVITY Refrain from sexual intercourse until genital lesions fully resolved

DIET N/A

PATIENT EDUCATION
• Sexual counseling
• Use of condoms
• Local wound care
• Treatment of all sexual partners with same regimen as index case

Chancroid

MEDICATIONS

DRUG(S) OF CHOICE
• Azithromycin 1 gm po single dose (more expensive than other treatments)
• Ceftriaxone 250 mg IM single dose
• Erythromycin base 500 mg qid x 7 days
Contraindications: Allergy to the medication
Precautions: Refer to manufacturer's profile of each drug
Significant possible interactions: Refer to manufacturer's profile of each drug

ALTERNATIVE DRUGS
• Amoxicillin-clavulanate 500 mg/125 mg (Augmentin) po tid x 7 days
• Ciprofloxacin 500 mg po bid for 7 days or other quinolone

FOLLOWUP

PATIENT MONITORING
• Patient followed until all clinical signs of infection resolved
• Baseline syphilis serology and at 3 months
• HIV testing at 3 months post-treatment

PREVENTION/AVOIDANCE Avoidance of sexual activity until ulcers resolved

POSSIBLE COMPLICATIONS
• Phimosis
• Balanoposthitis
• Rupture of buboes with fistula formation and scarring

EXPECTED COURSE/PROGNOSIS
• Full clinical resolution with appropriate treatment
• 5% relapse after treatment

MISCELLANEOUS

ASSOCIATED CONDITIONS
• Syphilis (concurrently in 5% of patients)
• HIV infection

AGE-RELATED FACTORS N/A
Pediatric: N/A
Geriatric: N/A
Others: HIV disease may affect treatment response

PREGNANCY Maternal to infant transmission has not been reported

SYNONYMS
• Soft chancre
• Ulcus molle

ICD-9-CM 0999.O

SEE ALSO N/A

OTHER NOTES Chancroid has been shown to be an established risk factor for acquisition of HIV infection

ABBREVIATIONS N/A

REFERENCES
• U.S. Department of Health and Human Services, Centers for Disease Control and Prevention: Sexually transmitted diseases treatment guideline. Morbidity and Mortality Weekly Report. Vol. 42, No. RR-14; 20-22, 1993
• Schulte JM, Schmid G: Recommendations for treatment of chancroid. Clin Infect Dis 1995;20(Suppl 1):539-546
• Trees DL, Morse SA: Chancroid and haemophilus ducreyi: an update. Clin Microbiol Rev 1995;8(3):357-375
Illustrations: N/A
Internet references: http://www.5mcc.com

Author(s)
Jeffery T. Kirchner, DO, FAAFP

Chickenpox

BASICS

DESCRIPTION A common, highly contagious, childhood exanthem characterized by the development of typical crops of vesicles on the skin and mucous membranes.
• The virus is spread by respiratory droplets or direct contact with vesicles or indirectly through freshly soiled articles
• Outbreaks tend to occur from January to May
• The usual incubation period is 14-16 days (range 11-21). Patients are infectious from 24 hours before appearance of the rash until the final lesions have crusted. Most people acquire chickenpox during childhood and develop long immunity.
System(s) affected: Skin/Exocrine, Nervous
Genetics: No known genetic pattern
Incidence/Prevalence in USA: Common
Predominant age: Peak incidence 5-9 years, but may occur at any age
Predominant Sex: Male = Female

SIGNS AND SYMPTOMS
• Prodromal symptoms - fever, malaise, anorexia, mild headache
• Characteristic rash - crops of "teardrop" vesicles on erythematous bases
• Lesions erupt in successive crops
• Progress from macule to papule to vesicle, then begin to crust
• Rash present in various stages of development
• Pruritic
• Usually begins on trunk, then spreads to face and scalp
• Minimal involvement of the extremities
• Lesions may be present on mucous membranes, oral and vaginal

CAUSES
• Human (alpha) herpesvirus 3 (varicella-zoster virus, V-Z virus), a member of the Herpesvirus group. (Reservoir: humans)

RISK FACTORS
• No prior history of varicella
• Immunosuppressed (especially children with leukemia/lymphoma in remission or on high-dose corticosteroids)

DIAGNOSIS

DIFFERENTIAL DIAGNOSIS
• Herpes simplex
• Herpes zoster
• Impetigo
• Coxsackievirus infection
• Papular urticaria
• Scabies
• Dermatitis herpetiformis
• Drug rash

LABORATORY
• Leukocyte count may be normal, low, or mildly increased
• Marked leukocytosis is suggestive of secondary infection
• Multinucleated giant cells on Tzanck smear from scrapings of vesicles
• Isolated virus from human tissue culture
Drugs that may alter lab results: N/A
Disorders that may alter lab results:
• Herpes zoster
• Herpes simplex

PATHOLOGICAL FINDINGS
• Skin lesions histologically identical to herpes simplex virus
• In fatal cases intranuclear inclusions can be found in the endothelium of blood vessels and most organs

SPECIAL TESTS
For complicated cases and epidemiologic studies:
• Visualization of the virus by EM
• Detection of viral antigen in smears by FA
• Detection of viral DNA by PCR

IMAGING N/A

DIAGNOSTIC PROCEDURES N/A

TREATMENT

APPROPRIATE HEALTH CARE
Outpatient except for complicating emergencies

GENERAL MEASURES
• Supportive/symptomatic treatment
• Good hygiene to avoid secondary infection

SURGICAL MEASURES N/A

ACTIVITY As tolerated. Children may return to school when lesions have scabbed over, temperature is normal and sense of well-being has returned.

DIET No special diet

PATIENT EDUCATION Griffith: Instructions for Patients; Philadelphia, 1994, W.B. Saunders Co.

Chickenpox

MEDICATIONS

DRUG(S) OF CHOICE
• Antipyretics for fever
• Avoid aspirin because of its link to Reye's syndrome
• Local and/or systemic antipruritic agents for itching
• In immunocompromised host, then varicella-zoster immune globulin (VZIG) available for passive immunization. VZIG must be given within 96 hours after exposure to be beneficial. After 4th day postexposure, wait for rash to develop then give acyclovir 500 mg/m2/day intravenously every 8 hours for 7 days.
• Acyclovir - decreases duration of fever and shortens time of viral shedding. Recommended for adolescents, adults and high-risk patients. Most beneficial if initiated early in the disease (≤ 24 hours).
   ◊ 2-16 yr: 20 mg/kg/dose (max. 800 mg/dose), qid for 5 days
   ◊ Adults: 800 mg, 5 times daily.
Contraindications: Hypersensitivity to the drug
Precautions: Possible renal insufficiency with acyclovir
Significant possible interactions: Concurrent administration of probenecid increases half-life. Increased effect with zidovudine (drowsiness, lethargy)

ALTERNATIVE DRUGS
• Famciclovir
• Vidarabine
• Interferon

FOLLOWUP

PATIENT MONITORING Usually none in mild cases. If complications occur, intensive supportive care may be required.

PREVENTION/AVOIDANCE
• Exposed, susceptible individuals considered infectious for 21 days
• Isolation of hospitalized patients
• Passive immunization with VZIG for immunocompromised
• Varicella-Virus vaccine (Varivax) - a live attenuated vaccine approved by the FDA for immunization of healthy individuals, 12 months and above, who have not had chickenpox. Duration of immunity is unknown
   ◊ 12m-12y: single dose 0.5 mL SC. Cumulative efficacy 70-90%
   ◊ 13y and above: two 0.5 mL SC doses 4-8 weeks apart. Efficacy 70%
• Vaccine recipients should avoid contact with immunocompromised people, and pregnant women who have never had chickenpox and their newborns, for up to 6 weeks after vaccination

POSSIBLE COMPLICATIONS
• Secondary bacterial infection - cellulitis, abscess, erysipelas, sepsis, septic arthritis/osteomyelitis, staphylococcal pyomyositis
• Pneumonia (20-30% of adults with chickenpox have lung involvement)
• Encephalitis (the most common CNS complication)
• Reye's syndrome
• Purpura
• Lymphadenitis
• Nephritis

EXPECTED COURSE/PROGNOSIS
• In the healthy child, chickenpox is rarely a serious disease and recovery is complete
• Confers long immunity
• Second attach rare, but subclinical infection common
• Infection latent and may recur years later as herpes zoster in adults (and sometimes in children)
• Fatalities rarely occur from complications

MISCELLANEOUS

ASSOCIATED CONDITIONS N/A

AGE-RELATED FACTORS
Pediatric:
• Neonates born to mothers who develop chickenpox 5 days before or 2 days after delivery are at risk for serious disease. Must give VZIG.
• Varicella bullosa seen mainly in children under two. Lesions appear as bullae instead of vesicles. Clinical course unchanged.
• Case-fatality (in USA) 2/100,000
• Most common cause of death: septic complications and encephalitis
Geriatric:
• Infection more severe than in children
• Latent varicella infection may reactivate and cause the exanthem shingles or zoster
• Case-fatality 30/100,000
• Most common cause of death: primary viral pneumonia
Others: N/A

PREGNANCY Risk of transplacental infection following maternal infection is 25%. Congenital malformations are seen in 5% when the fetus is infected during the 1st or 2nd trimester. There is an increased morbidity for women infected during pregnancy (e.g., pneumonia)

SYNONYMS
• Varicella

ICD-9-CM
052.9 Varicella without mention of complication

SEE ALSO
• Immunizations
• Herpes Zoster

OTHER NOTES N/A

ABBREVIATIONS
DNA = deoxyribonucleic acid
FA = direct fluorescent or immunofluorescent antibody test
EM = electron microscopy
PCR = polymerase chain reaction
VZIG = varicella-zoster immune globulin
VZV = varicella-zoster vaccine

REFERENCES
• Mandell GL, ed: Principles and Practice of Infectious Diseases. 4th Ed. New York, Churchill Livingstone, 1995
• Benenson, AS, ed: Control of Communicable Diseases Manual. 16th ed. Baltimore, United Book Press, Inc, 1995.
Illustrations: 6 available on CD-ROM
Internet references: http://www.5mcc.com

Author(s)
Vicente J. Arano, MD

Child abuse

BASICS

DESCRIPTION
• Emotional abuse: sustained, repetitive, inappropriate emotional response to the child's experience of emotion and its accompanying expressive behavior
• Psychological abuse: sustained, repetitive, inappropriate behavior which damages or substantially reduces the creative and developmental potential of crucially important mental faculties and mental processes of a child
• Physical abuse: (most frequent type) injury to a child caused by a caretaker for no apparent reason including reaction to unwanted behavior. The use of an instrument on any part of the body is abuse, i.e., belt.
• Sexual abuse: any contact or interaction between a child and another person in which the child is sexually exploited for the gratification or profit of the perpetrator. Offenders can be juveniles.
• Neglect: occurs when those responsible for meeting the basic needs of a child fail to do so
System(s) affected: Nervous, Reproductive, Endocrine/Metabolic; Skeletal, Gastrointestinal, Skin/Exocrine
Genetics: N/A
Incidence/Prevalence in USA: More than 1 million per year
Predominant age: 7 years old
Predominant sex: Male = Female

SIGNS AND SYMPTOMS
• Non-specific symptoms of abuse
  ◊ Behavior regression
  ◊ Anxiety, depression
  ◊ Sleep disturbances, night terrors
  ◊ Increased sex play
  ◊ School problems
  ◊ Self-destructive behaviors
• Physical abuse
  ◊ May be no physical signs
  ◊ Skin markings (lacerations, burns, ecchymoses, linear contusions)
  ◊ Contusions with definite shapes (coat hangers, belt buckles)
  ◊ Circular contusions on trunks or limbs (finger pressure points)
  ◊ Bites
  ◊ Cigarette burns on palms, extremities
  ◊ Immersion injuries with clearly demarcated lines
  ◊ Oral trauma (torn frenulum, loose teeth)
  ◊ Ear trauma (ear pulling)
  ◊ Eye trauma (hyphema, hemorrhage, hematomas)
  ◊ Abdominal blunt trauma
  ◊ Fractures
  ◊ Head trauma
• Sexual abuse
  ◊ Unequivocal abnormalities are found in a small number of children (2-8%)
  ◊ Abuse often consists of fondling, rubbing and other contacts not likely to produce detectable injuries
  ◊ Unexplained vaginal injuries or bleeding
  ◊ Pregnancy
  ◊ Sexually transmitted diseases
  ◊ Sexual promiscuity/prostitution

◊ Erythema and increased vascularity of the perihymenal tissues
◊ Increased friability of the posterior fourchette
◊ Hymenal attenuation and asymmetry, lacerations, especially if hymenal margin is altered
◊ Perianal lacerations, scars and fissures, circumferential edema (Tyre sign), delta-shaped abrasion
◊ May be no physical signs
• Neglect
◊ May be small, scrawny, dirty, with rashes
◊ Fearful or too trusting
◊ Clinging to or avoiding mother
◊ Flat or balding occiput
◊ Abnormal development or growth parameters

CAUSES Not well-defined

RISK FACTORS May be many, but poverty (5 times greater risk), parental substance abuse, lower educational status, maternal history of abuse and negative maternal attitude toward pregnancy appear to be strongly associated, history of parent(s) having been abused, mentally ill parent, parental isolation

DIAGNOSIS

DIFFERENTIAL DIAGNOSIS
• Physical trauma
  ◊ Accidental injury
  ◊ Bleeding disorders (e.g., classic hemophilia)
  ◊ Metabolic diseases (e.g., vitamin K deficiency)
  ◊ Congenital (type I Ehlers-Danlos syndrome)
  ◊ Salicylate toxicity
  ◊ Conditions with skin manifestations: Mongolian spots, Schönlein-Henoch purpura, purpura fulminans of meningococcemia, erythema multiforme, hypersensitivity vasculitis, platelet aggregation disorders, disseminated intravascular coagulation (DIC), phytophotodermatitis, car seat burns, staphylococcal scalded skin syndrome, chicken pox, impetigo, osteogenesis imperfecta, congenital syphilis
• Neglect
  ◊ Endocrinopathies (e.g., diabetes mellitus, diabetes insipidus, thyroid disorders, adrenal problems, pituitary problems)
  ◊ Constitutional
  ◊ GI (clefts, chalasia, gastroesophageal reflux, celiac disease, inflammatory bowel disease)
  ◊ Cystic fibrosis
  ◊ Liver disease
  ◊ Renal tubular acidosis
  ◊ CNS abnormalities
• Skeletal trauma
  ◊ Obstetrical trauma
  ◊ Prematurity
  ◊ Nutritional - metabolic defects (scurvy, rickets, mucolipidosis II, secondary hyperparathyroidism)
  ◊ Infection (congenital syphilis,

osteomyelitis)
  ◊ Osteogenesis imperfecta
  ◊ Infantile cortical hyperostosis
  ◊ Leukemia
  ◊ Histiocytosis X
  ◊ Metastatic neuroblastoma

LABORATORY
• Urinalysis, urine culture and sensitivity
• CBC
• Electrolytes, creatinine, BUN, glucose
• Some would add PT, PTT, bleeding time, platelet count, factor XIII, urine toxicology screen
Drugs that may alter lab results: Usually none
Disorders that may alter lab results: See Differential Diagnosis

PATHOLOGICAL FINDINGS
• Spiral fractures in non-ambulatory patients
• Chip fractures or bucket-handle fractures (classic for abuse)
• Epiphyseal - metaphyseal rib fractures in infants
• Rupture of liver and spleen in abdominal blunt trauma
• Retinal hemorrhages in shaken baby syndrome
• Abnormalities strongly suggesting sexual abuse include: Recent or healed lacerations of the hymen and vaginal mucosa, procto-episiotomy, bite marks
• The presence of sperm is a definitive finding of child abuse

SPECIAL TESTS
• Sexual abuse
  ◊ Wet mount for motile sperm and one fixed for cytopathology exam for sperm
  ◊ Tests for gonorrhea, chlamydia
  ◊ Serum pregnancy tests
  ◊ Rapid plasma reagin (RPR)
  ◊ Consider HIV testing (needs to be repeated in 6 months)
  ◊ Acid phosphatase test of secretions for sperm
  ◊ If the assault occurred within 72 hours of the examination, samples should be collected for the forensic laboratory (contact police investigator for proper protocol)
• Neglect
  ◊ Stool exam
  ◊ Calorie count
  ◊ Purified protein derivative (PPD) and anergy panel
  ◊ Sweat test
  ◊ Lead and zinc protoporphyrin levels

IMAGING
• Photographs
• Chest x-ray, skeletal survey (skull frontal and lateral, lateral thoracolumbar spine, frontal upper extremities to include shoulder girdle and hands, frontal lower extremities to include lower lumbar spine, pelvis and feet)
• In some hospitals a standard set of x-rays called a SNAT (suspected non-accidental trauma) series is defined
• Possible bone scan

DIAGNOSTIC PROCEDURES Consider photocolposcopy in sexual abuse

Child abuse

TREATMENT

APPROPRIATE HEALTH CARE
• Acute episodes, especially of sexual abuse, are often best managed in an emergency room equipped for collecting forensic specimens and maintaining "chain of evidence"
• Hospital admission for children with moderate to severe injuries, unstable neurologic or cardiovascular exams and those with acute psychological trauma
• If not hospitalized, a child should be sent to another relative or arrange for foster care if the suspected abuser lives with the child
• Counseling is imperative
• Mandatory reporting to Child Protective Authorities
• Counseling for entire family

GENERAL MEASURES
• After initial evaluation, consider referral to sexual assault center
• Always explain what the physical exam will involve and why certain procedures are necessary
• Examine child in a quiet, comfortable setting and allow child to choose who will be in the room
• To examine female genitalia, use dorsolithotomy position for older girls and the "frog leg" position for younger girls
• Examine anus of all young children in prone knee-chest position

SURGICAL MEASURES   As clinically indicated

ACTIVITY   As clinically indicated

DIET   As clinically indicated

PATIENT EDUCATION   Counsel family not to use negative terms such as "ruined," "violated," or "dirty" in reference to the child. The child's emotional reaction to abuse will be profoundly influenced by the responses of adult caretakers.

MEDICATIONS

DRUG(S) OF CHOICE   Antibiotics as indicated for treatment of documented sexually-transmitted disease
Contraindications: Refer to manufacturer's profile of each drug
Precautions: Refer to manufacturer's profile of each drug
Significant possible interactions: Refer to manufacturer's profile of each drug

ALTERNATIVE DRUGS   Other postcoital contraceptive drugs

FOLLOWUP

PATIENT MONITORING   Patient must be referred to the appropriate state protective services and followed as closely as clinically and psychologically indicated

PREVENTION/AVOIDANCE   Early detection of and intervention in dysfunctional families whenever possible

POSSIBLE COMPLICATIONS   Long-term physical and psychological damage

EXPECTED COURSE/PROGNOSIS
Without intervention, child abuse is a recurrent and escalating phenomenon

MISCELLANEOUS

ASSOCIATED CONDITIONS
• Failure-to-thrive
• Shortfalls in development
• Poor school performance
• Poor social skills
• Psychological illnesses

AGE-RELATED FACTORS
Pediatric: N/A
Geriatric: N/A
Others: N/A

PREGNANCY   Use of ethinyl estradiol and norgestrel (Ovral) reduces rate of pregnancy after rape to under 2% which is one-third the rate that would be expected without intervention. It is thought to work by making the uterine lining inhospitable to implantation and must be considered an abortifacient in this setting.

SYNONYMS
• Battered child syndrome
• SNAT

ICD-9-CM
999.5

SEE ALSO   N/A

OTHER NOTES   When documenting an examination on an allegedly or suspected abused child, especially in cases of possible sexual abuse, never record "findings not consistent with abuse" or "no evidence of abuse." Simply record findings and note that the findings neither exclude nor confirm allegations of abuse. The absence of physical findings does not indicate the child's history is incorrect.

ABBREVIATIONS
SNAT = suspected non-accidental trauma

REFERENCES
• Reece RM, ed: Pediatric Clinics of North America, Vol 37, No. 4. Philadelphia, W.B. Saunders Co, August 1990
• Rosenstein BJ, Fosarelli PD: Pediatric Pearls. Yearbook Medical Publishers, Inc, 1989:330-334
• Flaherty EG, Weiss H: Medical Evaluation of Abused and Neglected Children. American Journal of Diseases of Children 1990;144
• Muram D: Child Sexual Abuse. Obstetrics and Gynecology Clinics of North America 1992;19(1)
• Child Abuse and Neglect Statistical Fact Sheet. National Clearinghouse on Child Abuse Information, 1996
• Gibbons M, Vincent EC: Childhood Sexual Abuse. Amer Fam Phys 1994;49:125-136
• O'Hagan KP: Emotional and psychological abuse: Problems of definition. Child Abuse and Neglect 1995;19:4
Illustrations: 3 available on CD-ROM
Internet references: http://www.5mcc.com

Author(s)
Sumner T. McAllister, MD
Bruce T. Vanderhoff, MD

- 215 -

Chlamydia pneumoniae

 BASICS

DESCRIPTION
Chlamydia pneumoniae, an obligate intracellular bacteria, has been established as an important cause of adult respiratory disease including pneumonia, bronchitis, sinusitis and pharyngitis. There is no animal reservoir.

System(s) affected: Pulmonary
Genetics: No known genetic predisposition
Incidence/Prevalence in USA: Estimated incidence of 100 to 200 cases of pneumonia/100,000/year. Accounts for 6 to 12% of pneumonias and 3 to 6% of bronchitis cases. Studies to date have included relatively few geographic areas. Numbers do not necessarily apply to all areas. Incidence of subclinical infection much greater.
Predominant age: Uncommon in children under 5 years. Pneumonia more common in elderly.
Predominant sex: Male > Female (10-25% more)

SIGNS AND SYMPTOMS
• 70% to 90% of infections are mild or subclinical
• Onset often gradual with delayed presentation
• Sore throat and hoarseness may precede cough by a week or more, giving biphasic appearance to illness
• Cough (often prominent with scant sputum)
• Fever (usually early in illness)
• Sore throat
• Rhinitis
• Headache
• Malaise
• Hoarseness
• Sinus congestion
• Rales, rhonchi or wheezing
• Pharyngeal erythema
• Sinus tenderness

CAUSES
Infection with C. pneumoniae

RISK FACTORS
Outbreaks have occurred among groups of military recruits, university students, boarding school students and school children

 DIAGNOSIS

DIFFERENTIAL DIAGNOSIS
• Definite diagnosis requires positive serology or culture
• Consider other common bacterial respiratory pathogens, including Streptococcus, Bordetella, Hemophilus, Klebsiella, Mycoplasma and Legionella species

LABORATORY
• Leukocyte count usually normal or low
• Sedimentation rate often moderately elevated
• Sputum usually negative by gram stain and routine culture
Drugs that may alter lab results: Early treatment with tetracycline may blunt IgG antibody response
Disorders that may alter lab results: None known

PATHOLOGICAL FINDINGS
Not usually available

SPECIAL TESTS
• Most easily cultured in HL or HEp2 cells
• Complement fixation (CF) serology for Chlamydia widely available but cannot distinguish C. pneumoniae infection from C. psittaci
• Microimmunofluorescence (MIF) test, which is specific for C. pneumoniae, is available at some research institutions or commercially (from American Medical Laboratories, MRL Diagnostics)
• Every effort should be made to obtain paired sera. The convalescent sera should be obtained 3 weeks after disease onset.
• Four-fold antibody rise diagnostic of acute infection
• Presence of IgM antibody ($\geq$ 1:16) or of high IgG antibody titers ($\geq$ 1:512) by MIF suggests a recent or acute infection
• Polymerase chain reaction (PCR) from pharyngeal swab or bronchoalveolar lavage specimen

IMAGING
• Chest radiograph may be abnormal even in clinically mild disease
• Variable radiographic abnormalities include unilateral and bilateral infiltrates and pleural effusions

DIAGNOSTIC PROCEDURES
None

 TREATMENT

APPROPRIATE HEALTH CARE
• Usually outpatient
• Patients with severe pneumonia or coexisting illness may require hospitalization

GENERAL MEASURES
No specific general measures

SURGICAL MEASURES
N/A

ACTIVITY
Usually reduced during illness

DIET
No special diet

PATIENT EDUCATION
• Griffith HW: Instructions for Patients; Philadelphia, W.B. Saunders Co.
• For a listing of sources for patient education materials favorably reviewed on this topic, physicians may contact: American Academy of Family Physicians Foundation, P.O. Box 8418, Kansas City, MO 64114, (800)274-2237, ext. 4400

MEDICATIONS

DRUG(S) OF CHOICE
• Azithromycin (Zithromax) 500 mg on day 1, then 250 mg a day on days 2 through 5
or
• Clarithromycin (Biaxin) 500 mg po every 12 hours for 10-14 days
or
• Tetracycline 500 mg po qid for at least 14 days
or
• Doxycycline 100 mg po q 12 hours for at least 14 days
Contraindications:
• Tetracycline not for use in pregnancy or children < 8 years.
Precautions: Tetracycline may cause photosensitivity; sunscreen recommended.
Significant possible interactions:
• Tetracyclines may increase the anticoagulant effect of warfarin
• Broad-spectrum antibiotics may reduce the effectiveness of oral contraceptives; barrier method recommended.

ALTERNATIVE DRUGS
• Erythromycin base 250-500 mg qid for 14-21 days
• Beta-lactam (penicillin based) antibiotics and sulfisoxazole not effective

FOLLOWUP

PATIENT MONITORING
Weekly until well, for response to treatment and resolution of radiographic abnormalities

PREVENTION/AVOIDANCE
• Transmission presumably via respiratory secretions. Avoid infected persons.
• Hand washing

POSSIBLE COMPLICATIONS
• Reactive airway disease
• Erythema nodosum
• Otitis media
• Endocarditis
• Myocarditis
• Pericarditis
• Sarcoidosis
• Meningitis
• Reactive arthritis

EXPECTED COURSE/PROGNOSIS
• Resolution of cough and malaise often requires several weeks or longer
• Chronic bronchospastic disease has been reported following acute infection
• Persistent or relapsed symptoms may respond to second course of antibiotics

MISCELLANEOUS

ASSOCIATED CONDITIONS
• Chronic obstructive pulmonary disease
• HIV infection
• Cystic fibrosis

AGE-RELATED FACTORS
Pediatric: Usually milder disease in children
Geriatric: Usually more severe in older adults
Others: None known

PREGNANCY
• No known special risks
• Tetracyclines contraindicated

SYNONYMS
• TWAR

ICD-9-CM
078.89 Chlamydia pneumoniae

SEE ALSO
• Pneumonia, Mycoplasma
• Psittacosis

OTHER NOTES
• No significant seasonal variation
• Most cases occur sporadically, though intrafamilial spread also occurs
• Infection in debilitated or hospitalized patients can be severe
• Reinfection is possible
• Individuals have been reported who are persistently culture positive despite antibiotic treatment
• Country-wide epidemics of C. pneumoniae infections have been documented in the Scandinavian countries
• Found in atherosclerotic plaque in coronary arteries, carotid arteries and the aorta. Also associated with MI and stroke in seroepidemiologic studies. Role in atherogenesis in humans not established. Clinical significance not known.

ABBREVIATIONS N/A

REFERENCES
• Grayston JT, Campbell LA, Kuo CC, et al: A new respiratory tract pathogen: Chlamydia pneumoniae strain TWAR. J Infect Dis 1990;161:618-25
• Thom DH, Grayston JT: Infections with Chlamydia pneumoniae strain TWAR. In: Winterbauer RH, ed. Clinics in Chest Medicine 1991;12(2):245-56
Illustrations: N/A
Internet references: http://www.5mcc.com

Author(s)
David H. Thom, MD, PhD
J. Thomas Grayston, MD

Chlamydial sexually transmitted diseases

BASICS

DESCRIPTION The most common STD in USA is caused by Chlamydia trachomatis serovars D-K. Among the smallest prokaryotic organisms, these obligate intracellular, membrane bound organisms cause disease that is often asymptomatic to non-specific in presentation. It is difficult to diagnose both clinically, in the lab, and difficult to provide screening. The infection has serious sequelae and its transmission is difficult to control.
System(s) affected: Reproductive
Genetics: Unknown
Incidence/Prevalence in USA:
• Males 3-5% general medical population, 15-20% STD clinics
• Females 3-5% general medical population, 20% STD clinics
Predominant age: 15-25
Predominant sex: Male = Female

SIGNS AND SYMPTOMS The majority of women infected with Chlamydia trachomatis are asymptomatic, historical variables are typically not predictive of risk. Chlamydia trachomatis has a tropism for columnar or transitional epithelium with subsequent extension to the cervix, uterus, fallopian tubes and peritoneum in females, and epididymis in males, as well as rectal epithelial cells.
• Males
  ◊ Urethritis
  ◊ Epididymitis
  ◊ Proctitis
  ◊ Reiter's syndrome
• Females
  ◊ Cervicitis - typically mucopurulent
  ◊ Urethral syndrome
  ◊ Bartholinitis
  ◊ Endometritis
  ◊ Salpingitis/pelvic inflammatory disease (PID)
  ◊ Fitz-Hugh-Curtis perihepatitis syndrome
• Infants
  ◊ Conjunctivitis
  ◊ Pneumonitis
  ◊ Carriage-pharynx/GI tract

CAUSES Chlamydia trachomatis serovars D-K

RISK FACTORS
• Sexual promiscuity
• Lower socioeconomic groups
• Prevalence correlates inversely with age

DIAGNOSIS

DIFFERENTIAL DIAGNOSIS
• Neisseria gonorrhea
  ◊ Urethritis
  ◊ Proctitis
  ◊ Epididymitis
  ◊ Cervicitis
  ◊ PID
  ◊ Bartholin's abscess
  ◊ Perihepatitis
• Ureaplasma urealyticum
  ◊ Urethritis, epididymitis
  ◊ Reiter's disease
  ◊ PID
• Chlamydia trachomatis (Serovars Ll-3)
  ◊ Lymphogranuloma venereum
  ◊ Proctitis

LABORATORY
• Chlamydial culture - costly, requires 3-7 days, 70-90% sensitive
• Antigen detection - sensitivity 50-90+%
• Monoclonal antibody direct immunofluorescence, requires experienced lab technician
• ELISA determination of eluded chlamydial antigens
Drugs that may alter lab results: N/A
Disorders that may alter lab results: N/A

PATHOLOGICAL FINDINGS N/A

SPECIAL TESTS Polymerase chain reaction test is available. Highly sensitive and specific.

IMAGING N/A

DIAGNOSTIC PROCEDURES
• Specimen collection: cell scrapings (obtain with cytology brush) rather than inflammatory discharge will improve yield since this is an epithelial cell disease
• Transport media is imperative: sucrose-phosphate media supplemented with gentamicin, vancomycin, and nystatin

TREATMENT

APPROPRIATE HEALTH CARE
Outpatient care for virtually all problems

GENERAL MEASURES
• All patients should be evaluated for syphilis and gonorrhea by appropriate Gram stains, cultures and serology.
• Empirical therapies may be indicated
• Offer HIV counseling and testing
• Evaluation and treatment of sex partners - institute empirical treatment of women who are sex partners of men with non-gonococcal urethritis is recommended. Partners of women with mucopurulent cervicitis or salpingitis should also be empirically treated. Since Chlamydial co-infection occurs with gonorrheal disease, anti-chlamydial therapy should be instituted concomitantly.

SURGICAL MEASURES N/A

ACTIVITY Sexual abstention pending elucidation and treatment of underlying infection

DIET N/A

PATIENT EDUCATION
• Risk-reduction counseling
• Safe sex practices, such as barrier protection
• Serious sequelae of Chlamydial disease i.e., tubal infertility
• Stress need to finish entire course of antibiotics
• For a listing of sources for patient education materials favorably reviewed on this topic, physicians may contact: American Academy of Family Physicians Foundation, P.O. Box 8418, Kansas City, MO 64114, (800)274-2237, ext. 4400

MEDICATIONS

DRUG(S) OF CHOICE
• Urethritis, cervicitis, sexual partners of infected persons
  ◊ Doxycycline - 100 mg po bid x 7 days
  ◊ Azithromycin - 1 gm orally in a single dose
  ◊ Pregnant women - erythromycin base, 250 mg po qid x 14 days
• Chlamydial syndromes.
  ◊ Epididymitis - tetracycline, doxycycline, erythromycin for 10-14 days as above.
  ◊ Pelvic inflammatory disease - doxycycline for 10-14 days to cover the chlamydial component of PID (gonorrhea and anaerobic organisms must be treated as well; see CDC recommendations: ceftriaxone 250 mg IM once, cefoxitin, other 3rd generation cephalosporin, or a quinolone), erythromycin for 10-14 days may be needed in pregnant or tetracycline intolerant females to treat chlamydial component.
Contraindications:
• Tetracycline: not for use in pregnancy or children < 8 years.
Precautions:
• Tetracycline: may cause photosensitivity; sunscreen recommended.
Significant possible interactions:
• Tetracycline: avoid concurrent administration with antacids, dairy products, or iron.
• Broad-spectrum antibiotics: may reduce the effectiveness of oral contraceptives; barrier method recommended.
• Erythromycin: terfenadine (Seldane); ECG abnormalities

ALTERNATIVE DRUGS
• Erythromycin base - 500 po qid x 7 days
• Ofloxacin - 300 mg po bid x 7 days (contraindicated in pregnancy)

FOLLOWUP

PATIENT MONITORING
• Test of cure is not routine, although it is reasonable to retest women weeks to months after treatment
• Sexual partners need to be evaluated and treated empirically if necessary, to prevent passing the disease back and forth between partners. Partnerships with community health departments should be fostered.
• Non-resolution or recurrence of symptoms must be immediately reported to the physician
• Severe cases of urethritis/cervicitis as well as the chlamydial syndromes should be seen in followup after completion of therapy
• Up to 25% of asymptomatic patients screened for chlamydia may not return for treatment post-chlamydia culture results. Strategies must be developed to insure treatment can be instituted.

PREVENTION/AVOIDANCE
Target populations, where prevalence of disease is > 5%, that should be screened for Chlamydia trachomatis:
• Women with mucopurulent cervicitis
• Sexually active women < 20 years of age
• Women 20-24 years of age who meet either of the following criteria or women > 24 years of age who meet both criteria:
  ◊ Inconsistent use of barrier contraception
  ◊ New or more than one sex partner during the prior 3 months
• Patients attending the following clinics:
  ◊ Adolescent clinics and family planning clinics - all adolescents < 25 years of age
    ◊ STD clinics
    ◊ Abortion clinics
    ◊ Detention center clinics
    ◊ Prenatal clinics - third trimester testing so that treatment can be administered predelivery
• Women and men with anorectal pain, tenesmus, rectal discharge
• Men with testicular pain with or without urethral discharge

POSSIBLE COMPLICATIONS
Enhances transmission of HIV
• Males
  ◊ Transient oligospermia
  ◊ Post epididymitis urethral stricture (rare)
• Females
  ◊ Tubal infertility
  ◊ Tubal pregnancy
  ◊ Chronic pelvic pain

EXPECTED COURSE/PROGNOSIS
Prognosis good with early and compliant therapy. However, due to the asymptomatic nature of early disease and the population affected, symptomatic PID still accounts annually for 2.5 million outpatient visits and more than one quarter million hospitalizations.

MISCELLANEOUS

ASSOCIATED CONDITIONS
• Pelvic inflammatory disease, epididymitis, cervicitis, urethritis
• Other diseases caused by other chlamydial species:
  ◊ Psittacosis - Chlamydia psittaci
  ◊ Pneumonia - Chlamydia pneumoniae - Chlamydia trachomatis (infants)
  ◊ Lymphogranuloma venereum - Chlamydia trachomatis serovars L1-L3
  ◊ Trachoma - Chlamydia trachomatis serovars A-C

AGE-RELATED FACTORS
Pediatric: N/A
Geriatric: N/A
Others: Prevalence inversely proportional to age after onset of sexual activity

PREGNANCY   Perinatal acquisition may result in neonatal pneumonia and/or conjunctivitis. Tetracycline and ofloxacin contraindicated in pregnancy. Erythromycin should be used in this situation.

SYNONYMS N/A

ICD-9-CM
615 Inflammatory diseases of uterus, except cervix
616 Inflammatory diseases of cervix, vagina, and vulva

SEE ALSO
• Pelvic inflammatory disease (PID)
• Epididymitis
• Cervicitis
• Urethritis
• HIV infection & AIDS
• Gonococcal infections
• Syphilis

OTHER NOTES N/A

ABBREVIATIONS
• STD = sexually transmitted disease
• PID = pelvic inflammatory disease
• HIV = human immunodeficiency virus
• CBD = common bile duct

REFERENCES
• Stamm WE, Holmes K, et al: Chlamydia trachomatis Infections in the Adult. In: Sexually Transmitted Diseases. 2nd Ed. New York, McGraw-Hill, 1990
• Centers for Disease Control and Prevention: Sexually transmitted disease treatment guidelines. MMWR 1993.42 (no. RR-14): 50-52
• Hook EW III, et al: Use of cell culture and a rapid diagnostic assay for Chlamydia trachomatis screening. JAMA 1995;272(11):867
• Heath C, Heath J: Chlamydia trachomatis infection update. Am Fam Phys 1995;52:1455-1461
Illustrations: N/A
Internet references: http://www.5mcc.com

Author(s)
Richard M. Mandel, MD
Henry Arguinchona, MD

Cholangitis

BASICS

DESCRIPTION Bacterial inflammation of the bile duct system that is associated with obstructive biliary duct pathology. May be acute or chronic.
System(s) affected: Gastrointestinal
Genetics: N/A
Incidence/Prevalence in USA: N/A
Predominant age: 55-70 years, rare in children, more common in adults
Predominant sex: Female > Male

SIGNS AND SYMPTOMS
May have only one or two symptoms, and the abdominal exam may be unrevealing
• Right upper quadrant pain (RUQ), not severe
• Jaundice
• Chills and fever
• Shock
• CNS depression

CAUSES
• Biliary tract obstruction from:
  ◊ Stones
  ◊ Tumor (pancreatic, CBD, ampulla, metastatic)
  ◊ Benign strictures (postsurgical, PSC)
  ◊ Parasites (Ascaris)
  ◊ Pancreatitis
  ◊ Blood clots
• Reflux of small bowel bacteria
  ◊ Choledochoenterostomy
  ◊ "Sump syndrome"
• Other
  ◊ Cholecystitis
  ◊ Bacteriemia
  ◊ Surgical, radiographic, endoscopic manipulation

RISK FACTORS
• Cholelithiasis
• Endoscopic or surgical manipulation
• Foreign bodies, such as parasites

DIAGNOSIS

DIFFERENTIAL DIAGNOSIS
• Acute cholecystitis - pain and tenderness are invariably present. (May be very difficult to distinguish between cholangitis and acute cholecystitis).
• Pyogenic liver abscess
• Hepatitis
• Acute pancreatitis
• Perforated duodenal ulcer
• Pelvic inflammatory disease with peritonitis
• Kidney stones

LABORATORY
• Increasing WBC with left shift
• Hyperbilirubinemia - in 90%
• Alkaline phosphatase - increasing in 90%
• Positive blood culture - in 50% (gram negative aerobes, and some anaerobes)
Drugs that may alter lab results: N/A
Disorders that may alter lab results: N/A

PATHOLOGICAL FINDINGS
In acute toxic disease, pus under pressure in the common bile duct

SPECIAL TESTS
• Need to delineate underlying biliary tract abnormality
• Cholangiography is definitive test
• Percutaneous transhepatic cholangiography (PTC) or endoscopic retrograde cholangiopancreatography (ERCP)

IMAGING
Ultrasound will diagnose gallbladder stones and common bile duct size, but will demonstrate common bile duct calculi in less than 15%

DIAGNOSTIC PROCEDURES N/A

TREATMENT

APPROPRIATE HEALTH CARE Inpatient

GENERAL MEASURES Control sepsis, then evaluate with cholangiography and treat underlying biliary tract pathology

SURGICAL MEASURES
• Patients who do not respond to antibiotics and supportive care require emergency decompression of the biliary duct system. This may be accomplished by surgery, endoscopy, or transhepatic cholangiography.
• In case of obstruction secondary to stones, endoscopic papillotomy and stone extraction will drain the duct and may be definitive treatment of the underlying cause and is shown to reduce mortality

ACTIVITY As tolerated

DIET Nothing by mouth until acute phase is terminated

PATIENT EDUCATION For patient education materials favorably reviewed on this topic, contact: National Digestive Diseases Information Clearinghouse, Box NDDIC, Bethesda, MD 20892, (301)468-6344

MEDICATIONS

DRUG(S) OF CHOICE
• Antibiotic regimen should cover gram negative aerobes, enterococci, and anaerobes.
 ◊ Ampicillin 1 gm q6h IV (substitute ciprofloxacin in penicillin allergic patient) +
 ◊ Aminoglycoside (e.g., tobramycin, amikacin is an alternative but is expensive) +
 ◊ Metronidazole 500 mg q8h IV
Contraindications: Refer to manufacturer's profile of each drug
Precautions: Renal toxicity of aminoglycoside therapy; check peak and trough levels
Significant possible interactions: Refer to manufacturer's profile of each drug

ALTERNATIVE DRUGS   N/A

FOLLOWUP

PATIENT MONITORING   Requires careful monitoring of hemodynamic parameters

PREVENTION/AVOIDANCE
Cholangiography when indicated at time of cholecystectomy with endoscopic, radiographic, or surgical clearance of retained CBD stones

POSSIBLE COMPLICATIONS
• Most serious is hepatic abscess
• Sepsis
• Secondary sclerosing cholangitis

EXPECTED COURSE/PROGNOSIS
• Acute cholangitis - good
• Acute toxic cholangitis - mortality high

MISCELLANEOUS

ASSOCIATED CONDITIONS
• Choledocholithiasis
• Malignant tumors
• Benign strictures
• Biliary-enteric anastamosis
• Invasive procedures
• Foreign bodies
• Parasites
• Secondary sclerosing cholangitis

AGE-RELATED FACTORS
Pediatric: N/A
Geriatric: N/A
Others: N/A

PREGNANCY   N/A

SYNONYMS   N/A

ICD-9-CM   576.1 Cholangitis

SEE ALSO   Cholelithiasis

OTHER NOTES   N/A

ABBREVIATIONS   N/A

REFERENCES
• Nahrwold DL: Cholangitis. In: Sabiston DC, ed. Textbook of Surgery. 13th Ed. Philadelphia, W.B. Saunders Co., 1986
• Boeg JH, Way LW: Acute Cholangitis. Ann Surg 1980;191:264
• Pitt HA, Longmire WP Jr: Suppurative Cholangitis. In: Hardy JM, ed. Critical Surgical Illness. 2nd Ed. Philadelphia, W.B. Saunders Co., 1980
Illustrations: N/A
Internet references: http://www.5mcc.com

Author(s)
Leo C. Mercer, MD

Cholecystitis

BASICS

DESCRIPTION
Inflammation of the gallbladder occurring acutely or chronically, often secondary to previously asymptomatic gallstones.
System(s) affected: Gastrointestinal
Genetics: Increased prevalence in Native Americans and Caucasians, less prevalent in African Americans
Incidence/Prevalence in USA:
• Steady increase with age, varies in different ethnic groups. Percentage with gallstones (approximately half will develop symptoms over their lifetime):
◊ By age 30, 30% of Native Americans
◊ By age 60, 80% of Native Americans
◊ By age 60, 30% of Caucasians
◊ By age 60, 20% of African Americans
Predominant age: 5th and 6th decade
Predominant sex: Female > Male (2:1)

SIGNS AND SYMPTOMS
• Asymptomatic. 5-10% become symptomatic each year.
• Acute cholecystitis
◊ Abdominal pain - sudden onset, intense, in epigastrium or right upper quadrant, radiates to shoulder or back. Pathognomonic feature is "biliary colic" a pain rising over 2-3 minutes to a plateau of intensity that is maintained for > 20 minutes.
◊ Nausea and vomiting
◊ Recurrent attacks following meals by 1-6 hours, lasting > 12 hours until recovered, usually < 3 days
◊ Elevated temperature - mild to moderate
◊ Local tenderness, rarely diffuse
◊ Murphy's sign - inspiratory arrest elicited when palpating right upper quadrant while asking the patient for deep inhalation
◊ Palpable gall bladder - 5% of cases
• Common duct stone
◊ Jaundice in 50%
◊ Biliary colic 60%
◊ Fever and chills 30%
◊ Pruritus 10%
◊ Loose bowel movements, light color
◊ Mild to marked hepatomegaly > 80%
◊ Tenderness infrequent
◊ Palpable gall bladder 10%
◊ Gallstone ileus (rare)
◊ Gallstone > 3 cm fistulizes into bowel and obstructs at ileocecal area
◊ Antecedent pain, often over weeks with non-biliary colic
◊ Abdominal distension, mild tenderness
◊ Air in biliary passages on plain x-ray
◊ Intestinal obstruction at level of terminal ileum
• Pancreatitis
◊ Pain over upper abdomen
◊ Nausea and vomiting
• Empyema
◊ Phlegmon of obstructed gall bladder
◊ Insidious weight loss, mild wasting
◊ Gradual onset of occult infection signs, fever, anorexia
◊ Mass usually present
◊ Tenderness usually absent

• Chronic cholecystitis
◊ Associated with gallstones, often asymptomatic; 20% become symptomatic over 15-20 years
◊ Mild dyspepsia following fatty meals

CAUSES
• Gallstones - 90-95% of cases. As they migrate along the biliary passages, they may cause obstruction of cystic duct, leading to acute cholecystitis; obstruction of the common bile duct, causing jaundice, or obstruction of the pancreatic duct, causing pancreatitis.
• Gall bladder sludge - a viscous material, insoluble in bile that layers on sonogram, and occasionally produces cholecystitis, common duct obstruction or pancreatitis. Occurs in most pregnant women, most total parenteral nutrition, and most patients with rapid weight loss
• Acalculous cholecystitis - 5% of cases. Associated with severe stressful situations including cardiac surgery, multiple trauma. May be associated with ischemic damage to the gall bladder wall.
• Bacteria - usually do not initiate the inflammation but important in the complications of empyema and ascending cholangitis. In emphysematous cholecystitis, clostridia are probably responsible for both initiation and complications.
• Neoplasms and strictures of common bile duct - usually associated with cholangitis and pancreatitis.
• Ischemia - in patients with diabetes, but uncommon
• Torsion - lost fixation of gallbladder, uncommon

RISK FACTORS
• Cardiac surgery
• Trauma
• Biliary parasites
• Gallstones (see topic Cholelithiasis)
• Rapid weight loss
• Prolonged parenteral alimentation
• Pregnancy

DIAGNOSIS

DIFFERENTIAL DIAGNOSIS
Acute pancreatitis, ulcer, diverticulitis, pyelonephritis, pneumonitis, hepatic abscess, hepatic tumors, Irritable bowel disease, non-ulcer dyspepsia

LABORATORY
• Acute cholecystitis
◊ Leukocytosis - 12,000-15,000
◊ Liver tests usually abnormal; ALT, AST slightly elevated, alkaline phosphatase, GGT elevated with common duct obstruction
• Common duct stone
◊ High bilirubin in 50%, in 100% after 10 days
◊ Elevated alkaline phosphatase and gamma glutamyl transpeptidase (GGT) in 85%
◊ Positive blood culture in 15%
◊ Barely abnormal ALT, AST
◊ Elevated fasting bile salts

◊ Elevated WBC if infection
◊ Serum amylase may be elevated. If > 1000 units, concomitant pancreatitis should be considered.
Drugs that may alter lab results:
• Steroids
• Immunosuppressive drugs. These may mask leukocytosis and early signs of inflammation.
Disorders that may alter lab results:
• Old age, malnutrition
• Lymphoma, other immunocompromised states

PATHOLOGICAL FINDINGS   N/A

SPECIAL TESTS
99mTc Imino diacetic acid (HIDA) scan - highly sensitive (97%) for diagnosis of acute cholecystitis. HIDA derivatives are taken up by hepatocytes and excreted in bile and concentrated in gallbladder. Failure to see gallbladder in 1 hour is highly suspicious for acute cholecystitis. Usually abnormal in acalculous cholecystitis.

IMAGING
• Plain radiographs (upright)
◊ 20% of gallstones are radio-opaque
◊ Air cholangiogram if there is gallbladder-gut fistula
◊ Emphysematous cholecystitis - air in the gallbladder wall or in lumen
• Ultrasonography
◊ Best technique to diagnose gallstones (high sensitivity - 95%, and specificity - 98%)
◊ Best noninvasive imaging technique to diagnose acute cholecystitis. Findings include thick gall bladder wall (> 3 mm), gallbladder distension, sludge in lumen, pericholecystic fluid.
• CT scan
◊ No advantage over ultrasonography in gallstone/acute cholecystitis diagnosis
◊ Better than ultrasonography to detect enlargement of pancreas. Helpful in the diagnosis of abscess formation. Shows thickened gall bladder wall in cancer.
◊ Better than US for dilated common bile duct

DIAGNOSTIC PROCEDURES
• Ultrasound or CT scan often diagnostic
• Tc HIDA test during acute pain
• Endoscopic retrograde cholangiopancreatography (ERCP) - to see status of biliary and pancreatic ducts
• Percutaneous transhepatic cholangiography test (PTC) - gives more information about intrahepatic biliary system
• Laparotomy - if unable to make diagnosis by less invasive means

TREATMENT

APPROPRIATE HEALTH CARE
• Outpatient for patients with mild symptoms
• Inpatient - patients with biliary colic lasting for more than 6 hours and showing toxicity, jaundice, rigors, or requiring narcotics for pain
• Ascending cholangitis is a surgical emergency. If laparotomy is inappropriate, drainage can be obtained by ERCP or transhepatic cholangiography.
• Direct drainage of gallbladder by invasive radiologist occasionally required

GENERAL MEASURES
NPO, IV fluids, nasogastric suction

SURGICAL MEASURES
• Surgery (cholecystectomy) is the appropriate treatment for symptomatic cholecystitis. Best performed by laparoscopy if available, but a standard laparotomy is acceptable. Mortality rate - 0.1% in age < 50 years and 0.8% age > 50.
• If there is jaundice, exploration of the common bile duct is essential at open laparotomy, or by a separate ERCP. Mortality rate for laparotomy is 0.1% < 50 years and 0.8% > 50 years. In acute cholecystitis - early cholecystectomy is the general practice rather than delayed interval cholecystectomy (delay only if surgery is contraindicated)
• Laparoscopic cholecystostomy - rapidly replacing alternative surgical drainage procedure. If the patient is a poor risk, drainage of the gallbladder or biliary passages can be achieved by radiological or endoscopic techniques. This will allow control of infection and jaundice for several weeks or months.
• Dissolution therapy - infrequently used if laparoscopic cholecystectomy can be performed. Ursodeoxycholic acid (Actigall) in 10 mg/kg is the drug of choice. To be effective there must be a functioning gallbladder on oral cholecystography. Stones must be free of calcium. Many small stones have best prognosis to dissolve. An alternative drug is chenodeoxycholic acid (Chenodiol) 12-15 mg/kg/day.
• Other indications for emergency surgery include - toxic patient, doubtful diagnosis, perforation or abscess

ACTIVITY
As tolerated by the patient

DIET
• NPO during acute cholecystitis
• Fatty meals precipitate mild attacks. Avoid if possible.

PATIENT EDUCATION
National Digestive Diseases Information Clearinghouse, Box NDDIC, Bethesda, MD 20892, (301) 468-6344

MEDICATIONS

DRUG(S) OF CHOICE
• Mild attack
  ◊ Diclofenac 75 mg IV may abort early attack
  ◊ Ampicillin 4-6 gm/day or cefazolin (Ancef) 2-4 gm/day
• Severe attack - gentamicin 3-5 mg/kg/day and clindamycin 1.8-2.7 gm/day. A penicillin could be added if needed.
• The formation of gallstones during rapid weight loss after bariatric surgery or severe diets is prevented by ursodiol (ursodeoxycholic acid) 10 mg/kg/day
• Formation of gallstones in prolonged parenteral alimentation is prevented by daily feeding of 100 kcal or daily injection of cholecystokinin
Contraindications: Hypersensitivity reactions
Precautions:
• Nephrotoxicity, ototoxicity with aminoglycosides
• Adjust the dose according to creatinine clearance
Significant possible interactions: Refer to manufacturer's profile of each drug

ALTERNATIVE DRUGS
For acute cholecystitis - 3rd generation cephalosporins

FOLLOWUP

PATIENT MONITORING
Post cholecystectomy - follow through postoperative period

PREVENTION/AVOIDANCE
• Avoid risk factors when possible
• During rapid weight loss following bariatric surgery or very low calorie diets, ursodeoxycholic acid (ursodiol)10 mg/kg/day
• During total parenteral alimentation for more than one month, daily ingestion of 100 kcal, or injection of cholecystokinin

POSSIBLE COMPLICATIONS
Occur in about 5% cases of acute cholecystitis and include - perforation, abscess formation, fistula formation (intestine, colon, cutaneous), gangrene, empyema, cholangitis, hepatitis, pancreatitis, gallstone ileus, carcinoma

EXPECTED COURSE/PROGNOSIS
• In general the prognosis is good for gallbladder disease. Those who die during acute episodes are mainly due to other conditions, especially coronary artery disease.
• Symptomatic gallstones usually have recurrent symptoms in 3 to 6 months indicating need for future action
• After cholecystectomy, stones may recur in bile ducts

MISCELLANEOUS

ASSOCIATED CONDITIONS
• Pancreatitis
• Hemolytic anemias such as sickle cell disease, spherocytosis
• Cirrhosis, hypersplenism

AGE-RELATED FACTORS
Pediatric: N/A
Geriatric: Sometimes difficult to diagnose; complications more likely; cholecystectomy mortality rate higher
Others: N/A

PREGNANCY N/A

SYNONYMS N/A

ICD-9-CM
574.0 Calculus of gallbladder with acute cholecystitis
574.1 Calculus of gallbladder with other cholecystitis
575.0 Acute cholecystitis
575.1 Other cholecystitis (without mention of calculus)

SEE ALSO
• Cholelithiasis
• Cholangitis
• Choledocholithiasis
• Adenocarcinoma of the gallbladder
• Jaundice

OTHER NOTES
Lithotripsy - can be used in patients with chronic cholecystitis. Contraindications - stones greater than 25 mm, more than 3 stones, calcified stones, bile duct stones, poor general condition. Largely replaced by laparoscopic cholecystectomy.

ABBREVIATIONS N/A

REFERENCES
• Sleisenger MH, Fordtran JS, eds: Gastrointestinal Disease: Pathophysiology, Diagnosis, Management. 5th Ed. Philadelphia, W.B. Saunders Co., 1994
• Shiffman ML, Kaplan GD, Brinkman-Kaplan V, Vickers FF: Prophylaxis against gallstone formation with urosodeoxycholic acid in patients participating in a very-low-calorie diet program. Ann Int Med 1995;122:899-905
• Ransohoff DF, et al: Issues in cholecystectomy and management of common duct stones. Am J Gastroenterology 1994;Supple 89:S160-176
• Akriviadis EA, Hatzigavriel M, Kapnias D, et al: Treatment of biliary colic with diclofenac: a randomized double-blind, placebo-controlled study. Gastroenterology 1997;113:225-231
Illustrations: N/A
Internet references: http://www.5mcc.com

Author(s)
Frank L. Iber, MD

Choledocholithiasis

 BASICS

DESCRIPTION Stones in common bile duct (usually composed of cholesterol) that migrate from the gallbladder. Calcium bilirubinate stones may form de novo.
System(s) affected: Gastrointestinal
Genetics: N/A
Incidence/Prevalence in USA: 10-15% of patients with gallbladder stones discovered at time of cholecystectomy
Predominant age: Incidence increases with age
Predominant sex: Female > Male

SIGNS AND SYMPTOMS
• May be asymptomatic
• Biliary colic
• Common bile duct obstruction
• Cholangitis
• Pancreatitis
• Pain can't be differentiated from pain arising from gallbladder
• Epigastric pain
• Abdominal tenderness
• Pain unrelieved by antacids
• Anorexia, vomiting
• Dark urine
• Light colored feces
• Right upper quadrant tenderness
• Palpable gallbladder

CAUSES
• Increased biliary cholesterol secretion
• Chronic hemolytic states
• Hepatobiliary parasitism
• Duct stricture

RISK FACTORS
• Cholelithiasis
• Obesity
• Cirrhosis
• Chronic hemolysis
• Prior cholecystectomy

 DIAGNOSIS

DIFFERENTIAL DIAGNOSIS
• Biliary stricture
• Narrowed biliary - enteric anastomosis
• Sclerosing cholangitis
• Sphincter of Oddi dysfunction
• Biliary parasites
• Papillary stenosis
• Blood clots

LABORATORY
• Increasing WBC
• Increasing alkaline phosphatase
• Hypercholesterolemia (when associated with chronic cholestasis)
• Increased transaminases
• Hyperbilirubinemia
Drugs that may alter lab results: N/A
Disorders that may alter lab results: N/A

PATHOLOGICAL FINDINGS
• Dilated bile ducts
• Bile plugging
• Small bile duct proliferation
• Cholesterol gallstones

SPECIAL TESTS Nuclear medicine (PIPIDA), endoscopic retrograde cholangiopancreatography (ERCP), percutaneous transhepatic cholangiography (PTC)

IMAGING
• Intraoperative cholangiography - common bile duct filling defects
• Nuclear medicine cholescintigraphy
• Endoscopic cholangiography or PTC - common bile duct filling defects
• Endoscopic ultrasonography - can likely detect stones, but no therapeutic capability

DIAGNOSTIC PROCEDURES
• Ultrasound will reveal gallbladder stones - not reliable for common bile duct stones, but may reveal ductal dilatation over 75% of the time
• ERCP will visualize the common bile duct and other portions of the upper gastrointestinal tract and will allow for papillotomy plus stone extraction in majority of cases.

 TREATMENT

APPROPRIATE HEALTH CARE Inpatient

GENERAL MEASURES N/A

SURGICAL MEASURES
• In the elderly, ERCP and papillotomy with stone removal may prevent or delay the need for cholecystectomy
• Identification and removal of stones in the course of cholecystectomy
• If the gallbladder has been previously removed, ERCP, papillotomy plus stone extraction

ACTIVITY As tolerated

DIET Low fat may be helpful

PATIENT EDUCATION National Digestive Diseases Information Clearinghouse, Box NDDIC, Bethesda, MD 20892, (301)468-6344

Choledocholithiasis

MEDICATIONS

DRUG(S) OF CHOICE Antibiotics to treat gram negative aerobes and anaerobes. Selection based on culture and sensitivities. One useful specific regimen, for example: Cefoxitin, 2 grams intravenously perioperatively.
Contraindications: Refer to manufacturer's profile of each drug
Precautions: Refer to manufacturer's profile of each drug
Significant possible interactions: Refer to manufacturer's profile of each drug

ALTERNATIVE DRUGS N/A

FOLLOWUP

PATIENT MONITORING Routine postoperative care

PREVENTION/AVOIDANCE
• Operative cholangiography at time of cholecystectomy to identify common bile duct stones and then duct exploration or endoscopic sphincterotomy for their removal
• T-tube cholangiogram before removal of tube after operative bile duct exploration

POSSIBLE COMPLICATIONS
• Cholangitis - most frequent (60%)
• Bile duct obstruction
• Pancreatitis
• Biliary enteric fistula
• Hemobilia

EXPECTED COURSE/PROGNOSIS
Good prognosis if treated

MISCELLANEOUS

ASSOCIATED CONDITIONS
• Cholecystitis
• Cholangitis
• Periampullary diverticula

AGE-RELATED FACTORS
Pediatric: N/A
Geriatric: Prognosis guarded
Others: N/A

PREGNANCY Cholestasis of pregnancy may lead to choledocholithiasis

SYNONYMS
• Common bile duct stone
• Common bile duct calculi

ICD-9-CM
547.3 Calculus of bile duct with acute cholecystitis
574.5 Calculus of bile duct without mention of cholecystitis

SEE ALSO
• Cholangitis
• Cholecystitis
• Cholelithiasis
• Adenocarcinoma of the gallbladder
• Jaundice

OTHER NOTES N/A

ABBREVIATIONS
• ERCP = endoscopic retrograde cholangiopancreatography
• PTC = percutaneous transhepatic cholangiography

REFERENCES
• Nahrwold DL: The Biliary System. In: Sabisto DC, ed. Textbook of Surgery. Philadelphia, W.B. Saunders, 1986
• Jordan GL Jr: Choledocholithiasis. Curr Prob Surg 1982;19:723
Illustrations: N/A
Internet references: http://www.5mcc.com

Author(s)
Leo C. Mercer, MD

Cholelithiasis

BASICS

DESCRIPTION Cholesterol or pigmented stones formed and contained in the gallbladder
System(s) affected: Gastrointestinal
Genetics: N/A
Incidence/Prevalence in USA: 8-10% of population. Increased incidence in American Indians and Hispanics.
Predominant age: Increases with age - peak at sixth decade
Predominant sex: Female > Male (2:1)

SIGNS AND SYMPTOMS
• Mostly asymptomatic. 5-10% become symptomatic each year. Over lifetime, less than half of patients with gallstones develop symptoms.
• Episodic right upper quadrant or epigastric pain radiating to back (biliary colic)
• Nausea
• Vomiting
• Fatty food intolerance (not proven)
• Indigestion

CAUSES
• Production of bile supersaturated with cholesterol
• Decrease in bile content of either phospholipids or bile acids
• Biliary stasis
• Hemolytic diseases
• Biliary infection

RISK FACTORS
• Short gut syndrome
• Inflammatory bowel disease
• Multiparity
• Long term total parenteral nutrition
• Cirrhosis (for pigment stones)
• Hemolytic disorders - hereditary spherocytosis, sickle cell anemia
• Prosthetic cardiac valves
• Biliary parasites
• Rapid weight loss
• Childhood malignancy
• Native American descent
• Diabetes (for complications)
• Female gender

DIAGNOSIS

DIFFERENTIAL DIAGNOSIS
• Peptic ulcer
• Hepatitis, pancreatitis
• Coronary artery disease
• Appendicitis
• Pneumonia
• Gallbladder cancer
• Renal stones
• Blood clots
• Stricture
• Gallbladder polyps
• Biliary sludge

LABORATORY None
Drugs that may alter lab results: N/A
Disorders that may alter lab results: N/A

PATHOLOGICAL FINDINGS Gallstones

SPECIAL TESTS Hepatobiliary radionuclide scan

IMAGING
• Ultrasound (best technique to diagnose gallstones)
• Oral cholecystogram
• CT scan (no advantage over ultrasound)

DIAGNOSTIC PROCEDURES N/A

TREATMENT

APPROPRIATE HEALTH CARE Inpatient for surgical procedures

GENERAL MEASURES
• Treat only symptomatic gallstones
• Advise patient of presence of stones
• Observe asymptomatic stones
• Oral dissolution - only if surgery option not available (less than 25% of all patients eligible)

SURGICAL MEASURES
• Laparoscopic cholecystectomy
• Open cholecystectomy
• Direct contact dissolution - only for a small subset of patients - high recurrence rate
• Extracorporeal shock wave lithotripsy - role of this modality unclear and currently under study - not FDA approved
• Percutaneous cholecystostomy in high risk patients

ACTIVITY N/A

DIET Low fat diet may be helpful

PATIENT EDUCATION
• Seek medical attention if signs and symptoms develop
• Additional information available from: National Digestive Diseases Information Clearinghouse, Box NDDIC, Bethesda, MD 20892, (301)468-6344

MEDICATIONS

DRUG(S) OF CHOICE
• Analgesic for symptom relief
• Ursodiol (ursodeoxycholic acid, Actigall) 8-10 mg/kg/day bid-tid - for up to two years - oral dissolution
• Chenodiol (Chenix) 250 mg bid for 2 weeks; then increase by 250 mg increments until a dose of 13-16 mg/kg daily is reached or intolerance develops - oral dissolution
• Methyl tert-butyl ether - contact dissolution
Contraindications:
• Known allergy
• Acute cholecystitis - dissolution agents
• Severe abnormal liver function tests
• Non-functioning gallbladder
• Calcified (radiopaque) stones - relative
• Multiple stones
• Stones greater than 2 cm
• Stones that don't float on oral cholecystogram
Precautions:
• Monitor liver enzymes - may rise in up to 30% of patients
• Monitor serum cholesterol
• Methyl tert-butyl ether should only be used by one experienced with this contact dissolution method
• Observe for severe diarrhea
Significant possible interactions: N/A

ALTERNATIVE DRUGS
NSAID's may have a role in pain relief since prostaglandins are important in the development of pain
Note:
• Oral dissolution only effective for radiolucent (cholesterol) stones
• Ursodiol probably preferred over chenodiol as it has a lower incidence of adverse effects

FOLLOWUP

PATIENT MONITORING
• Medical attention if asymptomatic stones become symptomatic
• Patients on oral dissolution agents should be followed with liver enzymes, serum cholesterol and imaging studies

PREVENTION/AVOIDANCE
Use of ursodiol (Actigall) with rapid weight loss prevents stone formation

POSSIBLE COMPLICATIONS
• Acute cholecystitis (90-95% secondary to gallstones)
• Gallstone pancreatitis
• Acute cholangitis
• Common bile duct stones with obstructive jaundice
• Gallstone ileus
• Liver abscess
• Biliary-enteric fistula
• Peritonitis
• Gallbladder cancer

EXPECTED COURSE/PROGNOSIS
• Less than half of patients with gallstones will become symptomatic
• Cholecystectomy - mortality 0.5% elective, 3-5% emergency, morbidity less than 10% elective, 30-40% emergency
• 10-15% will have associated choledocholithiasis
• After cholecystostomy, stones may recur in bile duct

MISCELLANEOUS

ASSOCIATED CONDITIONS
90% of gallbladder carcinomas have gallstones

AGE-RELATED FACTORS
Pediatric:
• Uncommon before 10 years of age
• Associated with blood dyscrasia
Geriatric:
• Incidence increases with age
• Age alone should not alter therapy plan
Others: N/A

PREGNANCY
Attempt conservative therapy but surgery if indicated

SYNONYMS
Gallstones

ICD-9-CM
574.0 Calculus of gallbladder with acute cholecystitis
574.1 Calculus of gallbladder with other cholecystitis
574.2 Calculus of gallbladder without mention of cholecystitis
575.0 Acute cholecystitis
575.1 Other cholecystitis (without mention of calculus)

SEE ALSO
• Cholangitis
• Choledocholithiasis
• Cholecystitis
• Adenocarcinoma of the gallbladder
• Jaundice

OTHER NOTES
Laparoscopic cholecystectomy has become most frequently used procedure. (Lithotripsy can be considered in rare circumstances.)

ABBREVIATIONS
N/A

REFERENCES
• Hardy JD, ed: Hardy's Textbook of Surgery. 2nd Ed. Philadelphia, J.B. Lippincott, 1988
• Pitt HA, ed: The Surgical Clinics of North America. Vol. 70, No. 6. Philadelphia, W.B. Saunders, Dec, 1990
Illustrations: N/A
Internet references: http://www.5mcc.com

Author(s)
Gary B. Williams, MD

Cholera

BASICS

DESCRIPTION An acute infectious disease caused by Vibrio cholerae (El Tor type is responsible for current epidemic, the other type, classic, is found only in Bangladesh). (New serotype now in Bangladesh, India (0139). Important because of lack of efficacy of standard vaccine.) Characteristics include severe diarrhea with extreme fluid and electrolyte depletion, and vomiting, muscle cramps and prostration. Usual course: acute; chronic; relapsing.
• Clinical course is 3-5 days, and in the early stages a severely affected patient can lose one liter of fluid per hour
• Endemic areas: India; Southeast Asia; Africa; Middle East; Southern Europe; Oceania; South and Central America
System(s) affected: Gastrointestinal
Genetics: N/A
Incidence/Prevalence in USA: 0.01 cases/100,000. The few cases in the U.S. have been in returning travelers or associated with food brought into the country illicitly.
Predominant age: All ages
Predominant sex: Male = Female

SIGNS AND SYMPTOMS
• Abdominal discomfort
• Anorexia
• Anuria
• Apathy
• Cholera gravis
• Cyanosis
• Decreased skin turgor
• Dehydration
• Diarrhea, painless
• Distant heart sounds
• Diuresis, sudden
• Dysrhythmias
• Fever
• Hypotension
• Hypothermia
• Hypovolemic shock
• Increased or decreased bowel sounds
• Lethargy
• Listlessness
• Malaise
• Non-tender abdomen
• Oliguria
• Rice-water diarrhea
• Seizures
• Sunken eyes
• Tachycardia
• Thirst
• Vomiting
• Washerwoman's fingers
• Weak peripheral pulses
• Weakness

CAUSES
• Enterotoxin elaborated by gram-negative
• Vibrio cholera (O-group 1)
• Human host
• Contaminated food
• Contaminated water
• Contaminated shellfish

RISK FACTORS
• Traveling or living in epidemic areas
• Exposure to contaminated food or water
• Person-to-person transmission (rare)
• In endemic areas, children under age 5
• Attack more severe in blood group O as compared to AB
• Individual with low gastric acid secretion
• Gastrectomy
• Individuals on acid-suppressing medications

DIAGNOSIS

DIFFERENTIAL DIAGNOSIS Other causes of severe diarrhea and dehydration (e.g., Shigella, E. coli, viruses)

LABORATORY
• Stool culture - on selective media (thiosulfate citrate bile salts sucrose [TCBS])
• Typed antisera specific agglutination
• Dark field microscopy - characteristic vibrio motility in stool
• Increased vibriocidal antibodies in unimmunized individual
• Laboratory abnormalities of severe dehydration:
　◊ Acidemia
　◊ Acidosis
　◊ Hypokalemia
　◊ Hyponatremia
　◊ Hypochloremia
　◊ Hypoglycemia
　◊ Increased specific gravity
　◊ Polycythemia
　◊ Mild neutrophilic leukocytosis
Drugs that may alter lab results: N/A
Disorders that may alter lab results: N/A

PATHOLOGICAL FINDINGS
• Electron microscopy - organism adherent to mucosa
• Intact mucosa
• Increased cellularity of lamina propria
• Increased cellularity of mucosa
• Vascular congestion
• Lymphoid hyperplasia of Peyer's patches
• Lymphoid hyperplasia of mesenteric lymph nodes
• Lymphoid hyperplasia of spleen
• Cerebral edema
• Acute tubular necrosis
• Vacuolar hypokalemic nephropathy
• Pulmonary edema
• Hyaline membranes
• Bronchopneumonia
• Focal myocardial damage
• Lipid-depleted adrenals
• Tubularization of zona fasciculata

SPECIAL TESTS N/A

IMAGING
• Abdominal film - ileus
• Chest x-ray - microcardia

DIAGNOSTIC PROCEDURES Physical examination and medical history that includes recent travel

TREATMENT

APPROPRIATE HEALTH CARE
Outpatient for mild cases, inpatient for moderate or severe cases

GENERAL MEASURES
• Determination of the amount of fluid loss (may compare patient's previous weight to current weight)
• Rehydration therapy. Oral for mild to moderate cases. Patients with severe dehydration may require intravenous replacement.

SURGICAL MEASURES N/A

ACTIVITY Bedrest until symptoms resolved and strength returns

DIET Small, frequent meals when vomiting stops and appetite returns

PATIENT EDUCATION
• Centers for Disease Control. Traveler's Information Hotline: (404)332-4559 (available 24 hours via a touch-tone telephone).
• International Association for Medical Assistance to Travelers, 417 Center St., Lewiston, NY 14092, (716)754-4883

MEDICATIONS

DRUG(S) OF CHOICE
• Oral rehydration therapy
For mild disease:
◊ Oral rehydration solution (ORS) commercial brands available (Pedialyte, Rehydralyte, Resol, Ricelyte) or
◊ ORS formula from World Health Organization (WHO) - per liter:
- Sodium chloride 3.5 grams
- Potassium chloride 1.5 grams
- Glucose 20 grams
- Trisodium citrate 2.9 grams
• Parenteral rehydration
Severely dehydrated patients
◊ IV rehydration (Ringer's lactate) is followed by oral or nasogastric administration of glucose or sucrose-electrolyte solution
• Antibiotics
◊ For older children and adults - doxycycline (Vibramycin) - 300 mg once or 100 mg bid for 3 days or tetracycline 50 mg/kg/day for 3 days
◊ For young children - trimethoprim-sulfamethoxazole (SMX-TMP, Bactrim, Septra) 8 mg/kg trimethoprim plus 40 mg/kg sulfamethoxazole per day, divided q12h. This dosage is equivalent to 1 mL/kg of SMX/TMP suspension. Alternatively, furazolidone (Furoxone) 5-10 mg/kg/day divided q6h for 3 days.
◊ In pregnancy - furazolidone 100 mg qid x 7-10 days.

Contraindications:
• Tetracycline: not for use in pregnancy or children < 8 years.
• Furazolidone and alcohol may cause disulfiram-like reaction.

Precautions:
• Tetracycline: may cause photosensitivity; sunscreen recommended.

Significant possible interactions:
• Tetracycline: avoid concurrent administration with antacids, dairy products, or iron.

ALTERNATIVE DRUGS   N/A

FOLLOWUP

PATIENT MONITORING   Follow patient until symptoms resolved

PREVENTION/AVOIDANCE
• Water purification
• Careful food selection, e.g., no unpeeled raw fruits or vegetables, no raw or undercooked seafood
• Enteric precautions
• Tetracycline for contacts
• Natural infection confers long-lasting immunity
• Prophylactic vaccine
◊ 50% effective for 3 to 6 months
◊ Not recommended unless required by destination country, and if so, a single dose is sufficient
◊ Concomitant administration with yellow fever vaccine may result in reduced vaccine response to yellow fever
◊ Invariably associated with local side effects
◊ Systemic side effects of fever and malaise
◊ A new vaccine shows promise, but still in the testing stage

POSSIBLE COMPLICATIONS
• Hypovolemic shock
• Chronic biliary infection
• Up to 50% mortality with untreated shock
• Intermittent stool shedding

EXPECTED COURSE/PROGNOSIS
• Prompt oral or IV treatment can be lifesaving
• Appropriate disposal of human waste
• Antibiotic treatment reduces duration and infectivity of disease
• Mortality less than 1% with appropriate supportive care
• Increased mortality with untreated hypovolemic shock

MISCELLANEOUS

ASSOCIATED CONDITIONS   Increased risk of disease with gastric achlorhydria

AGE-RELATED FACTORS
Pediatric:
• Breast-feeding is protective against cholera
• Vaccine not recommended for children less than 6 months
Geriatric: N/A
Others: N/A

PREGNANCY   N/A

SYNONYMS
• Asiatic cholera
• Epidemic cholera
• Rice water diarrhea
• Cholera gravis

ICD-9-CM   001.9 Cholera, unspecified

SEE ALSO
• Oral rehydration
• Diarrhea, acute

OTHER NOTES   Centers for Disease Control does not expect a major outbreak of cholera in the U.S., but it has issued a "Cholera Preparedness Plan," outlining steps for proper surveillance, treatment, laboratory diagnosis, investigation of outbreaks, and public education

ABBREVIATIONS   N/A

REFERENCES)
• Mandell GL, ed: Principles and Practice of Infectious Diseases. 4th Ed. New York, Churchill Livingstone, 1995
• Warren KS, Mahmoud AA, eds: Tropical and Geographical Medicine. New York, McGraw-Hill, 1990
• Dhiman BR, Greenough CB III, eds: Cholera. New York, Plenum Medical Book Co., 1992
Illustrations: N/A
Internet references: http://www.5mcc.com

Author(s)
Abdulrazak Abyad, MD, MPH, AGSF

Chronic fatigue syndrome

BASICS

DESCRIPTION Chronic fatigue syndrome (CFS) is characterized primarily by profound fatigue, in association with multiple systemic and neuropsychiatric symptoms, lasting at least 6 months, severe enough to reduce/impair daily activity.
System(s) affected: Endocrine/Metabolic, Musculoskeletal
Genetics: N/A
Incidence/Prevalence in USA: 10/100,000
Predominant age: Young adult
Predominant sex: Female > Male (slightly)

SIGNS AND SYMPTOMS
- Fatigue (100%)
- Ability to date onset of illness (100%)
- Unexplained general muscle weakness (90%)
- Arthralgias (90%)
- Forgetfulness (90%)
- Inability to concentrate (90%)
- Emotional lability (90%)
- Myalgias (90%)
- Confusion (90%)
- Mood swings (90%)
- Low-grade fever (37.5-38.6°C) (85%)
- Irritability (85%)
- Prolonged fatigue lasting 24 hours after exercise (80%)
- Depression (80%)
- Headaches (76%)
- Photophobia (76%)
- Difficulty sleeping (76%)
- Allergies (70%)
- Vertigo (40%)
- Adenopathy (40%)
- Shortness of breath (33%)
- Chest pain (33%)
- Nausea (33%)
- Weight loss (30%)
- Hot flushes (30%)
- Palpitations (30%)
- Painful lymph nodes (30%)
- Gastrointestinal complaints (30%)
- Night sweats (25%)
- Weight gain (15%)
- Rash (15%)

CAUSES Unknown. Multiple immunologic abnormalities suggestive of viral reactivation syndrome have been reported, but no one source identified. Attention given most to herpes (EBV and HHV-6) and other enteroviruses, possibly in concert, possibly with environmental factors.

RISK FACTORS Unknown

DIAGNOSIS

DIFFERENTIAL DIAGNOSIS
- Malignancies
- Autoimmune disease
- Localized infection (occult abscess, etc.)
- Chronic or subacute bacterial disease (endocarditis)
- Lyme disease
- Fungal disease (histoplasmosis, coccidioidomycosis)
- Parasitic disease (amebiasis, giardiasis, helminths)
- HIV related disease
- Psychiatric disease
- Chronic inflammatory disease (sarcoidosis, Wegener's granulomatosis)
- Known chronic viral disease (chronic hepatitis)
- Neuromuscular disease (multiple sclerosis, myasthenia gravis)
- Endocrine disorder (hypothyroidism, Addison's, Cushing's, diabetes mellitus)
- Drug dependency or abuse (including prescription drugs)
- Iatrogenic (as from medication side effects)
- Toxic agent exposure
- Other known or defined systemic disease (chronic pulmonary, cardiac, hepatic, renal, or hematologic disease)
- Physiologic (inadequate or disrupted sleep, menopause, etc.)

LABORATORY
- Initial lab studies
  ◊ Chemistry panel
  ◊ CBC
  ◊ Urinalysis
  ◊ Thyroid function
- Additional studies
  ◊ ESR
  ◊ ANA
  ◊ VDRL
  ◊ Rheumatoid factor
  ◊ Purified protein derivative
  ◊ Serum cortisol
  ◊ HIV
  ◊ Immunoglobulin
  ◊ Epstein-Barr serology

Drugs that may alter lab results: N/A
Disorders that may alter lab results: N/A

PATHOLOGICAL FINDINGS N/A

SPECIAL TESTS None. Diagnosis of exclusion. History, physical exam normal.

IMAGING Experimental at present

DIAGNOSTIC PROCEDURES
To establish the diagnosis - 2 major criteria and at least 6 symptoms plus at least 2 physical signs; or at least 8 symptoms
- Major criteria:
  ◊ New onset fatigue lasting longer than 6 months with a 50% reduction in activity
  ◊ No other medical or psychiatric conditions that could cause symptoms
- Symptoms:
  ◊ Low grade fever
  ◊ Sore throat
  ◊ Painful cervical or axillary adenopathy
  ◊ Generalized muscle weakness
  ◊ Myalgias
  ◊ Headaches
  ◊ Migratory arthralgias
  ◊ Sleep disturbances (hypersomnia or insomnia)
  ◊ Neuropsychological complaints (one or more of: photophobia, visual scotomas, forgetfulness, irritability, confusion, difficulty concentrating, depression)
- Physical signs:
  ◊ Low grade fever (37.5-38.6°C)
  ◊ Pharyngitis (nonexudative)
  ◊ Cervical or axillary adenopathy

TREATMENT

APPROPRIATE HEALTH CARE
Outpatient

GENERAL MEASURES
- Because the cause of CFS is unknown and no specific therapy has shown consistent results, mainstay of therapy is supportive care
- A program of moderate exercise (with rest periods during exacerbations of the disease), a healthy diet, stress reduction, and support groups or counselling is likely to be beneficial and while not necessarily curative will help the patient cope with their disease
- Alternative therapies (chiropractic, homeopathy, acupuncture, enforced rest) helpful for some; no proven efficacy; may be worth trying
- Psychiatric symptoms often prominent but generally felt secondary rather than causative

SURGICAL MEASURES N/A

ACTIVITY As tolerated, but strenuous exercise tends to exacerbate symptoms in most

DIET No restrictions

PATIENT EDUCATION
- Support groups available. Contact CFS Association, 3521 Broadway, Suite 222, Kansas City, MO 64111, (816)931-4777
- CFIDS Association. P.O. Box 220398, Charlotte, NC 28222-0398
- International Chronic Fatigue Syndrome Society. P.O. Box 230108, Portland, OR 97223

MEDICATIONS

DRUG(S) OF CHOICE
• None
• Ampligen, essential fatty acid therapy, IV immune globulin, vitamin B12, and bovine liver extract (LEFAC) are used experimentally.
• Supportive therapy directed toward symptoms with NSAID's, antidepressants including fluoxetine, others including buspirone.
Contraindications: Refer to manufacturer's literature
Precautions: Refer to manufacturer's literature
Significant possible interactions: Refer to manufacturer's literature

ALTERNATIVE DRUGS N/A

FOLLOWUP

PATIENT MONITORING No consensus. Periodic re-evaluation appropriate for support, symptom relief, assessment for other cause.

PREVENTION/AVOIDANCE Unknown

POSSIBLE COMPLICATIONS
• Depression
• Socio-economic problems

EXPECTED COURSE/PROGNOSIS
• Indolent; waxes and wanes
• Generally very slow improvement over months or years

MISCELLANEOUS

ASSOCIATED CONDITIONS
Fibromyalgia (70% reported to meet criteria)

AGE-RELATED FACTORS
Pediatric: Reported in children
Geriatric: Reported in elderly
Others: N/A

PREGNANCY No information

SYNONYMS
• CFS
• Chronic Epstein-Barr syndrome
• Yuppie flu

ICD-9-CM 300.5 neurasthenia

SEE ALSO
• Epstein-Barr virus infections

OTHER NOTES Controversial topic, data often conflicting

ABBREVIATIONS N/A

REFERENCES
• Holmes GP, Kaplan JE, et al: Chronic Fatigue Syndrome: A Working Case Definition. Annals of Internal Medicine 1988;108, 387-389
• Klimas NG, et al: Immunologic Abnormalities in Chronic Fatigue Syndrome. J. Clinical Microbiology 1990;28(6),1403-1410
• English T: Skeptical of Skeptics. JAMA 1991;265(8):964,
• An information packet, for health care providers, is available from the CDC's Viral Diseases Division (404)639-1338
Illustrations: N/A
Internet references: http://www.5mcc.com

Author(s)
David Hanson, MD

Chronic obstructive pulmonary disease & emphysema

BASICS

DESCRIPTION Chronic obstructive pulmonary disease encompasses several diffuse pulmonary diseases including chronic bronchitis, asthma, cystic fibrosis, bronchiectasis, and emphysema. The term usually refers to a mixture of chronic bronchitis and emphysema.
• Chronic bronchitis is defined clinically by increased mucus production and recurrent cough present on most days for at least three months during at least two consecutive years.
• Emphysema is the destruction of interalveolar septa. The disease occurs in the distal or terminal airways and involves both airways and lung parenchyma.
System(s) affected: Pulmonary
Genetics:
• Chronic bronchitis is not a genetic disorder although some studies have hinted at a predisposition for development of this condition.
• A rare form of emphysema, antiprotease deficiency (due to alpha 1-antitrypsin deficiency), is an inherited disorder that is an expression of two autosomal codominant alleles.
Incidence/Prevalence in USA:
• 10-20% of adults; more than 60,000 deaths/year
• 8 million people have chronic bronchitis; 2 million people have emphysema
Predominant age: Over 40 years
Predominant sex: Male > Female

SIGNS AND SYMPTOMS
• Chronic bronchitis
  ◊ Cough
  ◊ Sputum production
  ◊ Frequent infections
  ◊ Intermittent dyspnea
  ◊ Pedal edema
  ◊ Plethora
  ◊ Cyanosis
  ◊ Wheezing
  ◊ Weight gain
  ◊ Diminished breath sounds
• Emphysema
  ◊ Minimal cough
  ◊ Scant sputum
  ◊ Dyspnea
  ◊ Often significant weight loss
  ◊ Occasional infections
  ◊ Barrel chest
  ◊ Minimal wheezing
  ◊ Use of accessory muscles of respiration
  ◊ Pursed lip breathing
  ◊ Cyanosis is slight or absent
  ◊ Breath sounds very diminished

CAUSES
• Cigarette smoking
• Air pollution
• Antiprotease deficiency
• Occupational exposure (i.e., firefighters)
• Infection possibly (viral)

RISK FACTORS
• Passive smoking (especially adults whose parents smoked)
• Severe viral pneumonia early in life
• Aging
• Ethyl alcohol (EtOH) consumption
• Airway hyperactivity

DIAGNOSIS

DIFFERENTIAL DIAGNOSIS Acute bronchitis, asthma, bronchiectasis, bronchogenic carcinoma, acute viral infection, normal aging of lungs, occupational asthma, chronic pulmonary embolism, sleep apnea, primary alveolar hypoventilation, chronic sinusitis

LABORATORY
• Chronic bronchitis
  ◊ Hypercapnia
  ◊ Polycythemia
  ◊ Hypoxia can be moderate to severe
• Emphysema
  ◊ Normal serum hemoglobin or polycythemia
  ◊ Normal PaCO2; unless FEV1 < 1 L/sec, then can be elevated
  ◊ Mild hypoxia
Drugs that may alter lab results:
Sedatives including alcohol
Disorders that may alter lab results:
Obesity, concurrent restrictive lung dysfunction, primary pulmonary hypertension, acute infections, anemia, pulmonary embolism sleep apnea, congestive heart failure

PATHOLOGICAL FINDINGS
• Chronic bronchitis
  ◊ Bronchial mucous gland enlargement
  ◊ Increased number of secretory cells in surface epithelium
  ◊ Thickened small airways from edema and inflammation
  ◊ Smooth muscle hyperplasia
  ◊ Mucus plugging
  ◊ Bacterial colonization of airways
• Emphysema
  ◊ Entire lung affected
  ◊ Bronchi usually clear of secretions
  ◊ Anthracotic pigment
  ◊ Alveoli enlarged with loss of septa
  ◊ Cartilage atrophy
  ◊ Bullae

SPECIAL TESTS
• Pulmonary function testing
  ◊ Decreased FEV1 with concomitant reduction in FEV1/FVC ratio
  ◊ Poor or absent reversibility to bronchodilators
  ◊ FVC may be normal or reduced
  ◊ Normal or increased total lung capacity
  ◊ Increased residual volume
  ◊ Diffusing capacity is normal or reduced
• Nocturnal oximetry

IMAGING
• Chronic bronchitis chest x-ray shows increased bronchovascular markings and cardiomegaly
• Emphysema chest x-ray shows small heart, hyperinflation, flat diaphragms and possibly bullous changes

DIAGNOSTIC PROCEDURES
• Pulmonary function tests
• ABGs
• Chest x-ray

TREATMENT

APPROPRIATE HEALTH CARE
• Outpatient treatment is usually adequate. However, hospitalization may be required for exacerbation, infection, or diagnostic procedures (i.e., transbronchial lung biopsy).
• Acute respiratory failure may require an intensive care unit and possibly a mechanical ventilator to support the patient

GENERAL MEASURES
• Smoking cessation
• Aggressive treatment of infections
• Treat any reversible bronchospasm
• Reduction of secretions through good pulmonary hygiene
• Cor pulmonale may necessitate use of home oxygen
• Pulmonary rehabilitation
• Appropriate vaccinations
• Adequate hydration

SURGICAL MEASURES
• Lung reduction surgery (selected cases)
• Lung transplantation (selected cases)

ACTIVITY As tolerated. Full activity should be encouraged.

DIET A well balanced, high protein diet is suggested. Low carbohydrates may benefit those with hypercarbia.

PATIENT EDUCATION
• Printed material is available from the National Jewish Hospital in Denver, Colorado. The local branch of the American Lung Association also has educational material.
• Coach patients in pulmonary rehabilitation

Chronic obstructive pulmonary disease & emphysema

MEDICATIONS

DRUG(S) OF CHOICE
• Theophylline - (Theo-Dur, Slo-bid, Unidur, Uniphyl) 400 mg/day. Increase by 100-200 mg in one to two weeks if necessary.
• Sympathomimetics - e.g., metaproterenol (Alupent), albuterol (Proventil, Ventolin), pirbuterol (Maxair), terbutaline (Brethaire). 1-2 puffs from the metered dose inhaler every 4-6 hrs. May be increased to every 3 hrs. Use of spacer device (aerochamber, inspirease) may be beneficial. (Up to 4 puffs recommended by some.) Long acting sympathomimetics - salmeterol (Serevent) to be considered.
• Anticholinergics - ipratropium (Atrovent). Two puffs (36 µg) 4 times daily. May take additional inhalations not to exceed 12 in 24 hrs.
• Corticosteroids - prednisone (Deltasone). Given orally 7.5-15 mg/day. Most useful in bronchitis with some reversibility.

Contraindications:
• Theophylline - hypersensitivity
• Sympathomimetics - cardiac arrhythmias associated with tachycardia; hypersensitivity
• Anticholinergics - hypersensitivity to atropine or its derivatives
• Corticosteroids - systemic fungal infections; hypersensitivity

Precautions:
• Theophylline - reduce dosage in patients with impaired renal or liver function; age over 55; CHF. Therapeutic drug level is 5-15 µg/mL (55.5-111 µmol).
• Rifampin - may cause a decrease in theophylline levels by increasing theophylline metabolism. Monitor serum theophylline level.
• Sympathomimetics - excessive use may be dangerous. May need to reduce dose in patients with cardiovascular disease, hypertension, hyperthyroidism, diabetes or convulsive disorders.
• Anticholinergics - narrow angle glaucoma, prostatic hypertrophy, bladder-neck obstruction
• Corticosteroids - may mask infection or predispose to infection, especially fungal; subcapsular cataracts; glaucoma; adrenocortical insufficiency; psychic derangements; gastrointestinal bleeding; diabetes mellitus, reactivation of tuberculosis

Significant possible interactions:
• Theophylline - lithium carbonate; propranolol; erythromycin; cimetidine; ranitidine; rifampin; ciprofloxacin
Addition of cimetidine, ciprofloxacin, or erythromycin will decrease theophylline clearance causing theophylline levels to rise. Careful monitoring of serum theophylline levels is warranted. (Note: cimetidine is now an OTC drug.)
• Sympathomimetics - other sympathomimetics, monoamine oxidase inhibitors or tricyclic antidepressants
• Anticholinergics - refer to manufacturer's profile
• Corticosteroids - NSAID's (indomethacin), aspirin, synthetic thyroid hormone

ALTERNATIVE DRUGS
• Theophylline may be given orally, intravenously or by rectal suppository
• Sympathomimetics may be given as aerosolized solution (albuterol, metaproterenol [Metaprel], isoetharine) when mixed with saline; orally (Alupent, Proventil, Brethine, Ventolin) or subcutaneously (terbutaline)
• Anticholinergics - atropine sulfate, glycopyrrolate. Ipratropium (Atrovent) now available in aerosolized solution and may be mixed with albuterol.
• Corticosteroids may be given intravenously (hydrocortisone, methylprednisolone) or inhaled (beclomethasone, flunisolide, triamcinolone acetonide)
• Home oxygen

FOLLOWUP

PATIENT MONITORING
• Severe or unstable patients should be seen monthly
• When stable, may be seen biannually
• Check theophylline level with each dose adjustment until the desired level (or result) is achieved, then check every 6-12 months
• With home oxygen, check arterial blood gasses yearly or with any change in condition. Monitor oxygen saturation (pulse oximetry) more frequently.
• Some patients only desaturate at night thereby only needing nocturnal oxygen
• Avoid travel at high altitude. Air travel with oxygen requires pre-arrangement.

PREVENTION/AVOIDANCE   Avoidance of smoking is the most important preventive measure. Passive smoke also has been shown to be harmful.

POSSIBLE COMPLICATIONS
• Infection is common
• Cor pulmonale, secondary polycythemia, bullous lung disease, acute or chronic respiratory failure, pulmonary hypertension, malnutrition

EXPECTED COURSE/PROGNOSIS
• The patient's age and post-bronchodilator forced expiratory volume (FEV1) are the most important predictors of prognosis. Young age and FEV1 > 50% predicted have a good prognosis. Older patients with more severe lung disease do worse.
• Supplemental oxygen, when indicated, has been shown to increase survival
• Smoking cessation is also important for an improved prognosis
• Malnutrition, cor pulmonale, hypercapnia and pulse > 100 indicate a poor prognosis

MISCELLANEOUS

ASSOCIATED CONDITIONS
• Lung cancer
• Coronary artery disease
• Peptic ulcer disease
• Chronic sinusitis
• Malnutrition
• Laryngeal carcinoma

AGE-RELATED FACTORS
Pediatric: Repeated childhood respiratory illnesses make COPD a greater risk
Geriatric: Relative risk is 1.2 to 2.3 times greater than in younger person
Others: Unusual under age 25 unless antiprotease deficiency is present. Incidence increases as age approaches 60.

PREGNANCY   N/A

SYNONYMS
• Bronchitis
• COLD (Chronic obstructive lung disease)
• OAD (Obstructive airways disease)
• COPD

ICD-9-CM
• 496 COPD
• 492.8 Emphysema

SEE ALSO
• Asthma
• Bronchitis, acute

OTHER NOTES
• Albuterol is also known as salbutamol
• Other important considerations for treatment include adequate hydration, supplemental oxygen, antibiotics when indicated, mucolytic agents, pulmonary rehabilitation, good pulmonary hygiene

ABBREVIATIONS
FVC = forced vital capacity
FEV1 = forced expiratory volume at 1 second
COPD = chronic obstructive pulmonary disease
ABG = arterial blood gases

REFERENCES   Fishman A: Pulmonary Diseases and Disorders. 2nd Ed. New York, McGraw-Hill Book Co., 1988
Illustrations: N/A
Internet references: http://www.5mcc.com

Author(s)
Alan J. Cropp, MD, FCCP

Cirrhosis of the liver

BASICS

DESCRIPTION Histologically cirrhosis is defined by the presence of fibrosis with regenerative nodules. Clinically cirrhosis presents with evidence of portal hypertension, i.e. ascites, variceal bleeding, hepatic encephalopathy.
System(s) affected: Gastrointestinal, Cardiovascular, Endocrine/Metabolic
Genetics: For hereditary hemochromatosis mutation on chromosome 6
Incidence/Prevalence in USA: Accounts for over 30,000 deaths per year
Predominant age: Etiology dependent
Predominant sex: Etiology dependent

SIGNS AND SYMPTOMS
• The onset of the disease is often insidious with:
  ◊ Fatigue
  ◊ Anorexia
  ◊ Nausea
  ◊ Abdominal discomfort and distention
  ◊ Weakness and malaise
• Signs and symptoms that are related to cirrhosis are those of complications:
  ◊ Hematemesis
  ◊ Encephalopathy
  ◊ Jaundice
  ◊ Hepatomegaly
  ◊ Splenomegaly
  ◊ Abdominal collateral circulation
  ◊ Ascites
  ◊ Gynecomastia
  ◊ Testicular atrophy
  ◊ Asterixis (liver flap)
  ◊ Palmar erythema
  ◊ Spider angiomas

CAUSES
• Alcoholic cirrhosis
• Chronic viral hepatitis, B (with/without D), C
• Wilson's disease
• Hemochromatosis
• Alpha 1-antitrypsin deficiency
• Cystic fibrosis
• Autoimmune chronic hepatitis with cirrhosis
• Primary biliary cirrhosis
• Secondary biliary cirrhosis
• Primary sclerosing cholangitis
• Cardiac cirrhosis
• Drug induced (other than alcohol)
• Inherited causes that may be present in infancy and childhood:
  ◊ Glycogen storage disease
  ◊ Galactosemia
  ◊ Fructose intolerance
  ◊ Tyrosinemia
  ◊ Acid cholesterol ester hydrolase deficiency

RISK FACTORS Included with Causes

DIAGNOSIS

DIFFERENTIAL DIAGNOSIS
• Depends on presentation
• Ascites - increased right heart pressure, hepatic vein thrombosis, peritoneal infection or malignancy, pancreatic disease, thyroid disease, lymphatic obstruction
• Other causes of UGI bleeding
• Other metabolic encephalopathies - renal, cardiopulmonary, drug.

LABORATORY
• Recognition of liver injury - elevated AST, elevated ALT; elevated alkaline phosphatase. Note: All liver injury tests may be normal.
• Functional impairment of the liver - elevated bilirubin, decreased albumin, elevated globulin, prolonged prothrombin time
• Etiologic screen for liver disease
  ◊ Ceruloplasmin (Wilson's disease)
  ◊ Iron, iron binding capacity, ferritin (hemochromatosis)
  ◊ Alpha fetoprotein (hepatocellular cancer)
  ◊ HBsAg (hepatitis B)
  ◊ Anti-HCV (hepatitis C)
  ◊ HCV RNA by PCR to confirm activity
  ◊ ANA (autoimmune hepatitis)
  ◊ Anti-smooth muscle antibody (autoimmune hepatitis)
  ◊ Anti-mitochondrial antibody (AMA) (primary biliary cirrhosis)
  ◊ Alpha 1-antitrypsin (deficiency)
  ◊ Serum protein electrophoresis (SPEP) - increased IgG with any liver disease; increased IgM with primary biliary cirrhosis (PBC)
Drugs that may alter lab results: N/A
Disorders that may alter lab results: N/A

PATHOLOGICAL FINDINGS
• Fibrosis and regenerative nodules; specific findings/patterns may indicate etiology
• Quantitative liver chemistry for iron, copper
• Special stains for iron, copper, bilirubin, collagen, alpha 1-antitrypsin, hepatitis B

SPECIAL TESTS
• Laparoscopic liver biopsy to reduce sampling error
• Cholangiography to rule out common duct obstruction and recognize sclerosing cholangitis
• Doppler ultrasound to indicate direction of flow in and patency of the portal and hepatic veins
• Visceral angiography to determine vascular anatomy, patency and collaterals
• Esophagogastroduodenoscopy to assess varices

IMAGING
• Ultrasound good for detecting bile duct dilatation and space occupying lesions. Cannot make diagnosis of cirrhosis based on ultrasound alone.
• CT, if ultrasound technically inadequate

DIAGNOSTIC PROCEDURES
• A liver biopsy establishes the diagnosis of cirrhosis
• Patterns of injury as well as special stains may identify a precise etiology such as alcoholic liver disease, hemochromatosis, alpha 1-antitrypsin deficiency, hepatitis B, primary biliary cirrhosis

TREATMENT

APPROPRIATE HEALTH CARE
Outpatient except for complicating emergencies:
• GI bleeding
• Hepatic encephalopathy
• Spontaneous bacterial peritonitis
• Unexplained decompensation
• Renal failure

GENERAL MEASURES
• Treatment designed to remove or alleviate underlying cause of cirrhosis, prevent further liver damage and prevent complications
• Phlebotomy for hemochromatosis
• Therapies involve drug treatment, dietary restrictions, rest, other supportive measures. Adequate protein intake for liver regeneration.

SURGICAL MEASURES
• Interventional
  ◊ Possible procedures for portal hypertension include - splenorenal or portacaval anastomosis, transjugular intrahepatic portal-systemic shunt
  ◊ Transplantation - in suitable candidate (substance free, motivated and adherent). Evaluate prior to major decompensation.

ACTIVITY Maintain as active as possible. With peripheral edema, leg elevation necessary.

DIET
• Adequate protein (1 gm/kg) and generous calories to help regenerate the liver
• In the presence of hepatic encephalopathy protein restriction is necessary
• In the presence of ascites salt restriction is necessary (2 gm or less/day)
• In the presence of hyponatremia (Na < 130 mEq [< 130 mmol]) fluid restriction is necessary (< 1 L)
• No alcohol

PATIENT EDUCATION
• Pamphlets are available through: American Liver Foundation, (800)223-0179
• Additional material: National Digestive Diseases Information Clearinghouse, Box NDDIC, Bethesda, MD 20892, (301)468-6344

MEDICATIONS

DRUG(S) OF CHOICE

• Large esophageal varices seen at endoscopy prior to clinical bleeding - nonselective beta blocker at a dose to decrease the resting pulse by 25%
• Ascites: spironolactone 100 mg up to 400 mg every day as a single dose. Takes three days before onset of action. Add furosemide 40-160 mg/day if needed. Loop diuretics may produce a rapid diuresis and subsequent intravascular volume depletion.
• Encephalopathy: lactulose (Cholac) 15-30 mL/day to produce 2-3 soft stools per day
• Spontaneous bacterial peritonitis (SBP): ampicillin plus aminoglycoside or cefotaxime alone as initial treatment; norfloxacin 400 mg/day or trimethoprim-sulfamethoxazole decreases risk for subsequent development of SBP after treatment
• Specific drug based on etiology
  ◊ Wilson's disease: penicillamine, 125-250 mg qid (give on empty stomach to avoid inactivation by metal binding)
  ◊ Autoimmune chronic hepatitis: corticosteroids with or without azathioprine
  ◊ Chronic hepatitis B and C: interferon
  ◊ PBC: ursodiol (ursodeoxycholic acid), 12-15 mg/kg/day in a bid dose
Contraindications: Refer to manufacturer's literature
Precautions: Refer to manufacturer's literature
Significant possible interactions: Refer to manufacturer's literature

ALTERNATIVE DRUGS
Ursodeoxycholic acid for cholestatic disease

FOLLOWUP

PATIENT MONITORING
• In a stable patient - yearly battery of liver tests. After 10 years, consider alpha-fetoprotein and imaging to detect hepatocellular carcinoma.
• In an unstable patient - tests may be repeated at weekly intervals
• Have patient monitor weight and maintain a daily diary

PREVENTION/AVOIDANCE
• Limit use of alcohol and other liver toxins
• No sharing of syringes
• Safer sex
• Screening of family members when a genetic disease is recognized
• Influenza and pneumococcal vaccines for cirrhosis patients exposed to crowds
• Liver test surveillance while on hepatotoxic drugs (e.g., INH)

POSSIBLE COMPLICATIONS
• Ascites
• Jaundice
• Coagulopathy
• Hepatic encephalopathy
• Bleeding esophageal varices
• Liver failure
• Carcinoma of the liver (uncommon)
• Susceptibility to infections
• Spontaneous bacterial peritonitis
• Renal failure

EXPECTED COURSE/PROGNOSIS
A function of ongoing hepatic injury as well as residual hepatic reserve. If a treatable cause is identified and intervention results in cessation of liver destruction, then the prognosis may be good.

MISCELLANEOUS

ASSOCIATED CONDITIONS
• Hepatitis
• Diseases and defects of the bile ducts
• Cystic fibrosis
• Heart failure
• Hepatocellular cancer

AGE-RELATED FACTORS
Pediatric: N/A
Geriatric: Cirrhosis is one of the leading causes of death for people over age 65
Others: N/A

PREGNANCY Cirrhosis may decompensate during pregnancy. Higher rates of spontaneous abortion, premature birth and perinatal death.

SYNONYMS N/A

ICD-9-CM
571.2 Alcoholic cirrhosis of liver
571.5 Cirrhosis of liver without mention of alcohol

SEE ALSO N/A

OTHER NOTES N/A

ABBREVIATIONS
PBC = Primary biliary cirrhosis
UGI = upper gastrointestinal
ANA = anti-nuclear antibody

REFERENCES
• Sampliner RE: The recognition of early liver disease. Hospital Practice 1989;53-56
• Schiff L, Schiff ER, eds: Diseases of the Liver. Philadelphia, J.B. Lippincott co., 1993
• Runyon BA: Care of patients with ascites. NEJM 1994;330:337-342
Illustrations: N/A
Internet references: http://www.5mcc.com

Author(s)
Richard E. Sampliner, MD

Claudication

BASICS

DESCRIPTION The feeling of muscle fatigue after a period of minimal exercise of an extremity. The feeling may progress to a cramp-like pain, usually in the calf muscles. It is always relieved by resting the extremity. It can be reproduced by undergoing a similar exercise pattern. It may occur in the arms, but is more common in the legs, calf > thigh.
System(s) affected: Cardiovascular, Musculoskeletal
Genetics: N/A
Incidence/Prevalence in USA: Common
Predominant age: Common in males > 55, females > 60
Predominant sex: Male > Female (4:1)

SIGNS AND SYMPTOMS
• May start gradually or suddenly
• Unable to walk distances
• Pain varies from muscle tiredness to a frank cramp in muscle group involved
• May be a loss of hair on toes
• Foot may show rubor on dependency
• Pedal pulses absent
• Popliteal pulse absent
• With thigh claudication, femoral pulse absent
• Absent pulses in the distal extremity, secondary to more proximal arterial occlusion. The occlusion is usually from an arterial plaque.

CAUSES
• Lower extremity claudication - blockage of superficial femoral artery, secondary to arteriosclerosis in 95% of cases
• Other causes of arterial blocks - embolus, popliteal entrapment, adventitious cystic disease of popliteal artery, thromboangiitis obliterans
• Thigh and hip claudication - blockage of aortic and iliac vessels
• Upper extremity claudication - similar blocks of subclavian, axillary, and brachial artery

RISK FACTORS
• Smoking
• Diabetes
• Hypertension
• Hyperlipidemia
• Obesity
• Preexisting heart disease

DIAGNOSIS

DIFFERENTIAL DIAGNOSIS
• Pseudoclaudication, sometimes secondary to some form of spinal stenosis, usually impinging on the cauda equina portion of the spinal cord. The pain in the legs is characteristically relieved by squatting or sitting. The latter relieves tension on spinal nerve roots.
• Osteoarthritis of hips and knees sometimes can be confused with claudication, but pain starts immediately on weight bearing.

LABORATORY N/A
Drugs that may alter lab results: None
Disorders that may alter lab results: Arterial calcinosis, often found in diabetics, will cause a falsely high ankle/arm index

PATHOLOGICAL FINDINGS N/A

SPECIAL TESTS
• Noninvasive vascular tests - pulse volume recordings. Measurement of blood pressure in the arm compared to pedal arterial pressures before and after exercise establish the diagnosis as well as the severity of occlusion. The patient with one to two block claudication will have an ankle/arm index of 0.7-0.4 with 1.0 being normal. If below 0.4, there is a major threat of losing part of the leg if left untreated. Pseudoclaudication does not affect the pulses in the extremity.

IMAGING
• Duplex ultrasound
• Intra-arterial arteriography

DIAGNOSTIC PROCEDURES
• Arteriography - when surgical correction is anticipated
• Noninvasive vascular tests

TREATMENT

APPROPRIATE HEALTH CARE
Outpatient, except for severe cases or advanced disease

GENERAL MEASURES
• Conservative measures: stop smoking, initiate walking and exercise program, control of hyperlipidemia
• Reduce risk factors

SURGICAL MEASURES
• Surgical treatment with bypass of arterial obstruction may be appropriate in selected cases
• Angioplasty

ACTIVITY Ambulatory

DIET None

PATIENT EDUCATION Prevention methods

MEDICATIONS

DRUG(S) OF CHOICE
• Aspirin - to reduce platelet aggregation: low dose 80 mg/day
• Pentoxifylline (Trental) - to decrease internal configuration of red cells - 400 mg bid-tid. Administer for at least 6-8 weeks to determine if therapy is effective.
Contraindications: Refer to manufacturer's literature
Precautions: Try to reduce risk factors first
Significant possible interactions: Refer to manufacturer's literature

ALTERNATIVE DRUGS
• Ticlopidine
• Vasodilators
• Calcium channel blockers
• Anticoagulants

FOLLOWUP

PATIENT MONITORING Peripheral non-invasive vascular studies every 6 months

PREVENTION/AVOIDANCE
• Institute walking program of 4-5 miles
• Avoid smoking

POSSIBLE COMPLICATIONS Only 10% of people without diabetes will progress to some amputation of the involved extremity

EXPECTED COURSE/PROGNOSIS
Gradual improvement in walking distance or progression of problem to gangrene, rest pain and/or tissue necrosis

MISCELLANEOUS

ASSOCIATED CONDITIONS Other manifestations of arteriosclerotic vascular disease - history of myocardial infarction(s), carotid disease, renal vascular hypertension

AGE-RELATED FACTORS
Pediatric: N/A
Geriatric: More common with advancing age
Others: N/A

PREGNANCY N/A

SYNONYMS N/A

ICD-9-CM
443.9

SEE ALSO
• Thromboangiitis obliterans (Buerger's disease)

OTHER NOTES N/A

ABBREVIATIONS N/A

REFERENCES Rutherford RB, ed: Vascular Surgery. 4th Ed. Philadelphia, WB Saunders Co, 1995
Illustrations: N/A
Internet references: http://www.5mcc.com

Author(s)
William V. Sharp, MD

Coarctation of the aorta

BASICS

DESCRIPTION A constriction (discrete or of varying lengths) of the aorta usually located just distal to the left subclavian artery at the junction of the ligamentum arteriosum
System(s) affected: Cardiovascular
Genetics: No Mendelian inheritance, but common in Turner's syndrome
Incidence/Prevalence in USA: 64/100,000 under 1 year of age
Predominant age: Usually diagnosed in infancy
Predominant sex: Male > Female (1.7:1)

SIGNS AND SYMPTOMS
• Headaches
• Exertional leg fatigue and pain
• Prominent neck pulsations
• Epistaxis
• Hypertension
• Pulse disparity
• Delayed, weak, or absent pulse
• Prominent left ventricular impulse
• Murmur (aortic stenosis or insufficiency, ventricular septal defect, rarely mitral valve)
• S4 systolic ejection click
• Bruit (coarctation, collaterals, patent ductus arteriosus)
• Cyanosis, rarely
• In infancy may also have heart failure, failure to thrive, irritability, tachypnea, and dyspnea
• Extensive collaterals develop from branches of the subclavian, internal mammary, superior intercostal, and axillary arteries

CAUSES
Congenital: Takayasu's arteritis, Turner's syndrome, multiple left-sided obstruction

RISK FACTORS
• Turner's syndrome
• Congenital left heart abnormalities

DIAGNOSIS

DIFFERENTIAL DIAGNOSIS
• Takayasu's arteritis
• Neurofibromatosis
• Pseudocoarctation (with or without hypertension, peripheral vascular disease)

LABORATORY N/A
Drugs that may alter lab results: N/A
Disorders that may alter lab results: N/A

PATHOLOGICAL FINDINGS
• Segmental tubular hypoplasia
• Discrete obstruction with medial thickening
• Distal aneurysm

SPECIAL TESTS
• Doppler examination of pulses reveals disparity
• Electrocardiogram may show left ventricular hypertrophy
• Blood pressures - all 4 extremities

IMAGING
• Chest x-ray may show rib notching, "3" sign, rarely cardiomegaly
• Echocardiography for coarctation and coexisting cardiac anomalies
• Transesophageal echocardiography
• Magnetic resonance imaging (MRI)

DIAGNOSTIC PROCEDURES
Cardiac catheterization and angiography: post-stenotic dilation

TREATMENT

APPROPRIATE HEALTH CARE Inpatient surgery

GENERAL MEASURES N/A

SURGICAL MEASURES
• Surgical correction or balloon angioplasty can be done in infancy if urgently needed. Best results when performed age 1-2 years.
• Surgery should be done in childhood and adulthood as soon as coarctation diagnosed to prevent late complications
• Three common surgical procedures for correction of coarctation include (1) end-to-end anastomosis, (2) patch aortoplasty (insertion of dacron patch), and, (3) subclavian flap procedure
• Balloon angioplasty of coarctation offers good results for primary treatment and for post-operative re-stenosis

ACTIVITY Exercise may exacerbate hypertension, but normal activity recommended after correction

DIET No special diet

PATIENT EDUCATION
• Discuss post-coarctation syndrome
• For patient education materials favorably reviewed on this topic, contact: American Heart Association, 7320 Greenville Avenue, Dallas, TX 75231, (214)373-6300

MEDICATIONS

DRUG(S) OF CHOICE
• Alprostadil (prostaglandin E1), patency of ductus arteriosus
• Antibiotic prophylaxis (for dental and/or invasive procedures) for life (even after correction)
• Antihypertensives if needed
• Preload and afterload reduction if heart failure develops
Contraindications: Refer to manufacturer's profile of each drug
Precautions:
• Lowering upper extremity blood pressure may cause hypoperfusion of lower extremities
• Lowering blood pressure not advised in pregnancy unless emergency
Significant possible interactions: Refer to manufacturer's profile of each drug

ALTERNATIVE DRUGS N/A

FOLLOWUP

PATIENT MONITORING Frequent post-operative followup for evidence of re-stenosis (check for hypertension and pulse disparities) and late complications

PREVENTION/AVOIDANCE Patients should be encouraged to have normal lifestyles and activities after coarctation correction

POSSIBLE COMPLICATIONS
• Most common with late or no correction
• Heart failure
• Aneurysm of circle of Willis, rupture possible
• Hypertension
• Rupture or dissection of aortic aneurysm
• Endarteritis or endocarditis (need antibiotic prophylaxis)
• Aortic valve disease (stenosis or insufficiency)
• Post coarctectomy syndrome: recurrence, hypertension, atherosclerotic heart disease, aneurysm at site of coarctectomy, progressive aortic stenosis and/or regurgitation

EXPECTED COURSE/PROGNOSIS
• Depends on age of repair and presence of other cardiac abnormalities
• Residual or restenosis (6-33%)
• Subsequent cardiac surgery (11%)
• Hypertension (25%)
• Survival after surgery: 10 years (91%), 20 years (84%), 30 years (72%)
• Uncorrected, 80% mortality before age 50

MISCELLANEOUS

ASSOCIATED CONDITIONS
• Bicuspid aortic valve (85%)
• Patent ductus arteriosus (65%)
• Ventricular septal defect (30-35%)
• Aortic stenosis and/or insufficiency
• Subvalvular aortic stenosis
• Mitral valve abnormalities (common)
• Transposition of great vessels or double outlet right ventricle
• Aneurysm of circle of Willis

AGE-RELATED FACTORS Greater risk of complications if correction is delayed beyond early childhood. Often diagnosis is delayed.
Pediatric: N/A
Geriatric: N/A
Others: N/A

PREGNANCY Uncorrected (or restenosis) coarctation carries high risk of aortic rupture or dissection and cerebral hemorrhage (aneurysm of circle of Willis rupture), but lower risk of pre-eclampsia than other forms of hypertension

SYNONYMS N/A

ICD-9-CM 747.1

SEE ALSO N/A

OTHER NOTES N/A

ABBREVIATIONS N/A

REFERENCES
• Hurst JW, et al: The Heart. 7th Ed. New York, McGraw-Hill, 1990
• Adams FH, Emmanouilides GC, Riemenschneider TA: Moss' Heart Disease in Infants, Children and Adolescents. 4th Ed. Baltimore, Williams & Wilkins, 1989
• Braunwalk E: Heart Disease. 4th Ed. Philadelphia, WB Saunders Co, 1992.
Illustrations: N/A
Internet references: http://www.5mcc.com

Author(s)
Karil Bellah, MD

Coccidioidomycosis

BASICS

DESCRIPTION Pulmonary fungal infection endemic to the Southwest USA. Can become progressive and involve extrapulmonary sites, including bone, CNS, and skin. Known as the "great imitator." Incubation period is 1 to 4 weeks after exposure.
System(s) affected: Pulmonary, Nervous, Musculoskeletal, Skin/Exocrine, Endocrine/Metabolic
Genetics: Unknown
Incidence/Prevalence in USA: 100,000 cases per year. (0.5% extrapulmonary)
Predominant age: All ages
Predominant sex: Male = Female

SIGNS AND SYMPTOMS
• Anorexia
• Arthralgias
• Chest pain
• Chills
• Confusion
• Cough, dry or productive
• Cyanosis
• Dyspnea
• Erythema nodosum
• Fatigue
• Fever
• Headache
• Hepatomegaly
• Hydrocephalus
• Hyperreflexia
• Malaise
• Night sweats
• Pleural friction rub
• Rash
• Sore throat
• Splenomegaly
• Tachycardia
• Tenosynovitis
• Toxic erythema
• Weight loss
• Note: Over half of cases are subclinical

CAUSES Coccidioides immitis, a soil fungus especially adapted to arid conditions. Liberated spores are inhaled when soil is disturbed: digging, construction sites, archaeological sites, dust storms, spelunking (exploring caves). Soil that lines rodent burrows is worst.

RISK FACTORS
• Certain groups are more prone to dissemination: immunocompromised hosts, pregnant women, African-Americans, Filipinos.
• CNS involvement more common in young white males
• Immunosuppression. Previously infected patients can experience relapse years later through the mechanism of cell-mediated immune deficiency.
• Diabetes mellitus
• AIDS

DIAGNOSIS

DIFFERENTIAL DIAGNOSIS
• Pneumonia, all etiologies
• Lung carcinoma
• Sarcoidosis
• Histoplasmosis, other fungi
• Lung abscess
• TB
• Lymphoma
• Meningitis
• Plus all other causes of cough, fever, fatigue
• Old granulomas can be mistaken for tumors

LABORATORY
• Skin test turns positive at 3 weeks to 3 months; may remain positive indefinitely; applying skin test will not interfere with serologies
• Serology - precipitin antibodies (IgM) rise within 2 weeks and disappear after 2 months; complement fixation antibodies (IgG) rise at 1-3 months; patients with mild symptoms may never develop detectable serology
• Culture of sputum, wound exudate, joint aspirate; unlikely to grow fungus in urine, blood, pleural fluid
Drugs that may alter lab results: Steroids may alter ability to react to skin testing
Disorders that may alter lab results: N/A

PATHOLOGICAL FINDINGS Fungal elements, spherules

SPECIAL TESTS Biopsy of affected tissue, e.g., lung nodule, skin lesion

IMAGING Chest x-ray findings include - normal, infiltrate(s), nodule(s), cavity, adenopathy mediastinal or hilar, pleural effusion

DIAGNOSTIC PROCEDURES If unable to establish diagnosis from skin testing and serologies - bronchoscopy, fine-needle biopsy, open lung biopsy, pleural biopsy, bone/skin/node biopsy

TREATMENT

APPROPRIATE HEALTH CARE
• Outpatient except in very severe cases
• Recommend referral to pulmonary or infectious disease specialist if drug treatment becomes imperative. Consider such treatment if IgG titers > 1:16, if disease persists without improvement over 6 weeks, or if skin test remains negative in the face of positive serology.

GENERAL MEASURES
• Cool mist humidifier for dry cough or sore throat
• Rest
• Supportive therapy

SURGICAL MEASURES N/A

ACTIVITY As tolerated

DIET No special diet

PATIENT EDUCATION For patient education materials favorably reviewed on this topic, contact: American Lung Association, 1740 Broadway, New York, NY 10019, (212)315-8700

MEDICATIONS

DRUG(S) OF CHOICE
• In mild cases, treat for symptomatic relief of cough with antitussives plus treat pleuritic pain with nonsteroidal anti-inflammatory agents
• For persistent, progressive, or disseminated disease the following drugs are indicated. However, dosing, whom to treat, and length of treatment is controversial.
◊ Amphotericin B: 0.5-1.0 mg/kg with a total cumulative dose of 2-4 gm
◊ Ketoconazole: 200-400 mg/day
◊ Fluconazole: 200-400 mg/day.
Fluconazole is also the treatment of choice for coccimeningitis with a usual dose of 800 mg/day.
Contraindications: Avoid steroids
Precautions: Amphotericin is highly nephrotoxic.
Significant possible interactions:
• Ketoconazole-H2 blockers: decrease absorption of ketoconazole (ketoconazole requires an acidic pH for absorption).
• Azole antifungals-terfenadine (Seldane) or astemizole (Hismanal): QT prolongation and ventricular arrhythmias

ALTERNATIVE DRUGS   N/A

FOLLOWUP

PATIENT MONITORING
• If skin test and serology are negative but index of suspicion is high, repeat every 2 weeks. With positive serologies, follow titers every 2 weeks until titers are dropping and patient has clinical improvement or resolution.
• Follow abnormal chest x-rays until findings are resolved or scarring process is complete

PREVENTION/AVOIDANCE
• Not contagious between host and contacts
• Cultures in lab are highly contagious via inhalation and lab personnel must be very cautious when handling specimens
• High risk populations (see Risk factors) should consider avoiding high risk activities, such as construction, archaeological digs, etc.)

POSSIBLE COMPLICATIONS
• Severe cases are fatal, especially if associated with meningitis. Can cause destruction of pulmonary tissue due to scarring, cavities, etc.
• Hemoptysis

EXPECTED COURSE/PROGNOSIS
• Most cases are self-limited, resolve within a few months. Progressive and disseminated disease can be difficult to eradicate.
• Prognosis poor if weak cell mediated immunity response or high IgG
• Relapse of extrapulmonary or disseminated disease is common.

MISCELLANEOUS

ASSOCIATED CONDITIONS   N/A

AGE-RELATED FACTORS
Pediatric: N/A
Geriatric: N/A
Others: N/A

PREGNANCY   Increased risk for dissemination, especially if contracted late in gestation

SYNONYMS
• Cocci
• Desert fever
• Posada-Wernicke disease
• Valley fever
• San Joaquin fever

ICD-9-CM
114.9 Coccidiomycosis, unspecified

SEE ALSO   N/A

OTHER NOTES   Travel history is essential when working up any pulmonary infection not responding to normal measures

ABBREVIATIONS   N/A

REFERENCES
• Isselbacher KJ, et al, eds: Harrison's Principles of Internal Medicine. 13th Ed. New York, McGraw-Hill, 1994
• Hedges E, Miller S: Coccidiomycosis: Office diagnosis and treatment. Amer Fam Phys 1990
Illustrations: N/A
Internet references: http://www.5mcc.com

Author(s)
Sandra Miller, MD

Colic, infantile

BASICS

DESCRIPTION Colic is an incompletely understood state of excessive crying seen in young infants who are otherwise well. A working definition - abnormal crying that lasts > 3 hours/day for at least 3 times/week.
Incidence/Prevalence in USA: 10,000/100,000 in some reports, as high as 25,000/100,000 in others
System(s) affected: Gastrointestinal, Nervous
Genetics: N/A
Predominant Age: 3 weeks of age to 3 months of age
Predominant Sex: Male = Female

SIGNS AND SYMPTOMS
• Rhythmic crying, paroxysmal
• No consolability
• Fist clenching
• Back arching
• Drawing up of infant's legs
• Excessive flatus

CAUSES
• Poorly understood
• Small percentage related to milk allergy

RISK FACTORS Physiologic predisposition in infant

DIAGNOSIS

DIFFERENTIAL DIAGNOSIS
• Any organic cause for excessive crying in infants (i.e. meningitis, sepsis, strangulated hernia, occult fracture)
• Entirely a clinical diagnosis

LABORATORY N/A
Drugs that may alter lab results: N/A
Disorders that may alter lab results: N/A

PATHOLOGICAL FINDINGS N/A

SPECIAL TESTS N/A

IMAGING N/A

DIAGNOSTIC PROCEDURES N/A

TREATMENT

APPROPRIATE HEALTH CARE
Outpatient management

GENERAL MEASURES
• Handling of the colicky infant in a calm and non-stimulating manner should be demonstrated
• Use of pacifier
• Use of gentle rhythmic motion (i.e., car rides)
• Use of music

SURGICAL MEASURES N/A

ACTIVITY N/A

DIET Removal of cow's milk from diet for a one week trial

PATIENT EDUCATION American Academy of Pediatrics, 141 Northwest Point Blvd., P.O. Box 927, Elk Grove Village, IL 60009-0927, (800)433-9016

MEDICATIONS

DRUG(S) OF CHOICE Simethicone may be useful in some cases
Contraindications: N/A
Precautions: N/A
Significant possible interactions: N/A

ALTERNATIVE DRUGS N/A

FOLLOWUP

PATIENT MONITORING Frequent outpatient visits as needed for parental reassurance and education

EXPECTED COURSE/PROGNOSIS
• Usually subsides by 3 months of age
• Prognosis not sufficiently investigated

PREVENTION/AVOIDANCE N/A

POSSIBLE COMPLICATIONS N/A

MISCELLANEOUS

ASSOCIATED CONDITIONS N/A

AGE-RELATED FACTORS
Pediatric: A problem of infancy
Geriatric: N/A
Others: N/A

PREGNANCY N/A
Others: N/A

SYNONYMS N/A

ICD-9-CM 789.0 abdominal pain

SEE ALSO N/A

OTHER NOTES N/A

ABBREVIATIONS N/A

REFERENCES Behrman RE, Kleigman RM: Nelson Textbook of Pediatrics. Philadelphia, WB Saunders Co, 1993
Illustrations: N/A
Internet references: http://www.5mcc.com

Author(s)
Jeryl Dansky, MD

Colorectal malignancy

BASICS

DESCRIPTION A malignant neoplasm arising from the luminal surface of the colon, rectum or anus.
• Adenocarcinoma - by far, most common histologic form, usually arising from benign adenoma. Unequally distributed, with 38% in proximal colon and 62% in distal colon or rectum.
• Carcinoid - uncommon, arising from enterochromaffin cells. Usually located in appendix or rectum; not likely to metastasize unless larger than 2 cm in diameter.
• Squamous cell carcinoma - uncommon form; located in the anal canal. Also called epidermoid or cloacogenic.
• Melanoma - rare; usually presents as pigmented lesion adjacent to dentate line
System(s) affected: Gastrointestinal
Genetics:
• Hereditary autosomal dominant in 5-10%; first-degree relative in 20%
• Ras oncogene mutations seen in 40-50% of adenocarcinoma; alterations of suppressor genes also seen in 75%, especially involving chromosomes 17,18
Incidence/Prevalence in USA: 155,000 new cases/year
Predominant age: Adenocarcinoma usually occurs in individuals > age 50 years with peak incidence in the seventh decade
Predominant sex: Male = Female

SIGNS AND SYMPTOMS
• Vary with location
• Early lesions are frequently asymptomatic
• Right-sided adenocarcinoma
  ◊ Anemia
  ◊ Pain and/or mass in right lower quadrant
  ◊ Occult blood in stool
  ◊ Change in appearance of stool (infrequent)
• Left-sided adenocarcinoma
  ◊ Change in bowel habits (may be constipation or diarrhea)
  ◊ Reduced caliber of stool
  ◊ Red blood mixed in stool
• Rectal adenocarcinoma
  ◊ Bright red rectal bleeding
  ◊ Tenesmus
  ◊ Mass on digital exam
• Carcinoid
  ◊ Often incidental finding
  ◊ Appendicitis-like if located in appendix
  ◊ Rectal bleeding
  ◊ Crampy abdominal pain
  ◊ Carcinoid syndrome; occurs with metastases to liver; includes facial flushing, abdominal cramps, diarrhea
• Squamous cell carcinoma
  ◊ Painful defecation
  ◊ Rectal bleeding
  ◊ Mass or ulcer in anal canal
  ◊ Non-healing anal fissure

CAUSES
• Undetermined; both genetic and environmental factors may contribute
• Environmental - high dietary animal fat, low dietary fiber

RISK FACTORS
• Adenocarcinoma
  ◊ Two-thirds of patients are over 50 years old
  ◊ Pancolonic ulcerative colitis, (2% per year after 10 years active disease)
  ◊ Familial polyposis (100%)
  ◊ Hereditary nonpolyposis colorectal cancer (family history)
  ◊ Benign adenomas (tubular 3%; villous 9-12%)
  ◊ Coexisting (synchronous) colon cancer (5%)
  ◊ Previous (metachronous) colon cancer (2-5%)
• Carcinoid
  ◊ Multiple endocrine adenopathy (MEA), rare
  ◊ Other organs with carcinoid (small bowel, bronchial)
• Squamous cell carcinoma
  ◊ Bowen's disease
  ◊ Paget's disease

DIAGNOSIS

DIFFERENTIAL DIAGNOSIS
• Strictures (ischemic, Crohn's, diverticulosis)
• Other neoplasms (prostatic carcinoma, lipoma, leiomyoma, sarcoma, others)
• Infectious/inflammatory lesions (ameboma, tuberculoma, hemorrhoids)
• Extrinsic masses (abscesses, cysts/pseudocysts, phlegmons)

LABORATORY
• Positive fecal occult blood test
• Anemia
• Urinary 5-hydroxyindoleacetic acid (5-HIAA); elevated in carcinoid
• Elevated plasma carcinoembryonic antigen (CEA)
Drugs that may alter lab results:
• Aspirin-containing medications and nonsteroidal anti-inflammatory drugs - positive fecal occult blood test
• Smoking - increased carcinoembryonic antigen
Disorders that may alter lab results:
• Peptic ulcer disease, ulcerative colitis, hemorrhoids, benign polyps - positive fecal occult blood test
• Renal failure - increased carcinoembryonic antigen

PATHOLOGICAL FINDINGS
• Adenocarcinoma
  ◊ May appear as ulcerated, polypoid, or fungating mass. May extend to local structures or metastasize by blood, lymphatics; staging of tumor reflects level of penetration.
  ◊ Duke's Stage A - mucosal involvement with or without submucosal extension
  ◊ Duke's Stage B1 - to muscularis propria but not through serosa
  ◊ Duke's Stage B2 - extends beyond serosa
  ◊ Duke's Stage C - regional nodes involved
  ◊ Duke's Stage D - distant metastases (liver, lung)
• Carcinoid
  ◊ Tend to be multicentric
  ◊ Metastasize by blood, lymphatics
• Squamous cell carcinoma
  ◊ Most are ulcerative but may vary greatly in size
  ◊ Metastasize to inguinal lymphatics

SPECIAL TESTS Carcinoembryonic antigen - usually elevated with bulky tumor or metastases

IMAGING
• Barium enema (air-contrast preferred) - may not be necessary if colonoscopy is complete and provides adequate diagnostic information
• Computed tomography - sometimes used to determine extent of pelvic or liver involvement; not usually necessary
• Transrectal ultrasound - may be useful in defining extent of involvement by small rectal lesions

DIAGNOSTIC PROCEDURES
• Anoscopy - useful for anal canal visualization, biopsies
• Proctoscopy/flexible sigmoidoscopy with biopsy - used for distal lesions when complementary barium enema available for proximal colon
• Colonoscopy with biopsy - for primary diagnosis, screening of high-risk patients and post-resection surveillance

Colorectal malignancy

TREATMENT

APPROPRIATE HEALTH CARE Inpatient

GENERAL MEASURES N/A

SURGICAL MEASURES
• Surgical procedures - radical resection of tumor with wide margins; includes segments of normal colon, mesentery, lymph nodes
• Right hemicolectomy for proximal tumors
• Left hemicolectomy for descending colon cancers
• Sigmoid colectomy for sigmoid cancers
• Abdominoperineal resection with colostomy for cancers of distal rectum (within 5-7 cm of dentate line)
• Preoperative or postoperative radiotherapy and chemotherapy: May improve outcome when used for rectal carcinoma
• For carcinoma of anus - combined chemotherapy (5-fluorouracil and mitomycin C) and radiotherapy. Convert to abdominoperineal resection for residual or recurrent tumor.

ACTIVITY Usually normal; may be slightly modified for patient with stoma

DIET Usually normal; avoidance of gas-producing foods may be helpful in ostomates (cabbage, beans, onions, alcoholic beverages)

PATIENT EDUCATION
• Facts on Colorectal Cancer, American Cancer Society, 1988
• National Cancer Institute, Dept. of Health And Human Services, Public Inquiries Section, Office of Cancer Communications, Building 31, Room 101-18, 9000 Rockville Pike, Bethesda, MD 20892, (301)496-5583,

MEDICATIONS

DRUG(S) OF CHOICE
• Steroids, somatostatin or methysergide may ameliorate symptoms of carcinoid syndrome
• Stage C adenocarcinoma - fluorouracil (5-FU) plus levamisole
Contraindications: Peptic ulcer disease (steroids)
Precautions: Refer to manufacturer's literature
Significant possible interactions: Refer to manufacturer's literature

ALTERNATIVE DRUGS N/A

FOLLOWUP

PATIENT MONITORING
• Adenocarcinoma (after remainder of colon is cleared of all lesions)
  ◊ Colonoscopy - annually x 2 years; then every 3 years
  ◊ Carcinoembryonic antigen test, liver chemistries, fecal occult blood test - every three months for 2 years; then every 6 months for 2 years; then annually
• Carcinoid:
  ◊ 5-HIAA every 6 months x 2 years, then annually
• Squamous cell carcinoma:
  ◊ Clinical evaluation every 4 months x 1 year, then annually
  ◊ Biopsy suspicious areas in anus, groin

PREVENTION/AVOIDANCE Colonic polyps should be removed, examined microscopically. If benign, surveillance colonoscopy should be performed every 3 years.

POSSIBLE COMPLICATIONS
• Following resections:
  ◊ Mortality 5-10%
  ◊ Wound infection 5-15%
  ◊ Anastomotic stricture/leak/abscess 2-5%
  ◊ Pneumonia 5-10%
  ◊ Urinary tract infection 5-20%
• During chemotherapy or radiation therapy:
  ◊ Stomatitis
  ◊ Proctitis/diarrhea
  ◊ Temporary loss of hair

EXPECTED COURSE/PROGNOSIS
• Adenocarcinoma: Overall 5-year survival is 55% but relates to tumor stage in individual patients
  ◊ Duke's A - 95%
  ◊ Duke's B1 - 85-90%
  ◊ Duke's B2 - 60-70%
  ◊ Duke's C - 15-25%
  ◊ Duke's D - 5%
• Carcinoid:
  ◊ Overall 5-year survival is 65%
  ◊ Relates to tumor stage as in adenocarcinoma
• Squamous cell carcinoma:
  ◊ Overall 5-year survival is 79%

MISCELLANEOUS

ASSOCIATED CONDITIONS Colonic carcinoid - multiple endocrine neoplasia types I, II

AGE-RELATED FACTORS
Pediatric: Adenocarcinoma of colon occurs rarely in children; prognosis is very poor
Geriatric: Coexistence of medical illness may complicate postoperative course
Others: N/A

PREGNANCY N/A

SYNONYMS N/A

ICD-9-CM
• 1540 Colorectal cancer
• 44144 Colectomy

SEE ALSO N/A

OTHER NOTES N/A

ABBREVIATIONS N/A

REFERENCES
• Silverman A, Desai TK, Dhar R, et al: Clinical Features, Evaluation, and Detection of Colorectal Cancer. Gastroenterology Clinics of North America 1988;17:713-25
• Twomey P, Burchell M, Strawn D, Guernsey J: Local Control in Rectal Cancer. A Clinical Review and Meta-analysis, Arch Surg 1989;124:1174-9
• Vogelstein B, Fearon ER, Hamilton SR, et al: Genetic Alterations During Colorectal-tumor Development. N Engl J Med 1988;319:525-32
• Craanen ME, Blok P, Offerhaus GT, Tygat GN: Recent developments in hereditary nonpolyposis colorectal cancer. Scand J Gastroenterol 1996;31(suppl 218):92-97
Illustrations: N/A
Internet references: http://www.5mcc.com

Author(s)
Wayne H. Schwesinger, MD

Common cold

BASICS

DESCRIPTION Inflammation of the nasal passages due to any number of respiratory viruses. Usually not serious; vast majority are self-treated.
System(s) affected: Pulmonary
Genetics: American Indians and Eskimos at higher risk than other ethnic groups and have more frequent complications such as otitis media; individuals with certain alpha-1-antitrypsin genotypes may be unusually susceptible to the common cold.
Incidence/prevalence in USA: Preschool children 6-10 colds/yr; kindergarten 12/yr; schoolchildren 7/yr; adolescents/adults 2-4/yr. National Ambulatory Survey: 31 episodes/100 persons/year (counting only colds that lead to medical attention or at least one day of restricted activity).
Predominant age: Children > adults
Predominant sex: Male = Female

SIGNS AND SYMPTOMS
• Nasal stuffiness and/or obstruction (80-100%)
• Sneezing (50-70%)
• Scratchy throat (50%)
• Cough (40%)
• Hoarseness (30%)
• Malaise (20-25%)
• Headache (25%)
• Fever > 100°F/37.7°C (0-1%)

CAUSES
• Usually due to one of 200 virus strains from six virus families; many strains present within the same geographic region or family
  ◊ Rhinovirus (> 200 serotypes)
  ◊ Influenza A, B, C viruses
  ◊ Parainfluenza viruses
  ◊ Respiratory syncytial viruses
  ◊ Coronaviruses
  ◊ Adenoviruses
  ◊ Certain ECHO viruses
• In 40% cases, no agent can be identified

RISK FACTORS
• Exposure to infected individuals
• Touching one's nose or conjunctiva with contaminated fingers

DIAGNOSIS

DIFFERENTIAL DIAGNOSIS
• Mumps
• Rubeola
• Allergic rhinitis
• Cytomegalovirus
• Epstein-Barr virus
• Mycoplasma pneumonia
• Influenza – systemic symptoms including myalgias, malaise, severe headache and ocular symptoms overshadow the respiratory complaints

LABORATORY
• CBC if symptoms persist for more than 10 days or with fever > 100°F (37.8°C)
• Nasal smear for eosinophilia may be useful in select individuals
Drugs that may alter lab results: N/A
Disorders that may alter lab results: N/A

PATHOLOGICAL FINDINGS
• Rhinovirus infects the ciliated epithelium lining the nose. Edema and hyperemia of nasal mucous membranes results.
• Exudation of serous and mucinous fluid containing immunoglobulins
• Histology: edema of subepithelial connective tissue, and a scanty cellular infiltrate containing neutrophils, plasma cells, lymphocytes, and eosinophils
• Rhinovirus causes a "non-destructive" inflammation of the mucous membranes, in contrast to influenza and parainfluenza which denude epithelium to the basement membrane

SPECIAL TESTS
In some centers, rapid antigen tests for various respiratory viruses are available for patients requiring hospitalization or for research purposes

IMAGING
Not indicated unless there is concern for bacterial superinfection of the sinuses, supraglottic region, trachea, or lungs

DIAGNOSTIC PROCEDURES
In rare cases, may want to attempt to culture virus from nasal washings or identify by ELISA or RIA methods

TREATMENT

APPROPRIATE HEALTH CARE
Outpatient self-care

GENERAL MEASURES
• Rest, fluids, and symptomatic measures
• Reassure that usual course is 6-10 days
• Humidify inspired air
• Discontinue tobacco and alcohol products (if not already done)
• In infants, clear nasal passages with a bulb syringe, position mattress at 45°, use saline nasal drops

SURGICAL MEASURES N/A

ACTIVITY
Up as tolerated with increased rest in the first few days

DIET
Encourage fluids

PATIENT EDUCATION
• Reassure that colds are ubiquitous and a normal part of human existence
• Spread is primarily via hand-to-hand transmission of virus contaminated nasal secretions; persons with colds touch their nose and eyes and then touch others
• Small-particle aerosols released in talking, coughing, and sneezing do not travel very far and contain only a low concentration of rhinovirus
• Rhinovirus survives for hours on the hands and hard surfaces, but does not survive long on porous surfaces such as tissues
• Individual susceptibility to colds, depends in large part, on pre-existing antibody levels
• Serum immunity lasts for years, but most individuals gain little protection against future colds due, in part, to the large number of viral serotypes and the antigenic drift that occurs over time in some viral types (rhinovirus, influenza)
• Educate about the expected course and symptomatic measures that can be used
• Advise patients to contact you if they develop dyspnea, productive cough, temperature > 102°F (38.9°C), or shaking chills

MEDICATIONS

DRUG(S) OF CHOICE
No cure or practical preventive measure documented. Medications targeting a particular symptom reduce the likelihood of adverse systemic effects
Topical decongestants (sympathomimetics)
• Reduce edema and swelling of the nasal mucosa, promote drainage, and reduce nasal airflow resistance. Preferred over oral because of minimal systemic effects. Sprays preferred over drops in ages > 6.
• oxymetazoline
  ◊ Adults and children ages 6-12: 0.05% solution, 2 or 3 sprays in each nostril bid
  ◊ Children ages 2-6: 0.025% solution, 2 or 3 drops in each nostril bid
  ◊ Rebound congestion (rhinitis medicamentosa) is unlikely if used < 5 days
Topical anticholinergics
Control rhinorrhea but do not relieve nasal congestion or sneezing
• ipratropium:
  ◊ Adults and children >11: 0.06% solution, 2 sprays to each nostril TID for 4 days
Oral decongestants (sympathomimetics)
Advantages over topical decongestants: longer duration of action, lack of local irritation and no risk of rhinitis medicamentosa
• Pseudoephedrine
  ◊ Adults: 60 mg q4-6h (120 mg sustained release q12h)
  ◊ Children ages 6-12: 30 mg q4-6h
  ◊ Children 2-5: 15 mg q4-6h
Antihistamines
• Histamine has not been shown to play a significant role in the common cold. Nevertheless, antihistamines are safe and effective in alleviating sneezing and rhinorrhea, but many dissenting opinions make their role adjunctive. Their perceived benefit may come from anticholinergic effects drying nasal and pharyngeal secretions and their sedative effects promote rest.
• Chlorpheniramine
  ◊ Adults: 4 mg q4-6h (or 8 mg tid, 12 mg bid)
  ◊ Children ages 6-12: 2 mg q4-6h
  ◊ Children ages 2-6: 1 mg q4-6h

Cough suppressants
- Codeine
  ◊ Adults: 10-20 mg q4-6h
  ◊ Children ages 6-12: 5-10 mg q4-6h
  ◊ Children ages 2-6: 2.5-5 mg q4-6h
- Dextromethorphan
  ◊ Adults: 10-30 mg q4-8h
  ◊ Children ages 6-12: 15 mg q6-8h
  ◊ Children ages 2-6: 2.5-7.5 mg q4-8h
- Cough of the common cold is most likely due to irritation of tracheobronchial receptors by post nasal drip of mucous and may benefit from decongestant therapy. If the cough is nonproductive, or interferes with sleep or normal activities, a cough suppressant is indicated.
- Codeine and dextromethorphan exhibit comparable efficacy. Common adverse effects include drowsiness and gastrointestinal upset.

Expectorants
- Though commonly employed in cold remedies, efficacy is not proven
- Example: guaifenesin
  ◊ Adults: 100-400 mg q4h
  ◊ Children ages 6-12: 100-200 mg q4h
  ◊ Children ages 2-5: 50-100 mg q4h

Contraindications: Oral decongestants are contraindicated in patients taking monoamine oxidase inhibitors and selegiline

Precautions:

Oral decongestants
- Affect all vascular beds and may increase blood pressure. They are cardiac stimulants and may result in arrhythmias. They may increase glucose levels in individuals with glucose intolerance or diabetes mellitus.
- Other adverse effects include headache, nervousness, sleeplessness, and dizziness
- Should be used with caution in patients taking guanethidine

Antihistamines
- Nasal blockage and sinus congestion may worsen

Cough suppressants
- The possibility of misuse and dependence is higher with codeine, but dextromethorphan abuse by adolescents has been reported

Expectorants
- Liquid expectorant preparations may contain high concentrations of alcohol
- Nausea, vomiting or abdominal pain are common adverse effects

Vitamin C
- Use is generally safe, but precipitation of urate, oxalate, or cystine stones has been seen, and urine glucose monitoring may be inaccurate in individuals taking large doses

Significant possible interactions: See manufacturer's literature

ALTERNATIVE DRUGS
- Many mouthwashes, gargles and lozenges are promoted to relieve the pain of sore throat. The demulcent effects of hard candy, gargling with warm saline, and the use of products containing anesthetics such as benzocaine or phenol, may all provide significant subjective relief of pain. Antibacterial gargles or lozenges are of no value in treating a viral illness.
- Aromatic oils such as menthol, camphor and eucalyptus, when applied topically or taken in a lozenge, produce a sensation of increased airflow in the absence of a significant change in airflow resistance.

Antivirals
- Interferon
  ◊ Prevents viral invasion of mucosa and can successfully prevent colds; side effects include nasal irritation or bleeding in about 10% of patients; may eventually be useful in groups that have close contact
- Zinc chloride
  ◊ Prevents viral replication in vitro, but the efficacy of zinc lozenges is unproven

Vitamin C (ascorbic acid)
- Doses of 1 gram or more have been advocated. Studies have failed to demonstrate a preventive effect of vitamin C and have shown only a modest (average 23%) reduction in the severity and duration of symptoms.

FOLLOWUP

PATIENT MONITORING Patients should contact their physician if they develop fever associated with systemic symptoms, difficulty breathing, dyspnea, and/or purulent drainage

PREVENTION/AVOIDANCE Frequent hand washing and avoiding touching the face may help prevent colds

POSSIBLE COMPLICATIONS
- Lower respiratory tract infection
- Bronchial hyperreactivity
- May lead to decompensation in patients with asthma and chronic lung disease
- Otitis media (2% of colds)
- Acute sinusitis (0.5% of colds)
- Pneumonia
- Rhinitis medicamentosa

EXPECTED COURSE/PROGNOSIS
Complete recovery expected within 3-10 days

MISCELLANEOUS

ASSOCIATED CONDITIONS
- Pharyngitis
- Sinusitis
- Bronchitis
- Bronchiolitis
- Pneumonia
- Croup
- Asthma

AGE-RELATED FACTORS
Pediatric:
- Medications are likely to produce adverse effects or toxicity in young children
- Incidence of colds is highest
Geriatric: Medications commonly produce adverse effects in the elderly
Others: N/A

PREGNANCY
- Decongestants: no clear association between drug use and congenital defects
- Antihistamines: no clear association between

drug use and congenital defects
- Codeine: indiscriminate use during pregnancy may pose a risk to the fetus

SYNONYMS
- URI
- Upper respiratory infection

ICD-9-CM
460 Acute nasopharyngitis (common cold)

SEE ALSO
- Pharyngitis
- Mumps
- Measles, rubeola
- Rhinitis, allergic
- Cytomegalovirus inclusion disease
- Epstein-Barr virus infections
- Pneumonia, mycoplasma
- Influenza

OTHER NOTES N/A

ABBREVIATIONS
- ELISA = enzyme linked immunosorbent assay
- RIA = radioimmunoassay
- URI = upper respiratory infection

REFERENCES
- Bryant BG, Lombardi TP: Cold, cough and allergy products. In: Covington CR, Lawson LC, Young LL, eds. Handbook of Nonprescription Drugs.10th Ed. Washington, D.C, American Pharmaceutical Association, 1993:89-115
- Gadomski A: Rational use of over-the-counter medications in young children. JAMA 1994;272:1063-1064
- Hemila H: Does vitamin C alleviate the symptoms of the common cold?-a review of current evidence. Scandinavian Journal of Infectious Diseases 1994;26(1):1-6
- Hendeles L: Efficacy and safety of antihistamines and expectorants in nonprescription cough and cold preparations. Pharmacotherapy 1993;13(2):154-158
- Hendeles L: Selecting a decongestant. Pharmacotherapy 1993;13(6 Pt2):129S-134S
- Hendley JO, Gwaltney JM Jr: Mechanisms of transmission of rhinovirus infections. Epidemiologic Reviews 1988;10:243-258
- Lowenstein SR, Parrino TA: Management of the common cold. Advances in Internal Medicine 1987;32:207-233
- Saroea HG: Common colds: Causes, potential cures, and treatment. Canadian Family Physician 1993;39:2215-2216, 2219-2220
- Smith MB, Feldman W: Over-the-counter cold medications. A critical review of clinical trials between 1950 and 1991. JAMA 1993;269(17):2258-2263
- Tyrrell DA: A view from the common cold unit. Antiviral Research 1992;18(2):105-125
Illustrations: N/A
Internet references: http://www.5mcc.com

Author(s)
Barcey T. Levy, PhD, MD
Michael W. Kelly, PharmD, MS

Complete atrioventricular (AV) canal

BASICS

DESCRIPTION The central atrioventricular (AV) portion of the cardiac septum and the contiguous mitral and tricuspid valves are abnormal, allowing for an unobstructed atrioventricular canal. Children with Down syndrome and this anomaly rapidly progress to pulmonary vascular obstructive disease (within 3 to 6 months).
• Rastelli classification:
  ◊ Type A: Common anterior AV valve leaflet is divided and attached to the crest of the ventricular septum by chordae
  ◊ Type B: Common anterior AV valve leaflet is divided and chordae tendineae from the midportions of the divided anterior leaflet are attached to the right ventricular medial papillary muscle
  ◊ Type C: Common anterior AV valve leaflet is undivided and not attached to the ventricular septum (free-floating leaflet)
System(s) affected: Cardiovascular
Genetics: No known genetic pattern
Incidence/Prevalence in USA: 1 in 250,000 live births; type A being the most common
Predominant age: Congenital, present at birth
Predominant sex: Female > Male

SIGNS AND SYMPTOMS
• Pulmonary congestion
• Congestive heart failure
• Low systemic arterial blood oxygen saturation
• Tachycardia
• Poor feeding
• Growth failure
• Mitral regurgitation
• Pulmonary vascular obstructive disease, and cyanosis (30% in the first 2-3 years)

CAUSES Defective development of the endocardial cushions

RISK FACTORS Unknown

DIAGNOSIS

DIFFERENTIAL DIAGNOSIS
• Atrial septal defect
• Ventricular septal defect
• Incomplete or intermediate AV canal
• Patent ductus arteriosus
• Mitral valve prolapse
• Secondary mitral regurgitation
• Pulmonary vascular obstructive disease
• Anomalous pulmonary venous return

LABORATORY Arterial blood gas
Drugs that may alter lab results: N/A
Disorders that may alter lab results: N/A

PATHOLOGICAL FINDINGS Low oxygen saturation in the arterial blood gas

SPECIAL TESTS
• Cardiac 2-D echo-Doppler showing anatomic defect, increased pulmonary pressures, mitral regurgitation, tricuspid regurgitation, right and left atrial and ventricular enlargements
• ECG - superior QRS axis, right ventricular hypertrophy (RVH), left ventricular hypertrophy (LVH), possibly peaked P waves

IMAGING
• Cardiac angiogram demonstrating AV canal and mitral and tricuspid regurgitation, left and right atrial and ventricular enlargement
• Chest x-ray showing increased pulmonary vasculature, left and right atrial and ventricular enlargement
• MRI offers excellent imaging of crux

DIAGNOSTIC PROCEDURES
• Pulmonary artery catheter showing prominent "V" waves, elevated pulmonary capillary wedge pressures, right atrial "step-up" in oxygen saturations
• Angiography

TREATMENT

APPROPRIATE HEALTH CARE Medical management (digoxin, diuretics, afterload reducers) either as an inpatient or an outpatient, dependent upon the patient's condition

GENERAL MEASURES Provide general treatment for congestive heart failure

SURGICAL MEASURES If pulmonary edema, growth failure and congestive heart failure is refractive in spite of optimal medical therapy, reparative surgery should be pursued as early as possible. Repair should be especially early in children with Down syndrome (approximately 3 months). Repair should be performed before 2 years of age to avoid the continued progression of pulmonary vascular obstructive disease. Patients more than 2 years of age can undergo repair if the pulmonary vascular resistance (PVR) does not exceed 8-10 units-meters squared. At a minimum, surgical correction includes closure of the interatrial and interventricular septal defects and suspension of the medial aspects of the left and right AV valve leaflets. Pulmonary artery banding might still be a possibility.

ACTIVITY As tolerated

DIET High calorie, low salt

PATIENT EDUCATION Instruct regarding travel to altitudes and plane travel causing potential hypoxia

MEDICATIONS

DRUG(S) OF CHOICE Digoxin, ACE inhibitors or isosorbide dinitrate plus hydralazine, furosemide, potassium supplementation
• Doses for term infants
◊ Digoxin - oral 30 µg/kg (digitalizing), then 10 µg/kg/24 hrs. Adjust to maintain levels within therapeutic range - 0.5-2.0 ng/mL (0.64-2.6 nmol/L)
◊ Captopril - 0.05-0.1 mg/kg/dose tid-qid
◊ Isosorbide dinitrate - refer to manufacturer's literature
◊ Hydralazine - 0.75-3.0 mg/kg/dose, increase as needed to maximum of 6 mg/kg/dose
◊ Furosemide - oral 2 mg/kg, increase as needed to maximum of 6 mg/kg
◊ Potassium - supplement patients who require furosemide. Maintenance dose is 2-3 mEq/kg/24 hours.
Contraindications: Profound systemic hypotension, worsening hypoxia and V/Q mismatch with treatment
Precautions: Refer to manufacturer's literature
Significant possible interactions: Refer to manufacturer's literature

ALTERNATIVE DRUGS Dobutamine or amrinone drips

FOLLOWUP

PATIENT MONITORING
• As indicated by clinical intervention and disease progression
• Serial measurements of arterial oxygen content
• Serial measurements of pulmonary vascular resistance

PREVENTION/AVOIDANCE Avoid
hypoxic embarrassment in environments of low oxygen tension

POSSIBLE COMPLICATIONS
• Refractive hypoxia secondary to progressive pulmonary vascular obstructive disease
• Cyanosis
• Polycythemia
• Growth failure
• Congestive heart failure/pulmonary edema
• Complications of surgery:
◊ Residual ventricular septal defect
◊ Residual left ventricular to right atrial shunting
◊ Complete AV block

EXPECTED COURSE/PROGNOSIS
• PVR less than 5:
◊ If undergoing reparative surgery, are at risk for an approximate 10% surgical mortality
◊ The majority of those surviving realize complete relief of their symptoms and will need no further treatment
• PVR between 5-13 undergoing surgery:
◊ Perioperative mortality approaches 33%
◊ Survivors realize functional class I or II (New York Heart Association [NYHA] classification)
• PVR greater than 5 who do not or can not undergo surgical intervention:
◊ Deterioration is progressive with death ranging from 2-16 years of age

MISCELLANEOUS

ASSOCIATED CONDITIONS
• Down syndrome. Very high percentage have complete atrioventricular canal lesions.
• Tetralogy of Fallot
• Unbalanced canal with left or right dominance

AGE-RELATED FACTORS
Pediatric: Surgical intervention before age 2 or before marked increase in PVR occurs
Geriatric: N/A
Others: N/A

PREGNANCY N/A

SYNONYMS N/A

ICD-9-CM 745.69 Endocardial cushion defects, other

SEE ALSO
• Atrial septal defect (ASD)

OTHER NOTES N/A

ABBREVIATIONS
AVC = atrioventricular canal
PVR = pulmonary vascular resistance
V/Q = ventilation-perfusion ratio

REFERENCES
• Brandenburg RO, Fuster V, Giuliani ER, McGoon DC: Cardiology: Fundamentals and Practice. Chicago, Year Book Medical Publishers, 1987
• Braunwald E, ed: Heart Disease: A Textbook of Cardiovascular Medicine. 4th Ed. Philadelphia, WB Saunders Co, 1992
Illustrations: N/A
Internet references: http://www.5mcc.com

Author(s)
David J. Framm, MD, FACC

Condyloma acuminata

BASICS

DESCRIPTION Condyloma acuminata are soft, skin colored, fleshy warts that are caused by the HPV (human papilloma virus). There are at least 60 known types of HPV and types 6, 11, 16, 18, 31, 33 have been associated with condyloma acuminata. The disease is highly contagious, can appear singly or in groups, small or large. They appear in the vagina, on the cervix, around the external genitalia and rectum and occasionally, the throat. The incubation period may be from 1-6 months.
System(s) affected: Skin/Exocrine, Reproductive
Genetics: N/A
Incidence/Prevalence in USA: Minimum of 10-20% of sexually active women may be infected with HPV. Studies in men suggest a similar prevalence.
Predominant Age: 15-30 years of age
Predominant Sex: Male = Female

SIGNS AND SYMPTOMS
• Tumors, soft, sessile
• Surface smooth to very rough
• Multiple fingerlike projections
• Perianal condylomata acuminatum usually rough and cauliflower-like
• Penile lesions often smooth and papular
• Penile lesions often occur in groups of three or four
• Male sites - frenulum, corona, glans, prepuce, meatus, shaft, scrotum
• Female sites - labia, clitoris, periurethral area, perineum, vagina, cervix (flat lesions)
• Pruritis
• Irritation
• Bleeding (result of trauma)
• Perianal area (both sexes)
• Subclinical HPV infection
• May be detected by Pap test

CAUSES Human papillomaviruses. These are circular double-stranded DNA molecules. There are over 60 HPV subtypes. The cause of common venereal warts are types 6 and 11. Cervical dysplasia and carcinoma in situ are likely caused by types 16, 18, 31, 33, and 34.

RISK FACTORS
• Young adult
• Sexually active
• Not using condoms
• Possibly subclinical infection
• Young age of commencing sexual activity
• Cigarette smoking
• Poor hygiene
• Pregnancy
• Caucasian
• History of genital warts

DIAGNOSIS

DIFFERENTIAL DIAGNOSIS
• Condyloma lata (flat warts of syphilis)
• Lichen planus
• Normal sebaceous glands
• Seborrheic keratosis
• Molluscum contagiosum
• Keratomas
• Scabies

LABORATORY Serologic test for syphilis - negative
Drugs that may alter lab results: N/A
Disorders that may alter lab results: N/A

PATHOLOGICAL FINDINGS
• Possible cervical dysplasia in females
• Benign
• Well organized basal layer
• Underlying infiltration of lymphocytes
• Plasma cells
• Hyperplastic epithelial changes
• Basement membrane intact
• Sometimes difficult to differentiate from squamous cell carcinoma

SPECIAL TESTS Acetowhitening: Subclinical lesions can be visualized by wrapping the penis with gauze soaked with 5% acetic acid for 5 minutes. Using a ten X hand lens or colposcope, warts appear as tiny white papules. A shiny white appearance of the skin represents foci of epithelial hyperplasia (subclinical infection).

IMAGING N/A

DIAGNOSTIC PROCEDURES
• Biopsy with highly specialized identification techniques (not clinically useful)
• Colposcopy, androscopy, anoscopy, Pap smear

TREATMENT

APPROPRIATE HEALTH CARE
Outpatient

GENERAL MEASURES
• Treatment determined by location and size of warts
• Small warts may be treated with topical applications
• Cryotherapy

SURGICAL MEASURES
• Larger warts require laser treatment or electrocoagulation
• Surgical excision for large warts

ACTIVITY No restrictions

DIET No special diet

PATIENT EDUCATION
• Explain preventive measures and chronic nature of the infection
• Numerous pamphlets on HPV, STD prevention, condom use
• Emphasize need for women to get regular Pap smears

Condyloma acuminata

MEDICATIONS

DRUG(S) OF CHOICE
• Cryotherapy - liquid nitrogen is applied to warts in 5-10 second bursts. Usually requires 2-3 weekly sessions.
• Podophyllin in tincture of Benzoin. Apply directly to warts. Leave on for 1-4 hours, then wash off. Repeat treatment every 7 days until gone
or
• Podofilox (Condylox) - for external warts. Apply to external warts every 12 hours (allowing to dry) for 3 consecutive days. May repeat after 4 days.
Contraindications:
• Podophyllin - do not use during pregnancy or on oral, cervical, urethral or perianal warts. Can use on small number of vaginal warts with careful drying after application.
• Cryotherapy - none
Precautions:
• Podophyllin - to minimize local and systemic reactions, wash treated areas 1-4 hours after application and use ointments to protect surrounding skin from contact with podophyllin
• Cryotherapy - none
• Electrocautery - don't use in patient with pacemaker
Significant Possible Interactions: N/A

ALTERNATIVE DRUGS
• External (penile and perianal)
  ◊ Podophyllin
  ◊ Podofilox (Condylox) self-treatment
  ◊ Trichloroacetic acid (TCA) - apply weekly
  ◊ Electrocautery, laser, intralesional interferon
• Urethral meatus
  ◊ Laser
  ◊ Podophyllin
  ◊ Topical fluorouracil
• Anal
  ◊ Trichloracetic acid (TCA) - apply weekly
  ◊ Topical fluorouracil
• Oral
  ◊ Electrocautery
  ◊ Surgery
  ◊ Laser

FOLLOWUP

PATIENT MONITORING
• Every 2 weeks for treatment until clear
• Pap test every 1 year for indefinite period
• Biopsy for persistent warts
• Monitor sex partners

PREVENTION/AVOIDANCE
• Use of condoms by infected men
• Use of condoms by male sexual partners of individuals who have been treated for HPV infection
• Abstinence by women until treatment completed
• Circumcision may prevent recurrence in some men

POSSIBLE COMPLICATIONS
• Cervical dysplasia
• Carcinoma - cervical (squamous or adenocarcinoma) penile or rectal
• Male urethral obstruction

EXPECTED COURSE/PROGNOSIS
• Warts clear with treatment or spontaneous regression
• Recurrence is common with all forms of therapy
• Asymptomatic infection persists indefinitely

MISCELLANEOUS

ASSOCIATED CONDITIONS
• 90% of cervical cancer contains evidence of HPV infection
• Gonorrhea
• Syphilis
• AIDS
• Chlamydia
• Other sexually transmitted disease

AGE-RELATED FACTORS Young adults, infants and children
Pediatric: N/A
Geriatric: N/A
Others: Venereal warts are increasing in an ever younger population. A recent study of 487 college women showed an infection rate of 48%.

PREGNANCY
• Warts often grow larger in pregnancy and regress spontaneously after delivery. Use cryotherapy.
• HPV can be transmitted to infant at time of delivery and cause laryngeal papillomas

SYNONYMS
• Genital warts
• Venereal warts
• Papilloma acuminatum

ICD-9-CM
078.1 Condyloma acuminatum

SEE ALSO N/A

OTHER NOTES N/A

ABBREVIATIONS N/A

REFERENCES Fitzpatrick TB, et al: Color Atlas and Synopsis of Clinical Dermatology. New York, McGraw-Hill, 1992
Illustrations: 2 available on CD-ROM
Internet references: http://www.5mcc.com

Author(s)
Robert B. Daigneault, MD, FAAP
Kay A. Bauman, MD, MPH

Congenital megacolon

 BASICS

DESCRIPTION
Congenital disease of the colon, characterized by functional obstruction and accumulation of feces and massive dilatation of colon

System(s) affected: Gastrointestinal, Nervous

Genetics: Familial 50 times base rate. Sometimes associated with Down syndrome.

Incidence/Prevalence in USA: 1 in 2000 to 5000 births (Caucasians 91%, Blacks 8%, Oriental 0.5%)

Predominant age: Infancy

Predominant sex:
• Males > Females for short segment (8:2)
• Males > Females for long segment (5:4)

SIGNS AND SYMPTOMS
• Stools in pellets or ribbons with pasty consistency
• Early infancy:
  ◊ Onset early in infancy, newborn fails to pass meconium in 24 to 48 hours after birth
  ◊ Obstipation
  ◊ Marked enlargement and distention of abdomen
  ◊ Colonic peristalsis visible
  ◊ Vomiting
  ◊ Palpable fecal mass
  ◊ Growth retardation (possible)
• Older infants:
  ◊ Failure to thrive
  ◊ Anorexia
  ◊ Lack of physiologic urge to defecate
  ◊ Empty rectum on digital examination
  ◊ Palpable colon
  ◊ Visible peristalsis
  ◊ Hypoalbuminemia

CAUSES
Congenital absence of Auerbach's and Meissener's autonomic plexuses in bowel wall - usually limited to the colon

RISK FACTORS
• Family history of Hirschsprung's disease
• Offspring risk if parent has short segment - 2%; if parent has long segment - up to 50%
• Sibling risk if male affected - female has 0.6% risk (short segment)
• Sibling risk if female affected - male has 18% risk (long segment)

 DIAGNOSIS

DIFFERENTIAL DIAGNOSIS
• Megacolon, secondary (to Chagas' disease)
• Megacolon, acquired, functional
• Functional constipation
• Hypoganglionosis
• Meconium plug syndrome
• Small left colon syndrome
• Meconium ileus

LABORATORY
Electrolytes, albumin, CBC, urinalysis, thyroid function

Drugs that may alter lab results: N/A

Disorders that may alter lab results: N/A

PATHOLOGICAL FINDINGS
• Congenital absence of Auerbach's and Meissner's autonomic plexuses in myenteric plexus of colon wall
• Obstruction may begin at anus, and may extend proximally to involve varying portions of the colon or terminal ileum
• Enormous dilatation and hypertrophy of all layers of involved colon
• Rectosigmoid aganglionosis
• Submucosal hypertrophied nerve bundles

SPECIAL TESTS
• Proctoscopy: Ampulla empty of feces
• Biopsy: Absence of ganglia in wall of narrowed rectum
• Ano-rectal manometry

IMAGING
• X-ray - barium enema shows:
  ◊ Large ovoid mass mottled by small, irregular gas shadows
  ◊ Dilatation of sigmoid colon above narrowed distal sigmoid or rectum
  ◊ Narrowed portion rippled or segmented
  ◊ Fluid levels within bowel
  ◊ Diaphragm elevated

DIAGNOSTIC PROCEDURES
• Suction aspiration biopsy of bowel wall
• Barium enema
• Proctosigmoidoscopy
• Large bowel wall biopsy
• Laparoscopy: Normal proximal colon dilatation
• Ano-rectal manometry: Internal sphincter relaxation failure

 TREATMENT

APPROPRIATE HEALTH CARE
Early work-up (ambulatory or hospital). Inpatient for surgery.

GENERAL MEASURES
• Treatment may be symptomatic or definitive
• May need emergency correction of fluid and electrolyte imbalance
• Removal of fecal accumulation - retention enemas of 3-4 ounces (90-120 mL) of mineral oil followed by repeated colonic irrigations with isotonic saline solution. Avoid use of other solutions, e.g., water, soapsuds enemas.

SURGICAL MEASURES
Surgery (inpatient) for colostomy at site in the colon proximal to aganglionic segment or resection of the aganglionic segment or bypass of the segment. Endorectal pull-through techniques may be utilized.

ACTIVITY
No restrictions

DIET
• Dictated by stage of disease
• Diet will not control the obstipation of Hirschsprung's
• Postoperative diet - standard for age

PATIENT EDUCATION
• After surgery instruct parents to detect and report dehydration, decreased urinary output, sunken eyes, poor skin turgor, vomiting, fever
• Encourage bonding with parents by having parents participate in child's care as much as possible
• Request enterotomy therapist to teach family

MEDICATIONS

DRUG(S) OF CHOICE
• None recommended for treatment
• Preliminary to surgery: Bowel prep with neomycin or nystatin
Contraindications: N/A
Precautions: N/A
Significant possible interactions: N/A

ALTERNATIVE DRUGS
• Metronidazole (Flagyl) for bowel preparation

FOLLOWUP

PATIENT MONITORING Closely until recuperated fully from surgical intervention

PREVENTION/AVOIDANCE N/A

POSSIBLE COMPLICATIONS
• Toxic enterocolitis, possibly fatal
• Bleeding and/or perforation

EXPECTED COURSE/PROGNOSIS
Guardedly favorable with surgery prior to onset of complications

MISCELLANEOUS

ASSOCIATED CONDITIONS
• Chagas' disease (secondary aganglionic megacolon may be a late complication of Chagas')
• Megacolon, acquired, functional usually begins in 3rd or 4th year of life
• Down syndrome
• Septal defects
• Tetralogy of Fallot
• Dandy-Walker syndrome
• Associated with anomalies 22% of the time, especially neurological, cardiovascular, urological, gastrointestinal

AGE-RELATED FACTORS
Pediatric: Occasionally infants have only mild or intermittent constipation with intervening bouts of diarrhea. These cases may not be diagnosed until later in infancy.
Geriatric: N/A
Others: N/A

PREGNANCY N/A

SYNONYMS
• Aganglionic megacolon
• Hirschsprung's disease
• Zer-Wilson's disease (total colonic aganglionosis)

ICD-9-CM
751.3 Hirschsprung's disease

SEE ALSO
• Constipation

OTHER NOTES Diagnosis must be made as early as possible to prevent toxic enterocolitis

ABBREVIATIONS N/A

REFERENCES
• Ryan ET, et al: J of Ped Surg 1992;1:76-81
• Walsh K, et al, eds: Pediatric Surgery. New York, Yearbook Medical Publishers, 1986
• Eastwood GL, Avunduk C, eds: Manual of Gastroenterology. Boston, Little, Brown, 1988
• Barakat AY, ed: Renal Disease in Children: Clinical Evaluation & Diagnosis. New York, Springer-Verlag, 1990
Illustrations: N/A
Internet references: http://www.5mcc.com

Author(s)
James A. Nard, MD

Congestive heart failure

BASICS

DESCRIPTION Congestive heart failure (CHF) is the principal complication of heart disease. It is a pathophysiologic state produced by an abnormality in cardiac pump function (either transient or prolonged). The heart is unable to transport blood in a sufficient flow to meet metabolic needs. CHF occurs at some time in all cases of severe heart disease.
• This produces a variety of clinical circumstances from acute left ventricular dysfunction (due to tachyarrhythmia, bradyarrhythmia, and acute myocardial infarction) to chronic left ventricular dysfunction (due to chronic volume/pressure overload as seen in valvular heart disease)
• Two physiologic components explain most of the clinical findings of CHF - most patients have findings consistent with both mechanisms:
  ◊ an inotropic abnormality resulting in diminished systolic emptying (systolic failure)
  ◊ a compliance abnormality in which the ability of the ventricles to accept blood is impaired (diastolic failure).
System(s) affected: Cardiovascular, Pulmonary
Genetics: N/A
Incidence/Prevalence in USA:
• Most common inpatient diagnosis for patients over 65
Predominant age: Varies by etiology of heart disease
Predominant sex:
• Male > Female - ages 40-75
• Male = Female - ages 75 and over

SIGNS AND SYMPTOMS
• Early and mild impairment:
  ◊ Basilar rales
  ◊ Positive hepatojugular reflux
  ◊ Faint S3 gallop
  ◊ Nocturia
  ◊ Dyspnea on exertion-cardinal sign of left heart failure
  ◊ Deteriorating exercise capacity
  ◊ Fatigue
  ◊ Difficulty breathing
  ◊ Weakness
  ◊ Tachypnea with mild exertion
• Moderate impairment:
  ◊ Nocturnal nonproductive cough
  ◊ Orthopnea
  ◊ Paroxysmal nocturnal dyspnea
  ◊ Wheezing, especially nocturnal in absence of history of asthma or infection (cardiac asthma)
  ◊ Anorexia
  ◊ Fullness to dull pain in RUQ
  ◊ Tachypnea at rest
  ◊ Anxiety
  ◊ Hepatomegaly with tenderness to palpation
  ◊ Cool extremities due to peripheral vasoconstriction
  ◊ Prominent rales over bases
  ◊ Right pleural effusion
  ◊ Edema
  ◊ Gallop rhythm
  ◊ Diastolic hypertension

  ◊ Elevated jugular venous pressure
  ◊ Cardiomegaly
• Severe impairment:
  ◊ Cerebral dysfunction
  ◊ Abdominal bloating (ascites)
  ◊ Cyanosis
  ◊ Hypotension
  ◊ Pulsus alternans
  ◊ Anasarca
  ◊ Frothy and/or pink sputum
  ◊ Increased P2
  ◊ Cardiac cachexia
  ◊ Cheyne-Stokes respirations

CAUSES
• Myocardial infarction
• Cardiomyopathy
  ◊ Alcoholic
  ◊ Viral
  ◊ Long-standing hypertension
  ◊ Drugs (e.g., cyclosporine)
• Valvular abnormalities
  ◊ Aortic stenosis or regurgitation
  ◊ Rheumatic heart disease (mitral and aortic valvular disease)
• Volume overload
• Cardiac depressants; negative inotropes (e.g., beta blockers)
• Arrhythmias, eg, atrial fibrillation
• High output states
  ◊ Hyperthyroidism

RISK FACTORS
• Iatrogenic inappropriate reduction of intensity of therapy
• Patient non-compliance
• Intercurrent arrhythmia, eg, atrial fibrillation
• Administration of drug with negative inotropic effects
• Inappropriate physical, emotional, or environmental stress
• Thyrotoxicosis, pregnancy, or any condition associated with increased metabolic demand

DIAGNOSIS

DIFFERENTIAL DIAGNOSIS
• Nephrotic syndrome: excluded by absence of history of asymptomatic edema, proteinuria in nephrotic range, and history of renal disease
• Cirrhosis: excluded by absence of stigmata of liver disease, and history of liver disease and its risk factors
• Left heart failure: findings of pulmonary congestion and diminished cardiac output appearing in patients with myocardial infarction, aortic and mitral valve disease, and hypertensive disease
• Right heart failure: findings of systemic vascular congestion (edema, ascites) appear in patients with cor pulmonale, tricuspid insufficiency, and most commonly in patients with uncorrected prolonged left heart failure
• Venous occlusive disease with subsequent peripheral edema

LABORATORY
• Lab findings - early and mild to moderate in severity
  ◊ Respiratory alkalosis
  ◊ Mild azotemia
  ◊ Decreased erythrocyte sedimentation rate
  ◊ Proteinuria (usually less than 1 gm/24 h that clears with treatment)
• Lab findings - severe
  ◊ Increased creatinine
  ◊ Hyperbilirubinemia in severe cases
  ◊ Dilutional hyponatremia with treatment in severe cases
Drugs that may alter lab results: N/A
Disorders that may alter lab results: N/A

PATHOLOGICAL FINDINGS
• Early and acute
  ◊ Firm lungs with microscopic revealing engorged capillaries with thickening of the alveolar septa with extravasation of red cells and edema fluid
  ◊ Liver is engorged, firm, and fluid-filled. Microscopic - reveals dilated central hepatic veins and sinusoids.
• Late and chronic
  ◊ Hemosiderin deposits in lungs
  ◊ "Nutmeg" liver with centrilobular necrosis
  ◊ Occasionally hemorrhagic nonbacterial enterocolitis with hemorrhagic necrosis secondary to mesenteric vasoconstriction

SPECIAL TESTS   N/A

IMAGING
• X-ray - mild changes: pulmonary artery wedge pressure = 18-23 mm Hg (2.4-3.1 kPa)
  ◊ Increased heart size
  ◊ Increased blood flow to the upper lobes
  ◊ Equalization of flow between the upper and lower lobes
• X-ray - moderate severe pulmonary artery wedge pressure = 20-25 mm Hg (2.7-3.3 kPa)
  ◊ Interstitial edema
  ◊ Kerley's B lines
  ◊ Perivascular edema
  ◊ Subpleural effusions
• X-ray - severe changes: pulmonary artery wedge pressure > 25 mm Hg (> 3.3 kPa)
  ◊ Alveolar edema
  ◊ Butterfly pattern of pulmonary edema

DIAGNOSTIC PROCEDURES
• Echocardiographic studies
• Cardiac catheterization, both right and left, for full diagnosis and prognosis

TREATMENT

APPROPRIATE HEALTH CARE Inpatient when severe

GENERAL MEASURES
• Immediate treatment of the heart failure
• Search for underlying correctable conditions
• Eliminate contributing factors when possible
• Supplemental oxygen
• Antiembolism stockings
• Fluid and sodium restriction. Education about this is imperative for long term control. Daily weights guide overall therapy.
• Identify and control underlying correctable conditions (e.g., acute MI, valvular disease, hyperthyroidism, but most commonly inadvertent salt and/or fluid overload)

SURGICAL MEASURES
• Heart valve surgery - possibly, if defective heart valve is responsible
• Cardiac transplantation - to be considered in patients (age < 55) without other disqualifying medical problems, who are developing CHF unresponsive to other therapeutic maneuvers, and who are felt to have a life expectancy of less than a year

ACTIVITY
• During severe stage, bed rest with elevation of head of bed and anti-embolism stockings to help control leg edema
• Gradual increase in activity with walking will help increase strength

DIET
• Sodium restriction (initially 4 gm sodium qd)
• Weight reduction diet if appropriate
• Low fat diet to retard coronary artery disease

PATIENT EDUCATION
• Printed patient information available from:
  ◊ American Heart Association, 7320 Greenville Avenue, Dallas, TX 75231, (214)373-6300
  ◊ American College of Cardiology, 911 Old Georgetown Road, Bethesda, MD 20814, (301) 897-5400

MEDICATIONS

DRUG(S) OF CHOICE
Diuretics, usually in combination with digitalis are used to initiate therapy. ACE inhibitors have become a mainstay of therapy. For acute pulmonary edema, IV morphine remains cornerstone of therapy.

• Digoxin
  ◊ Improves contractility, slows ventricular rate in atrial fibrillation
  ◊ May be harmful in acute MI, hypertrophic cardiomyopathy
  ◊ Loading dose should be sufficient to have early beneficial effect, especially in atrial fibrillation with a rapid rate, e.g., 0.5-1.0 mg IV/po, then another 1.0-1.5 mg in divided doses q4-6h
• Diuretics
  ◊ Furosemide (Lasix): IV or po, depending on severity of pulmonary congestion. May require continuous drip
  ◊ Metolazone (Zaroxolyn): excellent addition when furosemide does not seem to be sufficient
  ◊ Spironolactone: when used carefully, to avoid hyperkalemia. May be proper addition to difficult chronic cases.
• ACE Inhibitors
  ◊ Used to decrease afterload
  ◊ Improve general symptomatology and overall exercise capacity
• Beta blockers - carvedilol in appropriate doses (3.125 mg po bid for 2 weeks, then 6.25 mg bid for 2 weeks, increased to maximum 25 mg bid for class I to III CHF). This drug has been shown to improve longevity in CHF. It is started with close observation as outpatient.
• Vasodilators
  ◊ IV nitroglycerin may be of short-term benefit to decrease preload, afterload, and systemic resistance.
  ◊ Oral medications, e.g., hydralazine, prazosin, and Isosorbide dinitrate demonstrate tachyphylaxis
Contraindications: Refer to manufacturer's literature
Precautions: ACE inhibitors may produce hypotension on first use in volume depleted patients. Beta blockers may produce profound hypotension.
Significant possible interactions: Refer to manufacturer's literature

ALTERNATIVE DRUGS
• Sympathomimetic amines. Can be used in severe CHF unresponsive to above measures
  ◊ Dopamine and dobutamine have been successful for short periods in treatment
  ◊ Dobutamine can be used on an intermittent outpatient basis with intermittent infusion. However, in spite of possibly improving quality of life, reduces long-term survival.

FOLLOWUP

PATIENT MONITORING
• Variable depending on clinical circumstances. Initially every 2-3 weeks after patient stabilized.
• Closely follow - history and physical findings, chest x-ray, electrolytes, BUN, and creatinine

PREVENTION/AVOIDANCE Treatment of underlying disorders when possible

POSSIBLE COMPLICATIONS
• Electrolyte disturbance
• Atrial and ventricular arrhythmias
• Mesenteric insufficiency
• Protein enteropathy
• Digitalis intoxication

EXPECTED COURSE/PROGNOSIS
• Result of initial treatment is usually good, whatever the cause
• Long-term prognosis variable. Mortality rates range from 10% with mild symptoms to 50% with advanced, progressive symptoms.

MISCELLANEOUS

ASSOCIATED CONDITIONS See Causes

AGE-RELATED FACTORS
Pediatric: Usually associated with congenital heart disease
Geriatric: Medications may need dosage adjustment
Others: N/A

PREGNANCY If occurs, will require special care

SYNONYMS
• Heart failure
• Dropsy
• Circulatory failure
• Cardiac failure

ICD-9-CM 428.0 Congestive heart failure

SEE ALSO N/A

OTHER NOTES N/A

ABBREVIATIONS
CCF = congestive cardiac failure

REFERENCES
• Braunwald E, ed: Heart Disease: A Textbook of Cardiovascular Medicine. 4th Ed. Philadelphia, W.B. Saunders Co., 1992
• Harvey AM: The Principles and Practice of Medicine. 22nd Ed. Norwalk, CT, Appleton & Lange, 1988
Illustrations: 8 available on CD-ROM
Internet references: http://www.5mcc.com

Author(s)
Phil Lobstein, MD

Conjunctivitis

BASICS

DESCRIPTION Inflammation of palpebral and/or bulbar conjunctiva. Pink eye refers to non-Neisseria bacterial conjunctivitis.
System(s) affected: Nervous, Skin/Exocrine
Genetics: N/A
Incidence/Prevalence in USA: Unknown, but common
Predominant age: Depends on cause
Predominant sex: Male = Female

SIGNS AND SYMPTOMS
• General
  ◊ Conjunctival hyperemia
  ◊ Burning
  ◊ Foreign body sensation
  ◊ Pruritus
  ◊ Lacrimation
  ◊ Exudation and matting
  ◊ Chemosis
  ◊ Pseudoptosis
  ◊ Preauricular adenopathy
  ◊ Tarsal plate papillary hypertrophy
  ◊ Tarsal plate lymphoid follicles
  ◊ Pseudomembranous and membranes
  ◊ Photosensitivity
  ◊ Decreased acuity if there is complicating ulcer or keratitis
  ◊ Granulomas (rare)
• Bacterial
  ◊ Minimal pruritus
  ◊ Moderate tearing
  ◊ Profuse exudate, particularly Neisseria species
  ◊ Usually unilateral (or initially unilateral)
  ◊ Small tarsal plate papillae
  ◊ Neisseria species may cause chemosis
  ◊ Gram and Giemsa stain: Polymorphonuclear neutrophils (PMN's) and bacteria (gram negative intracellular diplococci with Neisseria species)
• Viral
  ◊ Minimal pruritus
  ◊ Profuse tearing
  ◊ Minimal exudate
  ◊ Often bilateral
  ◊ Preauricular adenopathy common
  ◊ Subconjunctival hemorrhage (acute hemorrhagic conjunctivitis)
  ◊ Associated viral systemic symptom (fever, myalgia, etc.)
  ◊ Tarsal plate follicles
  ◊ Pharyngeal follicles if associated pharyngitis
  ◊ Gram and Giemsa stain: Mononuclear cells (lymphocytes)
  ◊ Rare chemosis except with epidemic keratoconjunctivitis
  ◊ Subepithelial corneal opacities with epidemic keratoconjunctivitis
  ◊ Diffuse punctate corneal fluorescein uptake or dendrites with herpes simplex
  ◊ Typical zoster rash along ophthalmic branch of trigeminal nerve with varicella-zoster blepharoconjunctivitis
  ◊ Typical measles rash, Koplik's spots, etc. with measles
• Chlamydial
  ◊ Minimal pruritus

◊ Moderate to profuse tearing
◊ Profuse exudate (sometimes modest)
◊ Often bilateral
◊ Small tarsal plate papillae
◊ Tarsal plate follicles present
◊ Gram and Giemsa stain: PMN's, plasma cells, inclusion bodies, in trachoma large palely staining lymphoblastic cells
◊ Inclusion conjunctivitis commonly has preauricular adenopathy and large tarsal plate papillae and follicles. Occasionally associated genitourinary symptoms in young adults or history of bilateral conjunctivitis unresponsive to topical antibiotics.
◊ Lymphogranuloma venereum is rare and non-follicular (mostly granulomatous conjunctival) with large preauricular node (visible bubo)
◊ Trachoma rare in the USA (except American Indians of Southwest) and has 4 clinical stages
• Allergic
  ◊ Severe pruritus
  ◊ Moderate tearing
  ◊ No exudate
  ◊ Bilateral
  ◊ Chemosis very common
  ◊ Tarsal papillae
  ◊ Gram and Giemsa's stain: Eosinophils and basophils
  ◊ Allergic rhinoconjunctivitis has associated sneezing, rhinitis but if not of sufficient duration will not develop papillae
  ◊ Vernal conjunctivitis is recurrent in warm weather associated with large "cobblestone" papillae in those with history of atopic allergy
  ◊ Giant papillary conjunctivitis has similar appearance to vernal conjunctivitis with less pruritis and is seen in soft (and occasionally hard) contact lens use
• Chemical or irritative
  ◊ Tarsal follicles with conjunctivitis of topical medications
  ◊ Tearing and exudation depends on toxicity of chemical
  ◊ Chemosis common in post therapeutic irrigation
  ◊ Gram and Giemsa stain: PMN's if tissue necrosis

CAUSES
• Bacterial
  ◊ Staphylococcus aureus
  ◊ Streptococcus pneumoniae
  ◊ Haemophilus influenzae
  ◊ Neisseria gonorrhoeae
  ◊ Neisseria meningitidis
  ◊ Rarely other Streptococcal sp., pseudomonas, Branhamella catarrhalis, Coliforms, Klebsiella, Proteus, Corynebacterium diphtheriae, Mycobacterium tuberculosis, Treponema pallidum
• Viral
  ◊ Adenoviruses types 3, 4, 7 (pharyngitis with conjunctivitis)
  ◊ Adenoviruses types 8 and 19 (epidemic keratoconjunctivitis)
  ◊ Adenovirus 11, Coxsackie A24, enterovirus 70 (acute hemorrhagic conjunctivitis)
  ◊ Herpes simplex (primary and recurrent)
  ◊ Coxsackievirus type A28
  ◊ Molluscum contagiosum
  ◊ Varicella
  ◊ Herpes zoster

◊ Measles virus
• Chlamydial
  ◊ Chlamydia trachomatis (trachoma)
  ◊ Chlamydia oculogenitalis (inclusion conjunctivitis)
  ◊ Chlamydia lymphogranulomatis (lymphogranuloma venereum)
• Allergic
  ◊ Rhinoconjunctivitis (hay fever) - humoral
  ◊ Vernal conjunctivitis
  ◊ Giant papillary conjunctivitis
  ◊ Delayed (cellular)
  ◊ Autoimmune (Sjögren's, pemphigoid, Wegener's granulomatosis)
• Chemical or irritative
  ◊ Topical medication
  ◊ Home/industrial chemicals
  ◊ Wind
  ◊ Smoke
  ◊ Ultraviolet light
• Other
  ◊ Rickettsial, fungal, parasitic, tuberculosis, syphilis, Kawasaki disease
  ◊ Thyroid disease, gout, carcinoid, sarcoidosis, psoriasis, Stevens-Johnson syndrome, Ligneous conjunctivitis, Reiter's syndrome

RISK FACTORS Numerous, including trauma from wind, cold and heat, chemicals and foreign body

DIAGNOSIS

DIFFERENTIAL DIAGNOSIS
• Uveitis (iritis, iridocyclitis, choroiditis)
• Acute glaucoma
• Corneal disease or foreign body
• Canalicular obstruction (canaliculitis, dacryocystitis)
• Scleritis and episcleritis

LABORATORY
• Culture from conjunctiva
• Gram and Giemsa stain of the discharge or scrapings
Drugs that may alter lab results: N/A
Disorders that may alter lab results: N/A

PATHOLOGICAL FINDINGS   N/A

SPECIAL TESTS
• Cultivation on HeLa cells and neutralization tests for epidemic keratoconjunctivitis
• Bovin fixation and Papanicolaou stain for multinucleated giant cells of herpes simplex conjunctivitis. Also available, viral culture and immunofluorescence test for Herpes simplex.
• Immunofluorescent antibody tests for chlamydia serology
• Frei test for lymphogranuloma venereum

IMAGING   N/A

DIAGNOSTIC PROCEDURES
• Culture of exudate
• Smear and stain of exudate

TREATMENT

APPROPRIATE HEALTH CARE
Outpatient

GENERAL MEASURES
• Record acuity
• Fluorescein staining to detect ulcer, keratitis
• No patch
• See Medications
• Culture
• No topical steroids
• Ophthalmologic referral if ulcer, keratitis, suspected herpes or worsens after 24 hours of treatment
• Compresses - warm if infective, cold if allergic or irritative
• Remove purulent material and debris (may require frequent irrigation)
• Giant papillary allergic conjunctivitis requires discontinuing use of contact lenses

SURGICAL MEASURES   N/A

ACTIVITY   No restrictions

DIET   No restrictions

PATIENT EDUCATION
• Transmission route of infecting agent if contagious
• Demonstrate eye drop techniques
• Demonstrate ointment techniques

MEDICATIONS

DRUG(S) OF CHOICE
• Bacterial
  ◊ 0.3% tobramycin or gentamicin. As drops (1-2 gtts) instilled every 4 hours while awake for 5 days, as ointment qid.
  ◊ 10% sodium sulfacetamide. As drops (1-2 gtts) instilled every 4 hours while awake for 5 days, as ointment qid and hs (stings).
  ◊ Erythromycin ophthalmic ointment qid
  ◊ Systemic treatment for Neisseria species as other sites usually involved. Some authorities (with ophthalmology consult) add topical erythromycin.
• Viral
  ◊ Trifluridine 1% drops, 1 drop every 2 hours while awake, maximum 9 drops a day
  ◊ Acyclovir oral and topical for herpetic (wide range of doses, consult drug reference)
  ◊ Topical antibiotics to prevent bacterial superinfection or if diagnosis is in doubt
• Chlamydial
  ◊ Oral doxycycline 100 mg bid (3 weeks) for inclusion conjunctivitis

• Allergic
  ◊ Topical vasoconstrictor and/or antihistamine combination such as naphazoline 0.05% or antazoline (Albalon-A, Vasocon-A) 0.5%
  ◊ Oral antihistamine
  ◊ Topical cromolyn sodium (Opticrom) 2%, 4% qid starting 2 weeks before season. (Opticrom no longer imported into the U.S. Available in Canada, UK, and Europe in 2% solution.)

Contraindications:
• Tetracycline: not for use in pregnancy or children < 8 years.

Precautions:
• Tetracycline: may cause photosensitivity; sunscreen recommended.
• Vasoconstrictors make the eye appear less severely affected
• Avoid contamination of medication bottles by touching lids

Significant possible interactions:
• Tetracycline: avoid concurrent administration with antacids, dairy products, or iron.

ALTERNATIVE DRUGS
• Bacterial
  ◊ Polymyxin-gramicidin
  ◊ Neomycin-polymyxin B-bacitracin (Neosporin); 15% of people have hypersensitivity reaction to neomycin
  ◊ Chloramphenicol - warning, slight hematological risk)
  ◊ Ciprofloxacin
  ◊ Framycetin
  ◊ Norfloxacin
• Chlamydial
  ◊ Oral tetracycline or erythromycin (3 weeks) for inclusion conjunctivitis. Some authorities recommend topical tetracycline or erythromycin in addition.
• Allergic
  ◊ Numerous topical vasoconstrictors and antihistamines
  ◊ Numerous oral antihistamines

FOLLOWUP

PATIENT MONITORING   Referral if worse in 24 hours

PREVENTION/AVOIDANCE
• Avoid listed causes when possible
• Wash hands frequently

POSSIBLE COMPLICATIONS
• Bacterial
  ◊ Chronic marginal blepharitis
  ◊ Conjunctival scar if membrane developed
  ◊ Corneal ulcer or perforation
  ◊ Hypopyon
  ◊ Rare portal of entry for meningococcus
• Viral
  ◊ Corneal scars with herpes simplex
  ◊ Corneal scars, lid scars, entropion, misdirected lashes with Varicella-zoster
  ◊ Bacterial superinfection
• Chlamydial
  ◊ Clinical trachoma (not with inclusion

conjunctivitis)
• Allergic, chemical and others
  ◊ Bacterial superinfection

EXPECTED COURSE/PROGNOSIS
• Bacterial
  ◊ 10-14 days without treatment
  ◊ 2-4 days with treatment
• Viral
  ◊ 10 days for pharyngitis with conjunctivitis
  ◊ 3-4 weeks for epidemic keratoconjunctivitis
  ◊ 2-3 weeks for herpes simplex
• Chlamydial
  ◊ 3-9 months for untreated inclusion conjunctivitis
  ◊ 3-5 weeks for trachoma with treatment

MISCELLANEOUS

ASSOCIATED CONDITIONS   N/A

AGE-RELATED FACTORS
Pediatric: Neonatal conjunctivitis may be toxic, bacterial (genital tract bacteria or nosocomial) or chlamydial
Geriatric: More likely to have diseases or problems listed in Causes
Others: N/A

PREGNANCY   N/A

SYNONYMS   Pink eye

ICD-9-CM
• 372.5 Acute atopic conjunctivitis
• 372.14 Other chronic allergic conjunctivitis

SEE ALSO   Rhinitis, allergic

OTHER NOTES   N/A

ABBREVIATIONS
PMN = polymorphonuclear neutrophils

REFERENCES
• Rosen P, Barkin R: Emergency Medicine. 3rd Ed. St. Louis, Mosby, 1992
• Howes R: Emergency Clinics of North America 1988;6(I)
Illustrations: 1 available on CD-ROM
Internet references: http://www.5mcc.com

Author(s)
Charles W. Ricketson, MD, FRCPC

Constipation

BASICS

DESCRIPTION A combination of changes in the frequency, size, consistency, and ease of stool passage, which leads to an overall decrease in volume of bowel movements. Very subjective, each individual has their own threshold level.
System(s) affected: Gastrointestinal
Genetics: Unknown (the condition may be familial)
Incidence/Prevalence in USA:
• Higher at extremes of life, i.e., among infants/children and the elderly
• Common; affects a majority of persons during their lifetimes
Predominant age: All ages can be affected; more frequent at the extremes of life (infancy and old age)
Predominant Sex: Female > Male

SIGNS AND SYMPTOMS
• Less frequency of stooling than the patient perceives as "normal" (normal is 3-5 times/week)
• Harder stool than "normal"
• Smaller stools than normal (average < 35 grams/day is abnormal)
• Impaction of stool secondary to hardness
• Inspissated stool
• Lack of consistent urgency to stool
• Difficulty expelling feces from the rectum
• Painful evacuation of feces
• Lingering sense of incomplete emptying of the bowel
• Abdominal fullness or a feeling of malaise secondary to inadequate bowel evacuation
• Tenesmus

CAUSES
• Electrolyte abnormalities
  ◊ Hypercalcemia
  ◊ Hypokalemia
• Hormonal abnormalities
  ◊ Hypothyroidism
  ◊ Diabetes
• Congenital impediments, e.g., aganglionic megacolon (Hirschsprung's disease) or excessively elongate, redundant, capacious bowel (dolichocolon)
• Congenital or acquired neuromuscular bowel impairment ("pseudo-obstruction")
• Concomitant illness, injury, or debility
• Mechanical bowel impediment (obstruction or ileus, due to any cause)
• Inadequate fluid intake
• Side-effect of drugs (e.g., anticholinergic agents, opiates)
• Chronic abuse of laxatives or cathartics
• Psychiatric, cultural, emotional, environmental factors
• Painful fecal evacuation from anal disease (e.g., fissures)

RISK FACTORS
• Extremes of life (very young and very old)
• Neurosis
• Polypharmacy
• Sedentary life style or condition

DIAGNOSIS

DIFFERENTIAL DIAGNOSIS
• Congenital
  ◊ Hirschsprung's
  ◊ Hypoganglionosis
  ◊ Congenital dilation of the colon
  ◊ Small left colon syndrome
• Meconium ileus
• "Normal" stooling with anxious patient or parent
• Illnesses predisposing to constipation
  ◊ Dehydration
  ◊ Hypothyroidism
  ◊ Hypokalemia
  ◊ Hypercalcemia
• Other causes of abdominal pain

LABORATORY
• Only necessary when other disorders are being considered
  ◊ CBC to detect anemia that may indicate colorectal neoplasm
  ◊ Thyroid functions
  ◊ Electrolytes, glucose, calcium
Drugs that may alter lab results: N/A
Disorders that may alter lab results: N/A

PATHOLOGICAL FINDINGS
• None in common, "functional" constipation
• Paucity or absence of intramural enteric ganglia in certain cases of congenital or acquired megacolon
• Neuromuscular abnormalities in certain cases of "pseudo-obstruction"

SPECIAL TESTS
• In selected cases of long-standing constipation, timed measure of passage of ingested stool markers may help discern differing impediments
• Anorectal motility in patients with suspected Hirschsprung's or anorectal motility disorders

IMAGING
• Plain (KUB) film of the abdomen may help to discern the extent and nature of the problem
• Barium enema or barium swallow with small bowel follow through looking for anatomical defects (mass lesions, ileus)
• Cineradiography of passage of barium, instilled in, then expelled from the rectosigmoid segment ("defecography"), may help define evacuation disorders in selected cases

DIAGNOSTIC PROCEDURES
• Digital rectal exam to rule out a rectal mass, check for blood in the stool, and define stool consistency
• Sigmoidoscopy or colonoscopy is seldom required, unless needed to define an abnormality discovered by barium enema or when there is evidence of iron deficiency anemia or blood in the stool

TREATMENT

APPROPRIATE HEALTH CARE
Outpatient usually, except when investigation discloses an underlying lesion or obstruction that requires hospitalization

GENERAL MEASURES
• Attempt to eliminate medications that may cause or worsen constipation
• Increase fluid intake
• Modify diet
• Enemas if other methods fail

SURGICAL MEASURES N/A

ACTIVITY Encourage exercise

DIET
• If no anatomic abnormalities, increase fiber to approximately 15 gm/day (bran, fruit, green vegetables, and whole grain cereals and breads)
• Encourage liberal intake of fluids

PATIENT EDUCATION
• Define constipation and normal variations
• Occasional mild constipation is normal
• Instruction in consistent "bowel training" i.e., allowing adequate time for bowel evacuation in a quiet, unhurried environment; instruction in facilitating posture on commode, e.g., thighs flexed toward abdomen
• Parents sometimes needs more treatment/advice than the constipated child

MEDICATIONS

DRUG(S) OF CHOICE
• Hydrophilic colloids (bulk-forming agents; not really drugs)
  ◊ Psyllium (Konsyl, Metamucil, Perdiem)
  ◊ Methylcellulose (Citrucel)
  ◊ Polycarbophil (Mitrolan, Fibercon)
• Osmotic laxatives - appropriate for short-term use. The usual dose is 15 mL to 30 mL once or twice a day.
  ◊ Milk of magnesia
  ◊ Magnesium citrate
  ◊ Phosphate of soda
  ◊ Lactulose (Chronulac)
  ◊ Sorbitol
  ◊ Alumina-magnesia (Maalox, Mylanta)
• Stool softeners
  ◊ Docusate sodium (Colace) 100 mg bid
Contraindications:
• Any impediment to bowel transit, such as an obstructing lesion or ileus. Osmotic laxatives may result in overdistension or bowel perforation
• Any acute intra-abdominal inflammatory condition
• Renal and heart failure are relative contraindications
Precautions: Advise patient against chronic use of irritant and osmotic laxatives
Significant possible interactions:
• Magnesium containing laxatives
  ◊ Bind tetracyclines preventing their absorption
  ◊ Reduce the effectiveness of digitalis and phenothiazines
  ◊ Sodium polystyrene sulfonate (Kayexalate) bind and prevent neutralization of bicarbonate, leading to systemic alkalosis, which may be severe

ALTERNATIVE DRUGS
• Lubricants (e.g., mineral oil) are unpalatable to many patients, subject to leakage, and impose the risk of aspiration
• Emollient suppositories are useful, if at all, in allaying anorectal soreness
• Irritant cathartics (stimulants)
  ◊ Ricinoleic acid or castor oil (Neoloid); 30-60 mL/day
  ◊ Phenolphthalein (Ex-Lax, Modane)
  ◊ Bisacodyl (Dulcolax); 2-3 tabs swallowed whole or 1 suppository bid
• Motor and secretory properties
  ◊ Anthraquinones-senna (Senokot); 1-2 cap or 15-30 mL qhs
• Enemas (avoid soap suds - may lead to colitis)
  ◊ Phospho soda (Fleets)
• Suppositories
  ◊ Osmotic: sodium phosphate
  ◊ Lubricant: glycerin
  ◊ Stimulatory: bisacodyl
• Prokinetic agents

FOLLOWUP

PATIENT MONITORING What seems to be simple, "functional" constipation, if it persists, should be further investigated for a possible "organic" cause

PREVENTION/AVOIDANCE Because for some patients a tendency to constipation is habitual, instruction in proper diet, bowel training, and use of bulk-forming supplements must be reinforced

POSSIBLE COMPLICATIONS
• Acquired megacolon: in severe, long-standing cases
• Cathartic colon: repeated laxative abuse
• Fluid and electrolyte depletion: laxative abuse
• Rectal ulceration ("stercoral ulcer") related to recurrent fecal impaction

EXPECTED COURSE/PROGNOSIS
Constipation that is only occasional, brief, and responsive to simple measures is harmless. That which is habitual can be a lifelong nuisance.

MISCELLANEOUS

ASSOCIATED CONDITIONS Debility, either general, as in the aged, or that imposed by specific, underlying illness

AGE-RELATED FACTORS
Pediatric: Consider Hirschsprung's disease
Geriatric:
• Elderly persons, who have enjoyed regular bowel action throughout their lives, seldom suffer constipation due to age alone
• Persons with a lifelong tendency to constipation often encounter increasing difficulty with advancing age
• There is an increased incidence of colorectal neoplasms with age that may be associated with constipation.
Others: N/A

PREGNANCY Women with a tendency to constipation may find the condition more troublesome in the third trimester and require dietary adjustment and supplements

SYNONYMS
• Costive bowel
• Locked bowels

ICD-9-CM
564.0 constipation
564.7 megacolon, other than Hirschsprung's
564.8 Other specified functional disorders of intestine (includes atony of colon)
751.3 Hirschsprung's disease and other congenital functional disorders of colon

SEE ALSO
• Congenital megacolon

OTHER NOTES
Obstipation refers to intractable constipation

ABBREVIATIONS N/A

REFERENCES
• Rogers AI: Constipation In: Berk JE, Haubrich WS, eds. Gastrointestinal Symptoms: Clinical Interpretation. Philadelphia, B.C. Decker Inc., 1991
• Haubrich WS: Constipation. In: Berk JE, et al, eds. Bockus Gastroenterology. 4th Ed. Philadelphia, W.B. Saunders Co., 1985
• Devroede G: Constipation. In: Sleisenger MH, Fordtran JS, eds. Gastrointestinal Disease. 4th Ed. Philadelphia, W.B. Saunders Co., 1989
• Wald A: Approach to the patient with constipation. In: Yamada T, ed. Textbook of Gastroenterology. Vol. I. Philadelphia, J.B. Lippincott Co., 1991
• Nunez M, Robinson B: Management of Constipation in the Older Patient. J Florida MA 1991;78:12, 829-831
• Leonard-Jones JE: Clinical Management of Constipation, Pharmacology 1993;47(suppl1):216-223
• Goroll AH, May LA, Mulley AG: Approach to the Patient with Constipation. In Primary Care Medicine, Lippincott, 1987
Illustrations: N/A
Internet references: http://www.5mcc.com

Author(s)
David Frank, MD

Contraception

BASICS

DESCRIPTION Variety of practices designed to prevent. Most are designed to prevent pregnancy, to prevent implantation, to be spermicidal or to prevent sperm from reaching egg. Natural family planning aims to avoid coitus at the time of expected ovulation. Failure rates vary among methods. The most effective is permanent sterilization, either tubal sterilization in the female (by electrocautery, loops, clips, or ligation and excision) or vasectomy in the male. Neither should be considered reversible, but either may be reversed under certain circumstances. Surgical attempts at reversal are often unsuccessful.
• Reversible methods and approximate pregnancy rates (preg/100 women/year):
  ◊ Implantable contraceptive (Norplant) - 1
  ◊ Injectable contraceptive (Depo-Provera) - 1
  ◊ Oral contraceptives (the pill) - 3
  ◊ Intrauterine device (IUD) - 5
  ◊ Condom (rubber) - 12
  ◊ Diaphragm - 18
  ◊ Periodic abstinence - 20
  ◊ Spermicides alone - 21
  ◊ Female condom - 25
System(s) affected: Reproductive
Genetics: N/A
Incidence/Prevalence in USA:
• About two-thirds of women at risk for unwanted pregnancies use contraception
• Among individuals of reproductive age having regular coitus:
  ◊ Tubal sterilization 16.6%
  ◊ Vasectomy 7.0%
  ◊ Oral contraceptives 18.5%
  ◊ Condoms 8.8%
  ◊ Diaphragm 3.5%
  ◊ Intrauterine device 1.2%
  ◊ Natural family planning 1.0%
  ◊ Foam 0.6%
  ◊ Implantable contraceptive (Norplant) - N/A
  ◊ Injectable contraceptive (Depo-Provera) - N/A
Predominant age:
• Female - 11-52 years
• Male - any age after puberty
Predominant sex: Female. However, condom or vasectomy are the common male methods.

SIGNS AND SYMPTOMS N/A

CAUSES N/A

RISK FACTORS
• For pregnancy
  ◊ Any woman who is ovulating and having intercourse with a fertile male
    ◊ Young adolescents
    ◊ Socioeconomic factors - less access to medical care, or have limited knowledge about reproduction

DIAGNOSIS

DIFFERENTIAL DIAGNOSIS N/A

LABORATORY
• Female
  ◊ Cervical cytology
  ◊ Cultures for gonorrhea and Chlamydia
  ◊ Blood lipid studies (with family history of hyperlipidemia or coronary artery disease at a young age)
  ◊ Blood sugar (if suspected of having diabetes mellitus)
  ◊ Pregnancy test (if hormonal contraception is not initiated at time of menses)
• Male
  ◊ None needed except routine pre-operative studies prior to vasectomy
  ◊ Semen analysis showing no sperm after vasectomy. (Will require up to 15 ejaculations before aspermia is present for 3 consecutive studies.)
Drugs that may alter lab results: N/A
Disorders that may alter lab results: N/A

PATHOLOGICAL FINDINGS N/A

SPECIAL TESTS N/A

IMAGING N/A

DIAGNOSTIC PROCEDURES N/A

TREATMENT

APPROPRIATE HEALTH CARE
Outpatient

GENERAL MEASURES
Non-drug methods
• Latex condom
• IUD (2 currently available)
  ◊ Progestasert (change annually)
  ◊ Paragard (change every 10 years)
  ◊ Inserted by a practitioner who has been appropriately trained. Insert at menses to rule out pregnancy.
  ◊ Contraindicated in nulliparity or multiple sexual partners (because of the risk of PID). Not advisable in patients with heavy menses.
• Diaphragm
  ◊ Needs professional fitting
  ◊ Use largest size which can be inserted without discomfort or distortion
  ◊ Refit after childbirth or if weight changes by more than 10%
  ◊ Contraindicated in significant uterine prolapse

• Female condom (Reality)
  ◊ Available over-the-counter: package includes lubricant, instructions and diagrams
• Periodic abstinence
  ◊ Need accurate record of menstrual cycles for at least 12 months prior to use
  ◊ Fertile period calculated as shortest cycle minus 18 days to longest cycle minus 11 days; problem for women with variable cycle length
  ◊ Added effectiveness attained by observing cervical mucus (for disappearance of abundant clear mucus) and by observing basal temperature rise of about 1° for 3 days. Both usually indicate that ovulation has occurred.
• Permanent sterilization
  ◊ Tubal sterilization in the female (by electrocautery, loops, clips, or ligation and excision) - sometimes performed as an office procedure
  ◊ Vasectomy in the male

SURGICAL MEASURES N/A

ACTIVITY N/A

DIET N/A

PATIENT EDUCATION
• Condoms
  ◊ Use water-based lubricants
  ◊ Check for holes before using. Leave space at tip to act as reservoir for the semen. Withdraw from vagina before penis becomes flaccid. Use a spermicide in addition in order to increase effectiveness.
• Intrauterine device
  ◊ Check for the presence of the string frequently
• Diaphragm
  ◊ Before inserting, place one tablespoon of spermicidal gel or cream into the dome of diaphragm and line entire rim of the diaphragm with it
  ◊ Insert the diaphragm and check for proper placement
  ◊ Leave in for at least 8 hours after coitus - then remove and clean according to directions. Check for holes.
  ◊ If another act of coitus occurs before 8 hours, insert additional spermicidal gel or cream into vagina without displacing the diaphragm
• Female condom
  ◊ Use new condom for each sex act
  ◊ Insert properly so that inner ring is well into vagina and outer ring lies against vulva. Make sure that penis enters inside the sheath.
  ◊ Remove condom after intercourse being careful not to spill semen
• Oral contraception:
  ◊ Take pill daily at approximately same time
  ◊ If a pill is missed, take two the following day but use an additional method of protection, such as a barrier method, until next period
  ◊ If two periods are missed, seek medical care to rule out pregnancy. Do not stop pills if a period is missed.
• Medroxyprogesterone (Depo-Provera): return every 3 months for injection
• Norplant: should be replaced after 5 years of use. Requires surgical insertion and removal.
• Printed materials available from ACOG (1-800-673-8444)

Contraception

MEDICATIONS

DRUG(S) OF CHOICE
• Oral contraceptives
  ◊ Use sub-50 microgram estrogen dose to minimize side effects and risks (current pills contain 20, 30, or 35 mcg)
  ◊ Triphasics contain less total progestogen and therefore are less likely to affect lipid profile adversely
  ◊ All current pills contain ethinyl estradiol or mestranol as the estrogen
  ◊ The progestogen varies between manufacturers - all are derivatives of testosterone and slight differences in the molecule produce different biological effects. Newer progestogens are less androgenic and therefore should have less adverse effects on lipoproteins. However, there is concern about an increased risk of stroke with pills containing desogestrel, e.g., desogestrel-ethinyl estradiol (Desogen, Orthocept).
  ◊ Generics should be avoided because of uncertain or fluctuating dosage in each batch of pills. Choice of specific pill usually depends upon experiences and preferences of physician.
  ◊ If side effects occur, the pill may be changed. Reaction of patients to a particular pill differ and changing to eliminate side effects is by trial and error. Low dose progestogen-only pills have high pregnancy rates; avoid them except in lactating women.
• Spermicides
  ◊ All contain nonoxynol-9
  ◊ Choice depends upon preferences of user and local sensitization to bases. Foam or creams are preferable since they disperse well. Suppositories or tablets first must dissolve, making dispersal unpredictable.
• Implantable contraceptive - levonorgestrel (Norplant)
  ◊ 6 silastic tubes implanted into the upper arm by physician
  ◊ Effective for up to 5 years; after implantation do not require an active role by the patient
• Injectable contraceptive; medroxyprogesterone acetate (Depo-Provera)
  ◊ 150 mg IM q 3 months
  ◊ Contraceptive levels of hormone persist for up to 4 months (giving 2-4 week margin of safety)

Contraindications:
• Implantable or injectable contraceptives
  ◊ Active liver disease
  ◊ Thrombophlebitis
  ◊ Pregnancy
  ◊ Unexplained, abnormal, uterine bleeding
  ◊ Cholestatic jaundice
  ◊ Hyperlipidemia
• Oral contraceptives
  ◊ Same as implantable contraception plus noncompliance and estrogen dependent malignancies
  ◊ Relative contraindications are uterine leiomyomata, hypertension, insulin-requiring diabetes mellitus, and migraine headaches

Precautions: Refer to manufacturer's literature
Significant possible interactions:
• When these drugs needed, add a barrier method (or rarely, use a 50 mcg estrogen pill)
  ◊ Phenytoin (Dilantin) - induces microsomal liver enzymes causing accelerated metabolism of hormones with subsequent reduced blood levels. The same effect occurs in implantable contraception.
  ◊ Antibiotics - decreased enterohepatic circulation. Rifampin may also increase metabolism of oral contraceptives.

ALTERNATIVE DRUGS   N/A

FOLLOWUP

PATIENT MONITORING
• Annual pelvic exam and Pap smear
• Whenever side effects or problems occur
• Check for presence of IUD 1 month after insertion. If string is not found, use pelvic ultrasound to locate the device.
• Oral contraceptive users: 3 months after starting for hypertension; then annually

PREVENTION/AVOIDANCE   N/A

POSSIBLE COMPLICATIONS
• Oral contraceptives, serious
  ◊ Thromboembolism - stop method and treat the disorder. Do not resume oral contraception.
  ◊ Hypertension - stop method; do not resume
  ◊ MI - main risk in smokers, after age 35. Avoid in such patients.
• Oral contraceptives, minor
  ◊ Nausea/vomiting - take after eating
  ◊ Breakthrough bleeding - usually self-limited after 3 months. If not, change pill.
  ◊ Amenorrhea - rule out pregnancy, then either change to a different pill or add conjugated estrogen 0.3 mg for the first 10 days of pill package
  ◊ Cyclic weight gain - use smallest dose of estrogen available
  ◊ Breast tenderness - rare with low dose pill
  ◊ Depression - rare with low dose pill
  ◊ Chloasma - stop pill or cover with makeup
  ◊ Acne or hirsutism - change to a less androgenic progestogen
  ◊ Cholestatic jaundice - stop pill; do not restart
  ◊ Weight gain throughout cycle - use triphasic pill to minimize dose of progestogen or use newer progestogen
• Implantable contraceptive (Norplant)
  ◊ Amenorrhea - about 33% (if it persists for 2 months, rule out pregnancy)
  ◊ Irregular bleeding - about 33%
Note: Both are self-limited after about a year - inform patient of side effects before choosing this method
• Injectable contraceptive (Depo-Provera)
  ◊ Irregular bleeding during first few months
  ◊ Not readily reversible
  ◊ Amenorrhea - common after 1 year of use
  ◊ Weight gain

• IUD
  ◊ Pelvic inflammatory disease or salpingitis - remove IUD and start antibiotics
  ◊ Heavy bleeding and cramps - remove IUD.

EXPECTED COURSE/PROGNOSIS
• Pregnancy may occur with any method
  ◊ After permanent sterilization - pregnancy indicates failure of the procedure and need for reoperation; evaluate for tubal implantation.
  ◊ If IUD, remove the device if string visible. If string not seen, leave in place and account for device postpartum; slight increased risk of spontaneous abortion.
  ◊ With oral contraceptives - stop pill. No increase in rate of birth defects is expected except very slight chance of virilization in female fetus.
  ◊ With implantable contraceptive - remove implants

MISCELLANEOUS

ASSOCIATED CONDITIONS   N/A

AGE-RELATED FACTORS
Pediatric: Use of estrogen prior to pubertal growth spurt may lead to a reduction in ultimate height due to epiphyseal closure
Geriatric: Avoid high dose oral contraceptives for estrogen replacement therapy
Others: Healthy non-smokers may use oral contraceptives until age 50. When stopped, observe for menopause signs. Use other contraceptive method during this period.

PREGNANCY   See above

SYNONYMS
• Birth control
• Family planning

ICD-9-CM   None

SEE ALSO   N/A

OTHER NOTES
• Other benefits of oral contraception
  ◊ Decrease in the amount of menstrual flow and some protection against ovarian and endometrial cancer
  ◊ Relationship to breast cancer is uncertain; some suggest a slight increase in risk in certain groups

ABBREVIATIONS
PID = pelvic inflammatory disease

REFERENCES Speroff L, Glass RH, Kase NG: Clinical Gynecologic Endocrinology and Infertility. 5th Ed. Baltimore, Williams & Wilkins, 1994
Illustrations: N/A
Internet references: http://www.5mcc.com

Author(s)
Alvin Langer, MD

Cor pulmonale

BASICS

DESCRIPTION Disturbance in the pulmonary circulation resulting in right ventricular dysfunction
• Acute cor pulmonale - acute dilitation of the right ventricle secondary to pulmonary hypertension usually resulting from massive pulmonary embolism
• Chronic cor pulmonale - hypertrophy and dilitation of the right ventricle resulting from diseases of the pulmonary parenchyma and/or vascular system
System(s) affected: Cardiovascular, Pulmonary
Genetics: No known genetic pattern
Incidence/Prevalence in USA: 5-10% of organic heart diseases
Predominant age: > 45
Predominant sex: Male > Female

SIGNS AND SYMPTOMS
Depends on underlying disease process, but includes:
• Cough with or without sputum production
• Dyspnea, especially with exertion
• Jugular venous distention with prominent a- and v-waves
• Accentuated P2 and murmur of tricuspid regurgitation
• Right ventricular heave and S3 (usually late sign)
• Atypical chest pain, particularly if pulmonary artery dilitation is present
• Rhonchi and wheezing
• Hepatomegaly and ascites
• Cyanosis

CAUSES
• Disease affecting structure of the pulmonary tree
  ◊ Chronic obstructive pulmonary diseases
  ◊ Diffuse interstitial lung diseases: idiopathic pulmonary fibrosis, radiation induced fibrosis
  ◊ Pulmonary resection
  ◊ Granulomatous diseases: sarcoidosis, rheumatoid arthritis, systemic lupus erythematosus, eosinophilic granuloma
  ◊ Bronchiectasis
  ◊ Cystic fibrosis
  ◊ Malignant infiltration
• Diseases affecting the pulmonary vasculature
  ◊ Primary pulmonary hypertension
  ◊ Pulmonary embolism
  ◊ Pulmonary vascular disease secondary to systemic illness
  ◊ Intravenous drug abuse
• Diseases affecting thoracic cage function
  ◊ Obesity
  ◊ Kyphoscoliosis
  ◊ Neuromuscular diseases
  ◊ Sleep apnea
• Chronic hypoxia at high altitude

RISK FACTORS
• Tobacco abuse
• Living at high altitudes

DIAGNOSIS

DIFFERENTIAL DIAGNOSIS
• Primary disease of the left side of the heart
• Congenital heart disease

LABORATORY
• Hematocrit - frequently elevated
• pO2 - reduced
• pCO2 varies according to underlying disease
Drugs that may alter lab results: N/A
Disorders that may alter lab results: N/A

PATHOLOGICAL FINDINGS
• Evidence of underlying etiology
• Dilated, hypertrophic right ventricle

SPECIAL TESTS
ECG - often normal, but findings can include:
• RVH - most common in primary pulmonary hypertension
• Rightward axis
• Tall P wave, particularly in lead II
• Transient changes with hypoxia which may include:
  ◊ Rightward axis shift of 30°
  ◊ Right precordial T wave flattening or inversion
  ◊ ST depression in II, III and a VF
  ◊ Incomplete right bundle-branch block

IMAGING
• Chest x-ray - evidence of the primary disease, right atrial, ventricular and pulmonary artery enlargement
• Echocardiogram - right ventricular dimensions, assessment of tricuspid regurgitation and Doppler quantitation of pulmonary artery pressure

DIAGNOSTIC PROCEDURES Right heart catheterization for quantitation of ventricular and pulmonary pressures and exclusion of congenital heart disease as etiology of right heart failure

TREATMENT

APPROPRIATE HEALTH CARE
Outpatient

GENERAL MEASURES
• Vigorous antibiotic treatment of acute respiratory tract infections
• Avoidance of airway irritants (i.e., tobacco smoke) as well as sedatives and tranquilizers which may reduce respiratory effort
Appropriate treatment of underlying pulmonary disease, for example:
• Chronic obstructive pulmonary disease
  ◊ Bronchodilators
  ◊ Supplemental oxygen
  ◊ Vasodilators, diuretics and phlebotomy are possibly useful
  ◊ Digoxin with concomitant left ventricular failure
• Ventilatory abnormalities, i.e., sleep apnea
  ◊ CPAP (continuous positive airway pressure) or BiPAP (biphasic positive airway pressure)
  ◊ Progestins
  ◊ Tracheostomy
• Acute or chronic thromboembolic disease
  ◊ Appropriate anticoagulation

SURGICAL MEASURES N/A

ACTIVITY As tolerated

DIET Moderate salt restriction

PATIENT EDUCATION
• Diet restrictions
• Signs of edema to watch for
• Stress the need for adequate rest
• Referral to social service agency for home care help (oxygen, suctioning, etc.)
• Report any signs of infections to physician
• Avoid use of non-prescription medications, especially sedatives

MEDICATIONS

DRUG(S) OF CHOICE
• O2 at a flow rate adequate to restore O2 tensions to > 60 mm Hg (> 8.0 kPa) in the arterial blood. In patients with CO2 retention care must be taken not to supply so much O2 that the patient's hypoxic respiratory drive is inhibited.
• Bronchodilators - (e.g., metaproterenol, albuterol) on a regular dosing schedule of every six hours and more often if necessary
• Diuretics: (e.g., furosemide) for the relief of fluid retention. Dose as necessary.
• Vasodilators: (e.g., hydralazine, nifedipine, diltiazem, prazosin) may be tried if conventional measures fail. Success with these agents can only be measured if they are administered during invasive monitoring and is defined as a > 20% decrease in pulmonary vascular resistance associated with a decreased or unchanged pulmonary artery pressure and an increased or unchanged cardiac output. Monitoring for systemic hypotension during initiation of these medications is necessary.

Contraindications: Vary according to underlying disease, but generally sedatives and respiratory depressants should be avoided

Precautions: Diuretics - electrolytes should be monitored as excessive loss of potassium and chloride may result in profound metabolic alkalosis

Significant possible interactions: Refer to manufacturer's literature

ALTERNATIVE DRUGS
Digoxin 0.125-0.25 mg/day remains controversial for the treatment of right heart failure. Beneficial effects are not as apparent as in the treatment of left heart failure and electrolyte disturbances with resulting arrhythmias are of concern.

FOLLOWUP

PATIENT MONITORING Depends on the severity of the underlying disease and the extent of right heart failure as well as the medications being used in treatment

PREVENTION/AVOIDANCE Discontinue tobacco use

POSSIBLE COMPLICATIONS N/A

EXPECTED COURSE/PROGNOSIS
Depends on underlying disease and degree of pulmonary hypertension. Generally, a 10-50% 5 year mortality has been observed which improves with supplemental oxygen. In COPD with cor pulmonale, 3 year mortality can approach 30-50%.

MISCELLANEOUS

ASSOCIATED CONDITIONS Left heart failure

AGE-RELATED FACTORS
Pediatric: N/A
Geriatric: Metabolism of sedatives and narcotics may be slow, thus the respiratory drive of these patients may be affected for prolonged periods
Others: N/A

PREGNANCY Patient should be seen immediately by a cardiologist as the consequences of an increase in demand for output from the right heart may be quite severe

SYNONYMS N/A

ICD-9-CM
416.9 Cor pulmonale, chronic
415.0 Cor pulmonale, acute

SEE ALSO
• Congestive heart failure
• Cystic fibrosis
• Obesity
• Bronchiectasis

OTHER NOTES N/A

ABBREVIATIONS N/A

REFERENCES
• Brandenburg RO, Fuster V, Giuliani ER, McGoon DC: Cardiology: Fundamentals and Practice. Chicago, Year Book Medical Publishers, 1987
• McFadden ER, Braunwald E: Cor pulmonale. In: Braunwald E, ed. Heart Disease. 4th Ed. Philadelphia, WB Saunders Co, 1992
Illustrations: N/A
Internet references: http://www.5mcc.com

Author(s)
Robert Kowal, MD

Corneal ulceration

BASICS

DESCRIPTION Corneal ulcers represent an infection of the cornea by bacteria, virus or fungi as a result of breakdown in the protective epithelial barrier. If left untreated, corneal ulcers can result in blindness. Ulcerations may be central or marginal.
System(s) affected: Nervous
Genetics: None
Incidence/Prevalence in USA: Common
Predominant age: None
Predominant sex: Male = Female

SIGNS AND SYMPTOMS
• Eyelid and conjunctiva become inflamed
• Mucopurulent discharge
• The corneal epithelium will be absent with underlying ulceration and infiltration of the corneal stroma with leukocytes
• Foreign body sensation
• Blurred vision
• Light sensitivity
• Pain

CAUSES
• Corneal ulcers are predisposed by the presence of an entry to the external eye. Dry eye, burns, abrasion, contact lenses, inappropriate use of topical anesthetics, antibiotics, or anti-viral drops, immunosuppressant drugs, diabetes, immunodeficiency.
• Causative agents for foreign entry:
  ◊ Gram positive organisms (staphylococci, streptococci, and bacilli)
  ◊ Anaerobes (cocci, bacilli)
  ◊ Gram negative organisms (diplococcus, rods, and anaerobes)
  ◊ Pseudomonas
  ◊ Viruses such as herpes

RISK FACTORS
• Any abrasive injury
• Contact lenses (especially soft lenses)
• Chronic topical steroid use

DIAGNOSIS

DIFFERENTIAL DIAGNOSIS Identify infecting organisms

LABORATORY Culture the ulcer
Drugs that may alter lab results: Pretreatment with topical antibiotics or corticosteroids may delay diagnosis
Disorders that may alter lab results: N/A

PATHOLOGICAL FINDINGS Scrapings for Gram's and Giemsa's stain may demonstrate bacteria, yeast, or intranuclear inclusions which may aid in the diagnosis

SPECIAL TESTS N/A

IMAGING N/A

DIAGNOSTIC PROCEDURES Scrapings of the corneal ulcer may be necessary to identify the underlying organism. The sample should be plated onto the culture media directly.

TREATMENT

APPROPRIATE HEALTH CARE
• Outpatient or inpatient for severe ulcer or noncompliant patient
• All cases of corneal ulceration should be promptly referred to an ophthalmologist

GENERAL MEASURES
• Aggressive topical antibiotic treatment directed toward the causative agent should be instituted immediately while culture studies are pending
• Supplemental topical cycloplegia reduces the inflammation and aids in patient comfort
• Bandaging the eye should be avoided and topical steroids should never be used. Daily evaluation is necessary and prompt consultation with an ophthalmologist or corneal specialist is advised.

SURGICAL MEASURES N/A

ACTIVITY Reduced, until vision returns to normal and healing is complete

DIET No special diet

PATIENT EDUCATION Prevention of abrasions and proper handling of contact lenses can prevent recurrence of corneal ulcers

MEDICATIONS

DRUG(S) OF CHOICE
• Sulfacetamide 10% suspension (bacteriostatic) is only good for low grade conjunctival infections
• Topical gentamicin and tobramycin are effective against Pseudomonas, Enterobacter, Klebsiella, and aerobic gram negative organisms, while cephalosporins (e.g., cefazolin 50 mg/mL) may be effective against many gram negative organisms. The combination aminoglycoside and cephalosporin may be the most appropriate initial therapy.
• Topical quinolones, e.g., ciprofloxacin (Ciloxan) 0.3%, were recently introduced for ocular use. These may be treatment of choice for Pseudomonas infections.
• Fungal keratitis needs to be treated with parenteral amphotericin B for candida and aspergillus; clotrimazole, miconazole, econazole, and ketoconazole may also be required
Contraindications: Refer to manufacturer's profile of each drug
Precautions: Refer to manufacturer's profile of each drug
Significant possible interactions: Refer to manufacturer's profile of each drug

ALTERNATIVE DRUGS   N/A

FOLLOWUP

PATIENT MONITORING   The patient should be monitored at least daily

PREVENTION/AVOIDANCE   Avoid corneal abrasion or injury and improper contact lens handling

POSSIBLE COMPLICATIONS   Scarring of the cornea and loss of vision

EXPECTED COURSE/PROGNOSIS
• Corneal ulcerations should improve daily and heal with appropriate therapy
• If healing does not occur or the ulcer extends, then consideration should be given to an alternative diagnosis and treatment

MISCELLANEOUS

ASSOCIATED CONDITIONS   Chronic ulcerations may be associated with neurotrophic keratitis due to lack of fifth nerve innervation of the cornea. Individuals with thyroid disease, diabetes, immunosuppressive conditions are particularly at risk.

AGE-RELATED FACTORS
Pediatric: N/A
Geriatric: Ring ulceration more common
Others: N/A

PREGNANCY   N/A

SYNONYMS   N/A

ICD-9-CM   370.0 Corneal ulcer

SEE ALSO   N/A

OTHER NOTES   N/A

ABBREVIATIONS   N/A

REFERENCES   None
Illustrations: N/A
Internet references: http://www.5mcc.com

Author(s)
Robert M. Kershner, MD, FACS

Costochondritis

BASICS

DESCRIPTION Anterior chest wall pain associated with pain and tenderness of the costochondral and costosternal regions.
System(s) affected: Musculoskeletal
Genetics: Unknown
Incidence/Prevalence in USA: 10% of chest pain complaints. 15-20% of teenagers with chest pain.
Predominant age: 20-40
Predominant sex: Female

SIGNS AND SYMPTOMS
• Insidious onset
• History of overuse trauma
• History of unusual physical activity
• Often a history of recent upper respiratory infection
• Pain usually sharp in nature, sometimes pleuritic
• Pain involves multiple locations, the second through fifth costal cartilage most often involved
• Pain worse with movement and breathing
• Heat often provides relief of pain
• Chest tightness is often associated with the pain
• Pain sometimes radiates into arm
• Non-suppurative edema and tenderness at rib articulations
• Redness and warmth at sites of tenderness
• Self-limited course
• Often recurs

CAUSES
• Not fully understood
• Trauma
• Overuse

RISK FACTORS   Included with causes

DIAGNOSIS

DIFFERENTIAL DIAGNOSIS
• Cardiac
  ◊ Coronary artery disease
  ◊ Aortic aneurysm
  ◊ Mitral valve prolapse
  ◊ Pericarditis
  ◊ Myocarditis
• Gastrointestinal
  ◊ Gastroesophageal reflux
  ◊ Peptic esophagitis
  ◊ Esophageal spasm
  ◊ Gastritis
• Musculoskeletal
  ◊ Fibromyalgia
  ◊ Slipping rib syndrome - involves the lower ribs
  ◊ Costovertebral arthritis
  ◊ Painful xiphoid syndrome
  ◊ Rib trauma with swelling
  ◊ Thoracic disk compression
  ◊ Ankylosing spondylitis
  ◊ Epidemic myalgia
  ◊ Precordial catch syndrome
• Psychogenic
  ◊ Anxiety disorder
  ◊ Panic attacks
  ◊ Hyperventilation
• Respiratory
  ◊ Asthma
  ◊ Pneumonia
  ◊ Chronic cough
  ◊ Pneumothorax
• Other
  ◊ Herpes zoster
  ◊ Spinal tumor
  ◊ Metastatic cancer
  ◊ Substance abuse (cocaine)

LABORATORY The diagnosis of costochondritis is based on a complete and thorough history and physical examination. Laboratory exams should only be utilized if there is concern regarding other elements of the differential diagnosis. Erythrocyte sedimentation rate inconsistently elevated.
Drugs that may alter lab results: N/A
Disorders that may alter lab results: N/A

PATHOLOGICAL FINDINGS
Costochondral joint inflammation

SPECIAL TESTS None indicated for the diagnosis of costochondritis

IMAGING No imaging is indicated for the diagnosis of costochondritis. Chest x-ray normal.

DIAGNOSTIC PROCEDURES None

TREATMENT

APPROPRIATE HEALTH CARE
Outpatient therapy

GENERAL MEASURES Patient reassurance. Rest and heat.

SURGICAL MEASURES N/A

ACTIVITY As tolerated

DIET Regular

PATIENT EDUCATION Educate the patient in regards to the self-limited nature of the illness. Instruct patient on proper physical activity regimens to avoid overuse syndromes. Also stress the importance of avoiding sudden, significant changes in activity.

MEDICATIONS

DRUG(S) OF CHOICE Nonsteroidal anti-inflammatory drugs (NSAID's) such as aspirin, ibuprofen (Advil, Motrin), naproxen (Anaprox, Naprosyn, Aleve) or diclofenac (Voltaren). Other analgesics may be used as needed.
Contraindications:
• History of anaphylaxis to aspirin
• Peptic ulcer disease
• Renal insufficiency
Precautions:
• Peptic ulcers may occur with chronic use of nonsteroidal anti-inflammatory drugs
• Acute interstitial nephritis
• Drug accumulation with renal insufficiency
• Liver function abnormalities in up to 15% of patients
Significant possible interactions:
• NSAID's
◊ Albumin-bound drugs - displacement of either drug
◊ Warfarin - increased prothrombin time. Monitor prothrombin times closely and adjust warfarin dosage as needed. Monitor lithium levels and adjust lithium dosage as needed. May need to increase lithium dosage when non-steroidal anti-inflammatory drugs have been discontinued.
◊ Lithium - increased lithium plasma level
◊ Furosemide - decreased natriuretic effect and increased risk of acute renal failure secondary to decreased renal blood flow
◊ Propranolol - decreased anti-hypertensive effect

ALTERNATIVE DRUGS Acetaminophen

FOLLOWUP

PATIENT MONITORING Followup in one week

PREVENTION/AVOIDANCE Avoid activity which increases the pain

POSSIBLE COMPLICATIONS Incomplete attention to differential diagnosis or inappropriate interventions in a desire to ensure that a more life-threatening diagnosis is not missed

EXPECTED COURSE/PROGNOSIS
Self-limited illness

MISCELLANEOUS

ASSOCIATED CONDITIONS Upper respiratory infections

AGE-RELATED FACTORS
Pediatric: Special attention should be paid to psychogenic chest pain with children who perceive family discord
Geriatric: Often present with multiple problems capable of causing chest pain, making a thorough history and physical exam imperative.
Others: N/A

PREGNANCY Unknown

SYNONYMS
• Costosternal syndrome
• Parasternal chondrodynia
• Anterior chest wall syndrome
• Tietze's disease
• Tietze's syndrome
• Chondrocostal junction syndrome

ICD-9-CM 733.99

SEE ALSO N/A

OTHER NOTES N/A

ABBREVIATIONS N/A

REFERENCES
• Milov DE, Kantor RJ: Chest pain in teenagers. Postgraduate Medicine 1990; 88(5):145-154
• A report from ASPN: An exploratory report of chest pain in primary care. J Am Board Fam Prac 1990, 3:143-150
• Klinkman MS, Stevens D, Gorenflaw DW: Episodes of care for chest pain: A preliminary report. From MIRNET, J Fam Practice 1994;38(4):345-52
• Disla E, Rhim HR, Reddy A, Karten I, Taranta A: Costochondritis. a prospective analysis in an emergency department setting. Archives Int Med 1994:154(21):2466-2469
• Wise OM, Semble EL, Dalton CB: Musculoskeletal chest wall syndromes in patients with noncardiac chest pain: a study of 100 patients. Archives PMR 1992:73(2):147-149
Illustrations: N/A
Internet references: http://www.5mcc.com

Author(s)
Scott A. Fields, MD

Crohn's disease

BASICS

DESCRIPTION An idiopathic inflammatory disease of the small intestine (60%), the colon (20%) or both; involving all of the layers of the bowel, but most commonly involving the terminal ileum. It is a slowly progressive and recurrent disease with prominent involvement of multiple regions of the intestine with normal sections in between.
System(s) affected: Gastrointestinal
Genetics: 15% of patients have first-degree relatives with inflammatory bowel disease. Family members develop the disease with similar patterns and similar age of onset.
Incidence/Prevalence in USA:
• More common in Caucasians than African-Americans or Asians
• More common in Jews
• 20-100/100,000 prevalence
Predominant Age:
• Most cases 15-25 age of onset
• Second smaller peak in ages 55-65
Predominant Sex: Female > Male (slightly)

SIGNS AND SYMPTOMS
• All forms of Crohn's
◊ Diarrhea occurs at some time in most patients
◊ Abdominal pain occurs in about two-thirds
◊ Weight loss
◊ Abdominal tenderness often less than expected, in view of symptoms
◊ Abdominal mass (occasionally)
◊ Fistula - perirectal, bladder, skin, vagina
◊ Extraluminal disease (10%) skin, iritis, arthritis, sclerosing cholangitis
• Small bowel disease only
◊ Diarrhea prominent, at any time including nocturnal
◊ Vague abdominal pain frequent. Only half of patients with abdominal pain have associated tenderness, not relieved with evacuation and often aggravated by food.
◊ Intestinal obstruction in one-third. Cramping abdominal pain precedes for months.
◊ Bleeding occurs in 20%, rarely massive
◊ Perianal disease, including fistulae
◊ Internal fistulae
◊ Arthritis 5%
• Colon disease only
◊ Diarrhea prominent, at any time including nocturnal
◊ Hematochezia
◊ Abdominal pain in half the patients, often relieved by stooling
◊ Perianal disease in 40%, fistulae
◊ Weight loss prominent
◊ Megacolon occurs in about 10%
◊ Arthritis in 20%
◊ Intestinal obstruction occasional
• Colon and small bowel disease
◊ Intestinal obstruction much more common
◊ Arthritis 5%

CAUSES
• Idiopathic
• Aggravated by bacterial infection
• Aggravated by inflammatory cascade
• Aggravated by smoking cessation

RISK FACTORS
• More cigarette smokers than expected

DIAGNOSIS

DIFFERENTIAL DIAGNOSIS
• Colon disease
◊ Ulcerative colitis
◊ Ischemic colitis (older age group)
◊ Enteric pathogens: Amebiasis, Tuberculosis, Yersinia, Campylobacter, Gonorrhea, Clostridium difficile toxin, Shigella, Salmonella, LGV and non-LGV Chlamydia, Fungi(e.g., actinomycosis)
◊ Malignancy: Lymphoma, adenocarcinoma
◊ Caustic enemas (e.g., H2O2)
• Small bowel disease
◊ Enteric pathogens: Tuberculosis, Yersinia, Campylobacter, LGV and non-LGV Chlamydia, Fungi (e.g., actinomycosis), Chlamydial pelvic inflammation in women
◊ Lymphoma
◊ Drugs (e.g., NSAID's)
V Eosinophilic gastroenteritis

LABORATORY
• Elevated sedimentation rate
• Anemia common
• Albumin decreased in severe cases
• Serum electrolytes imbalance
• Specific nutrient deficiency: B12, fat soluble vitamins, folate
Drugs that may alter lab results: Sulfa drugs may lower folate after years of administration
Disorders that may alter lab results: All tests are non-specific, similar degrees of disease from other causes produce similar changes

PATHOLOGICAL FINDINGS
• Involvement of all layers of gut wall with inflammation in > 95% cases at least focal areas
• Skip areas in 80% (a normal segment between two involved segments)
• Granuloma in 15%
• Fat hypertrophy following mesenteric vessels in 50% of small bowel disease

SPECIAL TESTS
• Colonoscopy with ileoscopy and biopsy
• Mucosa ulceration, loss, undermining ulcers and distortion, with skip areas

IMAGING
• Barium x-rays - enema and small bowel
◊ Loss of smooth mucosa, undermined ulcers prominent
◊ Narrowed lumen in most involved segments of small bowel
◊ Fistulae from involved segment to other bowel loops, bladder, vagina or external
◊ Skip areas, multiple lesions common
◊ Failure to reflux into ileum on barium enema (not specific)
◊ Ulcers undermining mucosa
◊ Small bowel ulcerated wall
◊ Narrowed lumen
◊ Fistula to other parts of intestine

• Plain x-rays
◊ Of painful or distended abdomen (intestinal obstruction)
◊ Toxic patient with colon disease, toxic megacolon
◊ Evaluation of arthritis
◊ Sacroiliitis
• CT Scans
◊ Define thickening of bowel wall if lumen not narrowed
◊ Define abscess cavities associated with fistulae
◊ Identify extensive perirectal disease

DIAGNOSTIC PROCEDURES
• Ileoscopy and enteroscopy
• The constellation of barium-identified distribution of lesions, endoscopic findings, and biopsies usually establish the diagnosis
• Biopsies of gut mucosa of involved areas usually compatible with diagnosis, but not precisely diagnostic. Helps rule out other causes.

TREATMENT

APPROPRIATE HEALTH CARE
• Outpatient customary, inpatient for complications or special treatments
• Disease progresses with average patient requiring surgical treatment each 4 to 7 years

GENERAL MEASURES
• Attention to maintaining weight and nutrition
• Monitor severe cases for fat malabsorption
• Perirectal disease, sitz baths, soap and water after stooling, surgical drainage of perirectal abscesses, surgical treatment of recurrent fistulae if medical management fails
• Extracolonic disease (uveitis, arthritis, dermatitis, sclerosing cholangitis) managed as other diseases in that special area
• Folate supplements often needed

SURGICAL MEASURES
• Indications for surgery:
◊ Severe recurrent hemorrhage
◊ Inability to thrive
◊ Abscess
◊ Total or recurrent intestinal obstruction
◊ Toxicity of megacolon or extensive disease
◊ Symptomatic fistulae other than rectal
◊ Failure of ostomy to function after 1 or more years

ACTIVITY Full activity as tolerated

DIET
• Usually no restrictions
• If fat malabsorption, diminish fat in diet
• If strictures or recurrent obstruction, avoid highly fibrous substances
• If diarrhea prominent, increase dietary fiber (sometimes recommended), decrease fat

PATIENT EDUCATION An important part of management. Best information from Crohn's and Colitis Foundation of America Inc, 11th floor, Park Ave South, NY 10016, Phone (800)343-3637. Many free pamphlets, local chapters in major metropolitan areas, excellent inexpensive authoritative books. Joining local chapters recommended.

MEDICATIONS

DRUG(S) OF CHOICE
• Maintenance therapy
◊ Usually with mesalamine (5-aminosalicylic acid), methotrexate, or azathioprine (Imuran) prolongs remission and delays additional surgery
◊ Inducing a remission usually depends on prednisone or mesalamine enemas for rectal symptoms because the response is rapid
◊ Several delivery forms of mesalamine exist; each targets a different portion of the intestine. Select form appropriate to patient.
• Bringing acute exacerbations or complications under control
◊ Prednisone 20 to 40 mg/day. Response in 1-3 weeks, taper after 4-6 weeks.
◊ Sulfasalazine, or 5-aminosalicylic acid derivative. Increase dose each 4 days from 0.5 gm bid to 1 gm qid if tolerated. Response in 4 to 6 weeks.
• Rectal and left sided colon disease
◊ Mesalamine enema (5-aminosalicylic acid, 5-ASA, Rowasa) 2 gm 2-3 times daily
◊ Hydrocortisone (Cortenema) enema 2-3 times daily or suppositories for proctitis
• Predominantly perirectal disease with fistulae
◊ Metronidazole (Flagyl) 250 mg tid for max of 8 weeks
• Colon disease in sulfasalazine intolerant patient
◊ Mesalamine (5-ASA) preparations, enteric-coated: Asacol (800 mg tid), Claversal, Rowasa controlled release
◊ Olsalazine (Dipentum) 1 gm/day in two divided doses, increase up to maximum of 2 gm/day.
• Ileal disease
◊ Oral or IV steroids
◊ Mesalamine (Asacol)
Contraindications: Allergy to prescribed drugs
Precautions:
• Sulfasalazine may not be tolerated by the stomach at necessary dose since it frequently causes nausea, vomiting, and other gastrointestinal distress
• Allergies common
• Male sterility problem with chronic use
• Watch for thrombocytopenia and pancytopenia
Significant possible interactions: Folic acid supplements needed with mesalamine. Refer to manufacturer's profile of each drug.

ALTERNATIVE DRUGS
• Sulfasalazine least costly and well tolerated in 90% of patients. Similar effectiveness but better tolerance with the 5-aminosalicylic acid compounds.
• Metronidazole produces severe peripheral neuritis after months of treatment. Other antibiotics seem similar in action and may be used.
• Antibiotics
• Azathioprine (Imuran), mercaptopurine (6-mercaptopurine)

FOLLOWUP

PATIENT MONITORING
• Regular assessment (each 3-6 months if patient is stable) of symptoms, particularly status of weight, pain, diarrhea, hemoglobin and sedimentation rate
• Regular calculation of an activity index based upon:
1) loose stools/day
2) pain
3) general well being
4) systemic manifestations
5) use of antidiarrheal
6) presence of abdominal mass
7) hematocrit
8) change in body weight. Highly useful in following patients and making decisions to increase or diminish medications and/or hospitalize.
• Endoscopy and further images if there are changes in symptoms and signs
• Check liver tests yearly
• Check vitamin B12 level in those with ileal disease or ileal resection
• Check folate level in all on 5-aminosalicylate

PREVENTION/AVOIDANCE
• Ongoing care with available physician
• Use consultants for review and long term advice

POSSIBLE COMPLICATIONS
• Progression nearly certain - both expansion of old lesions and new lesions occur
• Recurrence after operation nearly certain, usually occurs in gut segment most proximal to anastomoses
• Fistulae occur about 15% of patients; perirectal, cutaneous, enterovaginal, enterovesicular are all seen
• Extraluminal disease occurs in 10% with skin, uveal tract, joint, and biliary tract disease most common. All are fairly specific in pattern, but do not parallel activity of the luminal disease.
• Extensive colon disease associated with increased risk of adenocarcinoma
• Colon perforation and massive bleeding
• Toxic megacolon

EXPECTED COURSE/PROGNOSIS
• Average patient has surgery each 7 years. After 4 surgeries may expect short-bowel syndrome.
• Expect disease to recur
• Majority of patients have normal life with work, children, full activities, but overall life is shortened

MISCELLANEOUS

ASSOCIATED CONDITIONS
• Viral gastroenteritis may be more devastating
• Arthritis of two types - similar to rheumatoid and spondylitis
• Variety of skin lesions, erythema nodosum, non-specific rashes, pyoderma gangrenosum
• Uveal tract disease rare but related
• Sclerosing cholangitis in about 10%, manifest from mild liver test abnormalities including pericholangitis on biopsy to full syndrome

AGE-RELATED FACTORS
Pediatric: Rare
Geriatric: N/A
Others: Occurs at any age

PREGNANCY
• Reversible male sterility after long time on sulfasalazine - folate defers
• No contraindications to pregnancy

SYNONYMS
• Granulomatous colitis
• Regional enteritis
• Regional ileitis
• Regional colitis
• Regional ileocolitis

ICD-9-CM
555.0 Regional enteritis, small intestine
555.1 Regional enteritis, large intestine
555.9 Regional enteritis, unspecified site

SEE ALSO
• Ulcerative colitis
• Diarrhea, acute
• Diarrhea, chronic
• Intestinal parasites
• Short-bowel syndrome
• Celiac disease

OTHER NOTES N/A

ABBREVIATIONS
LGV = lymphogranuloma venereum

REFERENCES
• Farmer RG, Hawk WA, Turnbull RB: Clinical patterns in Crohn's disease: a statistical study of 615 cases. Gastroenterology 1975;68,:627-38
• Stenson WF, MacDermott RP: Inflammatory Bowel Disease. In: Yamada T, ed. Textbook of Gastroenterology. Philadelphia, J.B. Lippincott Co., 1991
• Williams JG, Wong WD, Rothenberger DA, Goldberg SM: Recurrence of Crohn's disease after resection. British Journal of Surgery 1991;78:10-19
• Hanauer SB: Inflammatory bowel disease. NEJM 1996;334:841-847
Illustrations: 5 available on CD-ROM
Internet references: http://www.5mcc.com

Author(s)
Frank L. Iber, MD

Cryptococcosis

BASICS

DESCRIPTION Cryptococcus neoformans is a fungus which rarely causes disease in hosts with normal immune function. Cryptococcal meningitis is one of the more common AIDS-defining infections in HIV seropositive persons.
System(s) affected: Nervous, Pulmonary, Skin/Exocrine, Endocrine/Metabolic
Genetics: N/A
Incidence/Prevalence in USA: Accounts for 5-8% of opportunistic infections in AIDS patients
Predominant age: Generally adults
Predominant sex: Male > Female

SIGNS AND SYMPTOMS
• Cryptococcal meningitis
◊ Often insidious onset with subtle findings
◊ Frontal or temporal headache (80-95% of patients)
◊ Fever (60-80% of patients)
◊ Impaired mentation
◊ Seizures or focal neurologic signs are rare. May occur if cryptococcomas (granulomas) are present
◊ Meningismus usually absent (80% of patients)
• Pulmonary cryptococcus
◊ May be asymptomatic (32% of patients)
◊ Cough (54% of patients)
◊ Sputum
◊ Fever
◊ Hemoptysis
◊ May disseminate in immunosuppressed patients
• Disseminated cryptococcus
◊ Painless skin nodules (5-10% of patients). May occur as erythematous papules, vesicles, macules, or ulcers.
◊ The heart, bone, kidney, adrenals, eyes, prostate and lymph nodes may harbor infection with symptoms referable to affected organ

CAUSES The cryptococcus fungus is ubiquitous. No person to person transmission has been documented.

RISK FACTORS Immunosuppression which results in reactivation of latent infection (usually foci in lungs). Rarely, invasive infection may occur in normal hosts.

DIAGNOSIS

DIFFERENTIAL DIAGNOSIS
• In CNS disease - toxoplasmosis, lymphoma, AIDS dementia complex, progressive multifocal leukoencephalopathy, herpes encephalitis, other fungal disease
• In pulmonary disease - tuberculosis, histoplasmosis, coccidioidomycosis, Kaposi's sarcoma, lymphoma, pneumocystis
• In disseminated disease - tuberculosis, histoplasmosis, lymphoma, coccidioidomycosis

LABORATORY
• Latex agglutination assay of cryptococcal antigen in CSF, serum, urine. (False positives and false negatives have occurred but CSF cryptococcal antigen is positive in 95% of culture-proven positive cases.)
• India ink preparation of CSF (60% positive in non-AIDS patients; 75-85% positive in AIDS patients)
• Culture of CSF, sputum, blood, urine
Drugs that may alter lab results: N/A
Disorders that may alter lab results: In presence of rheumatoid factor, false positive latex agglutination tests have occurred

PATHOLOGICAL FINDINGS
Inflammation, granuloma formation (may caseate and cavitate), basilar meningitis with mucoid exudate

SPECIAL TESTS Lumbar puncture in cryptococcal meningitis: In non-AIDS patients - elevated opening pressure, elevated CSF protein, decreased glucose and lymphocytic pleocytosis. In AIDS patients - minimal pleocytosis, normal protein and glucose.

IMAGING
• In cryptococcal meningitis - CT of brain is negative unless focal cryptococcomas present
• In pulmonary cryptococcosis - chest x-ray may show nodules, mass lesions (with occasional cavitation), miliary spread, hilar adenopathy (10%), pleural effusions (less than 5%)

DIAGNOSTIC PROCEDURES Biopsies of skin lesions may be diagnostic

TREATMENT

APPROPRIATE HEALTH CARE Inpatient; outpatient for mild cases

GENERAL MEASURES N/A

SURGICAL MEASURES N/A

ACTIVITY As tolerated

DIET As tolerated

PATIENT EDUCATION Life-long antifungal medication required for suppression. In severely immune deficient patients, consider prophylaxis with fluconazole.

Cryptococcosis

MEDICATIONS

DRUG(S) OF CHOICE
• Amphotericin B at 0.5-1.0 mg/kg/day IV until patient is clinically improving (2-3 weeks). (Some experts add flucytosine but evidence for increased efficacy is lacking.)
• Fluconazole (Diflucan), an oral (or intravenous) anti-fungal agent is usually given after the patient has improved symptomatically on amphotericin B. Some experts recommend 400 mg/day po until a total of 8 weeks of primary therapy has been completed.
• Note: Studies comparing fluconazole vs. amphotericin B in initial treatment of cryptococcal meningitis are ongoing. Although the initial response is better with amphotericin B, there is some evidence that patients with less severe symptoms (normal mental status) may do well on initial fluconazole (400 mg per day) alone. This course would obviate the need for hospitalization.
Contraindications: Refer to manufacturer's profile of each drug
Precautions: With amphotericin B - permanent renal impairment may occur, hypokalemia, hypomagnesemia; during infusion - fever, chills, headache - pretreat with diphenhydramine, acetaminophen to decrease fever and chill. Add heparin 500 U and hydrocortisone 50 mg to IV amphotericin B to decrease phlebitis.
Significant possible interactions: Refer to manufacturer's literature

ALTERNATIVE DRUGS
• Liposomal amphotericin treatment is being studied
• For increased intracranial pressure: acetazolamide, mannitol, or steroids may be helpful

FOLLOWUP

PATIENT MONITORING
• Monitor clinical status
• Patients who fail treatment (for meningitis) may require intrathecal amphotericin
• Foci in the prostate may be difficult to eliminate

PREVENTION/AVOIDANCE
• Without suppression, relapse is common (50% in AIDS patients within one year)
• Fluconazole 200-400 mg po daily or amphotericin B 0.5-1.0 mg/kg/day given 3-5 times per week is recommended for lifelong suppression
• Avoid bird roosts
• Primary prophylaxis with fluconazole (200 mg/day) in selected patients with CD4 < 50 decreases the incidence of cryptococcosis, however, no change in mortality is seen

POSSIBLE COMPLICATIONS
• Cryptococcal infections are fatal unless treated
• Increased intracranial pressure

EXPECTED COURSE/PROGNOSIS
• Fatal without treatment
• No statistics available on survival

MISCELLANEOUS

ASSOCIATED CONDITIONS
• HIV infection
• AIDS

AGE-RELATED FACTORS
Pediatric: N/A
Geriatric: N/A
Others: N/A

PREGNANCY Amphotericin contraindicated in pregnancy except when treating cryptococcal meningitis

SYNONYMS Torulosis

ICD-9-CM 117.5 Cryptococcosis

SEE ALSO
• HIV infection & AIDS

OTHER NOTES N/A

ABBREVIATIONS
CSF = cerebrospinal fluid
AIDS = acquired immunodeficiency syndrome

REFERENCES
• White MH, Armstrong D: Cryptococcosis. Infect Dis Clin North Am 1994;8(2):383-398
• Powderly WG: Cryptococcal meningitis and AIDS. Clin Infect Dis 1993;17(5):837-842
• Quagliarello VJ, et al: Primary prevention of cryptococcal meningitis by fluconazole in HIV-infected persons. Lancet 1994;345:548-52
• Haubrich RM, et al: High dose fluconazole for treatment of cryptococcal disease in patients with human immunodeficiency virus infection. J Infect Dis 1994;170:238-44
Illustrations: 2 available on CD-ROM
Internet references: http://www.5mcc.com

Author(s)
Cynthia Gail Carmichael, MD

Cryptorchidism

BASICS

DESCRIPTION Incomplete or improper descent of one or both testicles. Normally, descent is in the 7th to 8th month of gestation. The cryptorchid testis may be palpable or non-palpable.
• Ectopic testes: Lies outside the normal path of descent. It may be located within the perineum, above the symphysis pubis, along the medial thigh or on the contralateral side.
• Incomplete descent: The testis lies along the normal path of descent but hasn't reached the scrotum
• Intra-abdominal: The testis has not moved into the inguinal canal due to lack of development of the processus vaginalis and gubernaculum
• Gliding testis: Seen in boys with a patent processus vaginalis and gubernaculum. The testis may be present in the canal or intra-abdominally
• Iatrogenic: A testis that was previously located in the scrotum, but after a hernia repair or some other surgery has become trapped in the scar
System(s) affected: Reproductive
Genetics: Occurrence of undescended testes in siblings as well as fathers suggests a genetic etiology
Incidence/Prevalence: 3% of full-term and 33% of premature newborn males
Predominant age: Premature newborns
Predominant sex: Male only

SIGNS AND SYMPTOMS One or both testicles in a site other than the scrotum. May be an isolated defect or associated with other congenital anomalies.

CAUSES
• Not fully known
• May involve alterations in mechanical factors (gubernaculum, length of vas deferens and testicular vessels, groin anatomy, epididymis, cremasteric muscles, and abdominal pressure), hormonal factors (gonadotropin, testosterone, dihydrotestosterone, and Mullerian inhibiting substance), and neural factors (ileoinguinal nerve and genitofemoral nerve)

RISK FACTORS Family history of cryptorchidism

DIAGNOSIS

DIFFERENTIAL DIAGNOSIS
• Retractile testis (hypermobile testis): A normally descended testis that ascends into the inguinal canal because of an active cremasteric reflex
• Atrophic testis: May occur as a result of neonatal torsion

LABORATORY N/A
Drugs that may alter lab results: N/A
Disorders that may alter lab results: N/A

PATHOLOGICAL FINDINGS Higher incidence of carcinoma in undescended testis and alterations in spermatogenesis

SPECIAL TESTS N/A

IMAGING Ultrasonography is able to detect testicles in the inguinal canal and pubic region in 70% of cases, but is only able to detect 20% of intra-abdominal testicles. CT scan findings in children are inconsistent.

DIAGNOSTIC PROCEDURES
• Physical exam
  ◊ Performed with child in sitting, standing and squatting positions with warm hands
  ◊ A Valsalva maneuver and applied pressure to lower abdomen may help identify the testes, especially a gliding testis
  ◊ Failure to palpate a testis after repeated exams suggests an intra-abdominal or atrophic testis
  ◊ An enlarged contralateral testis in the presence of a non-palpable testis suggests testicular atrophy/absence

TREATMENT

APPROPRIATE HEALTH CARE
Outpatient until surgery performed

GENERAL MEASURES
• Rule out retractile testis
• Most testicles will descend by age 6 months, if they are going to descend
• Administration of chorionic gonadotropin - may cause testicular descent in some boys. Reports of efficacy are inconsistent.

SURGICAL MEASURES
• Reasons to consider: Avoids torsion, averts trauma, decreases but does not eliminate risk of malignancy, and prevents further alterations in spermatogenesis
• Orchiopexy should be performed by age 1. Alterations in germ cell count in the cryptorchid testis have been identified by age 2.

ACTIVITY No restrictions

DIET No special diet

PATIENT EDUCATION Discuss with parents about causes, available treatments, and possible effects on patient's reproductive potential

MEDICATIONS

DRUG(S) OF CHOICE Chorionic gonadotropin (HCG): 500-1000 IU IM twice weekly for 5 weeks. Alternatively, 1500-2500 IU IM weekly for 3 doses, or every other day for 3 to 9 doses.
Contraindications: Contraindicated in patients with a clinically apparent inguinal hernia, those with a history of previous ipsilateral groin surgery or in ectopic testicles. Also refer to manufacturer's literature.
Precautions: May induce precocious puberty - discontinue drug, effects should reverse in 4 weeks
Significant possible interactions: Refer to manufacturer's literature

ALTERNATIVE DRUGS N/A

 FOLLOWUP

PATIENT MONITORING
Patients should be followed after surgery to evaluate testicular growth and when older be taught testicular self-examination

PREVENTION/AVOIDANCE No preventive measures known

POSSIBLE COMPLICATIONS
• Progressive failure of spermatogenesis, if left untreated. Even with orchiopexy, the fertility rate is still reduced, especially with bilateral undescended testicles. Spermatogenesis related to duration of cryptorchidism and the location of the testis. Abnormalities have also been identified in the contralateral descended testis, although less severe
• Higher risk (20-46 times) of testicular cancer (risk may remain despite orchiopexy)
• Hernia development (25%)

EXPECTED COURSE/PROGNOSIS
Disorder usually corrected with medical or surgical therapy, however; possible lifelong consequences

 MISCELLANEOUS

ASSOCIATED CONDITIONS
• Inguinal hernia
• Hemiscrotum
• Hydrocele
• Abnormalities of vas deferens and epididymis
• Klinefelter's syndrome
• Hypogonadotropic hypogonadism
• Germinal cell aplasia
• Mullerian inhibiting factor deficiency
• 5 alpha-reductase deficiency
• True hermaphrodite
• Prune belly syndrome
• Meningomyelocele
• Hypospadias
• Wilm's tumor

AGE-RELATED FACTORS
Pediatric: This problem is usually detectable at birth or soon thereafter. If surgery is to be the treatment, it should be performed during the first year of life.
Geriatric: N/A
Others: Puberty: If unilateral cryptorchidism is discovered at or after puberty, usual treatment is orchiectomy

PREGNANCY N/A

SYNONYMS
• Undescended testes

ICD-9-CM
752.5 Undescended testicle

SEE ALSO
• Hydrocele
• Meningomyelocele
• Wilms' tumor

OTHER NOTES N/A

ABBREVIATIONS
IU = international units

REFERENCES
• Cendron M, Keating MA, Huff DS, et al: Cryptorchidism, Orchidopexy and Infertility: Critical Long-Term Retrospective Analysis. J Urol 1989;142:559-62
• Guiney EJ, Corballo M, Malone PS: Laparoscopy and the Management of the Impalpable Testis. Br J Urol 1989;63:313
• Kogan S: Cryptorchidism. In: Kelalis PP, King LR, Belmar AB, eds. Clinical Pediatric Urology. Philadelphia, WB Saunders Co, 1992:1050-1083
• Merguerian PA, Ellsworth P: Current Management of Cryptorchidism. In: Rous SN, ed. Urology Annual. Vol. 7. New York, WW Norton & Co, 1993:287-308
Illustrations: N/A
Internet references: http://www.5mcc.com

Author(s)
Pamela I. Ellsworth, MD
William A. Primack, MD

Cushing's disease and syndrome

BASICS

DESCRIPTION Clinical abnormalities associated with chronic exposure to excessive amounts of cortisol (the major adrenocorticoid). The most frequent cause is prolonged use of exogenous glucocorticoids.
System(s) affected:
Endocrine/Metabolic, Musculoskeletal, Skin/Exocrine, Cardiovascular
Genetics:
• Multiple endocrine neoplasia type I
• Carney complex
Incidence/Prevalence in USA:
Uncommon
Predominant age: All ages
Predominant sex: Females > Males

SIGNS AND SYMPTOMS
• Moon face (facial adiposity)
• Increased adipose tissue in neck and trunk
• Central weight gain
• Emotional lability
• Hypertension
• Osteoporosis
• Purple striae on the skin
• Diabetes or glucose intolerance with fasting hyperglycemia and/or glycosuria
• Muscle weakness due to loss of muscle mass from increased catabolism
• Skeletal growth retardation in children
• Easy bruising
• Hirsutism

CAUSES
• Exogenous glucocorticoids and/or ACTH
• Endogenous ACTH-dependent hypercortisolism
  ◊ ACTH-secreting pituitary tumor
  ◊ Ectopic ACTH production (e.g., small-cell carcinoma of lung, bronchial carcinoid)
• Endogenous ACTH-independent hypercortisolism
  ◊ Adrenal adenoma
  ◊ Adrenal carcinoma
  ◊ Macro/micro nodular hyperplasia

RISK FACTORS
• Any medical problem requiring prolonged use of corticosteroids
• Pituitary tumor
• Adrenal mass
• Neuroendocrine tumor (e.g., bronchial carcinoid)

DIAGNOSIS

DIFFERENTIAL DIAGNOSIS
• Obesity, diabetes mellitus, hypertension
• Adrenogenital syndrome
• Hypercortisolism secondary to alcoholism (pseudo-Cushing's)

LABORATORY
• 24 hour urinary 17-Hydroxycorticosteroids and cortisol
• Plasma cortisol
• Plasma ACTH concentration
• Glycosuria (possible)
• Neutrophilia
• Lymphopenia
• Hyperglycemia
• Hyperlipidemia
• Hypokalemia
• Dynamic endocrine testing (e.g., dexamethasone suppression test)
Drugs that may alter lab results: Refer to lab test or drug reference
Disorders that may alter lab results: Refer to lab test reference

PATHOLOGICAL FINDINGS
• Hyalinization of basophilic cells (anterior pituitary) - Crooke's cell changes
• Muscular atrophy
• Nephrosclerosis

SPECIAL TESTS If ACTH-dependent, inferior petrosal sinus sampling for ACTH

IMAGING
• Chest films
• X-rays of the lumbar spine - osteoporosis is common
• If pituitary tumor suspected - pituitary MRI scan
• If adrenal disease suspected - CT scan
• If ectopic ACTH-secretion suspected - chest CT scan

DIAGNOSTIC PROCEDURES Not all tests indicated for every case. Choice of diagnostic procedure dependent on circumstances and judgment.

TREATMENT

APPROPRIATE HEALTH CARE Inpatient for surgical procedures

GENERAL MEASURES
• Depends on etiology. Surgery is the treatment of choice; persistent disease may require - radiation, drug therapy, or surgery
• Medical treatment with adrenocortical inhibitors
  ◊ Has not been too successful
  ◊ Should be used when other methods fail
  ◊ In consultation with a clinician having experience in their use

SURGICAL MEASURES
• Primary hypersecretion of ACTH
  ◊ Transsphenoidal microsurgery. Radiation therapy as an adjunct for patients not cured.
• Adrenocortical tumors
  ◊ Surgical removal when possible
  ◊ If adrenocortical carcinoma, prognosis is poor
• Ectopic ACTH production
  ◊ Removal of the neoplastic tissue
  ◊ Metastatic spread makes surgical cure unlikely/impossible
  ◊ Bilateral adrenalectomy

ACTIVITY Determined by patient's symptoms and form of treatment used

DIET
• Potassium supplements
• High protein diet

PATIENT EDUCATION
• Instructions on drug therapy, diet, activity
• Early treatment of infections
• Monitor weight daily
• Emotional lability prevention

Cushing's disease and syndrome

MEDICATIONS

DRUG(S) OF CHOICE
• Medications in treatment should be used in consultation with an endocrinologist
• Adjunctive management considerations
◊ Inhibit cortisol production - ketoconazole 400-600 mg twice daily (dosages higher than conventionally recommended)
◊ Glucocorticoid replacement following surgery. In most cases, can be discontinued by 3-12 months.
Contraindications: Refer to manufacturer's literature
Precautions: Refer to manufacturer's literature
Significant possible interactions: Refer to manufacturer's literature

ALTERNATIVE DRUGS
• Mitotane
• Aminoglutethimide
• Metyrapone

FOLLOWUP

PATIENT MONITORING
• Individualize depending on therapy
• Check regularly for signs of adrenal hypofunction

PREVENTION/AVOIDANCE
• Avoid excessive corticosteroid treatment when possible
• Comprehensive teaching to help patient cope with lifelong treatment (if needed)

POSSIBLE COMPLICATIONS
• Osteoporosis
• Increased susceptibility to infections
• Hirsutism
• Metastases of malignant tumors

EXPECTED COURSE/PROGNOSIS
• Usual course - chronic with cyclic exacerbations and rare remissions
• Guardedly favorable prognosis with surgery

MISCELLANEOUS

ASSOCIATED CONDITIONS Tumors of the pituitary; multiple endocrine neoplasia Type I, Carney complex

AGE-RELATED FACTORS
Pediatric: Rare in infancy and childhood. Most cases (under age 8) are due to malignant adrenal tumors.
Geriatric: N/A
Others: N/A

PREGNANCY Can cause exacerbation of Cushing's disease

SYNONYMS N/A

ICD-9-CM
255.0 Cushing's syndrome

SEE ALSO N/A

OTHER NOTES Pituitary ACTH excess due to a pituitary tumor causes what is called Cushing's disease

ABBREVIATIONS
CRH = corticotropin releasing hormone

REFERENCES
• Kaye TB, Crapo L: The Cushing syndrome. An update in diagnostic tests. Ann Intern Med 1990;112:434
• Flack MR, Oldfield EH, Cutle GB Jr, et al: Urine free cortisol in the high dose dexamethasone suppression test for the differential diagnosis of the Cushing syndrome. Ann Intern Med 1992;116:211
• Miller JW, Crapo L: The medical treatment of Cushing's syndrome. Endocrine Reviews 1993;14:443
• Young WF Jr: Cushing's syndrome. In: Rakel RE, ed. Conn's Current Therapy. New York, NY, W.B. Saunders Co., 1996
Illustrations: 4 available on CD-ROM
Internet references: http://www.5mcc.com

Author(s)
William F. Young, Jr., MD

Cutaneous drug reactions

BASICS

DESCRIPTION Cutaneous or mucocutaneous eruptions are the most common adverse reactions to oral or parenteral drug therapy. Reactions may be immunologically mediated (either IgE dependent or immune complex dependent).
• Non-immunologic reactions occur more commonly. The majority of reactions occur within one week of initiation of drug therapy but make occur up to 4 weeks after initiation of therapy.
• Maculopapular and urticarial eruptions are the most common but multiple morphologic types of reactions may occur
System(s) affected: Skin/Exocrine, Hemic/Lymphatic/Immunologic
Genetics: No known genetic inheritance pattern
Incidence/Prevalence:
• Three reactions per 1000 drug courses
• Approximately 120 million inpatient drug courses annually in the USA, therefore approximately 144/100,000
• Approximately 125 million Americans regularly use prescription drugs as outpatients; overall prevalence in this group is unknown
Predominant age: All ages affected
Predominant sex: Female > Male (specific ratio unknown)

SIGNS AND SYMPTOMS
(note: in order of frequency)
• Maculopapular eruptions (exanthems):
　◊ Most frequent cutaneous reaction
　◊ Maybe indistinguishable from viral exanthem
　◊ Erythematous macules and papules
　◊ Often confluent and symmetrical
　◊ Pruritus common
　◊ Mucus membranes, palms and soles maybe involved
　◊ Onset typically 7-10 days after initiation of drug: may last one to two weeks
• Urticaria:
　◊ Pruritic red wheals distributed anywhere on the body including mucous membranes
　◊ Individual lesions fade within 24 hours but new urticaria may develop
　◊ May be mediated by anaphylactic or accelerated IgE reactions, serum sickness or non-immunologic histamine reactions
　◊ Deep dermal and subcutaneous swelling constitute angioedema and when mucus membranes are involved, maybe life-threatening
• Acneform eruptions
　◊ Pustular lesions but unlike true acne, no comedones
• Eczematous reactions
　◊ Pruritic scale-like erythematous lesions typically on flexor surfaces of arms or legs

• Erythema multiforme
　◊ Target lesions
　◊ Bullous lesions
　◊ Mucous membrane involvement (Stevens-Johnson syndrome)
• Exfoliative erythroderma
　◊ Generalized erythema and scaling
　◊ Potentially life-threatening
• Fixed drug eruptions
　◊ Single or multiple round sharply defined dark red plaques
　◊ Appear shortly after drug exposure and reappear in the same location after drug ingestion Lesions can occur anywhere: glans penis common in men
　◊ Onset usually 2 hours after ingestion of drug
　◊ Some patients have a refractory period during which the drug fails to activate lesions
• Lichen planus like eruptions
　◊ Violaceous papules extensor wrist surfaces
　◊ Reticular pattern, buccal mucosa
• Lupus erythematosus-like reactions
　◊ Malar erythema
• Photosensitivity reaction
　◊ Phototoxic reactions within 24 hours of light exposure
　◊ Photoallergic reactions; less common
• Vasculitis
　◊ Petechiae or purpura concentrated on lower legs
• Vesiculobullous eruptions
　◊ Small isolated bullae, erythema multiforme, toxic epidermal necrolysis (potentially fatal)

CAUSES
• Acneform: OCP's, corticosteroids, iodinated compounds, hydantoins, lithium
• Erythema multiforme: Sulfonamides, penicillins, barbiturates, hydantoins, NSAID's, tetracycline, cefaclor, terbinafine
• Erythema nodosum: OCP's, sulfonamides, penicillins
• Fixed drug eruptions: OCP's, barbiturates, salicylates barbiturates, tetracycline, sulfonamides
• Lichenoid: Gold, antimalarials, tetracycline
• Photosensitivity: Phenothiazines, griseofulvin, sulfonamides, tetracycline
• Vasculitis: Thiazides, gold, sulfonamides, NSAID's, tetracycline
• Bullous: NSAID's, thiazides, barbiturates, captopril
• Skin necrosis: Warfarin

RISK FACTORS
Drug therapy, especially with sulfonamides, penicillins

DIAGNOSIS

DIFFERENTIAL DIAGNOSIS
• Viral exanthem: since maculopapular eruptions are the most common form of drug reaction these are often difficult to distinguish from viral exanthems. Presence of fever, lymphocytosis, and other systemic findings may help differentiate.
• Drug eruptions manifest as many types of dermatosis as previously listed; consider a primary dermatosis in the differential diagnosis. Resolution of the eruption upon withdrawal of a drug will help to clarify.

LABORATORY
• Routine laboratory tests generally nonspecific and usually not helpful
• Eosinophilia: Possible in certain allergic reactions but generally of little value clinically
Drugs that may alter lab results:
Procainamide, hydralazine - positive ANA
Disorders that may alter lab results: N/A

PATHOLOGICAL FINDINGS
• Pathological findings dependent upon type of reaction; may be nonspecific
• Punch biopsy sometimes helpful for fixed drug eruptions which show certain characteristic histological features, e.g., lichen planus-like or erythema multiforme

SPECIAL TESTS
• Skin testing (useful in IgE mediated reactions)
• IgG and IgM: hemagglutination assays can detect drug-specific antibodies, but not routinely useful

IMAGING N/A

DIAGNOSTIC PROCEDURES
• Detailed drug-use history including all OTC medicines, duration of therapy, medications used within the last four weeks
• Withdrawal of suspected offending agent and observation for resolution of rash
• Selective special testing for suspected IgE mediated reactions

TREATMENT

APPROPRIATE HEALTH CARE
• Urticaria, angioedema, or bullous lesions are all potentially more serious than other types of reactions therefore these patients should be seen as soon as possible for evaluation
• Consider inpatient treatment for anaphylactic reactions, Stevens-Johnson syndrome, extensive bullous reactions, or toxic epidermal (TEN) necrolysis

GENERAL MEASURES
• Discontinue suspected offending agent. In patients with multiple medications, the decision to discontinue each medication should be based on the likelihood of each individual medication causing the reaction (e.g., 7% for penicillins, sulfonamides) and the risk/benefit ratio of continuing each medication.
• Re-challenge with specific medications thought to have caused urticaria, angioedema, anaphylaxis, erythema multiforme, or other bullous lesions is potentially dangerous

SURGICAL MEASURES N/A

ACTIVITY
• No specific restrictions in general
• For acute eczematous or urticarial reactions with intense pruritus, tepid bathing and avoidance of activities resulting in perspiration may be helpful
• For toxic epidermal necrolysis, admit to burn unit

DIET No dietary restrictions

PATIENT EDUCATION Printed patient information is available from American Academy of Dermatology, 930 N. Meacham Rd., P.O. Box 4014, Schaumberg, IL 60168-4014; (708)330-0230

MEDICATIONS

DRUG(S) OF CHOICE
• Specific therapy depends on the type of drug eruption. Most require no specific therapy.
• Symptomatic therapy helpful for pruritus, xeroses, urticaria and angioedema
• For pruritus - antihistamines, e.g., diphenhydramine (Benadryl) 25-50 mg q6h, hydroxyzine (Atarax) 10-25 mg q6-8h)
• Anaphylaxis or widespread urticaria - epinephrine 1:1000, 0.01 mL per kilogram (0.3 mL maximum) subcutaneous
• For anaphylaxis, severe urticaria, erythema multiforme - corticosteroids parenterally as indicated by patient's condition; or on tapering po schedule (10-14 days). Therapy of toxic epidermal necrolysis controversial; majority do not favor use of systemic corticosteroids.
• Topical lubricants, emollients for eczematous reactions
• Topical corticosteroids (Group I-III) for limited eczematous type eruptions, or for lichenoid eruptions
• Systemic corticosteroids (for urticaria, angioedema, and anaphylaxis) - prednisone 40-60 mg/d for 5-10 days. Also useful in severe diffuse eczematous reactions.
Contraindications: Refer to manufacturer's information
Precautions: Refer to manufacturer's information
Significant possible interactions: Refer to manufacturer's information

ALTERNATIVE DRUGS N/A

FOLLOWUP

PATIENT MONITORING
• For urticarial, bullous, or erythema multiforme-like lesions, close patient followup is indicated to insure there is no progression
• Patients with systemic anaphylaxis or wide spread bullous lesions, including toxic epidermal necrolysis, should be admitted to hospital until condition improves
• Maintain at least telephone follow-up until eruption has completely cleared
• Label patient's chart with the suspected agent and the specific type of reaction

PREVENTION/AVOIDANCE
• Future avoidance of specific drugs and any analogs
• Be aware of any potential cross over reactions (i.e., 8-10% incidents of reactions of cephalosporins in patient's sensitized to penicillins and the cross-over for the anticonvulsive drugs hydantoin, barbiturates, and carbamazepine [Tegretol])
• Always question patient's about prior drug reactions, specific type of reaction, and use of OTC medicines

EXPECTED COURSE/PROGNOSIS
• Eruptions generally fade within days after removing offending agent
• Urticaria, angioedema, bullous reactions, are potentially more serious, even life-threatening

POSSIBLE COMPLICATIONS
• Anaphylaxis
• Laryngeal edema
• Possible associated bone marrow suppression
• Possible cross reaction to chemically similar agents with future exposure

MISCELLANEOUS

ASSOCIATED CONDITIONS N/A

AGE-RELATED FACTORS
Pediatric: May occur in this age group
Geriatric:
• Possibly more likely in this age group due to greater number of medications
• Severe systemic reactions less well tolerated
Others: N/A

PREGNANCY N/A

SYNONYMS
• Drug eruptions
• Dermatitis medicamentosa

ICD-9-CM
693.0

SEE ALSO N/A

OTHER NOTES N/A

ABBREVIATIONS
TEN = toxic epidermal necrolysis

REFERENCES
• Habif T: Clinical Dermatology. 3rd Ed. St. Louis, CV Mosby, 1996
• Fitzpatrick TB, et al, eds: Dermatology in General Medicine. 4th Ed. New York, McGraw-Hill, 1993
• Rovjeau JC, Stern RS: Severe adverse cutaneous reactions to drugs. New Engl J Med 1994;331:1272-1285
• Shiohara T: What is new in fixed drug eruption? Dermatol 1995;191:185-187
• Breathnach SM: Mechanisms of drug eruptions. Australian J of Dermatol 1995;36(3):121-127
• Stern RS, Steinberg LA: Epidemiology of adverse cutaneous reactions to drugs. Dermatol Clin 1995;13(3):681-688
• Mathelier-Fusade P, Leynadier F: The management of adverse drug reactions. Clin Reviews in Allergy and Immunology 1995;13(3):281-290
Illustrations: 37 available on CD-ROM
Internet references: http://www.5mcc.com

Author(s)
J. Randall Richard, MD

Cutaneous squamous cell carcinoma

BASICS

DESCRIPTION Malignant epithelial tumor arising from keratinocytes
System(s) affected: Skin/Exocrine
Genetics: N/A
Incidence/Prevalence in USA: Varies within geographic U.S. 32.3/100,000 for Caucasian males; 14.3/100,000 for Caucasian females
Predominant age: Elderly population
Predominant sex: Male > Female

SIGNS AND SYMPTOMS
• Occurs most commonly in chronically sun-exposed areas in light-skinned people e.g., scalp, neck, upper extremities, back of hands, superior surface of pinna
• Often develops in previously damaged skin, e.g., solar keratoses, actinic cheilitis
• In African Americans - equal frequency in sun-exposed and unexposed
• Tumors present often as small, firm nodules with indistinct margins or as plaques
• Surface may be smooth, verrucous or papillomatous
• Varying degrees of ulceration, erosion, crust, scale
• Color often red to red-brown to tan
• May appear white in areas of moisture
• May arise in chronic skin ulcers, e.g., venous stasis ulcers
• May arise in scars
• Can arise in skin damaged by radiation, x-rays, etc.
• Varies from slowly growing, locally invasive to aggressive tumor with propensity to metastasis
• On lip, often arises in patch of leukoplakia

CAUSES
• Exact mechanism not established, epidemiologic and experimental evidence suggests the following as causative agents
• Sunlight (solar radiation)
• Radiation exposure
• Inorganic arsenic exposure
• Exposure to coal tar, other oil and tar derivatives
• Immunosuppression by medications or disease

RISK FACTORS
• Older age
• Male
• Outdoor actinic exposure
• Irish-Scottish-British descent
• Fair complexion, fair hair
• Light blue or green eyes
• Poor tanning ability with tendency to burn

DIAGNOSIS

DIFFERENTIAL DIAGNOSIS
Keratoacanthoma, basal cell carcinoma, actinic keratosis, malignant melanoma

LABORATORY Requires biopsy for precise pathologic diagnosis
Drugs that may alter lab results: N/A
Disorders that may alter lab results: N/A

PATHOLOGICAL FINDINGS Abnormal epithelial cells extending into the dermis from the epidermis. Varying degrees of atypical appearance can be noted.

SPECIAL TESTS N/A

IMAGING N/A

DIAGNOSTIC PROCEDURES Surgical biopsy mandatory to ensure proper and precise diagnosis

TREATMENT

APPROPRIATE HEALTH CARE All outpatient unless extensive lesion

GENERAL MEASURES N/A

SURGICAL MEASURES
• Excisional surgery - appropriate for almost all squamous cell lesions
• Electrodesiccation and curettage - used for small lesions (generally < 1.0 cm) on flat surfaces, e.g., forehead, cheek. Requires training and expertise in electrosurgery.
• Indications for Moh's chemosurgery include: Recurrent tumor; larger, ill-defined lesions; presence of bone or cartilage invasion; multiple carcinomas; lesion in area of late radiation change. Requires referral to appropriately trained dermatologic surgeon.
• Radiation therapy - suitable for larger advanced lesions. Requires specialized training.

ACTIVITY Full activity

DIET No restrictions

PATIENT EDUCATION
• Instruct patient in skin self exam
• Appropriate sun avoidance measures, e.g., sunscreens, protective clothing
• Patient education materials available from American Cancer Society

MEDICATIONS

DRUG(S) OF CHOICE N/A
Contraindications: N/A
Precautions: N/A
Significant possible interactions: N/A

ALTERNATIVE DRUGS N/A

FOLLOWUP

PATIENT MONITORING After therapy, skin exam every month for 3 months, 6 months post-treatment, then yearly

PREVENTION/AVOIDANCE
• Sun-avoidance measures - sunscreens, hats, etc.
• Avoid contact with known carcinogenic compounds

POSSIBLE COMPLICATIONS
• Recurrence locally
• Metastatic disease

EXPECTED COURSE/PROGNOSIS
• About 90-95% cure rate with appropriate treatment
• Lesion equal to or greater than 2 cm more prone to recur
• Head and neck lesions have better prognosis

MISCELLANEOUS

ASSOCIATED CONDITIONS
• Xeroderma pigmentosum
• Albinism
• Chronic skin ulcers of the leg
• Chronic thermal burns
• Actinic keratosis (cutaneous horn)
• Bowen's disease

AGE-RELATED FACTORS
Pediatric: N/A
Geriatric: N/A
Others: N/A

PREGNANCY N/A

SYNONYMS
• Squamous cell carcinoma of the skin
• Epidermoid carcinoma
• Prickle cell carcinoma

ICD-9-CM
Code varies with location
173.3 (face)
173.4 (scalp, neck)
173.5 (trunk)
173.6 (upper limb)
173.7 (lower limb)
173.9 (site unspecified)

SEE ALSO N/A

OTHER NOTES N/A

ABBREVIATIONS N/A

REFERENCES
• Fitzpatrick TN, et al: Dermatology in General Medicine. New York, McGraw-Hill Book Company, 1987
• Friedman RJ, et al: Cancer of the Skin. Philadelphia, WB Saunders Co, 1991
Illustrations: 4 available on CD-ROM
Internet references: http://www.5mcc.com

Author(s)
John M. Little, MD

Cutaneous T cell lymphoma

BASICS

DESCRIPTION Cutaneous T cell lymphoma (mycosis fungoides) is an uncommon chronic lymphoma characterized by a malignant proliferation of T helper cells in the skin. In the late stage, the lymph nodes and viscera are affected.
Genetics: Evidence suggests increased frequency of HLA antigens Aw31 and Aw32
System(s) affected: Skin/Exocrine, Hemic/Lymphatic/Immunologic
Incidence/Prevalence in USA: 0.29 cases per 100,000 per year
Predominant age: Most cases occur in fifth and sixth decades, incidence increases with age
Predominant sex: Male > Female

SIGNS AND SYMPTOMS
- Skin eruption
  ◊ Patches (eczema-like rash)
  ◊ Plaques
  ◊ Tumors
  ◊ Pruritus
  ◊ Exfoliative erythroderma
  ◊ Ulcers of the skin
  ◊ Lymphadenopathy
  ◊ Hepatomegaly (late)
  ◊ Splenomegaly (late)

CAUSES   Unknown

RISK FACTORS
- HTLV-I
- Exposure to petrochemicals, metals and solvents
- Association with lymphomatoid papulosis

DIAGNOSIS

DIFFERENTIAL DIAGNOSIS
- Patches:
  ◊ Parapsoriasis
  ◊ Atopic eczema
  ◊ Nummular eczema
- Plaques:
  ◊ Parapsoriasis
  ◊ Psoriasis
- Tumors:
  ◊ Other primary skin cancers
  ◊ Internal malignancies metastatic to skin
- Exfoliative erythroderma:
  ◊ Psoriasis
  ◊ Atopic dermatitis
  ◊ Drug eruption

LABORATORY
- CBC with differential and platelets
- Total lymphocyte count
- Automated chemical profile
Drugs that may alter lab results: N/A
Disorders that may alter lab results: N/A

PATHOLOGICAL FINDINGS
- Skin biopsy:
  ◊ Epidermotropism of lymphocytes
  ◊ Pautrier's microabscesses of lymphocytes
  ◊ Widened, fibrotic papillary dermis
  ◊ Superficial band-like dermal infiltrate
  ◊ Occasionally granulomatous component

SPECIAL TESTS
- Sézary's cell preparation
- Electron microscopy
- HTLV-I serology
- Enzyme histochemistry
- DNA flow cytometry
- Immunophenotyping
- Immunogenotyping
- Molecular cytogenetics
- Polymerase chain reaction

IMAGING
- Chest x-ray
- CT scan of abdomen

DIAGNOSTIC PROCEDURES
- Skin biopsy - diagnostic procedure of choice
- Lymph node biopsy
- Bone marrow biopsy
- Liver biopsy

TREATMENT

APPROPRIATE HEALTH CARE The majority of patients can be managed on an outpatient basis

GENERAL MEASURES
- No disease-specific special measures
- Treatment should be individualized for each patient as in most cases this is a chronic slowly progressive disease

SURGICAL MEASURES   N/A

ACTIVITY   Fully active

DIET   No special diet

PATIENT EDUCATION   By physician on individual basis

MEDICATIONS

DRUG(S) OF CHOICE
• Therapy must be individualized. There is no universally accepted standard approach to treatment of this disease. The extent and the rapidity of progression of the disease dictates the aggressiveness of therapy.
• For early and less aggressive disease:
 ◊ Topical mechlorethamine (nitrogen mustard, Mustargen)
 ◊ PUVA or REPUVA (retinoids plus PUVA)
 ◊ Topical carmustine (BCNU)
• For more resistant disease:
 ◊ Electron beam therapy
 ◊ Combination therapy - interferon or retinoids plus phototherapy (UVA or UVB)
 ◊ Methotrexate
 ◊ Extracorporeal photochemotherapy (especially Sézary syndrome)
• For advanced and resistant disease:
 ◊ Systemic chemotherapy
 ◊ Interleukin-2
• Topical nitrogen mustard (Mustargen) (for early disease) in aqueous or ointment preparation applied once daily to entire skin surface avoiding genitalia
Contraindications: See manufacturer's profile of each drug
Precautions:
• Delayed hypersensitivity occurs in 50%
• Radiomimetic - patients should practice prudent sun avoidance
• Maintenance treatment required after clearing
Significant possible interactions: See manufacturer's profile of each drug

ALTERNATIVE DRUGS
• PUVA (psoralen and ultraviolet A light)
• Topical carmustine (BCNU)
• Total body electron beam therapy
• Localized orthovoltage x-ray therapy
• Interferon
• Retinoids (e.g., etretinate)
• Extracorporeal photochemotherapy
• Systemic chemotherapy

FOLLOWUP

PATIENT MONITORING Must be individualized

PREVENTION/AVOIDANCE N/A

POSSIBLE COMPLICATIONS Metastatic spread to organs other than skin

EXPECTED COURSE/PROGNOSIS
• The development of lymphadenopathy, tumors or cutaneous ulcerations during the course of the disease is associated with a median survival of 4 years
• The appearance of the third sign (irrespective of the order developed) is associated with a median survival of 1 year

MISCELLANEOUS

ASSOCIATED CONDITIONS N/A

AGE-RELATED FACTORS
Pediatric: N/A
Geriatric: N/A
Others: N/A

PREGNANCY N/A

SYNONYMS
• Mycosis fungoides
• Sézary's syndrome

ICD-9-CM
202.8 Other lymphomas

SEE ALSO
• HIV infection & AIDS

OTHER NOTES Sézary's syndrome is the leukemic variant of cutaneous T cell lymphoma. Characteristics include erythroderma, pruritus, adenopathy and circulating atypical cells with cerebriform nuclei.

ABBREVIATIONS
HTLV = Human T-lymphotropic virus

REFERENCES
• Edelson RL: J. Am Acad Derm 1980;2:89-106
• Braverman IM: Curr Prob Derm 1991;3 (6):184-227
Illustrations: 6 available on CD-ROM
Internet references: http://www.5mcc.com

Author(s)
Vera Y. Soong, MD

Cystic fibrosis

 BASICS

DESCRIPTION Generalized, autosomal recessive disorder of infants, children and young adults with widespread dysfunction of the exocrine glands. Characteristics include chronic pulmonary disease, pancreatic insufficiency, abnormally high levels of electrolytes in the sweat and less frequently biliary cirrhosis, diabetes mellitus.
System(s) affected: Pulmonary, Gastrointestinal, Endocrine/Metabolic, Reproductive
Genetics: Autosomal recessive, gene on chromosome 7. Linkage detection in families with known disease. Probes for direct detection available.
Incidence/Prevalence: The most common lethal genetic disease. Caucasians: 1 in 2000 births, lower in African-Americans, Native Americans and Asian ancestry.
Incidence in USA: In 1992 - 20/333.
Predominant age: Infants, children and young adults (oldest patient at time of diagnosis was 65)
Predominant sex: Male = Female

SIGNS AND SYMPTOMS
• Sweat gland secretions:
  ◊ Increased concentrations of sodium and chloride leading to hyponatremia, hypochloremia, arrhythmias
  ◊ Dehydration with heat and infections
• Respiratory:
  ◊ Wheezing
  ◊ Chronic cough
  ◊ Dyspnea
  ◊ Tachypnea
  ◊ Barrel chest
  ◊ Cyanosis
  ◊ Recurrent bronchitis and pneumonia leading to bronchiectasis
  ◊ Predominant flora - Staphylococcus aureus and Pseudomonas aeruginosa
  ◊ Digital clubbing
  ◊ Nasal polyposis
• Gastrointestinal:
  ◊ Meconium ileus
  ◊ Failure to thrive
  ◊ Distal intestinal obstruction syndrome (DIOS)
  ◊ Colonic strictures possible with high-dose enzyme replacement (>10,000 U lipase /kg/day)
  ◊ Chronic, recurrent abdominal pain
  ◊ Gastroesophageal reflux
  ◊ Voracious appetite prior to treatment
  ◊ Abdominal distension
  ◊ Hypoelectrolytemia and alkalosis
  ◊ Characteristically frequent, bulky, foul - smelling, pale stool with a high fat content
  ◊ Vitamin deficiencies (A,D,E,K)
  ◊ Rectal prolapse
• Others:
  ◊ Delayed weight gain during growth and development
  ◊ Retarded bone growth
  ◊ Delayed sexual development
  ◊ Males infertile

CAUSES Autosomal recessive genetic defect

RISK FACTORS Positive family history (rarely seen due to recessive nature)

 DIAGNOSIS

DIFFERENTIAL DIAGNOSIS
• Immunodeficiency
• Recurrent pneumonias
• Bronchiectasis
• Infertility
• Dyskinetic cilia
• Asthma

LABORATORY
• Elevation of sodium and chloride concentrations in sweat (quantitative pilocarpine iontophoresis sweat test)
• Genetic screening if sweat test inadequate (see Special Tests below)
• Stool trypsin and chymotrypsin absent or diminished
• 72 hour fecal fat excretion - increased fat in stool
• Decreased albumin, fat soluble vitamins
• CF gene screen (reference lab)
• Pseudomonas in respiratory secretions
Drugs that may alter lab results: N/A
Disorders that may alter lab results:
• Edema
• Hypoproteinemia
• Inadequate quantities of sweat to study

PATHOLOGICAL FINDINGS
• Lungs (major problem) - chronic inflammation, inspissated mucus, bronchiectasis with areas of fibrosis and atelectasis
• Pancreas - obstructed ducts, acini replaced by fibrotic tissue, cysts, amorphous eosinophilic concretions and thick mucus
• Liver - secretions obstruct biliary ducts; focal biliary cirrhosis
• Intestine - hypertrophied mucous glands
• Males - hypoplasia or atrophy of vas deferens

SPECIAL TESTS
• Pulmonary function studies (2-3 times a year)
• Sputum culture and sensitivity
• Exercise testing
• Response to bronchodilators - may show paradoxical drop
• In newborns - serum concentration of immunoreactive trypsin reported to be elevated and used as a means of newborn screening. Radioimmuno assay developed for use with dried blood spots that are routinely collected for newborn metabolic screening.
• Genetic testing to identify patient defect and analyze family for carrier status or prenatal diagnosis
• Echocardiogram

IMAGING Chest x-ray - hyperaeration, hilar adenopathy, occasional pneumothorax, bronchiectasis, blebs, increased involvement in right upper lobe

DIAGNOSTIC PROCEDURES Diagnosis made in presence of clinical symptoms and positive sweat test, gene screen

 TREATMENT

APPROPRIATE HEALTH CARE
• Outpatient usually
• Inpatient during infections or other crisis
• Homecare for IV antibiotics

GENERAL MEASURES
• Care by experienced physician and team (respiratory therapist, nurse, nutritionist, physical therapist, counsellor, social worker)
• Goals are to prevent and treat respiratory failure and pulmonary complications
• Postural drainage and chest physiotherapy - adjuncts include flutter valve and CPT vest (expensive)
• Pancreatic enzyme replacement
• Regular exercises for fitness
• Press for adequate growth through good nutrition - supplements may be needed
• Aerosol B2 agonists
• Antibiotics
• DNase - newly approved aerosolized mucolytic
• Oxygen therapy when needed
• Barium enemas or surgery for unrelieved meconium ileus (newborn)
• For fecal accumulation and intussusception in adults - enemas of diatrizoate sodium or Golytely per NG
• Insulin, if diabetes develops

SURGICAL MEASURES
• Surgery may be indicated for some complications
• Organ transplants possible for lung, liver, endocrine pancreas

ACTIVITY Physical conditioning to the extent possible for cardiorespiratory fitness (does not improve pulmonary function)

DIET
• Allow liberal salting of foods per patient preference
• High protein
• High calories (1.5 x recommended for general population)
• High fat (previously not recommended)
• Vitamin supplements (double RDA)

PATIENT EDUCATION Written information and support: Cystic Fibrosis Foundation, 6931 Arlington Road, Ste. 2000, Bethesda, MD 20814, (800)344-4823

Cystic fibrosis

MEDICATIONS

DRUG(S) OF CHOICE
• Oral antibiotics
◊ Cephalexin for Staphlococcal prophylaxis in infants not found to be indicated
◊ Ciprofloxacin for exacerbations; cautious use if < 10 years old
• Aerosolized antibiotics
◊ Tobramycin 80 mg tid. Higher doses being studied.
• IV antibiotics
◊ According to culture and sensitivity studies when ill with respiratory infections
◊ For pseudomonas infections - IV tobramycin, start with 10 mg/kg/24 hrs; peak 8-12 µg/mL (17-26 µmol/L); trough 1-2 µg/mL (2-4 µmol/L) plus IV ceftazidime or antipseudomonas penicillin.
◊ For staphylococcal infections - IV cephalothin (Keflin), other cephalosporin, based on sensitivity
• Other therapies
◊ Pancreatic enzyme replacements - dose 1500 units lipase/kg/meal. Distal colonic strictures possible with high doses.
◊ Bronchodilators, if response demonstrated
◊ Dornase alfa (DNase) nebulized daily
◊ Ibuprofen, regular use, may retard lung disease, but levels must be monitored
◊ Oxygen therapy for severe pulmonary insufficiency or hypoxemia
◊ Occasional assisted ventilation, controversial
◊ IPPB contraindicated
◊ Routine administration of annual influenza vaccine
Contraindications: Refer to manufacturer's literature
Precautions: Refer to manufacturer's literature. Higher dosages for shorter administration intervals usually required.
Significant possible interactions: Refer to manufacturer's literature

ALTERNATIVE DRUGS Other antipseudomonal antibiotic

FOLLOWUP

PATIENT MONITORING At least 3 times a year; cystic fibrosis center recommended

PREVENTION/AVOIDANCE
• In prenatal situations
◊ Genetic counseling
◊ Prenatal diagnosis for future pregnancies
• For complications
◊ For respiratory infections - maintain pertussis and measles immunity; annual influenza immunization
◊ Avoid general anesthetics. Consider epidural, spinal, or local.
◊ Good medical teamwork in the management of the multifaceted problems of the disease

POSSIBLE COMPLICATIONS
• Atelectasis
• Pneumothorax
• Hemoptysis
• Right heart failure
• Pulmonary hypertension
• Pulmonary emphysema
• Digital clubbing
• Hypertrophic pulmonary osteoarthropathy
• Diabetes
• Metabolic alkalosis
• Volume depletion
• Bleeding esophageal varices
• Symptomatic biliary cirrhosis
• Intestinal obstruction
• Females anovulatory (fertility rate about 80%)
• Numerous psychosocial aspects
• Malnutrition
• Retarded growth

EXPECTED COURSE/PROGNOSIS
• Largely dependent on pulmonary involvement
• Prognosis improving due to early detection and aggressive treatment
• Median survival is to age 29

MISCELLANEOUS

ASSOCIATED CONDITIONS See Complications

AGE-RELATED FACTORS
Pediatric: Diagnosis usually confirmed in infancy or early childhood but some go undetected until adolescence. Newborn screening methods are in development. Psychosocial considerations
Geriatric: N/A
Others: N/A

PREGNANCY If cystic fibrosis patient's condition (pulmonary and nutrition) good at start of pregnancy, usually returns to that level following birth. If these conditions are compromised before pregnancy, they may deteriorate following birth.

SYNONYMS
• CF

ICD-9-CM
277.0 Cystic fibrosis

SEE ALSO
• Bronchiectasis
• Asthma

OTHER NOTES
• Advise genetic counseling for at-risk individuals
• Encoded protein on long arm of chromosome 7 contains 1480 amino acids
• Multiple types of gene defects are possible (>500 defined)

ABBREVIATIONS
CF = cystic fibrosis
IPPB = intermittent positive pressure breathing

REFERENCES
• Tizzano F, Buchwald M: Cystic fibrosis: Beyond the gene to therapy. Jour of Pediatrics 1992;120;337-343
• Tizzano F, Buchwald M: Recent advances in cystic fibrosis research. Jour of Pediatrics 1993;122:985-988
• Schidlow DV, Taussig LM, Knowles MR: Cystic Fibrosis Foundation Conference Report on Pulmonary Complications of Cystic Fibrosis; Pediatric Pulmonology 1993;15:187-198
• Taussig LM: Cystic Fibrosis. New York, Thieme-Stratton Inc., 1984
Illustrations: N/A
Internet references: http://www.5mcc.com

Author(s)
Nancy N. Dambro, MD

Cytomegalovirus inclusion disease

BASICS

DESCRIPTION Infection with cytomegalovirus, a DNA virus belonging to the herpes family. All cytomegaloviruses have a propensity for remaining latent in humans. They cannot be propagated in laboratory animals or in most cell cultures.
• The disease occurs world-wide and may be transferred in several ways, including by human contact. Approximately four out of five people over age 35 have been infected with cytomegalovirus, usually during childhood or early adulthood. In most of these, the disease is mild and overlooked.
• CMV infection during pregnancy can be hazardous to the fetus and may lead to stillbirth, brain damage, birth defects or to severe neonatal illness
• The name derives from the infected cells that are large and bear intranuclear inclusions
• Infection may be in almost any organ, but the salivary glands are the most common site in children and the lungs in adults. This infection can occur congenitally, postnatally, or at any age
• Categories of CMV infections include:
  ◊ Congenital: These infections vary greatly from cytomegaloviremia in a normal infant to the cause of abortion, stillbirth, postnatal death from hemorrhage, anemia, liver or CNS damage.
  ◊ Acute infection in a normal host
  ◊ Infections in bone marrow transplant patients - usually pneumonia
  ◊ Infection in patients with AIDS - usually retinitis
  ◊ Infections in other immunocompromised patients - pulmonary, gastrointestinal, or renal disease
System(s) affected: Pulmonary, Skin/Exocrine, Nervous
Genetics: May be passed from mother to fetus
Incidence/Prevalence in USA:
• Common, but frequently asymptomatic
• Up to 90% of adults have been infected, almost all with inapparent disease. Infection seems to be more common in homosexual males.
Predominant age: All ages, peaks at < 3 months; 16-40 years, and 40-75 years
Predominant sex: Male > Female

SIGNS AND SYMPTOMS
• Congenital:
  ◊ Abortion
  ◊ Asymptomatic cytomegaloviremia
  ◊ Hemorrhage
  ◊ Anemia
  ◊ Jaundice
  ◊ Signs of CNS damage
• Acquired:
(Acute infection in a normal or immunocompromised host)
  ◊ May be asymptomatic
  ◊ Fatigue
  ◊ Nausea
  ◊ Vomiting
  ◊ Bone pain
  ◊ Chills
  ◊ Fever
  ◊ Diarrhea
  ◊ Jaundice
  ◊ Hepatomegaly
  ◊ Splenomegaly
  ◊ Dyspnea
• Infections in bone marrow transplant patients:
  ◊ Pneumonitis with cough, fever, chills, chest pain
• Infections in AIDS patients:
  ◊ Retinitis
  ◊ Esophageal, gastric, small bowel and colonic ulcerations
  ◊ Pneumonitis

CAUSES
• Infection with cytomegalovirus
• Reactivation of a latent process in patients who are immunosuppressed

RISK FACTORS
• HIV infection
• AIDS
• Organ transplantation (50% attack rate, depending on serologic status)
• Blood transfusion. A postperfusion syndrome may develop in 2 to 4 weeks in patients having fresh blood transfusions. Characteristics include fever lasting 2 to 3 weeks, hepatitis, with or without jaundice, atypical lymphocytosis similar to that of infectious mononucleosis, and a skin rash.
• Immunocompromised host
• Living in closed population
• Corticosteroid therapy
• Day care environment - infant or geriatric
• For congenital infection - maternal infection during pregnancy

DIAGNOSIS

DIFFERENTIAL DIAGNOSIS
• Congenital: Bacterial, viral, and protozoan infections, such as toxoplasmosis, rubella, syphilis
• Acquired: Viral hepatitis, infectious mononucleosis

LABORATORY
• Human fibroblastic cell culture inoculation may isolate the virus from urine, blood, other body fluids, or tissues
• Leukopenia
• Thrombocytopenia
• Increased lymphocytes
• Demonstration of CMV in secretions or tissues by immunofluorescence with commercially available monoclonal antibodies or by in situ hybridization
Drugs that may alter lab results: N/A
Disorders that may alter lab results: N/A

PATHOLOGICAL FINDINGS Giant cells with basophilic inclusion bodies

SPECIAL TESTS
• Human fibroblastic tissue cultures to isolate the virus
• Immunofluorescence techniques for virus demonstrations

IMAGING Skull film - intracranial calcifications

DIAGNOSTIC PROCEDURES
• Bronchoscopy in bone marrow transplant patients if suspicious of CMV pneumonia
• Buffy coat culture
• Endoscopic biopsy of gastrointestinal tract

TREATMENT

APPROPRIATE HEALTH CARE Inpatient for disseminated infection or CMV reactivation syndrome

GENERAL MEASURES Isolation

SURGICAL MEASURES N/A

ACTIVITY Bedrest

DIET No special diet

PATIENT EDUCATION N/A

MEDICATIONS

DRUG(S) OF CHOICE
• Cytomegalovirus immune globulin
• Antivirals, such as ganciclovir, relatively resistant to acyclovir. New oral agent with a limited role - famciclovir.
Contraindications: Refer to manufacturer's literature
Precautions: Refer to manufacturer's literature
Significant possible interactions: Refer to manufacturer's literature

ALTERNATIVE DRUGS N/A

FOLLOWUP

PATIENT MONITORING   Close followup in ICU (isolated) during infection with disseminated form

PREVENTION/AVOIDANCE   Avoid immunosuppression (when possible)

POSSIBLE COMPLICATIONS
• Chorioretinitis
• Encephalitis
• Mononucleosis
• Colitis
• Deafness
• Mental retardation

EXPECTED COURSE/PROGNOSIS
Disseminated form often fatal

MISCELLANEOUS

ASSOCIATED CONDITIONS
• Acquired immune deficiency syndrome (AIDS)
• Corticosteroid therapy
• Leukemia
• Lymphoma

AGE-RELATED FACTORS
Pediatric: May occur congenitally or postnatally
Geriatric: N/A
Others: N/A

PREGNANCY N/A

SYNONYMS
• Giant cell inclusion disease
• CID
• CMV
• Salivary gland virus disease

ICD-9-CM
078.5 Cytomegaloviral disease

SEE ALSO N/A

OTHER NOTES N/A

ABBREVIATIONS N/A

REFERENCES
• Mandell GL, ed: Principles and Practice of Infectious Diseases. 4th Ed. New York, Churchill Livingstone, 1995
• Onorato IM, et al: Epidemiology of Cytomegaloviral Infection: Recommendations for Prevention & Control. Rev Infect Dis 1985;7:479
• Cohen JI, Corey GR: Cytomegalovirus Infection in the Normal Host. Medicine 1985;64:100-114
Illustrations: 1 available on CD-ROM
Internet references: http://www.5mcc.com

Author(s)
Vance D. Rodgers, MD

Decompression sickness

BASICS

DESCRIPTION Metastatic dissolution of gas bubbles (usually nitrogen) into tissues caused by a relatively rapid decrease in the environmental pressure. Five types based on symptomatology:
• Limb bends - gas deposition in tissues causes a poorly-localized "pain-only" syndrome; may herald more serious disease.
• Cerebral bends - stroke-like picture due to paradoxical arterial gas embolism (via A-V or intracardiac shunt), denovo arterial gas formation, and/or cerebral edema.
• Spinal cord bends - transverse paresis caused by retrograde venous thrombosis with patchy necrosis and edema of the spinal cord; predilection for high lumbar nerve roots due to lack of collateral circulation.
• Inner ear bends - development of bubble formation and hemorrhage in labyrinthine fluid spaces and vasculature.
• Lung bends ("chokes") - excessive venous bubbles develop and release vasoactive substances causing pulmonary irritation and bronchoconstriction. The primary symptoms are substernal chest pain (worse with inspiration), dyspnea, and cough.
System(s) affected: Cardiovascular, Nervous, Musculoskeletal, Pulmonary
Genetics: N/A
Incidence/Prevalence in USA:
Uncommon, even in high-density diving areas and areas of caisson work
Predominant age: 20-29
Predominant sex: 95% males, although there is no evidence to suggest increased susceptibility based on sex.

SIGNS AND SYMPTOMS
• 95% present in 3-4 hours, but may be delayed for 24 hours or more
• Burning blebs (skin bends)
• Painful pruritic red rash ("cutis marmorata")
• Vague, poorly localized pain
• Headache
• Ataxia
• Delirium
• Coma
• Convulsions
• Confusion
• Patchy numbness
• Respiratory "chokes" in 2%
• Coughing paroxysm's (Behnke's sign)
• Arrhythmia
• Bradycardia or tachycardia
• Hypotension
• Tachypnea
• Subcutaneous emphysema along tendon sheaths (rare)
• Rapidly ascending paraplegia

CAUSES
• Rapid ascent from scuba diving (depth > 33 feet)
• Rapid ascent/decompression in an airplane
• Tunnel work = caisson disease
• Inadequate pressurization/denitrogenation when flying
• Flying to high altitude too soon after scuba diving

RISK FACTORS
• Prolonged dive at depth over 33 feet
• Obesity
• Multiple, repetitive scuba dives
• Cold water diving
• Poor physical conditioning
• Vigorous physical activity
• Dehydration
• Local injury
• Patent foramen ovale (for neurologic symptoms)

DIAGNOSIS

DIFFERENTIAL DIAGNOSIS
• Arterial gas embolism
• Traumatic injury to extremity
• Cerebrovascular accident
• Musculoskeletal strains
• Urticaria
• Malingering

LABORATORY
• ABGs - may show decreased pO_2, decreased pCO_2, and metabolic acidosis.
• CBC - increased hematocrit in severe cases due to dehydration. Thrombocytopenia.
• Coagulation tests - may see increased fibrin split products and increased prothrombin time
Drugs that may alter lab results: N/A
Disorders that may alter lab results: N/A

PATHOLOGICAL FINDINGS
• Skin lesions: painful, pruritic, blotchy red rash on torso, burning blebs on skin, lymphedema
• Joints: erythema and edema on the periarticular surfaces

SPECIAL TESTS EEG - irregular slowing with cerebral bends

IMAGING
• Chest x-ray - pneumothorax, mediastinal emphysema; +/- right heart enlargement. Plain x-ray or ultrasound - gas bubbles in joints, tendons, bursae muscles.
• CT scan - should be performed on all patients with history of trauma or neurologic signs

DIAGNOSTIC PROCEDURES "Test of pressure" = trial of recompression to 2.8 ATA/100% oxygen/10'

TREATMENT

APPROPRIATE HEALTH CARE Referral through Divers' Alert Network [DAN (919)684-8111] to nearest hyperbaric facility for recompression test. The specific treatment may vary from institution to institution, but is based on the procedures first established in the Armed Services (e.g., US Navy Table 6). Patients may be sent home when cutaneous symptoms only are present, if the appropriate response to therapy is observed in the emergency department.

GENERAL MEASURES
• 100% oxygen via tight nonbreathing mask
• Fluid resuscitation (avoid D5W or hypotonic IV solutions with cord injury). Despite the theoretical advantages of volume expanders (dextran, albumin, etc.), no experimental or clinical studies support their use since they are not without risk.
• Rapid referral to hyperbaric chamber facility
• Position recumbent or Trendelenburg (for cerebral symptoms)
• Transport via ground, low-altitude airplane, or aircraft pressurized to sea level

SURGICAL MEASURES N/A

ACTIVITY Bedrest when neurologic involvement present

DIET As tolerated

PATIENT EDUCATION Anyone who desires to perform scuba diving should be certified by an appropriate diving agency: NAUI, PADI, SSI, or YMCA. Sport divers who have not been diving for > 6 months should review diving principles/skills via a refresher course.

MEDICATIONS

DRUG(S) OF CHOICE 100% oxygen; diazepam 5-15 mg IV (IM absorption unpredictable) for inner ear decompression sickness. Symptoms of vertigo, nausea and vomiting may get significant relief. The use of steroids has been advocated by some for the assumed vasogenic edema seen in decompression sickness. This form of therapy remains controversial and not proven in controlled clinical trials. If steroids are prescribed, they should not be used for more than 4-5 days for neurological symptoms.
Contraindications: Hypersensitivity to benzodiazepines and acute narrow-angle glaucoma
Precautions: Administration of diazepam requires monitoring of the respiratory status, blood pressure and heart rate. Dosage reductions are required in the elderly and patients with hepatic dysfunction.
Significant possible interactions: Benzodiazepines potentiate the effects of other CNS depressants.

ALTERNATIVE DRUGS
• Adjunctive therapy:
  ◊ Digitalization for CHF/tachycardia
  ◊ Aminophylline NOT useful for "chokes"
  ◊ Roles of steroids and heparin not determined

FOLLOWUP

PATIENT MONITORING Symptomatic assessment for relapse/progression which occurs in 25%

PREVENTION/AVOIDANCE
• Follow decompression tables (Navy, NAUI, PADI) for diving to depth (> 33 feet) or use dive computers that calculate nitrogen content of various tissues
• Allow adequate time between diving and flying to altitude (24 hours)

POSSIBLE COMPLICATIONS
• Oxygen toxicity with seizures (infrequent and unpredictable)
• Neurologic sequelae for non-responders
• Long-term risk of aseptic necrosis

EXPECTED COURSE/PROGNOSIS
• Excellent for early symptomatic presentation, referral and treatment
• Related to duration and severity of symptoms prior to treatment
• Although recompression therapy is best administered early as possible, some patients may still benefit even at six to nine days after the incident, referral is critical, even if symptoms resolve, since 25% of patients will relapse

MISCELLANEOUS

ASSOCIATED CONDITIONS N/A

AGE-RELATED FACTORS
Pediatric: N/A
Geriatric: N/A
Others: N/A

PREGNANCY Pregnant patient with decompression sickness a priority as fetus may also be affected; no contraindication to recompression

SYNONYMS
• Bends
• Paretic bends
• Caisson disease

ICD-9-CM
993.3 Caisson disease

SEE ALSO Arterial gas embolism

OTHER NOTES
• The diagnosis may be difficult due to the variable clinical manifestations. The most important clue is recent decompression.
• 71% of nervous system decompression sickness present as skin or limb bends
• Limb bends with musculoskeletal complaints frequently diagnosed as malingering due to vague nature
• Only way to exclude the diagnosis in patient at risk is a negative test of pressure

ABBREVIATIONS
DCS = decompression sickness
NAUI = National Association for Underwater Instructors
PADI = Professional Association for Diving Instructors
SSI = Sport SCUBA Instructors
YMCA = Young Men's Christian Association
ATA = atmospheres absolute

REFERENCES
• Bove A, Davis JC: Diving Medicine. 2nd Ed. Philadelphia, W.B. Saunders Co., 1990
• Catron PW, Flynn ET: Adjuvant drug therapy for decompression sickness: A review. Undersea Biomed Res 1982;9:161-173
Illustrations: N/A
Internet references: http://www.5mcc.com

Author(s)
Jeffrey R. Welko, MD
Darell E. Heiselman, DO, FCCM, FACP, FACC, FCCP

Dementia

BASICS

DESCRIPTION A pathologic process defined as a persistent impairment of a prior level of intellectual functioning
• Dementia of the Alzheimer's type (DAT) is the most common form and characterized by a relentless deterioration of higher cortical functioning. The rate of deterioration is variable.
• Multi-infarct dementia (MID) occurs as a result of clinical or subclinical cerebral infarcts secondary to atherosclerosis. Deterioration is stepwise with periods of clinical plateaus.
• Sub-cortical dementia is accompanied by movement and gait disorders and characterized by psychomotor slowing
• Secondary dementias - also referred to as "reversible dementias" because the cognitive impairment may reverse with treatment of the primary disorder
System(s) affected: Nervous
Genetics:
• At least 15% of patients with DAT will report a positive family history
• Persons with Trisomy 21 (Down syndrome) who survive into their 20's and 30's will inevitably develop a progressive dementia
Incidence/Prevalence in USA:
• 0.5% between ages 60 and 64; 3.2% between ages 80-90
• 1480/100,000
• 1.2 million people in the U.S. have severe dementia and another 2.5 million have moderate illness; 10% of all persons over the age of 65 have clinically important dementia
Predominant age: Increasing incidence with increasing age. Can occur in younger persons secondary to trisomy 21 or AIDS.
Predominant sex: Male = Female

SIGNS AND SYMPTOMS
• Impaired short- and long-term memory
• Impaired abstract thinking
• Impaired judgment
• Aphasia
• Apraxia
• Agnosia
• Anomia
• Personality change, emotional outbursts, wandering, restlessness, hyperactivity
• Sleep disturbances
• Mood disturbances
• Urinary incontinence (usually late in DAT or normal pressure hydrocephalus)
• Fecal incontinence (late)
• Rigidity (especially with subcortical dementias)
• Tremor (especially with subcortical dementias)
• Hallucinations
• Delusions
• Overt paranoid behavior
• Weight loss
• Seizures

CAUSES
• DAT - genetic predisposition in > 15%
• MID - due to cerebral atherosclerosis or emboli with clinical or subclinical infarcts
• Cortical dementias - causes include parkinsonism, progressive supranuclear palsy, and Huntington's disease
• Secondary dementias - causes include hypothyroidism, vitamin B deficiency, normal pressure hydrocephalus, AIDS, syphilis, and various medications. The dementia will be accompanied by the other signs and symptoms characteristic of the primary disorder.

RISK FACTORS
• Increasing age
• Prevalence of atherosclerotic disease (MID)
• Trisomy 21 (Down syndrome)
• History of head trauma
• History of CNS infection

DIAGNOSIS

DIFFERENTIAL DIAGNOSIS
• Delirium
• Normal aging (age-associated memory impairment)
• Depression
• Schizophrenia
• Sensory deprivation states
• Chronic alcoholism
• Heat stroke
• Postsurgical and/or postanesthesia state

LABORATORY
Done primarily to rule out potentially reversible causes
• Thyroid function tests
• Syphilis serology
• Serum B12 and folate
• Complete blood count and screening metabolic profile
Drugs that may alter lab results: Thyroid hormone replacement and iodine preparations may affect thyroid function tests
Disorders that may alter lab results: False positive syphilis serology with acute infections, leprosy, subacute bacterial endocarditis, and autoimmune disorders

PATHOLOGICAL FINDINGS
• DAT - granulovesicular degeneration, neurofibrillary tangles, senile neuritic plaques, microvascular amyloid
• MID - old infarcts, atherosclerotic disease
• Cortical dementia - degeneration of nigrostriatal neurons

SPECIAL TESTS
• Mental status testing
• Neuropsychologic testing
• Electroencephalogram for patients with altered consciousness or associated seizures

IMAGING
• Head computed tomography if history suggestive of a mass, or focal neurologic signs or in patient with dementia of brief duration
• Magnetic resonance imaging (MRI) is more sensitive than computed tomography for detection of soft tissue lesions (small infarcts, mass lesions, atrophy of the brainstem, and other subcortical structures). MRI may also clarify ambiguous computed tomography findings.
• Isotope cisternography if suspicious of normal pressure hydrocephalus
• Positive emission tomography (PET) shows cortical hypometabolism

DIAGNOSTIC PROCEDURES N/A

TREATMENT

APPROPRIATE HEALTH CARE
• Outpatient except when complications warrant hospitalization
• Nursing home - if disease progresses to the point that long-term care becomes necessary

GENERAL MEASURES
• Daily schedules and written directions
• Support and education of caregivers
• Emphasis on nutrition, personal hygiene, personal safety (accident-proofing the home) and supervision
• Discussions with the family concerning advanced directives
• Socialization (adult day care)
• Sensory stimulation (prominent displays of clocks and calendars)
• Improvement in sleep hygiene
• Pharmacotherapy should be reserved for specific behavioral symptoms after nonpharmacologic therapy has failed

SURGICAL MEASURES N/A

ACTIVITY Fully active with direction and supervision

DIET No special diet

PATIENT EDUCATION
• The 36-Hour Day by Mace and Rabins
• Printed material available from the Alzheimer's Association, (800)621-0379

MEDICATIONS

DRUG(S) OF CHOICE
• Appropriately treat secondary causes, such as hypothyroidism or vitamin B12 deficiency
• With other causes, drugs are used to treat behavioral symptoms after nonpharmacologic therapy has failed

• Sun-downing, aggressive behavior: antipsychotics such as haloperidol (Haldol) 0.5-1.0 mg at bedtime or thioridazine (Mellaril) 10-25 mg bid are reasonable choices in a non-emergency situation
• Depression: nortriptyline (Pamelor) 20-50 mg or desipramine (Norpramin) 25 mg bid or the serotonin reuptake inhibitors sertraline (Zoloft), fluoxetine (Prozac), paroxetine (Paxil), fluvoxamine (Luvox)
• Sleep disturbance: Intermittent use of temazepam (Restoril) 15 mg, zolpidem (Ambien) 5 mg, trazodone (Desyrel) 25-50 mg, or chloral hydrate 500 mg at bedtime is occasionally warranted.
• Donepezil (Aricept) 5-10 mg every AM for mild to moderate DAT
• Tacrine (Cognex): 10-40 mg qid used to treat mild-moderate DAT (doses >100 mg/day appear to be associated with increased risk of hepatotoxicity). Increase dose in 40 mg/day increments every 6 weeks.

Contraindications:
• Antipsychotics (haloperidol, thioridazine) - severe depression; Parkinson's disease; hypo- or hypertension
• Tricyclic antidepressants (nortriptyline, desipramine) - acute recovery phase following myocardial infarction, acute narrow-angle glaucoma
• Acute active liver disease, active untreated peptic ulcers

Precautions:
• Hypnotics should not be used on a regular basis
• In the elderly, begin with small doses and increase slowly
• Lorazepam (Ativan) may produce paradoxical excitation or daytime drowsiness
• Triazolam (Halcion) can produce confusion and psychotic reactions in the elderly
• Antipsychotics
   ◊ Use with caution in patients with severe cardiovascular disorders because of the possibility of severe hypotension
   ◊ Tardive dyskinesia
   ◊ Neuroleptic malignant syndrome
   ◊ Lowered seizure threshold
   ◊ Monitor bone marrow function with CBC
• Tricyclic antidepressants (TCA)
   ◊ Anticholinergic effects
   ◊ Sedation, increased confusion
   ◊ May produce arrhythmia, sinus tachycardia, and prolong conduction time
   ◊ Lowered seizure threshold
• Benzodiazepines
   ◊ Dependence
   ◊ Sedation, increased confusion
   ◊ Respiratory depression
   ◊ Withdrawal symptoms
• Tacrine (Cognex)
   ◊ Use with caution in persons with a history of elevated liver function tests, neuromuscular disease, seizures or asthma
• Donepezil (Aricept) use with caution:
   ◊ If at risk for developing gastrointestinal ulcers
   ◊ In persons with sick sinus syndrome or other supraventricular cardiac conduction conditions
• Serotonin reuptake inhibitors
   ◊ Weight loss
   ◊ Possibly might decrease seizure threshold
   ◊ Dry mouth

   ◊ Tremor
   ◊ Nausea, vomiting, diarrhea
Significant possible interactions:
• Antipsychotics: lithium may induce extrapyramidal symptoms and disorientation
• Tricyclic antidepressants (TCA): monoamine oxidase inhibitors should not be administered with TCA. Antipsychotic administration, cimetidine and estrogens may increase the TCA concentration.
• Benzodiazepines: increased serum phenytoin concentration. Cimetidine may increase the benzodiazepine concentration.
• Tacrine (Cognex): decrease theophylline dose by 50%. Use with caution with anticholinergic medications and NSAID's.
• Serotonin reuptake inhibitors: do not use in combination with monoamine oxidase inhibitors; allow 6 weeks between stopping SSRI and starting MAO-I. May increase warfarin effect. Monitor lithium levels closely in those patients on lithium when a serotonin reuptake inhibitor is added.

ALTERNATIVE DRUGS
• Lithium carbonate
• Carbamazepine (Tegretol)

FOLLOWUP

PATIENT MONITORING
• Periodic mental status testing to assess progression and predict prognosis
• Periodic monitoring of nutritional status
• Periodic monitoring of the caregiver status to assess for caregiver stress
• Periodic assessment of the environment for safety
• Liver function tests with tacrine therapy

PREVENTION/AVOIDANCE N/A

POSSIBLE COMPLICATIONS
• Antipsychotic-induced extrapyramidal effects
• Falls
• Pressure sores
• Malnutrition
• Constipation
• Various infections

EXPECTED COURSE/PROGNOSIS
• DAT - a progressive disease with variable rates of progression, but inevitably leading to profound cognitive impairment
• MID - less likely to be progressive but cognitive improvement is unlikely
• Cortical dementias - treatment of the disease rarely has an effect on the cognitive deficit as cognitive impairment is generally a late component
• Secondary dementias - treatment of the underlying condition may lead to improvement

MISCELLANEOUS

ASSOCIATED CONDITIONS
• Depression
• Insomnia

AGE-RELATED FACTORS
Pediatric: N/A
Geriatric:
• In the elderly, begin drugs with small doses and increase slowly
• Drugs with a long half-life (fluoxetine, lorazepam, etc.) require closer monitoring in the elderly; it may be better to choose a drug with a shorter half-life (sertraline, paroxetine, temazepam)
Others: N/A

PREGNANCY N/A

SYNONYMS Senility

ICD-9-CM
290.0 Senile dementia, uncomplicated
290.10 Presenile dementia, uncomplicated
290.40 Arteriosclerotic dementia, uncomplicated
331.0 Alzheimer's disease

SEE ALSO
• Alzheimer's disease
• Parkinson's disease
• Huntington's chorea
• Stroke (Brain attack)
• Down's syndrome
• Hypothyroidism, adult
• Syphilis
• Creutzfeldt-Jakob disease
• Juvenile amaurotic familial idiocy
• Pellagra
• Pick's disease
• Wilson's disease

OTHER NOTES N/A

ABBREVIATIONS
DAT = dementia of Alzheimer's type
MID = multi-infarct dementia

REFERENCES
• NIH Consensus Conference on Differential Diagnosis of Dementing Diseases. JAMA 1987;258(23):3411-3416
• Diagnostic and Statistical Manual of Mental Disorders. 4th Ed., Washington, D.C., American Psychiatric Association, 1994
• Van Horn G: Dementia. The American Journal of Medicine 1987;83:101-110
Illustrations: N/A
Internet references: http://www.5mcc.com

Author(s)
Aubrey L. Knight, MD

Depression

BASICS

DESCRIPTION Depression results when a person experiences more frustration and anger than he or she can handle. Each person is capable of handling a different amount of frustration or anger. The result is an abnormal receptor-neurotransmitter relationship at the synapse mainly in the limbic system in the brain. The presynaptic receptors deal primarily with the storage, release and uptake of neurotransmitters. The primary neurotransmitters, both monoamines, are serotonin and norepinephrine. Dopamine has also been associated with depression. The available antidepressants, according to the latest theory, may increase the sensitivity of the post-synaptic receptor sites and decrease the presynaptic receptor sites. It is thought by some that the antidepressants may work by blocking the uptake of the neurotransmitters, thereby upgrading the synapse by having more available.
• Bipolar disorder has a prominent depressive phase, but is a different clinical entity that is treated differently from depression
System(s) affected: Nervous
Genetics: Possible defect on chromosome II or X
Incidence/Prevalence in USA: Estimated that 5-20% of population will experience a significant depression at some time
Predominant age:
• Bipolar - mean, 30 years
• Unipolar - mean, 40 years
Predominant sex: Female > Male

SIGNS AND SYMPTOMS
• Depressed mood
• Anhedonia
• Depression is probable when at least four of the following exist in addition to depressed mood or anhedonia:
  ◊ Poor appetite - either weight gain or loss (may eat or drink out of boredom or reasons other than appetite)
  ◊ Sleep disorder - either insomnia or hypersomnia
  ◊ Fatigue - tiredness is out of proportion to the amount of energy expended
  ◊ Psychomotor retardation or agitation (restlessness, irritability or withdrawal)
  ◊ Poor self image - self reproach, excessive guilt
  ◊ Difficulty in concentrating, poor memory, unable to make decisions
  ◊ Suicidal ideation. Sometimes when people begin to recover they gain enough energy to think about and sometimes to attempt suicide.

CAUSES
• Impaired synthesis of the neurotransmitters
• Increased breakdown or metabolism of the neurotransmitters
• Increased pump uptake of the neurotransmitters. When a person experiences anger or frustration these chemicals are released at the synapse. The action potential is passed on from neuron to neuron. Following this the neurotransmitter is (1) reabsorbed into the neuron where it is either destroyed by an enzyme or actively removed by a reuptake pump and stored until needed or (2) destroyed by monoamine oxidase (MAO) located in the mitochondria.
• Lack of these neurotransmitters causes certain types of depression, e.g., decreased norepinephrine causes dullness and lethargy, while decreased serotonin causes irritability, hostility and suicide ideation
• Environmental factors and learned behavior may effect neurotransmitters and/or have independent influence on depression

RISK FACTORS
• Females more likely to develop depressive illness than males
• Strong family history (depression, suicide, alcoholism, other substance abuse)
• Presence of chronic disease, especially multiple diseases
• Migraine headaches
• Back pain
• Chronic pain
• Recent myocardial infarction
• Peptic ulcer disease
• Insomnia
• Stressful situations
• Adolescence
• Advancing age
• Retirement
• Children with behavioral disorders, especially hyperactivity

DIAGNOSIS

DIFFERENTIAL DIAGNOSIS
• Organic brain diseases
• Endocrine diseases, such as hypothyroid and hyperthyroid diseases
• Diabetes mellitus
• Liver failure
• Renal failure
• Chronic fatigue syndrome
• Vitamin deficiency (pernicious anemia, pellagra)
• Medication side effects (many drugs cause or worsen depression)
• Medication overdose
• Medication abuse
• Withdrawal from medication
• Alcohol abuse
• Substance abuse
• Withdrawal from abused substance (alcohol, cocaine, marijuana)

LABORATORY Depression is a clinical diagnosis. Laboratory tests are used primarily to rule out other diagnoses.
Drugs that may alter lab results: All psychoactive drugs
Disorders that may alter lab results: Thyroid disease

PATHOLOGICAL FINDINGS N/A

SPECIAL TESTS
• ECG (diagnosis of arrhythmia, especially heart block)
• EEG

IMAGING CT or MRI of brain, if organic brain syndrome (OBS) included in differential

DIAGNOSTIC PROCEDURES
• Depression is primarily a clinical diagnosis that depends on skillfully eliciting family, social and psychosocial factors
• Validated standard rating scales can assist in identifying and following depressed patients
  ◊ Zungs Self-rating Depression Scale
  ◊ BDI - Beck's Depression Inventory
  ◊ CES-D Scale - Criteria for Epidemiologic Studies-depression Scale
  ◊ CDI - Children's Depression Inventory
  ◊ Yesavage's Geriatric Depression Scale

TREATMENT

APPROPRIATE HEALTH CARE
Outpatient

GENERAL MEASURES
• Psychotherapeutic interventions act synergistically with pharmacologic therapy.
• Use the correct medication
• Use the correct dosage
• Use the correct medication long enough
• ECT can be very effective in refractory cases

SURGICAL MEASURES N/A

ACTIVITY No restrictions

DIET No special diet

PATIENT EDUCATION
• Carefully teach about medications
• Consider referral to support groups
• Stress need for long-term treatment and followup
• Recommend reading for patients, e.g., How to Cope With Depression by DePaulo and Ablow; Depression is a Treatable Illness: A Patient's Guide, AHCPR Publications Clearinghouse
• Contact local support groups through National Depression Manic Depression Association (DMDA) (800)82-MDMDA

Depression

MEDICATIONS

DRUG(S) OF CHOICE
All of the below listed medications are equally efficacious for depression. Selection is based on side effects profile.
• Polycyclic (mostly tricyclic [TCA's]) antidepressants with sedating properties (also have anticholinergic properties, potential for fatal overdose):
◊ Amitriptyline (Elavil, Endep) 150-300 mg/day qhs
◊ Nortriptyline (Pamelor, Aventyl) 75-150 mg/day qhs (a metabolite of amitriptyline)
◊ Doxepin (Adapin, Sinequan) 150-300 mg/day qhs
◊ Trimipramine (Surmontil) 75-250 mg/day qhs
◊ Trazodone (Desyrel) 150-300 mg/day qhs
• Polycyclic antidepressants with activating properties (also have anticholinergic properties, insomnia, anxiety, potentially fatal overdose):
◊ Imipramine (Tofranil, Tipramine) 150-300 mg/day
◊ Desipramine (Norpramin, Pertofrane) 150-300 mg/day
◊ Protriptyline (Vivactil) 30-60 mg/day
• Selective serotonin reuptake inhibitors (can cause insomnia, anxiety, appetite suppression; overdose less likely to be fatal):
◊ Fluoxetine (Prozac) 20 mg/day q am
◊ Sertraline (Zoloft) 50-100 mg/day q am
◊ Paroxetine (Paxil) 10-30 mg/day q am
• Others:
◊ Venlafaxine (Effexor) 75-100 mg/day in divided doses. Increases effective serotonin and norepinephrine; can cause insomnia, anxiety, anorexia).
◊ Bupropion (Wellbutrin) 100-450 mg/day in divided doses) catecholamine reuptake inhibitor)
Contraindications: Refer to manufacturer's profile of each drug
Precautions:
• Decrease beginning dose by half for children and elderly
• Fluoxetine, sertraline, paroxetine best given in the morning
• Polycyclic antidepressant prescriptions should initially be written for small total amounts to prevent suicide (TCA's fatal with doses > 1-1.5 gm in adults)
• TCA's may produce arrhythmias and lower seizure threshold
• Venlafaxine - allow approximately two weeks washout of other medications before instituting therapy with venlafaxine
Significant possible interactions:
• Refer to manufacturer's profile of each drug
• Avoid nonprescription drugs containing pseudoephedrine, phenylephrine, or phenylpropanolamine (cold medicines)

ALTERNATIVE DRUGS
• Clomipramine (Anafranil) 100-250 mg/day (although primarily used to treat obsessive-compulsive disorder)
• MAO inhibitors - significant drug and food interactions limit their use

FOLLOWUP

PATIENT MONITORING
• See patient within 2 weeks after starting medication. The patient will probably not feel greatly improved at this visit.
• During followup visits evaluate side effects, dosage and effectiveness of the medication
• Follow about every 2 weeks until improvement begins. If treatment is adequate, the depression should improve within 4 weeks of initiating treatment.
• Follow every 3 months thereafter
• Explain to the patient that the treatment must continue even after improvement
• Plan to treat at least 6 months to 2 years. Longer in patients with family history of depression and the very young.

PREVENTION/AVOIDANCE See Causes and Risk factors

POSSIBLE COMPLICATIONS
• Suicide
• Failure to improve

EXPECTED COURSE/PROGNOSIS This is one of the most rewarding conditions to treat because, once you find the right drug and the right dose, you can almost guarantee the patient that he or she will improve

MISCELLANEOUS

ASSOCIATED CONDITIONS
• Manic depression (bipolar)
• Schizophrenia
• Schizo-affective disorders
• Psycho-physiological disorders
• Physical disorders
• Cyclothymic and grief reactions
• Alcoholism

AGE-RELATED FACTORS
Pediatric: Depression occurs in children
Geriatric: More common in elderly and difficult to precisely diagnose. Depression frequently coexists with dementia or delirium.
Others: N/A

PREGNANCY Caution in using psychoactive medications in pregnancy. Rely on psychotherapy and support groups until pregnancy is completed.

SYNONYMS Unipolar affective disorder

ICD-9-CM
• 311 Depressive disorder, not elsewhere classified
• 296.2 Major depressive disorder, single episode
• 296.3 Major depressive disorder, recurrent episode

SEE ALSO
• Obsessive compulsive disorder

OTHER NOTES
• Depression is the fourth most common reason to visit the family physician
• Like so many other medical illnesses with psychological symptoms, family, doctors and patients tend to try to overlook this condition because they feel they should be able to control it themselves
• Attention deficit syndromes are being treated with antidepressants. They may be more effective than methylphenidate (Ritalin) or amphetamines.

ABBREVIATIONS
OBS = organic brain syndrome
TCA = tricyclic antidepressant
TSH = thyroid stimulating hormone

REFERENCES
• Kavan MG: Screening for Depression. In AFP, Mar 1990 1990
• Diagnosis and Treatment (Quick reference guide for Physicians) AHCPR publication 93-0552
• Shererer SL, Adams GK: Nonpharmacologic aids in the treatment of depression. Amer Fam Phys;1993(2)
Illustrations: N/A
Internet references: http://www.5mcc.com

Author(s)
Dannen D. Mannschreck, MD

Dermatitis, atopic

BASICS

DESCRIPTION Chronic pruritic eczematous condition affecting characteristic sites. Associated with family history of atopy (asthma, allergic rhinitis, atopic dermatitis).
System(s) affected: Skin/Exocrine
Genetics: Genetic predisposition - family history positive in two-thirds of cases
Incidence/Prevalence in USA: Common; incidence 7-24/1000
Predominant age: Mainly childhood disease. Affects 5% of all children, usually starting after 2 months of age. Atopic dermatitis is present by age 5 in 90% of patients.
Predominant sex: Male = Female (females tend to have somewhat worse prognosis)

SIGNS AND SYMPTOMS
• Pruritus is the most common symptom
• Distribution of lesions
◊ Infants - trunk, face, and extensor surfaces
◊ Children - antecubital and popliteal fossae
◊ Adults - face, neck, upper chest, and genital areas
◊ In adults with limited distribution of lesions a history of childhood eczema is a clue to diagnosis
• Morphology of lesions
◊ Infants - erythema and papules; may develop oozing, crusting vesicles
◊ Children and adults - lichenification and scaling are typical with chronic eczema
◊ Family history of atopic dermatitis may be more useful than morphology in making the diagnosis
• Associated features
◊ Facial erythema, mild to moderate
◊ Perioral pallor
◊ Infraorbital fold (Dennie's sign/Morgan line)
◊ Dry skin
◊ Increased palmar linear markings
◊ Pityriasis alba (hypopigmented asymptomatic areas on face and shoulders)
◊ Keratosis pilaris

CAUSES Unknown. Genetically determined, non-allergic disease.

RISK FACTORS
• Skin infections
• Emotional stress
• Irritating clothes and chemicals
• Excessively hot or cold climate
• Food allergy in children (controversial)
• Exposure to tobacco smoke

DIAGNOSIS

DIFFERENTIAL DIAGNOSIS
• Photosensitivity rashes
• Contact dermatitis (especially if only the face is involved)
• Scabies
• Seborrheic dermatitis (especially in infants)
• Psoriasis or lichen simplex chronicus if only localized disease is present in adults
• Rare conditions of infancy: histiocytosis X, Wiskott-Aldrich syndrome, ataxia-telangiectasia syndrome
• Ichthyosis vulgaris

LABORATORY Serum IgE levels are frequently elevated
Drugs that may alter lab results: N/A
Disorders that may alter lab results: N/A

PATHOLOGICAL FINDINGS Epidermis is thickened and hyperkeratotic. Dermis shows perivascular inflammation.

SPECIAL TESTS None

IMAGING None

DIAGNOSTIC PROCEDURES Skin biopsy shows nonspecific eczematous changes. (Biopsy is rarely required since diagnosis is made on clinical grounds.)

TREATMENT

APPROPRIATE HEALTH CARE
Generally outpatient, using topical corticosteroids

GENERAL MEASURES
• Decrease stress if possible
• Avoid agents that may cause irritation (e.g., wool, perfumes)
• Minimize sweating
• Lukewarm (not hot) baths
• Minimize use of soap (superfatted soaps best)
• Frequent systemic lubrication with oil baths, moisturizers, etc. (use oil after soaking)
• Sun exposure may be helpful
• Humidify the house

SURGICAL MEASURES N/A

ACTIVITY No restrictions

DIET There is controversy regarding the role of food allergies and exacerbations of atopic dermatitis. Food allergies do not play a role in adult eczema. In infants and children the most common suspicious foods are eggs, milk, wheat and peanuts. Consider elimination diets (e.g., for 3-4 weeks) and food challenges. Also consider delaying introduction of the common suspicious foods until an infant is 6 months old.

PATIENT EDUCATION
• Eczema is not caused by nerves
• Eczema is not caused by an allergy
• Goal is control, not cure (although many patients will outgrow their disease)
• See also Epstein, E.: Common Skin Disorders. 4th Ed. Medical Economics, 1994

MEDICATIONS

DRUG(S) OF CHOICE
• Topical steroids achieve good control in 90% of patients
• In infants and children, use 0.5-1% topical hydrocortisone
• In adults, may use higher potency (over 1%) topical corticosteroids in areas other than face and skin folds
• Use short courses of higher potency corticosteroids for flares, then return to the lowest potency (creams preferred) that will control dermatitis
Contraindications: None
Precautions: Beware that chronic potent fluorinated corticosteroids use may cause striae or atrophy, especially in children. High potency topical corticosteroids may produce systemic effects if used for prolonged periods.
Significant possible interactions: None

ALTERNATIVE DRUGS
• Coal tar, e.g., tar-oil baths, topical tar at bedtime, etc.
• Antihistamines for pruritus (e.g., hydroxyzine, 10-25 mg at bedtime and prn)
• Plastic occlusion - in combination with topical medication, this promotes absorption and may be useful for secondary infection (e.g., erythromycin or dicloxacillin)
• For stubborn localized eczema, may use intralesional steroids
• For severe atopic dermatitis, consider systemic steroids for 1-2 weeks, e.g., prednisone 2 mg/day po (max 80 mg) initially, tapered over 7-14 days. Start topical steroids simultaneously to assist in rapid taper of oral steroids.

FOLLOWUP

PATIENT MONITORING
Individualize, depending on severity of disease

PREVENTION/AVOIDANCE
• Smallpox vaccine should be avoided because of risk of eczema herpeticum (see Possible Complications)

POSSIBLE COMPLICATIONS
• Cataracts are more common in patients with atopic dermatitis
• Skin infections (usually staphylococcus aureus); sometimes subclinical
• Eczema herpeticum - generalized vesiculopustular eruption caused by infection with herpes simplex or vaccinia virus. Patients are acutely ill and require hospitalization.
• Atrophy and/or striae if fluorinated corticosteroids are used on face or skin folds
• Systemic absorption may occur if large areas of skin are treated, particularly if high-potency medications and occlusion are combined

EXPECTED COURSE/PROGNOSIS
• Chronic disease that tends to burn out with age. 90% of patients have spontaneous resolution by puberty.
• Some adults may continue to have localized eczema, e.g., chronic hand or foot dermatitis, eyelid dermatitis, or lichen simplex chronicus

MISCELLANEOUS

ASSOCIATED CONDITIONS
• Asthma
• Allergic rhinitis
• Hyper-IgE syndrome (Job's syndrome) which is characterized by atopic dermatitis, elevated IgE, recurrent pyodermas, and decreased chemotaxis of mononuclear cells

AGE-RELATED FACTORS
Pediatric: More frequent
Geriatric: Relatively rare
Others: N/A

PREGNANCY N/A

SYNONYMS
• Eczema
• Disseminated neurodermatitis
• Atopic eczema
• Atopic neurodermatitis
• Constitutional dermatitis
• Besnier's prurigo

ICD-9-CM 691.8

SEE ALSO N/A

OTHER NOTES
If very resistant to treatment, search for a coexisting contact dermatitis

ABBREVIATIONS

REFERENCES
• Habif T: Clinical Dermatology. 3rd Ed. St. Louis, CV Mosby, 1996
• Fitzpatrick TB, et al, eds: Dermatology in General Medicine, 4th ed. New York, McGraw-Hill, 1993.
• Behrman RE, et al, eds: Nelson Textbook of Pediatrics. 15th ed. Philadelphia, 1996
Illustrations: 19 available on CD-ROM
Internet references: http://www.5mcc.com

Author(s)
Dennis E. Hughes, DO

Dermatitis, contact

BASICS

DESCRIPTION The cutaneous reaction to an external substance
• Primary irritant dermatitis is due to direct injury of the skin. It affects individuals exposed to specific irritants and generally produces discomfort immediately after exposure.
• Allergic contact dermatitis (ACD) affects only individuals previously sensitized to the contactant. It represents a delayed hypersensitivity reaction, requiring several hours for the cascade of cellular immunity to be completed to manifest itself.
System(s) affected: Skin/Exocrine
Genetics: Increased frequency of ACD in families with allergies
Incidence/Prevalence in USA: N/A
Predominant age: All ages
Predominant sex: Male = Female.
Variations due to differences in exposure to offending agents as well as normal cutaneous variations between male and female (eccrine and sebaceous gland function and hair distribution).

SIGNS AND SYMPTOMS
• Acute
  ◊ Papules, vesicles, bullae with surrounding erythema
  ◊ Crusting and oozing may be present
  ◊ Pruritus
• Chronic
  ◊ Erythematous base
  ◊ Thickening with lichenification
  ◊ Scaling
  ◊ Fissuring
• Distribution
  ◊ Where epidermis is thinner (eyelids, genitalia)
  ◊ Areas of contact with offending agent (e.g., nail polish)
  ◊ Palms and soles more resistant
  ◊ Deeper skinfolds spared
  ◊ Linear arrays of lesions
  ◊ Lesions with sharp borders and sharp angles - pathognomonic

CAUSES
• Plants
  ◊ Rhus-urushiol (poison ivy, oak, sumac)
  ◊ Primary contact - plant (roots/stems/leaves)
  ◊ Secondary contact - clothes/fingernails (not blister fluid)
• Chemicals
  ◊ Nickel - jewelry, zippers, hooks, watches
  ◊ Potassium dichromate - tanning agent in leather
  ◊ Paraphenylenediamine - hair dyes, fur dyes, industrial chemicals
  ◊ Turpentine - cleaning agents, polishes, waxes
  ◊ Soaps, detergents

• Topical medicines
  ◊ Neomycin - topical antibiotics
  ◊ Thimerosal (Merthiolate) - preservative in topical medications
  ◊ Anesthetics - benzocaine
  ◊ Parabens - preservative in topical medications
  ◊ Formalin - cosmetics, shampoos, nail enamel

RISK FACTORS
• Occupation
• Hobbies
• Travel
• Cosmetics
• Jewelry

DIAGNOSIS

DIFFERENTIAL DIAGNOSIS
• Based on clinical impression - appearance, periodicity, localization
• Groups of vesicles - herpes simplex
• Diffuse bullous or vesicular lesions - bullous pemphigoid
• Photo-distribution - phototoxic/allergic reaction to systemic allergen
• Eyelids - seborrheic dermatitis
• Scaly eczematous lesions - atopic dermatitis, nummular eczema, lichen simplex chronicus, stasis dermatitis, xerosis

LABORATORY N/A
Drugs that may alter lab results: N/A
Disorders that may alter lab results: N/A

PATHOLOGICAL FINDINGS
• Intercellular edema
• Bullae

SPECIAL TESTS Patch tests for allergic contact dermatitis (systemic corticosteroids or recent, aggressive use of topical steroids may alter results)

IMAGING N/A

DIAGNOSTIC PROCEDURES Patch test

TREATMENT

APPROPRIATE HEALTH CARE
Outpatient

GENERAL MEASURES
• Removal of offending agent
• Topical soaks with cool tap water, Burow's solution (1:40 dilution), or saline (1 tsp/pint water), or silver nitrate solution (25.5%)
• Lukewarm water baths - antipruritic
• Aveeno (oatmeal) baths
• Chronic - emollients (white petrolatum, Eucerin)

SURGICAL MEASURES N/A

ACTIVITY Stay active, but avoid overheating

DIET No special diet

PATIENT EDUCATION
• Avoidance of irritating substance
• Cleaning of secondary sources (nails, clothes)
• Fallacy of blister fluid spreading disease

MEDICATIONS

DRUG(S) OF CHOICE
• Topical
 ◊ Shake lotion of zinc oxide, talc, menthol 0.25%, phenol 0.5%
 ◊ Corticosteroids: high potency steroids, fluocinonide (Lidex) 0.05% ointment 3-4 times daily. Caution regarding face/skinfolds - use lower potency steroids and avoid prolonged usage.
 ◊ Calamine lotion
 ◊ Topical antibiotics for secondary infection (bacitracin, gentamicin, erythromycin)
• Systemic
 ◊ Antihistamine: hydroxyzine 25-50 mg qid, diphenhydramine 25-50 mg qid
 ◊ Corticosteroids: prednisone. Taper starting at 60-80 mg/d, tapered over 10-14 days.
 ◊ Antibiotics: erythromycin 250 mg qid if secondarily infected
Contraindications: N/A
Precautions:
• Drowsiness from antihistamines
• Local skin effects: atrophy, stria, telangiectasia from prolonged use of potent topical steroids
Significant possible interactions: N/A

ALTERNATIVE DRUGS Other topical antibiotics depending on organisms and sensitivity

FOLLOWUP

PATIENT MONITORING
• As necessary for recurrence
• Patch testing for etiology after resolved

PREVENTION/AVOIDANCE
Avoid causative agents. Use of protective gloves (with cotton lining) may be helpful.

POSSIBLE COMPLICATIONS
• Generalized eruption secondary to autosensitization
• Secondary bacterial infection

EXPECTED COURSE/PROGNOSIS
Self-limited, benign

MISCELLANEOUS

ASSOCIATED CONDITIONS N/A

AGE-RELATED FACTORS
Pediatric: Younger individuals - increased incidence of positive patch testing due to better delayed hypersensitivity reactions
Geriatric: Increased incidence of irritant dermatitis secondary to skin dryness
Others: N/A

PREGNANCY Usual cautions with medications

SYNONYMS Dermatitis Venenata

ICD-9-CM
• 692 Contact dermatitis and other eczema
• 692.9 Unspecified cause

SEE ALSO N/A

OTHER NOTES N/A

ABBREVIATIONS ACD = allergic contact dermatitis

REFERENCES
• Bondi E, Jegasothy B, Lazarus G: Dermatology, Diagnosis and Therapy. Norwalk, CT, Appleton & Lange, 1991
• Abel E, Farber E: Scientific American Inc., New York, 1985
Illustrations: 32 available on CD-ROM
Internet references: http://www.5mcc.com

Author(s)
Jeffrey A. Stearns, MD

Dermatitis, diaper

 BASICS

DESCRIPTION Diaper dermatitis is a rash occurring under the covered area of a diaper. The rash may be an irritant contact dermatitis, candidiasis, atopic dermatitis or seborrheic dermatitis.
System(s) affected: Skin/Exocrine
Genetics: N/A
Incidence/Prevalence in USA: Common
Predominant age: Infants
Predominant sex: Male = Female

SIGNS AND SYMPTOMS
• Irritant contact diaper dermatitis
  ◊ Prominent rash on buttocks and pubic skin
  ◊ Creases of skin are relatively spared
  ◊ Rash is dusky red and shiny
  ◊ Skin seems chapped
  ◊ Weeping, crusting, and excoriations are not prominent
• Candidiasis diaper rash
  ◊ Initial involvement of creases with rapid extension
  ◊ Color: bright red
  ◊ Accompanying edema
  ◊ Isolated satellite papules and pustules at margins of inflammatory plaques
  ◊ Excoriations are prominent
  ◊ Positive KOH preparation
  ◊ Positive cultures
• Atopic diaper dermatitis
  ◊ Distribution spares creases
  ◊ Genitalia frequently involved
  ◊ Itch-scratch cycle with excoriations are prominent
  ◊ Child scratches vigorously at night
  ◊ Weeping, crusting, excoriations sometimes present; secondary bacterial infection can occur
• Seborrheic diaper dermatitis
  ◊ Dusky-red patches and plaques deep within skin creases
  ◊ Non-intertriginous skin is relatively spared
  ◊ Weeping, crusting, excoriations - not prominent
  ◊ Other sites of seborrheic dermatitis are frequently present: retroauricular, axillary folds, scalp

CAUSES Irritation to skin from prolonged contact with urine or feces

RISK FACTORS
• Infrequent diaper changes
• Waterproof diapers
• Improper laundering
• Family history of dermatitis
• Hot, humid weather
• Recent treatment with oral antibiotics
• Diarrhea

 DIAGNOSIS

DIFFERENTIAL DIAGNOSIS
• Contact dermatitis
• Seborrheic dermatitis
• Candidiasis
• Atopic dermatitis
• Acrodermatitis enteropathica
• Letterer-Siwe disease
• Congenital syphilis

LABORATORY Culture will reveal candida, if present
Drugs that may alter lab results: N/A
Disorders that may alter lab results: N/A

PATHOLOGICAL FINDINGS Varying inflammation is the most prominent finding

SPECIAL TESTS
• KOH preparation
• Culture pustules if present

IMAGING N/A

DIAGNOSTIC PROCEDURES
• Culture lesions
• KOH preparation

 TREATMENT

APPROPRIATE HEALTH CARE
Outpatient

GENERAL MEASURES
• Expose the buttocks to air as much as possible
• Don't use waterproof pants during treatment - day or night. They keep skin wet and subject to rash or infection.
• Change diapers frequently - even at night if the rash is extensive
• Super absorbable diapers beneficial
• Discontinue using baby lotion, powder, ointment or baby oil (except zinc oxide)
• Zinc oxide ointment to the rash at the earliest sign of diaper rash, and 2 or 3 times a day thereafter (apply to clean, thoroughly dry skin)
• Use mild soap and pat dry

SURGICAL MEASURES N/A

ACTIVITY Protect from overheating

DIET No special diet

PATIENT EDUCATION N/A

MEDICATIONS

DRUG(S) OF CHOICE
• If candidiasis suspected or diaper rash persistent, use antifungal such as miconazole nitrate 2% cream, miconazole powder, econazole (Spectazole), clotrimazole (Lotrimin), or ketoconazole (Nizoral) cream, at each diaper change.
• If inflammation is prominent, consider very low potency steroid cream, such as hydrocortisone 0.5-1% tid along with an antifungal cream or and combination product such as clioquinol-hydrocortisone (Vioform-Hydrocortisone) cream
• If a secondary bacterial infection is suspected, use an anti-Staphylococcal oral antibiotic or mupirocin (Bactroban) ointment topically

Contraindications: N/A
Precautions: Avoid high or the moderate potency steroids often found in combination steroid-antifungal mixtures
Significant possible interactions: N/A

ALTERNATIVE DRUGS N/A

FOLLOWUP

PATIENT MONITORING Recheck weekly until clear, then at times of recurrence

PREVENTION/AVOIDANCE See General Measures

POSSIBLE COMPLICATIONS
• Secondary bacterial infection
• Secondary yeast infection

EXPECTED COURSE/PROGNOSIS
Quick complete clearing with appropriate treatment

MISCELLANEOUS

ASSOCIATED CONDITIONS
• Contact (allergic or irritant) dermatitis
• Seborrheic dermatitis
• Psoriasis
• Candidiasis
• Atopic dermatitis

AGE-RELATED FACTORS
Pediatric: Problem most common in this age group
Geriatric: Incontinence
Others: N/A

PREGNANCY N/A

SYNONYMS
• Diaper rash

ICD-9-CM
691.0 Diaper or napkin rash

SEE ALSO
• Dermatitis, contact
• Candidiasis
• Dermatitis, atopic
• Psoriasis

OTHER NOTES Two or more types of diaper dermatitis can exist concomitantly. If so, treat each accordingly.

ABBREVIATIONS N/A

REFERENCES
• Fitzpatrick T, et al, eds: Dermatology In General Medicine. 4th Ed. New York, McGraw-Hill, 1993
• Janniger CK, Thomas I: Diaper Dermatitis: An approach to prevention employing effective diaper care. Cutis 1993;52:153-55
• Habif T: Clinical Dermatology. 3rd Ed. St. Louis, CV Mosby, 1996
Illustrations: N/A
Internet references: http://www.5mcc.com

Author(s)
Dennis E. Hughes, DO

Dermatitis, exfoliative

BASICS

DESCRIPTION A generalized scaling eruption of the skin, either idiopathic in nature or secondary to underlying cutaneous or systemic disease
System(s) affected: Skin/Exocrine
Genetics: No known genetic pattern
Incidence/Prevalence in USA: Rare; estimated 1% of hospitalizations for skin disease
Predominant Age: 75% of patients are over age 40
Predominant sex: Male > Female (2:1)

SIGNS AND SYMPTOMS
• Fine generalized scales with mild erythema and lichenification of skin
• With acute onset and in early stages of exudative dermatitis, may have thin epidermis, erythema, and exudation with subsequent development of crusting
• Initial distribution is that of any underlying cutaneous disease, Subsequently, as exfoliative dermatitis further develops, this distribution is lost and the scaling is generalized.
• With no underlying cutaneous disease, the distribution initially favors the genital region, trunk, and head before generalizing
• Sensation of skin tightness
• Nail dystrophy
• Hair loss, with alopecia in up to 25%
• Pruritus
• Fever in 40-50%
• Chills
• Malaise/weakness
• Mucous membranes spared
• Anemia (both microcytic and macrocytic) in up to 65%
• Eosinophilia
• Nontender generalized lymphadenopathy
• Steatorrhea
• Hepatomegaly in 20-35%
• Splenomegaly when underlying lymphoma/leukemia present
• Gynecomastia
• Hypoproteinemia
• Dehydration
• High output cardiac failure
• Tachycardia
• Lymphadenopathy in 60% or more

CAUSES
• Idiopathic in up to 19% of cases
• 80% may occur in response to one of the following:
  ◊ Atopic dermatitis
  ◊ Colon carcinoma
  ◊ Contact dermatitis (10%)
  ◊ Drug eruptions (14%)
  ◊ Fungal disease with id reaction
  ◊ HIV infection
  ◊ Ichthyosiform dermatoses
  ◊ Leukemia
  ◊ Lichen planus
  ◊ Lung carcinoma
  ◊ Lymphoma - 15% of cases overall and 35-50% of patients over age 40
  ◊ Medications - sulfonamides and sulfones, penicillins, cephalosporins, anticonvulsants, NSAID's, codeine, heavy metals, INH, quinidine, captopril, iodine, antimalarials, Phenothiazines, methotrexate
  ◊ Multiple myeloma
  ◊ Mycosis fungoides
  ◊ Pemphigus foliaceus
  ◊ Photosensitivity reaction
  ◊ Pityriasis rosea
  ◊ Pityriasis rubra pilaris
  ◊ Psoriasis
  ◊ Pyoderma with id reaction
  ◊ Reiter's syndrome
  ◊ Scabies
  ◊ Seborrheic dermatitis
  ◊ Sézary syndrome
  ◊ Staphylococcal scalded skin syndrome
  ◊ Stasis dermatitis
  ◊ Systemic lupus erythematosus
  ◊ Toxic epidermal necrolysis

RISK FACTORS
• Underlying diseases as noted above
• Male sex
• Age greater than 40

DIAGNOSIS

DIFFERENTIAL DIAGNOSIS Acutely eczematous dermatoses such as contact dermatitis and drug eruptions should be considered

LABORATORY None diagnostic. May have elevated WBC with eosinophilia, anemia, elevated ESR, decreased albumin and electrolyte abnormalities
Drugs that may alter lab results: N/A
Disorders that may alter lab results: N/A

PATHOLOGICAL FINDINGS May have characteristics of the underlying cutaneous disease. Other changes are nonspecific: Hyperkeratosis, parakeratosis, acanthosis in the epidermis; and edema, vasodilation, perivascular infiltrates with lymphocytes, histiocytes, and eosinophils in the dermis.

SPECIAL TESTS None

IMAGING Chest x-ray and other imaging procedures as indicated to investigate any underlying disease process

DIAGNOSTIC PROCEDURES
• Careful history and physical exam
• Skin biopsy; lymph node biopsy and bone marrow biopsy as indicated to investigate an underlying disease process

TREATMENT

APPROPRIATE HEALTH CARE
Outpatient except in those cases with complications of secondary infection, dehydration, or heart failure

GENERAL MEASURES
• Withdrawal of any implicated medications or treatment of any identified underlying infection/disease
• Protection from development of hypothermia
• Cool colloid baths with oatmeal (Aveeno) - 1 cup in 10 inches [25.4 cm] water
• Local moisturizing ointments/lotions

SURGICAL MEASURES N/A

ACTIVITY As tolerated

DIET
• High protein. Increased fluid intake should be encouraged in those with more extensive skin involvement.
• Watch for folate iron deficiency in chronic cases

PATIENT EDUCATION
• Patients should avoid any identified etiologic agents
• Patients with underlying diseases that have caused exfoliative dermatitis can be educated regarding symptomatic treatment of the dermatitis and be advised that successful treatment of the underlying disease will usually also be successful for the exfoliative dermatitis
• Protection against hypothermia and dehydration and identification of signs of infection should be part of the education process
• Advise those patients, without an identified cause for the exfoliative dermatitis, that many cases spontaneously remit (exact number uncertain) and that medical therapy to control symptoms can be provided
• American Academy of Dermatology (708)330-0230

MEDICATIONS

DRUG(S) OF CHOICE
• Systemic corticosteroids initial dosage equivalent to prednisone 40 mg/day with increases in dosage by 20 mg/day if there is no response after 3-4 days at a given dose. Subsequently, dosage should be tapered to control symptoms.
• In addition, treatment specific to any underlying infection or disease should be provided
Contraindications: Psoriasis as the underlying cause of the exfoliative dermatitis
Precautions:
• Atopic dermatitis and seborrheic dermatitis as underlying causes
• Avoid coal tar treatment except with psoriasis, and then only use after 24-48 hours of hydration therapy
Significant possible interactions: Refer to manufacturer's literature

ALTERNATIVE DRUGS
• Antihistamines can be useful for pruritus and topical steroids can be used for more localized disease
• When psoriasis is the underlying cause, methotrexate, etretinate, phototherapy, or other treatments specific to this disease should be provided
• Photochemotherapy may be useful therapy for treating exfoliative dermatitis associated with mycosis fungoides
• Isotretinoin has been used when pityriasis rubra pilaris is the underlying cause
• Antibiotic or antifungal therapy as indicated for superinfection

FOLLOWUP

PATIENT MONITORING Patients should be monitored for response to therapy, development of complications, and for adverse effects related to therapy

PREVENTION/AVOIDANCE Known or suspected etiologic agents should be avoided

POSSIBLE COMPLICATIONS
• Infection
• Hypothermia
• Dehydration/electrolyte disturbances
• Heart failure
• Bacterial/fungal superinfection

EXPECTED COURSE/PROGNOSIS
• In patients with an identified underlying cause, the course and prognosis will parallel the primary disease
• For patients with idiopathic exfoliative dermatitis, the prognosis is poor with frequent recurrences or chronic symptoms requiring chronic steroid therapy

MISCELLANEOUS

ASSOCIATED CONDITIONS Any of the infections or diseases listed under causes

AGE-RELATED FACTORS
Pediatric: Less common, but may occur, associated with atopic dermatitis medications or the inherited dermatoses
Geriatric: N/A
Others: N/A

PREGNANCY N/A

SYNONYMS
• Erythroderma
• Pityriasis rubra

ICD-9-CM 695.89 Other specified erythematous conditions, other

SEE ALSO N/A

OTHER NOTES N/A

ABBREVIATIONS N/A

REFERENCES
• Fitzpatrick TB, et al, eds: Dermatology In General Medicine. 3rd Ed. New York, McGraw-Hill, 1987
• Moschella SL, Hurley HJ: Dermatology. 3rd Ed. Philadelphia, W.B. Saunders Co., 1992
• Domonkos AN, Arnold HL, Odom RB: Andrews' Diseases of the Skin. 8th Ed. Philadelphia, W.B. Saunders Co., 1990
• Sauer GC: Manual of Skin Diseases. Philadelphia, J.B. Lippincott Co., 1991
Illustrations: 4 available on CD-ROM
Internet references: http://www.5mcc.com

Author(s)
Carolyn Nine, MD
Mitchell S. King, MD

Dermatitis, herpetiformis

BASICS

DESCRIPTION Dermatitis herpetiformis is an intensely pruritic papulovesicular disease on extensor skin surfaces
System(s) affected: Skin/Exocrine
Genetics: High incidence of HLA B8/Dw3
Incidence/Prevalence in USA:
Uncommon. Prevalence not known and most likely varies with the race and ethnicity of the population studied.
Predominant age: 15-60, mean age of onset is in the fourth decade
Predominant sex: Male > Female (1.5:1)

SIGNS AND SYMPTOMS
• Symmetrical intensely pruritic, papulovesicular eruption
• Elbows and extensor forearms are the most common site of involvement
• Buttocks, knees, upper back, posterior neck and scalp also frequent
• Oral lesions in 33%
• Secondary excoriations may be prominent
• Burning or stinging feeling may be prominent

CAUSES   Unknown

RISK FACTORS
• Gluten-sensitive enteropathy
• Family history of dermatitis herpetiformis

DIAGNOSIS

DIFFERENTIAL DIAGNOSIS
• Scabies
• Erythema multiforme
• Bullous pemphigoid
• Transient acantholytic dermatosis
• Subcorneal pustular dermatosis
• Erythema elevatum diutinum
• Papular urticaria
• Eczema
• Tinea corporis
• Excoriations

LABORATORY   Abnormal thyroid function tests in 32%
Drugs that may alter lab results:
• Thyroid
• Steroids
Disorders that may alter lab results: N/A

PATHOLOGICAL FINDINGS
• Papillary dermal neutrophilic microabscesses
• Subepidermal vesicles

SPECIAL TESTS   Direct immunofluorescence reveals granular IgA deposition in the dermal papilla

IMAGING   Thyroid scan if indicated by physical exam

DIAGNOSTIC PROCEDURES   Skin biopsy

TREATMENT

APPROPRIATE HEALTH CARE
Outpatient

GENERAL MEASURES   No special measures

SURGICAL MEASURES   N/A

ACTIVITY   Fully active

DIET   Clinical improvement occurs with gluten-free diet

PATIENT EDUCATION   Contact American Academy of Dermatology, 930 N. Meacham Rd., P.O. Box 4014, Schaumber, IL 60168-4014, (708)330-0230

MEDICATIONS

DRUG(S) OF CHOICE Dapsone 50 mg per day will usually improve symptoms within 24 to 48 hours in adults. Average maintenance dose is 100 to 200 mg per day.

Contraindications: See manufacturer's profile of each drug

Precautions:
- Side effects of dapsone include:
  ◊ Hemolytic anemia
  ◊ Methemoglobinemia
  ◊ Toxic hepatitis
  ◊ Cholestatic jaundice
  ◊ Hypoalbuminemla
  ◊ Sensory and motor neuropathy
  ◊ Psychosis
  ◊ Infectious mononucleosis syndrome with fever and lymphadenopathy
  ◊ Agranulocytosis
  ◊ Aplastic anemia
  ◊ Exfoliative dermatitis
  ◊ Erythema multiforme
  ◊ Erythema nodosum
  ◊ Urticaria
  ◊ Dapsone is secreted in breast milk and will produce hemolytic anemia in infants
  ◊ Dapsone will produce a severe hemolytic anemia in patients with glucose-6-phosphate dehydrogenase (G6PD) deficiency

Significant possible interactions: See manufacturer's profile of each drug

ALTERNATIVE DRUGS
- Sulfapyridine; colchicine; prednisone

FOLLOWUP

PATIENT MONITORING
- Baseline CBC and liver function studies should be obtained
- G6PD should be quantified in Asians, blacks and those of southern Mediterranean descent
- CBC should be checked weekly for first month, monthly for the next five months and semi-annually thereafter
- Chemistry profile should be checked every six months
- Patient should be made aware of potential hemolytic anemia and the blue-gray discoloration associated with methemoglobinemia

PREVENTION/AVOIDANCE N/A

POSSIBLE COMPLICATIONS N/A

EXPECTED COURSE/PROGNOSIS
- Patients respond dramatically to dapsone
- Strict adherence to a gluten-free diet will produce improvement of clinical symptoms and a decrease in dapsone requirement in the majority of patients
- Occasional new lesions (2-3 per week) are to be expected and are not an indication for altering daily dosage

MISCELLANEOUS

ASSOCIATED CONDITIONS
- Gluten-sensitive enteropathy
- Hyperthyroidism
- Hypothyroidism
- Thyroid nodules
- Multi-nodular goiter
- Thyroid carcinoma
- Pernicious anemia
- Gastrointestinal lymphoma
- Glomerulopathy
- Immunologic disorders including systemic lupus erythematosus, Addison's disease, rheumatoid arthritis, ulcerative colitis, Raynaud's phenomenon, atopy, Sjögren's syndrome, vitiligo, and dermatomyositis have been reported to be associated with dermatitis herpetiformis

AGE-RELATED FACTORS
Pediatric: Dapsone dose must be adjusted
Geriatric: N/A
Others: N/A

PREGNANCY Data is inconclusive but suggests that dapsone is safe during pregnancy. It is recommended that adherence to a strict gluten-free diet, preferably for 6-12 months before conception be instituted in the hope of eliminating the need for dapsone during pregnancy.

SYNONYMS Duhring's disease

ICD-9-CM 694.0

SEE ALSO N/A

OTHER NOTES N/A

ABBREVIATIONS N/A

REFERENCES
- Zone JJ: Prob. in Derm. Vol. 3, No. 1:6-41
- Hall RP: The pathogenesis of herpetiformis: Recent advances. J. Am Acad. Derm 1987;16:1129-44
- Hall RP: Dermatitis herpetiformis. J Invest Dermatol 1992;99:873
Illustrations: N/A
Internet references: http://www.5mcc.com

Author(s)
Vera Y. Soong, MD

Dermatitis, seborrheic

 BASICS

DESCRIPTION Chronic, superficial, inflammatory condition affecting hairy regions of the body, especially scalp, eyebrows, and face. Mechanism of disease unknown.
System(s) affected: Skin/Exocrine
Genetics: Positive family history common
Incidence/Prevalence in USA: Common
Predominant age: Infancy, adolescence, and adulthood
Predominant sex: Male = Female

SIGNS AND SYMPTOMS
• Infants
　◊ Cradle cap - greasy scaling of scalp, sometimes with associated mild erythema
　◊ Diaper and/or axillary rash
　◊ Onset typically about age one month
　◊ Usually resolves by age 8-12 months
• Adults
　◊ Red, greasy, scaling rash in most locations, consisting of patches and plaques with indistinct margins
　◊ Red, smooth, glazed appearance in skin folds
　◊ Minimal pruritus
　◊ Chronic waxing and waning course
　◊ Bilateral and symmetrical
　◊ Most commonly located in hairy skin areas with numerous sebaceous glands, e.g., scalp and scalp margins, eyebrows and eyelid margins, nasolabial folds, ears and retroauricular folds, presternal area and mid-upper back

CAUSES
• Pityrosporum ovale (the cause of tinea versicolor) may be a contributing factor
• Genetic and environmental factors also contribute to disease, i.e., disease flares are common with any stress or illness
• Disease also seems to parallel increased sebaceous gland activity in infancy and adolescence or as a result of some acnegenic drugs

RISK FACTORS
• Parkinson's disease
• AIDS (disease severity correlated with progression of immune deficiency)
• Emotional stress

 DIAGNOSIS

DIFFERENTIAL DIAGNOSIS
• Atopic dermatitis - (distinction may be difficult in infants)
• Psoriasis - usually knees, elbows, nails will be involved. Scalp psoriasis will be more sharply demarcated than seborrhea, with crusted, infiltrated plaques rather than mild scaling and erythema.
• Candida
• Tinea cruris or capitis - suspect these when usual medications fail, or if there is hair loss
• Eczema of auricle or otitis externa
• Rosacea
• Discoid lupus erythematosus
• Histiocytosis X - may appear as seborrheic type eruption. Consider biopsy if usual therapies fail and especially if petechiae are noted.
• Dandruff (scalp only, noninflammatory)

LABORATORY N/A
Drugs that may alter lab results: N/A
Disorders that may alter lab results: N/A

PATHOLOGICAL FINDINGS Nonspecific changes of eczematous dermatitis. (Biopsy unnecessary unless there is a suspicion of histiocytosis X).

SPECIAL TESTS N/A

IMAGING N/A

DIAGNOSTIC PROCEDURES N/A

 TREATMENT

APPROPRIATE HEALTH CARE
Outpatient

GENERAL MEASURES
• Increase frequency of shampooing
• Sunlight in moderate doses may be helpful

SURGICAL MEASURES N/A

ACTIVITY Full activity

DIET No special diet

PATIENT EDUCATION Goal of treatment is control, rather than cure, of disease. Seborrheic dermatitis does not cause hair loss.

MEDICATIONS

DRUG(S) OF CHOICE
• Cradle cap:
 ◊ Frequent shampooing with a mild, non-medicated shampoo
 ◊ Remove thick scale by applying warm olive or mineral oil and then wash off several hours later with Dawn dishwashing detergent and a soft bristle toothbrush
 ◊ May use a coal tar shampoo or ketoconazole (Nizoral) shampoo if the non-medicated shampoo is ineffective
• Adults:
 ◊ Wash off all affected areas with antiseborrheic shampoos. Start with over-the-counter brands (Tegrin, Selsun Blue) and increase to more potent preparations (containing coal tar, sulfur, selenium or salicylic acid) if no improvement is noted.
 ◊ For dense scalp scaling, 10% Liquor Carbonic Detergens (LCD) in Nivea Oil may be used at bedtime, covering the head with a shower cap. This should be done nightly for 1-3 weeks.
 ◊ Ketoconazole (Nizoral) cream may be used to clear scales in other areas, followed by application of steroids to reduce inflammation. Begin with 1% hydrocortisone and advance to more potent (fluorinated) steroid preparations as needed. Avoid continuous use of the more potent steroids to reduce the risk of skin atrophy or systemic absorption (especially in infants and children).
 ◊ Once controlled, washing with zinc soaps or selenium lotion with periodic use of steroid cream will help maintain remission
• For secondary infections: Short course of erythromycin or dicloxacillin
Contraindications: None
Precautions: Fluorinated corticosteroids and higher concentrations of hydrocortisone (e.g., 2.5%) may cause atrophy or striae if used on the face or on skin folds
Significant possible interactions: None

ALTERNATIVE DRUGS N/A

FOLLOWUP

PATIENT MONITORING Every 2 to 12 weeks as necessary, depending on disease severity and degree of patient sophistication

PREVENTION/AVOIDANCE N/A

POSSIBLE COMPLICATIONS
• Skin atrophy or striae possible from fluorinated corticosteroids, especially if used on the face
• Glaucoma - can result from use of fluorinated steroids around the eyes
• Photosensitivity - occasionally caused by tars
• Herpes keratitis - rare complication of herpes simplex. Instruct patient to stop eyelid steroids if herpes simplex develops.

EXPECTED COURSE/PROGNOSIS
• In infants, seborrheic dermatitis usually remits after 6 to 8 months
• In adults, seborrheic dermatitis is usually chronic and unpredictable, with exacerbations and remissions. Disease is usually easily controlled with shampoos and topical steroids.

MISCELLANEOUS

ASSOCIATED CONDITIONS Parkinson's disease, AIDS (disease severity correlated with progression of immune deficiency)

AGE-RELATED FACTORS
Pediatric: Common in infants
Geriatric: N/A
Others: N/A

PREGNANCY N/A

SYNONYMS
• Seborrhea
• Cradle cap

ICD-9-CM 690

SEE ALSO
• Dermatitis, atopic
• Tinea capitis
• Tinea cruris

OTHER NOTES N/A

ABBREVIATIONS N/A

REFERENCES
• Janniger CK, Schwartz, RA: Seborrheic Dermatitis. American Family Physician 1995;52:149-155
• Janniger, CD: Infantile Seborrheic Dermatitis: An Approach to Cradle Cap. Cutis 1993;51:233-235
• Habif T: Clinical Dermatology. 3rd Ed. St Louis, CV Mosby, 1996
Illustrations: 3 available on CD-ROM
Internet references: http://www.5mcc.com

Author(s)
Dennis E. Hughes, DO

Dermatitis, stasis

 BASICS

DESCRIPTION
Chronic, noninflammatory edema of the lower leg accompanied by cycle of scratching, excoriations, weeping, crusting, and inflammation
System(s) affected: Skin/Exocrine
Genetics: Familial link probable
Incidence/Prevalence in USA: Common in patients over 50 years of age
Predominant age: Adult, geriatric
Predominant sex: Female > Male

SIGNS AND SYMPTOMS
• Violaceous (sometimes brown), erythematous colored lesions - due to deoxygenation of venous blood (postinflammatory hyperpigmentation)
• Distribution - medial aspect of ankle with frequent extension onto the foot and lower leg
• Noninflammatory edema precedes the skin eruption
• Stasis ulcers (frequently accompanies stasis dermatitis) secondary to cuts, bruises, excoriations to the weakened skin around the ankle
• Mild pruritus, pain (if ulcer present)

CAUSES
• Continuous presence of edema in ankles, usually present because of venous valve incompetency (varicose veins)
• Trauma to edematous, eczematized skin

RISK FACTORS
• Atopy
• Superimposition of itch-scratch cycle
• Trauma
• Previous deep vein thrombosis
• Previous pregnancy
• Prolonged medical illness
• Obesity
• Secondary infection
• Low-protein diet
• Old age

 DIAGNOSIS

DIFFERENTIAL DIAGNOSIS
• Other eczematous diseases such as:
  ◊ Atopic dermatitis
  ◊ Contact dermatitis (due to topical agents used to self-treat)
  ◊ Neurodermatitis

LABORATORY
Culture stasis ulcers if you decide to use antibiotics (use of antibiotics topically or systemically is controversial)
Drugs that may alter lab results: N/A
Disorders that may alter lab results: N/A

PATHOLOGICAL FINDINGS
Chronic inflammation

SPECIAL TESTS
Culture ulcer base or prurient crusted areas to determine whether secondary infection is present

IMAGING
N/A

DIAGNOSTIC PROCEDURES
N/A

 TREATMENT

APPROPRIATE HEALTH CARE
• Outpatient
• Inpatient for vein stripping or skin grafts

GENERAL MEASURES
• Reduce edema:
  ◊ Leg elevation - heels higher than knees, knees higher than hips
• Elastic bandage wraps - Ace bandages or Unna's paste boot (zinc gelatin) if lesions are dry or compression stockings (Jobst or non-fitted type)
  ◊ Diuretic therapy
• Treat infection:
  ◊ S. aureus or beta-hemolytic streptococcus, treat with oral antibiotics
  ◊ Gram-negative colonization, treat with topical antimicrobial agents (e.g., benzoyl peroxide, acetic acid, silver nitrate, or Hibiclens) or broad-spectrum topical antibiotics (e.g., neomycin or Polysporin)
• Debride the ulcer base of necrotic tissue

SURGICAL MEASURES
N/A

ACTIVITY
• Avoid standing still
• Stay active
• Elevate foot of bed unless contraindicated

DIET
No special diet. Lose weight, if overweight.

PATIENT EDUCATION
• Stress staying active to keep circulation and leg muscles in good condition. Walking is ideal.
• Keeping legs elevated while sitting or lying
• Don't wear girdles, garters, or pantyhose with tight elastic tops
• Don't scratch
• Elevate foot of bed with 2-4 inch blocks

MEDICATIONS

DRUG(S) OF CHOICE
• 5% aluminum acetate solution (Burow's) wet dressings and cooling pastes
• Topical triamcinolone 0.1% (Kenalog, Aristocort) cream/ointment tid or topical betamethasone
• Betamethasone valerate 0.1% (Valisone) cream/ointment/solution tid
• Topical antipruritic - pramoxine, camphor, menthol, doxepin
Contraindications: N/A
Precautions: Refer to manufacturer's literature
Significant possible interactions: N/A

ALTERNATIVE DRUGS
• Consider antibiotics on basis of culture results of exudate from ulcer craters
• Lubricants when dermatitis is quiescent
• Antipruritic medications

FOLLOWUP

PATIENT MONITORING   If Unna's boot is used - cut off and reapply boot once a week (restricts edema and prevents scratching)

PREVENTION/AVOIDANCE
• Avoid recurrence of edema with compression stockings
• Topical lubricants twice daily to prevent fissuring and itching

POSSIBLE COMPLICATIONS
• Secondary bacterial infection
• Deep vein thrombus
• Bleeding at dermatitis sites
• Squamous cell carcinoma in edges of long standing stasis ulcers
• Scarring, which in turn leads to further compromise to blood flow and increased likelihood of minor trauma

EXPECTED COURSE/PROGNOSIS
Chronic course with intermittent exacerbations and remissions

MISCELLANEOUS

ASSOCIATED CONDITIONS
• Varicose veins
• Other eczematous disease

AGE-RELATED FACTORS
Pediatric: N/A
Geriatric: Common in this age group
Others: N/A

PREGNANCY   N/A

SYNONYMS
• Gravitational eczema
• Varicose eczema
• Venous dermatitis

ICD-9-CM   454.1 Stasis dermatitis

SEE ALSO   Varicose veins

OTHER NOTES   N/A

ABBREVIATIONS   N/A

REFERENCES
• Prystowsky JH, Cohen PR: Venous stasis ulcers. In: Sams WM Jr, Lynch PR, eds. Principles and Practices of Dermatology. New York, Churchill Livingstone, 1990
• Fitzpatrick TB, et al, eds: Dermatology In General Medicine, 3rd Ed. New York, McGraw-Hill, 1987
• Sauer GC: Manual of Skin Diseases. 6th Ed. Philadelphia, J.B. Lippincott, 1991
Illustrations: 9 available on CD-ROM
Internet references: http://www.5mcc.com

Author(s)
Joseph A. Florence, MD

Diabetes insipidus

BASICS

DESCRIPTION Defective regulation of water balance secondary to decreased secretion of, or failure of response to, vasopressin
• Inadequate secretion of vasopressin may be due to loss of or malfunction of the neurosecretory neurons that make up the neurohypophysis (posterior pituitary)
• Insensitivity to vasopressin - a disorder of renal tubular function resulting in inability to respond to vasopressin in absorption of water
• Excessive water intake - (primary polydipsia) usually of functional origin
System(s) affected: Endocrine/Metabolic
Genetics: Familial cases of vasopressin deficiency have been reported (commonly autosomal dominant) but the disease is usually isolated, and often secondary to other disorders.
• Nephrogenic diabetes insipidus (insensitivity to vasopressin)- usually inherited (sex linked recessive), expressed in males, rarely in females
Incidence/Prevalence in USA: N/A
Predominant age:
• Vasopressin deficiency may occur at any age including infancy and childhood
• Nephrogenic diabetes insipidus is usually manifest in infancy
Predominant sex: Nephrogenic diabetes insipidus is encountered in males with rare exception, reflecting its X-linked recessive mode of inheritance

SIGNS AND SYMPTOMS
• Thirst/polydipsia
• Polyuria
• Nocturia
• Dehydration
• Headache
• Visual disturbance

CAUSES
• Inadequate secretion of vasopressin: a variety of pathological lesions may produce damage including tumors (craniopharyngioma, lymphoma, metastasis); infections (meningitis, encephalitis), trauma, granulomas (sarcoid, histiocytosis), or vascular disorders. Some are idiopathic or familial.
• Excessive water intake (psychogenic)
• Insensitivity to vasopressin: genetic defect in resorption of water in renal tubule (collecting ducts)
• Drugs: Lithium, demeclocycline, and methoxyflurane may produce nephrogenic diabetes insipidus

RISK FACTORS N/A

DIAGNOSIS

DIFFERENTIAL DIAGNOSIS
• Diabetes mellitus and other causes of polydipsia and polyuria
• Increased solute load for excretion as occurs with high salt intake
• Psychogenic polydipsia (ultimately impairs vasopressin secretion)
• Nephrogenic diabetes insipidus (differentiate from vasopressin deficiency by clinical trial of desmopressin [DDAVP])

LABORATORY
• Hypernatremia (presenting manifestation, particularly in infants and children)
• Inability to concentrate urine (measure by osmolality, rather than specific gravity)
• Urinary glucose (to rule out diabetes mellitus)
• Plasma vasopressin or urinary vasopressin following osmotic stimulus, such as fluid restriction or administration of hypertonic saline
Drugs that may alter lab results: Lithium, demeclocycline and methoxyflurane may produce vasopressin insensitivity
Disorders that may alter lab results: Hypokalemia and hypercalcemia alter ability to concentrate urine

PATHOLOGICAL FINDINGS
Degeneration and death of neurosecretory neurons in the neurohypophysis

SPECIAL TESTS
• Testing ability to concentrate urine in face of water deprivation should be done by measuring urine and plasma osmolality before and after a six hour period of thirst. This should be done during the day. It is not wise to do overnight thirst tests, particularly in children.
• The most valuable measurements are the urine/plasma osmolal ratio and plasma vasopressin concentrations. The results are sometimes difficult to interpret since low ratios may be found in patients with primary polydipsia. If results support the diagnosis, desmopressin should be administered to test renal concentrating ability.

IMAGING If the diagnosis of diabetes insipidus is made, appropriate studies for cause including imaging of the brain must be performed

DIAGNOSTIC PROCEDURES Fluid deprivation to concentrate urine

TREATMENT

APPROPRIATE HEALTH CARE Initial diagnosis and management may require hospitalization. Continuing care is provided on an outpatient basis with self-medication.

GENERAL MEASURES
• Control fluid balance and prevent dehydration
• Check weight daily
• Provide good skin and mouth care

SURGICAL MEASURES N/A

ACTIVITY Not restricted

DIET Normal with free access to fluids except that young infants with nephrogenic diabetes insipidus may benefit from low solute formula

PATIENT EDUCATION
• Administration and dosage of intranasal desmopressin
• Importance of having access to fluids as thirst dictates
• Wear a medical identification neck tag or bracelet

Diabetes insipidus

MEDICATIONS

DRUG(S) OF CHOICE
• Central (vasopressin deficient) diabetes insipidus - desmopressin (DDAVP) (a derivative of vasopressin) given intranasally two times daily in dosage necessary to control polyuria or polydipsia usually (10-25 µg) or 2-4 µg parenterally in 2 divided doses
• Nephrogenic diabetes insipidus - thiazide diuretics
Contraindications: Desmopressin should be used with caution in the immediate postoperative period for intracranial lesions because of possible cerebral edema
Precautions: Overdose of desmopressin may produce water intoxication in patients with excessive water intake
Significant possible interactions: See manufacturer's profile of each drug

ALTERNATIVE DRUGS
• Chlorpropamide (Diabinese) 250-500 mg/day reduces polyuria and polydipsia
• Clofibrate (Atromid-S) at a maximum dose of 1 gm tid also has an antidiuretic effect
• Hydrochlorothiazide 50 mg/day
Note: The effects of these alternate drugs are not as predictable as desmopressin

FOLLOWUP

PATIENT MONITORING
• Requires regular followup at intervals of 2-3 weeks initially and 3-4 months later
• Adjustment of treatment based on the urine and electrolyte concentrations and patient's symptoms

PREVENTION/AVOIDANCE Avoid
situations of marked increase in water loss. Take fluids as dictated by thirst with no water restriction.

POSSIBLE COMPLICATIONS
• Dilatation of urinary tract has been observed (probably secondary to large volume of urine)
• Complications of primary disease (tumor histiocytosis, etc.) should be anticipated
• In nephrogenic diabetes, there is an associated retardation of mental development in some patients (cause undetermined)
• Subnormal growth rate

EXPECTED COURSE/PROGNOSIS
• Condition is usually permanent, although an occasional case following trauma or tumor goes into permanent remission
• Prognosis of diabetes insipidus per se is good depending on underlying disorder
• Without treatment, dehydration can lead to confusion, stupor and coma

MISCELLANEOUS

ASSOCIATED CONDITIONS
• Infection (e.g., encephalitis, tuberculosis, syphilis)
• Tumors
• Xanthomatosis
• Pyelonephritis
• Renal amyloidosis
• Potassium depletion
• Sjögren's syndrome
• Sickle cell anemia
• Chronic hypercalcemia
• Wolfram syndrome (DIDMOAD)

AGE-RELATED FACTORS
Pediatric: Nephrogenic diabetes insipidus is usually manifest in infancy
Geriatric: N/A
Others: N/A

PREGNANCY N/A

SYNONYMS N/A

ICD-9-CM
253.5 Diabetes insipidus

SEE ALSO N/A

OTHER NOTES N/A

ABBREVIATIONS
• DI = diabetes insipidus
• DIDMOAD = diabetes insipidus, diabetes mellitus, optic atrophy and deafness

REFERENCES Robertson G: Posterior
Pituitary Hormones. In: Felig P, Baxter JD, Broadus AE, Frohman LA, eds. Endocrinology and Metabolism. New York, McGraw-Hill, 1995:385
Illustrations: N/A
Internet references: http://www.5mcc.com

Author(s)
William W. Cleveland, MD

Diabetes mellitus, insulin-dependent (IDDM or Type I)

BASICS

DESCRIPTION A chronic disease caused by pancreatic insufficiency (deficiency) of insulin production, resulting in hyperglycemia and end-organ complications such as accelerated atherosclerosis, neuropathy, nephropathy, and retinopathy. Features include:
• Patients insulinopenic and require insulin
• Prone to ketosis
• Usually of rapid onset
• Nutritional status - normal or thin
• Disease lability
• Response to oral drugs uncommon
• Seasonability: January-April are peak onset periods (children less than 6 years old have greater degree of seasonability)
System(s) affected: Endocrine/Metabolic
Genetics:
• Mode of genetic expression not clear
• Genes located on major histocompatibility complex on chromosome 6
• HLA DR3 and DR4 are individually associated with increased risk factor of 4; if carrying both susceptibility genes, relative risk factor increases to 12
• HLA B8 and B15 also associated with increased risk
Incidence/Prevalence: Incidence of 15 out of 100,000 per year. Racial predilection for Caucasian American. African-Americans have lowest overall incidence of Type I diabetes.
Predominant age: Mean age of onset 8-12 years, peaking in adolescence; onset about 1.5 years earlier in girls than boys. Rapid decline in incidence after adolescence.
Predominant sex: Male = Female

SIGNS AND SYMPTOMS
• Polyuria and polydipsia
• Polyphagia is classic, but not common
• Anorexia is commonly observed
• Weight loss (usually from 10-30%, and often almost devoid of body fat at time of diagnosis)
• Increased fatigue
• Decreased energy levels and lethargy
• Muscle cramps
• Irritability and emotional lability
• Vision changes, such as blurriness
• Altered school and work performance
• Headaches
• Anxiety attacks
• Chest pain and occasional difficult breathing
• Abdominal discomfort and pain
• Nausea
• Diarrhea or constipation

CAUSES
• The inherited defect causes an alteration in immunologic integrity, placing the beta cell at special risk for inflammatory damage. The mechanism of damage is autoimmune.
• Environmental factors include:
◊ Viruses (such as mumps, Coxsackie, CMV, and hepatitis viruses)
◊ Dietary factors - breast feeding may provide a degree of protection against the disease while diets high in dairy products are associated with increased risk
◊ Possible risk in diets high in nitrosamines

◊ Environmental toxins
◊ Emotional and physical stress

RISK FACTORS
• Certain HLA types (see above)
• Presence of a specific 64K protein which may be responsible for antibody formation
• Increased risk when either insulin-dependent or non-insulin dependent diabetes present in any first-degree relatives

DIAGNOSIS

DIFFERENTIAL DIAGNOSIS
• Benign renal glycosuria
• Glucose intolerance
• Type II (non-insulin-dependent) diabetes mellitus - a small number of children might have MODY (maturity-onset diabetes of the young)
• Infantile-onset diabetes mellitus
• Secondary diabetes
◊ Pancreatic disease (pancreatitis, cystic fibrosis)
◊ Hormonal disorders (pheochromocytoma, multiple endocrine adenomatosis)
◊ Inborn errors of metabolism (glycogen storage disease, Type I)
◊ Genetic disorders with insulin resistance (acanthosis nigricans)
◊ Hereditary neuromuscular disease
◊ Progeroid syndromes
◊ Obesity (Prader-Willi syndrome)
◊ Cytogenetic syndromes (trisomy 21, Klinefelter's and Turner's syndromes)
◊ Drug or chemical-induced glucose intolerance (see list below)
◊ Acute poisonings (salicylate poisoning can be associated with hyperglycemia and glycosuria, and may mimic diabetic ketoacidosis)

LABORATORY
• Blood glucose
• Electrolytes
• Venous pH
• U/A for glucose and ketones
• CBC (WBC may be elevated)
• Hemoglobin Alc level
• C-peptide insulin level
• Islet-cell antibodies
• T4 and thyroid antibodies
Drugs that may alter lab results:
• The following may cause hyperglycemia (particularly in patients prone to diabetes)
◊ Hormones: glucagon, glucocorticoids, growth hormone, epinephrine, estrogen and progesterone (oral contraceptives), thyroid preparations
◊ Drugs: thiazide diuretics, furosemide, acetazolamide, diazoxide, beta-blockers, alpha-agonists, calcium channel blockers, phenytoin, phenobarbital sodium, nicotinic acid, cyclophosphamide, l-asparaginase, epinephrine-like drugs (decongestants and diet pills), nonsteroidal anti-inflammatory agents, nicotine, caffeine, sugar-containing syrups, fish oils

Disorders that may alter lab results: See Differential Diagnosis

PATHOLOGICAL FINDINGS Inflammatory changes with lymphocytic infiltration around the Islets of Langerhans, or islet cell destruction

SPECIAL TESTS
• Oral glucose tolerance test (possibly with insulin levels, if diagnosis is questionable)
• Intravenous glucose test (for possible early detection of subclinical diabetes)
• Consider HLA-typing

IMAGING None indicated

DIAGNOSTIC PROCEDURES N/A

TREATMENT

APPROPRIATE HEALTH CARE
• Initial care: inpatient stabilization versus outpatient management, preferably in a diabetes unit where a team approach is used
• If in diabetic ketoacidosis (DKA): initially IV fluids and IV insulin until stable, then restore electrolyte and acid-base balance, correct hyperglycemia, prevent hypoglycemia and hypokalemia, risk of cerebral edema
• Remaining health care is done by the family at home. Encourage the child to do as much self-care as possible.

GENERAL MEASURES
• Overall "control" of carbohydrate metabolism for the very young child:
◊ Normoglycemia (adjusted for age) "tight" control with striving for blood glucose levels in range of 80-150 mg/dL (4.4-8.3 mmol/L) all the time, might be dangerous (risk of repeated hypoglycemia)
◊ Hemoglobin Alc level as close to the normal (nondiabetic) range as possible
• Overall good health
◊ Asymptomatic
◊ Normal appearance
◊ Try to keep lipid profile normal
• Normal growth and development
◊ Reach optimal height for genetic potential
◊ Appropriate and timely pubertal maturation
◊ Coping psychosocial development: Normal school or work attendance and performance. Normal future goals and career plans.
• Prevent acute complications
◊ Hypoglycemic insulin reactions
◊ Ketoacidosis
• Delay or prevent chronic complications

SURGICAL MEASURES N/A

ACTIVITY
• All normal activities, including full participation in sports activities
• Regular, rather than periodic, aerobic exercise is preferable

Diabetes mellitus, insulin-dependent (IDDM or Type I)

DIET Appropriate diabetes exchange (ADA) diet for age (carbohydrate-50%, protein-20%, fat-30%)

PATIENT EDUCATION
• Complete initial education and ongoing education for patient and family. Team approach is ideal, if available
• For a listing of sources for patient education materials favorably reviewed on this topic, physicians may contact: American Academy of Family Physicians Foundation, P.O. Box 8418, Kansas City, MO 64114, (800)274-2237, ext. 4400

MEDICATIONS

DRUG(S) OF CHOICE
• Insulin (U-100)
  ◊ Source: Human (Humulin) or pure pork
  ◊ Type: NPH, Lente, Regular, Ultralente, 70/30 premixture
• Insulin regimens (given subcutaneously)
  ◊ 2 dose: NPH/Lente and Regular often in a 2:1 ratio before breakfast and before supper). AM dose usually 1/2 to 2/3 of total daily insulin dose.
  ◊ 3 dose: NPH/Lente and regular before breakfast; supper dose of regular; and bedtime dose of NPH/Lente (this regimen may prevent the dawn or Somogyi phenomenon)
  ◊ 4 dose: regular insulin before breakfast, lunch, and supper, and NPH/Lente at bedtime
  ◊ Insulin pump (external) therapy: in select patients, giving basal hourly insulin, 50% of total daily needs; pre-meal boluses, before 3 meals and bedtime snack; all insulin given is regular insulin
Contraindications: None
Precautions: Avoid hypoglycemia, the dawn phenomenon, and Somogyi syndrome (rebound hyperglycemia)
Significant possible interactions:
• Beta-blockers may mask symptoms of hypoglycemia and delay return to normoglycemia

ALTERNATIVE DRUGS
• Oral hypoglycemics usually not indicated in Type I diabetes (unless an obese patient, who may have MODY; or a combination of Type I and Type II)
• Immunosuppressants
  ◊ Cyclosporine: reduces rate of autoimmune beta cell destruction, must be started in initial weeks after the diagnosis of diabetes is made (studies: at 1 year, 20% of cyclosporine-treated patients on no insulin, compared to 12-15% of placebo controls; after 1 year, progressive decline in beta cell function and loss of remission. Toxic side effects include renal disease, hypertension, lymphoma formation.
  ◊ Other interventional drugs being studied - azathioprine, steroids, nicotinamide

FOLLOWUP

PATIENT MONITORING
• Initially, frequent outpatient followup visits till stable; every 2-3 months thereafter. Monitor height, weight, sexual maturation.
• Daily home blood glucose monitoring with home blood glucose meter (One-Touch, Accuchek, Glucometer, Exactech, Answer, etc.) 3-4 times daily, with adjustment/supplementation of insulin dose based on blood glucose levels
• Periodic (about every 3 months) measurement of hemoglobin A1c to assess overall glycemic control
• Yearly measurement of serum lipids and thyroid function
• Regular review and update of dietary management. Adjust for increased caloric needs for age, level of physical activity, pubertal growth spurt, changes in weight.

PREVENTION/AVOIDANCE   None known

POSSIBLE COMPLICATIONS
• Microvascular disease (retinopathy, nephropathy, neuropathy)
• Hyperlipidemia
• Macrovascular disease (coronary and cerebral artery disease)
• Foot problems
• Hypoglycemia
• Diabetic ketoacidosis
• Excessive weight gain
• Psychologic problems related to chronic disease

EXPECTED COURSE/PROGNOSIS
• Initial remission or "honeymoon" phase with decreased insulin needs and easier overall control, usually lasts 3-6 months and rarely beyond a year
• Progression to "total diabetes" when endogenous insulin is insignificant; usually is gradual, but a major stress or illness may bring it on more acutely
• Current prognosis
  ◊ Increasing longevity and "quality of life" with careful blood glucose monitoring and improvement in insulin delivery regimens and systems
  ◊ At this time, probable reduced life expectancy, but this has improved dramatically over the past 20 years
  ◊ Continue to be optimistic about advances in understanding diabetes that may prevent or minimize complications

MISCELLANEOUS

ASSOCIATED CONDITIONS
• Other autoimmune diseases such as hypothyroidism and Addison's Disease (screening regularly for hypothyroidism particularly important in females, who have a much higher incidence of this already)
• Diabetes mellitus can also be seen as part of multiple endocrine adenomatosis

AGE-RELATED FACTORS
Pediatric: More prevalent in this age. Over the past 10 years, a larger percentage of very young children (less than 5 years of age) present with diabetes.
Geriatric: N/A
Others: N/A

PREGNANCY
• At the time of embryogenesis, hyperglycemia increases the incidence of congenital malformations. Hence, planning the pregnancy and tightly controlling the blood sugar before conception is important.
• It is now possible to have a safe pregnancy, with vaginal delivery of a term baby (with care by a physician skilled in managing pregnant diabetic patients)

SYNONYMS
• Childhood diabetes
• Brittle diabetes

ICD-9-CM
250.01 Diabetes mellitus without complications, juvenile
250.11 Diabetes with ketoacidosis, juvenile
250.41 Diabetes with renal manifestations, juvenile

SEE ALSO
• Diabetes mellitus, non-insulin dependent

OTHER NOTES   N/A

ABBREVIATIONS
MODY = maturity-onset diabetes of the young

REFERENCES
• Travis L, et al: Diabetes Mellitus in Children and Adolescents. Philadelphia, WB Saunders Co, 1987
• Pediatric and Adolescent Endocrinology. Pediatric Clinics of North America, Volume 34, Number 4, W.B. Saunders Co., August 1987
• Lebovitz HE, ed: Therapy for Diabetes Mellitus and Related Disorders. American Diabetes Association, Inc., 1991
• Clark CM, et al: Prevention and treatment of the complications of diabetes mellitus. New Engl J Med 1995;332(18):1210-1217
Illustrations: 16 available on CD-ROM
Internet references: http://www.5mcc.com

Author(s)
Robert M. Schultz, MD

Diabetes mellitus, non-insulin dependent (NIDDM)

BASICS

DESCRIPTION Non-ketosis prone hyperglycemia and glucose intolerance due to defects in insulin secretion and peripheral insulin action. Accounts for 80% of diabetic cases.
System(s) affected: Endocrine/Metabolic, Nervous, Renal/Urologic, Cardiovascular
Genetics: Strong polygenic familial susceptibility. Concordance is nearly complete in identical twins.
Incidence/Prevalence in USA:
• Incidence:
 ◊ 300/100,000 (males 230/100,000, females 340/100,000)
• Prevalence:
 ◊ 5,000/100,000
 ◊ More common in some groups such as Pima Indians with 35% prevalence
Predominant age: Typically occurs after age 40
Predominant sex: Female > Male in Caucasian populations

SIGNS AND SYMPTOMS
• Related to hyperglycemia and complications including nephropathy, neuropathy, and retinopathy
• Polyuria
• Polydipsia
• Polyphagia
• Weight loss
• Weakness
• Fatigue
• Frequent infections

CAUSES Genetic factors and obesity are important

RISK FACTORS
• Family history
• Gestational diabetes

DIAGNOSIS

DIFFERENTIAL DIAGNOSIS
• Insulin-dependent diabetes mellitus
• Pancreatic insufficiency
• Pheochromocytoma
• Cushing's syndrome
• Corticosteroid use
• "Stress" hyperglycemia

LABORATORY
• Fasting blood sugar (FBS) > 140 mg/dL (> 7.77 mmol/L) on two occasions
• Random plasma glucose ≥ 200 mg/dL (≥ 11 mmol/L) plus classic symptoms of DM (e.g., polydipsia, polyuria, polyphagia, weight loss)
• FBS < 140 mg/dL (< 7.77 mmol/L) plus sustained elevated plasma glucose during at least 2 oral glucose tolerance tests. The 2 hour sample and at least one other between 0 and 2 hours after 75 gram glucose dose should be ≥ 200 mg/dL (≥ 11 mmol/L). Do not do if FBS > 140 mg/dL (> 7.77 mmol/L).
• Hemoglobin A1c is elevated
Drugs that may alter lab results:
Corticosteroids can cause hyperglycemia
Disorders that may alter lab results:
Cushing's syndrome

PATHOLOGICAL FINDINGS N/A

SPECIAL TESTS Glucose tolerance test usually not necessary, except when diagnosing gestational diabetes

IMAGING N/A

DIAGNOSTIC PROCEDURES N/A

TREATMENT

APPROPRIATE HEALTH CARE Regular outpatient follow-up except for complicating emergencies such as severe hyperglycemia, hyperosmolar coma, and severe infections

GENERAL MEASURES
• Home monitoring of blood or urine glucose
• Regular examination for complications: retinopathy, neuropathy, nephropathy

SURGICAL MEASURES N/A

ACTIVITY Regular aerobic exercise can improve glucose tolerance and decrease medication requirements

DIET
• American Diabetes Association (ADA) provides dietary recommendations for NIDDM. The emphasis is on achieving glucose, lipid, and blood pressure goals. Mild caloric restriction is recommended to achieve mild to moderate weight loss (5-10 kg).
• Food choices are similar to Dietary Guidelines for Americans and the Food Guide Pyramid:
 ◊ 10-20% of calories from protein
 ◊ < 10% of calories each from saturated and polyunsaturated fat
 ◊ Remainder of calories from monounsaturated fat and carbohydrates, depending on individual patient factors
 ◊ Sugar is not specifically prohibited

PATIENT EDUCATION
• Education is critical for patients with NIDDM. Include information on the disease, medication treatment, self-monitoring, foot care, physical activity and diet management
• Support groups and classes certified by the ADA are recommended
• The ADA has prepared numerous patient education materials (430 North Michigan Ave. Chicago, IL 60611 or contact local ADA affiliate listed in white pages of telephone directory)

Diabetes mellitus, non-insulin dependent (NIDDM)

MEDICATIONS

DRUG(S) OF CHOICE
• First generation oral agents (avoid in elderly and renal failure):
  ◊ Tolbutamide 500-3000 mg/d in 2-3 doses
  ◊ Tolazamide 100-1000 mg/d in 1-2 doses
  ◊ Chlorpropamide 100-500 mg/d in 1 dose
• Second generation oral agents:
  ◊ Glyburide (Diabeta, Micronase) 1.25-20 mg/d in 1-2 doses (1st 10 mg in AM)
  ◊ Glipizide (Glucotrol) 2.5-40 mg/d in 1-2 doses (1st 20 mg in AM)
  ◊ Glipizide extended release tablets 5-20 mg/day in one dose
Note: All oral agents may be taken with meals except glipizide which should be taken 30 minutes before meals
• Insulin - regular, NPH, Lente, Ultralente in 1 or preferable 2-3 injections per day
• Combination of oral agents plus insulin useful occasionally. Some clinicians add an evening dose of intermediate acting insulin when oral agents fail to control blood glucose levels (e.g., fasting plasma glucose >180 or hemoglobin A1c > 1.5% above normal range). When 2 doses of insulin are required to control glucose levels, oral agents are probably best discontinued.

Contraindications:
• To oral agents: Insulin dependent diabetes mellitus, ketotic patient, pregnancy, history of allergy
• Use caution in liver or renal disease and acute infection or stress

Precautions:
• Warn patients of signs of hypo- and hyperglycemia
• Home glucose monitoring (1-4 times per day) is recommended for most patients taking insulin

Significant possible interactions:
• Drugs which potentiate oral hypoglycemics, e.g., salicylates, clofibrate, warfarin (Coumadin), chloramphenicol, ethanol
• Beta-blockers may mask symptoms of hypoglycemia and delay return to normoglycemia

ALTERNATIVE DRUGS
• Glimepiride: as monotherapy or in combination with insulin. Begin 1-2 mg q AM and increase by 1-2 mg each week to maximum 8 mg q AM. Usual dose range 1-4 mg.
• Troglitazone: Begin 200 mg once a day, increasing each 2 weeks to maximum 600 mg once a day in patients on insulin with poor glycemic control despite doses over 30/mg/day.
• Metformin: 500-850 mg bid-tid; can be used concurrently with a sulfonylurea to improve control/overcomes insulin resistance. Avoid metformin (in situations which increase risk for lactic acidosis): renal insufficiency, radiocontrast agents, surgery or acute illnesses such as liver disease, cardiogenic shock, pancreatitis or hypoxia. Use caution in CHF, alcohol abuse, elderly or with tetracycline.

• Acarbose: 25-100 mg tid at beginning of meals to decrease postprandial glucose peaks. Avoid use in renal insufficiency, inflammatory bowel disease, colonic ulceration or partial bowel obstruction.

FOLLOWUP

PATIENT MONITORING
• Frequency of followup depends on compliance and degree of metabolic control. Every two to four months is typical.
• Review of symptoms and home blood glucose levels
• Hemoglobin A1c
• Funduscopy
• Cardiopulmonary exam
• Foot exam for ulcers, arterial insufficiency, neuropathy
• After five years, perform yearly: Ophthalmologist exam, monitor for proteinuria and renal insufficiency

PREVENTION/AVOIDANCE
Avoidance of weight gain and obesity and maintenance of regular physical activity may prevent or delay NIDDM

POSSIBLE COMPLICATIONS
• Appear to be due to effects of diabetes mellitus on arterial walls in one form or another
• Peripheral neuropathy
• Proliferative retinopathy
• Nephropathy and chronic renal failure
• Atherosclerotic cardiovascular and peripheral vascular disease
• Hyperosmolar coma
• Gangrene of extremities
• Blindness
• Glaucoma
• Cataracts
• Skin ulceration
• Charcot joints

EXPECTED COURSE/PROGNOSIS
• Maintenance of normal blood sugar levels may delay or prevent complications of diabetes
• In susceptible individuals, complications begin to appear 10-15 years after onset, but can be present at time of diagnosis since NIDDM may go undetected for years

MISCELLANEOUS

ASSOCIATED CONDITIONS
• Hypertension is common (strict control may retard renal complications)
• Hyperlipidemia
• Impotence

AGE-RELATED FACTORS
Pediatric: Occasional cases of nonketosis-prone diabetes mellitus have been seen in children

Geriatric: NIDDM is common in the elderly and is a significant contributing factor to blindness, renal failure, and lower limb amputations
Others: NIDDM is generally of adult onset, appearing after age 40

PREGNANCY
Diabetes can cause significant maternal complications and fetal wasting. Intensive management by those skilled in this area has improved the outcome dramatically.

SYNONYMS
• Adult onset diabetes mellitus
• Type II diabetes mellitus
• Nonketotic diabetes mellitus
• NIDDM

ICD-9-CM
• 250.00 Diabetes mellitus
• 250.20 Diabetes with hyperosmolarity
• 250.40 Diabetes with renal manifestations
• 250.50 Diabetes with ophthalmic manifestations
• 250.60 Diabetes with neurological manifestations
• 250.70 Diabetes with peripheral circulatory manifestations
• 250.80 Diabetes with other specified manifestations
• 250.90 Diabetes with unspecified manifestations
• 5th digit 2 = uncontrolled

SEE ALSO N/A

OTHER NOTES N/A

ABBREVIATIONS
• NIDDM = Non-insulin dependent diabetes mellitus
• ADA = American Diabetic Association

REFERENCES
• Davidson MB: Diabetes mellitus. 3rd Ed. New York, Churchill Livingstone, 1991
• Karam JH: Diabetes mellitus: perspectives on therapy. Endocrinology and Metabolism Clinics of North America 1992;21(2)
• American Diabetes Association clinical practice recommendations 1997. Diabetes Care 1997;20(S1): S1-S70
Illustrations: 16 available on CD-ROM
Internet references: http://www.5mcc.com

Author(s)
David S. Gray, MD

Diabetic ketoacidosis (DKA)

BASICS

DESCRIPTION A true medical emergency secondary to absolute or relative insulin deficiency characterized by hyperglycemia, ketonemia, metabolic acidosis, and electrolyte depletion
System(s) affected: Endocrine/Metabolic
Genetics: N/A
Incidence/Prevalence in USA: 46 episodes/10,000 diabetic patients; 2 per 100 patient years of type 1 DM
Predominant age: 0-19 years of age
Predominant sex: Male = Female

SIGNS AND SYMPTOMS
• Polyuria
• Polydipsia
• Generalized weakness
• Malaise/lethargy
• Nocturia
• Nausea/vomiting
• Abdominal pain and tenderness
• Decreased bowel sounds
• Decreased perspiration
• Hypotension
• Hypothermia
• Decreased reflexes
• Coma
• Confusion
• Tachycardia
• Tachypnea
• Fever +/-
• Breath fruity, with acetone smell
• Dry mucous membranes
• Anorexia or increased appetite

CAUSES
• Insulin dependent diabetes mellitus (20-30% in newly diagnosed diabetics)
• Infarction (myocardial) 5-7%
• Infection (30-40%) usually respiratory or urinary
• Idiopathic (20-30%)
• Medication non-compliance
• CVA
• Trauma
• Surgery
• Emotional stress

RISK FACTORS
• Any condition that leads to an absolute or relative insulin deficiency
• History of corticosteroid therapy

DIAGNOSIS

DIFFERENTIAL DIAGNOSIS
• Hyperosmolar non-ketotic coma
• Alcoholic ketoacidosis
• Lactic acidosis
• Acute hypoglycemic coma
• Uremia

LABORATORY
• Blood sugar elevated (usually 250-800 mg/dL [13.88-44.4 mmol/L] range)
• Serum ketosis
• Urine ketosis
• Glycosuria
• Hyponatremia
• Hyperamylasemia
• Hypertriglyceridemia
• Hypercholesterolemia
• Increased BUN
• HCO_3 < 15 (< 15 mmol/L)
• Decreased calculated total body K+
• Metabolic acidosis on ABGs
• Increased serum osmolality
• Increased anion gap
Drugs that may alter lab results: N/A
Disorders that may alter lab results:
• With concomitant lactic acidosis, acetoacetate production may be inhibited in presence of high levels of beta hydroxybutyrate. The nitroprusside reaction, which measures only acetoacetate, may not be strongly positive.
• A very low serum sodium (< 110 mmol/L) suggests an artifact due to severe hypertriglyceridemia
• Severe acidosis gives artificially high K+ level
• Markedly increased serum ketones may cross react and cause a falsely high serum creatinine

PATHOLOGICAL FINDINGS N/A

SPECIAL TESTS
• ECG (especially if MI suspected). May also assist in evaluation of K+ status. Usually shows sinus tachycardia.
• Urine and blood cultures

IMAGING Chest x-ray to rule out pulmonary infection

DIAGNOSTIC PROCEDURES N/A

TREATMENT

APPROPRIATE HEALTH CARE
• Inpatient intensive care. This is a life threatening emergency.
• Goals are to increase rate of glucose utilization by insulin-dependent tissues, to reverse ketonemia and acidosis, and to correct the depletion of water and electrolytes.

GENERAL MEASURES
• IV Fluids adults: 1000 mL over first hour, then 500 mL/hr (approximately 7 mL/kg/hr) x 4 hrs or until dehydration improves, then 250 mL/hour (3.5 mL/kg/hr). Switch to D5 in 1/2 NS when serum glucose < 300 mg/dL (16.65 mmol/l). Expect to give 4-8 L/ first 24 hrs. (Some do not recommend initial IV bolus).
• Pediatric maintenance requirements: 100 mL/kg for first 10 kg, 50 mL/kg for second 10 kg and 20 mL/kg thereafter. Fluid deficit: (Multiply patient's body weight by percentage dehydration). Replace maintenance and deficit evenly over 48 hours.

SURGICAL MEASURES N/A

ACTIVITY Bedrest

DIET Nothing by mouth initially. Advance to pre-ketotic diet when nausea and vomiting are controlled.

PATIENT EDUCATION
• For prevention, careful control of blood glucose (usually HgA1c 7%)
• Monitor glucose carefully during periods of stress, infection, trauma etc.

MEDICATIONS:

DRUG(S) OF CHOICE
- Insulin-initiate infusion at 0.1U/kg/hr
- Potassium
- Bicarbonate
- Phosphate

Contraindications:
- No demonstrable clinical benefit from bicarbonate with a pH > 7.0.
- Hold K+ if > 5.5 (> 5.5 mmol/L)

Precautions:
- Double insulin if no response in serum glucose over first 2 hours
- Must continue insulin until serum bicarbonate and anion gap normalize
- Add dextrose to IV fluid when blood sugar < 300 mg/dL (16.65 mmol/L)
- If using bicarbonate, add 50 mg NaHCO3 to 1L 1/2 NS and give over 2 hours
- Delay K+ administration in patients with inadequate urine output or evidence of diabetic nephropathy
- If blood sugar does not fall by approximately 75 mg % q2h, increase insulin rate
- Taper IV insulin and start NPH/Reg insulin after acidosis clears and patient is eating

Significant possible interactions: For each 0.1 unit of pH, serum K+ will change by approximately 0.6 mEq (0.6 mmol/L) K in the opposite direction

ALTERNATIVE DRUGS N/A

FOLLOWUP

PATIENT MONITORING
- Monitor mental status, vital signs, urine output q 30-60 minutes until improved, then q2-4 h x 24 hrs
- Blood sugar q 1 hr until < 300 mg/dL (16.65 mmol/L), then q2-6h
- K+, HCO3, Na+, anion gap, q 2 hrs
- Phosphate, Ca++, Mg++, q4-6h

PREVENTION/AVOIDANCE
- Monitor glucose closely during stressful situations
- Careful insulin control

POSSIBLE COMPLICATIONS
- Cerebral edema
- Pulmonary edema
- Venous thrombosis
- Hypokalemia
- Myocardial infarction
- Acute gastric dilatation
- Late hypoglycemia
- Erosive gastritis
- Infection
- Respiratory distress
- Hypophosphatemia
- Mucormycosis

EXPECTED COURSE/PROGNOSIS
- DKA accounts for 14% of all hospital admissions for diabetes and for 16% of all diabetic related fatalities
- Overall mortality of 5-15%
- In children < 10 years old, DKA causes 70% diabetes related fatalities

MISCELLANEOUS

ASSOCIATED CONDITIONS Look for complications of chronic diabetes (nephropathy, neuropathy, retinopathy, etc.)

AGE-RELATED FACTORS
Pediatric:
- Occasionally children or adolescents with DKA exhibit marked mental deterioration, including development of coma 4-6 hrs after therapy has begun. Mortality is high.
  ◊ Diagnose by CT scan (cerebral edema)
  ◊ Treat with IV bolus of 1 gram mannitol/kg in 20% solution
  ◊ If no response, hyperventilation to a pCO2 of 28 mm Hg
Geriatric: Must be careful with renal status or congestive heart failure
Others: N/A

PREGNANCY Risk of fetal death with DKA during pregnancy is nearly 50%

SYNONYMS N/A

ICD-9-CM 250.1

SEE ALSO Diabetes mellitus, insulin-dependent (IDDM or Type I)

OTHER NOTES N/A

ABBREVIATIONS
NS = normal saline
ABG = arterial blood gases
D5 = 5% dextrose

REFERENCES
- Isselbacher KJ, et al, eds: Harrison's Principles of Internal Medicine. 13th Ed. New York, McGraw-Hill, 1994
- Bennett JC, Plum F, eds: Cecil Textbook of Medicine. 20th Ed. Philadelphia, W.B. Saunders Co., 1996
- Bell DS, et al: Diabetic ketoacidosis: Why early detection and aggressive treatment are crucial. Postgrad Med 1997;101(9):193-200
Illustrations: N/A
Internet references: http://www.5mcc.com

Author(s)
Stoney A. Abercrombie, MD

Diarrhea, acute

 BASICS

DESCRIPTION Diarrhea of abrupt onset in a healthy individual is most often related to an infectious process. A variety of symptoms are often observed, including frequent passage of loose or watery stools, fever, chills, anorexia, vomiting and malaise.
• Acute viral diarrhea - the most common form, usually occurs for 1-3 days, and is self-limited. It causes changes in the small intestine cell morphology such as villous shortening and an increase in the number of crypt cells.
• Bacterial diarrhea - may be suspected if there is a history of a similar and simultaneous illness in individuals who have shared contaminated food with the patient. Diarrhea developing within 12 hours of the meal is most likely due to ingestion of a preformed toxin.
• Protozoal infections - such as Giardia lamblia cause prolonged, watery diarrhea that often afflicts travelers returning from endemic areas where the water supply has been contaminated.
• Traveler's diarrhea - typically begins three to seven days after arrival in a foreign location and is generally quite acute
System(s) affected: Gastrointestinal, Endocrine/Metabolic
Genetics: N/A
Incidence/Prevalence: N/A
Predominant age: All ages
Predominant sex: N/A

SIGNS AND SYMPTOMS
• Loose liquidy stools +/- blood or mucus
• Fever
• Abdominal pain and distension
• Headache
• Anorexia
• Malaise
• Vomiting
• Myalgia
• With Giardia - cramping, pale-greasy stools, fatigue, weight loss, chronicity

CAUSES
• Bacterial
  ◊ E. coli
  ◊ Salmonella
  ◊ Shigella
  ◊ Campylobacter jejuni
  ◊ Vibrio parahaemolyticus
  ◊ Vibrio cholerae
  ◊ Yersinia enterocolitica
• Viral
  ◊ Rotavirus
  ◊ Norwalk virus
• Parasitic
  ◊ Giardia lamblia
  ◊ Cryptosporidium
  ◊ Entamoeba histolytica

RISK FACTORS
• Individual from an industrialized country visiting a developing country
• Immunocompromised host

 DIAGNOSIS

DIFFERENTIAL DIAGNOSIS
• Ulcerative colitis
• Crohn's disease
• Drugs (cholinergic agents, magnesium-containing antacids)
• Pseudomembranous colitis secondary to antibiotic use
• Diverticulitis
• Spastic (irritable) colon
• Fecal impaction
• Malabsorption
• Zollinger-Ellison syndrome
• Ischemic bowel
• Gastrinoma

LABORATORY
• CBC - increased WBC with a left shift may indicate an infectious process; decreased hemoglobin/hematocrit may indicate anemia from blood loss
• Serum electrolytes - increased sodium from dehydration, decreased potassium from diarrhea
• BUN, creatinine - elevated in dehydration
• pH - hyperchloremic acidosis
• Stool sample - occult blood (present in IBD, bowel ischemia, bacterial infections), fecal leukocytes (present in diarrhea caused by Salmonella, Campylobacter, Yersinia), bacterial culture and sensitivity (for Salmonella, Yersinia, Shigella, Campylobacter), ova and parasites, C. difficile toxin, Ziehl-Neelsen stain (for Cryptosporidium)
Drugs that may alter lab results: N/A
Disorders that may alter lab results: N/A

PATHOLOGICAL FINDINGS
• Viral diarrhea - changes in small intestine cell morphology that include villous shortening, increased number of crypt cells and increased cellularity of the lamina propria
• Bacterial diarrhea - bacterial invasion of colonic wall leads to mucosal hyperemia, edema and leukocytic infiltration

SPECIAL TESTS N/A

IMAGING Abdominal x-rays (flat plate and upright) are indicated in patients with abdominal pain or evidence of obstruction to rule out toxic megacolon and bowel ischemia

DIAGNOSTIC PROCEDURES
Sigmoidoscopy indicated in patients with bloody diarrhea or suspected pseudomembranous or ulcerative colitis

 TREATMENT

APPROPRIATE HEALTH CARE
Outpatient except for complicating emergencies (dehydration)

GENERAL MEASURES
• Replacement of lost fluid and electrolytes
• Clear liquids such as tea, broth, carbonated beverages (without caffeine) and rehydration fluids (e.g., Gatorade) to replace lost fluid
• Packets of rehydration salts (one packet to be diluted in one quart of water); drink until thirst is quenched; will help in replacing lost electrolytes. Treatment of choice for pediatric patients.

SURGICAL MEASURES N/A

ACTIVITY Bedrest

DIET
• During periods of active diarrhea, avoid coffee, alcohol, dairy products, most fruits, vegetables, red meats, and heavily seasoned foods
• After 12 hours with no diarrhea, begin by eating clear soup, salted crackers, dry toast or bread, and sherbet
• As stooling rate decreases, slowly add to diet, rice, baked potato, and chicken soup with rice or noodles
• As stool begins to retain shape, add to diet baked fish, poultry, applesauce, and bananas

PATIENT EDUCATION See guidelines in Prevention/Avoidance

MEDICATIONS

DRUG(S) OF CHOICE
• Loperamide, 4 mg followed by 2 mg capsule after each unformed stool, or bismuth subsalicylate, 30 mL every half hour until 8 doses, may be helpful in mild diarrhea
• If diarrhea persists and a bacterial or parasitic organism is identified, antibiotic therapy should be started:
◊ Giardia: metronidazole 250 mg tid for 5-10 days
◊ E. histolytica: metronidazole 500-750 mg tid for 10 days
◊ Shigella: trimethoprim-sulfamethoxazole 160 mg and 800 mg, respectively, bid for five days, or ciprofloxacin (Cipro) 500 mg bid for 10 days
◊ Campylobacter: erythromycin 250 mg qid for 5 days or ciprofloxacin (Cipro) 500 mg bid for 7 days
◊ C. difficile: metronidazole 250 mg tid for 10-14 days
◊ Traveler's diarrhea: trimethoprim-sulfamethoxazole one double strength tablet bid for 3 days or ciprofloxacin (Cipro) 500 mg bid for 3 days

Contraindications:
• Antibiotics are contraindicated in Salmonella infections unless caused by S. typhosa or the patient is septic
• Avoid alcoholic beverages with metronidazole due to possibility of disulfiram reaction

Precautions:
• Antiperistaltic agents (e.g., loperamide) should be used with caution in patients suspected of having infectious diarrhea or antibiotic associated colitis
• Doxycycline, sulfamethoxazole-trimethoprim, ciprofloxacin - may cause photosensitivity. Use sunscreen.

Significant possible interactions:
• Salicylate absorption from bismuth subsalicylate can cause toxicity in patients already taking aspirin containing compounds and may alter anticoagulation control in patients taking coumadin
• Ciprofloxacin and erythromycin increase theophylline levels

ALTERNATIVE DRUGS
• Doxycycline 100 mg bid for 3 days
• Diphenoxylate-atropine in nonpregnant adults
• Tinidazole or secnidazole for E. histolytica
• Vancomycin for C. difficile infections

FOLLOWUP

PATIENT MONITORING If diarrhea continues for three to five days with or without blood or mucus then consult physician

PREVENTION/AVOIDANCE
• Frequent oversights during foreign travel include brushing teeth with contaminated water, ingesting ice cubes, or eating cold salads or meats
• Avoid uncooked or undercooked seafood or meat, buffet meals left out for several hours, or food served by street vendors

POSSIBLE COMPLICATIONS
• Dehydration
• Sepsis
• Shock
• Anemia

EXPECTED COURSE/PROGNOSIS A
common problem that is rarely life-threatening if attention is given to maintaining adequate hydration

MISCELLANEOUS

ASSOCIATED CONDITIONS
• Diabetes mellitus
• Ileal resection
• Gastrectomy
• Hyperthyroidism

AGE-RELATED FACTORS
Pediatric:
• Rotavirus is a common cause of viral diarrhea in the winter months and is accompanied with vomiting
• Other etiologies include overfeeding, medications, cystic fibrosis and malabsorption
Geriatric: Watery diarrhea in elderly patient with chronic constipation may be caused by fecal impaction or obstructing neoplasm
Others: N/A

PREGNANCY Avoid dehydration since this may lead to preterm labor

SYNONYMS N/A

ICD-9-CM
558.9

SEE ALSO
• Cholera
• Botulism
• Food poisoning, bacterial

OTHER NOTES N/A

ABBREVIATIONS
IBD = inflammatory bowel disease

REFERENCES
• Hirschhorn N, Greenough WB: Progress in oral rehydration therapy. Scientific American 1991;264:5
• Dupont HL, Edelman R: Infectious diarrhea: From E.Coli to Vibrio. Patient Care, May 30,1991
Illustrations: N/A
Internet references: http://www.5mcc.com

Author(s)
Tejal Parikh, MD

Diarrhea, chronic

BASICS

DESCRIPTION The frequent passage of loose stools greater than 200 grams per day for more than 3 weeks. Understanding of the pathophysiology divides the cause into inflammatory diarrhea, osmotic diarrhea secretory diarrhea, intestinal dysmotility and factitious diarrhea.
System(s) affected: Gastrointestinal
Genetics:
• Celiac sprue may be familial
• Lactose intolerance - increased incidence in certain geographic regions
Incidence/Prevalence in USA: Unknown, but felt to be underdiagnosed, especially in celiac sprue
Predominant age: Determined by certain illnesses
Predominant Sex: Female > Male

SIGNS AND SYMPTOMS
• Frequent loose stools, fever, abdominal pain, weight loss, tenesmus,
plus
  ◊ Inflammatory: blood (must rule out colonic neoplasm)
  ◊ Osmotic: steatorrhea, azotorrhea, improves with fasting
  ◊ Secretory: large volumes, persists with fasting
  ◊ Altered intestinal motility: alternating diarrhea and constipation, passage of mucus and incomplete evacuation
  ◊ Factitious: peripheral edema, weakness, nausea

CAUSES
• Inflammatory diarrhea:
  ◊ Inflammatory bowel disease (ulcerative colitis and Crohn's disease)
  ◊ Radiation enterocolitis
  ◊ Eosinophilic gastroenteritis
  ◊ AIDS - mucosal and submucosal inflammation with possible impairment in absorption and excessive secretion
• Osmotic diarrhea
  ◊ Pancreatic insufficiency
  ◊ Bacterial overgrowth
  ◊ Celiac disease
  ◊ Lactase deficiency
  ◊ Whipple's disease
  ◊ Abetalipoproteinemia
  ◊ Short bowel syndrome
  ◊ Drugs (colchicine, neomycin, and para-aminosalicylic acid - nondigestible intraluminal solute that exerts an osmotic force increasing the intraluminal fluid overwhelming the colonic mucosal absorptive capacities
• Secretory diarrhea:
  ◊ Carcinoid syndrome
  ◊ Zollinger-Ellison syndrome
  ◊ Vasoactive intestinal peptide-secreting pancreatic adenomas
  ◊ Medullary carcinoma of thyroid
  ◊ Villous adenoma of rectum
  ◊ Microscopic colitis
  ◊ Choleraic diarrhea - excessive secretion of electrolytes

• Altered intestinal motility
  ◊ Irritable bowel syndrome
  ◊ Fecal impaction
  ◊ Neurologic diseases
  ◊ Diabetes - increased transit and possible bacterial overgrowth
• Factitious
  ◊ Laxative abuse
  ◊ Self induced (patient may add water or urine to stool)

RISK FACTORS
• Inflammatory: AIDS, infections, radiation
• Osmotic: infectious, abdominal surgery including cholecystectomy, resection gastric and small bowel, vagotomy, chronic alcohol abuse, Sorbitol, fructose, gluten
• Secretory: distal ileal surgery
• Altered intestinal motility: diabetes, fecal impaction or neurological diseases
• Factitious: laxatives

DIAGNOSIS

DIFFERENTIAL DIAGNOSIS
• Functional disorder
• Inflammatory bowel disease: look for systemic illness or extra-intestinal manifestations (arthritis, pyoderma gangrenosum, erythema nodosum, uveitis or vasculitis); consider Crohn's or ulcerative colitis
• Factitious: psychiatric disease or history of
• Irritable bowel syndrome: alternating diarrhea and constipation
• Tropical sprue
• TB enteritic
• Chronic radiation enterocolitis
• Colonic neoplasm

LABORATORY
• Stool ova and parasites
• Stool leukocytes
• Stool fat and osmolality, and occult blood
• Serum electrolytes and blood count
• serum Iron studies, vitamin B12, folate, vitamin D, PT, blood chemistry for albumin and cholesterol, serum carotene
• D-xylose absorption test
• Biopsies with esophagogastroduodenoscopy (EGD) or colonoscopy when performed
• Inflammatory diarrhea: blood or leukocytes in stool, hypoproteinemia (hypoalbuminemia and hypoglobulinemia)
• Factitious: hypokalemia
Drugs that may alter lab results: Screen for laxative abuse, e.g., phenolphthalein
Disorders that may alter lab results: Unspecified noninfectious gastroenteritis; psychiatric behavior in factitious diarrhea may contaminate stool study

PATHOLOGICAL FINDINGS
• When present, findings are those of the associated or underlying disease
• None seen in functional disorder

SPECIAL TESTS Inflammatory: colonic biopsies

IMAGING Barium enema, KUB
DIAGNOSTIC PROCEDURES
• Colonoscopy for inflammatory lesions and associated occult blood in stool or with iron deficiency
• If barium enema is negative and diarrhea persists, biopsies are required (to rule out microscopic colitis in which the mucosa may appear normal).
• Melanosis coli suggests cathartic abuse
• Thorough history and physical exam helpful

TREATMENT

APPROPRIATE HEALTH CARE Unless electrolyte abnormality, deconditioning or hypotensive, outpatient therapy is adequate

GENERAL MEASURES Fluids with electrolyte supplementation

SURGICAL MEASURES N/A

ACTIVITY Restricted only for the debilitated patient

DIET
• Abstain from gluten products, sorbitol, lactose-containing products
• In IBS, may need to add dietary supplements of hydrophilic colloids (e.g., psyllium or synthetic analogs) to normal bowel action

PATIENT EDUCATION
• Explain in simple terms of bowel physiology
• Reassure that normal frequency varies widely

MEDICATIONS

DRUG(S) OF CHOICE
• Efforts to increase stool consistency may be undertaken using psyllium or other hydrophilic agents
• In secretory diarrhea, opiates may help
• Diphenoxylate-atropine (Lomotil) 5-20 mg daily or loperamide (Imodium) 4-16 mg daily; given in doses calculated and timed according to the patient's individual needs. These agents may be contraindicated in infectious diarrheas because of possible organism enhancement of tissue.
• Kaolin-pectin (Kapectolin, Donnagel) 2-16 tablespoons daily, divided and timed according to individual need
• Specific agents include:
  ◊ Octreotide (Sandostatin) a analogue of somatostatin used in carcinoid syndrome
  ◊ Omeprazole: an H-K-ATPase inhibitor for use in Zollinger-Ellison syndrome
  ◊ Indomethacin: prostaglandin inhibitor used in medullary carcinoma of the thyroid and villous adenomas
  ◊ H1 and H2 receptor antagonists combination for systemic mastocytosis
  ◊ Cholestyramine (Questran) for bile salt malabsorption
  ◊ Lactase (Lactaid, Lactrase) for lactose intolerance
Contraindications: Any impediment to bowel transit, obstruction, ileus
Precautions: Excessive dosage may lead to obstipation
Significant possible interactions: N/A

ALTERNATIVE DRUGS N/A

FOLLOWUP

PATIENT MONITORING If diarrhea persists, further evaluation recommended

PREVENTION/AVOIDANCE Refrain from dietary or pharmacological agents that may precipitate a diarrhea event

POSSIBLE COMPLICATIONS Fluid and electrolyte abnormalities; malnutrition

EXPECTED COURSE/PROGNOSIS
Variable from a short (factitious and altered intestinal motility) and treatable course to a chronic illness (e.g., Crohn's, ulcerative colitis, etc.)

MISCELLANEOUS

ASSOCIATED CONDITIONS See Causes

AGE-RELATED FACTORS
Pediatric: Diarrhea secondary to dietary products, e.g., fructose and apple juice
Geriatric: Patients with life-long diarrhea may suffer increasing difficulty with advanced age
Others: N/A

PREGNANCY N/A

SYNONYMS
• Loose bowels
• The runs

ICD-9-CM
558.9 Other and unspecified noninfectious gastroenteritis

SEE ALSO N/A

OTHER NOTES N/A

ABBREVIATIONS
IBD = inflammatory bowel disease

REFERENCES
• Spiro HM: Diarrhea Diseases. In: Spiro HM, ed. Clinical Gastroenterology. 4th Ed. New York, McGraw-Hill, Inc., 1993:356-358
• Krejs GJ: Diarrhea. In: Wyngaarden JB, Smith HL, eds. Cecil Textbook of Medicine. 19th Ed. Philadelphia, W.B. Saunders Co., 1992:680-687
• Freidman LS, Isselbacher KJ: Chronic Diarrhea. In: Braunwald E, Isselbacher KJ, et al, eds. Harrison's Principles of Internal Medicine. 13th Ed. New York, McGraw-Hill, Inc., 1994:216-219.
• Fine KD, Krejs GJ, Fordtran JS: Diarrhea. In: Sleisenger MH, Fordtran JS, eds. Gastrointestinal Disease. 5th Ed. Philadelphia, W.B. Saunders Co., 1994:1043-1072
Illustrations: N/A
Internet references: http://www.5mcc.com

Author(s)
Guy W. Neff, MD
Samuel Sim, MD

Digitalis toxicity

BASICS

DESCRIPTION A condition that may result from digitalis overdosage, hypokalemia, advanced degenerative heart disease with conduction disturbances, or a combination of factors. Toxicity may develop even when serum levels are within normal range. Usual course - acute; chronic.
Genetics: No known genetic pattern
System(s) affected: Cardiovascular, Nervous, Gastrointestinal
Incidence/Prevalence in USA: Occurs in 5-23% of patients sometime during therapy
Predominant age: Middle age to elderly (40-75 years)
Predominant sex: Male = Female

SIGNS AND SYMPTOMS
• Abdominal pain
• Anorexia
• Bilateral central scotomata
• Bizarre mental symptoms in elderly patients
• Blurred vision
• Bradycardia
• Confusion
• Delirium
• Depression
• Diarrhea
• Disorientation
• Drowsiness
• Fatigue
• Hallucinations
• Halos around lights
• Headache
• Hypotension
• Impaired color vision
• Irregular pulse
• Lethargy
• Loss of visual acuity
• Mydriasis
• Nausea
• Neuralgia
• Nightmares
• Personality changes
• Photophobia
• Restlessness
• Vertigo
• Vomiting
• Weakness

CAUSES
• Alkalosis
• Cor pulmonale
• Hemodialysis
• Hypernatremia
• Hypokalemia
• Hypomagnesemia
• Hypothyroidism
• Myocarditis
• Overdosage
• Poisoning with plants containing cardiac glycosides, such as oleander, foxglove
• Procaine
• Quinidine
• Reserpine
• Steroids

RISK FACTORS
• Anoxia
• Catecholamines
• Diuretics
• Hypercalcemia
• Myocardial infarction
• Recent cardiac surgery
• Renal failure
• Suicide attempt

DIAGNOSIS

DIFFERENTIAL DIAGNOSIS
• Heart block
• Renal disease
• Other causes of life-threatening arrhythmia

LABORATORY
• Eosinophilia
• Increased digitalis level, especially if ≥ 4 ng/mL (≥ 5.1 nmol/L)
• Potassium - hyperkalemia with acute ingestion; hypokalemia with chronic ingestion of excess or chronic renal failure
Drugs that may alter lab results: Any digitalis drug
Disorders that may alter lab results: Many cardiac abnormalities

PATHOLOGICAL FINDINGS N/A

SPECIAL TESTS
• EKG (Note that no arrhythmia is unique to digitalis toxicity, thus any sudden change in cardiac rhythm suggests possible toxicity)
  ◊ Accelerated junctional rhythms
  ◊ Atrial flutter
  ◊ Atrial premature contractions
  ◊ Atrial tachycardia with AV block
  ◊ Bidirectional tachycardia
  ◊ Bundle branch block
  ◊ Junctional premature beats
  ◊ Sinus bradycardia
  ◊ Sinus bradycardia with junctional tachycardia
  ◊ Ventricular fibrillation
  ◊ Ventricular premature contractions
  ◊ Wenckebach's block with junctional premature beats
   ◊ P-R changes
   ◊ Q-T changes

IMAGING N/A

DIAGNOSTIC PROCEDURES N/A

TREATMENT

APPROPRIATE HEALTH CARE Inpatient - coronary care unit

GENERAL MEASURES
• Discontinue digitalis
• Pacemaker insertion for heart block
• Check serum electrolytes; maintain potassium in high-normal range
• Correct calcium and magnesium abnormalities
• Avoid quinidine, which may increase serum digoxin levels by displacing digoxin from its binding sites and by decreasing renal and nonrenal excretion
• Avoid beta-adrenergic blocking drugs and isoproterenol
• Procainamide may be used
• If the patient is hemodynamically stable with primarily enhanced vagal activity (1st or 2nd degree AV block) and if the peak digitalis effect has been reached, no acute therapy is required

SURGICAL MEASURES N/A

ACTIVITY Bedrest with monitoring

DIET Low salt, low fat

PATIENT EDUCATION Griffith, H.W.: Instructions for Patients; Philadelphia, W.B. Saunders Co.

Digitalis toxicity

MEDICATIONS

DRUG(S) OF CHOICE
• Fluid plus electrolyte therapy
• Correct acidity
• Digoxin Immune Fab (Digibind)
◊ Indicated for treatment of severe, life-threatening arrhythmias due to digoxin or digitoxin overdosage
◊ Obtain a digoxin level before administration - be aware that the digoxin level may be falsely high if measured < 6 hours after ingestion
◊ Do not draw another digoxin level for 4 days after digoxin antibody (Digibind) administration since drug's half-life is up to 20 hours in patients with normal renal function
◊ For adults and children ingesting an unknown amount of digoxin, administer 10 vials of digoxin Immune Fab in 50 mL of NS IV over 30 minutes. Observe response and administer an additional 10 vials if clinically indicated. Watch for volume overload in children
◊ For toxicity during chronic therapy: Adults, 15 vials digoxin Immune Fab in 50 mL NSS IV over 30 minutes; children, < 20 kg, 1 vial should suffice
• Lidocaine 50 to 100 mg IV (for ventricular arrhythmias), repeated in 3-5 minutes if needed, up to a total of 300 mg. Give no more than 300 mg in 1 hour. One protocol calls for an initial bolus of lidocaine followed by 20-50 mcg/kg/min infusion for maintenance.
Contraindications: Refer to manufacturer's literature
Precautions: Refer to manufacturer's literature
Significant possible interactions: Refer to manufacturer's literature

ALTERNATIVE DRUGS
• Phenytoin as alternative to lidocaine - 100 mg q 3-5 minutes up to 1000 mg
• Consider atropine, cholestyramine

FOLLOWUP

PATIENT MONITORING
• Close EKG monitoring, potassium and digitalis levels throughout total treatment
• Monitor kidney function

PREVENTION/AVOIDANCE
• Store digitalis safely
• Monitor for toxicity
• Fluid plus electrolyte therapy according to need as determined by periodic studies, particularly of potassium level
• If there is a documentable recent exposure, consider gastric decontamination by lavage and administer activated charcoal
• Symptomatic overdose patients might best be managed by a poison control center or toxicologist

EXPECTED COURSE/PROGNOSIS
Recovery likely if patient survives 24 hours

POSSIBLE COMPLICATIONS
• Death
• Conduction defects
• Life threatening rhythm disturbances

MISCELLANEOUS

ASSOCIATED CONDITIONS
• Chronic heart failure
• Acute pulmonary edema

AGE-RELATED FACTORS
Pediatric: N/A
Geriatric: Morbidity and mortality greater
Others: N/A

PREGNANCY N/A

SYNONYMS N/A

ICD-9-CM 972.1 poisoning by cardiotonic glycosides

SEE ALSO Ventricular tachycardia (VT)

OTHER NOTES N/A

ABBREVIATIONS
NS = normal saline

REFERENCES
• Carter BL, et al: Monitoring digoxin therapy in two long-term facilities. J Am Geriatr Soc 1981;29:263
• Beller GA, et al: Digitalis intoxication: a prospective clinical study with serum level correlations. N Engl J Med 1971;284:989
• Duhme DW, et al: Reduction of digoxin toxicity associated with measurement of serum levels. Ann Int Med 1974;80:516
• Marcus FI: Diagnosing digitalis intoxication. Hospital Med 1990;7:75
• Burroughs Wellcome Co: Digibind product information. Research Triangle Park, NC., 1991
Illustrations: N/A
Internet references: http://www.5mcc.com

Author(s)
Bruce T. Vanderhoff, MD
Bradley Kunz, MD

Diphtheria

BASICS

DESCRIPTION Acute respiratory tract infection caused by Corynebacterium diphtheriae, usually producing a membranous pharyngitis
• Incubation period 2 to 5 days. Infection usually occurs in fall and winter in temperate regions. In the tropics, seasonal trends are less distinct.
• Transmission by respiratory route from infected person or carrier. Humans are the only reservoir.
• Several forms occur:
  ◊ Membranous pharyngotonsillar diphtheria - the membrane is gray, adheres to the pharynx and is surrounded by erythema. The underlying mucosa bleeds when the membrane is removed.
  ◊ Nasal diphtheria - unilateral discharge
  ◊ Obstructive laryngotracheitis - complication when membrane descends into larynx or bronchial tree. When it breaks up in young children, total obstruction of the airway may occur.
  ◊ Cutaneous diphtheria - punched-out ulcer covered by gray membrane (particularly in tropics and among homeless). Peaks August to October in southern United States.
System(s) affected: Pulmonary, Skin, Cardiovascular, Nervous
Genetics: N/A
Incidence/Prevalence in USA: 1.6 in 100,000,000 for non-cutaneous form
Predominant age: Children less than 15 and poorly immunized adults. Diphtheria is a rare condition in the U.S. today. Recent outbreaks have occurred in the new independent states of the former Soviet Union.
Predominant sex: Male = Female

SIGNS AND SYMPTOMS
• Membranous pharyngotonsillar diphtheria:
  ◊ Initially, white to yellow membrane which is easily removed
  ◊ Adherent, whitish-gray, leathery membrane on tonsils or pharynx
  ◊ Removing membrane causes bleeding of mucosa
  ◊ Injected pharynx
  ◊ Membrane may become black due to hemorrhage
  ◊ Sore throat
  ◊ Cervical adenopathy with swelling
  ◊ Malaise and prostration
  ◊ Enlarged, tender cervical and submandibular lymph nodes
  ◊ May progress to edematous, swollen neck (bull neck)
  ◊ Paralysis of soft palate
  ◊ Low grade fever of 37.8-38.8°C (100-100.9°F)
  ◊ Thrombocytopenia and purpura
• Nasal diphtheria:
  ◊ Serosanguineous or seropurulent discharge and excoriations
  ◊ Often discharge is unilateral
  ◊ Often chronic, mild course

• Obstructive laryngotracheitis:
  ◊ Hoarseness
  ◊ Croupy cough
  ◊ Progresses to dyspnea and stridor
  ◊ Labored breathing
  ◊ Thick speech
• Cutaneous diphtheria:
  ◊ On skin, conjunctiva, vulva, vagina, penis
  ◊ Primary cutaneous diphtheria - starts as tender pustule on lower extremity and becomes deep, round, punched-out ulcer covered by grayish membrane
  ◊ Secondary infection of preexisting wound - purulent exudate, partial membrane

CAUSES Corynebacterium diphtheriae

RISK FACTORS
• Crowded living conditions
• Inadequate immunization. In the USA, 22-62% of people age 18 to 39 years and 41-84% of people over 60 years of age lack protective levels of antibody.
• Lower socioeconomic status
• Native Americans
• Alcoholism
• Travelers - outbreaks have occurred in the Ukraine and Russia

DIAGNOSIS

DIFFERENTIAL DIAGNOSIS
• Bacterial pharyngitis including group A streptococcus
• Viral pharyngitis
• Mononucleosis
• Oral syphilis
• Candidiasis
• Vincent's angina
• Acute epiglottitis

LABORATORY
• Gram-positive rods in the pathognomonic Chinese character configuration
• Moderate leukocytosis
• Thrombocytopenia
• Transient albuminuria
• Methylene-blue stains can assist in a presumptive diagnosis in experienced hands
• Culture from nose and throat beneath membrane and have plated on special media; inform lab that diphtheria is suspected
• Should test for toxigenicity of strain
Drugs that may alter lab results: If an antibiotic was used, then 5 or more days may be required for the culture to grow on Loeffler's medium
Disorders that may alter lab results: N/A

PATHOLOGICAL FINDINGS
• Pleomorphic gram-positive rods
• Necrotic epithelium
• Hyaline degeneration

SPECIAL TESTS
• Serial ECG's and cardiac enzymes to detect myocarditis
• Delayed peripheral nerve conduction velocities
• Culture on Loeffler's or tellurite medium is positive in 8 to 12 hours if not previously treated with an antibiotic. Laboratory must be alerted to use one of the special media.

IMAGING N/A

DIAGNOSTIC PROCEDURES
• Culture throat or lesions
• Smear of exudate for gram stain

TREATMENT

APPROPRIATE HEALTH CARE
• Inpatient, initially hospitalized in unit which can monitor cardiac and respiratory status. (Must act on presumptive diagnosis because therapy cannot wait for culture confirmation).
• Isolation until cultures on two consecutive days are negative. The first culture must be taken at least 24 hours after the cessation of antibiotic therapy.

GENERAL MEASURES
• Have intubation or tracheostomy readily available. For laryngeal disease, laryngoscopy is desirable. Intubation or tracheostomy should be considered early for laryngeal disease.
• Avoid hypnotics and sedatives while monitoring respiratory status
• Physical therapy in convalescence for range of motion exercises to prevent contractions

SURGICAL MEASURES N/A

ACTIVITY Bedrest (for at least 3 weeks until risk of developing myocarditis has passed)

DIET Liquid to soft as tolerated

PATIENT EDUCATION Explain aspects of illness and complications

Diphtheria

MEDICATIONS

DRUG(S) OF CHOICE
Both antitoxin and antibiotics are needed for non-cutaneous diphtheria
• Diphtheria antitoxin, equine: Use 20,000 to 40,000 units of antitoxin for laryngeal or pharyngeal disease of less than 48 hours duration, 40,000 to 60,000 units for nasopharyngeal lesions, 80,000 to 120,000 units for extensive disease of 3 or more days duration or swelling of the neck (bull neck). Administer antitoxin by IV infusion over 60 minutes and/or by intramuscular injection. Some experts recommend treating cutaneous disease with 20,000 to 40,000 units of antitoxin while others doubt its value when there are no signs of systemic disease. Antitoxin is obtained from the CDC.
• Erythromycin parenterally or orally, 40-50 mg/kg/day; maximum of 2 grams/day for 14 days
Contraindications: See Precautions
Precautions:
• Equine antitoxin: 7% of patients are sensitive to equine antitoxin and need desensitization. Always test for hypersensitivity to antitoxin prior to its administration.
◊ First, a drop of 1:100 dilution of antitoxin is placed on a scratch on the forearm. If negative, an interdermal skin test is done with 1:1000 dilution (0.02 mL).
◊ A positive reaction is the development of urticaria within 20 minutes of injection
◊ If no reaction, then repeat test with a 1:100 dilution. If person has a negative history for animal allergy, has not previously received animal serum and had a negative scratch test, then 1:100 dilution may be used initially.
Significant possible interactions: N/A

ALTERNATIVE DRUGS
• Penicillin G intramuscularly, 100,000 to 150,000 units/kg/day in four divided doses up to 600,000 units per day
• DL-carnitine 100 mg/kg/day given bid po in children for 4 days in myocarditis (experimental)

FOLLOWUP

PATIENT MONITORING
• ECG, cardiac enzymes and respiratory status. Serial ECG 2-3 times per week for 4-6 weeks to detect myocarditis.
• Elimination of the organism should be documented by three negative cultures at least 24 hours apart. The first culture should be at least 24 hours after the completion of antimicrobial therapy.
• During convalescence, patients should be immunized against diphtheria because infection does not necessarily confer immunity

PREVENTION/AVOIDANCE
• Prevention is by immunization:
◊ Children 6 weeks up to 7 years of age should receive doses at 2, 4, 6 and 15-18 months of age with 0.5 mL of DTaP vaccine IM If the pertussis component is contraindicated then pediatric DT should be used. A booster dose should be given at 4-6 years of age.
◊ Unimmunized persons 7 years of age or older should receive two doses of Adult Td 4-8 weeks apart with a third dose 6-12 months later. 0.5 mL of Td should be given IM.
◊ Subsequently, booster doses with Td should be given every 10 years to all individuals without a contraindication. An alternative strategy is a booster at age 11-12 or 14-16 years and a single adult booster at 50 years of age.
◊ Immunized individuals may develop diphtheria but their course is milder; immunization protects against the toxin, not infection or microbial carriage in the nose, pharynx or skin
◊ Disinfect all articles in contact with patient
◊ Close contacts should be cultured and given antibiotic prophylaxis regardless of immunization status. Previously immunized contacts should receive a booster of diphtheria toxoid. Unimmunized contacts should begin the series. Prophylaxis with erythromycin for 7 days.

POSSIBLE COMPLICATIONS
• Myocarditis (10-25% of patients) may occur early
• Cranial and peripheral neuropathy (2-6 weeks after onset)
• ECG abnormalities in two-thirds of patients, including: bundle branch block, tachycardia, atrial or ventricular fibrillation, extrasystoles
• Right sided heart failure
• Local paralysis of soft palate and posterior pharynx demonstrated by regurgitation of fluids through the nares
• Peripheral and cranial neuropathy affecting primarily motor nerve functions. Motor dysfunction starts proximally and extends distally. Usually slowly resolves.
• Guillain-Barré-like syndrome

EXPECTED COURSE/PROGNOSIS
• 5-10% mortality rate
• Prognosis guarded until recovery
• 5-10% chronicity

MISCELLANEOUS

ASSOCIATED CONDITIONS N/A

AGE-RELATED FACTORS
Pediatric: N/A
Geriatric: N/A
Others: N/A

PREGNANCY N/A

SYNONYMS N/A

ICD-9-CM
032 Diphtheria
032.0 Faucial diphtheria
032.1 Nasopharyngeal diphtheria
032.2 Anterior nasal diphtheria
032.3 Laryngeal diphtheria
032.8 Other specified diphtheria
032.81 Conjunctival diphtheria
032.82 Diphtheritic myocarditis
032.83 Diphtheritic peritonitis
032.84 Diphtheritic cystitis
032.85 Cutaneous diphtheria
032.89 Other
032.9 Diphtheria, unspecified

SEE ALSO N/A

OTHER NOTES N/A

ABBREVIATIONS N/A

REFERENCES
• Rakel RE, ed: Conn's Current Therapy 1997. Philadelphia, W.B. Saunders Co., 1997
• Red Book Report of the Committee on Infectious Diseases, 1997. Elk Grove Village, American Academy of Pediatrics, 1997
• Advisory Committee on Immunization Practices
Illustrations: N/A
Internet references: http://www.5mcc.com

Author(s)
Richard Kent Zimmerman, MD, MPH
Gregory A. Poland, MD

Disseminated intravascular coagulation (DIC)

BASICS

DESCRIPTION Generation of fibrin in the blood and consumption of procoagulants and platelets occurring in complications of obstetrics, (e.g., abruptio placenta), infection (especially gram-negative), malignancy and other severe illnesses
System(s) affected:
Hemic/Lymphatic/Immunologic
Genetics: Homozygous protein C or protein S deficiency
Incidence/Prevalence in USA: Unknown
Predominant age: None
Predominant sex: Male = Female

SIGNS AND SYMPTOMS
- Epistaxis
- Gingival bleeding
- Mucosal bleeding
- Hemoptysis
- Hematemesis
- Metrorrhagia
- Cough
- Dyspnea
- Confusion
- Disorientation
- Stool blood
- Hematuria
- Oliguria
- Fever
- Skin petechiae
- Purpura
- Ecchymosis
- Skin hemorrhagic necrosis
- Localized rales
- Tachypnea
- Pleural friction rub
- Retinal hemorrhages
- Anuria
- Thrombosis
- Stupor
- Peripheral cyanosis

CAUSES
- Coagulation disorder due to widespread activation of clotting mechanism
- Obstetric complications
- Infection
- Neoplasms
- Intravascular hemolysis
- Vascular disorders; thrombosis
- Snake bite
- Massive tissue injury
- Trauma
- Hypoxia
- Liver disease
- Infant and adult RDS
- Purpura fulminans
- Thermal injury

RISK FACTORS
- Pregnancy
- Prostatic surgery
- Head injury
- Inflammatory states

DIAGNOSIS

DIFFERENTIAL DIAGNOSIS
- Massive hepatic necrosis
- Vitamin K deficiency
- Thrombocytopenic purpura
- Hemolytic-uremic syndrome
- Primary fibrinolysis

LABORATORY
- Thrombocytopenia
- Increased partial thromboplastin time
- Increased prothrombin time
- Increased thrombin time
- Decreased fibrinogen
- Increased fibrin degradation product (FDP)
- Decreased antithrombin III
- Positive D-Dimer assay
- Increased bleeding time
- Schizocytosis
- Anemia
- Leukocytosis
- Increased lactate dehydrogenase (LDH)
- Increased BUN
- Decreased factor V
- Decreased or increased factor VIII
- Decreased factor X
- Decreased factor XIII
- Hemoglobinemia
- Hematuria
- Guaiac-positive stools
- Decreased protein C

Drugs that may alter lab results: N/A
Disorders that may alter lab results: N/A

PATHOLOGICAL FINDINGS N/A

SPECIAL TESTS N/A

IMAGING Chest x-ray: Bilateral perihilar soft density

DIAGNOSTIC PROCEDURES N/A

TREATMENT

APPROPRIATE HEALTH CARE Inpatient

GENERAL MEASURES
- Treat underlying condition e.g., evacuation of uterus in abruptio placenta. Broad-spectrum antibiotics for gram-negative sepsis.
- Replacement of blood loss
- Platelet concentrates
- Fresh frozen plasma
- Cryoprecipitate
- Antithrombin III concentrate

SURGICAL MEASURES N/A

ACTIVITY As tolerated

DIET No special diet

PATIENT EDUCATION Griffith, H.W.: Instructions for Patients; Philadelphia, W.B. Saunders Co.

MEDICATIONS

DRUG(S) OF CHOICE
• Anticoagulants (heparin) if clinical findings suggest developing thrombotic complications, but never after head injury
• Broad-spectrum antibiotics for sepsis
Contraindications:
• Head injury
• Hemorrhagic stroke
Precautions: Refer to manufacturer's literature
Significant possible interactions: Refer to manufacturer's literature

ALTERNATIVE DRUGS
For DIC associated with metastatic prostatic carcinoma, consider heparin, aminocaproic acid (Amicar). Do not use fibrinolytic inhibitors (Amicor) unless severe fibrinolysis is documented.

FOLLOWUP

PATIENT MONITORING Closely until much improved

PREVENTION/AVOIDANCE No preventive measures known

POSSIBLE COMPLICATIONS
• Acute renal failure
• Shock
• Cardiac tamponade
• Hemothorax
• Intracerebral hematoma
• Gangrene and loss of digits

EXPECTED COURSE/PROGNOSIS
Related to severity of cause of DIC

MISCELLANEOUS

ASSOCIATED CONDITIONS
Thromboembolic phenomena associated with venous thrombosis, thrombotic vegetations on the aortic heart valve, arterial emboli, neonatal purpura fulminans (homozygous protein C or protein S deficiency)

AGE-RELATED FACTORS
Pediatric: Neonatal purpura fulminans associated with DIC and protein C or protein S deficiency (homozygous)
Geriatric: N/A
Others: N/A

PREGNANCY N/A

SYNONYMS
• Consumptive coagulopathy
• Defibrination syndrome
• DIC

ICD-9-CM
286.6 Defibrination syndrome

SEE ALSO N/A

OTHER NOTES N/A

ABBREVIATIONS
RDS = respiratory distress syndrome
FDP = fibrin degradation products

REFERENCES
• Isselbacher KJ, et al, eds: Harrison's Principles of Internal Medicine. 13th Ed. New York, McGraw-Hill, 1994
• Stites DP, Stobo JD, Wells JV, eds: Basic and Clinical Immunology. 8th Ed. New York, Appleton & Lange, 1994
Illustrations: 2 available on CD-ROM
Internet references: http://www.5mcc.com

Author(s)
Stan G. Smith, MA, MB, FCFPC

Dissociative disorders

BASICS

DESCRIPTION A sudden change in state of consciousness, identity, motor behavior, thoughts, feelings and perception of external reality to such an extent that these functions do not operate congruently. Many pathologic symptoms can be found, but the patient experiences dysphoria, suffering, and maladaptive functioning. Disorders include:
• Dissociative amnesia
• Dissociative fugue
• Dissociative identity disorder
• Depersonalization disorder
• Dissociative disorder not otherwise specified (NOS). Authors may include somnambulism (sleep-walking disorder), conversion reactions, pseudo-epilepsy and (in some cultures) a variety of possession syndromes.
System(s) affected: Nervous
Genetics: N/A
Incidence/Prevalence in USA: 8-10% of the general psychiatrically ill. As many as 70% of young adults report short periods of dissociative experiences that are self-limiting and resolve spontaneously.
Predominant age: Adolescents and young to middle age adults; rare as a new illness in elderly. If untreated, may linger from childhood into adult and old age.
Predominant sex: Female > Male (2:1)

SIGNS AND SYMPTOMS
• All disorders share:
◊ Symptoms cause significant distress or impairment in social, occupational, or other important areas of functioning
◊ Symptoms are not due to the direct physiological effects of a substance (e.g., drug of abuse, a medication) or a general medical condition (e.g., temporal lobe epilepsy)
Dissociative amnesia:
• One or more episodes of inability to recall important personal information that is too extensive to be explained by ordinary forgetfulness
• Not occurring during another psychiatric illness and not due to effects of chemical substance (drug abuse or medication)
• Not due to a neurological or other medical condition (e.g., head trauma)
Dissociative fugue:
• Sudden unexpected travel away from home or one's customary place of work with an inability to recall one's past
• Confusion about personal identity or assumption of a new identity (partial or complete)
• Above symptoms do not occur exclusively during course of dissociative identity disorder
• Symptoms cause significant distress or impairment in social, occupational, or other important areas of functioning with activities of daily living
Dissociative identity disorder:
• Presence of two or more distinct identities or personality states (each with its own relatively enduring pattern of perceiving, relating to, and thinking about environment and self).
• At least two of these identities or personality states recurrently take control of the person's behavior
• Inability to recall important personal information (too extensive to be explained by ordinary forgetfulness)
• Reports of time distortion, lapses and discontinuities
• Experiencing voices from inside one's head
• Chronic headaches
• History of severe emotional or physical abuse as a child
• Referring to self as "he/she," "we," "us"
• Eating disorders
• Flashbacks
• Feelings of derealization
• Feelings of depersonalization
• Amnesia about important childhood events
• Personal objects and belongings that cannot be accounted for
• Disowning unrecalled behaviors
• Different handwriting styles
• Different signatures and names found in personal diary
• Sudden mood changes
• Sudden behavioral changes, i.e., from adult to young child
• Episodes of déjà vu
• Feeling controlled by "another person" from within
• Self-inflicted violence such as wrist cutting
Depersonalization disorder:
• Persistent or recurrent experiences of feeling detached from, and as if one is an outside observer of one's mental processes or body (e.g., feeling like one is in a dream)
• During the depersonalization experience, reality testing remains intact
• The depersonalization experience does not occur exclusively during the course of another mental disorder, such as schizophrenia, panic disorder, acute stress disorder or another dissociative disorder
Dissociative disorder NOS:
• Predominant feature is a dissociative symptom (i.e., a disruption in the usually integrated functions of consciousness, memory, identity, or perception of the environment) that does not meet the criteria for any specific dissociative disorder. Examples:
◊ Clinical presentations similar to dissociative identity disorder that fail to meet the full criteria for this disorder. Examples include a) there are not two or more distinct personality states or b) amnesia for important personal information does not occur
◊ Derealization unaccompanied by depersonalization in adults
◊ States of dissociation that occur in individuals who have been subjected to periods of prolonged and intense coercive persuasion (e.g., brainwashing, thought reform, or indoctrination while captive)
◊ Dissociative trance disorder: Single or episodic disturbances in the state of consciousness, identity, or memory that are indigenous to particular locations and cultures. Dissociative trance involves narrowing of awareness of immediate surroundings or stereotyped behaviors or movements that are experienced as being beyond one's control.
◊ Possession trance: Involves replacement of the customary sense of personality identity, attributed to the influence of a spirit, power, and associated with stereotyped "involuntary" movements or amnesia.
◊ Loss of consciousness, stupor, or coma not attributed to a general medical condition
◊ Ganser syndrome: The giving of approximate answers to questions (e.g., "2 plus 2 equals 5") when not associated with dissociative amnesia or dissociative fugue

CAUSES
• Physical, emotional, verbal, or sexual abuse in childhood
• Sudden and severe trauma or threat to one's psychological or physical integrity
• Sudden and unexpected exposure to watching others being killed or severely injured (as in an industrial or car accident)
• A preponderance of coping with trauma and internal or inter-personal conflicts by the use of dissociation
• Psychological/social support to cope with the trauma/abuse was not available

RISK FACTORS
• Exposure to neglect, abuse and trauma in one's childhood
• Tendency to cope with life stresses by excessively using an escape mechanism of day dreaming and/or dissociation

DIAGNOSIS

DIFFERENTIAL DIAGNOSIS
• Other mental/CNS disorder: Schizophrenia, depression, anxiety disorder, mania, obsessive/compulsive disorder, identity disorder, phobic disorders, eating disorders
• Other: Extreme sensory deprivation, epilepsy; early phases of dementia, encephalitis, head trauma, migraine, cerebral vascular disease, brain tumors
• Endocrinopathy: Hypoglycemia, hypothyroidism, hyperthyroidism
• Miscellaneous: Huntington's disease, carbon monoxide poisoning, mescaline intoxication, botulism, hyperventilation
• Obstructive sleep apnea, nocturnal myoclonus

LABORATORY Toxicology screening may be helpful
Drugs that may alter lab results: Lithium carbonate may produce hypothyroidism
Disorders that may alter lab results: Patients (especially those with dissociative identity disorder) may present with medical oddities such as fast healing of broken bones, radiographs resembling brain atrophy, brain infarcts, lupus, or abnormal pulmonary function tests.
A variety of symptoms (including blurred vision, nausea and vomiting, rapid heart beat, palpitation, extreme bradycardia, urinary frequency and urgency, extreme changes in levels of blood glucose) may lead to erroneous diagnosis

Dissociative disorders

SPECIAL TESTS EEG to rule out epilepsy and sleep disorders. Polysomnogram to rule out sleep apnea.

IMAGING CT scan and MRI of the head to rule out multiple infarct dementia, brain tumors, and some forms of encephalopathy

DIAGNOSTIC PROCEDURES
• Neuro-psychological testing is helpful in ruling out learning disabilities and cognitive deficits due to early dementia or borderline mental retardation
• Psychological testing helps identify specific psychiatric disorders, personality structure and dynamics
• Dissociation scales help assess the tendency to dissociate in daily living activities
• Sodium amytal interviews (narcoanalysis) and special interviews under hypnosis are useful in selected cases
• Clinician reviews patient's diary for handwriting and signature changes.

TREATMENT

APPROPRIATE HEALTH CARE
• Outpatient, individual psychotherapy
• At times of crisis: intensive hospital-based treatment (as a protection for patients with suicidal or homicidal impulses, and/or self-inflicted violence)
• Use inpatient care to verify diagnosis with special tests and begin treatment program that continues on outpatient basis
• Note: Treatment emphasis on progress in the adaptive functions with daily living activities, symptom alleviation, ego strengthening, prevent regressions

GENERAL MEASURES
• Individual psychotherapy plus behavior modification, narcoanalysis and narcosynthesis, hypnoanalysis and hypnotherapy
• Adjuncts: support groups, group therapy, expressive art therapy, occupational and recreational therapy
• Bibliotherapy and graphotherapy are useful

SURGICAL MEASURES N/A

ACTIVITY Based on patient's condition

DIET N/A

PATIENT EDUCATION
• Self-hypnosis, relaxation exercises and guided imagery
• Encourage patients to read about their condition and be inspired by others who have been diagnosed, treated, and recovered, e.g., "A Mind of My Own" by Chris Sizemore, published by W. Morrow, New York, 1989

MEDICATIONS

DRUG(S) OF CHOICE
No medications are specifically curative. The following have been helpful:
• Antidepressants: depression
• Benzodiazepines: anxiety and insomnia
• Propranolol 80-400 mg/day: flashbacks and other dissociative symptoms
• Neuroleptics (in low doses): self-abusive behavior. Thioridazine 10-200 mg/day; haloperidol 2-10 mg/day; chlorprothixene 3-200 mg/day, and perphenazine 4-22 mg/day or risperidone 1-4 mg/day.
• In severe agitation, droperidol 1-5 mg IM is effective in producing calm sleep and stopping agitation
• Mood swings, in dissociative disorders, do not respond to the use of lithium carbonate, carbamazepine or divalproex unless patient has co-morbid bipolar disorder
Contraindications: N/A
Precautions:
• Abuse potential of short-acting benzodiazepines
• Overdose/suicide potential with TCA's
• Very low doses of neuroleptics can be used without producing tardive dyskinesia (try to avoid higher doses).
Significant possible interactions: Avoid MAO inhibitors with TCA's or SSRI's

ALTERNATIVE DRUGS
• Buspirone for anxiety 30-80 mg/day
• Clomipramine, 75-200 mg/day or fluvoxamine 100-300 mg/day for obsessive-compulsive symptoms

FOLLOWUP

PATIENT MONITORING
• Outpatients: 1-4 hrs of psychotherapy per week to avoid hospitalization
• Inpatients: more intensive treatment, e.g. daily psychotherapy

PREVENTION/AVOIDANCE
• Child abuse prevention via parent education and community agency intervention
• Crisis intervention following individual trauma or disasters for prevention of chronic morbidity/disability

POSSIBLE COMPLICATIONS
Self-inflicted violence; suicide attempts; substance abuse and chemical dependency

EXPECTED COURSE/PROGNOSIS
• Natural history ranges from spontaneous improvement, in cases of dissociative amnesia, dissociative fugue, and depersonalization disorder, to acute and chronic morbidity in others
• Without treatment, dissociative identity disorder patient may have a healthy functioning facade, with episodes of depression, confusion, mood swings, etc. With age, intensity/frequency of dissociative experiences may decrease and crystallize around 1-2 major personality states.
• Effective treatment produces partial or full recovery for many patients

MISCELLANEOUS

ASSOCIATED CONDITIONS See Causes

AGE-RELATED FACTORS
Pediatric: Suspect abuse or neglect
Geriatric: Decrease in dissociative disorders. Medication side effects more likely.
Others: N/A

PREGNANCY N/A

SYNONYMS
• Hysterical neurosis, dissociative type
• Ganser's syndrome

ICD-9-CM
• 300.15 Dissociative disorder or reaction
• 301.50 Histrionic personality disorder

SEE ALSO N/A

OTHER NOTES N/A

ABBREVIATIONS N/A

REFERENCES
• Michelson LK, Ray WJ, eds: Handbook of Dissociation. New York, Plenum Press, 1996
• Torem MS: Medications in the treatment of dissociative identity disorder. Spira JL, ed. In: Treating Dissociative Identity Disorder. San Francisco, CA, 1996:99-132
• Steinberg M: Handbook for the assessment of dissociation, a clinical guide. American Psychiatric Press, 1995
Illustrations: N/A
Internet references: http://www.5mcc.com

Author(s)
Moshe S. Torem, MD, FAPA

Diverticular disease

BASICS

DESCRIPTION Diverticulosis of the colon and its varied clinical consequences. Diverticuli develop in people in countries eating a low fiber diet and are much more prevalent in western societies.
• Diverticula of colon: Herniation of the colon mucosa through the muscular layer, usually at the site of a perforating artery, lying between two layers of serosa in the mesentery. They are more common in the sigmoid and distal colon and increase in numbers with age.
• Diverticulitis: An abscess or peridiverticular inflammation initiated by the rupture of a mucosal microscopic abscess into the mesentery. Such infection may progress, fistulize into the genitourinary system, obstruct, or spontaneously resolve. Develops in about 5% of subjects with diverticulosis each year. Over a lifetime about half of patients with diverticulosis develop inflammation.
System(s) affected: Gastrointestinal
Genetics: No known genetic pattern
Incidence/Prevalence in USA:
• 2200-3000/100,000 (diverticulitis)
• Up to 20% in general population but increases progressively with age reaching up to 40%-50% in 6th-8th decade
Predominant age: Rare below 40 years, most common in 6th-8th decade
Predominant sex: Male = Female

SIGNS AND SYMPTOMS
• Diverticulosis
 ◊ Only 10-25% of subjects harboring diverticula will develop symptoms (possibly related to coexistent irritable bowel disease)
 ◊ Pain - due to tension in colonic wall, mostly in left lower quadrant, worse after eating, some relief following bowel movement or passage of flatus
 ◊ Diarrhea or constipation
 ◊ Palpable mass in left iliac fossa - firm, tender
 ◊ Abdomen may be distended and tympanitic
 ◊ Absent signs of peritoneal inflammation
 ◊ Melena, hematochezia if diverticula bleed
• Diverticulitis
 ◊ Pain - acute onset, mostly localized in left lower quadrant. Prominently associated with tenderness in same region.
 ◊ Fever with chills as severity increases
 ◊ Anorexia, nausea, vomiting
 ◊ Constipation or diarrhea
 ◊ Rebound tenderness, involuntary guarding, board-like rigidity
 ◊ Palpable mass - tender, firm, fixed
 ◊ Abdomen distended and tympanitic
 ◊ Bowel sounds depressed or could be exaggerated if obstruction ensues
 ◊ Dysuria, frequency if bladder involved
 ◊ Pneumaturia, fecaluria if colovesical fistula develops
 ◊ Rectal exam may reveal tenderness, induration, mass in the cul-de-sac
 ◊ Enterocutaneous, enterovaginal, and perirectal fistulae may be initial manifestation

CAUSES
• Causes are speculative/not clearly proven
• Defects in colonic motility and increased intraluminal pressure, partially brought about by too little fecal volume
• Colonic segmentation - nonpropulsive contractions producing isolated segments or little chambers with high pressure in them
• Low fiber diet - increases segmentation and causes higher intraluminal pressure
• Defects in colonic wall strength
• Cause of bleeding unclear, not related to diverticulitis. Right sided diverticula, though less common, account for 50% of all bleeding from diverticula.

RISK FACTORS
• Age over 40
• Low residue diet
• Previous diverticulitis
• Number of diverticuli in the colon

DIAGNOSIS

DIFFERENTIAL DIAGNOSIS
• Irritable bowel syndrome
• Lactose intolerance
• Carcinoma of distal colon
• Ulcerative colitis, Crohn's disease
• Angiodysplasia (for rectal bleed)
• Ischemic or infectious colitis
• Appendicitis
• Other gynecologic and urologic disorders

LABORATORY
• WBC count normal in diverticulosis, elevated with immature polymorphs in diverticulitis
• Hemoglobin low if bleeding is a symptom
• Sedimentation rate elevated in diverticulitis
• Urine analysis may reveal WBC's, RBC's, pus cells in fistula formation
• Urine culture - persistent infection in colovesical fistula
• Blood culture - positive in diverticulitis with generalized peritonitis
Drugs that may alter lab results:
• Steroids
• Other immunosuppressive drugs
Disorders that may alter lab results:
• Elderly patient
• Lymphomas, other immunocompromised states
• Severe malnutrition

PATHOLOGICAL FINDINGS
• Prediverticular state - myochosis (thickening of circular layer of muscle, shortening of tenia, restriction of lumen)
• Multiple diverticula - spastic colon diverticulosis, simple massed diverticulosis, right sided diverticulosis
• Solitary diverticulum - giant sigmoid diverticulum
• Diverticulitis - inflammation, necrosis, perforation
• Diverticulitis - earliest stage, rupture of a mucosal abscess into mesentery. Does not start with obstruction of the neck as does appendicitis.

SPECIAL TESTS
• 99mTc labeled RBC scan for bleeding (rarely used) and/or angiography
• Gallium or indium labeled leukocytes to localize abscess (rarely used)

IMAGING
• Plain film abdomen supine and upright - useful in peritonitis and perforation
• Barium enema - best means for diagnosis of diverticulosis. Less useful in diagnosis of diverticulitis.
• Diverticuli may be seen on endoscopy, but less sensitive than Barium enema.
• CT scan with or without rectal contrast - diagnostic for abscess, fistula, size and location of inflammatory mass
• Angiography - diagnostic as well as therapeutic in diverticular bleeding
• Fistulograms
• Spinal CT scan with bolus of IV contrast dye may demonstrate bleeding

DIAGNOSTIC PROCEDURES
• Colonoscopy and flexible sigmoidoscopy - helpful in diagnosis of diverticulosis and extremely valuable in differential diagnosis to prove or rule out cancer. Ulcerative or ischemic colitis can uniformly be diagnosed by these modalities.
• Cystoscopy - in colovesical fistula

TREATMENT

APPROPRIATE HEALTH CARE
• Diverticulosis - outpatient with fiber supplements to soften stools
• Outpatient diverticulitis (pain, tenderness, leukocytosis, but no toxicity or peritoneal signs)
• About 2% subjects require hospitalization for toxicity, septicemia, peritonitis or failure to resolve in a few days. About half of these will require surgery.
• Toxic patients require hospitalization and intravenous antibiotics at least until response

GENERAL MEASURES
• IV fluids, analgesics, nasogastric suction
• Indications for surgery - severe diverticulitis, perforation, abscess, fistula, severe diverticular bleeding (requiring more than 2,000 mL of blood in 24 hours), recurrent episodes

SURGICAL MEASURES
• Usual indication related to diverticulitis. Multiple attacks in 2 years, unhealing fistulae, abscess or toxicity may lead to surgery.
• Large pus collections are usually drained radiologically and when resolved, the most involved segment of the colon resected

ACTIVITY Fully active in diverticulosis, restricted activity in diverticulitis

Diverticular disease

DIET
• NPO during acute diverticulitis, progress to fluids, then to high fiber as normal bowel function returns
• All patients with diverticula should increase dietary fiber to high level through foods, and/or fiber supplement if appropriate

PATIENT EDUCATION
• Importance of high fiber diet and recognizing the symptoms of complications at early stage
• Additional material from:
National Digestive Diseases Information Clearinghouse, Box NDDIC, Bethesda, MD 20892, (301)468-6344

MEDICATIONS

DRUG(S) OF CHOICE
• Diverticulosis
◊ Pain syndromes may be treated with antispasmodics - hyoscyamine (Levsin) 0.125 mg or 2 each 4 hours; buspirone (BuSpar) 15-30 mg/day; or meperidine (Demerol) 100-150 mg/day along with high fiber diet
◊ Constipation and diarrhea, manage as indicated for irritable bowel disease
• Diverticulitis
◊ Oral treatment for mild disease - metronidazole (Flagyl) 250-500 mg q 8 hours and amoxicillin 500 mg q 8 hours combination, or ciprofloxacin 500 mg bid. Expect response within 3 days. Continue oral therapy for one week.
◊ More severe cases in hospital - gentamicin 3-5 mg/kg/day plus clindamycin 1.8-2.7 gm/day along with analgesic. Aminoglycoside dose varies with creatinine clearance.
• Diverticular bleeding
◊ Vasopressin 0.2-0.3 units/minute through selective intra-arterial catheter. Used when bleeding demonstrated at angiography.
Contraindications: Hypersensitivity reaction
Precautions:
• Avoid morphine and other opiates except for Demerol
• Watch for renal toxicity and ototoxicity with aminoglycosides
Significant possible interactions: Refer to manufacturer's profile of each drug

ALTERNATIVE DRUGS Tobramycin and metronidazole, 3rd generation cephalosporins

FOLLOWUP

PATIENT MONITORING
• Some physicians would not do any invasive studies; others have recommended repeat barium enema every 3 years if symptoms infrequent or absent, or following corrective surgery
• Colonoscopy, if needed based on above results

PREVENTION/AVOIDANCE High fiber diet, psyllium, agar, methylcellulose

POSSIBLE COMPLICATIONS
• Hemorrhage
• Perforation
• Peritonitis
• Bowel obstruction
• Abscess - paracolic, subhepatic, subphrenic
• Fistula - colovesical, colovaginal, colocutaneous

EXPECTED COURSE/PROGNOSIS
• Prognosis is good with early detection and treatment of the complications
• Of those with a first episode of diverticulitis who are successfully managed medically, up to 67% will not have subsequent attacks requiring hospitalization; 33% will recur. Two or three recurrences in 1-2 years is an indication to electively remove the involved segment of colon.
• Of those with diverticular bleeding, up to 20% will rebleed in a period of months to years

MISCELLANEOUS

ASSOCIATED CONDITIONS Often occurs in conjunction with spastic colon

AGE-RELATED FACTORS
Pediatric:
• Very rare
• When present, it is more aggressive and recurrent in young age
Geriatric:
• More common
• May sometimes be difficult to diagnose
Others: N/A

PREGNANCY Differentiate from ectopic pregnancy

SYNONYMS N/A

ICD-9-CM
• 562.10 Diverticulosis of colon without mention of diverticulitis
• 562.11 Diverticulitis of colon without mention of diverticulitis

SEE ALSO Irritable bowel syndrome

OTHER NOTES N/A

ABBREVIATIONS N/A

REFERENCES
• Rege RV, et al: Curr Probl Surg 1989;26, 133-89
• Sleisenger MH, Fordtran JS, eds: Gastrointestinal Disease. 5th Ed. Philadelphia, W.B. Saunders Co., 1994
Illustrations: N/A
Internet references: http://www.5mcc.com

Author(s)
Frank L. Iber, MD

Down syndrome

BASICS

DESCRIPTION A common form of mental retardation whose cause is unknown. All patients have extra chromosome 21 material; chromosome non-disjunction usually occurs in female meiosis. The syndrome occurs in all races with equal frequency.
• Trisomy 21: 90% of patients, an extra chromosome 21 is found in all cells
• Translocation 21: 5% of patients, extra chromosome 21q material is translocated to another chromosome, usually 13 or 15. For the 5% of translocation trisomies, 1/2 are new, 1/2 have a parental carrier.
• Mosaic 21: 5% of patients, 2 or more cell populations found, usually normal and trisomy 21. Clinical manifestations milder.
System(s) affected: Nervous, Cardiovascular, Skin/Exocrine
Genetics: As above. Extra chromosome comes from mother in > 90% of the cases.
Incidence/Prevalence in USA: 1 in 1000 births
Predominant age: Most identified at birth. Life-span shortened.
Predominant sex: Male = Female

SIGNS AND SYMPTOMS
• Infants and children
  ◊ Brachycephaly (100%)
  ◊ Hypotonia (80%)
  ◊ Posterior 3rd fontanel
  ◊ Small ears, +/- superior ear folds, +/- low set ears
  ◊ Mongoloid slant, eyes (90%)
  ◊ Epicanthic folds (90%)
  ◊ Brushfield's (speckled) spots of iris (50%)
  ◊ Esotropia (50%)
  ◊ Depressed nasal bridge
  ◊ Enlarged tongue (75%)
  ◊ Small chin
  ◊ Short neck
  ◊ Cardiac murmur (50%)
  ◊ Abnormal dermatoglyphics, including single palmar crease, distal palmar triradius, and absence of plantar whorl (ball of foot)
  ◊ Developmental delay, which may not be apparent in 1st year
  ◊ Mild-moderate instability of neck at C1-C2
• In adults
  ◊ Most findings milder, but brachycephaly remains
  ◊ Patients are retarded (IQ = 40-45) but usually personable and cooperative
  ◊ Most adults can care for their personal needs. Some have jobs, but all require a sheltered environment.
  ◊ A small percent of patients have some autistic features. A small percent of patients are non-verbal.

CAUSES
• Genetic - unequal chromosome division
• Genetic - translocation (5% of cases)

RISK FACTORS
• Increases with mother's age:
  ◊ 1/2000, age 20
  ◊ 1/200, age 35
  ◊ 1/100, age 37
  ◊ 1/20, age 45

DIAGNOSIS

DIFFERENTIAL DIAGNOSIS
• Minor familial anomalies such as Mongoloid slant, epicanthic folds and depressed nasal bridge, particularly in a child with hypotonia
• The presence of a whorl on the ball of the foot usually indicates a normal child

LABORATORY A chromosome test is definitive and should always be done because of the chance of translocation
Drugs that may alter lab results: N/A
Disorders that may alter lab results: N/A

PATHOLOGICAL FINDINGS Alzheimer's plaques found in 100% of brains after age 20

SPECIAL TESTS N/A

IMAGING Abdominal ultrasound for urinary tract anomalies in children with pyuria or fevers of unknown origin

DIAGNOSTIC PROCEDURES
• Cardiac echo in all children. A VSD/endocardial cushion defect may not be apparent at birth.
• X-ray of neck for minor trauma, or there is neck pain, long tract symptoms or breathing problems

TREATMENT

APPROPRIATE HEALTH CARE
• Genetic evaluation and counseling
• Cardiac evaluation and ECG
• Appropriate pediatric health care

GENERAL MEASURES
• Parents can usually adapt to a special child
• Most important is to address parental fears and treat the infant normally
• Infant stimulation programs recommended, but definitive proof of effectiveness is lacking

SURGICAL MEASURES N/A

ACTIVITY
• Fully active unless heart disease
• A controlled environment is needed for older children and adults

DIET No special diet. Programs suggesting megavitamin therapy have been disproved.

PATIENT EDUCATION
• National Down Syndrome Congress (800)232-NDSC
• Down syndrome Usenet list serv: listserv@vm1.nodak.edu
• Down syndrome WWW is available for more information, counseling: http://www.nas.com/downsyn

MEDICATIONS

DRUG(S) OF CHOICE N/A
Contraindications: N/A
Precautions: N/A
Significant possible interactions: N/A

ALTERNATIVE DRUGS Current enthusiasm for "neural enhancers", e.g., piracetam, a GABA analog, not proven, but under study

FOLLOWUP

PATIENT MONITORING
• 1 or 2 subsequent genetic visits to complete counseling and a visit at 1-2 years
• Follow cardiac status carefully
• Thyroid and possibly cardiac investigation if growth rate decreased

PREVENTION/AVOIDANCE
• Prenatal chorion villus biopsy at 9-10 weeks and amniocentesis at 13-15 weeks
• A low screening maternal serum alpha-fetoprotein (MSAFP, and abdominal triple screen at 14-16 weeks gestation finds 50-60% of cases
• Prenatal testing recommended for all pregnant females over 35, but this only impacts 25% of cases
• Recurrence:
  ◊ 1% for trisomy 21 if child has trisomy 21
  ◊ Is one-fifth to one-sixth for parents with a balanced translocation
  ◊ If the translocation is 12:21, the recurrence is 100%
  ◊ Increased recurrence in families with mosaic Down syndrome is not clear, but prenatal testing is recommended

POSSIBLE COMPLICATIONS
• Bowel obstruction (fistula, intestinal anomalies [10%])
• Hirschsprung's disease (3%)
• Thyroid disease (hypo-and hyperthyroidism 5-8%)
• Leukemia (0.5%)
• Congenital heart disease (50%) especially endocardial cushion defect, ventricular septal defect
• Alzheimer's disease

EXPECTED COURSE/PROGNOSIS
• Development is normal in the first year in about one-third of cases and mildly delayed in the rest
• Development slows after age 1 and language and cognition are moderately delayed
• The outcome and longevity may be dependent on congenital heart disease
• Some adult individuals can work in protected situations; a few largely independent
• Intestinal complications and congenital heart disease may be of immediate concern
• Hypothyroid disease occurs after 6 months when found, and diminished growth is the principal sign
• Clinical Alzheimer's disease in 1/3 of patients after age 35
• There is premature aging. Most patients die at 50-60, earlier if there is heart disease.

MISCELLANEOUS

ASSOCIATED CONDITIONS N/A

AGE-RELATED FACTORS
Pediatric: N/A
Geriatric: Seldom survive to geriatric age
Others: N/A

PREGNANCY Pregnancy is possible in patients with Down syndrome. The risk for Down syndrome in an infant is 50%.

SYNONYMS
• Trisomy 21
• Trisomy G
• Down's syndrome

ICD-9-CM
758.0 Down syndrome

SEE ALSO N/A

OTHER NOTES Mongolism is a term no longer used

ABBREVIATIONS N/A

REFERENCES
• Behrman RE, Kliegman RM, eds: Nelson Textbook of Pediatrics. 14th Ed. Philadelphia, W.B. Saunders Co., 1992
• Smith D: Recognizable Patterns of Human Malformation. 4th Ed. Philadelphia, W.B. Saunders Co., 1988
Illustrations: N/A
Internet references: http://www.5mcc.com

Author(s)
Paul J. Benke, MD, PhD

Dumping syndrome

 BASICS

DESCRIPTION Gastrointestinal symptoms resulting from rapid gastric emptying. Usually occurs following gastric surgery (gastrectomy, vagotomy, pyloroplasty).
System(s) affected: Gastrointestinal
Genetics: N/A
Incidence/Prevalence in USA: After vagotomy: 0.9% of proximal gastric vagotomy; 10-22% truncal vagotomy
Predominant age: Middle age to elderly
Predominant sex: Male = Female

SIGNS AND SYMPTOMS
Most common to least common:
• Abdominal discomfort, pain
• Diarrhea (postprandial)
• Bloating
• Nausea
• Palpitations
• Diaphoresis
• Weight loss
• Flushing
• Lightheadedness
• Confusion and syncope

CAUSES Multifactorial including:
• Rapid delivery of hyperosmolar material into intestine
• Supraphysiologic release of various peptides/vasoactive mediators
• Reactive hypoglycemia

RISK FACTORS Surgical drainage procedures, particularly gastrectomy; anti-ulcer surgery

 DIAGNOSIS

DIFFERENTIAL DIAGNOSIS
• Mechanical obstruction
• Gastroenteric fistula
• Celiac sprue
• Crohn's disease
• Pancreatic exocrine insufficiency
• Neuroendocrine tumors (e.g., carcinoid)

LABORATORY
• Postprandial hypoglycemia
• Anemia
• Hypoalbuminemia
Drugs that may alter lab results: Insulin
Disorders that may alter lab results: Diabetes mellitus

PATHOLOGICAL FINDINGS N/A

SPECIAL TESTS N/A

IMAGING
• Upper GI series - barium rapidly emptying from stomach
• Nuclear medicine gastric emptying study
• Endoscopy (exclude mechanical obstruction)

DIAGNOSTIC PROCEDURES N/A

 TREATMENT

APPROPRIATE HEALTH CARE
Outpatient except in rare circumstances

GENERAL MEASURES Dietary and medical management

SURGICAL MEASURES Surgery only if dietary and medical management unsuccessful and symptoms debilitating; variable results

ACTIVITY
• No restrictions
• Lying down after eating or when symptoms occur

DIET
• Low carbohydrate
• Frequent small meals with minimal liquid
• Drink fluids between meals only
• High protein diet
• Adequate caloric intake

PATIENT EDUCATION National Digestive Diseases Information Clearinghouse, Box NDDIC, Bethesda, MD 20892, (301)468-6344

MEDICATIONS

DRUG(S) OF CHOICE
• Octreotide (Sandostatin) 200-400 mcg/day subcutaneous, given in divided doses q8h. Can be very expensive.
• Pectin/guar gum
Contraindications:
• Hypersensitivity
Precautions: N/A
Significant possible interactions: Refer to manufacturer's literature

ALTERNATIVE DRUGS
Anticholinergics. Results generally disappointing.

FOLLOWUP

PATIENT MONITORING
Follow to be sure of adequate nutrition

PREVENTION/AVOIDANCE
• Eating frequent, small, dry meals that contain no refined carbohydrates
• Restrict fluids to between meals

POSSIBLE COMPLICATIONS
• Hypoglycemia
• Malnutrition
• Electrolyte disturbances including hypokalemia

EXPECTED COURSE/PROGNOSIS
Favorable

MISCELLANEOUS

ASSOCIATED CONDITIONS
• Peptic ulcer disease
• Reactive hypoglycemia
• Gastrectomy/vagotomy

AGE-RELATED FACTORS
Pediatric: N/A
Geriatric: N/A
Others: N/A

PREGNANCY N/A

SYNONYMS
Early postgastrectomy syndrome

ICD-9-CM
564.2 Postgastric surgery syndromes

SEE ALSO
• Peptic ulcer disease
• Peptic ulcer with hemorrhage
Peptic ulcer with penetration
• Diarrhea, chronic
• Hypoglycemia, nondiabetic

OTHER NOTES N/A

ABBREVIATIONS N/A

REFERENCES
• Sleisenger MH, Fordtran JS, eds: Gastrointestinal Disease: Pathophysiology, Diagnosis, Management. 5th Ed. Philadelphia, W.B. Saunders Co., 1994
• Spiro HW, ed: Clinical Gastroenterology. 4th Ed. New York, McGraw-Hill, 1993
Illustrations: N/A
Internet references: http://www.5mcc.com

Author(s)
Philip E. Jaffe, MD

Dupuytren's contracture

 BASICS

DESCRIPTION Contracture of the palmar fascia due to fibrous proliferation resulting in flexion deformities and loss of function. Similar change may rarely occur in plantar fascia. It usually appears simultaneously.
System(s) affected: Musculoskeletal
Genetics:
• Autosomal dominant with variable penetrance
• 10% of patients have a positive family history
Incidence/Prevalence in USA:
• Unknown
• Norway - 9% males and 3% females
Predominant age: 50
Predominant sex: Male > Female (ranges from 2:1 to 10:1)

SIGNS AND SYMPTOMS
• Unilateral or bilateral (50%)
• Right hand more frequent
• Ring finger more frequent
• Ulnar digits more affected than radial
• Mild pain early
• Later painless plaques or nodules in palmar fascia
• Extends into a cord-like band in the palmar fascia
• Skin adheres to fascia and becomes puckered
• Nodules can be palpated under the skin
• Digital fascia becomes involved as disease progresses
• Web space contractures
• Dupuytren's diathesis can involve plantar (Ledderhose's - 10%) and penile (Peyronie's - 2%) fascia
• Knuckle pads

CAUSES
• Unknown
• Ischemia to the fascia with oxygen free radical formation
• Possibly related to release of angiogenic basic fibroblast growth factor
• Related to microhemorrhage and release of growth factors

RISK FACTORS
• Smoking
• Alcohol intake
• Increasing age
• Male/Caucasian
• Diabetes mellitus (one-third affected, increases with time, usually mild)
• Epilepsy
• Chronic illness (e.g., pulmonary tuberculosis, liver disease)
• Hypercholesterolemia
• Liver disease
• HIV infection

 DIAGNOSIS

DIFFERENTIAL DIAGNOSIS
• Early for callosity
• Tendon abnormalities

LABORATORY N/A
Drugs that may alter lab results: N/A
Disorders that may alter lab results: N/A

PATHOLOGICAL FINDINGS
• Myofibroblasts
• First stage (proliferative) - increased myofibroblasts
• Second stage (residual) - dense fibroblast network
• Third stage (involutional) - myofibroblasts disappear

SPECIAL TESTS N/A

IMAGING MR can assess cellularity of lesions which correlate with higher recurrence after surgery

DIAGNOSTIC PROCEDURES N/A

 TREATMENT

APPROPRIATE HEALTH CARE
• Outpatient monitoring and physical therapy
• Inpatient if surgery indicated

GENERAL MEASURES
• Steroid injection for acute tender nodule
• Physiotherapy is ineffective alone
• Isolated involvement of palmar fascia can be followed
• Metacarpo-phalangeal (MP) joint involvement can be followed if flexion contracture is < 30 degrees

SURGICAL MEASURES
• Surgery - selective fascial ray release
  ◊ Indications: Any involvement of the proximal interphalangeal (PIP) joints. Hueston's table-top test, if positive, consider surgery (when the palm is placed on a flat surface, the digits can not be simultaneously placed fully on the same surface as the palm because of flexion contractures).
  ◊ May require skin grafts for wound closure with severe cutaneous shrinkage
  ◊ 80% have full range of movement if operated on early
  ◊ Continuous elongation technique is useful to prepare a severely contracted PIP joint for surgery. The digit can frequently be completely extended, however, will relapse if surgery not performed.
  ◊ Amputation of little finger, if severe and deforming

ACTIVITY
• No restrictions
• Physical therapy after surgery - started 3-5 days postsurgery (passive and active exercises, posterior dynamic extension splints)

DIET No special diet

PATIENT EDUCATION
• Avoid risk factors especially with a strong family history
• Regular follow-up by physician every 6 months-1 year

MEDICATIONS

DRUG(S) OF CHOICE Steroid injection for an acute tender nodule
Contraindications: N/A
Precautions: N/A
Significant possible interactions: N/A

ALTERNATIVE DRUGS Topical high-potency steroids - case report of improvement with clobetasol 0.1% bid and hs for 2-4 weeks

FOLLOWUP

PATIENT MONITORING Follow patient in early stages of disease

PREVENTION/AVOIDANCE None known. Avoid risk factors when possible.

POSSIBLE COMPLICATIONS
• Postsurgery development of reflex sympathetic dystrophy
• Postoperative recurrence or extension 46-80%
• Postoperative hand edema and skin necrosis
• Digital infarction

EXPECTED COURSE/PROGNOSIS
• Unpredictable, but usually slowly progressive
• Patients likely to have aggressive disease (one or more) < 40 at onset, knuckle pads, positive family history, bilateral disease involving radial side of hand
• Reports of clinical regression with continuous passive skeletal traction in extension and under a skin graft
• Recurrence rate after surgery is 10-34%
• Prognosis better for MP joint vs PIP joint after surgery

MISCELLANEOUS

ASSOCIATED CONDITIONS
• Alcoholism
• Epilepsy
• Diabetes mellitus
• Chronic lung disease
• Occupational hand trauma (vibration white finger)
• Shoulder-hand syndrome
• Status post myocardial infarction
• Hypercholesterolemia

AGE-RELATED FACTORS
Pediatric: N/A
Geriatric: Primarily in this age group
Others: N/A

PREGNANCY N/A

SYNONYMS N/A

ICD-9-CM
728.6 Contracture of palmar fascia (Dupuytren's)

SEE ALSO N/A

OTHER NOTES N/A

ABBREVIATIONS
MP = metacarpo-phalangeal
PIP = proximal interphalangeal

REFERENCES
• Attali P, Ink O, et al: Dupuytren's Contracture, Alcohol Consumption and Chronic Liver Disease. In Arch Intern Med 1987;147:1065-1067
• Hill N, Hurst L: Dupuytren's Contracture. Hand Clinics 1989;5(3):349-357
• Way LW: Current Surgical Diagnosis & Treatment. 8th Ed. Los Altos, CA, Lange, 1989
• Hueston JT: Repression of Dupuytren's contracture. J of Hand Surg 1992;17(4):453-457
• McFarlane RM: The current status of Dupuytren's disease. J of Hand Surg 1995;8(3):181-184
Illustrations: N/A
Internet references: http://www.5mcc.com

Author(s)
Jeffrey F. Minteer, MD

Dysfunctional uterine bleeding (DUB)

BASICS

DESCRIPTION Abnormal uterine bleeding, usually associated with anovulatory cycles, in the absence of other detectable organic lesions. This unit will deal only with women of reproductive age. Three major categories are:
• Estrogen breakthrough bleeding
• Estrogen withdrawal bleeding
• Progestin breakthrough bleeding
System(s) affected: Reproductive, Endocrine/Metabolic
Genetics: Unclear; tendency to have familial characteristics
Incidence/Prevalence in USA: Exact numbers not available, widespread prevalence, without specific geographic variation
Predominant age: 12-45
Predominant sex: Female only

SIGNS AND SYMPTOMS
• Uterine bleeding:
  ◊ Unrelated to menses
  ◊ In excess of normal menstrual flow
  ◊ Occurring in an irregular pattern
  ◊ Rarely painful
• Absence of:
  ◊ Other systemic symptoms
  ◊ Unusual bleeding from other areas
  ◊ Urinary or gastrointestinal irregularities
  ◊ Sustained aspirin or anticoagulant use
  ◊ Use of hormonal preparations
  ◊ Evidence of thyroid disease
  ◊ Galactorrhea
  ◊ Pregnancy (especially ectopic)
  ◊ Evidence for reproductive tract malignancy

CAUSES
• After Eisenberg:
  ◊ Midcycle spotting - caused by a decrease in estrogen at midcycle following ovulation
  ◊ Frequent menses - due to short follicular phase as a result of inappropriate feedback at pituitary/hypothalamic level
  ◊ Deficiency of luteal phase - associated with premenstrual spotting or polymenorrhea when luteal phase is suddenly shortened by prematurely decreased progesterone; due to corpus luteum insufficiency
  ◊ Prolonged corpus luteum activity - caused by persistent progesterone production - results in prolonged cycles or protracted episodes of bleeding
  ◊ Anovulation - production of estrogen unaccompanied by cyclic surges of luteinizing hormone (LH) or secretion of progesterone from the corpus luteum. 90% of all DUB is anovulatory. Usually seen at extremes of reproductive life.
  ◊ Other - uterine lesions, leiomyomata, polyps, carcinoma, vaginal infection, foreign body, ectopic pregnancy, hydatid mole, endocrine dysfunction (especially thyroid), blood dyscrasias

RISK FACTORS Listed with Causes

DIAGNOSIS

DIFFERENTIAL DIAGNOSIS
• Advanced liver disease
• Anabolic steroids
• Hematological disease (von Willebrand's, leukemia, thrombocytopenia)
• Hormonal imbalance
• Iatrogenic causes
• Intrauterine devices
• Medications (oral contraceptives, corticosteroids, hypothalamic depressants, anticholinergics, digitalis, anticoagulants
• Pregnancy (ectopic, incomplete miscarriage
• Thyroid disease
• Trauma
• Uterine cancer
• Uterine leiomyomas

LABORATORY
• Rarely necessary unless clinical picture suggests other endocrine or hematological disease, or if patient is perimenopausal
• Consider thyroid function tests, CBC, PT, PTT, workup for hirsutism, HCG (to rule out pregnancy and/or hydatid mole), prolactin (pituitary dysfunction)
Drugs that may alter lab results: N/A
Disorders that may alter lab results: N/A

PATHOLOGICAL FINDINGS Variable, depending on the disease process present. Pathological review of endometrial sampling specimens is mandatory in all patients.

SPECIAL TESTS Basal body temperature to document anovulation

IMAGING
• Ultrasound may be helpful in identifying ovarian cysts and uterine tumors
• Transvaginal ultrasound (TVUS) recently developed and may be useful in many circumstances. Consider TVUS if you suspect pregnancy, anatomic problems, polycystic ovarian syndrome. The ultrasonographer should have a great deal of experience with the technique.

DIAGNOSTIC PROCEDURES
• Careful history of bleeding, with graphic display of cycles often helpful
• Pelvic examination
• Pap smear
• Endometrial biopsy in selected patients:
  ◊ All patients over 35 years of age
  ◊ Obese patients
  ◊ Patients with diabetes mellitus
  ◊ Patients with hypertension
  ◊ Patients with suspected polycystic ovary syndrome
• Dilatation and curettage in those who have higher risk for endometrial hyperplasia and carcinoma (consider D&C more strongly over endometrial biopsy if the suspected diagnosis is endometritis, atypical hyperplasia, or carcinoma):
  ◊ Heavy, uncontrolled bleeding
  ◊ Histological examination is necessary, but biopsy is contraindicated
  ◊ Medical curettage fails

TREATMENT

APPROPRIATE HEALTH CARE Almost always outpatient; may need hospitalization for profuse bleeding and hemodynamic instability

GENERAL MEASURES See Medications

SURGICAL MEASURES
• Acute (profuse bleeding, hemodynamic instability):
  ◊ Dilatation and curettage
  ◊ Hysterectomy in selected (rare) cases
• Nonacute:
  ◊ Hysterectomy in selected patients if medical therapy fails
  ◊ Endometrial ablation in selected patients if medical therapy fails

ACTIVITY As tolerated

DIET Normal; include adequate iron

PATIENT EDUCATION
• Thorough yet easily comprehended explanation of diagnostic approach and plan of treatment is important. Many questions regarding fertility, cancer, and infectious disease.
• Discuss ways for patient to avoid prolonged stress or emotional turmoil
• American College of Obstetricians & Gynecologists (ACOG), 409 12th St., SW, Washington, DC 20024-2188, (800)762-ACOG

Dysfunctional uterine bleeding (DUB)

MEDICATIONS

DRUG(S) OF CHOICE
• Acute (heavy bleeding, unstable):
◊ Conjugated equine estrogens (25 mg intravenously) every 4 hours for a maximum of six doses
◊ When bleeding has stopped, induce shedding of the endometrium with 10 mg medroxyprogesterone qd for 10-13 days, or with oral contraceptive medication containing 35 mcg of ethinyl estradiol or equivalent
◊ Correct anemia with supplemental iron therapy
• Nonacute:
◊ Progestin: Medroxyprogesterone acetate 10 mg each day for 10-13 days
◊ Estrogen and progesterone (if bleeding when seen or bleeding continues with progesterone or with OCP's): Add 1.25 mg conjugated estrogens daily for days 1-25
◊ Oral contraceptives: Any preparation is usually adequate; initial therapy is one pill qid for 5-7 days. After withdrawal bleeding, may begin normal regimen, usually for at least 3 months or give medroxyprogesterone, 10 mg every day for 10 days every 30 days to regulate menses. Can add estrogen, conjugated (Premarin) 1.25 mg daily for 7 days during and in addition to regimen in order to stop intermenstrual bleeding.
◊ Prostaglandin synthetase inhibitors (e.g., naproxen sodium, mefenamic acid): Can decrease amount of blood loss
◊ Gonadotropin-releasing hormone agonists (induce hypoestrogenism and amenorrhea): Leuprolide acetate, nafarelin, goserelin
◊ Correct anemia with supplemental iron therapy
Contraindications: Therapy should not be instituted until a reasonable attempt at diagnosis has been made, and other causes of uterine bleeding have been considered. "Blind" hormonal therapy is ill-advised and potentially dangerous.
Precautions: Absence of withdrawal bleeding requires workup. Estrogens should not be administered to perimenopausal women or those at risk for endometrial cancer until endometrial hyperplasia and carcinoma have been excluded. Failure of a particular regimen should prompt thorough review of the diagnostic pathway before further steps are taken.
Significant possible interactions: Refer to manufacturer's profile of each drug

ALTERNATIVE DRUGS
• Progesterone:
◊ 100 mg IM progesterone in oil (an alternate to oral methylprogesterone). This works well for active bleeding. Not appropriate for cyclic therapy.
◊ Vaginal suppositories due to leakage and uncertain amount of effective medication should not be used
◊ "Natural" progesterone lozenges (sublingual/oral) have not be adequately studied for use with DUB and have questionable safety.
• Danazol [unlabeled use]: 200-400 mg/day. Much more expensive and may cause masculinization. Usually reserved for women planning to undergo endometrial ablation soon.

FOLLOWUP

PATIENT MONITORING All women treated for DUB with estrogens should maintain a menstrual calendar to document the pattern of bleeding abnormalities and their relation to therapy

PREVENTION/AVOIDANCE N/A

POSSIBLE COMPLICATIONS
• Anemia
• Adenocarcinoma of the uterus if prolonged unopposed estrogen stimulation in women with intact uterus
• Significant side effects of individual preparations. See manufacturer's printed information.

EXPECTED COURSE/PROGNOSIS
• Varies with pathophysiologic process
• In young women, most anovulatory cycles can be treated confidently and successfully with physiologically sound therapeutic regimens, without surgical intervention

MISCELLANEOUS

ASSOCIATED CONDITIONS Listed with Causes

AGE-RELATED FACTORS
Pediatric: N/A
Geriatric: Uterine bleeding in a postmenopausal female must be pursued as if there were carcinoma or other significant pathology present
Others: Early postpubertal females and those in their later reproductive years most often affected

PREGNANCY May confuse with ectopic pregnancy, hydatidiform mole

SYNONYMS N/A

ICD-9-CM
626.8 Disorders of menstruation and other abnormal bleeding from female genital tract, other

SEE ALSO
• Ectopic pregnancy
• Dysmenorrhea
• Menorrhagia

OTHER NOTES If DUB cannot be controlled with medical treatment, options besides hysterectomy are available. Among these are the ND:YAG laser or electrocautery of the endometrium with a ball-end resectoscope.

ABBREVIATIONS N/A

REFERENCES
• Anderson ABM, Haynes PJ, Guilleband J, Turnbull AC: Reduction of menstrual blood loss by prostaglandin synthetase inhibitors. Lancet 1976;1:774
• DeVore GR, Owens O, Kase N: Use of intravenous Premarin in the treatment of dysfunctional uterine bleeding - a double-blind randomized control study. Obstet Gynecol 1982;59:285
• Speroff L, Glass RH, Kase NG, eds: Clinical Gynecologic Endocrinology and Infertility. 5th Ed. Baltimore, Williams and Wilkins, 1994
• Cowan BD, Morrison JC: Management of abnormal genital bleeding in girls and women. N Engl J Med 1991;324:1710
• Apgar BS. Dysmenorrhea and dysfunctional uterine bleeding. Primary Care; Clinics in Office Practice. 1997;24: 161-178
• Goldfarb HA: A review of 35 endometrial ablations using ND:YASG laser for recurrent menorrhagia. Obstet Gynecol Clin 1990;79 (5pt1):833-835
Illustrations: N/A
Internet references: http://www.5mcc.com

Author(s)
Kurt Elward, MD, MPH

Dyshidrosis

 BASICS

DESCRIPTION
• Dyshidrotic eczema: Recurrent vesicular eruption primarily of the palms, soles and interdigital areas. The term pompholyx (Greek "bubble") is generally reserved for the cases of deep-seated pruritic vesicles (the so-called "sago grain" appearance). Generally associated with, but not caused by, hyperhidrosis.
• Lamellar dyshidrosis: A fine spreading exfoliation of the superficial epidermis in the same distribution as described above. Hyperhidrosis may or may not be associated.
System(s) affected: Skin/Exocrine
Genetics: N/A
Incidence/Prevalence in USA: 20/100,000
Predominant age: Usually < age 40
Predominant sex: Male = Female

SIGNS AND SYMPTOMS
• Dyshidrotic eczema
 ◊ Small superficial vesicles of the palms and soles and between the fingers and toes
 ◊ Scaling, fissures and lichenification may follow vesicle formation
 ◊ Burning and itching are common
 ◊ Bilateral and frequently symmetrical lesions
 ◊ Vesicles may sometimes coalesce to form larger vesicles or even bullae
 ◊ Vesicles may rupture leading to a fine scaling similar to tinea
• Lamellar dyshidrosis
 ◊ Small white macules which spread peripherally
 ◊ Central area begins to scale
 ◊ Desquamation of the horny layer of the skin that continues to spread

CAUSES
• Exact cause is not known
• May represent an id reaction especially to a dermatophyte infection
• Stress may play a role since dyshidrosis is more frequent in anxious individuals, and those with psychosocial stress
• Hyperhidrosis is not a cause, but is often associated with the disease

RISK FACTORS
• Atopic dermatitis
• Contact dermatitis
• Dermatophytosis
• Bacterial infections
• Foods
• Drugs, such as aspirin or other salicylates

 DIAGNOSIS

DIFFERENTIAL DIAGNOSIS
• Tinea manuum or pedis
• Id reaction
• Contact dermatitis
• Atopic dermatitis
• Drug reaction
• Dermatophytid
• Pustular psoriasis
• Seborrheic dermatitis
• Acrodermatitis continua
• Pustular bacterid

LABORATORY N/A
Drugs that may alter lab results: N/A
Disorders that may alter lab results: N/A

PATHOLOGICAL FINDINGS
• Dyshidrotic eczema: Reveals fine 1-2 mm spongiotic vesicles intraepidermally. Sweat ducts are not involved.
• Lamellar dyshidrosis: Exfoliation of the horny layer of the epidermis

SPECIAL TESTS N/A

IMAGING N/A

DIAGNOSTIC PROCEDURES
• Diagnosis is usually based on clinical exam
• Skin biopsy

 TREATMENT

APPROPRIATE HEALTH CARE
Outpatient

GENERAL MEASURES
• Avoidance of possible causative factors (see Risk factors)
• Though hyperhidrosis is not a cause, excessive sweating may increase pruritus and burning
• Moisturizers will give symptomatic relief of dry scaly lesions
• If feet involved:
 ◊ Wear shoes with leather soles rather than rubber (e.g., sneakers)
 ◊ Wear socks made of cotton instead of synthetic materials
 ◊ Remove shoes and socks whenever possible to allow sweat evaporation and to apply lubricants

SURGICAL MEASURES N/A

ACTIVITY
• Avoid, when possible, stress or excessive sweating (may be psychological or thermal sweating)
• Avoid excess detergents and water

DIET No restrictions

PATIENT EDUCATION
• Instructions on self-care, complications and avoidance
• Explain the association between stress and dyshidrosis and suggest counseling if appropriate

MEDICATIONS

DRUG(S) OF CHOICE
• Dyshidrotic eczema-mild cases
　◊ Topical steroids (medium to high potency), or
　◊ 5% salicylate in alcohol (provided salicylates are not a cause), or
• Dyshidrotic eczema-moderate to severe cases
　◊ A systemic corticosteroid such as short course of oral prednisone
　◊ Intramuscular ACTH or triamcinolone acetonide 40 mg
　◊ PUVA (psoralens and ultraviolet A) therapy is effective therapy (including mild cases)
• Lamellar dyshidrosis
　◊ Application of coal tar (Estar) preparations
　◊ Intramuscular corticosteroids
　◊ Keratolytics and moisturizers are sometimes helpful
Contraindications: Refer to manufacturer's profile of each drug
Precautions: Refer to manufacturer's profile of each drug
Significant possible interactions: Refer to manufacturer's profile of each drug

ALTERNATIVE DRUGS   N/A

FOLLOWUP

PATIENT MONITORING   As needed

PREVENTION/AVOIDANCE
• Control of emotional stress, avoid sweating
• Treatment for psychological factors, if appropriate

POSSIBLE COMPLICATIONS   Bacterial secondary infections

EXPECTED COURSE/PROGNOSIS
• Benign and without scarring
• Lesions will often resolve spontaneously, though faster with appropriate treatment
• Recurrence is the rule rather than the exception

MISCELLANEOUS

ASSOCIATED CONDITIONS   N/A

AGE-RELATED FACTORS
Pediatric: N/A
Geriatric: N/A
Others: N/A

PREGNANCY   N/A

SYNONYMS
• Pompholyx
• Cheiropompholyx
• Keratolysis exfoliativa

ICD-9-CM
705.81 Dyshidrosis

SEE ALSO   N/A

OTHER NOTES   N/A

ABBREVIATIONS   N/A

REFERENCES
• Domonkos AN, Arnold HL, Odom RB: Andrew's Diseases of the Skin. 8th Ed. Philadelphia, W.B. Saunders Co., 1990
• Fitzpatrick TB, et al, eds: Dermatology in General Medicine. 4th Ed. New York, McGraw-Hill, 1993
• Fitzpatrick TB: Color Atlas and Synopsis of Clinical Dermatology. 2nd Ed. New York, McGraw-Hill, 1992
• Sauer R: Manual of Skin Diseases. 6th Ed. Philadelphia, J.B. Lippincott, 1991
Illustrations: 2 available on CD-ROM
Internet references: http://www.5mcc.com

Author(s)
Scott A. Kincaid, MD

Dysmenorrhea

 BASICS

DESCRIPTION Pelvic pain occurring at or around the time of menses. Is a leading cause of absenteeism for women under age 30
• Primary dysmenorrhea - without pathological physical findings
• Secondary dysmenorrhea - pain occurring prior to or during menses, often more severe than primary, having a secondary pathologic (structural) cause
System(s) affected: Reproductive
Genetics: Not well studied
Incidence/Prevalence in USA:
• 40% of adult females have menstrual pain
• 10% are incapacitated for 1-3 days each month
Predominant age:
• Primary - teens to early 20's
• Secondary - 20's to 30's
Predominant sex: Female only

SIGNS AND SYMPTOMS
• Mild - pelvic discomfort or cramping or heaviness on first day of bleeding with no associated symptoms
• Moderate - discomfort occurring on first 2-3 days of menses and accompanied by mild malaise, diarrhea and headache
• Severe - intense, cramp-like pain lasting 2-7 days; often with gastrointestinal upset, back pain, thigh pain, and headache

CAUSES
• Primary:
  ◊ Elevated production (2-7 times normal) of prostaglandins and other mediators in the uterus which produce uterine ischemia through:
    -Platelet aggregation
    -Vasoconstriction
    -Dysrhythmic contractions with pressures higher than the systemic blood pressure
• Secondary:
  ◊ Congenital abnormalities of uterine or vaginal anatomy
  ◊ Cervical stenosis
  ◊ Pelvic infection
  ◊ Adenomyosis
  ◊ Endometriosis
  ◊ Pelvic tumors - especially leiomyomata

RISK FACTORS
• Primary:
  ◊ Nulliparity
  ◊ Positive family history
• Secondary:
  ◊ Pelvic infection
  ◊ Sexually transmitted diseases
  ◊ Endometriosis

 DIAGNOSIS

DIFFERENTIAL DIAGNOSIS
• Primary:
  ◊ History is characteristic
• Secondary:
  ◊ Pelvic or genital infection
  ◊ Complication of pregnancy
  ◊ Missed or incomplete abortion
  ◊ Ectopic pregnancy
  ◊ Uterine or ovarian neoplasm
  ◊ Endometriosis
  ◊ Urinary tract infection

LABORATORY Noncontributory except in case of acute infection, in which case white blood cell count may be elevated and blood or cervical cultures positive
Drugs that may alter lab results:
Antibiotics
Disorders that may alter lab results: N/A

PATHOLOGICAL FINDINGS
• Primary:
  ◊ None
• Secondary:
  ◊ Uterine enlargement
  ◊ Leiomyomata
  ◊ Ligamentous thickening
  ◊ Fixation of pelvic structures
  ◊ Endometritis
  ◊ Salpingitis

SPECIAL TESTS
• Primary - consider ultrasound to rule out secondary abnormalities
• Secondary - ultrasound or laparoscopy to define anatomy

IMAGING N/A

DIAGNOSTIC PROCEDURES
• Primary:
  ◊ History is characteristic
  ◊ Physical examination should be normal
• Secondary:
  ◊ History of onset at least 18-24 months after menarche
  ◊ Physical examination may reveal anatomic abnormalities or tenderness
  ◊ Laparoscopy (rarely needed)

 TREATMENT

APPROPRIATE HEALTH CARE
• Primary - outpatient
• Secondary - usually outpatient

GENERAL MEASURES
• Secondary dysmenorrhea - treatment of infections. Suppression of endometrium if endometriosis is suspected.
• General physical conditioning, exercise to raise endorphins
• Transcutaneous electrical nerve stimulator (TENS)

SURGICAL MEASURES If due to severe endometriosis, presacral neurectomy; adenomyosis, hysterectomy

ACTIVITY Normal

DIET Normal

PATIENT EDUCATION
• Reassure patient that primary dysmenorrhea is treatable with use of nonsteroidal anti-inflammatory agents prior to menses and/or oral contraceptives, and will usually abate with age and parity
• Refer to web site: www.5mcc for resources for patient education material

MEDICATIONS

DRUG(S) OF CHOICE
• Ibuprofen (Motrin, Advil, Nuprin) 400-600 mg every 4-6 hours,
or
• Naproxen sodium (Anaprox, Aleve) 550 mg every 12 hours,
or
• Aspirin 650 mg every 4-6 hours,
or
• Other nonsteroidal anti-inflammatory drugs
• Oral contraceptives
Contraindications:
• Platelet disorders
• Gastric ulceration or gastritis
• Thromboembolic disorders
• Vascular disease
• Contraindications to oral contraceptives
Precautions:
• GI irritation
• Lactation
• Coagulation disorders
• Impaired renal function
• Congestive heart failure
• Liver dysfunction
Significant possible interactions:
• Coumarin-type anticoagulants
• Aspirin with other NSAID's
• Methotrexate
• Furosemide
• Lithium

ALTERNATIVE DRUGS
• Nafarelin acetate 200-400 mg/day for endometriosis (will simulate menopause)
• Calcium channel blockers (nifedipine, others) in low doses; efficacy reported, but not FDA approved for this use
• Hydrocodone or tramadol (Ultram) for management of severe symptoms
• Other NSAIDs

FOLLOWUP

PATIENT MONITORING N/A

PREVENTION/AVOIDANCE
• Primary - choose a diet low in animal fats, dairy products and eggs. Increase vegetables, raw seeds and nuts to increase production of beneficial prostaglandins.
• Secondary - reduce risk of sexually-transmitted diseases

POSSIBLE COMPLICATIONS
• Primary - anxiety and/or depression
• Secondary - infertility from underlying pathology

EXPECTED COURSE/PROGNOSIS
• Primary - improves with age and parity
• Secondary - likely to require therapy based on underlying cause

MISCELLANEOUS

ASSOCIATED CONDITIONS N/A

AGE-RELATED FACTORS N/A
Pediatric: Onset with first menses raises probability of genital tract anatomic abnormality such as transverse vaginal septum, uterine anomalies
Geriatric: N/A
Others: N/A

PREGNANCY Consider ectopic pregnancy in differential diagnosis of pelvic pain with vaginal bleeding

SYNONYMS Menstrual cramps

ICD-9-CM
625.3 Dysmenorrhea

SEE ALSO Endometriosis

OTHER NOTES N/A

ABBREVIATIONS N/A

REFERENCES
• Dawood MY: Dysmenorrhea. In Clin Obstet Gynecol 1990;33(1):168-78
• Milson I, Hedner N, Mannheimer C: A comparative study of the effect of high-intensity transcutaneous nerve stimulation and oral naproxen on intrauterine pressure and menstrual pain in patients with primary dysmenorrhea. Am J Obstet Gynecol 1994;170(1 Pt 1):123-9
• Nigam S, Benedetto C, et al: Increased concentrations of eicosanoids and platelet-activating factor in menstrual blood from women with primary dysmenorrhea. Eicosanoids 1991;4(3):137-31
• Jacobson J, Harris S, Bullingham R: Low dose intranasal nafarelin for the treatment of endometriosis. Acta Obstet Gynecol Scand 1994;73:144-150
• Smith RP: Cyclic pelvic pain and dysmenorrhea. Obstet Gynecol Clin North Am. 20(4):753-764
Illustrations: N/A
Internet references: http://www.5mcc.com

Author(s)
Janice E. Daugherty, MD

Dyspareunia

BASICS

DESCRIPTION Recurrent and persistent genital pain associated with intercourse, in either the male or female. Dyspareunia may be due to organic, emotional or psychogenic causes.
• Primary: Present throughout one's sexual history
• Secondary: Arising from some specific event or condition, e.g., menopause, drugs
• Superficial: Difficulty or pain at or near the introitus or vaginal barrel associated with penetration
• Deep: Pain after penetration located at the cervix or lower abdominal area
• Complete: Present under all circumstances
• Situational: Occurring selectively with specific situations
System(s) affected: Reproductive
Genetics: N/A
Incidence/Prevalence in USA:
• Most women who are sexually active will experience dyspareunia at some time in their lives. Approximately 15% (4-40%) of adult women will have dyspareunia on a few occasions during a year. About 1-2% of women will have painful intercourse on a more than occasional basis.
• Male prevalence unknown
Predominant age: All ages
Predominant sex: Female > Male

SIGNS AND SYMPTOMS Varying degrees of pelvic/genital pressure, aching, tearing and/or burning

CAUSES
• Disorders of vaginal outlet
  ◊ Hymenal ring abnormalities
  ◊ Postmenopausal atrophy
  ◊ Decreased lubrication
  ◊ Episiotomy scars
  ◊ Vulvar vestibulitis/vulvodynia
  ◊ Infections
  ◊ Trauma
  ◊ Adhesions
  ◊ Clitoral irritation
  ◊ Vulvar papillomatosis
• Disorders of vagina
  ◊ Infections
  ◊ Masses or tumors
  ◊ Decreased lubrication
  ◊ Pelvic relaxation resulting in rectocele, uterine prolapse or cystocele
  ◊ Inflammatory or allergic response to foreign substance
  ◊ Abnormality of vault due to surgery or radiation
  ◊ Congenital malformations
• Disorders of pelvic structures
  ◊ Pelvic inflammatory disease
  ◊ Endometriosis
  ◊ Malignant or benign tumors of the uterus
  ◊ Ovarian pathology
  ◊ Pelvic adhesions
  ◊ Prior pelvic fracture
  ◊ Levator ani myalgia
  ◊ Pelvic venous congestion

• Disorders of the gastrointestinal tract
  ◊ Inflammatory bowel disease
  ◊ Crohn's disease
  ◊ Diverticulitis
  ◊ Constipation
  ◊ Hemorrhoids
  ◊ Fistulas
• Disorders of the urinary tract
  ◊ Interstitial cystitis
  ◊ Ureteral or vesical lesions
• Male
  ◊ Genital muscle spasm
  ◊ Infection and irritation of penile skin
  ◊ Cancer of penis
  ◊ Penile anatomy disorders
  ◊ Prostate infections and enlargement
  ◊ Infection of seminal vesicles
  ◊ Testicular disease
  ◊ Torsion of spermatic cord
  ◊ Musculoskeletal disorders of pelvis and lower back
  ◊ Urethritis
• Psychologic disorders
  ◊ Fear
  ◊ Anxiety
  ◊ Phobic reactions
  ◊ Conversion reactions
  ◊ Hostility towards partner
  ◊ Psychological trauma

RISK FACTORS
• Diabetes
• Estrogen deficiency
• Alcohol/marijuana consumption
• Menopause
• Medroxyprogesterone use

DIAGNOSIS

DIFFERENTIAL DIAGNOSIS
• Vaginismus

LABORATORY
• Gonorrhea culture
• Wet mount
• Chlamydia culture
• Herpes culture
• Urine analysis
• Urine culture
• Pap smear to assess estrogen status
Drugs that may alter lab results: N/A
Disorders that may alter lab results: N/A

PATHOLOGICAL FINDINGS Dependent on etiology

SPECIAL TESTS N/A

IMAGING
• Voiding cystourethrogram if urinary tract involvement
• Gastrointestinal contrast studies if GI symptoms

DIAGNOSTIC PROCEDURES
• Colposcopy and biopsy if vaginal/vulvar lesions
• Laparoscopy if complex deep penetration pain
• Cystoscopy if urinary tract involvement
• Sigmoidoscopy if GI involvement

TREATMENT

APPROPRIATE HEALTH CARE
Outpatient

GENERAL MEASURES
• The first step in treatment is to educate the patient and partner as to the nature of the problem and reassure them the problem can be solved
• Organic causes can generally be identified during the initial evaluation and specific treatment initiated
• Once organic causes have been ruled out, individual and/or couple behavioral therapy should be initiated
• Behavioral therapy
  ◊ Designed to systemically desensitize to intercourse through a series of interventions over a period of weeks
  ◊ Interventions range from muscle relaxation and mutual body massage to sexual fantasies and erotic massage, with the ultimate goal of intercourse and sexual responsiveness
• Individual therapy
  ◊ Indicated to help the patient deal with intrapsychic issues and assess the role of the partner
• Couple therapy
  ◊ Indicated to help resolve interpersonal problems
  ◊ May involve short-term structured intervention or sexual counseling
  ◊ Referral for long-term therapy may be necessary

SURGICAL MEASURES Should be avoided

ACTIVITY Routine

DIET Regular; a high-fiber diet may help if constipation is the cause

PATIENT EDUCATION Patient education models, information on sexual arousal techniques, Kegel exercise information (Instructions for Patients, Griffith, H.W., W.B. Saunders Co., Philadelphia; Our Bodies, Ourselves, Boston Women's Health Collective, Simon & Schuster, New York)

MEDICATIONS

DRUG(S) OF CHOICE Dependent on the etiology. May include antibiotics for infection, estrogen for vaginal atrophy, analgesics for pain, and lubricants for dryness.
Contraindications: Refer to manufacturer's profile on each drug
Precautions: Refer to manufacturer's profile on each drug
Significant possible interactions: Refer to manufacturer's profile on each drug

ALTERNATIVE DRUGS N/A

FOLLOWUP

PATIENT MONITORING Dependent on therapy. Every 6-12 months once resolved.

PREVENTION/AVOIDANCE Avoidance of alcohol and tobacco products

POSSIBLE COMPLICATIONS N/A

EXPECTED COURSE/PROGNOSIS The majority of cases will respond to treatment

MISCELLANEOUS

ASSOCIATED CONDITIONS Vaginismus

AGE-RELATED FACTORS
Pediatric: N/A
Geriatric: The incidence increases dramatically in the postmenopausal woman who is not receiving HRT primarily because of vaginal atrophy. Over half of all sexually active women will report dyspareunia.
Others: N/A

PREGNANCY The episiotomy has been associated with dyspareunia. Some studies show the incidence is decreased in women who have had midline episiotomy when compared with those who have had a mediolateral episiotomy.

SYNONYMS N/A

ICD-9-CM
• 302.76 Psycho-sexual dysfunction with functional dyspareunia
• 625.0 Pain and other symptoms associated with female genital organs, dyspareunia
• 608.89 Male

SEE ALSO
• Balanitis
• Endometriosis
• Pelvic inflammatory disease
• Sexual dysfunction
• Vaginismus
• Vulvovaginitis, estrogen deficient
• Vulvovaginitis, candidal
• Vulvovaginitis, bacterial

OTHER NOTES N/A

ABBREVIATIONS N/A

REFERENCES
• Sciarra J: Obstetrics and Gynecology. Philadelphia, J.B. Lippincott Co., 1991
• Steege JF, Ling FW: Dyspareunia: A special type of chronic pelvic pain. Obstet-Gynecol Clin North Am 1993;20(4):779-793
Illustrations: N/A
Internet references: http://www.5mcc.com

Author(s)
Scott T. Henderson, MD

Dyspepsia, functional

 BASICS

DESCRIPTION An ill-defined condition characterized by the presence of chronic intermittent symptoms of epigastric pain and fullness, early satiety, nausea and/or vomiting without mucosal lesions or other structural abnormalities of the gastrointestinal tract
System(s) affected: Gastrointestinal
Genetics: N/A
Incidence/Prevalence in USA: Common, affecting 15-20% of patients referred to gastroenterologists
Predominant Age: Adults, but can be seen in children
Predominant Sex: Females > Males

SIGNS AND SYMPTOMS
• Belching
• Aerophagia, gaseousness, abdominal distension
• Borborygmus
• Epigastric pain, gnawing or burning; eating may improve or worsen symptoms
• Substernal pain, gnawing or burning
• Anorexia, nausea, or vomiting
• Change in bowel habits
• Abdominal tenderness
• No anatomic abnormalities

CAUSES
• Often unknown, may be of several different etiologies
• Evanescent ulcers (20-30% go on to develop ulcers)
• Gastric motility disorder
• Adverse drug effects
• Helicobacter pylori may be causative in some patients

RISK FACTORS
• Other functional disorders
• Anxiety
• Depression

 DIAGNOSIS

DIFFERENTIAL DIAGNOSIS
• Gastroesophageal reflux
• Cholecystitis
• Peptic ulcer disease
• Gastric cancer
• Esophageal spasm
• Malabsorption syndromes
• Pancreatic disease
• Irritable bowel syndrome
• Aerophagia
• Ischemia heart disease
• Diabetes mellitus
• Thyroid disease
• Connective tissue disorders
• Conversion disorder

LABORATORY
• CBC
• Chemistry panel
• Stool for occult blood
Drugs that may alter lab results: Too many to list
Disorders that may alter lab results: N/A

IMAGING
• Recommended in:
  ◊ Patients over 45 years of age at onset of symptoms
  ◊ Patients with symptoms and signs suggesting more serious disease
  ◊ Patients who need added reassurance
  ◊ Younger patients who do not respond rapidly to empiric treatment
• Usual:
  ◊ Endoscopy, or
  ◊ Upper GI series
• Sometimes:
  ◊ Barium enema
  ◊ Gallbladder studies (e.g., ultrasound or oral cholecystogram)

SPECIAL TESTS
• Esophageal manometry (rarely needed)
• 24-hour intra-esophageal pH monitoring (rarely needed)

PATHOLOGICAL FINDINGS None (by definition)

DIAGNOSTIC PROCEDURES
• Careful history and physical
• Normal studies of esophagus, stomach and duodenum (particularly in patients over 45)

 TREATMENT

APPROPRIATE HEALTH CARE
Outpatient

GENERAL MEASURES
• Supportive measures
  ◊ Reassurance
  ◊ Do not overinvestigate
  ◊ Dietary changes (see below)
  ◊ Elevate head of bed (where applicable)
  ◊ Maintain ideal body weight
  ◊ Explore psychological issues

SURGICAL MEASURES N/A

ACTIVITY
• Stress reduction
  ◊ Relaxation techniques
  ◊ Physical exercise
  ◊ Reflux precautions where applicable

DIET
• Avoid foods known to exacerbate symptoms
• Frequent small meals
• Avoid regular and decaffeinated coffee
• Avoid tea, cocoa, chocolate
• Avoid heavy alcohol use
• Avoid cigarette smoking
• Avoid aspirin containing compounds and NSAID's

PATIENT EDUCATION N/A

MEDICATIONS

DRUG(S) OF CHOICE
• 60% of patients improve with placebo
• Acid reduction drugs - H2 antagonists
• Antacids
Precautions:
• H2 antagonist dosage should be adjusted in patients with renal disease
• Calcium containing antacids may precipitate the formation of kidney stones
Contraindications:
• Magnesium containing antacids should be avoided in patients with significant renal dysfunction
Significant possible interactions:
• H2 blockers interact with drugs metabolized by, and affecting the liver
• Antacids compete with digoxin, iron salts, tetracycline, fluoroquinolones, and other drugs for absorption from the stomach

ALTERNATIVE DRUGS
• Gastric motility drugs
  ◊ Metoclopramide; although side effects are significant
  ◊ Cisapride (Propulsid)
  ◊ Erythromycin
• Proton pump inhibitors
  ◊ Omeprazole
  ◊ Lansoprazole

FOLLOWUP

PATIENT MONITORING
• Usual duration of medication is 4 weeks, then 2 weeks intermittently for exacerbations. If chronic medication use is needed, should do imaging to rule out serious pathology.
• Continuing observation to provide support and reassurance
• Minimize diagnostic studies unless disabling symptoms persist or new problems arise

PREVENTION/AVOIDANCE Continued
health habits suggested under Treatment (i.e., avoid activities known to exacerbate problems, maintain healthy lifestyle, continue stress reduction techniques)

POSSIBLE COMPLICATIONS
Undiagnosed serious pathology

EXPECTED COURSE/PROGNOSIS
Long-term or chronic symptoms with periods that are symptom free

MISCELLANEOUS

ASSOCIATED CONDITIONS Other
functional bowel disorders

AGE-RELATED FACTORS
Pediatric: Look for family system dysfunction
Geriatric: Cancer risk is higher
Others: N/A

PREGNANCY May exacerbate

SYNONYMS
• Non-ulcer dyspepsia
• Moynihan's dyspepsia
• Pseudo-ulcer dyspepsia
• Phantom ulcer
• Non-organic dyspepsia
• Nervous dyspepsia

ICD-9-CM
536.8 dyspepsia and other specified disorders of function of stomach

SEE ALSO
• Irritable bowel syndrome
• Gastritis

OTHER NOTES N/A

ABBREVIATIONS N/A

REFERENCES Talley NJ: Non-ulcer
dyspepsia: Current approaches to diagnosis and management. Am Fam Phys 1993;47:1407-1416
Illustrations: N/A
Internet references: http://www.5mcc.com

Author(s)
K. Patricia McGann, MD, MSPH

Dysphagia

 BASICS

DESCRIPTION The sensation of difficulty swallowing. This is a disorder of esophageal transport and is a symptom of an underlying process. The problem is commonly divided into oropharyngeal and esophageal types.
System(s) affected: Gastrointestinal
Genetics: N/A
Incidence/Prevalence in USA: N/A
Predominant age: All ages
Predominant sex: Male = Female

SIGNS AND SYMPTOMS
• Oropharyngeal type
  ◊ Choking with swallowing
  ◊ Coughing with swallowing
  ◊ Weak voice
  ◊ Aspiration pneumonia
  ◊ Weight loss
• Esophageal type
  ◊ Pressure sensation in mid-chest (patient may localize pathology to correct anatomic site)
  ◊ Symptoms should distinguish whether dysphagia is for solids or liquids or both
  ◊ Aspiration pneumonia
  ◊ Weight loss
  ◊ Symptoms of GERD
  ◊ Longer time required to eat meals (patient unconsciouisly chews food more thoroughly)

CAUSES
• In children
  ◊ Malformations - congenital (esophageal atresia, choanal atresia)
  ◊ Malformations - acquired (corrosive or herpetic esophagitis)
  ◊ Neuromuscular/neurologic - delayed maturation, cerebral palsy, muscular dystrophy
  ◊ Gastroesophageal reflux disease
• In adults
  ◊ Structural - tumors (cancer or benign), strictures (peptic, chemical, trauma, radiation), rings & webs, extrinsic compression (goiter)
  ◊ Gastroesophageal reflux disease
  ◊ Neuromuscular - achalasia, diffuse esophageal spasm, scleroderma, myasthenia gravis

RISK FACTORS
• Children - hereditary and/or congenital malformations
• Adults - age > 50 years, when cancer of the esophagus is more likely
• Smoking
• Long history of gastroesophageal reflux disease
• Medications (quinine, potassium chloride, vitamin C, tetracycline, nonsteroidal anti-inflammatory drugs, and others)

 DIAGNOSIS

DIFFERENTIAL DIAGNOSIS
• Cardiac chest pain
• Globus hystericus

LABORATORY N/A
Drugs that may alter lab results: N/A
Disorders that may alter lab results: N/A

PATHOLOGICAL FINDINGS
• Squamous cell or adenocarcinoma
• Barrett's metaplasia
• Fibrous tissue of a ring, web or stricture
• Acute or chronic inflammatory change
• Heterotopic gastric mucosa (inlet patch)

SPECIAL TESTS
• In infants/children
  ◊ Observe sucking/eating
  ◊ Attempt to pass nasogastric tube to assess esophageal patency
    ◊ X-ray neck and chest
    ◊ Contrast x-ray
    ◊ Endoscopy
• In adults
  ◊ X-ray of neck and chest
  ◊ Endoscopy
  ◊ Barium cine/video esophagogram
  ◊ Ambulatory, 24 hour pH testing

IMAGING
• X-ray: chest, neck, abdomen
• Contrast x-ray: esophogram, cine-esophogram, modified cine-esophogram (cookie swallow)
• CT scan of chest

DIAGNOSTIC PROCEDURES
• Endoscopy with biopsy
• Esophageal manometry (altered by anticholinergics [propantheline], calcium channel blockers [nifedipine], nitrates [nitroglycerin], prokinetics [metoclopramide, cisapride], sedatives [diazepam])
• Esophageal pH monitoring (altered by anticholinergics [propantheline], H2 receptor antagonists [cimetidine], proton pump inhibitors [omeprazole], prokinetics [cisapride])

 TREATMENT

APPROPRIATE HEALTH CARE
• Outpatient for those conditions where the patient is able to maintain nutrition and where there is little risk of complication
• Hospitalization may be required for either infants or adults where dysphagia is associated with total or near total obstruction of the esophageal lumen
• Endoscopy and/or esophageal dilatation may be needed for stenoses
• Surgery may be needed in either benign or malignant processes

GENERAL MEASURES
• Determine esophageal patency to exclude inflammation
• Ensure airway and pulmonary function
• Exclude cardiac disease
• Assess nutritional status

SURGICAL MEASURES
• Esophageal dilatation (pneumatic or bougie)
• Esophageal stent; laser for late cancer

ACTIVITY No restriction

DIET Varies from nothing by mouth to near normal, depending on the degree of obstruction.

PATIENT EDUCATION
• Counsel on avoiding irritating drugs
• Counsel on chewing, consistency of food
• In infants/children - discuss underlying problem and therapy for recurrent aspiration
• In adults - discuss etiology and therapy (need for repeat dilatations). Speech therapy may be helpful in teaching swallowing techniques.

Dysphagia

MEDICATIONS

DRUG(S) OF CHOICE
• For spasms:
 ◊ Nitrates
 ◊ Calcium channel blockers (nifedipine [Procardia]10-30 mg tid)
• For esophagitis:
 ◊ Antacids
 ◊ H2-blockers (cimetidine [Tagamet], ranitidine [Zantac], nizatidine [Axid], famotidine [Pepcid])
 ◊ Proton pump inhibitors (omeprazole [Prilosec], lansoprazole [Prevacid]), in case of H2-blocker failure
 ◊ Prokinetic agents (metoclopramide [Reglan], cisapride [Propulsid])

Contraindications:
• Anticholinergics - obstructive uropathy, glaucoma, myasthenia gravis, achalasia
• Nitrates - early myocardial infarction, severe anemia, increased intracranial pressure

Precautions: May need to use liquid forms of medications

Significant possible interactions: Refer to manufacturer's profile of each drug

ALTERNATIVE DRUGS N/A

FOLLOWUP

PATIENT MONITORING The type of reassessment and frequency of follow-up is related to the specific etiology of the dysphagia

PREVENTION/AVOIDANCE
• Very hot or very cold foods may worsen.
• Observe feeding of infants closely for aspirations - have suction available
• Advise for correction of poorly fitting dentures in adults or elderly
• Avoid drinking alcohol with meals

POSSIBLE COMPLICATIONS
• Aspiration
• Esophageal "asthma"
• Pneumonia
• Barrett's esophagus
• Death

EXPECTED COURSE/PROGNOSIS
Course and prognosis varies with the specific diagnosis (cancer - poor; esophageal peptic stricture - good)

MISCELLANEOUS

ASSOCIATED CONDITIONS
• Esophageal carcinoma
• Gastroesophageal reflux disease
• Dysphagia lusoria
• Achalasia
• Symptomatic diffuse esophageal spasm
• Scleroderma
• Myasthenia gravis
• CVA

AGE-RELATED FACTORS
Pediatric: Congenital malformations
Geriatric:
• Poor dentition and/or dentures
• Drug induced
Others: N/A

PREGNANCY N/A

SYNONYMS N/A

ICD-9-CM
787.2 Symptoms involving digestive system

SEE ALSO Gastroesophageal reflux disease

OTHER NOTES This is a symptom of an abnormal process. A search for the etiology is of great importance.

ABBREVIATIONS
GERD = gastroesophageal reflux disease

REFERENCES
• Silverman A, Roy CC: Pediatric Clinical Gastroenterology. St. Louis, C.V. Mosby Co, 1983
• Just RJ, Castell DO: Diagnostic Approach to the Patient with Dysphagia, Contemporary Internal Medicine 1993;5(6):68
• Pope CE: Motor Disorders. In: Sleisenger MH, Fordtran JS, eds. Gastrointestinal Disease. 5th Ed. Philadelphia, W.B. Saunders Co., 1994
• Ravick WJ, Hendoix TR: Disorders of Swallowing. In Stobo JD, Hellmann DB, Ladenson PW, Petty BG, Traill TA The Principles and Practice of Medicine, 23rd ed, 1996
Illustrations: N/A
Internet references: http://www.5mcc.com

Author(s)
Duane C. Roe, MD

Eclampsia (toxemia of pregnancy)

BASICS

DESCRIPTION The presence of seizure activity in an obstetric patient with the syndrome of hypertension, edema, and proteinuria (pre-eclampsia), in a patient without underlying neurological disease. Nearly all postpartum cases occur within 24 hours of delivery.

System(s) affected: Reproductive, Nervous, Hemic/Lymphatic/Immunologic

Genetics: There does seem to be some genetic predisposition. The single-gene model best explains the frequency of about 25%, but multifactorial inheritance is also possible.

Incidence/Prevalence IN USA:
• Unclear; incidence varies, but preeclampsia has been reported to complicate 5% of all deliveries
• 0.5-2% of preeclamptic patients will progress to eclampsia. With improved monitoring and prepartum care, this number has decreased in recent years.

Predominant age: Most of the cases occur in younger women because of the higher incidence of preeclampsia in younger (nulliparous) women. However, older (> 40 years), preeclamptic patients have 4 times the incidence of seizures compared with patients in their 20's.

Predominant sex: Female only

SIGNS AND SYMPTOMS
• Tonic-clonic seizure activity (focal or generalized)
• Headache, visual disturbance and epigastric or right upper quadrant pain often precedes seizure
• Seizures may occur once or repeatedly
• Postictal coma, cyanosis (variable)
• Temperatures > 39°C consistent with CNS hemorrhage
• Disseminated intravascular coagulation (DIC), thrombocytopenia, liver dysfunction, renal failure associated
• Proteinuria
• Up to 30% may not have edema, 20% may not have proteinuria
• Normal blood pressure - however, normal blood pressure, even in "response" to treatment, does not rule out potential for seizures
• Hemoconcentration - predisposition to pulmonary and or cerebral edema with fluid therapy. There is actually an excess of extracellular fluid that is inappropriately distributed to the extracellular spaces.

CAUSES
• Exact cause of seizures remains unclear
• Trophoblastic tissue seems to be required, and somehow results in widespread vasospasm
• Severe cerebral vasoconstriction; hemorrhages occur due to failure of the constriction to limit perfusion pressure in the capillaries, with consequent rupture and vasogenic cerebral edema and ring hemorrhages

RISK FACTORS
• Young nulliparous woman
• Nulliparity age > 35
• Obstetric conditions associated with abundance of chorionic villi (multifetal gestation, trophoblastic disease, erythroblastosis)
• Preexisting hypertension or renal disease
• Strong family history of preeclampsia-eclampsia
• Poor prenatal care prevents early detection and treatment of preeclampsia, thereby increasing the risk of progression to eclampsia
• Pregnancy weight gain over 30 pounds
• Tobacco use was associated with a lower risk of preeclampsia/eclampsia of unknown cause

DIAGNOSIS

DIFFERENTIAL DIAGNOSIS
• Epilepsy
• Cerebral tumors
• Ruptured cerebral aneurysm
• Until other causes are proven, however, all pregnant women with convulsions should be considered to have eclampsia

LABORATORY
• CBC/platelets
• 24 hour urine for protein/creatinine
• Liver function testing (LDH, AST)
• Uric acid
• Electrolytes
• BUN

Drugs that may alter lab results: Concurrent treatment with Dilantin, barbiturates (not with magnesium)

Disorders that may alter lab results: N/A

PATHOLOGICAL FINDINGS Cerebral edema, hyperemia, focal anemia, thrombosis, and hemorrhage; cerebral lesions account for 40% of eclamptic deaths

SPECIAL TESTS EEG, cerebral spinal fluid studies (CSF) - rarely useful in management

IMAGING Computed tomography can evaluate for mass lesions, infarct, hemorrhages, but is rarely used when usual clinical picture is present. Should be considered if focal findings persist or uncharacteristic signs/symptoms present.

DIAGNOSTIC PROCEDURES
• No additional procedures generally applicable
• EEG may vary from posterior slow waves to status epilepticus, but is rarely useful
• Cerebral spinal fluid studies are of no value unless other causes (e.g., meningitis) are seriously considered in differential diagnosis

TREATMENT

APPROPRIATE HEALTH CARE
• Inpatient, with parenteral access for medications and availability for invasive monitoring if necessary
• Adequacy of newborn care facilities should be considered and transport arranged for newborn if needed

GENERAL MEASURES
• Control of convulsions, correction of hypoxia and acidosis, lowering blood pressure, steps to effect delivery as soon as convulsions are controlled
• See Medications

SURGICAL MEASURES
• If fetal distress is evident or maternal condition at high risk of deterioration in spite of medical therapy, Cesarean section may be indicated. Patient is still at some risk for post partum eclampsia, hovever.

ACTIVITY Bedrest

DIET Nothing by mouth until stable, then usual seizure precautions; low salt diet commonly recommended

PATIENT EDUCATION
• Explain to the patient and partner/family what has happened and the need for the prompt actions necessary to ensure the safety of the mother and infant
• Additional materials from: American College of Obstetricians & Gynecologists, 409 12th St., SW, Washington, DC 20024-2188, (800)762-ACOG

MEDICATIONS

DRUG(S) OF CHOICE
Recent randomized trials: magnesium sulfate superior to phenytoin in treatment and prevention of eclampsia and probably more effective and safer than diazepam
• Protocol of Parkland Hospital as described in Williams' Obstetrics (1989): Control of convulsions with magnesium sulfate, 4 grams as a 20% solution intravenously at a rate of 0.5-1 gram per minute. Follow with 10 grams of 50% magnesium sulfate solution, one-half injected into each buttock. If convulsions persist after 15 minutes, give up to 2 grams additional intravenously as a 20% solution at a rate not to exceed 1 gram/minute. Every four hours thereafter, repeat 5 grams of 50% solution IM. Prior to administration, must ensure that:
a) patellar reflex is present
b) respirations are not depressed
c) urine output has been at least 25 cc/hr
• Many others give magnesium intravenously (as proposed by Zuspan et al.). One method is to provide the initial 4-6 grams intravenously, followed by an infusion of 1-3 grams/hour, with the amount given gauged on the basis of the neurological exam, particularly the patellar reflex. Levels of 6-8 mEq/L (3-4 mmol/L) are felt to be "therapeutic." There is little evidence that any one route is preferable, although one advantage may be that intravenous administration can be immediately discontinued if necessary.
• Fluid therapy: Ringer's lactate with 5% dextrose at 60-120 mL/hr, with careful attention to fluid-volume status. Invasive monitoring may be needed. Earlier transfusion may be considered due to attenuated intravascular volume and hemoconcentration.

Contraindications:
• Previous sensitivity/intolerance to a specific drug
• Avoid diuretics which can decrease the already lowered intravascular volume
• Hyperosmotic agents are dangerous due to capillary leakage

Precautions: Careful monitoring of neurological status, urine output, respirations, and fetal status

Significant possible interactions:
Combinations of medications may cause respiratory depression. Calcium carbonate (1 gram administered slowly IV) can reverse magnesium-induced respiratory depression.

ALTERNATIVE DRUGS
• Benzodiazepines, e.g., diazepam 2 mg/min until resolution or 20 mg given, or lorazepam 1-2 mg/min up to total of 10 mg, or phenytoin 18-20 mg/kg at a rate of 20-40 mg/min, or phenobarbital 100 mg/min to a total of 20 mg/kg given
• Nifedipine may be added to magnesium sulfate, but is not yet standard therapy (Austral N Zeal J OBstet Gynecol 1994;34: 144-48)

FOLLOWUP

PATIENT MONITORING
Blood pressure, neurological examination, condition of fetus

PREVENTION/AVOIDANCE
• Adequate prenatal care
• Good control of preexisting hypertension
• Recognition and treatment of preeclampsia

POSSIBLE COMPLICATIONS
• 56% have transient deficits including cortical blindness
• Most women do not have long-term sequelae from eclampsia
• Death from toxemia or its complications
• Death of fetus

EXPECTED COURSE/PROGNOSIS
• 25% of eclamptic women will have hypertension in subsequent pregnancies, but only 5% of these will be severe, and only 2% will be eclamptic again
• Eclamptic, multiparous women may be at higher risk for subsequent essential hypertension
• Multiparous women with eclampsia have higher mortality in subsequent pregnancies than primiparous women
• Racial factors are unclear, since the higher incidence of essential hypertension in blacks may predispose them to higher rates of hypertension postpartum, rather than a history of eclampsia

MISCELLANEOUS

ASSOCIATED CONDITIONS None

AGE-RELATED FACTORS
Pediatric: Essential for adequate neonatal care/facilities
Geriatric: N/A
Others: Younger patients have highest incidence, but most likely related to the fact that younger patients represent largest numbers of primigravidas

PREGNANCY By definition, a complication of pregnancy

SYNONYMS
• Pregnancy-associated seizures
• Toxemic seizures

ICD-9-CM
• 642.4 Mild or unspecified pre-eclampsia
• 642.5 Severe pre-eclampsia
• 642.6 Eclampsia
• 642.9 Unspecified hypertension complicating pregnancy, childbirth, or the puerperium
• 780.3 Convulsions

SEE ALSO Preeclampsia

OTHER NOTES N/A

ABBREVIATIONS N/A

REFERENCES
• Cunningham FG, MacDonald PC, Gant NF, eds: Williams' Obstetrics. 19th Ed. Norwalk, CT, Appleton and Lange, 1993
• Chesley LC, Annitto JE, Cosgrove RA: Long-term follow-up study of eclamptic women: sixth periodic report. Am J Obst Gyneco 1976;124:446
• American College of Obstetrics and Gynecology. Technical bulletin, Number 91, 1986
• Lucas MJ, Leveno KJ, Cunningham FG. A comparison of magnesium sulfate with phenytoin for the prevention of preeclampsia. N Engl J Med 1995;333: 201-5
• Lindheimer MD. Preeclampsia-eclampsia 1996: preventable? Have disputes on its treatment been resolved? Current Opinion in Nephrology and Hypertension. 1996:5: 452-58
Illustrations: N/A
Internet references: http://www.5mcc.com

Author(s)
Kurt Elward, MD, MPH

Ectopic pregnancy

BASICS

DESCRIPTION Extrauterine pregnancy - any pregnancy existing outside the confines of the uterine cavity
• Tubal pregnancy - pregnancy existing within the different portions of the fallopian tubes, i.e., ampullary (55%), isthmic (25%), fimbrial (17%), interstitial (cornual) (2%)
• Ovarian pregnancy - pregnancy existing within the confines of an ovary
• Abdominal pregnancy - pregnancy existing in the abdominal (peritoneal) cavity, most commonly within the cul-de-sac. Occasionally it may implant on the intestines, pelvic side-walls, omentum, or even on the surfaces of the liver or spleen.
• Cervical pregnancy - pregnancy is implanted in the substance of the cervix below the level of the internal os
• Intraligamentary pregnancy - after a tubal pregnancy ruptures, the surviving embryo secondarily implants within the confines of the anterior and posterior leaves of the broad ligament
System(s) affected: Reproductive
Genetics: N/A
Incidence/Prevalence in USA:
• 88,000 cases in 1987
• 16.8 per 1000 pregnancies (live birth, legally induced abortions, and ectopic pregnancies)
Predominant age: Over 40% occurred in women between ages 20 and 29
Predominant sex: Female only

SIGNS AND SYMPTOMS
• Tubal pregnancy:
    ◊ Pelvic pain
    ◊ Amenorrhea followed by irregular vaginal bleeding
    ◊ Abdominal tenderness
    ◊ Adnexal tenderness or mass
    ◊ Tenesmus
    ◊ Shoulder pain
    ◊ Syncope
    ◊ Passage of decidual cast
• Ovarian pregnancy:
    ◊ Pain and cramps
    ◊ Pelvic mass
    ◊ Vaginal bleeding after a period of amenorrhea
    ◊ Clinical shock after rupture
• Abdominal pregnancy:
    ◊ History suggestive of tubal abortion or rupture
    ◊ Pregnancy complicated by unusual gastrointestinal symptoms
    ◊ Fetal movements very marked or painful
    ◊ Easy palpation of the fetal parts or movements
    ◊ Pregnancy described by a multipara as "different"
    ◊ False labor near term
    ◊ High lying fetus in abnormal presentation, often transverse
    ◊ Displacement of a firm, long cervix
    ◊ Palpation of the fetal parts through the vaginal fornix
    ◊ Unusually loud vascular souffle

• Cervical pregnancy:
    ◊ A soft and disproportionately enlarged cervix equal to or greater than the uterine corpus (hourglass effect)
    ◊ Extrusion of dark tissue through the external os
    ◊ Continuous vaginal bleeding after amenorrhea
• Intraligamentary pregnancy:
    ◊ History suggestive of tubal abortion or rupture
    ◊ Unilateral pelvic mass associated with pain

CAUSES
• Tubal pregnancy:
    ◊ Previous tubal pregnancy
    ◊ Pelvic inflammatory disease
    ◊ Endometriosis
    ◊ Previous tubal surgery
    ◊ Salpingitis isthmica nodosa
    ◊ Pelvic adhesions
    ◊ Pelvic tumors
• Ovarian pregnancy:
    ◊ Implantation of the fertilized ovum on the ovarian surface
    ◊ Tubal abortion with secondary implantation of the embryo on the tubal surface
• Abdominal pregnancy:
    ◊ Tubal abortion with secondary implantation
    ◊ Uteroperitoneal fistula following rupture of cesarean section or myomectomy scars
    ◊ External transmigration theory
    ◊ Menstrual regurgitation of a fertilized ovum theory
• Cervical pregnancy:
    ◊ Unreceptive endometrium to implantation due to infection
    ◊ Uterine myomas
    ◊ Atrophic endometrium
    ◊ Septate uterus
    ◊ Presence of intrauterine device (IUD)
    ◊ Scarring of the endometrium
    ◊ Oral contraceptive use
• Intraligamentary pregnancy:
    ◊ Rupture of a tubal pregnancy and secondary implantation between the anterior and posterior leaves of the broad ligament

RISK FACTORS
• Previous tubal surgery
• Previous pelvic inflammatory disease
• Pelvic adhesions
• Previous tubal pregnancy
• Previous uterine surgery
• Use of an intrauterine device
• History of endometritis
• Recipients of assisted reproductive technologies, e.g., in-vitro fertilization and embryo transfer

DIAGNOSIS

DIFFERENTIAL DIAGNOSIS
• Uterine abortion
• Appendicitis
• Salpingitis
• Ruptured corpus luteum cyst
• Cornual myoma or abscess
• Ovarian tumor
• Endometrioma
• Cervical cancer
• Cervical phase of uterine abortion
• Placenta previa

LABORATORY
• Urine pregnancy test
• Human chorionic gonadotropin (HCG) - serial quantitative serum beta
• Serial blood counts to quantify blood loss
• Serum progesterone level
Drugs that may alter lab results: N/A
Disorders that may alter lab results: N/A

PATHOLOGICAL FINDINGS
• Tubal pregnancy:
    ◊ Presence of chorionic villi within the tubal wall
• Ovarian pregnancy (Spiegelberg's criteria):
    ◊ The pregnancy must occupy the position of the ovary
    ◊ The pregnancy must be connected to the uterus by the utero ovarian ligament
    ◊ The ipsilateral oviduct must be normal
    ◊ The pregnancy sac must show the presence of ovarian tissue
• Abdominal pregnancy - primary form:
    ◊ Both ovaries and oviducts must be normal
    ◊ There is no uteroperitoneal fistula
    ◊ Attachment of the conceptus is exclusively to the peritoneal surface
• Abdominal pregnancy - secondary form:
    ◊ Fetal or placental tissue is found within the abdominal cavity beyond the ovaries or oviducts
• Cervical pregnancy:
    ◊ Chorionic villi are implanted within the substance of the uterine cervix below the level of the internal os
    ◊ The uterine cavity above the internal os is free of the products of conception
• Intraligamentary pregnancy:
    ◊ The products of conception are within the confines of the broad ligament

SPECIAL TESTS
• Culdocentesis
• Endometrial biopsy and/or dilatation and curettage

IMAGING
• Vaginal and abdominal ultrasonography
• CT scan
• MRI
• Endovaginal color Doppler flow imaging

DIAGNOSTIC PROCEDURES
• Laparoscopy
• Laparotomy

Ectopic pregnancy

TREATMENT

APPROPRIATE HEALTH CARE
• Outpatient for most evaluation and treatment
• Outpatient surgery for unruptured tubal pregnancy
• Inpatient surgery for unstable hemodynamic conditions after resuscitation

GENERAL MEASURES N/A

SURGICAL MEASURES
• Laparotomy is required for ovarian, abdominal, and intraligamentary pregnancy
• Careful curettage, packing of the cervix and uterine cavity, bilateral internal iliac artery ligations, or even hysterectomy may be necessary as treatment for cervical pregnancy
• Unruptured tubal pregnancy may be treated by salpingostomy
• Unruptured tubal pregnancy of less than 4 cm. diameter may be treated through laparoscopy. With methotrexate, best results obtainable when unruptured tubal pregnancy is less than 2 cm diameter or HCG less than 1000 mIU/mL, and before ultrasound evidence of fetal heart beats.

ACTIVITY Variable

DIET Variable

PATIENT EDUCATION American College of Obstetricians & Gynecologists (ACOG), 409 12th St., SW, Washington, DC 20024-2188, (800)762-ACOG

MEDICATIONS

DRUG(S) OF CHOICE
• Methotrexate as primary treatment for unruptured tubal pregnancy and for persistent disease after salpingotomy
• Methotrexate as supplementary treatment for retained placenta after delivery of the fetus in abdominal pregnancy
• Dosage: Methotrexate 1 mg/kg IM every other day with leucovorin 0.1 mg/kg IM in between. Maximum of 4 doses of methotrexate or methotrexate x 1 without leucovorin, at 50 mgm per square meter of body surface area; may repeat once if unsatisfactory response.
Contraindications: Pregnant women with psoriasis
Precautions: Methotrexate has toxic effects on the hematologic, renal, gastrointestinal, pulmonary, and neurologic systems
Significant possible interactions: Refer to manufacturer's profile of each drug

ALTERNATIVE DRUGS Dactinomycin

FOLLOWUP

PATIENT MONITORING
• Serial serum quantitative ß-HCG until level drops to near zero
• Followup pelvic ultrasonogram for persistent or recurrent masses
• Followup imaging studies for retained placenta in abdominal pregnancy, e.g., ultrasonography, CT scan, and MRI

PREVENTION/AVOIDANCE
• Reliable contraception
• Repeat tubal pregnancies occur in about 12%. For patient who becomes pregnant again, use ultrasound to verify intrauterine pregnancy.

POSSIBLE COMPLICATIONS
• Hemorrhage and hypovolemic shock
• Infection
• Loss of reproductive organs after complicated surgery
• Infertility
• Urinary and/or intestinal fistulas after complicated surgery
• Need for blood transfusions with its hazards
• Disseminated intravascular coagulation

EXPECTED COURSE/PROGNOSIS With early diagnosis and treatment, rupture unlikely to occur

MISCELLANEOUS

ASSOCIATED CONDITIONS N/A

AGE-RELATED FACTORS
Pediatric: N/A
Geriatric: N/A
Others: N/A

PREGNANCY N/A

SYNONYMS
• Extrauterine pregnancy
• Tubal pregnancy
• Ovarian pregnancy
• Abdominal pregnancy
• Cervical pregnancy
• Intraligamentary pregnancy

ICD-9-CM 633 Ectopic pregnancy

SEE ALSO
• Abortion, spontaneous

OTHER NOTES N/A

ABBREVIATIONS N/A

REFERENCES
• Herbst AL, Mishell DR, Stenchever MA, Droegemueller W: Comprehensive Gynecology. 2nd Ed. St. Louis, The C.V. Mosby Co., 1992
• Durfee RB, Pernoll ML: Early Pregnancy Risks In: Pernoll M, Benson RC, eds. Current Obstetric and Gynecologic Diagnosis and Treatment. 7th Ed. Norwalk, CT, Appleton and Lange, 1991
• Kurman RJ, ed: Blaustein's Pathology of the Female Genital Tract. 3rd Ed. New York, Springer-Verlag, 1987
• Novak ER, Woodruff JD: Novak's Gynecologic and Obstetric Pathology With Clinical and Endocrine Relations. 8th Ed. Philadelphia, W.B. Saunders Co., 1979
• Stovall TG, Ling FW: Single dose methotrexate, an expanded clinical trial. Am J OB-GYN 1993;168:1759-1765
• Stovall TG, Ling FW: Gonadotrophin in screening for ectopic pregnancy. Human Repro 1992;7:723-725
• Wolf GC, et al: Completely non-surgical management of ectopic pregnancies. Gynecol-Obstet Invest 1994;37:232-235
• Kadar N, et al: The discriminatory HCG zone for endovaginal sonography, a prospective randomized study. Fertil Steril 1994;61:1016-1020
• Emerson DS, et al: Diagnostic efficacy of endovaginal color Doppler flow imaging in an ectopic pregnancy screening. Radiology 1992;183:413-420
• Pellerito JS, et al: Ectopic pregnancy: Evaluation with endovaginal color flow imaging. Radiology 1992;183:407-411
Illustrations: N/A
Internet references: http://www.5mcc.com

Author(s)
Albert T. Shiu, MD, FACOG

Ejaculatory disorders

BASICS

DESCRIPTION Premature ejaculation: Inability to constantly control the ejaculatory reflex is a common sexual disorder affecting all age groups. Definition criteria vary, e.g., inability to maintain an erection of sufficient duration to satisfy a partner, or ejaculation that occurs before individual wants it to. Natural biological response is to ejaculate within 2 minutes after vaginal penetration. Ejaculatory control is an acquired behavior that increases with experience.
• Retarded ejaculation: A rare condition in which erection is normal, or prolonged, but ejaculation does not occur
• Retrograde ejaculation: The valve at the base of the bladder fails to close during ejaculation and the ejaculate is forced backward into the bladder. Erection and sexual pleasure are usually not diminished.
System(s) affected: Reproductive, Nervous
Genetics: No known genetic pattern
Incidence/Prevalence: Premature ejaculation is common (particularly in the adolescent)
Predominant age: All age groups
Predominant sex: Male only

SIGNS AND SYMPTOMS
• Ejaculation occurring before individual wishes
• Ejaculation does not occur following normal erection (including masturbation)

CAUSES
• Peripheral neuropathy
• Premature ejaculation
  ◊ Adolescence
  ◊ Fear of sexually transmitted disease
  ◊ Anxiety
  ◊ Psychological factors
  ◊ Guilty feelings about sex
  ◊ Interpersonal maladaptation (marital problems, unresponsiveness of mate)
  ◊ Close proximity of other persons in the household (e.g., mother-in-law)
• Retarded ejaculation
  ◊ Rarely may be due to underlying painful disorder, e.g., prostatitis, seminal vesiculitis
  ◊ Usually psychogenic
  ◊ Diabetes mellitus
  ◊ Some drugs may impair ejaculation, e.g., thioridazine, mesoridazine, antihypertensives, beta-blockers, certain antidepressants
• Retrograde ejaculation
  ◊ Prostatectomy
  ◊ Surgery on the neck of the bladder
  ◊ Extensive pelvic surgery
  ◊ Retroperitoneal lymph node dissection for testicular cancer (also can produce failure of emission)
  ◊ Neurologic disorders, e.g., multiple sclerosis
  ◊ Drugs, e.g., amoxapine, desipramine, imipramine

RISK FACTORS Listed with Causes

DIAGNOSIS

DIFFERENTIAL DIAGNOSIS N/A

LABORATORY
• Laboratory test results are usually normal
• Post-ejaculate urinalysis will confirm retrograde ejaculation when infertility is a concern
Drugs that may alter lab results: N/A
Disorders that may alter lab results: N/A

PATHOLOGICAL FINDINGS N/A

SPECIAL TESTS N/A

IMAGING N/A

DIAGNOSTIC PROCEDURES Detailed sexual history

TREATMENT

APPROPRIATE HEALTH CARE
Outpatient

GENERAL MEASURES
• Identification of any medical cause (even if not reversible) helps patient accept condition
• Improve partner communication
• Reduce performance pressure through reassurance
• Use sensate focus therapy
• Techniques to learn ejaculatory control, e.g., coronal squeeze technique or start-and-stop technique
• Use of a variety of resources may be necessary, e.g., psychiatrists, psychologists, sex therapists, vascular surgeons, urologists, endocrinologists, neurologists
• If drugs are a possible cause, consider discontinuing or changing dosage
• Retrograde ejaculation may be helped if intercourse occurs when bladder is full

SURGICAL MEASURES N/A

ACTIVITY No restrictions

DIET No special diet

PATIENT EDUCATION N/A

MEDICATIONS

DRUG(S) OF CHOICE None
Contraindications: N/A
Precautions: N/A
Significant possible interactions: N/A

ALTERNATIVE DRUGS N/A

FOLLOWUP

PATIENT MONITORING As needed depending on type of therapy

PREVENTION/AVOIDANCE N/A

POSSIBLE COMPLICATIONS
Psychological impact on some males - signs of severe inadequacy, self-doubt, additional anxiety and guilt

EXPECTED COURSE/PROGNOSIS
Usually curable with therapy

MISCELLANEOUS

ASSOCIATED CONDITIONS
• Neurological disorders, e.g., multiple sclerosis
• Prostatitis
• Psychological disorders
• Interpersonal disorders

AGE-RELATED FACTORS
Pediatric: N/A
Geriatric: Age alone does not cause ejaculation problems
Others: N/A

PREGNANCY N/A

SYNONYMS
• Premature ejaculation
• Retarded ejaculation
• Retrograde ejaculation
• Inhibited orgasm in males

ICD-9-CM
• 608.89 ejaculation painful
• 306.59 ejaculation psychogenic
• 302.75 ejaculation premature

SEE ALSO N/A

OTHER NOTES N/A

ABBREVIATIONS N/A

REFERENCES
• Yaffe M, Fenwick E: Sexual Happiness: A Practical Approach. New York, H. Holt & Co., 1988
• Stine CC, Collins M: Male sexual dysfunction. Prim Care 1989;16:1031
• Walsh PC, Gittes RF, Perlmutter AD, eds: Campbell's Urology. 6th Ed. Philadelphia, W.B. Saunders Co., 1992
• Segraves RT: Effects of psychotropic drugs on human erection and ejaculation. Arch Gen Psych 1989;46:275-284
Illustrations: N/A
Internet references: http://www.5mcc.com

Author(s)
Mark D. Thomas, MD

Encephalitis, viral

BASICS

DESCRIPTION Acute inflammation of the brain caused by viral invasion or by a viral-mediated inflammatory response in the brain following an acute, systemic infection. Meningeal, spinal cord, and peripheral nerve involvement may accompany encephalitis. Most cases of viral encephalitis are rare complications of common systemic viral infections. Post-viral encephalitis usually occurs via immune-mediated mechanisms and has onset 2-12 days after the primary viral infection.

System(s) affected: Nervous
Genetics: N/A
Incidence/Prevalence in USA:
Uncommon; total of 903 cases reported to Centers for Disease Control and Prevention in 1992. Estimated 20,000 cases per year overall, most of which are mild. HSV encephalitis estimated incidence 1 in 250,000 per year. Seasonal variation:
• Arthropod-borne diseases (e.g., arboviruses, Colorado tick fever) are predominantly spring and summer
• Enteroviruses peak in late summer
• Mumps and varicella prevalent in spring
• Most others (e.g., herpes simplex virus) are not seasonal
Predominant age: Age extremes at highest risk, especially for herpes simplex encephalitis
Predominant sex: None

SIGNS AND SYMPTOMS
• Nonspecific symptoms (malaise, fever, rhinorrhea) may precede neurologic symptoms
• Meningeal involvement is signified by stiff neck and headache
• Photophobia, lethargy progressing to coma, seizures, and focal neurologic deficits may be observed
• Progression is variable; may be rapid or follow a more indolent course

CAUSES
• Endemic
  ◊ Herpes simplex virus types 1 and 2
  ◊ Epstein-Barr virus
  ◊ Varicella-zoster virus
  ◊ Adenovirus
  ◊ Rabies
  ◊ Dengue
  ◊ Benign lymphocytic choriomeningitis V
  ◊ Infectious mononucleosis
  ◊ California virus
  ◊ Japanese B encephalitis
  ◊ Russian spring-summer encephalitis
  ◊ Murray Valley
• Epidemic
  ◊ Arboviruses (e.g., St. Louis encephalitis, eastern equine encephalitis, western equine encephalitis, Venezuelan equine encephalitis)
  ◊ Enteroviruses (most commonly Coxsackie B viruses)
  ◊ Mumps
  ◊ Varicella-zoster
  ◊ Influenza
  ◊ HTLV III (HIV)

RISK FACTORS
• Many of the agents produce more severe disease in newborns and the elderly
• Travel to endemic areas
• Exposure to vectors (e.g., mosquitoes)
• HIV positivity

DIAGNOSIS

DIFFERENTIAL DIAGNOSIS
• Bacterial infection
  ◊ Meningitis
  ◊ Brain abscess
  ◊ Tuberculosis
  ◊ Cat-scratch disease
• Rickettsial infection
  ◊ Rocky Mountain spotted fever
  ◊ Ehrlichiosis
• Spirochetal infection
  ◊ Syphilis
  ◊ Lyme disease
  ◊ Leptospirosis
• Other infectious agents
  ◊ Free-living amoeba (Naegleria, Acanthamoeba)
  ◊ Toxoplasmosis
• Intracranial hemorrhage
• Intracranial tumor
• Trauma
• Thromboembolism
• Systemic lupus erythematosus
• Toxic ingestion
• Hypoglycemia

LABORATORY
• Standard laboratory studies (CBC, serum chemistries) are usually normal or nonspecifically abnormal
• Cerebrospinal fluid examination is essential
  ◊ White cell count usually increased (10-2000 cells/mm3) but may be normal, especially in immunocompromised host; neutrophils predominate early, then see shift to mononuclear cells
  ◊ Red cell count usually normal (more likely elevated in herpes simplex infections)
  ◊ Protein may be normal or mildly elevated
  ◊ Glucose may be normal or mildly decreased
Drugs that may alter lab results: Steroid therapy may mask CSF inflammatory findings
Disorders that may alter lab results: Immunocompromised patients may have normal CSF findings

PATHOLOGICAL FINDINGS
• Varies according to etiology
• Usually have prominent perivascular inflammation
• Swelling and degenerative changes of neural elements
• Negri bodies may be seen in brain, conjunctiva, and skin from the base of the neck in rabies patients

SPECIAL TESTS
• Electroencephalographic findings are usually abnormal, with slowing or epileptiform activity present. Temporal lobe abnormalities, particularly periodic lateralized epileptic form discharges (PLEDS), should suggest a diagnosis of HSV encephalitis.
• Most viral encephalitis cases have specific diagnosis made by measurement of acute and convalescent (2-3 weeks) serum antibody concentrations for the specific pathogen. A four-fold change in titer is suggestive of the diagnosis.
• CSF antibody index can be used to ascertain specific central nervous system production of antibody against the infecting agent: Serum and CSF IgG antibody and serum and CSF albumin concentrations are determined. Infection may be suggested by a higher specific antibody: albumin ratio in CSF than in serum.
• Antigen detection in CSF by polymerase chain reaction has been useful in cases of HSV and enteroviral disease, but is available only in some academic centers
• Enteroviruses may be recovered from CSF viral culture about 60% of cases, but most other viral agents are present in too low quantities to be detected by these techniques

IMAGING Imaging studies (CT scan, MRI, brain scan) may be normal early; later, nonspecific abnormalities are seen. Again, temporal lobe pathology suggests the diagnosis of HSV.

DIAGNOSTIC PROCEDURES Brain biopsy may be useful in certain cases, particularly to identify treatable causes

TREATMENT

APPROPRIATE HEALTH CARE Inpatient with symptomatic and supportive therapy as needed

GENERAL MEASURES
• Maintenance of adequately respiratory and circulatory support
• Control cerebral edema if necessary (hyperventilation, osmotic diuresis)
• Anticonvulsant as needed
• Monitor for SIADH

SURGICAL MEASURES N/A

ACTIVITY As indicated by clinical condition

DIET As indicated by clinical condition. May need fluid restriction for SIADH or cerebral edema.

PATIENT EDUCATION Advice to travelers to specific areas (e.g., Japan for Japanese encephalitis, Africa for many arthropod-borne infections)

MEDICATIONS

DRUG(S) OF CHOICE
• Acyclovir [30 mg/kg/day for adults; 1500 mg/m2/day for children] for HSV infections
• No specific antiviral therapy for other etiologies
Contraindications: None
Precautions: Not approved for pregnant women, but benefits probably outweigh risks to fetus
Significant possible interactions: N/A

ALTERNATIVE DRUGS
Vidarabine (adenine arabinoside) for acyclovir-resistant HSV; has been used in combination with acyclovir

FOLLOWUP

PATIENT MONITORING Intracranial pressure monitoring may be needed for severe cases

PREVENTION/AVOIDANCE Use of appropriate insect repellants

POSSIBLE COMPLICATIONS
• Varies with etiologic agent
• HSV encephalitis has highest morbidity and mortality of the common viral encephalitides (untreated mortality 70%; < 5% of survivors have normal neurologic function)

EXPECTED COURSE/PROGNOSIS
• Prognosis generally difficult to predict; somewhat based on infecting agent (e.g., HSV severe, varicella mild)
• With HSV, therapy is more beneficial if initiated early, prior to onset of coma

MISCELLANEOUS

ASSOCIATED CONDITIONS N/A

AGE-RELATED FACTORS
Pediatric:
• Children more commonly symptomatic from arboviral infection than are adults
• Neonatal - newborns at higher risk for severe HSV and enteroviral CNS disease
Geriatric: May also be at risk for severe disease
Others: N/A

PREGNANCY Risk of HSV infection in an infant delivered vaginally to a mother with a primary genital infection is approximately 40%; drops to 3-5% in reactivation genital lesions. Enteroviruses may be transmitted transplacentally to fetus; cause of neonatal disease if mother infected just prior to delivery.

SYNONYMS N/A

ICD-9-CM
047.9 Unspecified viral meningitis
049.9 Unspecified non-arthropod-borne viral diseases of central nervous system

SEE ALSO
• Adenovirus infections
• Epstein-Barr virus infections
• Herpes simplex
• Herpes zoster
• Meningitis, viral

OTHER NOTES N/A

ABBREVIATIONS
HSV = herpes simplex virus
SIADH = syndrome of inappropriate antidiuretic hormone secretion

REFERENCES
• Whitley RJ: Viral encephalitis. New Engl J Med 1990;323:242
• Griffin DE, Johnson RT: Encephalitis, myelitis, and neuritis. In: Mandell GL, et al, eds. Principles and Practice of Infectious Diseases. 4th Ed. New York, Churchill Livingstone, 1995
Illustrations: N/A
Internet references: http://www.5mcc.com

Author(s)
Bernhard L. Wiedermann, MD
Elizabeth A. Frankel, MD

Encopresis

BASICS

DESCRIPTION The regular passage of fecal material into clothes or other inappropriate places by a child older than four years of age
System(s) affected: Gastrointestinal
Genetics: Unknown
Incidence/Prevalence in USA: 1.3% of all children > 4 years of age
Predominant age: 70% have onset before 5 years of age
Predominant sex: Males > Females 1.5:1.

SIGNS AND SYMPTOMS
• Constipation usually accompanies encopresis (there is a subgroup of children who do not have constipation)
• Unrecognized constipation and/or stool retention often precedes the symptom presented to the care provider
• Large amount of fecal material on abdominal, pelvic or rectal exam
• Pasty stool found on underclothes
• Fecal or foul odor surrounds the child
• Often intermittent periumbilical pain
• Occasional passage of a voluminous stool
• History of painful bowel movements
• Some children seem shy and withdrawn; others show acting out or aggressive behavior
• Some have had psychotherapy
• Some have had recurrent urinary tract infections

CAUSES
Many events precipitate constipation and hence encopresis
• Psychologic
  ◊ Difficulty with toilet training
  ◊ Resistance to using toilet facilities, such as school bathrooms or outdoor toilets during camping trips
• Anatomic
  ◊ Anal fissure or painful defecation
  ◊ Muscle hypotonia
  ◊ Slow intestinal motility
  ◊ Aganglionic megacolon or Hirschsprung's disease
  ◊ Spinal cord defects or injuries
  ◊ Anal stenosis
  ◊ Anterior displacement of the anus: anogenital index (the distance from the posterior aspect of the vagina or scrotum to the anus divided by the full distance to the tip of the coccyx) > 0.34 females/> 0.45 males
  ◊ Post surgical stricture of anus or rectum
  ◊ Pelvic mass
  ◊ Neurofibromatosis
• Dietary or metabolic
  ◊ Lack of fiber
  ◊ Excessive protein or milk intake
  ◊ Inadequate water intake
  ◊ Hypothyroidism

RISK FACTORS
• Boys are more often affected
• Difficulty with bowel training
• Unresolved fecal retention and impaction

DIAGNOSIS

DIFFERENTIAL DIAGNOSIS
• Not difficult when brought to provider's attention
• Suspect when exam detects soiling of underclothes, as the problem is often not mentioned by mother or child
• Must look for underlying treatable causes of the constipation

LABORATORY
• Urinalysis and urine culture may be indicated
• Thyroid function studies
Drugs that may alter lab results: N/A
Disorders that may alter lab results: N/A

PATHOLOGICAL FINDINGS N/A

SPECIAL TESTS N/A

IMAGING Abdominal plain films are occasionally necessary if an impaction is suspected but not detected by abdominal or rectal examination

DIAGNOSTIC PROCEDURES
• Detailed history and complete physical exam including neurological examination of lower extremities and genital area and a digital rectal examination usually is sufficient for a diagnosis
• History of constipation prior to one month of age is almost always present with aganglionic megacolon and that history would warrant a barium enema and/or rectal biopsy

TREATMENT

APPROPRIATE HEALTH CARE Hospital admission and abdominal x-ray may be necessary to insure complete removal of impaction

GENERAL MEASURES
• Anticipatory guidance relative to toilet training beginning at 18 months
• The impaction must be eliminated before starting maintenance treatment
• Avoid redevelopment of an impaction
• Avoid frequent and repeated digital examinations, enemas, and suppositories
• Biofeedback training can be used as alternative therapy or when conventional therapy has been unsuccessful
• Child to sit on toilet twice a day at the same times each day for 10-15 minutes and 10-15 minutes after a meal

SURGICAL MEASURES N/A

ACTIVITY Unrestricted

DIET
• Avoid excessive milk, bananas, apples, gelatin
• Increase fiber

PATIENT EDUCATION
• Your Child's Health by Barton D. Schmitt, M.D.
• Education and demystifying the process
• Careful and full explanation of the treatment plan
• Allay the guilt and avoid punishment for soiling

MEDICATIONS

DRUG(S) OF CHOICE
Remove stool impaction: (before starting maintenance treatment program)
• Give 1 ounce of mineral oil the first day
• On the next day, give 1-3 enemas till clear; this may need to be repeated on 1-2 subsequent days
  ◊ First give an oil retention enema
  ◊ Follow the oil retention enema with hypophosphate enemas, e.g., sodium phosphate (Fleet's) 1 ounce (28.4 gm) per 20 pounds (9.1 kg) of body weight, or
  ◊ Normal saline enemas - 2 tsp table salt per quart (946 mL) of warm water and give 2 ounces (60 mL) per year of age to a maximum of 16 ounces (480 mL)
  ◊ A bisacodyl (Dulcolax) suppository can be inserted to assist the evacuation
• Alternative: give an oral solution of polyethylene glycol (Colyte, Nulytely) at 20 mL/kg/hr for 4 hours on 2 consecutive days. Nulytely is a newer, equally effective and more palatable preparation.
Maintenance treatment
• Up to 6 months or more to keep stool slippery or soft, and for child to develop regular bowel habit
• Give mineral oil (at least 2 tablespoons each day) mixed with cold orange juice to help it go down
• Fiber or other hydrophilic agents may be used to soften the stool - lactulose, methylcellulose (Citrucel), psyllium (Metamucil, Perdiem), polycarbophil (Mitrolan), malt soup extract (Maltsupex) and fiber wafers; adjust dose to keep the stool soft.
• Multivitamins must be given between mineral oil doses to ensure absorption of the fat soluble vitamins (A,D,E,K)
Contraindications: Refer to manufacturer's profile of each drug
Precautions: Avoid bedtime doses of mineral oil to decrease risk of aspiration
Significant possible interactions: Refer to manufacturer's profile of each drug

ALTERNATIVE DRUGS N/A

FOLLOWUP

PATIENT MONITORING
• Continue the maintenance treatment program for at least 6 months and maybe for as long as 1-2 years
• Visits every 4-10 weeks for support and to ensure compliance
• Telephone availability to prevent problems and adjust doses
• Redevelopment of impaction must be removed as above
• Counselling and/or referral for associated psychosocial issues

PREVENTION/AVOIDANCE
• Optimal feeding practices
• Normal bowel function and recommendations for bowel training
• Early detection of problems
• Use of dark Karo syrup and fiber for hard stools
• Prompt treatment of perianal dermatitis to avoid painful defecation
• Look for signs of relapse which include large caliber stools, decrease in frequency of defecation, soiling

POSSIBLE COMPLICATIONS
• Excessive enemas or suppositories may cause colitis
• Perianal dermatitis
• Anal fissure

EXPECTED COURSE/PROGNOSIS
• Usually responds well though relapses may occur
• Children with psychosocial or emotional problems which preceded the encopresis are more recalcitrant to treatment

MISCELLANEOUS

ASSOCIATED CONDITIONS
• Perianal dermatitis
• Urinary tract infections

AGE-RELATED FACTORS
Pediatric: N/A
Geriatric: N/A
Others: N/A

PREGNANCY N/A

SYNONYMS
Soiling

ICD-9-CM
787.6 Incontinence of feces

SEE ALSO Constipation

OTHER NOTES N/A

ABBREVIATIONS N/A

REFERENCES
• Hatch TF: Encopresis and constipation in children. Pediatric Clinics of N Am 1988;35(2):257-78
• Schmitt BD: Soiling with constipation. Parent handout in Clinical Reference Systems, Ltd., 1989
• Olness K, McParland F, Piper L: Biofeedback: A new modality in the management of children with fecal soiling. J Pediatrics 1980;96:505-509
• Iwata G, Iwai N, Nagashima M, Fukata R: New biofeedback therapy in children with encopresis. Europ J Pediatr Surg 1995;5:231-234
Illustrations: N/A
Internet references: http://www.5mcc.com

Author(s)
Burris Duncan, MD

Endocarditis, infective (part 1)

BASICS

DESCRIPTION A disease resulting from infection primarily of the valvular endocardium and occasionally the mural endocardium
• Acute endocarditis: Aggressive course, usually caused by more virulent organisms, such as Staphylococcus aureus, group B streptococcus, may not have underlying valve lesion
• Subacute endocarditis: Indolent course, usually caused by alpha-hemolytic streptococci, enterococci (usually in setting of underlying structural valve disease)
• Endocarditis in intravenous drug abusers: Commonly involves the tricuspid valve. Staphylococcus aureus is the most common infecting organism.
• Early prosthetic valve endocarditis: Occurs within 60 days of valve implantation. Staphylococci, gram-negative bacilli and Candida are common infecting organisms.
• Late prosthetic valve endocarditis: Occurs 60 days or longer after valve implantation. Staphylococcus epidermidis, alpha-hemolytic streptococci and enterococci are common infecting organisms.
System(s) affected: Cardiovascular and others
Genetics: Unknown
Incidence/Prevalence in USA: 1.7-4.2/100,000; 0.32-1.3/1000 hospital admissions
Predominant age: All ages
Predominant sex: Male > Female (slightly)

SIGNS AND SYMPTOMS
• Fever, may be high, low or absent. May be only symptom in prosthetic valve endocarditis.
• Night sweats, chilly sensation
• Malaise, myalgia, joint pain
• Back pain, may be severe
• Anorexia, weight loss
• Stiff neck
• Delirium, headache
• Paralysis, hemiparesis, aphasia
• Numbness, muscle weakness
• Cold extremity with pain
• Bloody urine, may be gross or microscopic
• Bloody sputum, from septic pulmonary emboli
• Petechiae
• Conjunctival hemorrhage
• Hemorrhagic or necrotic pustule
• Pain of finger tip, or toe tip (subjective symptom of Osler node)
• Chest pain, shortness of breath, cough
• Pallor
• Roth spot
• Osler node
• Janeway lesion
• Heart murmur, may be absent
• Neck vein distention
• Gallops
• Rales
• Cardiac arrhythmia
• Pericardial rub
• Pleural friction rub
• Splenomegaly

CAUSES
• Staphylococcus aureus is a causative organism in all types of endocarditis, especially acute endocarditis and endocarditis seen in IV drug abusers
• Acute endocarditis
  ◊ Staphylococcus aureus
  ◊ Streptococcus groups A, B, C, G
  ◊ Haemophilus influenzae
  ◊ Haemophilus parainfluenzae
  ◊ Streptococcus pneumoniae
  ◊ Staphylococcus lugdunensis
  ◊ Enterococcus species
  ◊ Neisseria gonorrhoeae
• Subacute endocarditis
  ◊ Alpha-hemolytic streptococci (viridans streptococci)
  ◊ Streptococcus bovis
  ◊ Enterococcus species (E. faecalis, E. faecium, E. durans)
  ◊ Haemophilus aphrophilus and paraphrophilus
  ◊ Actinobacillus actinomycetemcomitans
  ◊ Cardiobacterium hominis
  ◊ Eikenella corrodens
  ◊ Kingella kingae
  ◊ Staphylococcus aureus
• Endocarditis in intravenous drug-abusers
  ◊ Staphylococcus aureus
  ◊ Pseudomonas aeruginosa
  ◊ Pseudomonas cepacia
  ◊ Other gram-negative bacilli
  ◊ Enterococcus species
  ◊ Candida species
• Early prosthetic valve endocarditis
  ◊ Staphylococcus aureus
  ◊ Staphylococcus epidermidis
  ◊ Gram-negative bacilli
  ◊ Candida species
  ◊ Aspergillus species
• Late prosthetic valve endocarditis
  ◊ Alpha-hemolytic streptococci (viridans streptococci)
  ◊ Enterococcus species
  ◊ Staphylococcus epidermidis
  ◊ Candida species
  ◊ Aspergillus species
• Culture-negative endocarditis
  ◊ 5-10%
  ◊ Patients on antibiotics
  ◊ Bartonella quintana (homeless people)
  ◊ Bartonella henselae (cat owners)
  ◊ Brucella
  ◊ Fungi
  ◊ Coxiella burnetii (Q fever)
  ◊ Chlamydia trachomatis
  ◊ Chlamydia psittaci

RISK FACTORS
• Conditions predisposed to development of endocarditis
  ◊ Prosthetic cardiac valves, including bioprosthetic and homograft valves
  ◊ Previous bacterial endocarditis, even in the absence of heart disease
  ◊ Most congenital cardiac malformations
  ◊ Rheumatic and other acquired valvular dysfunction, even after valvular surgery
  ◊ Hypertrophic cardiomyopathy
  ◊ Mitral valve prolapse with valvular regurgitation
  ◊ Indwelling intravascular devices
• Dental or surgical procedures that may cause transient bacteremia leading to endocarditis in susceptible hosts
  ◊ Dental procedures known to produce gingival irritation, including professional cleaning
  ◊ Tonsillectomy and/or adenoidectomy
  ◊ Surgical operations that involve intestinal or respiratory mucosa
  ◊ Bronchoscopy with a rigid bronchoscope
  ◊ Sclerotherapy for esophageal varices
  ◊ Esophageal dilatation
  ◊ Gallbladder surgery
  ◊ Cystoscopy
  ◊ Urethral dilatation
  ◊ Urethral catheterization if urinary tract infection is present
  ◊ Urinary tract surgery if urinary tract infection is present
  ◊ Prostatic surgery
  ◊ Incision and drainage of infected tissue
  ◊ Vaginal hysterectomy
  ◊ Vaginal delivery in the presence of infection

DIAGNOSIS

DIFFERENTIAL DIAGNOSIS
• Brain abscess
• Cerebral embolus especially in a young person
• Cerebral hemorrhage with fever
• Connective tissue diseases
• Fever of unknown origin
• Glomerulonephritis
• Intra-abdominal infections
• Meningitis
• Myocardial infarction
• Osteomyelitis
• Pericarditis
• Purulent meningitis
• Rheumatic fever
• Salmonellosis
• Tuberculosis
• Septic pulmonary infarcts

LABORATORY
• Positive blood cultures taken at different times
• 2-dimensional echocardiography, not always positive for vegetations (transesophageal echocardiography has high sensitivity)
• Leukocytosis in acute endocarditis
• Anemia in subacute endocarditis
• Elevated erythrocyte sedimentation rate
• Decreased C3, C4, CH50 in subacute endocarditis
• Hematuria, microscopic or macroscopic
• Rheumatoid factor in subacute endocarditis
• Serologies for Chlamydia, Q fever (Coxiella) and Bartonella may be useful in "culture-negative" endocarditis

Drugs that may alter lab results:
Antibiotics may make blood cultures falsely negative

Disorders that may alter lab results:
• Endocarditis caused by fungi, Chlamydia trachomatis, Chlamydia psittaci, Coxiella burnetii, Bartonella species may be associated with negative blood cultures
• Prolonged incubation of blood cultures is needed in endocarditis caused by fastidious organisms, e.g., HACEK organisms (Haemophilus species, Actinobacillus actinomycetemcomitans, Cardiobacterium hominis, Eikenella corrodens, Kingella species), Brucella species

PATHOLOGICAL FINDINGS
• Vegetations on the affected endocardium are composed of platelets, fibrin and colonies of micro-organisms. Destruction of valvular endocardium, perforation of valve leaflets, rupture of chordae tendineae, abscesses of myocardium, rupture of sinus of Valsalva, pericarditis may occur.
• Emboli and/or infarction may be found in different body organs. Abscesses and micro-abscesses may be found in different organs. Kidneys may show embolic and/or immune-complex glomerulonephritis.

SPECIAL TESTS N/A

IMAGING
• Pulmonary ventilation perfusion scan may be useful in right-sided endocarditis
• Computerized axial tomographic scan may be useful in locating abscesses

DIAGNOSTIC PROCEDURES
• Transesophageal echocardiography may be useful, especially in prosthetic or bioprosthetic valve endocarditis
• Cardiac catheterization may be indicated to ascertain the degree of valvular damage
• Aortic root injection may be useful when aortic root abscess or rupture of sinus of Valsalva is suspected

Duke criteria for diagnosis of infective endocarditis.
• For the diagnosis of infective endocarditis:
◊ 2 major criteria, or
◊ 1 major and 3 minor criteria, or
◊ 5 minor criteria
<u>Major criteria</u>
• 1. Positive blood culture for infective endocarditis
◊ Typical microorganism for infective endocarditis from 2 separate blood cultures
- Viridans streptococci,† Streptococcus bovis, HACEK†† group, or
- Community acquired Staphylococcus aureus or enterococci, in the absence of a primary focus, or
◊ Persistently positive blood culture, defined as recovery of a microorganism consistent with infective endocarditis from:
- A) Blood cultures drawn more than 12 hours apart, or
- B) All of 3 or a majority of 4 or more separate blood cultures, with first and last drawn at least 1 hour apart
• 2. Evidence of endocardial involvement
◊ Positive echocardiogram for infective endocarditis
- A) Oscillating intracardiac mass, on valve or supporting structures, or in the path of regurgitant jets, or on implanted material, in the absence of an alternative anatomic explanation, or
- B) Abscess, or
- C) New partial dehiscence of prosthetic valve, or
◊ New valvular regurgitation (increase or change in pre-existing murmur not sufficient
<u>Minor criteria</u>
• 1. Predisposition: predisposing heart condition or intravenous drug use
• 2 Fever ≥ 38.0°C (100.4°F)
• 3. Vascular phenomena: major arterial emboli, septic pulmonary infarcts, mycotic aneurysm, intracranial hemorrhage, conjunctival hemorrhage, Janeway lesions
• 4. Immunologic phenomena: glomerulonephritis, Osler's nodes, Roth spots, rheumatoid factor
• 5. Microbiologic evidence: positive blood culture, but not meeting major criterion as noted previously††† or serologic evidence of active infection with organism consistent with infective endocarditis
• 6. Echocardiogram: consistent with infective endocarditis but not meeting major criterion as previous noted

---

† Including nutritional variant strains
†† HACEK = Haemophilus spp, Actinobacillus actinomycetemcomitans, Cardiobacterium hominis, Eikenella spp, Kingella kingae
††† Excluding single positive cultures for coagulase-negative staphylococci and organisms that do not cause endocarditis

Endocarditis, infective (part 2)

TREATMENT

APPROPRIATE HEALTH CARE
• Initial hospitalized care
• Intensive care may be needed in critically ill patients
• Outpatient home intravenous antibiotic therapy may be utilized in selected patients who are stable and reliable

GENERAL MEASURES
• Treatment for congestive heart failure if it occurs
• Oxygen treatment may be indicated
• Hemodialysis may be used in patients who develop renal failure

SURGICAL MEASURES
• Cardiac surgery to replace infected valve may be performed before antibiotic treatment course is completed when:
  ◊ There is evidence of congestive heart failure due to valve incompetence,
or
  ◊ Multiple major systemic emboli have occurred,
or
  ◊ The infection is caused by resistant organisms, e.g., fungus, Pseudomonas aeruginosa,
or
  ◊ There is dehiscence of infected prosthetic valve,
or
  ◊ There is relapse of prosthetic valve endocarditis,
or
  ◊ There is persistent bacteremia despite antibiotic treatment

ACTIVITY
• Bedrest is indicated initially
• Ambulation when clinically improved

DIET No special diet

PATIENT EDUCATION
• Instruct patient regarding importance of dental hygiene
• Emphasize to patient that it is important to take antibiotic prophylaxis when undergoing certain dental/surgical procedures
• Give the patient an AHA wallet card listing antibiotic regimens for prophylaxis. Obtain the AHA wallet card, 78-1003 (CP), from local chapters of American Heart Association.

MEDICATIONS

DRUG(S) OF CHOICE
• Endocarditis due to penicillin-susceptible viridans streptococci and Streptococcus bovis: Aqueous crystalline penicillin G 10-20 million U/24 h IV in 4-6 equally divided doses, plus gentamicin [see Other Notes] for 2 weeks (6 weeks for prosthetic valve endocarditis). In patients with native valve endocarditis: Those older than 65 years of age, those with impairment of the eighth nerve or of renal function, or those with central nervous system involvement, use aqueous crystalline penicillin G only, in the same dosage alone for 4 weeks.
• Endocarditis due to enterococci: Aqueous crystalline penicillin G 20-40 million U/24 h in 6 equally divided doses, plus gentamicin (see Other Notes) for 4-6 weeks (6 weeks for prosthetic valve endocarditis). Test the enterococcal strain in vitro for high-level resistance to gentamicin and streptomycin (minimal inhibitory concentration [MIC] > 2000 µg/mL). Use streptomycin, 1 gm IM every 24 hours, instead of gentamicin if there is high-level resistance to gentamicin and not to streptomycin.
• Endocarditis of native valve due to Staphylococcus: Oxacillin or nafcillin 2 g IV every 4 h for 6 weeks. For the first 3-5 days, gentamicin (see Other Notes) may be added.
• Prosthetic valve endocarditis due to staphylococci: Vancomycin 15 mg/kg (usual dose 1 g) IV infused over 1 h every 12 h, plus rifampin 300 mg po every 8 h, both for 6 weeks, plus gentamicin (see Other Notes) for the first 2 weeks
• Endocarditis due to HACEK organisms (Haemophilus species, Actinobacillus actinomycetemcomitans, Cardiobacterium hominis, Eikenella corrodens, Kingella kingae) - ceftriaxone 2 gm IM or IV every 24 h for 4 weeks

Contraindications: For patients who are allergic to penicillin, use alternative drugs

Precautions:
• In patients with renal impairment, dosage adjustment should be made for penicillin G, oxacillin, gentamicin, cefazolin, vancomycin
• Rapid infusion of vancomycin (less than one hour) may cause "red-neck syndrome", an intense redness or rash over the upper half of the body. This is due to histamine release and not an allergic reaction. It will disappear when the rate of infusion is reduced.

Significant possible interactions:
• The combination of vancomycin and gentamicin may cause increased incidence of renal toxicity
• Rifampin may increase the requirement for coumarin oral anticoagulant and oral hypoglycemic agents

ALTERNATIVE DRUGS
• For patients who are allergic to penicillin
  ◊ Endocarditis due to penicillin-susceptible viridans streptococci and Streptococcus bovis: ceftriaxone 2 g IM or IV every 24h (not to be used in patients with immediate type hypersensitivity to penicillin), or vancomycin 15 mg/kg (usual dose 1 g) IV infused over 1 h every 12 h for 4 weeks (6 weeks for prosthetic valve endocarditis)
  ◊ Endocarditis due to enterococci: Desensitization to penicillin should be considered. Vancomycin 15 mg/kg (usual dose 1 g) IV infused over 1 h every 12 h, plus gentamicin (see Other Notes) for 4-6 weeks (6 weeks for prosthetic valve endocarditis).
  ◊ Endocarditis of native valve due to Staphylococcus: Cefazolin 2 gm IV every 8 h (not to be used in patients with immediate-type hypersensitivity to penicillin), or vancomycin 15 mg/kg (usual dose 1 g) IV infused over 1 h every 12 h, for 6 weeks

FOLLOWUP

PATIENT MONITORING
• Gentamicin blood levels should be performed if used for more than 5 days, and in patients with renal dysfunction. Peak gentamicin level should be around 3 µg/mL and trough less than 1 µg/mL.
• Vancomycin blood levels should be performed in patients with renal dysfunction. Desired peak level is 30-45 mcg/mL and trough less than 10 mcg/mL.
• Twice weekly BUN and serum creatinine should be performed while the patient is receiving gentamicin
• Consider audiometry baseline and follow-up during long-term aminoglycoside therapy

PREVENTION/AVOIDANCE
• Dental caries should be treated while the patient is being treated for endocarditis
• Patients should maintain good oral hygiene
• Antibiotic prophylaxis should be given to the patient who is undergoing dental or surgical procedures that may cause transient bacteremia
• Standard antibiotic regimen for dental/oral/upper respiratory tract procedures: (May be used in patients with prosthetic valves)
  ◊ Amoxicillin 2 g orally one h before procedure
  ◊ For patients who are allergic to penicillin: clindamycin 300 mg orally 1 h before a procedure
• Alternate antibiotic regimens for dental/oral/upper respiratory tract procedures
  ◊ For patients unable to take oral medications: Ampicillin 2.0 g IV (or IM) 30 minutes before procedure
  ◊ For patients who are allergic to penicillin: Clindamycin 300 mg IV 30 minutes before a procedure
• Standard antibiotic regimen for genitourinary/gastrointestinal procedures
  ◊ Ampicillin 2.0 g IV (or IM) plus gentamicin 1.5 mg/kg IV (or IM) (not to exceed 120 mg) 30 minutes before procedure
  ◊ For patients who are allergic to penicillin: vancomycin 1.0 g IV infused over one hour plus gentamicin 1.5 mg/kg IV (or IM) (not to exceed 120 mg); complete infusion 30 minutes before procedure
• Alternate oral regimen for moderate-risk patients undergoing genitourinary/gastrointestinal procedures
  ◊ Amoxicillin 2.0 g orally one hour before procedure or ampillicin 2 g IV (or IM) 30 minutes before procedure
  ◊ For patients who are allergic to penicillin: vancomycin 1.0 g IV infused over 1 hour; complete infusion 30 minutes before procedure

POSSIBLE COMPLICATIONS
• Congestive heart failure
• Ruptured valve cusp
• Sinus of Valsalva aneurysm
• Aortic root abscesses
• Myocardial abscesses
• Myocardial infarction
• Pericarditis
• Cardiac arrhythmia
• Meningitis
• Cerebral emboli
• Brain abscesses
• Ruptured mycotic aneurysm
• Septic pulmonary infarcts
• Splenic infarcts
• Arterial emboli and infarcts
• Arthritis
• Myositis
• Glomerulonephritis
• Acute renal failure
• Mesenteric infarct

EXPECTED COURSE/PROGNOSIS
• In staphylococcal endocarditis, fever and positive blood cultures may persist up to 10 days after appropriate treatment started
• In streptococcal endocarditis, there should be clinical response within 48 hours of antibiotic treatment and blood cultures should be negative soon after antibiotic treatment is started
• Prognosis depends largely on the possible complications

MISCELLANEOUS

ASSOCIATED CONDITIONS
Most patients who have tricuspid valve endocarditis are intravenous drug abusers or have indwelling IV lines

AGE-RELATED FACTORS
Pediatric: N/A
Geriatric: Prognosis is worse in elderly people
Others: N/A

PREGNANCY
Gentamicin should be used with caution; avoid use if possible

SYNONYMS
• Bacterial endocarditis
• Infectious endocarditis
• Subacute bacterial endocarditis
• Subacute infective endocarditis
• Acute bacterial endocarditis
• Acute infective endocarditis

ICD-9-CM
421.0 Endocarditis/ABE
421.9 Endocarditis/SBE
996.61 Prosthetic valve endocarditis:

SEE ALSO
• Bartonella infections
• Brucellosis

OTHER NOTES
• Gentamicin dosing: 3 mg/kg/day in divided doses every 8-12 hours, depending on renal function and results of peak/trough measures.

ABBREVIATIONS
IE = Infective endocarditis
ABE = Acute bacterial endocarditis
SBE = Subacute bacterial endocarditis

REFERENCES
• Francoli P, Etienne J, Hoigne R, et al: Treatment of streptococcal endocarditis with a single daily dose of ceftriaxone sodium for 4 weeks. Efficacy and outpatient treatment feasibility. JAMA 1992;267:264-267
• Watanakunakorn C, Burkert T: Infective endocarditis at a large community teaching hospital, 1980-1990. A review of 210 episodes. Medicine 1993;72:90-102
• Watanakunakorn C: Staphylococcus aureus endocarditis at a community teaching hospital, 1980 to 1991. An analysis of 106 cases. Arch Inter Med 1994;154:2330-2335
• Wilson WR, Karchner AW, Dajani AS, et al: Antibiotic treatment of adults with infective endocarditis due to streptococci, enterococci, staphylococci, and HACEK microorganisms. JAMA 1995;274:1706-1713
• Durack DT, Lukes AS, Bright DK, et al: New criteria for diagnosis of infective endocarditis: Utilization of specific echogradiographic findings. Am Jour Med 1994;96:200-209
• Dajani AS, Taubert KA, Wilson W, et al: Prevention of bacterial endocarditis. Recommendations by the American Heart Association. JAMA 1997;277:1744-1800
Illustrations: 2 available on CD-ROM
Internet references: http://www.5mcc.com

Author(s)
Chatrchai Watanakunakorn, MD, FACP, FCCP

Endometriosis

 BASICS

DESCRIPTION Heterotopic islands of uterine mucosa (endometrium) found in many locations.
• Pelvic sites - peritoneal surfaces (bladder, cul-de-sac, pelvic side walls, broad ligaments, uterosacral ligaments, fallopian tubes, and uterus), lymph nodes, ovaries, bowel
• Distant sites - vagina, cervix, abdominal wall, arm, leg, pleura, lung, diaphragm, kidneys, spleen, gallbladder, nasal mucous membranes, spinal canal, stomach, breast
System(s) affected: Reproductive
Genetics: N/A
Incidence/Prevalence in USA:
8-30/100,000; may be as high as 50% in women of reproductive age (probable range 8-30%)
Predominant age: Women of reproductive age
Predominant Sex: Female only

SIGNS AND SYMPTOMS
• Infertility (30-40% of patients with endometriosis)
• Dyspareunia
• Dysmenorrhea
• Dyschezia
• Chronic pelvic pain
• Premenstrual spotting
• Spontaneous abortion
• Luteinized unruptured follicle syndrome

CAUSES
• Retrograde menstruation (Sampson's theory)
• Lymphatic/vascular metastases (Halban's theory)
• Direct implantation
• Coelomic metaplasia (coelomic epithelium undergoes metaplasia forming functioning endometrium)

RISK FACTORS
• Hereditary/genetic predisposition
• Personality traits (achieving, egocentric, overanxious, perfectionist, intelligent, underweight - but validity of these observations lacking)
• Delayed childbearing
• Luteinized unruptured follicle syndrome (granulosa/theca cells undergo luteinization but actual follicular rupture fails to occur, thereby predisposing to limited progesterone secretion into peritoneal cavity thus allowing refluxed endometrial cells to implant and proliferate)

 DIAGNOSIS

DIFFERENTIAL DIAGNOSIS Differential diagnosis of pelvic pain include all causes of acute abdomen including complications of intrauterine pregnancy and extrauterine, urinary tract infection, irritable bowel syndrome, ulcerative colitis, Crohn's disease, pelvic adhesions, acute salpingitis, ruptured ovarian cyst, and other conditions

LABORATORY No special value, but CA-125 levels may be elevated
Drugs that may alter lab results: N/A
Disorders that may alter lab results: N/A

PATHOLOGICAL FINDINGS Biopsy of endometriotic lesions usually demonstrate both endometrial glands and stroma

SPECIAL TESTS CA-125

IMAGING
• Vaginal/abdominal ultrasound (identify only endometriomas of ovaries)
• MRI for pelvic masses (endometriomas)
• Hysterosalpingography for tubal occlusion proximally or distally and periadnexal adhesions

DIAGNOSTIC PROCEDURES
Laparoscopy

 TREATMENT

APPROPRIATE HEALTH CARE Diagnose and treat "early" to prevent sequelae such as infertility and pelvic pain

GENERAL MEASURES N/A

SURGICAL MEASURES
• At the time of laparoscopy, attempt laser vaporization or fulguration of implants, drainage/resection of ovarian endometriomas, and lysis of pelvic adhesions
• Consider uterosacral ligament laser vaporization/fulguration for presacral neurectomy for severe pelvic pain or dysmenorrhea. Microsurgery or in-vitro fertilization (IVF) or gamete intrafallopian tube transfer (GIFT) may be necessary in cases where laparoscopic surgery followed by superovulation induction with human menopausal gonadotropins (Pergonal), pure follicle-stimulating hormone (Metrodin) and artificial intrauterine insemination have failed to achieve pregnancy.

ACTIVITY Activity may be limited depending upon severity of pelvic pain

DIET No special diet

PATIENT EDUCATION
• Prevention of disease difficult but may be maintained in quiescent state with oral contraceptive agents
• Printed materials available from The American Fertility Society, 2140 11th Ave South, Suite 200, Birmingham, AL 35205-2800, (205)933-8494

MEDICATIONS

DRUG(S) OF CHOICE
• Gonadotropin-releasing hormone (GnRH) agonists such as
  ◊ Nafarelin (Synarel) intranasal 400 µg/day divided as 2 inhalations/day, one in each nostril. If patient continues with menses after 2 months of treatment, dose may be increased to 800 µg
  ◊ Leuprolide acetate (Lupron, Depo-Lupron) 0.5-1.0 mg/day or 3.75-7.5 mg/month, respectively
  ◊ Goserelin (Zoladex) implant 3.6 mg subcutaneously every 4 weeks for 6 months
• Maintenance:
  ◊ 6-9 months of therapy followed by "active" attempts at pregnancy or maintenance therapy with oral contraceptive agents
  ◊ Calcium supplementation 1000-1500 mg/day is recommended when using GnRH analog therapy to prevent calcium loss as women become severely hypoestrogenic

Contraindications: Any contraindication to the drug itself or of hypoestrogenemia

Precautions:
• Calcium loss secondary to hypoestrogenemia
• Hot flashes secondary to hypoestrogenemia
• Paresthesias of face and upper extremities
• Contraception measures should be used by sexually active women since ovulation may not be suppressed even if menses cease

Significant possible interactions: Refer to manufacturer's literature

ALTERNATIVE DRUGS
• Danazol (Danocrine) 400-800 mg/day for 6-9 months
• Medroxyprogesterone (Provera) 30 mg/day for 6-9 months
• Megestrol (Megace) 40 mg/day for 6-9 months
• "Continuous" oral contraceptives, e.g., norgestrel-ethinyl estradiol (Lo/Ovral, Ovral) until childbearing is desired

FOLLOWUP

PATIENT MONITORING
• Monitor serum estradiol levels until less than 10 pg/mL (37 pmol/L) when using GnRH analogs
• Monitor patient's pain response with history and physical exams every 8-12 weeks
• Monitor size of ovarian endometriomas with ultrasound every 8-12 weeks
• May need additional surgery depending upon patient's fertility and/or pelvic pain

PREVENTION/AVOIDANCE
• Pregnancy seems to have a temporary ameliorating effect upon the course of the disease
• Endometriosis is generally a recurring disorder that may persist even into early menopause

POSSIBLE COMPLICATIONS
• Infertility/subfertility
• Sterility
• Chronic pelvic pain
• Total abdominal hysterectomy and bilateral salpingo-oophorectomy

EXPECTED COURSE/PROGNOSIS
• Pregnancy should occur, but depends upon the severity of the disease
• Signs and symptoms generally regress with the onset of the menopause, but can usually be controlled during the reproductive years

MISCELLANEOUS

ASSOCIATED CONDITIONS
• Pelvic endometriosis is rarely associated with endometrioid carcinoma of the ovary
• Hematuria with bladder involvement
• Rectal bleeding with bowel involvement
• Hemoptysis with lung involvement

AGE-RELATED FACTORS
Pediatric: N/A
Geriatric: Endometriosis may persist even during early menopause and may be exacerbated with estrogen replacement therapy
Others:
• Endometriosis of the intramural portion of the fallopian tube may cause isthmic proximal tubal obstruction and infertility
• Infertility may not only be related to anatomical disruption of pelvic structures but to liberation of peritoneal macrophages which can predispose to gamete phagocytosis
• Immune disorders such as production of anti-endometrial antibodies can also be associated with reproductive dysfunction

PREGNANCY Refer to board certified reproductive endocrinologist or gynecologist with expertise in infertility

SYNONYMS Endometriosis externa

ICD-9-CM
• 617.1 Endometriosis of uterus
• 617.3 Endometriosis of pelvic peritoneum

SEE ALSO
• Appendicitis
• Ectopic pregnancy

ABBREVIATIONS N/A

OTHER NOTES Educate female patients of reproductive age as to the signs and symptoms of pelvic endometriosis

REFERENCES Speroff L, Glass RH, Kase NG: Endometriosis and Infertility. In: Brown CL, ed. Clinical Gynecologic Endocrinology and Infertility. 5th Ed. Baltimore, Williams & Wilkins, 1994
Illustrations: N/A
Internet references: http://www.5mcc.com

Author(s)
Nicholas J. Spirtos, DO

Enuresis

BASICS

DESCRIPTION
Involuntary urination
• Nocturnal enuresis: involuntary urination during sleep more than once a month in girls over 5 and in boys over 6 years of age
• Day-time enuresis: involuntary urination during waking hours
• Primary enuresis: the child who has never been completely continent for an extended (3-6 month) period
• Secondary enuresis: the return of the involuntary loss of urinary control after an extended period of urinary continence.

System(s) affected: Renal/Urologic, Nervous

Genetics: In some families, there appears to be an inheritance which follows an autosomal dominant pattern with a penetrance of 90% and the marker has been identified on chromosome 13q

Incidence/Prevalence in USA:
Approximately 10% of children

Predominant age: Occurs in 40% of three year olds, 10% of six year olds, 3% of 12 year olds, and 1% of 18 year olds

Predominant sex: Male > Female

SIGNS AND SYMPTOMS
• Important historical information includes age, primary or secondary incontinence, nocturnal or diurnal or both, voiding pattern (intermittently continent or wet all the time), any delay in developmental milestones, toilet training techniques
• Inability to keep from urinating while asleep at least once per month
• Diurnal enuresis may be associated with frequency, dysuria, or activities that cause an increase in intra-abdominal pressure
• Some children may be withdrawn and shy and some may show aggressive behaviors; both may be secondary to the enuresis and not primary behaviors
• Stress factors such as intrafamilial discord, significant life events, psychosocial or emotional problems may be present

CAUSES
• Primary enuresis
  ◊ Growing evidence that some enuretic children lack a normal increase in nocturnal ADH secretion resulting in an amount of urine which exceeds the bladder capacity
  ◊ Nocturnal enuresis alone rarely has a psychiatric, neurologic or anatomic basis (reduced bladder capacity is usually functional, not anatomic)
  ◊ Reduced bladder capacity (normal capacity is 2 oz at birth and increases 1 oz per year of age up to 12 oz) and/or frequent uninhibited contractions (maturational lag or persistent infantile pattern)
  ◊ Recent reports suggest enuretic children have a lower morning level of vasopressin
  ◊ Some suggestion that food allergies may influence bladder capacity
  ◊ Spinal cord malformations are rarely found

• Secondary enuresis and/or diurnal enuresis
  ◊ Bacteriuria
  ◊ Inability to concentrate urine due to insufficient anti-diuretic hormone or to renal tubular defect
  ◊ Glucosuria
  ◊ Pelvic mass such as pregnancy
  ◊ Spinal cord malformations are still rare but a careful examination of the lower back for signs of spinal dysrhaphia and a thorough neurologic examination of lower extremities and genital area is mandatory

RISK FACTORS
• History of one parent having been enuretic gives 44% occurrence rate in offspring
• History of both parents having been enuretic gives a 77% occurrence rate in their offspring
• First born child

DIAGNOSIS

DIFFERENTIAL DIAGNOSIS
• Diabetes insipidus
• Diabetes mellitus
• Renal tubular defects
• Spinal cord malformations or tumors; particularly suggestive in the case of secondary enuresis and with diurnal enuresis

LABORATORY
• Urinalysis including specific gravity, glucose, protein, microscopic exam
• Urine culture
• Tests for pregnancy if history indicates

Drugs that may alter lab results: N/A
Disorders that may alter lab results: N/A

PATHOLOGICAL FINDINGS Usually none

SPECIAL TESTS Estimation of bladder size: Have the child hold urine until the urge is unbearable. Then measure urine in a measuring cup.

IMAGING
• Renal ultrasound, intravenous pyelogram, or voiding cystourethrogram are necessary only if urinary tract infections are associated with the enuresis
• Historical information and/or abnormal physical findings may suggest the need for spinal x-rays or imaging studies of the cord

DIAGNOSTIC PROCEDURES
Observation of the child's urinary stream for caliber and projectile force may be helpful

TREATMENT

APPROPRIATE HEALTH CARE
Outpatient

GENERAL MEASURES
• Anticipatory guidance relative to toilet training beginning by 18 months
• Counseling and behavior modification
• Treatments which are free from side effects can be started when child is toilet trained
• Secondary or diurnal enuresis needs more investigation and other treatments appropriate to the identified etiology
• Encourage daytime fluids and encourage less frequent urination to help increase bladder size
• Discourage any fluids during the 2 hours prior to bedtime
• Protect the bed from urine by covering the mattress with plastic, have the child wear extra thick underwear (not diapers), and put a towel on the bed in the area of the child's bottom
• Encourage the child to take responsibility for the problem
• Encourage the child to get up to urinate during the night but parents should not awaken the child to urinate
• When enuresis occurs, the child should rinse pajamas and underwear and the towel
• Do not punish the child for wet nights, but act sympathetically
• Heap praise on the child for dry nights. A calendar for gold stars or happy faces can be used as an incentive.
• Bladder stretching exercises may be helpful
• Self-awakening or hypnotherapy programs may be helpful
• Bed-wetting alarms have the greatest rate of success (70%) and the lowest rate of relapse (30%)

SURGICAL MEASURES   N/A

ACTIVITY   No restrictions

DIET   No fluids for 2 hours prior to bedtime

PATIENT EDUCATION
• Inform parents and the patient that most children overcome the problem between ages 6 and 10, and in only a very few cases does the problem persist beyond 16 years of age
• Since enuresis is self-limiting, potential harmful treatments should be avoided

MEDICATIONS

DRUG(S) OF CHOICE Tricyclic antidepressants - such as imipramine, 1-2 mg/kg q hs to maximum of 50 mg, or desipramine. Initial success is offset by a high relapse rate resulting in an overall success rate after withdrawal of only 40%.
Contraindications: Refer to manufacturer's profile of each drug
Precautions:
• Imipramine can cause arrhythmias or conduction blocks. Obtain an ECG prior to starting this drug.
• Imipramine is one of the leading causes of childhood drug-related deaths in the US; usually from accidental overdose
Significant possible interactions: Refer to manufacturer's profile of each drug

ALTERNATIVE DRUGS
• Desmopressin (DDAVP)
◊ An analogue of vasopressin, has been used in children over 6 years of age in an initial dose of 20 mcg intranasally at bedtime
◊ The dose may be adjusted upward to a maximum of 40 mcg
◊ The success rate is high, but the relapse rate is also high on withdrawal of the drug
◊ A recent report on the use of desmopressin tablets in children and adolescents is of interest

FOLLOWUP

PATIENT MONITORING Frequent visits are necessary for support and encouragement

PREVENTION/AVOIDANCE No preventive measures known

POSSIBLE COMPLICATIONS Urinary tract infection

EXPECTED COURSE/PROGNOSIS
• Self-limiting problem
• By age 4-5 years, only 12% of children will not have complete urinary control. These 12% convert to complete control at a rate of 15% per year. By puberty, only 2-3% have not achieved complete control.

MISCELLANEOUS

ASSOCIATED CONDITIONS
• Psychosocial problems
• Institutionalization

AGE-RELATED FACTORS
Pediatric: N/A
Geriatric: N/A
Others: N/A

PREGNANCY N/A

SYNONYMS
• Bed-wetting
• Primary nocturnal enuresis

ICD-9-CM 307.6, 788.3

SEE ALSO N/A

OTHER NOTES N/A

ABBREVIATIONS N/A

REFERENCES
• McLorie GA, Husmann DA: Incontinence and enuresis. Pediatr Clinics of N Am 1987;34:1159-1174
• Rutherford A: Enuresis: its diagnosis and management. A general practice perspective. Aust Fam Phys 1988;17(9):749-754
• Starfield: Enuresis: its pathogenesis and management. Clin Pediatr 1972;11(6):343-350
• Stenberg A, Lackgren G: Desmopressin tablets in the treatment of severe nocturnal enuresis in adolescents. Pediatr 1994;94(6):841-846
• Willie S, Aili M, Harris A, Aronson S: Plasma and urinary levels of vasopressin in enuretic and non-enuretic children. Scandinavian Jour Urology & Nephrology 1994;28(2):119-122
• Willie S: Primary nocturnal enuresis in children. Scandinavian Jour Urology & Nephrology Suppl 1994;156:1-48
• Eiberg H, Berendt I, Mohr J: Assignment of dominant inherited nocturnal enuresis to chromosome13q. Nature Genetics 1995;75:354-434
• Mark SD, Frank JD: Nocturnal enuresis. Brit Jour Urology 1995;75:427-434
Illustrations: N/A
Internet references: http://www.5mcc.com

Author(s)
Burris Duncan, MD

Eosinophilic pneumonias

 BASICS

DESCRIPTION
Eosinophilic pneumonias are characterized by eosinophilic lung infiltrates with or without peripheral blood eosinophilia. They are classified as acute or chronic and can be either idiopathic or secondary to other causes.
• Included are:
◊ Löffler's syndrome (simple pulmonary eosinophilia)
◊ Allergic bronchopulmonary aspergillosis (ABPA)
◊ Drug-induced pulmonary eosinophilia
◊ Tropical pulmonary eosinophilia
◊ Chronic or prolonged pulmonary eosinophilia
◊ The hypereosinophilic syndrome
◊ Churg-Strauss syndrome (polyarteritis nodosa) or allergic angiitis
System(s) affected: Pulmonary
Genetics: No known genetic pattern
Incidence/Prevalence in USA: Rare
Predominant age: Any age
Predominant sex: Male = Female (male in 4th decade; female in 6th decade)

SIGNS AND SYMPTOMS
• Low grade fever
• Symptoms may be mild or life-threatening
• Cough
• Chills
• Hypoxia
• Hepatomegaly
• Dyspnea
• Wheezing
• Anorexia
• Decreased localized breath sounds
• Mucoid sputum
• Tachycardia

CAUSES
• Idiopathic (though hypersensitivity suspected) in one third of cases
• Drugs/toxins (penicillin, nitrofurantoin, isoniazid, chlorpropamide, sulfonamides, antituberculosis therapy (PAS), gold, aspirin, hydralazine)
• Tropical
◊ Parasites
◊ Toxocara larvae
◊ Filariae
◊ Nematodes (Strongyloides, Ascaris, Ancylostoma
• Aspergillus fumigatus (asthmatic pulmonary eosinophilia)
• Systemic vasculitis

RISK FACTORS
• Patients with chronic disorders, e.g., asthma, cystic fibrosis
• Living or traveling in certain geographical areas, e.g., India, Ceylon, Burma, Malaysia, Indonesia, tropical Africa, South America, South Pacific

 DIAGNOSIS

DIFFERENTIAL DIAGNOSIS
• Tuberculosis
• Sarcoidosis
• Hodgkin's disease
• Other lymphoproliferative disorders
• Eosinophilic granuloma of the lung
• Desquamative interstitial pneumonitis
• Hypereosinophilic syndrome
• Wegener's granulomatosis

LABORATORY
• Findings determined by etiology
• Leukocytosis
• Eosinophilia in peripheral blood
• A. fumigatus found in sputum
• Positive filarial complement fixation
• Elevated IgE levels
• Increased WBC
• Elevated ESR
• Stool examination for parasites
Drugs that may alter lab results: N/A
Disorders that may alter lab results: N/A

PATHOLOGICAL FINDINGS
• Lung
◊ Alveolar eosinophilic filling
◊ Septal eosinophilic infiltration
◊ Septal plasma cell infiltration

SPECIAL TESTS
• High resolution chest CT
• Bronchoscopy with broncho alveolar lavage
• Lung biopsy when diagnosis uncertain or clinical course is severe (rare)
• Pulmonary function studies

IMAGING
Chest x-ray - migratory infiltrates, small pleural effusion; transient infiltrates

DIAGNOSTIC PROCEDURES
History and physical exam with particular emphasis on drug intake, recent travel to tropical areas, and systemic symptoms

 TREATMENT

APPROPRIATE HEALTH CARE
Outpatient for milder cases. More severe cases may require inpatient care.

GENERAL MEASURES
• Evaluate for secondary causes
• Mild cases may require no specific therapy
• Coughing and deep breathing exercises to clear secretions
• Discontinuing offending drug
• Treatment of underlying parasite infestation

SURGICAL MEASURES   N/A

ACTIVITY   As tolerated.

DIET   High calorie, high protein, soft diet

PATIENT EDUCATION   Information about activity, diet, symptoms of recurrence

MEDICATIONS

DRUG(S) OF CHOICE
• Corticosteroid therapy. In chronic pulmonary eosinophilia, 20-40 mg prednisone daily. In Churg-Strauss syndrome may require large doses e.g., 40-60 mg of prednisone daily. Withdrawal should be possible after recovery. In chronic conditions, treatment should continue for 6-12 months.
• Treat asthma, if present
• Piperazine for Ascaris infestation
• Diethylcarbamazine [available only from the manufacturer] 6-8 mg/kg orally in 3 divided doses a day for 10-14 days for tropical pulmonary eosinophilia
• Appropriate vermifuges for helminthic infections
Contraindications: Refer to manufacturer's literature
Precautions: Refer to manufacturer's literature
Significant possible interactions: Refer to manufacturer's literature

ALTERNATIVE DRUGS
In Churg-Strauss syndrome, cases resistant to corticosteroid therapy, adding azathioprine or cyclophosphamide may be helpful

FOLLOWUP

PATIENT MONITORING
Physical examinations and chest x-rays until resolved

PREVENTION/AVOIDANCE
None

EXPECTED COURSE/PROGNOSIS
• Excellent in the milder forms
• Corticosteroid therapy is dramatically effective in more severe cases
• Relapse is rare

POSSIBLE COMPLICATIONS
• Some patients may show evidence of small airways dysfunction
• Delay in treatment of tropical pulmonary eosinophilia may result in irreversible pulmonary fibrosis

MISCELLANEOUS

ASSOCIATED CONDITIONS
• Asthma
• Hypersensitivity pneumonitis
• Wegener's granulomatosis

AGE-RELATED FACTORS
Pediatric: N/A
Geriatric: More morbidity, probably due to decreased lung capacity and likelihood of concomitant diseases
Others: N/A

PREGNANCY
N/A

SYNONYMS
• Löffler's syndrome
• Pulmonary infiltrates with eosinophilia syndrome (PIE)

ICD-9-CM
518.3 eosinophilic pneumonia

SEE ALSO
N/A

OTHER NOTES
N/A

ABBREVIATIONS
N/A

REFERENCES
Idiopathic eosinophilic pneumonias: Acute and chronic. In Kelly NW (ed): Textbook of Internal Medicine. New York, Lippincott-Raven, 1997
Illustrations: N/A
Internet references: http://www.5mcc.com

Author(s)
George E. Kikano, MD

Epididymitis

 ## BASICS

DESCRIPTION Inflammation of the epididymis resulting in scrotal pain, swelling and induration of the posterior-lying epididymis, and eventual scrotal wall edema, involvement of the adjacent testicle, and hydrocele formation
System(s) affected: Reproductive
Genetics: N/A
Incidence/Prevalence in USA: Common
Predominant age: Usually younger sexually active men or older men with urinary infection, but may also rarely occur in prepubertal boys
Predominant sex: Male only

SIGNS AND SYMPTOMS
• Scrotal pain, sometimes extending to the groin region, may begin relatively acutely over several hours
• Urethral discharge or symptoms of urinary tract infection, such as frequency of urination, dysuria, cloudy urine, or hematuria
• Initially, only the posterior-lying epididymis, usually the lowermost tail section, will be very tender and indurated
• Elevation of the testes/epididymis improves the discomfort
• Entire hemiscrotum becomes swollen, the testis becomes indistinguishable from the epididymis, the scrotal wall becomes thick and indurated, and reactive hydrocele may occur
• Fever and chills occur with severe infection and abscess formation

CAUSES
• Younger than age 35
  ◊ Usually chlamydia or Neisseria gonorrhea
  ◊ Look for serous urethral discharge (chlamydia) or purulent discharge (gonorrhea)
• Older than age 35
  ◊ Coliform bacteria usually, but sometimes Staphylococcus aureus or epidermidis
  ◊ Often associated with distal urinary tract obstruction
  ◊ Tuberculosis, if sterile pyuria and nodularity of vas deferens
  ◊ Sterile urine reflux after transurethral prostatectomy
  ◊ Granulomatous reaction following bacillus Calmette-Guerin (BCG) intravesical therapy for superficial bladder cancer
• Prepubertal boys
  ◊ Usually coliform bacteria
  ◊ Evaluate for underlying congenital abnormalities, such as vesicoureteral reflux or ectopic ureter

RISK FACTORS
• Urinary tract infection, particularly prostatitis
• Indwelling urethral catheter
• Urethral instrumentation or transurethral surgery
• Urethral stricture

 ## DIAGNOSIS

DIFFERENTIAL DIAGNOSIS
• Epididymal congestion following vasectomy
• Testicular torsion
• Torsion of appendix testis
• Mumps orchitis
• Testicular tumor
• Testicular trauma
• Epididymal cyst
• Spermatocele
• Hydrocele
• Varicocele

LABORATORY Pyuria on urinalysis, leukocytosis, gram stain urethral discharge
Drugs that may alter lab results: N/A
Disorders that may alter lab results: N/A

PATHOLOGICAL FINDINGS
• Gross and microabscesses
• Organisms reach the epididymis through the lumen of the vas deferens
• Interstitial congestion
• Fibrous scarring

SPECIAL TESTS N/A

IMAGING Ultrasound of scrotum, radionuclide scan

DIAGNOSTIC PROCEDURES Scrotal exploration or aspiration of epididymis (rarely performed)

 ## TREATMENT

APPROPRIATE HEALTH CARE
• Outpatient, usually
• Inpatient, if septic or if surgery is scheduled

GENERAL MEASURES
• Scrotal elevation
• Ice pack
• Spermatic cord block with local anesthesia in severe cases

SURGICAL MEASURES
• Aspiration of hydrocele to assist examination of scrotal contents and relieve discomfort
• Vasostomy to drain infected material
• Scrotal exploration, if uncertain whether this is epididymitis or testicular torsion
• Drainage of abscesses, epididymectomy, or epididymo-orchiectomy in severe cases not responding to antibiotics

ACTIVITY Bedrest for minimum of 1-2 days

DIET No restrictions, but force fluids

PATIENT EDUCATION
• Limit activity, immobilize scrotal contents
• Stress completing course of antibiotics, even when asymptomatic

MEDICATIONS

DRUG(S) OF CHOICE
- Younger than age 35 for chlamydia
  ◊ Doxycycline 100 mg po bid for 10 days
or
  ◊ Tetracycline 500 mg po qid for 10 days
- Older men with bacteriuria
  ◊ Trimethoprim-sulfamethoxazole (Bactrim, Septra) double strength po bid for 10-14 days
  ◊ Ciprofloxacin (Cipro) 500 mg po bid for 10-14 days
  ◊ Ofloxacin (Floxin) 300 mg po bid for 12-14 days
  ◊ Norfloxacin (Noroxin) 400 mg po bid for 10-14 days
- Analgesia
  ◊ Nonsteroidal anti-inflammatory drug (e.g., naproxen or ibuprofen) for mild to moderate pain
  ◊ Acetaminophen-codeine or oxycodone-acetaminophen for moderate to severe pain
- Septic or toxic patient
  ◊ Third generation cephalosporin (ceftriaxone 1-2 gm IV/IM every 24 hours)
  ◊ Aminoglycoside (gentamicin 1 mg/kg IV/IM every 8 hours, adjusted for renal function) after a loading dose of 2 mg/kg
Contraindications: None
Precautions: Refer to manufacturer's profile of each drug
Significant possible interactions: Refer to manufacturer's profile of each drug

ALTERNATIVE DRUGS
- Other aminoglycosides or third generation cephalosporin depending on specific pathogen
- Add rifampin (rifampicin) or vancomycin as required

FOLLOWUP

PATIENT MONITORING Office visits until all signs of infection have cleared

PREVENTION/AVOIDANCE
- Vasectomy or vasoligation during transurethral surgery
- Antibiotic prophylaxis for urethral manipulation
- Early treatment of prostatitis
- Avoid vigorous rectal examination with acute prostatitis

POSSIBLE COMPLICATIONS
- Recurrent epididymitis
- Infertility
- Fournier's gangrene (necrotizing synergistic infection)

EXPECTED COURSE/PROGNOSIS
- Pain improves within 1-3 days, but induration may take several weeks/months to completely resolve
- If bilateral involvement, sterility may result

MISCELLANEOUS

ASSOCIATED CONDITIONS
- Prostatitis
- Urethritis

AGE-RELATED FACTORS
Pediatric:
- Bacteremia from Haemophilus influenzae infection may produce acute epididymitis
- In adolescent males, must rule out acute testicular torsion
Geriatric: Diabetic patients with sensory neuropathy may have little pain despite severe infection/abscess
Others: N/A

PREGNANCY N/A

SYNONYMS
Epididymo-orchitis

ICD-9-CM
604 Orchitis and epididymitis

SEE ALSO N/A

OTHER NOTES
- Syphilis, brucellosis, blastomycosis, coccidioidomycosis, and cryptococcosis are rare causes of epididymitis
- Non-bacterial epididymitis and epididymo-orchitis are not rare. Cause is not clear, but may be secondary to retrograde extravasation.

ABBREVIATIONS N/A

REFERENCES Berger RE: Urethritis and epididymitis. Semin Urol 1983;1:139
Illustrations: N/A
Internet references: http://www.5mcc.com

Author(s)
Peter T. Nieh, MD

Epiglottitis

BASICS

DESCRIPTION   Acute inflammation of the supraglottic structures with inflammation of the epiglottis, vallecula, aryepiglottic folds and arytenoids
System(s) affected: Pulmonary
Genetics: N/A
Incidence/Prevalence in USA: Incidence has decreased dramatically since the introduction of the Haemophilus b vaccine
Predominant age:
• 3-7 years most common, though any age can be affected
• Generally older than typical croup patient
• Infrequent in adults
Predominant sex: Male = Female

SIGNS AND SYMPTOMS
• Sudden onset and fulminating course
• Fever
• Dysphagia, drooling
• Sore throat
• Cervical adenopathy
• Respiratory distress
• "Tripod" position (sitting propped up on hands with head forward and tongue out)
• Muffled voice/cry (vs. hoarseness in croup)
• Minimal cough (vs. barky cough in croup)
• Toxic appearance/shock (occasionally, due to associated septicemia)
• Stridor softer and less prominent than croup
• Usually no history of prodromal upper respiratory infection (vs. positive history in croup)
• Bacteremia
• Hypoxia. A late symptom usually not present unless totally obstructed.

CAUSES
• Haemophilus influenzae in children
• Haemophilus influenzae and Group A Streptococcus in adults

RISK FACTORS   N/A

DIAGNOSIS

DIFFERENTIAL DIAGNOSIS
• Viral croup (laryngotracheobronchitis)
• Sepsis
• Aspirated foreign body
• Bacterial tracheitis (pseudomembranous croup)
• Peritonsillar abscess
• Retropharyngeal abscess
• Diphtheria in an unimmunized patient

LABORATORY
• Blood culture (positive in over 90%). See under Diagnostic Procedures - should not visualize/swab epiglottis except in controlled environment, i.e., operating room. Blood tests also contraindicated until airway secured.
• Epiglottic swab culture (positive in 70%)
Drugs that may alter lab results: N/A
Disorders that may alter lab results: N/A

PATHOLOGICAL FINDINGS   N/A

SPECIAL TESTS   N/A

IMAGING
• Neck radiographs are contraindicated if epiglottitis is suspected, due to danger of sudden complete airway obstruction
• Chest radiographs are indicated for endotracheal tube placement. Pneumonia can occur as a complication.

DIAGNOSTIC PROCEDURES
• Visualization of epiglottis with tongue depressor is contraindicated due to danger of sudden complete airway obstruction
• Controlled visualization of epiglottis at intubation in operating room is diagnostic
• Lumbar puncture is indicated if there is clinical suspicion of meningitis
• In adult, indirect laryngoscopy is generally safe

TREATMENT

APPROPRIATE HEALTH CARE
Hospitalize during acute illness

GENERAL MEASURES
• Each institution should have emergency protocol involving a team of emergency room physicians, pediatricians, anesthesiologists, surgeons, pediatric intensivists, and pediatric ICU nurses (principles are similar for pediatric and adult patients)
• Call anesthesiologist to bedside
• Have equipment for intubation and needle cricothyrotomy or percutaneous tracheostomy at bedside
• Notify OR
• Notify pediatric surgery or ENT for standby in OR in case tracheostomy becomes necessary
• Keep patient quiet, calm, sitting up (in parent's arms)
• Avoid venipuncture, blood gases, oxygen masks, intravenous lines, injections, monitors, and radiographs
• Avoid sedation
• Avoid racemic epinephrine
• Avoid examining the pharynx
• Transport patient and parent together to OR in a wheelchair
• Intubate all patients, preferably in OR under controlled circumstances by experienced anesthesiologist with surgery or ENT on standby for emergency tracheostomy
• Tracheostomy not indicated unless intubation unsuccessful
• Tape airway securely in place and use a bite block if indicated
• Splint elbows and restrain arms to avoid self-extubation
• Use humidity in a tent and avoid T-piece (traction increases risk of accidental extubation)
• CPAP, mechanical ventilation, and sedation usually unnecessary
• Pay attention to supervision and pulmonary toilet/suctioning to minimize risk of endotracheal tube plugs

SURGICAL MEASURES   See General Measures

ACTIVITY   N/A

DIET   IV fluid initially, then nasogastric feedings while intubated

PATIENT EDUCATION   Reassurance about treatment and outcome

MEDICATIONS

DRUG(S) OF CHOICE Cefotaxime 100 mg/kg/day divided q 6 hours IV or ceftriaxone 75 mg/kg/day divided q 12 hours IV. Start promptly after blood and epiglottic cultures are obtained.
Contraindications: Refer to manufacturer's profile
Precautions: Refer to manufacturer's profile
Significant possible interactions: Refer to manufacturer's profile

ALTERNATIVE DRUGS
• Ampicillin 100 mg/kg/day divided q 6 hours IV and chloramphenicol 100 mg/kg/day divided q 6 hours. Follow levels. May stop chlorophenicol only if H. influenzae B sensitive to ampicillin.
• Steroids and racemic epinephrine of no benefit
• Antipyretics if necessary

FOLLOWUP

PATIENT MONITORING
• Serial exams to detect secondary foci of infection
• Follow swallowing ability and presence of an air leak around endo/nasotracheal tube
• Followup laryngoscopy prior to extubation (advocated by some)
• Observe in ICU for 24 hours following extubation

PREVENTION/AVOIDANCE
• H. influenzae vaccine is effective though not 100% protective
• Rifampin prophylaxis (20 mg/kg once daily for 4 days, maximum daily dose 600 mg) for all household and day care contacts. Family and close contacts may be asymptomatic carriers of H. influenza

POSSIBLE COMPLICATIONS
• Pneumonia, meningitis, cervical adenitis, septic arthritis, pericarditis, cellulitis (rare)
• Septic shock (in about 1%)
• Pneumothorax, pneumomediastinum (very rare)
• Death from asphyxia

EXPECTED COURSE/PROGNOSIS
• Most can be extubated after 24 to 48 hours
• Morbidity and mortality is low with appropriate intervention

MISCELLANEOUS

ASSOCIATED CONDITIONS N/A

AGE-RELATED FACTORS
Pediatric: N/A
Geriatric: N/A
Others: N/A

PREGNANCY N/A

SYNONYMS Supraglottitis

ICD-9-CM
• 464.30 Acute Epiglottitis without mention of obstruction
• 464.31 Acute Epiglottitis with mention of obstruction

SEE ALSO N/A

OTHER NOTES N/A

ABBREVIATIONS N/A

REFERENCES
• Gerber AC, Pfenningerm J: Acute epiglottitis: Management during intubation and hospitalization. Intensive Care Med 1986;12:407-411
• Vernon DD, Ashok PS: Acute epiglottitis in children: A conservative approach to diagnosis and management. Crit Care Med 1986;14:23-25
• Blanc VF, Duquenne P, Charest J: Acute epiglottitis: An overview. Acta Anaesthesial Belg 1986;37:171-178
Illustrations: N/A
Internet references: http://www.5mcc.com

Author(s)
Diane Neddenriep, MD

Epistaxis

BASICS

DESCRIPTION Hemorrhage from nostril, nasal cavity or nasopharynx
• Anterior bleed: Originates from anterior nasal cavity, usually Little's area (Kiesselbach's plexus) on septum just above posterior end of nasal vestibule. Second most common is anterior end of inferior turbinate.
• Posterior bleed: Originates from posterior nasal cavity or nasopharynx usually under the posterior half of the inferior turbinate or the roof of the nasal cavity
System(s) affected: Pulmonary
Genetics: N/A
Incidence/Prevalence in USA: Unknown
Predominant age: Less than 10 years and over 50 years
Predominant sex: Male = Female

SIGNS AND SYMPTOMS Usually nostril hemorrhage, however cases of posterior bleed may be asymptomatic or present with hemoptysis, nausea, hematemesis or melena

CAUSES
• Idiopathic (most common)
• Traumatic/blunt - nose picking (epistaxis digitorum), low humidity, foreign body
• Infection - upper respiratory, acute/chronic rhinitis, acute/chronic sinusitis
• Vascular abnormalities - sclerotic vessels of age, hereditary hemorrhagic telangiectasia, arteriovenous malformation
• Neoplasm
• Hypertension (usually in combination with another cause)
• Coagulopathy - hereditary (e.g., hemophilia), therapeutic or adverse effect of drugs, blood dyscrasias, leukemias, thrombocytopenia or platelet dysfunction
• Septal perforation
• Septal deviation (one side is overexposed to dry air)
• Bleeding originating in a sinus (fracture, tumor)
• Endometriosis (nasal ectopic endometrium)

RISK FACTORS Included in Causes

DIAGNOSIS

DIFFERENTIAL DIAGNOSIS Epistaxis is a symptom or a sign, not a disease. Less than 10% are caused by neoplasm or coagulopathy.

LABORATORY CBC, crossmatch for hypovolemic shock or anemia
Drugs that may alter lab results: N/A
Disorders that may alter lab results: N/A

PATHOLOGICAL FINDINGS N/A

SPECIAL TESTS As indicated for unusual causes

IMAGING Sinus films (rarely)

DIAGNOSTIC PROCEDURES
Angiography (rarely)

TREATMENT

APPROPRIATE HEALTH CARE
• Outpatient (usually). Inpatient for severe hemorrhage.
• Elderly patient with posterior bleeds and balloon or packing usually requires admission

GENERAL MEASURES
• Resuscitation as indicated
• Sedation, analgesic, antihypertensive or anticoagulant reversal as needed
• Patient should be gowned and sitting, if stable. Gown, gloves, and eye protection for examiner.
• Attempt to locate bleeding site using headlamp, suction, nasal speculum and help of assistant. Clear nasal cavity of blood with suction, forceps withdrawal of clot or patient blowing nose. If bleeding has stopped, rub suspicious areas with wet cotton tipped applicator to identify site. Diffuse ooze or multiple sites suggests systemic cause. In cases of posterior bleed try to identify as either roof or low posterior site since each has different arterial supply (will be important if arterial ligation is necessary).
• Locating the bleeding site may be difficult if patient presents with bilateral bleed. Usually there is only one bleeding site and the blood appears on the other because of (1) septal perforation, (2) obstruction of the affected side by pinching or packing or (3) there is a posterior bleed and blood passes behind the nasal septum. Clues are the side on which bleeding started and a careful examination using suction, headlamp and speculum.

• Anterior bleed:
◊ Place pledget soaked in vasoconstrictor and local anesthetic in cavity and pinch nostril for several minutes to stop bleeding by direct pressure
◊ Remove pledget and visualize vessel. Cauterize with silver nitrate stick directly on vessel with firm pressure for 30 seconds.
◊ Alternative chemical cautery includes bead of chromic acid or 25% trichloracetic acid. Larger vessels respond better to thermal cautery or bipolar electrocautery. Avoid indiscriminate cauterization of a large area.
◊ If unsuccessful, apply second dose of anesthetic and place anterior pack using 1/2 x 72 inch ribbon gauze impregnated with petroleum jelly (Vaseline). Use bayonet forceps and nasal speculum to insert in folding layers as far back as possible. Press each layer firmly down on the last in one continuous strip with the folded ends alternating front and back. The average nasal cavity will accommodate the full length if properly placed. Tape 2x2 gauze over nostril as drip catch and to prevent packing end from falling out of nostril.
• Posterior bleed:
◊ Traditional posterior packing as described in ENT texts has been replaced by various balloon systems. However it is very effective if balloon systems fail to control bleeding.
◊ Balloon systems include single large balloon with or without central tube for airway. They usually come in 3 or 4 sizes and right or left. Other systems provide a small (10 cc) posterior balloon and larger (30 cc) anterior balloon. After local anesthesia, the tube is placed in the affected nostril and is passed to the nasopharynx as one would a nasogastric tube. Then inflate the posterior balloon with air or water (see manufacturer's directions) and pull forward to press upon the posterior area. Then inflate the anterior balloon (see note under Complications) . A very effective method uses a 10 to 14 Fr Foley catheter. Place tip of Foley through the nostril to nasopharynx or upper oropharynx. Visualize through mouth avoiding placement in hypopharynx. Inflate balloon 7 to 15 cc. Pull forward until balloon wedges in posterior passage. Have assistant maintain gentle traction and place catheter along mid-section of lateral wall of nasal cavity. Insert anterior pack described above. Maintain catheter traction and stretch slightly. Place umbilical cord clamp on catheter across nostril against anterior pack so that elasticity of catheter compresses balloon against anterior pack. Protect facial skin from clamp by padding with 2x2 gauze. Drape rest of catheter over ear and tape in place.
• Intractable bleed:
◊ Bilateral packing is sometimes required to achieve adequate compression
◊ Bleeding from roof may be controlled by placing double balloon system with small anterior pack placed above anterior balloon. Inflation then raises pack to place pressure on roof.
◊ Intractable bleed will require surgical arterial ligation (ideally after visual identification of bleeding site to define appropriate arterial supply). Alternative is angiographic selective arterial embolization.

SURGICAL MEASURES
• Arterial ligation for intractable bleeding

ACTIVITY Bedrest with head at 45 to 90 degrees

DIET No alcohol or hot liquids

PATIENT EDUCATION Demonstrate proper pinching pressure techniques

MEDICATIONS

DRUG(S) OF CHOICE
• Vasoconstrictor: Cocaine 4%, phenylephrine 0.25%, xylometazoline 0.1%, epinephrine l:1000
• Anesthetic: Cocaine 4%, lidocaine laryngeal spray, lidocaine jelly 2%, lidocaine solution 4%, lidocaine viscous 2%
• Some experts suggest systemic antibiotics and decongestants to prevent sinusitis with packs or balloons
• Consider iron supplementation for patients with considerable blood loss
Contraindications: Allergy to any component
Precautions:
• Hypertension, coronary artery disease with epinephrine
• Large doses of cocaine in children
Significant possible interactions: Refer to manufacturer's profile of each drug

ALTERNATIVE DRUGS Numerous other topical anesthetics and vasoconstrictors

FOLLOWUP

PATIENT MONITORING Hemodynamics and blood loss as indicated. Packs or balloons removed in 24 to 36 hours.

PREVENTION/AVOIDANCE Liberal application of petroleum jelly (Vaseline) to nostril to prevent drying and picking. Humidification at night. Cut fingernails.

POSSIBLE COMPLICATIONS
• Sinusitis
• Double balloon systems tend to migrate posteriorly, if anterior balloon breaks, patient may obstruct airway with migrated posterior balloon. Prevent by placing umbilical cord clamp across end of tubing at nostril after inflation.
• Septal hematoma or abscess from excessive trauma during packing
• Septal perforation secondary to aggressive cauterization
• External nasal deformity secondary to pressure necrosis from the anterior component of posterior packing
• Mucosal pressure necrosis secondary to high balloon inflation pressures
• Cocaine, lidocaine toxicity
• Vasovagal episode during packing

EXPECTED COURSE/PROGNOSIS
Good results with proper treatment

MISCELLANEOUS

ASSOCIATED CONDITIONS In the elderly - hypertension, atherosclerosis and conditions that decrease platelets and clotting functions

AGE-RELATED FACTORS
Pediatric: More likely anterior bleed
Geriatric: More likely posterior bleed
Others: N/A

PREGNANCY N/A

SYNONYMS Nosebleed

ICD-9-CM 784.7 Epistaxis

SEE ALSO N/A

OTHER NOTES N/A

ABBREVIATIONS N/A

REFERENCES
• Votey R, Dudley JP: Emergency ear, nose and throat procedures. Emerg. Clin. NA 1989;7(1)117-154
• Perretta LJ, et al: Emergency evaluation and management of epistaxis. Emerg. Clin. NA 1987;5(2)265-277
• Wong, Jafek: Pediatric Otorhinolaryngology. Appleton-Century-Crofts,1989
Illustrations: N/A
Internet references: http://www.5mcc.com

Author(s)
Charles W. Ricketson, MD, FRCPC

Epstein-Barr virus infections

BASICS

DESCRIPTION EBV is tropic for B lymphocytes which apparently are infected in the oropharynx through salivary exchange; infected B cells then circulate in the blood and are distributed to the bone marrow and lymphoreticular system. The virus can also be found in infected epithelial cells of the buccal mucosa, salivary glands, tongue and endocervix. Within the oropharynx both parotid ductal epithelium and pharyngeal squamous epithelial cells harbor EBV DNA and are sites of viral replication and release. This suggests that chronic epithelial replication brings about continuous reinfection of B lymphoid cells. Immune T cell responses to latently infected B cells account for the clinical findings.
• Epstein-Barr virus (EBV) infections acquired early in life are asymptomatic or associated with non-specific symptoms suggesting upper respiratory infections.

System(s) affected:
Hemic/Lymphatic/Immunologic
Genetics: N/A
Incidence/Prevalence in USA:
• Incidence is about 60/100,000 persons
• College students: 5,000/100,000 persons
• Worldwide in distribution, but clinical IM is observed predominantly in countries with advanced socio-hygienic conditions
Predominant Age:
• Older children, adolescents and young adults
• By young adult life, 60-90% of persons are antibody positive
Predominant Sex: Male = Female

SIGNS AND SYMPTOMS
• May begin abruptly or insidiously
• In adults, the temperature may rise to 103°F (39.4°C) and gradually falls over a variable period of 7-10 days; in severe cases temperature elevations of 104-105° F (40.0-40.6°C) may persist for 2 weeks
• Children usually have a low-grade fever or may be afebrile
• Diffuse hyperemia and hyperplasia of oropharyngeal lymphoid tissue
• Gelatinous, grayish-white exudative tonsillitis persists for 7-10 days in 50%
• Petechiae develop at the border of the hard and soft palates in 33%
• Tender lymphadenopathy (cervical nodes are most commonly enlarged)
• Axillary, epitrochlear, popliteal, inguinal, mediastinal and mesenteric nodes may be affected
• Lymph node enlargement subsides over days or weeks
• Splenomegaly in 50%
• Abnormal hepatic enzymes in 80% of patients for several weeks after onset. Hepatomegaly in 15-20%.
• Pneumonitis
• Chest pain (myocarditis and pericarditis)
• Hilar adenopathy may be observed in IM cases having extensive lymphoid hyperplasia
• Neurologic (rare)
 ◊ Aseptic meningitis
 ◊ Bell's palsy
 ◊ Meningoencephalitis
 ◊ Guillain-Barré syndrome
 ◊ Transverse myelitis
 ◊ Cerebellar ataxia
 ◊ Acute psychosis
• Hematologic (rare)
 ◊ Thrombocytopenia, slight to moderate, early in illness
 ◊ Hemolytic anemia with marked neutropenia during early weeks of disease
 ◊ Aplastic anemia
 ◊ Agammaglobulinemia
• Skin manifestations (3-16%)
 ◊ Erythematous macular or maculopapular rash
 ◊ Petechial and purpuric exanthems have been reported
 ◊ Rash location - trunk and upper arms; occasionally the face and forearms involved
 ◊ Urticarial lesions on the abdomen, arms, legs

CAUSES The Epstein-Barr virus, a member of the herpesvirus (DNA virus) group.

RISK FACTORS
• Age
• Socio-hygienic level
• Geographic location

DIAGNOSIS

DIFFERENTIAL DIAGNOSIS
• Streptococcal pharyngitis and tonsillitis
• Diphtheria
• Blood dyscrasias
• Rubella
• Measles
• Viral hepatitis
• Cytomegalovirus
• Toxoplasmosis

LABORATORY
• Lymphocytes and atypical lymphocytes
 ◊ Increased numbers of lymphocytes and atypical lymphocytes (may be up to 70% of leukocytes) in peripheral blood
 ◊ In the first week after onset of illness, the white blood cell count is normal or moderately decreased. By the second week, lymphocytosis develops with more than 10% atypical lymphocytes. Such cells vary in size and shape with indented, oval or horseshoe-shaped nuclei and basophilic, vacuolated, foamy cytoplasm.
 ◊ During early illness, atypical lymphocytes are B cells transformed by EBV; later, the atypical cells are primarily T cells having immunoregulatory function
• Antibodies
 ◊ Heterophil antibodies in 80-90% of adults.
 ◊ The responsible heterophile antibody is an IgM response which appears during the first or second week of illness and persists for 3-6 months. Sheep cell agglutinins are not specific for IM and may occur in other conditions including serum sickness, infectious hepatitis, rubella, leukemia and Hodgkin's disease; low titers may also be found in normal healthy individuals.
 ◊ Differential absorption techniques distinguish these agglutinins from EBV heterophile antibodies. In general, the agglutinin titer is higher in IM than in other disorders; an unabsorbed heterophile titer greater than 1:128 and 1:40 or higher after absorption is significant.
• Specific antibodies to EBV-associated antigens
 ◊ Develop regularly in IM
 ◊ Viral capsid (VCA)-specific IgM and IgG are present early in illness; VCA-IgM responses disappear after several months whereas VCA-IgG antibodies persist for life.
 ◊ Antibodies to EBV early antigen (EA) complexes, associated with viral replication, are present in 70-80% of patients during acute disease and usually disappear after 6 months
 ◊ Antibodies to the EBV nuclear antigen complex (EBNA) appear slowly and develop 1-6 months after onset
Drugs that may alter lab results: N/A
Disorders that may alter lab results: Atypical lymphocytes are not specific for Epstein-Barr infections and may be present in other clinical conditions including rubella, infectious hepatitis, allergic rhinitis, asthma and primary atypical pneumonia. In IM, increased numbers of atypical forms are present in peripheral blood whereas in other disorders the quantitative percentage is usually less.

PATHOLOGICAL FINDINGS
• Widespread focal and perivascular aggregates of mononuclear cells are found throughout the body
• Mononuclear infiltrations involve lymph nodes, tonsils, spleen, lungs, liver, heart, kidneys, adrenal glands, skin and central nervous system
• Bone marrow hyperplasia develops regularly and small granulomas may be present; these are non-specific and have no prognostic significance
• A polyclonal B cell proliferative response is characteristic of IM. Relatively few circulating lymphocytes are infected by EBV and represent less than 0.1% of circulating mononuclear cells in acute illness.

SPECIAL TESTS N/A

IMAGING Ultrasound, splenomegaly

DIAGNOSTIC PROCEDURES See under Laboratory

TREATMENT

APPROPRIATE HEALTH CARE
Outpatient usually

GENERAL MEASURES
• The treatment is chiefly supportive
• During acute stage, rest in bed

SURGICAL MEASURES
• With profound thrombocytopenia, refractory to corticosteroid therapy, splenectomy may be necessary.

ACTIVITY
• Decided on an individual basis during convalescence
• Excess exertion, heavy lifting and participation in contact sports are prohibited during acute illness and also in the presence of splenomegaly. Rupture of the spleen may be fatal if not recognized and requires blood transfusions, treatment for shock, and splenectomy.

DIET
• Maintain adequate fluid intake
• Low fat, high carbohydrate diet
• Avoid alcohol for 6-8 months

PATIENT EDUCATION
Reassurance and support

MEDICATIONS

DRUG(S) OF CHOICE
• Antimicrobial agents (usually a penicillin) if throat culture is positive for Group A, beta-hemolytic streptococci. Avoid ampicillin because of rash that occurs with ampicillin in mononucleosis.
• Aspirin and warm saline gargles for the pain of pharyngeal involvement and enlarged lymph nodes
• Codeine or meperidine, for unrelieved pain
• Corticosteroids
   ◊ With severe pharyngo-tonsillitis with oropharyngeal edema and airway encroachment, a short course of corticosteroids may be utilized. Prednisone or its equivalent is used. Start with an initial dosage of 10-15 mg qid for 2 days. Decrease by 5 mg daily so that steroid treatment is discontinued in approximately 10 days.
   ◊ Considered for patients with marked toxicity or major complications (e.g., hemolytic anemia, thrombocytopenic purpura, neurologic sequelae, myocarditis, pericarditis and severe

generalized dermatologic lesions).
Contraindications: Steroids not recommended for mild, uncomplicated IM
Precautions: Refer to manufacturer's literature
Significant Possible Interactions: Refer to manufacturer's literature

ALTERNATIVE DRUGS N/A

FOLLOWUP

PATIENT MONITORING
• Avoid contact sports, heavy lifting, and excess exertion until the spleen and liver have returned to normal size.
• Eliminate alcohol or exposure to other hepatotoxic drugs until liver function studies return to normal
• Patients should be monitored closely on an outpatient basis during the first 2-3 weeks after onset of symptoms. Thereafter patients may be followed for an additional month or so, until all symptoms have subsided.
• Rarely, laboratory results resolve more slowly and symptoms including malaise, fatigue, intermittent sore throat and lymphadenopathy may persist for several months

PREVENTION/AVOIDANCE N/A

POSSIBLE COMPLICATIONS
• Airway obstruction
• Hematologic or neurologic complications
• Toxemia
• Splenic rupture (rare)
• Hypersensitivity skin rash
   ◊ Develops 7-10 days after initiation of ampicillin treatment; this generalized erythematous maculopapular eruption occurs mainly over the trunk and extremities, including palms and soles
   ◊ Rash persists for approximately one week; desquamation may continue for several days
   ◊ Hypersensitivity skin rashes may also develop in IM cases with the use of ampicillin analogues such as amoxicillin and certain other penicillins, including methicillin.

EXPECTED COURSE/PROGNOSIS
• Most IM cases in young adult age groups are mild or moderate in severity
• Acute symptoms usually last 2-3 weeks and patients recover uneventfully over 4-8 weeks

MISCELLANEOUS

ASSOCIATED CONDITIONS
• Infectious mononucleosis (IM): the symptomatic primary EBV infection seen in otherwise healthy older children, adolescents and young adults. Clinical features are variable in severity and duration; in children the disease is generally mild, whereas in

adults it is more severe and protracted. The incubation period is 30-50 days.
• X-linked lymphoproliferative syndrome (Duncan's disease)
• Lymphoproliferative syndromes due to EBV infections in transplant patients
• Lymphomas (B cell lymphoblastic, T cell)
• Lymphocytic interstitial pneumonitis
• Hairy leukoplakia of the tongue and central nervous system lymphomas in AIDS patients
• Burkitt's lymphoma
• Nasopharyngeal carcinoma
• Parotid carcinoma
• Hodgkin's disease

AGE-RELATED FACTORS
Pediatric:
• Infection during infancy and childhood usually subclinical and inapparent
• Clinical IM more common in older children and young adults
Geriatric: Heterophile positive IM has been reported in an elderly patient 5 weeks following blood transfusion
Others: N/A

PREGNANCY One large prospective study of pregnant women failed to demonstrate evidence of any intrauterine EBV infection. However, rare birth defects considered to be due to congenital EBV infection have been reported; such defects include cataracts, hypotonia, cryptorchidism and micrognathia.

SYNONYMS N/A

ICD-9-CM 075 Infectious mononucleosis

SEE ALSO N/A

OTHER NOTES N/A

ABBREVIATIONS
IM = infectious mononucleosis
EBNA = Epstein-Barr nuclear antigen

REFERENCES
• Niederman JC, McCollum RW, Henle G, Henle W: Infectious mononucleosis: clinical manifestations in relation to EB virus antibodies. JAMA 1968;203:205-208
• Miller G, Niederman JC, Andrews LL: Prolonged oropharyngeal excretion of Epstein-Barr virus after infectious mononucleosis. New Engl J Med 1973;288:229-232
• Rickinson AB, Yao QY, Wallace LE: The Epstein-Barr virus as a model of virus-host interactions. Br Med Bull 1985;41:75-79
• Miller G, Katz BZ, Niederman JC: Some recent developments in the molecular epidemiology of Epstein-Barr virus infection. Yale J Biol Med 1986;60:307-316
• Straus SE, Tosato G, Meier J: Epstein-Barr virus infections: biology, pathogenesis, and management. Ann Int Med 1993;118(1):45-58
Illustrations: N/A
Internet references: http://www.5mcc.com

Author(s)
James C. Niederman, MD

Erectile dysfunction

BASICS

DESCRIPTION Dissatisfaction with size, rigidity, or duration of erection. Male sexual dysfunction encompasses an even larger group of complaints and disorders of arousal, desire, orgasm, sensation, and relationship. Transient periods of impotence occur in about half of adult males and are not considered dysfunctional.
System(s) affected: Reproductive, Nervous, Cardiovascular, Renal/Urologic
Genetics: Rarely related to chromosomal disorders
Incidence/Prevalence in USA: Erectile failure involves about 10% of men, but is underreported by patients
Predominant Age:
• Patients with psychologic, gender, and primary organic problems often present themselves for help between adolescence and the third decade
• Patients with relationship problems, but concerned mainly about physical problems, tend to seek care in the sixth decade
• Most patients with physical problems are in the seventh and eighth decade, but rarely seek help
Predominant Sex: Male only

SIGNS AND SYMPTOMS
• Reduction of erectile size and rigidity
• Inability to maintain erection
• Inability to achieve erection
• Reduced body hair
• Thyromegaly
• Gynecomastia
• Testicular atrophy or absence
• Deformed penis
• Peripheral vascular disease
• Neuropathy

CAUSES
• Endocrine
• Neurologic
• Vascular
• Medication
• Psychological
• Structural

RISK FACTORS
• Prior pelvic surgery
• Medication use
• Risk factors for disorders listed in Causes

DIAGNOSIS

DIFFERENTIAL DIAGNOSIS
• Endocrine
    ◊ Low or high thyroxine
    ◊ Low testosterone
    ◊ High prolactin
    ◊ Diabetes
    ◊ High estrogen effect
    ◊ Renal failure
    ◊ Zinc deficiency
• Neurological
    ◊ Central
    ◊ Spinal
    ◊ Peripheral
• Vascular
    ◊ Arterial insufficiency
    ◊ Cavernosal insufficiency
    ◊ Venous insufficiency
• Medication
    ◊ Many types, e.g., beta-blockers, thiazides
• Psychological
    ◊ Depression
    ◊ Schizophrenia
    ◊ Relationship disorders
    ◊ Personality disorders
    ◊ Anxiety
• Structural
    ◊ Microphallus
    ◊ Chordee and Peyronie's disease
    ◊ Cavernosal scarring
    ◊ Phimosis
    ◊ Hypospadias
    ◊ Postsurgical sequelae

LABORATORY
• CBC
• Glucose
• K+
• Na+
• Albumin
• BUN/creatinine
• TSH
• Prolactin
• Testosterone
Drugs that may alter lab results: N/A
Disorders that may alter lab results: N/A

PATHOLOGICAL FINDINGS Most men over age 55 will have some test abnormality or risk factor, but it is not necessarily the cause of the patient's impotence

SPECIAL TESTS
• 24 hour urine zinc
• Dorsal nerve somatosensory evoked potentials
• Sacral evoked response
• Penile-brachial blood pressures
• Aortogram
• Selective pudendal angiogram
• Dynamic cavernosography
• Nocturnal penile tumescence (NPT) testing
• Penile blood pressure

IMAGING Doppler, angiogram, cavernosogram

DIAGNOSTIC PROCEDURES Response to papaverine or alprostadil injection

TREATMENT

APPROPRIATE HEALTH CARE Since erectile dysfunction is multifactorial, evaluation by a generalist in an outpatient setting

GENERAL MEASURES
• Early use of penile implants is now discouraged because of success with vacuum erectile devices, sensate focus therapy and injection therapy
• Improve partner communication
• Reduce performance pressure
• Use sensate focus therapy
• Try vacuum erectile device
• Use of psychiatrists, psychologists, sex therapists, vascular surgeons, urologists, endocrinologists, neurologists, plastic surgeons, etc., often necessary for refractory cases

SURGICAL MEASURES N/A

ACTIVITY No restrictions

DIET Control diabetes if present

PATIENT EDUCATION The New Male Sexuality by Bernie Zilbergeld, Ph.D., Bantam Books, 1992; and problem-specific handouts

Erectile dysfunction

MEDICATIONS

DRUG(S) OF CHOICE
• If hypogonadism present, testosterone cypionate 200 mg IM every two weeks
• If hyperprolactinemia present, bromocriptine 2.5 mg bid up to 40 mg/day
• To induce erection
  ◊ Intracavernous injection of a solution containing phentolamine 0.5-1.0 mg and papaverine 30 mg per mL, starting with 0.1 mL or
  ◊ Alprostadil (Caverject) 10-20 µg/mL; inject into the dorsolateral aspect of proximal third of the penis. Do not exceed 60 mg dose. Do not use more than 3 times a week or more than once in 24 hours. Patient to notify physician if erection lasts > 6 hours for immediate attention.
  ◊ Alprostadil (Muse) urethral suppository 125 mg, 250 mg, 500 mg, and 1000 mg pellets. Maximum of 2 uses in 24 hours.

Contraindications:
• Injections should be avoided in patients with bleeding disorders, patients with sickle cell disease or trait, and in patients with penile deformities.
• Avoid use in patients with known allergies to constituents

Precautions:
• With testosterone, watch for urinary retention, acne, sodium retention and gynecomastia
• With bromocriptine, watch for self-limited nausea, vomiting
• With injection therapy, watch for priapism, fibrosis, hypotension and nausea
• With urethral suppositories, watch for penile pain and irritation, as well as testicular pain. No reports yet of priapism.

Significant possible interactions: N/A

ALTERNATIVE DRUGS
Use vacuum erection device before injections

FOLLOWUP

PATIENT MONITORING
Meet with patient and, if possible, his partner, as required by cause, therapy, and response

PREVENTION/AVOIDANCE
Since erectile dysfunction is multifactorial, referral to a sex therapist or couples therapist may help to speed recovery and prevent future problems

POSSIBLE COMPLICATIONS
Specific to therapy

EXPECTED COURSE/PROGNOSIS
• Given that the majority of patients have unspecified causes of their erectile disorders, vacuum erection device, injection therapy and penile implant have improved the outlook greatly
• Expect 20% failure rate of vacuum erection device, high drop-out rate from injection therapy, and a 10-30% non-use rate for penile implants
• Spontaneous cure rate is about 15%
• Early studies indicate a response rate of 65% for urethral alprostadil compared to 85-90% for the injection

MISCELLANEOUS

ASSOCIATED CONDITIONS
see above

AGE-RELATED FACTORS
Pediatric: N/A
Geriatric: Aging alone is not a cause of impotence
Others: N/A

PREGNANCY
N/A

SYNONYMS
Impotence

ICD-9-CM
• 302 Sexual disorders
• 302.7 Psychosocial dysfunction
• 302.70 Psychosocial dysfunc nos
• 302.71 Inhibited sexual desire
• 302.72 Inhibited sex excitement
• 302.79 Psychosocial dysfunc nec
• 302.8 Psychosocial dis nec
• 302.89 Psychosexual dis nec
• 302.9 Psychosexual dis nos
• V41.7 Sexual function problem
• 607.84 Impotence, organic origin

SEE ALSO
• Priapism

OTHER NOTES
N/A

ABBREVIATIONS
N/A

REFERENCES
• Montague D: Disorders of Male Sexual Dysfunction. Boca Raton, Year Book Medical Publishers, 1988
• Wagner G, Green R: Impotence. New York, Plenum Press, 1981
• Segraves RT, Schoenberg HW: Diagnosis and Treatment of Erectile Disturbances. New York, Plenum Medical Book Company, 1985
• Block B: Erectile Dysfunction Decision Support System. Chapel Hill, Health Sciences Consortium, 1995
Illustrations: N/A
Internet references: http://www.5mcc.com

Author(s)
Bruce Block, MD

Erysipelas

 BASICS

DESCRIPTION Bacterial cellulitis involving the superficial skin lymphatics usually due to group A streptococcus. Usually acute, but a chronic recurrent form also exists.
System(s) affected: Skin/Exocrine
Genetics: N/A
Incidence/Prevalence in USA: Unknown
Predominant age: Usually infants and adults over 40. Greatest in elderly (> 75 years).
Predominant sex: Male = Female

SIGNS AND SYMPTOMS
• Prodrome of malaise, fever and chills
• Headache, vomiting are prominent
• Arthralgias
• Pruritus
• Skin discomfort
• Vesicles
• Facial redness
• Acute onset of erythema
• Begins as erythematous patch
• Sharply demarcated raised border
• Center of lesion defervesces as periphery spreads
• Desquamation and vesicle formation can occur
• Face is the most common area involved, especially nose and ears
• Chronic form may recur hours to years after initial episode
• Chronic form usually recurs at site of the previous infection
• Fever is usually the differentiating factor among similar skin manifestations

CAUSES
Group A beta-hemolytic streptococcus

RISK FACTORS
• Operative wounds
• Fissured skin (especially at the nose and ears)
• Any inflamed skin
• Traumatic wounds/abrasions
• Leg ulcers/stasis dermatitis
• Chronic diseases (diabetes, malnutrition, nephrotic syndrome)
• Immunocompromised or debilitated individual

 DIAGNOSIS

DIFFERENTIAL DIAGNOSIS
• Erysipeloid (little toxicity)
• Contact dermatitis (no fever)
• Angioneurotic edema (no fever)
• Scarlet fever (usually more widespread without edema)
• Lupus (of the face, less fever, positive antinuclear antibodies)
• Polychondritis (of the ear)
• Dermatophytid
• Tuberculoid leprosy

LABORATORY
• Leukocytosis (usually > 15,000)
• Strep may be cultured from exudate or from non-involved sites
• Antistreptolysin (ASO), streptozyme, anti-DNAse may be helpful
• Blood culture
Drugs that may alter lab results: N/A
Disorders that may alter lab results: N/A

PATHOLOGICAL FINDINGS
• Edema
• Vasodilation and enlarged lymphatics
• Infiltration of polymorphonuclear leukocytes, lymphocytes and other inflammatory cells
• Endothelial cell swelling
• Gram positive cocci

SPECIAL TESTS N/A

IMAGING N/A

DIAGNOSTIC PROCEDURES None

 TREATMENT

APPROPRIATE HEALTH CARE
Outpatient

GENERAL MEASURES
• Symptomatic treatment of aches and fever
• Adequate fluid intake
• Local treatment with cold compresses

SURGICAL MEASURES N/A

ACTIVITY Bedrest with activity based on severity of illness

DIET No special diet

PATIENT EDUCATION Importance of completing medication regimen prescribed

MEDICATIONS

DRUG(S) OF CHOICE
• Penicillin V (Pen VK) for at least ten days (improvement in 24-48 hours). Children: 25-50 mg/kg/day divided q6h; Adults: 250-500 mg/dose q6h.
• Parenteral antibiotics are recommended for severe or complicated cases (1-2 million units every 4-6 hours)
• In chronic recurrent infections some authors recommend lower dose daily maintenance/prophylactic treatment after the acute infection resolves
Contraindications: Penicillin allergy
Precautions: Refer to manufacturer's profile of each drug
Significant possible interactions: Refer to manufacturer's profile of each drug

ALTERNATIVE DRUGS
• Erythromycin. Children: 30-40 mg/kg/day divided q6h; adults: 250 mg/dose q6h.
• Cephalosporins

FOLLOWUP

PATIENT MONITORING Patients should be treated until all symptoms and skin manifestations have resolved

PREVENTION/AVOIDANCE
• Maintenance antibiotics for chronic recurrent cases
• Men who shave within five days of facial erysipelas are more likely to have a recurrence
• In recurrent cases, search for other possible source of streptococcal infection (e.g., tonsils, sinuses, teeth, toenails, etc.)

POSSIBLE COMPLICATIONS
• Bacteremia
• Scarlet fever
• Pneumonia
• Abscess
• Embolism
• Gangrene
• Meningitis
• Sepsis
• Death

EXPECTED COURSE/PROGNOSIS
• Adequate treatment results in full recovery
• Chronic edema/scarring can result from chronic recurrent cases
• Rarely elephantiasis may result from chronic recurrent cases
• Untreated cases sometimes will resolve spontaneously

MISCELLANEOUS

ASSOCIATED CONDITIONS N/A

AGE-RELATED FACTORS
Pediatric:
• Group B strep may be a cause in neonates/infants
• Abdominal involvement more common in infants
• Face, scalp, and leg common in older children
Geriatric:
• Fever may not be as prominent
• More prone to complications
• High output cardiac failure may occur in debilitated patients with underlying cardiac disease
• Face and lower extremity most common areas
Others: N/A

PREGNANCY N/A

SYNONYMS
• Saint Anthony's fire
• Ignis sacer

ICD-9-CM
035 Erysipelas

SEE ALSO N/A

OTHER NOTES Patients on systemic steroids may be more difficult to diagnose since signs and symptoms of the infection may be masked by anti-inflammatory action of the steroids

ABBREVIATIONS N/A

REFERENCES
• Fitzpatrick TB, et al: Color Atlas and Synopsis of Clinical Dermatology. 2nd Ed. New York, McGraw-Hill, 1992
• Sauer R: Manual of Skin Diseases. Philadelphia, J.B. Lippincott, 1985
• Domonkos AN, Arnold HL, Odom RB: Andrew's Diseases of the Skin. 8th Ed. Philadelphia, W.B. Saunders Co., 1990
• Wherle PF, Tops FH Sr: Communicable and Infectious Diseases. St. Louis, C.V. Mosby, 1981
• Fitzpatrick TB, et al, eds: Dermatology in General Medicine. 3rd Ed. New York, McGraw-Hill, 1987
Illustrations: N/A
Internet references: http://www.5mcc.com

Author(s)
Scott A. Kincaid, MD

Erythema multiforme

BASICS

DESCRIPTION An acute, self-limited hypersensitivity reaction involving the skin and mucous membranes
• Erythema multiforme minor - milder form characterized by a pleomorphic rash with or without involvement of one mucous membrane site
• Erythema multiforme major - severe, with extensive skin and mucous membrane involvement. It may involve multiple organ systems as complications of the disease, and is commonly referred to as Stevens-Johnson Syndrome.
System(s) affected: Skin/Exocrine
Genetics: Possible association with HLA-B15
Incidence/Prevalence in USA: Uncertain; estimated 1% of outpatient visits
Predominant Age: Peak incidence in 20's and 30's; rare under age 3 and over age 50
Predominant sex: Male > Female (3:2)

SIGNS AND SYMPTOMS
• Variable and nonspecific prodrome, often with features of upper respiratory tract infection
• Sudden onset, rapidly progressive, symmetrical pleomorphic rash on palms, soles, dorsum of hands and extensor surface of extremities and face
• Mucous membrane vesicles/ulceration in 20-45% of cases
• Classic skin rash is "target lesion" consisting of central erythema or purpura, with or without vesiculation, surrounded by normal appearing skin and an outer ring of erythema
• Burning sensation to skin/mucous membranes
• Pruritus usually absent
• Corneal ulcerations

CAUSES
Idiopathic in up to 50% of cases. The remaining 50% may represent a hypersensitivity response to one of the following:
• Viral infections - particularly herpes simplex; also Epstein-Barr, Coxsackie, echovirus, varicella, mumps and poliovirus
• Bacterial infections - especially Mycoplasma pneumoniae; also brucellosis, diphtheria, Yersinia, tuberculosis, tularemia, and gonorrhea
• Protozoan infections
• Collagen vascular disease
• Medications - especially sulfonamides, penicillins, anticonvulsants, salicylates
• Vaccines - tetanus/diphtheria (Td), bacillus Calmette-Guérin (BCG), oral polio vaccine (OPV)
• Malignancy
• Pregnancy
• Premenstrual hormonal changes
• Consumption of beer
• Reiter's syndrome
• Sarcoidosis

RISK FACTORS
• Previous history of erythema multiforme
• Male sex

DIAGNOSIS

DIFFERENTIAL DIAGNOSIS
• Urticaria
• Necrotizing vasculitis
• Drug eruptions
• Contact dermatitis
• Pityriasis rosea
• Secondary syphilis
• Ringworm
• Pemphigus vulgaris
• Pemphigoid
• Dermatitis herpetiformis
• Herpes gestationis
• Septicemia
• Serum sickness
• Viral exanthems
• Rocky Mountain spotted fever
• Collagen vascular diseases
• Mucocutaneous lymph node syndrome
• Meningococcemia
• Lichen planus
• Behçet's syndrome
• Recurrent aphthous ulcers
• Herpetic gingivostomatitis
• Granuloma annulare

LABORATORY None
Drugs that may alter lab results: N/A
Disorders that may alter lab results: N/A

PATHOLOGICAL FINDINGS Epidermal necrolysis is characteristic. Spongiosis, intracellular edema, vacuolar changes at the dermal-epidermal junction, edema and extravasated erythrocytes in the dermis may also be seen on biopsy specimen.

SPECIAL TESTS None

IMAGING N/A

DIAGNOSTIC PROCEDURES Skin biopsy

TREATMENT

APPROPRIATE HEALTH CARE
Outpatient, except in those cases with severe extensive skin involvement (see Stevens-Johnson syndrome) or with oral involvement precluding oral intake, in whom dehydration may occur

GENERAL MEASURES
• Withdrawal of any implicated medications or treatment of any identified underlying infection/disease
• For mild cases, symptomatic treatment is sufficient. For more severe cases, meticulous wound care and use of Burow's solution or Domeboro solution dressings.
• Oral lesions can be treated with mouthwashes with warm saline, or a solution of diphenhydramine, Xylocaine, and Kaopectate to provide symptomatic relief and oral hygiene, and to facilitate oral intake

SURGICAL MEASURES N/A

ACTIVITY As tolerated

DIET As tolerated. Increased fluid intake should be encouraged in those with more extensive skin involvement.

PATIENT EDUCATION Patients should be reassured that the disease is self-limited. Recurrences are possible. Encourage avoidance of any identified etiologic agent.

MEDICATIONS

DRUG(S) OF CHOICE Systemic corticosteroids, initial dosage equivalent to prednisone 1-2 mg/kg/day with subsequent tapering. (Particularly useful in rapidly evolving or more severe cases). Treatment specific to any underlying infection or disease should be provided.
Contraindications: Any infectious process in which use of steroids would be contraindicated
Precautions: Refer to manufacturer's profile of each drug
Significant possible interactions: Refer to manufacturer's profile of each drug

ALTERNATIVE DRUGS Acyclovir may be given to suppress recurrent herpetic disease if this is identified as the underlying cause

FOLLOWUP

PATIENT MONITORING The disease is self-limited, however, during the course of the illness patients should be followed closely for development of severe disease or complications

PREVENTION/AVOIDANCE
• Known or suspected etiologic agents should be avoided
• Acyclovir may help prevent herpes-related erythema multiforme
• Tamoxifen has been shown to prevent premenstrual related disease

POSSIBLE COMPLICATIONS
• Progression to Stevens-Johnson syndrome or toxic epidermal necrolysis
• Secondary infections
• Dehydration/electrolyte disturbances
• Ophthalmic complications of corneal ulcerations or iritis

EXPECTED COURSE/PROGNOSIS
• Rash evolves over 1-2 weeks and subsequently resolves within 2-3 weeks, generally without scarring or sequelae
• Following resolution there may be some post-inflammatory hyperpigmentation
• Risk of recurrence may be as high as 37%

MISCELLANEOUS

ASSOCIATED CONDITIONS
• Any of the infections or diseases listed under Causes
• Stevens-Johnson syndrome and toxic epidermal necrolysis are more severe forms of the disease

AGE-RELATED FACTORS
Pediatric: More severe forms of the disease tend to occur in younger males. Rare under age 3 years.
Geriatric: Rare over age 50 years
Others: N/A

PREGNANCY Reported as a possible etiologic condition

SYNONYMS Erythema exudativum multiforme

ICD-9-CM 695.1 erythema multiforma

SEE ALSO
• Stevens-Johnson syndrome
• Urticaria
• Dermatitis, contact
• Pityriasis rosea
• Tinea corporis
• Pemphigus vulgaris
• Herpes gestationis
• Dermatitis, herpetiformis
• Serum sickness

OTHER NOTES Because it is an immunologic reaction, drug related erythema multiforme will not occur until 7-14 days after exposure to the offending agent, unless the patient has had the medication previously

ABBREVIATIONS N/A

REFERENCES
• Fitzpatrick TB, et al, eds: Dermatology in General Medicine. 3rd Ed. New York, McGraw-Hill, 1987
• Moschella SL, Hurley HJ: Dermatology. 3rd Ed. Philadelphia, W.B. Saunders Co., 1992
• Domonkos AN, Arnold HL, Odom RB: Andrews' Diseases of the Skin. 8th Ed. Philadelphia, W.B. Saunders Co., 1990
Illustrations: 4 available on CD-ROM
Internet references: http://www.5mcc.com

Author(s)
Marc LeDuc, MD
Mitchell S. King, MD

Erythema nodosum

BASICS

DESCRIPTION Clinical pattern of multiple, bilateral, cutaneous, inflammatory, non-ulcerating, non-scarring eruptions that undergo characteristic color changes ending in temporary bruise-like areas. Occurs most commonly on the extensor surface of the shins, less common on thighs and forearms. It is often idiopathic, but may be seen as a response to a variety of clinical entities. Will usually subside in 3 to 6 weeks without scarring or atrophy.
System(s) affected: Skin/Exocrine
Genetics: N/A
Incidence/Prevalence in USA: Unknown
Predominant age: 20-30 years
Predominant sex: Female > Male (3:1)

SIGNS AND SYMPTOMS
• Raised, warm, tender, brightly erythematous nodules located on anterior shins
• Can also occur on any area with subcutaneous fat
• Diameter 1-15 cm
• Fever, malaise, chills
• Arthralgias
• Bluish discoloration late in course
• Hilar adenopathy
• Episcleral lesions
• Eruptions often preceded by URI symptoms

CAUSES
• Idiopathic
• Bacterial - streptococcal infections, tuberculosis, leprosy, Yersinia enterocolitica, tularemia, Campylobacter, salmonella, Shigella, gonorrhea
• Sarcoid
• Drugs - sulfonamides, oral contraceptives, bromides
• Pregnancy
• Deep fungal - dermatophytes, coccidioidomycosis, histoplasmosis, blastomycosis
• Viral/chlamydial - infectious mononucleosis, lymphogranuloma venereum, paravaccinia
• Enteropathies - ulcerative colitis, Crohn's disease
• Malignancies - lymphoma/leukemia, sarcoma, post radiation therapy

RISK FACTORS Listed with Causes

DIAGNOSIS

DIFFERENTIAL DIAGNOSIS
• Superficial thrombophlebitis
• Cellulitis
• Septic emboli
• Erythema induratum (cold, ulcerating nodules on calves)
• Nodular vasculitis (warm, ulcerating nodules)
• Weber-Christian disease (violaceous, scarring nodules)
• Lupus panniculitis
• Cutaneous polyarteritis nodosa
• Sarcoidosis granulomata
• Lymphoma

LABORATORY
• Elevated erythrocyte sedimentation rate
• CBC: mild leukocytosis
• Throat culture, ASO titers
• Stool culture and leukocytes if indicated
• Skin testing for mycobacteria if indicated
Drugs that may alter lab results:
Antecedent antibiotics may affect cultures
Disorders that may alter lab results: N/A

PATHOLOGICAL FINDINGS
• Septal panniculitis
• Neutrophilic infiltrate in septa of fat tissue, early in course
• Mononuclear cells and histiocytes predominate, late in course
• Lower dermis/subcutis involvement and septal fibrosis may occur

SPECIAL TESTS N/A

IMAGING Chest x-ray for hilar adenopathy or infiltrates

DIAGNOSTIC PROCEDURES Deep skin excisional biopsy including subcutaneous fat. Usually not necessary.

TREATMENT

APPROPRIATE HEALTH CARE
Outpatient

GENERAL MEASURES
• Wet dressings (hot soaks and topical medications are not useful)
• Discontinue potentially causative drugs
• Treat underlying disease

SURGICAL MEASURES N/A

ACTIVITY
• Bedrest, keep legs elevated
• Elastic wraps or support stockings may be helpful if patients want to be up and around

DIET No restrictions

PATIENT EDUCATION
• Lesions will resolve over a few months
• No scarring is anticipated
• Joint aches and pains may persist
• Less than 20% recur

MEDICATIONS

DRUG(S) OF CHOICE
• Medication usually more effective after initial onset versus with chronic disease
• Recurrence is common following cessation of therapy
• Nonsteroidal anti-inflammatory drugs (NSAID's):
 ◊ Aspirin: 325 mg 8-12 per day; use enteric coated to decrease GI upset. Titrate to blood levels.
 ◊ Indomethacin: 75-150 mg per day, divided tid
 ◊ Naproxen (Naprosyn): 500-1000 mg per day, divided bid

Contraindications:
• Active or recent peptic ulcer disease
• History of NSAID's hypersensitivity

Precautions:
• Gastrointestinal upset/bleeding
• Fluid retention
• Dose reduction in elderly, especially those with renal disease, diabetes, heart failure
• May mask fever
• NSAID's may elevate liver function tests

Significant possible interactions:
• May blunt antihypertensive effects of diuretics and beta-blockers
• NSAID's can elevate plasma lithium levels
• Caution advised with naproxen or any highly protein-bound drug since it may compete for albumin binding and elevate levels
• NSAID's can cause significant elevations in and prolongation of methotrexate levels

ALTERNATIVE DRUGS
• Potassium iodide 400-900 mg daily, divided bid-tid
• Corticosteroids only in very severe, refractory cases
• Other NSAIDs

FOLLOWUP

PATIENT MONITORING
Monthly followup or as dictated by underlying disorder

PREVENTION/AVOIDANCE
N/A

POSSIBLE COMPLICATIONS
Vary according to underlying disease. None expected from lesions of erythema nodosum.

EXPECTED COURSE/PROGNOSIS
• Individual lesions resolve over 3-6 week course
• Total time course of 6-12 weeks, but may vary with etiologic disease if present
• Joint aches and pains may persist for years
• Lesions do not scar
• One or more recurrences in 12-14% of cases; these occur over variable periods, averaging several years, seen most often with sarcoid, streptococcal infection, pregnancy, and oral contraceptives

MISCELLANEOUS

ASSOCIATED CONDITIONS
See Causes

AGE-RELATED FACTORS
Pediatric: Incidence equal male and female
Geriatric: N/A
Others: N/A

PREGNANCY
May have repeat outbreaks during pregnancy

SYNONYMS
Dermatitis contusiformis

ICD-9-CM
695.2 Erythema nodosum

SEE ALSO
N/A

OTHER NOTES
• Lofgren's syndrome (erythema nodosum and hilar adenopathy) is seen with multiple etiologies and does not exclusively indicate sarcoid
• Clinical variant of erythema nodosum migrans (subacute nodular migratory panniculitis) is often unilateral with nodules fewer in number, smaller in size and longer lasting, often extending radially by division into smaller nodules

ABBREVIATIONS
N/A

REFERENCES
• Kannuksela M: Clinics in Dermatology. October-December 1986:88-95
• Fitzpatrick TB, et al, eds: Dermatology in General Medicine. 3rd Ed. New York, McGraw-Hill, 1987
• Habif T: Clinical Dermatology. 3rd Ed. St. Louis, CV Mosby, 1996
Illustrations: 3 available on CD-ROM
Internet references: http://www.5mcc.com

Author(s)
Bruce T. Vanderhoff, MD
Sumner T. McAllister, MD

Erythroblastosis fetalis

BASICS

DESCRIPTION Hemolytic anemia of the fetus or newborn caused by transplacental transmission of maternal antibody. When severe, the anemia can result in extramedullary hematopoiesis, secondary organ dysfunction, heart failure, hydrops, and death. The name erythroblastosis refers to the presence of immature erythrocytes in the peripheral blood from accelerated hematopoiesis.

System(s) affected:
Hemic/Lymphatic/Immunologic, Cardiovascular, Nervous

Genetics: Can occur when the fetus inherits a paternal blood group antigen lacking in the mother. The Rh D antigen is most frequently implicated. (For more on inheritance of Rh antigens, see Rh incompatibility.)

Incidence/Prevalence in USA:
• Uncommon
• About 9% of pregnancies have an Rh-negative mother with an Rh-positive fetus
• With Rho(D) immune globulin prophylaxis, risk of sensitization is reduced to less than 1% of susceptible pregnancies

Predominant age: Fetus and newborn
Predominant sex: Male = Female

SIGNS AND SYMPTOMS
• Pallor
• Respiratory distress
• Hepatomegaly
• Splenomegaly
• Ascites
• Hypotension/shock
• Edema/anasarca/hydrops
• Jaundice of newborn
• Purpura/bleeding problems
• Fetal death in utero

CAUSES
• Maternal isoimmunization to Rh antigen by transfusion of Rh-positive blood
• Maternal isoimmunization from exposure to fetal Rh antigens in prior pregnancy or current pregnancy
• Maternal isoimmunization to other blood group antigens (Kell, Duffy, Kidd, M, S, Diego, etc.) is unusual but may cause serious disease

RISK FACTORS
• Prior transfusion with incompatible blood
• Any Rh-positive pregnancy in Rh-negative woman
• Without prophylactic immunotherapy (Rh immune globulin), risk of Rh sensitization is up to 16% during or after term pregnancy, about 3% for spontaneous abortion and 5-6% for surgical abortion
• Sensitization by exposure to fetal blood can occur also with ectopic pregnancy, amniocentesis, chorionic villus sampling, placental trauma or manipulation, placental abruption
• Prophylaxis with Rh immune globulin greatly reduces but does not eliminate the risk

DIAGNOSIS

DIFFERENTIAL DIAGNOSIS
• Fetal blood loss anemia
• Twin-to-twin transfusion
• Arteriovenous or cardiac malformations
• Hereditary hemolytic anemias
• Drug-induced hemolytic anemia
• Nonimmune fetal hydrops
• Hemolysis from intrauterine infection (syphilis, toxoplasmosis, CMV, others)

LABORATORY
• Positive indirect Coombs test (antibody screen) during pregnancy
• Positive direct Coombs test in fetus or newborn
• Anemia in fetus or newborn
• Reticulocytosis
• Nucleated RBC's on differential count
• Hyperbilirubinemia (indirect bilirubin)
• Thrombocytopenia

Drugs that may alter lab results: Prior administration of Rho(D) immune globulin may lead to weakly (false) positive indirect Coombs test in mother and direct Coombs test in infant

Disorders that may alter lab results: N/A

PATHOLOGICAL FINDINGS
• Erythroid hyperplasia of bone marrow
• Extramedullary hematopoiesis
• Hepatomegaly
• Splenomegaly
• Cardiac enlargement
• Pulmonary hemorrhages
• Enlargement, edema of placenta

SPECIAL TESTS
• Elevated amniotic fluid bilirubin (delta OD 450)
• Paternal blood typing may exclude pregnancy from being at risk

IMAGING
• Ultrasonography can demonstrate hepatomegaly, abdominal enlargement, ascites, or signs of hydrops
• Doppler flow studies of fetus are experimental in assessing degree of anemia
• Fetus may be severely affected without hydrops; ultrasound poor at predicting need for intervention

DIAGNOSTIC PROCEDURES
• Amniocentesis
• Umbilical cord blood sampling

TREATMENT

APPROPRIATE HEALTH CARE
• Affected pregnancies usually managed at the tertiary care level because of the specialized, somewhat hazardous treatment measures involved
• Delivery should occur in an institution capable of performing exchange transfusion even if only mild involvement of infant is expected
• Infants with moderate or severe disease require neonatal intensive care

GENERAL MEASURES
• See Patient Monitoring
• Depending on severity of involvement, treatment of infant may include:
  ◊ Phototherapy
  ◊ Transfusion after delivery
  ◊ Exchange transfusion
  ◊ Diuretics and digoxin for hydrops
  ◊ Early delivery
  ◊ Intrauterine transfusion. Intravascular approach via the umbilical vein is becoming preferred over the intraperitoneal approach and appears to be more effective.

SURGICAL MEASURES N/A

ACTIVITY N/A

DIET N/A

PATIENT EDUCATION Griffith: Instructions for Patients, 5th Ed. Philadelphia, W.B. Saunders Co., to photocopy for patient

MEDICATIONS

DRUG(S) OF CHOICE N/A
Contraindications: N/A
Precautions: N/A
Significant possible interactions: N/A

ALTERNATIVE DRUGS
• Diuretics, inotropic agents, etc., may be used in addition to transfusion to manage heart failure in the newborn
• Promethazine, immune serum globulin, corticosteroids, and plasmapheresis have been tried as alternatives to invasive treatments but have not been effective

FOLLOWUP

PATIENT MONITORING
• Antibody titer measured every few weeks during pregnancy. A titer of 1:16 or greater indicates need for further testing.
• Periodic amniocentesis for photometric determination of amniotic fluid bilirubin levels in pregnancies with elevated antibody titers. Results estimate the extent of fetal hemolysis and the need for cord blood sampling.
• Percutaneous umbilical blood sampling (PUBS, cordocentesis) for fetal blood type, hematocrit, reticulocyte count, presence of erythroblasts
• Fetal heart rate testing/ultrasonography to assess fetal status
• Amniocentesis for fetal lung maturity

PREVENTION/AVOIDANCE
• Rho(D) Immune Globulin (RhIG, RhoGAM, Gamulin Rh) given prophylactically to unsensitized, Rh-negative pregnant women at risk. Usually at 28-32 weeks gestation and at birth if infant is Rh positive (see Rh incompatibility topic).
• Artificial insemination with sperm from antigen-negative donor for isoimmunized woman married to antigen-positive man

POSSIBLE COMPLICATIONS
• Fetal distress requiring emergent delivery
• Fetal death in utero
• Disseminated intravascular coagulation (DIC)
• Pregnancy loss from umbilical blood sampling
• Pregnancy loss from intrauterine transfusion
• Asphyxia
• Neonatal hemolytic anemia, mild to severe
• Neonatal anemia from hematopoietic suppression after intrauterine transfusion
• Pulmonary edema
• Congestive heart failure
• Shock
• Neonatal jaundice, mild to severe
• Kernicterus

EXPECTED COURSE/PROGNOSIS
• 50% of affected infants have mild disease and require no treatment (or treatment of anemia and jaundice only after delivery), and can be delivered at or near term
• 30% have moderate disease with anemia and hepatomegaly. They require close followup of the pregnancy for signs of deterioration which may require early delivery after 32-34 weeks or intrauterine transfusion prior to that age. After delivery exchange transfusion is likely to treat anemia and hyperbilirubinemia.
• 20% have fetal hydrops, require intrauterine transfusion and delivery as early as 32-34 weeks
• Disease severity tends to worsen in successive affected pregnancies
• Hydrops is associated with poorer prognosis
• Without treatment overall perinatal mortality is 30%
• With appropriate monitoring and treatment most infants do well, even those requiring intrauterine transfusion
• Fortunately, with universal screening for Rh sensitization and widespread use of Rh immune globulin in 3rd trimester and/or birth have made disease relatively rare

MISCELLANEOUS

ASSOCIATED CONDITIONS N/A

AGE-RELATED FACTORS
Pediatric: Exclusively affects fetus and neonate
Geriatric: N/A
Others: N/A

PREGNANCY N/A

SYNONYMS
• Erythroblastosis neonatorum
• Hemolytic disease of the newborn
• Congenital anemia of the newborn
• Immune hydrops fetalis
• Icterus gravis neonatorum

ICD-9-CM
773.0 Rh hemolytic disease in fetus or newborn
773.1 ABO hemolytic disease in fetus or newborn
773.2 Other hemolytic disease in fetus or newborn
773.3 Isoimmune hydrops fetalis
773.4 Isoimmune kernicterus
773.5 Isoimmune late anemia

SEE ALSO
• Rh incompatibility
• Anemia, autoimmune hemolytic

OTHER NOTES N/A

ABBREVIATIONS N/A

REFERENCES
• Cunningham FG, MacDonald PC, Gant NF, eds: Williams' Obstetrics. 19th Ed. Norwalk, CT, Appleton and Lange, 1993
• Scott JR, et al, eds: Danforth's Obstetrics and Gynecology. 7th Ed. Philadelphia, J.B. Lippincott, 1994
• Duerbeck NB, Seeds JW: Rhesus Immunization in Pregnancy: A Review. Obstetrical and Gynecological Survey 1993;48(12):801-810
• Oski FA: Principles and Practices of Pediatrics. 2nd Ed. J.B. Lippincott Co., 1994
• Merenstein GB, Gardner SL: Handbook of Neonatal Intensive Care. 3rd Ed. St. Louis, Mosby, 1993
Illustrations: N/A
Internet references: http://www.5mcc.com

Author(s)
Donald A. F. Nelson, MD

Esophageal tumors

BASICS

DESCRIPTION
• Carcinomas - begin in the esophagus (primary) and usually occur in the lower third. Types: Squamous cell carcinoma; adenocarcinoma (may now account for more than 25% of esophageal cancer). At the time of diagnosis, 80% have metastases to the lymph nodes.
• Benign neoplasms - rare. Types: Leiomyoma (most common), papilloma, and fibrovascular polyps.
System(s) affected: Gastrointestinal
Genetics: No known genetic pattern
Incidence/Prevalence in USA:
• Squamous cell: 3-15/100,000 males; 3-4/100,000 females (highest incidence in Blacks)
• Adeno: Rising incidence (vast majority have Barrett's esophagus)
Predominant age: > 50 years (peak incidence 50-60)
Predominant sex: Male > Female (2.6:1)

SIGNS AND SYMPTOMS
• Progressive dysphagia for solids over weeks to months
• Progressive weight loss
• Regurgitation and aspiration are common (especially at night)
• Cachexia
• Supraclavicular lymphadenopathy
• Esophageal obstruction
• Hiccups
• Cough
• Hoarseness
• Gastrointestinal blood loss

CAUSES
Unknown. Most esophagus cancers are primary, but some spread from other body parts.

RISK FACTORS
• Smoking
• Excess alcohol consumption
• Head and neck tumors
• Nitrates in foods
• Lye stricture
• Achalasia
• Tylosis
• Plummer-Vinson syndrome (anemia and esophageal web)
• Coexisting primary oro-pharyngeal carcinoma
• Barrett's metaplasia (develops in 10-40% of patients with chronic gastroesophageal reflux)

DIAGNOSIS

DIFFERENTIAL DIAGNOSIS
• Benign causes of dysphagia, achalasia
• Motility disorders of the esophagus
• Extrinsic esophageal compression secondary to mediastinal/pulmonary disease

LABORATORY
• Esophageal biopsy/brushing
• Anemia
Drugs that may alter lab results: N/A
Disorders that may alter lab results: N/A

PATHOLOGICAL FINDINGS
• Location - 20% in upper third, 30% in middle third, 50% in lower third
• Elevated plaques
• Ulceration
• Strictures

SPECIAL TESTS
Esophagoscopy

IMAGING
• Barium swallow - stenosing lesion
• CT scan - valuable for looking for metastases
• X-ray of the upper-intestinal tract may show pneumonitis, pleural effusion, lung abscess
• Endoscopic ultrasound - staging (most accurate)

DIAGNOSTIC PROCEDURES
• Esophagoscopy with biopsy
• Brush cytology (> 95% positive)
• Bronchoscopy - distortion of the bronchial lumen, blunting of the carina, or intrabronchial tumor
• Once tumor is identified, liver function studies and ultrasonography and/or CT scan for evidence of liver metastases
• Endoscopic ultrasound is most sensitive and specific test to determine local spread

TREATMENT

APPROPRIATE HEALTH CARE
• Inpatient occasionally
• Home care or extended-care facility following definitive treatment

GENERAL MEASURES
• Palliative therapeutic options include: surgery, radiotherapy, chemotherapy, laser photocoagulation, photodynamic therapy, dilation, placement of endoluminal prosthesis (stent) or combination of these methods. The specific choice will depend on the extent of the tumor and symptoms and the individual patient's state of health.

SURGICAL MEASURES
• Majority of tumors are not resectable for cure at time of presentation
• Important to stage the lesion before determining treatment plan
• Strictures may be dilated for temporary relief
• Prior to surgery - average patient requires nutritional and pulmonary preparation, e.g., feeding tube with formula diet and respiratory therapy
• Endoluminal prosthesis may be attempted for patients who have failed other methods of palliation

ACTIVITY
Adjusted to patient's ability

DIET
• Soft to liquid
• High calorie supplements (usually liquid)

PATIENT EDUCATION
For patient education materials favorably reviewed on this topic, contact: National Cancer Institute, Dept. of Health And Human Services, Public Inquiries Section, Office of Cancer Communications, Building 31, Room 101-18, 9000 Rockville Pike, Bethesda, MD 20892, (301)496-5583

MEDICATIONS

DRUG(S) OF CHOICE
• Chemotherapy in selected patients
• Analgesics
• Antacids, H2 receptor antagonist, or proton pump inhibitors when gastroesophageal reflux symptoms co-exist
• Metoclopramide or cisapride if gastric emptying problems coexist (frequently paraneoplastic)
Contraindications: Refer to manufacturer's literature
Precautions: Refer to manufacturer's literature
Significant possible interactions: Refer to manufacturer's literature

ALTERNATIVE DRUGS   N/A

FOLLOWUP

PATIENT MONITORING   Individualized to follow results of preoperative and postoperative treatment

PREVENTION/AVOIDANCE
• Avoid tobacco, excess alcohol, corrosive chemicals
• Endoscopic surveillance of those at high risk (Barrett's, esophagus, head and neck cancer)

EXPECTED COURSE/PROGNOSIS
• Overall 5-year survival 5%; in squamous cell carcinoma with uninvolved lymph nodes 15-20%
• Death rate following resection or bypass is 10-15%

POSSIBLE COMPLICATIONS
• Metastases to anterior jugular, supraclavicular, subdiaphragmatic lymph nodes, liver, lungs
• Complications from surgical procedures (anastomotic leak or stricture, fistula formation, empyema, malnutrition)
• Radiation can cause esophageal perforation, stricture, fistula, esophagitis, pneumonitis, myelitis, and pulmonary fibrosis
• Toxicities of chemotherapy - nausea, vomiting, hair loss, gastroenteritis, hematopoietic and immune depression
• Tubes can become blocked or dislodged
• Aspiration from esophageal obstruction

MISCELLANEOUS

ASSOCIATED CONDITIONS
• Barrett's metaplasia
• Head and neck cancer
• Achalasia

AGE-RELATED FACTORS
Pediatric: N/A
Geriatric: Most common in males over 60
Others:
• Uncommon under age 50
• Definitive treatment is standard regardless of age
• Symptomatic therapy requires dose adjustment for very old and very young

PREGNANCY   N/A

SYNONYMS
• Esophagus squamous cell carcinoma
• Esophagus adenocarcinoma

ICD-9-CM   150 malignant neoplasm of esophagus

SEE ALSO   Gastroesophageal reflux

OTHER NOTES   N/A

ABBREVIATIONS   N/A

REFERENCES
• Chabner BA, Collins JM: Cancer Chemotherapy: Principles and Practice. Philadelphia, J.B. Lippincott Co., 1990
• Livstone EM: General considerations of tumors of the esophagus. In: Berk JE, ed. Bockus' Gastroenterology. 4th Ed. Philadelphia, W.B. Saunders Co., 1985
Illustrations: N/A
Internet references: http://www.5mcc.com

Author(s)
Philip E. Jaffe, MD

Failure to thrive (FTT)

BASICS

DESCRIPTION Failure to thrive is a symptom (rather than a disease) characterized by disproportionate failure to gain weight in comparison to height due to caloric insufficiency (or under utilization of ingested food) without obvious etiology.
System(s) affected: Endocrine/Metabolic, Musculoskeletal, Nervous
Genetics: No consistent genetic pattern
Incidence/Prevalence in USA:
• Not known
• 3-5% of pediatric in-patient admissions are for evaluation of failure to thrive (FTT). It is a common and difficult diagnostic problem.
Predominant age: Usually 6-12 months; almost all are under 3-5 years
Predominant sex: Male = Female

SIGNS AND SYMPTOMS
• Weight low for age
• Growth chart shows significant deceleration of weight gain
• Difficult personality, feeding and sleep problems
• Apathetic and withdrawn, or watchful and alert
• Poor hygiene
• Signs of inflicted trauma
• Primary caretaker characteristics - psychosocial problems, often depressed
• Family characteristics - unstable, disturbed

CAUSES
• Organic etiology: less than 20%, usually gastrointestinal or neurologic. Includes some infants who were profoundly premature
• Environmental deprivation: about 70%, of which one-third are simple educational problems, such as incorrect feeding
• Normal, small children (about 10%) not truly FTT

RISK FACTORS
• Parent with psychosocial problems
• Premature or sick newborn
• Infant with physical deformity
• Unstable, disturbed family

DIAGNOSIS

DIFFERENTIAL DIAGNOSIS Any condition of sufficient severity to cause failure to gain weight adequately, including child abuse and/or neglect

LABORATORY
• Routine laboratory work-up should be kept to a minimum
    ◊ CBC
    ◊ Sedimentation rate
    ◊ Urinalysis
    ◊ Urine culture
    ◊ Chemical profile, including BUN, calcium, phosphorus
• Other studies dictated by results of history and physical examination, such as thyroid profile, pituitary studies
Drugs that may alter lab results: NA
Disorders that may alter lab results: Various blood chemistries may be altered by malnutrition regardless of cause

PATHOLOGICAL FINDINGS   N/A

SPECIAL TESTS   N/A

IMAGING
• Skeletal survey if there is suspicion or evidence of physical abuse
• X-rays for bone age (wrist film)

DIAGNOSTIC PROCEDURES
• Careful, detailed history and physical examination are most important
• Observation of infant and his or her interaction with caretakers and environment essential
• If suspicious of Turner's syndrome, a karyotype is indicated. Buccal smears were previously the test of choice but are no longer considered appropriate.
• Carefully plotted growth curves, including weight, height, and head circumference

TREATMENT

APPROPRIATE HEALTH CARE
Outpatient, except inpatient when all other attempts to improve have failed

GENERAL MEASURES
• Admission to inpatient setting
• Use of few sympathetic primary caretakers in hospital
• Provision of stimulation, cuddling, affection as inpatient or outpatient

SURGICAL MEASURES   N/A

ACTIVITY   No restrictions

DIET Provision of balanced, high caloric diet on both a scheduled and ad lib basis, 150-200 kcal/kg/day

PATIENT EDUCATION Depends on etiology of FTT. When environmental deprivation is established, attempts to re-educate in a non-punitive way is essential.

MEDICATIONS

DRUG(S) OF CHOICE None; routine vitamin supplementation
Contraindications: N/A
Precautions: N/A
Significant possible interactions: N/A

ALTERNATIVE DRUGS N/A

FOLLOWUP

PATIENT MONITORING
• When etiology is organic, followup depends on particular disease involved
• When environmental deprivation is established, extremely close followup, both at home and in office is essential. If family fails to comply, child protection authorities must be notified and foster care may be necessary.

PREVENTION/AVOIDANCE Stable home life with caring parents

POSSIBLE COMPLICATIONS N/A

EXPECTED COURSE/PROGNOSIS
Long-term prognosis of children with FTT due to environmental deprivation is not encouraging. Many children remain small, most demonstrate developmental and educational deficiencies and personality disorders. Only one-third are ultimately normal.

MISCELLANEOUS

ASSOCIATED CONDITIONS N/A

AGE-RELATED FACTORS N/A
Pediatric: N/A
Geriatric: N/A
Others: N/A

PREGNANCY N/A

SYNONYMS N/A

ICD-9-CM 783.4

SEE ALSO
• Turner's syndrome
• Down's syndrome

OTHER NOTES N/A

ABBREVIATIONS FTT = failure to thrive

REFERENCES
• Sills RH: Failure to Thrive. In: Stockman JA, ed. Difficult Diagnosis in Pediatrics. Philadelphia, W.B. Saunders Co., 1990
Illustrations: N/A
Internet references: http://www.5mcc.com

Author(s)
Kurt J. Wegner, MD

Fecal impaction

BASICS

DESCRIPTION
Incomplete evacuation of feces, leading to formation of a large, firm, immovable mass of stool in the rectum (70%), sigmoid flexure (20%) or proximal colon (10%). The rectosigmoid colon dilates to accommodate the mass, which, in turn, is not pliable enough to pass through the disproportionately small anal canal by the patient's weak defecation effort. Impacted stool may exist as a single mass (stercolith) or as a composite of small, rounded fecal particles (scybalum).

System(s) affected: Gastrointestinal
Genetics: Fecal impaction of the cecum may be seen in cystic fibrosis
Incidence/Prevalence in USA:
• General population - 1% (1000/100,000)
• Children - 1.5%
• Nursing home residents - 30%
Predominant age: Over age 60
Predominant sex: No sex preponderance in adults. Among children, 75% are boys.

SIGNS AND SYMPTOMS
• Fecal incontinence, interpreted as "diarrhea"
• Postprandial abdominal pain
• Tenesmus
• Colic
• Nausea, vomiting
• Anorexia, weight loss
• Dehydration
• Headache
• General malaise
• Agitation; confusion
• Fever to 39.4°C (103°F)
• Tachycardia
• Tachypnea
• Urinary frequency, incontinence
• Large mass of stool palpable in lower left quadrant and rectal vault

CAUSES
• Diet lacking in fiber
• Drugs (stimulant laxatives, opiates, benzodiazepines, tricyclic antidepressants, phenothiazines, antihypertensives, sucralfate, iron)
• Local or generalized neurogenic bowel disorders (e.g., stroke, parkinsonism, spinal cord lesions)
• Painful rectal conditions inhibiting voluntary defecation, (e.g., anal fissure, hemorrhoids)
• Neoplastic or inflammatory obstructing lesions (e.g., rectal bezoars)
• Hypothyroidism
• Hypokalemia
• Hypercalcemia
• Excess of gastrointestinal inhibitory hormones (prolactin, endorphins, glucagon, secretin)

RISK FACTORS
• Institutionalization
• Psychogenic illness
• Immobility, inactivity
• Pica
• Chronic renal failure; renal transplant recipients

DIAGNOSIS

DIFFERENTIAL DIAGNOSIS
• Irritable bowel syndrome
• Gastroenteritis, colitis
• Diverticulitis
• Appendicitis
• Carcinoma of the colon

LABORATORY
• Leukocytosis to 15,000 WBC/cu.mm
• Hyponatremia
• Hypokalemia
• Stool may be positive for occult blood
• Anemia, due to blood loss
Drugs that may alter lab results: N/A
Disorders that may alter lab results: N/A

PATHOLOGICAL FINDINGS   N/A

SPECIAL TESTS
Sigmoidoscopy may be used to clarify the nature of a rectosigmoid mass beyond digital reach

IMAGING
• Plain abdominal radiography identifies masses of stool or signs of obstruction if digital exam unrevealing
• Barium enema can differentiate feces from tumor

DIAGNOSTIC PROCEDURES   N/A

TREATMENT

APPROPRIATE HEALTH CARE
Outpatient

GENERAL MEASURES
• Manual fragmentation and extraction of fecal mass (after lubrication with lidocaine jelly) by physician or nurse
• More proximal masses can be disimpacted with water jet directed through fiberoptic sigmoidoscope
• Enemas - containing 20% water soluble contrast material (Gastrografin, Hypaque) may further fragment stool bolus
• For complete evacuation after partial fragmentation - bisacodyl suppositories or enemas with mineral oil, tap water or sodium phosphate
• Ensure minimum fluid intake of 1.5-2.0 liters/day (may use poorly absorbed isosmotic solution of polyethylene glycol, e.g., Golytely, Colyte)

SURGICAL MEASURES
Laparotomy - necessary only in extreme cases

ACTIVITY   Increased activity important

DIET   High fiber

PATIENT EDUCATION
• Avoid catharsis
• No hot water, soap or hydrogen peroxide enemas! They may burn or irritate rectal mucosa, causing bleeding.

MEDICATIONS

DRUG(S) OF CHOICE None
Contraindications: Avoid lactulose, since colonic distention can result from its bacterial fermentation
Precautions: N/A
Significant possible interactions: N/A

ALTERNATIVE DRUGS N/A

FOLLOWUP

PATIENT MONITORING
• Less than one bowel movement every other day suggests impaction
• Periodic rectal exam

PREVENTION/AVOIDANCE
• Establish regular, consistent toilet time by evoking gastrocolic reflex
• Maintain high fiber diet
• Reinforce exercise
• Install user-friendly commodes
• Use hydrophilic mucilloids (Metamucil) or stool-wetting agents (Colace) as needed
• Consider biofeedback; bowel training
• Periodic enemas, if indicated
• Periodic polyethylene glycol

POSSIBLE COMPLICATIONS
• Complications of impaction
  ◊ Urinary tract obstruction
  ◊ Recurrent urinary tract infections
  ◊ Intestinal obstruction
  ◊ Spontaneous perforation of colon
  ◊ Stercoral ulceration
  ◊ Hernia
  ◊ Volvulus
  ◊ Megacolon
  ◊ Rectal prolapse
  ◊ Pneumothorax
  ◊ Hypoxia
  ◊ Hypovolemic shock
  ◊ Iliac occlusion
• Complications of disimpaction
  ◊ Sepsis
  ◊ Hypotension
  ◊ Instrumental perforation
  ◊ Bleeding
  ◊ Postoperative obstruction

EXPECTED COURSE/PROGNOSIS
• Reimpaction likely, if bowel program not followed
• Prognosis poor for perforation with peritonitis
• Mortality with impaction and obstruction highest in very young and very old (up to 16%)

MISCELLANEOUS

ASSOCIATED CONDITIONS Pulmonary aspiration

AGE-RELATED FACTORS
Pediatric: Habitual neglect of defecation urge, because of interference with play, may promote impaction
Geriatric:
• Measure thyroid function, electrolyte activity and urea nitrogen levels in elderly patients presenting with impaction
• Much more likely to occur in patients over 80
Others: N/A

PREGNANCY Impaction can produce dysfunctional labor, dystocia

SYNONYMS Terminal reservoir syndrome

ICD-9-CM 560.39 Impaction of intestine, other

SEE ALSO
• Constipation
• Encopresis
• Diarrhea, chronic

OTHER NOTES Electrohydraulic lithotripsy has been used to safely remove large calcified fecaliths

ABBREVIATIONS N/A

REFERENCES
• Sleisenger MH, Fordtran JS, eds: Gastrointestinal Disease. 5th Ed. Philadelphia, W.B. Saunders, 1994
• Minaker KL, Harari D: Constipation in the elderly. Hospital Practice 1995;30:67-76
Illustrations: N/A
Internet references: http://www.5mcc.com

Author(s)
Richard Viken, MD

Fertility problems

BASICS

DESCRIPTION Failure to conceive after one year of unprotected intercourse
System(s) affected: Reproductive, Endocrine/Metabolic
Genetics: N/A
Incidence/Prevalence in USA: 10-15% of all couples
Predominant age: Increases with age, e.g., ages 30-34: 14% infertile, ages 35-39: 20% infertile, ages 40-45: 25% infertile
Predominant sex: N/A

SIGNS AND SYMPTOMS
• Thorough history and physical should be performed on each partner
• Genital/pelvic infection (e.g., pelvic inflammatory disease) often associated with an obstruction of reproductive tract
• Endocrine dysfunction (e.g., hypothyroidism, hypogonadism, abnormal puberty) often associated with abnormalities of ovulation or spermatogenesis
• Sexual dysfunction (e.g., premature ejaculation) may contribute to the problem
• Anovulatory cycles are frequently irregular, without premenstrual symptoms nor dysmenorrhea. Some patients may have features (e.g., hirsutism) suggestive of polycystic ovarian syndrome.
• Endometriosis is often associated with cyclic premenstrual pain and dysmenorrhea

CAUSES
• Most couples have more than one factor
• Male factors 30-40%
• Ovulation factors 15%
• Cervical/uterine factors 10%
• Tubal/peritoneal factors 25-30%
• Immunologic factors 5%
• Psychogenic/nutritional/metabolic factors 5%

RISK FACTORS Multiple - see under Causes

DIAGNOSIS

DIFFERENTIAL DIAGNOSIS Only basic elements of evaluation and diagnosis will be discussed here. Most of the tests of spermatogenesis and ovulation should be repeated at least once if abnormal.

LABORATORY
• Semen analysis, normal values are:
  ◊ Volume 2-6 mL
  ◊ pH 7-8
  ◊ Viscosity - liquefies within one hour
  ◊ Count - 20 million or greater
  ◊ Motility - 50% or more
  ◊ Morphology - 60% or more
• Post coital test
  ◊ Evaluates sperm/cervical mucus interaction
  ◊ Cervical mucus is aspirated with a tuberculin syringe from the os after intercourse during the fertile period
  ◊ If 10 or more sperm with directional movement are seen per high-power field of a microscope, the result is good. Sperm with shaking motion suggest sperm antibody.
• Basal body temperature charting
  ◊ Assesses ovulation and adequacy of the luteal phase
  ◊ Morning temperature should rise about one degree Fahrenheit at the time of ovulation and remain elevated for 13-14 days
• Serum progesterone
  ◊ Assesses ovulation and corpus luteum function
  ◊ A level of 15 or greater correlates with normal corpus luteum function
  ◊ Should be obtained on approximately day 21 of a 28 day menstrual cycle
• Endometrial biopsy
  ◊ Obtain on day 25-27 of a 28 day cycle
  ◊ Assesses ovulation, function of the corpus luteum, and normalcy of the endometrium
• The following tests are useful to evaluate underlying causes of anovulation or low sperm counts:
  ◊ Thyroid stimulating hormone and prolactin (elevations associated with suppressed gonadal function)
  ◊ Testosterone (decreased in primary gonadal failure)
  ◊ Follicle stimulating hormone (FSH) and luteinizing hormone (LH) (elevated in primary gonadal failure, decreased in hypopituitarism)

Drugs that may alter lab results:
• Semen abnormalities can be caused by:
  ◊ Cimetidine
  ◊ Spironolactone
  ◊ Furadantin
  ◊ Sulfasalazine
  ◊ Marijuana
  ◊ Chemotherapeutic agents
  ◊ Cocaine
  ◊ Occupational/environmental hazards

Disorders that may alter lab results:
• Polycystic ovarian disease
• Endometriosis
• Severe hypospadias
• Retrograde ejaculation (often associated with diabetes)
• Varicocele
• Testicular injury (e.g., surgery, mumps, trauma)
• Occupational/environmental hazards

PATHOLOGICAL FINDINGS N/A

SPECIAL TESTS Multiple tests (e.g., hamster egg penetration assay) are available to study specific aspects of reproduction, but are used only by fertility specialists, and available in only specialized labs

IMAGING Hysterosalpingogram (HSG) - evaluates tubal patency and uterine contour. This procedure may have some therapeutic benefit.

DIAGNOSTIC PROCEDURES
Laparoscopy - should be deferred until basic evaluation is complete

TREATMENT

APPROPRIATE HEALTH CARE
Outpatient evaluation, with attention to the emotional support of the couple

GENERAL MEASURES
• Dispel myths and provide accurate information
• Simultaneously evaluate and counsel both partners
• Find and correct causes of infertility
• Provide information on adoption when appropriate
• Consider donor insemination for refractory abnormalities of semen analysis

SURGICAL MEASURES
• Consider varicocele repair for abnormal semen analysis
• Consider laparotomy for tubal anastomosis, lysis of adhesions, and correction of tubal obstruction

ACTIVITY
• Males with low sperm counts should avoid hot tubs/saunas (decreased spermatogenesis with elevated scrotal temperature)
• If the male has low sperm counts, intercourse should be timed to occur approximately every 36 hours during the fertile period. Delay of intercourse beyond 7 days also adversely affects semen quality.

DIET N/A

PATIENT EDUCATION
• RESOLVE, 5 Water St, Arlington, MA 02174
• Fertility Research Foundation, 1430 Second Avenue, Suite 103, New York, NY 10021, (212)744-5500
• American College of Obstetricians & Gynecologists, 409 12th St, SW, Washington, DC 20024-2188, (800)762-ACOG

MEDICATIONS

DRUG(S) OF CHOICE
• Clomiphene citrate: Indicated for induction of ovulation. Typical dose - 50 mg daily x 5 days. This estrogen antagonist binds to receptors in the hypothalamus and stimulates increased release of gonadotropin releasing hormone (GnRH), leading to increased secretion of follicle stimulating hormone (FSH) and luteinizing hormone (LH) from the pituitary.
• Bromocriptine: Indicated for treatment of anovulation associated with hyperprolactinemia and normal head CT scan or microadenomas. Dose - 1.25-2.5 mg/day. Increase slowly as tolerated to maximum of 15 mg/day.

Contraindications:
• Clomiphene - hyperprolactinemia, pituitary failure, ovarian cysts
• Bromocriptine - pituitary macroadenomas

Precautions:
• Clomiphene - hyperstimulation syndrome, multiple pregnancy, blurred vision, diplopia. Pelvic exams are useful to rule out ovarian enlargement. Cervical mucus may be scant and require estrogen supplementation.
• Bromocriptine - headaches, visual field defects, and diabetes insipidus may occur during pregnancy of patients with macroadenomas

Significant possible interactions:
• Clomiphene - none
• Bromocriptine - alcohol, antihypertensives, tricyclic antidepressants, phenothiazines

ALTERNATIVE DRUGS
All used for induction of ovulation
• Human chorionic gonadotropin
• menotropins; human menopausal gonadotropin (hMG)
• GnRH analogs

FOLLOWUP

PATIENT MONITORING See under Diagnosis

PREVENTION/AVOIDANCE Prevention of sexually transmitted disease and subsequent pelvic inflammatory disease

POSSIBLE COMPLICATIONS
• Plural gestation with ovulation induction
• Ectopic pregnancy following tubal re-anastomosis

EXPECTED COURSE/PROGNOSIS
• About half of couples conceive during the second year of unprotected intercourse
• If the couple has been infertile for four or more years, the prognosis tends to be poor

MISCELLANEOUS

ASSOCIATED CONDITIONS Increasing tubal damage associated with pelvic inflammatory disease and IUD use

AGE-RELATED FACTORS
• Increasing anovulation with increasing age
• Increased disease burden with age from diseases like endometriosis, and cumulative exposure to environmental/occupational hazards
Pediatric: N/A
Geriatric: N/A
Others: N/A

PREGNANCY N/A

SYNONYMS N/A

ICD-9-CM
• Male infertility 606.9
• Female infertility 628.9

SEE ALSO N/A

OTHER NOTES N/A

ABBREVIATIONS N/A

REFERENCES Speroff L, Glass R., Kase N: Clinical Gynecologic Endocrinology and Infertility. 5th Ed. Baltimore, Williams & Wilkins, 1994
Illustrations: N/A
Internet references: http://www.5mcc.com

Author(s)
John Freeman, MD

Fever of unknown origin (FUO)

BASICS

DESCRIPTION Defined in 1961 by Petersdorf and Beeson as: Temperature greater than 38.3°C on several occasions during a period of at least 3 weeks and having an uncertain diagnosis after 1 week's evaluation in a hospital
• Various criteria have been proposed: Fever greater than 38.3°C (101°F) on at least four occasions over a 14 day period and illness of 14 days duration without an obvious cause
System(s) affected: Endocrine/Metabolic
Genetics: N/A
Incidence/Prevalence in USA: No data on actual incidence
Predominant age: All ages
Predominant sex: Dependent on etiology

SIGNS AND SYMPTOMS
• Fever does not present as the only manifestation of a disease. The type and pattern of fever is of little help in making the diagnosis.
• Constitutional symptoms that almost always accompany a fever: headache, myalgia, malaise

CAUSES
• Infection
  ◊ Abdominal abscesses
  ◊ Mycobacterial infection
  ◊ Cytomegalovirus
  ◊ Endocarditis/pericarditis
  ◊ Sinusitis
  ◊ HIV
  ◊ Renal
  ◊ Osteomyelitis
  ◊ Catheter infections
  ◊ Amebic hepatitis
  ◊ Wound infections
  ◊ Other miscellaneous infections
• Neoplasms
  ◊ Lymphoma
  ◊ Leukemia
  ◊ Solid tumors (hypernephroma)
  ◊ Hepatoma
  ◊ Atrial myxoma
  ◊ Colon cancer
• Collagen vascular disease
  ◊ Giant cell arteritis
  ◊ Polyarteritis nodosa
  ◊ Rheumatic fever
  ◊ Systemic lupus erythematosus
  ◊ Rheumatoid arthritis
  ◊ Polymyalgia rheumatica
• Other causes
  ◊ Granulomatous diseases
  ◊ Pulmonary emboli
  ◊ Drug fever
  ◊ Thermoregulatory disorders
  ◊ Endocrinologic diseases
  ◊ Occupational causes
  ◊ Periodic fever
  ◊ Factitious/fraudulent fever
  ◊ Cerebrovascular accident
  ◊ Cirrhosis
  ◊ Alcoholic hepatitis
  ◊ Other

RISK FACTORS
• Recent travel
• Exposure to biologic or chemical agents
• Persons in AIDS risk group
• Elderly persons
• Drug abuse
• Immigrants

DIAGNOSIS

DIFFERENTIAL DIAGNOSIS See Causes

LABORATORY
• CBC - leukopenia, anemia, thrombocytopenia/thrombocytosis
• C-reactive protein
• Sedimentation rate - elevated
• Liver function tests (especially alkaline phosphatase) - evidence of inflammation, obstruction or infiltrative disease
• Blood cultures (not to exceed 6)
• Urinalysis and urine culture
Drugs that may alter lab results: N/A
Disorders that may alter lab results: N/A

PATHOLOGICAL FINDINGS Dependent on etiology

SPECIAL TESTS
• Tuberculin skin test - may not be helpful if anergic or acute infection. If test negative, repeat in 2 weeks.
• Sputum and urine cultures for tuberculosis
• Gastric washing for tuberculosis
• Serologic tests - Epstein-Barr, hepatitis, syphilis, Lyme disease, Q fever, cytomegalovirus, amebiasis/coccidiomycosis
• HIV antibody test
• Serum protein electrophoresis - if immunologic etiology suspected
• Thyroid function tests - if thyroiditis suspected
• Rheumatoid factor and antinuclear antibody test - if collagen vascular disease suspected

IMAGING
• Chest x-ray
• Abdominal films
• Sinus x-rays - if clinically indicated
• Bone scan - if osteomyelitis or metastatic disease suspected
• CT scan or MRI of abdomen and pelvis (plus directed biopsy, if indicated) - if infectious process or mass lesions suspected
• 67-gallium or Tc-sulfur colloid scan - if infectious process or tumor suspected
• Ultrasound of abdomen and pelvis (plus directed biopsy, if indicated) - if mass lesions, renal obstruction or gallbladder/biliary tree pathology suspected
• Echocardiogram - if cardiac valve lesions, atrial myxomas or pericardial effusion suspected (transthoracic vs transesophageal)
• Ventilation/perfusion scan - if pulmonary emboli suspected
• Indium-labeled leukocyte scanning - if inflammatory process suspected

DIAGNOSTIC PROCEDURES
• Bone marrow - if granulomatous disease, infection or malignancy suspected
• Liver biopsy - if granulomatous disease suspected
• Temporal artery biopsy - if giant cell arteritis suspected
• Lymph node, muscle or skin biopsy - if clinically indicated
• Spinal tap - if clinically indicated
• Exploratory laparotomy - if otherwise unsuccessful in determining etiology

TREATMENT

APPROPRIATE HEALTH CARE
• Outpatient
• Hospitalization reserved for ill and debilitated and also in those in which factitious fever has been ruled out or an invasive procedure is indicated

GENERAL MEASURES
• Attempt to determine etiology before initiating therapy
• Avoid therapeutic trials unless as a last resort and only if therapy is reasonably specific
• "Shotgun" approaches are condemned since they do not solve the problem, obscure the clinical picture and have effects

SURGICAL MEASURES N/A

ACTIVITY Ambulatory primarily

DIET With temperature elevations, patients will have increased caloric and fluid demands

PATIENT EDUCATION Maintain an open line of communication between physician and patient/family as the workup progresses; the extended time required in establishing a diagnosis can be frustrating for all parties

MEDICATIONS

DRUG(S) OF CHOICE
• Dependent on diagnosis. In up to a fifth of patients, the cause of the fever will not be identified in spite of a thorough work up. If the patient has symptoms with the fever or continues to decline, a therapeutic trial may be indicated.
◊ Antipyretics such as acetaminophen or aspirin
◊ Nonsteroidal anti-inflammatory drugs such as indomethacin or naproxen
◊ Steroid trial based on patient's history
◊ Antibiotic trial based on patient's history
Contraindications: Aspirin should be avoided in children because of the risk of Reye's syndrome
Precautions: If a steroid trial is initiated, the physician must be aware the patient may have a relapse after treatment or if certain conditions (such as tuberculosis) have been undiagnosed, the therapy may have deleterious effects
Significant possible interactions: Refer to manufacturer's literature

ALTERNATIVE DRUGS   N/A

FOLLOWUP

PATIENT MONITORING   If the etiology of the fever continues to elude the physician, a history and physical examination along with screening laboratory studies should be repeated. Special attention should be paid to travel, occupational, sexual, and drug exposure.

PREVENTION/AVOIDANCE   N/A

POSSIBLE COMPLICATIONS   Dependent on etiology

EXPECTED COURSE/PROGNOSIS
• Dependent on etiology and age
◊ HIV infected patients have highest mortality
◊ One year survival rates reflecting deaths due to all causes:
91% < 35 year olds
82% 35-64 year olds
67% > 64 year olds

MISCELLANEOUS

ASSOCIATED CONDITIONS   N/A

AGE-RELATED FACTORS
Pediatric:
• Infections and collagen-vascular diseases most likely etiology
• Inflammatory bowel disease common etiology in older children and adolescents
• Has a better prognosis than in non-pediatric cases
Geriatric:
• Most common causes are acute leukemia, Hodgkin's lymphoma, intra-abdominal infections, tuberculosis and temporal arteritis
• Signs and symptoms in the elderly are much more nonspecific
• Co-existing diseases and numerous medications may cloud features
• Mortality rates are higher in the elderly
Others: Consider factitious fever in young female health care workers

PREGNANCY   Fever is known to increase the risk of neural tube defects and trigger preterm labor

SYNONYMS   N/A

ICD-9-CM
780.6 Pyrexia of unknown origin
778.4 Pyrexia of unknown origin in newborn
659.2 Pyrexia of unknown origin during labor
672 Pyrexia of unknown origin during puerperium

SEE ALSO
• Arthritis, juvenile rheumatoid (JRA)
• Atrial myxoma
• Colorectal malignancy
• Cytomegalovirus inclusion disease
• Endocarditis, infective (part 1)
• Endocarditis, infective (part 2)
• Giant cell arteritis
• Granulomatous disease of childhood, chronic
• Hepatitis, alcoholic
• Hepatoma
• HIV infection & AIDS
• Leukemia
• Osteomyelitis
• Polyarteritis nodosa
• Polymyalgia rheumatica
• Pulmonary embolism
• Rheumatic fever
• Sinusitis
• Stroke (Brain attack)
• Systemic lupus erythematosus (SLE)

OTHER NOTES   N/A

ABBREVIATIONS
PUO = pyrexia of unknown origin

REFERENCES
• Wong SY, Lam MS: Pyrexia of unknown origin - approach/management. Singapore Med J 1995;36:204-208
• Cunha BA: Fever of unknown origin. Infect Dis Clin NA 1996;10:111-127
• Knockaert DC, Dujardin KS, Bobbaers HJ: Long-term follow-up of patients with undiagnosed fever of unknown origin. Arch Int Med 1996;156:618-620
Illustrations: N/A
Internet references: http://www.5mcc.com

Author(s)
Scott T. Henderson, MD

Fibrocystic breast disease

BASICS

DESCRIPTION Fibrocystic breast disease is a generalized term for benign breast disorders such as lumps and pain. It is, however, a misnomer since it has neither a well-defined set of symptoms, nor a clear etiology. The term benign breast disease is preferred. Benign lumps are usually smooth, regular, and mobile. The following classifications are useful:
• Lumps:
  ◊ Physiologic nodularity - lumps vary with the phase of the menstrual cycle, common in young women
  ◊ Mastoplasia - a ropy, thickening of the breast tissue, most common in the upper outer quadrant, persists throughout the menstrual cycle
  ◊ Cysts - distended, fluid filled masses caused by an imbalance between secretion and absorption in the breast lobule, common in the decade preceding menopause
  ◊ Fibroadenoma - benign solid tumor, smooth margins, mobile, most common tumor in teenagers and young women, may occur at any age after thelarche
  ◊ Phyllodes tumors - painless, solid, smooth, lobular, bulky; stromal hyperplasia; 10% are malignant
• Nipple discharge
  ◊ Although considered one of the warning signs for breast cancer, 90% of patients with nipple discharge have benign disease
  ◊ Bilateral duct ectasia - most common cause of nipple discharge; benign inflammatory condition; bilateral, sticky, multicolored discharge; usually has to be expressed
  ◊ Bilateral galactorrhea-prolactin-secreting pituitary tumors - usually in association with amenorrhea; drugs (isoniazid, methyldopa, thiazides, reserpine, tricyclic antidepressants, BCP's); trauma; hypothyroidism
  ◊ Unilateral intraductal papilloma - spontaneous discharge from one duct. Carcinoma must be excluded.
• Pain
  ◊ Cyclical mastodynia - hormonal, an exaggeration of the normal premenstrual tenderness
  ◊ Non-cyclical - sclerosing adenosis, cysts, chest wall muscle spasm, costochondritis, fibromyalgia, neuritis, stress, referred pain
• Inflammatory conditions
  ◊ Fat necrosis - a solid lump with or without pain that can mimic carcinoma
  ◊ Superficial phlebitis of the thoracoepigastric vein (Mondor's disease) - local tenderness and induration
  ◊ Mastitis/abscess - exquisite pain and tenderness, erythema (common), not always a definite mass, common with lactation and squamous metaplasia of lactiferous ducts (Zuska's disease), usually caused by staphylococcal organisms

• Growth disorders
  ◊ Accessory nipples (polythelia)
  ◊ Absence of the breast (amastia)
  ◊ Absence of the nipple (athelia)
  ◊ Hypoplasia (often associated with hypoplasia of the thorax and pectoral muscles, and abnormalities of the hand, i.e., Poland's syndrome)
  ◊ Gigantomastia: occurs during puberty and pregnancy
  ◊ Gynecomastia: occurs in men in association with puberty, senescence, liver disease, and testicular tumors, and medications such as digoxin and cimetidine
System(s) affected: Skin/Exocrine
Genetics:
• Little is known about the genetic aspects of benign breast disease
• Family history of cysts common
Incidence/Prevalence in USA: Unknown. It is estimated that at least 50% of women have benign breast symptoms during their lifetime.
Predominant age:
• Symptoms tend to occur in menstruating women
• Mastoplasia - most common in women from mid 20's to 55 years of age
• Cysts - usually seen in women in their 40's
• Cyclical mastodynia - common in menstruating women
• Non-cyclical pain - can occur at any age after breast development
Predominant sex: Female > Male (almost exclusively)

SIGNS AND SYMPTOMS
• Asymptomatic
• Breast pain
• Breast tenderness
• Pain subsides after menses
• Smooth masses
• Tense masses
• Fluctuant masses
• Bilateral masses
• Breast engorgement
• Breast thickening
• Nipple discharge

CAUSES
• The etiology of benign breast disease is unknown
• Possible causes:
  ◊ Luteal phase defect in progesterone
  ◊ Increased estrogen (17 beta estradiol)
  ◊ Hyperprolactinemia
  ◊ End organ hypersensitivity to estrogen
  ◊ Sensitivity to methylxanthines
  ◊ Dietary fat intake

RISK FACTORS
• Unknown
• The effect of consumption of methylxanthine-containing substances, e.g., coffee, tea, cola, and chocolate is controversial

DIAGNOSIS

DIFFERENTIAL DIAGNOSIS
• Lumps - breast cancer
• Skin changes - breast cancer, eczema
• Pain - costochondritis, chest wall muscle spasm, neuralgia, anxiety, depression, breast cancer, angina pectoris, gastroesophageal reflux, Pancoast tumor

LABORATORY Prolactin, TSH (if galactorrhea), aspiration cytology or biopsy of discrete mass
Drugs that may alter lab results: N/A
Disorders that may alter lab results: N/A

PATHOLOGICAL FINDINGS Hyperplasia of breast epithelium or stroma, adenosis, microcysts, macrocysts, duct ectasia (plasma cell mastitis), apocrine metaplasia

SPECIAL TESTS N/A

IMAGING
• Mammography
  ◊ Signs of malignancy include irregular mass, clustered masses, calcifications, architectural distortion, dilated duct
  ◊ May be normal in presence of malignancy
• Ultrasonography
  ◊ Useful for differentiating cystic from solid lesions

DIAGNOSTIC PROCEDURES
• Fine needle aspiration and biopsy - allows differentiation of cystic and solid lesion. Cells sent for cytology can diagnose cancer with a high degree of accuracy. Low morbidity.
• Core needle biopsy - usually not indicated for fibrocystic disease. Useful in diagnosis of a large cancer.
• Excisional biopsy - indicated for all solid lumps that are not clearly benign

TREATMENT

APPROPRIATE HEALTH CARE
Outpatient. May be inpatient for biopsy or surgery.

GENERAL MEASURES
• Evaluate to be certain there is no malignancy by means of imaging and diagnostic procedures
• Pain rarely severe or disabling
• Frequently resolves spontaneously
• Reassure patient there is no malignancy
• Cold compresses may be helpful
• Well fitting, supportive brassiere (worn night and day)

SURGICAL MEASURES
Possibly excision (under local anesthesia) of benign fibroadenoma or phyllode tumors, and fat necrosis lesions

ACTIVITY
No restrictions. Avoid activities that may cause trauma to the breasts.

DIET
Abstention from methylxanthines (coffee, tea, chocolate)

PATIENT EDUCATION
• American College of Obstetricians & Gynecologists, 409 12th St., SW, Washington, DC 20024-2188, (800)762-ACOG
• Booklet on Breast Self Examination from Primary care and Care and Cancer, 17 Prospect St., Huntington, NY 11743, (516)424-8900
• National Cancer Institute, (800)4-CANCER

MEDICATIONS

DRUG(S) OF CHOICE
• For cyclical pain and swelling unresponsive to general measures - spironolactone (Aldactone) 10 mg bid premenstrually may be helpful or vitamin A 150,000 IU daily for 3 months; vitamin E 300-600 IU a day for 3 months; oral contraceptives
• For more severe disease - danazol (Danocrine) 100-200 mg per day or bromocriptine 2.5 mg bid for 3 months may be useful, but side effects and expense limit their usefulness

Contraindications: Refer to manufacturer's literature
Precautions: Refer to manufacturer's literature
Significant possible interactions: Refer to manufacturer's literature

ALTERNATIVE DRUGS N/A

FOLLOWUP

PATIENT MONITORING
• Patients with fibrocystic change may have an increased risk of malignancy
• If there is no atypia on biopsy the risk is only minimally increased
• Patients need to be assessed with clinical examination, radiological studies, and, sometimes, biopsy to be certain a given lump is not malignant
• Followup times are variable depending on the clinical situation. A young patient in whom physiological nodularity is suspected should be observed through one menstrual cycle.
• Mammograms should be obtained at age 35, at least every 1-2 years after age 40, and yearly after age 50
• Ultrasound is useful to differentiate cysts from solid lesions, but is not used for screening
• Aspiration cytology is useful for diagnosis of cysts and solid lesions. The false positive rate ranges from 0-5.8%, and the false negative rate from 1.7-22%.
• When physical examination, mammography, and needle aspiration are used in combination, detection rates for breast cancer range from 93-100%

PREVENTION/AVOIDANCE
Avoiding caffeine may reduce breast pain

POSSIBLE COMPLICATIONS
• Fibrocystic change can make physical examination and mammograms difficult to interpret
• Atypical hyperplasia may lead to cancer

EXPECTED COURSE/PROGNOSIS
Benign, chronic, recurring, intermittent

MISCELLANEOUS

ASSOCIATED CONDITIONS
Breast carcinoma

AGE-RELATED FACTORS
Pediatric: Biopsy in children should be avoided since a developing breast bud may be inadvertently removed
Geriatric: Not as common in this age group
Others: Prophylactic mastectomy for pain is rarely indicated since many patients have underlying psychiatric problems

PREGNANCY N/A

SYNONYMS
• Chronic cystic mastitis
• Adenosis
• Benign breast disease
• Mammary dysplasia
• Fibrocystic disease

ICD-9-CM 610.1 diffuse cystic mastopathy

SEE ALSO N/A

OTHER NOTES N/A

ABBREVIATIONS N/A

REFERENCES
• Grundfest-Broniatowski S, Esselstyn CBE Jr: Controversies in Breast Disease: Diagnosis and Management. New York, Marcel Dekker, Inc., 1988
• Harris JR, Hellman S, Henderson IC, Kinne DW: Breast Diseases. Philadelphia, J.B. Lippincott Co., 1987
• Technical Bulletin. American College of Obstetricians & Gynecologists, #156, June 1991
Illustrations: N/A
Internet references: http://www.5mcc.com

Author(s)
John Freeman, MD

Fibromyalgia

BASICS

DESCRIPTION Extremely common pain phenomenon occurring in a defined pattern, reproduced by pressure on "trigger points"
System(s) affected: Musculoskeletal
Genetics: N/A
Incidence/Prevalence in USA: 3 in 100
Predominant age: 18-70
Predominant sex: Female > Male

SIGNS AND SYMPTOMS
• Pressure manually applied to specific sites, referred to as "trigger points" reproduce the patient's symptoms:
　◊ Temporalis - above the ear
　◊ Anterior to tragus of ear
　◊ Scalenus capitis
　◊ Sternocleidomastoid
　◊ Low anterior neck
　◊ Pectoralis minor
　◊ Manubriosternal
　◊ Anterior and posterior axillary folds
　◊ Trapezius ridge
　◊ Upper rhomboids
　◊ Lower rhomboids
　◊ Iliac crest
　◊ Mid-buttocks
　◊ Mid-rectus femoris
　◊ Mid-vastus lateralis
　◊ Quadriceps insertion - at the patella
　◊ Humeral epicondyles (many investigators would diagnose fibromyalgia, while some prefer epicondylitis) and negative tenderness at "neutral sites" (e.g., scapula, glabella)
• Other signs and symptoms
　◊ Typically insidious in onset
　◊ Pain is increased in the morning, with weather changes, anxiety, stress
　◊ Pain improved by mild physical activity or vacations (stress-relieving situations) Non-restorative sleep, with early morning awakening in an unrefreshed state.
　◊ Abnormal non-rapid eye movement (non-REM) stage IV sleep
　◊ Generalized fatigue or tiredness
　◊ Anxiety
　◊ Chronic headache
　◊ Irritable bowel syndrome
　◊ Subjective, non-confirmable complaints of swelling or numbness, not associated with objective neurologic findings
　◊ Depression
　◊ Reduced physical endurance
　◊ Decreased social interaction

CAUSES
• Loss of non-REM stage IV sleep
• Stress
• Trauma

RISK FACTORS
• Sleep disturbance
• Trauma
• Depression
• Weather changes

DIAGNOSIS

DIFFERENTIAL DIAGNOSIS
• Hypothyroidism
• Psychogenic rheumatism
• Muscle strain/sprain
• Muscle disease
• Polymyalgia rheumatica
• Temporal arteritis

LABORATORY
• Normal Westergren erythrocyte sedimentation rate
• Normal creatine phosphokinase and aldolase
• Normal TSH, T3 resin uptake and T4
• Normal complete blood count, renal and liver function
Drugs that may alter lab results:
Steroids
Disorders that may alter lab results: N/A

PATHOLOGICAL FINDINGS None

SPECIAL TESTS Thermography
(controversial)

IMAGING N/A

DIAGNOSTIC PROCEDURES The
clinical history and physical examination

TREATMENT

APPROPRIATE HEALTH CARE
Outpatient

GENERAL MEASURES Electroprobe,
electrical stimulation, ultrasound, hot packs, conditioning, increasing social interactions and general conditioning exercises

SURGICAL MEASURES N/A

ACTIVITY Fully active. However, the pain of
fibrositis may be so distracting as to reduce attentiveness, predisposing to error and accident.

DIET No restrictions

PATIENT EDUCATION Printed material:
Rothschild, B.: Diagnosing and treating fibrositis and fibromyalgia. Geriatric Consultant, 9(5/6):26-28, 1990

Fibromyalgia

MEDICATIONS

DRUG(S) OF CHOICE
• Nonsteroidal anti-inflammatory drugs (NSAID's) may provide non-narcotic symptomatic pain relief
• Sleep restorative without interfering with stage IV sleep:
Reinforce discontinuation if paradoxical effect, memory loss, thought process changes, or behavior changes.
◊ Amitriptyline (Elavil) 10 mg 2 po hs prn, increased gradually to 50 mg
◊ Cyclobenzaprine (Flexeril) 10 mg tid prn
◊ Zolpidem (Ambien) 5 mg po hs prn, increased to 10 mg
◊ Temazepam (Restoril) 15 mg po hs prn, increased to 30 mg
◊ Flurazepam (Dalmane) 15 mg po hs prn, increased to 30 mg (note: Significant "hangover" potential secondary to long half-life)
◊ Triazolam (Halcion) 0.125 mg po hs prn increased gradually to 0.5 mg (use is controversial)
Contraindications: Drug allergy, suicide potential
Precautions:
• NSAID's - refer to manufacturer's literature
• Others - observe for grogginess or aberrant behavior, discontinue if it occurs. Psychological and/or physical dependence may occur. However, if the patient is nonfunctional without them, long-term use is reasonable.
Significant possible interactions:
• NSAID's - refer to manufacturer's literature
• Others - digoxin, phenytoin, MAO inhibitors

ALTERNATIVE DRUGS
Trazodone (Desyrel) 50 mg po hs prn

FOLLOWUP

PATIENT MONITORING
• For efficacy at 2-4 weeks
• For medication side effects every 3-6 months

PREVENTION/AVOIDANCE
• Adequate sleep
• General conditioning exercises

POSSIBLE COMPLICATIONS
• Chronicity
• Fibromyalgia is allegedly a greater source of work loss and dysfunction than rheumatoid arthritis

EXPECTED COURSE/PROGNOSIS
• With resolution of sleep disturbance, may resolve totally
• Aggressive physical therapy is critical in those who do not respond
• Approximately 5% do not respond to any form of therapeutic intervention. Hypnosis may be attempted in that group.

MISCELLANEOUS

ASSOCIATED CONDITIONS So common almost any disease can be associated with it

AGE-RELATED FACTORS
Pediatric: Uncommon
Geriatric: Common; polypharmacy may be part of the problem
Others: N/A

PREGNANCY Limits therapeutic approach to physical therapy modalities

SYNONYMS
• Fibrositis
• Myofascial pain syndrome

ICD-9-CM
729.1 Fibromyositis

SEE ALSO
• Irritable bowel syndrome
• Chronic fatigue syndrome

OTHER NOTES Perhaps the most common cause of neck or back pain in this patient population and most common rheumatologic problem in general

ABBREVIATIONS N/A

REFERENCES
• Rothschild BM, Martin L: Paleopathology: Diseases in the Fossil Record. London, CRC Press, 1993
• Rothschild BM: Fibromyalgia: An explanation for the aches and pains of the 90's. Comprehensive Therapy 1991;17(6):9-14
• Rothschild BM: Diagnosing and treating fibrositis and fibromyalgia. Geriatric Consultant 1990;9(5/6):26-28
• Vu J, Rothschild BM: Retrospective assessment of fibromyalgia therapeusis. Comprehensive Therapy, 1994
• Yunus M, Masi AT, Calabro JJ, Miller KA, Feigenbaum SL: Primary fibromyalgia (fibrositis): Clinical study of 50 patients with matched normal controls. Semin Arthritis Rheum 1981;11:151-171
• Wolfe F, Smythe HA, Yunus MB, Bennett RM, et al: The American College of Rheumatology criteria for the classification of fibromyalgia. Arthritis Rheum 1990;33:160-172
Illustrations: N/A
Internet references: http://www.5mcc.com

Author(s)
Bruce M. Rothschild, MD

Folliculitis

BASICS

DESCRIPTION Inflammation of hair follicles, often due to microbes or chemical irritation. May be superficial or deep.
System(s) affected: Skin/Exocrine
Genetics: No known genetic pattern
Incidence/Prevalence in USA: Common (no statistics available)
Predominant age: All ages
Predominant sex: Male > Female

SIGNS AND SYMPTOMS
• Characteristic lesions are yellow or gray pustules surrounded by erythema and pierced by a hair
• Lesions are commonly grouped
• Lesions may occur on any body surface. Common on scalp, beard area, and limbs.
• Patients are usually afebrile and without systemic symptoms
• Nontender or slightly tender
• May be pruritic

CAUSES
• Staphylococcus aureus - most common agent
• Pseudomonas aeruginosa - occurs in bathing suit areas of users of hot tubs and saunas
• Candida albicans - occurs in patients on immunosuppressants or long-term antibiotic therapy. May also occur on the back of hospitalized, febrile patients.
• Dermatophyte fungi - uncommon, but may occur in beard area
• Exposure to various agents - such as hydrocarbons, and some drugs (such as iodides)

RISK FACTORS
• Abrasion
• Injury
• Nearby surgical wounds or draining abscesses
• Tight clothing (jeans folliculitis)
• Poor hygiene
• Exposure to hydrocarbons
• Use of hot tubs or saunas
• Immunodeficiency
• Diabetes mellitus

DIAGNOSIS

DIFFERENTIAL DIAGNOSIS
• Ingrown hairs (especially in the beard area of black males who shave)
• Keratosis pilaris (follicular papules on extensor surfaces of extremities in atopic individuals)
• Contact dermatitis
• Tinea
• Acne
• Pustular miliaria
• Flat warts
• Molluscum contagiosum

LABORATORY
• Gram stain - look for gram positive cocci
• KOH preparation - look for budding yeast or hyphae
• Culture
Drugs that may alter lab results: N/A
Disorders that may alter lab results: N/A

PATHOLOGICAL FINDINGS Suppurative inflammation

SPECIAL TESTS N/A

IMAGING N/A

DIAGNOSTIC PROCEDURES Biopsy may be required in resistant cases, or if diagnosis is in doubt

TREATMENT

APPROPRIATE HEALTH CARE
Outpatient

GENERAL MEASURES
• Cleanse area bid with antibacterial soap (e.g., Dial)
• Shampoo daily with Selsun Blue for lesions on scalp
• Apply moist heat to allow the lesion to drain
• Change razor blade daily
• Avoid use of topical oils
• Avoid exposure to causative factors

SURGICAL MEASURES N/A

ACTIVITY Fully active

DIET No special diet

PATIENT EDUCATION As listed under General Measures

MEDICATIONS

DRUG(S) OF CHOICE
• Staphylococcus aureus
 ◊ Dicloxacillin (Dycill, Dynapen, Pathocil) 250 mg po qid for 10 days
 ◊ Erythromycin 250 mg po qid for 10 days
• Pseudomonas aeruginosa
 ◊ Ciprofloxacin (Cipro) 500 mg po bid for 10 days (other quinolones may be used alternatively)
 ◊ Ofloxacin 400 mg bid
Contraindications:
• History of hypersensitivity to the antibiotic
• Quinolone antibiotics are contraindicated in pregnancy and pediatrics
Precautions: Refer to manufacturer's literature
Significant possible interactions:
• Ciprofloxacin and ofloxacin - antacids, sucralfate, oral anticoagulants, theophylline, caffeine, probenecid
• Erythromycin - theophylline, oral anticoagulants, carbamazepine, corticosteroids, digoxin, ergot alkaloids, cyclosporine, phenytoin, terfenadine, astemizole

ALTERNATIVE DRUGS
• Mupirocin (Bactroban) topical therapy to affected area three times a day
• First generation cephalosporins for Staph. aureus
• Pseudomonas: A third generation cephalosporin; e.g. ceftazidime and cefoperazone, aminoglycoside or ticarcillin

FOLLOWUP

PATIENT MONITORING
• One return visit in 2 weeks if symptoms abate
• Resistant cases should be followed every 2 weeks until cleared

PREVENTION/AVOIDANCE
• Good personal hygiene, avoid sharing towel or washcloth. Discard any dressings carefully.
• Avoidance of causative factors
• Find and treat family members or friends who may be a source of reinfection

POSSIBLE COMPLICATIONS May occasionally progress to furuncles

EXPECTED COURSE/PROGNOSIS
• Usually resolves with treatment
• May recur in Staph. carriers. Mupirocin may be required on nares of patient to treat carrier state. Family carriers may also need to be treated.
• Resistant or severe cases may warrant testing for diabetes mellitus or immunodeficiency

MISCELLANEOUS

ASSOCIATED CONDITIONS
• Diabetes mellitus
• Immunodeficiency

AGE-RELATED FACTORS
Pediatric: N/A
Geriatric: N/A
Others: N/A

PREGNANCY Pruritic folliculitis of pregnancy is a rare disorder that resolves spontaneously after delivery

SYNONYMS Sycosis

ICD-9-CM 704.8 other specified diseases of hair and hair follicles

SEE ALSO N/A

OTHER NOTES N/A

ABBREVIATIONS N/A

REFERENCES Habif T: Clinical Dermatology. 3rd Ed. St. Louis, CV Mosby, 1996
Illustrations: N/A
Internet references: http://www.5mcc.com

Author(s)
Michelle D. Kimmel, MD

Food allergy

BASICS

DESCRIPTION Food allergy is a hypersensitivity reaction which is caused by certain foods. Adverse reactions after food ingestion may be caused by immunologic mechanisms, such as the classic IgE allergic response, or by non-immunologic mediated mechanisms.

System(s) affected:
Hemic/Lymphatic/Immunologic, Gastrointestinal, Skin/Exocrine, Pulmonary, Nervous

Genetics: In family members with a history of food hypersensitivity, the probability of food allergy in subsequent siblings may be as high as 50%

Incidence/Prevalence in USA:
• The incidence of IgE mediated food allergy has been estimated to range from 1-7% of the population
• In children up to 4 years of age the incidence is between 8-16%
• Only about 3-4% of children over 4 years of age have persisting food allergy. Therefore, it is frequently a transient phenomena.

Predominant age: All ages, but more common in infants and children
Predominant sex: Male > Female (2:1)

SIGNS AND SYMPTOMS
• Gastrointestinal (system usually affected)
  ◊ More common: Nausea, vomiting, diarrhea, abdominal pain, occult bleeding, flatulence, bloating
  ◊ Less common: Malabsorption, protein losing enteropathy, eosinophil-gastroenteritis, and colitis
• Dermatologic
  ◊ More common: Urticaria/angioedema, atopic dermatitis, pallor or flushing
  ◊ Less common: Contact rashes
• Respiratory
  ◊ More common: Allergic rhinitis, asthma and bronchospasm, cough, serous otitis media
  ◊ Less common: Pulmonary infiltrates (Heiner's syndrome), pulmonary hemosiderosis
• Neurologic
  ◊ Less common: Hyperkinesis, tension-fatigue syndrome, migraine headaches, syncope
• Other symptoms:
  ◊ Systemic anaphylaxis, vasculitis
  ◊ Suspected manifestations include enuresis, proteinuria and arthropathy
  ◊ Growth retardation

CAUSES
• Any food or ingested substance can cause allergic reactions. Most commonly implicated foods include cow's milk, egg whites, wheat, soy, peanut, fish, tree nuts (walnut and pecan), shellfish, melons, sesame seeds, sunflower seeds, chocolate.
• Several food dyes and additives can elicit allergic-like reactions

RISK FACTORS
• Persons with allergic or atopic predisposition are at increased risk of hypersensitivity reaction to foods
• Family members with a history of food hypersensitivity

DIAGNOSIS

DIFFERENTIAL DIAGNOSIS
• A careful history is necessary to document a temporal relationship with the manifestations of suspected food hypersensitivity
• The gastrointestinal, dermatologic, respiratory, neurologic or other systemic manifestations may mimic a variety of clinical entities

LABORATORY
• Eosinophilia in either blood or tissue suggests atopy
• Epicutaneous (prick or puncture) allergy skin tests are useful in documenting IgE mediated immunologic hypersensitivity. In most clinical situations, the allergy skin tests are good for screening. An oral challenge should be completed to accurately determine the clinical hypersensitivity. The overall agreement between allergy skin testing and oral food challenge is approximately 60% (i.e., a positive skin test showing a positive challenge reaction to a particular food).
• Radioallergosorbent (RAST) test can also detect specific IgE antibodies to offending foods. In certain laboratories, the RAST test was almost as accurate as a skin test in predicting positive oral challenges.
• Leukocyte histamine release and assays for circulating immune complexes are predominantly research procedures and are of limited use in clinical practices. Assays for IgG and IgG 4 subclass antibodies are commercially available. There are no convincing data that these tests are reliable for the diagnosis of food allergy.
• The provocative injection and sublingual provocative tests are both highly controversial and have been proven to be useless for the diagnosis of food allergy
• The leukocytotoxic assay is an unproven diagnostic procedure and is not useful for the diagnosis of allergy

Drugs that may alter lab results: N/A
Disorders that may alter lab results: N/A

PATHOLOGICAL FINDINGS Acute and chronic rectal inflammation

SPECIAL TESTS Stool exam, mucus, eosinophilia

IMAGING Upper GI series for gastric antral inflammation, in rare cases

DIAGNOSTIC PROCEDURES
• Elimination and challenge test
  ◊ The best procedure for confirming food allergy
  ◊ First, the suspected food is eliminated from the diet for 1-2 weeks
  ◊ The patient's symptoms are monitored. If the patient's symptoms disappear or substantially improve, an oral challenge with the suspected food should be performed under medical supervision.
  ◊ Optimally, this challenge should be performed in a double-blind, placebo controlled manner
  ◊ Most allergic reactions will occur within 30 minutes to 2 hours after the challenge, although late reactions have also been described, which may occur from 12-24 hours

TREATMENT

APPROPRIATE HEALTH CARE
Outpatient

GENERAL MEASURES
• Avoidance of the offending food is the most effective mode of treatment for patients with food allergies
• Those patients with exquisite and severe allergy hypersensitivity to a food should be more cautious in their avoidance of that food. They should carry epinephrine for self-administration in the event that the offending food is ingested unknowingly, and a subsequent immediate reaction develops.
• Immunotherapy or hyposensitization with food extracts by various routes, including subcutaneous immunotherapy or sublingual neutralization are not recommended since the success with these methods have not been proven in controlled scientific studies

SURGICAL MEASURES N/A

ACTIVITY No restrictions

DIET As determined by tests

PATIENT EDUCATION
• Patients should be counselled by a dietician to be sure that they maintain a nutritionally sound diet, in spite of avoiding those foods to which patient is sensitive
• Patient support - Food Allergy Network, 4744 Holly Ave., Fairfax, VA 22030-5647, 703-691-3179

MEDICATIONS

DRUG(S) OF CHOICE
• Symptomatic treatment, e.g., antihistamine
• The use of cromolyn has been suggested, but is not practical for use in most patients with food allergy
• Recent studies have suggested the use of ketotifen, which is a mast cell stabilizer. This drug is not available in the United States.
Contraindications: N/A
Precautions: N/A
Significant possible interactions: N/A

ALTERNATIVE DRUGS N/A

FOLLOWUP

PATIENT MONITORING As needed

PREVENTION/AVOIDANCE Avoidance of offending food

POSSIBLE COMPLICATIONS
• Anaphylaxis
• Angioedema
• Bronchial asthma
• Enterocolitis
• Eczematoid lesions

EXPECTED COURSE/PROGNOSIS
• Most infants will outgrow their food hypersensitivity by 2-4 years. It may be possible to reintroduce the offending food cautiously into the diet (particularly helpful when the food is one that is difficult to avoid).
• Adults with food hypersensitivity (particularly to milk, fish, shellfish or nuts) tend to maintain their allergy for many years

MISCELLANEOUS

ASSOCIATED CONDITIONS N/A

AGE-RELATED FACTORS
Pediatric: N/A
Geriatric: N/A
Others: N/A

PREGNANCY N/A

SYNONYMS
• Allergic bowel disease
• Dietary protein sensitivity syndrome

ICD-9-CM
693.1 Dermatitis due to food taken internally
692.5 Contact dermatitis and other eczema due to food in contact with the skin
995.60 Anaphylactic shock or reaction due to food

SEE ALSO
• Celiac disease
• Irritable bowel syndrome
• Pyloric stenosis
• Epiglottitis

OTHER NOTES N/A

ABBREVIATIONS N/A

REFERENCES
• Sampson HA: Adverse Reactions to Foods. In Allergy Principles and Practice. 4th Ed. New York, C.V. Mosby Co., 1993
• Chandra RK, ed: Food Allergy. Clin Rev Allergy/Immu 1995;13:291-376
• Metcalf DD, et al, eds: Food Allergy, Adverse Reactions to Foods and Food Additives. New York, Blackwell Scientific, 1991
Illustrations: N/A
Internet references: http://www.5mcc.com

Author(s)
Stanley Fineman, MD

Food poisoning, bacterial

BASICS

DESCRIPTION
A variety of related illnesses resulting from ingestion of food contaminated with bacteria capable of causing disease. The illness may be produced by bacterial infection itself (salmonellosis, shigellosis) or by toxins produced by the bacteria (Staphylococcus aureus, Clostridium perfringens, Bacillus cereus).
System(s) affected: Gastrointestinal
Genetics: N/A
Incidence/Prevalence in USA: Poor reporting overall. Estimated 6.3 million cases/year. 1 in 10 Americans with foodborne diarrhea/year. Approximate incidence is 2,500/100,000.
Predominant age: All ages
Predominant sex: Male = Female

SIGNS AND SYMPTOMS
Suspect when multiple persons become ill after eating the same meal. Timing and type of clinical presentation can aid in establishing etiology.
• Nausea, vomiting 1-8 hours after meal (S. aureus, B. cereus)
• Cramps, diarrhea 8-16 hours after meal (C. perfringens, B. cereus)
• Fever, cramps, diarrhea 18-72 hours after meal (Campylobacter jejuni, Yersinia enterocolitica, E. coli, Vibrio parahaemolyticus, Shigella and Salmonella species)
• Bloody diarrhea without fever 3-5 days after meal (verotoxigenic E. coli, occasionally C. jejuni)
• Pseudoappendicitis (Y. enterocolitica)
• Sepsis, meningitis (Listeria monocytogenes, Shigella and Salmonella species)
• Occasional metastatic foci of infection (arthritis, L monocytogenes, Salmonella, etc.)

CAUSES
• S. aureus (preformed enterotoxin)
• B. cereus (preformed enterotoxin)
• C. perfringens (enterotoxin elaborated in gut)
• C. jejuni (tissue invasion)
• Y. enterocolitica (tissue invasion)
• E. coli (enterotoxigenic, verotoxigenic [hemorrhagic], and tissue invasive forms)
• V. parahaemolyticus (toxin elaboration, possibly invasion)
• Shigella species (tissue invasion)
• Salmonella species (tissue invasion)
• L. monocytogenes (tissue invasion)

RISK FACTORS
Ingestion of:
• High protein foods: egg salad, cream-filled pastries, poultry, ham - S. aureus
• Cereals, fried rice, dried foods and herbs, meats, vegetables - B. cereus
• Meats, gravies, dried foods, vegetables - C. perfringens
• Under-cooked poultry, meat, raw dairy products - C. jejuni
• Under-cooked pork, other meat and dairy products - Y. enterocolitica
• Raw vegetables and other foods, contaminated water - E. coli
• Raw and cooked seafood - V. parahaemolyticus
• Raw vegetables, egg salads, contaminated water - Shigella
• Under-cooked eggs, poultry, dairy products, meat - Salmonella
• Under-cooked meat, dairy products, and many other foods - L. monocytogenes

DIAGNOSIS

DIFFERENTIAL DIAGNOSIS
• Infectious gastroenteritis of any kind
• Inflammatory bowel disease
• Appendicitis and other acute surgical abdominal processes
• Hepatitis

LABORATORY
Culture of stool most reliable. Laboratory must be specifically notified of diagnostic considerations for most pathogens except Salmonella and Shigella.
Drugs that may alter lab results: Prior or concomitant antibiotic therapy may eliminate pathogen from stool
Disorders that may alter lab results: N/A

PATHOLOGICAL FINDINGS
Only present in invasive or colitic syndromes

SPECIAL TESTS
Sigmoidoscopy (occasionally needed)

IMAGING
N/A

DIAGNOSTIC PROCEDURES
• Stool culture
• Epidemiologic investigation
• Culture of suspected food source if available

TREATMENT

APPROPRIATE HEALTH CARE
Usually outpatient management sufficient. Hospitalization for septicemias or focal infections, severe electrolyte imbalance or dehydration.

GENERAL MEASURES
• Most are self-limited syndromes and do not require specific therapy
• Oral solutions for rehydration. Intravenous fluid and electrolyte replacement if necessary for more severe dehydration (particularly in the elderly).
• For infants, rehydration products (e.g., Pedialyte) provides adequate fluid and electrolyte replacement. Don't use for more than 1 to 2 days without clinical reassessment of nutritional needs.

SURGICAL MEASURES
N/A

ACTIVITY
Bedrest for comfort if needed during the acute phase

DIET
Eliminate contaminated food. Bland diet during recovery. Nothing by mouth, if needed, for excessive vomiting or diarrhea.

PATIENT EDUCATION
• Avoidance of raw or under-cooked foods
• Proper food storage and preparation techniques such as refrigeration
• Instruction on prevention if patient traveling to foreign countries

MEDICATIONS

DRUG(S) OF CHOICE For septicemias and focal infections, antibiotic therapy may be indicated (e.g., ampicillin plus aminoglycoside for listeriosis)
Contraindications:
• Avoid antiperistaltic agents in colitic (bloody diarrhea) syndromes since they may increase the chance of dissemination
• Antiemetics may be given but are usually unnecessary
Precautions: N/A
Significant possible interactions:
Digoxin toxicity with electrolyte imbalance, exacerbation of diuretic effects

ALTERNATIVE DRUGS N/A

FOLLOWUP

PATIENT MONITORING Individualized based on degree of dehydration and electrolyte imbalance, or signs of sepsis. Serious disturbances require hospitalization, frequent vital signs, strict recording of input and output with appropriate fluid replacement.

PREVENTION/AVOIDANCE
• No ingestion of raw seafood, meats, or poultry
• Avoid any unpasteurized dairy products
• Clean thoroughly any food preparation area in contact with causative items
• Ensure proper cooling of any prepared foods not immediately consumed

POSSIBLE COMPLICATIONS
• Cardiovascular collapse
• Arrhythmias from electrolyte disturbance
• Septicemias or other metastatic infections
• Hypoglycemic seizures or coma

EXPECTED COURSE/PROGNOSIS
Resolution of signs and symptoms over a few days in most cases

MISCELLANEOUS

ASSOCIATED CONDITIONS N/A

AGE-RELATED FACTORS
Pediatric:
• Day care center outbreaks may occur. Perhaps at higher risk of complications from antiperistaltic drugs.
• Newborns and infants are a high risk for mortality and complications
• Shigellosis is a rare cause of chronic vaginal discharge in young girls
Geriatric:
• Nursing home outbreaks may occur
• Significant cause of mortality
Others: N/A

PREGNANCY Perinatal salmonellosis, listeriosis, and campylobacteriosis may secondarily infect newborn with severe consequences of sepsis and meningitis

SYNONYMS N/A

ICD-9-CM
003.0 Salmonella gastroenteritis
004.0 Shigella dysenteriae
004.9 Shigellosis, unspecified
005.0 Staphylococcal food poisoning
005.1 Botulism
005.9 Food poisoning, unspecified
008.0 Escherichia coli intestinal infection

SEE ALSO
• Diarrhea, acute
• Eosinophilic gastroenteritis
• Intestinal parasites
• Salmonella infection
• Typhoid fever
• Brucellosis
• Botulism
• Dehydration
• Hypokalemia
• Appendicitis

OTHER NOTES N/A

ABBREVIATIONS N/A

REFERENCES
• Mandell GL, Douglas RG Jr, Bennett JE: Principles and Practice of Infectious Diseases. 4th Ed. New York, Churchill Livingstone, 1995
• Roberts D: Sources of infection: Food. Lancet 1990;336:859
Illustrations: N/A
Internet references: http://www.5mcc.com

Author(s)
Bernhard L. Wiedermann, MD

Fragile X syndrome

BASICS

DESCRIPTION Fragile X syndrome is the most common known genetic cause of mental retardation. As a result, it is the most common form of familial mental retardation. This condition received its name from the cytogenetic marker at which a "fragile site" is seen on the long arm of the X chromosome (Xq27.3). It is associated with abnormal increase in CGG repeats in the untranslated region of the FMR-1 gene in both carriers and affected individuals. Affected individuals also exhibit hypermethylation at the fragile site.

System(s) affected: Nervous, Reproductive, Musculoskeletal

Genetics:
• The pattern of inheritance is X-linked, however, this condition is seen in both sexes. Males usually more severely affected than females.
• The specific factors controlling the expression of genes at the fragile X site are not fully understood
• 80% of males with the fragile X chromosome will be affected with moderate to severe mental retardation, with 20% unaffected and defined as transmitting males
• Only one third of the female carriers will have mental retardation, and their degree of handicap usually is less severe. Females may demonstrate emotional problems.

Incidence/Prevalence in USA: Affected males = 1/1250 and transmitting males 1/5000 which gives an overall male prevalence of 1/1000. Affected females = 1/2000 and an overall female carrier rate of 1/700. Based on these estimates, 1/850 people carry the fragile X chromosome.

Predominant age: Life-long condition

Predominant sex: Males usually more severely affected, but females demonstrate a higher carrier rate

SIGNS AND SYMPTOMS
• The signs and symptoms seen in the "classic" case of fragile X syndrome may be diagnostic; however, the clinical presentation is extremely varied, is age-dependent, and sex-influenced. Blacks are also less likely to show the characteristic features.
• Early childhood:
    ◊ Global developmental delay with speech and language severely affected
    ◊ Overgrowth
    ◊ Autistic-like behaviors
• Postpubertal males (affected)
    ◊ Mental retardation (100%)
    ◊ Connective tissue dysplasia which may present as:
        - Macro-orchidism (> 95%)
        - Long, thin face (60-65%)
        - Prominent jaw (60-65%)
        - Large ears (> 7.0 cm) (60-65%)
        - Midface hypoplasia (50-60%)
        - Prominent forehead (40%)
        - Large, fleshy hands (30%)
        - Unusual dermatoglyphics

CAUSES Transmission of affected X chromosome

RISK FACTORS
• Transmitting males are intellectually normal and pass the affected chromosome to all of their daughters, the latter who may have affected sons
• Affected females transmit the affected chromosome to their offspring on a 50/50 chance basis
• To date, one affected male has been reported to have transmitted the permutation to his daughter

DIAGNOSIS

DIFFERENTIAL DIAGNOSIS
• Fragile X syndrome should be considered in patients (male or female) with mental retardation of unknown etiology
• Many male children will present primarily with speech delay or overgrowth and may have been misdiagnosed as having cerebral gigantism (Soto's) syndrome
• Approximately 5% of children diagnosed as autistic and mentally retarded have fragile X syndrome
• Males or females with significant learning disabilities with speech and language deficits
• Familial pattern of MR
• Persuasive developmental disorder
• Significant learning disability
• FRAXE - cytogenetically positive/DNA negative

LABORATORY Molecular genetic testing (DNA) is the diagnostic test of choice. Molecular studies can identify full mutations, mosaic patterns, and carrier states in intellectual normal males and females.

Drugs that may alter lab results: N/A
Disorders that may alter lab results: N/A

PATHOLOGICAL FINDINGS N/A

SPECIAL TESTS Affected patients are in need of educational and psychological evaluation for the development of learning programs

IMAGING N/A

DIAGNOSTIC PROCEDURES N/A

TREATMENT

APPROPRIATE HEALTH CARE Affected individuals will usually require life-long adult supervision and should be referred to the local mental retardation board for case management

GENERAL MEASURES Early detection allows initiation of pre-school intervention programs

SURGICAL MEASURES N/A

ACTIVITY Full activity

DIET No special diet

PATIENT EDUCATION
• The patient and the family should receive genetic evaluation and counseling
• Patient and family could contact: The National Fragile X Foundation, (800)688-8765

MEDICATIONS

DRUG(S) OF CHOICE Folic acid 20 mg qd, has been reported anecdotally to improve behavior and attention span in prepubertal males. No statistical benefit has been observed in children or adults during double-blind studies.
Contraindications: N/A
Precautions: N/A
Significant possible interactions: N/A

ALTERNATIVE DRUGS N/A

FOLLOWUP

PATIENT MONITORING General health maintenance

PREVENTION/AVOIDANCE Genetic counseling and evaluation of at-risk family members and pregnancies. Prenatal diagnosis is available.

POSSIBLE COMPLICATIONS Learning and/or behavioral problems (which are more frequent among female patients)

EXPECTED COURSE/PROGNOSIS
• Males with a full mutation may require life-long adult supervision
• Among affected males and females, life-span is generally not affected
• Among males, intellect manifests early plateauing which causes a decline in IQ scores
• Females are less affected and may have mild to moderate mental retardation
• Approximately 1/3 of affected females manifest learning disabilities

MISCELLANEOUS

ASSOCIATED CONDITIONS
• Speech and language problems
• Developmental delay
• Mental retardation
• Maladaptive behavior
• Attention deficit disorder/hyperactivity disorder (ADHD)
  ◊ Is found with greater frequency among individuals with neuropsychological dysfunction
  ◊ Treatment for ADHD among the mentally retarded is not unlike that for the "normal" population
  ◊ Data indicates overuse of psychoactive substances to aid caretakers

AGE-RELATED FACTORS
Pediatric: N/A
Geriatric: N/A
Others: N/A

PREGNANCY Patient and family should receive genetic evaluation and counseling as prenatal diagnosis is available

SYNONYMS
• Martin-Bell syndrome
• Marker X syndrome
• X-linked mental retardation

ICD-9-CM
758.9 Conditions due to anomaly of unspecified chromosome

SEE ALSO
• Down syndrome
• Mental retardation
• Attention deficit hyperactivity disorder
• Autism

OTHER NOTES Extensive family history is mandatory

ABBREVIATIONS ADHD = attention deficit disorder/hyperactivity disorder

REFERENCES
• Simensen RJ, Rogers RC: Fragile X Syndrome. Amer Fam Phys 1989;39(5):185-193
• Special Issue: X-Linked Mental Retardation-6. American Journal of Medical Genetics 1994;51:4
Illustrations: N/A
Internet references: http://www.5mcc.com

Author(s)
Richard J. Simensen, PhD
Gene S. Fisch, PhD

Frostbite

BASICS

DESCRIPTION A localized complication of exposure to cold, resulting in diminished blood flow to the affected part (especially hands, face or feet). Dehydration, enzymatic destruction and ultimately cell death occurs. In severe cases, deep tissue freezing may occur with damage to underlying blood vessels, muscles and nerve tissue.
System(s) affected: Endocrine/Metabolic, Skin/Exocrine
Genetics: N/A
Incidence/Prevalence in USA:
Approximately 4,800/year
Predominant age: All ages
Predominant sex: Male = Female

SIGNS AND SYMPTOMS
• Injured area first appears cold, hard, white and is anesthetic to touch. Progresses to blotchy-red, swollen and painful regions after rewarming.
• Loss of cutaneous sensation
• Numbness
• Throbbing pain
• Paresthesia
• Excessive sweating
• Joint pain
• Pallor
• Subcutaneous edema
• Hyperemia
• Blistering
• Blue discoloration
• Skin necrosis
• Gangrene

CAUSES
• Prolonged exposure to cold
• Refreezing thawed extremities

RISK FACTORS
• Impaired cerebral function
• Under the effects of alcohol or drug abuse
• Underlying psychiatric disturbance
• Ambient temperature less than 0°F (-17.8°C)
• Smoker
• Elderly
• Raynaud's phenomenon

DIAGNOSIS

DIFFERENTIAL DIAGNOSIS Frostnip - superficial damp cold injury

LABORATORY
• Hemoconcentration
• Decreased hepatic function
Drugs that may alter lab results: N/A
Disorders that may alter lab results: N/A

PATHOLOGICAL FINDINGS
• Ice crystallization in the intravascular extracellular space
• Atrophy
• Fibroblastic proliferation
• Skin necrosis

SPECIAL TESTS ECG - bradycardia, atrial fibrillation, atrial flutter, ventricular fibrillation, diffuse T wave inversion

IMAGING N/A

DIAGNOSTIC PROCEDURES
Consider Doppler studies

TREATMENT

APPROPRIATE HEALTH CARE
Outpatient or inpatient, depending on severity

GENERAL MEASURES
• Emergency measures for patient without pulse or respiration. Such measures may include CPR and internal warming with warm IV's and warm oxygen (see hypothermia)
• Prevent refreezing. May be necessary to keep frostbitten part frozen until patient can be transported to a care facility.
• Treat for hypothermia
• Cautious rewarming. May immerse frozen body part for several minutes in water no hotter than 40-42°C (104-107°F).
• Keep patient dry. If conscious, give warm fluids with high sugar content.
• Amputation not to be considered until it is definite that tissues are dead. May take about 3 weeks to know if the tissue is permanently injured.
• Prevention of infection, once treatment begins
• Ongoing whirlpool therapy for cleansing and debridement
• Prevention of damage to other body parts

SURGICAL MEASURES N/A

ACTIVITY
• As tolerated, protect injured body parts
• Initiate physical therapy once healing progresses sufficiently

DIET
• As tolerated
• Warm oral fluids

PATIENT EDUCATION
• Local library
• Exposure protection
• Early signs and symptoms of frostbite

MEDICATIONS

DRUG(S) OF CHOICE
• Warm IV fluids via central venous pressure (CVP) line
• Heated oxygen
• For myxedema coma - Levothyroxine 500 µg IV plus 300 mg hydrocortisone
• Tetanus toxoid
• For severe pain - analgesics or narcotics
• Antibiotics may be required for infection
• Maintenance - gastric lavage, peritoneal dialysis, hemodialysis, and mediastinal lavage if needed (using warmed fluids)
Contraindications: Refer to manufacturer's profile of each drug
Precautions: Refer to manufacturer's profile of each drug
Significant possible interactions: Refer to manufacturer's profile of each drug

ALTERNATIVE DRUGS
Consider nifedipine or pentoxifylline

FOLLOWUP

PATIENT MONITORING
• Preferably electronic probe for temperature monitoring (rectal or vascular)
• Followup for physical therapy progress, infection, other complications

PREVENTION/AVOIDANCE
• Dress in layers with appropriate cold weather gear. Cover exposed areas and extremities appropriately.
• Proper preparation for trips to cold climates. Avoid alcohol.

POSSIBLE COMPLICATIONS
• Hyperglycemia
• Acidosis
• Refractory arrhythmias
• Tissue loss. Distal parts of an extremity may undergo spontaneous amputation.
• Gangrene
• Death

EXPECTED COURSE/PROGNOSIS
• Anesthesia and bullae may occur
• The affected areas will heal or mummify without surgery. The process may take 6-12 months for healing. Patient may be sensitive to cold and experience burning and tingling.

MISCELLANEOUS

ASSOCIATED CONDITIONS
Alcohol and/or drug abuse

AGE-RELATED FACTORS
Pediatric: Loss of epithelial growth centers
Geriatric:
• Associated disease states increase mortality
• Periarticular osteoporosis complicates
• More prone to hypothermia
Others: N/A

PREGNANCY
Acidosis

SYNONYMS
• Dermatitis congelationis
• Frostnip
• Environmental injuries

ICD-9-CM
991.3

SEE ALSO
• Hypothermia

OTHER NOTES
N/A

ABBREVIATIONS
N/A

REFERENCES
• Rakel RE, ed: Textbook of Family Practice. 5th Ed. Philadelphia, W.B. Saunders Co., 1995
• Berkow R, et al, eds: Merck Manual. 16th Ed. Rahway, NJ, Merck Sharp & Dohme, 1992
• Kelly KJ, Glaeser P, Rice TB, Wendelberger KJ: Profound accidental hypothermia and freeze injury of the extremities in a child. In Critical Care Medicine. Baltimore, Williams & Wilkins, 1990
• Urschel JD: Frostbite: Predisposing factors and predictors of poor outcome. In Trauma. Baltimore, Williams & Wilkins, 1990
• Mills WF, et al: Cold Injury: A Collection of Papers. Alaska Med 1993;35(1)
Illustrations: N/A
Internet references: http://www.5mcc.com

Author(s)
Timothy Robinson, DO
Richard B. Birrer, MD

Frozen shoulder

BASICS

DESCRIPTION Adhesive capsulitis which restricts shoulder motion in all directions. The disorder may complicate other inflammatory shoulder disorders.
System(s) affected: Musculoskeletal
Genetics: N/A
Incidence/Prevalence in USA: Unknown
Predominant age: Middle aged and elderly
Predominant sex: Female > Male

SIGNS AND SYMPTOMS
• Decreased range of motion in all directions sometimes bilaterally
• Diffuse shoulder tenderness

CAUSES Alteration in the axillary fold of the shoulder capsule, chronic bursitis, trauma

RISK FACTORS
• Sedentary workers
• Immobilization
• Diabetes
• Peripheral vascular disease

DIAGNOSIS

DIFFERENTIAL DIAGNOSIS
• Infection
• Degenerative arthritis
• Pancoast's tumor
• Chronic posterior dislocation

LABORATORY N/A
Drugs that may alter lab results: N/A
Disorders that may alter lab results: N/A

PATHOLOGICAL FINDINGS Morphologic changes of fibrosis and fibroplasia without inflammation

SPECIAL TESTS N/A

IMAGING
• Arthrogram (if used) - decreased redundancy in axillary folds and obliteration of the space in axillary region
• MRI - to evaluate rotator cuff

DIAGNOSTIC PROCEDURES N/A

TREATMENT

APPROPRIATE HEALTH CARE
Outpatient

GENERAL MEASURES
• Prophylactic physiotherapy
• Passive manipulation under general anesthesia and injection of steroids (controversial)
• Application of heat
• Lastly, operative arthrotomy of the anterior inferior hanging axillary fold and subscapularis tendon
• Gentle passive and active assisted range-of-motion to tolerance

SURGICAL MEASURES N/A

ACTIVITY No restrictions. Passive exercise of the shoulder. Avoid forceful manipulation of the shoulder joint during exercises.

DIET No restrictions

PATIENT EDUCATION Techniques for passive exercise

MEDICATIONS

DRUG(S) OF CHOICE
• NSAID's
• Corticosteroid injections (controversial)
Contraindications: Those of NSAID's
Precautions: Refer to manufacturer's literature
Significant possible interactions: Refer to manufacturer's literature

ALTERNATIVE DRUGS N/A

FOLLOWUP

PATIENT MONITORING As needed

PREVENTION/AVOIDANCE Stretching, both active and passive

POSSIBLE COMPLICATIONS N/A

EXPECTED COURSE/PROGNOSIS
Persistence in exercise program shows improvement in motion and decreased pain over 6-18 weeks

MISCELLANEOUS

ASSOCIATED CONDITIONS N/A

AGE-RELATED FACTORS
Pediatric: N/A
Geriatric: N/A
Others: N/A

PREGNANCY N/A

SYNONYMS Adhesive capsulitis

ICD-9-CM 726.0

SEE ALSO N/A

OTHER NOTES N/A

ABBREVIATIONS N/A

REFERENCES
• Rakel RE, ed: Textbook of Family Practice, 5th Ed. Philadelphia, W.B. Saunders Co., 1995
• Parker RD, et al: Frozen Shoulder Part I, Orthopedics 1989;12(6)
Illustrations: N/A
Internet references: http://www.5mcc.com

Author(s)
Richard W. Cohen, MD

Furunculosis

 BASICS

DESCRIPTION Acute abscess of a hair follicle due to infection by Staphylococcus aureus. Spreads away from hair follicle into surrounding dermis.
System(s) affected: Skin/Exocrine
Genetics: Unknown
Incidence/Prevalence in USA:
• Uncommon in children unless immunodeficiency state present (i.e., can appear in young girls with hyperimmunoglobulin E-Staphylococcal syndrome [Job's syndrome])
• Increase in frequency after puberty
Predominant age: Adolescents and young adults. Uncommon in young children unless immunodeficiency state present (i.e., can appear in young girls with hyperimmunoglobulin E-staphylococcal syndrome [Job's syndrome]).
Predominant sex: Males = Females

SIGNS AND SYMPTOMS
• Painful erythematous papules/nodules (1-5 cm) with central pustulation
• Located only in hirsute sites of body, especially areas prone to friction or minor trauma (i.e., underneath belt, anterior thighs)
• May be singular or multiple
• No fever or systemic symptoms
• Tender red perifollicular swelling, terminating in discharge of pus and necrotic plug
• Pus usually drains spontaneously

CAUSES Pathogenic strain of Staphylococcus aureus

RISK FACTORS
• Carriage of pathogenic strain of Staphylococcus in nares, skin, axilla, and perineum
• Rarely, polymorphonuclear leukocyte defect or hyperimmunoglobulin-E/Staphylococcus abscess syndrome
• Diabetes mellitus, malnutrition, alcoholism
• Primary immunodeficiency disease (chronic granulomatous disease, Chediak-Higashi syndrome, C3 deficiency, C3 hypercatabolism, transient hypogammaglobulinemia of infancy, immunodeficiency with thymoma, Wiskott-Aldrich syndrome)
• Secondary immunodeficiency (leukemia, leukopenia, neutropenia, therapeutic immunosuppression)

 DIAGNOSIS

DIFFERENTIAL DIAGNOSIS
• Folliculitis
• Pseudofolliculitis
• Carbuncles
• Ruptured epidermal cyst
• Hidradenitis suppurativa

LABORATORY Culture of abscess material
Drugs that may alter lab results:
Antibiotics
Disorders that may alter lab results: N/A

PATHOLOGICAL FINDINGS
Histopathologically - perifollicular necrosis containing fibrinoid material and neutrophils. At deep end of necrotic plug, in subcutaneous tissue, is a large abscess with a gram stain positive for small collections of staph aureus.

SPECIAL TESTS None except for immunoglobulin levels in rare cases

IMAGING N/A

DIAGNOSTIC PROCEDURES Culture of abscess material

 TREATMENT

APPROPRIATE HEALTH CARE
Outpatient

GENERAL MEASURES
• Moist, warm compresses (provides comfort, encourages localization/pointing/drainage) 30 minutes, 4 times a day
• If pointing or large, incise and drain
• Consider packing to promote drainage
• Routine culture not necessary for localized abscess in non-diabetic patients with normal immune system
• Systemic antibiotics usually unnecessary, unless extensive surrounding cellulitis or fever
• If recurrent, problem usually related to chronic skin carriage of particular strain of Staphylococcus in nares or on skin. Treatment goals are to 1) decrease or eliminate pathogenic strain or 2) in very difficult cases, implant less aggressive strain.
• Suppression of pathogenic strain
  ◊ Culture nares, skin, axilla, perineum
  ◊ Begin therapeutic antibiotic doses
  ◊ Wash entire body and fingernails (with nailbrush) daily for 1-3 weeks with povidone-iodine (Betadine), hisachlorophene (Hibiclens), or Phisohex soap (all can cause dry skin)
  ◊ After shower ointments
  ◊ Sanitary practices - change towels, washcloths and sheets daily; clean shaving instruments; avoid nose-picking; change wound dressings frequently
• Replacement of pathogenic strain with nonpathogenic strain (502A bacterial interference)
  ◊ Culture nose and lesions to document pathogenic strain
  ◊ Culture family members if disease involves them
  ◊ Treat patient and infected household members with antibiotics
  ◊ Discontinue topical/oral antibiotics 48 hours then inoculate anterior nares with Staphylococcus aureus 502A (stock bacteria) (tilt head back, swab each anterior nares with 2 soaked cotton swabs of culture while patient sniffs material into nares and nasopharynx)
  ◊ Followup 1 month later; repeat process if abscesses not controlled

SURGICAL MEASURES N/A

ACTIVITY Avoid contact sports (i.e., wrestling) if active lesions. Otherwise no restrictions.

DIET Unrestricted

PATIENT EDUCATION Refer to: Habif T: Clinical Dermatology. 3rd Ed. St. Louis, CV Mosby, 1996

MEDICATIONS

DRUG(S) OF CHOICE
• If abscesses multiple, if lesions have marked surrounding inflammation, or if immunocompromised
  ◊ Obtain culture and place on antibiotics for at least 14 days
  ◊ Cloxacillin (Tegopen) or dicloxacillin (Dynapen, Pathocil) 250 mg qid, or
  ◊ Erythromycin (E-mycin, PCE) 250-500 tid
• Suppression of pathogenic strain
  ◊ Dicloxacillin or cloxacillin 250 mg qid x 21 days
  ◊ Erythromycin 250-500 mg tid (if penicillin allergic) x 21 days
  ◊ If above fails - begin 1-3 month course of antibiotics. May need to add rifampin 600 mg q day x 10 days
  ◊ After showering - bacitracin ointment or mupirocin to both anterior nares with cotton swab tid-qid x > 14 days
• Replacement of pathogenic strain
  ◊ Treat patient and infected household members with dicloxacillin 250 mg qid or if child/infant with 50 mg/kg/day qid x 7-10 days
Contraindications:
• Cloxacillin and dicloxacillin - penicillin allergy
• Erythromycin, mupirocin - hypersensitivity
Precautions:
• Cloxacillin and dicloxacillin - anaphylactic reaction
• Erythromycin - cautious use in patients with impaired hepatic function; GI side effects especially abdominal cramping; pregnancy category B. Increased cardiac toxicity with terfenadine (Seldane), astemizole
Significant possible interactions:
Erythromycin - increases theophylline and carbamazepine levels; decreases warfarin clearance

ALTERNATIVE DRUGS
• Resistant strains of Staph. aureus: first generation cephalosporins, clindamycin, ciprofloxacin + rifampin (rifampicin), cotrimoxazole + rifampicin
• If known or suspected impaired neutrophil function (i.e., impaired chemotaxis, phagocytosis, superoxide generation), add vitamin C 500 mg/day for 30 days (prevents oxidation of neutrophils)
• If fail with antibiotic regimens
  ◊ May try oral pentoxifylline 400 mg tid for 2-6 months
  ◊ Contraindications - recent cerebral and/or retinal hemorrhage; intolerance to methylxanthines (i.e., caffeine, theophylline)
  ◊ Precautions - prolonged prothrombin time and/or bleeding; if on warfarin, frequent monitoring of prothrombin time

FOLLOWUP

PATIENT MONITORING
Instruct patient to see physician if compresses unsuccessful

PREVENTION/AVOIDANCE
Patient education regarding self care (see General Measures section. Treatment and prevention are interrelated.)

POSSIBLE COMPLICATIONS
• Scarring
• Bacteremia
• Metastatic seeding (i.e., septal/valve defect, arthritic joint)

EXPECTED COURSE/PROGNOSIS
• Self-limited (usually drains pus spontaneously and will heal with or without scarring within several days)
• Recurrent/chronic lasting for months or years

MISCELLANEOUS

ASSOCIATED CONDITIONS
• Usually normal immune system
• Diabetes mellitus
• Polymorphonuclear leukocyte defect (rare)
• Hyperimmunoglobulin-E/staphylococcal abscess syndrome (rare)
• See Risk Factors for others

AGE-RELATED FACTORS
Pediatric: N/A
Geriatric: N/A
Others: Most common after puberty. Clusters have been reported in teenagers living in crowded quarters.

PREGNANCY N/A

SYNONYMS
• Boils

ICD-9-CM
680.9 Carbuncle and furuncle, unspecified site

SEE ALSO
• Folliculitis
• Hidradenitis suppurativa

OTHER NOTES
• If abscess culture grows gram negative bacteria or fungus then consider polymorphonuclear neutrophil (PMN) leukocyte function defect
• Hydradenitis suppurativa is a particular form of furunculosis
• Can order Staphylococcus aureus 502A from American Type Culture Collection, Rockville, Md.

ABBREVIATIONS N/A

REFERENCES
• Sams WM Jr, Lynch P: Principles and Practice of Dermatology. New York, Churchill Livingstone, 1990
• du Vivier A: Dermatology in Practice. Philadelphia, J.B. Lippincott Co., 1990
• Habif T: Clinical Dermatology. 3rd Ed. St. Louis, CV Mosby, 1996
• Levy R, Schlaeffer F: Successful treatment of a patient with recurrent furunculosis by vitamin C. International J of Dermatology 1993;32(11):832-834
• Wahba-Yahav AV: Intractable chronic furunculosis: Prevention of recurrence with pentoxifylline. Acta Dermato-Venereologica 1992;72(6):461-462
Illustrations: 4 available on CD-ROM
Internet references: http://www.5mcc.com

Author(s)
W. Paul Slomiany, MD

Galactorrhea

BASICS

DESCRIPTION Milky nipple discharge. Galactorrhea technically does not include serous, purulent, or bloody nipple discharge.
System(s) affected:
Endocrine/Metabolic/Reproductive
Genetics: N/A
Incidence/Prevalence in USA: 1-50% of non-pregnant, reproductive-aged women (studies vary widely)
Predominant age: Reproductive ages (15-50)
Predominant sex: Almost exclusively female

SIGNS AND SYMPTOMS
• Milky nipple discharge
• May also have signs/symptoms of associated conditions (e.g., hypothyroidism, Cushing's disease, acromegaly, fibrocystic breast disease)
• May also have signs/symptoms of pituitary enlargement (e.g., headache, visual field loss)

CAUSES
• Physiologic (pregnancy and up to 6 months after delivery or after stopping breast-feeding)
• Prolactin producing pituitary adenoma
• Medications (e.g., opioids, tricyclics, metoclopramide, verapamil, phenothiazines, alpha-methyldopa, isoniazid, estrogens, reserpine, butyrophenones)
• Oral contraceptive pill withdrawal
• Hypothyroidism
• Chest wall conditions (e.g., herpes zoster, post-thoracotomy, fibrocystic changes)
• Postoperative state (any major surgery, but especially oophorectomy)
• Chiari-Frommel (idiopathic galactorrhea more than 6 months postpartum)
• Idiopathic
• Miscellaneous causes (e.g., sarcoid, renal failure, Cushing's disease, cirrhosis, head trauma, lupus, multiple sclerosis or other pituitary or hypothalamic disease)

RISK FACTORS   Listed with Causes

DIAGNOSIS

DIFFERENTIAL DIAGNOSIS
• Non-milky discharge (e.g., serous) - consider fibrocystic disease
• Purulent discharge - consider mastitis
• Bloody discharge - rule out breast malignancy

LABORATORY
• Blood chemistries and pregnancy test
• Check prolactin level and thyroid functions in all galactorrheic patients
• Check FSH/LH if also amenorrheic
• Check growth hormone (GH) and adrenal steroids, if clinically suspect acromegaly or Cushing's disease
Drugs that may alter lab results: See medications listed under Causes. Most of these cause galactorrhea by causing hyperprolactinemia.
Disorders that may alter lab results: See disorders listed under Causes

PATHOLOGICAL FINDINGS   None, unless pituitary resection needed (very rare)

SPECIAL TESTS   Formal visual field testing if pituitary adenoma suspected

IMAGING
• Pituitary MRI if prolactin even minimally elevated, or if any other reason to suspect pituitary disease clinically
• CT only if MRI not available. Avoid "coned-down" or plain tomograms of pituitary as they are relatively insensitive.

DIAGNOSTIC PROCEDURES   Usually limited to history, physical exam, blood work and imaging as described above

TREATMENT

APPROPRIATE HEALTH CARE
Outpatient unless pituitary resection needed (very rare)

GENERAL MEASURES
• Treat underlying causes as indicated; galactorrhea by itself is not harmful
• Other reasons to treat include symptom management (if symptoms cause patient anxiety), fertility restoration (if amenorrheic), to cause growth retardation or regression of adenoma, or to prevent osteoporosis (if estrogen deficient)
• "Watchful waiting" is often most appropriate
• Discontinue offending medications, if any
• Pituitary macroadenomas warrant treatment even if asymptomatic

SURGICAL MEASURES   Large adenomas may be treated with x-ray therapy (variable success, 50% risk of panhyperpituitarism at 5 years) or transsphenoidal adenoma removal (variable success, recurrence common)

ACTIVITY   No restrictions

DIET   No restrictions

PATIENT EDUCATION
• Discussion of treatment rationale and risks
• Discussion of symptoms of complications of growing pituitary adenoma (e.g., central headache, visual field loss)

MEDICATIONS

DRUG(S) OF CHOICE Bromocriptine (Parlodel) if hyperprolactinemic. Start low at 1.25 mg or 2.5 mg daily, then increase as tolerated over several weeks to 2.5 mg tid. Higher doses sometimes required for prolactinoma regression. Start first dose of bromocriptine with night meal.
Contraindications: Uncontrolled hypertension, sensitivity to any ergot alkaloids, preeclampsia
Precautions:
• Nausea (often dose limiting)
• Orthostasis
• Drowsiness
• Lightheadedness and syncope
• Hypertension (rare)
• Seizures (rare)
• Acute psychosis (rare)
Significant possible interactions:
Phenothiazines, butyrophenones, other drugs listed under Causes

ALTERNATIVE DRUGS
• Intravaginal bromocriptine
• Sustained release bromocriptine (Parlodel SRO)
• Intramuscular bromocriptine (Parlodel LAR)
• New dopamine agonists (cabergoline, quinagolide)

FOLLOWUP

PATIENT MONITORING
• Depends on etiology
• If hyperprolactinemic, check prolactin level every 6-12 months, formal visual field testing yearly, and MRI in 1 year and then every 2-5 years, depending on clinical course

PREVENTION/AVOIDANCE N/A

POSSIBLE COMPLICATIONS
• Depends on underlying cause
• If pituitary adenoma, there is risk of permanent visual field loss

EXPECTED COURSE/PROGNOSIS
• Depends on underlying cause
• Symptoms tend to recur after discontinuation of bromocriptine

MISCELLANEOUS

ASSOCIATED CONDITIONS See Causes

AGE-RELATED FACTORS
Pediatric: N/A
Geriatric: N/A
Others: N/A

PREGNANCY Adenomas can grow dramatically during pregnancy. Most galactorrhea during pregnancy is physiologic.

SYNONYMS
• Disordered lactation
• Nipple discharge

ICD-9-CM 676.6 Galactorrhea

SEE ALSO
• Hyperprolactinemia
• Pituitary basophilic adenoma
• Pituitary chromophobe adenoma

OTHER NOTES Can occur in males, but usually not unless/until they are extremely hyperprolactinemic

ABBREVIATIONS N/A

REFERENCES
• Kleinberg DL, Noel GH, Frantz G: Galactorrhea: A study of 235 cases including 48 with pituitary tumors. N Engl J Med 1977;296:589
• Yen SSC, Jaffe RB, eds: Reproductive Endocrinology. 3rd Ed. Philadelphia, W.B. Saunders Co., 1991
• Sarapura V, Schlaff WD: Recent advances in the understanding of the pathophysiology and treatment of hyperprolactinemia. Curr Opin in OB & Gyn 1993;5:360-367
• Molitch ME: Pathologic hyperprolactinemia. Endocrinology and Metabolism Clinics of North America 1992;21(4):877-901
• Katz E, Adash E: Hyperprolactinemia disorders. Clinical Ob and Gyn 1990;33(3):622-639
• Jones TH: The management of hyprolactinemia. Brit J of Hosp Med 1995;53(8):374-378
• New drugs for hyprolactinemia. Drug and Therapeutics Bulletin 1995;33(9):65-67
Illustrations: N/A
Internet references: http://www.5mcc.com

Author(s)
Geoffrey R. Swain, MD

Gastric malignancy

BASICS

DESCRIPTION Gastric malignancy may occur anywhere in the stomach. Over the last 20 years the incidence of adenocarcinoma of the proximal stomach and the gastroesophageal junction has risen while the incidence of distal cancers has remained unchanged or decreased slightly. Infiltration to lymph nodes, omentum, lungs and liver is rapid. Uncommon in U.S. natives.
System(s) affected: Gastrointestinal
Genetics:
• 2 to 4 times more common in first degree relatives
• More common in people with blood group A
Incidence/Prevalence in USA:
7/100,000; 22,800 new cases per year
Predominant age: Over 55 (2/3 over age 65)
Predominant sex: Male > Female (1.6:1)

SIGNS AND SYMPTOMS
• Chronic non-colicky abdominal pain (especially in epigastrium) ranging from postprandial fullness to severe steady pain
• Anorexia
• Pain unrelieved by antacids
• Pain exacerbated by food
• Pain relieved by fasting
• Dysphagia
• Nausea and vomiting
• Constipation
• Early satiety

CAUSES Unknown. Probably arises from a non-specific mucosal injury. Possible association with H. pylori infection. Probable association with food preservatives (e.g., nitrates, sulfites).

RISK FACTORS
• Diet rich in additives (smoked, pickled or salted foods; highly spiced oriental foods)
• Achlorhydria
• Atrophic gastritis/intestinal metaplasia
• Pernicious anemia
• Prior gastric resection
• Smoking/tobacco abuse
• Ethnic background: Hispanic, Japanese, Chilean, Costa Rican. First or second generation Japanese, Chilean or Costa Rican in the United States.
• Polyps or dysplasia anywhere in alimentary canal
• Helicobacter pylori infection (possible)
• Familial polyposis
• Barrett's esophagus
• Low consumption of fruits and vegetables

DIAGNOSIS

DIFFERENTIAL DIAGNOSIS
• Gastric lymphoma
• Peptic ulcer with or without hemorrhage
• Eosinophilic gastroenteritis
• Giant hypertrophic gastritis (Ménétrier's disease)
• Carcinoma of the colon
• Functional dyspepsia
• Carcinoma of body or tail of the pancreas
• Angiodysplasia of the colon
• GI sarcoidosis
• Small intestinal lymphoma
• Crohn's disease

LABORATORY
• Positive stool guaiac for blood
• Hemoglobin less than 12 g/dL (1.86 mmol/L)
• Hematocrit less than 35 (0.35)
• Albumin less than 3 g/dL (30 g/L)
Drugs that may alter lab results: N/A
Disorders that may alter lab results:
Pernicious anemia may cause a false positive pentagastrin test

PATHOLOGICAL FINDINGS
• Adenocarcinomas 90% (75% ulcerative gastric carcinomas, 10% polypoid, 15% diffuse infiltrative scirrhous [linitis plastica])
• Gastric lymphomas 6%
• Gastric sarcomas less than 4%
• Gastric leiomyosarcoma < 2%

SPECIAL TESTS Pentagastrin test - stomach pH less than 6

IMAGING Double contrast upper GI study - barium filling defect, endoscopy, endoscopic ultrasound, CT scan

DIAGNOSTIC PROCEDURES Upper endoscopy for direct visualization, cytology and biopsy, endoscopic ultrasound is most accurate preoperative staging tool

TREATMENT

APPROPRIATE HEALTH CARE Inpatient
GENERAL MEASURES
• Surgical excision of the tumor with resection of the local lymph nodes offers the only chance for cure. Even patients who are not felt to have a curable lesion should be offered an attempt at surgical reduction of the tumor since it offers the best form of palliation and improves the likelihood of benefit if chemotherapy and/or radiation therapy is administered. Exception is early (superficial) gastric cancer where nonsurgical ablation (usually endoscopic) may be curative. Gastric cardia tumors may be effectively palliated by nonsurgical means.
• Radiation therapy is of little benefit due to the radioresistancy of gastric tumors and the high doses of radiation required. It does have use in the palliation of pain.

SURGICAL MEASURES
• Radical subtotal gastrectomy with gastrojejunostomy or gastroduodenostomy is the usual treatment of choice. A large part of the stomach along with the greater and lesser omentum is removed en bloc. At times a splenectomy and distal pancreatectomy are also performed. Direct extensions are also excised.
• Total gastrectomy is indicated only if necessary to remove the local lesion
• Local excision for palliation of incurable lesion by resection of bleeding area or area of obstruction

ACTIVITY Adjusted to patient's ability

DIET Dependent on the surgical procedure. Supplemental feedings or total parenteral nutrition (TPN) may be necessary to ensure adequate caloric intake.

PATIENT EDUCATION
• Contact local American Cancer Society
• Cancer Research Institute Helpbook: What to Do If Cancer Strikes. FDR Station, Box 5199, New York, NY 10150-5199

MEDICATIONS

DRUG(S) OF CHOICE
• Chemotherapy has little activity in the treatment of gastric malignancy. Multiple combinations have been tried. The following combinations may offer some palliation or possible prolongation of life:
◊ Fluorouracil
◊ Fluorouracil + leucovorin
◊ Fluorouracil + doxorubicin ± methotrexate
◊ Fluorouracil + doxorubicin + mitomycin
◊ Etoposide + fluorouracil + cisplatin
◊ Etoposide + cisplatin ± doxorubicin
◊ Etoposide + leucovorin + fluorouracil
◊ Fluorouracil + epirubicin + carmustine
Note: Dosing of these agents is patient specific; refer to Drug Evaluations Annual. American Medical Association, 1996 or other sources

Contraindications:
• 5-fluorouracil: Poor nutritional state, depressed bone marrow function, serious infections, major surgery in last month
• Doxorubicin: Preexisting myelosuppression, impaired cardiac function
• Mitomycin-C: Platelet count less than 75,000/mm3, leukocyte count less than 3000/mm3, serum creatinine greater than 1.7 mg/dL (150 µmol/L), coagulation disorders, serious infections

Precautions:
• Myelosuppression can occur with any of these agents
• Fluorouracil: Stomatitis, gastrointestinal injury, alopecia
• Doxorubicin: Stomatitis, gastrointestinal injury, alopecia, cardiac toxicity
• Mitomycin-C: Renal toxicity, hypercalcemia, gastrointestinal injury, cardiac toxicity
• Etoposide: Peripheral neuropathy, mucositis, hepatic damage
• Methotrexate: Stomatitis, mucositis, gastrointestinal damage, pulmonary infiltrates and fibrosis
• Epirubicin: cardiac toxicity
• Cisplatin: Ototoxicity, renal tubular damage, hypomagnesemia, hypokalemia, hypocalcemia, hemorrhagic cystitis

Significant possible interactions:
• Cisplatin: Aminoglycosides may potentiate nephrotoxicity and ototoxicity
• Loop diuretics may potentiate ototoxicity

ALTERNATIVE DRUGS
• Ondansetron (Zofran), dronabinol (Marinol), metoclopramide (Reglan), and others for nausea control

FOLLOWUP

PATIENT MONITORING
Routine, frequent followup is necessary to monitor disease state, assess treatments, monitor for recurrence/metastasis, and assess nutritional status

PREVENTION/AVOIDANCE
• Insufficient data to establish that screening would decrease mortality in US population
• Screening may be of benefit in high prevalence areas

POSSIBLE COMPLICATIONS
• Metastatic disease (especially hepatic, cerebral and pulmonary)
• Anemia (especially pernicious)
• Pyloric stenosis

EXPECTED COURSE/PROGNOSIS
• The prognosis for gastric carcinoma is not optimistic. Since most lesions do not produce symptoms until late in their course, gastric carcinomas are usually advanced at the time of diagnosis. Surgery offers the only chance for a cure.
• Overall 5 year relative survival rate 18% (if local disease 57%, regional spread 19%, distant spread 2%)
• Early gastric cancers are usually detected as incidental findings or when screening endoscopy is performed in endemic areas. Five year survival rate is > 40% depending on specific staging and tumor differentiation.

MISCELLANEOUS

ASSOCIATED CONDITIONS
• Predisposed by giant hypertrophic gastritis (Ménétrier's disease)
• Predisposed by intestinal metaplasia of the stomach
• Atrophic gastritis
• H. pylori

AGE-RELATED FACTORS
Pediatric: Rare
Geriatric: Prevalence greater
Others: N/A

PREGNANCY
Gastric cancer is rarely diagnosed in pregnancy. Prognosis is poor if diagnosed.

SYNONYMS
Linitis plastica

ICD-9-CM
• 151 Malignant neoplasm of stomach
• 150.0 cardia
• 151.1 pylorus
• 151.2 pyloric antrum
• 151.3 fundus of stomach
• 151.4 body of stomach
• 151.5 lesser curvature, unspecified
• 151.6 greater curvature, unspecified
• 151.8 other specified sites of stomach
• 151.9 stomach, unspecified

SEE ALSO
Esophageal tumors

OTHER NOTES
• Patients in lower socioeconomic classes are at greater risk of developing gastric tumors
• Migrants from high incidence areas (such as Iceland, Chile or Japan) to low incidence areas maintain an increased risk while their offspring have an occurrence rate that corresponds to the new location

ABBREVIATIONS
N/A

REFERENCES
• Isselbacher KJ, et al, eds: Harrison's Principles of Internal Medicine. 13th Ed. New York, McGraw-Hill, 1994
• Sawyers JL: Gastric carcinoma. Curr Prob Surg 1995;32:105-178
• Fuchs CS, Mayer RJ: Gastric carcinoma. NEJM 1995;333:32-41
Illustrations: N/A
Internet references: http://www.5mcc.com

Author(s)
Scott T. Henderson, MD

Gastritis

BASICS

DESCRIPTION Inflammatory reaction in the stomach; typically involves the mucosa, seldom the full thickness of the stomach wall
• Patchy erythema of gastric mucosa: a common endoscopic finding; usually insignificant
• Erosive gastritis: a reaction to mucosal injury by a noxious chemical agent, e.g., drugs (especially NSAID's) or alcohol
• Reflux gastritis: a reaction to protracted reflux exposure to bile and pancreatic juice, usually associated with a defective pylorus; typically limited to the prepyloric antrum
• Hemorrhagic gastritis (stress ulceration): a reaction to hemodynamic disorder, viz., hypovolemia or hypoxia (as in shock). Also, very common in intensive care units (ICU).
• Infectious gastritis: commonly associated with Helicobacter pylori (possibly causative, maybe opportunistic); viral infection, usually as a component of systemic infection, is common; significant infection by other specific microbes is rare
• Gastric mucosal atrophy, sometimes called atrophic gastritis: frequent, in varying degrees, in the elderly; invariable in primary (pernicious) anemia
System(s) affected: Gastrointestinal
Genetics: Unknown (except, probably, for gastric mucosa atrophy)
Incidence/Prevalence in USA: N/A
Predominant age: All ages; an estimated 60% of persons older than 60 years harbor H. pylori in their gastric mucosa, but in only a small fraction is this significant
Predominant sex: Male = Female

SIGNS AND SYMPTOMS
• Nondescript epigastric distress, often aggravated by eating
• Anorexia
• Nausea, with or without vomiting
• Significant bleeding is unusual except in hemorrhagic gastritis
• Hiccups

CAUSES
• Alcohol
• Aspirin and other nonsteroidal anti-inflammatory drugs
• Bile reflux
• Pancreatic enzyme reflux
• Stress (hypovolemia or hypoxia)
• Radiation
• Staphylococcus aureus exotoxins
• Bacterial infection (ex: helicobacter pylori)
• Viral infection
• Pernicious anemia
• Gastric mucosal atrophy
• Portal hypertension gastropathy

RISK FACTORS
• Age over 60
• Exposure to potentially noxious drugs or chemical agents
• Hypovolemia, hypoxia (shock)
• Candidal autoimmune

DIAGNOSIS

DIFFERENTIAL DIAGNOSIS
• Functional gastrointestinal disorder
• Peptic ulcer disease
• Linitis plastica
• Viral gastroenteritis
• Pancreatic disease
• Gastric cancer (elderly)

LABORATORY Usually unremarkable, except when blood loss results in anemia
Drugs that may alter lab results:
Antibiotics or omeprazole may affect urea breath test for H. pylori
Disorders that may alter lab results: N/A

PATHOLOGICAL FINDINGS Acute or chronic inflammatory infiltrate in gastric mucosa, often with distortion or erosion of adjacent epithelium. Presence of H. pylori may be confirmed.

SPECIAL TESTS
• 13C-urea breath test for H. pylori (not widely available)
• Serologic test available for H. pylori (office and clinical laboratory)
• Gastric acid analysis may be abnormal but is not a reliable indicator of gastritis

IMAGING Nuclear scintigraphy not done clinically

DIAGNOSTIC PROCEDURES
Gastroscopy, usually with biopsy, is essential for a precise diagnosis

TREATMENT

APPROPRIATE HEALTH CARE
Outpatient, except for severe hemorrhagic gastritis

GENERAL MEASURES
• No specific therapy for gastritis (with the exception of H. pylori infection)
• Parenteral fluid and electrolyte supplements required if vomiting prevents food intake
• Consider discontinuing NSAIDs or adding misoprostol

SURGICAL MEASURES N/A

ACTIVITY Usually no restriction

DIET Restriction, if any, depends on severity of symptoms (e.g., light, soft diet); avoid caffeine

PATIENT EDUCATION
• Explanation, reassurance
• Smoking cessation

MEDICATIONS

DRUG(S) OF CHOICE
• Antacids - best given in liquid form, 30 mL 1 hour after meals and at bedtime; useful mainly as an emollient
• H2 receptor antagonists e.g., cimetidine (Tagamet) - "priming" dose of 300 mg IV, then a steady infusion of 37.5-75 mg per hour, dissolved in the running fluid. Patients less severely ill - oral cimetidine 300 mg q6h (or ranitidine [Zantac] or famotidine [Pepcid] or nizatidine [Axid]). Not shown to be clearly superior to antacids.
• Sucralfate (Carafate) 1 g q4-6h on an empty stomach. Rationale uncertain, but empirically helpful.
• Prostaglandins, e.g., misoprostol (Cytotec), can help allay gastric mucosal injury, suggested dosage of 100-200 µg qid
• To eradicate H. pylori:
◊ "Triple therapy" is advised – bismuth (as Pepto-Bismol) 30 mL liquid or 2 tablets qid for 4 weeks plus metronidazole 250 mg qid for the first week, plus tetracycline 250 mg qid or amoxicillin 250 mg tid for 2-4 weeks
or
◊ "Dual therapy" with omeprazole 20 mg bid plus amoxicillin 500 mg qid for 2 weeks
Contraindications: Hypersensitivity to the drug(s)
Precautions:
• If bismuth is prescribed, warn patient of black stools
• Refer to manufacturer's profile of each drug
Significant possible interactions: Refer to manufacturer's profile of each drug

ALTERNATIVE DRUGS N/A

FOLLOWUP

PATIENT MONITORING
Gastroscopy should be repeated after 6 weeks if gastritis has been severe or if symptomatic response to treatment has not been achieved

PREVENTION/AVOIDANCE
• Patients should be warned of known or potentially injurious drugs or chemical agents
• Patients liable to hypovolemia or hypoxia (especially patients confined to an intensive care ward) should receive prophylactic therapy

POSSIBLE COMPLICATIONS
Bleeding from extensive mucosal erosion or ulceration

EXPECTED COURSE/PROGNOSIS
• Most cases clear spontaneously when the cause has been identified and allayed
• Recurrence of H. pylori infection may require a repeated course of treatment

MISCELLANEOUS

ASSOCIATED CONDITIONS
• Gastric or duodenal peptic ulcer
• Primary (pernicious) anemia
• Portal hypertension

AGE-RELATED FACTORS
Pediatric: Gastritis rarely occurs in infants or children
Geriatric: Persons over 60 often harbor apparently harmless H. pylori infection
Others: N/A

PREGNANCY N/A

SYNONYMS
• Erosive gastritis
• Reflux gastritis
• Hemorrhagic gastritis
• Acute gastritis

ICD-9-CM 535.5 (unless otherwise specified)

SEE ALSO N/A

OTHER NOTES N/A

ABBREVIATIONS
NSAID's = nonsteroidal anti-inflammatory drugs

REFERENCES
• Richardson CT: Gastritis. In: Wyngaarden JB, Smith LH Jr, eds. Cecil Textbook of Medicine. Philadelphia, W.B. Saunders Co., 1988:689-692
• Graham DY, Malaty HM, Evans G, et al: Epidemiology of Helicobacter pylori in an asymptomatic population in the US. Gastroenterology 1991;100:1495-1501
• Zinner MJ, Rypins EB, Martin LR, et al: Misoprostol versus antacid titration for preventing stress ulcers in postoperative surgical ICU patients. Ann Surg 1989;210:590-595
Illustrations: N/A
Internet references: http://www.5mcc.com

Author(s)
Douglas M. Hoy, MD

Gastroesophageal reflux disease

BASICS

DESCRIPTION Reflux of gastroduodenal contents into the esophagus with or without esophageal inflammation
System(s) affected: Gastrointestinal
Genetics: N/A

Incidence/Prevalence in USA: Increasing; recent Gallup surveys reveal 65% of adults have suffered heartburn and 24% have had symptoms for more than 10 years. 17% of adults use indigestion aids at least once weekly, and only 24% of sufferers have consulted a physician. Children affected 1/300-1000; 30-80% of pregnant women report heartburn.
Predominant age: All ages
Predominant sex: Male = Female

SIGNS AND SYMPTOMS
• Heartburn (pyrosis) 70-85%
• Regurgitation 60%
• Dysphagia (suggests possible stricture) 15-20%
• Angina-like chest pain 33%
• Bronchospasm (asthma) 15-20%
• Laryngitis (dysphonia)
• Chronic cough
• Globus sensation
• In infants: Recurrent emesis, failure to thrive, apnea syndrome

CAUSES
• Inappropriate relaxation of lower esophageal sphincter (LES) (idiopathic, food- or drug-related)
• Pregnancy (progestational hormones cause decreased LES pressure)
• Scleroderma (reduced esophageal motility and incompetent LES)
• Chalasia of infancy
• Delayed gastric emptying (impaired acid clearance)
• Acid hypersecretion (e.g., Zollinger-Ellison syndrome)
• Heller's myotomy for achalasia (30% develop reflux)

RISK FACTORS
• Foods that lower LES pressure (high-fat content, yellow onions, chocolate, peppermint)
• Foods that irritate esophageal mucosa (citrus fruits, spicy tomato drinks)
• Hiatal hernia - acid trapping
• Cigarette smoking
• Excessive alcohol
• Coffee
• Medications that lower LES pressure (e.g., theophylline, anticholinergics, progesterone, calcium channel blockers (nifedipine, verapamil), alpha adrenergic agents, diazepam, meperidine
• Indwelling nasogastric tube
• Chest trauma
• In children: Down syndrome, mental retardation, cerebral palsy, repaired tracheoesophageal fistula
• Eradication of H. pylori infection (resulting in increased acid production, loss of acid buffering, etc.)

DIAGNOSIS

DIFFERENTIAL DIAGNOSIS
• Infectious esophagitis (candida, herpes, HIV, cytomegalovirus)
• Chemical esophagitis (lye ingestion)
• Radiation injury
• Crohn's disease of esophagus
• Angina pectoris
• Esophageal carcinoma
• Pill-induced esophagitis (e.g., doxycycline, ascorbic acid, quinidine, potassium chloride, bisphosphonates, etc.)
• Achalasia
• Ulcer disease

LABORATORY N/A
Drugs that may alter lab results: N/A
Disorders that may alter lab results: N/A

PATHOLOGICAL FINDINGS
• Acute inflammation (especially eosinophils)
• Hyperplasia (thickening) of the basal zone of the epithelium seen in 85%
• Lengthening of vascular channels within vascular papillae so that they approach the luminal surface
• Barrett's epithelial change - gastric columnar epithelium (intestinal metaplasia) migrates upward into the distal esophagus; may be associated with strictures and peptic ulceration; dysplasia and malignant transformation

SPECIAL TESTS
• Esophageal pH monitoring (antacids, H2 blockers, proton pump inhibitors and other antisecretory agents can give false negative pH monitoring)
• Esophageal manometry (anticholinergics, theophylline, calcium channel blockers, meperidine, diazepam may give falsely low LES pressure on manometry)
• Acid perfusion (Bernstein) test
• Gastric analysis (exclude gastric hypersecretion)

IMAGING
• Barium swallow: Presence of a sliding hiatal hernia appears to be a predictor of reflux esophagitis; mucosal irregularity due to inflammation and edema; prominent longitudinal folds, erosions, ulcers; smoothly tapered strictures; pseudodiverticula
• Radionuclide scintigraphy

DIAGNOSTIC PROCEDURES
Endoscopy:

Grade	Finding	% Patients with grade
0	Normal	20-40
I	Erythema, friability	20-30
II	Nonconfluent erosions	20-30
III	Confluent erosions, exudate	5-10
IV	Ulceration, stricture	5

• Barrett's change suspected when salmon-colored mucosa extends > 2 cm above normal squamocolumnar junction (seen in up to 10%).
• Mucosal biopsy
• Cytology for Barrett's dysplasia (flow cytometry useful adjunct when available)
• Metoclopramide or cisapride may give falsely negative gastric emptying results

TREATMENT

APPROPRIATE HEALTH CARE
• Outpatient diagnosis (typical heartburn history has a positive predictive value of > 80% and warrants empiric therapy in absence of alarm symptoms)
• Inpatient if surgery indicated.

GENERAL MEASURES
• Elevate head of bed, avoid lying down directly after meals
• Avoid stooping, bending, tight-fitting garments
• Avoid drugs causing decreased LES pressure
• Weight loss
• Avoid voluntary eructation
• Stepped therapy
  ◊ Phase I: lifestyle and diet modifications plus antacids or OTC H2 blockers
  ◊ Phase II: H2 blockers in prescription doses
  ◊ Phase III: (1) high-dose H2 blocker or proton pump inhibitor (e.g., omeprazole or lansoprazole) or (2) H2 blockers or proton pump inhibitor plus cisapride
  ◊ Phase IV: surgery

SURGICAL MEASURES Phase IV of stepped therapy (see General Measures)

ACTIVITY Full activity

DIET Avoid chocolate, peppermint, onions, high-fat foods, alcohol, tobacco, coffee, citrus juices

PATIENT EDUCATION Patient educational materials available from Digestive Diseases Clearinghouse, Suite 600, 1555 Wilson Blvd., Rosslyn, VA 22209, (212)685-3440

Gastroesophageal reflux disease

MEDICATIONS

DRUG(S) OF CHOICE
• Mild to moderate disease: H2 blockers in equipotent oral doses, e.g., cimetidine (Tagamet) 800 mg bid or 400 mg qid or ranitidine (Zantac) 150 bid or famotidine (Pepcid) 20 mg bid or nizatidine (Axid) 150 mg bid or cisapride (Propulsid) 10-20 mg qid (before meals and at bedtime). Expected endoscopic healing rates 30-50% at 6 weeks, 50-80% at 12 weeks.
• Erosive esophagitis: Omeprazole (Prilosec) 20 mg qd or lansoprazole (Prevacid) 30 mg qd, or higher dose H2 receptor antagonist (e.g., ranitidine 150 mg qid or famotidine 40 mg bid) with or without cisapride for up to 12 weeks
• Severe disease (refractory to initial therapy): Omeprazole (Prilosec) 20-40 mg daily or lansoprazole (Prevacid) 30 mg qd; or higher-dose H2 blockers (e.g., ranitidine 150 mg qid)

Contraindications: Known hypersensitivity to H2 blockers, omeprazole, lansoprazole, cisapride

Precautions:
• Dose reduction of H2 blockers for renal failure
• Avoid cimetidine when potentially interacting drugs are co-administered (or closely monitor prothrombin time or serum theophylline levels, etc.)
• Cisapride should be used with caution with antifungal imidazole agents (e.g., ketoconazole, fluconazole, etc.) and erythromycin as prolonged QT intervals may occur

Significant possible interactions:
• Cimetidine interacts with > 60 drugs (e.g., theophylline, warfarin, phenytoin, lidocaine). Refer to manufacturer's profile.
• Omeprazole
  ◊ May prolong the elimination of diazepam, warfarin and phenytoin
  ◊ Prolonged PPI use associated with hypergastrinemia and potential for carcinoid tumors of the stomach (experimental data)
• Sedative effects of alcohol or benzodiazepines may be accelerated by cisapride
• Avoid anticholinergics with cisapride

ALTERNATIVE DRUGS
• Antacids; alginates e.g., alumina-magnesium (Gaviscon)
• Metoclopramide (Reglan) 5-10 mg before meals used adjunctively with H2 blockers (neuropsychiatric side effects in 30% limits its usefulness)
• Bethanechol (Urecholine) adjunct with H2 blocker (cholinergic side effects)

FOLLOWUP

PATIENT MONITORING Follow symptomatically; repeat endoscopy at 6-12 weeks for poor symptomatic response; annual endoscopy and biopsy for Barrett's esophagus (to detect dysplasia)

PREVENTION/AVOIDANCE
• Long-term maintenance therapy with H2 blockers along with lifestyle and diet modifications to prevent symptomatic relapse
• Peptic strictures may require periodic dilatation (although frequency of dilatation is reduced by PPI maintenance)
• Omeprazole 20 mg daily or lansoprazole 15 mg daily, effective (both approved for chronic maintenance in severe GERD)
• Antireflux surgery should be considered for patients with severe disease in lieu of chronic drug therapy (laparoscopic approach rapidly gaining acceptance)
• Annual (or every other year) endoscopy, biopsy and cytology to detect dysplasia in Barrett's epithelium

POSSIBLE COMPLICATIONS
• Peptic stricture (10-15%)
• Hemorrhage (3%)
• Barrett's esophagus (10%)
• Pulmonary or ear, nose, throat complications (5-10%)
• Noncardiac chest pain
• Adenocarcinoma from Barrett's epithelium

EXPECTED COURSE/PROGNOSIS
• Majority of patients respond well to antisecretory or prokinetic therapy
• Symptoms and esophageal inflammation often return promptly when treatment withdrawn
• Relapse prevention therapy with H2 blockers/proton pump inhibitor often requires the full healing dose be maintained
• Antireflux surgery (e.g., fundoplication) for complications or "refractory" disease; excellent short-term results but long-term followup is relatively limited
• Regression of Barrett's epithelium does not routinely occur despite aggressive medical or surgical therapy
• Cost effectiveness of longterm maintenance therapy has been shown

MISCELLANEOUS

ASSOCIATED CONDITIONS
• Reflux-induced asthma
• Pulmonary aspiration
• Chronic cough/throat clearing
• Loss of dental enamel
• Halitosis
• Laryngitis
• Globus sensation
• Vocal cord granulomas

AGE-RELATED FACTORS
Pediatric:
• Reflux symptoms usually resolve by 18 mo
• Vomiting, weight loss, failure to thrive more common than heartburn
• Positional treatment = use of infant seat for 2-3 hours after meals; thickened feedings
• Drug treatment = antacids or liquid H2 blockers (e.g., Zantac syrup)
• Surgery for severe symptoms (apnea, choking, persistent vomiting) successful in 85-95%
Geriatric: Complications more likely
Others: N/A

PREGNANCY
• Heartburn (when first experienced): 52% 1st trimester, 24% 2nd trimester, 9% 3rd trimester
• Tends to recur in subsequent pregnancies
• Symptomatic therapy includes multiple small meals, avoid lying down for 2-3 hours after meals, elevating the head of the bed at night
• Antacids or H2 blockers are probably safe in the 2nd trimester

SYNONYMS
• Reflux esophagitis
• Peptic esophagitis
• Barrett's esophagus
• Symptomatic hiatal hernia

ICD-9-CM
530.1 Esophagitis
750.6 Hiatal hernia
787.1 Heartburn

SEE ALSO
• Peptic ulcer disease
• Esophageal tumors

OTHER NOTES
Alkaline (bile) reflux accounts for up to 15% of Barrett's esophagus and severe esophagitis; promotility agent or surgery may be required in this setting

ABBREVIATIONS
• LES = lower esophageal sphincter
• GER = gastroesophageal reflux
• GERD = gastroesophageal reflux disease
• PPI = proton pump inhibitor

REFERENCES
• Fennerty MB, Sampliner RE, Garewal HS: Barrett's oesphagus - cancer risk, biology and therapeutic management. Ailment Pharmacol Ther 1993;7:339-345
• DeVault KR, Castell DO: Guidelines for the diagnosis and treatment of gastroesophageal reflux disease. Arch Intern Med 1995;155:2165-2173
• Labenz J, Blum AL, Bayerdorffer E, et al: Curing Helicobacter pylori infection in patients with duodenal ulcer may provoke reflux esophagitis. Gastroenterology 1997;112:1442-1447
• Zagari M, Villa KF, Freston JW: Proton pump inhibitors versus H2-receptor antagonists for the treatment of erosive gastroesophageal reflux disease: a cost-comparison study. Am J Managed care 1995;1:247-255
• Gotley DC, Smithers BM, Rhodes M, et al: Laparoscopic Nissen fundoplication-200 consecutive cases. Gut 1996;38:487-491
• Kahrilas PJ: Gastroesophageal reflux disease. JAMA 1996;276:983-986
Illustrations: N/A
Internet references: http://www.5mcc.com

Author(s)
James H. Lewis, MD, FACP, FACG

Giant cell arteritis

BASICS

DESCRIPTION A systemic granulomatous, predominantly, large vessel arteritis, most commonly affecting the branches of the cranial arteries, (but may involve other aortic branches), seen primarily in the elderly. Frequently associated with polymyalgia rheumatica (PMR).
System(s) affected:
Hemic/Lymphatic/Immunologic, Cardiovascular
Genetics: May be important, several family clusters have been identified
Incidence/Prevalence in USA: More common in northern latitudes (15-30/ 100,000 person over 50/year) vs. southern latitudes (less than 2/100,000 in some series). Primarily Caucasian, Northern European descent.
Predominant age: 60 years or older (very rare under 50). Incidence increases with age.
Predominant sex: Female > Male (2:1)

SIGNS AND SYMPTOMS
• Onset may be abrupt or insidious over months
• Local
  ◊ Headache (usually unilateral temporal, may be generalized or occipital) seen in 2/3 of patients
  ◊ Jaw/tongue "claudication" upon mastication (fairly specific)
  ◊ Visual disturbances early - amaurosis fugax, scotoma, diplopia); late - ischemic optic neuritis, blindness
  ◊ Scalp tenderness
  ◊ Swollen, red temporal artery
  ◊ Decreased temporal artery pulse (may be increased early)
  ◊ Sore throat, cough (10%)
  ◊ Neurologic manifestations - TIA, stroke, peripheral neuropathy, mononeuritis multiplex (3%)
• Systemic
  ◊ Polymyalgia rheumatica - seen in 40-60%
  ◊ Fever (low grade) - 15% with FUO
  ◊ Fatigue/malaise
  ◊ Weight loss/anorexia
  ◊ Arthralgias, myalgias, arthritis

CAUSES
• Etiology unknown
• Possibly immunologic mechanism

RISK FACTORS
• Age over 50
• Presence of polymyalgia rheumatica

DIAGNOSIS

DIFFERENTIAL DIAGNOSIS
• Cerebral vasculitides
• Other causes of headache (tumor, sinusitis, cervical or temporomandibular joint arthritis)
• Cerebral vascular insufficiency
• Other connective tissue disease
• Retinal detachment or other causes of loss of vision
• Septic arteritis

LABORATORY
• ESR (Westergren) usually greater than 50 (may be over 100)
• ESR may be normal in 10% of patients
• Elevated alkaline phosphatase over 1.5 x normal (unusual)
• Elevated aspartate aminotransferase (AST) over 1.5 x normal (unusual)
• Anemia - mild to moderate, normochromic/normocytic
• Mild leukocytosis
• Mild thrombocytosis
Drugs that may alter lab results:
Prednisone
Disorders that may alter lab results:
• Tumor, infarction, serum protein abnormalities all raise the ESR.

PATHOLOGICAL FINDINGS
• Inflammatory infiltrate (either mononuclear cells or granulomas with giant multinucleated cells) seen in the intima and media of large vessels with resultant disruption of the internal elastic lamina. Lesions may be isolated (i.e., skip lesions)
• Biopsy may not show evidence of active arteritis. However, changes of healing arteritis or vasculitis supports the diagnosis of GCA. If clinically active disease (headache, jaw claudication, elevated ESR), treat as GCA and use high dose steroids.

SPECIAL TESTS
• Temporal artery biopsy

IMAGING Temporal arteriography (in selected cases)

DIAGNOSTIC PROCEDURES
• Temporal artery biopsy
  ◊ Minimum 2.5 cm segment of vessel with serial sections
  ◊ Within 96 hours of starting steroids
  ◊ If negative, must consider biopsy of contralateral artery (may increase yield up to 10-14%)

TREATMENT

APPROPRIATE HEALTH CARE
• Inpatient (or outpatient surgery) initially for temporal artery biopsy. Outpatient subsequently.
• If there is a high index of suspicion, immediately institute corticosteroid therapy while arranging temporal artery biopsy

GENERAL MEASURES N/A

SURGICAL MEASURES
• Temporal artery biopsy

ACTIVITY Ambulatory ad lib

DIET
• Appropriate salt restriction
• Adequate calcium intake (1500 mg/day)
• Watch serum glucose

PATIENT EDUCATION
• Precautions regarding steroid use, especially osteoporosis
• Exacerbation of disease with medication dose adjustment
• Adrenal suppression - patients should get medical alert bracelet or neck tag

MEDICATIONS

DRUG(S) OF CHOICE
• Prednisone - early:
  ◊ 60 mg prednisone/d; divided dose initially, then single morning dose (never use every other day steroids)
  ◊ Begin slow taper after 6 weeks if asymptomatic and ESR decreased (occasionally patient may not normalize ESR)
• Prednisone - taper:
  ◊ Taper initially by 5 mg every 2 weeks to dose of 25 mg. Then slow taper by 2.5 mg decrements every 2-4 weeks to a dose of 10-15 mg if above guidelines are met. (Must be individualized).
  ◊ Continue 10-15 mg daily for several months-year, with periodic attempts to taper (i.e., every 3-6 months) by 1 or 2 mg
  ◊ Use symptoms and ESR to help guide taper
  ◊ Average time to disease remission 3-4 years, range 1-10 years

Contraindications:
• Systemic fungal infections, although physician must evaluate risks and benefits.
• Relative contraindications: Avoid, if possible, in patients with congestive heart failure, diabetes mellitus, systemic fungal or bacterial infection (must treat infection concurrently if steroids are necessary).

Precautions:
• Long term steroid use
  ◊ Associated with several potentially severe adverse effects, including: Increased susceptibility to infection, glucose intolerance, adrenal suppression, muscle wasting, osteoporosis, peptic ulcer disease, sodium and water retention, cataracts, avascular necrosis, GI bleeding, psychosis, weight gain
  ◊ Use lowest possible dose for shortest duration
  ◊ Upon discontinuing, if the patient has received long-term therapy, taper slowly to avoid Addisonian crisis. May need temporary stress dose steroids for surgical procedures, accidents or severe infections.

Significant possible interactions: Refer to manufacturer's literature

ALTERNATIVE DRUGS
Cytotoxic agents only if patient cannot use steroids (brittle diabetes mellitus, severe osteoporosis, congestive heart failure, etc.) or fails to respond to steroids

FOLLOWUP

PATIENT MONITORING
• ESR - repeat at monthly intervals initially and while tapering, then every 3 months
• Follow visual/constitutional symptoms monthly initially, then as needed

PREVENTION/AVOIDANCE   N/A

POSSIBLE COMPLICATIONS
• Complications related to steroids
• Exacerbation of disease during therapy or taper

EXPECTED COURSE/PROGNOSIS
• With early treatment, resolution of symptoms and preservation of vision
• Average length of disease 3-4 years
• With no treatment, high risks of blindness and stroke
• Occasionally ESR elevation not related to GCA activity and cannot be used to monitor and/or adjust treatment

MISCELLANEOUS

ASSOCIATED CONDITIONS
Polymyalgia rheumatica

AGE-RELATED FACTORS
Pediatric: Does not occur in this age group
Geriatric: Incidence increases with age (twice as common in patients over 80 as it is in 50-59 age group)
Others: N/A

PREGNANCY   N/A

SYNONYMS
• Temporal cell arteritis

ICD-9-CM   446.5 giant cell arteritis

SEE ALSO
• Polymyalgia rheumatica
• Fibrositis
• Polymyositis/dermatomyositis
• Depression
• Headache, tension
• Headache, cluster

OTHER NOTES
Westergren ESR is preferable. If other ESR used (i.e., Wintrobe or ZSR) then cannot use the listed guidelines for abnormalities.

ABBREVIATIONS
GCA = Giant cell arteritis
TA = temporal arteritis

REFERENCES
• Hunder GG: Giant Cell Arteritis and Polymyalgia Rheumatica. In: Kelly WN, Harris ED, Ruddy S, Sledge CB, eds. Textbook of Rheumatology. 4th Ed. p1123-1132, Philadelphia, W.B. Saunders Co., 1997
• Hunder GG, et al: The American College of Rheumatology 1990 Criteria for the Classification of Giant Cell Arteritis. In Arthritis Rheum 1990;33:1122-1128
Illustrations: N/A
Internet references: http://www.5mcc.com

Author(s)
Bridget T. Walsh, DO
Eric P. Gall, MD

Giardiasis

BASICS

DESCRIPTION   Intestinal infection caused by the protozoan parasite, Giardia lamblia. Infection results from ingestion of the cysts that excyst into trophozoites which colonize the small intestine and cause the symptoms. The cycle is continued when the trophozoites encyst in the small intestine and water, food, or hands are contaminated by feces of the infected person. Most infections result from fecal-oral transmission or ingestion of contaminated water, less commonly from contaminated food.
System(s) affected: Gastrointestinal
Genetics: N/A
Incidence/Prevalence in USA: 5% of patients with stools submitted for ova and parasite exams. Overall prevalence is lower and variable.
Predominant age: All ages, but most common in early childhood
Predominant sex: Slightly more common in males

SIGNS AND SYMPTOMS
• Approximately 25-50% of infected persons are symptomatic
• Chronic diarrhea (lasting more than 5-7 days and frequently weeks)
• Abdominal bloating
• Flatulence
• Loose, greasy, foul-smelling stools
• Weight loss
• Nausea
• Lactose intolerance

CAUSES   Protozoan parasite (Giardia lamblia) infection acquired through fecal-oral transmission or ingestion of contaminated water, less commonly from contaminated food

RISK FACTORS
• Day care centers
• Male homosexuality
• Wilderness camping

DIAGNOSIS

DIFFERENTIAL DIAGNOSIS
• Includes other etiologies of small intestinal diarrhea
• Infectious causes include cryptosporidiosis, isosporiasis
• Other causes of malabsorption includes celiac sprue, tropical sprue, bacterial overgrowth syndromes, Crohn's ileitis
• Irritable bowel is suspected when diarrhea is not accompanied by weight loss

LABORATORY
• Stool for ova and parasites, repeated 3 times if necessary. Cysts are seen in fixed or fresh stools and occasionally, trophozoites are found in fresh diarrheal stools.
• Fluorescent antibody and ELISA tests of fecal specimens are available
Drugs that may alter lab results: A number of drugs interfere with stool exams
Disorders that may alter lab results: N/A

PATHOLOGICAL FINDINGS   Intestinal biopsy shows flattened, mild lymphocytic infiltration and trophozoites on the surface.

SPECIAL TESTS   String test (Enterotest). A gelatin capsule on a string is swallowed and left in the duodenum for several hours or overnight.

IMAGING   N/A

DIAGNOSTIC PROCEDURES
Esophagogastroduodenoscopy with biopsy and sample of small intestinal fluid.

TREATMENT

APPROPRIATE HEALTH CARE
Outpatient for mild cases, inpatient if symptoms are severe

GENERAL MEASURES
• Medical therapy for all infected individuals
• Fluid replacement if dehydrated

SURGICAL MEASURES   N/A

ACTIVITY   As tolerated

DIET   Good nutrition, low lactose, low fat

PATIENT EDUCATION   Avoidance of risk factors

Giardiasis

MEDICATIONS

DRUG(S) OF CHOICE
• Metronidazole (Flagyl) 250 mg tid for 5-7 days
Contraindications: Both are relatively contraindicated in pregnancy, especially first trimester
Precautions:
• Rare toxic psychosis with quinacrine
• Theoretical risk of carcinogenesis with metronidazole
Significant possible interactions: Occasional disulfiram reaction with metronidazole

ALTERNATIVE DRUGS
• Furazolidone 8 mg/kg/day tid for 10 days (slightly less effective, but commonly used in pediatrics because it is well tolerated)
• Paromomycin (Humatin), a nonabsorbable aminoglycoside which is probably less effective, but commonly recommended in pregnancy because of theoretical risk of teratogenicity of other agents
• Tinidazole is effective when given as a single dose. It is the treatment of choice in much of Europe, but is not available in the US.
• Quinacrine 100 mg tid for 5-7 days. Was the treatment of choice for giardiasis, but is no longer available commercially in the US.
• Albendazole 400 mg daily for 5 days. Antihelminthic drug which is as effective as metronidazole and better tolerated.

FOLLOWUP

PATIENT MONITORING
Symptoms, weight, stool exams

PREVENTION/AVOIDANCE
Good hand washing when caring for diapered children, water purification when camping

POSSIBLE COMPLICATIONS
Those of malabsorption and weight loss

EXPECTED COURSE/PROGNOSIS
Untreated giardiasis lasts for weeks. Patients usually (90%) respond to treatment within a few days and most of the non-responders or relapses respond to a second course with the same or a different agent.

MISCELLANEOUS

ASSOCIATED CONDITIONS
Hypogammaglobulinemia and possibly IgA deficiency. The diarrhea is more severe and prolonged in these patients.

AGE-RELATED FACTORS
Pediatric: Most common in early childhood
Geriatric: N/A
Others: N/A

PREGNANCY
Concern for potential teratogenicity of medications. Consult infectious disease specialist or gastroenterologist for symptomatic disease.

SYNONYMS N/A

ICD-9-CM 007.1 Giardiasis

SEE ALSO N/A

OTHER NOTES
G. lamblia is also called G. duodenalis, G. intestinalis

ABBREVIATIONS N/A

REFERENCES
• Fedorak RN, Rubinoff MJ: Basic Investigation of a Patient with Diarrhea. In: Field M, ed. Diarrheal Diseases. New York, Elsevier Science Publishing Co., Inc., 1991
• Adam R.D: The Biology of Giardia spp. Microbiol, Rev 1991;55:706-732
• Hill DR: Giardia lamblia. In: Mandel GL, Douglas RG, Bennett JE, eds. Principles and Practice of Infectious Diseases. 4th Ed. New York, Churchill Livingstone, 1995
• Ortega I, Adam RD: Giardia: overview and update. In press, Clinical Infectious Dis, 1997
Illustrations: N/A
Internet references: http://www.5mcc.com

Author(s)
Rodney D. Adam, MD

Gilbert's disease

BASICS

DESCRIPTION Mild chronic or intermittent unconjugated hyperbilirubinemia (not due to hemolysis) with otherwise normal liver function
System(s) affected:
Hemic/Lymphatic/Immunologic
Genetics: A gene defect resulting in reduced bilirubin UDP-glucuronosyltransferase-1 appears to be necessary but not sufficient for Gilbert's syndrome.
Incidence/Prevalence in USA: About 7% of the population
Predominant age: Present from birth, but most often presents in the second or third decade of life; heterozygous for single abnormal gene
Predominant sex: Male > Female (2-7:1)

SIGNS AND SYMPTOMS No significant symptoms have been attributed to this disorder, although a variety of nonspecific symptoms have been described. There are no abnormal physical findings other than occasional mild jaundice

CAUSES The hyperbilirubinemia results from impaired hepatic bilirubin clearance (approximately 30% of normal). Hepatic bilirubin conjugation (glucuronidation) is reduced, though this is likely not the only defect.

RISK FACTORS None

DIAGNOSIS

DIFFERENTIAL DIAGNOSIS Hemolysis, ineffective erythropoiesis (megaloblastic anemias, certain porphyrias, thalassemia major, sideroblastic anemia, severe lead poisoning, congenital dyserythropoietic anemias), cirrhosis, chronic persistent hepatitis, pancreatitis or biliary tract disease

LABORATORY
• Bilirubin: less than 6 mg/dL (103 μmol/L) and usually less than 3 mg/dL (51 μmol/L), virtually all unconjugated
• CBC with peripheral smear is normal
• Reticulocyte count is normal
• Liver function tests (SGOT, SGPT, alkaline phosphatase, GGT) are normal
• Fasting and postprandial serum bile acids are normal
• Up to 60% of patients have clinically insignificant mild hemolysis which frequently can only be detected with sophisticated red cell survival studies
Drugs that may alter lab results:
Bilirubin level may be raised by nicotinic acid and lowered by phenobarbital
Disorders that may alter lab results:
Bilirubin levels increase during fasting, and may increase during a febrile illness

PATHOLOGICAL FINDINGS None

SPECIAL TESTS None

IMAGING N/A

DIAGNOSTIC PROCEDURES
• A liver biopsy is not usually needed to exclude other diagnoses
• Some clinicians recommend confirming the diagnosis by reducing daily caloric intake to 400 kcal for 48 hours, which results in a two to threefold increase in unconjugated bilirubin

TREATMENT

APPROPRIATE HEALTH CARE
Outpatient. The most important treatment is to make a positive diagnosis of Gilbert's disease to reassure the patient and prevent further unnecessary procedures

GENERAL MEASURES None

SURGICAL MEASURES N/A

ACTIVITY Full activity

DIET Normal

PATIENT EDUCATION Reassure the patient that the condition is benign with no known sequelae

MEDICATIONS

DRUG(S) OF CHOICE N/A
Contraindications: N/A
Precautions: N/A
Significant possible interactions: N/A

ALTERNATIVE DRUGS N/A

FOLLOWUP

PATIENT MONITORING If history, physical examination, and laboratory tests are normal, see the patient on two or three further occasions during the ensuing 12 to 18 months. If the patient develops no symptoms, reticulocytosis or new liver function abnormalities, make the diagnosis of Gilbert's disease.

PREVENTION/AVOIDANCE N/A

POSSIBLE COMPLICATIONS No known complications

EXPECTED COURSE/PROGNOSIS The disorder is benign with an excellent prognosis

MISCELLANEOUS

ASSOCIATED CONDITIONS Gilbert's disease may be part of a spectrum of hereditary disorders which includes types I and II Crigler-Najjar syndrome

AGE-RELATED FACTORS
Pediatric: It is rare for the disorder to be diagnosed before puberty
Geriatric: N/A
Others: N/A

PREGNANCY The relative fasting that may occur with morning sickness can elevate the bilirubin level

SYNONYMS Gilbert's syndrome

ICD-9-CM 277.4

SEE ALSO
• Crigler-Najjar syndrome

OTHER NOTES N/A

ABBREVIATIONS N/A

REFERENCES
• Okolicsanyi L, Fevery J, Billing B, et al: How should mild, isolated unconjugated hyperbilirubinemia be investigated? Sem Liver Dis 1983;3(1):36-41
• Watson KJR, Gollan JL: Gilbert's syndrome. Bailliere's Clin Gastroenterol 1989;3(2):337-55
• Bosma PJ, Choudhury JR, Bakker C, et al: The genetic basis of the reduced expression of bilirubin UDP-glucuronosyltransferase-1 in Gilbert's syndrome. NEJM 1995;333:1171-5
Illustrations: N/A
Internet references: http://www.5mcc.com

Author(s)
Robert A. Marlow, MD, MA

Gingivitis

BASICS

DESCRIPTION Inflammation of the gingiva, one of the forms of significant oral infections
• Others forms of oral infection:
◊ Periodontitis - progression of gingivitis to connective tissue and alveolar bone
◊ Vincent's angina (trench mouth, necrotizing ulcerative gingivitis, fusospirochetosis) - fusiform bacillus or spirochete infection
◊ Glossitis - inflammation of the tongue (see separate title on this subject)
System(s) affected: Gastrointestinal
Genetics: No known genetic pattern
Incidence/Prevalence: Pandemic, 90% of the population affected
Predominant age: Mostly adult
Predominant sex: Male = Female

SIGNS AND SYMPTOMS
• Mouth odor (bad breath)
• Gum swelling (painless)
• Gum redness
• Change of normal gum contours
• Gum bleeding when flossing or brushing
• Edema of interdental papillae
• Narrow band of bright red inflamed gum surrounding neck of tooth
• Vincent's angina - ulcers, fever, malaise, regional lymphadenopathy, pain

CAUSES
• Noncontagious
• Inadequate plaque removal
• Blood dyscrasias
• Reaction to oral contraceptives
• Vincent's - fusiform bacillus or spirochete infection
• Allergic reactions
• Endocrine disturbances, i.e., pregnancy, menses
• Chronic debilitating disease

RISK FACTORS
• Diabetes mellitus
• Malocclusion
• Poor dental hygiene
• Mouth breathing
• Faulty dental restoration
• HIV positive

DIAGNOSIS

DIFFERENTIAL DIAGNOSIS
• Gingivitis of diabetes mellitus
• Gingivitis of pregnancy
• Desquamative gingivitis
• Gingivitis in leukemia
• Phenytoin gingivitis
• Pericoronitis
• HIV

LABORATORY Smear to identify causative agent
Drugs that may alter lab results: N/A
Disorders that may alter lab results: N/A

PATHOLOGICAL FINDINGS
• Acute or chronic inflammation
• Broken crepuscular epithelium
• Hyperemic capillaries
• Polymorphonuclear infiltration
• Papillary projections in subepithelial tissue
• Fibroblasts

SPECIAL TESTS N/A

IMAGING N/A

DIAGNOSTIC PROCEDURES N/A

TREATMENT

APPROPRIATE HEALTH CARE
Outpatient

GENERAL MEASURES
• Remove irritating factors (plaque, calculus, faulty dentures)
• Good oral hygiene
• Regular dental check-ups
• No smoking
• Warm saline rinses twice daily
• Prophylaxis by dental hygienist

SURGICAL MEASURES N/A

ACTIVITY No restrictions

DIET Assure adequate vitamins and minerals

PATIENT EDUCATION Printed patient information available from: American Dental Association, 211 E. Chicago Avenue, Chicago, IL 60611, (800)621-8099

MEDICATIONS

DRUG(S) OF CHOICE
• Antibiotics, e.g., penicillin V, pediatric dose 25-50 mg/kg/day divided q6h; adult dose 250-500 mg q6h, or
• Erythromycin - pediatric dose 30-40 mg/kg/day divided q6h; adult dose 250 mg q6h
• Topical corticosteroids e.g., triamcinolone in orabase)
Contraindications: Allergy to antibiotics
Precautions: Erythromycin frequently causes significant gastrointestinal upsets
Significant possible interactions: Refer to manufacturer's literature

ALTERNATIVE DRUGS
Other antibiotics according to culture or smear

FOLLOWUP

PATIENT MONITORING
Until clear

PREVENTION/AVOIDANCE
• Good oral hygiene, daily brushing and flossing
• Cleaning by a dentist or hygienist every 6 months or sooner

POSSIBLE COMPLICATIONS
Severe periodontal disease

EXPECTED COURSE/PROGNOSIS
• Usual course - acute; relapsing; intermittent; chronic
• Prognosis - generally favorable, responds well to appropriate treatment

MISCELLANEOUS

ASSOCIATED CONDITIONS
• Periodontitis
• Glossitis

AGE-RELATED FACTORS
Pediatric: Mild cases common in children and usually requires no treatment
Geriatric: More frequent in this age group (due more to lifelong accumulation, rather than increased susceptibility)
Others: N/A

PREGNANCY Characteristics - hyperplasia, pedunculated gingival growths, pyogenic granuloma

SYNONYMS Denture sore mouth

ICD-9-CM 523.1 Chronic gingivitis

SEE ALSO Glossitis

OTHER NOTES N/A

ABBREVIATIONS N/A

REFERENCES Berkow, R., et al. (eds.): Merck Manual, 16th Ed. Rahway, NJ, Merck Sharp & Dohme, 1992
Illustrations: 1 available on CD-ROM
Internet references: http://www.5mcc.com

Author(s)
Thomas Lewis, DDS

Glaucoma, chronic open-angle

BASICS

DESCRIPTION A precise definition of "glaucoma" is difficult to find. It is believed (although not without controversy) that sufficiently high intraocular pressure will result in damage to the optic nerve and ultimately loss of visual field and visual acuity. Glaucoma is a disease of pressure; adequate lowering of intraocular pressure almost always stops optic nerve damage.
• In chronic open-angle glaucoma, aqueous secretion by the ciliary body is normal, and its flow between the lens and the iris through the pupil into the anterior chamber is normal; however, the trabecular meshwork does not permit adequately rapid egress of aqueous with a resultant pressure elevation
System(s) affected: Nervous
Genetics: N/A
Incidence/Prevalence: Glaucoma affects approximately 4% of the population above the age of 40, with over 90% of these glaucomas being COAG
Predominant age: Over age 40, but can occur at any age.
Predominant sex: Male = Female

SIGNS AND SYMPTOMS None, until far advanced; then, gradual painless visual loss

CAUSES
• Impaired outflow through the trabecular meshwork (most common)
• Obstruction to the outflow from Schlemm's canal and the aqueous veins created by elevated orbital venous pressure (as in AV malformations, orbital congestion due to thyroid disease, etc.)
• Too much aqueous secretion (extremely rare)

RISK FACTORS
• Positive family history
• Diabetes mellitus
• African-American ancestry

DIAGNOSIS

DIFFERENTIAL DIAGNOSIS
• Vascular occlusive disease
• Severe anemia
• Hemodynamic crisis in past
• Cerebral neoplasia

LABORATORY N/A
Drugs that may alter lab results: N/A
Disorders that may alter lab results: N/A

PATHOLOGICAL FINDINGS
Ophthalmoscopic - optic nerve head damage

SPECIAL TESTS N/A

IMAGING N/A

DIAGNOSTIC PROCEDURES
• IOP recording - elevated
• Visual field testing - loss
• Characteristic optic nerve damage

TREATMENT

APPROPRIATE HEALTH CARE
Outpatient

GENERAL MEASURES
• Treatment of COAG is directed at lowering the intraocular pressure so that a healthy IOP to optic nerve perfusion pressure gradient is restored
• The disease cannot be cured. Control can be obtained by decreasing the rate of aqueous secretion, by increasing the rate of aqueous outflow, or by a combination of the two.
• Usually medical therapy is able to lower the IOP sufficiently to protect the optic nerve from progressive damage and ultimate visual field damage and visual loss
• Early detection and adequate treatment can prevent visual loss in virtually every case.

SURGICAL MEASURES
• When medical therapy not successful, laser or conventional surgery (trabeculectomy) is indicated.

ACTIVITY No limitations

DIET No special diet

PATIENT EDUCATION
• Necessity for periodic IOP checks and eye exams
• For patient education materials favorably reviewed on this topic, contact:
◊ Foundation for Glaucoma Research, 490 Post Street, Suite 830, San Francisco, CA 94102, (415)986-3162
◊ American Academy of Ophthalmology, 655 Beach Street, San Francisco, CA 94109, (415)561-8500

MEDICATIONS

DRUG(S) OF CHOICE
Medications can be used singly or in combination to achieve the desired reduction of IOP. Begin with a single agent, then add a 2nd or 3rd in a stepwise fashion.
Topical
• Reduction of aqueous secretion
  ◊ Beta-adrenergic blocking agents (timolol, betaxolol, levobunolol, carteolol, metipranolol)
  ◊ Adrenergic agents (epinephrine, and dipivefrin, the "pro-drug" of epinephrine; apraclonidine)
  ◊ Carbonic anhydrase inhibitors (dorzolamide)
• Increase aqueous humor outflow (cholinergic agents)
  ◊ Direct-acting cholinergic agents (pilocarpine, carbamylcholine) "fool" the eye into believing that acetylcholine has been administered
  ◊ Indirect acting cholinergic agents (physostigmine, demecarium bromide, echothiophate iodide, and isoflurophate [DFP]) are all cholinesterase inhibitors
Systemic
• Reduction of aqueous secretion
  ◊ Acetazolamide (Diamox)
  ◊ Dichlorphenamide [sulfonamide]
  ◊ Methazolamide [sulfonamide]

Contraindications:
• The non-selective beta-adrenergic blocking agents (timolol, levobunolol, carteolol, metipranolol) are relatively contraindicated for patients with asthma/obstructive airway disease
• Carbonic-anhydrase inhibitors are contraindicated with history of sensitivity to sulfonamides

Precautions:
• Sympathomimetic agents - used with caution in patients with cardiovascular disease
• Carbonic anhydrase inhibitors - used with caution in patients with a history of nephrolithiasis, myeloproliferative disorders, respiratory acidosis, severely compromised lung capacity, diabetes mellitus, hepatic disease (especially cirrhosis), history of sulfonamide sensitivity
• Beta-adrenergic blocking agents are contraindicated in patients with a history of asthma/COPD, and must be used with caution with patients with marginal cardiac output, bradycardia, and patients using calcium channel blockers.

Significant possible interactions:
• Cholinesterase inhibitors - with the administration of general anesthesia. Should a depolarizing agent such as succinylcholine be used for intubation, these patients will not be able to metabolize this agent and will be respirator-dependent until the systemic activity of cholinesterase is restored, i.e., 3 weeks. Deaths have been reported from this unfortunate complication.
• Carbonic anhydrase inhibitors - may decrease excretion of some drugs (e.g., amphetamines, procainamide, quinidine, tricyclic antidepressants). May potentiate salicylate toxicity secondary to systemic acidosis.
• Beta-adrenergic antagonists have been associated with death in patients also on calcium channel blockers

ALTERNATIVE DRUGS N/A

FOLLOWUP

PATIENT MONITORING
• Every 3-4 months for life
• Chronic carbonic anhydrase inhibitor therapy requires periodic monitoring of the blood count for evidence of reduction in the hemoglobin, hematocrit, and white blood cell count as well as K+ wasting

PREVENTION/AVOIDANCE N/A

POSSIBLE COMPLICATIONS N/A

EXPECTED COURSE/PROGNOSIS
• Lifetime IOP control
• Excellent visual prognosis, unless diagnosis delayed until disorder far advanced or in end-stages

MISCELLANEOUS

ASSOCIATED CONDITIONS Diabetes mellitus

AGE-RELATED FACTORS
Pediatric: N/A
Geriatric: N/A
Others: N/A

PREGNANCY N/A

SYNONYMS Chronic simple glaucoma

ICD-9-CM
365.11 Primary open angle glaucoma
377.14 Glaucomatous atrophy (cupping) of optic disc

SEE ALSO N/A

OTHER NOTES N/A

ABBREVIATIONS
COAG = chronic open-angle glaucoma
IOP = intraocular pressure

REFERENCES Hoskins HD, Kass M, eds: Becker-Shaffer's Diagnosis and Therapy of the Glaucomas. 6th Ed. St. Louis, C.V. Mosby, 1989
Illustrations: N/A
Internet references: http://www.5mcc.com

Author(s)
Barton L. Hodes, MD

Glaucoma, primary angle-closure

BASICS

DESCRIPTION Primary angle-closure glaucoma results from obstruction of aqueous humor outflow through the trabecular meshwork by peripheral iris apposition to the cornea with consequent elevation in intraocular pressure (IOP). The underlying mechanism is pupillary block, in which aqueous egress through the pupil is limited causing forward iris displacement. Angle-closure glaucoma can occur in subacute, acute, and chronic forms and is associated with an anatomically narrow anterior chamber angle; the angle comprises the peripheral iris, anterior ciliary body, trabecular meshwork, and peripheral cornea and can only be observed with a special examination technique called gonioscopy. In its acute form, primary angle-closure glaucoma is an ophthalmic emergency with a natural history of severe visual loss.
System(s) affected: Nervous
Genetics: Polygenic inheritance; first degree relatives have a 2-5% lifetime risk
Incidence/Prevalence in USA:
• 100 cases/100,000 population
• 500/100,000 (Blacks and Asians more common than Caucasians)
Predominant Age: 55-70
Predominant Sex: Female > Male

SIGNS AND SYMPTOMS
• Subacute
  ◊ Dull ache in or around one eye
  ◊ Mildly blurred vision
  ◊ Symptoms occur when watching TV or movies in dark room, reading, or when fatigued. Relieved by sleep or rest.
  ◊ Normal intraocular pressure (10-23 mmHg)
  ◊ Shallow anterior chamber
  ◊ Iris bombé
  ◊ Intermittent peripheral anterior synechiae
  ◊ Enlarged pupil
• Acute
  ◊ Ocular pain
  ◊ Blurred vision
  ◊ Lacrimation
  ◊ Halos around lights
  ◊ Frontal headache
  ◊ Nausea and vomiting
  ◊ Symptoms likely to occur with times of emotional stress and with activities as for subacute form
  ◊ Elevated intraocular pressure (usually 40-80 mm Hg)
  ◊ Corneal microcystic edema
  ◊ Lid edema, conjunctival hyperemia, and circumcorneal injection
  ◊ Fixed mid-dilated pupil, often oval
  ◊ Shallow anterior chamber often with inflammatory reaction
• Chronic
  ◊ May have symptoms of subacute form or may be asymptomatic
  ◊ Multiple peripheral anterior synechiae
  ◊ Normal or elevated intraocular pressure
  ◊ Increased cup to disc ratio
  ◊ Normal pupil

CAUSES Predisposing ocular anatomy

RISK FACTORS
• Small cornea
• Hyperopia
• Shallow anterior chamber
• Eskimo ancestry
• Female sex
• Use of antidepressants or other drugs with cholinergic inhibition
• Cataract
• Iris and ciliary body cysts

DIAGNOSIS

DIFFERENTIAL DIAGNOSIS
• Neovascular glaucoma
• Absolute glaucoma
• Malignant glaucoma
• Plateau iris syndrome
• Miotic induced glaucoma
• Phacomorphic glaucoma
• Anterior uveitis

LABORATORY None
Drugs that may alter lab results: N/A
Disorders that may alter lab results: N/A

PATHOLOGICAL FINDINGS
• Corneal stromal and epithelial edema
• Endothelial cell loss
• Iris stromal necrosis
• Anterior subcapsular cataract (glaukomflecken)
• Optic disc congestion, cupping
• Optic nerve atrophy

SPECIAL TESTS Gonioscopy

IMAGING N/A

DIAGNOSTIC PROCEDURES Careful ophthalmic examination including indentation gonioscopy and tonometry

TREATMENT

APPROPRIATE HEALTH CARE
• For acute form - inpatient admission from office or emergency room
• Other forms - outpatient
• Ophthalmology consultation

GENERAL MEASURES
• For acute form
  ◊ Intravenous access for administering medications is helpful, antiemetics may be necessary
  ◊ Definitive treatment is laser iridotomy once the attack is broken, intraocular pressure has normalized, and intraocular inflammation has subsided

SURGICAL MEASURES
• Peripheral iridectomy
• Argon or Nd:YAG laser iridotomy (procedure of choice for subacute and chronic forms)
• Argon laser genioplasty

ACTIVITY For acute form - bedrest until attack subsides

DIET Usual for patient

PATIENT EDUCATION
• Usually patients need bilateral treatment since second eye is at risk for same disease process
• For patient education materials favorably reviewed on this topic, contact:
  ◊ Foundation for Glaucoma Research, 490 Post Street, Suite 830, San Francisco, CA 94102, (415)986-3162
  ◊ American Academy of Ophthalmology, 655 Beach Street, San Francisco, CA 94109, (415)561-8500

MEDICATIONS

DRUG(S) OF CHOICE
• For acute form: (a combination of the following)
◊ Hyperosmotic agents - oral 50% glycerin 0.1-1.5 g/kg or oral isosorbide dinitrate 1.5-2.0 g/kg, and/or intravenous mannitol 20% 1-2 g/kg over 45 minutes
◊ Carbonic anhydrase inhibition - acetazolamide (Diamox) 500 mg IV plus 500 mg po, then 250 mg po q6h prn; dorzolamide 2% eyedrops q8h.
Note: Use of the intravenous and oral agents above is sometimes necessary prior to the use of eye drops in order to lower the IOP enough to permit intraocular penetration.
◊ Beta-blockers - timolol (Timoptic) 0.5% q12h or levobunolol (Betagan) 0.5% q12h or betaxolol (Betoptic) 0.5% q12h
◊ Miotics - pilocarpine 2-4% one dose. In complicated cases with multiple mechanisms, miotics may paradoxically worsen the condition. Hence, they must be used with caution. See Contraindications.
◊ Corticosteroid - prednisolone acetate (Pred Forte) 1% q4-6h
◊ Other - apraclonidine (Iopidine) 0.5% or 1% q8h; also, latanoprost (Xalatan) 0.005% q24h
• For subacute and chronic forms:
◊ Treatment is surgical
Contraindications: With history of recent intraocular surgery, possibility of malignant glaucoma is increased and miotics may be contraindicated
Precautions:
• Timolol, levobunolol, and betaxolol, use with caution in patients with chronic heart failure or chronic obstructive pulmonary disease
• Mannitol, use with caution in patients with chronic heart failure or renal failure
• Acetazolamide, use with caution in patients with history of nephrolithiasis or metabolic acidosis
Significant possible interactions:
Acetazolamide may accelerate potassium loss and metabolic acidosis in patients on other diuretics

ALTERNATIVE DRUGS As above

FOLLOWUP

PATIENT MONITORING
• Subacute and chronic forms, check tonometry and gonioscopy initially every 3 months after laser iridotomy, follow visual fields every 6-12 months
• Acute form, discharge after laser iridotomy and intraocular pressure are controlled and follow as with the chronic form
• Consider frequent serum electrolytes while on mannitol
• Semi-annual CBC while on acetazolamide

PREVENTION/AVOIDANCE Prophylactic laser treatment of second eye

POSSIBLE COMPLICATIONS
• Chronic corneal edema
• Corneal fibrosis and vascularization
• Iris atrophy
• Cataract
• Lens subluxation
• Optic atrophy
• Malignant glaucoma
• Central retinal vein occlusion

EXPECTED COURSE/PROGNOSIS
• Varies with delay of patient presentation and severity of attack
• Preceding chronic angle-closure may have caused optic atrophy
• Recurrence is quite rare following peripheral iridotomy or iridectomy and implies a rare variant known as the iris plateau syndrome

MISCELLANEOUS

ASSOCIATED CONDITIONS
• Cataract
• Microphthalmos
• Hyperopia

AGE-RELATED FACTORS
Pediatric: Rare
Geriatric: Secondary angle closure glaucoma can be caused by many common eye conditions in the elderly including cataract, ocular surgery and diabetes
Others: N/A

PREGNANCY N/A

SYNONYMS
• Acute glaucoma
• Narrow angle glaucoma

ICD-9-CM
• 365.20 Primary angle-closure glaucoma, unspecified
• 365.02 Borderline glaucoma, anatomical narrow angle

SEE ALSO Glaucoma, chronic open-angle

OTHER NOTES
• Medications (higher risk) that may exacerbate angle-closure glaucoma:
◊ Systemic or topical anticholinergics
◊ Topical sympathomimetics
◊ Antihistamines
◊ Phenothiazines
◊ Antidepressants
• Medications (lower risk) that may exacerbate angle-closure glaucoma:
◊ Benzodiazepine
◊ Carbonic anhydrase inhibitors
◊ CNS stimulants (including cocaine)
◊ MAO inhibitors
◊ Systemic sympathomimetics
◊ Theophylline
◊ Vasodilators

ABBREVIATIONS
NAG = narrow angle glaucoma

REFERENCES
• Ritch R, Shields MB, Krupin T: The Glaucomas. St. Louis, C.V. Mosby, 1989
• Fraunfelder FT, Roy FH: Current Ocular Therapy 3. 3rd Ed. Philadelphia, W.B. Saunders Co., 1990
Illustrations: N/A
Internet references: http://www.5mcc.com

Author(s)
Robert G. Fante, MD

Glomerulonephritis, acute

BASICS

DESCRIPTION An immunologic response to an infection (usually streptococcal) which damages the renal glomeruli. It can be initiated by other bacterial and viral infections. This is an immune complex, hypocomplementemic glomerulonephritis. Most common in children. Characterized by diffuse inflammatory changes in the glomeruli and clinically by the abrupt onset of hematuria with red blood cell casts, and mild proteinuria. Accompanied in many cases by hypertension, edema, and azotemia.
System(s) affected: Renal/Urologic
Genetics: No known genetic pattern
Incidence/Prevalence in USA:
20/100,000/year (1-2% of pyoderms and 8% of streptococcal infections in children; occurs with impetigo in the late summer and with streptococcal pharyngitis in the winter)
Predominant age:
• 60% of cases in children 2-12 years old
• Only 10% older than 40 years of age
Predominant sex: Male > Female (60:40)

SIGNS AND SYMPTOMS
• Classic findings of acute nephritis
  ◊ Hematuria (100%)
  ◊ Oligoanuria (52%)
  ◊ Edema (85%)
  ◊ Hypertension (82%)
  ◊ Hypocomplementemia (C3) (83%)
  ◊ Gross hematuria (30%), tea-colored urine
  ◊ Edema of face and eyes in the am and feet and ankles in the afternoons and evenings
  ◊ Fever (rare)
• Other signs and symptoms
  ◊ Pharyngitis
  ◊ Respiratory infection
  ◊ Scarlet fever
  ◊ Dark urine
  ◊ Weight gain
  ◊ Abdominal pain
  ◊ Anorexia
  ◊ Back pain
  ◊ Pallor
  ◊ Impetigo

CAUSES
• Follows group A beta-hemolytic streptococcus infection
• "Nephritogenic" strains of strep - groups 1, 4, 11, 12, 49 "Red Lake", 55, 60
• Unusual to have a second attack - protective immunity to nephritogenic antigen
• Cases of "postinfective" glomerulonephritis have also been reported from pneumococcus, staphylococcus, meningococcus, chickenpox, and hepatitis
• Streptococcal infection precedes renal lesions by 1-3 weeks
• Pharyngitis precedes renal lesions by 1-2 weeks (types 1, 2, 4, 12)
• Impetigo - (types 49, 55, 57) usually precedes throat or otitis media infection by 2-4 weeks

RISK FACTORS
• 15% occurrence rate after infection with nephritogenic strain
• Endemic with cyclic epidemics
• Subclinical cases 20 times more common
• Streptococcal infection (e.g., scarlet fever or erysipelas) can be associated with rheumatic fever or acute glomerulonephritis, rarely both

DIAGNOSIS

DIFFERENTIAL DIAGNOSIS
• Membranoproliferative glomerulonephritis
• Other postinfective glomerulonephritis
• Systemic lupus erythematosus
• IgA nephropathy
• Anaphylactoid purpura
• Rapidly progressive glomerulonephritis

LABORATORY
• Streptococcal tests (Streptozyme) that include many antigens are most sensitive (+ or -) for screening but not quantitative
• Antistreptolysin O (ASO) - quantitative titer. Increased in 60-80% of cases. Increase begins 1-3 weeks, is highest 3-5 weeks, normal in 6 months. ASO titer is unrelated to severity, duration or prognosis of renal disease.
• Red blood cells casts on urinalysis:
  ◊ destroyed by centrifugation
  ◊ disintegrate in urine, particularly alkaline urine
• Characteristically, red blood cells from glomerular bleeding are distorted while those from lower urinary tract have normal morphology
• U/P creatinine > 40, decreased renin
• Culture throat and skin lesions for streptococcus
• C3 and C4 complements are best for evaluation
• Streptozyme
• Hypertriglyceridemia
• Proteinuria
• Decreased glomerular filtration rate
• Uremia
• Increased serum creatinine
• Anemia
• ANA to rule out systemic lupus erythematosus
Drugs that may alter lab results: N/A
Disorders that may alter lab results: N/A

PATHOLOGICAL FINDINGS
• On renal biopsy
  ◊ Diffuse proliferative and exudative glomerulonephritis
  ◊ Electron microscopy - subepithelial deposits
  ◊ Immunofluorescence - C3 in almost all cases, some with IgG and IgM

SPECIAL TESTS N/A

IMAGING X-rays and/or ultrasound are not necessary to make the diagnosis

DIAGNOSTIC PROCEDURES
• If progressive, consider renal biopsy. Biopsy usually not indicated.

TREATMENT

APPROPRIATE HEALTH CARE
• Most patients can be safely followed as outpatients
• Inpatient usually until blood pressure and creatinine normalized and edema begins to recede

GENERAL MEASURES
• Decrease salt: no-added salt diet until edema and hypertension clear
• Decrease fluids to insensible losses plus 2/3 of the urine output until diuresis
• Control hypertension with diuretics
• Dialysis: peritoneal dialysis or hemodialysis for symptomatic azotemia, unresponsive hyperkalemia, intractable acidosis, diuretic resistant pulmonary edema

SURGICAL MEASURES N/A

ACTIVITY Can return to full activity after clinically improved. May have increased hematuria after exercise for up to two years.

DIET
• "No-added" salt diet until edema, hypertension, and azotemia clear
• Restrict protein in presence of azotemia and metabolic acidosis
• Avoid high potassium foods

PATIENT EDUCATION National Kidney Foundation, 30 E. 33rd Street, Suite 1100, New York, NY 10016, (212)889-2210

MEDICATIONS

DRUG(S) OF CHOICE
• Hyperkalemia
◊ No potassium in IV fluids until hyperkalemia resolves
◊ Sodium polystyrene sulfonate (Kayexalate) resin: 1 gm/kg in 10% sorbitol, pr or po
◊ If acidosis present, treat as indicated below
◊ Hypocalcemia with symptomatic hyperkalemia: 0.5 cc/kg 10% calcium gluconate IV over 30 minutes
◊ Hypocalcemia with asymptomatic hyperkalemia: oral calcium carbonate (Tums) 1-2 gm calcium/day. (Tums have 650 mg calcium/tablet)
• Pulmonary edema
◊ Oxygen
◊ Furosemide (Lasix)
◊ Digitalization is not effective
• Peripheral edema
◊ Furosemide 1-2 mg/kg/dose given bid-tid po or IV
◊ Treatment with diuretics decreases the duration and severity of edema and hypertension
• Acidosis
◊ Sodium bicarbonate 1-2 mEq/kg/dose (1-2 mmol/kg/dose) IV over 30 minutes to correct acidosis
• Strep infection
◊ Give penicillin for 10 days (po if possible)
◊ Erythromycin in penicillin allergic patients
• Hypertension
◊ Control with diuretics (furosemide 0.5-1 mg/kg IV or 2 mg/kg po bid or tid) and vasodilators (hydralazine [Apresoline] 0.25-1.0 mg/kg qid or nifedipine 0.25 mg/kg po prn or qid)
Contraindications: Refer to manufacturer's literature
Precautions: Refer to manufacturer's literature
Significant possible interactions: Refer to manufacturer's literature

ALTERNATIVE DRUGS N/A

FOLLOWUP

PATIENT MONITORING
• Depends on severity of disease
• Urinalysis at 2, 4 and 8 weeks and 4, 6 and 12 months
• Stop followup when urinalysis is normal
• Monitor blood pressure each visit
• Monitor serum creatinine at 2, 6, and 12 months
• C3 complement should be normal by 6 weeks

PREVENTION/AVOIDANCE Treat streptococcal infections aggressively

POSSIBLE COMPLICATIONS
• Hypertensive retinopathy
• Hypertensive encephalopathy
• Rapidly progressive glomerulonephritis
• Abnormal urinalysis may persist for years (microhematuria)
• Chronic renal failure (rare)
• Nephrotic syndrome (approximately 10%)
• Marked decline in glomerular filtration rate (rare)

EXPECTED COURSE/PROGNOSIS
• Usually self-limited to 2-3 weeks
• Immediate mortality < 0.5%
• Long-term: excellent in children; almost all patients recover completely.
• May have more morbidity in adults or in those with pre-existing renal lesions
• Microscopic hematuria may persist for 24 months (or longer with complete recovery)
• Proteinuria persists for up to 3 months
• Symptoms can be exacerbated by a intercurrent illness but rarely after 12 months
• Urine may be darker (microscopic hematuria) after strenuous exercise

MISCELLANEOUS

ASSOCIATED CONDITIONS N/A

AGE-RELATED FACTORS
Pediatric: Common in children ages 2-16
Geriatric: N/A
Others: N/A

PREGNANCY N/A

SYNONYMS
• Acute nephritic syndrome
• Postinfectious glomerulonephritis
• Acute post-streptococcal glomerulonephritis

ICD-9-CM
580 Glomerulonephritis, acute

SEE ALSO
• Glomerulonephritis, membranous
• Hyperkalemia
• Renal failure, acute
• Hypocalcemia
• Hypertensive emergencies

OTHER NOTES N/A

ABBREVIATIONS N/A

REFERENCES
• Brenner B, Rector F: The Kidney. 5th Ed. Philadelphia, W.B. Saunders Co., 1995
• Holliday M., Barratt T, Avner E: Pediatric Nephrology. 3rd Ed. Baltimore, Williams & Wilkins, 1993
Illustrations: N/A
Internet references: http://www.5mcc.com

Author(s)
Watson C. Arnold, MD

Glossitis

BASICS

DESCRIPTION Acute or chronic inflammation of the tongue either as a primary disease or symptom of systemic disease
System(s) affected: Gastrointestinal
Genetics: N/A
Incidence/Prevalence in USA: Common
Predominant age: All ages
Predominant sex: Male > Female

SIGNS AND SYMPTOMS
• Reddened tip and edges of tongue (with pellagra, anemia, excess smoking)
• Fiery red, swollen, ulcerated tongue (pellagra)
• Tongue smooth and pale (anemias)
• Ulcers (herpetic or aphthous lesions, streptococcal infection, erythema multiforme, pemphigus)
• White patches (candidiasis, syphilis, leukoplakia, lichen planus, mouth breathing)
• Denuded smooth areas (geographic tongue)
• Painful tongue (anemia, pellagra, viral)
• Hairy tongue (follows antibiotic therapy, fever or excessive use of mouthwashes with peroxide)
• Tenderness, pain, swelling of the tongue (infections or trauma)
• Burning, painful tongue (candidiasis, anemia, diabetes, malignancies)
• Non-painful solitary ulcerations (malignancy)
• Painful combination of ulcers, nodules, linear fissures (herpetic geometric glossitis in HIV)
• Malignancy - painless red and/or white lesions

CAUSES
• Systemic:
  ◊ Malnutrition with avitaminosis (e.g., B group)
  ◊ Anemia (pernicious, iron deficiency)
  ◊ Skin diseases (e.g., lichen planus, erythema multiforme, aphthous lesions, Behçet's syndrome, pemphigus vulgaris, syphilis)
  ◊ HIV (candidiasis, HSV, loss of papillae)
• Local:
  ◊ Infections (viral, candidiasis, tuberculosis, streptococcal)
  ◊ Trauma (ill-fitting dentures, burns, convulsive seizures)
  ◊ Primary irritants (alcohol, tobacco, hot foods, spices, excessive peppermint, citrus)
  ◊ Sensitization (chemical irritants, e.g., dyes, mouth wash, toothpaste, systemic drugs)
  ◊ Malignancy

RISK FACTORS
• Low socioeconomic status
• Poor nutrition
• Dentures
• Smoking
• Smokeless tobacco
• Alcoholism
• Anxiety, stress
• Depression
• Advancing age
• Immunocompromised state

DIAGNOSIS

DIFFERENTIAL DIAGNOSIS
• Systemic:
  ◊ Avitaminosis (particularly B group, e.g., pellagra)
  ◊ Anemia (pernicious, iron deficiency)
  ◊ Skin diseases (e.g., lichen planus, erythema multiforme, aphthous lesions, Behçet's syndrome, pemphigus vulgaris, syphilis)
  ◊ HIV
• Local:
  ◊ Infections (viral, candidiasis, tuberculosis, streptococcal)
  ◊ Trauma (ill-fitting dentures, burns, convulsive seizures)
  ◊ Primary irritants: alcohol, tobacco, hot foods, spices
  ◊ Sensitization (chemical irritants, e.g., dyes, mouth wash, toothpaste, systemic drugs)
  ◊ Malignancy (95% are squamous cell)
  ◊ Geographic tongue (also known as migratory glossitis) - benign, but recurrent

LABORATORY
• CBC
• Serologic tests for syphilis
• Chemical profile
• Tests for vitamin B12 deficiency
• Postprandial glucose
• Smear and culture lesions when indicated
Drugs that may alter lab results: N/A
Disorders that may alter lab results: N/A

PATHOLOGICAL FINDINGS Varies
according to underlying causes

SPECIAL TESTS
• Biopsy solitary lesions that do not respond to treatment in one week
• 10% KOH scrapings for suspected candidiasis

IMAGING N/A

DIAGNOSTIC PROCEDURES
• Biopsy
• KOH scrapings

TREATMENT

APPROPRIATE HEALTH CARE
Outpatient

GENERAL MEASURES
• Avoid any possible sensitizing irritants or agents
• Specific therapy for oral infections (see Medications)
• Local treatment (see Medications)
• Analgesics when needed
• Request dental evaluation
• Scrupulous oral hygiene

SURGICAL MEASURES N/A

ACTIVITY No restrictions unless there is a systemic infection

DIET Bland or liquid diet

PATIENT EDUCATION Griffith: Instructions for Patients; Philadelphia, W.B. Saunders Co. 5th ed., 1994

MEDICATIONS

DRUG(S) OF CHOICE
• For candidiasis:
◊ Nystatin oral suspension 400,000 units (4 mL) to 600,000 units qid for 10 days as an oral rinse, then swallowed
• For oral infections:
◊ Oral penicillin V
◊ Multivitamins (vitamin B-complex, vitamin E)
◊ Iron (if deficient)
• Local treatment:
◊ Mouth rinse with 2% lidocaine viscous, 1 tablespoon before each meal and every 3 hours if needed for pain
◊ Mouth wash of 1/2 teaspoon sodium bicarbonate in 8 oz (240 mL) warm water qid
◊ Mouth rinse with carbamide peroxide (Gly-Oxide) 10% 0.5 mL or 10 drops qid (expectorate after use) for irritation, aphthous ulcers
◊ Triamcinolone (Kenalog) in dental paste (Orabase): Compound triamcinolone 0.1% in emollient dental paste applied to specific lesions, especially aphthous ulcers
◊ 50/50 mixture of kaolin-pectin and diphenhydramine (Benadryl) as mouth rinse (coats and topically anesthetizes)
Contraindications: Refer to manufacturer's literature
Precautions: Depressed gag reflex with lidocaine viscous. Decreased sensitivity to hot/cold liquids.
Significant possible interactions: Refer to manufacturer's literature

ALTERNATIVE DRUGS
• For candidiasis:
◊ Clotrimazole - 10 mg oral lozenges 5 times a day for 10 days
or
◊ Ketoconazole - one 200 mg tablet (for children 1/4 tablet) orally once a day

FOLLOWUP

PATIENT MONITORING
• Re-visits periodically when needed until healing occurs
• If lesions do not heal, biopsy is indicated

PREVENTION/AVOIDANCE
• Evaluation of nutritional status including B-vitamin deficiencies, anemias
• Cessation of tobacco use (including "smokeless")
• Assess for irritation from teeth, dentures

POSSIBLE COMPLICATIONS
• Lymphadenopathy
• Chronicity

EXPECTED COURSE/PROGNOSIS
• Prompt improvement when cause can be identified and treated
• Aphthous ulcers, erythema multiforme and hairy tongue often recur

MISCELLANEOUS

ASSOCIATED CONDITIONS
• Diabetes mellitus
• HIV infection

AGE-RELATED FACTORS
Pediatric: Median rhomboid glossitis is a developmental lesion causing a rhomboid-shaped, smooth, reddish, nodular area on the dorsal surface of the back portion of the middle third of the tongue. This type of glossitis is innocuous and requires no treatment.
Geriatric: Many patients with glossitis are postmenopausal or elderly
Others: N/A

PREGNANCY N/A

SYNONYMS N/A

ICD-9-CM 529 Glossitis

SEE ALSO
• HIV infection & AIDS
• Vitamin deficiency
• Candidiasis

OTHER NOTES Some symptoms of glossitis have no organic cause. Treat symptoms and reassure regarding malignancy.

ABBREVIATIONS N/A

REFERENCES
• Pondborg JJ: Atlas of Diseases of the Oral Mucosa. 4th Ed. Philadelphia, W.B. Saunders Co., 1986
• Scully C, et al: Oral manifestations of HIV-infection and their management: More common lesions. Oral Surg, Oral Med & Oral Path 1991;71:158-166
• Nally F: Diseases of the Tongue. The Practitioner (Brit) 1991;235:65-71
• Cohen PR, et al: Geometric glossitis. Southern Med Jour 1995;88(12):1231-1235
• Kretzschmar JL, Kretzschmar DP: Common oral conditions. Amer Fam Phys 1996;54(1):225-234
Illustrations: 1 available on CD-ROM
Internet references: http://www.5mcc.com

Author(s)
J. Randall Richard, MD

Gonococcal infections

BASICS

DESCRIPTION Gonorrhea is a purulent inflammation of mucous membrane surfaces caused by a sexually transmitted microorganism, Neisseria gonorrhoeae. Virtually any mucous membrane can be infected. Occasionally the organism may become blood-borne causing a syndrome comprised of combinations of any of the following features: Fever, skin lesions, arthralgias/tenosynovitis, and septic arthritis.
• Hematogenous dissemination may also lead to endocarditis, or rarely, meningitis
• In women, salpingitis, local extension from the endocervical canal to the fallopian tubes is common. The ovaries may be involved with abscess formation. The entire complex of upper genital tract infection in women is referred to as pelvic inflammatory disease (PID).
• In men, the epididymis may become infected with extension to the testicle
• An asymptomatic carrier state can occur in both sexes
System(s) affected: Reproductive, Musculoskeletal, Nervous, Cardiovascular, Skin/Exocrine
Genetics: Individuals with congenital deficiency of the late components of the complement cascade (C 7,8,9) are prone to develop dissemination of local gonococcal infections
Incidence/Prevalence in USA: In 1992 - 204/100,000 people
Predominant age: 15-29
Predominant sex: Male > Female (symptomatic disease)

SIGNS AND SYMPTOMS
• Adolescent and adult males:
  ◊ Scant to copious purulent urethral discharge (98%)
  ◊ Dysuria (98%)
  ◊ Testicular pain (1%)
  ◊ Asymptomatic urethral infection (incidence of about 1%)
  ◊ Urethral stricture
• Adolescent and adult females without PID:
  ◊ Asymptomatic cervical infection (approximately 20%)
  ◊ Endocervical discharge (on pelvic exam) (96%)
  ◊ Vaginal discharge
  ◊ Dysuria
  ◊ Bartholin's gland abscess
• Adolescent and adult females with PID:
  ◊ Dysmenorrhea
  ◊ Metromenorrhagia
  ◊ Lower abdominal pain and tenderness
  ◊ Fever
  ◊ Cervical traction tenderness
  ◊ Palpable, tender fallopian tubes and/or ovaries
  ◊ Abdominal rebound tenderness
  ◊ Infertility
  ◊ Chronic pelvic pain

• Either sex, if receptive partner in anal intromission:
  ◊ Rectal discharge: purulent or bloody
  ◊ Tenesmus
  ◊ Rectal burning or itching
  ◊ Asymptomatic rectal infection
• Either sex, other syndromes:
  ◊ Pharyngeal infection - asymptomatic infection (98%), sore throat, exudative pharyngitis (< 1%)
  ◊ Eye infection (rare) - purulent discharge, conjunctivitis, chemosis, eyelid edema, corneal ulceration
  ◊ Disseminated syndromes - fever; chills; arthralgias (small joints); synovial sheath tenderness and swelling (hands and/or feet); painful skin lesions (pustular, red, tender); septic arthritis (usually asymmetric, polyarticular, and mainly involving elbows, knees and more distal joints; manifested by joint pain, swelling, erythema, and induration)
  ◊ Endocarditis - rapid cardiac valve destruction, high fevers
  ◊ Meningitis - meningeal signs, headache, skin lesions, fever, altered mental status
• Infants and children
  ◊ Eye infection (rare - because of routine ocular prophylaxis in the USA)
  ◊ Pneumonia (of the newborn) - fever, infiltrate on chest x-ray
  ◊ Vulvovaginitis - vaginal discharge
  ◊ Rectal infection
  ◊ Pharyngeal infection
  ◊ Meningitis
  ◊ Other forms of disseminated infection - fever, chills, arthralgias, synovial sheath tenderness and swelling, skin lesions, septic arthritis, endocarditis

CAUSES Neisseria gonorrhoeae (gonococcus)

RISK FACTORS
• Sexual exposure to an infected individual without barrier protection (condom)
• Multiple sexual partners
• Infant - passage through the infected birth canal of the mother
• Children - sexual abuse by infected individual
• Auto-inoculation (finger to eye)
• For PID - use of intrauterine devices

DIAGNOSIS

DIFFERENTIAL DIAGNOSIS
• Chlamydia infections (may mimic all aspects of gonococcal infections except disseminated syndromes)
• Urinary tract infections
• Vaginitis caused by other infectious agents (yeast, trichomonas, bacterial vaginosis)

LABORATORY
• Gram stain of exudate from infected mucosal surface
• Demonstration of pairs or clumps of Gram-negative kidney-shaped diplococci associated with the cytoplasm of polymorphonuclear leukocytes. The adjacent surfaces are slightly concave.
• Sensitivity of urethral smear in symptomatic male ≥95%
• Sensitivity of endocervical smear in infected woman = 40-60%
• Culture of exudate on selective medium (Thayer-Martin or Martin-Lewis, containing antibiotics to inhibit other microorganisms). Demonstration of typical organisms by Gram-stain morphology and growth on selective media constitutes a "presumptive" diagnosis of gonococcal infection. Culture should always be done in women because of low sensitivity of the smear, and in suspected cases of child abuse.
• Sensitivity of blood culture in disseminated disease - 50%
• Sensitivity of joint fluid culture in septic arthritis - 50%
Drugs that may alter lab results: Prior administration of even small amounts of many commonly available antibiotics may render a culture falsely negative
Disorders that may alter lab results: N/A

PATHOLOGICAL FINDINGS
• Exudate consisting of polymorphonuclear leukocytes is typical
• In PID - loss of ciliated columnar epithelium from the fallopian tubes. Tubes, pelvic mesentery, and ovaries may be bound together with dense fibrosis and abscess formation.

SPECIAL TESTS
• Confirmation of the isolate as the gonococcus by standard sugar fermentation tests, enzymatic tests or DNA probes. Important in medicolegal situations such as rape or child abuse since other Neisseria, which are normal inhabitants of mucosal surfaces, may look like gonococcus on Gram-stained smear.
• Testing for antimicrobial susceptibility. ß-lactamase production and chromosomally mediated resistance to penicillin and/or tetracycline are becoming more common. Although routine ß-lactamase testing of N. gonorrhoeae has been recommended by the U.S. Public Health Service, the need for such routine testing is questionable if current therapy guidelines are observed.

IMAGING Pelvic ultrasound or CT scan may demonstrate thick, dilated fallopian tubes or abscess formation

DIAGNOSTIC PROCEDURES
• Culdocentesis may demonstrate free purulent exudate, and provide material for gram staining and culture
• Gram staining material from unroofed skin lesions of disseminated disease may sometimes show typical organisms

Gonococcal infections

TREATMENT

APPROPRIATE HEALTH CARE
• Outpatient for uncomplicated infection, with contact notification and contact treatment
• Hospitalization for hematogenously disseminated infection
• Hospitalization for pneumonia or eye infection in infants
• Hospitalization for women with PID if they cannot take oral medications, if significant tubo-ovarian abscess is present or if the patient is pregnant

GENERAL MEASURES
• Abstain from sexual activity until after followup examination, plus testing and treatment of partner(s)
• Serologic test for syphilis
• Encouragement to obtain testing for HIV infection

SURGICAL MEASURES N/A

ACTIVITY Fully active for uncomplicated disease

DIET No special diet

PATIENT EDUCATION
• Discuss sexually transmitted diseases and methods of prevention
• Discuss HIV infection and risks; encourage patient and partner(s) to be tested

MEDICATIONS

DRUG(S) OF CHOICE
Treatment of adults:
• Uncomplicated N. gonorrhoeae infection of urethra, cervix, rectum, and/or pharynx: Initial single dose of ceftriaxone 125 mg IM or cefixime 400 mg po or ofloxacin 400 mg po or ciprofloxacin 500 mg po plus an agent with activity against chlamydia, e.g., doxycycline 100 mg po bid x 7 days or azithromycin 1.0 g po as a single dose
Note: In pregnancy, ceftriaxone is the treatment of choice. Erythromycin 500 mg po qid x 7 days is an alternative anti-chlamydia agent for use in pregnancy. In the absence of pregnancy, ofloxacin 300 mg po bid x 7 days is another alternative anti-chlamydia therapy. Alternative parenteral agents for therapy of gonococcal infections include other 3rd generation cephalosporins and spectinomycin.
• PID - outpatients regimens (see citations for treatment of hospitalized patients)
  ◊ Regimen A: Cefoxitin 2g IM + probenecid 1g po or ceftriaxone 250 mg IM plus doxycycline 100 mg po bid x 14 days
  ◊ Regimen B: Ofloxacin 400 mg po bid x 14 days plus clindamycin 450 mg po qid x 14 days or metronidazole 500 mg po bid x 14 days

• Disseminated infections
  ◊ Dermatitis-arthritis complex: Initiate therapy with ceftriaxone 1g IV daily. With clinical improvement, complete of 7-10 days of therapy with cefixime 400 mg po bid, ciprofloxacin 500 mg po bid, or other agents to which the infecting organism has been proven fully susceptible.
  ◊ Meningitis: Ceftriaxone 1-2g IV q 12 hours for 10-14 days
  ◊ Endocarditis: Ceftriaxone 1-2g IV q 12 hours for 4 weeks
Note: Parenteral penicillin G can be used to treat disseminated infection if full susceptibility is documented. Other third generation cephalosporins also can be substituted for ceftriaxone for parenteral therapy.
• Sex contacts of persons with gonococcal infections should undergo clinical evaluation and undergo treatment comparable to that recommended for uncomplicated infection
Treatment of infants and children < 45 kg:
(Patients >45 kg should receive adult dosing)
• Uncomplicated genital, pharyngeal, rectal, or conjunctival infection and infants born to mothers with untreated gonorrhea
  ◊ Ceftriaxone 25-50 mg/kg IV or IM in single daily dose x 7 days; 10-14 days in the setting of meningitis; 4 weeks in the setting of endocarditis
  ◊ Cefotaxime 25 mg/kg IV or IM q 12 hours for comparable durations
Contraindications: Fluoroquinolones and tetracyclines such as doxycycline are contraindicated in pregnancy
Precautions: Refer to manufacturer's profile of each drug
Significant possible interactions: Refer to manufacturer's profile of each drug

ALTERNATIVE DRUGS If organisms are not penicillin-resistant, IV aqueous crystalline penicillin G may be substituted for IV cephalosporins in complicated disease. (Note: Some penicillin resistance is now due to penicillinase production.) Oral ampicillin or amoxicillin plus probenecid may be substituted for cephalosporins in uncomplicated disease, also after laboratory confirmation of absence of resistance to penicillin.

FOLLOWUP

PATIENT MONITORING Retesting to document cure is not necessary if one of the recommended regimens is used unless symptoms persist or there is concern about poor compliance with therapy

PREVENTION/AVOIDANCE
• For recurrence: No sexual intercourse until culture results known/partner(s) tested and treated
• For prevention of initial infection: Condoms offer partial protection

POSSIBLE COMPLICATIONS
• Urethral stricture in men
• Infertility in women
• Corneal scarring after eye infections
• Destruction of joint articular surfaces
• Destruction of cardiac valves, particularly aortic
• Death from congestive heart failure or meningitis

EXPECTED COURSE/PROGNOSIS With adequate, early therapy complete cure and return to normal function is the rule

MISCELLANEOUS

ASSOCIATED CONDITIONS Other sexually transmitted infections such as chlamydia infections, syphilis, HIV infection, hepatitis B, herpes and vaginal infections in women

AGE-RELATED FACTORS
Pediatric: N/A
Geriatric: N/A
Others: N/A

PREGNANCY PID during pregnancy may be associated with fetal loss, or premature labor and delivery

SYNONYMS
• GC
• Clap

ICD-9-CM
098 Gonococcal infections
098.0 Acute, lower genitourinary tract
614.9 Unspecified inflammatory disease of female pelvic organs and tissue

SEE ALSO
• Chlamydial sexually transmitted diseases
• Pelvic inflammatory disease (PID)
• Syphilis

OTHER NOTES N/A

ABBREVIATIONS
• GC = gonococcal
• PID = pelvic inflammatory disease

REFERENCES
• Centers for Disease Control and Prevention (CDC). 1993, Sexually transmitted diseases treatment guidelines. Morbidity Mortality Weekly Report 42(Supplement RR-14):47-83
• Handsfield HH, Sparling FR: Neisseria gonorrhoeae. In: Mandell GL, Bennett JE, Dolin R, eds. Principles and Practice of Infectious Diseases, 4th Ed. New York, Churchill Livingstone, 1995:1409-1926
Illustrations: 1 available on CD-ROM
Internet references: http://www.5mcc.com

Author(s)
Leonard N. Slater, MD

Gout

BASICS

DESCRIPTION Inflammatory reaction to urate crystals in joints, bones and subcutaneous structures. Initially, a hyperacute arthritis which may progress to a chronic arthritis. Rarely it may present as a chronic arthritis. Recognition of the crystals in fluid is pathognomonic.
• Primary gout - the most common: underexcretion or overproduction of uric acid
• Secondary gout - related to myeloproliferative diseases or their treatment, therapeutic regimens producing hyperuricemia, renal failure, renal tubular disorders, lead poisoning, hyperproliferative skin disorders, enzymatic defects (e.g., deficient hypoxanthine guanine phosphoribosyltransferase, glycogen storage diseases)
System(s) affected: Musculoskeletal, Endocrine/Metabolic, Renal/Urologic
Genetics: N/A
Incidence/Prevalence in USA: 100/100,000. Under age 18: rare; age 18-44: 3; age 45-64: 21; age over 65: 35
Predominant age: 30-60
Predominant sex: Male > Female (20:1)

SIGNS AND SYMPTOMS
• Hyperacute onset (within 24 hours) of severe pain, swelling, redness, and warmth in one or two joints (75% are monoarticular)
• Soft tissue redness, swelling, warmth
• Exquisite tenderness
• Propensity for first MTP joint, symptomatic in 50% of initial attacks; eventually in 75%
• Acute untreated attacks last 2-21 days
• Attack may be isolated, more often repetitive, 2nd attack may not occur for years
• Recurrent attacks last longer and occur more frequently with each recurrence
• Intracritical period - absence of inflammation (until the chronic or tophaceous phase occurs)
• Rarely polyarticular - proximal interphalangeal, distal interphalangeal, metacarpal phalangeal, wrist, knee, ankle, midtarsal joints, heel
• Migratory polyarthritis is a rare presentation
• 50% of untreated patients develop a chronic arthritis within 3-42 years
• Inflammatory synovial effusion
• Subcutaneous or intraosseous nodules (20%), referred to as tophi - may affect ears (antihelix), extensor aspects of peripheral joints (e.g., olecranon), rarely fingertips, cornea, aorta, spine or even intracranial
• Subcutaneous nodules may have a creamy (urate) discharge
• Fever, chills
• Carpal tunnel syndrome
• Kidney stones

CAUSES
• Hyperuricemia
• Dietary excess (e.g., anchovies, sardines, sweetbreads, kidney, liver and meat extracts)
• Inborn errors of metabolism
• Lead poisoning (Saturnine gout from moonshine)
• Kidney disease
• Hemoproliferative disorders

RISK FACTORS
• Ethanol ingestion
• Family history
• Polynesian extraction (e.g., Samoan gout)
• Medications - aminophylline, caffeine, corticosteroids, cytotoxic drugs, diazepam, diphenhydramine, diuretics, L-dopa, dopamine, epinephrine, ethambutol, methaqualone, alpha-methyl dopa, nicotinic acid, probenecid (low dose), pyrazinamide, salicylates (< 10/dL blood levels), sulfinpyrazone (low dose), vitamins B12 and C.
• Diuretics may be responsible for 20% of secondary gout
• Ketosis
• Surgery or trauma
• Obesity (50%)
• Hypertension (50%)
• Vascular disease
• Diabetes
• Renal failure
• Hypothyroidism
• Hyperparathyroidism; hypoparathyroidism
• Hyperlipidemia types II, IV, V
• Paget's disease
• Hyperproliferative skin disorders (e.g., psoriasis)
• Lymphoproliferative disorders
• Calcium pyrophosphate deposition disease
• Sarcoidosis
• Hemolytic anemia
• Hemoglobinopathies
• Pernicious anemia
• Radiation treatment
• Type I glycogen storage disease
• Down syndrome
• Gut sterilization by antibiotics

DIAGNOSIS

DIFFERENTIAL DIAGNOSIS Infectious arthritis, pseudogout (calcium pyrophosphate deposition disease), type IIa hyperproteinemia, amyloidosis, multicentric reticulohistiocytosis, hyperparathyroidism, spondyloarthropathy, rheumatoid arthritis (rarely)

LABORATORY
• WBC usually elevated with left shift during acute attacks
• ESR usually elevated during acute attacks
• Hyperuricemia may be present, although not diagnostic
Drugs that may alter lab results:
• Intra-articular steroids - many have inherent birefringence, which will cause confusion on synovial fluid analysis
• Hyperuricemia - induced by drugs that reduce effective circulating blood volume (induced by low dose aspirin, probenecid or sulfinpyrazone)
• Cyclosporine - induced renal insufficiency
Disorders that may alter lab results:
Alcoholism, sarcoidosis, lead poisoning, kidney failure, psoriasis, hemoglobinopathy

PATHOLOGICAL FINDINGS
• Urate crystals in synovial membrane (98% of specimens processed entirely anhydrously [urate is water soluble])
• Tophus in 29% of individuals with untreated gout of 5 years duration, in 74% of individuals with untreated gout of 40 years duration

SPECIAL TESTS
• Synovial fluid white blood cell count is usually inflammatory (10,000-70,000 cells/dL), but may have as few as 1,000 WBC/dL
• Wet mounts of synovial fluid reveal negatively birefringent urate crystals on polarizing exam
• Gout crystals may be identified in asymptomatic joints

IMAGING
• X-ray is usually normal in the first year of uncontrolled disease.
• X-ray in chronic gout reveals "punched-out" erosions (lytic areas) often with periosteum overgrowing the erosion ("overhanging edge" sign). This is highly suggestive, but may also be caused by amyloidosis, type IIa hyperlipoproteinemia, and by multicentric reticulohistiocytosis.
• X-ray erosions with preservation of joint space is similarly characteristic. X-ray rarely reveals intraosseous lytic areas (tophi).
• Bone scan reveals increased nuclide concentration at affected sites

DIAGNOSTIC PROCEDURES
• Arthrocentesis with polarizing optical examination
• Biopsy of synovial membrane or subcutaneous nodule, processing the specimen anhydrously (urate is water soluble) and examining with polarizing optics

TREATMENT

APPROPRIATE HEALTH CARE
Outpatient, except for consideration of associated joint infection or for therapeutic unresponsiveness

GENERAL MEASURES
• Control the acute attack of gout
• Addressing the underlying cause

SURGICAL MEASURES N/A

ACTIVITY Affected joint(s) at rest until hyperacute phase is controlled

DIET Reduce ingestion of fat, alcoholic beverages, sardines, anchovies, liver, sweetbreads

PATIENT EDUCATION
• Arthritis Foundation pamphlet on gout
• Rothschild, BM.: Hyperuricemia in the elderly. Geriatric Consultant, 4:14-16, 31, 1985.

Gout

MEDICATIONS

DRUG(S) OF CHOICE
- Acute attack
  ◊ A NSAID at full dosage for 2-5 days
  ◊ When acute attack is controlled, reduce dose by 1/4 - 1/2
- Chronic treatment
  ◊ Initiate when acute attack controlled (unless kidneys at risk because of unusual uric acid load)
  ◊ Generally not pursued unless recurrent attacks or evidence of tophaceous or renal disease
  ◊ Any contributing medication regimens are first altered and any predisposing medical conditions/habits addressed
  ◊ Patient is tested for uric acid excretion (<600 mg/day while on purine free diet or <800 mg/day on unrestricted diet implies hypoexcretor)
  - Hypoexcretor: probenecid is initiated at 500 mg qd and increased by 500 mg at monthly intervals, until the uric acid is lowered to normal range or at least 2 mg/dL (0.12 mmol/L) less than the levels during which attacks are noted. (Maximum dose 2-3 g/day.) Urinary alkalinization and recommendation of ingestion of copious amounts of fluid are adjunctive.
  - Hyperexcretor, tophaceous or renal disease are present: allopurinol, initiated at 100 mg qd and increased by 100 mg weekly, to a maximum of 600 mg per day.

Contraindications:
- Related to medicinal control of the acute attack:
  ◊ Peptic ulcer disease
  ◊ Psychosis
  ◊ Severe headache
  ◊ Pregnancy
  ◊ Concomitant anticoagulant use
  ◊ Presence of a blood dyscrasia
- Related to probenecid control of the underlying hyperuricemia:
  ◊ Uric acid overproduction
  ◊ Uric acid stones
  ◊ Renal impairment
  ◊ Concomitant salicylates
- Related to allopurinol control of the underlying hyperuricemia:
  ◊ Bone marrow suppression
  ◊ Liver disease
  ◊ Concomitant cytotoxic drugs
  ◊ Diuretics may require increased amount of allopurinol

Precautions:
- Probenecid and allopurinol may themselves predispose to acute gouty attacks. Use low dose NSAID for 6-24 mos to reduce risk.
- Reduce NSAID dosage in presence of renal or liver disease
- Reduce cytotoxic drug dose in presence of allopurinol
- With allopurinol risk of skin rash

Significant possible interactions:
- Related to medicinal control of the acute attack:
  ◊ Anticoagulants
  ◊ Anti-diabetic agents
  ◊ Anticonvulsants
  ◊ Lithium
- Related to probenecid control of the underlying hyperuricemia:
  ◊ Antibiotics
  ◊ Antidiabetic agents
  ◊ Thiopental
  ◊ Ketamine
  ◊ NSAID's
  ◊ Lorazepam
  ◊ Rifampin
  ◊ Antagonized by pyrazinamide, salicylates
- Related to allopurinol control of the underlying hyperuricemia:
  ◊ Mercaptopurine (requires reduction of chemotherapy dose to 1/3 of usual dose)
  ◊ Azathioprine
  ◊ Methotrexate
  ◊ Possibly cyclophosphamide
  ◊ Anticoagulants
  ◊ Antidiabetic agents

ALTERNATIVE DRUGS
- Related to control of the acute attack:
  ◊ Colchicine, a controversial toxic agent which must be taken within 24 hours of onset of the acute attack to be effective; IV preferred 2 mg, followed by 1 mg q6h for 2 doses; do not repeat in less than 3 days
  ◊ Intra-articular long-acting (depot) corticosteroid (if infection definitely ruled out)
- Related to control of the underlying hyperuricemia in the hypoexcretor:
  ◊ Sulfinpyrazone, initiated at 400 mg qd
  ◊ ACTH 40-80 IU IM

FOLLOWUP

PATIENT MONITORING
- Related to medicinal control of the acute attack and suppressing attacks:
  ◊ Adjusting therapeutic regimen if no significant clinical response to therapy within 3 days of its initiation.
  ◊ CBC, renal and hepatic blood testing and urinalysis at 1 wk, 6 wks and every 3 months
- Related to control of the underlying hyperuricemia:
  ◊ CBC, uric acid level, renal and hepatic blood testing, and urinalysis at monthly intervals (with dosage/regimen modification) until desired serum uric acid level achieved

PREVENTION/AVOIDANCE   Avoidance of exacerbating medications/diets/habits

POSSIBLE COMPLICATIONS
- Increased susceptibility to infection
- Urate nephropathy
- Uric acid nephropathy
- Renal stones
- Nerve/spinal cord impingement
- Recognition of urate crystals does not preclude concomitant infectious arthritis

EXPECTED COURSE/PROGNOSIS
- With early treatment, total control
- If recurrent attacks, successful uric acid adjustment (requiring lifelong use of uricosuric or allopurinol medication) usually effective

- During the first 6-24 months of uricosuric or allopurinol therapy, acute gout may occur

MISCELLANEOUS

ASSOCIATED CONDITIONS
- Myeloproliferative disorders
- Lymphoproliferative disorders
- Ethanolism
- Hyperlipidemia
- Obesity
- Hypertension
- Diabetes
- Lesch-Nyhan syndrome - chorea, spasticity, self-mutilation in childhood

AGE-RELATED FACTORS
Pediatric: Onset in this age group identifies gout secondary to an inborn error of metabolism or underlying disease process
Geriatric: Usually related to medications
Others: N/A

PREGNANCY   Usual pregnancy precautions

SYNONYMS   N/A

ICD-9-CM
274.0 Gouty arthropathy
274.1 Gouty nephropathy
274.11 Uric acid nephrolithiasis
274.81 Gouty tophi of ear
984.9 Toxic effect of unspecified lead compound

SEE ALSO
- Alcoholism
- Anemia, sickle cell

OTHER NOTES   N/A

ABBREVIATIONS
MP = metatarsal phalangeal
NSAID = nonsteroidal anti-inflammatory drug

REFERENCES
- Yu TF: Gout. In: Katz W, ed. Diagnosis and Management of Rheumatic Diseases. Philadelphia, J.B. Lippincott, 1988
- Kelley WN, Harris ED Jr, Ruddy S, Sledge CB: Textbook of Rheumatology. Philadelphia, W.B. Saunders Co., 1993
- Rothschild BM: Crystalline Arthritis: Gout. Fairlawn, CT, Clinical AV, 1982
- Rothschild BM, Heathcote GM: Characterization of gout in a skeletal population sample. Amer J Phys Anthrol 1995;98:529-525
Illustrations: 2 available on CD-ROM
Internet references: http://www.5mcc.com

Author(s)
Bruce M. Rothschild, MD

Granuloma annulare

BASICS

DESCRIPTION   Chronic, self-limited inflammation of the skin exhibited by annularly arranged papules
• Localized granuloma annulare - the more common form consists of a solitary group of flesh colored papules that gradually involute centrally to form circles or semi-circles
• Disseminated granuloma annulare - occurs less often and consists of widespread lesions with the same characteristics as localized type
System(s) affected: Skin
Genetics: Not specified, although a familial incidence has been noted among siblings, twins, and successive generations
Incidence/Prevalence in USA: Not specified
Predominant age:
• Localized granuloma annulare - children and young adults
• Disseminated granuloma annulare - adults in 4th to 7th decades
Predominant sex: Females > Males (2:1)

SIGNS AND SYMPTOMS
• Papular, circular or semi-circular lesions
• Papules usually found on dorsal surface of hands, fingers, feet, extensor aspects of arms and legs, trunk
• Subcutaneous nodules seen on palms, legs, buttocks, scalp
• Papules can perforate
• Lesions may be pruritic on rare occasions, but usually asymptomatic

CAUSES   Unknown

RISK FACTORS
• Diabetes mellitus
• Positive family history
• Rheumatoid arthritis

DIAGNOSIS

DIFFERENTIAL DIAGNOSIS
• Papular lesions
  ◊ Necrobiosis lipoidica
  ◊ Cutaneous amyloidosis
  ◊ Annular elastolytic granuloma
  ◊ Papular sarcoid
  ◊ Lichen planus
  ◊ Tinea
  ◊ Tuberculoid (TT) or borderline tuberculoid (BT) leprosy
  ◊ Erythema migrans
  ◊ Verruca plana
  ◊ Majocchi granuloma
  ◊ Appendageal hamartomas, e.g., eruptive syringomata
• Subcutaneous nodules
  ◊ Rheumatoid nodules

LABORATORY   If disseminated form, check blood sugar. Also rheumatoid factor if symptoms of RA present.
Drugs that may alter lab results: N/A
Disorders that may alter lab results: N/A

PATHOLOGICAL FINDINGS   Palisading granuloma with histiocytes and epithelial cells surrounding a central zone of altered collagen in the mid to upper dermis

SPECIAL TESTS   N/A

IMAGING   N/A

DIAGNOSTIC PROCEDURES
• Inspection of skin usually reveals diagnosis
• Skin scraping to rule out fungi can be done
• If diagnosis is in doubt, skin biopsy can be performed

TREATMENT

APPROPRIATE HEALTH CARE
Outpatient

GENERAL MEASURES   Treatment is not always satisfactory.

SURGICAL MEASURES   N/A

ACTIVITY   Full activity

DIET   American Diabetic Association guidelines when associated with diabetes

PATIENT EDUCATION   If patient has disseminated form, papules may be accentuated by sun exposure

MEDICATIONS

DRUG(S) OF CHOICE
• Localized form - intralesional triamcinolone acetonide, 5 mg/mL injected into the elevated border only. A 30 gauge needle is used. May be repeated at monthly intervals.
• Topical steroids with occlusion or incorporated in tape are occasionally useful for localized form
• Disseminated form - dapsone 100 mg qd or bid; PUVA or REPUVA
Contraindications: Dapsone should not be given to patients with G6PD deficiency
Precautions: See manufacturer's profile of each drug
Significant possible interactions: See manufacturer's profile of each drug

ALTERNATIVE DRUGS
• Localized form may respond to cryosurgeryy, but atrophy possible
• For disseminated form isotretinoin 80 mg qd is used in refractive cases
• Niacinamide 1.5 gm qd or potassium iodide is recommended by some

FOLLOWUP

PATIENT MONITORING Depends on nature of treatment; generally two week intervals while undergoing treatment

PREVENTION/AVOIDANCE Avoid sun-exposure in patients with disseminated form if association with light

POSSIBLE COMPLICATIONS None

EXPECTED COURSE/PROGNOSIS
Lesions disappear without scarring in 75% of patients in two years. 40% of patients experience recurrences

MISCELLANEOUS

ASSOCIATED CONDITIONS
• Diabetes mellitus is mainly associated with disseminated granuloma annulare but the frequency is unknown. Likewise, some patients with rheumatoid arthritis have developed granuloma annulare.
• Can be associated with other granulomatous disease, such as, necrobiosis lipoidica, rheumatoid nodules and sarcoidosis

AGE-RELATED FACTORS
Pediatric: N/A
Geriatric: Disseminated form is more common in older patients
Others: N/A

PREGNANCY N/A

SYNONYMS N/A

ICD-9-CM 695.89 Other specified erythematous conditions, other

SEE ALSO N/A

OTHER NOTES N/A

ABBREVIATIONS N/A

REFERENCES
• Habif T: Clinical Dermatology. 3rd Ed. St Louis, Mosby, 1996
• Hurwitz S: Clinical Pediatric Dermatology. 2nd Ed. Philadelphia, W.B. Saunders Co., 1993
• Fitzpatrick TB, et al: Color Atlas and Synopsis of Clinical Dermatology. 3rd Ed. New York, McGraw-Hill, 1997
Illustrations: 6 available on CD-ROM
Internet references: http://www.5mcc.com

Author(s)
Gary J. Silko, MD

Granuloma, pyogenic

BASICS

DESCRIPTION Benign, solitary mass that involves exposed areas such as distal extremities and face as well as the oral cavity (most frequently the gingiva)
System(s) affected: Skin/Exocrine, Gastrointestinal
Genetics: N/A
Incidence/Prevalence: Unknown
Predominant age: Any, most frequently children and second to fifth decades
Predominant sex: Slight predilection for females

SIGNS AND SYMPTOMS
• Sessile or pedunculated
• Granular, smooth or slightly nodular
• Soft
• May be ulcerated, bleeding easily
• Red, purple, or brown in color
• Ranges from a few millimeters to 2-3 centimeters in diameter

CAUSES
• Thought to be an over-reaction to minor trauma
• May be related to hormonal changes in pregnancy

RISK FACTORS
• Pregnancy
• Intraoral trauma or surgery

DIAGNOSIS

DIFFERENTIAL DIAGNOSIS
• Peripheral ossifying granuloma
• Giant cell granuloma
• Odontogenic fibroma
• Kaposi's sarcoma
• Malignant melanoma
• Angiolymphoid hyperplasia with eosinophilia
• Metastatic carcinoma
• IN AIDS patients, bacillary angiomatosis, deep mycoses

LABORATORY N/A
Drugs that may alter lab results: N/A
Disorders that may alter lab results: N/A

PATHOLOGICAL FINDINGS
• Micro-small, endothelial lined vascular spaces
• Micro- loose or dense connective tissue stroma
• Micro- acute and chronic inflammatory cells
• Micro- no true granuloma formation
• Micro- abundant mitotic activity

SPECIAL TESTS N/A

IMAGING N/A

DIAGNOSTIC PROCEDURES Excisional biopsy

TREATMENT

APPROPRIATE HEALTH CARE
Outpatient

GENERAL MEASURES
• Occasional spontaneous resolution
• Good oral hygiene

SURGICAL MEASURES
• Surgical excision of lesion (with cleaning of adjacent teeth if lesion is gingival)
• May recur if inadequately excised

ACTIVITY As tolerated

DIET As tolerated

PATIENT EDUCATION Patient should avoid trauma to the area following excision

MEDICATIONS

DRUG(S) OF CHOICE None
Contraindications: N/A
Precautions: N/A
Significant possible interactions: N/A

ALTERNATIVE DRUGS N/A

FOLLOWUP:

PATIENT MONITORING As needed

PREVENTION/AVOIDANCE Good oral hygiene

POSSIBLE COMPLICATIONS
Recurrence. After removal or destruction of a solitary lesion, multiple satellite lesions can form around the original treatment site.

EXPECTED COURSE/PROGNOSIS
Complete resolution expected with adequate excision.

MISCELLANEOUS

ASSOCIATED CONDITIONS N/A

AGE-RELATED FACTORS N/A
Pediatric: N/A
Geriatric: N/A
Others: N/A

PREGNANCY Lesion also occurs in pregnant women, and is known as "pregnancy tumor"

SYNONYMS
• Pregnancy tumor
• Granuloma gravidum

ICD-9-CM
686.1 Pyogenic granuloma
522.6 Maxillary alveolar ridge
528.9 Oral mucosa

SEE ALSO N/A

OTHER NOTES N/A

ABBREVIATIONS N/A

REFERENCES
• Wood NK, Goaz PW: Differential Diagnosis of Oral Lesions. St. Louis, C.V. Mosby, 1985
• Ash MM: Oral Pathology. Philadelphia, Lea & Febiger, 1986
Illustrations: 3 available on CD-ROM
Internet references: http://www.5mcc.com

Author(s)
Laurene L. Howell, MD
Gregg W. Suits, MD

Guillain-Barré syndrome

BASICS

DESCRIPTION The most common cause of acute neuromuscular paralysis. An acute ascending motor weakness usually beginning with paresthesias in fingers and toes, sometimes leading to respiratory failure from respiratory muscle paralysis. Sensory involvement common, autonomic neuropathy variable. Infection commonly precedes syndrome by 1-3 weeks.
Incidence/Prevalence in USA:
0.6-1.9/100,000 annually, non-seasonal, non-epidemic
System(s) affected: Nervous
Genetics: Recurrent form - chronic relapsing polyneuropathy shows correlation with HLA-Aw30 and HLA-Aw31
Predominant age: All ages
Predominant sex: Male > Female (1.5:1)

SIGNS AND SYMPTOMS
• Progressive weakness of all 4 limbs, usually ascending and symmetric
• Hypotonia or areflexia
• Sensory involvement
• Bulbar variant: dysphagia, dysarthria, and drooling with descending weakness
• Pain is common, especially shoulders, thighs, lumbar region
• Miller-Fisher syndrome (variant): ataxia, ophthalmoplegia, areflexia
• Respiratory muscle paralysis (in 25%)
• Autonomic neuropathy with labile BP and arrhythmias a cause of death

CAUSES
• Autoimmune destruction of myelin and/or axon
• 66% associated with antecedent infection, especially Campylobacter jejuni, also Mycoplasma pneumoniae, CMV, EBV, HIV
• Vaccinations: especially swine flu vaccine and rabies vaccine (but not other influenza vaccine)
• Malignancies (lymphomas especially Hodgkin's)
• Surgery
• Drugs - gold, penicillamine, streptokinase, captopril, danazol, IV heroin, IV gangliosides

RISK FACTORS
Antecedent infection, especially Campylobacter jejuni, which is associated with a worse course and with residual disability

DIAGNOSIS

DIFFERENTIAL DIAGNOSIS
• Spinal cord syndromes especially post-infectious transverse myelitis
• Neuropathies - porphyria, vasculitis (SLE, PAN), heavy metals and other toxins, alcohol, diphtheria, B12 or folate deficiency, hereditary neuropathies, malignant infiltration of nerves
• Neuromuscular junction - Eaton-Lambert, botulism, myasthenia gravis
• Muscle - polymyositis
• CNS - brainstem CVA or encephalitis, polio, cauda equina syndrome
• Metabolic - disorders of K+, hypophosphatemia
• Functional

LABORATORY
• CSF: elevated protein (in 90% of patients) with normal pressure and without WBC's (>10 WBC/mcL in CSF suggests associated HIV). CSF protein may be normal the first week.
Drugs that may alter lab results: N/A
Disorders that may alter lab results: N/A

PATHOLOGICAL FINDINGS
• Demyelination and/or axonal degeneration of peripheral nerves
• Inflammatory cell infiltration of nerves

SPECIAL TESTS N/A

IMAGING Gadolinium-enhanced MRI of lumbosacral spine shows enhancement of cauda equina nerve roots in 95% of typical patients

DIAGNOSTIC PROCEDURES
Nerve conduction studies in association with CSF are the best tests for diagnosing/confirming GBS but are unreliable for following patient.
• Nerve conduction studies
  ◊ Conduction block
  ◊ Prolonged distal latencies
  ◊ Decreased CMAP amplitude
  ◊ Decreased motor conduction velocities
  ◊ F-wave abnormalities
• Lumbar puncture

TREATMENT

APPROPRIATE HEALTH CARE
• Hospitalization with elective intubation for impending respiratory failure
• IVIG or plasmapheresis for all patients too weak to walk

GENERAL MEASURES
• Serial measurements of vital capacity: ICU for VC < 20 mL/kg (1.5 L), intubation for VC < 1L or clinical signs of impending respiratory failure. Peak flow machines inappropriate (measure air flow resistance not respiratory muscle strength). Oxygen saturation normal until respiratory failure already present.
• ICU and intubation if necessary for difficulty swallowing/aspiration from bulbar palsy
• EKG monitoring for associated arrhythmias. Tachyarrhythmias - usually do not require treatment. Bradyarrhythmias - atropine; sinus arrest and complete heart block - temporary pacemaker.
• BP monitoring:
  ◊ Hypertension: small doses beta-blockers; avoid vasodilators including calcium channel blockers which may cause hypotension
  ◊ Hypotension: mechanical treatments (Trendelenburg and colloid infusion)
• Prevention of complications of prolonged immobilization and ventilation: pneumonia, decubitus ulcers, contractures, thromboembolism
• Pain is common and recalcitrant: muscular - analgesics and NSAIDs, neuropathic - carbamazepine, amitriptyline, TENS
• Constipation/ileus from autonomic neuropathy - use laxatives, enemas, cisapride (Propulsid)
• Depression - antidepressants, frequent reminders that full recovery is the rule

SURGICAL MEASURES Tracheostomy for prolonged intubation

ACTIVITY No limitation. Physical therapy to prevent contractures.

DIET No special diet. Enteral feedings if intubated.

PATIENT EDUCATION N/A

MEDICATIONS

DRUG(S) OF CHOICE
• No specific drug treatment for GBS. Plasmapheresis and IVIG equally effective and no benefit if both used
• Plasmapheresis shows clear benefit, especially early. Early relapses respond to repeat plasmapheresis.
• Immune globulin, intravenous (IVIG): 0.4 g/kg/d over 5 days or 1 g/kg/d x 2 days
Contraindications: IVIG in IgA deficiency if the IVIG preparation contains IgA.
Precautions:
• Plasmapheresis: hypotension usually responds to volume infusion; plasmapheresis can cause sepsis and severe autonomic instability.
• IVIG: fever and flushing improve with slowing of infusion rate, aseptic meningitis and acute renal failure have been reported
Significant possible interactions: None

ALTERNATIVE DRUGS
• Steroids by themselves are ineffective and possibly deleterious

FOLLOWUP

PATIENT MONITORING Physical rehabilitation to regain muscle strength

PREVENTION/AVOIDANCE N/A

POSSIBLE COMPLICATIONS
• Paralysis
• Respiratory failure; mechanical ventilation
• Hypo- or hypertension
• Cardiac arrhythmias
• Ileus
• Aspiration
• Urinary retention
• Psychiatric problems including depression

EXPECTED COURSE/PROGNOSIS
• Variable course in time and severity
  ◊ Worst case: tetraplegia within 24 hours with incomplete recovery after 18 months or longer
  ◊ Best case: mild difficulty walking with recovery within weeks
  ◊ Usual: peak weakness in 10-14 days, recovery in weeks to months. Average time on respirator (without treatment) 50 days.
• 50% complete recovery
• 33% permanent neurologic sequelae
• 15% significant, permanent damage
• 10% relapse before full recovery
• 2-5% relapse after full recovery
• 5% die of complications; most often dysautonomia
• Rapid progression with mainly motor neuropathy associated with prolonged ventilation and permanent disability
• After IVIG or plasmapheresis, initial improvement may be followed by relapse because of persistent active disease. Repeat treatment causes improvement. Relapses may also occur months to years after resolution of disease, often from chronic inflammatory demyelinating polyneuropathy (CIDP), which may respond to chronic IVIG therapy.
• Further recovery of nerve function after 2 years is unlikely

MISCELLANEOUS

ASSOCIATED CONDITIONS Chronic inflammatory demyelinating polyneuropathy (CIDP)

AGE-RELATED FACTORS
Pediatric: Disease tends to be milder
Geriatric: N/A
Others: N/A

PREGNANCY No data

SYNONYMS
• Ascending paralysis
• Acute idiopathic polyneuritis
• Acute immune mediated polyneuritis (AIMP)
• Landry-Guillain-Barré
• Acute polyneuropathy
• Infectious idiopathic polyneuropathy
• Laundry's ascending paralysis
• Acute segmentally demyelinating polyradiculoneuropathy

ICD-9-CM 357.0

SEE ALSO N/A

OTHER NOTES N/A

ABBREVIATIONS
GBS = Guillain-Barré syndrome

REFERENCES
• Adams RD, Victor M: Principles of Neurology. 5th Ed. New York, McGraw-Hill, 1993
• Rees J: Guillain-Barre Syndrome. Drugs 1995; 49(6):912-920
• Rees J: Campylobacter Jejuni infection and Guillain Barré Syndrome. NEJM 1995; 333(21):1374-9
• Kleyweg RP, van der Meche FGA: Treatment related fluctuations in Guillain-Barré syndrome after high-dose immunoglobulins or plasma-exchange. Jour Neurology, Neurosurgery & Psychiatry 1991; 54(11): 957-960
• Randomized trial of plasma exchange, intravenous immunoglobulin. Lancet 1997; 349(9047): 225-30
• Gorson KC, Ropper AH, Murielloma, Blair R: Prospective evaluation of MRI lumbosacral/nerve root... Neurology 1996; 47(3): 813-7
• Dematteis JA: Guillain-Barré syndrome. Am Fam Phy 1996; 54(1): 197-200
Illustrations: N/A
Internet references: http://www.5mcc.com

Author(s)
Hetty B. Hall, MD

Gynecomastia

BASICS

DESCRIPTION A benign glandular enlargement of the male breast that is generally bilateral (may be asymmetric, or rarely, unilateral)
- Type I: Benign adolescent hypertrophy
  ◊ Physiologic discoid subacute mass
  ◊ Resolves spontaneously
- Type II: Physiologic gynecomastia
  ◊ Generalized enlargement to greater degree
- Type III:
  ◊ Obesity simulates gynecomastia
- Type IV:
  ◊ Pectoral muscle hypertrophy

System(s) affected: Skin/Exocrine, Endocrine/Metabolic
Genetics: Some instance of familial gynecomastia may be inherited as a male-limited autosomal trait
Incidence/Prevalence in USA: 38-64% of pubertal males; rare except when drug-induced
Predominant age: Puberty; and over the age of 65 (especially with a weight gain)
Predominant sex: Male only

SIGNS AND SYMPTOMS
- Usually asymptomatic
- May be painful and tender if it has developed rapidly (drug-induced, refeeding gynecomastia)

CAUSES
- Physiologic - transient in neonatal boys and at puberty
- Exposure to a high level of estrogen compared to testosterone concentration
- Tumors - estrogen secreting, gonadotropin secreting and prolactin secreting pituitary adenomas
- Drug-induced (hormones, marijuana, digitalis, spironolactone, cimetidine, ketoconazole, cytotoxic drugs, antihypertensives, sedatives, antidepressants, amphetamine)
- Systemic disorders - cirrhosis, thyrotoxicosis, renal failure
- Androgen production deficiency
- Androgen resistant syndromes
- Trauma
- Idiopathic

RISK FACTORS
- Klinefelter's syndrome
- Obesity
- Testicular failure
- Recovery from prolonged severe illness associated with malnutrition and weight loss (refeeding gynecomastia)
- Family history
- Peutz-Jeghers syndrome
- Male pseudohermaphroditism

DIAGNOSIS

DIFFERENTIAL DIAGNOSIS
- Obesity with increase in adipose tissue
- Carcinoma of the male breast
- Lipomas
- Neurofibromas

LABORATORY
- Laboratory evaluation rarely indicated
- Human chorionic gonadotropin levels - high levels may lead to finding a choriocarcinoma or other hCG-secreting tumor
- Plasma testosterone and luteinizing hormone measurements - help diagnose hypogonadism
- Serum estradiol
- Serum prolactin
- Liver function
- Others if clinically indicated e.g., thyroid function, chromosomal analysis
Drugs that may alter lab results: N/A
Disorders that may alter lab results:
- Cirrhosis
- Thyrotoxicosis
- Renal failure

PATHOLOGICAL FINDINGS
- Dense, periductal hyaline, collagenous connective tissue
- Hyperplastic ductal lining
- Plasma cell infiltrate

SPECIAL TESTS Full endocrine investigations may be indicated

IMAGING CT, ultrasonography (rarely indicated)

DIAGNOSTIC PROCEDURES
- History and physical exam to determine possible etiology
- Biopsy, if suspicious

TREATMENT

APPROPRIATE HEALTH CARE
Outpatient

GENERAL MEASURES
- Correct underlying disorder
- Withdrawal of causative drug if feasible
- Observation with reassurance that problem is transient

SURGICAL MEASURES
- Biopsy if suspicious for cancer
- Subcutaneous mastectomy for severe, persistent cases or those with psychological concerns

ACTIVITY No restrictions

DIET
- No special diet
- If obesity a problem, weight loss diet

PATIENT EDUCATION N/A

MEDICATIONS

DRUG(S) OF CHOICE None
Contraindications: N/A
Precautions: N/A
Significant possible interactions: N/A

ALTERNATIVE DRUGS N/A

FOLLOWUP

PATIENT MONITORING
• Every 3-6 months for physiologic gynecomastia
• Until well for non-physiologic gynecomastia

PREVENTION/AVOIDANCE In men taking estrogen for prostate cancer - low dose radiation prior to institution of diethylstilbestrol

POSSIBLE COMPLICATIONS
• Nipple inversion may occur following subcutaneous mastectomy
• Asymmetry of breasts

EXPECTED COURSE/PROGNOSIS
• Physiologic gynecomastia clears without treatment (may take up to 2 years)
• Drug withdrawal cures
• Other causes - outcome depends on etiology
• Little change in Type III without substantial weight loss
• Good results with subcutaneous mastectomy

MISCELLANEOUS

ASSOCIATED CONDITIONS Listed with Causes

AGE-RELATED FACTORS
Pediatric:
• Transient gynecomastia seen in neonatal boys
• At puberty, may be observed in 38-64% of boys
Geriatric: Drug induced form more common
Others: N/A

PREGNANCY N/A

SYNONYMS Male breast hypertrophy

ICD-9-CM 611.1

SEE ALSO
• Klinefelter's syndrome

OTHER NOTES N/A

ABBREVIATIONS N/A

REFERENCES
• Becker KL, ed: Principles and Practice of Endocrinology and Metabolism. Philadelphia, J.B. Lippincott Co., 1990
• Holder TM, Ashcroft KW, eds: Pediatric Surgery. 2nd Ed. Philadelphia, W.B. Saunders Co., 1993
• Mahoney CP: Adolescent gynecomastia. Differential diagnosis and management. Pediatr Clin North Am 1990;37:1389
Illustrations: N/A
Internet references: http://www.5mcc.com

Author(s)
Timothy L. Black, MD, FACS, FAAP

Headache, cluster

BASICS

DESCRIPTION Attacks of severe, unilateral headache typically localized in periorbital area and temple associated with ipsilateral lacrimation, rhinorrhea, ptosis, miosis, and nasal congestion. Individual attacks last 30-180 minutes and occur 1-6 times per day. Two forms exist: episodic with attack phases lasting 4-12 weeks, followed by a cluster-free interval of generally 6 months to years duration; and chronic, with a cluster-free interval of less than 1 week in a 12 month period of time.
System(s) affected: Nervous
Genetics: Unknown
Incidence/Prevalence in USA: 0.5-1% of adult population
Predominant age: Mean age of onset: 30 years in men, later in women
Predominant sex: Male > Female (6:1)

SIGNS AND SYMPTOMS
• Sudden onset of severe headache
• Headache reaches crescendo within 15 minutes, lasts < 3 hours
• Pain is unilateral, oculo-temporal or oculo-frontal; rare in other locations
• Severe, piercing, boring, exploding, penetrating (occasionally throbbing) pain
• Ipsilateral partial Horner's syndrome (ptosis and miosis)
• Lacrimation (84%)
• Injected conjunctiva (58%)
• Ptosis (57%)
• Nasal stuffiness (48%)
• Rhinorrhea (43%)
• Bradycardia (43%)
• Nausea (40%)
• Perspiration (26%)
• Restlessness and agitation during attacks
• Attacks may occur at same time for consecutive days; frequently an attack occurs within 90 minutes of falling to sleep (corresponding to first REM sleep)

CAUSES
Unknown, perhaps:
• Disruption of circadian rhythm based on hypothalamus
• Disturbed autoregulation of cerebral arteries
• Disorder of serotonin metabolism or transmission in CNS
• Disorder of histamine concentrations or receptors

RISK FACTORS
• Male gender
• Age > 30 years
• Small amounts of vasodilators, such as, alcohol or nitroglycerine
• Occasional relationship to previous head trauma or surgery

DIAGNOSIS

DIFFERENTIAL DIAGNOSIS Diagnosis generally made through careful history. Differential includes other head and neck pathology, migraine, trigeminal and other facial neuralgias, chronic paroxysmal hemicrania (probably a cluster variant), temporal arteritis, pheochromocytoma.

LABORATORY Not useful except to rule out differential diagnosis
Drugs that may alter lab results: N/A
Disorders that may alter lab results: N/A

PATHOLOGICAL FINDINGS N/A

SPECIAL TESTS N/A

IMAGING Generally of little value except in atypical presentations or those unresponsive to therapy

DIAGNOSTIC PROCEDURES N/A

TREATMENT

APPROPRIATE HEALTH CARE
Outpatient except in patient at suicidal risk

GENERAL MEASURES
• During cluster periods, avoid alcohol, bright lights and glare, excessive emotion and stress as these may precipitate attacks
• Avoid narcotic analgesics, especially oral preparations
• Tobacco (high predilection for tobacco abuse in this population) may make patients more refractory to therapy

SURGICAL MEASURES Radiofrequency trigeminal gangliolysis in carefully selected refractory patients with strictly unilateral attacks

ACTIVITY
• Avoid self-injury during bouts of excruciating pain
• Vigorous physical activity at first symptom may abort attack in some
• Compression of ipsilateral carotid or temporal artery may reduce pain in some. Caution exercised in recommending carotid massage in patient at risk for occult carotid disease.

DIET
• During cluster phase, alcohol even in small amounts frequently precipitates attacks
• Rarely, specific foods may trigger attacks

PATIENT EDUCATION
• Focus on the validity, natural history, and pathology of the condition
• Advise patient to avoid known precipitants
• Assist patient with learning self-treatment methods
• Provide supportive relationship and follow-up
• Avoid high altitudes

MEDICATIONS

DRUG(S) OF CHOICE
- General information
  ◊ Prophylactic therapy is paramount
  ◊ Avoid pain therapy for acute attacks, especially narcotic analgesics
  ◊ Assess cardiovascular risk before instituting vasoactive drugs, such as, ergotamine or sumatriptan
- Acute attacks
  ◊ Oxygen 100% at 7-10 liters for 10-15 minutes administered through a tight-fitting face mask with patient in sitting position and breathing at normal respiratory rate
  ◊ Sumatriptan (Imitrex) 6 mg subcutaneous, maximum of 12 mg per 24 hours with at least 1 hour between injections
  ◊ Dihydroergotamine mesylate (DHE 45) 1 mg IM or IV. May teach self-administration with SC.
- Prophylaxis (to shorten cluster period or prevent expected attacks):
  ◊ Verapamil 80 mg PO qid spaced evenly through waking hours
  ◊ Lithium carbonate (Eskalith) 300 mg 2-4 times a day
  ◊ Methysergide (Sansert) 4-10 mg daily divided doses tid or qid. More useful in younger patient in early stage of disease.
  ◊ Ergotamine timed to be at peak serum level during anticipated attack, e.g., 2 mg rectal or 1-2 mg oral 2 hours before. This is especially useful to prevent nocturnal attacks.
  ◊ Prednisone, various schedules, e.g., 60-80 mg PO for 7 days followed by rapid tapering over 6 days or 40 mg/day for 5 days tapered over 3 weeks. This therapy is initiated while other long-term agent is being employed, such as, verapamil or lithium.

Contraindications: Refer to manufacturer's literature

Precautions: Refer to manufacturer's literature

Significant possible interactions: Refer to manufacturer's literature

ALTERNATIVE DRUGS
- Acute attack:
  ◊ Lidocaine intranasal instillation of 1 mL of 4% topical solution slowly on same side as symptoms. Position patient supine with head extended 45 degrees and rotated 40 degrees to the side of pain. May need to premedicate with 1-2 drops of intranasal 0.5% phenylephrine for nasal stuffiness.
- Prophylaxis
  ◊ Indomethacin up to 150 mg per day in divided doses. Absolute responsiveness in chronic paroxysmal hemicrania (CPH) and useful in female cluster patients.
  ◊ Nifedipine 40-120 mg/day
  ◊ Nimodipine up to 240 mg/day
  ◊ Combinations of verapamil and lithium with or without ergotamine may be useful when single drug therapy is ineffective
  ◊ Histamine desensitization done at certain major headache centers

FOLLOWUP

PATIENT MONITORING
- To anticipate cluster bouts and initiate early prophylaxis
- Monitor for adverse medication response and side-effects
- Monitor for unmasking of outlying cardiovascular disorder
- Education for patient and family

PREVENTION/AVOIDANCE
- Alcohol, nitroglycerine, and some foods can induce cluster attack
- Disturbances in sleep cycle can induce attacks (sleep cycle disruption common due to anticipation and occurrence of nocturnal attacks)
- Strong emotions, anger, excessive physical activity may induce attacks
- Tobacco may slow responsiveness to medication
- Narcotics may expedite transformation of episodic cluster to chronic cluster

POSSIBLE COMPLICATIONS
- Self-injury during attack
- Side-effects of medication including unmasking of coronary heart disease
- Potential for drug abuse

EXPECTED COURSE/PROGNOSIS
- Recurrent attacks
- Prolonged remissions
- Possibility of transformation of episodic cluster to chronic cluster and occasionally chronic cluster to episodic cluster

MISCELLANEOUS

ASSOCIATED CONDITIONS
- Significantly higher incidence of peptic ulcer and coronary heart disease (males)
- Prior history of migraine frequently in female patients
- Increased risk of suicide

AGE-RELATED FACTORS
Pediatric: Very rare cases reported
Geriatric: N/A
Others:
- With age - more likely to begin in women, often in peri- or post-menopausal years
- Characteristic appearance - "leonine" face, thickened skin, above average height, more likely to have hazel eye color, and be heavy smokers. No evidence of specific psychologic type.

PREGNANCY
Very rare in pregnancy

SYNONYMS
- Migrainous neuralgia
- Sphenopalatine neuralgia
- Histamine cephalalgia

ICD-9-CM
346.2 Variants of migraine (including cluster and histamine)
784.0 Headache

SEE ALSO
- Headache, tension
- Migraine

OTHER NOTES N/A

ABBREVIATIONS N/A

REFERENCES
- Cady RK, Fox AW, eds: Treating the Headache Patient. New York, Marcel Dekker, 1995
- Dechant KC, Clissol SP: Sumatriptan (review). Drugs 1992;43:776-98
- Dalessio DJ, Silberstein SD: Wolff's Headache and Other Head Pain. 6th Ed. New York, Oxford University Press, 1993
- Raskin NH: Headache. 2nd Ed. New York, Churchill Livingstone, 1988
Illustrations: N/A
Internet references: http://www.5mcc.com

Author(s)
Roger Cady, MD

Headache, tension

BASICS

DESCRIPTION Tension headache can be divided into two types:
• Episodic - usually associated with some stressful event, is of moderate intensity, self-limited, and usually responds to nonprescription preparations
• Chronic - often recurring daily, bilateral location, usually occipito-frontal and associated with contracted muscles of the neck and scalp
System(s) affected: Musculoskeletal
Genetics: 40% have a positive family history for headache
Incidence/Prevalence in USA: Common
Predominant age: 60% have onset after age 20 (unusual to begin after age 50)
Predominant sex: Female > Male

SIGNS AND SYMPTOMS
• Bilateral headache in 90%
• Located fronto-occipital or generalized
• Dull, pressing or band-like
• Intensity varies throughout the day
• Often present upon arising or shortly thereafter
• Chronic headaches have a duration greater than 5 years in 75% of patients
• Insomnia
• Teeth grinding
• Not aggravated by physical activity
• Difficulty concentrating
• Muscular tightness or stiffness in neck, occipital and frontal regions

CAUSES
• Poor posture
• Stress and/or anxiety
• Depression (found in 70% of those with daily headache)
• Low platelet serotonin
• Cervical osteoarthritis
• Intramuscular vasoconstriction

RISK FACTORS
• Obstructive sleep apnea
• Medications
• Excess caffeine

DIAGNOSIS

DIFFERENTIAL DIAGNOSIS
• Cervical spondylosis
• TMJ syndrome
• Caffeine-dependency
• Non-prescription analgesic dependency
• Depression
• Head injury
• Severe anemia or polycythemia
• Uremia and hepatic disorders
• Toxic effects from drugs or fumes
• Dental disease
• Paget's disease of bone
• Chronic sinusitis
• Refractive error
• Hypertension
• Hypoxia
• Temporal arteritis
• Migraine
• Lesions of the eye or middle ear
• Lesions of the oral cavity

LABORATORY
• CBC
• SMAC-20
• Thyroid studies
• ESR in anyone over 50 years of age
Drugs that may alter lab results: N/A
Disorders that may alter lab results: Chronic hepatitis, renal and thyroid conditions

PATHOLOGICAL FINDINGS Normal neurological examination, furrowed brow, tense masseter muscle, tight muscles in the scalp and neck

SPECIAL TESTS N/A

IMAGING
• X-rays of cervical spine
• Head CT or MRI necessary only when headache pattern has recently changed or there is a positive finding on neurological exam

DIAGNOSTIC PROCEDURES NA

TREATMENT

APPROPRIATE HEALTH CARE
Outpatient setting

GENERAL MEASURES
• Relief measures - use relaxation routines; rest in quiet, dark room with cold washcloth over eyes; hot bath or shower; massaging back of neck and temples
• Biofeedback training offers a nonpharmacologic alternative which is often beneficial

SURGICAL MEASURES N/A

ACTIVITY Encourage physical fitness, range of motion and strengthening exercises for the neck

DIET No demonstrated link between diet and tension headache

PATIENT EDUCATION
• Life style changes to minimize stress. Suggest patient seek counseling, if appropriate.
• Encourage relaxation techniques, aerobic exercise, assertiveness training
• Patient information available from the National Headache Foundation, 5252 N. Western Ave., Chicago, IL 60625, (800)843-2256

Headache, tension

MEDICATIONS

DRUG(S) OF CHOICE
• Acute attack - nonsteroidal anti-inflammatory drugs (NSAID's):
  ◊ Naproxen sodium (Naprosyn, Aleve) 500 mg/bid
  ◊ Fenoprofen calcium (Nalfon) 600 mg/day (200 mg q 4-6 hours)
  ◊ Ibuprofen (Motrin, Advil) 400 mg/tid
  ◊ Ketoprofen (Orudis) 50 mg/tid
• Prophylaxis for chronic tension headache - antidepressants
  ◊ Amitriptyline (Elavil) 50-100 mg/day
  ◊ Desipramine (Norpramin) 50-100 mg/day
  ◊ Imipramine (Tofranil) 50-100 mg/day
  ◊ Nortriptyline (Pamelor) 25-50 mg/day

Contraindications:
• NSAID's and antidepressants, in general, not suitable for use in children
• Antidepressants should not be used concomitantly with MAO inhibitors

Precautions:
• Do not use antidepressants in presence of acute myocardial infarction
• Avoid over dependence on nonprescription caffeine-containing preparations
• Use NSAID's with precaution in patients with history of previous peptic disease

Significant possible interactions:
Antidepressants and alcohol create accentuated depression

ALTERNATIVE DRUGS
• Beta blockers - prophylaxis (select one):
  ◊ Propranolol (Inderal LA) 80 mg/daily
  ◊ Nadolol (Corgard) 40 mg/daily
  ◊ Atenolol (Tenormin) 50-100 mg/daily
• Combination agent - prophylaxis
  ◊ Isometheptene - dichloralphenazone - acetaminophen (Midrin) one capsule tid
• Other NSAIDs

FOLLOWUP

PATIENT MONITORING
A warm, nonjudgmental, understanding relationship with the physician is the best predictor for a successful treatment program

PREVENTION/AVOIDANCE
• Physical therapy
• Biofeedback and relaxation therapy
• Cervical traction
• Injection of trigger points

POSSIBLE COMPLICATIONS
• Undue reliance on non-prescription caffeine-containing analgesics
• Dependence/addiction to narcotic analgesics
• GI bleed from NSAID use
• Risk of addiction to analgesics
• Risk of epilepsy is four times that of the general population

EXPECTED COURSE/PROGNOSIS
• Usually follows a chronic course when life stressors are not changed
• Most cases are intermittent and should not interfere with work or normal life span

MISCELLANEOUS

ASSOCIATED CONDITIONS
10% of patients with tension headache also have migraine headache

AGE-RELATED FACTORS
Pediatric: 15% will have onset at age less than 10 years
Geriatric: Onset of new headache in the elderly is always worrisome and cause for careful study
Others: Unusual for tension-type headaches to begin after age 50

PREGNANCY
No documented relationship

SYNONYMS
• Muscle contraction headache
• Cephalgia

ICD-9-CM
307.81 Tension headache

SEE ALSO
N/A

OTHER NOTES
N/A

ABBREVIATIONS
N/A

REFERENCES
• Bonica JJ: The Management of Pain. 2nd Ed. Philadelphia, Lea and Febiger, 1990
• Perchalsji JJ: Managing the Patient with Chronic Daily Headache. Family Practice Recertification 1994;16(11):34-42.
• Smith R: Chronic Headaches in Family Practice. JABFP 15(6):589-599
Illustrations: N/A
Internet references: http://www.5mcc.com

Author(s)
Don McHard, MD

Hearing loss

BASICS

DESCRIPTION Complete or partial hearing loss that may involve the middle ear (mechanical, conductive) or the inner ear (nerve, sensorineural)
System(s) affected: Nervous
Genetics: Both types may be on a genetic basis
Incidence/Prevalence in USA:
• 140/100,000/year (134 adults, 6 school age children)
• 3,494 (cases/100,000), with 3,333 for adults and 161 for school age children
Predominant age: All ages, but more common in elderly
Predominant sex: Male = Female

SIGNS AND SYMPTOMS Obvious difficulty hearing, with possible association of other symptoms such as tinnitus, dizziness, pain, and fullness

CAUSES
• Conductive
  ◊ Cerumen impaction
  ◊ Perforation of tympanica membrane
  ◊ Middle ear fluid (serous otitis media)
  ◊ Acute otitis media
  ◊ Adhesive otitis media
  ◊ Damage to ossicles (trauma, infection, etc.)
  ◊ Tympanosclerosis (thickening of drum that may produce fixation)
  ◊ Otosclerosis (new bone growth that produces stapes fixation)
  ◊ Cholesteatoma (growth of skin into middle ear)
  ◊ Middle ear tumor (glomus, etc.)
  ◊ Congenital problems (atresia, ossicular fixation, etc.)
  ◊ Temporal bone fracture, injuries
• Sensorineural
  ◊ Acoustic tumor
  ◊ Meniere's disease
  ◊ Noise induced (industrial, recreational, occupational)
  ◊ Hereditary
  ◊ Congenital
  ◊ Viral (relatively common, esp. mumps)
  ◊ Ototoxicity (ASA, quinine, gentamicin, kanamycin, etc.)
  ◊ Syphilis - hearing loss, tinnitus, dizzy
  ◊ Presbycusis (hearing loss related to aging)
  ◊ Temporal bone injury, fracture
  ◊ Metabolic (hypothyroid, etc.)
  ◊ Perilymphatic (inner ear) fistula (usually secondary to pressure changes or trauma)
  ◊ Autoimmune disease

RISK FACTORS Nasal allergy and other causes of eustachian tube obstruction; exposure to loud noise levels; use of ototoxic antibiotics; prematurity; heredity (otosclerosis)

DIAGNOSIS

DIFFERENTIAL DIAGNOSIS
• In conductive loss, must rule out cholesteatoma
• In sensorineural loss, must rule out acoustic tumor

LABORATORY N/A
Drugs that may alter lab results: N/A
Disorders that may alter lab results: N/A

PATHOLOGICAL FINDINGS N/A

SPECIAL TESTS
• Audiometry including pure tone and speech testing, and impedance (middle ear pressure) testing. Both types of hearing loss may fluctuate, making audiometric results variable from test to test. Marked conductive loss in one ear may be difficult to exclude (mask) when testing opposite ear.
• Otoscopy with operating microscope (sometimes necessary to see small superior, attic perforation, indicating a cholesteatoma)

IMAGING
• CT scan (not routinely needed) is useful to demonstrate tumors and cholesteatoma of the temporal bone
• MRI scan is more useful to show acoustic and other cerebellopontine angle tumors (usually produce a sensorineural hearing loss)

DIAGNOSTIC PROCEDURES
• Exploratory tympanotomy sometimes necessary to confirm presence of middle ear fluid, tumor, etc.
• Underlying conditions are identified primarily on basis of history of hearing loss, otoscopy, and hearing test (audiometry)
• FTA or equivalent
• Sed rate for autoimmune disease

TREATMENT

APPROPRIATE HEALTH CARE
Outpatient

GENERAL MEASURES
• Conductive (mechanical)
  ◊ Cerumen: Remove with suction and irrigation (not if perforation is present). Don't direct water against drum but against canal wall. Manipulation with wire curette may help.
  ◊ Tympanic membrane perforation: Surgical correction
  ◊ Serous otitis (primarily in children). Treat underlying conditions. Use decongestants, antibiotics. Urge inflation of eustachian tube (hold nose and blow).
  ◊ Adhesive otitis: Looks like perforation. Treat eustachian tube problem. May need surgery.

◊ Damage to ossicles: Don't manipulate. Refer to otolaryngologist.
◊ Tympanosclerosis: Drum has white plaques. Treat only if hearing loss is present.
◊ Otosclerosis: Suspect on basis of history of onset, early in life, that is progressive, with positive family history of hearing loss. Consider surgery. Refer to otolaryngologist.
◊ Cholesteatoma: Identify by perforation that is located near margin of drum. Refer to otolaryngologist.
◊ Middle ear tumor: May see through drum. Most commonly will be glomus tumor, which has red color and may cause pulsation. Significant problem, needs prompt referral to otolaryngologist.
◊ Congenital deformity: Don't attribute all hearing loss in children to infections and middle ear fluid. Refer to otolaryngologist.
◊ Temporal bone injury: If limited, may only involve middle ear. Drum likely to appear blue. Refer to otolaryngologist.
• Sensorineural (nerve)
◊ Acoustic tumor: Most significant type of hearing loss. Very important to diagnose promptly. Suspect when unilateral hearing loss and tinnitus (with or without dizziness) are present. Needs much higher degree of suspicion on part of primary care physician. Refer to otolaryngologist.
◊ See topic on Meniere's disease
◊ Noise damage: The most common cause of hearing loss in this country. Very frequent on occupational basis, and has the attention of federal government (OSHA regulations). Also occurs secondary to sports and recreation (hunting, use of guns, loud music, chain saws, shop tools). Needs much greater level of recognition at primary care level. Refer to otolaryngologist.
◊ Hereditary/congenital: Needs immediate recognition early in life, so that if significant, hearing aids can be placed. Rarely, surgery may be effective.
◊ Viral: A relatively common cause of permanent hearing loss, frequently unilateral, e.g., mumps
◊ Ototoxic (medication): Needs much more recognition at primary care level. Suspect when hearing loss, and perhaps dizziness and tinnitus come on during course of treatment with certain antibiotics (and many other medications). See Medications.
◊ Syphilis: Treat with high dose penicillin given intravenously, as well as steroids
◊ Presbycusis: No specific treatment available, but important to provide hearing rehabilitation. This includes counseling patient to avoid factors that may cause further loss (noise exposure, ototoxic drugs). Emphasize development of lip reading skills, and counseling family to pronounce words clearly, face patient when speaking, etc. Offer hearing aid trial when patient is a suitable candidate.
◊ Temporal bone injury: No treatment available specifically for hearing loss unless middle ear is involved
◊ Metabolic: Treatment of specific problem (e.g. hyperlipidemia, hypothyroid)
◊ Perilymphatic fistula: Diagnosis based on history of injury to ear including barotrauma during diving. Treatment is early exploration to confirm fistula in round or oval window of middle ear, with repair of fistula. Refer to otolaryngologist.

◊ Total or near total sensorineural hearing loss: Cochlear implant (electronic device inserted into mastoid and inner ear)
◊ Autoimmune sensorineural hearing loss: Steroids and chemotherapy. Refer to otolaryngologist.

SURGICAL MEASURES
See General Measures

ACTIVITY
• Patients having perforation of the ear drum or ventilation tube in place should be advised not to swim or allow water to enter the ear
• Patients having hearing loss secondary to noise exposure should be advised to avoid loud noise, or to use suitable protection (ear plugs or ear muffs)

DIET
Patients whose hearing loss is due to Meniere's disease should avoid excessive use of salt

PATIENT EDUCATION
See information under other headings

MEDICATIONS

DRUG(S) OF CHOICE
• Cerumen impaction - it is frequently helpful to soften the wax prior to removing it. triethanolamine polypeptide oleate-condensate (Cerumenex) is popular, but should not be used in the presence of a perforation, and may produce a skin reaction. A good alternative is simply to place, or have the patient place mineral oil in the ear canal overnight prior to wax removal. Hexachlorophene (pHisoHex) and topical docusate sodium (Colace) are also useful to soften very hard wax.
• Acute otitis media - erythromycin or amoxicillin
• Chronic otitis media with purulent drainage - neomycin-polymyxin B-hydrocortisone (Cortisporin) otic drops (or an equivalent) placed into the ear canal (3-6 drops bid)
• Serous otitis media - decongestant, e.g., phenylephrine - phenylpropanolamine - guaifenesin (Entex) and erythromycin
• Sudden sensorineural hearing loss with no apparent cause - steroid therapy in high dosage form (80 mg/day of prednisone, or equivalent steroid) may be helpful
Contraindications: History of sensitivity to any of the antibiotics referred to above
Precautions: Avoid the temptation of over-diagnosing "red ear" and using antibiotics without a well thought out diagnosis
Significant possible interactions: Refer to manufacturer's literature

ALTERNATIVE DRUGS
• Acute otitis media - cefaclor
• Chronic ear infection with drainage - ear drops and powder containing ciprofloxacin. Gentamicin drops is another alternative.

FOLLOWUP

PATIENT MONITORING
Hearing testing (audiometry) is the primary means of monitoring patient progress

PREVENTION/AVOIDANCE
• Impaired eustachian tube function (serous otitis media, acute otitis media) - improve tubal function with treatment of allergic and sinus disease. Treat upper respiratory infections (URI) promptly and aggressively if ear problems are frequent.
• Sensorineural hearing loss due to noise exposure (or any type of nerve deafness) - advise against excessive noise exposure; recommend ear plugs/ear muffs
• Nerve deafness due to ototoxic medications may be prevented by the avoidance, or careful use of drugs known to be ototoxic (consider audiometric monitoring if used). The most frequently implicated antibiotics are gentamicin, kanamycin, neomycin, vancomycin, and streptomycin. Other implicated drugs include lidocaine, morphine, digitalis, quinidine, and furosemide. Use of these drugs cannot always be avoided. Be more suspicious of the possibility that a given medication might be ototoxic, and when hearing loss is a problem, to prescribe with care.
• Serious nerve deafness resulting from CNS disease (meningitis, lues) may be prevented by thorough treatment of the primary problem
• If URI present, avoid flying or diving

POSSIBLE COMPLICATIONS
• Middle ear problems may progress to chronic ear problems (perforations, cholesteatoma)
• Cholesteatoma is capable of producing major complications including permanent loss of hearing, balance problems, facial nerve paralysis, meningitis, lateral sinus thrombosis, and brain abscess. Glomus tumors and acoustic tumors must be identified, or major CNS complications may result.
• Meniere's disease may proceed to total and permanent hearing loss if not treated, and may occur in spite of treatment
• Severe nerve deafness, particularly associated with tinnitus may produce such an emotional impact on the patient that suicide may occur. Treat the patient with empathy and understanding, offer help even if it seems limited. Encouragement and followup care are extremely helpful in managing these patients.

EXPECTED COURSE/PROGNOSIS
Sensorineural hearing loss is usually permanent, but in a few instances, may be improved, cured or have progression halted

MISCELLANEOUS

ASSOCIATED CONDITIONS
Noise, allergy, sinus disease, trauma, heredity, ototoxicity, CNS infections (meningitis, lues), age, hyperlipidemia, hypothyroid, barotrauma and autoimmune disease

AGE-RELATED FACTORS
Pediatric: Eustachian tube problems and secondary middle ear problems are more common in infants and small children, usually becoming less frequent by approximately age 10
Geriatric: Presbycusis is common and is made worse by noise exposure and other factors
Others: N/A

PREGNANCY
Otosclerosis may become active during pregnancy

SYNONYMS
N/A

ICD-9-CM
Cerumen: 380.4; perforation: 389.02 and 384.21; serous otitis media: 381.10 and 389.03; acute otitis media: 382.00 and 389.03; adhesive otitis media: 389.03 and 385.13; ossicular damage: 389.03 and 872.72; tympanosclerosis:385.03 and 389.03; otosclerosis: 387.0; cholesteatoma: 384.22; glomus tumor of middle ear: 212.0; congenital conductive loss: 744.04, 744.02, and 389.03; temporal bone fracture with conductive hearing loss: 384.21, 389.02, and 801.01; acoustic neuroma: 225.1; Meniere's disease: 386.01; noise related sensorineural hearing loss (SNHL): 388.12; hereditary SNHL:389.8, V19.2; congenital SNHL: 389.18 and 744.3; viral SNHL: 389.18 and 079.9; ototoxic SNHL: 389.18 and 960.6; luetic SNHL: 094.86; age related SNHL (presbycusis): 388.01; temporal bone injury with SNHL: 951.5; perilymphatic fistula with SNHL: 386.41 and 389.18

SEE ALSO
N/A

OTHER NOTES
N/A

ABBREVIATIONS
SNHL = sensorineural hearing loss

REFERENCES
DeWeese DD, Saunders WH, Schuller DE, Schleuning AJ: Otolaryngology-Head and Neck Surgery. 7th Ed. St. Louis, C.V. Mosby Company, 1988:445-477
Illustrations: N/A
Internet references: http://www.5mcc.com

Author(s)
Gale Gardner, MD, FACS

Heat exhaustion & heat stroke

BASICS

DESCRIPTION A continuum of increasingly severe heat illnesses caused by dehydration, electrolyte losses, and failure of the body's thermoregulatory mechanisms
• Heat exhaustion is an acute heat injury with hyperthermia due to dehydration
• Heat stroke is extreme hyperthermia with thermoregulatory failure and profound central nervous system dysfunction
System(s) affected: Endocrine/Metabolic, Nervous
Genetics: N/A
Incidence/Prevalence in USA: Dependent on predisposing conditions in combination with environmental factors
Predominant age: More likely in children or elderly
Predominant sex: Male = Female

SIGNS AND SYMPTOMS
• Heat Exhaustion
 ◊ Fatigue and lethargy
 ◊ Weakness
 ◊ Dizziness
 ◊ Nausea, vomiting
 ◊ Myalgias
 ◊ Headache
 ◊ Profuse sweating
 ◊ Tachycardia
 ◊ Hypotension
 ◊ Lack of coordination
 ◊ Agitation
 ◊ Intense thirst
 ◊ Hyperventilation
 ◊ Paresthesias
 ◊ Core temperature elevated but < 103°F (< 39.4°C)
• Heat Stroke
 ◊ Exhaustion
 ◊ Confusion, disorientation
 ◊ Coma
 ◊ Hot, flushed, dry skin
 ◊ Core temperature > 105°F (> 40.5°C)

CAUSES Failure of heat-dissipating mechanisms or an overwhelming heat stress leading to a rise in core temperature, dehydration and salt depletion

RISK FACTORS
• Poor acclimatization to heat or poor physical conditioning
• Salt or water depletion
• Obesity
• Acute febrile or gastrointestinal illnesses
• Chronic illnesses - uncontrolled diabetes or hypertension, cardiac disease
• Alcohol and other substance abuse
• High heat and humidity, poor air circulation in environment
• Heavy, restrictive clothing

DIAGNOSIS

DIFFERENTIAL DIAGNOSIS
• Other causes of elevated temperature, dehydration or circulatory collapse
 ◊ Febrile illnesses, sepsis
 ◊ Drug-induced fluid loss
 ◊ Cardiac arrhythmia or infarction
 ◊ Acute cocaine intoxication
 ◊ Malignant hyperthermia (an autosomally inherited disorder of skeletal and cardiac muscle in which patients have abnormal muscle metabolism on exposure to halothane or skeletal muscle reactants)

LABORATORY
• Used primarily to detect end-organ damage
• Electrolytes, urinalysis
• Creatinine, blood urea nitrogen
• Liver enzymes
• Complete blood count
• Increased urine specific gravity
• Results of above studies yield hypernatremia, hyperchloremia, hemoconcentration
Drugs that may alter lab results: Diuretics
Disorders that may alter lab results: N/A

PATHOLOGICAL FINDINGS Only those associated with major organ system failure

SPECIAL TESTS N/A

IMAGING N/A

DIAGNOSTIC PROCEDURES Rectal temperature monitoring

TREATMENT

APPROPRIATE HEALTH CARE Emergency treatment - best in a hospital setting

GENERAL MEASURES
• Rapid cooling - remove clothing, wet patient down, ice packs
• Fluid and electrolyte replacement with hypotonic oral fluids or IV 0.5-1.0 liter normal saline
• Consider central venous pressure monitoring

SURGICAL MEASURES N/A

ACTIVITY Rest with legs elevated

DIET
• Cool or cold clear liquids only (non-carbonated)
• Avoid caffeine
• Unrestricted sodium

PATIENT EDUCATION
• Stress the importance of proper conditioning and acclimatization
• Instruct patients to recognize heat stress signs and symptoms
• Maintain as much skin exposure as possible in hot, humid conditions, while using proper sun block protection
• Avoid dehydration with proper fluids during activity or exercise - 8 oz fluid intake for every 15 minutes of moderate exercise

MEDICATIONS

DRUG(S) OF CHOICE No medications are required in the initial management. Use isotonic saline solution to rehydrate.
Contraindications: N/A
Precautions: N/A
Significant possible interactions: N/A

ALTERNATIVE DRUGS N/A

 ## FOLLOWUP

PATIENT MONITORING
• Rectal temperature monitoring - cooling may be discontinued when the core temperature drops to 102°F (38.9°C) and stabilizes
• Heat stroke patients may require airway management, hemodynamic monitoring and careful fluid and electrolyte administration and monitoring
• Consider central venous pressure monitoring

PREVENTION/AVOIDANCE Most important factor in preventing heat stress is adequate fluid replacement. Allow acclimatization to hot weather through proper conditioning and activity modification. Dress appropriately with loose-fitting, open weave, light-colored clothing.

POSSIBLE COMPLICATIONS
• May involve failure of any major organ system
• Cardiac arrhythmias or infarction
• Pulmonary edema, adult respiratory distress syndrome
• Coma, seizures
• Acute renal failure
• Rhabdomyolysis
• Disseminated intravascular coagulation
• Hepatocellular necrosis

EXPECTED COURSE/PROGNOSIS
• Good when mental function is not altered and when serum enzymes are not elevated. Recovery is within 24-48 hours in most cases.
• The mortality rate for heat stroke (10-80%) is directly related to the duration and intensity of hyperthermia as well as to the speed and effectiveness of diagnosis and treatment

 ## MISCELLANEOUS

ASSOCIATED CONDITIONS N/A

AGE-RELATED FACTORS
Pediatric: Children are more susceptible
Geriatric: Elderly are more susceptible
Others: N/A

PREGNANCY May be more prone to volume depletion with heat stress

SYNONYMS
• Heat illness
• Heat injury
• Hyperthermia
• Heat collapse
• Heat prostration

ICD-9-CM
• 992.5 Heat exhaustion
• 992.0 Heat stroke

SEE ALSO Hyperthermia, malignant

OTHER NOTES N/A

ABBREVIATIONS N/A

REFERENCES)
• Mellion MB, Shelton GL: Safe exercise in the heat and heat injury. In: Mellion MB, Walsh AR, Shelton GL, eds. The Team Physician's Handbook. Philadelphia, Hanley & Belfus, 1990:59-69
• Hubbard RW, Armstrong LE: Hyperthermia: new thoughts on an old problem. Phys Sportsmed 1989;17(6):97-113
• Knochel JP: Heatstroke and related heat stress disorders. Disease-A-Month 1989;35(5):301-377
• Brouchama A: Heat stroke: a new look at an ancient disease. Int Care Med 1995;21(8):623-625
Illustrations: N/A
Internet references: http://www.5mcc.com

Author(s)
Scott A. Fields, MD

Hemochromatosis

 BASICS

DESCRIPTION A hereditary disorder in which the small intestine absorbs excessive iron. Since the body lacks any way to excrete iron, the excess is stored in glands and muscle, such as the liver, pancreas, and heart. Over the years, the involved organs begin to fail.
System(s) affected: Endocrine/Metabolic
Genetics: Autosomal recessive; acquired; HLA-A3; HLA-B14; HLA-B7
Incidence/Prevalence in USA:
3 cases/1000 people (heterozygote frequency 1 in 10) - the most common abnormal gene in the US population
Predominant age: Present from birth, but symptoms usually present in the fifth and sixth decades
Predominant sex: Male = Female (clinical signs are more frequent in men (8:1 male to female ratio)

SIGNS AND SYMPTOMS
• Weakness (83%)
• Abdominal pain (58%)
• Arthralgia (43%)
• Loss of libido or potency (38%)
• Amenorrhea (22%)
• Dyspnea on exertion (15%)
• Neurologic symptoms (6%)
• Hepatomegaly (83%)
• Increased skin pigmentation (75%)
• Loss of body hair (20%)
• Splenomegaly (13%)
• Peripheral edema (12%)
• Jaundice (10%)
• Gynecomastia (8%)
• Ascites (6%)
• Testicular atrophy
• Hepatic tenderness
• Diabetes mellitus symptoms

CAUSES
• The mechanism for increased iron absorption in the face of excessive iron stores is unknown. Iron metabolism appears normal in this disease except for a higher level of circulating iron.
• Iron overload may be due to thalassemia, sideroblastic anemia, liver disease, excess iron intake, chronic transfusion

RISK FACTORS
• The disease is a genetic disorder. Some variables influence the age of onset and severity of symptoms
• Intake of iron, especially from vitamin supplements. These may contain large amounts of iron as well as vitamin C, which enhances iron absorption
• Alcohol increases the absorption of iron (as high as 41% of patients with symptomatic disease are alcoholic)
• Loss of blood delays the onset of symptoms, such as blood loss in women because of menstruation and pregnancy.

 DIAGNOSIS

DIFFERENTIAL DIAGNOSIS
• Repeated transfusions
• Hereditary anemias with ineffective erythropoiesis
• Alcoholic cirrhosis
• Porphyria cutanea tarda
• Atransferrinemia
• Excessive ingestion of iron (rare)

LABORATORY
• Transferrin saturation (serum iron concentration divided by total iron-binding capacity x 100): greater than 70% is virtually diagnostic of iron overload; 50% or higher warrants further evaluation
• Serum ferritin: greater than 300 µg/L for men and 120 µg/L for women
• Urinary iron
• Increased urine hemosiderin
• Hyperglycemia
• Decreased FSH
• Decreased LH
• Decreased testosterone
• Increased SGOT
• Hypoalbuminemia
Drugs that may alter lab results: Iron supplements, transfusions may elevate serum iron
Disorders that may alter lab results: Inflammatory reactions, other forms of liver disease, certain tumors (e.g., acute granulocytic leukemia), rheumatoid arthritis may elevate serum ferritin

PATHOLOGICAL FINDINGS
• Increased hepatic parenchymal iron stores
• Hepatic fibrosis and cirrhosis with hepatomegaly
• Pancreatic enlargement
• Excess hemosiderin in liver, pancreas, myocardium, thyroid, parathyroid, joints, skin
• Cardiomegaly
• Joint deposition of iron

SPECIAL TESTS After diagnosis established, consider oral glucose tolerance test to rule out diabetes and echocardiogram to rule out cardiomyopathy

IMAGING CT scan, MRI, and magnetic susceptibility measurement (MSM) are being studied for measuring body iron, but have not yet reached validation and general availability

DIAGNOSTIC PROCEDURES Liver biopsy for stainable iron is the standard for diagnosis. Presence or absence of cirrhosis can also be ascertained.

 TREATMENT

APPROPRIATE HEALTH CARE
Outpatient

GENERAL MEASURES
• Removal of excess iron by repeated phlebotomy once or twice weekly to establish and maintain a mild anemia (hematocrit of 37-39%)
• When the patient finally becomes iron deficient, a lifelong maintenance program of 4-6 phlebotomies a year to keep storage iron normal

SURGICAL MEASURES N/A

ACTIVITY Full activity unless significant heart disease

DIET
• An iron-poor diet is not of significant benefit
• Avoid alcohol, iron-fortified foods, and iron-containing supplements
• Restrict vitamin C to small doses between meals
• Tea chelates iron and may be drunk with meals

PATIENT EDUCATION
• Hemochromatosis Research Foundation, Inc., P.O. Box 8569, Albany, NY 12208
• Iron Overload Diseases Association, Inc., 433 Westwind Dr., North Palm Beach, FL 33408

MEDICATIONS

DRUG(S) OF CHOICE None. Only when phlebotomy is not feasible or in the presence of severe heart disease should the iron-chelating agent deferoxamine (Desferal) be considered.
Contraindications: N/A
Precautions: N/A
Significant possible interactions: N/A

ALTERNATIVE DRUGS None

FOLLOWUP

PATIENT MONITORING
• Measure hematocrit before each phlebotomy - skip phlebotomy if hematocrit is less than 36%
• Schedule an additional phlebotomy when hematocrit is greater than 40%
• When anemia becomes refractory, repeat transferrin saturation and serum ferritin to confirm depletion of iron stores
• When iron stores are depleted, 4 to 6 phlebotomies a year should keep iron stores normal
• During maintenance therapy, measure transferrin saturation and serum ferritin yearly
• Liver biopsy to assess iron stores when serum iron transferrin and ferritin results have not normalized

PREVENTION/AVOIDANCE Family members should be screened

POSSIBLE COMPLICATIONS
• Cirrhosis
• Hepatoma (only in patients with cirrhosis)
• Diabetes mellitus
• Cardiomyopathy
• Arthritis
• Hypogonadism

EXPECTED COURSE/PROGNOSIS
• Patients diagnosed before cirrhosis develops and treated with phlebotomy have a normal life expectancy
• Life expectancy is reduced in patients with cirrhosis, diabetes mellitus, and patients that require longer than 18 months of phlebotomy therapy to return iron stores to normal

MISCELLANEOUS

ASSOCIATED CONDITIONS See Possible complications

AGE-RELATED FACTORS
Pediatric: Although rare, iron overload can occur even as early as 2 years of age. The disorder can be diagnosed before iron overload is clinically apparent
Geriatric: N/A
Others: N/A

PREGNANCY Avoid iron supplements

SYNONYMS
• Bronze diabetes
• Troisier-Hanot-Chauffard syndrome

ICD-9-CM 275.0 Disorders of iron metabolism

SEE ALSO N/A

OTHER NOTES Most patients with hemochromatosis go undiagnosed. Since treatment with phlebotomy will prevent all complications when begun early, the diagnosis of hemochromatosis should be considered much more frequently by physicians

ABBREVIATIONS N/A

REFERENCES
• Crosby WH: Hemochromatosis: Current concepts and management. Hosp Pract (Off) 1987;22(2):173-7, 181-92
• Smith LH: Overview of hemochromatosis. West J Med 1990153:296-308
• Kumar A, Riely CA: Inherited liver diseases in adults. West J Med 1995;163:382-386
Illustrations: 1 available on CD-ROM
Internet references: http://www.5mcc.com

Author(s)
Robert A. Marlow, MD, MA

Hemophilia

 BASICS

DESCRIPTION
• Hemophilia A and hemophilia B are clinically indistinguishable, inherited bleeding disorders due to a deficiency of coagulant factor VIII (hemophilia A) or factor IX (hemophilia B)
• Disease severity is determined by percent of coagulant factor present. Less than 2% factor activity is severe, 2-5% factor activity is moderate, 6-25% factor activity is mild. Those with greater than 25% factor activity rarely may fail to clot after major trauma or surgery.
System(s) affected:
Hemic/Lymphatic/Immunologic
Genetics: Both hemophilia A and hemophilia B are X-linked, recessive
Incidence/Prevalence in USA:
• Hemophilia A - 10 in 100,000 males
• Hemophilia B - 2 in 100,000 males
Predominant age:
• Both are congenital conditions
• Severe disease generally noted at birth or in first year
• Mild disease may not be diagnosed until young adulthood
Predominant sex: Females are generally asymptomatic carriers. Rare exceptions occur from consanguinity within families, concomitant Turner's syndrome, or extremely disproportionate lyonization resulting in the preponderance of cells in the carrier female containing the X chromosome with the hemophilic gene.

SIGNS AND SYMPTOMS
• Bleeding into soft tissues, muscles, and weight-bearing joints
• Bleeding occurs hours to days after injury, can involve any organ, and can continue for hours to days
• Compartment syndromes and ischemic nerve damage from large hematomas
• Repeated bleeding into a joint causes osteoarthritis, articular fibrosis, and joint ankylosis
• Hematuria
• CNS bleeding, usually post-traumatic

CAUSES Congenital

RISK FACTORS Positive family history. Can predict risk to offspring using simple Mendelian genetics for an X-linked recessive disorder.

 DIAGNOSIS

DIFFERENTIAL DIAGNOSIS
• Von Willebrand's disease
• Vitamin K deficiency (factor IX is vitamin K dependent)
• Other factor deficiencies, afibrinogenemia, dysfibrinogenemia, fibrinolytic defects, platelet disorders

LABORATORY
• Activated partial thromboplastin time (PTT) is prolonged while platelet count, and prothrombin time are normal
• Bleeding time is prolonged in 15-20% of patients with hemophilia A
• PTT is corrected when mixed with normal plasma
• Hemophilia A - diagnostic test is low factor VIII.
• Hemophilia B - diagnostic test is low factor IX
Drugs that may alter lab results: Recent aspirin use will increase bleeding time, leading to confusion with Von Willebrand's disease
Disorders that may alter lab results: N/A

PATHOLOGICAL FINDINGS
• Synovial hemosiderosis
• Articular cartilage degeneration
• Thickening of periarticular tissues
• Bony hypertrophy

SPECIAL TESTS Hemophilia A - carrier detection compares the ratio of factor VIII to von Willebrand's factor protein and is predictive in up to 95% of cases. Molecular diagnosis is preferred for carrier testing.

IMAGING N/A

DIAGNOSTIC PROCEDURES N/A

 TREATMENT

APPROPRIATE HEALTH CARE
• Outpatient
• Home infusion therapy
• Inpatient for infusions following significant bleeding episodes

GENERAL MEASURES
• Avoid aspirin or aspirin-containing drugs
• Treat early. Symptoms often precede obvious bleeding.
• An uncomplicated, soft tissue bleeding or an early hemarthrosis requires a single infusion to 20-30% activity
• More extensive hemarthrosis or retroperitoneal bleeding requires bid infusions for 72 or more hours to 25-50% activity
• Life-threatening bleeding into the CNS requires maintaining levels greater than 50% activity for 2 weeks
• Major surgery requires greater than 50% activity preoperatively, continued for 1-2 weeks postoperatively
• Orthopedic care and physical therapy to prevent contractures and maintain joint mobility
• Vaccinate against hepatitis B at time of diagnosis
• Maintain good dental care
• Annual evaluation in a comprehensive hemophilia center
• Consideration for three times weekly prophylaxis in severe factor VIII deficiency

SURGICAL MEASURES N/A

ACTIVITY
• Attempt to lead as normal a life as possible
• Restrict activities in proportion to the degree of factor deficiency, but maintaining a trim physical condition is important

DIET No special diet

PATIENT EDUCATION
• Teach patient and family about signs and symptoms to watch for
• Genetic counseling
• Home care with self administered replacement therapy is often used
• Printed patient information available from: National Hemophilia Foundation, 110 Green Street, Room 406, New York, NY, 10012, (212)219-8180

Hemophilia

MEDICATIONS

DRUG(S) OF CHOICE
• Hemophilia A: Recombinant or monoclonal factor VIII is treatment of choice for hemophilia A patients who are HIV negative and who have had minimal prior concentrate exposure.
◊ Requires plasma products enriched in factor VIII [cryoprecipitate, factor VIII concentrate]
◊ 1 unit of factor VIII (the amount in 1 mL of plasma) will raise the plasma level of the recipient by 2% per kilogram of body weight
◊ To calculate amount of factor VIII needed: Number units needed = [(desired percent activity minus current percent activity) times (body weight in kilograms)] divided by 2% per unit per kilogram
◊ For example: 70 kg man with 5% activity needs to be taken to 25% activity. Equation for number units needed: [(25% - 5%) x (70 kg)] / 2% per kg = [(25 - 5) x (70)] / 2 = 700 units needed
◊ Half-life of factor VIII is 8-12 hours, therefore need to infuse at least bid to maintain a chosen factor VIII level, and tid when tight control of the level is needed
• Hemophilia B: Monoclonal antibody purified factor IX is treatment of choice for hemophilia B patients who are HIV negative and who have had minimal prior concentrate exposure.
◊ Fresh frozen plasma may be used for mild patients. Generally requires about 10-20 mL/kg bid. There is danger of volume overload.
◊ Factor IX concentrate for moderate to severe hemorrhage and patients to undergo surgery. One unit/kg will raise levels 1%
Contraindications: None
Precautions: Hemophilia B - some factor IX concentrates contain trace amounts of activated vitamin K-dependent factors and therefore are thrombogenic and carry a risk for thromboembolism
Significant possible interactions: N/A

ALTERNATIVE DRUGS
• Desmopressin should be used in mild hemophilia to transiently raise factor VIII levels. A convenient intranasal preparation is now available
• Aminocaproic acid (epsilon-aminocaproic acid, EACA) can be used for minor dental work following a single factor VIII infusion. Aminocaproic acid greatly enhances the risk of thromboembolism and should be used with caution with factor IX concentrates.
• Patients with inhibitors to factor VIII may require intensive plasmapheresis, large doses of concentrate, infusion of prothrombin complex concentrates (by-passing products), or porcine factor VIII

FOLLOWUP

PATIENT MONITORING Regular evaluations every 6 to 12 months include a musculoskeletal evaluation, an inhibitor screen, liver tests, and tests for antibodies to hepatitis viruses and human immunodeficiency virus (HIV)

PREVENTION/AVOIDANCE Genetic counseling

POSSIBLE COMPLICATIONS
• Factor VIII and IX preparations and transfusions result in viral hepatitis, chronic liver disease, and acquired immunodeficiency syndrome (AIDS). However, recent advances in factor VIII concentrate preparation should prevent future HIV infection and hepatitis B and C.
• Hemophilia A - 10-20% of patients develop inhibitors to factor VIII, typically those with severe disease receiving multiple transfusions. Type I (high responders) inhibitors to factor VIII rapidly neutralize factor VIII and prevent effective transfusion therapy. Type II (low responders) inhibitors are low-titer and may respond to higher than normal doses of factor VIII.

EXPECTED COURSE/PROGNOSIS
• Repeated hemarthroses result in eventual deformity and crippling
• Survival is normal for those with mild disease, and mortality is increased 2 to 6 fold in those with moderate to severe disease, primarily due to complications of infection
• Median life expectancy with this condition peaked in late 1970's at 68 years, and is now declining due to the AIDS epidemic
• Up to 70% are HIV seropositive, especially those with severe disease, and 4% with severe disease develop AIDS. Younger patients whose treatment began since the mid-late 80's are largely HIV negative and are not expected to be exposed by modern replacement products. The proportion of HIV positive hemophiliacs is therefore declining.

MISCELLANEOUS

ASSOCIATED CONDITIONS None

AGE-RELATED FACTORS
Pediatric: Mean age of onset of symptoms is 1.5 years for severe disease (often noted in first year), 3.0 years for moderate disease, and 5.0 years for mild disease
Geriatric: N/A
Others: N/A

PREGNANCY
• The vast majority of females are asymptomatic carriers, although an occasional carrier will bleed at time of surgery. They require no specific treatment during pregnancy or delivery.
• Prenatal diagnosis previously required sampling fetal blood for coagulant activity. Newer prenatal detection schemes detect an identifiable restriction fragment length polymorphism or a gene deletion or rearrangement in a sample of chorionic villus or from fluid obtained at amniocentesis.

SYNONYMS
• Hemophilia A
• Factor VIII deficiency
• Classic hemophilia
• Hemophilia B
• Factor IX deficiency
• Christmas disease

ICD-9-CM
286.0 Hemophilia A
286.1 Hemophilia B

SEE ALSO N/A

OTHER NOTES Recombinant factor VIII is available. It has biologic activity and clinical efficacy comparable to plasma factor VIII, while posing no risk of transmitting hepatitis viruses or HIV. There are factor VIII and factor IX concentrates prepared from human plasma using a monoclonal antibody method plus either heat or detergent treatment of the concentrate. These monoclonal-prepared concentrates have the lowest risk for hepatitis B and essentially no risk for HIV infection.

ABBREVIATIONS N/A

REFERENCES
• Jones PK, Ratnoff OD: The changing prognosis of classic hemophilia (factor VII "deficiency"). Ann Int Med 1991;114(8):641-8
• Schwartz RS, et al: Human Recombinant DNA-Derived Antihemophilic Factor (Factor VIII) in the Treatment of Hemophilia A. N Engl J Med 1990;323(26):1800-5
Illustrations: N/A
Internet references: http://www.5mcc.com

Author(s)
W. Paul Bowman, MD

Hemorrhoids

 BASICS

DESCRIPTION Varicosities of the hemorrhoidal venous plexus. Usual course - acute; chronic; relapsing.
• External hemorrhoids are located below the dentate line and covered by squamous epithelium
• Internal hemorrhoids are located above the dentate line
System(s) affected: Gastrointestinal, Cardiovascular
Genetics: No known genetic pattern
Incidence/Prevalence in USA: Common
Predominant age: Adults, although may occur at any age
Predominant sex: Male = Female

SIGNS AND SYMPTOMS
• Rectal bleeding
• Anal protrusion
• Anal pain (with ulceration or thrombosis)
• Pruritus
• Constipation
• Straining with defecation
• Bowel incontinence
• Dilated hemorrhoidal veins
• Hematochezia
• Stool mucus
• Sensation of incomplete evacuation of the rectum
• Anal fissure
• Anal infection
• Anal ulceration
• Hemorrhoidal prolapse
• Hemorrhoidal strangulation
• Anemia (rare)
• Hemorrhoidal thrombosis

CAUSES Dilated veins of hemorrhoidal plexus

RISK FACTORS
• Pregnancy
• Colon malignancy
• Liver disease
• Portal hypertension
• Constipation
• Occupations that require prolonged sitting
• Loss of muscle tone in old age, rectal surgery, episiotomy, anal intercourse
• Obesity

 DIAGNOSIS

DIFFERENTIAL DIAGNOSIS N/A

LABORATORY N/A
Drugs that may alter lab results: N/A
Disorders that may alter lab results: N/A

PATHOLOGICAL FINDINGS N/A

SPECIAL TESTS N/A

IMAGING N/A

DIAGNOSTIC PROCEDURES
• Ano-rectal examination including anoscopy
• Sigmoidoscopy
• Inspection following straining at stool

 TREATMENT

APPROPRIATE HEALTH CARE
All of these treatments, except surgical, are outpatient with recovery and freedom from symptoms within 48 hours

GENERAL MEASURES
• Mild symptoms or prevention:
   ◊ Avoid prolonged sitting at stool
   ◊ Avoid straining
   ◊ Avoid constipation through stool softeners
   ◊ Use soap and water for cleanup after stool
• For pain, sitz baths with soapy water, or hypertonic epson salts (cup per 2 quarts of water)

SURGICAL MEASURES
• Indications
   ◊ Persisting and soiling bleeding
   ◊ Prolapsed internal hemorrhoids
   ◊ Poor anal hygiene due to prolapsed hemorrhoids
   ◊ Persistent pain
• Treatments
   ◊ For severe pain:
     - Incision of thrombosed hemorrhoid
   ◊ Severe protruding hemorrhoids:
     - Rubber band ligation (internal hemorrhoids only)
     - Injection therapy (suitable for one or two)
     - Cryosurgery or laser surgery for external hemorrhoids
   ◊ Prolapsed rectum
     - Requires surgical correction
   ◊ Surgical resection - for major external or internal hemorrhoids

ACTIVITY
• No restrictions
• Encourage physical fitness
• Avoid prolonged sitting and straining on the toilet

DIET High fiber

PATIENT EDUCATION Explain recurrence benignity, need for good diet, exercise and stooling health

MEDICATIONS

DRUG(S) OF CHOICE
- Prevention:
  ◊ Fiber supplements
  ◊ Stool softeners
- Pain:
  ◊ Analgesic sprays or ointments - benzocaine (Hurricaine), dibucaine (Nupercainal)
- Pruritus:
  ◊ Hydrocortisone (Anusol-HC; Cortifoam) ointment
- Bleeding:
  ◊ Astringent suppositories (Preparation H)
  ◊ Hydrocortisone (Anusol; Cortifoam) ointment

Contraindications: Refer to manufacturer's literature

Precautions: Refer to manufacturer's literature

Significant possible interactions: Refer to manufacturer's literature

ALTERNATIVE DRUGS N/A

FOLLOWUP

PATIENT MONITORING As needed, depending on treatment

PREVENTION/AVOIDANCE
- Avoid constipation
- Lose weight, if overweight
- Avoid prolonged sitting on the toilet
- Avoid prolonged sitting at work. Get up and move around periodically.

POSSIBLE COMPLICATIONS
- Thrombosis
- Secondary infection
- Ulceration
- Anemia (rare)
- Incontinence

EXPECTED COURSE/PROGNOSIS
- Spontaneous resolution
- Recurrence

MISCELLANEOUS

ASSOCIATED CONDITIONS
- Liver disease
- Pregnancy
- Portal hypertension
- Constipation

AGE-RELATED FACTORS
Pediatric:
- Uncommon in infants and children. Look for underlying cause, e.g., venacaval or mesenteric obstruction, cirrhosis, portal hypertension.
- Occasionally, as in adults, hemorrhoids may result from chronic constipation, fecal impaction and straining at stool. Surgery is rarely required.

Geriatric: Common in elderly along with rectal prolapse

Others: N/A

PREGNANCY Common in pregnancy. Usually resolves after pregnancy. No treatment required, unless extremely painful.

SYNONYMS Piles

ICD-9-CM
455.6 hemorrhoids, nos

SEE ALSO
- Colorectal malignancy
- Portal hypertension
- Portal vein thrombosis

OTHER NOTES N/A

ABBREVIATIONS N/A

REFERENCES
- Fazio VW: Anorectal Disorders. In Gastroenterology Clinics of North America, Philadelphia, W.B. Saunders Co., 1987
- Guthri, JF: The Current Management of Hemorrhoids. Pract Gastroenterol 1987;11:56

Illustrations: N/A

Internet references: http://www.5mcc.com

Author(s)
Frank L. Iber, MD

Hepatic encephalopathy

BASICS

DESCRIPTION Altered mental and neuromotor functioning associated with acute or chronic liver disease and/or portal systemic shunting of blood. The prominent features are mild to marked forgetfulness, impaired arousability, and a "flapping tremor" (asterixis).
System(s) affected: Gastrointestinal, Nervous
Genetics: Unknown
Incidence/Prevalence in USA:
• Occurs in 1/3 cases of cirrhosis
• Occurs in all cases of fulminant hepatic failure
• Present in nearly half of patients who reach the stage of liver disease requiring transplantation
Predominant age: Parallels that of fulminant liver disease with peak in the 40's, and cirrhosis with peak in late 50's. May occur at any age.
Predominant sex: Male = Female (reflecting the underlying liver disease)

SIGNS AND SYMPTOMS
• Ages 10-60
◊ Prominent signs of underlying liver disease (50%), jaundice most common, ascites second most common
◊ Gastrointestinal hemorrhage with hematemesis or melena (20%)
◊ Systemic infection, urinary tract or pulmonary (20%)
◊ Four stages of confusion and obtundity described. (1) forgetfulness, disturbance in nocturnal sleep, daytime drowsiness, (2) mild confusion but arousability, (3) arousable, but markedly confused, limited orientation and thought content, (4) unarousable.
◊ Asterixis prominent in stages 2, 3
◊ Handwriting and hand coordination deteriorated in stages 1, 2
◊ Tremor prominent in stage 2
◊ Psychotic thoughts infrequent
◊ Reflexes symmetrically hyperactive
◊ Tremor and asterixis not observed in ocular muscles
◊ Mental and neurological signs change rapidly (over 6 to 12 hours)
• Age over 60
◊ Signs of underlying liver disease diminished (25%)
◊ Confusion more prominent
◊ Precipitating gastrointestinal hemorrhage or infection less often identified
◊ Remains in stage 1 or 2 for many days
◊ Progression slower
• Age under 10
◊ Signs of underlying liver disease prominent, usually fulminant hepatic failure or extremely advanced cirrhosis
◊ Progression through the stages very rapid, often 6 to 12 hours
◊ Precipitating cause frequently not identified

CAUSES
• Shunting of intestinal blood through the severely diseased liver without the intervention of viable liver cells
• Shunting of such blood through collateral circulation or surgically constructed portacaval shunts
• Thus hepatic coma may occur in extremely advanced acute liver disease (fulminant hepatic failure) or following portacaval shunting or transjugular intrahepatic portal shunt (TIPS). However, it is most common in long standing cirrhosis of the liver with spontaneous shunting of intestinal blood through collaterals.
• Failure of liver to detoxicate agents noxious to CNS, e.g., ammonia, mercaptans, fatty acids
• Increased aromatic and reduced branched chain amino acids in blood
• Precipitation of acute event, search for:
◊ New overt or occult infection including spontaneous peritonitis
◊ Potassium, magnesium or other electrolyte depletion
◊ Use of opiate, sedative, tranquilizer, drugs
◊ Gastrointestinal bleeding

RISK FACTORS
• Advancing age is the most prominent risk factor
• Viral hepatitis
• Drug hepatotoxicity (acetaminophen, halothane, carbon tetrachloride, yellow phosphorus)
• Surgical portacaval shunts including TIPS (transjugular intrahepatic portal systemic shunt)
• Pregnancy
• Herpesvirus

DIAGNOSIS

DIFFERENTIAL DIAGNOSIS
• Head trauma, concussion, subdural hematoma
• Alcohol withdrawal syndrome
• Toxic confusion due to medication
• Toxic confusion due to illicit drug use
• Meningitis
• Metabolic encephalopathy related to anoxia, hypoglycemia, hypokalemia, hypo- or hypercalcemia, uremia

LABORATORY
• Screening blood, sputum and urine cultures to identify infection
• Hematology to identify anemia and signs of infection
• Standard biochemistry profile to identify hypokalemia, bilirubinemia, altered calcium status, hypomagnesemia, urea, hypoglycemia
• Arterial blood gases
• Liver tests to evaluate severity of underlying liver disease
• Prothrombin and partial thromboplastin time
• Venous ammonia (elevated in 70% of liver coma)
• Toxicology screen for illicit drugs

Drugs that may alter lab results:
• Infusion of amino acid solutions may affect ammonia level
• Opiate administration - producing severe constipation may affect ammonia level
Disorders that may alter lab results:
• Uremia may affect ammonia level
• Rapid and severe tissue breakdown, massive burns, trauma or infection may affect ammonia level

PATHOLOGICAL FINDINGS
• Brain edema in 100% of fatal cases
• Glial hypertrophy in chronic encephalopathy

SPECIAL TESTS
• Electroencephalogram shows symmetrical slowing of basic (alpha) rhythm in common with other forms of metabolic encephalopathy
• Visually-evoked potential specific in stages 2, 3 and 4

IMAGING
• Useful only to rule out other diagnoses
• CT scan of head most useful
• Brain MRI shows increased glutamine in basal ganglia

DIAGNOSTIC PROCEDURES
• Clinical setting and findings adequate in 80% of cases
• Venous ammonia of great aid in patients with chronic liver disease when the clinical findings are confusing
• EEG is useful to a limited extent, but findings are similar in other forms of metabolic encephalopathy
• Treatment response often confirms diagnosis

TREATMENT

APPROPRIATE HEALTH CARE
• Outpatient for stages 1 and 2 when diagnosis is clear and if recurrent can be managed satisfactorily
• Stage 3 or 4 requires inpatient management
• Stage 3 or 4 in fulminant hepatic failure is a strong indication for evaluation for liver transplantation. Transfer to a transplant center should be considered.

GENERAL MEASURES
• Identify and treat vigorously precipitating causes - gastrointestinal bleed, infection, sedative drugs, or electrolyte imbalance are most common
• Stage 2 or higher - attention to adequate fluid intake, and at least 1000 kcal (4.19 MJ) of food daily
• Give Fleet's enema to all patients without diarrhea
• Clumsiness and poor judgment prominent. Be sure patient has the care needed to avoid falls, cuts on broken glass, smoking burns, machinery or auto accidents.
• Avoid sedative or opiate medications. Benzodiazepine sedatives and opiate derivatives such as Lomotil have caused liver coma.

SURGICAL MEASURES N/A

ACTIVITY
• As tolerated
• Avoid driving and machinery

DIET
• Integrate with needs of underlying liver disease
• Lower total protein. Stage 1 - avoid protein gluttony. Stage 2 - limit red meat and consume small portions of all other protein foods, total protein for day 50-60 grams. Stage 3 - consume 40 gram protein or vegetable protein diet (about 20 grams). Stage 4 - consume 10 or fewer grams of protein. For all stages at least 1000 kcal (4.19 MJ) ingested daily.
• As coma improves, increase dietary protein as tolerated

PATIENT EDUCATION
• Include family in education
• Dietician instruction in eating lower protein diets, avoid protein bingeing
• Avoid unnecessary sedative or antianxiety medications and opiates
• Recognition of early signs and to get treatment promptly
• Pamphlets (quite good for family) - American Association for the Study of Liver Diseases, 6900 Grove Road, Thorofare, NJ 08086, (609)848-1000)

MEDICATIONS

DRUG(S) OF CHOICE
• Lactulose (Cephulac) syrup 30 mL of 50% solution four times daily. Diminish to bid when 3 or more bowel movements a day occur daily.
• If stage 4 is present, worsening occurs, or no improvement in 2 days, add antibiotics. Amoxicillin 4 gm/day is suitable. Neomycin 1-4 gm/day in 4 divided doses may be used if renal status is good.
• Antacids as needed
Contraindications:
• Total ileus
• Hypersensitivity reaction
Precautions:
• Potassium depletion
• Electrolyte imbalance
• Renal failure
Significant possible interactions: Refer to manufacturer's profile of each drug

ALTERNATIVE DRUGS
• Any antibiotic affecting intestinal flora such as:
  ◊ Metronidazole or vancomycin in refractory cases
  ◊ Dopamine agonists, e.g., bromocriptine have been tried
  ◊ Branched-chain amino acids IV
  ◊ Flumazenil

FOLLOWUP

PATIENT MONITORING
• To optimize treatment a trail-making test should be followed (provided by Cephulac makers). Apply to Stage 1 and 2 patients to determine how much maintenance treatment and diet needed. Should be run daily at first and then at each visit when changes in drugs and diet are made.
• Patients with changed findings should be seen twice weekly
• Stable patients should be seen monthly
• Trail-making test performed at each office visit

PREVENTION/AVOIDANCE
• Avoid unessential medications, particularly opiates, sedatives
• Avoid protein binges

POSSIBLE COMPLICATIONS
• Recurrence
• Stable, chronic, impaired status
• With many recurrences, permanent basal ganglion injury (non-Wilsonian hepatolenticular degeneration)
• Hepatorenal syndrome
• Acute tubular necrosis
• Bleeding
• Disseminated intravascular coagulation
• Bacteremia
• Shock

EXPECTED COURSE/PROGNOSIS
• In acute or fulminant
  ◊ With adequate aggressive treatment, disappears without residue or recurrence
• In chronic liver disease
  ◊ Coma returns
  ◊ With each recurrence it becomes more and more difficult to treat
  ◊ Plateau of maximum improvement shows a decrement over several years, such that the degree of improvement with treatment is less and less. Eventual 80% mortality.

MISCELLANEOUS

ASSOCIATED CONDITIONS
• Liver disease
• Rarely with portacaval shunt with normal liver function

AGE-RELATED FACTORS See under
Signs and symptoms
Pediatric: N/A
Geriatric: N/A
Others: N/A

PREGNANCY May occur as a complication
of pregnancy

SYNONYMS
• Hepatic coma
• Liver coma

ICD-9-CM 572.2 Hepatic encephalopathy

SEE ALSO N/A

OTHER NOTES N/A

ABBREVIATIONS N/A

REFERENCES
• Gammal SH, et al: Hepatic encephalopathy. Med Clin North Am 1989;73:793-813
• Jones EA, et al: Ann Intern Med 1989;110:532-46
• Chapman RW, et al: Liver transplantation for acute liver failure. Lancet 1990;335(8680):32-35
Illustrations: N/A
Internet references: http://www.5mcc.com

Author(s)
Frank L. Iber, MD

Hepatitis, viral

BASICS

DESCRIPTION A group of systemic infections involving the liver with common clinical manifestations; caused by different viruses with typically distinctive epidemiological patterns

System(s) affected: Gastrointestinal

Genetics: Some predisposition to immunologic manifestations; DR4 - positive increase with concurrent immunologic disease

Incidence/Prevalence in USA:
• HAV - 33% of Americans have antibodies; 125,000-200,000 infections/yr; 70% symptomatic
• HBV - 140,000-320,000 infections/year; 1-1.25 million chronically infected; >500,000 carriers (10% of infected). Post-transfusion HBV<1% of blood recipients.
• HCV - 16% of sporadic hepatitis: 35,000-180,000 new infections year ; 3.9 million chronically infected (85% of infected)
• HDV - present in 1% of HBV
• HEV - unknown
• HGV - 0.3% of acute viral hepatitis; 900-2,000 infections/yr; found in 2% of nonA, nonB chronic hepatitis. Frequent co-infection with HCV. In cryptogenic cirrhosis, HGV present in 12%; clinical significance unclear.

Predominant age: HAV rare in infants; susceptibility increases with age. HBV, HCV, HEV occur in all ages.

Predominant sex: Fulminant HBV: Male > Female (2:1)

SIGNS AND SYMPTOMS
• Fever (60%); unusual with HBV and HCV
• Malaise (67%)
• Nausea (80%)
• Anorexia (54%)
• Jaundice (in adults, 62%); 66% of HCV anicteric
• Dark urine (84%)
• Abdominal pain (56%)
• Fatigue (major complaint in HCV)
• Headache
• Meningismus (occasional)
• Vomiting

CAUSES
• Multiple viruses possible
• HAV and HEV transmitted enterically (fecal-oral); parenteral route rare
• Maximum infectivity 2 weeks before jaundice
• May be endemic in institutions
• HBV transmitted sexually or by blood products including infection acquired perinatally; also enterically. HDV coinfection increases HBV severity.
• HCV transmitted through blood or its products; in 40%, mode unknown
• HDV identified only with HBV infection
• HGV has similar patterns to HCV

RISK FACTORS
• Health care workers/other occupational risks
• Hemodialysis
• Recipients of blood and/or blood products
• IV drug users (53% of new infections); individuals with tattoos
• Sexually active homosexual males
• Household exposure
• Intimate exposure
• Positive needlestick
• Transplanted organs

DIAGNOSIS

DIFFERENTIAL DIAGNOSIS Infectious mononucleosis, primary or secondary hepatic malignancy, ischemic hepatitis, drug-induced hepatitis, alcoholic hepatitis, autoimmune hepatitis, Wilson's disease

LABORATORY
• Marked elevation of AST/ALT (acute hepatitis, particularly ALT, 400-several thousand U/L); HCV may have normal ALT; AST/ALT ratio =>1 associated with cirrhosis in chronic HCV
• Mild elevation of alkaline phosphatase
• Bilirubin from normal to markedly elevated; with elevation, conjugated and unconjugated fractions usually increased
• Serological markers to identify viruses

```
-------------------------------
Diagnosis    Biochemical markers
HAV:
  A, R          Anti-HAV IgM
  P             Anti-HAV IgG
HBV:
  A, E          HBsAg
  A             Anti-HBc IgM,
                   HBsAg, HBeAg
  C             HBsAg, +/- HBeAg
HCV:
  A,C,Rcv       Anti-HCV (ELISA)
HDV:
  A             HDAg, Anti-HDV IgM
  P             Anti-HDV IgG
HEV:            Test not available
HGV:            PCR-RNA
-------------------------------
A-acute infection, R-recent in
fection, C-chronic infection
P-previous infection, E-early/
carrier state, Rcv-Recovered
```

• For severe hepatitis, measure PT and PTT, albumin, electrolytes, glucose and CBC
• If HBV chronic, confirm by HBV-DNA titer
• Patients with severe HBV infection should be tested for coinfection with HDV
• HBeAg indicates high infectivity (horizontal and vertical transmission)
• Persistence > 10 weeks indicates probable chronic liver disease
• Acute, ongoing HCV, confirm by other markers, RIBA, esp. HCV-RNA (for chronic HCV); >viral titers in genotypes 1a, 1b than 2, 3
• In early acute HCV infection, anti-HCV may be negative; may need retest in 3-6 months

• HCV antibodies (ELISA, RIBA) are sensitive markers for patients with chronic HCV, but not sensitive enough for detection of asymptomatic carriers (blood donors)
• Chronic HCV, may find (+) ANA, ASMA, LKMA
• Subtyping HCV genotypes using RIBA may be useful

Drugs that may alter lab results: N/A
Disorders that may alter lab results: N/A

PATHOLOGICAL FINDINGS Liver biopsy in persistent or chronic disease shows wide range of histologic changes (variable inflammation and/or necrosis, cholestasis, steatosis, fibrosis, cirrhosis or chronic active hepatitis. Clinical course does not predict severity of histopathologic changes.

SPECIAL TESTS Liver biopsy usually needed for determining type and extent of liver injury in persistent disease and to exclude other diseases. Also, usually necessary prior to start of interferon alfa treatment.

IMAGING Usually not of diagnostic importance. Ultrasound may demonstrate ascites or exclude obstruction.

DIAGNOSTIC PROCEDURES
• History; exposure source; exclude drugs
• Tenderness on fist percussion over the liver; may be hepatomegaly
• Jaundice may or may not be present
• Serum "liver function tests" often elevated before bilirubin increases; measure aminotransferases in acute illnesses when there is no evident cause
• Serum biochemical markers for each virus, diagnosis in 90% of patients

TREATMENT

APPROPRIATE HEALTH CARE
• Outpatient care usual
• Segregation helpful for food handlers with HAV, or health care workers with HBV or HCV

GENERAL MEASURES
• Correct: coagulation defects, fluid and electrolytes, acid-base imbalance, hypoglycemia, impairment of renal function
• Report acute cases to public health dept

SURGICAL MEASURES Consider liver transplantation in fulminant acute hepatitis/end-stage liver disease (HCV)

ACTIVITY As tolerated

DIET Adequate calories; balanced nutrition

PATIENT EDUCATION
• Proper use and disposal of needles
• Proper hygiene, particularly food handlers
• HBV sexually transmitted; HCV sexual transmission low, but does occur

MEDICATIONS

DRUG(S) OF CHOICE
• Interferon alfa-2b (IFN, Intron A) or Interferon alfa-2a (Roferon-A)(HCV), or with ribavirin (Virazole) 1 g/day (HCV; induces remission (25-50% in HBV; 40% in HCV); decreases abnormal aminotransferase concentrations in chronic HBV/HCV. May be used safely post-transplant.
• Amantadine (Symmetrel) or rimantadine (Flumadine) may be useful in HCV non-responders (to IFN) - 100 mg bid for 6 mo. Famciclovir (Famvir) 500 mg tid has been used for HBV.
• Corticosteroids: In cholestatic HAV, a short course may shorten illness, but may be most effective in milder disease
Contraindications: Interferon: platelet count < 50,000. Mouse immunoglobulin, egg protein or neomycin allergy. Corticosteroids may add to morbidity/increased mortality.
Precautions:
• Other disorders of coagulation, myelosuppression, seizures, depression (esp. suicide ideation), pregnancy, fertile age group, lactation.
• Increased serum triglycerides may occur during IFN therapy; may cause abnormal ALT. Measure HCV-RNA to assess response in such patients.
• Psychiatric evaluation may be prudent prior to IFN treatment in chronic HCV
Significant possible interactions: Refer to manufacturer's profile of each drug

ALTERNATIVE DRUGS
Lamivudine 100 mg daily for chronic hepatitis B

FOLLOWUP

PATIENT MONITORING
• Serial measurement of serum AST/ALT
• Appropriate serum viral markers useful for evaluation of recovery or progression
• Liver biopsies in chronic disease
• Monitor for metabolic complications
• WBC, platelets with interferon alpha therapy
• Chronic HBV, HBV-DNA valuable for prediction of favorable response to IFN. High pretreatment ALT and low pretreatment HBV-DNA associated with favorable response.
• With HCV, quantitative serum HCV-RNA levels monitor response and post-treatment relapse (if negative after 3 months, sustained response likely)

PREVENTION/AVOIDANCE
• General
  ◊ Screen blood products
  ◊ Proper disposal of needles
  ◊ Good sanitation, hygiene

• HAV
  ◊ Immune globulin (passive immunization) - 0.02 mL/kg IM (given 1-2 weeks after exposure prevents illness in 80-90%). With prolonged exposure give q 5 months. Also use for close contacts, day care staff/children (if case occurs), institutions with multiple cases, travelers to areas of high prevalence (with 3 week lead time, use vaccine).
  ◊ Hepatitis A vaccine (Havrix, Vaqta) 0.5 mL dose IM in children > 2 yrs; 1.0 mL in adults IM; 2nd dose 6-12 mo later for >8 yrs. Separate syringe site from immune globulin. Use for travelers, day-care staff/children, custodial facility employees, sewage workers, military, homosexual men, food handlers, Native Americans/Alaskan natives.
• HBV
  ◊ Hepatitis B vaccine: 3 injections - 0.5 mL(2.5 mcg)/dose age < 11 yrs; 11-19 yrs 0.5 mL (5.0 mcg); > 20 yrs 1.0 mL (10 mcg) 1 mo and 6 mo apart
  ◊ High risk groups, use hepatitis B human immune globulin within 24 hr of exposure (0.06 mL/kg IM)
  ◊ HBV screening in pregnant women; vaccinate all infants at birth. Schedule: 3 injections - birth, 2 mo, 6-18 mo. Children/adolescents may start series anytime, but complete by age 11-12 yrs.
• HCV: No specifics on prevention/avoidance
• HDV: Preventing HBV will prevent HDV
• HEV: No specifics on prevention/avoidance
• HGV: Recommendations same as for HCV

POSSIBLE COMPLICATIONS
Acute or subacute necrosis, chronic active or chronic hepatitis, cirrhosis, hepatic failure; hepatocellular carcinoma (HBV, HCV)

EXPECTED COURSE/PROGNOSIS
• Varies with causative virus
• Severity of hepatic encephalopathy best predictor of poor survival in hepatic failure
• HAV may cause mild disease at times, often no jaundice; no chronic liver disease; mortality < 1%; lifetime immunity usual with recovery. 3 rare variants: relapsing, cholestatic, fulminant.
• HBV (mortality 1%) and HDV (with icterus, mortality 2-20%) more severe symptoms; often leads to persistent/chronic liver disease, cirrhosis, liver failure, hepatocellular carcinoma (HCC); more severe problems if impaired immune function. Follow treatment with HBV-DNA levels.
• In HCV, regardless of severity, >80% progress to chronic hepatitis, 20-50% to cirrhosis, and some, liver failure. Typically slow progression 10-30 years. May progress to HCC, but IFN may decrease HCC risk. Association with type II AI. Chronic HCV unlikely to clear HCV-RNA spontaneously. HCV after needlestick, usually sustained IFN response. Final phase HCV rare cause of fulminant hepatic failure.
• Alcohol may be factor for HCC in chronic HCV
• Chronic HDV, 70% develop cirrhosis; low incidence of HCC
• HEV does not result in chronic disease

MISCELLANEOUS

ASSOCIATED CONDITIONS
• Arthritis, urticaria, immune complex nephritis (particularly membranous glomerulopathy), anemias (including aplastic anemia), dermatitis and cardiomyopathy (usually with HBV, rare with HCV). HCV implicated in sporadic form of idiopathic mixed cryoglobulinemia, porphyria cutanea tarda, polyarteritis nodosa.
• HIV-HCV: more severe course

AGE-RELATED FACTORS
Pediatric: HAV milder; usually anicteric; may be unrecognized. HBV more acute, less prolonged, less complications, but may become chronic.
Geriatric: N/A
Others: Alcohol abuse a major factor for chronic liver disease from HBV and HCV. Measure viral biochemical markers in patients with alcoholic liver disease (esp. anti-HCV).

PREGNANCY
• Test, in later gestation, for HBsAg
• HBV transmitted vertically (< 10%) as well as perinatally and produces carrier state in 30%. Give HBIg 0.5 mL and HBV vaccine (Recombivax HB; separate sites) within 12 hrs of birth followed by HBV vaccine, 0.5 mL IM at ages 1 and 6 months. Check HBsAg and HBsAb at age 1
• HCV vertical transmission increased in HIV

SYNONYMS N/A

ICD-9-CM 070.10 HAV without coma; 070.30 HBV without coma; 070. 51 HCV without coma; 070.32 chronic HBV without HDV without coma; 070.54 chronic HCV without coma

SEE ALSO Immunizations

OTHER NOTES N/A

ABBREVIATIONS PCR = polymerase chain reaction; HCC = hepatocellular carcinoma; AI = autoimmune hepatitis

REFERENCES
• Alter MJ, Mast EE: The epidemiology of viral hepatitis in the U.S. Gastroenterol Clin North Am 1994; 23:437-455
• Seeff LP: Natural history of hepatitis, type C. Semin Gastrointest Dis, 1995;6:20
Illustrations: N/A
Internet references: http://www.5mcc.com

Author(s)
Douglas H. Sandberg, MD

Hepatoma

BASICS

DESCRIPTION Primary malignant tumor of liver arising from hepatic parenchymal cells (hepatocytes), blood vessels or cholangioles within the liver, excluding gallbladder and biliary passages. With the exception of fibrolamellar type almost always associated with an underlying liver disease, usually cirrhosis.
System(s) affected: Gastrointestinal
Genetics: No known genetic pattern
Incidence/Prevalence in USA:
• 1-5 new cases per 100,000 of population per year
• Among known cirrhotics, 2-5 cases/100/year
Predominant age: 6th-8th decade (mean age 55-62 years) in USA and western countries. Among immigrants from Asia and Africa occurs 2-3 decades earlier.
Predominant sex: Male > Female (3-4:1)

SIGNS AND SYMPTOMS
• Early curable stage
  ◊ Paraneoplastic syndrome - feminization, precocious puberty
  ◊ Palpable nodule on liver
  ◊ Age 2 to 6 years - abdominal mass in liver, abdominal pain, irregular hepatomegaly
• Usual adult manifestations
  ◊ Known cirrhosis or prominent clinical signs of cirrhosis - 80%
  ◊ Abdominal pain - 80%, right upper quadrant, dull ache to severe, aggravated by jolting
  ◊ Hepatomegaly - 80-90%, irregular, nodular, firm to hard, tender
  ◊ Weight loss, 30%
  ◊ Hepatic arterial bruit, 20%
  ◊ Friction rub - rare, more common in metastatic liver disease
  ◊ Nausea, vomiting
  ◊ Fever - 10-50%, low grade, intermittent
  ◊ Paraneoplastic manifestations - hypertrophic osteoarthropathy, carcinoid syndrome, feminization, polycythemia
  ◊ Hemoperitoneum, most common tumor cause
  ◊ Unexplained deterioration of stable cirrhosis
  ◊ Budd-Chiari syndrome
  ◊ Blockage of portal vein, inferior vena cava, renal veins

CAUSES
• Cirrhosis - accounts for 60 to 80% of cases. Alcoholic cirrhosis most important in western world. Reported risk of hepatoma in alcoholic cirrhosis is 3-10% with micronodular pattern.
• Hepatitis B virus infection - associated with > 70% of cases worldwide. Most important factor in Africa and Asia but less important in western countries. In USA, HBsAg is positive in 20% cases of this tumor.
• Hepatitis C virus infection - 50-70% of HBsAg negative patients are positive for anti-HCV antibody, an important factor in hepatoma patients not due to HBV infection. Particular problem in Orientals.

• Mycotoxins (aflatoxins) - metabolite of fungus Aspergillus flavus that contaminates foods. Two series, B1 and derivatives and G1 and derivatives. B1 being the most potent carcinogen, important in Sub-Saharan Africa and Southeast Asia, no significant role in USA.
• Vinyl polymer, but not the finished product, produces angiosarcoma

RISK FACTORS
• Primary liver disease - cirrhosis, chronic active hepatitis
• HBsAg positivity, anti-HCV antibody
• Chronic use of oral contraceptives
• Hemochromatosis
• Alpha-1-antitrypsin deficiency
• Primary biliary cirrhosis
• Metabolic disorders (tyrosinemia, Niemann-Pick disease)
• Clonorchiasis, gallstones, choledochal cysts - cholangiocarcinoma

DIAGNOSIS

DIFFERENTIAL DIAGNOSIS
• Early asymptomatic tumor - underlying liver conditions, e.g., cirrhosis, chronic hepatitis; benign liver nodules, hamartoma, hemangioma, metastatic adenocarcinoma, gallstones, or gallbladder polyp
• Late symptomatic tumor with hepatomegaly - hepatic cyst, adenoma, hemangioma, abscess, metastatic malignancy of liver, cirrhosis with activity, infarction of liver, fatty infiltration, thrombosis of hepatic veins, portal vein, inferior vena cava, active viral hepatitis, alcoholic hepatitis
• Ruptured tumor - all causes of acute abdomen, traumatic hemoperitoneum

LABORATORY
• Erythrocytosis, elevated Ca, low glucose
• Liver function test abnormalities
• Tumor markers
  ◊ Alpha fetoprotein (AFP) - single most important lab test for screening and diagnosis of hepatoma - 70%. Negative in angiosarcoma, cholangiocarcinoma and fibrolamellar carcinoma. Level > 400 ng/mL (> 400 µg/L) is diagnostic, level does not correlate with prognosis.
  ◊ Other markers - des-gamma-carboxyprothrombin, gamma glutamyl transferase, carcinoembryonic antigen (CEA), variant alkaline phosphatase, isoferritins
Drugs that may alter lab results:
Hypoglycemic agents, calcitonin, vitamin D
Disorders that may alter lab results:
Acute or chronic hepatitis, germ cell tumors, pregnancy. All cause slight elevation of AFP.

PATHOLOGICAL FINDINGS
• Nodular - 75%, usually in cirrhotic liver
• Massive - common in children and non-cirrhotic livers, more prone to rupture
• Diffuse - rare, a large part of liver is involved
• Hepatocellular origin - most commonly multicentric, well differentiated, usually superimposed on underlying cirrhosis. Almost always produces bile. Anaplastic form often difficult to be certain of cell of origin or differentiate from metastatic malignancy.
• Fibrolamellar - single nodule, non-cirrhotic, extensive fibrous stroma
• Cholangiocarcinoma - multicentric, most often mixed with hepatocellular elements
• Angiosarcoma

IMAGING
• Plain x-ray - useful to demonstrate metastatic involvement to lung and bone
• Ultrasound - best diagnostic imaging technique, capable of detecting tumor < 1 cm, and may be positive when AFP is normal. Has been useful in serially following cases of cirrhosis to identify hepatocellular cancer when under 2 cm and curable.
• CT scan - valuable in determining extrahepatic spread of the disease
• MRI - helpful in delineating the details of tumor, and invasion of vessels
• Hepatic arteriography - mostly done to see the anatomy of hepatic vessels and extent of tumor while considering resection, embolization, dearterialization or intra-arterial infusion of cytotoxic agents. Most useful in detecting angiosarcoma, separating benign vs. malignant.
• Lipiodal angiography and CT - lipiodal is readily taken up by tumor cells, this technique can detect even millimeter sized lesions. Lipiodal also serves as a vehicle to deliver chemotherapeutic or radioactive agents to the tumor.
• Gallium scans - 90% of hepatocellular carcinoma and 60% of other types of liver cell tumors take up and retain gallium for up to 48 hours

DIAGNOSTIC PROCEDURES
• Liver biopsy - recommended for all tumors and particularly small nodules detected on serial ultrasound
• Fine needle aspiration - under ultrasonography, may be difficult to determine cell origin when anaplastic, unable to diagnose fibrolamellar and angiosarcoma due to too small a sample of tissue
• Laparoscopy - to visualize the extent of tumor, to see whether non-tumorous liver is cirrhotic, peritoneal spread, and obtain diagnostic biopsy
• Exploratory laparotomy with operative biopsy, commonly used in children

TREATMENT

APPROPRIATE HEALTH CARE Inpatient initially

GENERAL MEASURES Precautions to avoid falls, attention to nutrition

SURGICAL MEASURES
• Surgery is lobectomy, liver segmentectomy or whatever required for complete removal
• Repeated alcohol injection of involved tumor sites under ultrasound guidance shrinks tumor mass and prolongs survival and improves quality of life
• Infarcting the tumor by radiological injection of its arterial supply does not prolong survival
• Liver transplantation curative in cancer with cirrhosis with 15% alive at 3 years
• Incidental hepatomas < 2 cm found at transplant do not influence survival.

ACTIVITY As tolerated

DIET High calorie, low protein diet

PATIENT EDUCATION Important for prevention; abstinence from alcohol and IV drugs, vaccination against HBV

MEDICATIONS

DRUG(S) OF CHOICE Only for unresectable hepatoma patients. Doxorubicin (Adriamycin) 60-75 mg/m2 every 3 weeks. Dose can be repeated depending on the response. Only partial response in 25% cases.
Contraindications:
• Cardiomyopathy
• Poor hepatic reserves (bilirubin > 2.0)
Precautions: Neutropenia with nadir at 10-14 days, septicemia, cardiotoxicity (25%) if cumulative dose > 550 mg/m2, hepatotoxicity
Significant possible interactions: N/A

ALTERNATIVE DRUGS
• Fluorouracil (5-FU), cyclophosphamide, methotrexate have been used but no promising results
• Immunotherapy: Radiolabeled antibodies like 131-I-antiferritin have been used. Can be used in conjunction with doxorubicin (Adriamycin), still experimental.
• Intra-arterial injection of 131-I Lipiodol or Lipiodol/Adriamycin, not in common use

FOLLOWUP

PATIENT MONITORING
• After successful resection there is high risk for recurrence
• Check AFP every 3 months
• Ultrasound every 4-6 months

PREVENTION/AVOIDANCE
• Prevention against HBV infection/cirrhosis
  ◊ General education regarding risks of exposure to HBV and precautions to avoid this
  ◊ Vaccination in high risk individuals - nurses, doctors, dialysis unit staff, lab technicians
  ◊ Vaccination of all children
  ◊ Abstinence from alcohol, IV drugs, homosexual behavior
  ◊ Persistent HBV and HCV infections eradicated with alpha interferon
• Screening and early diagnosis
  ◊ Early diagnosis to detect asymptomatic tumor (< 3 cm) at a potentially curable stage has been emphasized. The only screening test available so far is AFP testing which can detect 70-80% of tumors < 3 cm when used in conjunction with serial high resolution sonography.
  ◊ AFP should be done every 6 months in high risk individuals (cirrhosis, chronic active hepatitis) along with annual ultrasound. In moderate risk subjects (HBsAg positive but asymptomatic), AFP should be done yearly followed by ultrasound if it is abnormal.
  ◊ Patients exposed to 10 or more years of vinyl chloride polymerization should have q 6 months sonography. New nodules should be promptly biopsied.

POSSIBLE COMPLICATIONS Rupture, hemoperitoneum, liver failure, cachexia, metastases to other organs

EXPECTED COURSE OF PROGNOSIS
• Unresectable symptomatic tumors
  ◊ Grave prognosis, seldom live more than 6 months
  ◊ After liver transplantation - 2 year survival rate 15-20%
  ◊ After chemotherapy or chemoimmunotherapy, only partial remission in one quarter of cases
  ◊ Direct necrosis with alcohol injection
  ◊ Chemoembolization
• Resectable asymptomatic tumors
  ◊ Surgery is curative in > 70% of children without cirrhosis and in > 40% of adults without cirrhosis
  ◊ Surgery is curative in > 70% of cirrhosis when tumor nodules less than 2 cm; curative < 10% of the time if 3 cm or greater
  ◊ Liver transplantation curative in cancer with cirrhosis with 15% of patients alive at 3 years

MISCELLANEOUS

ASSOCIATED CONDITIONS
• Infections - chronic hepatitis B, hepatitis C, Delta hepatitis, clonorchiasis and schistosomiasis
• Primary liver diseases - alcoholic cirrhosis, primary biliary cirrhosis
• Metabolic diseases - Alpha1-antitrypsin deficiency, hemochromatosis, Wilson's disease, tyrosinemia

AGE-RELATED FACTORS Can occur in all age groups
Pediatric: Second most common tumor in first year of life following Wilms' tumor. High cure rate.
Geriatric: N/A
Others: N/A

PREGNANCY N/A

SYNONYMS
• Hepatocellular carcinoma
• Liver cancer
• Fibrolamellar carcinoma
• Cholangiocarcinoma

ICD-9-CM
155.0 Malignant neoplasm of liver, primary

SEE ALSO N/A

OTHER NOTES
• In Africa and Southeast Asia:
  ◊ Incidence of hepatoma is high - 15-20 cases/100,000/year
  ◊ Age group is younger - 3rd and 4th decade
  ◊ Male to female ratio is high - 6:1 to 7:1
  ◊ Aflatoxin and HBV are the major factors and cirrhosis is less important
  ◊ Course is more progressive and fulminant
  ◊ Tumors are mostly at unresectable stage at first presentation

ABBREVIATIONS
• HBsAg = hepatitis B surface antigen
• HCV = hepatitis C virus
• HBV = hepatitis B virus
• AFP = alphafetoprotein

REFERENCES
• Zakim D, Boyer TD: Hepatology, A Textbook of Liver Disease. 3rd Ed. Philadelphia, W.B. Saunders Co., 1995
• McIntyre N, Benhamou JP, Bircher J, Rizzota M, Rodes J: Oxford Text of Clinical Hepatology, Oxford Medical Publication, 1991
Illustrations: 1 available on CD-ROM
Internet references: http://www.5mcc.com

Author(s)
Frank L. Iber, MD

Hepatorenal syndrome

BASICS

DESCRIPTION An acute, functional and progressive reduction in renal blood flow and glomerular filtration rate (GFR) secondary to intense renal cortical vasoconstriction in the setting of decompensated cirrhosis. Other etiologies for renal failure in cirrhosis must be absent to diagnose hepatorenal syndrome (HRS). HRS may be classified as (1) type 1 HRS with a rapidly progressive decline in GFR (< 2 weeks); or (2) type II HRS which is not as rapidly progressive (> 2 weeks).

System(s) affected: Gastrointestinal, Nervous, Endocrine/Metabolic, Hemic/Lymphatic/Immunologic, Renal/Urologic

Genetics: Not important except as risk for liver disease (e.g., infantile or autosomal recessive polycystic kidney disease or alpha-1-antitrypsin deficiency, etc.)

Incidence/Prevalence in USA: Unknown (clear cut differentiation between hepatorenal syndrome and acute tubular necrosis [ATN] or pre-renal state not always made). Estimate: 32-41/100 admitted to the hospital for cirrhosis with ascites develop HRS at 2 and 5 years. One other study in patients with cirrhosis and ascites: 18% and 39% at 1 and 5 years.

Predominant Age: Usually > 4th decade (increased incidence of alcoholic cirrhosis) but may occur at any age

Predominant Sex: Male > Female (increased incidence and prevalence of alcoholic cirrhosis)

SIGNS AND SYMPTOMS
• Oliguria in the setting of cirrhosis
• Jaundice, ascites, encephalopathy
• GI bleeding
• Poor nutritional status
• Splenomegaly
• Spider angioma
• Peripheral vasodilatation
• Tachycardia and bounding pulse often present with HRS. Almost always develops during a hospitalization, not on admission.

CAUSES End stage liver disease from alcohol or toxins, viral hepatitis, fulminant hepatic failure, malignancy or any other injury which leads to cirrhosis (e.g., schistosoma) with accompanying risk factors

RISK FACTORS
• Any reduction of effective blood volume in cirrhosis including:
  ◊ Excessive diuresis and gastrointestinal blood loss (e.g., variceal bleeding)
  ◊ Excessive diarrhea (lactulose-induced)
  ◊ Bacteremia
  ◊ Reduction in venous return with tense ascites
  ◊ Vomiting; GI bleeding
  ◊ Protein-calorie malnutrition, especially with alcoholic cirrhosis

DIAGNOSIS

DIFFERENTIAL DIAGNOSIS
• For abrupt onset of oliguria in cirrhosis
  ◊ Volume contraction
  ◊ Cardiac failure (possibly alcoholic cardiomyopathy)
  ◊ Acute vasomotor nephropathy
  ◊ Obstruction
  ◊ Interstitial nephritis (drug-induced)

LABORATORY
• Azotemia in the setting of cirrhosis with appropriate spot urine values (consistent with tubular function): Na+ < 10 mEq/L, FeNa < 1%; urine/plasma creatinine > 30:1; osmolality mild to moderate concentrating ability (400-600 mOsm/kg/water). All reversible causes should be ruled out (e.g., pre-renal; obstruction).
• Urinalysis - absence of ATN casts; < 500 mg/dL protein
• Lack of improvement in renal function following diuretic withdrawal and expansion of plasma volume with 1.5 L of normal saline
• Minor criteria: urine volume < 500 cc/day; urine red cells < 50 hpf; serum sodium < 130 mcg/L

Drugs that may alter lab results: N/A
Disorders that may alter lab results: N/A

PATHOLOGICAL FINDINGS
• Liver: cirrhosis or acute fulminant failure
• Kidneys: would function if transplanted into hosts without liver disease, a functional renal derangement only

SPECIAL TESTS Xenon 133 washout curves show a profound reduction in renal cortical perfusion (historic interest)

IMAGING Renal ultrasound shows normal kidneys without obstruction

DIAGNOSTIC PROCEDURES Though experimental presently, renal duplex Doppler ultrasonography appears to have predictive value in separating cirrhotics who will develop HRS from those who won't based on resistive index

TREATMENT

APPROPRIATE HEALTH CARE
Maintenance of volume status in cirrhosis

GENERAL MEASURES
• Supportive
  ◊ Avoid iatrogenic events that precipitate HRS
  ◊ Diagnose and treat correctable causes of azotemia in cirrhosis: volume expanders (100 gm albumin in 500 cc normal saline) should always be tried if possible, left ventricular function maximized if possible, relief of urinary obstruction when present
• Other
  ◊ Large volume paracentesis
  ◊ Dialysis is only indicated as ancillary support for patients awaiting liver transplant
  ◊ Head-out water immersion and LaVeen shunts of dubious value
  ◊ Acute liver failure with HRS may reverse if the liver regenerates

SURGICAL MEASURES Liver transplantation when feasible is the only curative treatment. The observed 3 month to estimated 6 months to 1 year survival in patients with transjugular intrahepatic portosystemic stent-shunts is improved. LeVeen shunt may provide similar benefit.

ACTIVITY Bedrest

DIET N/A

PATIENT EDUCATION In alcoholic cirrhosis, abstention from alcohol is essential and may prevent further deterioration of cirrhosis

MEDICATIONS

DRUG(S) OF CHOICE Low dose dopamine may provide temporary benefit. Not curative.
Contraindications: N/A
Precautions:
• Avoid NSAID's, demeclocycline, aminoglycosides or other nephrotoxins
• Judicious use of loop diuretics
• Avoid iatrogenic volume contraction in cirrhotic inpatients
Significant possible interactions: Refer to manufacturer's literature

ALTERNATIVE DRUGS N/A

 FOLLOWUP

PATIENT MONITORING N/A

PREVENTION/AVOIDANCE See Risk Factors

POSSIBLE COMPLICATIONS Death

EXPECTED COURSE/PROGNOSIS
• Grave without liver transplant in chronic cirrhosis or without regeneration of the liver in acute fulminant failure
• If a liver transplant is performed, actuarial patient survival after transplant is less in patients with preceding hepatorenal syndrome
• The patient may be supported with hemodialysis and transjugular portosystemic stent-shunt prior to organ availability for transplant

 MISCELLANEOUS

ASSOCIATED CONDITIONS See Causes and Differential Diagnosis

AGE-RELATED FACTORS
Pediatric: See Genetics
Geriatric: N/A
Others: N/A

PREGNANCY May be associated with HRS if liver failure occurs during pregnancy

SYNONYMS
• Renal failure of cirrhosis
• Functional renal failure of cirrhosis
• Hepatic nephropathy
• Heyd's syndrome
• Oliguric renal failure of cirrhosis
• Hemodynamic renal failure of cirrhosis

ICD-9-CM
572.4 Hepatorenal syndrome
997.4 Hepatorenal syndrome, resulting from a procedure

SEE ALSO
• Acetaminophen poisoning
• Renal failure, acute (ARF)
• Cirrhosis of the liver
• Hepatitis, viral
• Schistosomiasis of the liver, chronic

OTHER NOTES N/A

ABBREVIATIONS
HRS = hepatorenal syndrome

REFERENCES
• Celeb H, Dondy E, Celikes H: Renal blood flow detection with Doppler ultrasonography in patients with hepatic cirrhosis. Arch Int Med 1997;157:564-566
• Arroyo V, Gines P, Gerbes AL et al: Definition and diagnostic criteria of refractory ascites and hepatorenal syndrome in cirrhosis. Hepatology 1996;23:164-176
• Roberts LR, Kamath PS: Ascites and hepatorenal syndrome; pathophysiology and management. Mayo Clin Proc 1996;71:874881
• Van Roey G, Moore K: The hepatorenal syndrome. Pediatr Nephrol 1996;10:100-107
• Brensing KA, Textor J, Strunk H, et al: Transjugular intrahepatic portosystemic stent-shunt for hepatorenal syndrome. Lancet 1997;349:697-698
• Henriksen JH: Cirrhosis: Ascites and hepatorenal syndrome. recent advances in pathogenesis. J of Hepatology 1995;23:(S-1)25-30
Illustrations: N/A
Internet references: http://www.5mcc.com

Author(s)
Gregory W. Rutecki, MD

Herpangina

BASICS

DESCRIPTION Infectious disease caused by Coxsackievirus group A. Characteristics - fever of short duration, typical vesicular or ulcerated lesions in the post pharynx or on the soft palate. Usual course - acute.
System(s) affected: Metabolic/digestive
Genetics: N/A
Incidence/Prevalence: N/A
Predominant age: 3 months-16 years
Predominant sex: Male = Female

SIGNS AND SYMPTOMS
• Anorexia
• Drooling
• Sore throat
• Fever
• Malaise
• Irritability
• Listlessness
• Local pain
• Emesis
• Backache
• Headache
• Coryza
• Diarrhea
• Bilateral discrete vesicles, gray base
• Erythematous parchory
• Vesicles may rupture ulcers to form ulcers
• Posterior pharynx location - pharynx, tonsils, soft palate, little involvement of anterior 2/3 of mouth

CAUSES
• Coxsackievirus A
• Coxsackievirus B

RISK FACTORS Contact with infected person

DIAGNOSIS

DIFFERENTIAL DIAGNOSIS
• Herpes simplex - multiple ulcers on lips and anterior mouth. Diagnose with Herpes culture.
• Drug reactions - cutaneous lesions often present (urticaria, erythema multiforme)
• Recurrent aphthous stomatitis
  ◊ Buccal, labial, alveolar, mucosal ulcers
  ◊ Recurrent crops
  ◊ Few systemic symptoms
• Lichen planus - painful ulcer, white "lacey" pattern on mucosa or may have cutaneous lesions which are purple and pruritic

LABORATORY
• Slight leukocytosis (< 50%)
• Positive viral culture - mouth washings, stool
Drugs that may alter lab results: N/A
Disorders that may alter lab results: N/A

PATHOLOGICAL FINDINGS N/A

SPECIAL TESTS
• Complement fixation
• Hemagglutinin inhibition tests

IMAGING N/A

DIAGNOSTIC PROCEDURES N/A

TREATMENT

APPROPRIATE HEALTH CARE
Outpatient

GENERAL MEASURES
• Self-limited
• Palliative and supportive
• Hydration

SURGICAL MEASURES N/A

ACTIVITY No restrictions

DIET Clear liquids

PATIENT EDUCATION N/A

MEDICATIONS

DRUG(S) OF CHOICE
• Analgesics - acetaminophen, NSAID's
• Topical anesthetics
• Mouthwash - aqueous solution of 1% dyclonine and 1% diphenhydramine (Benadryl) in 50% attapulgite (Kaopectate)
• 2% viscous lidocaine solution
Contraindications: N/A
Precautions: N/A
Significant possible interactions: N/A

ALTERNATIVE DRUGS N/A

FOLLOWUP

PATIENT MONITORING Hydration

PREVENTION/AVOIDANCE Avoid contact with infected individual

POSSIBLE COMPLICATIONS
• Exanthem
• Meningitis
• Myocarditis
• Encephalitis

EXPECTED COURSE/PROGNOSIS
Complete recovery

MISCELLANEOUS

ASSOCIATED CONDITIONS N/A

AGE-RELATED FACTORS
Pediatric: N/A
Geriatric: N/A
Others: N/A

PREGNANCY N/A

SYNONYMS N/A

ICD-9-CM
074.0 Herpangina

SEE ALSO
• Herpes simplex

OTHER NOTES N/A

ABBREVIATIONS N/A

REFERENCES Bondi J, Jegasothy B, Lazarus G: Dermatology, Diagnosis and Therapy. Norwalk, CT, Appleton & Lange, 1991
Illustrations: N/A
Internet references: http://www.5mcc.com

Author(s)
Jeffrey A. Stearns, MD

Herpes eye infections

BASICS

DESCRIPTION Infections of the eye caused by one of the herpesviruses. Herpes simplex (HSV) types 1 and 2 or varicella-zoster virus. These infections may affect the eyelids and surrounding skin and may also cause conjunctivitis, keratitis, uveitis, as well as retinitis or optic neuritis. These viruses establish latent infections and eye involvement is most often from reactivation of latent viruses. Epstein-Barr virus may cause conjunctivitis or keratitis in infectious mononucleosis. Cytomegalovirus, which is also a herpesvirus, can cause a severe retinitis in immunocompromised patients with AIDS.
System(s) affected: Nervous, Skin/Exocrine
Genetics: No genetic pattern
Incidence/Prevalence in USA:
• HSV - 500,000 cases per year; 1/10,000 infants born with neonatal HSV
• Zoster - 300,000 new cases per year
Predominant age:
• HSV may affect any age
• Zoster usually affects older people
Predominant sex: Male = Female

SIGNS AND SYMPTOMS
Varies according to the virus and the ocular structures involved
• Eye pain
• Red eye (usually unilateral)
• Photophobia
• Tearing
• Decreased vision
• Skin/eyelid rash and pain
• Fever (varicella-zoster or infectious mononucleosis)
• Malaise (varicella-zoster or infectious mononucleosis)

CAUSES
• Primary infections:
  ◊ Neonatal HSV, usually HSV-2
  ◊ Primary ocular HSV, usually HSV-1
• Recurrent infections:
  ◊ Reactivation of HSV or herpes zoster virus (HZV) from trigeminal ganglion
• Reactivating factors:
  ◊ Fever
  ◊ Ultraviolet light
  ◊ Cold wind
  ◊ Systemic illness
  ◊ Menstruation
  ◊ Emotional stress
  ◊ Local trauma
  ◊ Immunosuppression

RISK FACTORS
• Family members/close contact with HSV
• History of varicella infection

DIAGNOSIS

DIFFERENTIAL DIAGNOSIS
• Viral conjunctivitis of other cause
• Bacterial keratoconjunctivitis
• Adult inclusion (chlamydial) conjunctivitis
• Allergic conjunctivitis
• Corneal abrasion
• Recurrent corneal erosion
• Toxic conjunctivitis
• Fungal keratitis
• Iritis/uveitis
• Scleritis

LABORATORY
• Laboratory tests are usually not required unless diagnosis in doubt
• Viral culture from cornea, conjunctiva, or skin; fluorescent antibody; polymerase chain reaction (PCR)
• Giemsa stain of corneal or skin lesion scrapings for multinucleated giant cells
Drugs that may alter lab results: N/A
Disorders that may alter lab results: N/A

PATHOLOGICAL FINDINGS
• Vesicular skin rash
• Zoster rash follows dermatome, does not cross midline and involves upper eyelid
• Dendritic keratitis
• HSV dendrites stain with fluorescein
• Large geographic corneal ulcers may occur
• Corneal stromal inflammation, opacity and neovascularization may occur
• Decreased corneal sensation
• Uveitis
• Secondary glaucoma

SPECIAL TESTS
• Fluorescein staining of the cornea - positive staining with HSV
• Rose bengal staining of cornea - positive with zoster and HSV
• Corneal sensation - usually decreased
• Slit-lamp exam
• Measure intraocular pressure
• Dilated funduscope exam
• Evaluate zoster patients under age 40 for immunodeficiency

IMAGING N/A

DIAGNOSTIC PROCEDURES As above

TREATMENT

APPROPRIATE HEALTH CARE
• Outpatient
• Hospitalize if severe systemic spread for IV therapy

GENERAL MEASURES
• Warm compresses to skin lesions
• Gentle debridement of corneal epithelial lesions

SURGICAL MEASURES Occasionally, débridement of involved epithelium

ACTIVITY As tolerated

DIET Regular

PATIENT EDUCATION American Academy of Ophthalmology

MEDICATIONS

DRUG(S) OF CHOICE
Skin and eyelid lesions:
• Prophylactic topical antibiotic ointment, such as bacitracin or erythromycin bid for 1-2 weeks
• Trifluorothymidine (Viroptic) 1% drops or vidarabine 3% ointment 5 times per day if eyelid margin involved
• Zoster - acyclovir 800 mg po 5 times per day for 10 days; useful if started within 7 days of onset and active lesions are present
• Severe or persistent zoster - hospitalize; acyclovir 5-10 mg/kg IV q 8 hours for 5-10 days
• For postherpetic neuralgia in herpes zoster:
  ◊ Consider prednisone 60 mg po for 3-7 days and taper off over the next 1-2 weeks
  ◊ Cimetidine 400 mg po bid during prednisone treatment
  ◊ Consider antidepressant such as amitriptyline 25 mg po tid
Corneal disease:
• HSV epithelial disease:
  ◊ Trifluorothymidine 1% drops 9 times per day or vidarabine 3% ointment 5 times per day; taper over 10-21 days based on response
  ◊ Cycloplegia with scopolamine 0.25% or cyclopentolate 1% drops tid
• Stromal keratitis or uveitis (without epithelial disease):
  ◊ Cycloplegia with scopolamine 0.25% or cyclopentolate 1% drops tid
  ◊ Topical steroid such as prednisolone acetate 1% drops qid
  ◊ Trifluorothymidine 1% drops qid for prophylaxis while on topical steroids
Optic neuritis, chorioretinitis, or cranial nerve involvement with zoster:
• Acyclovir 5-10 mg/kg IV q 8 hours for 1 week
• Prednisone 60 mg po for 3-7 days and taper over the next 1-2 weeks

Herpes eye infections

Secondary glaucoma
• Aqueous humor suppressant such as timolol 0.5% drops bid or methazolamide 50 mg po bid or tid

Neurotrophic ulcer or persistent epithelial disease:
• Consider reducing or discontinuing topical antivirals to avoid toxicity
• Preservative-free lubricant ointment
• Erythromycin 3% ophthalmic ointment q hs or bid
• Consider patching or tarsorrhaphy

Contraindications:
• Topical steroids are contraindicated with active corneal epithelial disease
• Acyclovir is contraindicated in pregnancy
• Prednisone should not be used in immunocompromised patients

Precautions:
• Topical antiviral agents are toxic and may cause an allergic reaction; substitution with another agent may be tried
• Topical steroids can raise intraocular pressure
• Acyclovir dosage should be reduced in renal insufficiency
• See manufacturer's literature for additional precautions

Significant possible interactions: See manufacturer's literature

ALTERNATIVE DRUGS
• Idoxuridine 0.5% ointment or 0.1% drops 5 times per day is more toxic than the other antivirals, but may be substituted if allergic reaction develops to others
• Topical acyclovir ointment to skin lesions - effectiveness uncertain
• Medroxyprogesterone 1% drops in place of other steroids if corneal thinning
• Capsaicin 0.025% cream tid to 6 times per day for months to years for post-herpetic neuralgia
• Nonsteroidal anti-inflammatory agents po for scleritis associated with zoster

 FOLLOWUP

PATIENT MONITORING
• Size of epithelial defect
• Vision
• Corneal opacity
• Anterior chamber inflammation
• Intraocular pressure

PREVENTION/AVOIDANCE
• Avoid close contact with patients with active lesions
• Herpes zoster virus can be spread to individuals who have not had chicken pox
• Avoid known precipitating factors for recurrent HSV
• Topical steroids alone do not reactivate the virus, but may exacerbate spontaneous recurrences
• Very slow taper of topical steroids over many months for corneal epithelial disease
• Antiviral prophylaxis while on topical steroids
• Varicella vaccination prior to infection

POSSIBLE COMPLICATIONS
• Corneal neovascularization and scarring resulting in poor vision
• Neurotrophic ulcer with perforation
• Secondary bacterial or fungal infection
• Secondary glaucoma from uveitis or steroid treatment
• Necrotizing interstitial keratitis
• Corneal transplant may be required
• Post-herpetic neuralgia with zoster
• Vision loss from optic neuritis or chorioretinitis
• Systemic involvement

EXPECTED COURSE/PROGNOSIS
• Neonatal primary HSV often disseminated with high mortality rate, 37% have vision worse than 20/200
• Primary HSV in children and adults often asymptomatic; overt disease usually self-limited
• Recurrent ocular HSV:
  ◊ Skin lesions in clusters last for 5-7 days
  ◊ HSV epithelial disease - without treatment, 40% resolve without sequelae; with treatment, 90-95% resolve without complication
  ◊ HSV stromal keratitis usually resolve in weeks to months with some scarring; neovascularization increases risk for severe scarring
• Ocular varicella - may produce a keratitis; usually self-limited, but with occasional complications
• Herpes zoster ophthalmicus
  ◊ Dermatitis 8-14 days acute phase with subsequent scarring possible
  ◊ Conjunctivitis, episcleritis and scleritis may occur
  ◊ Two-thirds of patients develop keratitis and decreased corneal sensation
  ◊ Uveitis occurs in about 40%
  ◊ Neurotrophic keratitis occurs in one-half; most recover sensation in 2-3 months
  ◊ Secondary glaucoma occurs in 10%
  ◊ Post-herpetic neuralgia in 20-40%; usually longer lasting in older patients
• Recurrence common for HSV and HZO

MISCELLANEOUS

ASSOCIATED CONDITIONS
• Immunosuppression
• AIDS
• Malignancy

AGE-RELATED FACTORS
Pediatric: Neonatal HSV often systemic and life-threatening
Geriatric: Zoster more common in older age groups
Others: Consider immunodeficiency in zoster patients under age 40

PREGNANCY
• May increase recurrence
• Avoid systemic steroids, acyclovir and other medications contraindicated in pregnancy
• Pregnant women who have not had chicken pox should especially avoid contact with patients with active zoster

SYNONYMS
• Herpes simplex keratitis
• Herpes zoster ophthalmicus
• Herpetic keratitis or keratouveitis

ICD-9-CM
• 054.40 herpes simplex (HSV) with ophthalmic complications
• 053.2 herpes zoster (HZV) with ophthalmic complications

SEE ALSO Conjunctivitis

OTHER NOTES N/A

ABBREVIATIONS
• HSV = herpes simplex virus
• HZV = herpes zoster virus
• HZO = herpes zoster ophthalmicus
• VSV = varicella-zoster virus (synonym for HZV)

REFERENCES
• Albert DM, Jakobiec FA, eds: Principles and Practice of Ophthalmology. Philadelphia, W.B. Saunders Co., 1994
• Cullom RD Jr, Chang B, eds: The Wills Eye Manual - Office and Emergency Room Diagnosis and Treatment of Eye Diseases. 2nd Ed. Philadelphia, J.B. Lippincott Co., 1994
• Pepose JS, Holland GN, Wilhelmus KR. Ocular Infection and Immunity. St. Louis, Mosby, 1996
Illustrations: N/A
Internet references: http://www.5mcc.com

Author(s)
Thomas W. Hejkal, MD, PhD

Herpes gestationis

BASICS

DESCRIPTION A rare dermatopathic, immune-mediated and self-limited eruption most often occurring during mid-pregnancy
• Onset is in second trimester of pregnancy with remission after delivery except for some postpartum flares. May recur in subsequent pregnancies.
• Characterized by pruritic polymorphous vesicles, papules, and/or bullae often located in peri-umbilical or other truncal areas. May affect the buttocks, forearms, palms, or soles; less frequently scalp and face may be involved. Clustered vesicles may coalesce to form bullae, rupture to form crusts, then heal with hyperpigmentation.
• Mucous membranes are spared but intestinal mucosa may have celiac-like lesions without significant clinical malabsorption
System(s) affected: Skin/Exocrine, Reproductive
Genetics: Genetic predisposition possible, suggested by increased HLA-A1, -B8, and -DR3 antigens in affected women
Incidence/Prevalence in USA: Rare; 1 per 4000-50,000 pregnancies
Predominant age: Child-bearing years
Predominant sex: Female only

SIGNS AND SYMPTOMS Intensely pruritic papules and/or vesicles, occurring first in peri-umbilical area and spreading more generally

CAUSES
• Unknown but immune alterations suspected
• Not caused by herpes virus

RISK FACTORS
• Episode in prior pregnancy
• Herpes simplex does not increase risk

DIAGNOSIS

DIFFERENTIAL DIAGNOSIS
• Other pruritic conditions of pregnancy
  ◊ Besnier's prurigo gestationis with excoriated papules and no vesicles; usually limited to extensor surface of extremities
  ◊ Papular urticarial papules and plaques of pregnancy (PUPPP syndrome) which has urticarial plaques and small papules with a narrow, pale halo and no vesicles
  ◊ Impetigo herpetiformis has sterile pustules, not vesicles, and may involve mucous membranes, groin, and inner thighs
  ◊ Papular dermatitis of pregnancy
• Non-pregnancy conditions to consider
  ◊ Dermatitis herpetiformis (much more chronic and more often in middle-aged males)
  ◊ Bullous pemphigoid
  ◊ Toxic drug eruption including erythema multiforme

LABORATORY
• Tzanck smear negative
• Herpes simplex virus culture negative
• Peripheral eosinophilia may be present
Drugs that may alter lab results: N/A
Disorders that may alter lab results: N/A

PATHOLOGICAL FINDINGS
• Subepidermal vesicle often with eosinophils and edema of dermal papillae
• Acantholysis is rare
• Inflammation surrounds superficial and deep dermal vessels

SPECIAL TESTS Biopsy with direct immunofluorescence shows intense deposition of C3 (100%) and IgG (30-40%) along basement membrane. Serum may have circulating IgG antibasement membrane autoantibodies (10-20%) by indirect immunofluorescence; if not, half have herpes gestationis (HG) factor (a protein that fixes complement to basement membrane in-vitro human skin preparations).

IMAGING N/A

DIAGNOSTIC PROCEDURES Biopsy

TREATMENT

APPROPRIATE HEALTH CARE
Outpatient

GENERAL MEASURES
• Differentiate from herpes virus infection
• Relieve pruritus
• Prevent secondary infection
• Soothing compresses such as Domeboro or Burrow's solution may help relieve itching

SURGICAL MEASURES N/A

ACTIVITY As tolerated

DIET No special diet

PATIENT EDUCATION
• Educate about difference between this and herpes virus infection
• Inform of possible fetal risks and possibility of limited disease in newborn

MEDICATIONS

DRUG(S) OF CHOICE
• Topical steroids and antihistamines for mild pruritus
• Most will require systemic corticosteroids in doses of 20-60 mg/day (at the minimum effective dose) through first month postpartum

Contraindications: Weigh risk of aggravating hyperglycemia, potential effects on maternal and fetal bone, increased susceptibility to infections versus benefit of relieving pruritus, and resolving the lesions

Precautions:
• Use prednisone cautiously in patients with immune impairment, diabetes, or thrombophlebitis
• If prednisone has been used over several weeks, taper when discontinuing to prevent cortisol deficiency

Significant possible interactions:
Methylprednisolone may enhance toxicity of erythromycin

ALTERNATIVE DRUGS Pyridoxine

FOLLOWUP

PATIENT MONITORING Watch for secondary bacterial infection

PREVENTION/AVOIDANCE
• Avoid other people with infections, since there is susceptibility of open skin lesions and decreased resistance secondary to corticosteroids
• Some authorities recommend cesarean section when mother is known to be infected
• Avoid scalp monitors if disease involves maternal genitalia
• Use of estrogens or progesterone may trigger flare-up

POSSIBLE COMPLICATIONS
• Secondary bacterial infection
• Excess systemic medication in pregnancy
• Fetal deaths
• Premature births
• Fetal growth retardation
• Conjunctivitis
• Keratitis
• Cataracts
• Shock
• Transient herpes gestationis in the neonate

EXPECTED COURSE/PROGNOSIS
• Spreads during 2nd-3rd trimester
• Remits after delivery
• Often flares in puerperium
• Tends to recur in subsequent pregnancies
• Systemic steroids may suppress new lesions, relieve pruritus, and dampen course; fetal outcome may be worsened

MISCELLANEOUS

ASSOCIATED CONDITIONS
• Pregnancy
• Hydatidiform mole
• Choriocarcinoma

AGE-RELATED FACTORS
Pediatric:
• Has been associated with preterm birth (22%) and still birth (< 10%)
• Rare cases of transient neonatal herpes gestationis are usually mild and resolve spontaneously; these are probably from passive transfer of antibasement membrane antibodies and HG factor
Geriatric: N/A
Others: N/A

PREGNANCY By definition, a condition of pregnancy and puerperium

SYNONYMS
• Dermatitis gestationis
• Pemphigoid gestationis

ICD-9-CM
• 646.80 (unspecified relation to delivery)
• 646.83 (antepartum)

SEE ALSO N/A

OTHER NOTES Uncommon intrauterine infections are associated with microcephaly intracranial calcification and chorioretinitis

ABBREVIATIONS N/A

REFERENCES
• Pritchard JA, MacDonald PC, Gant NF, eds: Williams Obstetrics. Norwalk, CT, Appleton-Century-Crofts, 1985
• Zone JJ, Provost T: Bullous Disease. In: Moschella SL, ed. Dermatology. Philadelphia, W.B. Saunders Co., 1985
• Roger D, et al: Specific pruritic diseases of pregnancy. Arch Dermatol. 1994:130:734-739
• Borradori L, Saura J: Specific dermatoses of pregnancy. Arch Dematol 1994;130:778-780
Illustrations: N/A
Internet references: http://www.5mcc.com

Author(s)
Arthur R. Slaughter, MD

Herpes simplex

BASICS

DESCRIPTION Viral disease with many manifestations, usually seen as painful vesicles that often occur in clusters on skin, cornea, or mucous membranes; may occur as encephalitis, pneumonia, or disseminated infection.
Usual course of primary disease is 2 weeks; duration of recurrences varies; viral shedding in recurrence is briefer than with primary disease. Newborns or individuals with immune compromise are at risk for major morbidity or mortality.
System(s) affected: Skin/Exocrine, Nervous
Genetics: N/A
Incidence/Prevalence in USA:
• 29.2/100,000 office visits/year
• Widespread; 0.65-20% of adults may be excreting HSV1 or HSV2 at any given time
• Prevalence of antibodies varies from 30% in higher socioeconomic strata to 100% in lower socioeconomic strata; 20,000-70,000/100,000
Predominant age: All ages
Predominant sex: Male = Female

SIGNS AND SYMPTOMS

• Vesicles - usually cluster and open as painful ulcerated lesions, often with erythematous base
• Primary disease classic variations include:
◊ Herpetic whitlow: localized primary infection on a finger with intense itching and pain, followed by vesicles that may coalesce with swelling, erythema, and may mimic pyogenic paronychia; neuralgia and axillary adenopathy sometimes; heals over 2-3 weeks without incision. Primary inoculation of other abraded skin can occur (e.g., herpes gladiatorum in wrestlers).
◊ Primary herpetic gingivostomatitis and pharyngitis: first infection with HSV1 usually in early childhood; incubation from 2-12 days, then fever, sore throat, pharyngeal edema and erythema; small vesicles develop on pharyngeal and oral mucosa, rapidly ulcerate and increase in number to involve soft palate, buccal mucosa, tongue, floor of mouth, and often lips and cheeks; tender gums may bleed; fetid breath, cervical adenopathy; fever, general toxicity, poor oral intake, and drooling contribute to dehydration; autoinoculation of other sites may occur; resolves in 10-14 days with slower resolution of adenopathy
◊ Primary genital herpes: see Herpes, genital topic
◊ Primary herpes keratoconjunctivitis: by HSV1 usually; can present as unilateral conjunctivitis with regional adenopathy, as blepharitis with vesicles on lid margin, as keratitis with dendritic lesions or with punctate opacities; lasts 2-3 weeks but systemic involvement prolongs process
◊ Eczema herpeticum: diffuse pox-like eruption complicating atopic dermatitis; one cause of Kaposi's varicelliform eruption; sudden appearance of lesions in typical atopic areas (upper trunk, neck, head); high fever, local edema, adenopathy, umbilicated

vesicles develop hemorrhagic crust or become pustular; appear in crops for up to a week; significant fluid or blood loss and secondary bacterial infections can cause fatality; similar serious inoculations can occur with severe burn patients and go unrecognized under the eschar.
◊ Neonatal herpes simplex: perinatal primary infection is life-threatening and usually acquired by vaginal birth of infected mother; fetal risk and neonatal risk are greater in mothers with primary genital herpes infection since shedding is more prolonged and the inoculum is greater; incubation from 5-7 days usually (rarely 4 weeks); cutaneous, mucous membrane, or ocular signs in only 70%; congenital infection via prenatal transplacental virus transfer may present with jaundice, hepatosplenomegaly, DIC, encephalitis, seizures, temperature instability, chorioretinitis, and/or conjunctivitis with or without skin vesicles; neurologic morbidity worse with HSV2 than with HSV1 in neonates; fatal hepatic or adrenal necrosis may occur
• Recurrent diseases from endogenous reactivation include:
◊ Herpes labialis: recurrent lesions on lips with HSV1, usually less than one recurrence per six months, but 5-25% may have more than one attack per month; precipitating events may be sunlight, fever, trauma, menses, stress; prodrome of pain, burning, itching may last 6-48 hrs before vesicles appear, often at vermilion border with increased pain; will ulcerate and crust within 48 hrs; heals within 8-10 days generally; may have local adenopathy
◊ Ocular herpes: may recur as keratitis, blepharitis, or keratoconjunctivitis; may have dendritic ulcers, decreased corneal sensation, less visual acuity; uveitis may cause permanent visual loss
◊ Recurrent genital herpes (herpes progenitalis): see Herpes, genital topic

CAUSES Herpes simplex virus, a DNA virus of two major types: HSV1 and HSV2; most often HSV1 is associated with oral lesions and HSV2 with genital lesions but reverse occurs also

RISK FACTORS

• Immune compromise (brief as with occurrence of other illness or stress, or more chronic as with chemotherapy, malignancy, or AIDS)
• Newborns - if exposed to actively infected mother via birth canal or if exposed to case in nursery (insufficient maternal passive antibody transfer); risk greatest for neonate of mother with active primary H. simplex infection
• Prior HSV infection
• Sexual intercourse with infected person (condoms can help prevent but location of some lesions may permit spread even with condoms)
• Occupational exposure (medical/dental risk more for HSV1 whitlow and general community to HSV2 whitlow)

DIAGNOSIS

DIFFERENTIAL DIAGNOSIS
• Impetigo - straw-colored vesicles that crust
• Aphthous stomatitis - grayish, shallow erosions with ring of hyperemia, usually only anterior in mouth and lips
• Herpes zoster - unilateral dermatome distribution
• Syphilitic chancre - usually painless ulcer
• Herpangina - vesicles predominate on anterior tonsillar pillars, soft palate, uvula and oropharynx but not more anteriorly on lips or gums (usually caused by group A Coxsackievirus)
• Stevens-Johnson syndrome
• Other causes of Kaposi's varicelliform eruption are varicella and Coxsackievirus A16

LABORATORY
• Tzanck smear shows multinucleated giant cells often with intranuclear inclusions (scrape material from lesion onto slide, fix with ethanol or methanol, stain with Giemsa or Wright preparation; alternatively spray slide with cytological fixative and stain as for Pap smear)
• Herpes simplex virus culture - only half of true positives available in 2 days; rest may take 6 days or longer to be positive; not considered as reasonable means to follow activity of recurrent disease near labor and delivery
Drugs that may alter lab results: N/A
Disorders that may alter lab results:
Varicella (herpes zoster) has identical findings on Tzanck smear

PATHOLOGICAL FINDINGS
Multinucleated giant cells with 2-15 nuclei per cell with eosinophilic inclusion bodies within nuclei; intraepithelial edema (ballooning degeneration) and intracellular edema; brain biopsy (in encephalitis) has hemorrhagic necrosis of gray and white matter with acute and chronic inflammation, thrombosis and fibrinoid necrosis of parenchymal vessels, and intranuclear inclusions in astrocytes, oligodendroglia, and neurons

SPECIAL TESTS
• Clinically available antibody tests do not reliably distinguish between HSV-1 and HSV-2, but initially high titers or less than a fourfold rise of titers between acute and convalescent sera may help rule-out a primary infection
• IgM HSV antibodies may appear in first 4 weeks of life in infected infants

IMAGING N/A

DIAGNOSTIC PROCEDURES
• Occasionally biopsy is needed
• Screen for other sexually transmitted diseases with primary genital herpes

TREATMENT

APPROPRIATE HEALTH CARE
Outpatient

GENERAL MEASURES
• Limited skin lesions (as in recurrent herpes labialis) may benefit from early unroofing of vesicles and application of Campho-Phenique
• Intermittent cool moist dressings with Domeboro or Burow's solution
• Inability to void from severe periurethral lesions may be remedied by pouring a cup of warm water over genitals while urinating or sitting in a warm bath to urinate
• Children with gingivostomatitis may require IV hydration
• Extensive skin disease (as with neonates or with eczema herpeticum) may require vigorous volume replacement

SURGICAL MEASURES N/A

ACTIVITY No restrictions

DIET Avoid acidic foods with gingivostomatitis

PATIENT EDUCATION
• Avoid contact with immunocompromised
• Wash hands often
• Genital herpes: avoid sexual contact while disease is active; discuss condom benefits and limits and reinforce benefits of mutually monogamous sexual relations.
• Reassure and reduce stigma

MEDICATIONS

DRUG(S) OF CHOICE
• Acyclovir (Zovirax)
For certain indications, consider valacyclovir or famcyclovir
  ◊ Primary genital herpes: 200 mg po q4h x 5 doses daily for 10 days
  ◊ Recurrent genital herpes: 200 mg po q4h x 5 doses daily for 5 days; for chronic suppression in persons with frequent recurrences - 400 mg bid
  ◊ Neonatal herpes simplex or encephalitis: 10 mg/kg IV over 1 hour q8h x 10-14 days
  ◊ Primary herpes gingivostomatitis, recurrent herpes labialis and other HSV skin infections: 200 mg po q4h x 5 doses daily for 10 days
• Pencyclovir (Denavir)
  ◊ Oroherpes recurrence: 1% cream q2h while awake for 4 days
• Valacyclovir (Valtrex): better bioavailability orally than acyclovir, is converted to acyclovir; indicated for use only in immunocompetent
  ◊ Primary genital herpes: 1 gm po BID for 10 days
  ◊ Recurrent genital herpes: 500 mg po bid for 5 days; chronic suppression 500 mg po bid
• Famciclovir (Famvir) - is converted to

pencyclovir, with longer intracellular half-life and higher levels than acyclovir
  ◊ Primary genital herpes: 250 mg po tid for 10 days
  ◊ Recurrent genital herpes: 125 mg po bid for 5 days; chronic suppression 250 mg po bid
Contraindications: Acyclovir, valacyclovir, or famciclovir: Hypersensitivity or intolerance
Precautions:
• Reduce dosage in renal insufficiency for acyclovir, valacyclovir and famciclovir
• Acyclovir may produce encephalopathic reactions, particularly in the elderly
• Valacyclovir: Thrombotic thrombocytopenia purpura/hemolytic uremic syndrome (TTP/HUS) reported in some immunocompromised persons in trials on high doses (8 grams daily) for CMV suppression
• Pregnancy - see Miscellaneous section
Significant possible interactions:
Probenecid with IV acyclovir, possibly probenecid with valacyclovir can reduce renal clearance and elevate antiviral drug levels

ALTERNATIVE DRUGS
• Foscarnet: Drug of choice for acyclovir-resistance in immunocompromised persons with systemic HSV; 40 mg/kg IV q8h (assume valacyclovir and famciclovir resistance also if acyclovir resistance occurs)
• Other topicals:
  ◊ Ophthalmic preparations for herpes keratoconjunctivitis: Acyclovir, vidarabine (Vira-A), idoxuridine and trifluorothymidine; refer to ophthalmologist
  ◊ n-Docosanol 10% cream - undergoing phase III clinical trials for recurrent herpes labialis
  ◊ Cidofovir gel (Forvade) - for mucocutaneous, acyclovir-resistant simplex in AIDS patients

FOLLOWUP

PATIENT MONITORING Observe for disappearance of lesions and resolution of systemic manifestations

PREVENTION/AVOIDANCE See Patient Education

POSSIBLE COMPLICATIONS Herpes encephalitis - brain biopsy may be needed for diagnosis; herpes pneumonia; aseptic meningitis; herpes viremia

EXPECTED COURSE/PROGNOSIS
Good for treatment of recurrent episodes. Expect frequent recurrences.

MISCELLANEOUS

ASSOCIATED CONDITIONS Erythema multiforme

AGE-RELATED FACTORS
Pediatric: Previously described
Geriatric: Decreased immunological competence of old age may increase risk
Others: N/A

PREGNANCY
• Acyclovir for HSV in pregnancy is recommended for severe or complicated disease; contact manufacturer/CDC registry (1-800-722-9292- ext 58465 if acyclovir used in pregnancy.
• Risk of viral shedding at delivery from asymptomatic recurrent genital HSV low (~1.6%); not predicted by monitoring cultures
• Attack rate for neonatal HSV is 41% if primary maternal genital HSV present at time of delivery and about 4% for recurrent genital HSV at time of delivery. Avoid fetal scalp electrodes if maternal history of genital HSV.
• C-section indicated if any active genital lesions (or prodrome) are present during labor; consider if primary genital herpes occurred within 4 wks of expected delivery
• Obtain HSV cultures (urine, stool, CSF, eyes, throat) of neonates exposed to primary maternal genital HSV at delivery; treat with acyclovir if clinically ill, cultures positive, CSF abnormal
• Neonates with possible exposure to HSV with signs of infection: lethargy, poor feeding, fever, or lesions; admit, culture; treat immediately with IV acyclovir if HSV illness suspected

SYNONYMS N/A

ICD-9-CM
• 054.0 Eczema herpeticum
• 771.2 Neonatal herpes simplex
• 054.9 Herpes labialis

SEE ALSO Herpes, genital

OTHER NOTES N/A

ABBREVIATIONS N/A

REFERENCES
• Dwyer DE, Cunningham AL: Herpes simplex virus infection in pregnancy. Ballieres Clin Obstet Gynaecol 1993;7:75-105
• Hirsch MS: Herpes simples virus. In: Mandell GL, et al, eds. Principles and Practice of Infectious Diseases. New York, Churchill Livingstone, 1990
• Easterbrook P, Wood MJ: Successors to acyclovir. J Antimicrob 1994;34:307-311
• Drugs for non-HIV viral infections. The Medical Letter 1997;39:69-76
Illustrations: 18 available on CD-ROM
Internet references: http://www.5mcc.com

Author(s)
Arthur R. Slaughter, MD

Herpes zoster

BASICS

DESCRIPTION A disease usually presenting as a painful unilateral dermatomal eruption. Zoster results from reactivation of varicella-zoster (chickenpox) virus that has been dormant in the dorsal root ganglia.
System(s) affected: Skin/Exocrine, Nervous
Genetics: N/A
Incidence/Prevalence in USA:
• 215/100,000/year; incidence is increasing as population ages
• Occurs in 10-20% of the population at some time
• Active herpes zoster 23.9/100,000
• Post herpetic neuralgia 86/100,000
Predominant age: Increasing incidence with aging. 80% of cases occur in persons over age 20 years (2-3 per 1000 age 20 to 50; 10 per 1000 > 80 years).
Predominant sex: Male = Female

SIGNS AND SYMPTOMS
• Prodromal phase (sensations over involved dermatome prior to rash)
  ◊ Tingling
  ◊ Itching
  ◊ Boring or knifelike pain
• Acute phase
  ◊ Constitutional symptoms
  ◊ Fatigue
  ◊ Malaise
  ◊ Headache
  ◊ Low-grade fever
  ◊ Dermatomal rash
  ◊ Weakness (1% may have weakness in distribution of rash; herpes zoster motoricus)
  ◊ Initially erythematous and maculopapular that evolves rapidly to grouped vesicles
  ◊ Vesicles become pustular and/or hemorrhagic in 3 to 4 days
  ◊ Resolution of rash with crusts separating by 14 to 21 days
  ◊ Possible sine herpete (zoster without rash)
• Chronic phase
  ◊ Postherpetic neuralgia (15% overall; increases dramatically with age)
  ◊ A small percentage (1-5%) may affect the motor nerves causing weakness (herpes zoster motoricus), e.g., facial nerve (Ramsay Hunt syndrome), spinal motor radiculopathies

CAUSES Reactivation of dormant varicella-zoster (chicken pox) virus in dorsal root ganglia or gasserian ganglia

RISK FACTORS
• Increasing age
• Compromised cell-mediated immunity in immunosuppressed patients or patients with malignancy (especially leukemia and lymphoma)
• Spinal surgery
• Spinal cord radiation

DIAGNOSIS

DIFFERENTIAL DIAGNOSIS
• Rash - herpes simplex virus, Coxsackievirus, contact dermatitis, superficial pyoderma
• Pain - cholecystitis, pleuritis, myocardial infarction

LABORATORY
• Rarely necessary
• Viral culture
• Tzanck smear (does not distinguish from herpes simplex and false negatives occur)
• Monoclonal antibody tests
• Blood mononuclear cell testing for viral DNA (research tool)
Drugs that may alter lab results: N/A
Disorders that may alter lab results: N/A

PATHOLOGICAL FINDINGS
• Multinucleated giant cells with intralesional inclusion
• Lymphatic infiltration of sensory ganglia with focal hemorrhage and nerve cell destruction

SPECIAL TESTS N/A

IMAGING N/A

DIAGNOSTIC PROCEDURES Biopsy for direct immunofluorescence testing (rarely done)

TREATMENT

APPROPRIATE HEALTH CARE
Outpatient unless disseminated or occurring as complication of serious underlying disease requiring hospitalization

GENERAL MEASURES
• Wet dressings with tap water or 5% aluminum acetate (Burow's) applied 30 to 60 minutes 4-6 times per day
• Lotions such as calamine

SURGICAL MEASURES N/A

ACTIVITY No restrictions

DIET No special diet

PATIENT EDUCATION
• Duration of rash is 2-3 weeks
• Potential for dissemination and worrisome signs (constitutional illness signs and spreading rash)
• Potential postherpetic neuralgia

MEDICATIONS

DRUG(S) OF CHOICE
• Antiviral agents, if initiated early (within 48-72 hours of rash) are of benefit in relieving symptoms and speeding resolution of rash. Postherpetic neuralgia is probably reduced when antiviral agents prescribed in acute phase of zoster. Clearly indicated for zoster associated with serious underlying condition and in ophthalmic zoster.
• Antiviral
◊ Acyclovir (Zovirax) 800 mg every 4 hours (5 doses daily) for 7-10 days
◊ Famciclovir 500 mg po tid for 7 days
◊ Valacyclovir 1000 mg po tid for 7 days
• Pain medications (acetaminophen, codeine, nonsteroidal anti-inflammatory drugs)
• Silver sulfadiazine (Silvadene) topically for secondarily infected rash
Contraindications: Refer to manufacturer's profile of each drug
Precautions:
• Monitor renal function when using acyclovir
• Acyclovir - pregnancy category C
• Refer to manufacturer's profile of each drug
Significant possible interactions:
• Acyclovir-probenecid: may inhibit excretion of acyclovir

ALTERNATIVE DRUGS
• Sorivudine
• Vidarabine

FOLLOWUP

PATIENT MONITORING Symptom dependent

PREVENTION/AVOIDANCE
• Varicella vaccines currently available will theoretically reduce zoster incidence in the future
• Vaccines are being tested for prevention of herpes zoster in individuals previously infected with wild VZ virus
• Zoster patients may transmit virus causing varicella (chickenpox) to susceptible persons

POSSIBLE COMPLICATIONS
• Postherpetic neuralgia
• Ocular involvement with facial zoster
• Meningoencephalitis
• Cutaneous dissemination
• Superinfection of skin lesions
• Hepatitis
• Pneumonitis
• Peripheral motor weakness
• Segmental myelitis
• Cranial nerve syndromes especially ophthalmic and facial (Ramsay Hunt syndrome)
• Corneal ulceration
• Guillain-Barré syndrome

EXPECTED COURSE/PROGNOSIS
• Resolution of rash within 14 to 21 days
• Postherpetic neuralgia defined as pain persisting at least one month after rash has healed
• Postherpetic neuralgia incidence increases dramatically with age (4% age 30-50; 50% over age 80 years)

MISCELLANEOUS

ASSOCIATED CONDITIONS
Immunocompromise including HIV infection, transplant recipients, and malignancies

AGE-RELATED FACTORS
Pediatric:
• Occurs rarely in children (primarily immunosuppressed)
• Has been reported in infants primarily infected in utero
Geriatric:
• Increased incidence and prevalence
• Increased incidence of postherpetic neuralgia
Others: Consider HIV infection in young patients with zoster

PREGNANCY Can occur during pregnancy

SYNONYMS Shingles

ICD-9-CM 053.9 (site specific codes not listed; preferred by Medicare)

SEE ALSO
• Chickenpox
• Herpes simplex
• Herpes eye infections
• Bell's palsy

OTHER NOTES Corticosteroid efficacy to prevent postherpetic neuralgia remains controversial. Capsaicin, transcutaneous electrical nerve stimulation (TENS) and low dose amitriptyline are the current treatment(s) of choice for postherpetic neuralgia.

ABBREVIATIONS N/A

REFERENCES
• Lancaster T, et al: Primary care management of acute herpes zoster: systematic review of evidence from randomized controlled trials. British Jour of General Practice 1995; 45(390):39-45
• Donahue JG, et al: The Incidence of Herpes Zoster. Arch Intern Med 1995;155:1605
• Tyring S, et al: Famciclovir for the Treatment of Acute Herpes Zoster: Effects on Acute Disease and Postherpetic Neuralgia. Annals of Internal Medicine 1995;123:89
Illustrations: 8 available on CD-ROM
Internet references: http://www.5mcc.com

Author(s)
Larry W. Halverson, MD

Herpes, genital

BASICS

DESCRIPTION Herpes simplex virus (usually HSV-2) infection involving the genital organs
• Primary genital herpes - initial infection with herpes simplex. No previous antibodies to HSV, involves genitalia.
• First-episode (non-primary) genital herpes - prior infection with a herpes simplex serotype, first genital involvement
• Recurrent (secondary) genital herpes - reactivation of latent herpes virus infection, usually previous genital involvement
System(s) affected: Nervous, Skin/Exocrine, Reproductive
Genetics: N/A
Incidence/Prevalence in USA:
• 50-200/100,000 (300,000 - 700,000 cases/year)
• 10,000-30,000/100,000 people
Predominant age: 18-40
Predominant sex: Female > Male

SIGNS AND SYMPTOMS
• 60-70% of patients infected with HSV-2 are asymptomatic or do not recognize clinical manifestations of disease
• Primary genital herpes
  ◊ Fever
  ◊ Headache
  ◊ Malaise
  ◊ Myalgia
  ◊ Burning genital pain
  ◊ Dysuria (female)
  ◊ Dyspareunia
  ◊ Sacral paresthesia
  ◊ Inguinal adenopathy
  ◊ Aseptic meningitis in 30%
  ◊ Occasional urinary retention
  ◊ Vesicles, on an edematous erythematous base, which ulcerate, crust over, and resolve spontaneously within 21 days. Vesicles persist longer on dry skin.
  ◊ Bilateral lesions, primarily affecting the external genitalia: female - labia majora/minora, inner thighs, vaginal mucosa, cervix, perianal skin; male - penile glans, penile shaft, urethra
• Non-primary - first episode genital herpes
  ◊ Burning genital pain
  ◊ Vesicles, on a non-edematous erythematous base, which ulcerate, crust over, and resolve spontaneously within 14-17 days
• Non-primary - recurrent genital herpes
  ◊ Prodromal symptoms - burning, numbness, tingling, paresthesia of genitals at site of previous lesions which occur approximately 24 hours prior to the eruption of new vesicles
  ◊ Burning genital pain
  ◊ Vesicles, on a non-edematous erythematous base, which ulcerate, crust over, and resolve spontaneously within 7-10 days
  ◊ Unilateral lesions

CAUSES
• Herpes simplex virus - double stranded DNA
• Type 1 (HSV-1) - 10-30%
• Type 2 (HSV-2) - 70-90%

RISK FACTORS
• Primary inoculation
  ◊ Sexual activity - number of lifetime partners, duration of sexual activity, and past history of STD's
  ◊ Fomites - wet towels (rare)
• Transmission:
  ◊ Incubation period - 1-45 days (mean 5.8)
  ◊ Male to female transmission greater than female to male
  ◊ Annual risk for susceptible female acquiring disease from an infected male partner is 10-30%; for susceptible male from infected female approximately 5%
  ◊ Patients without HSV-1 antibody are at greater risk for acquiring HSV-2 infection than those with HSV-1 antibody
  ◊ Greater than 50% of new cases result from transmission via asymptomatic shedding
  ◊ Risk of asymptomatic shedding is highest within 1 year of occurrence of first episode of genital herpes, in HSV-2 infection, and in women with frequent symptomatic episodes
  ◊ Daily therapy with oral acyclovir has been shown to suppress subclinical shedding of HSV-2, but no data currently exists on the influence of acyclovir treatment on transmission
• Triggers (recurrent) - genital trauma, menses, intercurrent infection, emotional stress, sunlight

DIAGNOSIS

DIFFERENTIAL DIAGNOSIS
• Primary syphilis
• Chancroid
• Lymphogranuloma venereum
• Atypical genital warts
• Scabies
• Molluscum contagiosum
• Allergic contact dermatitis
• Trauma
• Candidiasis
• Herpes zoster
• Behçet's syndrome
• Stevens-Johnson syndrome
• Inflammatory bowel disease
• Granuloma inguinale
• Folliculitis
• Ulcerative balanitis
• Neoplasia

LABORATORY
• Viral tissue culture: swab vesicle fluid/ulcer
• Tzanck prep: Sensitivity = 40-50% compared to culture; multinucleated giant cells.
• Pap smear
• Serology: ELISA, direct fluorescent assay (DFA), radioimmunoassay (RIA) and complement fixation. Do not reliably discriminate between HSV-1 and HSV-2. Sensitivity = 80% compared to culture. Primary herpes - 4 x increase acute/convalescent titer; recurrent herpes - no increase in acute/convalescent titer.
Drugs that may alter lab results:
Calcium agglutinate swabs may be toxic to HSV and are not recommended for culture; use cotton or dacron tipped swabs instead

Disorders that may alter lab results:
Varicella-zoster will give identical Tzanck prep results

PATHOLOGICAL FINDINGS
• Histopathologic-cytopathic changes
  ◊ Intracellular edema of epithelial cells
  ◊ Nuclear margination of chromatin
  ◊ Formation of Cowdry type A intranuclear inclusions
  ◊ Cell fusion into multinucleated giant cells
• Pathologic stages:
  ◊ Primary mucocutaneous infection
  ◊ Acute ganglionic infection
  ◊ Establishment of latency
  ◊ Ganglionic reactivation
  ◊ Recurrent infection

SPECIAL TESTS Type specific serologic assays - Immunodot, Western Blot and monoclonal antibody blocking RIA - do discriminate between HSV-1 and HSV-2 infections, but are generally available only in research settings

IMAGING N/A

DIAGNOSTIC PROCEDURES N/A

TREATMENT

APPROPRIATE HEALTH CARE
Outpatient, self-care

GENERAL MEASURES
• Cool compresses (Burow's solution 4-6 times a day); ice packs to perineum; sitz baths
• Local perineal hygiene
• Analgesics - NSAID's
• Topical anesthetics - lidocaine

SURGICAL MEASURES N/A

ACTIVITY
• Avoid intercourse in the presence of symptomatic genital lesions
• Appropriate rest if systemic manifestations (primary) are present

DIET N/A

PATIENT EDUCATION Herpes Resource Center ASHA/HRC, P.O. Box 13827, Research Triangle Park, North Carolina 27709-9940, HRC Hotline (919)361-8488; web: http://sunsite.unc.edu./ASHA/phone/telher.html

MEDICATIONS

DRUG(S) OF CHOICE
• Acyclovir (Zovirax)
  ◊ Primary or 1st episode: 200 mg po 5 times per day for 7-10 days or 400 mg tid for 10 days

◊ Severe local or disseminated disease: 5 mg/kg IV every 8 hours for 7 days

◊ Encephalitis: 10 mg/kg IV, every 8 hours for 10 days

◊ Recurrent episodes: 200 mg po 5 times/day x 5 days (or 400 mg tid x 5 days, or 800 mg bid x 5 days)

◊ Chronic suppression: recommended for frequent (≥6/year) or disabling recurrences: 400 mg po bid (or 200 mg po 3-5 times/day) - appears safe and efficacious for at least 6 years duration of therapy

◊ HIV infection: 400 mg po 3-5 times/day until clinical resolution attained

Contraindications: Allergy to acyclovir

Precautions:
• Acyclovir

◊ Not approved for routine use in pregnancy

◊ Drug is excreted in breast milk

◊ Modify dose in patients with significant renal insufficiency

◊ Acyclovir resistance (in conjunction with famciclovir and valacyclovir resistance) occurs mostly in HIV infected patients

Significant possible interactions:
• Acyclovir

◊ Methotrexate - use with caution in patients who have had a neurologic reaction to intrathecal methotrexate

◊ Interferon - acyclovir is synergistic in vitro with interferon. Clinical significance is unknown. Use with caution in patients with prior neurological reactions to interferon.

◊ Probenecid - will decrease renal excretion, increase serum concentration

ALTERNATIVE DRUGS
• Acyclovir topical ointment - less effective
• Foscarnet - 40 mg/kg IV every 8 hours in severe disease with proven or suspected acyclovir resistant strains
• Vidarabine - 10 mg/kg/day infused over 10 hours; benefits HIV patients with HSV-1 infection failing acyclovir and foscarnet therapy
• Famciclovir (Famvir)

◊ Metabolized to penciclovir, inhibits viral replication

◊ Activity/side effects similar to acyclovir

◊ First episode genital - 250 mg po tid for 5 days (not FDA approved)

◊ Recurrent - 125 mg po bid for 5 days

◊ Chronic suppression - 125-500 mg po daily (not FDA approved)
• Valacyclovir (Valtrex)

◊ Metabolized to acyclovir and valine

◊ May cause thrombotic thrombocytopenia purpura/homolytic uremic syndrome in immunocompromised patients

◊ First episode genital - 1 g po bid x 10 days

◊ Recurrent - 500 mg bid for 5 days

FOLLOWUP

PATIENT MONITORING
• Acute episode - followup if complications
• Latent infection - annual pap smear; careful exam of pregnant women during prenatal visits and at onset of labor

PREVENTION/AVOIDANCE
• Condoms/spermicide in sexual activity
• Avoid multiple sexual partners
• Avoid stress when possible

POSSIBLE COMPLICATIONS
• Vaginal discharge
• Secondary bacterial infection
• Urinary retention
• Aseptic meningitis
• Transmission to neonate
• Increased risk for HIV infection

EXPECTED COURSE/PROGNOSIS
• Resolution of signs/symptoms: Primary in 14-21 days; first episode - non-primary 14-17 days; recurrent 7-10 days
• Latent infection - recurrences in 80% of patients within 1 year of initial HSV-2 infection; immunocompetent patients average 3-4/year
• Infection in immunocompromised individual - prolonged severe local or disseminated disease is common

MISCELLANEOUS

ASSOCIATED CONDITIONS
• Herpes labialis
• Syphilis
• Gonorrhea
• Non-gonococcal urethritis/cervicitis
• Genital warts (HPV)
• AIDS (HIV)
• Trichomoniasis

AGE-RELATED FACTORS
Pediatric:
• Genital lesions in prepubertal child is suggestive of sexual abuse
• Neonatal infection occurs in 10-20/100,000 live births (1500-2000 cases annually) and results in death or significant neurologic impairment in 85% of individuals. Most neonatal infections result from asymptomatic viral shedding from past maternal infection.
• High risk infant - begin acyclovir 30 mg/kg/day IV every 8 hours for 10-14 days
• Low risk infant - if asymptomatic - culture eyes, nasopharynx, mouth at 24-36 hours old and observe
Geriatric: N/A
Others: N/A

PREGNANCY
• Primary/1st episode genital herpes infection associated with increased rate of spontaneous abortion (45%) and preterm labor (35%)
• Greatest risk for neonatal infection occurs with primary or non-primary first episode genital herpes infection of the mother at time of delivery (30% transmission rate) enhanced by prolonged rupture of membranes, use of fetal scalp electrode, presence of lesions on cervix, and premature infant
• Low risk - recurrent asymptomatic HSV shedding in mother (3%)

• Infants born to mothers with high titer of neutralizing antibodies are at low risk of infection
• Cesarean section is indicated if herpetic genital lesions are present during labor
• Any lesion suspicious for genital herpes during pregnancy should be cultured
• Routine surveillance cultures for women with a history of genital herpes are indicated only at the time of labor
• Acyclovir therapy:

◊ Not approved for routine use in pregnancy

◊ It has been used by some clinicians during the last 1-2 weeks of pregnancy to avoid activation of lesions, and in the third trimester to treat life-threatening infections, both without apparent complications of therapy

◊ In women with recurrent genital herpes, oral acyclovir prophylaxis from 37 weeks gestation may be more cost-effective than cesarean delivery in preventing neonatal infection

◊ Pregnant women receiving acyclovir: report to CDC/ Wellcome Registry 800-722-GLAXO, x38465

SYNONYMS Herpes genitalis

ICD-9-CM 054.10 Genital herpes, unspecified

SEE ALSO Herpes simplex

OTHER NOTES N/A

ABBREVIATIONS N/A

REFERENCES
• U.S. Department of Health and Human Services, Centers for Disease Control and Prevention: Sexually transmitted diseases treatment guideline. Morbidity and Mortality Weekly Report 1993;42;RR-14:22-26
• Overall JC: Herpes simplex virus infection of the fetus and newborn. Pediatric Annals 1994;3:131-136
• McGrath BJ, Newman CL: Genital herpes simplex infections in patients with AIDS. Pharmacotherapy 1994;5:529-542
• Thomas DL, Quinn TC: Serologic testing for sexually transmitted diseases. Infect Dis Clin of NA 1993;7(4):793-802
• Lavole SR, Kaplowitz LG: Management of genital herpes infections. Seminars in Dermatology 1994;4:248-256
• Clark JL, Tatum NO, Noble SL: Management of genital herpes. Am Fam Phys 1995;51:175-182
• Patel R, Barton SE: Antiviral chemotherapy in genital herpes simplex virus infections. Internat J of STD & AIDS 1995;6:320-328
 Slomka MJ: Seroepidemiology and control of genital herpes. Communicable Disease Report. CDR Review 1996;6:R41-R45
• Randolph AG, Hartshorn RM: Acyclovir prophylaxis in late pregnancy to prevent neonatal herpes - a cost-effective analysis. Obstet-Gynecol 1996;88:603-610
Illustrations: N/A
Internet references: http://www.5mcc.com

Author(s)
Gary Levine, MD

Hiccups

BASICS

DESCRIPTION Sudden, involuntary, contraction of the inspiratory muscles (predominantly the diaphragm) terminated by abrupt closure of the glottis stopping the inflow of air and producing the characteristic sound.
System(s) affected: Pulmonary, nervous
Genetics: N/A
Incidence/Prevalence in USA: Self limited hiccups are extremely common; intractable hiccups are rare
Predominant age: All ages (including fetus)
Predominant sex: Male > Female (4:1)

SIGNS AND SYMPTOMS Hiccup attacks usually occur at brief intervals and last only a few seconds or minutes. Bouts lasting more than 48 hours often imply an underlying physical or metabolic disorder. Intractable hiccups may occur continuously for months or years. Hiccups usually occur with a frequency of 4 to 60 per minute.

CAUSES
• Pathophysiologic significance is unknown; hiccups have been associated with more than 100 underlying disorders.
• Results from stimulation of one or more limbs of the hiccup reflux arc (vagus and phrenic nerves) with a "hiccup center" located in the upper spinal cord
• In men greater than 90% have an organic basis while in women a psychogenic cause is more likely
• Specific underlying causes include:
  ◊ Alcoholism
  ◊ CNS lesions (brainstem tumors, vascular lesions, Parkinson's disease)
  ◊ Diaphragmatic irritation (tumors, pericarditis, eventration, splenomegaly, hepatomegaly, peritonitis)
  ◊ Hair, insect or foreign body irritating tympanic membrane
  ◊ Pharyngitis, laryngitis
  ◊ Mediastinal and other thoracic lesions (pneumonia, aortic aneurysm, tuberculosis, myocardial infarction, lung cancer)
  ◊ Esophageal lesions (reflux esophagitis, achalasia, Candida esophagitis, carcinoma, obstruction)
  ◊ Gastric lesions (ulcer, distention, cancer)
  ◊ Hepatic lesions (hepatitis, hepatoma)
  ◊ Pancreatic lesions (pancreatitis, pseudocysts, cancer)
  ◊ Inflammatory bowel disease
  ◊ Cholelithiasis, cholecystitis
  ◊ Prostatic disorders
  ◊ Appendicitis
  ◊ Postoperative, abdominal procedures
  ◊ Toxic metabolic causes (uremia, hyponatremia, gout, diabetes)
  ◊ Drug induced (dexamethasone, methylprednisolone, benzodiazepines, alpha methyldopa)
  ◊ Psychogenic causes (hysterical neurosis, grief, malingering)
  ◊ Idiopathic

RISK FACTORS
• General anesthesia
• Post-operative state
• Irritation of the vagus nerve branches
• Structural, vascular, infectious or traumatic CNS lesions

DIAGNOSIS

DIFFERENTIAL DIAGNOSIS See Causes (burping [eructation] may be confused with hiccups)

LABORATORY N/A
Drugs that may alter lab results: N/A
Disorders that may alter lab results: N/A

PATHOLOGICAL FINDINGS N/A

SPECIAL TESTS N/A

IMAGING Fluoroscopy is useful to determine if one hemidiaphragm is dominant

DIAGNOSTIC PROCEDURES N/A

TREATMENT

APPROPRIATE HEALTH CARE
• Outpatient (usually)
• Inpatient (if elderly, debilitated or intractable hiccups)

GENERAL MEASURES
• Treat any specific underlying cause when identified.
  ◊ Dilate esophageal stricture or obstruction
  ◊ Remove hair or foreign body from ear canal
  ◊ Angostura bitters for alcohol induced hiccups
  ◊ Catheter stimulation of pharynx for operative and post-operative hiccups
  ◊ Anti-fungal treatment for Candida esophagitis
  ◊ Correct electrolyte imbalance
• Simple home remedies
  ◊ Swallowing a spoonful of sugar
  ◊ Sucking on a hard candy or swallowing peanut butter
  ◊ Holding breath and increasing pressure on diaphragm (Valsalva maneuver)
  ◊ Tongue traction
  ◊ Lifting the uvula with a cold spoon
  ◊ Drinking from the far side of a glass
  ◊ Inducing fright
  ◊ Smelling salts
  ◊ Rebreathing into a paper (not plastic) bag
  ◊ Sipping ice water
• Medical measures
  ◊ Relief of gastric distention (gastric lavage, nasogastric aspiration, induced vomiting)
  ◊ Counterirritation of the vagus nerve (supraorbital pressure, carotid sinus massage, digital rectal massage), to be used with caution
  ◊ Respiratory center stimulants (breathing 5% carbon dioxide)
  ◊ Phrenic nerve block of dominant hemidiaphragm; phrenic crush, transection
  ◊ Psychiatric (hypnosis, behavioral modification)
  ◊ Miscellaneous (cardioversion, acupuncture)

SURGICAL MEASURES N/A

ACTIVITY As tolerated

DIET Avoid gastric distension from overeating, carbonated beverages, aerophagia

PATIENT EDUCATION See General Measures

Hiccups

MEDICATIONS

DRUG(S) OF CHOICE
Possible drug remedies:
• Baclofen, a GABA analog, 5-10 mg tid (best choice)
• Chlorpromazine 25-50 mg IV
• Haloperidol 2-12 mg IM
• Phenytoin 200 mg IV then 100 mg qid
• Metoclopramide 5-10 mg qid
• Nifedipine 10-20 mg qd-tid
• Amitriptyline 10 mg tid
Contraindications: Refer to manufacturer's literature (baclofen is not recommended in patients with stroke or other cerebral lesions)
Precautions: Refer to manufacturer's literature (abrupt withdrawal of baclofen should be avoided)
Significant possible interactions: Refer to manufacturer's literature

ALTERNATIVE DRUGS
• Amantadine, carbidopa-levodopa in Parkinson's disease
• Steroid replacement in Addison's disease
• Antifungal agent in Candida esophagitis
• Ondansetron in carcinomatosis with vomiting

FOLLOWUP

PATIENT MONITORING   Until hiccups cease

PREVENTION/AVOIDANCE
• Correct underlying cause
• Maintenance drug therapy (e.g., baclofen 5-10 mg tid; phenytoin 100 mg qid; valproic acid 15 mg/kg undivided doses; nifedipine 10-20 mg qd-tid; metoclopramide 10 mg qid)

POSSIBLE COMPLICATIONS
• Inability to eat
• Weight loss
• Exhaustion, debility
• Insomnia
• Cardiac arrhythmias
• Wound dehiscence
• Death (rare)

EXPECTED COURSE/PROGNOSIS
• Hiccups often cease during sleep
• Most acute benign hiccups resolve with home remedies or spontaneously
• Intractable hiccups may last for years and decades
• Hiccups have persisted despite bilateral phrenic nerve transection

MISCELLANEOUS

ASSOCIATED CONDITIONS   See Causes

AGE-RELATED FACTORS
Pediatric: May persist from fetal state
Geriatric: Can be a serious problem among the elderly
Others: N/A

PREGNANCY   Fetal hiccups noted as rhythmic fetal movements (confirmed sonographically), fetal hiccups often recur in subsequent pregnancies

SYNONYMS
• Hiccoughs
• Singultus

ICD-9-CM
786.8 Hiccough

SEE ALSO   N/A

OTHER NOTES   N/A

ABBREVIATIONS   N/A

REFERENCES
• Lewis JH: Hiccups: Reasons and remedies. In: Lewis JH, ed. A Pharmacologic Approach to Gastrointestinal Disorders. Baltimore, Williams & Wilkins, 1994
• Lewis JH: Hiccups. In: Rakel RE, ed. Conn's Current therapy. Philadelphia, WB Saunders Co, 1996;11-16
Illustrations: N/A
Internet references: http://www.5mcc.com

Author(s)
James H. Lewis, MD, FACP, FACG

Hidradenitis suppurativa

BASICS

DESCRIPTION Acute, tender, cyst-like abscesses in apocrine gland bearing skin (axillae, anogenital area, pubes, areolae, also apocrine glands scattered around umbilicus, scalp, trunk and face). In chronic cases, fibrotic sinus tracts develop with intermittent drainage and periodic acute abscesses.
Genetics: Unknown
System(s) affected: Skin/Exocrine
Incidence/Prevalence in USA: Common
Predominant age: Late puberty through age 40, commonly 30-40.
Predominant sex: Female (perianal) > Male (axillary)

SIGNS AND SYMPTOMS
• Papules (dome-shaped) 1-3 cm in size
• Nodules (dome-shaped) 1-3 cm in size
• Larger lesions fluctuant
• Distribution - Apocrine glands as above with axillae and groin most common
• Multiple recurrences at the same site
• Healing sites accompanied by scarring and sinus tracts
• Comedones may be present
• Associated arthritis (rare)

CAUSES
• Blockage of pilosebaceous units to which apocrine glands are attached. This activity occurs (acne-like) after hormone stimulation beginning with puberty.
• Blockage of apocrine follicles may possibly be caused by embryologic malformation of apocrine duct, compression of the duct due to sweat retention, or bacterial infection
• May be part of "follicular occlusive triad"; acne conglobata, dissecting cellulitis of scalp, hidradenitis suppurativa)

RISK FACTORS
• Obesity
• African American
• Female
• Acne
• Diabetes Mellitus
• Hypercholesterolemia
• Low basal metabolic rate

DIAGNOSIS

DIFFERENTIAL DIAGNOSIS
• Furunculosis. Differentiate by specific culture and also by the response to specific antibiotics.
• Inflammatory bowel disease with anogenital fistula (may also coexist with hidradenitis suppurativa

LABORATORY Culture of exudate from lesion: Staphylococci, Streptococci, E. Coli, Proteus with chronic condition, usually not anaerobes. Increasing antibiotic resistance. Normocytic anemia with chronic cases.
Drugs that may alter lab results: N/A
Disorders that may alter lab results: N/A

PATHOLOGICAL FINDINGS Acute and chronic inflammation, multiple comedones, sinus tracts when recurrent

SPECIAL TESTS Culture discharge from lesion(s)

IMAGING N/A

DIAGNOSTIC PROCEDURES Incision and drainage of lesion(s) with biopsy

TREATMENT

APPROPRIATE HEALTH CARE
Generally outpatient

GENERAL MEASURES
• Symptomatic treatment acute lesions
• Prevent new lesions
• Local cleansing (germicidal soap)
• Improve environmental factors that cause follicular blockage

SURGICAL MEASURES
• Incision and drainage of lesions
• Consider excisional surgery (draining lesions are not contraindications for surgery)
  ◊ Remove sinus tracts
  ◊ Exteriorization with curettage and electrodesiccation
• Treatment for severe, intractable cases: excision and skin graft
• CO2 laser stripping with healing by secondary intention

ACTIVITY Fully active

DIET No restrictions

PATIENT EDUCATION
• Minimize heat exposure and sweating
• Reduce weight if obese
• Avoid constrictive clothing
• Medication precautions

MEDICATIONS

DRUG(S) OF CHOICE
• Antibiotics; sometimes for 2 or more months:
◊ Tetracycline 250 mg qid or 500 mg tid, or
◊ Minocycline (Minocin) 100 mg bid po, or
◊ Clindamycin 2% lotion or neomycin cream topically to control odor.
◊ Erythromycin 1-1.5 gm qd po
◊ Doxycycline 100 mg bid 7-14 days
◊ Other antibiotics depending on culture
• Consider oral retinoids
◊ Isotretinoin (Accutane) 40-80 mg/day po for 4 months. No Accutane during pregnancy (highly teratogenic). Still frequent recurrences.
• Birth control pills (female only), if antibiotic therapy fails
◊ Low-dose progesterone BCPs (e.g., Norinyl, Ortho-Novum, Enovid)
• Consider steroids
◊ Injection of lesions with depot-type steroids (e.g., triamcinolone)
◊ Consider brief course of systemic corticosteroids

Contraindications: Tetracycline - pregnancy, children < 8 years

Precautions:
• Tetracycline - use sunscreen (SPF 15 or better) to avoid phototoxicity.
• Review professional literature before prescribing birth control pills or Accutane

Significant possible interactions:
• Tetracycline - do not take dairy products, antacids, or iron preparations within 2 hours of tetracycline dose.

ALTERNATIVE DRUGS N/A

FOLLOWUP

PATIENT MONITORING Revisits monthly, or more often if needed

PREVENTION/AVOIDANCE
• Minimize heat exposure and sweating
• Lose weight if overweight
• Avoid constrictive clothing/frictional trauma
• Avoid underarm antiperspirants and deodorants

POSSIBLE COMPLICATIONS
• Lymphedema
• Contracture formation at the sites of lesions
• Squamous cell carcinoma may develop in indolent sinus tracts
• Disseminated infection - unusual
• Restricted limb mobility
• Urethral/rectal fistula
• Anemia
• Arthritis
• Amyloidosis
• Renal failure
• Interstitial keratitis

EXPECTED COURSE/PROGNOSIS
• Individual lesions (with or without drainage) heal slowly in 10-30 days
• Recurrences may last for several years
• Rare spontaneous resolution
• Relentlessly progressive scarring and sinus tracts

MISCELLANEOUS

ASSOCIATED CONDITIONS
• Acne
• Perifolliculitis capitis abscedens et suffodiens (dissecting cellulitis of scalp)
• Obesity with associated diabetes mellitus, atopy, acanthosis nigrans

AGE-RELATED FACTORS
Pediatric: Rarely occurs before puberty (1 case reported in a 2 year old)
Geriatric: Rare after menopause
Others: Common late puberty through age 40

PREGNANCY No Accutane treatment during pregnancy

SYNONYMS N/A

ICD-9-CM
705.83 Hidradenitis

SEE ALSO
• Furunculosis
• Folliculitis

OTHER NOTES
• Some patients develop only two or three papules per year. Others develop new lesions and drain as rapidly as old ones resolve.
• Although 50% of patients receiving Accutane, in doses similar to those for acne, obtain appreciable improvement, relapse occurs quickly upon discontinuing

ABBREVIATIONS N/A

REFERENCES
• Moschella SL, Hurley HJ: Dermatology. 3rd Ed. Philadelphia, W.B. Saunders, 1992
• Lynch PJ: Dermatology for the House Officer. 3rd Ed. Baltimore, Williams & Wilkins, 1994
• Bell BA, Ellis H: Hydradenitis Suppurativa. Journal of the Royal Society of Medicine 1978;71:511-515
• Sauer GC: Manual of Skin Diseases. 6th Ed. Philadelphia, J.B. Lippincott, 1991
• Orkin M, ed: Dermatology. Los Altos, CA, Lange Medical Publishers, 1991
• Lapins J, Marcusson JA, Emtestam L: Surgical treatment of chronic hidradenitis suppurativa: CO2 laser stripping-secondary intention technique. British J of Dermatol 1994 131:551-556
Illustrations: N/A
Internet references: http://www.5mcc.com

Author(s)
Paul J. Jaster, MD

Hip fracture

BASICS

DESCRIPTION   Fracture of the head or neck of the femur, usually as the result of a fall
• Types
 ◊ Neck, subcapital or transcervical
 ◊ Intertrochanteric
 ◊ Subtrochanteric; usually caused by more severe trauma and has higher incidence in males than the other types
System(s) affected: Musculoskeletal
Genetics: No known genetic factor
Incidence/Prevalence in USA:
• 200,000 patients per year over the age of 65 have fracture of hips
• In women over age 75, there is a 1% incidence per year
Predominant age: 80% occur in those over age 60
Predominant sex: Female > Male

SIGNS AND SYMPTOMS
• Pain in hip. If severe, it usually indicates a displaced fracture. Mild pain usually occurs in non-displaced fractures.
• Pain in knee. Pain is referred from hip and may occur in absence of hip pain.
• External rotation of leg
• Shortening of leg

CAUSES
• Falls
• Motor vehicle trauma
• Spontaneous in pathologic conditions

RISK FACTORS
• Osteoporosis, usually post menopausal
• Metastatic cancer
• Neurological disease
• Severe renal disease with secondary hyperparathyroidism
• Use of long-acting sedatives and hypnotics in the elderly

DIAGNOSIS

DIFFERENTIAL DIAGNOSIS   Rule out primary or metastatic malignancy

LABORATORY   Routine pre-operative laboratory including CBC, chemical profile, electrolytes
Drugs that may alter lab results: N/A
Disorders that may alter lab results: N/A

PATHOLOGICAL FINDINGS
Osteoporosis

SPECIAL TESTS   N/A

IMAGING
• X-rays - AP and "frog leg" lateral of hip
• X-ray AP pelvis to rule out pelvis fracture as cause of pain. Also provides information regarding appearance of opposite side.
• X-ray remainder of femur to include knee
• X-ray any other tender or painful area as other fractures are common and symptoms may be ignored with severe pain of hip fracture
• CT or MRI scans are not routinely indicated as the diagnosis is usually obvious from plain radiographs

DIAGNOSTIC PROCEDURES   N/A

TREATMENT

APPROPRIATE HEALTH CARE
• Treat as semi-emergency
• During transportation to hospital, gentle traction of the leg, especially Buck's traction 5# will help relieve discomfort. This can be maintained in bed, but requires close observation of circulation and skin changes.

GENERAL MEASURES
• Medical evaluation to have patient in best possible condition before surgery
• Surgery is almost always indicated. Older patients do not tolerate long periods of bed confinement.
• Protect pressure points to avoid decubitus ulcers, especially on the sacrum, heels and malleoli

SURGICAL MEASURES
• A hip prosthesis or pins are used in neck fractures. Nails or screws with side plates are used in intertrochanteric fractures. For subtrochanteric fractures, a nail with a long side plate, or intermedullary hip screws, or reconstructive rods may be used.

ACTIVITY
• Patients should be up (for toilet, and prevention of deep vein thrombosis and decubiti) as soon as possible after surgery, usually the next day
• Ambulate as soon as possible after surgery, e.g., with use of a walker. Close supervision by an experienced therapist necessary.

DIET   No special diet

PATIENT EDUCATION   Refer to physical therapy for walking instructions; usually non-weight bearing for several weeks at least

MEDICATIONS

DRUG(S) OF CHOICE Analgesics, as indicated. Drug of choice might be morphine sulfate 2-10 mg q3h prn with change to oral opioids as soon as possible.
Contraindications: Associated head injury or severe respiratory disease
Precautions: Dosage should be lower in older people to avoid respiratory problems
Significant possible interactions: Refer to manufacturer's literature

ALTERNATIVE DRUGS N/A

FOLLOWUP

PATIENT MONITORING
• X-rays of the hip taken prior to discharge from the hospital and every 8-12 weeks afterward until healed
• Monitor postoperative physical therapy for full recovery

PREVENTION/AVOIDANCE
• Prophylactic treatment for osteoporosis
• Avoid long-acting sedatives and hypnotics in the elderly
• Use walking canes or walkers if patient has unsteady gait
• Have older people use proper chair for sitting. Should not allow hip flexion greater than 90 degrees since rising from this position requires external rotation of the extremity with subsequent torsional forces which can cause fracture.
• Use sturdy rails in showers, bathrooms, stairs, or ramps

POSSIBLE COMPLICATIONS
• Mental deterioration. Present in 90% of older patients for varying periods of time after surgery. Usually subsides, but may persist due to pre-existing arteriosclerosis.
• Infection. More common in comminuted fractures and patients with diabetes. Surgical implants should be left in place and antibiotics given as indicated by culture and sensitivity. Some require the wound to be opened and drained.
• Aseptic necrosis of femoral head. Occurs in 25-30% of femoral neck fractures. Treatment requires a prosthetic replacement in older patients.
• Phlebitis. Prophylaxis with warfarin (Coumadin) to keep INR 2.0-2.5 or protime 15-18 scc - for at least 4 weeks; or enoxaparin (Lovenox) 30 mg SQ q12h beginning 12 hours after surgery and continuing until patient is mobile
• Nonunion
  ◊ In case of neck fractures, a prosthetic replacement is indicated
  ◊ In the intertrochanteric fracture, a bone graft, usually with replacement of the nail and plate, is indicated

EXPECTED COURSE/PROGNOSIS
• Hip fractures remain a serious injury in older people. There is a 15-20% three month mortality in trochanteric fractures and 10% in neck fractures.
• Sixty-five percent of patients can be expected to return to their former state of health

MISCELLANEOUS

ASSOCIATED CONDITIONS
• Osteoporosis
• Metastatic malignancy

AGE-RELATED FACTORS
Pediatric: N/A
Geriatric: Hip fractures common in geriatric age group
Others: N/A

PREGNANCY N/A

SYNONYMS
• Subcapital fracture
• Trochanteric fracture
• Femoral neck fracture

ICD-9-CM
820. Fracture of neck of femur (use appropriate modifier)

SEE ALSO
• Osteoporosis

OTHER NOTES None

ABBREVIATIONS N/A

REFERENCES
• Clinical Orthopedics #218, May, 1987; Symposium of hip fractures; pp. 2-104
• Bentley G: Impacted Fracture of the Neck of the Femur. Bone & Joint Surgery 1968, 50:B:551
• Sarmiento A, et al: Avoidance of Complications. Clinical Orthopedics 1967;53:47
Illustrations: N/A
Internet references: http://www.5mcc.com

Author(s)
Furnie W. Johnston, MD
R. Bruce Hall, MD

Hirsutism

BASICS

DESCRIPTION Excessive male-pattern hair growth due to increased androgenic hormones
• Often accompanied by menstrual irregularities
• Extreme androgenic effects (deep voice, clitorimegaly, balding) is known as virilization
System(s) affected: Endocrine/Reproductive
Genetics: Multifactorial
Incidence/Prevalence in USA: 8% of adult women
Predominant age: Postpubertal females
Predominant sex: Postpubertal females

SIGNS AND SYMPTOMS
• Hair thickens and darkens in "male" pattern - beard, moustache, chest hair
• Usually accompanied by irregular menses and anovulation
• Usually accompanied by acne
• May be accompanied by infertility
• Onset is usually gradual

CAUSES
• Excessive androgenic effects:
  ◊ Excess hormone production from the ovary or adrenal gland
  ◊ Increased peripheral sensitivity to androgens
  ◊ Decreased sex hormone binding globulin
• Causes with persistent anovulation:
  ◊ Polycystic ovary disease
  ◊ Hypothyroidism
  ◊ Hyperprolactinemia
• Ovarian causes:
  ◊ Polycystic ovaries
  ◊ Ovarian tumors
  ◊ Premature ovarian failure
• Adrenal causes:
  ◊ Tumor (rare)
  ◊ Cushing's (rare)
  ◊ Late onset congenital adrenal hyperplasia

RISK FACTORS
• Family history
• Anovulation

DIAGNOSIS

DIFFERENTIAL DIAGNOSIS All hirsutism is from relative excess of androgen. This can be produced by the ovaries, the adrenals, or caused indirectly by other hormone imbalances. A specific etiology is often not found.
• Excess ovarian androgen production (testosterone level)
• Excess adrenal androgen production (DHEAS [dehydroepiandrosterone sulfate])
• Late onset congenital adrenal hyperplasia (17 hydroxyprogesterone [17-OHP])
• Hypothyroidism (TSH)
• Hyperprolactinemia (prolactin level)
• Ovarian tumor (testosterone > 200)
• Adrenal tumor (DHEAS > 700)
• Idiopathic - possibly through peripheral conversion - no good test available
• Anabolic steroid use in performance athletes
• Cushing's disease - very rare

LABORATORY
• Basic workup - total testosterone, DHEAS, 17-OHP, TSH, prolactin
• If testosterone > 200, need ovarian tumor workup
• If DHEAS > 700, need adrenal tumor workup
• LH/FSH ratio is elevated in 75% of polycystic ovarian disease
• If testosterone, DHEAS or 17 OHP are elevated, but not in tumor range, treat
Drugs that may alter lab results: N/A
Disorders that may alter lab results: N/A

PATHOLOGICAL FINDINGS N/A

SPECIAL TESTS
• Some do endometrial biopsy if > 35 years old
• If strong suspicion of Cushing's disease, can do dexamethasone suppression test. Give 1 mg dexamethasone po at PM and draw plasma cortisol at 8:00 am. If cortisol > 5, borderline; if > 10, abnormal.
• If 17-OHP is 300-800, do ACTH (Cortrosyn) test (ACTH 0.25 mg IV and check 17-OHP at 0 and 1 hour)
• Some do 3 alpha-androstanediol glucuronide to check for peripheral conversion - but not a good test and doesn't change therapy
• If DHEAS is high, but not in tumor range, can do low dose dexamethasone test (0.5 mg dexamethasone qid x 5 days, then recheck DHEAS and testosterone - they will decrease if androgens are adrenal and won't if they are ovarian)

IMAGING
• If testosterone > 200 or DHEAS > 700, need CT of ovaries or adrenals
• Ultrasound can image polycystic ovaries as a supplement to clinical diagnosis

DIAGNOSTIC PROCEDURES N/A

TREATMENT

APPROPRIATE HEALTH CARE
Outpatient

GENERAL MEASURES
• Treatment is slow and often lifelong
• If patient desires pregnancy, ovulation induction may be necessary
• Provide contraception as needed
• Encourage patient to maintain ideal weight
• Treat accompanying acne

SURGICAL MEASURES N/A

ACTIVITY No special activity

DIET No special diet

PATIENT EDUCATION
• Hormonal treatment stops further hair growth but will not usually reverse present hair
• Treatment takes 6-24 months and may be life long
• Cosmetic measures include - plucking, bleaching, shaving, electrolysis and cover up cosmetics
• Electrolysis should be by a licensed professional

Hirsutism

MEDICATIONS

DRUG(S) OF CHOICE
After tumor has been ruled out:
- Hormonal therapy - the goal is to:
  ◊ Decrease androgens
  ◊ Increase sex steroid binding globulin (SBG)
  ◊ Increase testosterone clearance
  ◊ Decrease LH
- Oral contraceptives:
  ◊ Any brand is effective - monophasics and triphasics both work
  ◊ Estrogen dominant pills (e.g., Ortho brands) will increase SBG
  ◊ Progesterone dominant pills (e.g., Wyeth brands) will increase clearance of testosterone
  ◊ Estrogen and progesterone can be given separately
  ◊ Medroxyprogesterone (Depo-Provera) IM every 3 months
- Chronic dexamethasone therapy:
  ◊ Can be used in late onset congenital adrenal hyperplasia (0.5 mg qhs), but oral contraception also effective

Contraindications: Avoid giving medications in pregnancy
Precautions: N/A
Significant possible interactions: N/A

ALTERNATIVE DRUGS
- Antiandrogenic drugs (often used when workup is negative and oral contraceptives not helping. They have low efficacy and many side effects):
  ◊ Spironolactone: up to 200 mg/day - onset of action is slow, side effects include menorrhagia, contraindicated in pregnancy
  ◊ Cyproterone: orphan drug not routinely available - usually combined with estrogen - contraindicated in pregnancy. Monitor for LFTs.
  ◊ Flutamide: 250 mg tid - nonsteroidal antiandrogen. Monitor for LFTs. Need concurrent oral contraceptives.
  ◊ Ketoconazole: 400 mg day - avoid with terfenadine, astemizole, triazolam, cisapride
  ◊ Leuprolide (Lupron): lowers LH - side effects of menopause
  ◊ Danazol: lowers LH - side effects of menopause
  ◊ Metformin: experimentally decreases insulin secretion which decreases androgen production in polycystic ovaries

FOLLOWUP

PATIENT MONITORING Monitor for known side effects of medications

PREVENTION/AVOIDANCE
- Tumor must be ruled out before beginning therapy
- As hormone balance improves, fertility may increase - provide contraception as needed
- Patients desiring pregnancy may need fertility intervention such as ovulation induction
- Women with late onset congenital adrenal hyperplasia may be carriers for the severe early onset childhood disease - counsel
- Avoid quackery and unlicensed electrolysis
- Prolonged amenorrhea may, over time, put the patient at risk for endometrial hyperplasia or carcinoma
- There is an increased incidence of diabetes in polycystic ovarian disease

POSSIBLE COMPLICATIONS
- Dysfunctional uterine bleeding and anemia
- Androgenic excess may adversely affect lipid status, cardiac risk and bone density
- Poor self image/shame

EXPECTED COURSE/PROGNOSIS
- Excellent with long term therapy for halting further hair growth
- Moderate to poor for reversing current hair growth

MISCELLANEOUS

ASSOCIATED CONDITIONS
- Acne
- Infertility
- Obesity
- Hyperinsulinemia

AGE-RELATED FACTORS
Pediatric: N/A
Geriatric: Can occur after menopause if peripheral conversion of estrogen is poor
Others: N/A

PREGNANCY
- May have related infertility
- If pregnancy occurs, must discontinue known contraindicated drugs
- Pregnancy outcome is related to underlying cause of hirsutism

SYNONYMS N/A

ICD-9-CM 704.1 Hirsutism

SEE ALSO
- Fertility problems
- Acne vulgaris
- Obesity
- Polycystic ovarian disease
- Hyperprolactinemia
- Hypothyroidism, adult

OTHER NOTES N/A

ABBREVIATIONS
LFTs = liver function tests

REFERENCES
- Speroff L, Glass R, Kase N: Clinical Gynecologic Endocrinology and Infertility. 5th Ed. Williams & Wilkins, Baltimore, 1994
- Franks S: Polycystic ovarian disease. NEJM 1995;333(13):853-868
Illustrations: 1 available on CD-ROM
Internet references: http://www.5mcc.com

Author(s)
Laura L. Novak, MD

Histoplasmosis

BASICS

DESCRIPTION Fungal infection with Histoplasma capsulatum, a dimorphic soil-dwelling saprophyte that has multiple clinical manifestations. Initial infection in the normal host is often asymptomatic. Other manifestations include a self-limited flu-like syndrome, mediastinal fibrosis, scar tissue residual, chronic cavitary disease in those with obstructive lung disease and disseminated histoplasmosis which is more frequent in the immunocompromised host and infants.
• H. capsulatum has worldwide distribution; the most endemic region in North America is the central U.S. The fungus exists in mycelial form in nature and in yeast phase when exposed to mammalian temperatures. Spores may remain active for up to ten years. Exposure to bird or bat excrement promotes growth of the fungus for unexplained reasons.
• Chronic pulmonary histoplasmosis - usually occurs in white males with obstructive lung disease and apical bullous lung pathology. These patients exhibit evidence of an indolent infectious process.
• Disseminated histoplasmosis infection in the immunocompromised is a rare opportunistic infection which may mimic sepsis syndrome and progress to multiple organ system failure
System(s) affected: Pulmonary, Gastrointestinal, Skin/Exocrine, Hemic/Lymphatic/Immunologic
Genetics: None known
Incidence/Prevalence in USA:
• Infection in endemic areas is virtually 100%; few patients develop active disease; approximately 500,000 new infections in the U.S./yr
• Occurrence in AIDS patients is 2%-5%
• Disseminated histoplasmosis occurs in < 0.05% of infections, one-third of these are infants < 1 year old, in adults there is an increased prevalence with age > 60 years
Predominant age:
• None in acute histoplasmosis
• Infants < 1 year old are at higher risk for disseminated histoplasmosis
Predominant sex:
• Acute histoplasmosis - Male = Female
• Disseminated histoplasmosis - Male > Female (5-10:1)

SIGNS AND SYMPTOMS
• Primary infection in the normal host is usually asymptomatic
• 1% immunocompetent individuals with low-level exposure develop symptoms
• 99% subclinical infection
• Arthralgia-erythema nodosum-erythema multiforme is associated with acute infection
• Low grade fever, anorexia, weight loss, night sweats, and productive cough are associated with chronic infections

CAUSES Dimorphic fungus Histoplasma capsulatum

RISK FACTORS
• Spelunking
• Cleaning chicken coops
• Excavation near bird roosts
• Demolition or remodeling of old buildings
• Exposure to decayed wood or dead trees
• Performing routine activities in areas with high accumulation of bird droppings
• Immunosuppression

DIAGNOSIS

DIFFERENTIAL DIAGNOSIS
• Atypical pneumonia and viral pneumonitis
• Other fungal diseases such as blastomycosis, coccidioidomycosis
• Other granulomatous diseases such as M. tuberculosis and sarcoidosis
• Pneumoconiosis
• Lymphoma
• Malignancies associated with hilar lymphadenopathy

LABORATORY
• For disseminated histoplasmosis in AIDS patients, urinary and blood histoplasmosis
• Polysaccharide antigen detection is a rapid test for diagnosis and for monitoring relapse
• Complement fixation may be negative approximately 30% in acute histoplasmosis and 50% in disseminated histoplasmosis
• Immunodiffusion test may be negative in approximately 50% of patients with acute histoplasmosis. Maximum positivity of test occurs 4-6 weeks after exposure.
• Complement fixation antibodies at titers 1:8 or 1:16 are presumptive for diagnosis, > 1:32 is strongly supportive as is an acute 4-fold titer rise. Determining the presence of H and M bands may be helpful.
• For chronic histoplasmosis and disseminated disease, cultures of sputum, bronchoalveolar lavage, bone marrow, lymph nodes, blood, liver and cerebrospinal fluid may be positive. Demonstration of characteristic organisms by silver stain on biopsy and bronchoalveolar lavage and bronchial washing specimens is diagnostic.
Drugs that may alter lab results: N/A
Disorders that may alter lab results:
• Serologic tests may be falsely negative early in infection or in the immunocompromised
• False positive results may occur with tuberculosis and other fungal diseases
• Slow clearance of antibodies may identify patients with past Histoplasmosis infection who now present with a different disease
• False positive complement fixation titers may occur after histoplasmin skin antigen testing
• False positive H. capsulatum polysaccharide antigen test may occur with patients with disseminated blastomycosis and coccidiomycosis

PATHOLOGICAL FINDINGS Poorly formed caseating granulomas on biopsy or bronchoscopy specimens with identification of characteristic yeast forms by methenamine silver stain

SPECIAL TESTS
• Determine the presence of urinary H. capsulatum antigen
• Bronchoscopy
• Liver and bone marrow biopsies

IMAGING
• Routine chest roentgenogram may reveal focal mid-lung field infiltrates (27%), hilar or mediastinal adenopathy (25%) or both (30%). May see miliary or diffuse pattern with disseminated disease following large antigen load.
• If indicated, CAT scan of chest to differentiate mediastinal fibrosis from mediastinal granuloma

DIAGNOSTIC PROCEDURES
• Serologic blood work
• Bronchoscopy with bronchoalveolar lavage and transbronchial biopsy
• Liver and bone marrow biopsies for suspected disseminated disease
• Mediastinoscopy for lymph node biopsy

TREATMENT

APPROPRIATE HEALTH CARE
• Usually outpatient
• Disseminated histoplasmosis requires hospitalization for initial treatment

GENERAL MEASURES 99% of acute primary histoplasmosis resolve spontaneously; symptomatic treatment only

SURGICAL MEASURES N/A

ACTIVITY Avoid high risk exposures

DIET No restrictions

PATIENT EDUCATION Extended treatment needs in chronic cavitary histoplasmosis; maintenance therapy in AIDS

MEDICATIONS

DRUG(S) OF CHOICE
• Disseminated histoplasmosis
  ◊ Amphotericin B - test dose is 1 mg followed by 0.25 mg/kg/dose, which may be slowly increased to 0.5 mg/kg/dose. Cumulative dose to 1-2 gm (at least 35 mg/kg is indicated)
  ◊ Ketoconazole or itraconazole for mild disease
    - Ketoconazole: Induction therapy with 400 mg/day for 3 days, then maintenance therapy 200 mg or 400 mg a day
    - Itraconazole: Induction therapy with 200 mg twice a day for 3 days, then 200 mg once or twice daily

- AIDS patients
  ◊ Itraconazole for mild disease: Induction therapy with 600 mg/day for 3 days, then 400 mg/day. Drug of choice for primary and maintenance therapy is itraconazole. Ketoconazole is not effective in AIDS-related histoplasmosis. Maintenance therapy with itraconazole 400 mg/day or amphotericin-B 50-100 mg weekly (1 mg/kg).
- Chronic cavitary histoplasmosis
  ◊ Amphotericin-B for severe or moderately severe disease, 2.0-2.5 g cumulative
  ◊ Ketoconazole or itraconazole for mild disease
    - Ketoconazole: Induction therapy with 400 mg/day for 3 days, then maintenance therapy 200 mg or 400 mg/day
    - Itraconazole: Induction therapy with 200 mg twice daily for 3 days, then 200 mg once or twice daily
- Acute pulmonary histoplasmosis
  ◊ Amphotericin B for severe or moderately severe disease; test dose is 1 mg followed by 0.25 mg/kg/dose which may be slowly increased to 0.5 mg/kg/dose. Cumulative dose at least 35 mg/kg.
  ◊ Ketoconazole or itraconazole for mild disease
    - Ketoconazole: Induction therapy with 400 mg/day for 3 days, then maintenance therapy 200 mg or 400 mg/day
    - Itraconazole: Induction therapy with 200 mg twice daily for 3 days, then 200 mg once or twice daily
- Duration of treatment
  ◊ Optimal duration of treatment with antifungals has not been established
  ◊ Disseminated histoplasmosis - 6 months course
  ◊ Chronic cavitary histoplasmosis - at least 12 months course with stable chest roentgenogram findings over 3-6 months
  ◊ Acute pulmonary histoplasmosis - 2-3 month course
  ◊ AIDS-related or relapsed - chronic, lifelong, maintenance therapy
- Mediastinal granuloma
  ◊ Can mimic fibrosing mediastinitis, may respond to treatment with amphotericin B
- Fibrosing mediastinitis
  ◊ Has no active infection present and is not treatable

Contraindications: No contraindications to treatment in patients with progressive cavitary disease or disseminated histoplasmosis. The latter has a mortality rate of 80% if untreated.

Precautions:
- Amphotericin B
  ◊ Dosage probably does not need to be adjusted for creatinine clearance
  ◊ It is nephrotoxic. Renal function must be monitored closely. Monitor electrolytes, especially potassium and magnesium.
  ◊ Rigors can be prevented by pre-infusion meperidine. Fever and chills can be diminished by pre-infusion dose of acetaminophen plus diphenhydramine.
- Ketoconazole
  ◊ Is associated with gastrointestinal upset
  ◊ May inhibit testosterone synthesis and should be used with caution in patients with underlying hepatic dysfunction

Significant possible interactions:
- Expected benefits outweigh possible risks.
- Ketoconazole
  ◊ Requires an acid environment for dissolution. If the patient requires antacid or H2 blockade, administer at least 2 hours after dose of ketoconazole
  ◊ Co-administration of terfenadine may cause cardiac arrhythmias
  ◊ May increase cyclosporine levels
  ◊ May decrease Rifampin and INH levels as well as ketoconazole levels
  ◊ May increase phenytoin levels
- Itraconazole
  ◊ Rifampin levels may decrease itraconazole to undetectable levels
  ◊ May increase digoxin levels
  ◊ Questionable effect on cyclosporine levels
- Fluconazole
  ◊ May increase cyclosporine levels
  ◊ May increase warfarin effect
  ◊ Questionable effect of Rifampin on fluconazole

ALTERNATIVE DRUGS Fluconazole has not been approved for histoplasmosis therapy. Fluconazole is undergoing investigational studies in its use for chronic pulmonary and disseminated histoplasmosis. Preliminarily, fluconazole doses of 400 mg/day or higher may be necessary for therapeutic outcome.

FOLLOWUP

PATIENT MONITORING Renal function and liver chemistries every 1-2 months for chronic therapy patients; chestx-ray to evaluate therapy response at regular intervals

PREVENTION/AVOIDANCE Maintenance therapy is required in AIDS

POSSIBLE COMPLICATIONS
- Bronchial, tracheal or esophageal obstruction secondary to adenopathy, broncholithiasis
- Pulmonary, splenic and hepatic calcifications, rarely pericarditis, pleurisy or effusion
- CNS histoplasmosis (rare): Chronic meningitis or intracranial histoplasmosis
- Endocarditis involving aortic or mitral valves
- Pericardial effusions (sterile exudates) not thought to be secondary to hematogenous spread
- Fibrosing mediastinitis can cause stenosis of vascular and bronchial structures within the mediastinum causing pulmonary hypertension, superior vena cava syndrome and bronchial obstruction
- Acute renal failure and hepatic dysfunction secondary to medications
- Amphotericin induced hypokalemia
- Relapse occurring in the immunocompromised or inadequately treated patient with disseminated histoplasmosis

EXPECTED COURSE/PROGNOSIS
- Primary histoplasmosis - 99% resolve spontaneously

- The prognosis for chronic cavitary pulmonary histoplasmosis is determined by the loss of lung parenchyma and pulmonary function
- Treatment of disseminated disease in AIDS/non-AIDS cases does improve outcome with ketoconazole having > 80% success rate and amphotericin B being 60-100% successful. Despite maintenance therapy, AIDS patients, have 10-50% relapse rate.

MISCELLANEOUS

ASSOCIATED CONDITIONS
- Disseminated histoplasmosis is an opportunistic infection in the immunocompromised host
- HIV infection

AGE-RELATED FACTORS
Pediatric: 1/3 of cases of disseminated histoplasmosis occur in infants < 1 year old
Geriatric: Increased incidence of disseminated histoplasmosis in males during 6th and 7th decades
Others: N/A

PREGNANCY No increased incidence

SYNONYMS N/A

ICD-9-CM 115.9 Histoplasmosis, unspecified

SEE ALSO N/A

OTHER NOTES N/A

ABBREVIATIONS N/A

REFERENCES
- Dismukes WE, Cloud G, Bowles C, et al: Treatment of blastomycosis and histoplasmosis with ketoconazole. Ann Intern Med 1985;103:861-872
- Como JA, Dismukes WE: Oral azole drugs as systemic antifungal therapy. N Engl J Med 1994;330:263-272
- Wheat JL, Connolly-Stringfield P, Kohler RB, et al: Histoplasma capsulatum polysaccharide antigen detection in diagnosis and management of disseminated histoplasmosis in patients with acquired immunodeficiency syndrome. Am J Med 1989;87:396-400
- Wheat JL, Connolly-Stringfield PA, Baker RL, et al: Histoplasmosis in the acquired immune deficiency syndrome: clinical findings diagnosis and treatment, and review of the literature. In Medicine 1990;69:361-374
- Wheat J: Histoplasmosis: recognition and treatment. Clin Infect Dis. (suppl) 1994;1:S19-27
Illustrations: 1 available on CD-ROM
Internet references: http://www.5mcc.com

Author(s)
Robert P. Baughman, MD

HIV infection & AIDS

BASICS

DESCRIPTION A chronic infection with variable course (requiring about 10 years from the time of infection for 50% of persons to develop AIDS). HIV infects cells with CD4 receptors, most notably the CD4 lymphocytes (also called T4 or T helper cells). Infection causes cell death and a decline in immune function resulting in opportunistic infections, malignancies, and neurologic problems. These opportunistic conditions define the acquired immunodeficiency syndrome (AIDS). As of 1/1/93 all HIV infected persons with < 200 CD4 cells are categorized as AIDS. HIV appears to have direct effects on the central nervous system, the GI tract and other systems.

System(s) affected:
Hemic/Lymphatic/Immunologic, Nervous, Pulmonary, Gastrointestinal
Genetics: Unclear
Incidence/Prevalence in the USA: >
500,000 AIDS cases; > 300,000 deaths
Predominant age: Young adults - 25-44
Predominant sex: Male > Female

SIGNS AND SYMPTOMS
• Acute infection: Mononucleosis-like syndrome with fever, rash, myalgia, and malaise a self-limited syndrome occurring about 6-8 weeks postinfection, associated with the development of HIV antibody
• Asymptomatic infection: Follows initial infection; variable duration
• Persistent generalized lymphadenopathy: Characteristics - lymph node enlargement 1 cm or greater in two or more extra-inguinal sites. Adenopathy persists longer than 3 months.
• Other diseases:
◊ Constitutional: Fever lasting more than one month, involuntary weight loss of more than ten percent baseline weight, persistent diarrhea, skin rash, severe chronic fatigue
◊ Neurologic disease: Dementia, myelopathy or peripheral neuropathy not explained by other illness
◊ Secondary infectious disease:
- AIDS-defining opportunistic infections: Pneumocystis carinii pneumonia; chronic cryptosporidial diarrhea; cerebral toxoplasmosis; extra -intestinal Strongyloides; isosporiasis; esophageal, bronchial/pulmonary candidiasis; cryptococcosis; histoplasmosis; coccidioidomycosis; disseminated mycobacterial disease; cytomegalovirus disease; chronic mucocutaneous or disseminated herpes simplex; progressive multifocal leukoencephalopathy.
- Other specified infections: Oral hairy leukoplakia, dermatomal zoster, nocardioses, tuberculosis (pulmonary), recurrent salmonella bacteremia, oral candidiasis.
◊ Secondary cancers: Kaposi's sarcoma, non-Hodgkin's lymphoma, and primary brain lymphoma, invasive cervical cancer.
• Other conditions not classified above that may be attributed to HIV infection: idiopathic thrombocytopenic purpura, seborrheic dermatitis, chronic lymphoid interstitial pneumonitis, alopecia, and renal disease.
• 1993 revised classification: For HIV infection and expanded surveillance case definition for AIDS among adolescents and adults (from MMWR)
• Categories:

A	B	C
Asymptomatic or persistent general lympho-denopathy	Symptomatic; not category A or C conditions	AIDS indicator conditions

(includes acute [primary] infection)
• CD4 cell categories:

1	2	3
≥ 500/µg	200-499/µg	< 200/µg
A1, B1, C1†	A2, B2, C2†	A3†, B3†, C3†

(† = expanded AIDS surveillance case definition)
• Conditions: Included in the AIDS surveillance case definition
◊ Candidiasis of bronchi, trachea, or lungs
◊ Candidiasis, esophageal
◊ Cervical cancer, invasive
◊ Coccidioidomycosis, disseminated or extrapulmonary
◊ Cryptococcosis, extrapulmonary
◊ Cryptosporidiosis, chronic intestinal (> 1 month duration)
◊ Cytomegalovirus disease (other than liver, spleen or nodes)
◊ HIV encephalopathy
◊ Herpes simplex: chronic ulcer(s) (> than 1 month duration) or bronchitis pneumonitis, or esophagitis
◊ Histoplasmosis, disseminated or extrapulmonary
◊ Isosporiasis, chronic intestinal (> 1 month duration)
◊ Kaposi's sarcoma
◊ Lymphoma, Burkitt's (or equivalent term)
◊ Lymphoma, immunoblastic (or equivalent term)
◊ Lymphoma, primary in brain
◊ Mycobacterium avium complex or M. kansasii, disseminated or extrapulmonary
◊ Mycobacterium tuberculosis, any site (pulmonary or extrapulmonary)
◊ Mycobacterium, other species or unidentified species, disseminated or extrapulmonary
◊ Pneumocystis carinii pneumonia
◊ Progressive multifocal leukoencephalopathy
◊ Salmonella septicemia, recurrent
◊ Toxoplasmosis of brain
◊ Wasting syndrome resulting from HIV infection

CAUSES
• Human immunodeficiency virus (HIV); a retrovirus

RISK FACTORS
• Sexual activity
• Injection drug use
• Recipients of blood products: Highest risk 1975 to 3/1985
• Hemophiliacs who received pooled plasma
• Children of HIV-infected women:
◊ 30% of the these children during pregnancy will be infected without treatment
◊ Breast feeding is a possible route of transmission
◊ Prenatal, intrapartum and postpartum zidovudine significantly decreases the risk of HIV transmission from mother to child (from 29% to 8%)
• Needle stick (estimate 1 in 250 for hollow needles)
◊ Postexposure treatment with zidovudine, lamivudine, and indinavir for significant exposures (MMWR 1996)

DIAGNOSIS

DIFFERENTIAL DIAGNOSIS Screen for HIV infection when there is prolonged illness without ready explanation.

LABORATORY
• ELISA
◊ Sensitivity and specificity > 98%
◊ Reported as reactive or non-reactive. Reactive tests should be repeated. Confirm repeatedly reactive tests by another test (most commonly the Western Blot).
• Western blot
◊ Test results are positive, negative, or indeterminate (indeterminate tests result from non-specific reactions of HIV-negative sera with some HIV proteins)
◊ The CDC recommends reaction with two of the following three bands as criteria for positivity: P24; gp41, and gp 120/160. If the test is indeterminate, repeat test in 3-6 months.
Drugs that may alter lab results: N/A
Disorders that may alter lab results: N/A

SPECIAL TESTS As indicated by suspicion of opportunistic infection or HIV-associated condition.

IMAGING N/A

DIAGNOSTIC PROCEDURES N/A

TREATMENT

APPROPRIATE HEALTH CARE
Outpatient setting. Consultation with infectious disease or HIV specialist prior to onset of acute situations.

GENERAL MEASURES
• The initial visit:
◊ Past medical history including STD's and TB with dates and treatment
◊ Review of systems to include fever, chills, diarrhea, weight loss, fatigue, adenopathy, oral sores, cough, shortness of breath, dyspnea on exertion, visual changes, headaches, skin rash, neurologic changes, sinusitis, odynophagia
◊ Social history
◊ Physical examination, with PAP smear

◊ Immunization review (pneumococcal, influenza, and Td recommended in adults. OPV contraindicated in children [use IPV]).

◊ Studies: CBC with differential and platelets; SMAC; RPR; CD4 absolute count and %lymphocytes CD4; hepatitis B sAg and sAb; chest x-ray; PPD with control; HIV-1 RNA viral quantitation (viral load); toxoplasmosis IgG, CMV IgG, Pap smears in females
• Patients with CD4<500 or CD4 >500 and viral burden >10,000-30,000 copies/mL will benefit from antiretroviral treatment. Combination antiretroviral therapy has contributed to a 13% decline in AIDS deaths in the 1st half of 1996 as compared with 1995.
• Patients with CD4<200 or with oral candidiasis or other signs of significant immune suppression should receive Pneumocystis carinii prophylaxis
• Patients with CD4<100 and toxoplasmosis IgG should receive toxoplasmosis prophylaxis.
• Patients with CD4<75 should receive prophylaxis against Mycobacterium avium complex (MAC)

SURGICAL MEASURES N/A

ACTIVITY Encourage regular exercise.

DIET
• Encourage good nutrition
• Avoid raw eggs, unpasteurized milk and other potentially contaminated foods
• May require vitamin supplementation

PATIENT EDUCATION
• Provide frank, complete, non-judgmental information on the routes of transmission (primarily sexual and needle sharing). Teach HIV infected how to minimize risk to others.
• Pre-printed and additional information material is available from a wide variety of sources including: National AIDS Hotline - (800)342-2437 [Spanish (800)342-7432]
• National Institute of Health AIDS Clinical Trials Group (800)874-2572. Information on AIDS/HIV clinical trials.
• American Foundation for AIDS Research: (212)719-0033; new treatments and research

MEDICATIONS

DRUG(S) OF CHOICE
• Nucleoside reverse transcriptase inhibitors:
  ◊ Didanosine (ddI, Videx)
  ◊ Lamivudine (3TC, Epivir)
  ◊ Stavudine (d4T, Zerit)
  ◊ Zalcitabine (ddC, Hivid)
  ◊ Zidovudine (AZT, Retrovir)
• Protease inhibitors:
  ◊ Indinavir (Crixivan)
  ◊ Nelfinavir (Viracept)
  ◊ Ritonavir (Norvir)
  ◊ Saquinavir (Invirase)
• Non-nucleoside reverse transcriptase inhibitors:
  ◊ Nevirapine (Viramune)
  ◊ Delaviridine (Rescriptor)

• Current standard of care requires the use of 3 drugs to attempt to prevent the emergence of resistance. Goal of therapy is to reduce viral load (ideally to < 400) copies/mL and delay immunodeterioration.
Contraindications: Significant drug interactions
Precautions: Antiretroviral drugs have significant toxicities; refer to specific drug information
Significant possible interactions: Antiretroviral drugs, especially the protease inhibitors have potentially life-threatening interactions; refer to specific drug information

ALTERNATIVE DRUGS N/A

FOLLOWUP

PATIENT MONITORING
• Frequency determined largely by the patient's clinical and psychological status and by the need to monitor drug toxicity and immune function
• Recheck CD4 counts and viral load at least every 3 months depending on stage of illness and medical regimen
• Check at subsequent visits:
  ◊ Complete, careful physical exam
  ◊ Complete review of systems especially focused on neurologic symptoms (CNS infection, malignancy, or dementia), visual changes (CMV retinitis), diarrhea, fever, night sweats, shortness of breath, dyspnea on exertion (early P. carinii pneumonia), and odynophagia (esophageal candidiasis)

PREVENTION/AVOIDANCE When possible: avoid unscreened blood products; avoid unprotected sexual intercourse; use condoms; avoid injection drug abuse; avoid contact with fluids of HIV infected

POSSIBLE COMPLICATIONS
• Immunodeficiency
• Opportunistic infections
• Neuropsychiatric symptoms
• HIV-associated malignancies

EXPECTED COURSE/PROGNOSIS
When HIV infection leads to AIDS, life expectancy is two to three years. AIDS defining opportunistic infections usually do not develop until CD4<200. In HIV infection, CD4 counts decline at a rate of 50-80/year with more rapid decline as counts drop below 200. The newer retroviral regimens may delay or reverse immune dysfunction

MISCELLANEOUS

ASSOCIATED CONDITIONS
• Syphilis: May be more aggressive in HIV-infected persons. Definitive treatment for syphilis in HIV infected persons is

controversial; consult with an STD specialist.
• Tuberculosis is co-epidemic with HIV. HIV infection changes the management of TB; should test all persons with TB for HIV, or if not tested, should treat with multiple drugs as if HIV-infected.

AGE-RELATED FACTORS
Pediatric: Progresses more rapidly in infants
Geriatric: Progresses more rapidly in age >50
Others: N/A

PREGNANCY Consistent standards of care not yet evolved. There appears to be an increased risk of bacterial pneumonia during pregnancy and some increased risk of premature birth in HIV-infected women. Zidovudine has been shown to decrease the risk of HIV transmission to infants. Many are using combination antiretroviral therapy during pregnancy.

SYNONYMS
• Acquired immune deficiency syndrome

ICD-9-CM
042 Human immunodeficiency virus infection with specified conditions
043 Human immunodeficiency virus causing other specified conditions
044 Other HIV infection

OTHER NOTES Increased risk of cervical cancer in HIV-infected women. Perform pap smears at least every 6 months.

SEE ALSO
• Pneumonia, Pneumocystis carinii (PCP)
• Kaposi's sarcoma
• Candidiasis
• Candidiasis, mucocutaneous
• Cytomegalovirus inclusion disease
• Tuberculosis
• Cryptococcosis
• Idiopathic thrombocytopenic purpura (ITP)

ABBREVIATIONS N/A

REFERENCES
• Cohen P, Sande M, Volberding P: The AIDS Knowledge Base. Waltham, MA, The Medical Publishing Group, 1996
• Abrams D, Grieco M, McMeeking A: AIDS/HIV Treatment Directory. New York, American Foundation for AIDS Research (quarterly)
• Sande M, Volberding P: The Medical Management of AIDS. 4th Ed. Philadelphia, W.B. Saunders Co., 1996
• MMWR Vol45#22, June 7, 1996:468-471
Illustrations: 39 available on CD-ROM
Internet references: http://www.5mcc.com

Author(s)
Kevin Carmichael, MD

Hodgkin's disease

BASICS

DESCRIPTION Malignant disease of the lymphoid tissue, caused by malignant transformation of an uncertain progenitor cell to the pathognomonic Reed-Sternberg cell. Disease spreads to the contiguous lymphoid tissue, and eventually to non-lymphoid tissue.
• The Rye classification is based on pathologic findings:
  ◊ Nodular sclerosis - most common
  ◊ Mixed cellularity - 2nd most common
  ◊ Lymphocyte depletion
  ◊ Lymphocyte predominance

Incidence/Prevalence in USA:
3.5/100,000. Incidence: 7,900/year in 1993. Overall incidence is lower in economically underdeveloped countries.

System(s) affected:
Hemic/Lymphatic/Immunologic

Genetics:
• First degree relatives - 3 times risk
• Siblings of younger patients - 7 times risk

Predominant age: Bimodal, with peaks at ages 20 and 70

Predominant sex: Male > Female

SIGNS AND SYMPTOMS
• Enlarged lymph nodes (painless)
• Fever (Pel-Ebstein fever)
• Night sweats
• Weight loss > 10%
• Fatigue
• Anorexia

CAUSES Unknown

RISK FACTORS
• Immunodeficiency (acquired and inherited)
• Autoimmune diseases
• HIV infection

DIAGNOSIS

DIFFERENTIAL DIAGNOSIS
• Other lymphomas
• Infectious lymphadenopathy
• Other solid tumor metastases
• Sarcoidosis
• Autoimmune diseases
• AIDS/HIV infection
• Drug reaction

LABORATORY
• CBC with differential
• Chemistry profile
• ESR
• Liver function tests
• Renal function tests

Drugs that may alter lab results:
Phenytoin may produce pseudolymphoma

Disorders that may alter lab results: N/A

PATHOLOGICAL FINDINGS
• Reed-Sternberg cell (RS cell) - bilobed or multi-lobed with prominent inclusion nucleoli
• Diffuse infiltrate of lymphocytes with obliteration of lymph nodes
• Large round reticular cells

SPECIAL TESTS N/A

IMAGING
• Chest x-ray
• CT of chest, abdomen, and pelvis
• Role of MRI still evolving
• Lymphangiogram
• Gallium scan, bone scan (used infrequently)
• Abdomen ultrasound

DIAGNOSTIC PROCEDURES
• Lymph node biopsy - needle aspiration not sufficient
• Exploratory laparotomy with splenectomy in individual cases
• Bone marrow biopsy - especially if stage B
• Liver biopsy in individual cases

TREATMENT

APPROPRIATE HEALTH CARE
• Inpatient or outpatient for staging
• Initial staging is critical to therapy
  ◊ Stage I - single node group
  ◊ Stage II - two or more node groups on same side of diaphragm
  ◊ Stage III - node groups on both sides of diaphragm
  ◊ Stage IV - dissemination involving extra-lymphatic organs (not the spleen which is considered lymphoid tissue)
  ◊ Subclassified "A" - asymptomatic disease in any stage
  ◊ Subclassified "B" - symptomatic disease in any stage with: 10% weight loss, night sweats, or fever not otherwise explained
  ◊ Subclassified "X" - bulky disease (widening of mediastinum by more than one-third or > 10 cm nodal mass)

GENERAL MEASURES
• Treatment is aimed for cure with minimum toxicity
• Treatment can be radiation alone, chemotherapy alone, or combination therapy based on staging and tumor burden
• Stages I and II - typically radiation therapy alone, unless bulky disease
• Stage III A - mainly with radiation therapy
• Stages III B and IV - chemotherapy, and also radiation if bulky disease
• Autologous bone marrow transplant for patients who fail chemotherapy

SURGICAL MEASURES N/A

ACTIVITY As tolerated

DIET No restrictions

PATIENT EDUCATION
• Discuss gonadal side effects of therapy, and consider sperm banking for males
• Risks of secondary malignancy
• For patient education materials on this topic, contact: Leukemia Society of America, 733 3rd Avenue, New York, NY 10017, (212)573-8484

MEDICATIONS

DRUG(S) OF CHOICE
• Note: Must be monitored by experienced oncologist
• MOPP chemotherapy - 4 week cycles
  ◊ Mechlorethamine (nitrogen mustard, Mustargen) 6.0 mg/m2 IV on days 1 and 8
  ◊ Vincristine (Oncovin) 1.4 mg/m2 IV on days 1 and 8
  ◊ Procarbazine 100 mg/m2 po on days 1 through 14 (avoid vanilla, cheese and wine when taking procarbazine)
  ◊ Prednisone 40 mg/m2 po on days 1 through 14. Use in cycles 1 and 4.
• ABVD chemotherapy - 4 week cycles
  ◊ Doxorubicin (Adriamycin) 25 mg/m2 IV days 1 and 15
  ◊ Bleomycin 10 mg/m2 IV days 1 and 15
  ◊ Vinblastine 6.0 mg/m2 IV days 1 and 15
  ◊ Dacarbazine 375 mg/m2 IV days 1 and 15
• Note: Recently people have advocated alternating cycles with MOPP/ABVD to minimize toxicity. Repeat cycles at least 6 times if blood counts permit.
Contraindications: As in general for chemotherapy
Precautions: Chemotherapy toxicity, bone marrow suppression
Significant possible interactions: Refer to manufacturer's literature

ALTERNATIVE DRUGS N/A

FOLLOWUP

PATIENT MONITORING CBC, hydration status

PREVENTION/AVOIDANCE
Pneumococcal vaccine (Pneumovax), if splenectomy is planned for staging

POSSIBLE COMPLICATIONS
• After chemotherapy and radiation therapy, may develop secondary malignancies
• Sterility, and gonadal dysfunction
• Hypothyroidism - particularly with radiation therapy error
• Bone marrow suppression
• Immunosuppressed infections
• Anemia
• Idiopathic thrombocytopenic purpura and thrombotic thrombocytopenic purpura
• Coronary artery disease
• Pulmonary fibrosis

EXPECTED COURSE/PROGNOSIS
• 75% overall survival
• Stage I - 90% 5 year
• Stage II - 90% 5 year
• Stage III - 75% 10 year
• Stage IV - 66% 10 year
• Symptomatic (class B) - prognosis worse
• Asymptomatic (class A) - prognosis better

MISCELLANEOUS

ASSOCIATED CONDITIONS T-cell infections

AGE-RELATED FACTORS
Pediatric: Increased risk for males
Geriatric: Usually presents in a more advanced stage
Others:
• Increased incidence of nodular-sclerosis pathologic classification in younger groups
• In HIV - usually presents more advanced

PREGNANCY
• Following treatment, if fertility is maintained, pregnancy can be normal
• Pregnancy is not known to have a negative impact on the course of Hodgkin's disease
• Hodgkin's is not known to adversely affect the pregnancy or fetus IF treatment can be postponed until delivery
• The risk of disease progression if treatment is delayed during pregnancy is variable. Management must be individualized.

SYNONYMS Malignant lymphoma

ICD-9-CM
201.9x Hodgkin's disease, unspecified
201.7x Hodgkin's disease, lymphocyte depletion
201.6x Hodgkin's disease, mixed cellularity
201.5x Hodgkin's disease, nodular sclerosis
201.4x Hodgkin's disease, lymphocyte predominance
Fifth digit:
0 - Unspecified site
1 - Head, face, neck nodes
2 - Intra-thoracic nodes
3 - Intra-abdominal nodes
4 - Axillary and arm nodes
5 - Inguinal and leg nodes
6 - Pelvic nodes
7 - Spleen involved
8 - Multiple site nodes

SEE ALSO
• Lymphoma, non-Hodgkin's

OTHER NOTES N/A

ABBREVIATIONS N/A

REFERENCES
• Urba WJ, Longo DL: Hodgkin's disease. N Engl J Med 1992;326(10):678-87
• Weinshel EL, Peterson BA: Review in CA - A cancer Journal for Clinicians 1993;43:327-346
Illustrations: N/A
Internet references: http://www.5mcc.com

Author(s)
Raghu Ram, MD

Hordeolum (stye)

 BASICS

DESCRIPTION
The common term "stye" refers to any inflammation or infection of the eyelid margin involving the hair follicles of the eyelashes (external hordeolum), meibomian glands (internal hordeolum), or granulomatous infection of the meibomian glands (chalazion)
System(s) affected: Skin/Exocrine
Genetics: No known genetic pattern
Incidence/Prevalence in USA: Extremely common
Predominant age: None
Predominant sex: Male = Female

SIGNS AND SYMPTOMS
• Redness of the margin of the eyelid with scaling, collection of discharge
• Localized inflammation of the eyelashes
• Patients may experience itching or scaling of the eyelids, chronic redness, eye irritation leading to localized tenderness and pain

CAUSES
• The most common causes of eyelid infections are staphylococcal, although other organisms may also be involved
• Seborrhea can predispose to infections of the eyelid

RISK FACTORS
• Predisposing blepharitis (low grade infections of the eyelid margin)
• Poor eyelid hygiene
• Contact lens wearers
• Application of make-up

 DIAGNOSIS

DIFFERENTIAL DIAGNOSIS
• Blepharitis
• Eyelid neoplasms

LABORATORY
Culture of the eyelid margins is usually not necessary
Drugs that may alter lab results: None
Disorders that may alter lab results: None

PATHOLOGICAL FINDINGS
Bacterial contamination and white cells in eyelid discharge

SPECIAL TESTS
None

IMAGING
None

DIAGNOSTIC PROCEDURES
History and eye examination

 TREATMENT

APPROPRIATE HEALTH CARE
Outpatient

GENERAL MEASURES
• Warm compresses to the area of inflammation can help increase blood supply and potentiate spontaneous drainage
• Good personal hygiene with attention to cleansing the eyelids on a daily basis to prevent recurrent infections
• Application of an antibiotic ointment (such as erythromycin) to the margin of the eyelid after proper cleansing. (Except children under 12, where there is a risk of blurred vision and amblyopia.) Helps reduce bacterial proliferation.

SURGICAL MEASURES
If the infection becomes localized to a single gland, incision, drainage, and curettage is sometimes necessary. This is an in-office procedure with a local anesthetic.

ACTIVITY
No restrictions

DIET
No special diet

PATIENT EDUCATION
• The patient should be instructed in proper cleansing of the eyelids using a solution of tap water and baby shampoo or a commercially prepared hypoallergenic cleanser
• The stye should not be squeezed

MEDICATIONS

DRUG(S) OF CHOICE
• Erythromycin ophthalmic ointment
• Occasionally use of an aminoglycoside ophthalmic ointment such as gentamicin may be necessary if refractory to simpler treatment
Contraindications: None
Precautions: None
Significant possible interactions: None

ALTERNATIVE DRUGS None

 FOLLOWUP

PATIENT MONITORING The patient should be seen within several weeks to assess the effectiveness of therapy

PREVENTION/AVOIDANCE Eyelid hygiene

POSSIBLE COMPLICATIONS None expected. An internal hordeolum, if untreated, may lead to generalized cellulitis of the lid.

EXPECTED COURSE/PROGNOSIS
Responds well to treatment, but tends to recur in some patients

 MISCELLANEOUS

ASSOCIATED CONDITIONS
• Acne
• Seborrhea

AGE-RELATED FACTORS
Pediatric: N/A
Geriatric: N/A
Others: N/A

PREGNANCY N/A

SYNONYMS
• Internal hordeolum
• External hordeolum
• Chalazion hordeolum
• Zeisian sty
• Meibomian sty

ICD-9-CM
373.1 Hordeolum
373.2 Chalazion
373.0 Blepharitis

SEE ALSO N/A

OTHER NOTES N/A

ABBREVIATIONS N/A

REFERENCES None
Illustrations: N/A
Internet references: http://www.5mcc.com

Author(s)
Robert M. Kershner, MD, FACS

Horner's syndrome

 BASICS

DESCRIPTION Horner's syndrome is caused by interruptions of the sympathetic nerve supply to the eye and results in miosis, ptosis, and absence of sweating of the ipsilateral face and neck
• Peripheral lesion - distal to superior cervical ganglion
• Central lesion - proximal to superior cervical ganglion
Genetics: Some autosomal dominant familial incidence
System(s) affected: Nervous, Skin/Exocrine
Incidence/Prevalence in USA: Unknown
Predominant age: May occur at any age
Predominant sex: Male = Female

SIGNS AND SYMPTOMS
• Ptosis (drooping of the eyelid)
• Miosis (narrowing of the pupil of the eye)
• Anhidrosis
• Enophthalmos is sometimes found
• Iris (in congenital Horner's) reduced - pigmentation, blue-gray, mottled of the affected eye
• Loss of ciliospinal reflex

CAUSES
• Interruption of the sympathetic nerve fibres that originate in the hypothalamus and travel down to the lateral part of the brain stem to exit in the thoracic area. These fibers synapse in the cervical sympathetic ganglia and the postganglionic fibers travel to the eye along the wall of the carotid and ophthalmic arteries.
• Idiopathic

RISK FACTORS
• Apical bronchogenic carcinoma
• Aneurysm of the carotid or subclavian artery
• Injuries to the carotid artery high in the neck
• Congenital Horner's syndrome
• Dissection of the carotid arteries
• Cluster headaches, approximately 20% of which have an accompanying ipsilateral Horner's syndrome. The syndrome may outlast the headaches.
• Carotid artery occlusion, approximately 15% of patients with carotid artery occlusion develop ipsilateral Horner's syndrome - may occur without evidence of cerebral ischemia, neck injuries or operative procedures
• Syringomyelia
• Inflammatory process

 DIAGNOSIS

DIFFERENTIAL DIAGNOSIS Neurological diseases

LABORATORY N/A
Drugs that may alter lab results: N/A
Disorders that may alter lab results: N/A

PATHOLOGICAL FINDINGS
• Brainstem lesion
• Massive hemisphere lesion
• Cervical cord lesion
• Root lesion
• Sympathetic chain lesion

SPECIAL TESTS
• Instillation of 4% solution of cocaine into conjunctival sac produces dilatation of the pupil in Horner's syndrome caused by a central sympathetic pathways lesion. (Response is absent in peripheral sympathetic lesion.)
• Instillation of 1:1000 solution of epinephrine into conjunctival sac produces dilatation of the pupil in Horner's syndrome caused by a peripheral sympathetic lesion

IMAGING CT/MRI of the brain, chest, spinal cord

DIAGNOSTIC PROCEDURES Spinal tap - occasionally indicated in addition to above.

 TREATMENT

APPROPRIATE HEALTH CARE Inpatient or outpatient, depending upon cause

GENERAL MEASURES
• Search for tumor or other compressive lesion is indicated for any patient who develops Horner's syndrome
• Horner's syndrome in itself does not produce any disability or require treatment
• Treatment is management of the underlying condition

SURGICAL MEASURES N/A

ACTIVITY Disease dependent

DIET Disease dependent

PATIENT EDUCATION N/A

MEDICATIONS

DRUG(S) OF CHOICE Therapy appropriate for the underlying disease
Contraindications: N/A
Precautions: N/A
Significant possible interactions: N/A

ALTERNATIVE DRUGS N/A

FOLLOWUP

PATIENT MONITORING Disease dependent

PREVENTION/AVOIDANCE None known

EXPECTED COURSE/PROGNOSIS Variable with cause

POSSIBLE COMPLICATIONS Chronic pupillary constriction

MISCELLANEOUS

ASSOCIATED CONDITIONS
• Wallenberg's syndrome
• Pancoast's tumor
• C8 radiculopathy

AGE-RELATED FACTORS
Pediatric: N/A
Geriatric: N/A
Others: N/A

PREGNANCY N/A

SYNONYMS
• Bernard-Horner syndrome
• Bernard's syndrome
• Cervical sympathetic syndrome
• Oculosympathetic syndrome

ICD-9-CM 337.9 Horner's syndrome

SEE ALSO N/A

OTHER NOTES N/A

ABBREVIATIONS N/A

REFERENCES Pryce-Phillips W, Murray TJ: Essential Neurology. New York, Scientific American Medicine, 1991
Illustrations: N/A
Internet references: http://www.5mcc.com

Author(s)
Stan G. Smith, MA, MB, FCFPC

Huntington's disease

BASICS

DESCRIPTION An inherited disease characterized by dementia and chorea that has a gradual onset and slow progression. Symptoms usually don't develop until after 30 years of age. By the time of diagnosis the patient has usually reproduced and passed the disease to another generation.
System(s) affected: Nervous
Genetics: Autosomal dominant; genetic marker on chromosome 4
Incidence/Prevalence in USA: 4-8 cases/100,000 people in the U.S.
Predominant age: Young adult (16-40); middle age (40-75)
Predominant sex: Male = Female

SIGNS AND SYMPTOMS
• Chorea
• Dysphagia
• Dysarthria
• Impaired recent memory
• Impaired judgment
• Intellectual decline
• Emotional disturbances
• Depression
• Anxiety
• Delusions
• Aggressiveness
• Urinary incontinence
• Bowel incontinence
• Weight loss
• Hypotonia
• Gait disturbance
• Postural instability
• Hyperkinesia
• Abnormal eye movements
• Facial twitching
• Emotional lability
• Apathy
• Withdrawal
• Dementia
• Bradykinesia
• Rigidity
• Hypertonia
• Clonus
• Mania
• Hallucinations
• Delusions
• Paranoia
• Schizophrenia
• Impulsiveness
• Hostility
• Agitation
• Primitive reflexes

CAUSES Hereditary genetic mutation on short arm of chromosome number 4, specifically, an expanded run of cytosine-adenine-guanine (CAG) repeats

RISK FACTORS Family history is a definite risk factor. Although a small percent of patients with DNA-proven Huntington's disease will have a negative family history.

DIAGNOSIS

DIFFERENTIAL DIAGNOSIS
• Movement disorder - hereditary
  ◊ Huntington disease
  ◊ Hereditary nonprogressive chorea
  ◊ Neurocanthocytosis
  ◊ Wilson's disease
  ◊ Ataxia-telangiectasia
  ◊ Lesch-Nyhan syndrome
  ◊ Hallervorde-Spatz disease
  ◊ Fahr's disease
• Movement disorder - secondary
  ◊ Infections/immunologic
    - Sydenham chorea
    - Encephalitis
    - Systemic lupus erythematosus
    - Tertiary syphilis
  ◊ Drug induced
    - Levodopa
    - Anticonvulsants
    - Anticholinergics
    - Cimetidine
    - Isoniazid
  ◊ Metabolic and endocrine
    - Chorea gravidarum
    - Hyperthyroidism
    - Birth control pills
    - Hyperglycemic nonketoic encephalopathy
  ◊ Vascular
    - Hemichorea/hemiballism with subthalamic nucleus lesion
    - Periarteritis nodosa
• Movement disorder - unknown etiology
  ◊ Senile chorea
  ◊ Essential chorea
  ◊ Parkinson's disease
• Dementia
  ◊ Alzheimer's disease
  ◊ Creutzfeldt-Jacob
  ◊ Pick disease
• Emotional and perceptual disorders
  ◊ Bipolar disorder
  ◊ Schizophrenia
• Abnormal behavior
  ◊ Alcoholism
  ◊ Anti-social personality disorder

LABORATORY
• Decreased endogenous gamma-aminobutyric acid (GABA)
• Decreased glutamic acid decarboxylase
• Decreased choline-acetyltransferase
Drugs that may alter lab results: N/A
Disorders that may alter lab results: N/A

PATHOLOGICAL FINDINGS
• Gross - cerebral atrophy
• Gross - atrophic caudate nucleus
• Gross - atrophic putamen
• Gross - ventricular enlargement
• Gross - atrophic globus pallidus
• Gross - atrophic frontal lobes
• Gross - atrophic parietal lobes
• Gross - cortical atrophy
• Micro - loss of small neurons of striatum with fibrillary gliosis
• Micro - loss of small neurons with fibrillary gliosis in ventrolateral thalamic nucleus
• Micro - loss of small neurons with fibrillary gliosis in substantia nigra
• Electron microscopy - membranous whorls
• Electron microscopy - increased numbers of dense synaptic vesicles in presynaptic nerve terminals

SPECIAL TESTS Presymptomatic detection of the disease via genetic linkage analysis is possible; but widespread testing awaits the resolution of social and ethical considerations

IMAGING
• CT or MRI - cerebral atrophy and atrophy of caudate nucleus
• Positron emission tomography (PET) - reduced glucose utilization
• Head CT - enlarged lateral ventricle

DIAGNOSTIC PROCEDURES N/A

TREATMENT

APPROPRIATE HEALTH CARE
Outpatient

GENERAL MEASURES
• Genetic counseling
• Symptomatic treatment (dopamine receptor blocking drugs), such as phenothiazines or haloperidol
• Consider electroconvulsive therapy (ECT) for drug-resistant depression
• Speech and occupational therapy

SURGICAL MEASURES N/A

ACTIVITY Full activity as long as possible

DIET No special diet, but soft diet with liquid supplements may be needed.

PATIENT EDUCATION
• Counseling for offspring
• Newsletter and printed information available from: Huntington's Disease Society of America, 140 W. 22nd St, 6th Flr, New York, NY 10011-2420, phone (212)242-1968; fax (212)243-2443

Huntington's disease

MEDICATIONS

DRUG(S) OF CHOICE For dyskinesia and/or behavioral problems: Haloperidol (Haldol) 1 mg bid and increased every 3 or 4 days until satisfactory response. Suggested daily maximum 10 mg.
Contraindications: Refer to manufacturer's literature
Precautions: Extrapyramidal reactions, tardive dyskinesia may occur. Can be treated with anticholinergic medication.
Significant possible interactions: Do not administer with meperidine due to possibility of serotonin syndrome.

ALTERNATIVE DRUGS
• Presynaptic dopamine-depleting agents
• Reserpine
• Tetrabenazine
• Postsynaptic dopamine antagonists
• Tricyclic antidepressants
• Antipsychotics

FOLLOWUP

PATIENT MONITORING Periodically for behavioral changes

PREVENTION/AVOIDANCE Genetic counseling

POSSIBLE COMPLICATIONS
• Choking
• Subdural hematoma
• Chorea
• Personality changes
• Dementia
• Death
• Suicide

EXPECTED COURSE/PROGNOSIS Poor, progressive impairment, fatal outcome within 20 years

MISCELLANEOUS

ASSOCIATED CONDITIONS N/A

AGE-RELATED FACTORS
Pediatric: Usually does not occur until after puberty
Geriatric: Usually fatal before geriatric age group; but onset is after age 50 in 20%
Others: About 20% of relatives at 1-in-2 risk of inheriting Huntington's disease from an affected parent now accept the offer of presymptomatic testing

PREGNANCY N/A

SYNONYMS
• Chronic progressive hereditary chorea
• Huntington's chorea

ICD-9-CM 333.4 Huntington's disease

SEE ALSO Wilson's disease

OTHER NOTES N/A

ABBREVIATIONS N/A

REFERENCES
• Adams RD, Victor M: Principles of Neurology. 5th Ed. New York, McGraw-Hill, Inc., 1993
• Mendez MF: Huntington's disease: Update and review of neuropsychiatric aspects. Int J Psychiatry Med 1994;24:189-208
• Ranen NG, et al: ECT as a treatment for depression in Huntington's disease. J Neuropsychiatry Clin Neurosci 1994;6:154-159
• Bundey S: Few psychological consequences of presymptomatic testing for Hunntington's disease. Lancet 1997;349:4
Illustrations: N/A
Internet references: http://www.5mcc.com

Author(s)
Richard Viken, MD

Hydrocele

BASICS

DESCRIPTION
Hydrocele is a collection of fluid within the scrotum.
• Communicating hydrocele: Associated with a patent processus vaginalis, has associated indirect inguinal hernia
• Non-communicating hydrocele: Infantile type - no communication, frequent spontaneous resolution. Adult type - no communication, infrequent resolution.
• Hydrocele of the cord: Distal portion of processus vaginalis has closed, mid-portion patent and fluid filled, proximal portion may be open or closed
• Acute hydrocele: Acute fluid collection resulting from an acute process within the tunica vaginalis

System(s) affected: Reproductive
Genetics: Unknown
Incidence/Prevalence in USA: Estimated to be 1% of adult males; prevalence 1000/100,000
Predominant age: Childhood
Predominant sex: Male only

SIGNS AND SYMPTOMS
• Swelling in scrotum or inguinal canal
• Demonstrated fluctuation in size (communicating hydrocele)
• Usually not painful
• Sensation of heaviness in scrotum
• Pain radiating to back (occasionally)
• Fluid collection in scrotum that transilluminates

CAUSES
• Closure of processus vaginalis trapping peritoneal fluid (non-communicating)
• Closure of distal processus, trapping fluid in mid portion of processus vaginalis (hydrocele of cord)
• Failure of closure of processus vaginalis (communicating hydrocele)
• Infection
• Tumors
• Trauma
• Ipsilateral renal transplantation

RISK FACTORS
• Ventriculoperitoneal shunt
• Exstrophy of the bladder
• Ehlers-Danlos syndrome
• Peritoneal dialysis

DIAGNOSIS

DIFFERENTIAL DIAGNOSIS
• Indirect inguinal hernia
• Orchitis
• Epididymitis
• Traumatic injury to testicle
• Torsion of testicle or torsion of appendix testes

LABORATORY N/A
Drugs that may alter lab results: N/A
Disorders that may alter lab results: N/A

PATHOLOGICAL FINDINGS Patent processus vaginalis in communicating hydroceles

SPECIAL TESTS N/A

IMAGING
• Abdominal x-ray - may be useful to distinguish incarcerated hernias from hydrocele (rarely needed)
• Inguino-scrotal ultrasound - should be able to demonstrate presence of bowel, e.g., distinguish incarcerated hernia in child from a hydrocele of the cord
• Testicular nuclear scan or doppler ultrasound - to distinguish testicular torsion

DIAGNOSTIC PROCEDURES N/A

TREATMENT

APPROPRIATE HEALTH CARE
• Outpatient surgery
• Observation in early infancy until definite communication demonstrated or until 1-2 years of age

GENERAL MEASURES N/A

SURGICAL MEASURES
• Inguinal approach with ligation of processus vaginalis and drainage of hydrocele sac in children. (In hydrocele of cord, sac can be completely removed.)
• Scrotal approach with drainage of hydrocele and resection of tunica vaginalis in adults
• In adults no therapy is needed unless hydrocele causes discomfort or unless there is a significant underlying cause such as tumor
• Jaboulay-Winkelmann procedure (for thick hydrocele sac) - hydrocele sac wrapped posteriorly around cord structures
• Lord procedure (for thin hydrocele sac) - radial sutures used to gather hydrocele sac posterior to testis and epididymis
• Aspiration of hydrocele should not be done (with possible exception of postoperative hydrocele)

ACTIVITY Full activity after surgery

DIET For age

PATIENT EDUCATION N/A

MEDICATIONS

DRUG(S) OF CHOICE N/A
Contraindications: N/A
Precautions: N/A
Significant possible interactions: N/A

ALTERNATIVE DRUGS N/A

FOLLOWUP

PATIENT MONITORING
• Follow at 3 month intervals until decision for/against surgery made
• Postoperative, follow up at 2-4 weeks and then at 2-3 month intervals until resolution of any postoperative (traumatic) hydrocele

PREVENTION/AVOIDANCE N/A

POSSIBLE COMPLICATIONS
• Postoperative traumatic hydrocele common. Usually resolves spontaneously.
• Injury to vas deferens or spermatic vessels
• Suture granuloma
• Hematoma
• Wound infection

EXPECTED COURSE/PROGNOSIS
Recovery should be rapid and complete

MISCELLANEOUS

ASSOCIATED CONDITIONS
• Ehlers-Danlos syndrome
• Exstrophy of bladder
• Indirect inguinal hernia
• Hydrocephalus with ventriculo-peritoneal shunt
• Peritoneal dialysis

AGE-RELATED FACTORS
Pediatric: In communicating hydrocele consider contralateral inguinal exploration
Geriatric: N/A
Others: N/A

PREGNANCY N/A

SYNONYMS N/A

ICD-9-CM 603.9

SEE ALSO N/A

OTHER NOTES N/A

ABBREVIATIONS N/A

REFERENCES
• Gillenwater JY, Grayhach JT, Howards SS, Duckett J: Adult & Pediatric Urology. 2nd Ed. Philadelphia, Marby Year Book, 1991
• Holder TM, Ashcraft KW: Pediatric Surgery. 2nd Ed. Philadelphia, W.B. Saunders Co., 1993
• Kelalis PP, King LR, Belman AB: Pediatric Urology. 3rd Ed. Philadelphia, W.B. Saunders Co., 1992
• Resnick MI, Kursh ED: Current Therapy in Genito-Urinary Surgery. 2nd Ed. St. Louis, Mosby-Year Book, 1992
Illustrations: N/A
Internet references: http://www.5mcc.com

Author(s)
Timothy L. Black, MD, FACS, FAAP
James P. Miller, MD, FACS, FAAP

Hydronephrosis

BASICS

DESCRIPTION
Unilateral or bilateral dilatation of the urinary tract at any level secondary to intrinsic and/or extrinsic obstruction to urine flow. May also be functional.
System(s) affected: Renal/Urologic
Genetics: Unknown
Incidence/Prevalence in USA:
• Children 2 in 100
• Adults 3.8 in 100
Predominant age: All ages. Bimodal peaks: congenital and over age 60.
Predominant sex:
• Age 0 - 20 years: Male = Female
• Age 20 to 60 years: Female > Male
• Age greater than 60 years: Male > Female

SIGNS AND SYMPTOMS
• Varies with acute or chronic presentation
• Chronic hydronephrosis may be completely asymptomatic
• "Colic" referred to vulva or to testicle (lithiasis) with acute obstruction
• Change in urine output (anuria, polyuria, intermittent variation in urine volume)
• Hesitancy
• Dribbling
• Urinary tract infections
• Decreased force of urine or interrupted stream
• Nocturia
• Abdominal mass
• Frequency and urgency
• Thirst
• Hypertension (may be accelerated)
• Edema
• After relief - post obstructive diuresis
• Abdominal mass
• Epididymitis
• Acute or chronic urinary retention
• Residual urine

CAUSES
• Intrinsic, congenital
  ◊ Stenosis (ureteral, urethral and meatal)
  ◊ Adynamic ureter
  ◊ Spinal cord defects, e.g., spina bifida
  ◊ Duplication of the ureter
  ◊ Ureterocele
• Intrinsic, acquired
  ◊ Renal lithiasis
  ◊ Neoplasm (renal, ureteral or bladder)
  ◊ Papillary necrosis with sloughed papilla
  ◊ Ureterocele
  ◊ Trauma
  ◊ Blood clot
  ◊ Fungus ball
  ◊ Granuloma (tuberculosis)
  ◊ Neurogenic bladder
  ◊ Other nervous system diseases - tabes dorsalis, multiple sclerosis, diabetes mellitus, traumatic spinal cord injury
  ◊ Anticholinergics
  ◊ Phimosis, Ureteral valve, Polyp or stricture
  ◊ Schistosomiasis (hematobium)
  ◊ Wegener's granulomatosis
  ◊ Psychogenic polydipsia
  ◊ Imperforate hymen

• Extrinsic
  ◊ Retroperitoneal-neoplasm, blood, abscess, fibrosis, aneurysm
    ◊ Crohn's disease
    ◊ Lymphocele, hydrocele
    ◊ Gynecologic - gravid uterus, endometriosis, pelvic inflammatory disease, abscess, cyst, iatrogenic-ureteral injury during surgery, gynecologic malignancy, uterine prolapse
    ◊ Sjögren's syndrome (pseudolymphoma)
• Functional or non-mechanical - congenital
  ◊ Mega-ureter
  ◊ Prune belly syndrome
  ◊ Extra renal pelvis
• Functional or non-mechanical - other
  ◊ Diabetes insipidus
  ◊ Diuretics
  ◊ Pregnancy
  ◊ Vesico-ureteral reflux
  ◊ Postobstructive residual
  ◊ Postsurgical: post ureteral anastomosis
  ◊ Progestational agents

RISK FACTORS
• Radiation
• Prostatic hypertrophy and/or malignancy
• Renal lithiasis
• Methysergide
• Analgesic abuse (papillary necrosis, transitional cell carcinoma)
• Sickle cell anemia (papillary necrosis)
• Diabetes mellitus (papillary necrosis)
• Bleeding diathesis
• Anticholinergics
• See Causes

DIAGNOSIS

DIFFERENTIAL DIAGNOSIS See Causes

LABORATORY
• May be completely normal
• Azotemia
• Hyperkalemia
• Metabolic acidosis (with and without anion gap)
• Hypernatremia (nephrogenic diabetes insipidus)
• Urine analysis - hematuria, crystals, bacteriuria
• Decreased urine concentrating ability
• Polycythemia (rare)
• Anemia of chronic renal disease
Drugs that may alter lab results:
Nephrotoxins may aggravate azotemia (nonsteroidal anti-inflammatory drugs, immunosuppressants, aminoglycosides, iodinated contrast, anticholinergics)
Disorders that may alter lab results: N/A

PATHOLOGICAL FINDINGS
• Thin renal cortex
• Renal tubular atrophy
• Medullary destruction

SPECIAL TESTS
• Kidney and urinary bladder (KUB)
• Voiding cystourethrogram
• Measurement post void residual
• Ultrasound prostate with rectal transducer and biopsy if nodule found
• Prostatic specific antigen, acid phosphatase (malignancy)
• Prenatal sonography
• Rectal examination in males age > 50

IMAGING
• Ultrasound - abnormal renal function, cortical thinning, ureteral dilatation
• IVP with tomograms (normal renal function): Renal pelvis dilatation
• Renal flow scan, diuretic renogram
• CT scan; MRI
• Pulsed and color Doppler
• Diuretic enhanced duplex Doppler sonography

DIAGNOSTIC PROCEDURES
• To determine location and etiology:
  ◊ Cystoscopy/retrograde pyelography
  ◊ Antegrade pyelography
  ◊ Loopography (obstruction with ureteral diversion)

TREATMENT

APPROPRIATE HEALTH CARE
Outpatient

GENERAL MEASURES
• Females: Pelvic pap smear for potential gynecologic malignancy. Appropriate work-up for recurrent urinary tract infections.
• Males: Anatomic study of the urinary tract for any urinary tract infection, appropriate review of systems and digital rectal exam for prostatic hypertrophy. Prostatic specific antigen, acid phosphatase, rectal transducer ultrasound of prostate for prostatic enlargement.
• Relief of obstruction for preservation of renal function
  ◊ Foley catheter for prostatic hypertrophy
  ◊ Transurethral resection of the prostate gland for prostatic hypertrophy
  ◊ Nephrostomy tube
  ◊ Pyeloplasty
  ◊ Surgical diversion of ureters
  ◊ Ureteral stents
  ◊ Percutaneous nephrolithotomy (lithiasis)
  ◊ Basket capture (lithiasis)
  ◊ Lithotripsy (lithiasis with or without stent and percutaneous nephrolithotomy)
  ◊ Nephrectomy
• Neurogenic hydronephrosis
  ◊ Frequent voiding
  ◊ Double voiding
  ◊ Suprapubic pressure
  ◊ Intermittent catheterization
  ◊ Cholinergics
  ◊ Surgical reimplantation of ureters
  ◊ Antibiotics, when needed for infection

- Uremia
  - ◊ Dialysis
  - ◊ Hyperkalemia (calcium, Kayexalate, insulin and glucose)
  - ◊ Treat acidosis (1-2 teaspoons sodium bicarbonate tid or Shohl's solution)
  - ◊ Treat hypocalcemia (calcium acetate tablets 1-3 with meals; vitamin D - dihydrotachysterol 0.2 mg po every day)

SURGICAL MEASURES N/A

ACTIVITY Fully active

DIET
- If not uremic, no restriction
- When uremic - protein, salt, potassium restriction as needed
- For stone-formers, increased oral fluids

PATIENT EDUCATION
Printed material available from National Kidney Foundation, 30 East 33rd St., Ste. 1100, New York, New York, 10016 (800)622-9010. "What Everyone Should Know About Kidneys and Kidney Disease" (Order #01-01 BP English, #01-02 BP Spanish)

MEDICATIONS

DRUG(S) OF CHOICE
- Lithiasis - treatment is stone-specific:
  - ◊ Hypercalciuric calcium oxalate - hydrochlorothiazide 25-50 mg po every day to decrease urine calcium excretion
  - ◊ Uric acid nephrolithiasis - acutely alkalinize urine to pH ≥ 6.5 with sodium bicarbonate, chronic allopurinol 100-300 mg po every day

Contraindications: Allergy to drug
Precautions: N/A
Significant possible interactions: N/A

ALTERNATIVE DRUGS N/A

FOLLOWUP

PATIENT MONITORING
- Imaging procedure of choice depending on etiology of hydronephrosis (IVP, renal scan, cystoretrogrades, ultrasound)
- Metabolic studies for nephrolithiasis
- Appropriate cancer screening if applicable

PREVENTION/AVOIDANCE
- Avoid anticholinergics when obstruction present
- Avoid dehydration with lithiasis

POSSIBLE COMPLICATIONS
- Urinary tract infection from instrumentation
- Fibrosis from radiation for pelvic malignancy
- Obstruction from stone fragments on lithotripsy
- Postoperative bleeding

EXPECTED COURSE/PROGNOSIS
- Contingent on relief of obstruction and residual renal function
- Excellent course and prognosis with relief of obstruction and restoration of normal renal function
- Nonmechanical ureteropelvic junction (UPJ) obstruction has a good prognosis
- Reflux with pyelonephritis worsens prognosis significantly

MISCELLANEOUS

ASSOCIATED CONDITIONS See causes

AGE-RELATED FACTORS
Pediatric: Hydronephrosis most often congenital
Geriatric: In males, most often due to prostatic enlargement
Others: N/A

PREGNANCY Frequent temporary cause of hydronephrosis

SYNONYMS
- Urinary tract obstruction
- Obstructive uropathy
- Obstructive nephropathy
- Postrenal insufficiency
- Caliectasis
- Pyelectasis
- Ureterectasis

ICD-9-CM
753.2 congenital
 591 other

SEE ALSO
- Renal failure, acute (ARF)
- Renal failure, chronic
- Prostatic hyperplasia, benign (BPH)

OTHER NOTES N/A

ABBREVIATIONS N/A

REFERENCES
- Koga BA: Disorders of the ureter & ureteropelvic junction. In: Tanagho EA, McAnich JE, eds. Smith's General Urology. 14th Ed. Los Altos, CA, Lange Medical Publications, 1995
- King LR: Hydronephrosis: When is obstruction not obstruction? Urol Clin North Am 1995;22:31-42
- Peters CA: Urinary Tract Obstruction in Children. J Urol 1995;154:1874-1883
- Middleton RG: Prostate cancer: are we screening and treating too much? Ann Inter Med 1997;126:465-467
- Bomalaski MD: Vesicoureteral reflux and ureteropelvic junction obstruction: association, treatment options and outcome. J Urol 1997;157:969-974
- Gottlieb RH: Renal sonography: can it be used selectively in the setting of an elevated serum creatinine level? Am J Kid Dis 1997;29:362-367
Illustrations: N/A
Internet references: http://www.5mcc.com

Author(s)
Gregory W. Rutecki, MD

Hypercalcemia associated with malignancy

BASICS

DESCRIPTION The most common cause of hypercalcemia diagnosed in a hospital setting is malignancy, often heralding the patient's demise. Because of the extremely poor prognosis, it must be differentiated from other, more treatable, entities.
System(s) affected: Endocrine/Metabolic, Musculoskeletal, Nervous, Gastrointestinal
Genetics: N/A
IncidencePrevalence in USA: Occurs in 5-10% of cancer patients
Predominant age: N/A
Predominant sex: N/A

SIGNS AND SYMPTOMS
• Severity of symptoms depends on calcium level, rapidity of onset of hypercalcemia, state of hydration, and underlying malignancy
• Anorexia, nausea
• Polyuria, dehydration
• Lethargy, stupor, coma

CAUSES
• Solid tumors:
◊ 80% have increased levels of nephrogenous cyclic AMP, reflecting activity of ectopic parathormone-related peptide(s). True ectopic PTH production is exceedingly rare.
◊ Lung cancer (25% of cases usually squamous, less common are adenocarcinoma and large cell, rarely small cell)
◊ Squamous carcinoma of head, neck, esophagus, female genital tract (20% of cases)
◊ Renal cell carcinoma (8% of cases)
• Myeloma, lymphoma, breast cancer with osseous metastases, and others:
◊ Nephrogenous cyclic AMP is reduced, reflecting suppression of PTH by nonparathyroid hypercalcemia
◊ Factors implicated include interleukin-1, prostaglandins (E series), transforming growth factors alpha and beta, tumor necrosis factor, lymphotoxin, colony stimulating factor
◊ Direct resorption of bone by metastatic tumor (controversial)
◊ 1-alpha hydroxylase activity of some lymphomas, causing tumoral production of 1,25-dihydroxyvitamin D

RISK FACTORS
• Dehydration
• Immobilization

DIAGNOSIS

DIFFERENTIAL DIAGNOSIS
(not including benign familial hypercalcemia)
• Vitamins A and D
• Immobilization
• Thyrotoxicosis
• Addison's disease
• Milk alkali syndrome
• Inflammatory disorders
• Neoplastic-related disorders
• Sarcoidosis, TB, and other granulomatous diseases
• Thiazides, lithium; theophylline and aspirin toxicity
• Rhabdomyolysis
• AIDS
• Paget's disease, parenteral nutrition, parathyroid disease

LABORATORY
• Serum calcium: Total calcium level depends on binding proteins. Adjusted calcium can be estimated by:
Ca(adj) = Ca(tot) −0.8 x (albumin −4)
• Ionized calcium: Physiologically most important, affected by pH. May be measured directly if specimen is collected under anaerobic conditions and analyzed promptly.
• PTH assay: "Intact" molecule (especially two-site, noncompetitive) methods have greatest specificity, almost always suppressed, in malignancy. If elevated in a cancer patient, suspect concomitant hyperparathyroidism.
• PTH-related peptide: Assays now are clinically available; often elevated in hypercalcemia of malignancy (see above)
• 25-hydroxyvitamin D: May be elevated in vitamin D intoxication
• 1,25-dihydroxyvitamin D: Elevated in up to 50% of hypercalcemic patients with lymphoma
Drugs that may alter lab results: Lithium, thiazide diuretics, vitamin D preparations can all increase serum calcium
Disorders that may alter lab results: N/A

PATHOLOGICAL FINDINGS N/A

SPECIAL TESTS Staging techniques as necessary to determine extent of malignancy

IMAGING If there is laboratory evidence of primary hyperparathyroidism, imaging (such as ultrasound, CT, MRI, or nuclear parathyroid scans) may be required in patients with previous neck surgery, prior to re-exploration

DIAGNOSTIC PROCEDURES N/A

TREATMENT

APPROPRIATE HEALTH CARE Inpatient

GENERAL MEASURES
• Treatment of underlying malignancy
• Maintain hydration, encourage oral fluids; intravenous saline diuresis

SURGICAL MEASURES N/A

ACTIVITY Avoid bed rest or immobilization as much as possible

DIET No special diet

PATIENT EDUCATION N/A

MEDICATIONS

DRUG(S) OF CHOICE
• Loop diuretics - use only after adequate hydration
• Calcitonin: 4-8 IU/kg SC or IM every 8-12 hours. Intramuscular route preferred if patient is dehydrated. Nontoxic, acts in 12-24 hours, minor but uncomfortable side effects include nausea, flushing, cramps. "Escape" phenomenon may be antagonized by steroids.
• Plicamycin (mithramycin): 25 µg/kg IV over several hours. Very effective. Onset < 12 hours, peak effect 48-72 hours, duration 3-9 days. Toxicity - nausea, thrombocytopenia, hepatic and renal toxicity.
• Biphosphonates currently available: disodium etidronate. 7.5 mg/kg IV daily for 3-7 days. Efficacy similar to plicamycin but less toxic. Long-term use over several months may cause osteopenia and fractures. Pamidronate (Aredia) recently approved; 60-90 mg IV, single dose. Newer agents being developed and tested.
• Glucocorticoids: (40-60 mg/day prednisone or equivalent). Most effective in vitamin D intoxication, may be helpful in myeloma, lymphoma and other granulomatous disorders. Usually not effective in solid tumors.
• Oral phosphates: 1-2 gm/day neutral phosphates, 4 divided doses. Modest hypocalcemic effect, but significant GI distress.
• Intravenous phosphate - should be avoided because of calcium-phosphate precipitation in tissues, risk of severe hypotension
• Gallium nitrate: 100-200 mg/m2/day for 5-7 days. Dilute in 1000 mL 5% dextrose and infuse continuously over 24 hours.
Contraindications: Refer to manufacturer's literature
Precautions: Refer to manufacturer's literature
Significant possible interactions: Refer to manufacturer's literature

ALTERNATIVE DRUGS Listed above

FOLLOWUP

PATIENT MONITORING Frequent serum calcium and electrolyte determinations, expect relapse

PREVENTION/AVOIDANCE Encourage adequate hydration and activity, especially in multiple myeloma

POSSIBLE COMPLICATIONS N/A

EXPECTED COURSE/PROGNOSIS
Median survival after diagnosis of tumoral hypercalcemia depends on the type and extent of the malignancy, but usually indicates a poor prognosis

MISCELLANEOUS

ASSOCIATED CONDITIONS N/A

AGE-RELATED FACTORS N/A
Pediatric: N/A
Geriatric: N/A
Others: N/A

PREGNANCY N/A

SYNONYMS Tumoral hypercalcemia

ICD-9-CM
275.4 Disorders of calcium metabolism

SEE ALSO N/A

OTHER NOTES N/A

ABBREVIATIONS N/A

REFERENCES Marcus R, ed: Endocrinology and Metabolism Clinics of North America-Vol. 18, No. 3, September 1989:778-828
Illustrations: N/A
Internet references: http://www.5mcc.com

Author(s)
James H. Rudick, MD, FACP

Hypercholesterolemia

 BASICS

DESCRIPTION Serum cholesterol > 200 mg/dL (5.18 mmol/L). High risk 240 mg/dL (6.22 mmol/L) or more.
• High density lipoprotein fraction of cholesterol (HDL) - protective, low density lipoprotein (LDL) - atherogenic
System(s) affected: Endocrine/Metabolic, Gastrointestinal, Cardiovascular
Genetics: Heterozygous familial. Hypercholesterolemia, 1 in 500 cases. Autosomal dominant hypercholesterolemia 1 in 1 million.
Incidence/Prevalence in USA: 120 million people with cholesterol 200 mg/dL (5.18 mmol/L) or more, 60 million with 240 mg/dL (6.22 mmol/L) or more
Predominant age: Prevalence increases with age
Predominant sex: Male > Female

SIGNS AND SYMPTOMS
• Corneal arcus before 50
• Xanthomata
• Xanthelasma
• Arterial bruits
• Claudication
• Angina pectoris
• Stroke
• Myocardial infarction

CAUSES
• Primary
  ◊ Diet
  ◊ Heredity
  ◊ Obesity
  ◊ Sedentary life-style
  ◊ Stress
• Secondary
  ◊ Hypothyroidism
  ◊ Diabetes mellitus
  ◊ Nephrotic syndrome
  ◊ Obstructive liver disease
  ◊ Progestins
  ◊ Anabolic steroids
  ◊ Diuretics except indapamide (Lozol)
  ◊ Beta blockers except those with intrinsic sympathomimetic activity (ISA)
  ◊ Some immunosuppressants

RISK FACTORS
• Obesity
• Heredity

 DIAGNOSIS

DIFFERENTIAL DIAGNOSIS N/A

LABORATORY
• High density lipoprotein fraction of cholesterol (HDL), low density lipoprotein (LDL), triglycerides must be checked fasting
• Cholesterol is considered elevated if > than 200 mg/dL (5.18 mmol/L)
• T4 and TSH initially because hypothyroidism may cause hypercholesterolemia
Drugs that may alter lab results:
Caffeine may increase cholesterol
Disorders that may alter lab results:
• Hypothyroidism
• Nephrotic syndrome
• Obstructive liver disease

PATHOLOGICAL FINDINGS N/A

SPECIAL TESTS N/A

IMAGING N/A

DIAGNOSTIC PROCEDURES N/A

 TREATMENT

APPROPRIATE HEALTH CARE
Outpatient, except for complicating emergencies, e.g., myocardial infarction

GENERAL MEASURES
• Requires intervention: HDL less than 30 mg/dL (0.78 mmol/L), LDL greater than 160 mg/dL (4.14 mmol/L)
• Cholesterol 200-240 mg/dL (5.18-6.22 mmol/L) without coronary artery disease or two risk factors (male, smoking, HDL less than 35 mg/dL [0.91 mmol/L], severe obesity, diabetes, hypertension, strong family history) - prudent diet and recheck in one year
• Cholesterol 200-240 mg/dL (5.18-6.22 mmol/L) with coronary artery disease or two or more risk factors (as above) - lipoprotein analysis with further action based on HDL and LDL
• Cholesterol over 240 mg/dL (6.22 mmol/L) - lipoprotein analysis with further action based on HDL and LDL

SURGICAL MEASURES N/A

ACTIVITY Aerobic exercise at least 30 minutes, three times weekly. Important for increasing HDL, lowering total cholesterol, and losing weight.

DIET
• Reduce all dietary fats. Olive oil should be preferentially used.
• Increase fiber, increase intake of fruits, vegetables, whole grains, and garlic
• Emphasize, vegetarian, meatless, eggless, cheeseless meals, with poultry, fish, and nonfat milk or yogurt
• Minimal daily alcohol use may increase HDL
• Dietary adherence to low fat and cholesterol generally may be expected to result in a 10% LDL reduction

PATIENT EDUCATION American Heart Association publications

MEDICATIONS

DRUG(S) OF CHOICE
• Indications for initiating medications:
  ◊ No coronary heart disease (CHD) and fewer than 2 risk factors: if after 6 months of diet, exercise, LDL ≥ 190
  ◊ No CHD, but 2 or more risk factors: if after 6 months diet, exercise, LDL ≥ 160
  ◊ CHD: if after 6-12 weeks diet, exercise, LDL ≥ 130
• HMG-CoA reductase inhibitors (statins): Fluvastatin, lovastatin, pravastatin, simvastatin 5-80 mg per day, taken in single or divided doses with meals. Most suggest taking in evening. Effects: 25-45% LDL decrease (fluvastatin least, simvastatin greatest), decreases triglycerides. Atorvastatin (Lipitor)10-40 mg, recently released may be taken any time of day, may decrease LDL 60%, also raises HDL and lowers triglycerides.
• Cholestyramine (Questran) or colestipol (Colestid) bile acid binding resins. One to six packets per day taken qd, bid, or tid. Effect: 15-30% fall in LDL.
• Nicotinic acid: 500 mg to 3 gm taken one to three times daily with meals in timed release formulation to minimize side effects. Effect: 15-30% LDL lowering, decreases triglycerides. Hepatic dysfunction more common in patients who take sustained release niacin than in those who take immediate release form. Best to start with low doses and increase as tolerated.

Contraindications:
• Cholestyramine - complete biliary obstruction
• Nicotinic acid - hepatic dysfunction, acute peptic ulcer, diabetes mellitus.
• HMG-CoA reductase inhibitors - active liver disease, pregnancy

Precautions:
• HMG-CoA reductase inhibitors - liver function tests every three months during the first 15 months and periodically thereafter. Myositis with markedly elevated creatine kinase (CK) may occur. Cataract formation in excess has not been proven.
• Cholestyramine - gradually increase dose on weekly basis to minimize GI side effects (particularly constipation, flatulence)
• Colestipol or cholestyramine should be mixed with fruit juice or stirred into a pulpy fruit before administration. The powder should not be taken in its dry form since it may cause esophageal or GI blockage. Resins may increase triglycerides.
• Nicotinic acid - blood glucose and liver function tests must be monitored during early stages of therapy to insure no deleterious effect. Generalized flushing after dosage may be blocked by 325 aspirin 30 minutes before niacin.

Significant possible interactions:
• Cholestyramine - other drugs taken less than one hour before or within six hours after may be bound and not absorbed as well. Fat soluble vitamins A, D, E and K absorption may be impeded.
• Nicotinic acid and HMG-CoA reductase inhibitors - concomitant gemfibrozil, niacin, or immunosuppressives increase possibility of myositis (with water soluble pravastatin the least likely to cause this)

ALTERNATIVE DRUGS N/A

FOLLOWUP

PATIENT MONITORING
• While on medication, monitor cholesterol, HDL, LDL, triglycerides, liver enzymes (on statins, niacin) every 6 weeks until goal LDL reached, then every 6 months
• Cholesterol less than 200 - repeat in 5 years

PREVENTION/AVOIDANCE Prudent diet and weight control for all

POSSIBLE COMPLICATIONS Coronary heart disease, cerebrovascular disease, generalized arteriosclerosis

EXPECTED COURSE/PROGNOSIS
• 1% decrease in cholesterol results in 2% decreased risk of coronary heart disease
• Goals: LDL < 130, unless known coronary disease, then < 100.

MISCELLANEOUS

ASSOCIATED CONDITIONS
• Hypertension
• Obesity
• Diabetes mellitus
• Smoking
• Hypothyroidism

AGE-RELATED FACTORS
Pediatric:
• Screening every five years beginning as early as 12. (Childhood screening is controversial because no studies have shown a clear link between hypercholesterolemia in childhood to hypercholesterolemia in adulthood. Furthermore, the risks of reducing cholesterol in childhood are not known.)
• If total cholesterol greater than 170 mg/dL (4.40 mmol/L), check HDL and LDL levels. If LDL is 110-125 mg/dL (2.85-3.24 mmol/L) = moderate risk, if LDL is greater than 125 mg/dL (3.24 mmol/L) = high risk.
Geriatric: The benefit of cholesterol reduction in preventing coronary disease diminishes steadily beyond age 70
Others: N/A

PREGNANCY Fetal nutritional demands may alter diet and drug treatment

SYNONYMS N/A

ICD-9-CM
272.0 Pure hypercholesterolemia

SEE ALSO
• Hypothyroidism, adult

OTHER NOTES N/A

ABBREVIATIONS N/A

REFERENCES
• National Cholesterol Education Program. Arch Intern Med 1988;148:36-69
• Peters W: Drug Therapy to Lower Cholesterol. In Practical Cardiology 1988;38-47
• Havel RJ, Rapaport E: Management of primary hyperlipidemia. New Engl J Med 1995;332(22):1491-1498
• Shepherd J: Prevention of CHD with pravastatin in men with hypercholesterolemia, NEJM 1995;220:1302-1307
• Scandinavian simvastatin study group: Randomized trial of cholesterol lowering in 4,444 patients with CHD. Lancet 1994;344:1383-1389
Illustrations: 5 available on CD-ROM
Internet references: http://www.5mcc.com

Author(s)
John Z. Carter, MD

Hyperemesis gravidarum

BASICS

DESCRIPTION Persistent vomiting in a pregnant woman that interferes with fluid and electrolyte balance, as well as nutrition. Usually associated with the first 8 to 20 weeks of pregnancy. Believed to have biomedical and behavioral aspects. Associated with high estrogen levels. Symptoms usually begin about 2 weeks after first missed period.
System(s) affected: Gastrointestinal, Reproductive, Endocrine/Metabolic
Genetics: Unknown
Incidence/Prevalence in USA:
• 2% of pregnancies have electrolyte disturbances
• 50% of pregnancies have at least some gastrointestinal disturbance
Predominant age: 21-31
Predominant sex: Female only

SIGNS AND SYMPTOMS
• Hypersensitivity to smell
• Alteration in taste
• Nausea
• Vomiting with retching
• Acidosis
• Decreased urine output
• Volume depletion
• Fatigue
• Starvation

CAUSES
• Unknown
• May be psychological factors
• Hyperthyroidism
• Hyperparathyroidism
• Gestational hormones
• Liver dysfunction
• Autonomic nervous system dysfunction

RISK FACTORS
• Trophoblastic activity
• Gonadotropin production stimulated
• Altered gastrointestinal function
• Various odors
• Taste or sight of food
• Hyperthyroidism
• Hyperparathyroidism
• Obesity
• Multiple gestations
• Nulliparity
• Liver dysfunction

DIAGNOSIS

DIFFERENTIAL DIAGNOSIS
• Other common causes of vomiting must be considered:
  ◊ Gastroenteritis
  ◊ Gastritis
  ◊ Reflux esophagitis
  ◊ Peptic ulcer disease
  ◊ Cholelithiasis
  ◊ Cholecystitis
  ◊ Pyelonephritis
  ◊ Anxiety

LABORATORY
• Electrolytes decreased
• Urinalysis - glucosuria, albuminuria, granular casts and hematuria (rare)
• Increased uric acid
• Reduced protein
Drugs that may alter lab results: None likely
Disorders that may alter lab results: N/A

PATHOLOGICAL FINDINGS Fatty degeneration of the liver; renal tubular damage; heart damage; petechial brain hemorrhages

SPECIAL TESTS None indicated for the diagnosis of hyperemesis gravidarum

IMAGING No imaging is indicated for the diagnosis of hyperemesis gravidarum

DIAGNOSTIC PROCEDURES Only indicated if it is necessary to rule out other diagnoses

TREATMENT

APPROPRIATE HEALTH CARE
• Outpatient therapy
• In some severe cases, inpatient parenteral or enteral volume and nutrition repletion may be indicated

GENERAL MEASURES
• Patient reassurance
• Bedrest
• If dehydrated, IV fluids. Repeat if there is a recurrence of symptoms following initial improvement.

SURGICAL MEASURES N/A

ACTIVITY As tolerated after improvement

DIET
• Nothing by mouth for first 24 hours if patient is ill enough to require hospitalization
• For outpatient: A diet rich in carbohydrates and protein, such as fruit, cheese, cottage cheese, eggs, beef, poultry, vegetables, toast, crackers, rice. Limit intake of butter. Patients should avoid spicy meals and high fat foods.

PATIENT EDUCATION
• Attention should be given to psychosocial issues such as possible ambivalence about the pregnancy
• Patients should be instructed to take small amounts of fluid frequently to avoid volume depletion

MEDICATIONS

DRUG(S) OF CHOICE
• Pyridoxine 10-30 mg daily IV. Not always effective, but not harmful.
• Antihistamines (e.g., diphenhydramine [25-50 mg q4-6h] or dimenhydrinate, or doxylamine)
• Phenothiazines (e.g., promethazine or prochlorperazine)
• Meclizine 25 mg q6h
Contraindications: All medications taken during pregnancy should balance the risks and benefits both to the mother and the fetus
Precautions:
• Phenothiazines - associated with prolonged jaundice, extrapyramidal effects, hyper- or hyporeflexia in newborns
• Meclizine - associated with cleft palate in newborns
Significant possible interactions: Refer to manufacturer's profile of each drug

ALTERNATIVE DRUGS Avoid all drugs if possible

FOLLOWUP

PATIENT MONITORING
• Follow up on a daily basis for weight monitoring in severe cases
• Special attention should be given to monitoring for ketosis, hypokalemia, or acid-base disturbances due to hyperemesis

PREVENTION/AVOIDANCE Anticipatory guidance in first and second trimester regarding dietary habits in hopes of avoiding volume and nutritional depletion

POSSIBLE COMPLICATIONS
• Patients with greater than a 5% weight loss are associated with intrauterine growth retardation and fetal anomalies
• Hemorrhagic retinitis
• Liver damage
• CNS deterioration, sometimes to coma

EXPECTED COURSE/PROGNOSIS
• Self-limited illness with good prognosis if patient's weight is maintained at greater than 95% of the pre-pregnancy weight
• With complication of hemorrhagic retinitis, mortality rate is 50%

MISCELLANEOUS

ASSOCIATED CONDITIONS
Hyperthyroidism

AGE-RELATED FACTORS N/A
Pediatric: N/A
Geriatric: N/A
Others: N/A

PREGNANCY Problem is confined to early pregnancy

SYNONYMS Morning sickness

ICD-9-CM
• 643.0 for uncomplicated hyperemesis gravidarum less than 22 weeks
• 643.1 for severe hyperemesis gravidarum with metabolic disturbance

SEE ALSO N/A

OTHER NOTES N/A

ABBREVIATIONS N/A

REFERENCES
• Gross S, Librach C, Cecetti A: Maternal weight loss associated with hyperemesis gravidarum: A predictor of fetal outcome. Am. J. Obstet. Gynecol 1989;160:906-909
• Abell T, Riely C: Hyperemesis gravidarum. Gastrointestinal Clinics NA 1992;21(4):835-849
• Kousen M: Treatment of nausea and vomiting in pregnancy. Amer Fam Phys 1993;48(7):1279-1284
• Deuchair N: Vomiting in pregnancy: a review of the problem with particular regard to psychological and social aspects. Br J Obstet & Gynaecol 1995;102(1):6-8
• Naef RW, Chauhan SP, Roach H, Roberts WE, Trows KH, Morrison R: Treatment of hyperemesis gravidarum in the home: an alternative to hospitalization. J Perinatology 1995;15(4):289-292
Illustrations: N/A
Internet references: http://www.5mcc.com

Author(s)
Scott A. Fields, MD

Hyperkalemia

BASICS

DESCRIPTION
A common electrolyte disorder with plasma potassium concentration > 5.0 mEq/L (5.0 mmol/L). Four major causes:
• Increased load - either endogenous from tissue release or exogenous from a high intake which is usually in association with impaired excretion
• Decreased excretion - due to decreased glomerular filtration rate
• Cellular redistribution - shifting of intracellular (which is the major store of potassium) to extracellular space
• Factitious - related to improper collection or transport of blood sample

System(s) affected: Endocrine/Metabolic, Cardiovascular, Nervous
Genetics: N/A
Predominant age: N/A
Incidence/Prevalence in USA: Common
Predominant sex: Male = Female

SIGNS AND SYMPTOMS
• Cardiac - most important, dominating, and frequent symptoms
  ◊ Peaked T wave
  ◊ Flattened p wave
  ◊ Prolonged p-Q interval
  ◊ Widened QRS complex
  ◊ Sine wave
  ◊ Ventricular fibrillation
  ◊ Cardiac arrest
• Neuromuscular
  ◊ Numbness
  ◊ Weakness
  ◊ Flaccid paralysis

CAUSES
• Pseudohyperkalemia
  ◊ Hemolysis (most common)
  ◊ Thrombolysis
  ◊ Leukocytosis
  ◊ Infectious mononucleosis
  ◊ Familial
  ◊ Procedural technical error (ischemic blood draw due to tight, prolonged tourniquet application)
• Redistribution
  ◊ Acidosis
  ◊ Insulin deficiency
  ◊ Beta blockade due to beta blocking drugs
  ◊ Digitalis intoxication
  ◊ Succinylcholine
  ◊ Arginine hydrochloride/lysine hydrochloride
  ◊ Periodic paralysis
  ◊ Fluoride intoxication
  ◊ Exercise with heavy sweating
• Excessive endogenous potassium load
  ◊ Hemolysis
  ◊ Rhabdomyolysis
  ◊ Internal bleeding
• Excessive exogenous potassium load
  ◊ Parenteral administration
  ◊ Excess in diet
  ◊ Overdose of potassium supplements

• Diminished potassium excretion
  ◊ Decreased glomerular filtration rate (acute or far-advanced chronic renal failure)
  ◊ Decreased mineral corticoid activity
  ◊ Defect in tubular secretion (renal tubular acidosis II and IV)
  ◊ Drugs - nonsteroidal anti-inflammatory agents, cyclosporine, potassium sparing diuretics

RISK FACTORS
• Impaired urinary excretion
• Acidemia
• Massive cell breakdown
• Use of potassium sparing diuretics
• Excess potassium supplementation

DIAGNOSIS

DIFFERENTIAL DIAGNOSIS
• Cardiac arrhythmias
• Hypocalcemia

LABORATORY
Potassium greater than 5.0 mEq/L (5.0 mmol/L)
Drugs that may alter lab results: N/A
Disorders that may alter lab results:
• Acidemia - potassium shifts from intracellular to extracellular space in effort to buffer acid load. Once acidemia is corrected, the potassium may return to normal or even become decreased.
• Insulin deficiency

PATHOLOGICAL FINDINGS N/A

SPECIAL TESTS
• Cortisol and aldosterone levels to check for mineralocorticoid deficiency when other causes are ruled out
• ECG changes usually evolve as potassium rises above 6.0 mEq/L

IMAGING N/A

DIAGNOSTIC PROCEDURES N/A

TREATMENT

APPROPRIATE HEALTH CARE
Inpatient with cardiac monitoring if ECG changes are present or potassium is greater than 6.0 mEq/L (6.0 mmol/L)

GENERAL MEASURES
• Discontinue any K-sparing drugs or dietary K
• Major goal is to find the cause of hyperkalemia
• If hyperkalemia is severe, treat first, then do diagnostic investigations

SURGICAL MEASURES N/A

ACTIVITY Bedrest

DIET
80 mEq (80 mmol) or less of potassium per 24 hours

PATIENT EDUCATION Consult with dietician

Hyperkalemia

 MEDICATIONS

DRUG(S) OF CHOICE
• Dextrose (1 ampule of D50) and insulin, 10 units of regular subcutaneous). Temporary shift of potassium intracellularly taking effect in the first 30 minutes but only lasting a short time.
• Sodium bicarbonate, 50-100 mEq [50-100 mmol], in conjunction with the pH. Effects are temporary.
• Sodium polystyrene sulfonate (Kayexalate) 30-60 grams by mouth or by rectum. Effective in 1-4 hours and is a definitive treatment. May repeat q6h if necessary.
• Calcium gluconate, 1 ampule, is cardio-protective only and should only be used when ECG changes are present
• Hemodialysis when other measures are not effective
Contraindications: None
Precautions: Sodium bicarbonate and Kayexalate provide a sodium load that may exacerbate fluid overload in cardiac or renal failure patients
Significant possible interactions: See manufacturer's profile of each drug

ALTERNATIVE DRUGS N/A

 FOLLOWUP

PATIENT MONITORING Serial renal panels until correction complete

PREVENTION/AVOIDANCE Diet and oral supplement compliance

POSSIBLE COMPLICATIONS
• Life threatening cardiac arrhythmias
• Hypokalemia

EXPECTED COURSE/PROGNOSIS Full resolution with correction of the underlying etiology. Reduction of plasma potassium should begin within the first hour of initiation of treatment.

 MISCELLANEOUS

ASSOCIATED CONDITIONS
• Renal failure
• Mineralocorticoid deficiency

AGE-RELATED FACTORS
Pediatric: N/A
Geriatric: Increased risk for hyperkalemia in this age group due to decreases in renin and aldosterone
Others: N/A

PREGNANCY N/A

SYNONYMS N/A

ICD-9-CM 276.7 Hyperkalemia

SEE ALSO N/A

OTHER NOTES N/A

ABBREVIATIONS N/A

REFERENCES
• Isselbacher KJ, et al, eds: Harrison's Principles of Internal Medicine. 13th Ed. New York, McGraw-Hill, 1994
• Brenner BM, Rector FC Jr: The Kidney. 5th Ed. Philadelphia, W.B. Saunders Co., 1995
Illustrations: N/A
Internet references: http://www.5mcc.com

Author(s)
K. Shashi Kant, MD
Patricia Anderson, MD

Hypernatremia

BASICS

DESCRIPTION Water content of body fluid is deficient compared to sodium content (serum Na > 150 mEq/L [150 mmol/L])
• Significant hypernatremia (serum Na > 160 mEq/L [160 mmol/L]) - may not indicate total body sodium content
• Hypertonicity - increased solutes in extracellular fluid (ECF) which do not cross cell membranes, e.g., sodium, mannitol or glucose. Shifts water from intracellular fluid (ICF) to ECF.
• Hyperosmolality - increased solutes e.g., urea or alcohol, which freely cross all membranes or glucose which does not cross cell membranes. May be present without hypertonicity.
System(s) affected: Endocrine/Metabolic
Genetics: No known genetic pattern. Some diabetes insipidus (DI) may be hereditary.
Incidence/Prevalence in USA: Common in the elderly (e.g., 1% of hospitalized patients over age 65); also may occur with diarrhea in infants
Predominant age: N/A
Predominant sex: Male = Female

SIGNS AND SYMPTOMS
• Severity of symptoms usually correlate with the extent of hyperosmolality
• Primary neurological - thirst, restlessness, irritability, disorientation, delirium, coma, convulsions
• Dry mouth and mucous membranes
• Lack of tears and decreased salivation
• Flushed skin
• Fever
• Oligo/anuria
• Hyperventilation
• Hyperreflexia
• Brain hemorrhage
• Thirst is the primary protection against hypertonicity

CAUSES
• Sodium excess - total body sodium increased
   ◊ Oral - improperly mixed infant formula, salt given as "punishment" or as a prank, sea water ingestion
   ◊ IV - NaCl or NaHCO3 during cardiopulmonary resuscitation, intrauterine NaCl for abortion
• Water deficit - total body sodium normal
   ◊ Decreased intake: e.g., thirst, decreased access to water
   ◊ Increased urine water loss, e.g., diabetes insipidus
   ◊ Increased insensible water loss, e.g., fever, hyperventilation, hypermetabolic state
• Hypotonic fluid loss - total body sodium decreased
   ◊ Loss of fluid containing sodium - without adequate water replacement
• Urinary loss
   ◊ Osmotic diuretics
   ◊ Diabetes mellitus
   ◊ Diuresis from acute tubular necrosis (ATN) or from relief of acute urinary obstruction
• GI loss
   ◊ Diarrhea, especially in children
• Insensible loss
   ◊ Sweat
   ◊ Newborns under radiant warmers

RISK FACTORS
• Children
• Elderly
• Comatose patients

DIAGNOSIS

DIFFERENTIAL DIAGNOSIS
• Diabetes insipidus
• Hyperosmotic coma
• Salt ingestion
• Hypertonic dehydration

LABORATORY
• Serum Na > 150 to 170 mEq/L (> 150-170 mmol/L) - usually dehydration
• Serum Na > 170 mEq/L (> 170 mmol/L) - usually diabetes insipidus
• Serum Na > 190 mEq/L (> 190 mmol/L) - usually chronic salt ingestion
• Diabetes insipidus
   ◊ Urine osmolality less than serum osmolality
   ◊ Urine sodium usually low
   ◊ Polyuria
   ◊ Neurogenic vs. nephrogenic diabetes insipidus
• Hyperosmolar coma
   ◊ Blood sugar elevated
   ◊ Decreased urine output
   ◊ Increased urine osmolality
• Salt ingestion
   ◊ Increased urine Na
   ◊ Increased urine osmolality
• Hypertonic dehydration
   ◊ Decreased urine sodium
   ◊ Increased urine osmolality
Drugs that may alter lab results: A variety of medications may raise or lower sodium levels. Refer to a laboratory test reference.
Disorders that may alter lab results: N/A

PATHOLOGICAL FINDINGS N/A

SPECIAL TESTS
• Water deprivation (with diabetes insipidus urine osmolality does not increase when hypernatremic)
• Antidiuretic hormone (ADH) stimulation (with nephrogenic diabetes insipidus urine osmolality does not increase after ADH or DDAVP)

IMAGING CAT scan or MRI in diabetes insipidus - to rule out craniopharyngioma, tumor or median cleft syndrome

DIAGNOSTIC PROCEDURES History, physical, laboratory studies, family history for NDI

TREATMENT

APPROPRIATE HEALTH CARE Inpatient (many patients are already hospitalized and hypernatremia develops after admission)

GENERAL MEASURES
• Water replacement orally, if patient conscious
• Treat hypovolemia first, then treat hypernatremia
• Calculated water deficit (liters) = [(0.6 x wt) x (Na - 140)] ÷ 140
   Note: wt = weight in kilograms
   Na = current serum sodium
• Dialysis - especially with serum Na > 200 mEq/L (200 mmol/L)

SURGICAL MEASURES N/A

ACTIVITY Bedrest until stable or underlying condition resolved or controlled

DIET
• Assure proper nutrition during acute phase
• After resolution of acute phase, may want to consider sodium restricted diet for patient
• Severe salt restriction in nephrogenic diabetes insipidus

PATIENT EDUCATION Patients with nephrogenic diabetes insipidus must avoid salt and drink large amounts of water

MEDICATIONS

DRUG(S) OF CHOICE
• Hypovolemia
  ◊ Isotonic saline (normal saline or Ringer's lactate) 10-20 mL/kg IV over 1-2 hrs. May repeat if 10% or greater dehydration.
  ◊ Isotonic fluids: 5% dextrose with half-normal saline until urine output established
• Hypernatremia
  ◊ Hypotonic fluids (NaCl or dextrose 5% in water)
  ◊ Decrease serum sodium by 0.5 mEq/L/hour (0.5 mmol/L/hour) or by no more than 20 mEq/L/day (20 mmol/L/day). Allows idiogenic osmoles to resolve (mostly taurine in brain cell water).
  ◊ Hypocalcemia may occur during correction of hypernatremia. Add calcium (50 mg/kg 10% calcium gluconate) to IV fluids.
  ◊ Acidosis is often present in severely dehydrated patients. Add sodium bicarbonate, 50 mEq/L, to IV fluids. If both acidosis and hypocalcemia are present simultaneously, correct the calcium deficit first.
  ◊ Potassium and phosphate, if needed
• Neurogenic diabetes insipidus (DI)
  ◊ Desmopressin (DDAVP) acetate: adults 10-40 μg intranasally in 1-3 divided doses; children 5-30 μg in a single evening dose or in 2 divided doses. Oral DDAVP now available - dosage varies.
  ◊ May use 2.5 dextrose in water if giving large volumes of water in DI or NDI to avoid glycosuria
• Nephrogenic diabetes insipidus (NDI)
  ◊ Chlorothiazide: 10 mg/kg/dose given bid
  ◊ Chlorpropamide: 100-250 mg each morning
Contraindications: Refer to manufacturer's literature
Precautions:
• Rapid correction of hypernatremia can cause pulmonary edema. Hypocalcemia often occurs during correction.
• In diabetes insipidus - high rates of dextrose 5% in water can cause hyperglycemia and glucose induced diuresis
Significant possible interactions: Refer to manufacturer's literature

ALTERNATIVE DRUGS
Consider nonsteroidal anti-inflammatories in nephrogenic diabetes insipidus

FOLLOWUP

PATIENT MONITORING
• For patient in an acute setting, frequent re-examinations
• Electrolytes frequently
• Urine osmolality and urine output in DI
• Ensure adequate calories are ingested. Patients may ingest so much water that they feel full and do not eat.
• Daily weights

PREVENTION/AVOIDANCE
• Treatment or prevention of underlying cause
• Avoid preparing infant formula at home, and never add salt to any commercial infant formula

POSSIBLE COMPLICATIONS
• CNS thrombosis or hemorrhage
• Seizures
• Mental retardation
• Hyperactivity
• Chronic hypernatremia - over two days duration has higher mortality
• Serum sodium > 180 mEq/L (> 180 mmol/L) - often have residual CNS damage

EXPECTED COURSE/PROGNOSIS
Most recover but rate of neurological impairment is high

MISCELLANEOUS

ASSOCIATED CONDITIONS
Disorders listed under Causes

AGE-RELATED FACTORS N/A
Pediatric:
• May occur in low birth weight newborns
• May result from incorrect preparation of infant formula
Geriatric:
• More common in the elderly hospitalized patient, resulting in a higher morbidity or mortality
• Hypernatremia may be caused by administration of loop diuretics
Others: N/A

PREGNANCY N/A

SYNONYMS N/A

ICD-9-CM
270.6 disorders of urea cycle metabolism

SEE ALSO Diabetes insipidus

OTHER NOTES N/A

ABBREVIATIONS DI = diabetes insipidus

REFERENCES
• Brenner BM, Rector FC Jr: The Kidney. 5th Ed. Philadelphia, W.B. Saunders Co., 1995
• Holliday MA, Barratt TM, Avner ED: Pediatric Nephrology. 3rd Ed. Baltimore, Williams & Wilkins, 1994
• Kokko J, Tannen R: Fluid and Electrolytes. 2nd Ed. Philadelphia, W.B. Saunders Co., 1989
Illustrations: N/A
Internet references: http://www.5mcc.com

Author(s)
Watson C. Arnold, MD

Hyperparathyroidism

BASICS

DESCRIPTION Hyperparathyroidism represents a loss in control of the body's normal regulatory feedback mechanism on the parathyroid glands and their ability to maintain a normal serum calcium
• Primary hyperparathyroidism - direct hyperfunction of the parathyroid glands due to either glandular hyperplasia or adenoma
• Secondary hyperparathyroidism - usually found in chronic renal disease or vitamin D deficient states which cause hyperplasia of all four glands and associated increase in activity
• Multiple endocrine neoplasia (MEN syndromes) - disease states with associated endocrine malfunctions with parathyroid gland hyperplasia leading to a hyperparathyroid state
• Parathyroid carcinoma - extremely rare
System(s) affected: Endocrine/Metabolic
Genetics: N/A
Incidence/Prevalence in USA:
• Rare in children
• Male adults 60 years or older - 100 cases/100,000
• Female adults 60 years or older - 300-400 cases/100,000
• All-age adjusted incidence - 42 cases/100,000
• Prevalence all ages - 250 cases/100,000 population
Predominant age: Age greater than 50
Predominant sex: Females > Males (4:1)

SIGNS AND SYMPTOMS
• "Painful bones, renal stones, abdominal groans and psychic moans." You must think of it to diagnose it.
• Renal:
  ◊ Nephrolithiasis
  ◊ Nephrocalcinosis
  ◊ Reduced glomerular filtration rate
  ◊ Thirst
  ◊ Polydipsia
  ◊ Polyuria
• Gastrointestinal:
  ◊ Abdominal distress
  ◊ Gastroduodenal ulcer
  ◊ Pancreatitis
  ◊ Pancreatic calcification
  ◊ Constipation
  ◊ Vomiting
  ◊ Anorexia
  ◊ Weight loss
• Skeletal:
  ◊ Bone pain and tenderness
  ◊ Cystic bone lesions
  ◊ Skeletal demineralization
  ◊ Spontaneous fracture
  ◊ Vertebral collapse
  ◊ Osteoporosis
• Mental:
  ◊ Fatigue
  ◊ Apathy
  ◊ Anxiety
  ◊ Depression
  ◊ Psychosis
• Neurologic:
  ◊ Somnolence
  ◊ Coma
  ◊ Diffuse EEG abnormalities
• Neuromuscular:
  ◊ Muscle fatigue
  ◊ Weakness
  ◊ Hypotonia
• Cardiovascular:
  ◊ Hypertension
  ◊ Short QT interval
• Articular/periarticular:
  ◊ Arthralgia
  ◊ Gout
  ◊ Pseudogout
  ◊ Periarticular calcification
• Ocular:
  ◊ Band keratopathy
  ◊ Conjunctivitis
  ◊ Conjunctival calcium deposits

CAUSES
• Primary hyperparathyroidism
  ◊ Caused by usually one but sometimes multiple parathyroid gland hyperplasia or adenomatous changes which cause an unregulated increase of parathyroid hormone (PTH) production and release, causing increase in serum calcium
• Secondary hyperparathyroidism
  ◊ Seen most often in chronic renal failure because of adaptive parathyroid gland hyperplasia and hyperfunction
  ◊ Renal parenchymal loss resulting in hyperphosphatemia
  ◊ Impaired calcitriol production leading to hypocalcemia
  ◊ General skeletal and renal resistance to PTH for reasons unknown

RISK FACTORS
• Age greater than 50
• Female
• Occurs more frequently in temperate than tropical climates
• Higher incidence in people exposed to therapeutic low dose radiation

DIAGNOSIS

DIFFERENTIAL DIAGNOSIS
• Other causes of elevated serum calcium level must be excluded
• Due to increased PTH:
  ◊ Ectopic hyperparathyroidism
  ◊ Bronchogenic carcinoma
  ◊ Carcinoma of the kidney
• Nonparathyroid causes:
  ◊ Malignancy - breast carcinoma, multiple myeloma, lymphoma, leukemia, prostate cancer, Paget's disease
  ◊ Granulomatous disease - sarcoidosis, tuberculosis, berylliosis, histoplasmosis, coccidiomycosis
  ◊ Drugs - thiazide diuretics, furosemide, vitamin D intoxication, vitamin A excess, lithium, milk alkali syndrome, exogenous calcium intake
  ◊ Endocrine - hyperthyroidism, hypothyroidism, acute adrenal insufficiency, vipoma, pheochromocytoma
  ◊ Familial hypocalciuric hypercalcemia
  ◊ Immobilization

LABORATORY
• Elevated serum calcium greater than 10.2 mg/dL (2.55 mmol/L) on 3 successive measurements
• Elevated serum immunoreactive parathyroid hormone (iPTH) levels
• Low serum phosphate levels, less than 2.5 mg/dL (0.81 mmol/L)
• Elevated serum chloride levels
• Decreased serum CO2
• Hyperchloremic metabolic acidosis
• Increase in urinary cyclic AMP
Drugs that may alter lab results: N/A
Disorders that may alter lab results: N/A

PATHOLOGICAL FINDINGS
• Parathyroid hyperplasia - all parathyroid glands with cellular changes
• Parathyroid adenoma - only one gland usually with cellular changes
• Parathyroid carcinoma - cellular changes consistent with malignancy, i.e., cellular atypia, lymph node changes

SPECIAL TESTS Immunoassay directed against intact PTH molecule

IMAGING
• Neck ultrasonography
• Thallium technetium scanning
• Magnetic resonance imaging
• CT scanning with and without contrast

DIAGNOSTIC PROCEDURES
• Percutaneous needle biopsy aspiration for cytology and PTH determination
• Open surgical removal with frozen section diagnosis

TREATMENT

APPROPRIATE HEALTH CARE
Outpatient usually. Inpatient for surgery or for treatment of underlying cause.

GENERAL MEASURES
• A few patients with mild asymptomatic hypercalcemia due to hyperparathyroidism may not be candidates for surgery and may be managed conservatively. Avoiding dehydration is the most important treatment.

SURGICAL MEASURES
• Surgical removal of diseased gland is only proven curative therapy for hyperparathyroidism (subtotal resection)
• In preoperative and immediately postoperative patients, large fluid intake is indicated to help prevent formation of renal stones
• Open neck surgical exploration advocated approach
• Removal of obviously diseased gland with biopsies of other glands to make sure physiologically viable
• Total resection of all four glands with transplantation of normal gland to forearm advocated by some
• Special attention must be made during exploration and removal of parathyroid glands for ectopic gland in the neck area
• Postoperative course needs special attention paid to airway and risk of airway compromise
• Monitoring renal functions closely

ACTIVITY As tolerated

DIET As indicated by condition of patient

PATIENT EDUCATION
• Educate about medications
• Importance of periodic lab exams

 MEDICATIONS

DRUG(S) OF CHOICE
• Furosemide (Lasix) may be helpful in well hydrated individuals who are hypercalcemic
• Estrogens, e.g., conjugated estrogens (Premarin), estradiol (Estrace, Estraderm) are indicated in postmenopausal females with hyperparathyroidism
Contraindications: Avoid diuretics in individuals who are hypercalcemic
Precautions: Refer to manufacturer's literature
Significant possible interactions: Refer to manufacturer's literature

ALTERNATIVE DRUGS N/A

 FOLLOWUP

PATIENT MONITORING
• Postoperatively
  ◊ Monitor renal function closely
  ◊ Potential precipitous fall in serum calcium resulting in development of transient tetany

PREVENTION/AVOIDANCE N/A

POSSIBLE COMPLICATIONS
• Skeletal damage (pathologic fractures)
• Renal damage
• Urinary tract infections
• "Parathyroid poisoning"
• Hypertension
• From surgery:
  ◊ Hypoparathyroidism
  ◊ Recurrent laryngeal nerve damage
  ◊ Bleeding
  ◊ Infection
  ◊ Unsuccessful surgery (5%)

EXPECTED COURSE/PROGNOSIS
• Postoperative course requires following of serum calcium to make sure hyperparathyroid state does not redevelop
• Prognosis is excellent in primary hyperparathyroidism with resolution of many of the preoperative symptoms
• Secondary hyperparathyroidism carries a poor prognosis because of the primary disease state of chronic renal failure

 MISCELLANEOUS

ASSOCIATED CONDITIONS Multiple endocrine neoplasia (MEN) syndromes

AGE-RELATED FACTORS
Pediatric: N/A
Geriatric:
• Common in the elderly
• More likely to have a secondary disease
• May cause confusion and be interpreted as senile dementia
Others: N/A

PREGNANCY Rarely occurs during pregnancy

SYNONYMS N/A

ICD-9-CM
• Primary hyperparathyroidism - 252.0
• Ectopic - 259.3
• Secondary hyperparathyroidism in chronic renal disease - 588.8

SEE ALSO N/A

OTHER NOTES N/A

ABBREVIATIONS PTH = parathyroid hormone

REFERENCES
• Arnaud CD: The parathyroid glands, hypercalcemia, and hypocalcemia. In: Wyngaarden JB, Smith LH, eds. Cecil Textbook of Medicine. 18th Ed. Philadelphia, W.B. Saunders Co., 1988
• Clark O, Quan-Yank D: Primary hyperparathyroidism: a surgical perspective. In Endocrinology and Metabolism Clinics of North America 1989;18(3):701-715
Illustrations: 3 available on CD-ROM
Internet references: http://www.5mcc.com

Author(s)
Patrick J. McCarville, MD

Hyperprolactinemia

BASICS

DESCRIPTION An abnormal elevation in serum prolactin level
System(s) affected: Endocrine/Metabolic, Reproductive, Nervous
Genetics: N/A
Incidence/Prevalence in USA: 1% to 50% of non-pregnant, reproductive-aged women (studies vary widely). Less common in men.
Predominant age: Reproductive ages (15-50)
Predominant sex: Female > Male

SIGNS AND SYMPTOMS
• Galactorrhea (milky nipple discharge), oligomenorrhea, amenorrhea, infertility, male impotence
• May also have signs/symptoms of associated conditions (e.g., hypothyroidism, Cushing's disease, acromegaly, fibrocystic breast disease)
• May also have signs/symptoms of pituitary enlargement (e.g., headache, visual field loss)

CAUSES
• Physiologic (pregnancy and up to 6 months after delivery or after stopping breast-feeding)
• Prolactin producing pituitary adenoma
• Medications (e.g., opioids, tricyclics, metoclopramide, verapamil, phenothiazines, alpha-methyldopa, isoniazid, estrogens, reserpine, butyrophenones
• Oral contraceptive pill withdrawal
• Hypothyroidism
• Chest wall conditions (e.g., herpes zoster, post-thoracotomy, fibrocystic changes)
• Postoperative state (any major surgery, but especially oophorectomy)
• Idiopathic
• Miscellaneous causes (e.g., sarcoid, renal failure, Cushing's disease, cirrhosis, head trauma, lupus, multiple sclerosis or other pituitary or hypothalamic disease)

RISK FACTORS   Listed with Causes

DIAGNOSIS

DIFFERENTIAL DIAGNOSIS Since hyperprolactinemia is defined by the abnormal lab result, the differential is limited to lab error

LABORATORY
• Elevated prolactin level
• Evaluate thyroid functions in all hyperprolactinemic patients. Check FSH/LH if also amenorrheic. Consider blood chemistries and pregnancy test.
• Check growth hormone and adrenal steroids if clinically suspect acromegaly or Cushing's disease
Drugs that may alter lab results: See medications listed under Causes
Disorders that may alter lab results: See disorders listed under Causes

PATHOLOGICAL FINDINGS None, unless pituitary resection needed (very rare)

SPECIAL TESTS Formal visual field testing if pituitary adenoma suspected

IMAGING Pituitary MRI if prolactin even minimally elevated. CT only if MRI not available. Avoid "coned-down" or plain tomograms of pituitary as they are relatively insensitive.

DIAGNOSTIC PROCEDURES Usually limited to history, physical exam, blood work and imaging as described above

TREATMENT

APPROPRIATE HEALTH CARE
Outpatient unless pituitary resection needed (very rare)

GENERAL MEASURES
• Discontinue offending medications, if any
• Treat underlying causes as indicated; isolated hyperprolactinemia is rarely harmful
• Other reasons to treat include symptom management (e.g., galactorrhea causing patient anxiety), fertility restoration (if amenorrheic), to cause growth retardation or regression of a pituitary adenoma, or to prevent osteoporosis (if estrogen deficient)
• "Watchful waiting" is often most appropriate, but pituitary macroadenomas warrant treatment even if asymptomatic
• Large adenomas may be treated with X-ray therapy (variable success, 50% risk of panhyperpituitarism at 5 years) or transsphenoidal adenoma removal (variable success, recurrences common).

SURGICAL MEASURES See General Measures

ACTIVITY No restrictions

DIET No restrictions

PATIENT EDUCATION
• Discussion of treatment rationale and risks
• Discussion of symptoms of complications of growing pituitary adenoma (e.g., central headache, visual field loss)

Hyperprolactinemia

MEDICATIONS

DRUG(S) OF CHOICE Bromocriptine (Parlodel). Start low at 1.25 mg or 2.5 mg daily, then increase as tolerated over several weeks to 2.5 mg tid. Doses up to 30 mg daily are occasionally required for tumor regression, after which lower doses can be used for maintenance. First dose taken with evening meal.
Contraindications: Uncontrolled hypertension, sensitivity to any ergot alkaloids, preeclampsia
Precautions:
• Nausea
• Orthostasis
• Drowsiness
• Lightheadedness and syncope
• Hypertension (rare)
• Seizures (rare)
• Acute psychosis (rare)
• Pregnancy
Significant possible interactions:
Phenothiazines, butyrophenones, others drugs listed under Causes

ALTERNATIVE DRUGS
• Intravaginal bromocriptine
• Sustained release bromocriptine (Parlodel SRO)
• Intramuscular bromocriptine (Parlodel LAR)
• New dopamine agonists (cabergoline, quinagolide)

FOLLOWUP

PATIENT MONITORING Depends on etiology. Consider prolactin level every 6 to 12 months, formal visual field testing yearly, and MRI in one year and then every 2 to 5 years, depending on clinical course.

PREVENTION/AVOIDANCE N/A

POSSIBLE COMPLICATIONS Depends on underlying cause. If pituitary adenoma, risk permanent visual field loss.

EXPECTED COURSE/PROGNOSIS
Depends on underlying cause. Tends to recur after discontinuation of bromocriptine.

MISCELLANEOUS

ASSOCIATED CONDITIONS See Causes

AGE-RELATED FACTORS
Pediatric: N/A
Geriatric: N/A
Others: N/A

PREGNANCY Pituitary adenomas can grow dramatically during pregnancy

SYNONYMS N/A

ICD-9-CM
611.6 galactorrhea not associated with childbirth
259.9 Unspecified endocrine disorder

SEE ALSO
• Galactorrhea
• Pituitary basophilic adenoma
• Pituitary chromophobe adenoma

OTHER NOTES Symptomatic hyperprolactinemia occurs rarely in males. Males require very high levels of prolactin in order to develop symptoms.

ABBREVIATIONS N/A

REFERENCES
• Kleinberg DL, Noel GH, Frantz G: Galactorrhea: A study of 235 cases including 48 with pituitary tumors. N Engl J Med 1977;296:589
• Yen SSC, Jaffe RB, eds: Reproductive Endocrinology. 3rd Ed. Philadelphia, W.B. Saunders Co., 1991
• Sarapura V, Schlaff WD: Recent advances in the understanding of the pathophysiology and treatment of hyperprolactinemia. Curr Opin in Ob & Gyn 1993;5:360-367
• Molitch ME: Pathologic hyperprolactinemia. Endocrinology and Metabolism Clinics of North America 1992;21(4):877-901
• Katz E, Adash E: Hyperprolactinemia disorders. Clinical Ob and Gyn 1990;33(3):622-639
• Jones TH: The management of hyprolactinemia. Brit J of Hosp Med 1995;53(8):374-378
• New drugs for hyprolactinemia. Drug and Therapeutics Bulletin 1995;33(9):65-67
Illustrations: N/A
Internet references: http://www.5mcc.com

Author(s)
Geoffrey R. Swain, MD

Hypersensitivity pneumonitis

BASICS

DESCRIPTION Hypersensitivity pneumonitis (extrinsic allergic alveolitis) is a diffuse inflammatory disease of the lung caused by repeated inhalation of dust constituted of animal proteins, plant proteins or reactive inorganic compounds. Regardless of the etiologic inhalant, most forms share common features:
• Involvement of peripheral airways, alveoli and interstitium
• Mononuclear cell infiltration of interstitium with granuloma formation and increased alveolar macrophage activity
• Precipitating antibodies against offending dust without complement activation
• Normal IgE and eosinophil levels in chronic form. May present as either acute or sub-acute to chronic progressive pneumonitis.
System(s) affected: Pulmonary
Genetics:
• Not related to:
  ◊ Atopic predisposition
  ◊ Blood type
  ◊ HLA type
Incidence/Prevalence in USA:
• National prevalence unknown
• 1-8% of farmers and 6-15% of pigeon breeders develop related pneumonitis
Predominant age: All ages, but tends to occur in adults because of occupation related exposure
Predominant sex: Male = Female

SIGNS AND SYMPTOMS
• Acute hypersensitivity pneumonitis - the following occur within 6 hours of exposure to the offending antigen and may mimic an acute infectious pneumonia:
  ◊ Fever up to 40°C
  ◊ Cough
  ◊ Dyspnea
  ◊ Malaise
  ◊ Body aches
  ◊ Rare hemoptysis or sputum production
  ◊ Hypoxia
  ◊ Fine, mid- to end-inspiratory crackles in chest
• Chronic hypersensitivity pneumonitis - chronic progressive condition without acute exacerbation:
  ◊ Chronic cough
  ◊ Dyspnea and exercise limitation
  ◊ Anorexia and weight loss
  ◊ Fatigue
  ◊ Progressive hypoxia and cyanosis
  ◊ Clubbing
  ◊ Fine, mid- to end-inspiratory crackles in chest
  ◊ Cor pulmonale with right heart failure

CAUSES
• Exposure to dust capable of inciting immune response, for example:
  ◊ Farmer's lung (Thermophilic actinomycetes)
  ◊ Air conditioner lung (Thermophilic actinomycetes)
  ◊ Bagassosis (Thermophilic actinomycetes)
  ◊ Bird breeder's lung (avian protein and blood)
  ◊ Rat handler's lung (rat urine and protein)
  ◊ Isocyanate lung (toluene diisocyanate [TDI], methylene diisocyanate [MDI] exposure)
  ◊ Washing powder lung (Bacillus subtilis enzymes)

RISK FACTORS
• Intensity of exposure
• Size (1-5 micron particles reach deep into lung)
• Smokers at lower risk than non-smokers

DIAGNOSIS

DIFFERENTIAL DIAGNOSIS
• Acute hypersensitivity pneumonia:
  ◊ Acute infectious pneumonia
  ◊ Influenza
  ◊ Adenovirus
  ◊ Mycoplasma
  ◊ Pyogenic bacteria
  ◊ Pneumocystis carinii
  ◊ Fungus
• Chronic hypersensitivity pneumonia:
  ◊ Tuberculosis
  ◊ Sarcoidosis
  ◊ Pneumoconiosis
  ◊ Scleroderma
  ◊ Rheumatoid lung
  ◊ Lupus erythematosus
  ◊ Eosinophilic granuloma
  ◊ Lymphangitic carcinomatosis
  ◊ Fungal infections
  ◊ Pneumocystis carinii pneumonia
  ◊ Drug reactions
  ◊ Hemosiderosis
  ◊ Idiopathic pulmonary fibrosis

LABORATORY
• Leukocytosis with polymorphonuclear predominance in acute form
• Non-specific elevation of immunoglobulins and erythrocyte sedimentation rate
• Positive rheumatoid test and mononucleosis spot test
• Negative blood, sputum, throat cultures
Drugs that may alter lab results:
Bronchodilators alter lung function
Disorders that may alter lab results:
Asthma or atopy may lead to eosinophilia or increased IgE levels and confuse picture

PATHOLOGICAL FINDINGS
• Acute hypersensitivity pneumonitis:
  ◊ Alveolar walls infiltrated by polymorphs, lymphocytes, macrophages, plasma cells
  ◊ Eosinophils are rare
  ◊ Alveolar space contains proteinaceous exudate and edema
  ◊ Alveolar capillaries with fibrin/platelet thrombi, but no vasculitis
• Chronic hypersensitivity pneumonitis:
  ◊ Alveolitis and interstitial inflammation with lymphocytes, plasma cells and histiocytes with non-caseating granulomas
  ◊ Focal granulomatous inflammation of bronchioles
  ◊ Interstitial fibrosis and honeycombing in severe cases

SPECIAL TESTS
• Serum IgG precipitating antibodies to offending agent. Note: 40-50% of non-hypersensitive individuals with high exposure have positive precipitating antibodies.
• Skin testing: Standardized agents poorly available and of limited use
• Inhalation challenge testing can cause severe reactions and therefore is usually not performed except in specialized, in-hospital units
• Pulmonary function studies demonstrate:
  ◊ Reduced lung volume
  ◊ Impaired gas transfer
  ◊ Forced expiratory volume (FEV) 1, forced vital capacity (FVC) and FEV1/FVC ratio may be normal early on and then drop with the development of chronic airway obstruction
  ◊ Forced expiratory flow (FEF) 25-75 and flows near residual volume may be reduced
  ◊ Decreased lung compliance
• Bronchoalveolar lavage
  ◊ Acute form with neutrophils and lymphocytes
  ◊ Chronic form with high lymphocytes (60%) mostly T-cells of CD-8 type
  ◊ Differentiate from sarcoid which has mostly T-cells of CD-4 type
• Lung biopsy
  ◊ Rarely needed if treatment and avoidance of exposure results in improvement (see Pathological Findings)

IMAGING
• Acute hypersensitivity pneumonitis on chest roentgenography:
  ◊ 30-40% abnormal chest roentgenogram
  ◊ Diffuse interstitial infiltrate with hazy background
  ◊ Fine nodular shadows from 1-3 mm in size
  ◊ Linear striated shadows
  ◊ Occasional lower lobe consolidation
  ◊ Resolution between attacks
• Chronic hypersensitivity pneumonitis on chest roentgenography:
  ◊ Reticulonodular pattern
  ◊ Linear shadows and nodules change from fine to coarse pattern with progression of disease
  ◊ No hilar adenopathy, pleural effusion, or pneumothorax
  ◊ Upper lobe predominance in 40-50% of cases with ring shadows and bronchiectasis

DIAGNOSTIC PROCEDURES
• Lung biopsy rarely needed for diagnosis
• Role of CT scan is unclear

TREATMENT

APPROPRIATE HEALTH CARE
Outpatient except for acute pneumonitis cases and admission for workup (bronchial alveolar lavage [BAL], lung biopsy, challenge studies)

GENERAL MEASURES
Avoidance of offending antigen

SURGICAL MEASURES
N/A

ACTIVITY
Full activity, unless advanced disease

DIET
Normal

PATIENT EDUCATION
• Stress pathogenesis and critical importance of avoidance of allergen
• Stress risk of irreversible lung damage with continued exposure
• Note that chronic exposure may lead to a loss of acute symptoms with exposure, i.e., patient may lose awareness of exposure-symptom relationship
• Printed patient information available from: American Lung Association, 1740 Broadway, New York, NY 10019, (212)315-8700

MEDICATIONS

DRUG(S) OF CHOICE
• Avoidance is primary therapy
• Corticosteroids: Prednisone, 2 mg/kg/day or 60 mg/m2/day, or other comparable corticosteroid. Initial course of one to two weeks with progressive withdrawal of medication. Alternate day therapy if exposure cannot be discontinued may help, but may not prevent progression.
Contraindications: Refer to manufacturer's literature
Precautions:
• Observation for side effects:
 ◊ Immunosuppression
 ◊ Salt and water retention
 ◊ Osteoporosis
 ◊ Acne
 ◊ Hirsutism
 ◊ Behavioral changes
 ◊ Weight gain/appetite increase
Significant possible interactions: In patients with renal or cardiovascular disease a corticosteroid with minimal sodium retention should be chosen

ALTERNATIVE DRUGS
• Bronchodilators may symptomatically improve patients
• Oxygen may be needed in advanced cases

FOLLOWUP

PATIENT MONITORING
Initial followup should be weekly to monthly depending upon severity and course

PREVENTION/AVOIDANCE
Antigens must be avoided to stop process

POSSIBLE COMPLICATIONS
• Progressive interstitial fibrosis with end-stage lung disease
• Cor pulmonale and right heart failure

EXPECTED COURSE/PROGNOSIS
• Excellent prognosis with reversal of pathologic findings with effective treatment of early disease
• Stabilization of severe, advanced disease with avoidance and anti-inflammatory medication

MISCELLANEOUS

ASSOCIATED CONDITIONS
N/A

AGE-RELATED FACTORS
Pediatric: N/A
Geriatric: N/A
Others: N/A

PREGNANCY
Avoidance of antigen in early pregnancy. Avoidance and medication in later pregnancy.

SYNONYMS
• Extrinsic allergic alveolitis
• Allergic interstitial pneumonitis

ICD-9-CM
495.9

SEE ALSO
N/A

OTHER NOTES
In acute form, consider other toxic, non-hypersensitivity related conditions such as silo-filler's lung

ABBREVIATIONS
N/A

REFERENCES
• Sharma OP: Hypersensitivity pneumonitis. Disease-a-Month 1991;37(7):409-71
• Krumpe PE, Lum CCQ, Cross CE: Approach to the patient with diffuse lung disease. Med Clin North Am 1988;72(5):1225-1246
Illustrations: N/A
Internet references: http://www.5mcc.com

Author(s)
Nancy N. Dambro, MD

Hypertension, essential

BASICS

DESCRIPTION Hypertension is defined as a sustained elevated blood pressure (systolic blood pressure of 140 mm Hg or greater and/or diastolic blood pressure of 90 mm Hg or greater). Also conceptually includes the blood pressure level at which the benefits of action exceed those of inaction. Hypertension is a strong risk factor for cardiovascular disease.
System(s) affected: Cardiovascular
Genetics: Blood pressure levels are strongly familial but no clear genetic pattern has been discerned. The strong familial risk for cardiovascular diseases should be concomitantly considered.
Incidence/Prevalence in USA: 50 million (1988-1991 NHANES III); 20% of the U.S. population
Predominant age: Essential (primary, benign, idiopathic) hypertension usually has its onset in the 20's to 30's
Predominant sex: Males > Females (males tend to run higher pressures than females but more importantly have a significantly higher risk of cardiovascular disease at any given blood pressure)

SIGNS AND SYMPTOMS
• Hypertension should be considered asymptomatic except in extremes or after related cardiovascular complications develop
• Headache can be seen especially with higher blood pressures. This is often present on awakening and occipital in nature.
• Retinopathy - narrowed arteries, AV nicking, copper or silver wiring of retinal arterioles
• Increased A2 heart sound

CAUSES
• Over 90% of hypertension has no identified cause. These can be labeled essential or primary hypertension.
• Secondary causes of hypertension include four areas:
• Renal parenchymal
  ◊ Glomerulonephritis
  ◊ Pyelonephritis
  ◊ Polycystic kidneys
• Endocrine
  ◊ Primary hyperaldosteronism
  ◊ Pheochromocytoma
  ◊ Hyperthyroidism
  ◊ Cushing's syndrome
• Vascular
  ◊ Coarctation
  ◊ Renal artery stenosis
• Chemical
  ◊ Oral contraceptives
  ◊ NSAID's
  ◊ Decongestants
  ◊ Antidepressants
  ◊ Sympathomimetics
  ◊ Many industrial chemicals
  ◊ Corticosteroids
  ◊ Ergotamine alkaloids
  ◊ Lithium
  ◊ Cyclosporine

RISK FACTORS
• Family history
• Obesity
• Alcohol
• Excess dietary sodium
• Stress
• Physical inactivity

DIAGNOSIS

DIFFERENTIAL DIAGNOSIS Secondary hypertension (because of the low incidence of reversible secondary hypertension, special tests should be considered only if the history, physical, or basic laboratory evaluation indicates the possibility)

LABORATORY
• Hemoglobin and hematocrit or CBC
• Complete urinalysis (sometimes reveals proteinuria)
• Potassium, calcium and creatinine
• Cholesterol
• Fasting blood glucose
• Uric acid
Drugs that may alter lab results:
Numerous drugs and foods interfere with catecholamine measurements in considering pheochromocytoma
Disorders that may alter lab results: N/A

PATHOLOGICAL FINDINGS
• Late complications include
  ◊ Stroke
  ◊ Retinal vascular narrowing, hemorrhages, exudates, papilledema
  ◊ Left ventricular hypertrophy
  ◊ Congestive heart failure
  ◊ Ischemic heart disease
  ◊ Proteinuria and nephrosclerosis

SPECIAL TESTS
• Only if history, physical or lab indicates
  ◊ IVP and renal arteriogram
  ◊ Plasma catecholamines, urinary metanephrines/vanillylmandelic acid
  ◊ Plasma renin
  ◊ Aortogram
  ◊ ECG

IMAGING
• If history or physical indicate
  ◊ Chest x-ray
  ◊ Ultrasonography
  ◊ IVP
  ◊ Provocative renal nuclear scans (e.g., captopril renogram)
  ◊ Digital subtraction arteriography
  ◊ Angiogram

DIAGNOSTIC PROCEDURES
• Renal biopsy if renal parenchymal disease is suspected
• A presumptive diagnosis of hypertension can be made if the average of at least three blood pressure measurements exceeds either 90 mm Hg diastolic or 160 mm Hg systolic, assuming proper resting conditions, cuff size and application are maintained

• The Joint National Committee on Detection, Evaluation, and Treatment of High Blood Pressure (JNC): Recommends a good history and physical exam with emphasis on:
  ◊ Family history of hypertension and cardiovascular disease
  ◊ Personal past history of cardiovascular, cerebrovascular and renal disease as well as diabetes
  ◊ Previous elevated blood pressures
  ◊ Previous treatments
  ◊ History of weight gain, exercise activities, sodium intake, fat intake and alcohol use
  ◊ Symptoms suggesting secondary hypertension
  ◊ Psychosocial and environmental factors affecting blood pressure
  ◊ Other cardiovascular risk factors such as obesity, smoking, hyperlipidemia, and diabetes
  ◊ Funduscopic exam for arteriolar narrowing, arteriovenous compression, hemorrhages, exudates, and papilledema
  ◊ Complete cardiac and peripheral pulse exam. Compare radial and femoral pulse for differences in volume and timing.
  ◊ Abdominal exam for masses and bruits. Listen high in the flanks over the kidneys.

TREATMENT

APPROPRIATE HEALTH CARE
Outpatient

GENERAL MEASURES
• Goal blood pressures should be individualized based on risk factors but generally treat to diastolic < 90 mm Hg (< 12 kPa) and systolic < 160 mm Hg (< 21.3 kPa)
• Weight reduction for obese patients may significantly lower blood pressures
• Smoking cessation is an important part of a cardiovascular risk reduction program
• Biofeedback and relaxation exercises have been shown to reduce blood pressures

SURGICAL MEASURES N/A

ACTIVITY Normal activity with an appropriate aerobic fitness program

DIET
• Some patients will respond to a reduced salt diet
• Alcohol consumption should be reduced to less than 1 ounce per day
• Decrease saturated fats and increase monounsaturated fats
• Potassium and calcium should be considered although absolute effect uncertain

PATIENT EDUCATION
• Emphasize asymptomatic nature of hypertension and importance of lifetime treatment
• Review risk factors for cardiovascular disease with emphasis on comprehensive preventive program
• Printed Aids for High Blood Pressure Education, NIH Publication No. 301-251-1222

MEDICATIONS

DRUG(S) OF CHOICE
Hydrochlorothiazide and propranolol are most proven to prevent cardiovascular sequelae. ACE inhibitors should be used in patients with diabetes or CHF. Alpha adrenergic agents might benefit males with BPH. Beta blockers might benefit patients with ischemic heart disease or migraine. Calcium channel blockers could be considered in patients with migraine or asthma.

First line choices include the following categories and their representatives:
- Diuretics
  ◊ Hydrochlorothiazide 6.25-50 mg qd
  ◊ Chlorthalidone 12.5-50 mg qd
  ◊ Indapamide 1.25-5 mg qd
- Alpha adrenergic agents
  ◊ Prazosin 1-10 mg bid
  ◊ Terazosin 1-20 mg qd
  ◊ Doxazosin 1-16 mg qd
- ACE inhibitors
  ◊ Captopril 25-300 mg bid
  ◊ Enalapril 2.5-20 mg qd
  ◊ Fosinopril 10-80 mg qd
  ◊ Lisinopril 5-20 mg qd
  ◊ Ramipril 2.5-20 mg qd
  ◊ Quinapril 10-80 mg qd
  ◊ Benazepril 10-40 mg qd
- Angiotensin II receptor blocker
  ◊ Losartan 25-100 mg in 1 or 2 doses
- Calcium channel blockers
  ◊ Diltiazem, sustained release, 180-360 mg qd
  ◊ Felodipine 5-20 mg qd
  ◊ Nicardipine 20-40 mg tid
  ◊ Nifedipine, sustained release, 30-120 mg qd
  ◊ Nitrendipine 5-40 mg qd (not available in U.S.)
  ◊ Verapamil, sustained release, 120-480 mg qd
  ◊ Amlodipine 2.5-10 mg qd
- Beta blockers
  ◊ Acebutolol 400-800 mg qd
  ◊ Atenolol 25-100 mg qd
  ◊ Metoprolol 50-200 mg qd
  ◊ Nadolol 40-320 mg qd
  ◊ Penbutolol 20-40 mg qd
  ◊ Pindolol 5-30 mg bid
  ◊ Propranolol 40-240 mg/day, divided bid
  ◊ Timolol 10-40 mg daily, divided bid
  ◊ Betaxolol 5-40 mg qd
  ◊ Bisoprolol 2.5-20 mg qd

Contraindications:
- Diuretics may worsen gout and diabetes
- Beta blockers are relatively contraindicated in reactive airway disease, heart failure, and heart block. Diabetes and peripheral vascular disease are relative contraindications.
- Diltiazem or verapamil should be used cautiously with heart failure or block

Precautions: See manufacturer's profile of each drug

Significant possible interactions: See manufacturer's profile of each drug

ALTERNATIVE DRUGS
Many may be added to the above for combination therapy
- Centrally acting adrenergic inhibitors
  ◊ Clonidine 0.1-1.2 mg bid or weekly patch 0.1 mg/day to 0.3 mg/day
  ◊ Guanabenz 4-32 mg bid
  ◊ Guanfacine 1-3 mg qd
  ◊ Methyldopa 250-2000 mg bid
- Peripherally acting adrenergic inhibitors
  ◊ Guanadrel 5-75 mg daily, divided bid
  ◊ Guanethidine 10-50 mg qd
  ◊ Reserpine 0.1-0.25 mg qd
  ◊ Labetalol 100-900 mg bid
- Vasodilators
  ◊ Hydralazine 25-150 mg bid
  ◊ Minoxidil, rarely used due to adverse effects
- Loop diuretics (for patients with volume overload)
  ◊ Furosemide 20-320 mg qd
  ◊ Bumetanide 0.5-2 mg qd
  ◊ Ethacrynic acid 25-100 mg qd
- Potassium sparing diuretics
  ◊ Generally used in patients who have developed hypokalemia with thiazide diuretics
  ◊ Amiloride 5-10 mg qd
  ◊ Spironolactone 25-100 mg qd
  ◊ Triamterene 50-150 mg qd

FOLLOWUP

PATIENT MONITORING
- Once stable, patients should be revaluated at least every 3 to 6 months
- Review compliance, effectiveness and adverse reactions
- Quality of life issues should be considered, including sexual function
- At least annual evaluation of urinalysis, creatinine and potassium are appropriate, generally as part of a screening laboratory panel

PREVENTION/AVOIDANCE
Diet, exercise, reduce stress, stop smoking, little or no alcohol, compliance in taking medications

POSSIBLE COMPLICATIONS
- Congestive heart failure
- Renal failure
- Myocardial infarction
- Stroke
- Hypertensive heart disease

EXPECTED COURSE/PROGNOSIS
Good with adequate control

MISCELLANEOUS

ASSOCIATED CONDITIONS
See list in Causes

AGE-RELATED FACTORS
Pediatric:
- Blood pressure should be measured during routine examinations
- Hypertension can accompany a wide variety of acute and chronic illnesses in this age group
Geriatric: Isolated systolic hypertension more common in this group. Therapy has been shown to be effective although adverse reactions to medications are more frequent.
Others: N/A

PREGNANCY
Elevated blood pressures during pregnancy may be either chronic hypertension or pregnancy induced preeclampsia. Maternal and fetal mortality benefit from treatment. See topic on preeclampsia. Some medications may adversely affect the fetus.

SYNONYMS
- Benign hypertension
- Idiopathic hypertension
- Familial hypertension
- High blood pressure
- Chronic hypertension
- Genetic hypertension

ICD-9-CM
401.1 Essential hypertension, benign

SEE ALSO
Hypertensive emergencies
- Polycystic kidney disease

OTHER NOTES
N/A

ABBREVIATIONS
N/A

REFERENCES
- Kaplan NM: Clinical Hypertension. 6th Ed. Baltimore, Williams & Wilkins, 1994
- McMahon FG: Management of Essential Hypertension. New York, Futura Publishing, 1990
- The Fifth Report of the Joint National Committee on the Detection, Evaluation, and Treatment of High Blood Pressure. In Arch Intern Med 1993;153:154-183
Illustrations: 5 available on CD-ROM
Internet references: http://www.5mcc.com

Author(s)
David E. Burtner, MD

Hypertensive emergencies

BASICS

DESCRIPTION Terminology describing hypertensive emergencies can be confusing. Terms such as "hypertensive crisis," "malignant hypertension," "hypertensive urgency," "accelerated hypertension" and "severe hypertension" are all used in the literature and often overlap. Some definitions include a specific diastolic or systolic blood pressure reading, while others emphasize an acute change in the blood pressure or the presence of specific clinical syndromes.
• Severe hypertension is defined as a diastolic blood pressure of 115 mm Hg (15.3 kPa) or greater. Patients with severe hypertension may or may not have a hypertensive emergency.
• A hypertensive emergency occurs when an acute elevation of blood pressure causes rapid and progressive end-organ damage, particularly in the cardiovascular, renal and central nervous systems.
System(s) affected: Cardiovascular, Nervous, Pulmonary, Renal/Urologic
Genetics: N/A
Incidence/Prevalence: Less than 1% of patients with hypertension
Predominant age: Young or middle-aged patients with known hypertensive disease
Predominant sex: Male > Female

SIGNS AND SYMPTOMS
• Hypertension
• Headache
• Nausea, vomiting
• Seizure
• Retinopathy
• Visual disturbances
• Chest pain
• Shortness of breath, dyspnea, orthopnea
• Focal neurologic deficits
• Stupor, coma
• Pulmonary edema
• Hemorrhage
• Thrombosis
• Embolus
• Acute renal failure
• Abdominal pain

CAUSES
• Decongestants, appetite suppressants, steroids (including oral contraceptives), MAO inhibitors in combination with certain foods or drugs, and drugs of abuse such as cocaine or amphetamine
• Withdrawal from antihypertensives, especially clonidine (Catapres)
• Withdrawal from CNS depressants
• Eclampsia/preeclampsia
• Thrombotic thrombocytopenic purpura (TTP)
• Pheochromocytoma
• Idiopathic hypertension
• Renal disease
• Severe burns
• Postoperative hypertension

RISK FACTORS
• History of hypertension
• Drug abuse
• Non-compliance with medications

DIAGNOSIS

DIFFERENTIAL DIAGNOSIS Other CNS pathology

LABORATORY
• Urinalysis and renal function tests (red cell casts, hematuria, proteinuria are all common)
• Urine drug screen in selected patients
• Blood count and smear may indicate microangiopathic hemolytic anemia, thrombocytopenia
• Serum electrolytes (may indicate hypokalemic alkalosis)
• Calcium, glucose, uric acid and lipid profiles
• Subsequent work-up for renal artery stenosis or pheochromocytoma in selected patients
Drugs that may alter lab results: N/A
Disorders that may alter lab results: N/A

PATHOLOGICAL FINDINGS Extreme blood pressure elevations can overwhelm the autoregulatory mechanisms for organ blood flow resulting in damage to the arteriolar and capillary beds. This process produces organ hemorrhages and edema from the leakage of blood and fluid.

SPECIAL TESTS
• Electrocardiography may reveal ischemia or left ventricular hypertrophy
• Funduscopic examination may reveal papilledema, exudates or hemorrhages

IMAGING
• Chest radiographs:
  ◊ May show pulmonary edema and cardiomegaly due to congestive heart failure
  ◊ Mediastinal widening and blunting of the aortic knob consistent with a dissecting aneurysm
• Head CT
  ◊ Assess the patient with CNS symptoms for intracranial bleed

DIAGNOSTIC PROCEDURES
• Blood pressure - measured with an appropriately sized cuff, and two or more readings from both arms should be averaged before the blood pressure is accepted as elevated
• Sphygmomanometer is recommended

TREATMENT

APPROPRIATE HEALTH CARE
Intensive care unit

GENERAL MEASURES
• Comfortable environment, which may lower the blood pressure
• General goal is to lower the mean arterial pressure by approximately 20-25% or reduce diastolic pressure to 100-110 mm Hg (13.3-14.6 kPa) over one hour
• If ongoing end-organ damage is thought to be secondary to the hypertensive state, prompt treatment with intravenous medication is indicated. Monitor patient closely so that a rapid fall in blood pressure can be avoided.
• Optimally, an arterial catheter is used to monitor blood pressure
• Intravenous infusion pump
• Mean arterial pressure is approximately one-third of the sum of twice the diastolic pressure plus the systolic pressure

SURGICAL MEASURES N/A

ACTIVITY Bedrest

DIET Low sodium when tolerated

PATIENT EDUCATION
• Importance of medication compliance
• Lack of symptoms with hypertension until organ damage occurs

MEDICATIONS

DRUG(S) OF CHOICE The drug(s) used depends on the end organs affected and the patient's clinical status. All medications are IV unless otherwise indicated.
DRUGS:
• Nitroprusside (Nipride, Nitropress) infusion 0.5-10 µg/kg/min; contraindicated in pregnancy
• Hydralazine bolus 5-15 mg; preferred in pregnancy
• Diazoxide (Hyperstat) infusion 7.5-30 mg/min
• Labetalol (Normodyne, Trandate) bolus 20-80 mg q10-15 minutes; infusion 0.5-2.0 mg/min
• Nitroglycerin (NTG) infusion 5-100 µg/min
• NTG 0.4 mg SL tablet. Repeat q5min if needed. Consider IV infusion after 3 doses.
• Trimethaphan (Arfonad) infusion 0.5-5 mg/min
• Propranolol (Inderal) 2-4 mg/hr
• Phentolamine (Regitine) bolus 5-10 mg q5-15 minutes
• Oral clonidine: oral loading dose of 0.2 mg followed by 0.1 mg per hour until blood pressure has been lowered or a total dose of 0.8 mg has been administered

DISEASE STATES:
- Hypertensive encephalopathy
  ◊ Nitroprusside infusion or
  ◊ Diazoxide infusion or
  ◊ Labetalol
- Central nervous system events
  ◊ Nitroprusside infusion (treat only if diastolic pressure > 130 mm Hg [> 17.3 kPa])
- Myocardial ischemia
  ◊ Nitroglycerin infusion or
  ◊ Labetalol or
  ◊ Oral nifedipine
- Congestive heart failure
  ◊ Nitroprusside infusion or
  ◊ Nitroglycerin infusion
- Aortic dissection
  ◊ Nitroprusside and propranolol infusions or
  ◊ Trimethaphan and propranolol infusions
- Renal failure
  ◊ Nitroprusside infusion or
  ◊ Labetalol
- Pheochromocytoma
  ◊ Phentolamine or
  ◊ Labetalol or
  ◊ Nitroprusside infusion
- Antihypertensive withdrawal
  ◊ Labetalol or
  ◊ Phentolamine
- Interactions between MAO inhibitors and foods or drugs
  ◊ Phentolamine or
  ◊ Labetalol
- Eclampsia/preeclampsia
  ◊ Hydralazine
- Severe hypertension (hypertensive urgencies) without acute end-organ damage. Treatment is controversial. Some authorities recommend no emergent treatment. If treatment is elected, may use:
  ◊ Oral nifedipine or
  ◊ Oral clonidine

Contraindications:
- Diazoxide: not recommended for patients with suspected myocardial ischemia, congestive heart failure or aortic dissection
- Labetalol: not recommended for patients with asthma, chronic obstructive lung disease, congestive heart failure, heart block, cardiogenic shock or severe bradycardia (due to its beta-blockade property)
- Nitroprusside: not recommended in pregnancy

Precautions:
- Nitroprusside: when IV nitroprusside is continued for more than 48-72 hours, or the patient has compromised renal function, plasma thiocyanate levels should be monitored. Use with clonidine has caused myocardial infarction.
- Diazoxide and hydralazine: may produce reflex tachycardia with increased myocardial oxygen consumption (can be prevented by pretreatment with intravenous propranolol). Use with caution in suspected myocardial infarction.
- Topical clonidine has a slow onset of action and is generally not useful in hypertensive emergencies
- Oral/SL nifedipine (Adalat, Procardia) may cause serious adverse effects such as cerebral vascular ischemia, stroke, or severe hypotension and should probably not be used for hypertensive emergencies

Significant possible interactions: N/A

ALTERNATIVE DRUGS Dopamine-1 receptor agonists (investigational) may preserve renal function better than other agents.

 FOLLOWUP

PATIENT MONITORING
- Monitor closely to avoid a rapid fall in blood pressure
- Begin oral therapy as soon as possible after control achieved with IV medications

PREVENTION/AVOIDANCE
Counsel patient on importance of compliance with antihypertensive treatment and dangers of abrupt stoppage of medication

POSSIBLE COMPLICATIONS
- Abrupt lowering of the blood pressure may result in inadequate cerebral or cardiac blood flow, leading to stroke or myocardial ischemia
- Authorities have questioned whether the benefits of aggressive treatment outweigh the risks in patients with severe hypertension but no end-organ damage. No studies have proven that aggressive treatment reduces the risk of long-term morbidity or mortality from hypertensive urgencies.

EXPECTED COURSE/PROGNOSIS
- The blood pressure should return to normal levels within 24 hours

 MISCELLANEOUS

ASSOCIATED CONDITIONS
- Chronic renal failure
- Renovascular hypertension
- Acute glomerulonephritis
- Renal vasculitis

AGE-RELATED FACTORS
Pediatric: Usually associated with renal disease. May present with abdominal pain.
Geriatric: N/A
Others: N/A

PREGNANCY Hydralazine is drug of choice since nitroprusside decreases placental blood flow and cyanide metabolite crosses the placenta and is therefore relatively contraindicated in pregnancy. Treat eclampsia.

SYNONYMS
- Hypertensive crisis
- Severe hypertension
- Malignant hypertension
- Accelerated hypertension

ICD-9-CM
401.0 Malignant hypertension
405.01 Malignant hypertension due to renal artery stenosis
437.2 Hypertensive encephalopathy
642 Hypertension complicating a pregnancy, childbirth, or puerperium

SEE ALSO
- Hypertension, essential
- Eclampsia
- Preeclampsia
- Pheochromocytoma

OTHER NOTES N/A

ABBREVIATIONS
MAO = monoamine oxidase

REFERENCES
- Gifford R: Management of Hypertensive Crisis. J Amer Med Soc 1991;226:829-835
- Calhoun DA, Oparil S: Treatment of hypertensive crisis. N Engl J Med 1990;323:1177-83
- The 1988 report of the Joint National Committee on Detection, Evaluation, and Treatment of High Blood pressure. Arch Intern Med 1988;148:1023-38
- Haber E, Slater E: Hypertensive Emergencies in High Blood Pressure. In: Rubenstein E, Federman DD, eds. Scientific American Medicine, Scientific American Inc., 1978-1992
- Williams GH: Hypertensive Vascular Disease. In: Braunwald E, ed. Harrison's Principles of Internal Medicine. 12th Ed. New York, McGraw-Hill, 1991
- Graber MA: Emergency Medicine. In: Graber MR, et al, eds. The Family Practice Handbook. St Louis, Mosby-Yearbook, 1994
- Abdelwahab W, Frishman W, Landau A: Management of hypertensive urgencies and emergencies. J Clin Pharmacol 1995;35:747-762
- Murphy C: Hypertensive emergencies. Advances and Updates in Cardiovascular Emergencies 1995;13:973-1007
- Grossman E, Messerli FH, Grodzicki T, et al: Should a moratorium be placed on sublingual nifedipine capsules given for hypertensive emergencies and pseudoemergencies? JAMA 1996; 276: 1328-1331
Illustrations: N/A
Internet references: http://www.5mcc.com

Author(s)
John Guisto, MD
Arthur Sanders, MD

Hyperthyroidism

BASICS

DESCRIPTION
The reaction to excess production of thyroid hormone. Types of hyperthyroidism include:
• Graves' disease (GD) - the most common form - an autoimmune disease. Thyroid stimulating immunoglobulins (TSI's) of the IgG class are produced and bind to thyrotropin (TSH) receptors on the thyroid gland. The TSI's mimic the action of TSH and cause excess secretion of thyroxine (T4) and triiodothyronine (T3). Goiter and ophthalmopathy are common characteristics.
• Toxic multinodular goiter - occurs late in life. Nodules are insidious and almost never malignant. No ophthalmopathy or localized myxedema present.
• Toxic uninodular goiter - solitary nodule with autonomous function. Almost always benign.
• Other causes are rare and include TSH-secreting, pituitary tumors, surreptitious ingestion of T4 or T3, functioning trophoblastic tumors, and iodine-induced hyperthyroidism

System(s) affected: Endocrine/Metabolic
Genetics: Unknown
Incidence/Prevalence in USA: 1:1000 in women, 1:3000 in men
Predominant age: Any age, peaks in 3rd and 4th decades
Predominant sex: Female > Male

SIGNS AND SYMPTOMS
• In adults
 ◊ Nervousness (85%)
 ◊ Increased sweating (70%)
 ◊ Heat intolerance (70%)
 ◊ Palpitations and tachycardia (75%)
 ◊ Dyspnea (75%)
 ◊ Fatigue and weakness (60%)
 ◊ Weight loss (52%)
 ◊ Increased appetite (40%)
 ◊ Exophthalmos (34%)
 ◊ Goiter (87%)
 ◊ Tremor (65%)
 ◊ Warm and moist skin (72%)
 ◊ Emotional lability
• In children
 ◊ Linear growth acceleration
 ◊ Ophthalmic abnormalities more common

CAUSES
• Graves' disease - autoimmune disease
• Toxic multinodular goiter - iodine deprivation followed by iodine repletion
• Toxic uninodular goiter - unknown

RISK FACTORS
• Positive family history
• Female sex
• Other autoimmune disorders
• Iodide repletion after iodide deprivation

DIAGNOSIS

DIFFERENTIAL DIAGNOSIS
• Anxiety
• Malignancy
• Diabetes
• Pregnancy
• Menopause
• Pheochromocytoma

LABORATORY
• T3 - Radioimmunoassay (RIA) > 200 ng/mL
• T4 - RIA >12.5 µg/dL (161 nmol/L)
• Free thyroxine index (FTI) >12
• TSH - below normal
• Radioiodine uptake (RIU) - high in Graves' disease, high or normal in toxic nodules
Drugs that may alter lab results:
• Anabolic steroids
• Androgens
• Estrogens
• Heparin
• Iodine containing compounds
• Phenytoin
• Rifampin
• Salicylates
• Thyroxine
Disorders that may alter lab results:
• A variety of non-thyroidal illnesses can alter T4 and T3 with little effect on TSH
• FTI permits correction of misleading results caused by pregnancy and estrogens

PATHOLOGICAL FINDINGS
• Graves' disease - hyperplasia
• Toxic nodules - nodule formation

SPECIAL TESTS
Immunoradiometric assays

IMAGING
Thyroid scans using radioiodine: diffuse in GD, focal in toxic nodule

DIAGNOSTIC PROCEDURES N/A

TREATMENT

APPROPRIATE HEALTH CARE
• Outpatient except for treatment of thyroid storm, a life-threatening condition, which may cause heart failure, fever, and mania

GENERAL MEASURES
Antithyroid drugs, therapeutic radioiodine, beta blockers for tachycardia and tremor

SURGICAL MEASURES
Rarely, subtotal thyroidectomy

ACTIVITY
Modify activity according to disease severity

DIET
Sufficient calories to prevent weight loss

PATIENT EDUCATION
Importance of compliance with drug therapy

MEDICATIONS

DRUG(S) OF CHOICE
Initial treatment
• Propylthiouracil (PTU)
◊ Adults (preferred in elderly, those with cardiac disease, thyroid storm, and pregnant and lactating women) 100-900 mg/day po given tid. No more than 300 mg/day during pregnancy. Radioiodine often first choice.
◊ Children age > 10, 150-300 mg/day po given tid or 5-7 mg/kg/day
◊ Children age 6-10, 50-150 mg/day po given tid or 5-7 mg/kg/day
• Methimazole (Tapazole)
◊ Adults 15-60 mg/day po given once daily.
◊ Children 6-10, 0.4 mg/kg/day po once daily
Maintenance with antithyroids
• PTU
◊ Adults 50-600 mg/day given bid po
◊ Children 50 mg bid po (or 1/2-2/3 of initial dose)
• MMI
◊ Adults 5-30 mg/day po given daily. No more than 20 mg/day during pregnancy.
◊ Children 0.2 mg/kg/day po given daily
Thyrotoxic crisis
• PTU (preferred over MMI)
◊ Adults 15-20 mg po q4h during the first day (as an adjunct to other therapies)
◊ Neonates 10 mg/kg/day po given q4h
Additional drugs:
• Radioiodine therapy - sodium iodine131 (Iodotope I-131). Dosage calculation: estimated thyroid weight multiplied by 80 μCi/g divided by 24 hour radioiodine uptake
• Beta blocker - propranolol (Inderal) 40-240 mg daily po
Contraindications:
• Radioiodine therapy - pregnancy and nursing
• Propranolol - congestive heart failure, asthma, chronic bronchitis, pregnancy, hypoglycemia
Precautions:
• PTU and MMI - may cause dermatitis agranulocytosis or hepatotoxicity
• Radioiodine therapy often causes permanent hypothyroidism and may cause fetal hypothyroidism or malformation if administered during pregnancy
Significant possible interactions: Oral anticoagulants may be potentiated by PTU

ALTERNATIVE DRUGS
Ipodate sodium (Oragrafin) - 0.5 g qid po

FOLLOWUP

PATIENT MONITORING
• Repeat thyroid tests twice a year
• CBC and liver function tests when appropriate
• Therapy with antithyroids continues 3-12 months
• After radioiodine therapy, thyroid function tests at 6 weeks, 12 weeks, 6 months and annually thereafter if euthyroid

PREVENTION/AVOIDANCE   N/A

POSSIBLE COMPLICATIONS
• Hypoparathyroidism, recurrent laryngeal nerve damage, and hypothyroidism with subtotal thyroidectomy
• Development of hypothyroidism after radioiodine treatment
• Visual loss or diplopia due to severe ophthalmopathy
• Localized pretibial myxedema at any time
• Cardiac failure in the elderly with underlying heart disease
• Muscle wasting; proximal muscle weakness

PREVENTION/AVOIDANCE   N/A

EXPECTED COURSE/PROGNOSIS   With
precise diagnosis and adequate treatment, prognosis is good

MISCELLANEOUS

ASSOCIATED CONDITIONS   Other
autoimmune diseases and Down syndrome

AGE-RELATED FACTORS
Pediatric: Neonates treated with antithyroids 2-3 months. Most children treated with antithyroids.
Geriatric:
• Characteristic symptoms and signs may be absent in elderly
• Harder to diagnose
• Cardiac failure more likely
Others: N/A

PREGNANCY
• Treat with small doses of PTU due to increased risk of spontaneous abortion and premature delivery in hyperthyroid pregnant women
• Avoid treatment induced hypothyroidism
• Symptoms may be confusing
• Thyrotoxicosis often improves during pregnancy and relapses postpartum
• Radioiodine therapy absolutely contraindicated

SYNONYMS   Thyrotoxicosis

ICD-9-CM
• 242.0 toxic diffuse goiter
• 242.9 thyrotoxicosis without mention of goiter or other cause

SEE ALSO   N/A

OTHER NOTES   N/A

ABBREVIATIONS
• TSI = thyroid stimulating immunoglobulins
• TSH = thyroid stimulating hormone
• T4 = thyroxine
• T3 = triiodothyronine
• RIA = radioimmunoassay
• FTI = free thyroxine index
• RIU = radioiodine uptake
• PTU = propylthiouracil
• MMI = methimazole

REFERENCES
• Bardin CW, ed: Current Therapy in Endocrinology and Metabolism. 5th Ed. St. Louis, Mosby, 1994
• Degroot LJ, ed: Endocrinology. 3rd Ed. Philadelphia, W.B. Saunders Co, 1995
• DeGroot LW, Larsen PR, Hennemann G: The Thyroid and its Diseases, 6th Ed. Churchill, Livingston, 1996
Illustrations: 2 available on CD-ROM
Internet references: http://www.5mcc.com

Author(s)
Richard P. Levy, MD

Hypertriglyceridemia

BASICS

DESCRIPTION Triglycerides (TG) are fatty molecules of long-chain fatty acids and glycerol. The hypertriglyceridemias are a heterogeneous family of disorders due to disturbances in synthesis and/or degradation of triglycerides rich plasma lipoprotein.
• Normal triglycerides is less than 100 mg/dL (1.13 mmol/L) in children and less than 150 mg/dL (1.70 mmol/L) in adults.
• Borderline hypertriglyceridemia: 250-500 mg/dL (2.83-5.65 mmol/L)
• Distinct hypertriglyceridemia: More than 500 mg/dL (5.65 mmol/L)
• Physiology: The major triglycerides containing lipoproteins are:
  ◊ Chylomicron: In post prandial state from absorption of dietary fat from the gut.
  ◊ Very low density lipoprotein (VLDL): In fasting state endogenous synthesis from carbohydrates and fatty acid in the liver.
  ◊ Intermediate density lipoprotein (IDL): From degradation of chylomicron and VLDL.
• Classification: Hypertriglyceridemia falls into one of the following groups based on the lipoprotein pattern
  ◊ Type I: Markedly elevated chylomicron. Presents with high triglyceridemia and minimally elevated cholesterol. Usually present in childhood. Clinically associated with abdominal pain due to pancreatitis, eruptive xanthoma, hepatosplenomegaly and lipemia retinalis. The risk for atherosclerosis is not increased. The causes are either primary (autosomal recessive due to lipoprotein lipase or apo-C deficiency) or secondary, i.e., SLE and dysgammaglobulinemia.
  ◊ Type II-A: Elevated LDL. Presenting with high cholesterol. See separate topic on Hypercholesterolemia.
  ◊ Type II-B: Elevated LDL and VLDL. Presents with high cholesterol and high triglycerides. The risk for atherosclerosis is strong. The primary disorder includes several genetic disorders. Secondary causes include hypothyroidism, liver and kidney disease, porphyria, multiple myeloma.
  ◊ Type III: Elevated IDL (dysbetalipoproteinemia). Presents with high cholesterol and triglycerides. Majority of patients with primary disorder are homozygous for apoprotein E2. Secondary causes are hypothyroidism and dysgammaglobulinemia.
  ◊ Type IV: Elevated VLDL. Presents with high triglycerides and minimally elevated cholesterol. In some, the risk for atherosclerosis is increased.
  ◊ Type V: Elevated chylomicrons and VLDL. Presents with very high triglycerides and high cholesterol. Genetic form is autosomal recessive due to LPL or apo-C deficiency. There is increased risk of atherosclerosis.
Note: Above classification is only descriptive and provides little insight into the genetic and mechanism of the disorder. The plasma lipoprotein change with time in any individual, a phenomenon to be expected because of the precursor-product relationship in the metabolism of VLDL and LDL and effect of diet on VLDL. A single disease state can lead to several different lipoprotein patterns and a single lipoprotein phenotype can be caused by multiple disease state.
System(s) affected: Endocrine/Metabolic, Gastrointestinal, Cardiovascular
Genetics:
• Familial hypercholesterolemia: autosomal dominant
• Polygenic hypercholesterolemia: polygenic
• Familial hypertriglyceridemia: autosomal dominant
• Familial combined hyperlipidemia: autosomal dominant
• Familial dysbetalipoproteinemia: autosomal recessive
• LPL and apo-C deficiency: autosomal recessive
Incidence/Prevalence in USA:
• Familial combined hyperlipidemia - 1-2%
• Familial hypertriglyceridemia - 1-2%
• Familial dyslipoproteinemia - 1/10,000
Predominant age: N/A
Predominant sex: Male > Female

SIGNS AND SYMPTOMS
• Pancreatitis (TG over 1000)
• Chylomicronemia syndrome (TG over 2,000)
  ◊ Memory loss/dementia
  ◊ Dyspnea
  ◊ Headache/vertigo
  ◊ Eruptive xanthoma
  ◊ Lipemia retinalis
  ◊ Hepatosplenomegaly
  ◊ Lymphadenopathy
  ◊ Peripheral neuropathy/paresthesia
• Atherosclerosis

CAUSES
• Primary
  ◊ Sporadic
  ◊ Genetic
• Secondary
  ◊ Condition associated with hypertriglyceridemia: Obesity, diabetes mellitus, pregnancy, uremia/dialysis, hypothyroidism, nephrotic syndrome, acromegaly, Cushing's syndrome, systemic lupus erythematosis, dysgammaglobulinemias, glycogen storage Type I, lipodystrophy
  ◊ Drugs associated with hypertriglyceridemia: Alcohol, estrogen, birth control pill, beta blockers, diuretics, glucocorticoid, isotretinoin/retinoid, bile acid binding resins cause a modest (<10%) elevation in some patients with Type II hyperlipidemia.

RISK FACTORS
• Genetic susceptibility
• Obesity
• Diabetes
• Alcoholism
• Exacerbated by medical illness and/or drug (see secondary causes)

DIAGNOSIS

DIFFERENTIAL DIAGNOSIS Primary versus secondary

LABORATORY
• Turbid and milky serum
• Measurement of fasting plasma lipids
Drugs that may alter lab results: N/A
Disorders that may alter lab results:
• In TG induced pancreatitis, both serum and urinary amylase concentration may be normal due to interference of the plasma lipids or some other inhibitor with the assay
• TG may interfere with hemoglobin measurement, while bilirubin may be artificially elevated
• Pseudohyponatremia may result from very high TG

PATHOLOGICAL FINDINGS
• Atherosclerosis
• Pancreatitis
• In chylomicronemia syndrome - lipid laden macrophage (foam cell) infiltration of visceral organs, bone marrow and skin.

SPECIAL TESTS
• HDL cholesterol measurement (inversely related to TG)
• Apoprotein B measurement (may define a subset of mild hypertriglyceridemia patients at excess risk for CHD)
• Genetic testing for apoprotein E2

IMAGING
• Pancreatitis - CT of pancreas
• Atherosclerosis - doppler, angiography

DIAGNOSTIC PROCEDURES
• TG measured after a fast of 12-14 hours in:
  ◊ Any individual with total cholesterol level of ≥ 240 mg/dL (6.22 mmol/L)
  ◊ Any individual with HDL-C < 35 mg/dL (0.91 mmol/L)
  ◊ Patients with acute pancreatitis, signs and symptoms of chylomicronemia syndrome and lactescence plasma
  ◊ Individuals with past and present history of atherosclerosis, family history of premature arteriosclerosis
  ◊ Individuals with 2 or more CHD risk factors; a disease or medications which raise triglycerides

TREATMENT

APPROPRIATE HEALTH CARE
Outpatient usually. Inpatient, if underlying disorder warrants.

GENERAL MEASURES
• A thorough search for correctable secondary causes and treating an underlying illness or removing an incriminated drug
• In case of primary hypertriglyceridemia, screening the other family members
• Treatment is indicated in distinct hypertriglyceridemia to prevent acute pancreatitis and in mild hypertriglyceridemia to prevent CAD in patients with high risk, strong family or personal history of atherosclerosis.
• Treatment of severe hypertriglyceridemia associated with pancreatitis - hospitalization, elimination of dietary fat; if diabetic, continuous IV infusion of insulin

SURGICAL MEASURES N/A

ACTIVITY Usually no restrictions. Exercise is important.

DIET Weight reduction to ideal body weight with AHA Step I Diet (50-55% carbohydrate, less than 30% fat)

PATIENT EDUCATION
• Smoking cessation
• Elimination of alcohol

MEDICATIONS

DRUG(S) OF CHOICE
• Gemfibrozil (Lopid)
  ◊ Reduces triglycerides by 20-70%
  ◊ Decrease hepatic VLDL synthesis and increase VLDL metabolism
  ◊ Dosage: 600 mg bid
• Nicotinic acid
  ◊ Reduces triglycerides by 20-50%
  ◊ Inhibit hepatic VLDL synthesis
  ◊ Dosage: 1-3 g/day
Contraindications: Refer to manufacturer's literature
Precautions:
• Gemfibrozil
  ◊ Side effects - upper and lower GI side effects (usually mild and are the most frequent adverse effects), cholelithiasis, myalgia, hepatotoxicity
  ◊ May increase the incidence of myopathy/rhabdomyolysis if given with HMG-CoA reductase inhibitors
• Nicotinic acid
  ◊ Side effects - flushing and pruritus (prostaglandin mediated and alleviated by ASA)
  ◊ Upper GI discomfort and peptic ulcer disease (PUD)
  ◊ Hepatotoxicity (more with sustained release preparation)
  ◊ Hyperuricemia and gout, hyperglycemia, toxic amblyopia
Significant possible interactions:
Gemfibrozil with warfarin - enhanced anticoagulation effect; monitor PT closely following addition or withdrawal of gemfibrozil

ALTERNATIVE DRUGS
• HMG-CoA reductase inhibitors (lovastatin [Mevacor], pravastatin [Pravachol], simvastatin [Zocor], fluvastatin [Lescol]) lower triglycerides 10-20%
• Fish oil
• Clofibrate (Atromid-S)

FOLLOWUP

PATIENT MONITORING
• Fasting lipid profile
• Liver function test, CPK, CBC diff
• Target goals
  ◊ For pancreatitis - TG < 500 mg/dL (< 5.65 mmol/L)
  ◊ For CHD - primary prevention: TG < 200 mg/dL (< 2.26 mmol/L); secondary intervention: TG < 150 mg/dL (< 1.70 mmol/L)

PREVENTION/AVOIDANCE Covered in other headings

POSSIBLE COMPLICATIONS
• Acute pancreatitis
• Atherosclerosis

EXPECTED COURSE/PROGNOSIS
• Good in secondary disorder if the underlying causes are eliminated
• In primary, may need life-long treatment

MISCELLANEOUS

ASSOCIATED CONDITIONS
• Mostly associated with low HDL cholesterol
• May be associated with hypercholesterolemia

AGE-RELATED FACTORS
Pediatric: In severe cases only, diet is recommended
Geriatric: N/A
Others: N/A

PREGNANCY All drugs are contraindicated during pregnancy

SYNONYMS
• Hyperlipidemia
• Chylomicronemia syndrome

ICD-9-CM
• 272.4 Hyperlipidemia
• 272.3 Type I or V hyperlipidemia (chylomicronemia syndrome)
• 272.1 Hypertriglyceridemia - type IV
• 272.2 Type III, Type II-B, hyperlipoproteinemia
• 272,0 Type II-A

SEE ALSO Hypercholesterolemia

OTHER NOTES N/A

ABBREVIATIONS
• AHA = American Heart Association
• CAD = coronary artery disease
• HDL = high density lipoprotein
• IDL = intermediate density lipoprotein
• LDL = low density lipoprotein
• LPL = lipoprotein lipase
• PUD = peptic ulcer disease
• TG = triglycerides
• VLDL = very low density lipoprotein

REFERENCES
• NIH consensus conference, triglycerides, HDL and coronary heart disease. JAMA 1993;269:505-510
• Henkin Y, Kreisberg RA: Hypertriglyceridemia: Current concepts of a controversial issue. In: Mazzaferri EL, Kreisberg RA, eds. Advances in Endocrinology and Metabolism. St. Louis, C.V. Mosby, 1993
Illustrations: 5 available on CD-ROM
Internet references: http://www.5mcc.com

Author(s)
Reza Moattari, MD

Hypochondriasis

BASICS

DESCRIPTION Hypochondriasis is a mental disorder associated with an excessive worry about one's health and a preoccupation with a variety of symptoms whereby the person is convinced he/she is suffering from some sort of disease. Patients suffering from this condition mostly seek medical attention searching for the physician that will diagnose them with a physical illness to explain their symptoms. This often leads to a variety of excessive work-ups, including many repetitive and expensive lab tests and diagnostic procedures. Even though these are necessary to rule out some serious physical disease, this diagnosis should not be made by exclusion alone, but should also be made by using inclusive criteria as mentioned below.

System(s) affected: Nervous

Genetics: Some studies show an increase prevalence of hypochondriasis in families, especially among identical twins and first degree relatives.

Incidence/Prevalence in USA:
• Some studies point out that hypochondriasis is present in 3-14% of patients seen by primary care physicians.
• Some surveys show that 10-20% of the general population worry about illness from time to time. About 45% of patients seen by mental health professional worry about illness from time to time.

Predominant age: The peak incidence is believed to happen during the fourth or fifth decade of life, although all age groups can be affected, including children, adolescents, and the elderly.

Predominant sex: It is found equally in men and women; however, women tend to seek help more often than men

SIGNS AND SYMPTOMS
• Preoccupation with fears of having, or the idea that one has, a serious disease based on the person's misinterpretation of bodily symptoms
• The preoccupation persists despite appropriate medical evaluation and reassurance
• The belief is not of delusional intensity (as in delusional disorder, somatic type) and is not restricted to a circumscribed concern about appearance (as in body dysmorphic disorder).
• The preoccupation causes clinically significant distress impairment in social, occupational, or other important areas of functioning.
• The duration of the disturbance is at least 6 months
• The preoccupation is not better accounted for by generalized anxiety disorder, obsessive-compulsive disorder, panic disorder, a major depressive episode, separation anxiety, or another somatoform disorder.

CAUSES
• Biological: There is some evidence suggesting that patients with hypochondriasis may be born with a tendency to amplify somatic sensations and that they have lower threshold and a lower tolerance of physical discomfort
• Life events: Medical diseases may predispose a patient to hypochondriasis, such as certain patients being highly sensitive to certain physical symptoms following an acute stroke, myocardial infarction, intensive treatment following malignant illness, organ transplantation, etc. These may be experienced by the patient or by a close family member or friend.
• Childhood events: The experience of numerous or serious actual medical illnesses during one's childhood may predispose the individual to hypochondriasis later on in life.
• Psychological: Many authors view hypochondriasis as the patient's psychodynamic defense against guilt, shame, low self-esteem, and a narcissistic over-indulgence with one's self. Other authors view it as the patient's way of seeking attention by overly identifying with the sick role which offers the patient a way to alleviate symptoms of anxiety and seek reassurance.
• Socio-cultural: Some societies and cultures view mental symptoms in a pejorative and stigmatized way, blaming the patient for his/her illness, however, if the patient has physical symptoms and a bona fide medical diagnosis, he/she are treated with greater empathy, dignity, and respect and are not blamed for causing their illness.

RISK FACTORS Exposure to life-threatening medical conditions and procedures in one's childhood, adolescence, or in adult life

DIAGNOSIS

DIFFERENTIAL DIAGNOSIS
• Any patient suffering from hypochondriasis, as with any other psychiatric disorder is not immune from developing a medical/organic disease. Such organic diseases as those affecting many organ systems like connective tissue diseases, autoimmune diseases, as well as more focused single-organ type diseases must always be considered as a possibility in these patients.
• Underlying depressive disorders
• Schizophrenia
• Delusional disorders
• Conversion disorder
• Anxiety disorder
• Panic disorder
• Obsessive-compulsive disorder
• Factitious disorder with physical symptoms
• Somatization disorder
• Chronic pain disorder
• Body Dysmorphic disorder
• Malingering
• Munchausen syndrome

LABORATORY
• Lab tests are used to rule out organic diseases
Drugs that may alter lab results: N/A
Disorders that may alter lab results: N/A

PATHOLOGICAL FINDINGS N/A

SPECIAL TESTS N/A

IMAGING N/A

DIAGNOSTIC PROCEDURES
• Thorough mental status examination
• Psychological testing is used to rule out other psychiatric disorders and specifically confirm the diagnosis of hypochondriasis

TREATMENT

APPROPRIATE HEALTH CARE
Outpatient

GENERAL MEASURES
• Treatment of choice is individual psychotherapy delivered on an outpatient basis
• Many patients do better with supportive psychotherapy and behavior modification focused on the alleviation of their symptoms
• Group therapy: Some patients do better in a group setting where they get social support and interaction with others
• Reassuring the patient by repeating lab tests is only short-lived and does not solve the underlying problem

SURGICAL MEASURES N/A

ACTIVITY Regular exercise in moderation

DIET Good nutrition

PATIENT EDUCATION Providing cognitive knowledge about the condition strengthens the patient's intellectual capacities and provides a structure for better response to somatic symptoms, cognitive behavioral and other psychotherapeutic interventions.

MEDICATIONS:

DRUG(S) OF CHOICE
• No specific drug is known to cure hypochondriasis
• Anti-depressants and anti-anxiety medications are most successful in patients who have a preponderance of anxiety and depressive symptoms
• The SSRI group (selective serotonin reuptake inhibitors) are most helpful and have to be used selectively based on patient's tolerance to side effects
• Select patients with a preponderance of obsessive-compulsive symptoms have responded to such drugs as clomipramine 50-150 mg/day or fluoxetine 20-80 mg/day or fluvoxamine 100-300 mg/day

Contraindications:
• Avoid medications that patient is allergic to
• Avoid medications with many side effects
• Avoid medications with known drug interactions

Precautions: Avoid long term use of narcotics and other addictive medication

Significant possible interactions: N/A

ALTERNATIVE DRUGS
• Lithium carbonate: 300-900 mg/day with an optimal blood level of 0.5-0.9 mEq/L
• Divalproex: 500-2000 mg/day or 15-60 mg/kg/day with an optimal plasma level of 50-100 µg/mL

FOLLOWUP

PATIENT MONITORING
• Patients should be seen on a regular basis in the primary care physician's office or with a psychotherapist
• Appointments should be scheduled regardless of whether the patient has new symptoms or not
• Avoid the use of long hospitalizations and unnecessary lab work-ups
• Avoid statements such as, "Call me if you have a problem" or "Make an appointment only if you have a problem"
• Provide reassurance by careful listening to the patient's concerns. Allow the patient to talk about psychosocial issues.
• Provide a safe environment for empathic listening and understanding

PREVENTION/AVOIDANCE N/A

POSSIBLE COMPLICATIONS
• Risks of repeated and unnecessary lab and diagnostic procedures
• Narcotic and other drug addictions

EXPECTED COURSE/PROGNOSIS
• The natural history of this condition is usually chronic
• It has fluctuations in the intensity with periods of relative remission and exacerbation of acuity that may create destruction in the patient's life
• Prognosis varies depending on the patient's personality structure, education, social support system, intelligence, and motivation for change
• Many psychiatrists consider this condition to have a poor prognosis for psychoanalytic treatment

MISCELLANEOUS

ASSOCIATED CONDITIONS N/A

AGE-RELATED FACTORS
Pediatric: Early childhood exposure to serious medical illness and diagnostic procedures predisposes these patients to develop hypochondriasis in adult life
Geriatric: Elderly patients usually have a higher frequency for chronic medical illness which may co-exist with hypochondriasis and complicates the treatment of hypochondriasis
Others: N/A

PREGNANCY N/A

SYNONYMS
• Hypochondriacal neurosis
• Hypochondria

ICD-9-CM 300.7 Hypochondriasis

SEE ALSO N/A

OTHER NOTES N/A

ABBREVIATIONS N/A

REFERENCES
• Barsky AJ, Klerman GL: Overview: hypochondriasis, bodily complaints, and somatic styles. Am J Psychiatry 1983;140:273-283
• Barsky AJ, Cleary PD, Sarnie MD, Klerman GL: The course of transient hypochondriasis. Psychiatry 1993;150:484-488
• Brown HN, Vaillant GE: Hypochondriasis. Arch Intern Med 1981;141:723-726
• Diagnostic and Statistical Manual of Mental Disorders (DSM-IV). 4th Ed. Washington, DC, American Psychiatric Association, 445-469, 1994
• Ford CV: Dimensions of somatization & hypochondriasis. Neurol Clin 1995;13:241-253
• Ford CV: The Somatizing Disorders. Psychosomatic 1986;27:327-337
• Kellner R: Psychotherapeutic strategies in hypochondriasis: a clinical study. Am J Psychother 1982;36:146-157
• Kellner R: Prognosis of treated hypochondriasis: a clinical study. Acta Psychiatr Scand 1983;67-69&79
• Kellner R: Hypochondriasis and somatization. JAMA 1987;258:2718-2722
• Kenyon FE: Hypochondriacal states. Br J Psychiatry 1976;129:1-14
• Smith GR: Somatization disorder: In the Medical Setting. Washington, DC, National Institute of Mental Health, 1990
Illustrations: N/A
Internet references: http://www.5mcc.com

Author(s)
Moshe S. Torem, MD, FAPA

Hypoglycemia, diabetic

BASICS

DESCRIPTION An abnormally low concentration of glucose in the circulating blood of a diabetic. A side effect of insulin and/or sulfonylurea treatment in the course of normal treatment of diabetes mellitus.
System(s) affected: Endocrine/Metabolic
Genetics: No known genetic pattern
Incidence/Prevalence in USA:
• Most type I diabetics experience hypoglycemia. Tightly controlled type I often experience hypoglycemia weekly.
• Type II diabetics experience hypoglycemia much less frequently than type I diabetics
• Most common in type I diabetics
• Common in type II diabetic patients treated with oral agents and/or insulin
• Uncommon in diabetics treated with diet and exercise alone
Predominant age: All ages
Predominant sex: Male = Female

SIGNS AND SYMPTOMS
• Adrenergic hypoglycemia signs and symptoms include:
◊ Pallor
◊ Tremulousness
◊ Nervous anxiety
◊ Irritability
◊ Tachycardia
◊ Diaphoresis
◊ Weakness
• Neuroglycopenic hypoglycemia signs and symptoms include:
◊ Diplopia
◊ Lethargy
◊ Inability to concentrate or remember
◊ Confusion
◊ Behavior change
◊ Paresthesias
◊ Hunger
◊ Seizure
◊ Coma

CAUSES
• Loss of the hormonal counter-regulatory mechanism in glucose metabolism
• Diet - too little food (skipping a meal)
• Medication - too much insulin (improper dose or timing)
• Erratic absorption of insulin or oral hypoglycemics
• Adverse reaction from other medications
• Exercise - unplanned or excessive exercise
• Alcohol consumption
• Vomiting or diarrhea

RISK FACTORS
• Two or three times more common in the "tight control" patient (according to data from the Diabetes Control and Complications Trial).
• Most type 1 diabetics experience hypoglycemia. Type 2 diabetics experience hypoglycemia much less frequently unless insulin is used. Uncommon in those treated with diet and exercise alone.
• Greater than 5 years duration of diabetes
• Elderly patient
• Renal disease
• Liver disease
• Congestive heart failure
• Hypothyroidism
• Hypoadrenalism
• Gastroenteritis
• Starvation
• Alcoholism

DIAGNOSIS

DIFFERENTIAL DIAGNOSIS
• Gastrointestinal dysfunction causing postprandial hypoglycemia or alimentary reactive hypoglycemia
• Hormonal deficiency states (hormonal reactive hypoglycemia)
• Idiopathic reactive hypoglycemia
• Hypoglycemia of sepsis
• Islet cell tumors
• Factitious hypoglycemia from surreptitious injection of insulin

LABORATORY
• Plasma glucose ≤ 45 mg/dL (≤ 2.5 mmol/L) or less
• "Suspect" low when plasma glucose is between 45 and 60 mg/dL (2.5 and 3.33 mmol/L)
• In children plasma glucose ≤ 40 mg/dL (≤ 2.22 mmol/L)
Drugs that may alter lab results: N/A
Disorders that may alter lab results: N/A

PATHOLOGICAL FINDINGS N/A

SPECIAL TESTS Chronic hypoglycemia is evidenced by a low glycohemoglobin level

IMAGING N/A

DIAGNOSTIC PROCEDURES
• History
• Physical exam
• Plasma, or whole blood glucose

TREATMENT

APPROPRIATE HEALTH CARE
• Outpatient except for complicating emergencies (coma, unapparent cause, long acting oral hypoglycemic)
• Admit the patient if:
◊ There is any doubt of the cause
◊ Expectation of prolonged hypoglycemia
◊ Inability of the patient to drink

GENERAL MEASURES
• Education is the mainstay of prevention
• Any sugar-containing food or beverage which can be rapidly absorbed e.g., unsweetened juices, Lifesavers candies, glucose tabs

SURGICAL MEASURES N/A

ACTIVITY Rest until glucose is normal

DIET Avoid extra calories without changing the source of the problem - excess insulin or oral hypoglycemic

PATIENT EDUCATION
• Most important measure is prevention
• Educate patients, their relatives and close friends
• Teach home glucose monitoring and self-adjustment for insulin therapy, diet control, and exercise regimen

MEDICATIONS

DRUG(S) OF CHOICE
• General
◊ Oral administration of small molecule sugars (saccharose/glucose)
◊ Approximately 60-90 calories repeated every 15 minutes until blood sugar is 100 mg/dL (5.55 mmol/L) or more
◊ It takes about 15 minutes for the carbohydrates to be digested and to enter the blood stream as glucose
• In patients with loss of consciousness at home
◊ Administer glucagon IM or subcutaneous in the deltoid or anterior thigh:
◊ If under 5 years old, give 0.25 to 0.50 mg
◊ Older child (5-10 years old) give 0.50 to 1 mg
◊ Over 10 years old, give 1 mg
• If emergency medical personnel are present or patient hospitalized
◊ Give one-half amp 50% dextrose every 5-10 minutes until the patient awakens
◊ Then feed orally and/or administer 5% dextrose intravenously at a level that will maintain the blood glucose at a level above 100 mg/dL.
◊ Patients with hypoglycemia secondary to oral hypoglycemics should be monitored for 24-48 hours since hypoglycemia may recur after apparent clinical recovery
Contraindications: None
Precautions: Refer to manufacturer's literature
Significant possible interactions:
• Treatment may cause hyperglycemia (called Somogyi phenomenon)
• Clearance of certain oral hypoglycemics from plasma may be prolonged in persons with liver disease

ALTERNATIVE DRUGS
Acarbose, a potent alpha-glucosidase inhibitor slows the absorption kinetics of dietary carbohydrates by reversible competitive inhibition of alpha-glucosidase activity, and so reduces the post-prandial blood glucose increment and insulin response

FOLLOWUP

PATIENT MONITORING
Home glucose monitoring

PREVENTION/AVOIDANCE
• Educating patients, family and close friends
• Maintaining a routine schedule of diet, medication and exercise
• Regular blood-glucose testing
• Wearing a medical alert identification bracelet or necklace

POSSIBLE COMPLICATIONS
• Diabetic shock
• Permanent neurological damage

EXPECTED COURSE/PROGNOSIS
Full recovery is usual depending on the rapidity of diagnosis and treatment

MISCELLANEOUS

ASSOCIATED CONDITIONS
• Autonomic dysfunction
• Neuropathies
• Cardiomyopathies

AGE-RELATED FACTORS
Pediatric: Significance of hypoglycemia in infants of diabetic mothers remains to be defined
Geriatric: Often not diagnosed in the elderly
Others: N/A

PREGNANCY With hypoglycemic reactions during pregnancy the fetus is less likely to be hypoglycemic because of active transport of glucose across the placenta

SYNONYMS
• Low blood sugar
• Insulin reaction
• Insulin shock
• Reactive hypoglycemia

ICD-9-CM
251.2 Hypoglycemia (spontaneous)
251.0 Coma
251.2 Reactive

SEE ALSO
• Diabetes mellitus, insulin-dependent (IDDM or Type I)
• Diabetes mellitus, non-insulin dependent (NIDDM)

OTHER NOTES
• The tighter the diabetic control the greater the importance of home glucose monitoring to avoid hypoglycemia
• In patients receiving beta blockers, the drug will mask tachycardia, but not the sweating

ABBREVIATIONS N/A

REFERENCES
• Schwartz S: Management of Diabetes Mellitus. 2nd Ed. Oklahoma, Essential Medical Information Systems, Inc., 1991
• Cahill G: Hypoglycemia. New York, Scientific American Medicine, 1992
• American Diabetes Association Clinical Education Program: Diabetes Care 1994
• Krall LP, Beaser RS, eds: Joslin Diabetes Manual. 12th Ed. Philadelphia, Lea and Febiger, 1989
• Diabetes Control and Complications Trial (DCCT), 1994
Illustrations: N/A
Internet references: http://www.5mcc.com

Author(s)
Joseph A. Florence, MD

Hypoglycemia, nondiabetic

BASICS

DESCRIPTION Hypoglycemia is an abnormally low blood glucose level. Occurs often in diabetic patients (covered under a separate topic) and has a less common appearance in nondiabetic patients.
• Reactive hypoglycemia - in response to a meal, specific nutrients, or drugs. May occur within 2-3 hours after a meal, or later. Also seen after gastrointestinal surgery (in association with dumping syndrome in some patients).
• Spontaneous (fasting) hypoglycemia - may be associated with a primary condition, e.g., hypopituitarism, Addison's disease, myxedema, or in disorders related to liver malfunction, and renal failure. If hypoglycemia presents as a primary manifestation, other disorders to consider include hyperinsulinism and extrapancreatic tumors.
System(s) affected: Endocrine/Metabolic
Genetics: Some aspects may involve genetics (e.g., hereditary fructose intolerance)
Incidence/Prevalence in USA: Unknown
Predominant age: Older adult
Predominant sex: Female > Male

SIGNS AND SYMPTOMS
• Central nervous system (CNS); these symptoms predominate if glucose dropping gradually:
    ◊ Headache
    ◊ Confusion
    ◊ Visual disturbances
    ◊ Palsy
    ◊ Changes in personality
    ◊ Convulsions
    ◊ Coma
• Heart
    ◊ Palpitations
    ◊ Hypotension
• Gastrointestinal
    ◊ Hunger
    ◊ Nausea
    ◊ Belching
• Adrenergic; these symptoms are more prominent in acute drop in glucose (as in insulin reaction)
    ◊ Sweating
    ◊ Anxiety
    ◊ Tremulousness
    ◊ Dizziness
    ◊ Diaphoresis
    ◊ Nervousness

CAUSES
• Reactive causes:
    ◊ Meals (high in refined carbohydrates)
    ◊ Certain nutrients, e.g., fructose, galactose, leucine
    ◊ Drugs or alcohol (e.g., sulfonylureas, salicylates) can cause excess glucose utilization or deficient glucose production; surreptitious drug use - injection of insulin or taking oral hypoglycemics
    ◊ Gastrointestinal surgery
    ◊ Unknown

• Spontaneous causes:
    ◊ Hepatic disease
    ◊ Islet cell tumor
    ◊ Extrapancreatic tumor
    ◊ Exercise
    ◊ Fever
    ◊ Pregnancy
    ◊ Renal glycosuria
    ◊ Large tumor
    ◊ Ketotic hypoglycemia of childhood
    ◊ Adrenal insufficiency
    ◊ Hypopituitarism
    ◊ Enzyme deficiency

RISK FACTORS Listed with Causes

DIAGNOSIS

DIFFERENTIAL DIAGNOSIS
• CNS disorders
• Psychogenic

LABORATORY
• Lab studies best done when patient is symptomatic
• Measurement of blood and plasma glucose
• C-peptide measurement
• Check liver studies, serum insulin, cortisol
Drugs that may alter lab results: Many drugs can affect levels. Refer to a drug or laboratory reference.
Disorders that may alter lab results: N/A

PATHOLOGICAL FINDINGS   N/A

SPECIAL TESTS
• Plasma glucose overnight fasting - < 60 mg/dL (< 3.33 mmol/L)
• Plasma glucose 72-hour fasting - < 45 mg/dL (< 2.5 mmol/L) for females and < 55 mg/dL (< 3.05 mmol/L) for males
• Oral glucose tolerance - < 50 mg/dL (< 2.78 mmol/L)
• IV tolbutamide test - normal
• Insulin radioimmunoassay - elevated insulin levels if islet cell tumor present

IMAGING   Abdominal CT or ultrasound to rule out abdominal tumor

DIAGNOSTIC PROCEDURES
• Overinterpretation of glucose tolerance tests may lead to an overdiagnosis of hypoglycemia. More than 1/3 of normal patients have hypoglycemia with or without symptoms during a 4 hour tolerance test.
• For definitive diagnosis - patient should have (1) documented occurrence of low blood glucose levels
(2) symptoms that occur when the blood glucose is low
(3) evidence that the symptoms are relieved specifically by the ingestion of sugar or other food
(4) identification of the particular type of hypoglycemia

TREATMENT

APPROPRIATE HEALTH CARE
Outpatient except for severe cases. May also be inpatient for testing.

GENERAL MEASURES
• Oral carbohydrate for alert patient without drug overdose (2-3 tablespoons of sugar in glass of water or fruit juice, 1-2 cups of milk, a piece of fruit, soda cracker)
• If patient unable to swallow, glucagon IM or subcutaneously
• In hypoglycemia caused by drugs or certain nutrients, avoid or control the causative agents
• In hypoglycemia following meals - try high protein diet with restricted carbohydrates
• Avoid stress
• "Nonhypoglycemic hypoglycemia" or "pseudohypoglycemia"
    ◊ Many patients (often females, ages 20-45) present with the diagnosis of reactive hypoglycemia (self-diagnosed or overinterpretation of tests)
    ◊ Symptoms usually pertain to chronic fatigue and somatic complaints (stress often has a role in these symptoms)
    ◊ Management is difficult. Listening is important. Dietary changes, e.g., 120 gm carbohydrate diet, low in simple sugars can be recommended.
    ◊ Counseling - for stress or other problems may be useful

SURGICAL MEASURES   If islet cell tumor (insulinoma) - surgery is the treatment of choice. If it is inoperable, drug therapy may relieve symptoms.

ACTIVITY   May need to revise exercise routine

DIET
• High protein, low carbohydrate
• Frequent small feedings (6) instead of 2-3 larger meals
• Avoid fasting

PATIENT EDUCATION
• Instructions about fasting tests and interpretations of results
• Dietary instruction
• Counseling for stress, if appropriate
• Recognition of early symptoms of hypoglycemia and how to take corrective action

MEDICATIONS

DRUG(S) OF CHOICE
• Once an established diagnosis is made, drug therapy appropriate to the underlying disorder
• In patient unable to swallow - glucagon IM or subcutaneously. If no response, give IV glucose. For serious hypoglycemia, give IV bolus of 25-50 g of 50% glucose solution followed by a constant infusion of glucose until the patient can take by mouth.
• Insulinoma - see separate topic in book
• Postsurgical gastrectomy patients unresponsive to diet changes may benefit from propantheline which delays gastric emptying
Contraindications: Refer to manufacturer's literature
Precautions: Refer to manufacturer's literature
Significant possible interactions: Refer to manufacturer's literature

ALTERNATIVE DRUGS   N/A

FOLLOWUP

PATIENT MONITORING
• Dependent on type and severity of symptoms, and treatment of underlying cause
• Hypoglycemia from sulfonylurea can last for days

PREVENTION/AVOIDANCE
• Follow dietary and exercise guidelines
• Patient recognition of early symptoms and taking corrective action

POSSIBLE COMPLICATIONS   If tumor removed (insulinoma), some surgical risk involved

EXPECTED COURSE/PROGNOSIS
Favorable, with recognition and appropriate treatment

MISCELLANEOUS

ASSOCIATED CONDITIONS
• Insulinoma
• Severe liver disease
• Alcoholism
• Adrenocortical insufficiency
• Myxedema
• Malnutrition (patients with renal failure)
• Gastrointestinal surgery
• Panhypopituitarism
• Addison's disease

AGE-RELATED FACTORS
Pediatric: Usually divided into 2 syndromes (1) transient neonatal hypoglycemia and (2) hypoglycemia of infancy and childhood
Geriatric: More likely to have underlying disorders or be using causative drugs
Others: N/A

PREGNANCY   N/A

SYNONYMS
• Postprandial hypoglycemia
• Functional hypoglycemia
• Idiopathic hypoglycemia
• Alimentary hypoglycemia
• Postgastrectomy hypoglycemia
• Alcohol-induced hypoglycemia
• Factitious hypoglycemia
• Iatrogenic hypoglycemia
• Exogenous hypoglycemia

ICD-9-CM   251.2 Hypoglycemia, unspecified

SEE ALSO   Insulinoma

OTHER NOTES   N/A

ABBREVIATIONS   N/A

REFERENCES
• Foster DW, Rubenstein AH: Hypoglycemia. In: Braunwald E, Isselbacher KJ, Petersdorf RG, et al, eds. Harrison's Principles of Internal Medicine. 13 Ed. New York, McGraw-Hill, 1994:2000-2006
• Richardson CT: Zollinger-Ellison syndrome. In: Wyngaarden JB, Smith LH, Bennett JC, eds. Cecil: Textbook of Medicine. 19th Ed. Philadelphia, W.B. Saunders Co., 1992:665-667
Illustrations: N/A
Internet references: http://www.5mcc.com

Author(s)
Guy W. Neff, MD
Samuel Sim, MD
Ann Neff, MD

Hypokalemia

BASICS

DESCRIPTION Hypokalemia occurs when serum potassium (K) concentration is below the normal range, commonly 3.5-5.0 mEq/L (3.5-5.0 mmol/L).
System(s) affected: Endocrine/Metabolic, Nervous, Musculoskeletal, Renal/Urologic
Genetics:
• Some familial disorders are rare causes of hypokalemia
  ◊ Familial hypokalemic periodic paralysis
  ◊ Congenital adrenogenital syndromes
  ◊ Liddle's syndrome
  ◊ Familial interstitial nephritis
Incidence/Prevalence in USA: Common
Predominant age: N/A
Predominant sex: Male = Female

SIGNS AND SYMPTOMS
• Neuromuscular (most prominent manifestations) - skeletal muscle weakness (may range from mild weakness to total paralysis, including respiratory muscles); may lead to rhabdomyolysis in severe cases. Smooth muscle involvement may lead to gastrointestinal hypomotility producing ileus and constipation.
• Cardiovascular - ventricular arrhythmias, hypotension, cardiac arrest
• Renal - polyuria, nocturia due to impaired concentrating ability
• Metabolic - hyperglycemia

CAUSES
• General causes
  ◊ Decreased intake (uncommon): anorexia nervosa, deficient diet in alcoholics
  ◊ Gastrointestinal loss: vomiting, diarrhea, laxative abuse, fistulas, villous adenoma, ureterosigmoidostomy
  ◊ Intracellular shift of K (since only 2% of total body K is extracellular, hypokalemia can occur in the presence of normal total body K in those conditions that favor translocation of K from the extracellular to the intracellular compartment): metabolic alkalosis, insulin excess, beta adrenergic catecholamine excess (acute stress, intake of B2 agonists), hypokalemic periodic paralysis, intoxications (theophylline, barium, toluene)
• Renal potassium loss
  ◊ Drugs: diuretics, penicillin antibiotics, aminoglycosides
  ◊ Mineralocorticoid excess states: primary hyperaldosteronism, secondary hyperaldosteronism (congestive heart failure, cirrhosis, nephrotic syndrome, malignant hypertension, renin-producing tumors), Bartter's syndrome, congenital adrenogenital syndromes, exogenous mineralocorticoids (glycyrrhizic acid in licorice, carbenoxolone, steroids in nasal sprays), Liddle's syndrome
  ◊ Glucocorticoid excess states: Cushing's syndrome, exogenous steroids, ectopic ACTH production
  ◊ Renal tubular acidosis (RTA)
  ◊ Leukemia
  ◊ Magnesium depletion

RISK FACTORS Any disorder or medication regimen requiring potassium supplementation

DIAGNOSIS

DIFFERENTIAL DIAGNOSIS Spurious hypokalemia which occurs when blood with a high WBC count (> 100,000/mm3) is allowed to stand at room temperature (WBC's extract K from plasma)

LABORATORY Serum potassium < 3.5 mEq/L (< 3.5 mmol/L)
Drugs that may alter lab results: N/A
Disorders that may alter lab results: Leukemia and other conditions with high WBC

PATHOLOGICAL FINDINGS
• Vacuolization of proximal and distal renal tubular cells
• In severe hypokalemia, necrosis of cardiac and skeletal muscle

SPECIAL TESTS
• ECG - flattening or inversion of T waves, increased prominence of U waves, depression of ST segment, ventricular ectopia
• Work-up for etiology - excessive renal K loss is present when urinary K is in excess of 20 mEq/day in the presence of hypokalemia. In the patient with excessive renal K loss and hypertension (HTN), plasma renin and aldosterone levels should be determined to differentiate adrenal from non-adrenal causes of hyperaldosteronism. If HTN is absent and the patient is acidotic, RTA should be considered. If HTN is absent and serum pH is normal to alkalotic, a high urine chloride (> 10 mEq/day) (> 10 mmol/day) suggests hypokalemia secondary to diuretics or Bartter's syndrome and a low urine chloride (< 10 mEq/day) (< 10 mmol/day) suggests vomiting as the probable cause.

IMAGING If there is evidence of mineralocorticoid excess (see Special tests), proceed with CT scan of adrenal glands

DIAGNOSTIC PROCEDURES N/A

TREATMENT

APPROPRIATE HEALTH CARE
• Hypokalemia is usually not an emergency. For asymptomatic patients being treated with oral replacement, outpatient followup is sufficient.
• Patients with cardiac manifestations will require intravenous replacement with cardiac monitoring in an intensive care setting

GENERAL MEASURES
• Treatment of the underlying cause, if hypokalemia is mild
• When hypokalemia is severe, potassium replacement is necessary

SURGICAL MEASURES N/A

ACTIVITY No restrictions

DIET In mild hypokalemia (K = 3.0-3.5 mEq/L) (K = 3.0-3.5 mmol/L) not caused by GI losses, dietary supplementation may be sufficient. Potassium-rich foods include oranges, bananas, cantaloupes, prunes, raisins, dried beans, dried apricots, and squash.

PATIENT EDUCATION
• Instructions for diet
• If potassium supplementation is necessary, stress need for compliance

MEDICATIONS

DRUG(S) OF CHOICE
• For non-emergent conditions (serum K > 2.5 mEq/L [K > 2.5 mmol/L], no cardiac manifestations), oral therapy is preferred and doses of 40-120 mEq/day (40-120 mmol/day) are usually adequate. Potassium chloride is suitable for all forms of hypokalemia. Other K salts may be indicated if there is a coexisting disorder: Potassium bicarbonate or bicarbonate precursor (gluconate, acetate, or citrate) in metabolic acidosis or phosphate in phosphate deficiency.
• For emergent situations (serum K < 2.5 mEq/L [< 2.5 mmol/L], arrhythmias), intravenous replacement is indicated. The rate of administration should not exceed 20 mEq/hour (20 mmol/hour) and maximum recommended concentration is 60 mEq/L (60 mmol/L) of saline for peripheral administration. Central may give higher concentration.
• In non-emergent situations, intravenous K should be given only when oral administration is not feasible (e.g., vomiting, postoperative state). In this setting, rate should not exceed 10 mEq/hour and concentration should not exceed 40 mEq/L.
Contraindications: None
Precautions:
• Any form of K replacement carries the risk of hyperkalemia
• Serum K should be checked more frequently in groups at higher risk: Elderly, diabetics, and patients with renal insufficiency
• Patients receiving digitalis and patients with diabetic ketoacidosis in whom intracellular shift in K is expected after insulin therapy is initiated must have more aggressive replacement
Significant possible interactions:
Concomitant administration of K sparing diuretics (spironolactone, triamterene, amiloride) magnify the risk of hyperkalemia

ALTERNATIVE DRUGS   None

FOLLOWUP

PATIENT MONITORING
• Patients receiving intravenous therapy should have their serum K level checked frequently (q4-6 h)
• Patients requiring potassium supplements should have serum potassium studied at intervals dictated by calculation of patient compliance

PREVENTION/AVOIDANCE   Patients
being started on diuretics should be advised to increase their dietary K intake (see Diet)

POSSIBLE COMPLICATIONS
Hyperkalemia

EXPECTED COURSE/PROGNOSIS   The
ease of correction of hypokalemia and the need for prolonged treatment rests on the primary cause. If this can be eliminated (e.g., resolution of diarrhea, discontinuation of diuretics, removal of adrenal tumor), hypokalemia is expected to resolve and no further treatment is indicated.

MISCELLANEOUS

ASSOCIATED CONDITIONS   N/A

AGE-RELATED FACTORS   N/A
Pediatric: Not common in this age group, but may occur in chronic gastrointestinal loss or secondary to hyperadrenalism
Geriatric:
• Diuretic therapy, diarrhea and chronic laxative abuse are most common causes for hypokalemia in this age group
• May need to correct magnesium depletion
Others: N/A

PREGNANCY   Treatment is same

SYNONYMS   N/A

ICD-9-CM   276.8 Hypokalemia

SEE ALSO   N/A

OTHER NOTES   N/A

ABBREVIATIONS
RTA = renal tubular acidosis
K = potassium

REFERENCES
• Raymond KH, Kunau RT Jr: Hypokalemic states. In: Maxwell MH, Kleeman CR, Narins RG, eds. Clinical Disorders of Fluid and Electrolyte Metabolism. New York, McGraw-Hill, 1987:519-546
• Gabow PA, Peterson LN: Disorders of potassium metabolism. In: Schrier RW, ed. Renal and Electrolyte Disorders. Boston, Little, Brown and Company, 1986:207-250
Illustrations: N/A
Internet references: http://www.5mcc.com

Author(s)
K. Shashi Kant, MD

Hypokalemic periodic paralysis

BASICS

DESCRIPTION Episodic weakness associated with low serum potassium (K+) levels.
• Two forms exist:
  ◊ Familial hypokalemic periodic paralysis; the more common form (HPP) is usually inherited as an autosomal dominant trait
  ◊ Hypokalemic periodic paralysis with thyrotoxicosis (TPP); rarer, usually affects Asian males.
System(s) affected: Endocrine/Metabolic, Nervous, Musculoskeletal
Genetics: Autosomal dominant (HPP)
Incidence/Prevalence in USA: Not known (rare)
Predominant age: Onset of disease in late childhood or adolescence (HPP), early adulthood (TPP). Onset of disease after age 35 extremely rare.
Predominant sex:
• Male > Female (3:1) (HPP)
• Male > Female (20:1) (TPP)

SIGNS AND SYMPTOMS
• Episodic attacks of limb muscle weakness which last from a few hours to several days
• Typical attack comes on during sleep which was preceded by strenuous exercise
• Attacks also provoked by high carbohydrate or high sodium (Na+) meals
• Cold, stress, alcohol, diuretics, insulin, or epinephrine may also exacerbate attack
• Strength between attacks usually normal
• After years of prolonged, frequent attacks patient may develop persistent proximal weakness
• Myalgias
• Proximal weakness greater than distal weakness
• Muscles of the eyes, face, tongue, pharynx, larynx, diaphragm, and sphincters rarely involved
• Deep tendon reflexes hypoactive
• Sensation preserved

CAUSES
• Exact pathogenesis unknown
• Abnormality is in the muscle membrane
• A calcium channel mutation due to an abnormal gene on chromosome 1q 31-32 has been identified (HPP only)
• Contractile apparatus normal
• Defect may be related to increased Na+ "leak" across membrane into cell
• Na+ leak reduces electrical potentials across muscle membrane (prolonged depolarization), muscle will not propagate action potential and will not contract
• As cell membrane Na+, K+-ATPase pump tries to move Na+ out of cell, extracellular K+ is brought into cell due to K+-Na+ exchange
• Pathogenesis of HPP and TPP may be different since thyroid hormone doesn't worsen HPP

RISK FACTORS
• Male
• Age under 35
• Family history (HPP)
• Asian (TPP)

DIAGNOSIS

DIFFERENTIAL DIAGNOSIS
• Hyperkalemic periodic paralysis (adynamia episodica)
• Paramyotonia congenita
• Normokalemic periodic paralysis
• Barium poisoning
• Hyperventilation
• Secondary hypokalemia (laxative or diuretic use, diarrhea, vomiting, renal or adrenal disease, clay ingestion)
• Myasthenia gravis
• Guillain-Barré syndrome
• Tick paralysis
• Cataplexy
• Sleep paralysis
• Presyncope
• "Drop attacks"
• Akinetic epilepsy

LABORATORY
• Hallmark is low serum K+ (as low as 1.8 mEq/L [1.8 mmol/L])
• Urine K+ normal
• Elevated T3, T4, free thyroid index, and decreased TSH (TPP only)
Drugs that may alter lab results: N/A
Disorders that may alter lab results: N/A

PATHOLOGICAL FINDINGS
• Muscle biopsy may show atrophy, centrally placed vacuoles of sarcoplasm
• Electronmicroscopy studies show vacuoles are due to progressive dilatation of sarcoplasmic reticulum

SPECIAL TESTS
• With mild hypokalemia electrocardiogram (ECG) may show S-T depression, flattened T waves, presence of U waves
• With severe hypokalemia ECG may show peaked P waves, prolonged P-R interval, widened QRS
• Electromyography not helpful (usually normal between attacks)

IMAGING Thyroid scans using radioiodine (TPP only)

DIAGNOSTIC PROCEDURES
Provocative testing (50 to 100 g oral glucose with 2 to 4 g oral sodium followed by exercise, or 50 to 100 g oral glucose with 10-20 IU subcutaneous insulin) may be required. Patient should have cardiac monitoring during testing.

TREATMENT

APPROPRIATE HEALTH CARE
• Severe hypokalemia or weakness - inpatient with cardiac monitoring
• Mild hypokalemia or weakness - outpatient with close follow up

GENERAL MEASURES May rarely need respiratory support

SURGICAL MEASURES N/A

ACTIVITY As tolerated

DIET
• Avoid high carbohydrate, high sodium foods
• K+ rich fruit of dubious benefit

PATIENT EDUCATION N/A

Hypokalemic periodic paralysis

 MEDICATIONS

DRUG(S) OF CHOICE
• Acute attack
◊ Oral potassium chloride, 0.2 to 0.4 mEq/kg (0.2-0.4 mmol/kg), repeated every 15 to 30 min depending on response of ECG, serum K+, muscle strength (usual dose: 40 mEq [40 mmol])
◊ In life-threatening situation or if vomiting give intravenous (IV) KCl in mannitol [5% glucose or normal saline IV may worsen situation]. Bolus 0.1 mEq/kg (0.1 mmol/kg) every 5 to 10 min; monitor ECG, serum K+. (Usual dose: 15 mEq [15 mmol] over 15 minutes then 10 mEq/hr [10 mmol/hr] if peripheral IV, up to 60 mEq/hr [60 mmol/hr] if central IV and cardiac monitoring.)
• Prevention of attacks in HPP
◊ Oral KCl
◊ Acetazolamide (Diamox), 125 to 1000 mg/d divided qd to bid
• Prevention of attacks in TPP
◊ Treat underlying thyrotoxicosis with beta-adrenergic blocking agents (propranolol [Inderal] and others)
◊ Acetazolamide contraindicated

Contraindications:
• Acetazolamide - marked hepatic or renal dysfunction, hypersensitivity, adrenal failure, hyperchloremic acidosis, low serum Na+, K+
• Propranolol - cardiogenic shock, sinus bradycardia, 2nd or 3rd degree AV block, congestive heart failure, bronchial asthma

Precautions:
• Infusion of IV KCl must be monitored to avoid inadvertent infusion of large and potentially fatal doses
• Peripheral intravenous KCl infusion rates greater than 10 mEq/h (10 mmol/h) may be painful
• Acetazolamide - drowsiness or paresthesias at high doses
• Propranolol - impaired hepatic or renal function

Significant possible interactions:
• Acetazolamide - high dose aspirin
• Propranolol - reserpine, verapamil, aluminum hydroxide, phenytoin, rifampin, chlorpromazine, cimetidine, theophylline

ALTERNATIVE DRUGS
• Acute attack
◊ None
• Prevention of attacks in HPP
◊ Triamterene (Dyrenium) 25 to 100 mg/d
◊ Spironolactone (Aldactone) 25 to 100 200 mg/d
• Prevention of attacks in TPP
◊ Propylthiouracil, radioactive ablation of the thyroid

 FOLLOWUP

PATIENT MONITORING
• Follow serum K+, electrolytes (if on acetazolamide)
• Follow thyroid function tests (if on propranolol or propylthiouracil)

PREVENTION/AVOIDANCE See Medication (prevention of attacks) and Diet

POSSIBLE COMPLICATIONS Cardiac arrhythmias, respiratory collapse

EXPECTED COURSE/PROGNOSIS
• Frequency of attacks usually lessens with age
• After years of prolonged, frequent attacks patient may develop persistent proximal weakness

 MISCELLANEOUS

ASSOCIATED CONDITIONS
Hyperthyroidism with hypokalemic periodic paralysis with thyrotoxicosis, TPP

AGE-RELATED FACTORS
Pediatric: Onset of disease in late childhood or adolescence
Geriatric: Onset of disease after age 25-35 extremely rare; frequency of attacks usually lessens with age
Others: N/A

PREGNANCY N/A

SYNONYMS
• Paroxysmal myoplegia

ICD-9-CM 359.3 Hypokalemic familial periodic paralysis

SEE ALSO
• Hypokalemia
• Hyperthyroidism
• Myasthenia gravis
• Guillain-Barré syndrome

OTHER NOTES N/A

ABBREVIATIONS
• K+ = potassium
• Na+ = sodium
• ATPase = adenosine triphosphatase
• HPP = hypokalemic periodic paralysis (familial)
• TPP = thyrotoxic hypokalemic periodic

REFERENCES
• Barch R, Furman RE: Pathophysiology of myotonia and periodic paralysis. In: Asbury AK, McKhann GM, McDonald WI, eds. Diseases of the Nervous System, Clinical Neurobiology. 2nd Ed. Philadelphia, W.B. Saunders Co., 1992
• Ptacek LJ, Griggs RC: Periodic paralysis. In: Isselbacher KJ, Wilson JD, et al, eds. Harrison's Principles of Internal Medicine. 13th Ed. New York, McGraw Hill, 1994
• Stedwell R, Allen KM, Binder LS: Hypokalemic paralysis: A review of the etiologies, pathophysiology, presentation, and therapy. Am J Emerg Med 1992;10:143-148
• Sterns RH, Narins RG: Disorders of potassium balance. In: Stein JH, ed. Internal Medicine. 4th Ed. Boston, Little Brown & Co, 1994
• Ober KP: Thyrotoxic periodic paralysis in the United States: Report of 7 cases and review of the literature. Medicine 1992;71(3):109-120
• Jurkat-Rott K, Lehmann-Horn F, et al: A calcium channel mutation causing hypokalemic periodic paralysis. Human Molecular Genetics 1994;3(8):1415-1419
• Hoffman EP: Voltage-gated ion channelopathies: inherited disorders caused by abnormal sodium, chloride, and calcium regulation in skeletal muscle. Annual Review of Medicine 1995;46:431-441
• Lehmann-Horn F, Rüdel A: Channelopathies: the nondystrophic myotonias and periodic paralyses. Seminars in Pediatric Neurology 1996;3(2):122-139
• Ko GTC, Chow CC, Yeung HHL, et al: Thyrotoxic periodic paralysis in a Chinese population. QJ Med 1996;89:463-468
Illustrations: N/A
Internet references: http://www.5mcc.com

Author(s)
Chris Vincent, MD

Hyponatremia

BASICS

DESCRIPTION
Defined as a plasma sodium concentration < 135 mEq/L (< 135 mmol/L)
• Hypovolemic hyponatremia - there is a decrease in total body water (TBW) and a greater decrease in total body sodium. The extracellular fluid (ECF) volume is decreased. Orthostatic hypotension and other changes consistent with hypovolemia are present.
• Euvolemic hyponatremia - there is an increase in TBW with a normal total body sodium. The ECF volume is minimally to moderately increased but there is no edema.
• Hypervolemic hyponatremia - there is an increase in total body sodium and a greater increase in TBW. The ECF is increased markedly and there is edema.
• Redistributive hyponatremia - there is a shift of water from the intracellular compartment to the extracellular compartment with a resultant dilution of sodium. TBW and total body sodium are unchanged. This occurs with hyperglycemia.
• Pseudohyponatremia - there is a dilution of the aqueous phase by excessive proteins or lipids. TBW and total body sodium are unchanged. This occurs in hypertriglyceridemia or multiple myeloma.
System(s) affected: Endocrine/Metabolic
Genetics: N/A
Incidence/Prevalence in USA: Described as the most common electrolyte disorder seen in a general hospital population. A recent study of hospitalized patients found an incidence of 1% and a prevalence of 2.5%.
Predominant age: All ages
Predominant sex: Male = Female

SIGNS AND SYMPTOMS
• Lethargy
• Disorientation
• Generalized weakness
• Muscle cramps
• Anorexia
• Hiccups
• Nausea and vomiting
• Agitation or delirium
• Stupor
• Coma
• Depressed deep tendon reflexes
• Hypothermia
• Positive Babinski responses
• Cheyne-Stokes respiration
• Pseudobulbar palsy
• Seizures
• Orthostatic hypotension
• Cranial nerve palsies

CAUSES
• Hypovolemic hyponatremia (extrarenal loss of sodium)
  ◊ Gastrointestinal loss - vomiting, diarrhea
  ◊ Third spacing - peritonitis, pancreatitis, burns, rhabdomyolysis
  ◊ Skin loss - burns, sweating, cystic fibrosis
  ◊ Lung loss - bronchorrhea
• Hypovolemic hyponatremia (renal loss of sodium)
  ◊ Salt losing nephritis

  ◊ Mineralocorticoid deficiency
  ◊ Diuretic
  ◊ Bicarbonaturia - renal tubular acidosis, metabolic alkalosis
  ◊ Ketonuria or anion gap acidosis
  ◊ Partial urinary tract obstruction
  ◊ Osmotic diuresis
• Euvolemic hyponatremia
  ◊ Hypothyroidism
  ◊ Pure glucocorticoid deficiency
  ◊ Drugs
  ◊ Stress
  ◊ Syndrome of inappropriate antidiuretic hormone release (SIADH). Causes include pulmonary and central nervous system disorders.
• Hypervolemic hyponatremia
  ◊ Nephrotic syndrome
  ◊ Cirrhosis
  ◊ Congestive heart failure
  ◊ Renal failure
• Redistributive hyponatremia
  ◊ Hyperglycemia
  ◊ Mannitol infusion
• Pseudohyponatremia
  ◊ Hypertriglyceridemia
  ◊ Multiple myeloma

RISK FACTORS
Excessive fluid intake

DIAGNOSIS

DIFFERENTIAL DIAGNOSIS
See Causes

LABORATORY
• Serum sodium less than 135 mEq/L (135 mmol/L)
• Plasma osmolality
• Urine sodium
• BUN
• Creatinine
• Hypovolemic hyponatremia
  ◊ Plasma osmolality low
  ◊ BUN/creatinine ratio greater than 20/1
  ◊ Urine sodium > 20 mEq/L (> 20 mmol/L) - renal loss
  ◊ Urine sodium < 10 mEq/L (< 10 mmol/L) - extrarenal loss
  ◊ Serum potassium > 5.0 mEq/L (> 5 mmol/L) - consider mineralocorticoid deficiency
• Euvolemic hyponatremia
  ◊ Plasma osmolality low
  ◊ BUN/creatinine ratio less than 20/1
  ◊ Urine sodium > 20 mEq/L (> 20 mmol/L)
• Hypervolemic hyponatremia
  ◊ Plasma osmolality low
  ◊ Urine sodium < 10 mEq/L (< 10 mmol/L) in nephrotic syndrome, CHF, cirrhosis
  ◊ Urine sodium > 20 mEq/L (> 20 mmol/L) in acute and chronic renal failure
• Redistributive hyponatremia
  ◊ Plasma osmolality normal or high
  ◊ Glucose or mannitol levels elevated
• Pseudohyponatremia
  ◊ Plasma osmolality normal
  ◊ Triglyceride or protein levels elevated

Drugs that may alter lab results: N/A
Disorders that may alter lab results: N/A

PATHOLOGICAL FINDINGS N/A

SPECIAL TESTS
For euvolemic hyponatremia a thyroid stimulating hormone (TSH) to rule out hypothyroidism and a one-hour cosyntropin stimulation test to rule out adrenal insufficiency

IMAGING
• CT of head if pituitary problem suspected or if SIADH from CNS problem suspected
• Chest x-ray to rule out pulmonary pathology if SIADH diagnosed

DIAGNOSTIC PROCEDURES N/A

TREATMENT

APPROPRIATE HEALTH CARE
• Inpatient treatment mandatory if acute hyponatremia or symptomatic
• Inpatient treatment advised if asymptomatic and serum sodium less than 125 mEq/dL

GENERAL MEASURES
• Assess all medications patient is taking
• Institute seizure precautions

SURGICAL MEASURES N/A

ACTIVITY
Varies according to patient mental status

DIET
• Euvolemic hyponatremia - water restriction to 1000 cc/day
• Hypervolemic hyponatremia - water and sodium restriction
• Hypovolemic hyponatremia - isotonic saline
• Redistributive or pseudohyponatremia - treat underlying cause

PATIENT EDUCATION N/A

Hyponatremia

MEDICATIONS

DRUG(S) OF CHOICE
• Severe symptomatic hyponatremia: The use of hypertonic saline (3%) is clearly indicated only in patients who are both severely symptomatic and have sodium concentrations less than 120 mEq/L (120 mmol/L). Three percent saline should be used at a rate of 1 cc/kg/hr. This will raise the serum sodium level by approximately 1 mEq/L/hr (1 mmol/L/hr). The hypertonic saline infusion should only continue until a serum sodium of 120 mEq/L (120 mmol/L) is reached or the patient becomes asymptomatic. Avoid correction by more than 12 mEq/L/day (12 mmol/day).
• Chronic hyponatremia: If hyponatremia does not improve with fluid restriction or other appropriate treatment, consider using demeclocycline. In doses of 600-1200 milligrams per day, the drug produces a nephrogenic diabetes insipidus.
• Maintenance: Clinical judgment

Contraindications: Demeclocycline can cause nephrotoxicity in patients with liver disease

Precautions:
• Demeclocycline - photosensitivity and nausea can occur
• Three percent saline-rapid correction of severe symptomatic hyponatremia has been associated with central pontine myelinolysis (CPM). This neurologic disorder induces loss of myelin and supportive structures in the pons and occasionally in other areas of the brain. CPM is seen one to several days after rapid correction of serum sodium and is characterized by gradual neurologic deterioration.

Significant possible interactions:
Demeclocycline - oral anticoagulants, oral contraceptives, penicillin

ALTERNATIVE DRUGS   N/A

FOLLOWUP

PATIENT MONITORING
• Serum sodium level should be monitored when clinically indicated. If three percent saline is used the sodium level should be checked hourly.
• Volume status should be monitored if 3% or 0.9% saline is used

PREVENTION/AVOIDANCE   Dependent on underlying condition

POSSIBLE COMPLICATIONS
• Occult tumor may present with SIADH
• Hypervolemia if saline used
• Central pontine myelinolysis

EXPECTED COURSE/PROGNOSIS   With recognition and proper treatment a return to normal serum sodium and resolution of neurologic symptoms is expected. Prognosis is dependent on underlying condition.

MISCELLANEOUS

ASSOCIATED CONDITIONS
• Hypothyroidism
• Hypopituitarism
• Adrenocortical hormone deficiency

AGE-RELATED FACTORS   N/A
Pediatric: N/A
Geriatric: N/A
Others: N/A

PREGNANCY   N/A

SYNONYMS   N/A

ICD-9-CM   276.1 Hyposmolality and/or hyponatremia

SEE ALSO   N/A

OTHER NOTES   N/A

ABBREVIATIONS
• TBW = total body water
• ECF = extracellular fluid
• SIADH = syndrome of inappropriate antidiuretic hormone

REFERENCES   Schrier RW: Renal and Electrolyte Disorders. 3rd Ed. Boston, Little brown and Co., 1986
Illustrations: N/A
Internet references: http://www.5mcc.com

Author(s)
Peter Kozisek, MD

Hypoparathyroidism

 BASICS

DESCRIPTION Deficiency of parathyroid hormone (PTH) from disease, injury or congenital malfunction of the parathyroid glands. Manifested as hypocalcemia producing neuromuscular symptoms ranging from paresthesia to tetany.
• Classifications:
◊ Hypoparathyroidism (follows accidental removal or damage to parathyroid glands during surgery; may be transient or permanent)
◊ Idiopathic (parathyroids absent or atrophied)
◊ Pseudohypoparathyroidism (no PTH deficiency, but target organs do not respond to its action)
System(s) affected: Endocrine/Metabolic, Nervous, Musculoskeletal
Genetics: Idiopathic hypoparathyroidism may have a genetic component
Incidence/Prevalence in USA: All forms are rare
Predominant age: All ages
Predominant sex: Male = Female

SIGNS AND SYMPTOMS
• Chronic hypocalcemia may be asymptomatic
• Neuromuscular excitability as carpopedal spasm
• Increased deep tendon reflexes
• Chvostek's sign: hyperirritability of the facial nerve when tapped
• Trousseau's sign: carpopedal spasm within 2 minutes of inflating a blood pressure cuff over systolic pressure
• Dysphagia
• Organic brain syndrome
• Psychosis
• Mental deficiency (children)
• Tetany (paresthesias, pain, difficulty walking, laryngospasm, stridor, cyanosis, seizures)
• Dry hair
• Brittle fingernails
• Dry, scaly skin
• Cataracts
• Cardiac arrhythmias

CAUSES
• Idiopathic
◊ DiGeorge syndrome
◊ Congenital absence
◊ Late onset, autoimmune
• Postsurgical (may be transient)
• Infiltrative - metastatic carcinoma and others
• Irradiation
• Hypomagnesemia
• Alcohol

RISK FACTORS
• Neck surgery
• Neck trauma
• Head and neck malignancies

 DIAGNOSIS

DIFFERENTIAL DIAGNOSIS
• Rickets and osteomalacia
• Candidiasis
• Pseudohypoparathyroidism
• Addison's disease
• Pernicious anemia

LABORATORY
• Serum total and ionized calcium - decreased
• Serum phosphorus - increased (> 5.4 mg/dL [> 1.74 mmol/L])
• RIA (radioimmunoassay) for parathyroid hormone - decreased
Drugs that may alter lab results: Corticosteroids
Disorders that may alter lab results: Other hormonal disorders; hypoalbuminuria

PATHOLOGICAL FINDINGS
• Complete or almost complete replacement of parathyroid gland parenchymal tissue by fat
• Brain blood vessels calcified

SPECIAL TESTS
• ECG - increased Q-T and S-T intervals (due to hypocalcemia)
• Serum beta-carotene (normal)
• D-xylose absorption
• 72 hour stool fat
• Slit-lamp - may show early posterior lenticular cataract formation

IMAGING
• X-ray:
◊ Increased bone density
◊ Tooth roots absent
◊ Calcification of cerebellum, choroid plexus, cerebral basal ganglia

DIAGNOSTIC PROCEDURES N/A

 TREATMENT

APPROPRIATE HEALTH CARE
• Inpatient for work-up
• Inpatient for tetany
• Outpatient followup

GENERAL MEASURES
• Transient forms of hypoparathyroidism may not require treatment
• Acute attack hypoparathyroid tetany
◊ Is life-threatening and requires immediate IV treatment to raise calcium levels
◊ Verify adequate airway is present
◊ If patient is awake, breathing into paper bag can help raise serum calcium levels also
◊ Seizure prevention
◊ May require tracheostomy
• Maintenance
◊ Lifelong calcitriol and calcium
◊ Maintain serum calcium in the low normal range 8.5-9 mg/dL (2.12-2.25 mmol/L)
◊ Skin softeners for scaly skin
◊ Adequate control requires careful attention to avoid overtreatment or undertreatment

SURGICAL MEASURES N/A

ACTIVITY As tolerated

DIET No special diet

PATIENT EDUCATION
• Careful and detailed instructions about maintenance therapy
• Importance of periodic blood chemical evaluations
• Signs and symptoms of overtreatment and undertreatment to watch for

Hypoparathyroidism

MEDICATIONS

DRUG(S) OF CHOICE
• For tetany:
  ◊ Immediate IV calcium gluconate 10-20 mL of 10% solution given slowly until tetany ceases
  ◊ Calcium salts orally as soon as possible, 1-2 g daily
  ◊ Oral vitamin D (ergocalciferol) 500 IU/day
or
  ◊ Calcitriol - pediatric dose: 0.04-0.08 μg/kg/24 hr. Adult dose: 0.25 μg/24 hr. Then 0.25 μg qod. Adjust based on calcium and phosphorus levels.
• Maintenance:
  ◊ Calcium - 1-2 g daily in divided doses
  ◊ Oral vitamin D or calcitrol
  ◊ If associated endocrinopathies - appropriate hormone replacement
  ◊ Thiazide diuretic - for some patients to increase phosphate excretion and decrease calcium excretion
Contraindications: Refer to manufacturer's literature
Precautions: Refer to manufacturer's literature
Significant possible interactions: Refer to manufacturer's literature

ALTERNATIVE DRUGS N/A

FOLLOWUP

PATIENT MONITORING
• Outpatient after tetany
• Periodic blood chemical evaluations

PREVENTION/AVOIDANCE Care in surgical procedure that may cause damage to parathyroid glands

POSSIBLE COMPLICATIONS
• Neuromuscular symptoms (reversible)
• Cataracts
• Basal ganglia calcifications
• If condition starts early in childhood - stunting of growth, malformation of teeth, mental retardation
• Hypothyroidism
• Parkinsonian symptoms
• Ossification of the paravertebral ligaments
• Complications of overtreatment or undertreatment
• Institutionalized due to permanent mental damage

EXPECTED COURSE/PROGNOSIS
• Course - acute, chronic
• Transient hypoparathyroidism following surgery is reversible
• Fair outlook with diagnosis and treatment

MISCELLANEOUS

ASSOCIATED CONDITIONS
• DiGeorge's syndrome
• Addison's disease
• Mucocutaneous candidiasis

AGE-RELATED FACTORS
Pediatric:
• May occur in premature infants
• Congenital absence of parathyroids
• May appear later in childhood as idiopathic
Geriatric: Hypocalcemia fairly common in the elderly and may be due to multiple abnormalities
Others: N/A

PREGNANCY N/A

SYNONYMS Parathyroid tetany

ICD-9-CM 252.1 Hypoparathyroidism

SEE ALSO N/A

OTHER NOTES N/A

ABBREVIATIONS N/A

REFERENCES
• Wilson JD, Foster DW, eds: Williams Textbook of Endocrinology. 8th Ed. Philadelphia, W.B. Saunders Co., 1992
• Scriver CR, et al: The Metabolic Base of Inherited Disease. 7th Ed. New York, McGraw-Hill, 1995
• Guise TA, Mundy GR: Evaluation of hypocalcemia in children and adults. J Clin Endo & Metab 1995;80:1473-1478
Illustrations: N/A
Internet references: http://www.5mcc.com

Author(s)
Richard P. Levy, MD

Hypopituitarism

 BASICS

DESCRIPTION Generalized condition caused by partial or total failure of the pituitary gland's vital hormones - ACTH, TSH, LH, FSH, GH, prolactin (PRL)
System(s) affected: Endocrine/Metabolic, Reproductive, Skin/Exocrine, Nervous, Gastrointestinal, Musculoskeletal
Genetics: Some pituitary defects are congenital
Incidence/Prevalence in USA: Relatively rare
Predominant age: Occurs in adults and children. In children it causes dwarfism and pubertal delay.
Predominant sex: Male = Female

SIGNS AND SYMPTOMS
• Usually starts with hypogonadism or gonadotropin failure (decreased FSH and LH)
• Signs of hypofunction of target glands
• Secondary amenorrhea
• Impotence
• Infertility
• Decreased libido
• Diabetes insipidus (rare)
• Lethargy
• Tiredness
• Sensitivity to cold
• Anorexia
• Nausea
• Abdominal pain
• Lactation failure
• Retarded growth
• Failure of secondary sexual characteristics to develop
• Mental aberrations
• Headache
• Visual field defects
• Blindness

CAUSES
• Lesions or tumors of the anterior pituitary gland (intrasellar or extrasellar)
• Congenital defects
• Pituitary apoplexy
• Hypophysectomy
• Infiltrative diseases (e.g., sarcoidosis, histoplasmosis X)
• Sometimes idiopathic
• Lymphocytic hypophysitis
• Irradiation
• Accidental or surgical trauma
• Hypothalamic disease

RISK FACTORS
• Trauma
• Pregnancy and delivery

 DIAGNOSIS

DIFFERENTIAL DIAGNOSIS
• Primary hypothyroidism
• Anorexia nervosa
• Chronic liver disease
• Myotonia dystrophica
• Addison's disease
• Primary psychosis
• Primary hypogonadism

LABORATORY
• Confirms hormonal deficiencies
• Radioimmunoassay of pituitary and target gland hormones
• Provocative tests
Drugs that may alter lab results: Any hormone
Disorders that may alter lab results:
• Cushing's syndrome
• Addison's disease
• Hyperthyroidism
• Hypothyroidism

PATHOLOGICAL FINDINGS
• Destruction of anterior pituitary
• Atrophy of adrenal cortex, thyroid, gonads

SPECIAL TESTS
• Careful testing for smell
• Visual field examination by quantitative perimetry

IMAGING
• X-rays - chest, skull, hands, wrists (for bone age)
• CT or MRI

DIAGNOSTIC PROCEDURES N/A

 TREATMENT

APPROPRIATE HEALTH CARE
• Outpatient
• Inpatient for surgery when hypopituitarism is due to a pituitary tumor

GENERAL MEASURES
• Hormonal replacement
• Exercise program to rehabilitate
• Wear medical identification

SURGICAL MEASURES
• Surgery for pituitary tumor

ACTIVITY Encourage active physical exercise program

DIET High calorie, high protein

PATIENT EDUCATION
• Wear medical identification bracelet or necklace
• In patient with documented ACTH deficiency, stress need for additional cortisone at time of any major physical stress (e.g., fever above 101°F [38.3°C]; acute illness)

MEDICATIONS

DRUG(S) OF CHOICE
• Replacement of hormones secreted by the target glands:
◊ Hydrocortisone
◊ Thyroxine
◊ Androgen or cyclic estrogen
◊ Human growth hormone (for treating dwarfism)
◊ Dosages and administration schedule vary according to age and sex, refer to manufacturer's literature
Contraindications: Refer to manufacturer's literature
Precautions: Refer to manufacturer's literature
Significant possible interactions: Refer to manufacturer's literature

ALTERNATIVE DRUGS   N/A

FOLLOWUP

PATIENT MONITORING   3 and 12 month evaluations for post-treatment hormonal status. For patients with pituitary tumors include visual fields, thyroid and adrenal function, sellar computerized imaging.

PREVENTION/AVOIDANCE   None

POSSIBLE COMPLICATIONS
• Blindness
• Adrenal crisis
• Long-term medications

EXPECTED COURSE/PROGNOSIS
• Course - acute, chronic
• Variable, but guardedly favorable with replacement therapy
• If due to postpartum necrosis, may have complete or partial recovery

MISCELLANEOUS

ASSOCIATED CONDITIONS
• Childhood hypopituitarism
• Sheehan's syndrome
• Hypothyroidism
• Kallman's syndrome

AGE-RELATED FACTORS
Pediatric: Hypopituitarism in this age group leads to dwarfism due to lack of growth hormone
Geriatric: More difficult to diagnose
Others: N/A

PREGNANCY
• Severe postpartum hemorrhage can lead to hypopituitarism
• Lymphocytic hypophysitis may be triggered by pregnancy

SYNONYMS
• Pituitary cachexia
• Hypopituitarism syndrome
• Simmond's syndrome or disease
• Panhypopituitarism

ICD-9-CM
253.2 panhypopituitarism

SEE ALSO   N/A

OTHER NOTES   N/A

ABBREVIATIONS   N/A

REFERENCES
• Sheehan H, Summers VK: The syndrome of hypopituitarism. Q.J. Med 1949;42:319
• Vance M: Hypopituitarism. N Eng J Med 1994;330:1651
Illustrations: N/A
Internet references: http://www.5mcc.com

Author(s)
William F. Young, Jr., MD

Hypothermia

BASICS

DESCRIPTION Hypothermia occurs when a core (rectal, tympanic or esophageal) temperature falls below 35°C (95°F). It may take several hours or several days to develop. As the body temperature falls, all organ system are affected; cerebral blood flow decreases and the metabolic rate declines rapidly. Patients who have been immersed for as long as 45 minutes in very cold water and appear to be dead have still been resuscitated.
System(s) affected: Endocrine/Metabolic, Cardiovascular, Nervous, Skin/Exocrine
Genetics: N/A
Incidence/Prevalence in USA: Estimates vary widely due to lack of pathological evidence, and that hypothermia is usually considered a secondary cause in diagnosing disorders
Predominant age: Very young and the elderly
Predominant sex: Male = Female

SIGNS AND SYMPTOMS
• Mild (34-35°C)
  ◊ Lethargy
  ◊ Mild confusion
  ◊ Shivering
  ◊ Loss of fine motor coordination
  ◊ Increased pulse and blood pressure
  ◊ Peripheral vasoconstriction
• Moderate (30-34°C)
  ◊ Delirium
  ◊ Bradycardia
  ◊ Hypotension
  ◊ Hypoventilation
  ◊ Cyanosis
  ◊ Arrhythmias
  ◊ Semicoma and coma
  ◊ Muscular rigidity
  ◊ Generalized edema
  ◊ Slowed reflexes
• Severe (< 30°C)
  ◊ Very cold skin
  ◊ Rigidity
  ◊ Apnea
  ◊ No pulse - ventricular fibrillation or asystole
  ◊ Areflexia
  ◊ Unresponsive
  ◊ Fixed pupils

CAUSES
• Decreased heat production
• Increased heat loss
• Impaired thermoregulation

RISK FACTORS
• Malnutrition
• Cold water immersion
• Homeless
• Outdoor workers
• Trauma victims
• Alcohol consumption
• Mental illness
• Drug intoxication (barbiturates, phenothiazines, cyclic antidepressants, parasympatholytics, benzodiazepines, narcotics)

• Endocrinopathies (hypothyroidism, hypopituitarism, hypoadrenalism, hypoglycemia)
• Hypothalamic and CNS dysfunction
• Sepsis
• Cardiovascular disease
• Bronchopneumonia
• Hepatic failure
• Uremia
• Extensive skin disease
• Excessive fluid loss

DIAGNOSIS

DIFFERENTIAL DIAGNOSIS
• Cerebrovascular accidents
• Intoxication
• Drug overdose
• Complications of diabetes, hypothyroidism, hypopituitarism

LABORATORY
• Arterial blood gases (reported in the uncorrected form)
• Complete blood and platelet counts
• Toxicology screen
• Serum electrolytes
• Prothrombin time
• Partial thromboplastin time
• Fibrinogen levels
• Blood culture
• BUN/creatinine
• Glucose
• Amylase
• Liver function studies
• Thyroid function tests
• Serum cortisol
• Cardiac enzymes
Drugs that may alter lab results: Refer to laboratory test reference
Disorders that may alter lab results: Refer to laboratory test reference

PATHOLOGICAL FINDINGS
• Moderate dilation of right heart
• Pulmonary edema

SPECIAL TESTS
• Temperature measure - with special thermometers that can record low temperatures and measure core temperatures. Oral temperatures are of no value.
• Electrocardiogram - slowing of sinus rate with T-wave inversion, QT-interval prolongation, hypothermic J waves (Osburn waves) characterized by a notching of the QRS complex and ST segment
• Thyroid and pituitary function tests

IMAGING
X-rays of the cervical spine, chest, abdomen, if appropriate

DIAGNOSTIC PROCEDURES
History of prolonged exposure to cold may make the diagnosis obvious, but hypothermia may be overlooked, especially if patient is comatose

TREATMENT

APPROPRIATE HEALTH CARE Inpatient (emergency room or intensive care)

GENERAL MEASURES
• Establish ABC's of basic life support; establish airway, intubate if necessary. Give warm humidified oxygen (42-46°C). Correct metabolic acidosis.
• Evaluate for frostbite
• Rewarming
  ◊ Dependent on severity of hypothermia
  ◊ Rate of rewarming should be 0.5-2°C/hour. More rapid rewarming can cause ventricular fibrillation and hypovolemic shock.
• With all patients
  ◊ Remove wet garments
  ◊ Protect against heat loss and wind chill
  ◊ Maintain horizontal position
  ◊ Monitor core temperature and cardiac rhythm
• Mild hypothermia
  ◊ Passive rewarming (wrap in heated blanket or clothing)
  ◊ Administration of heated (43°C) IV solutions (D5NS)
  ◊ Warm fluids may be given if fully alert
• Moderate hypothermia
  ◊ Active external rewarming
  ◊ Heated blankets; heating pads
  ◊ Radiant heat sources
  ◊ Alcohol-circulating blankets
• Severe hypothermia
  ◊ Active internal (core) rewarming
  ◊ Peritoneal dialysis
  ◊ Gastrointestinal, colonic, or bladder lavage with warm fluids (43°)
  ◊ Heated intravenous fluids
  ◊ Heated humidified oxygen
  ◊ Thoracic cavity lavage (43°)
  ◊ Extracorporeal blood rewarming
• Cardiac arrhythmias
  ◊ Atrial fibrillation and sinus bradycardia are common, but patients usually convert to normal sinus rhythm with rewarming
  ◊ Transient type ventricular arrhythmias should not be treated. If treatment is required, bretylium is recommended.
  ◊ If cardiac pacing required, preferable to use external noninvasive pacemaker
• Sepsis bacterial infections
  ◊ In infants - signs may not be evident, initiate treatment with broad-spectrum antibiotic until culture results are available
  ◊ Older children and adults - if no signs, can usually wait for culture results
  ◊ Diabetic adults - consider prophylactic antibiotic coverage

SURGICAL MEASURES N/A

ACTIVITY Bedrest. Because of the cold, heart is irritable and susceptible to arrhythmias. Take special care in moving and transporting.

DIET Warm fluids only, if alert and able to swallow

Hypothermia

PATIENT EDUCATION
• Preventive measures to avoid recurrence
• If due to inadequate clothing or housing, refer patient to a social service agency
• Accidental hypothermia, NIH publication, No. 93-1464

MEDICATIONS

DRUG(S) OF CHOICE
• For sepsis or bacterial infection - antibiotics
• If ventricular fibrillation requires treatment, bretylium, 5 mg/kg, may be helpful. Magnesium sulfate, 100 mg/kg, is also effective.
• For hypoglycemia, D50W at a dose of 1 mg/kg IV
• Thiamine, 100 mg IV, should be given to any alcoholic or cachectic patient
• Naloxone, 2.0 mg IV, should be given to any patient with a depressed level of consciousness
• Levothyroxine 150-500 µg IV for hypothermic myxedema
• For severe acidosis - sodium bicarbonate
Contraindications:
• Medications, including epinephrine, lidocaine and procainamide can accumulate to toxic levels if used repeatedly in severely hypothermic patients
• Routine use of steroids, barbiturates or antibiotics have not been shown to increase survival or decrease postresuscitative damage
Precautions:
• If the patient fails to respond to the initial three defibrillation attempts or initial drug therapy, subsequent defibrillations or additional boluses of medication should be avoided until core temperature > 30°C. When temperature > 30°C, IV medications are indicated, but at longer than the standard intervals.
• Avoid vasopressors because of arrhythmogenic potential and delayed metabolism
• To prevent fluid overload, IV fluids should be slowly administered because of the decreased cardiac output
• Avoid lactated Ringer's solution because of decreased lactate metabolism
Significant possible interactions: Use all drugs cautiously because metabolism and renal elimination are impaired and once rewarming has occurred, there is mobilization of depot stores

ALTERNATIVE DRUGS N/A

FOLLOWUP

PATIENT MONITORING
• During acute episode
◊ Lab work repeated frequently (with particular attention to electrolytes and glucose)
◊ Continuous cardiac monitoring
◊ Urinary output monitoring
◊ Temperature monitoring
◊ Follow blood gases, both corrected and uncorrected
• Following acute episode
◊ Continued therapy for any underlying disorder

PREVENTION/AVOIDANCE
• Appropriate clothing for cold weather, with particular attention to head, feet and hand coverings
• If walking or climbing in cold climate, carry survival bags lined with space blankets for use if stranded or injured
• Avoid alcohol, especially if anticipating exposure to cold weather
• Alertness to early symptoms and initiating preventive steps, e.g., drinking warm fluids
• Adequate heat in the home
• Review patient's medications that may predispose to hypothermia (e.g., neuroleptics, sedatives, hypnotics, tranquilizers) and decrease dosage or discontinue if appropriate and feasible
• Referral of patient to social service agency for help with adequate housing, heat or clothing

POSSIBLE COMPLICATIONS
• Cardiac arrhythmias
• Hypotension secondary to marked vasodilatation of rewarming
• Pneumonia (aspiration and broncho)
• Pulmonary edema
• Pancreatitis
• Peritonitis
• Gastrointestinal bleeding
• Acute tubular necrosis
• Intravascular thromboses
• Metabolic acidosis
• Gangrene of extremities

EXPECTED COURSE/PROGNOSIS
• Mortality rates are decreasing for hypothermia due to increased recognition and advanced therapy. Mortality usually dependent upon the severity of underlying cause of hypothermia.
• In previously healthy individuals, recovery is usually complete
• Mortality rate in healthy patients < 5%
• Mortality rate in patients with co-existing illness > 50%

MISCELLANEOUS

ASSOCIATED CONDITIONS
• Congestive heart failure
• Hypothyroidism
• Hypopituitarism
• Uremia
• Addison's disease
• Ketoacidosis
• Pulmonary infection
• Sepsis
• Brain injury, tumor
• Diabetes

AGE-RELATED FACTORS
Pediatric:
• All infants are at increased risk of hypothermia because of their limited ability to produce heat when placed in a cold environment. This is particularly true during the first 12 hours of life and in asphyxiated infants. Newborns should be placed under a radiant heat source and the amniotic fluid dried off.
• A child's body temperature drops faster than an adult's when immersed in cold water. This may increase tolerance of the heart's arrhythmias.
Geriatric:
• Older adults have a lower metabolic rate and it is more difficult for them to maintain normal body temperature when environment drops below 18°C
• Aging also impairs the ability to detect temperature changes
• This population also has increased incidence of diseases that decrease heat production, increase or impair thermoregulation
Others: N/A

PREGNANCY Controlled hypothermia in the operating suite is safe during pregnancy, especially with cerebrovascular surgery

SYNONYMS Accidental hypothermia

ICD-9-CM
• 991.6 Accidental
• 995.89 Anesthetic
• 778.2-778.3 Newborn
• 780.9 Not associated with low environmental temperature

SEE ALSO
• Frostbite
• Near drowning

OTHER NOTES N/A

ABBREVIATIONS N/A

REFERENCES
• Cassel CK, Riesenberg DE, Sorensen LB, Walsh JR, eds: Geriatric Medicine. 2nd Ed. New York, Springer-Verlag, 1990
• Callahm ML, ed: Current Therapy in Emergency Medicine. Philadelphia, B.C. Decker Inc., 1987
• Danzl DT, Pozos R: Accidental hypothermia. New Engl J Med 1994;331:1756-1760
Illustrations: N/A
Internet references: http://www.5mcc.com

Author(s)
Scott T. Henderson, MD

Hypothyroidism, adult

BASICS

DESCRIPTION A clinical state resulting from decreased circulating levels of free thyroid hormone or from resistance to hormone action. Myxedema connotes severe hypothyroidism.
System(s) affected: Endocrine/Metabolic
Genetics:
• No known genetic pattern for idiopathic primary hypothyroidism
• Hypothyroidism may be associated with Type II autoimmune polyglandular syndrome, which is associated with HLA-DR3, DR4
• Secondary hypothyroidism frequently results from treatment for Graves disease, which may be familial
Incidence/Prevalence in USA:
• 5-10/1000 in general population
• Over age 65, increases to 6-10% of women, 2-3% of men
Predominant age: Over 40
Predominant sex: Female > Male, 5-10:1

SIGNS AND SYMPTOMS
• Symptoms
  ◊ Onset may be insidious, subtle
  ◊ Weakness, fatigue, lethargy
  ◊ Cold intolerance
  ◊ Decreased memory
  ◊ Hearing impairment
  ◊ Constipation
  ◊ Muscle cramps
  ◊ Arthralgias
  ◊ Paresthesias
  ◊ Modest weight gain (10 pounds [4.5 kg])
  ◊ Decreased sweating
  ◊ Menorrhagia
  ◊ Depression
  ◊ Hoarseness
  ◊ Carpal tunnel syndrome
• Signs
  ◊ Dry, coarse skin
  ◊ Dull facial expression
  ◊ Coarsening or huskiness of voice
  ◊ Periorbital puffiness
  ◊ Swelling of hands and feet
  ◊ Bradycardia
  ◊ Hypothermia
  ◊ Reduced systolic blood pressure
  ◊ Increased diastolic blood pressure
  ◊ Reduced body and scalp hair
  ◊ Delayed relaxation of deep tendon reflexes
  ◊ Macroglossia
  ◊ Dilutional hyponatremia
  ◊ Anemia (usually normochromic, normocytic)
  ◊ Enlarged heart on chest x-ray (often due to pericardial effusion)

CAUSES
• Post-ablative follows radioactive iodine therapy or thyroid surgery. Delayed hypothyroidism may develop in patients treated with thioamide drugs (propylthiouracil, methimazole) 4 to 25 years later.
• Primary hypothyroidism may develop as a result of autoimmune thyroiditis, or be idiopathic
• With goiter, most commonly due to autoimmune disease, such as Hashimoto's thyroiditis; or heritable biosynthetic defects, iodine deficiency (rare in the US), or drug induced (iodides, lithium, phenylbutazone, aminosalicylic acid)
• Suprathyroid hypothyroidism, may be due to deficiency of thyrotropin-releasing hormone (TRH) from the hypothalamus or thyroid-stimulating hormone (TSH) from the pituitary
• Transient hypothyroidism may result from silent thyroiditis (most common in post partum period) and subacute granulomatous thyroiditis

RISK FACTORS
• Risk increases with increasing age
• Autoimmune diseases

DIAGNOSIS

DIFFERENTIAL DIAGNOSIS
• Nephrotic syndrome
• Chronic nephritis
• Neurasthenia
• Depression
• Euthyroid sick syndrome
• Congestive heart failure
• Primary amyloidosis
• Dementia from other causes

LABORATORY
• Total serum thyroxine (T4) - decreased
• T3 resin uptake - increased
• TSH (radioimmunoassay) - elevated
• Free T4 index (= T3 resin uptake x total serum T4) - low
• In severe hypothyroidism, anemia, elevated cholesterol, CPK, LDH, AST, hyponatremia
Drugs that may alter lab results:
• Thyroid supplement
• Cortisone
• Dopamine
• Phenytoin
• Estrogen or androgen therapy in excess of replacement
• Amiodarone
• Salicylates
Disorders that may alter lab results:
• Any severe illness
• Pregnancy
• Chronic protein malnutrition
• Hepatic failure
• Nephrotic syndrome

PATHOLOGICAL FINDINGS Thyroid may be small, atrophic or enlarged

SPECIAL TESTS Radioimmunoassay

IMAGING None necessary

DIAGNOSTIC PROCEDURES Elevated TSH (greater than 20 μU/mL [3-20 mIU/L]) is diagnostic of primary thyroid failure

TREATMENT

APPROPRIATE HEALTH CARE Outpatient except for complicating emergencies (coma, hypothermia)

GENERAL MEASURES Goals of treatment are to restore and maintain a euthyroid state

SURGICAL MEASURES N/A

ACTIVITY As tolerated

DIET
• High-bulk diet may be helpful to avoid constipation
• Low fat diet for obese patients

PATIENT EDUCATION
• Importance of compliance with thyroid replacement therapy
• Need for lifelong treatment
• Report to physician any signs of infection, heart problems
• Signs of thyrotoxicity

Hypothyroidism, adult

MEDICATIONS

DRUG(S) OF CHOICE
• Levothyroxine (Synthroid, Levothroid)
◊ 50-100 µg/day. Increase by 25 µg/day every 4-6 weeks until TSH is in normal range.
◊ Dosage requirements may vary with age, sex, residual secretory capacity of thyroid gland, other drugs being taken by patient, intestinal function
◊ Elderly patients may require lower dose because clearance is decreased

Contraindications:
• Thyrotoxic heart disease
• Uncorrected adrenocorticoid insufficiency

Precautions:
• Start with lower doses in the elderly and patients with heart disease
• Diabetic patients may need readjustment of hypoglycemic agents with institution of thyroxine
• Dosage of oral anticoagulants may need adjustment; monitor prothrombin time while initiating treatment

Significant possible interactions:
• Oral anticoagulants
• Insulin
• Oral hypoglycemics
• Estrogen
• Oral contraceptives
• Cholestyramine
• Ferrous sulfate may decrease absorption when taken concomitantly

ALTERNATIVE DRUGS
None currently recommended

FOLLOWUP

PATIENT MONITORING
• Every 6 weeks until stabilized, then every 6 months
• Follow cardiac status closely in older patients

PREVENTION/AVOIDANCE N/A

POSSIBLE COMPLICATIONS
• Treatment induced congestive heart failure in people with coronary artery disease
• Myxedema coma - life threatening complication of hypothyroidism
• Increased susceptibility to infection
• Megacolon
• Organic psychosis with paranoia
• Adrenal crisis with vigorous treatment of hypothyroidism
• Infertility
• Hypersensitivity to opiates
• Overtreatment over long periods can lead to bone demineralization

EXPECTED COURSE/PROGNOSIS
• With early treatment, striking transformations in approved appearance and mental function. Return to normal state is the rule.
• Relapses will occur if treatment is interrupted
• If untreated, may progress to myxedema coma

MISCELLANEOUS

ASSOCIATED CONDITIONS
• Hyponatremia
• Anemia
• Idiopathic adrenocorticoid deficiency
• Diabetes mellitus
• Hypoparathyroidism
• Myasthenia gravis
• Vitiligo
• Hypercholesterolemia
• Mitral valve prolapse
• Depression
• Rapid cycling bipolar disorder

AGE-RELATED FACTORS
Pediatric: N/A
Geriatric:
• Characteristic signs and symptoms frequently changed or absent. Hypothyroidism is common in elderly. Diagnosis based on laboratory criteria.
• Replacement therapy is usually about two thirds of the dose used in young adults.
Others: N/A

PREGNANCY
• Replacement therapy may need adjustment. TSH levels should be monitored monthly during first trimester.
• Postpartum - check TSH levels at about 6 weeks
• Painless subacute thyroiditis may occur in the post partum period leading to transient hypothyroidism lasting about 3 months. Treatment with replacement therapy may be warranted. Up to 30% of these individuals develop permanent hypothyroidism.

SYNONYMS Myxedema

ICD-9-CM
• 244 Acquired hypothyroidism
• 244.0 Postsurgical hypothyroidism
• 244.2 Iodine hypothyroidism

SEE ALSO
• Thyroiditis
• Hyperthyroidism

OTHER NOTES
• Surgical procedures
◊ Hypothyroid patients (mild to moderate) tolerate surgery with mortality and complications similar to euthyroid patients
◊ If surgery is elective, render patient euthyroid prior to procedure
◊ If surgery is urgent, proceed with the procedure with individualized replacement therapy preoperatively and postoperatively

ABBREVIATIONS N/A

REFERENCES
• Barzel US: Hypothyroidism: diagnosis and management. Clin Geriatric Med 1995;11(2):239-249
• Ridgway EC: Modern concepts of primary thyroid gland failure. Clin Chemistry 1996;42(1)179-182
• Rudy DR, Tzagournis M: In: Rakel R, ed. Textbook of Family Medicine. 5th Ed. Philadelphia, WB Saunders Co, 1995:1099-1102
Illustrations: N/A
Internet references: http://www.5mcc.com

Author(s)
Barbara A. Majeroni, MD

Id reaction

BASICS

DESCRIPTION   A localized or generalized autosensitization skin reaction to a primary infection (fungi most often, sometimes unknown) at a site distant to a primary infection
• Most commonly the "id" reaction occurs on the hands with an acute dermatophytosis of the feet
System(s) affected: Skin/Exocrine
Genetics: N/A
Incidence/Prevalence in USA: Unknown, but common
Predominant age: All ages beyond infancy
Predominant sex: Male = Female

SIGNS AND SYMPTOMS
• Dyshidrotic-like, pruritic vesicular eruptions most commonly involving the sides of the fingers
• May occur as generalized eruptions
• May be accompanied by generalized adenopathy, splenomegaly, anorexia, and fever
• Generalized reaction may be seen with tinea capitis

CAUSES   Autosensitization to blood-borne circulating antigens at sensitized areas of skin

RISK FACTORS
• Tinea of the feet or hands
• Fungal infection elsewhere on the skin

DIAGNOSIS

DIFFERENTIAL DIAGNOSIS   Dyshidrotic eczema

LABORATORY
• Absence of fungal infection at site of reaction
• Definite fungal infection at a distant site
Drugs that may alter lab results: N/A
Disorders that may alter lab results: N/A

PATHOLOGICAL FINDINGS
• Vesicles in the upper dermis
• Lack of inflammation
• Acanthosis
• Increased granular cell layer

SPECIAL TESTS   Positive trichophytin skin test. Not very useful.

IMAGING   N/A

DIAGNOSTIC PROCEDURES   Potassium hydroxide (KOH) prep

TREATMENT

APPROPRIATE HEALTH CARE
Outpatient

GENERAL MEASURES   "Id" reaction will resolve with appropriate treatment of underlying primary infection

SURGICAL MEASURES   N/A

ACTIVITY   Fully active

DIET   No special diet

PATIENT EDUCATION
To prevent fungal infections of the feet:
   ◊ Good personal hygiene
   ◊ Wearing rubber or wooden sandals in community showers or bathing places
   ◊ Careful drying between the toes after showering or bathing
   ◊ Changing socks frequently
   ◊ Applying drying or dusting powder

MEDICATIONS

DRUG(S) OF CHOICE Appropriate medications to treat primary infection
Contraindications: Refer to manufacturer's profile of each drug
Precautions: Refer to manufacturer's profile of each drug
Significant possible interactions: Refer to manufacturer's profile of each drug

ALTERNATIVE DRUGS Systemic steroids bring about prompt clearing of the autoeczematous lesions, but will cause the underlying, original disease to heal more slowly

FOLLOWUP

PATIENT MONITORING Followup until original infection is resolved

PREVENTION/AVOIDANCE Prompt treatment of infections

POSSIBLE COMPLICATIONS Secondary bacterial infection may occur

EXPECTED COURSE/PROGNOSIS
• Resolution, with adequate treatment of primary disorder
• Recrudescence if treatment is inadequate

MISCELLANEOUS

ASSOCIATED CONDITIONS Primary fungal infection

AGE-RELATED FACTORS
Pediatric: N/A
Geriatric: N/A
Others: N/A

PREGNANCY N/A

SYNONYMS
• Dermatophytid
• Trichophytid

ICD-9-CM 692.89 Id reaction (due to bacteria)

SEE ALSO
• Tinea pedis
• Tinea corporis

OTHER NOTES Not all dyshidrotic eruptions are "id" reactions

ABBREVIATIONS N/A

REFERENCES Habif T: Clinical Dermatology. 3rd Ed. St. Louis, CV Mosby, 1996
Illustrations: 1 available on CD-ROM
Internet references: http://www.5mcc.com

Author(s)
Jose R. Parker, MD

Idiopathic hypertrophic subaortic stenosis (IHSS)

BASICS

DESCRIPTION This entity was the first known form of the hypertrophic cardiomyopathies (HCM) with the characteristic finding of inappropriate (disproportionate to the hemodynamic load) myocardial hypertrophy
• IHSS is characterized by a dynamic pressure gradient in the subaortic area leading clinically to both:
  ◊ Diastolic dysfunction with impaired ventricular filling and elevated atrial filling pressures producing dyspnea
  ◊ Systolic dysfunction with limitation of cardiac output response to exercise, exertional syncope, and secondary left ventricular hypertrophy
• Diagnosis usually is made by recognition of signs associated with outflow obstruction, but symptoms are predominantly characterized by diastolic dysfunction
System(s) affected: Cardiovascular
Genetics:
• Autosomal dominant with > 50% penetrance
• Evidence of disease (usually milder) is found in 25% of first degree relatives. Relatives usually do not have outflow obstruction, exhibit only localized hypertrophy, and are asymptomatic.
Incidence/Prevalence in USA:
Uncommon
Predominant age: Most commonly presents in third decade (disease of young adulthood), but occurs from newborns to elderly
Predominant sex: Male = Female

SIGNS AND SYMPTOMS
• Dyspnea: mainly a result of diastolic dysfunction and initially exertional in onset (50-90%)
• Angina pectoris (50-90%)
• Syncope: exertional (50-90%)
• Presyncope: exertional (50-90%)
• Fatigue (50-90%)
• Palpitations (50-90%)
• Paroxysmal nocturnal dyspnea (50%)
• Double apical impulse due to prominent atrial system
• PMI displaced laterally
• Rapidly rising bifid carotid pulse
• Prominent S4
• S2 variable splitting (depending on degree of outflow obstruction)
• Harsh systolic crescendo-decrescendo murmur best heard between apex and left sternal border
• Murmur: increases and lengthens with Valsalva, standing, amyl nitrite; decreases with sudden squatting, lying down, passive leg raising, isometric handgrip

CAUSES Thickened septum impinging on the anterior mitral valve leaflet during systole causing outflow obstruction

RISK FACTORS Family history of HCM

DIAGNOSIS

DIFFERENTIAL DIAGNOSIS
• Fixed outflow obstruction such as aortic stenosis (AS). In AS the carotid pulse is slow-rising and reduced in volume versus the rapid-rising bifid pulse of IHSS. Bedside hemodynamic maneuvers (Valsalva, etc.) also help to differentiate.

LABORATORY N/A
Drugs that may alter lab results: N/A
Disorders that may alter lab results: N/A

PATHOLOGICAL FINDINGS
• Distinctive pattern of left ventricular (LV) hypertrophy - localized disproportionate hypertrophy of the LV septum with the ratio of septal to free wall thickness > 1.3:1 without anatomic evidence of pressure overload
• Dilated atria
• Increased LV mass and small chamber sizes
• Mural plaque of LV outflow tract
• Mitral valve thickening
• Anatomic variants:
  ◊ Apical form; not associated with intraventricular gradients
  ◊ Localized mid-ventricular obstructive form
• Disorganization and disarray septal muscle bundles
• Abnormal intramural coronary arteries

SPECIAL TESTS
• Electrocardiogram: Common findings (50-90%)
  ◊ Non-specific ST-T wave abnormalities
  ◊ Left ventricular hypertrophy
• Electrocardiogram: Less common findings (< 50%)
  ◊ Prominent and abnormal Q waves in anterior precordial and lateral limbs lead, simulating myocardial infarction
  ◊ P-wave abnormalities indicating left atrial enlargement
  ◊ Short PR interval with QRS morphology suggestive of pre-excitation without clear evidence of pre-excitation (rare in IHSS)
  ◊ Holter findings - frequent ventricular arrhythmias with up to 25% revealing ventricular tachycardia
  ◊ Atrial fibrillation - late finding and poor prognostic sign

IMAGING Chest x-ray - variable findings from normal cardiac size to cardiomegaly, none of which is pathognomonic

DIAGNOSTIC PROCEDURES
• Echocardiography
  ◊ Asymmetric septal hypertrophy with septal to free wall ratio > 1.3:1
  ◊ Abnormal systolic anterior leaflet motion of the mitral valve
  ◊ Left ventricular hypertrophy
  ◊ Left atrial enlargement
  ◊ Small ventricular chamber size with increased contractility
  ◊ Partial systolic closure of aortic valve in mid-systole
  ◊ Mitral valve prolapse
  ◊ Mitral regurgitation by Doppler

◊ Decreased mid-aortic flow coincident with systolic anterior leaflet motion of mitral valve by Doppler
• Radionuclide
  ◊ Thallium scintigraphy with stress at times reveals positive defects in setting of arteriographically normal coronary arteries
• Cardiac catheterization and angiocardiography
  ◊ Hemodynamic measurement documents degree and lability of outflow obstruction, and diastolic characteristics of left ventricle
  ◊ Angiocardiography documents left and right ventricular anatomy and coronary arterial anatomy

TREATMENT

APPROPRIATE HEALTH CARE
Outpatient usually. Inpatient for studies and/or surgery.

GENERAL MEASURES
• Therapy based on pathophysiology, namely interventions to reduce ventricular contractility or increase ventricular volume, ventricular compliance, and outflow tract dimensions
• Digitalis glycosides are contraindicated except for atrial fibrillation with uncontrolled response
• Nitrates and sympathomimetic amines (e.g., isoproterenol) are contraindicated except with concomitant coronary heart disease
• Diuretics are relatively contraindicated because of their effect on ventricular volume and left ventricular myotomy

SURGICAL MEASURES
Left ventricular myomectomy - done only in setting of severe symptoms refractory to therapy in those patients with outflow gradient > 50 mm Hg (> 6.65 kPa), either at rest or with provocation. 95% successful in abolishing gradient with 70% of patients having marked symptomatic improvement for at least 5 years.

ACTIVITY
• Strenuous exercise, especially competitive sports, should not be undertaken because of high risk of sudden death. Younger patients with little or no functional impairment have the greatest risk of sudden death.
• Sports participation by patients with IHSS is not permitted if any of the following are present: Marked left ventricle hypertrophy, significant outflow gradient, significant supraventricular and/or ventricular arrhythmias, or history of sudden death in relatives with hypertrophic cardiomyopathy

DIET No special diet, but may need to reduce caloric intake, due to reduced activity

PATIENT EDUCATION
• Activity restrictions
• Refer for psychosocial counseling if appropriate (patient and family may suffer from restricted life-style and chronic disease problems)
• Recommend family learn cardiopulmonary resuscitation methods

MEDICATIONS

DRUG(S) OF CHOICE
• Propranolol (Inderal)
◊ May decrease outflow obstruction: Some evidence suggests that it may increase ventricular compliance. No clear evidence that it reduces incidence of sudden death.
◊ 1/3 to 2/3 of patients experience symptomatic improvement
◊ May titrate up to dose of 320 mg/day to obtain clinical effect provided patient tolerates dose
• Verapamil (Calan, Isoptin, Verelan)
◊ Alternative to therapy with propranolol
◊ May have better effect on exercise performance
◊ Decrease in outflow gradient due to depression of cardiac contractility
◊ Improves diastolic filling by improved diastolic relaxation
• Amiodarone (Cordarone)
◊ Limited use in treating ventricular arrhythmias because of documented pro-arrhythmic effects in HCM
◊ Only to be used in patients with ventricular tachycardia associated with hemodynamic compromise. Use of drug is to be guided by initial and followup electrophysiological studies.
Contraindications:
• Verapamil:
◊ Major side effects include depression of impulse formation and A-V block, negative inotropism, and vasodilatation - all of which can result in hypotension, shock, pulmonary edema, and death
◊ Therefore, relatively contraindicated for use in patients with increased left ventricle end diastolic pressure (LVEDP), paroxysmal nocturnal dyspnea (PND), orthopnea, and/or in patients with sinus node disease and A-V block (unless there is an appropriate pacing device)
Precautions: See manufacturer's profile of each drug
Significant possible interactions: See manufacturer's profile of each drug

ALTERNATIVE DRUGS
• Diltiazem
• Disopyramide

FOLLOWUP

PATIENT MONITORING Yearly when symptoms and pharmacologic regimens become stable

PREVENTION/AVOIDANCE
• Avoid strenuous exercise, especially competitive sports
• Avoid rapid standing
• Avoid inotropic drugs and diuretics
• Use antitussives for infections that are accompanied by a cough

POSSIBLE COMPLICATIONS
• Sudden death
• Congestive heart failure
• Arrhythmia
• Atrial fibrillation with mural thrombosis formation
• Infective mitral endocarditis

EXPECTED COURSE/PROGNOSIS
• Annual mortality rate - 4% a year (sudden death most common reason)
• Chronic illness with restricted life-style

MISCELLANEOUS

ASSOCIATED CONDITIONS
• Mitral regurgitation
• Essential hypertension
• Mitral valve prolapse
• Angina pectoris

AGE-RELATED FACTORS
Pediatric:
• IHSS being recognized with increasing frequency
• Children may be asymptomatic. Evaluation of a heart murmur may disclose IHSS.
Geriatric: Occurrence is more frequent with increasing age. Female prevalence is greater in this age group.
Others: N/A

PREGNANCY N/A

SYNONYMS
• Hypertrophic obstructive cardiomyopathy (HOCM)
• Muscular subaortic stenosis

ICD-9-CM 425.1

SEE ALSO N/A

OTHER NOTES Genetic counseling may be appropriate

ABBREVIATIONS
• HCM = hypertrophic cardiomyopathy
• AS = aortic stenosis
• LV = left ventricle
• PMI = Point of maximal impulse

REFERENCES
• Braunwald E, ed: Heart Disease: A Textbook of Cardiovascular Medicine. 4th Ed. Philadelphia, W.B. Saunders Co., 1992
• Maron BJ, et al: Sudden death in hypertrophic cardiomyopathy. A profile of 78 patients. Circulation 1982;65:1388
Illustrations: N/A
Internet references: http://www.5mcc.com

Author(s)
Peter Kozisek, MD

Idiopathic thrombocytopenic purpura (ITP)

 BASICS

DESCRIPTION A decrease in the circulating number of platelets (< 100,000 per microliter) in absence of toxic exposure or a disease associated with a low platelet count. It occurs as a secondary effect of peripheral platelet destruction as well as decreased platelet production. It is a diagnosis of exclusion.
• Acute ITP - a disease of childhood which usually follows an acute infection and has spontaneous resolution within 2 months. Platelet counts < 20,000. This is a common disorder.
• Chronic ITP - a disease which persists after 6 months without a specific cause. Usually seen in adults and persists for months to years. Platelet count typically 30,000-80,000.
System(s) affected:
Hemic/Lymphatic/Immunologic
Genetics: No known genetic pattern
Incidence/Prevalence in USA: 1 in 10,000
Predominant age:
• Acute ITP - children ages 2-9 years old
• Chronic ITP - 20-50 years old
Predominant sex:
• Acute ITP - Male = Female
• Chronic ITP - Female > Male (3:1)

SIGNS AND SYMPTOMS
• Post traumatic bleeding at 40,000-60,000 platelet count
• Petechial hemorrhages
• Purpura
• Bruising tendency
• Gingival bleeding
• Gastrointestinal bleeding
• Mucocutaneous hemorrhages
• Menometrorrhagia
• Menorrhagia
• Recurrent epistaxis
• Neurological symptoms secondary to intracerebral bleeding
• Non-palpable spleen (absence of splenomegaly is an essential diagnostic criterion)
• Spontaneous bleeding < 20,000 platelet count

CAUSES IgG autoantibodies on platelet surface

RISK FACTORS
• Acute infection
• Age
• Cardiopulmonary bypass
• Hypersplenism
• Antiphospholipid antibody syndrome
• Preeclampsia
• HIV infection

 DIAGNOSIS

DIFFERENTIAL DIAGNOSIS
• Drug induced immune thrombocytopenia. Over 150 drugs have been implicated.
• Infections
• Acute leukemia
• Thrombotic thrombocytopenia purpura (TTP)
• Hemolytic uremic syndrome
• Factitious: "platelet clumping on the peripheral smear"
• Thrombocytopenia secondary to sepsis
• Myelodysplastic syndrome, particularly in the older patient
• Decreased production in marrow: malignancy, drugs, viruses, megaloblastic anemia
• Post transfusion
• Isoimmune neonatal purpura
• Disseminated intravascular coagulation (DIC)
• Alcohol induced

LABORATORY
• Decreased platelet count: 5,000-75,000
• Relative lymphocytosis and slight eosinophilia
• Prolonged bleeding time (not useful in the presence of thrombocytopenia)
• Anemia
• PT, PTT normal
Drugs that may alter lab results: N/A
Disorders that may alter lab results: N/A

PATHOLOGICAL FINDINGS
• Peripheral smear shows normal red and white cells with diminished but large platelets
• Marrow reveals abundant megakaryocytes with normal erythroid and myeloid precursors

SPECIAL TESTS
• Peripheral smear
• Platelet associated antibody (PA-IgG)

IMAGING CT of head to rule out intracranial bleeding

DIAGNOSTIC PROCEDURES Bone marrow aspiration/biopsy

 TREATMENT

APPROPRIATE HEALTH CARE
• Outpatient management unless patient at risk for bleeding (platelet count < 20,000)
• Admit patients with active bleeding

GENERAL MEASURES
• Specific treatment usually not necessary unless count is < 100,000; possibly < 30,000 with chronic ITP
• Platelet transfusions for significant bleeding

SURGICAL MEASURES Splenectomy in patients who fail medical therapy. Be sure to administer pneumococcal vaccine at least 2 weeks prior to splenectomy.

ACTIVITY Minimal activity to prevent injury or bruising. Avoid contact sports.

DIET No special diet

PATIENT EDUCATION Avoidance of ASA and other platelet inhibiting drugs

Idiopathic thrombocytopenic purpura (ITP)

MEDICATIONS

DRUG(S) OF CHOICE
• Acute ITP: prednisone 1-2 mg/kg/day for 4 weeks, then taper. If refractory, consider splenectomy.
• Chronic ITP: prednisone 60 mg/day for 4-6 weeks, then taper. May require repetition. If ineffective at non-toxic doses, consider splenectomy. Prednisone may then be effective. If still refractory, consider alternate drugs.
Contraindications: Do not administer gamma globulin if patient has IgA deficiency
Precautions: Refer to manufacturer's literature
Significant possible interactions: Anaphylaxis in patients with IgA deficiency who have IgA auto-antibodies

ALTERNATIVE DRUGS
• Acute ITP: Immune globulin, intravenous (IVIG, gamma globulin) 1-2 gm/kg single dose or 400 mg/kg/day for 5 days. Minor adverse reactions - chills, nausea, headache, joint pains in 2-7%. If this occurs, slow the rate of infusion. Gamma globulin may be effective alone or as a pretreatment to facilitate platelet transfusion. May delay need for splenectomy.
• Chronic ITP: high doses of intravenous gamma globulin in emergencies
• Azathioprine or cyclophosphamide as single agents; either at doses of 2 mg/kg/day for 1-6 months
• Vincristine or vinblastine
• Danazol 200-400 mg bid
• Plasmapheresis
• Interferon
• rho(D) immune globulin 250 IU (50 µg/kg) as a single dose or in two divided doses given over 2 days; indications for use:
 ◊ Children with acute or chronic ITP
 ◊ Adults with chronic ITP
 ◊ ITP secondary to HIV infection

FOLLOWUP

PATIENT MONITORING
• Frequent platelet counts, daily to weekly, depending on severity and treatment
• Follow clinical status of hemostasis

PREVENTION/AVOIDANCE Avoid medications (when feasible) that inhibit platelet function (such as aspirin), or those that suppress bone marrow

POSSIBLE COMPLICATIONS
• 1% mortality due to intracranial hemorrhage
• Severe blood loss
• Corticosteroid adverse effects
• Pneumococcal infections if patient must have splenectomy. Use pneumococcal vaccine.

EXPECTED COURSE/PROGNOSIS
• Acute ITP:
 ◊ 80-85% completely recover within 2 months
 ◊ 15% proceed to chronic ITP
• Chronic ITP:
 ◊ 10-20% recover spontaneously
 ◊ Remainder with diminished platelets for months to years
 ◊ May see spontaneous remissions (5%) and relapses

MISCELLANEOUS

ASSOCIATED CONDITIONS
• Acute ITP:
 ◊ Varicella
 ◊ Other viral infections
• Chronic ITP:
 ◊ HIV
 ◊ Graves' disease
 ◊ Hashimoto's thyroiditis
 ◊ Sarcoidosis
 ◊ Systemic lupus erythematosus
 ◊ Autoimmune hemolytic anemia (Evans' syndrome)

AGE-RELATED FACTORS
Pediatric:
• The acute form is primarily a childhood disease
• Better prognosis than adults
Geriatric: ITP is uncommon in this age group; look for other cause of low platelet count
Others: N/A

PREGNANCY
• Patient in labor should receive intravenous gamma globulin due to risk to the infant
• Platelet autoantibodies cross the placenta and may cause neonatal thrombocytopenia. Consider prednisone 10-20 mg/day for 10-14 days prior to delivery.
• Preeclampsia may cause thrombocytopenia unrelated to ITP

SYNONYMS
• Postinfectious thrombocytopenia
• Immune thrombocytopenic purpura
• Werlhof's disease

ICD-9-CM 287.3 Primary thrombocytopenia

SEE ALSO N/A

OTHER NOTES N/A

ABBREVIATIONS N/A

REFERENCES
• Diagnosis and treatment of idiopathic thrombocytopenia purpura. American Society of Hematology ITP practice guideline panel. Amer Fam Phys 1996;54:2437-2447
• Schrier SL: Disorder of hemostasis and coagulation. Scientific American Medicine. New York, Scientific American 1993;5(6):14-21
• George JN, El-harake MA, Raskob GE: Chronic idiopathic thrombocytopenia purpura. N Engl J Med 1994;331:1207-1210
• Kirchner JT: Acute and chronic immune thrombocytopenia purpura. Post Grad Med 1992;92:112-126
Illustrations: N/A
Internet references: http://www.5mcc.com

Author(s)
Jeffery T. Kirchner, DO, FAAFP
Robert H. Scott, MD

Immunizations

BASICS

DESCRIPTION For the prevention of certain diseases.
Specific indications include:
Hepatitis B
• Infants (birth, 1 month and 6 months of age)
• Healthcare workers
• Laboratory personnel who might be exposed to the virus
• Intravenous drug users
• Male homosexuals
• Patients with a sexually transmitted disease
Pneumococcal
• All persons over age 65
• All patients prior to splenectomy
• Patients with chronic liver, heart, lung or renal disease
• Patients with diabetes mellitus, HIV, asplenia
Influenza
• All persons over age 65
• Healthcare workers
• Patients with chronic heart, lung or renal disease (may begin at 6 months of age)
• Patients with diabetes mellitus, HIV
Diphtheria, tetanus, acellular pertussis (pediatric)
• All children starting at age 2 months
• May be given up to the 7th birthday
• DTaP recommended over DTP
Diphtheria and tetanus (pediatric)
• Children < 7 years who cannot take DTaP
Tetanus and diphtheria (adult)
• Booster at ages 11-12 or 14-16 and either every 10 years thereafter or a single booster dose at age 50
Measles, mumps and rubella
• Children at age 12 to 15 months and again between 4 and 6 years (or 11 to 12 years)
• Adults (especially medical personnel and daycare workers) without prior immunization or uncertain immunizations born after 1957
• International travelers
• College students - 2 doses total if not previously vaccinated
Varicella
• Children at age 12 to 18 months (1 dose)
• Catch-up vaccination for children 18 months to 12 years (1 dose) without history of chickenpox
• Vaccination approved for persons ≥ 13 years without history of chickenpox (2 doses)
• Health care workers without a previous history of chickenpox
Polio
• All children starting at 2 months of age
• Adults previously immunized who will travel to areas where polio is prevalent
• Unimmunized adults should receive the inactivated IPV vaccine
• Polio vaccine options: OPV, IPV, or sequential (2 doses of IPV followed by 2 OPV doses)
    ◊ AAFP recommends patient provider choice among the OPV, IPV, and sequential schedules
    ◊ ACIP accepts the OPV, IPV, and sequential schedules, but recommends the sequential schedule

Haemophilus influenzae type b
• All children starting at 2 months of age
Hepatitis A
• Travelers to higher risk countries
• Patients with chronic liver disease
• Certain high-risk communities and ethnic groups, e.g., Native American/Alaskan
• Homosexual males
• Street drug users
• Laboratory personnel who might be exposed
System(s) affected:
Hemic/Lymphatic/Immunologic
Genetics: N/A
Incidence/Prevalence in USA: N/A
Predominant age: N/A
Predominant sex: N/A

SIGNS AND SYMPTOMS N/A

CAUSES N/A

RISK FACTORS N/A

DIAGNOSIS

DIFFERENTIAL DIAGNOSIS N/A

LABORATORY N/A
Drugs that may alter lab results: N/A
Disorders that may alter lab results: N/A

PATHOLOGICAL FINDINGS N/A

SPECIAL TESTS N/A

IMAGING N/A

DIAGNOSTIC PROCEDURES N/A

TREATMENT

APPROPRIATE HEALTH CARE N/A

GENERAL MEASURES
• Informed patient consent should discuss consequences of specific diseases and risks of immunizations - Vaccine Information Statements should be used
• Antipyretics (acetaminophen) are useful for the fever which may accompany immunizations

SURGICAL MEASURES N/A

ACTIVITY No restrictions after immunization

DIET No specific restrictions after immunization

PATIENT EDUCATION Report adverse events promptly. Minor redness, swelling, and or soreness at the site of injections can be expected; ice packs and acetaminophen may be helpful.

```
---IMMUNIZATION SCHEDULE-------------------------------------
      <------- months -------->  <------ years ----->
      0  1  2  4  6  12  15  18  4-6  11-12 14-16 65+
-------------------------------------------------------------
Hep B 1->2----->  3------------>              R
DTaP†       1  2  3   4-------->        5††
Td                                           1-----> and q 10 yrs
Hib         1  2  3   4-------->
Polio       1  2     3-------->        4
MMR                  1--->              2   or 2
Var                  1------->                R
INFL                                              1 yearly
PNEU                                              1 once
-------------------------------------------------------------
Dash (-->) indicate range of acceptable ages for vaccination
†DTaP Preferred over DTP
††Not needed if previous vaccine given after the 4th birthday
R = Review immunizations/administer needed primary series
```

MEDICATIONS

DRUG(S) OF CHOICE

```
--IMMUNIZATION DOSES----------
Agent        Dose (mL)   Route
--------------------------------
DTP           0.5         IM
MMR           0.5         SQ
Polio (OPV)   0.5         PO
Polio (IPV)   0.5         SQ
HBv†          ††          IM
Hib           0.5         IM
Influenza     0.5         IM
Td and DT     0.5         IM
Pneumococcal  0.5         IM
Varicella     0.5         SQ
--------------------------------
```

†Newborns of hepatitis B surface antigen positive mothers should also receive HBIG
††Variable

```
--TETANUS WOUND PROPHYLAXIS---
   (for Td and TIG)
               Prior tetanus
Type of        immunizations
 wound        ----------------
              Uncertain  | ≥3
              or <3 doses| doses
              Td    TIG  | Td‡
--------------------------------
Clean†        Yes   No   | 10
Dirty††       Yes   Yes  | 5
Puncture      Yes   Yes  | 5
Major†††      Yes   Yes  | 5
--------------------------------
```

For example, an adult with a puncture wound and 2 prior doses of tetanus toxoid should receive both Td and TIG.
‡TIG not needed; give Td if years indicated have passed since last immunization
†Clean: Minor wound
††Dirty: Contaminated with dirt, feces, or saliva
†††Major: Burn, frostbite, crush injury

Contraindications:
• Anaphylaxis to thimerosal: DTP, DT, TD, PRP-OMP, multi-dose vials of HbOC, influenza, and some brands of pneumococcal vaccine contraindicated
• Anaphylaxis to neomycin: MMR, DTP, Hib, OPV, IPV, varicella contraindicated
• Anaphylaxis to streptomycin: OPV, IPV contraindicated
• Anaphylaxis to previous dose
• Encephalopathy within 7 days after DTP: Give DT for next dose(s)
• Pregnancy: MMR, varicella
• Known, active, untreated tuberculosis: varicella contraindicated
• Anaphylaxis to eggs: influenza
• Other
  ◊ Immunocompromised patients should, in general, not receive live viral vaccines (MMR, varicella and OPV), although patients with HIV may receive MMR
  ◊ Persons with unavoidable (e.g., household) contact with the immunocompromised should not receive OPV (give IPV)

Precautions:
DTaP
• Suspected neurologic disease: Delay immunization until clarified
• Fever of ≥ 40.5°C (105°F) within 48 hours after previous DTP/DTaP
• Collapse or shock-like state (hypotonic-hyporesponsive episode) within 48 hours after DTP/DTaP
• Seizure within 3 days after DTP/DTaP
• Persistent, inconsolable crying lasting ≥ 3 hrs within 48 hours after DTP/DTaP
• The following are NOT contraindications and DTaP may be given if present:
  ◊ Family history of convulsions: Pre-treat with acetaminophen and after DTaP q4h for 24 hrs
  ◊ Family history of SIDS
  ◊ Family history of adverse event following DTaP/DTP
  ◊ Temperature < 40.5°C (105°F) following a prior DTaP/DTP
Varicella
• Avoid salicylates for 6 weeks
Significant possible interactions:
Avoid MMR and varicella vaccine within 3-11 months after gamma globulin (see ACIP)

ALTERNATIVE DRUGS None

FOLLOWUP

PATIENT MONITORING
• None routinely needed
• Hepatitis: Measure antibody (anti-HBs) response after HBv for healthcare workers, immunocompromised persons and offspring of hepatitis B carriers

PREVENTION/AVOIDANCE N/A

POSSIBLE COMPLICATIONS
Fever, malaise, local reactions (redness, pain) are most common. Rarely, allergic reactions, febrile seizures. Some believe DTP causes encephalopathy rarely.

EXPECTED COURSE/PROGNOSIS Most
patients develop antibodies

MISCELLANEOUS

ASSOCIATED CONDITIONS N/A

AGE-RELATED FACTORS
Pediatric: Most vaccines are given before entry into school. Do not delay DTaP immunization of the preterm infant unless specific contraindications exist.
Geriatric: Pneumococcal, influenza, and tetanus are needed in older age groups
Others: N/A

PREGNANCY MMR and varicella should not be routinely given to pregnant women or women who are planning pregnancy within 3 months (MMR) or next 1 month (varicella).

SYNONYMS
• Vaccinations
• Inoculations

ICD-9-CM
V05.9 Healthy person receiving prophylactic inoculation or vaccination

SEE ALSO
• Chickenpox
• Diphtheria
• Hepatitis, viral
• Influenza
• Measles, rubella
• Measles, rubeola
• Pertussis
• Pneumonia, bacterial
• Poliomyelitis
• Mumps
• Tetanus

OTHER NOTES
• PPD may be given at same time as MMR and/or OPV or wait 4 weeks after immunization to do skin test
• Culture-proven pertussis provides immunity; use DT instead of DTP
• Haemophilus disease: Immunity not provided when child under 2 years; administer Hib as if no disease has occurred
• Combination vaccines are available

ABBREVIATIONS
DTaP = pediatric diphtheria, tetanus toxoids, and acellular pertussis vaccine
DT = pediatric diphtheria and tetanus toxoids
Td = adult diphtheria and tetanus toxoids
TIG = tetanus immune globulin
HBv = hepatitis B vaccine
HBIG = hepatitis B immune globulin
OPV = trivalent oral polio vaccine
IPV = enhanced inactivated polio vaccine
HbOC = Hib vaccine (hibTITER)
PRP-OMP = Hib vaccine (PedvaxHIB)
PRP-T = Hib vaccine (ActHIB, OmniHIB)
MMR = measles, mumps, and rubella vaccine
Hib = conjugated Haemophilus influenzae type b vaccine
INF = influenza vaccine
PNEU = pneumococcal vaccine
PPD = purified protein derivative
VZIG = varicella-zoster immune globulin
Var = varicella zoster vaccine

REFERENCES
• Advisory Committee on Immunization Practices (ACIP)
• Red Book 1997 Report of the Committee on Infectious Diseases. American Academy of Pediatrics, 1997
• American Academy of Family Physicians
Illustrations: N/A
Internet references: http://www.5mcc.com

Author(s)
Richard Kent Zimmerman, MD, MPH
Richard D. Clover, MD

Immunodeficiency diseases

 BASICS

DESCRIPTION
Disorders associated with disruption of the integrity of the immune system resulting in a wide spectrum of illnesses
• May be primary or secondary and involve any or all of the system's cells and their products (T cells, B cells, monocytes, macrophages, etc.) their receptors, metabolic pathways and products which are normally involved in health maintenance and protection
• Primary
◊ Combined immunodeficiencies, e.g., severe combined immunodeficiency (SCID), adenosine deaminase (ADA) deficiency, and reticular dysgenesis
◊ Antibody deficiencies, e.g., X-linked agammaglobulinemia, IgA deficiency, Ig deficiency with increased IgM (hyper-IgM syndrome), common variable immunodeficiency (CVID) and transient hypogammaglobulinemia of infancy
◊ Other well-defined syndromes, e.g., Wiskott-Aldrich syndrome (eczema, thrombocytopenia and repeated infections), ataxia telangiectasia (cerebellar ataxia, oculocutaneous telangiectasia and immunodeficiency) and DiGeorge's syndrome (isolated T cell deficiency)
◊ Associated syndromes e.g., Down syndrome, chronic mucocutaneous candidiasis, hyper-IgE syndrome, chronic granulomatous disease, partial albinism and WHIM syndrome (warts, hypogammaglobulinemia, infection, myelokathexis [retention of leukocytes in a hypercellular marrow]), phagocytic defects with early onset of periodontal disease.
◊ Complement deficiencies
• Secondary
◊ AIDS
◊ Other infections, malignancies, malnutrition, protein-losing enteropathy, drugs, and chronic stress
System(s) affected:
Hemic/Lymphatic/Immunologic
Genetics: Included in Description
Incidence/Prevalence in USA:
• 1 in every 500 (including IgA deficiency) born with an immune system defect
• Many more will acquire a defect which may be transient or permanent
Predominant age:
• All ages. Children most likely to present with primary or inherited deficiencies.
• Number of newborns with AIDS increasing. In part associated with: (1) increased premature infant survival, (2) improved treatment and care of other primary diseases, (3) use of immunosuppressive agents.
Predominant sex: Male > Female

SIGNS AND SYMPTOMS
• Common features
◊ Unusual susceptibility to infection. Frequency and severity vary with type of defect.
◊ Malignancies, especially lymphoreticular
◊ Increased tendency toward autoimmune disorders
◊ Weight loss
◊ Fever
• More specific features
◊ Combined T and B cell deficiencies associated with severe fungal, bacterial and viral infections. Enzyme deficiencies may be involved.
◊ T cell deficiencies may be acquired (as with the human immunodeficiency virus) or congenital with wide spectrum manifestations. Children with DiGeorge's syndrome show cardiac defects, micrognathia, hypertelorism and hypocalcemic tetany.
◊ B cell or immunoglobulin deficiency syndromes may be associated with chronic sinusitis, recurrent respiratory infection, chronic diarrheal disease, rheumatoid arthritis, systemic lupus erythematosus (SLE), atopy, splenomegaly, anemia, recurrent pneumococcal pneumonia and meningococcal meningitis
◊ Chronic giardiasis, fever of unknown origin and malabsorption should cause suspicion of immunodeficiency
◊ Miscellaneous syndromes include chronic mucocutaneous candidiasis, fatal Epstein-Barr virus infection, and complement component deficiencies

CAUSES
• Primary immunodeficiency diseases
◊ Faulty genes and gene products resulting in inherited defects of the immune system including: antibody, cellular, phagocytic cytokine production, and complement deficiencies
◊ Manifested by infections soon after birth but may not be expressed clinically until later in life
• Secondary immunodeficiency diseases
◊ Treatment with immunosuppressive agents
◊ Nutritional deficiencies
◊ Use of drugs and exposure to chemicals should be considered
◊ X-ray treatment
◊ IgA deficiency associated with phenytoin or penicillamine
◊ Thymoma associated with hypogammaglobulinemia
◊ Viruses e.g., HIV-1 and HIV-2

RISK FACTORS
• Family history
• Almost anything less than good health practices
• Drug abuse and parenteral blood exposure
• Sexual lifestyle
• Aging

 DIAGNOSIS

DIFFERENTIAL DIAGNOSIS
• Must consider all immunodeficiency disorders
• Careful history and physical will direct proper search

LABORATORY
• High percentage of immunodeficiencies will be discovered by a CBC with a differential smear and immunoglobulin levels including: IgG, IgA, IgM and IgE. IgG subclasses should be included.
• Further assays include mononuclear cell populations which may be quantified
• Total lymphocyte a good screen
• Functional evaluation by skin testing (anergy battery) and antibody levels to common viruses and bacterial toxins
• Complement levels
• Phagocyte function
• Specific cytokine function
• Additional specific tests for suspected acquired causes for immunodeficiencies (AIDS, chronic diarrhea, malignancy, drugs, etc.)
Drugs that may alter lab results: N/A
Disorders that may alter lab results: N/A

PATHOLOGICAL FINDINGS
Vary with type of deficiency and resultant disease(s)

SPECIAL TESTS N/A

IMAGING
• MRI helpful in evaluation of CNS lesions associated with toxoplasmosis
• Techniques and technology continue to improve dramatically

DIAGNOSTIC PROCEDURES
• Careful history and physical
• Try to deduce whether infections associated with T cell response inadequacies (fungal and other opportunistic infections) or lack of B cell (antibodies) response or both

 TREATMENT

APPROPRIATE HEALTH CARE
• Outpatient or inpatient management appropriate to clinical problem

GENERAL MEASURES
• Depends mainly on complexity of the immune deficiency
• Bone marrow transplant with donor T cell engraftment in severe abnormalities of T cell function. Best done at referral research centers.
• Intravenous immunoglobulin - for patients deficient in IgG. Not appropriate for treatment for Ig deficiency other than IgG, but may be helpful in the hyper-IgM syndrome.

SURGICAL MEASURES N/A

ACTIVITY As appropriate

DIET Severe immunodeficiencies require sterile conditions

PATIENT EDUCATION Printed patient information available from: Immune Deficiency Foundation, 25 West Chesapeake Ave. Room 206, Rowson, MD 21204

MEDICATIONS

DRUG(S) OF CHOICE
• Antibiotics with appropriate spectra for infecting organism(s). Ketoconazole reported to be effective in some chronic fungal infections.
• Enzyme replacement therapy for ADA deficiency
• Autologous genetically corrected T cells with normal ADA gene
• Zidovudine (AZT) reduces rate of maternal transmission of HIV
• Combination drug therapy in HIV
• Recombinant interleukin-2 conjugated with polyethylene glycol (PEG), promising
Contraindications: Refer to manufacturer's literature
Precautions:
• Multidisciplinary input in order
• Refer to manufacturer's literature
Significant possible interactions: Refer to manufacturer's literature

ALTERNATIVE DRUGS N/A

FOLLOWUP

PATIENT MONITORING
• Children with SCID must remain in controlled environment, exposure to any pathogen may result in death
• IgG levels monitored and maintained in common variable hypogammaglobulinemia
• Meticulous instruction and checks for infections

PREVENTION/AVOIDANCE Genetic counseling for primary cases

POSSIBLE COMPLICATIONS
• Autoimmune disorders
• Serum sickness reactions to gamma globulin treatment
• Malignancies
• Overwhelming infection
• Fatal graft-versus-host disease following blood transfusions in SCID patients

EXPECTED COURSE/PROGNOSIS
Related closely to type and degree of immunodeficiency

MISCELLANEOUS

ASSOCIATED CONDITIONS N/A

AGE-RELATED FACTORS
Pediatric: Depends on specific immunodeficiency disorder
Geriatric: Depends on specific immunodeficiency disorder
Others: N/A

PREGNANCY AIDS transmission

SYNONYMS N/A

ICD-9-CM 279.3

SEE ALSO
• HIV infection & AIDS

OTHER NOTES
• Research opportunities:
  ◊ Continue studies at the cellular, cytokine, and molecular level
  ◊ Continue to develop techniques of replacing gene and gene products where deficiencies are either inherited or acquired
  ◊ Expand acquired immunodeficiency research and the addressing of clinical and social problems
  ◊ AIDS vaccine evaluation group

ABBREVIATIONS N/A

REFERENCES
• NIAID Task Force on Immunology and Allergy
• Isselbacher KJ, et al, eds: Harrison's Principles of Internal Medicine. 13th Ed. New York, McGraw-Hill, 1994
• Lichtenstein L, Fauci A: Current Therapy in Allergy, Immunology and Rheumatology. Toronto, B.C. Decker, Inc., 1988
• Stiehm ER, Blaese RM: Pediatric Research. Vol. 33, No. 1 (suppl)/Jan, 1993
• Immune Deficiency Foundation Clinical Updates, Littleton, CO
• Cunningham-Rundles C, et al: Brief Report - Enhanced Humoral Immunity in Common Variable Immune-Deficiency with Polyethyleneglycol-conjugated interleukin-2. NEJM 1995;331(14):918-921
Illustrations: N/A
Internet references: http://www.5mcc.com

Author(s)
J. Harlan Dix, MD, FACP

Impetigo

BASICS

DESCRIPTION A superficial, intraepidermal, unilocular, vesiculopustular infection. Typically begins as erythematous tender papule that rapidly progresses through a vesicular to a honey-crusted stage. Still debated as to relative importance of staphylococci versus streptococci. Cultures now give over 80% with Staphylococcus aureus alone or combined with group A beta-hemolytic streptococci. Change over past 10 years to predominately Staph. aureus.
• Bullous impetigo: Staphylococci impetigo that progress rapidly to small to large flaccid bulla. No lymphadenopathy.
• Folliculitis: Considered by some to be Staphylococci aureus impetigo of the hair follicle
• Ecthyma: A deeper, ulcerated, impetigo infection often with lymphadenitis
System(s) affected: Skin/Exocrine
Genetics: N/A
Incidence/Prevalence in USA: Unreported
Predominant age: 2-5 years
Predominant sex: Male = Female

SIGNS AND SYMPTOMS
• May be slow and indolent or rapidly spreading
• Tender red macule or papule as early lesion
• Thin roofed vesicle to bullae - usually nontender
• Pustules
• Weeping shallow red ulcer
• Honey-colored crusts
• Most frequent on face around mouth and nose, or at site of trauma
• Satellite lesions
• Often multiple sites
• Bullae on buttocks, trunk, face

CAUSES
• Coagulase positive staphylococci - pure culture about 50-90%. More contagious via contact.
• Beta-hemolytic streptococci - pure culture only about 10% of the time
• Mixed infections of streptococci and staphylococci common. Data suggest increasing importance of staphylococci over past 10 years.
• Direct contact or insect vector
• Can be contamination at trauma site

RISK FACTORS
• Warm, humid environment
• Tropical or subtropical climate
• Summer or fall season
• Minor trauma, insect bites, etc.
• Poor hygiene, epidemics, during war, etc.
• Familial spread
• Poor health with anemia and malnutrition
• Complication to pediculosis, scabies, chickenpox, eczema
• Contact dermatitis (Rhus)

DIAGNOSIS

DIFFERENTIAL DIAGNOSIS
• Nonbullous:
  ◊ Chickenpox
  ◊ Herpes
  ◊ Folliculitis
  ◊ Erysipelas
  ◊ Insect bites
  ◊ Severe eczematous dermatitis
  ◊ Scabies
  ◊ Tinea corporis
• Bullous:
  ◊ Burns
  ◊ Pemphigus vulgaris
  ◊ Bullous pemphigoid
  ◊ Stevens-Johnson syndrome

LABORATORY
None usually required
• Culture - taken from the base of lesion after removal of crust. Blood agar grows both staphylococci and group A streptococci
• ASO titer - can be weak positive for streptococci (not usually done)
• Streptozyme - positive for streptococci (not usually done)
Drugs that may alter lab results: N/A
Disorders that may alter lab results: Streptococci pharyngitis will alter streptococci enzyme tests

PATHOLOGICAL FINDINGS N/A

SPECIAL TESTS Cultures as listed under Laboratory

IMAGING N/A

DIAGNOSTIC PROCEDURES N/A

TREATMENT

APPROPRIATE HEALTH CARE Outpatient

GENERAL MEASURES Removal of crusts, cleanliness with gentle washing 2-3 times daily

SURGICAL MEASURES N/A

ACTIVITY No restrictions

DIET No special diet

PATIENT EDUCATION Good hygiene important to prevent possible spread

MEDICATIONS

DRUG(S) OF CHOICE
Note: Increasing incidence of Staphylococcus resistant to erythromycin may make the following suggestions inaccurate in your community.
• Nonbullous (minor spread, treat 7 days; widespread, treat 10 days); bullous (treat 10 days)
  ◊ Erythromycin base - adults 1 gm/day divided doses q6h in adults. Pediatric 30-40 mg/kg/d q6h.
  ◊ Mupirocin (Bactroban) topical ointment apply tid, 7-10 days (nonbullous only)
  ◊ Dicloxacillin - adult 250 mg qid. Pediatric 12-25 mg/kg/d divided q6h.
Contraindications: Drug allergy
Precautions: Refer to manufacturer's profile of each drug
Significant possible interactions:
• Erythromycin with theophyllines, astemizole, terfenadine (Seldane), and other drugs
• Refer to manufacturer's profile of each drug

ALTERNATIVE DRUGS
Oral doses:
• 1st generation cephalosporins - children
  ◊ Cephalexin: 25-50 mg/kg/24 h divided q6h
  ◊ Cefaclor: 20-40 mg/kg/24 h divided q8h
  ◊ Cephradine: 25-50 mg/kg/24 h divided q6-12h
  ◊ Cefadroxil: 30 mg/kg/24 h divided bid
• 1st generation cephalosporins - adults
  ◊ Cephalexin: 250 mg qid
  ◊ Cefaclor: 250 mg tid
  ◊ Cephradine: 500 mg bid
  ◊ Cefadroxil: 1 gm/day in divided doses
• Amoxicillin-clavulanate acid
  ◊ Adult: 250 mg tid
  ◊ Pediatric: 20-40 mg/kg/day of amoxicillin divided q8h
• Vancomycin
• Clindamycin
• Ciprofloxacin plus rifampin (rifampicin)

FOLLOWUP

PATIENT MONITORING If not clear within 7-10 days, culture the lesions

PREVENTION/AVOIDANCE Close attention to family hygiene, particularly hand washing

POSSIBLE COMPLICATIONS
• Ecthyma
• Erysipelas
• Post-streptococcal acute glomerulonephritis
• Deep cellulitis
• Bacteremia

EXPECTED COURSE/PROGNOSIS
• Complete resolution in 7-10 days with treatment
• Antibiotic treatment will not prevent or halt glomerulonephritis as it will with rheumatic fever

MISCELLANEOUS

ASSOCIATED CONDITIONS
• Malnutrition and anemia
• Crowded living conditions
• Poor hygiene
• Neglected minor trauma

AGE-RELATED FACTORS
Pediatric: Impetigo neonatorum may occur by nursery contamination
Geriatric: N/A
Others: N/A

PREGNANCY N/A

SYNONYMS
• Pyoderma
• Impetigo contagiosa
• Impetigo vulgaris
• Fox impetigo

ICD-9-CM 684 Impetigo

SEE ALSO N/A

OTHER NOTES N/A

ABBREVIATIONS N/A

REFERENCES
• Isselbacher KJ, et a, eds: Harrison's Principles of Internal Medicine. 13th Ed. New York, McGraw-Hill, 1994
• Dagan R: Impetigo in childhood: changing epidemiology and new treatments. Pediatric Annals 1993;22(4):235-240
• Grossman KL, Rasmussen JE: Recent advances in pediatric infectious diseases and their impact on dermatology. J Am Acad Derm 1991;24(3):379-389
Illustrations: 7 available on CD-ROM
Internet references: http://www.5mcc.com

Author(s)
William H. Billica, MD

Inappropriate secretion of antidiuretic hormone

BASICS

DESCRIPTION A form of hyponatremia with inappropriately elevated urine osmolality and no discernible stimulus for ADH release. Total body sodium levels may be normal or near normal. Total body water is usually increased. Associated with an underlying disorder, e.g., neoplasm, pulmonary disorder, or central nervous system disease.
System(s) affected: Endocrine/Metabolic
Genetics: No known genetic pattern
Incidence/Prevalence in USA: Rare
Predominant age: Common in the elderly
Predominant sex: N/A

SIGNS AND SYMPTOMS
- Usually neurological
- Lethargy
- Restlessness
- Confusion
- Edema (rare)
- Anorexia
- Nausea/vomiting
- Headache
- Irritability
- Decreasing reflexes
- Seizures
- Coma
- Asymptomatic

CAUSES
- Oat cell carcinoma of the lung
- Drugs (vincristine, narcotics, thiazide diuretics, cyclophosphamide, carbamazepine, barbiturates, morphine, chlorpropamide, nicotine, beta-adrenergic agents, general anesthetics, oxytocin)
- Ectopic ADH production
- Hodgkin's disease
- Hypothyroidism
- Idiopathic
- Infectious diseases
- Lupus erythematosus
- Meningitis
- Myocardial infarction
- Myxedema
- Pancreatic carcinoma
- Pneumonia
- Porphyria
- Positive-pressure breathing
- Pulmonary tuberculosis
- Rocky Mountain spotted fever
- Tumor - bronchogenic carcinoma
- Vascular diseases

RISK FACTORS
- Patient with causative disorder
- Use of predisposing drugs
- Elderly patient
- Postoperative
- Institutionalized patient

DIAGNOSIS

DIFFERENTIAL DIAGNOSIS
- Postoperative:
1) caused by non-osmotic release of ADH
2) affects women more than men
3) ADH increased by pain and narcotics.
- Postprostatectomy syndrome:
1) irrigating solution must be non-conducting (i.e., electrolyte free)
2) D5W absorbed
- Psychotic polydipsia:
1) active therapy rarely needed
2) diuresis occurs when intake stopped
3) intake usually over 10 L/day
4) interaction with other psychotropic drugs.
- Acute (usually in children):
1) swallowing water during swimming
2) diluted formula
3) tap water enemas.
- Drug induced:
1) oxytocin infusion - given in D5W during labor (oxytocin has antidiuretic effect)
2) cyclophosphamide - usually with IV administration
3) chlorpropamide (oral hypoglycemic agent)
4) carbamazepine - central ADH release
5) vincristine - central SIADH
6) nonsteroidal anti-inflammatory drugs (NSAID's) - decreased renal prostaglandins
- Diuretic drug induced:
1) usually thiazide
2) vasopressin increased by decreasing EABV
3) usually elderly patients or in bulimia
4) correct slowly
- Tumor induced
1) bronchogenic carcinoma (secretes ADH-like substance)
2) unexplained persistent hyponatremia may indicate a tumor
- Pulmonary:
1) tuberculosis - secretes ADH
2) mechanical ventilation - increased intrathoracic pressure, decreased cardiac output, causes decreased EABV, causes increased ADH
3) asthma, acute respiratory failure, pneumonia
- CNS/hypothalamic irritation:
1) meningitis
2) Rocky Mountain spotted fever
3) encephalitis
4) trauma - especially after CNS surgery
- Endocrine:
1) Addison's disease
2) hypothyroid
- Factitious hyponatremia
1) caused by increased serum glucose, cholesterol or proteins
- Other:
1)"Appropriate" ADH secretion and hyponatremia with decreased effective arterial blood volume, e.g., congestive heart failure, nephrotic syndrome, cirrhosis

LABORATORY
- BUN low or normal
- Creatinine low or normal
- Urine osmolality 200+ mOsmol/kg
- Urinary Na concentration > 20 mEq/L (> 20 mmol/L)
- Elevated serum concentration ADH
- Normal adrenal and renal function
- Uric acid low
Drugs that may alter lab results: N/A
Disorders that may alter lab results: N/A

PATHOLOGICAL FINDINGS N/A

SPECIAL TESTS Oral water-loading test may be helpful in diagnosis in some patients. Response to water-load will be impaired in SIADH.

IMAGING N/A

DIAGNOSTIC PROCEDURES N/A

TREATMENT

APPROPRIATE HEALTH CARE
Outpatient or inpatient depending on severity of symptoms or underlying cause

GENERAL MEASURES
- Mildly symptomatic
  ◊ Patient has serum Na > 125 mEq/L (> 125 mmol/L)
  ◊ Restrict fluid to 800-1000 mL/day
- Acute (less than 48 hours duration)
  ◊ Hypertonic saline
  ◊ Water diuresis
- Symptomatic (seizure, coma)
  ◊ High mortality due to cerebral edema if serum Na < 120 mEq/L (< 120 mmol/L)
  ◊ Decrease oral free water to 2/3 maintenance
  ◊ Increase oral salt
  ◊ Correct serum Na deficit. (mEq sodium deficit = desired sodium minus actual sodium times 0.5 times weight [kg])
  ◊ Increase serum sodium slowly with hypertonic saline by 0.5 mEq/L /hour until it reaches 120 mEq/L

SURGICAL MEASURES N/A

ACTIVITY As tolerated

DIET May need increased salt or decreased water intake depending on cause

PATIENT EDUCATION Diet and fluid restrictions

MEDICATIONS

DRUG(S) OF CHOICE
• Water diuresis - furosemide (Lasix) plus hourly sodium chloride and potassium chloride replacement - requires frequent monitoring. Treatment of choice for acute management.
• Demeclocycline - blocks ADH at renal tubule - produces nephrogenic diabetes insipidus. (Dosage for long term management: 600-1200 mg/day. Onset of action is within one week, therefore not best for acute management).
• Lithium - blocks ADH at renal tubule - has the problem of lithium toxicity, antianabolic effects especially in cirrhosis and congestive heart failure
• Hypertonic (3%) saline
  ◊ Increase serum Na by 10-12 mEq/L (10-12 mmol/L) every 24 hrs
  ◊ Increase serum Na ± 5% over first few hours
  ◊ Increase serum Na to only 120 mEq/L (120 mmol/L), acutely
  ◊ Increase serum Na by 0.5 mEq/hr (0.5 mmol/hr)

Contraindications: Avoid fluids in congestive heart failure, nephrotic syndrome or cirrhosis

Precautions:
• Too rapid correction can cause:
  ◊ Congestive heart failure
  ◊ Subdural and intracerebral hemorrhage
  ◊ Permanent CNS damage, especially with serum Na < 120 mEq/L (< 120 mmol/L)
  ◊ Demyelination syndrome

Significant possible interactions: Refer to manufacturer's literature

ALTERNATIVE DRUGS N/A

FOLLOWUP

PATIENT MONITORING
• Careful, continuous, clinical and laboratory monitoring of the hyponatremic state during acute phase
• For chronic management, monitor underlying cause as needed

PREVENTION/AVOIDANCE
• Search for cause of SIADH, if unknown
• Monitor electrolytes in postoperative patients to determine if fluid intake needs restriction
• Reducing or changing medications, if a drug is the cause
• Life-long restriction of fluid intake

POSSIBLE COMPLICATIONS
• Central pontine myelinolysis:
  ◊ Chronic hyponatremia - usually < 120 mEq/L (< 120 mmol/L)
  ◊ Too rapid correction - > 12 mEq/L/day (> 12 mmol/day)

EXPECTED COURSE/PROGNOSIS
Dependent on underlying cause

MISCELLANEOUS

ASSOCIATED CONDITIONS Listed with Causes

AGE-RELATED FACTORS
Pediatric: N/A
Geriatric: Most common in this age group
Others: N/A

PREGNANCY N/A

SYNONYMS
• SIADH
• Syndrome of inappropriate secretion of ADH

ICD-9-CM 276.9

SEE ALSO Hyponatremia

OTHER NOTES N/A

ABBREVIATIONS N/A

REFERENCES
• Brenner BM, Rector FC Jr: The Kidney. 5th Ed. Philadelphia, W.B. Saunders Co., 1995
• Kokko JM: Fluid and Electrolytes. 3rd Ed. Philadelphia, W.B. Saunders Co., 1996
Illustrations: N/A
Internet references: http://www.5mcc.com

Author(s)
Watson C. Arnold, MD

Influenza

 BASICS

DESCRIPTION An acute, usually self-limited, viral, febrile, infection caused by influenza virus types A and B. It is marked by inflammation of the nasal mucosa, pharynx, conjunctiva, and respiratory tract. Outbreaks occur almost every winter with varying degrees of severity.
• The influenza virus displays antigenic shift (variation) which leads to strains of the virus to which there is little immunologic resistance in the population and may result in pandemics. The influenza virus displays minor antigenic variation called drift.
System(s) affected: Respiratory
Genetics: N/A
Incidence/Prevalence in USA:
250,000-500,000 new cases each year. Attack rates in healthy children are 10-40% each year.
Predominant age:
• Incidence: highest in school-aged children (3 months-16 years); young adult (16-40 years)
• Morbidity: highest in elderly (> 75 years) and concurrent medical illnesses, such as lung disease
Predominant sex: Male = Female

SIGNS AND SYMPTOMS
Sudden onset of:
• High Fever
• Myalgia (sometimes severe and lasting for days)
• Sore throat/pharyngitis
• Nonproductive cough
• Headache
• Cervical lymphadenopathy
• Chills
• Nasal congestion
• Malaise
• Rhinorrhea
• Sinusitis
• Sneezing
• Conjunctivitis

CAUSES Orthomyxovirus (influenza antigenic types A and B) that are transmitted person-to-person, usually by the airborne route

RISK FACTORS
• For contracting disease:
 ◊ Patients in semi-closed environments such as nursing homes
 ◊ Students, prisoners
 ◊ Crowded, close environments during times of epidemics
• For complications
 ◊ Chronic pulmonary diseases
 ◊ Cardiovascular diseases including valvular problems and congestive heart failure
 ◊ Metabolic diseases
 ◊ Hemoglobinopathies
 ◊ Malignancies
 ◊ Pregnancy, especially in the 3rd trimester
 ◊ Neonates, elderly
 ◊ Immunosuppression

 DIAGNOSIS

DIFFERENTIAL DIAGNOSIS
• Respiratory viral infections including RSV, parainfluenza, adenovirus, enterovirus
• Atypical Mycoplasma pneumonia
• Q fever
• Viral or streptococcal tonsillitis
• Infectious mononucleosis
• Coxsackievirus infections
• Chlamydia

LABORATORY
• Rapid antigen test
• Culture of nasopharyngeal swab or aspirate
• Lymphopenia
• Leukocytosis may signal complications
Drugs that may alter lab results: N/A
Disorders that may alter lab results: N/A

PATHOLOGICAL FINDINGS Inflammation of respiratory tract

SPECIAL TESTS N/A

IMAGING
• Chest x-ray
 ◊ Usually normal unless secondary infection
 ◊ Basilar streaking
 ◊ Patchy infiltrate - mild disease

DIAGNOSTIC PROCEDURES
• Tissue culture of nasopharyngeal swab or aspirate
• Rapid ELISA antigen test
• History and physical examination - close attention to epidemiology (e.g., current outbreak in community). Contact CDC at (404)332-4555 or health department to determine type.

 TREATMENT

APPROPRIATE HEALTH CARE
Outpatient except for treatment of severe complications or treatment of those in high risk groups

GENERAL MEASURES
• Symptomatic treatment (saline nasal spray, analgesic gargle)
• Cool-mist, ultrasonic humidifier to increase moisture of inspired air
• Modified respiratory isolation techniques
• Hospitalized patients may require oxygen or ventilatory support
• Avoid smoking

SURGICAL MEASURES N/A

ACTIVITY As tolerated. Hospitalized individuals should have contact isolation with strict hand washing procedures.

DIET Increase fluid intake

PATIENT EDUCATION
• For a listing of sources for patient education materials favorably reviewed on this topic, physicians may contact: American Academy of Family Physicians Foundation, P.O. Box 8418, Kansas City, MO 64114, (800)274-2237, ext. 4400
• Educate high-risk patients about prevention

MEDICATIONS

DRUG(S) OF CHOICE
• Amantadine and rimantadine are effective only for influenza A
◊ Recommended for patients with pneumonia, severe disease or at high risk for complications. 100 mg twice per day orally for 3-5 days. It shortens duration of fever, systemic and respiratory symptoms by about 50%. Effective if administered within the first 48 hours.
◊ The amantadine dose should be decreased in the elderly and for those with impaired renal function (see manufacturer's guidelines).
◊ The rimantadine dose should be decreased for elderly nursing home residents and those with either liver or severe renal impairment.
◊ See manufacturer's guidelines for children's dosages. Rimantadine is not approved for influenza in children.
• Antipyretics
◊ Acetaminophen. For fever control in children.
◊ Aspirin should not be used in children under 16 years due to risk of Reye's syndrome
• Appropriate antibiotics
◊ If complicating bacterial infection
Contraindications: Nursing mothers; pregnancy unless benefits outweigh risks
Precautions:
• Amantadine and rimantadine
◊ May cause mild CNS symptoms (e.g., lightheadedness, insomnia, anxiety) which are dose related and clear with discontinuation. It might impair ability to perform hazardous activities or to drive a motor vehicle. Amantadine causes more CNS side effects than rimantadine.
◊ May potentiate underlying seizure disorders and exacerbate epilepsy; EEG abnormalities are increased
◊ Cautious use if uncontrolled psychosis or severe psychoneurosis
◊ Observe patients with congestive heart failure for deterioration (amantadine)
◊ Patients > 65 years old or with renal impairment should receive a reduced dose
◊ Those being treated with amantadine or rimantadine should avoid contact with unaffected individuals taking either drug for prophylaxis
Significant possible interactions:
Increased atropine-like effects may occur if amantadine is given concurrently with anticholinergic drugs (e.g., antihistamines). May interact with CNS stimulants as well.

ALTERNATIVE DRUGS
• Ribavirin reported to be effective against types A and B and when given as aerosol, not orally
• Ibuprofen or other NSAIDs for symptomatic relief

FOLLOWUP

PATIENT MONITORING In mild cases, usually no follow-up required. Follow moderate or severe cases until symptoms resolved and any complications are treated effectively.

PREVENTION/AVOIDANCE
• Incubation period is 1 to 4 days; infected persons are most contagious during period of peak symptoms
• Polyvalent influenza vaccine
◊ Recommended for all adults age 65 and over
◊ Recommended for high risk individuals: chronic pulmonary disease, cardiovascular disease, immunosuppression, hemoglobinopathies, renal diseases, metabolic disease, diabetes, HIV, long term aspirin therapy, asplenia, alcoholism
◊ Recommended for health care providers, home care providers, staff and residents of nursing homes and other chronic care facilities, homeless, public safety workers and close contacts of high risk individuals
◊ Should be administered in the Fall prior to influenza season
◊ Some side effects possible, e.g., fever and mild, local reaction at vaccination site.
◊ Two vaccines: Whole and split virus
- Split vaccine for children < 13 years old; adults may receive either vaccine.
- Dose is 0.5 IM except for children < 3 years old. Children 6 through 35 months old should receive 0.25 mL.
- Single dose/year except for children < 9 years old who should receive 2 doses the first year that they receive influenza vaccine (1 month apart)
- Vaccine contraindications: Anaphylaxis to eggs (do skin testing first)
- 2 weeks after immunization before protection occurs
• Amantadine and rimantadine:
◊ May be used prophylactically in high risk groups (that have not been vaccinated or need additional control measures) during epidemics of influenza A (ineffective against influenza B). It should not be considered as a substitute for vaccination unless vaccine contraindicated.
◊ Take for duration of outbreak, if no vaccine given. Discontinue after 14 days if used in addition to vaccine.
◊ Prophylactically during influenza season for those with contraindications to vaccine
◊ Prophylactically for staff and residents in nursing home outbreaks of influenza type A
◊ Protective efficacy about 80% for type A influenza virus only

EXPECTED COURSE/PROGNOSIS
Favorable

POSSIBLE COMPLICATIONS
• Otitis media
• Pneumonia
• Reye's syndrome
• Rhabdomyolysis
• Post-influenza asthenia
• Acute sinusitis
• Croup
• Apnea in neonates
• Bronchitis
• Death

MISCELLANEOUS

ASSOCIATED CONDITIONS Bacterial pneumonia

AGE-RELATED FACTORS
Pediatric: Reye's syndrome is a rare and severe complication associated with aspirin use. Do not give aspirin to children with influenza; use acetaminophen.
Geriatric:
• Elderly are more likely to have complications
• Immunization recommended for all individuals over age 65
Others: N/A

PREGNANCY
• Women with medical problems that place them at risk from complications of influenza should receive influenza vaccine regardless of trimester
• ACIP recommends vaccinating all women beyond first trimester of pregnancy during influenza season
• Amantadine is contraindicated in pregnant women

SYNONYMS
• Flu
• Grip
• Acute catarrhal fever

ICD-9-CM 487 Influenza

OTHER NOTES Persons with HIV infection should get annual influenza vaccination, however the antibody response to the vaccine may be low in persons with advanced HIV-related illnesses

SEE ALSO N/A

ABBREVIATIONS N/A

REFERENCES
• Report of the Committee on Infectious Diseases, 1997, Elk Grove Village, American Academy of Pediatrics, 1997
• Prevention and control of influenza. Recommendations of the Immunization Practices Advisory Committee (ACIP). MMWR; 46(RR-9):1997
• Mandell GL, ed: Principles and Practice of Infectious Diseases. 4th Ed. New York, Churchill Livingstone, 1995
Illustrations: N/A
Internet references: http://www.5mcc.com

Author(s)
Richard Kent Zimmerman, MD, MPH

Insect bites & stings

BASICS

DESCRIPTION Arthropods affect man by being pests, inoculating poison, invading tissue, or transmitting disease. Inoculation of poison may occur as either a bite or a sting. This discussion is limited to the irritative, poisonous, allergic effects of these pests.
• Harmful arthropods of the U.S. include:
◊ Bees: Bumblebees, sweat bees, honeybees
◊ Wasps: Hornets, wasps
◊ Ants: Fire ants, harvester ants
◊ Brown recluse spider
◊ Black widow spider
◊ Hobo spiders
◊ Scorpions
◊ Mosquitoes
◊ Flies: Deer, horse, black, stable, and biting midges
◊ Lice: Body, head, pubic
◊ Bugs: Kissing, bed, wheel
◊ Fleas: Human, cat, dog
◊ Mites: Itch mite (scabies), red bugs (chiggers)
◊ Ticks
◊ Caterpillars: Puss, browntail, buck
◊ Centipedes
• Characteristic reactions include:
◊ Local tissue irritation, inflammation and destruction
◊ Systemic effects related to inoculated poisons
◊ Allergic reactions: Immediate or delayed
System(s) affected: Skin/Exocrine
Genetics: N/A
Incidence/Prevalence in USA:
Widespread (seasonal and regional variance)
Predominant age: All ages
Predominant sex: Male = Female

SIGNS AND SYMPTOMS
• Local reactions:
◊ Erythema
◊ Pain
◊ Heat
◊ Swelling
◊ Itching
◊ Blisters
◊ Secondary infection - cellulitis, abscess
◊ Necrosis
◊ Ulceration
◊ Drainage
• Toxic reactions: Non-antigenic
◊ Nausea
◊ Vomiting
◊ Headache
◊ Fever
◊ Diarrhea
◊ Lightheadedness
◊ Syncope
◊ Drowsiness
◊ Muscles spasms
◊ Edema
◊ Convulsions
• Systemic reactions: Allergic
◊ Itching eyes
◊ Facial flushing
◊ Generalized urticaria
◊ Dry cough
◊ Chest/throat constriction
◊ Wheezing
◊ Dyspnea
◊ Cyanosis
◊ Abdominal cramps
◊ Diarrhea
◊ Nausea
◊ Vomiting
◊ Vertigo
◊ Chills/fever
◊ Stridor
◊ Shock
◊ Loss of consciousness
◊ Involuntary bowel/bladder action
◊ Frothy sputum
◊ Respiratory failure
◊ Cardiovascular collapse
◊ Death
• Delayed reaction:
◊ Serum-sickness-like reactions
◊ Fever
◊ Malaise
◊ Headache
◊ Urticaria
◊ Lymphadenopathy
◊ Polyarthritis
• Unusual reactions:
◊ Encephalopathy
◊ Neuritis
◊ Vasculitis
◊ Nephrosis
◊ Extreme fear/anxiety

CAUSES
• Local tissue inflammation and destruction from poison
• Allergic reaction from previous sensitization
• Toxic reaction from large inoculation of poison

RISK FACTORS
• Living environment
• Climate
• Season
• Clothing
• Lack of protective measures
• Perfumes, colognes
• Previous sensitization
• Young or elderly at more risk

DIAGNOSIS

DIFFERENTIAL DIAGNOSIS
• Local reaction: Infection, cellulitis, dermatoses, punctures, foreign bodies
• Toxic reaction: Chemical exposure/ingestion, medications, IV drug abuse, environmental, plants
• Allergic reaction: Medications, illicit drugs, foods, topical products, environmental, plants, chemicals

LABORATORY Leukocytosis,
thrombocytopenia, hypofibrinogenemia, abnormal coagulation, DIC, proteinuria, hemoglobinemia, hemoglobinuria, myoglobinemia, myoglobinuria, and azotemia are uncommon but possible manifestations in severe reactions

Drugs that may alter lab results: N/A
Disorders that may alter lab results: N/A

PATHOLOGICAL FINDINGS
Inflammation, ulceration, vesiculation, pustulation, rupture, eschar, swelling

SPECIAL TESTS N/A

IMAGING N/A

DIAGNOSTIC PROCEDURES N/A

TREATMENT

APPROPRIATE HEALTH CARE
• Outpatient or inpatient, depending on individual response to injury
• Hospitalize for severe systemic reactions with threatened airway obstruction, bronchospasm, hypotension, severe angiodermatitis or pain

GENERAL MEASURES
• First aid measures, local treatment, activate emergency services in severe reactions. If history of allergy or large envenomations, don't wait to seek emergency care.
• Use ANA kit and over-the-counter antihistamines, if available and required
• Local (depending on severity)
◊ Remove stinger (scrape it out - don't squeeze with tweezer)
◊ Cleanse wound
◊ Ice packs to bite or sting site (alternate 10 minutes on/10 minutes off)
◊ Elevation of affected part
◊ Rest the affected area
◊ Debride ulcers
◊ Drain abscesses
• Systemic (depending on severity, and type of reaction); home use - Epi-Pen
◊ Adequate airway (intubation, tracheostomy) - if needed to by-pass obstruction
◊ Oxygen (4-6 L/min) - if needed for respiratory distress
◊ Hospitalize and observe 24-48 hours

SURGICAL MEASURES Optimal
treatment of necrotic spider bites is not well defined. Surgical repair may be required of severe ulcerative lesions, but not until primary necrotizing process is complete.

ACTIVITY Rest to limit spread of poison

DIET No special diet; nothing by mouth if severe systemic reaction

PATIENT EDUCATION
• Protective measures, ANA kit use, risks
• Individuals with known sensitivity should wear medical identification (bracelet, tag) or carry a card

MEDICATIONS

DRUG(S) OF CHOICE
• Local (depending on severity)
◊ Analgesics
◊ Antihistamines - diphenhydramine (Benadryl) 25-50 mg qid
◊ Steroids topical or oral - prednisone 20-40 mg/day
◊ Antibiotics
• Systemic (depending on severity and type of reaction)
◊ Epinephrine [1:1000] subcutaneous: to combat urticaria, wheezing, angioedema - child 0.01 mL/kg, adult 0.3-0.5 mL
◊ Diphenhydramine: 25-50 mg IV or IM, to combat urticaria, wheezing, angioedema
◊ Aminophylline: adult 500 mg IV over 20-30 minutes, child 7.5 mg/kg, if needed for bronchospasm
◊ IV fluids (Ringer's lactate): if needed for hypotension, hypovolemia
◊ Dopamine: 200 mg in 250 mL at 5 mcg/kg/min - to correct vascular collapse. Titrate to maintain systemic blood pressure over 90 mm Hg.
◊ Hydrocortisone: 100-250 mg IV, if needed for severe urticaria or spider bite
◊ Tetanus prophylaxis and antibiotics: if indicated
◊ Diazepam (Valium): 5-10 mg, if needed for severe muscle spasms
◊ Morphine or meperidine (Demerol): if needed for pain
• Anti-venoms (e.g., Black Widow spider, scorpion) are available and appropriate in certain cases based on availability and identification of organism
Contraindications: Refer to manufacturer's literature
Precautions:
• Dosing appropriate to age
• If severe reaction, don't delay treatment
• Severe vascular collapse may require central pressure monitor
Significant possible interactions: Refer to manufacturer's literature

ALTERNATIVE DRUGS
Other antihistamines, e.g., loratadine, terfenadine, etc.

FOLLOWUP

PATIENT MONITORING
Followup wound care

PREVENTION/AVOIDANCE
• Avoid re-exposure in known hypersensitive individuals
• Prescribe anaphylactic (ANA kit) or Epi-Pen, if indicated
• Educate on risks of increasing anamnestic responses in future
• Consider desensitization with immunotherapy in severe cases

POSSIBLE COMPLICATIONS
• Infection
◊ Bacterial
◊ Arthropod associated diseases with tick, fly, bug and mosquito bites, e.g., lyme borreliosis, rickettsial disease (Rocky Mountain spotted fever), arborviral encephalitis, malaria, leishmaniasis, trypanosomiasis, dengue
• Scarring
• Drug reactions
• Multisystem failure
• Death

EXPECTED COURSE/PROGNOSIS
• Minor reactions - excellent
• Severe reactions - excellent with early, appropriate treatment

MISCELLANEOUS

ASSOCIATED CONDITIONS N/A

AGE-RELATED FACTORS
Pediatric: More at risk
Geriatric: More at risk
Others: N/A

PREGNANCY
Not a contraindication to appropriate management

SYNONYMS N/A

ICD-9-CM
• 989.5 Insect sting
• 910.-919. (injury superficial by site, plus 4th digit 0-9 for subdivision)

SEE ALSO N/A

OTHER NOTES N/A

ABBREVIATIONS N/A

REFERENCES
• Tintinalli JE, Krome RL, eds: Emergency Medicine. New York, McGraw-Hill, 1988
• Schroeder SA, Krupp MA, Tierne, LM, McPhee SJ, eds: Current Medical Diagnosis and Treatment. Norwalk, CT, Appleton & Lange, 1989
• MMWR: Necrotic arachnidism-Pacific Northwest, 1988-1996. 1996;Vol45:No 21
• Isselbacher KJ, et al, eds: Harrison's Principles of Internal Medicine. 13th Ed. New York, McGraw-Hill, 1994
Illustrations: 11 available on CD-ROM
Internet references: http://www.5mcc.com

Author(s)
Robert L. Weston, MD

Insomnia

BASICS

DESCRIPTION Difficulty in falling asleep or maintaining sleep, intermittent wakefulness, early morning awakening or a combination of these. Can be:
• Transient - due to a life crisis, bereavement, change in environment or concomitant illness
• Chronic - associated with medical and psychiatric conditions or drug intake.
System(s) affected: Nervous
Genetics: N/A
Incidence/Prevalence in USA: Affects an estimated 35% of the adult population. One of the most frequent complaints in primary care practice.
Predominant age: Elderly
Predominant sex: Male = Female

SIGNS AND SYMPTOMS
• Perceived reduction in sleeping time
• Initial insomnia - difficulty initiating sleep at usual time
• Middle insomnia - wakefulness during the usual sleep cycle, "tossing and turning"
• Terminal insomnia - early awakening
• Daytime sleepiness and napping
• Tiredness
• Anticipatory anxiety

CAUSES
• Medical illnesses - arthritis, fibromyalgia, hyperthyroidism, gastro-esophageal reflux disease, duodenal ulcer, Alzheimer's disease and other dementias, restless leg syndrome, sleep apnea, respiratory diseases, and all painful conditions (e.g., muscle cramps)
• Psychiatric illnesses - mostly depression, classically associated with early morning awakening, but can also be manifested by initial or middle insomnia
• Anxiety
• Schizophrenia
• Manic disorders
• Drug induced insomnia - alcohol, caffeine, nicotine
• Nonprescription drugs - diet aids, decongestants, cough preparations
• Prescribed drugs - steroids, theophylline, phenytoin (Dilantin), levodopa (Sinemet, Dopar)
• Obstructive sleep apnea
• Jet lag (transient)
• Heavy smoking

RISK FACTORS
• Chronic illnesses
• Age over 50
• Multiple drug intake
• Obesity

DIAGNOSIS

DIFFERENTIAL DIAGNOSIS N/A

LABORATORY N/A
Drugs that may alter lab results: N/A
Disorders that may alter lab results: N/A

PATHOLOGICAL FINDINGS N/A

SPECIAL TESTS Diagnosis can be confirmed by the use of polysomnography, particularly if sleep apnea is suspected. This is generally not necessary or practical.

IMAGING N/A

DIAGNOSTIC PROCEDURES Insomnia is a self-reported condition

TREATMENT

APPROPRIATE HEALTH CARE
Outpatient

GENERAL MEASURES
• Transient insomnia
  ◊ Lasts less than three to four weeks
  ◊ Reassurance and supportive counseling are appropriate treatment modalities
• Chronic insomnia
  ◊ Address the underlying cause: Pain, drugs, depression
  ◊ Avoid alcohol after 5 PM or within 6 hours of retiring because of secondary rebound stimulation
  ◊ Patient should be encouraged to avoid daytime napping and to develop bedtime rituals conducive to sleep
  ◊ A thorough review of the patient's habits, drug intake, diet, and exercise pattern may uncover correctable causes of insomnia
  ◊ Prescribe hypnotics only if the above strategies fail

SURGICAL MEASURES N/A

ACTIVITY
• No restriction
• A daily exercise routine is helpful. Avoid exercise close to bedtime.

DIET
• Avoid caffeine
• Avoid heavy, late night snacks (sometimes a light snack before bedtime may help)
• Avoid alcohol after 5 PM or within 6 hours of retiring, because of secondary rebound stimulation

PATIENT EDUCATION
• Explain sleep patterns and sleep hygiene
• Show limitations and noxious effects of drugs used for insomnia
• Incorporation of appropriate dietary and exercise protocol

MEDICATIONS

DRUG(S) OF CHOICE
- Analgesics as indicated for pain
- Benzodiazepines for insomnia (3 currently used in the U.S.)
  ◊ Flurazepam (Dalmane), 15-30 mg, long half life, elderly might benefit from smaller dose
  ◊ Temazepam (Restoril), 15 mg one to two hours before bedtime
  ◊ Triazolam (Halcion), shortest half life, 0.125 mg to 0.25 mg, smaller dose recommended for the elderly. Useful as part of treatment regimen for jet lag.
- Tricyclic antidepressants
  ◊ Widely used for insomnia associated with depression
  ◊ Preferred agent is amitriptyline (Elavil) because of its marked sedative effect. A typical starting dose is 50-100 mg at bedtime.
- Non-benzodiazepine agent
  ◊ Zolpidem (Ambien), 10 mg for adults and 5 mg for the elderly/debilitated.

Contraindications:
- Pregnancy and lactation
- Psychoses
- Acute narrow angle glaucoma
- Significant liver disease
- Depressed patient who may be suicide risk

Precautions:
- All benzodiazepines can cause paradoxical, agitated states, anterograde amnesia, and rebound insomnia
- Flurazepam may cause incoordination ataxia and impairment of intellectual functions
- Triazolam has been associated with withdrawal psychosis and seizures in some patients after abrupt cessation, psychological dependence, physical dependence
- Amitriptyline can cause constipation and orthostatic hypotension
- Zolpidem, although generally well-tolerated, should be used with the same precautions taken with other sedative hyponotics. Most common reported side effects are drowsiness, dizziness, headache.

Significant possible interactions:
- Alcohol may potentiate the CNS effects of the benzodiazepines
- Digoxin serum concentrations may be increased
- Levodopa efficacy may be reduced

ALTERNATIVE DRUGS
- Diphenhydramine (Benadryl) has been used to induce sleep in the elderly, but it may also cause confusion and "hangover"
- Chloral hydrate (Noctec), 250-500 mg, is favored by some clinicians since it does not cause tolerance or withdrawal. The nightly dose is 250-500 mg.
- Melatonin, a pineal hormone. Marketed as a dietary supplement. There is some evidence that controlled-release melatonin improves sleep quality in a selected elderly population. Not FDA approved. Appears useful for jet lag. Has mild hypnotic effect. No adverse effects have been reported, but controlled studies are lacking.

FOLLOWUP

PATIENT MONITORING
- Need for benzodiazepines to be reassessed periodically. Avoid standing prescriptions.
- Followup as needed depending on individual patient. Refer for psychosocial counseling, if appropriate.

PREVENTION/AVOIDANCE
Avoidance, when possible, of all possible causes

POSSIBLE COMPLICATIONS
- Transient insomnia becomes chronic
- Increased daytime sleepiness

EXPECTED COURSE/PROGNOSIS
Should resolve with time. Treatment of underlying symptoms helpful.

MISCELLANEOUS

ASSOCIATED CONDITIONS
- Obstructive sleep apnea
- Drug or alcohol addiction and dependence

AGE-RELATED FACTORS
Pediatric: N/A
Geriatric:
- Exert caution when prescribing benzodiazepines or other sedative-hypnotics to the elderly
- Educate older patients about age-related sleep changes
Others: N/A

PREGNANCY
Transient insomnia occurs due to discomfort in sleeping positions

SYNONYMS
Sleeplessness

ICD-9-CM
780.50 Sleep disturbance, unspecified
780.51 Insomnia with sleep apnea
780.52 Other insomnia

SEE ALSO
- Sleep apnea
- Depression
- Anxiety

OTHER NOTES
L-Tryptophan - formerly widely used - no longer available as a single ingredient

ABBREVIATIONS
N/A

REFERENCES
- Rakel R, ed: Textbook of Family Practice. 5th Ed. Philadelphia, W.B. Saunders Co., 1995
- Goldman HH: Review of General Psychiatry. 4th Ed. Norwalk, CT, Appleton & Lange, 1995
- Bahrat RS, Nakra MD, et al: Insomnia in the Elderly. Amer Fam Phys 1991;477-483
- The Medical Letter on Drugs and Therapeutics. Vol 35, Issue 895, April 30, 1993
- The Medical Letter on Drugs and Therapeutics. Vol 37, Issue 962, November 24, 1995
- Maczaj M: Pharmalogical treatment of insomnia. Drugs 1993;45(1):44-55
- Garfinkel D, Laudon M, Nof D, Zisapel N: Improvement of sleep quality in elderly people by controlled-release melatonin. Lancet 1995;346(8974):541-544
- Dockhorn RJ, Dockhorn DW: Zolpidem in the treatment of short-term insomnia: a randomized placebo-controlled trial. Clin Neuropharmacol 1996;19(4):333-340
Illustrations: N/A
Internet references: http://www.5mcc.com

Author(s)
Michel J. Dodard, MD

Insulinoma

BASICS

DESCRIPTION Insulinomas are tumors of the pancreatic beta cells of the islets of Langerhans. They are usually very small with 70% measuring less than 1.5 cm. They are usually single and benign with only 10-15% being malignant and only 10% being multiple tumors. Their malignant potential is not as clinically important as their functional ability to secrete insulin, which leads to symptomatic hypoglycemia.
• The symptomatic hypoglycemia is secondary to persistent, absolute, or relative hyperinsulinemia that is unresponsive to normal feedback mechanisms
• The hypoglycemic episodes are irregular, recurrent, and tend to increase in frequency and severity over time
• Hypoglycemic episodes are especially likely to occur when fasting or after exercise
• Pancreatic beta cells secrete both insulin and C-peptide
• Whipple's triad is the basis for the clinical diagnosis of insulinomas.
    ◊ Symptomatic fasting or postexercise hypoglycemia
    ◊ Low blood glucose levels less than 50 mg/dL (2.78 mmol/L) during symptoms.
    ◊ Resolution of symptoms when treated with oral or IV glucose
• Laboratory diagnosis is based on inappropriately high serum insulin and C-peptides during periods of low blood glucose (shows oversecretion and endogenous origin)
• Awareness is the key to early diagnosis
System(s) affected: Endocrine-Metabolic, Cardiovascular, Nervous, Gastrointestinal
Genetics: No known genetic pattern unless part of MEN 1 syndrome
Incidence/Prevalence in USA: Annual incidence of 1 in 1.25 million persons
Predominant age:
• Rare less than 20 years old
• 20% of cases in adults under 40 years old
• 40% of cases in adults between 40 and 60 years old
• 40% or cases in adults over 60 years old
Predominant sex: 60% of cases occur in males

SIGNS AND SYMPTOMS
Due to hypoglycemia
• Neurological
    ◊ Apathy
    ◊ Irritability
    ◊ Confusion
    ◊ Disorientation
    ◊ Delirium
    ◊ Coma
    ◊ Convulsions
    ◊ Diplopia
    ◊ Blurred vision
    ◊ Vertigo
    ◊ Inarticulate speech
    ◊ Tremor
    ◊ Dizziness
    ◊ Hallucinations
• Cardiovascular
    ◊ Palpitations
    ◊ Tachycardia
    ◊ Angina
    ◊ Sweating
• Gastrointestinal
    ◊ Hunger
    ◊ Abdominal discomfort
    ◊ Nausea
    ◊ Vomiting
    ◊ Weight gain

CAUSES   Etiology unknown

RISK FACTORS
• Male
• Older than 40
• MEN 1 syndrome

DIAGNOSIS

DIFFERENTIAL DIAGNOSIS
• Medications
    ◊ Inappropriate insulin
    ◊ Sulfonylureas
    ◊ Beta-blockers
    ◊ Salicylates
    ◊ Quinine
• Very rare causes
    ◊ Nesidioblastosis
    ◊ Large sarcomas
    ◊ Hepatocellular carcinoma
• Reactive hypoglycemia

LABORATORY
• Document low blood sugar during symptoms
• RIA of serum insulin and C-peptide (inappropriately elevated during symptoms)
• Insulin/glucose ratio much greater than normal of 0.4 or less
• Malignant tumors may secrete B-HCG
Drugs that may alter lab results: N/A
Disorders that may alter lab results: N/A

PATHOLOGICAL FINDINGS
• Usually small and single
• Malignant tumors tend to be larger and multiple
• Metastases are found in the liver or regional lymph nodes (distant metastases rare)
• Tumors evenly distributed throughout the pancreas (1/3 in head, 1/3 in body, 1/3 in tail)

SPECIAL TESTS
• Fast for 72 hours or until symptoms develop. When symptomatic, determine insulin, C-peptide, and glucose levels.
• Provocative testing
    ◊ IV calcium gluconate (15 mg/kg of elemental calcium) over 4 hours determining insulin and glucose levels
    ◊ Tolbutamide bolus (1 gram after an overnight fast) and determine insulin and glucose levels at 150 minutes
    ◊ C-peptide suppression with 0.1 unit/kg of insulin and determine C-peptide and glucose levels

IMAGING
• Selective mesenteric angiography (detects 52-85%)
• Preoperative CT (detects 70%)
• Endoscopic ultrasound
• Preoperative ultrasound (detects 22-63%)
• Intraoperative ultrasound (detects 86%)
• Somatostatin analogue I123 labeled TyR 3-octreotide

DIAGNOSTIC PROCEDURES
• Document high insulin/glucose ratio during symptoms
• 72 hour fast
• Portal venous sampling
• Intraoperative ultrasound
• Intraoperative palpation

TREATMENT

APPROPRIATE HEALTH CARE
Treatment is primarily surgical; medical treatment for surgically incurable lesions

GENERAL MEASURES
• Closely observe for severe hypoglycemic symptoms
• Attempt to increase glucose levels
• Attempt to decrease insulin levels
• Keep a ready glucose source available

SURGICAL MEASURES
• Enucleation if tumor is superficial
• Partial pancreatectomy if tumor is deep-seated or invasive

ACTIVITY   Avoid exercise

DIET Frequent high carbohydrate meals and snacks

PATIENT EDUCATION   N/A

MEDICATIONS

DRUG(S) OF CHOICE
• To decrease insulin secretion
◊ Diazoxide 100-150 mg po q8h (3-8 mg/kg daily in 2 or 3 divided doses)
◊ Octreotide acetate (long acting analog of somatostatin); 50-100 mcg SQ bid, increase as needed to control symptoms
• To increase glucose levels
◊ Oral or IV glucose
◊ IM or SQ glucagon
• For metastatic disease
◊ Streptozocin
◊ Fluorouracil

Contraindications: Refer to manufacturer's literature

Precautions:
• Strenuous exercise
• Prolonged fasts
• May need diuretic to counteract the sodium and fluid retention of diazoxide

Significant possible interactions: Refer to manufacturer's literature

ALTERNATIVE DRUGS
• Octreotide acetate. Continue treatment until surgery or lifelong if tumor is unresectable.
• Dacarbazine (DTIC, 5-dimethyltriazenoimidazole-4-carboxamine) for metastatic disease
• To increase glucose levels
◊ Corticosteroids
◊ Propranolol
◊ Phenytoin

FOLLOWUP

PATIENT MONITORING
Watch for recurrence of hypoglycemic symptoms

PREVENTION/AVOIDANCE
N/A

POSSIBLE COMPLICATIONS
• From surgery
◊ Pancreatitis
◊ Pancreatic leaks
◊ Fistulae
◊ Peritonitis
◊ Abscess
◊ Pseudocysts

EXPECTED COURSE/PROGNOSIS
Excellent if tumor solitary, benign, and completely resected

MISCELLANEOUS:

ASSOCIATED CONDITIONS
MEN 1 syndrome

AGE-RELATED FACTORS
Pediatric: N/A
Geriatric: N/A
Others: N/A

PREGNANCY
N/A

SYNONYMS
• Beta cell tumor
• Beta cell adenoma
• Nesidioblastoma

ICD-9-CM
157.4 Malignant neoplasm of the islets of Langerhans
211.7 Benign tumor of the islets of Langerhans

SEE ALSO
Hypoglycemia, nondiabetic

OTHER NOTES
• 8% of patients with MEN 1 syndrome have insulinomas
• Insulinomas associated with MEN 1 syndrome tend to be multiple tumors and present at an earlier age

ABBREVIATIONS
N/A

REFERENCES
• Mozell E, Woltering E, Stenzel P, Rosch J, O'Dorisio T: Functional endocrine tumors of the pancreas: clinical presentation, diagnosis, and management. Curr Prob Surg 1990;27:335-47
• Goode AW: Insulinoma. J R Soc Med 1989;82:383-4
• Modlin IM, Lewis JJ, Ahlman H, Bilchik AJ, Kumar RR: Management of unresectable malignant endocrine tumors of the pancreas. Surg Gynecol & Obstet 1993;176:507-18
• Correnti S, Liverani A, Antonini G, Paganelli MT, Mercati U: Intraoperative ultrasonography for pancreatic insulinomas. Hepato-Gastroenterology 1996;43:207-211
Illustrations: N/A
Internet references: http://www.5mcc.com

Author(s)
Rick Ricer, MD

Intestinal obstruction

BASICS

DESCRIPTION Intestinal obstruction exists where there is a failure, reversal or impairment of the normal transit of intestinal contents. Obstructions may be partial or complete and are manifested by abdominal pain, emesis and obstipation.
System(s) affected: Gastrointestinal
Genetics: Unknown
Incidence/Prevalence in USA: Accounts, for approximately 20% of all admissions for acute abdominal conditions
Predominant age: N/A
Predominant sex: Male = Female

SIGNS AND SYMPTOMS
• Abdominal pain - diffuse, poorly localized abdominal cramping at intervals of 5 to 15 minutes
• Emesis - usually occurs immediately after obstruction of bowel. More frequent in proximal obstruction. Unusual in colon obstruction until small bowel distention occurs.
• Obstipation - common symptom. May pass contents distal to obstruction especially in high intestinal obstruction. Pain followed by explosive diarrhea often seen in partial obstruction.
• Inspection - with or without distention (a late finding), less likely in proximal obstructions
• Auscultation - high pitched bowel sounds, peristaltic rushes
• Palpation - tenderness, mass, presence of peritoneal signs (these suggest strangulation)
• Rectal examination - may reveal fecal impaction. Occult blood may suggest colon malignancy.

CAUSES
• Luminal lesions
  ◊ Impactions
  ◊ Gallstones
  ◊ Meconium in newborns
  ◊ Intussusception in infants
• Intrinsic lesions
  ◊ Congenital (e.g., atresia and stenosis, imperforate anus, duplications, Meckel's diverticulum)
  ◊ Trauma
  ◊ Inflammatory (e.g., Crohn's disease, diverticulitis, ulcerative colitis, radiation, toxic [ingestions]
  ◊ Neoplastic (most common etiology of colon obstruction)
  ◊ Miscellaneous (e.g., endometriosis)
• Extrinsic lesions
  ◊ Adhesions (most common etiology of small bowel obstruction)
  ◊ Hernia and wound dehiscence
  ◊ Masses (e.g., annular pancreas, anomalous vasculature, abscess and hematoma, neoplasms)
  ◊ Volvulus
  ◊ Neuromuscular defect (e.g., megacolon, neuro/myopathic motility disorders)

RISK FACTORS
• Previous abdominal and/or pelvic surgery
• Hernia
• Chronic constipation
• Cholelithiasis
• Inflammatory bowel disease
• Ingested foreign bodies - pica, enteric potassium tablets, etc.
• Diverticular disease

DIAGNOSIS

DIFFERENTIAL DIAGNOSIS Adynamic ileus

LABORATORY
• WBC: Slight rise (15,000/mm3). Significant increases associated with strangulation.
• Hematocrit: Moderate rise associated with extracellular fluid loss
• Renal: Urine specific gravity 1.025-1.030 and rise in BUN and creatinine due to extracellular volume loss
• Amylase: May be elevated. Unreliable as an indicator of obstruction or strangulation.
• Blood gases: May be normal. Late changes are those of acidosis.
• No single or series of laboratory studies are useful in diagnosis of intestinal strangulation
Drugs that may alter lab results: N/A
Disorders that may alter lab results: N/A

PATHOLOGICAL FINDINGS
• Edema of mucosa
• Hypersecretion
• Necrosis

SPECIAL TESTS N/A

IMAGING
• Abdominal and chest radiographs
  ◊ Distention of small bowel or colon
  ◊ Air-fluid levels (may be seen in ileus, gastroenteritis, constipation)
  ◊ Lack of colon gas
  ◊ Free intraperitoneal air (strangulation with perforation)
  ◊ "Bird beak" lesion in colonic volvulus
  ◊ Foreign body visualization
• Contrast studies
  ◊ Barium enema useful for diagnosis of colonic obstruction and may be therapeutic in intussusception
  ◊ Barium or Gastrografin orally may differentiate obstruction from ileus
  ◊ Enteroclysis may identify site of small bowel obstruction

DIAGNOSTIC PROCEDURES
• Rigid proctoscopy. May be therapeutic in sigmoid volvulus.
• Flexible sigmoidoscopy

TREATMENT

APPROPRIATE HEALTH CARE
• Inpatient
• Treatment directed at early gastrointestinal decompression, correction of fluid and electrolyte abnormalities, timely operative intervention, surgical/GI consultation required

GENERAL MEASURES
• Nasogastric suction
• Foley catheter
• Swan-Ganz catheter or other central monitor, if required
• Intravenous fluids: Normal saline/Ringer's solution with potassium supplementation as required
• Antibiotic use controversial in absence of sepsis, but prophylactic antibiotics probably appropriate

SURGICAL MEASURES
• Timing of operative intervention critical, must correct electrolytes, volume quickly prior to surgery
• Surgical procedures:
  ◊ Closed bowel procedures: lysis of adhesions, reduction of intussusception, reduction of volvulus, reduction of incarcerated hernia
  ◊ Enterotomy for removal of bezoars, foreign bodies, gallstones
  ◊ Resection of bowel for obstructing lesions, strangulated bowel
  ◊ Bypasses of intestine around obstruction
  ◊ Enterocutaneous fistulae proximal to obstruction: colostomy, cecostomy

ACTIVITY Bedrest

DIET NPO

PATIENT EDUCATION N/A

MEDICATIONS

DRUG(S) OF CHOICE Surgeon's choice for prophylaxis
Contraindications: N/A
Precautions: N/A
Significant possible interactions: N/A

ALTERNATIVE DRUGS N/A

FOLLOWUP

PATIENT MONITORING Follow weekly postoperatively for 2-8 weeks

PREVENTION/AVOIDANCE N/A

POSSIBLE COMPLICATIONS
• Slow return of bowel function
• Higher risk of subsequent obstruction
• Sepsis

EXPECTED COURSE/PROGNOSIS
Usually excellent prognosis. In general, mortality from intestinal obstruction ranges from < 1% to > 20% depending upon etiology, bowel viability, co-morbidities, etc.

MISCELLANEOUS

ASSOCIATED CONDITIONS N/A

AGE-RELATED FACTORS
Pediatric:
• Different etiologies of obstruction in childhood
  ◊ Duodenal malformations
  ◊ Jejunoileal atresia
  ◊ Malrotation and midgut volvulus
  ◊ Meconium ileus
  ◊ Necrotizing enterocolitis
  ◊ Hirschsprung's disease
  ◊ Intussusception
  ◊ Duplications
  ◊ Meckel's diverticulum
  ◊ Imperforate anus
Geriatric:
• Colon neoplasms more common
• Chronic constipation/impactions more common
Others: N/A

PREGNANCY N/A

SYNONYMS N/A

ICD-9-CM 569+

SEE ALSO N/A

OTHER NOTES Rectal examination showing occult blood may represent colon malignancy as etiology of the obstruction

ABBREVIATIONS N/A

REFERENCES Sleisenger MH, Fordtran JS, eds: Gastrointestinal Disease: Pathophysiology, Diagnosis, Management. 5th Ed. Philadelphia, W.B. Saunders Co., 1994
Illustrations: N/A
Internet references: http://www.5mcc.com

Author(s)
Leo C. Mercer, MD

Intestinal parasites

BASICS

DESCRIPTION
• The class of infectious agents called parasites is divided into two parts:
◊ Protozoa are single cell animals which characteristically divide and multiply within the host, are usually direct fecal-oral in transmission, and do not cause an eosinophilia
◊ Helminths (worms) are multi-cellular animals and with rare exceptions (i.e., Strongyloides stercoralis, Hymenolepis nana) do not multiply within the host and are often associated with some degree of eosinophilia. The level of eosinophilia is associated with the degree of mucosal invasiveness. The worms have a limited life span within the host and without reinfection would eventually die on their own.
• Not all of the parasites that start out by ingestion in the bowel will remain in the bowel. Some are invasive and some do not release their infective forms into the bowel. This later group, including Toxoplasma gondii, Echinococcus, Trichinella spiralis will not be covered in this topic.
• Most worms require either a prolonged incubation period outside the host before being infectious or need a specific vector for transmission. A notable exception to this rule is Enterobius vermicularis (pinworm), the eggs of which are infectious shortly after being passed, so auto-infection occurs readily.
• Direct person-to-person transmission is uncommon
• The likelihood of acquiring an intestinal parasite depends on several factors - the presence of the specific infectious agent, an appropriate "vector" or mode of transmission, and a host who is susceptible to the infectious agent. The world-wide distribution of parasites is determined by geographic factors, socio-economics, age, and crowding with poor food preparation and a break in the standard of water and personal sanitation being the major factors.
System(s) affected: Gastrointestinal
Genetics: Genetic factors play a minor role in the acquisition, pathogenesis and clearance of these infections
Incidence/Prevalence in USA:
• From laboratory statistics: 5-30% general population
• From day care surveys: Asymptomatic 20-30%; symptomatic 50-80%
• Intestinal protozoa account for the majority of parasitological findings in North America (most considered to be non-pathogenic)
• In a random sampling, at least one parasite would be found in the stools of 5-10% of all people. If Blastocystis hominis were included in this accounting, 20-30% of specimens examined in parasitology will be positive.
• Helminths are considerably rarer and are highly dependent on population demographics and prior geographic exposure risk factors. In general, less than 10% of all parasitology reports include a helminth.

Predominant age: Pediatric
Predominant sex: Male = Female

SIGNS AND SYMPTOMS
• Diarrhea
• Abdominal pain/tenderness
• Excessive gas - bloating, eructation, flatulence, borborygmi
• Nausea or vomiting
• Weight loss and anorexia
• Dysentery, i.e., bleeding (rare, but associated with Entamoeba histolytica, Balantidium coli)
• Pruritus ani (E. vermicularis, Trichuris trichiura, S. stercoralis, tapeworms)
• Passing a worm or a worm segment
• Increased bowel sounds
• Peri-rectal or vulvar rash

CAUSES
• Protozoan pathogens:
◊ Giardia lamblia
◊ Entamoeba histolytica
◊ Cryptosporidium
◊ Isospora belli
◊ Balantidium coli
◊ Cyclospora cayetanensis
◊ Microsporida
• Possible protozoan pathogens:
◊ Dientamoeba fragilis
• Probable non-pathogenic protozoa
◊ All other Entamoeba
◊ Endolimax nana
◊ All other intestinal flagellates
• Helminthic pathogens - nematodes (roundworms):
◊ Enterobius vermicularis
◊ Trichuris trichiura
◊ Ascaris lumbricoides
◊ Hookworm (Necator americanus, Ancylostoma duodenale)
◊ Strongyloides stercoralis
◊ Capillaria philippinensis
◊ Trichostrongylus sp
• Helminthic pathogens - trematodes (flukes)
◊ Fasciolopsis buski
◊ Clonorchis sinensis
◊ Opisthorchis viverrini
◊ Heterophyes heterophyes
◊ Fasciola hepatica
◊ Paragonimus westermani
◊ Schistosoma mansoni
◊ S. japonicum
◊ S. hematobium
◊ S. mekongi
• Helminthic pathogens - cestodes (tapeworms)
◊ Taenia saginata
◊ Taenia solium
◊ Diphyllobothrium latum
◊ Hymenolepis nana
◊ Hymenolepis diminuta
◊ Dipylidium caninum

RISK FACTORS
• Age (children)
• Low socioeconomic status
• Poor sanitation - personal, food, water
• International travel
• Crowding - day care centers, institutional care
• Intercurrent medical conditions, pregnancy, gastric hypoacidity, immunosuppression (AIDS)

DIAGNOSIS

DIFFERENTIAL DIAGNOSIS
• Other intestinal infections
• Food poisoning
• Malabsorption
• Inflammatory bowel disease
• Hemorrhoids
• Rectal fissures

LABORATORY
• Examination of a single stool specimen collected into a preservative (i.e., sodium acetate formalin [SAF]), well mixed to fix and preserve all elements, will provide an accurate diagnosis in 90% of patients. Additional specimens will need to be examined for greater diagnostic accuracy.
• Newer techniques of lab exam of stool specimens (such as monoclonal antibodies, other antigen detection techniques, DNA detection) are exciting developments but currently provide little practical advantage over routine techniques. These techniques are needed to differentiate E. histolytica from E. dispas
• Serology - for specific infections, especially if they do not produce a patent infection in the bowel (i.e., no eggs or parasites released into the stool), or if low numbers of parasites makes the diagnosis difficult. These tests are rarely indicated and are usually available only through referral centers.
Drugs that may alter lab results: Use of antibiotics, oil based laxatives, and the presence of barium in the stool may make a parasitological diagnosis difficult or impossible
Disorders that may alter lab results: N/A

PATHOLOGICAL FINDINGS
• Majority of intestinal parasites are not invasive and produce no or non-specific changes in the histology of the bowel
• Invasive amebiasis of the bowel produces a classical endoscopic and histological picture of ulceration and inflammation in the colon
• Protozoa and helminths may be seen in bowel biopsies

SPECIAL TESTS
• Special techniques for the detection of Cryptosporidium, Isospora belli, Cyclospora, and microsporidia often require that the laboratory be informed of the "risk" profile of the patient before these tests will be done
• Pinworm paddles provide a greater diagnostic yield when Enterobius vermicularis is being considered. Multiple tests (5) may be needed to exclude the diagnosis of pinworms.
• Parasite culture is possible for a few organisms - Giardia lamblia, Entamoeba histolytica, Strongyloides stercoralis, but are rarely indicated and are usually available only in referral laboratories
• String tests and upper bowel intubations are rarely needed to diagnose the upper intestinal parasites

• Rarely, a biopsy will demonstrate the presence of an invasive helminth on tissue section. Worms can be extremely difficult to diagnose in this manner, usually needing the expertise of a tissue parasite pathologist. The other parasites may be visualized on the mucosa or in the mucous layer.

IMAGING Diagnostic radiology rarely needed. Exception is for invasive infections such as amebiasis where colitis, amebomas and liver abscesses may be demonstrated by the appropriate techniques.

DIAGNOSTIC PROCEDURES
• Invasive diagnostic procedures are rarely needed or indicated
• With hemorrhagic colitis and a possible diagnosis of invasive amebiasis, sigmoidoscopy will reveal a muco-purulent colitis with ulceration. A scraping from an ulcer, promptly examined by microscopy, will reveal the motile hematophagous trophozoites of E. histolytica.
• Upper intestinal endoscopy can yield fluid to be examined for Giardia lamblia and Strongyloides stercoralis, as can impression smears and biopsies obtained with the endoscope

TREATMENT

APPROPRIATE HEALTH CARE
Outpatient except for rare surgery or inpatient medical treatment

GENERAL MEASURES
• Therapy must be assessed in the best interest of the patient. Not all patients need to be treated with drugs.
• Symptomatic treatment is indicated for patient comfort once specific therapy has been initiated
• Bowel paralyzing drugs, for diarrhea caused by invasive organisms, are relatively contraindicated

SURGICAL MEASURES
• Surgical procedures play little role in treatment except when amebic liver abscesses need to be drained, e.g., multiple or large abscesses not responding to medical management, or threatened rupture, especially left lobe abscesses. Drainage of such abscesses is often accomplished by directed catheter placement in radiology, with surgical back-up as required.
• Surgery may be required if bowel or other organ obstruction occurs, as can be seen with Ascaris lumbricoides migration

ACTIVITY As tolerated

DIET
• Nutritional support may be required
• Many patients during and following bowel infections, especially when infected with Giardia lamblia, will experience irritable bowel syndrome and/or lactose intolerance. The majority of these patients will respond to a lactose free diet, reduction of caffeine intake, and an increase in dietary fiber.

PATIENT EDUCATION
• Educating the patient is important to reduce the risk of reinfection or transmission
• Education will depend on the parasite, host characteristics and the environment that the two interact in

MEDICATIONS

DRUG(S) OF CHOICE
• Protozoa
  ◊ Entamoeba histolytica asymptomatic needs individual assessment
  ◊ Entamoeba histolytica symptomatic intestinal - iodoquinol or diloxanide furoate
  ◊ Entamoeba histolytica invasive disease - iodoquinol or diloxanide furoate. Plus metronidazole, alone or dehydroemetine or emetine plus chloroquine phosphate.
  ◊ Giardia lamblia - metronidazole or tinidazole or furazolidone or quinacrine. Note: albendazole, available in US only from manufacturer, may have activity against G. lamblia.
  ◊ Cryptosporidium - none proven effective
  ◊ Isospora belli protozoa - trimethoprim-sulfamethoxazole
  ◊ Balantidium coli - tetracycline or iodoquinol or metronidazole
  ◊ Cyclospora - possibly sulfamethoxazole-trimethoprim
  ◊ Microsporidia - albendazole (some species)
• Helminths
  ◊ Nematodes (except Strongyloides and Trichostrongylus) - mebendazole or pyrantel pamoate or piperazine citrate or albendazole (available in US only from manufacturer)
  ◊ Strongyloides and Trichostrongylus - thiabendazole or albendazole (available in US only from manufacturer)
  ◊ Cestodes - praziquantel or niclosamide
  ◊ Trematodes - niclosamide or praziquantel
Contraindications: Refer to manufacturer's profile of each drug
Precautions: Refer to manufacturer's profile of each drug
Significant possible interactions: Refer to manufacturer's profile of each drug

ALTERNATIVE DRUGS N/A

FOLLOWUP

PATIENT MONITORING Repeat examination, to ensure clearance, should be timed taking into account: The life cycle of the parasite (how long would it take to regenerate and become patent) and the risk of reinfection, as well as the specific test likely to find the parasite (stool, pinworm paddle, culture, serology)

PREVENTION/AVOIDANCE The specific nature of the infection often dictates the specific methods needed to avoid reinfection. This usually involves matters of personal, food and/or water sanitation.

POSSIBLE COMPLICATIONS See specific text on individual parasite

EXPECTED COURSE/PROGNOSIS See specific text on individual parasite

MISCELLANEOUS

ASSOCIATED CONDITIONS N/A

AGE-RELATED FACTORS
Pediatric: Most common age group affected
Geriatric: Illness may cause more severe debilitation
Others: AIDS - susceptibility to infection

PREGNANCY Some of these infections can be particularly serious in pregnancy. Many of the drugs are contraindicated in pregnancy.

SYNONYMS N/A

ICD-9-CM 129 Intestinal parasitism, unspecified

SEE ALSO N/A

OTHER NOTES N/A

ABBREVIATIONS N/A

REFERENCES
• MacPherson DW: Intestinal Parasites. In: Rakel RE, ed. Conn's Current Therapy. Philadelphia, W.B. Saunders Co., 1990:486-92
• Abramowicz M, ed: Drugs for parasitic infections. In The Medical Letter. New York, The Medical Letter Inc. 1995, Vol. 37:97-108
• Mandell GL, ed: Principles and Practice of Infectious Diseases. 4th Ed. New York, Churchill Livingstone, 1995
Illustrations: N/A
Internet references: http://www.5mcc.com

Author(s)
D. W. MacPherson, MD, MSc (CTM), FRCPC
T. C. Yang, MD, FRCPC

Intussusception

BASICS

DESCRIPTION Invagination of a portion of intestine into itself (may involve any part of small intestine, ileocolic [95%], or colo-colic)
System(s) affected: Gastrointestinal
Genetics: N/A
Incidence/Prevalence in USA:
1.5-4/1000 live births
Predominant age: 5-10 months (65% are less than one year of age)
Predominant sex: Male > Female (3:2) - male preponderance is more notable in older infants

SIGNS AND SYMPTOMS
• Vomiting (80-100%)
• Blood per rectum - currant-jelly stools (65%-95%) highest percent in infants
• Intermittent, colicky abdominal pain (almost all children)
• Lethargy (22%) (more pronounced with longer duration of illness)
• Palpable mass (16-41%)
• Diarrhea (7%)
• Prolapse of intussusception through anus (3%)
• Fever
• Extreme pallor in some

CAUSES
• Children
  ◊ Marked hypertrophy of Peyer's patches (92-98%)
  ◊ Lead point in 2%-8% (polyp, Meckel's diverticulum, duplication cyst, ectopic pancreas, lymphoma, Henoch-Schönlein purpura, lipoma, carcinoma)
  ◊ Allergic reactions, diet changes, changes in intestinal activity may be other causes
  ◊ Possible adenovirus or rotavirus infection
• Adults
  ◊ Virtually always associated with lead point

RISK FACTORS
• Henoch-Schönlein purpura
• Leukemia
• Lymphoma
• Cystic fibrosis
• Recent upper respiratory infection (21%)
• Recent operation (1-24 days previously)

DIAGNOSIS

DIFFERENTIAL DIAGNOSIS
• Adhesive band small bowel obstruction
• Appendicitis
• Gastroenteritis

LABORATORY
• Electrolytes
• CBC
• Urinalysis
• Stool guaiac
Drugs that may alter lab results: N/A
Disorders that may alter lab results: N/A

PATHOLOGICAL FINDINGS
• Hyperplasia of Peyer's lymphatic patches of terminal ileum (92%) with or without mesenteric lymphadenopathy
• Recognizable lead point (see list in Causes) (2-8%)

SPECIAL TESTS   N/A

IMAGING
• Ultrasound
• Plain film - flat and upright abdominal films may suggest the diagnosis

DIAGNOSTIC PROCEDURES
• Contrast enema (barium, water soluble contrast or air)
• Abdominal ultrasound

TREATMENT

APPROPRIATE HEALTH CARE Inpatient until resolved

GENERAL MEASURES
• IV fluid resuscitation
• Foley catheter (if child severely dehydrated)
• Nasogastric tube
• Antibiotics useful only if necrotic bowel present
• Non-operative care:
  ◊ Hydrostatic/pneumatic reduction of intussusception (50-80% success)
  ◊ Barium column should be 40-42 inches high
  ◊ Enema continued as long as progress is made. Bowel may be drained and the enema repeated.
  ◊ Pneumatic reduction pressure should not exceed 120-140 mm Hg (16-18.6 kPa)

SURGICAL MEASURES
• Right lower quadrant incision
• Gentle manipulation by pushing intussusception (not pulling)
• If unable to reduce or non-viable bowel, segmental resection with re-anastomosis
• Enterotomy if lead point suspected
• Incidental appendectomy commonly done

ACTIVITY As tolerated after reduction

DIET Liquids started after abdominal distension resolves and bowel function returns

PATIENT EDUCATION Instruct family on possibility of recurrence (5-13%)

MEDICATIONS

DRUG(S) OF CHOICE N/A
Contraindications: N/A
Precautions: N/A
Significant possible interactions: N/A

ALTERNATIVE DRUGS N/A

 FOLLOWUP

PATIENT MONITORING Office visit one week after discharge

PREVENTION/AVOIDANCE N/A

POSSIBLE COMPLICATIONS
• Bowel perforation during attempted reduction
• Prolonged ileus
• Adhesions with intestinal obstruction
• Incisional hernia
• Ischemic intestine requiring second operation
• Electrolyte abnormality
• Anemia
• Pleural effusion
• Sepsis
• Recurrence

EXPECTED COURSE/PROGNOSIS
• Mortality should not exceed 1-2%
• Possible recurrence (5-13%) after hydrostatic reduction
• Possible recurrence (3%) after operative reduction

 MISCELLANEOUS

ASSOCIATED CONDITIONS
• Schönlein-Henoch purpura
• Cystic fibrosis

AGE-RELATED FACTORS
Pediatric:
• Usually no lead point
• Postoperative intussusception (1-24 days postoperatively) is virtually always in small bowel and only rarely can be reduced hydrostatically
Geriatric: 90% have lead point
Others: N/A

PREGNANCY N/A

SYNONYMS N/A

ICD-9-CM
560.0 Intussusception

SEE ALSO
• Intestinal obstruction
• Cystic fibrosis
• Schönlein-Henoch purpura

OTHER NOTES N/A

ABBREVIATIONS N/A

REFERENCES
• Pang .C: Intussusception revisited: Clinicopathologic analysis of 261 cases, with emphasis on pathogenesis. Southern Medical J 1989;82(2):215-228
• Skipper RP, Boeckman R, Klein R: Childhood intussusception. SGO 1990;171:151-153
• Welch KJ, Randolph JG, Ravitch MM, et al, eds: Pediatric Surgery, 4th Ed. Chicago, Year Book Medical Publishers, 1986
• West KW, Stephens B, Rescorla FJ, et al: Postoperative intussusception: Experience with 36 cases in children. Surgery 1988;104:781-787
Illustrations: N/A
Internet references: http://www.5mcc.com

Author(s)
Timothy L. Black, MD, FACS, FAAP
James P. Miller, MD, FACS, FAAP

Iron deficiency anemia

BASICS

DESCRIPTION Anemia due to decreased iron stores. Poor iron utilization and poor iron re-utilization (e.g., anemia of chronic disease) are also due to iron deficiency, but iron stores are not depleted. Onset may be acute with rapid blood loss, or chronic with poor diet or slow blood loss. This is the most common cause of anemia in the U.S.
System(s) affected:
Hemic/Lymphatic/Immunologic
Genetics: No known genetic pattern
Incidence/Prevalence in USA: It affects 10-30% of the adult population
Predominant age: All ages
Predominant sex: Female > Male

SIGNS AND SYMPTOMS
• Asymptomatic, initially
• Cheilosis
• Dyspnea on exertion
• Fatigue
• Tachycardia
• Palpitation
• Underlying GI ulceration, neoplasm, uterine disorders, bleeding varices
• Headache
• Inability to concentrate
• Irritability
• Listlessness
• Neuralgic pain
• Pallor
• Peripheral paresthesias
• Pica (dirt, paint, ice)
• Spoon-shaped, brittle nails
• Susceptibility to infection
• Vasomotor disturbances

CAUSES
• Blood loss (e.g., menses, GI bleed)
• Poor iron intake
• Poor iron absorption (e.g., postgastrectomy)
• Increased demand for iron (e.g., infancy, adolescence, pregnancy)
• Hookworm infestation
• Gastric carcinoma

RISK FACTORS See Causes

DIAGNOSIS

DIFFERENTIAL DIAGNOSIS
• Defective iron utilization (e.g., thalassemia, sideroblastosis, G6PD deficiency)
• Defective iron re-utilization (e.g., infection, inflammation, cancer, other chronic diseases)
• Hypoproliferation (e.g., decreased erythropoietin from hypothyroidism, renal failure, etc.)

LABORATORY
• Stainable iron in bone marrow aspiration is the gold standard
• Low serum ferritin is best non-invasive test in adults, but may miss some deficient patients since ferritin is an acute phase reactant. Fe/TIBC (transferrin ratio) is no longer recommended since it is less sensitive and less specific than ferritin.
• Peripheral smear usually shows hypochromia and microcytosis, but may be normal
• Hemoglobin is usually lower than 12 g/dL, but patients with higher premorbid hemoglobin (such as smokers and patients with chronic hypoxemia) may be anemic at higher Hgb levels
• Low RBC count helps to distinguish from thalassemia where count is normal or high
• Ovalocytosis and anemia unresponsive to iron suggest thalassemia trait
• Low MCV may be absent in mild anemia, or hidden by population of larger cells (e.g., reticulocytes or macrocytes)
• An empiric trial of iron at 3 mg/kg/day may be the best way to diagnose decreased iron stores in infants and children, if reticulocytes elevated in 7-10 days, or Hgb increased > 1.0 g/dL after 4 weeks
Drugs that may alter lab results: Iron supplements or multivitamin-mineral preparations that contain iron
Disorders that may alter lab results:
• Ferritin elevated by acute liver disease, cirrhosis, Hodgkin's disease, acute leukemia, solid tumors, fever, acute inflammation, renal dialysis
• Hemoglobin may be elevated by smoking or chronic hypoxemia, thereby hiding anemia if standard anemia limits are used

PATHOLOGICAL FINDINGS
• Absent marrow iron stores
• Marrow - hyperplastic, micronormoblastic

SPECIAL TESTS
• Cause of iron loss - stool guaiac testing, GI endoscopy, stool for O & P, clotting studies
• Rule-out thalassemia - review prior CBC's for persisting mild anemia and marked ovalomicrocytosis, Hgb A2, Hgb F, family history, high or high normal RBC count
• Rule-out G6PD deficiency - assay at least 6 weeks after last drop in Hgb
• Rule-out poor re-utilization - trial of iron (oral or parenteral), bone marrow aspiration and iron stain
• Rule-out gastric carcinoma, especially in the elderly

IMAGING GI endoscopy to discover occult bleeding sites

DIAGNOSTIC PROCEDURES
• Bone marrow aspiration
• Sigmoidoscopy
• Gastroscopy
• Colonoscopy

TREATMENT

APPROPRIATE HEALTH CARE
Outpatient

GENERAL MEASURES
• Search for cause and correct it. There can be no excuse for not searching for a bleeding site.
• Avoid transfusions except in rare instances

SURGICAL MEASURES N/A

ACTIVITY Patients with hypoxemia, low cardiac output or angina may require reduced activity prescriptions

DIET
• Limit milk to 1 pint a day (adults)
• Emphasize protein- and iron-containing foods (meat, beans, leafy green vegetables)
• Increase dietary fiber to decrease likelihood of constipation during iron replacement therapy
• No milk, other dairy product, antacid, or tetracycline within two hours of drug dosage

PATIENT EDUCATION For patient education materials contact: National Heart, Lung & Blood Institute, Communications & Public Information Branch, National Institutes of Health, Building 31, Room 41-21, 9000 Rockville Pike, Bethesda, MD 20892, (301)251-1222

Iron deficiency anemia

 MEDICATIONS

DRUG(S) OF CHOICE Ferrous sulfate 300 mg tid on an empty stomach one hour before meals is an ideal dose that provides 180 mg of elemental iron a day. Dose can be reduced as needed for GI symptoms, which affect 15% of patients on standard iron therapy. Or the dose can be taken with meals, which may reduce the delivery of iron by 50%. People with a moderate anemia (Hgb = 10 g/dL) need only 1500-2000 mg of elemental iron replacement. Reducing the amount of iron per dose as much as necessary to abate symptoms will make parenteral iron therapy unnecessary in almost all cases. Special iron formulations and compounds are very expensive and reduce symptoms only to the degree that they reduce delivery of iron. Liquid iron preparations are useful for children with a recommended dose of 3 mg/kg/day given in a single dose. Consider parenteral iron for patients with malabsorption.

Contraindications:
• Antacids concomitantly
• Tetracycline concomitantly

Precautions:
• Iron preparations cause black bowel movements
• Iron overdose is highly toxic. Patients should be instructed to keep tablets out of the reach of small children.

Significant possible interactions:
• Allopurinol
• Antacids
• Penicillamine
• Tetracyclines
• Vitamin E

ALTERNATIVE DRUGS N/A

 FOLLOWUP

PATIENT MONITORING Regularly after return to normal (in order to detect recurrences)

PREVENTION/AVOIDANCE
• Good nutrition with adequate iron intake
• Correction of gynecologic or other problems causing excess blood loss

POSSIBLE COMPLICATIONS Neglecting to identify hidden bleeding points, particularly a bleeding malignancy

EXPECTED COURSE/PROGNOSIS
Curable with iron therapy if the underlying cause can be discovered and cured

 MISCELLANEOUS

ASSOCIATED CONDITIONS N/A

AGE-RELATED FACTORS
Pediatric: Frequent problem in infants whose major source of nutrition is cow's milk
Geriatric: Accounts for 60% of anemias in people over 65
Others: N/A

PREGNANCY Common during pregnancy unless iron supplements are included in the diet

SYNONYMS
• Anemia of chronic blood loss
• Hypochromic, microcytic anemia
• Chlorosis

ICD-9-CM 280.9 iron deficiency anemia, unspecified

SEE ALSO N/A

OTHER NOTES N/A

ABBREVIATIONS N/A
• Hgb = hemoglobin
• TIBC = total iron binding capacity

REFERENCES
• Lee RG, Bithell TC, et al: Wintrobe's Clinical Hematology. 9th Ed. Philadelphia, Lea & Febiger, 1993
• Williams WJ, Beutler E, Erslev AJ, et al, eds: Hematology. 4th Ed. New York, McGraw-Hill, 1990
Illustrations: N/A
Internet references: http://www.5mcc.com

Author(s)
Bruce Block, MD

Iron toxicity, acute

BASICS

DESCRIPTION Acute iron overload due to accidental or intentional ingestion. Acute symptoms are characterized by vomiting, diarrhea, mild lethargy, upper abdominal pain, pallor, and hyperglycemia with more severe clinical findings including cyanosis, stupor, acidosis, hematemesis, shock, and coma.
System(s) affected: Gastrointestinal, Cardiovascular, Hemic/Lymphatic/Immunologic
Genetics: N/A
Incidence/Prevalence in USA: 3699 cases reported in 1988 along with 15,977 cases of intoxication with iron-fortified vitamins; leading cause of poisoning mortality of children in the US
Predominant age:
• Children most frequently involved (in 1984, 1337 out 1738 iron poisoning cases were reported in children < 6 years of age)
• From 1988-92, approximately 17% of children's deaths reported to poison control centers in the U.S. were iron poisonings
Predominant sex: N/A

SIGNS AND SYMPTOMS
• 0.5 to 2 hours - vomiting, hematemesis, abdominal pain, diarrhea, lethargy, shock, acidosis, and coagulopathy
• Apparent recovery may contribute to a false sense of security after initial ingestion, observe patient closely
• 2 to 12 hours - profound shock, severe acidosis, cyanosis and fever
• 12 to 48 hours - symptoms may recur and can include pulmonary edema, shock, acidosis, convulsions, anuria, hyperthermia, and death
• 2 to 6 weeks - if patient survives, pyloric or antral stenosis, hepatic cirrhosis and CNS damage can be seen

CAUSES
• Excessive iron ingestion - the average human lethal dose is 200 to 250 mg of elemental iron per kg of body weight (equivalent to about 230 ferrous sulfate based on 60 mg of elemental iron per tablet)
• Toxicity is likely following 60 mg/kg of elemental iron ingestion

RISK FACTORS
Access to iron products by children resulting in accidental ingestion

DIAGNOSIS

DIFFERENTIAL DIAGNOSIS
If unknown iron ingestion
• Gastritis
• Small bowel obstruction
• Drug intolerance/overdose
• Alcohol toxicity
• Viral illness
• Diabetic ketoacidosis

LABORATORY
• CBC
• Electrolytes and glucose
• Serum iron; total iron binding capacity (TIBC) (may not be available in some hospitals)
• PT/INR (prothrombin time /International Normalized Ratio) and activated partial thromboplastin time (APTT)
• Serum bicarbonate
• Liver function tests in severe overdose
Drugs that may alter lab results:
Deferoxamine can falsely lower serum iron unless a reducing agent is added to the specimen. Should obtain a free iron concentration.
Disorders that may alter lab results:
TIBC rises factitiously in the presence of high iron levels

PATHOLOGICAL FINDINGS None (by definition)

SPECIAL TESTS N/A

IMAGING Abdominal and chest x-ray

DIAGNOSTIC PROCEDURES Abdominal x-ray to evaluate for tablets in the gut

TREATMENT

APPROPRIATE HEALTH CARE
• Emergency room for acute ingestion
• Inpatient for severe ingestion
• Supportive treatment

GENERAL MEASURES
• Maintain proper airway, respiration and circulation
• Assess the amount of iron ingested
• Hemodialysis, peritoneal dialysis, and exchange transfusion have also be used in lethal overdoses
• Explore psychological issues if an intentional ingestion

SURGICAL MEASURES N/A

ACTIVITY N/A

DIET N/A

PATIENT EDUCATION
• Prevention counseling on proper storage of iron products out of the reach of children
• Educational material from poison control centers may be available to use
• An informative poster is available, at no charge, from the Department of Health and Human Services, 5600 Fishers Lane (HFI-40), Rockville, MD 20857

MEDICATIONS

DRUG(S) OF CHOICE
• Decontamination with syrup of ipecac [1-12 years: 15 mL; adult: 30 mL] if a patient has recent iron ingestion and is a candidate for emesis. Contraindications are signs of oral pharyngeal/esophageal irritation, a depressed gag reflex, or CNS excitation/depression. Controversy exists as to whether to give ipecac to children < 6 mo of age.
• Criteria for emesis/lavage:
  ◊ > 20 mg/kg ingested
  ◊ Symptomatic
  ◊ Adults
• Gastric lavage, using tepid water, may be indicated in patients who are comatose or at risk for convulsing
• Whole bowel irrigation with a solution containing polyethylene glycol (Colyte, GoLYTELY) electrolyte lavage, gives rapid diarrhea with relatively little fluid and electrolyte imbalance; (children: 25 mL/kg/h; adults: 1.5-2 L/h); indicated when radiographic evidence of iron past the pylorus or if tablets persist in the GI tract after other attempts of decontamination. End point: clear rectal effluent, disappearance of radiopacities.
• If serum iron exceeds TIBC or peak serum iron is > 300 mcg/dL, administer IV deferoxamine, 15 mg/kg/hr, for not more than 24 hrs to chelate iron and prevent it from entering into chemical reactions. Serum iron levels drop usually within 12 to 48 hours.
Contraindications: Deferoxamine is relatively contraindicated in patients with severe renal disease or anuria, primary hemochromatosis
Precautions: Deferoxamine may cause flushing of skin, urticaria, hypotension and shock with rapid IV injections
Significant possible interactions: N/A

ALTERNATIVE DRUGS N/A

 FOLLOWUP

PATIENT MONITORING
• Negative KUB
• Serum iron concentration
• CBC, electrolytes, serum bicarbonate, blood glucose, serum iron, and TIBC
• Some patients' urine will turn a characteristic vin rose color after treatment (previously this was used as a diagnostic test of significant iron poisoning)

PREVENTION/AVOIDANCE
• Keep prescription and over-the-counter iron products/vitamins out of reach of children
• Keep syrup of ipecac on hand in case of accidental acute ingestion

POSSIBLE COMPLICATIONS 2-4 weeks
after severe ingestion has resulted in pyloric or antral stenosis, hepatic cirrhosis and CNS damage

EXPECTED COURSE/PROGNOSIS
Depends on amount ingested and length of time patient exposed

 MISCELLANEOUS

ASSOCIATED CONDITIONS N/A

AGE-RELATED FACTORS
Pediatric: For a 2 year old, the average lethal dose of elemental iron is 3 grams
Geriatric: N/A
Others: N/A

PREGNANCY N/A

SYNONYMS Iron poisoning

ICD-9-CM
964.0 poisoning by iron and its compounds

SEE ALSO N/A

OTHER NOTES N/A

ABBREVIATIONS TIBC - total iron binding capacity

REFERENCES
• Aisen P, Cohen G, Kang JO: Iron Toxicosis. Int Rev Exp Pathol 1990;31:1-46
• Iron, Poisondex Toxicologic Management, 1974-1997 Micromedex Inc. Vol 92
• FDA Medical Bulletin 1995; 25.3. Washington, DC, Federal Food & Drug Administration, 1995
• Thompson DF: Reassessment of measuring total iron binding capacity in acute iron overdose. Ann Pharmacother 1994;28:63-66
• Chyka PA, Butler AY, Holley JE: Serum iron concentrations and symptoms of acute poisoning in children. Pharmacotherapy 1996;16:105301058
Illustrations: N/A
Internet references: http://www.5mcc.com

Author(s)
Julienne K. Kirk, PharmD

Irritable bowel syndrome

BASICS

DESCRIPTION Altered bowel habits, abdominal pain, gaseousness, in the absence of organic pathology (divided into four types):
• Alternating diarrhea with constipation
• Diarrhea predominant
• Constipation predominant
• Upper abdominal bloating and discomfort
System(s) affected: Gastrointestinal
Genetics: Unknown, but more common in families of patients
Incidence/Prevalence in USA:
• Unknown, but 50% of gastrointestinal visits, and second to upper respiratory infection as cause for lost workdays
• At least 15% of population (uncommon in children and early teens)
Predominant age:
• Late 20's, rarely in late teens
• If over age 40, other disease more likely
Predominant sex:
• Female > Male (2:1) in the US
• In other parts of the world - Male > Female

SIGNS AND SYMPTOMS
• All present in most patients but not with every episode
• Abdominal pain, usually lower quadrant, relieved by defecation
• Mucus in stools
• Constipation
• Diarrhea
• Distention
• Upper abdominal discomfort after eating
• Straining for normal consistency stools
• Urgency of defecation
• Feelings of incomplete evacuation
• Scybalous stools
• Nausea, vomiting (rarely)

CAUSES Unknown but patients show some gut motility abnormalities with increased response to stress and stimulants, and increase in the 3 cycles/minute smooth muscle contractions

RISK FACTORS
• Other members of the family with the same or similar gastrointestinal disorder
• History of childhood sexual abuse
• Sexual or domestic abuse in women

DIAGNOSIS

DIFFERENTIAL DIAGNOSIS
• Inflammatory bowel syndromes
• Lactose intolerance
• Infections (Giardia lamblia, Entamoeba histolytica, Salmonella, Campylobacter, Yersinia, Clostridium difficile)
• Diverticula
• Cathartic use
• Magnesium containing antacids
• Celiac sprue
• Pancreatic insufficiency
• Depression
• Somatization
• Adenocarcinoma of the colon
• Villous adenoma
• Endocrine tumors
• Hypo/hyperthyroidism
• Diabetes mellitus
• Radiation damage to colon or small bowel

LABORATORY
• As needed to rule out other pathology
  ◊ ESR
  ◊ CBC
  ◊ Stool for ova, parasites and culture
Drugs that may alter lab results: N/A
Disorders that may alter lab results: N/A

PATHOLOGICAL FINDINGS All labs normal except for sigmoidoscopy

SPECIAL TESTS Not needed for diagnosis

IMAGING
• Barium enema, if indicated is usually normal
• Small bowel series

DIAGNOSTIC PROCEDURES
Sigmoidoscopy (often normal), can show spasm that reproduces pain and increase mucosal folds

TREATMENT

APPROPRIATE HEALTH CARE
Outpatient

GENERAL MEASURES
• Heat to abdomen can help
• Biofeedback may help
• Reduce stress

SURGICAL MEASURES N/A

ACTIVITY As normal

DIET
• Increase fiber
• Avoid - large meals; spicy, fried, fatty foods; milk products

PATIENT EDUCATION
• Many materials available nationally and locally
• Stress the organicity of the disease versus any psycho-social interpretation
• Teach patient to avoid problem stimulants

MEDICATIONS

DRUG(S) OF CHOICE
• Use from among this list according to need or response
  ◊ Bulk producing agents - psyllium containing products (Metamucil) 1 tbsp bid or tid
  ◊ Constipating agents (if diarrhea is significant) - loperamide (Imodium) 4 mg initial dose, then 2 mg after each unformed stool or Diphenoxylate-atropine (Lomotil) 2.5-5.0 mg (1-2 tablets) after each unformed stool
  ◊ Antispasmodics/anticholinergics - dicyclomine (Bentyl) 10-20 mg bid to qid or lactase (Lactaid) 1-3 caplets ac for lactose intolerance
  ◊ Anticholinergics/sedatives - chlordiazepoxide-clidinium (Librax) 1 or 2 ac and qhs; phenobarbital-hyoscyamine-atropine-hyoscine (Donnatal) 1 or 2 tablets ac and hs; amitriptyline HCL (Elavil) 25-50 mg qhs
  ◊ Antiflatulents - simethicone (Mylicon) 2 or 4 tablets pc and hs
  ◊ For milk intolerance - lactase capsules or tablets; 1-2 tablets prior to ingesting milk products
Contraindications: Refer to manufacturer's profile of each drug
Precautions: Refer to manufacturer's profile of each drug
Significant possible interactions: Refer to manufacturer's profile of each drug

ALTERNATIVE DRUGS   N/A

FOLLOWUP

PATIENT MONITORING   As needed for symptoms

PREVENTION/AVOIDANCE   See Diet

POSSIBLE COMPLICATIONS   N/A

EXPECTED COURSE/PROGNOSIS
• No progression to cancer or inflammatory disease
• Expect recurrences, when under stress, throughout life. Frequency lessens as age increases.

MISCELLANEOUS

ASSOCIATED CONDITIONS
• Migraine
• Bladder frequency
• Nocturia
• Urgency
• Fecal incontinence
• Myalgia
• Dyspareunia
• Depression
• Stress incontinence

AGE-RELATED FACTORS   N/A
Pediatric: N/A
Geriatric: N/A
Others: N/A

PREGNANCY   Anecdotal information implies that irritable bowel syndrome gets worse in pregnancy. But there are no increased risks to fetus or mother.

SYNONYMS
• Mucous colitis
• Spastic colon
• Irritable colon

ICD-9-CM
564.1 Irritable colon

SEE ALSO   N/A

OTHER NOTES   Must not give patients the impression that this is a psychiatric illness

ABBREVIATIONS   N/A

REFERENCES
• Read NW, ed: Irritable Bowel Syndrome. London, Grune and Stratton, 1991
• Rakel R, ed: Textbook of Family Practice. 5th Ed. Philadelphia, W.B. Saunders Co., 1995
Illustrations: N/A
Internet references: http://www.5mcc.com

Author(s)
S. Shevaun Duiker, MD

Kaposi's sarcoma

 BASICS

DESCRIPTION   A neoplasm characterized by vascular tumors of skin and viscera in several different forms:
• Indolent (classic) Kaposi's sarcoma (KS)
• African (endemic) KS
• AIDS-related (epidemic) KS
• Form associated with immunosuppressive medications
System(s) affected: Skin/Exocrine
Genetics: Unknown
Incidence/Prevalence in USA:
• Indolent/lymphadenopathic - rare
• In AIDS patients - common
Predominant age: 16-75
Predominant sex: Male > Female

SIGNS AND SYMPTOMS
• Indolent Kaposi's
  ◊ Multicentric red-blue violaceous tumors on the skin
  ◊ Tender skin tumors
  ◊ Pruritic skin tumors
  ◊ In older men, lesions appear first on toes or legs
• African (endemic) Kaposi's
  ◊ Usually involves skin, viscera or lymph nodes
• In Kaposi's associated with HIV infection (epidemic)
  ◊ Skin lesions widely disseminated, on the face, arms, trunk
  ◊ Lesions on mucous membranes
  ◊ Lesions in lymph nodes
  ◊ Lesions in viscera

CAUSES   A herpes virus desnigated "Kaposi's sarcoma herpes virus" (KSHV) or human herpes virus type 8 (HHV8) has been strongly linked to KS. Samples from KS lesions have been found to contain DNA sequences idential with KSHV, and KSHV can be propagated from skin lesions of patients with KS.

RISK FACTORS
• HIV infection
• Living in endemic area (especially Zaire or Uganda)
• Immunosuppressant medications
• Transplantation and chemotherapy

 DIAGNOSIS

DIFFERENTIAL DIAGNOSIS   Bacillary angiomatosis, granuloma faciale, vascular proliferation and purpuric lesions

LABORATORY   Nothing specific
Drugs that may alter lab results: N/A
Disorders that may alter lab results: N/A

PATHOLOGICAL FINDINGS
• Micro - proliferation of atypical spindle cells
• Micro - proliferation of vascular channels
• Micro - large hyperchromic nuclei
• Micro - spindle-shaped perivascular cells
• Micro - hemosiderin laden macrophages

SPECIAL TESTS   Tissue examination

IMAGING   CT scan (chest, abdomen) may assess visceral involvement

DIAGNOSTIC PROCEDURES
• Biopsy of skin or lymph node
• Bronchoscopy with biopsy
• Liver biopsy

 TREATMENT

APPROPRIATE HEALTH CARE
• Outpatient
• Outpatient surgery

GENERAL MEASURES
• If KS due to immunosuppressant medications, eliminate or reduce medication dosage
• If KS is HIV-related, optimize anti-HIV therapy to reduce HIV viral load
• Treatment is otherwise determined by extent of the disease
• Observation
• Radiotherapy (electron beam) or x-ray therapy 1000 to 2000 rads
• Systemic chemotherapy, immunotherapy, or anti-viral therapy

SURGICAL MEASURES
• Cryotherapy
• Intralesional chemotherapy or immunotherapy
• Surgical excision

ACTIVITY   Remain active as long as possible

DIET   No special diet

PATIENT EDUCATION   N/A

Kaposi's sarcoma

 MEDICATIONS

DRUG(S) OF CHOICE
• Chemotherapy (should be given only by those with experience in this area)
  ◊ Doxorubicin
or
  ◊ Bleomycin
or
  ◊ Vinblastine
or
  ◊ Vincristine
or
  ◊ Danunorubicin
or
  ◊ Interferon - parenteral or intralesional
Note: Both doxorubicin and danunorubicin are available and approved for use in liposomal forms
Contraindications: Refer to manufacturer's literature
Precautions: Refer to manufacturer's literature. Myelosuppression with chemotherapy.
Significant possible interactions: Refer to manufacturer's literature

ALTERNATIVE DRUGS
• Uncontrolled studies have reported that some individuals have responded to anti-herpes medications such as foscarnet and ganciclovir
• Several clinical studies are underway using newer agents including 9-cis-retinoic acid

 FOLLOWUP

PATIENT MONITORING
In HIV patients with KS, other opportunistic infections must be aggressively treated

PREVENTION/AVOIDANCE
Safe sex practices

POSSIBLE COMPLICATIONS
Aggressive form affects at least 1/3 of HIV infected patients

EXPECTED COURSE/PROGNOSIS
• Improved HIV treatments may result in improved HIV-related KS survival
• Indolent form - 10 year survival

MISCELLANEOUS

ASSOCIATED CONDITIONS
• AIDS
• HIV infection

AGE-RELATED FACTORS
Pediatric: N/A
Geriatric: Indolent form most likely to occur in men in this age group
Others: N/A

PREGNANCY N/A

SYNONYMS
• Endotheliosarcoma
• Multiple, idiopathic hemorrhagic sarcoma

ICD-9-CM
173.9 Malignant neoplasm of the skin

SEE ALSO HIV infection & AIDS

OTHER NOTES N/A

ABBREVIATIONS
KS = Kaposi's sarcoma

REFERENCES
• Groopman JE, Scadden DT: Interferon therapy for Kaposi's sarcoma associated with the acquired immunodeficiency syndrome: A proposal for uniform evaluation, response, and staging criteria. J Clin Oncol 1989;7:1201
• Abrams D, Grieco M, McMeeking A: AIDS/HIV Treatment Directory. New York, American Foundation for AIDS Research (updated 4 times yearly)
• Cesarman E: Kaposi's sarcoma-associated herpes-like DNA sequences in AIDS-related body cavity-based lymphomas. NEJM 1995;332(18):1186-1191
• Moore PS, Chang Y: Detection of a herpesvirus-like DNA sequence in Kaposi's sarcoma in patients with and without HIV infection. NEJM 1995;331:1181-1185
Illustrations: 9 available on CD-ROM
Internet references: http://www.5mcc.com

Author(s)
R. Scott Gorman, MD

Kawasaki syndrome

BASICS

DESCRIPTION An acute, distinct, self-limited, febrile disease of children which is notable for vasculitis of coronary blood vessels with potential dilation, aneurysms, thrombosis, rupture, or myocardial ischemia.

System(s) affected: Cardiovascular, Gastrointestinal, Hemic/Lymphatic/Immunologic, Musculoskeletal, Nervous, Pulmonary, Renal/Urologic, Skin/Exocrine

Genetics: Increased incidence of HLA-Bw 22 in Japanese patients; increased incidence of HLA-Bw 51 in US Caucasians and in Jewish, Israeli patients. Slight increase in siblings of cases. Worldwide, affects all races, but most prevalent in Japan.

Incidence/Prevalence in USA:
Worldwide, affects all races but most prevalent in Japan. In the US, the annual incidence rate is 0.6 cases/100,000 children under 5 years old. Seasonal variation - increased in winter and spring. Increased outbreaks at 2-3 year intervals.

Predominant age: 1-5 years; 50% are < 2 years old, 80% are < 5 years old. Seldom seen after 8 years of age.

Predominant sex: N/A

SIGNS AND SYMPTOMS
• Fever for 5 days or more
◊ Fever is high (103-105°F [39.4-40.5°C]) and unresponsive to antibiotics
◊ May be prolonged (2-3 weeks with average duration of 11 days)
• Polymorphous rash
◊ May be maculopapular, scarlatiniform, morbilliform, erythema marginatum, or rarely vesiculopustular
◊ Frequently confluent in the perineum where it desquamates
• Bilateral conjunctival suffusion
◊ Nonpurulent
• Changes of lips and oral cavity
◊ Reddening of lips in the acute stage which crack, fissure and bleed in the subacute phase
◊ Strawberry or erythematous tongue
◊ Diffuse injection of oral and pharyngeal mucosa without exudate
• Acute, nonpurulent cervical lymphadenopathy
◊ Lymph nodes 1 cm or greater in diameter
◊ Generalized lymphadenopathy usually absent
• Extremity changes
◊ Reddened palms and soles on days 3-5
◊ Indurative edema of hands and feet on days 4-7
◊ Membranous desquamation from fingertips in convalescent phase
• Other organ system involvement:
◊ Cardiovascular
- Acutely may have tachycardia (disproportionate to fever), gallop rhythms, and ECG changes suggestive of myocarditis
- Pericarditis, often subclinical
- Coronary artery and other medium-sized arterial aneurysms

◊ Gastrointestinal
- Anorexia
- Vomiting or diarrhea
- Acute, acalculous cholecystitis may present as a right upper quadrant mass and pain
- Pancreatitis
◊ Renal
- Nephritis
- Urethritis
◊ Pulmonary
- Pneumonitis, atelectasis, or pleural effusions
◊ Joints
- Arthritis of wrists, knees, and ankles may appear in third week of illness
◊ Neurologic
- Irritability
- Aseptic meningitis
- Peripheral neuropathies

CAUSES
• Unknown
• Microbial agent is favored because of acute, self-limited course and community-wide outbreaks
◊ Leading theory is that a staphylococcal or streptococcal superantigen, in the appropriate host, stimulates T cell populations which in turn cause activation of immune responses directed against endothelial cell antigens

RISK FACTORS Environmental - exposure to rug shampoo and residing in close proximity to bodies of water have been inconsistently associated risk factors in large epidemics

DIAGNOSIS

DIFFERENTIAL DIAGNOSIS
• Staphylococcal scalded skin syndrome
• Toxic shock syndrome
• Stevens-Johnson syndrome
• Reiter's syndrome
• Juvenile rheumatoid arthritis
• Scarlet fever
• Measles
• Rubella
• Roseola
• Epstein-Barr virus infections
• Mycoplasma infection
• Leptospirosis
• Lyme disease
• Rocky Mountain spotted fever
• Toxoplasmosis
• Acrodynia
• Drug reactions
• Other vasculitides

LABORATORY
• Anemia (normochromic, normocytic)
• Leukocytosis (12,000-40,000 cells/mm3) with immature forms
• Elevated CRP, ESR, and alpha1-antitrypsin concentrations
• Platelet counts rise in subacute phase and peak in convalescent at 750,000-1,500,000
• Mildly elevated serum liver enzymes and bilirubin
• CSF pleocytosis may be seen

Drugs that may alter lab results: N/A
Disorders that may alter lab results: N/A

PATHOLOGICAL FINDINGS
• During acute stage, neutrophilic infiltrates involving pericardium, myocardium, endocardium, and vascular endothelium may be present
• Necrosis may develop and result in aneurysmal dilatation of medium-sized arteries
• Mononuclear infiltration predominates in the second week of illness, gradually resolving with or without fibrosis
• In addition to cardiac involvement, arteritis may also develop in lungs, kidneys, gastrointestinal tract, and other organs

SPECIAL TESTS
• Quantitative serum immunoglobulins
• ANA, RF, VDRL, immune complexes, complement levels

IMAGING
• Electrocardiogram may show ischemia, arrhythmias
• Echocardiogram may show cardiomyopathy, pericardial effusion, coronary artery dilatation or aneurysms
• Radiography including angiography

DIAGNOSTIC PROCEDURES
• No laboratory study proves diagnosis; diagnosis rests on clinical features and exclusion of other illnesses in differential diagnosis
• Diagnosis of typical syndrome requires fever of at least 5 days' duration, plus 4 of the following 5 criteria:
◊ Mucous membrane changes
◊ Extremity changes
◊ Cervical lymphadenopathy of at least 1 cm in size
◊ Rash
◊ Conjunctival suffusion
• Atypical cases occur with incomplete clinical findings; frequency of coronary artery aneurysms may be higher in this subset of patients

TREATMENT

APPROPRIATE HEALTH CARE When seen acutely, most children are hospitalized for diagnostic evaluation and supportive care. Older children with mild disease may be managed on an outpatient basis.

GENERAL MEASURES
• Antibiotics are given until bacterial etiologies are excluded
• Once KS is suspected, all patients need a cardiac evaluation, including electrocardiogram and echocardiogram
• Diuretics, inotropic agents, and pacemakers may be required for myocarditis

SURGICAL MEASURES Aortocoronary artery bypass surgery for symptomatic patients with severe stenotic lesions (> 75% occluded)

ACTIVITY May be limited if cardiac involvement

DIET IV fluids may be needed if fever and irritability make feeding difficult

PATIENT EDUCATION N/A

MEDICATIONS

DRUG(S) OF CHOICE
• Aspirin: 80-100 mg/kg/day during the febrile phase. When child is afebrile, continue with low, single dose (5 mg/kg/day, to maximum of 80 mg) therapy for antithrombotic effects until active disease subsides.
• Immune globulin, intravenous (IVIG) 2 gm/kg at the time diagnosis is made (preferably within the first 10 days of illness) lowers the risk of coronary artery aneurysms and may shorten the duration of the acute phase. Retreatment is occasionally considered if clinical response is incomplete, although this has not been well studied.
Contraindications: Corticosteroids may increase the chance of aneurysm formation and should be avoided except in exceptional cases
Precautions: High dose salicylate therapy can cause tinnitus and hepatitis
Significant possible interactions: Aspirin therapy is associated with Reye's syndrome in children who develop viral infections, particularly influenza B and varicella. Influenza vaccination is recommended for children requiring aspirin therapy during influenza season, and aspirin should probably be discontinued if influenza or varicella infection occurs.

ALTERNATIVE DRUGS
• Dipyridamole, 4 mg/kg/d, is sometimes administered if coronary artery abnormalities develop
• Fibrinolytic agents (urokinase) for coronary artery thrombosis
• Alprostadil (prostaglandin E1) for peripheral artery ischemia
• Heparin followed by warfarin for large or multiple nonobstructive or obstructive aneurysms

FOLLOWUP

PATIENT MONITORING
• Monitor platelet count and acute phase reactant along with clinical course; when all return to normal, aspirin can be stopped
• Repeat ECG and echocardiogram at 3 and 8 weeks if initial studies are normal; may need further studies (e.g., angiography) if abnormal

PREVENTION/AVOIDANCE N/A

POSSIBLE COMPLICATIONS
• 20% of untreated patients develop coronary artery aneurysms in convalescent phase. Risk factors include:
  ◊ Male sex
  ◊ Age < 1 year old
  ◊ Fever > 2 weeks
  ◊ Elevated ESR for > 4 weeks
• Ischemic heart disease risk factors include:
  ◊ Aneurysms > 8 mm
  ◊ Diffuse or saccular aneurysm
  ◊ Fever > 21 days
  ◊ Steroid therapy
  ◊ Age > 2 years old
• Mortality 0.5%, related to cardiovascular disease

EXPECTED COURSE/PROGNOSIS
• Usually self-limited
• Only potentially permanent sequelae involve cardiovascular system
• Unknown but possible increased risk of atherosclerotic heart disease in adulthood

MISCELLANEOUS

ASSOCIATED CONDITIONS None

AGE-RELATED FACTORS
Pediatric: See Description
Geriatric: N/A
Others: N/A

PREGNANCY N/A

SYNONYMS
• Mucocutaneous lymph node syndrome
• Infantile polyarteritis

ICD-9-CM 446.1 Kawasaki disease

SEE ALSO
• Polyarteritis nodosa
• Toxic shock syndrome

OTHER NOTES N/A

ABBREVIATIONS KS = Kawasaki syndrome

REFERENCES
• Feigin RD, et al: Kawasaki disease. In: Oski FA, et al, eds. Principles and Practice of Pediatrics. 2nd Ed. Philadelphia, J.B. Lippincott Co.,1994
• American Academy of Pediatrics. Kawasaki disease. In: Peter G, ed. 1994 Red Book: Report of the Committee on Infectious Diseases. 23rd Ed. Elk Grove Village, IL, Academy of Pediatrics, 1994
• Wortmann DW, Nelson AM: Kawasaki syndrome. Rheum Dis Clin N Amer 1990;16:363
Illustrations: 2 available on CD-ROM
Internet references: http://www.5mcc.com

Author(s)
Bernhard L. Wiedermann, MD
Elizabeth A. Frankel, MD

Keloids

BASICS

DESCRIPTION Abnormally large overgrowth of fibrous tissue (scar) occurring as a result of trauma or irritation that does not subside with time
System(s) affected: Skin/Exocrine
Genetics:
• 5-15 time more common in blacks and Asians than Caucasians. In all races, more darkly pigmented individuals are at higher risk.
• Both autosomal dominant and autosomal recessive familial inheritance have been reported
Incidence/Prevalence in USA: Largely unknown, but does affect 4-16% of the black and Hispanic population
Predominant age: N/A
Predominant sex: Male = Female

SIGNS AND SYMPTOMS
• Pain
• Tenderness
• Hyperesthesia
• Pruritus
• Firm, smooth, elevated scar with sharply demarcated borders
• Initially may be pale or mildly erythematous
• Older lesion hypo- or hyperpigmented
• Scar extends beyond margins of the initial wound
• Over period of years, keloids continue to grow and may develop claw-like projections

CAUSES
• Surgical wound
• Burn injury
• Acne scar
• Insect bite
• Folliculitis barbae

RISK FACTORS
• Family history of keloids
• Dark skin pigment
• Certain locations on the body, e.g., deltoids, chest, earlobes
• Pregnancy
• Adolescence

DIAGNOSIS

DIFFERENTIAL DIAGNOSIS
• Hypertrophic scar (usually spontaneously regress; do not cross wound margins)
• Dermatofibroma
• Infiltrating basal cell carcinoma (consider small punch biopsy)

LABORATORY N/A
Drugs that may alter lab results: N/A
Disorders that may alter lab results: N/A

PATHOLOGICAL FINDINGS Histology shows whorl-like arrangements of hyalinized collagen bundles with pressure thinning of papillary dermis and minimal elastic tissue

SPECIAL TESTS N/A

IMAGING N/A

DIAGNOSTIC PROCEDURES Biopsy, if unable to differentiate

TREATMENT

APPROPRIATE HEALTH CARE
Outpatient

GENERAL MEASURES
• Intralesional corticosteroid injections - cause atrophy and are most successful therapy
• Pressure helpful for prevention. Pressure bandages must maintain 24 mm Hg, and should be worn for 6-12 months. Bandages should not be removed for more than 30 minutes/day.
• Radiation - no advantage over other methods, therefore use only if all other methods fail, and then use in conjunction with steroids
• Topical agents - (e.g., retinoic acid, vitamin E, antineoplastic agents, silicone gel) no evidence to support efficacy

SURGICAL MEASURES
• Surgery - high recurrence rate, therefore used only for debulking of large keloids or if a lesion is unresponsive to steroid injections alone
• Laser surgery - no evidence of efficacy

ACTIVITY Full activity

DIET No special diet

PATIENT EDUCATION Stress possibility of recurrence despite adequate treatment

MEDICATIONS

DRUG(S) OF CHOICE
• Triamcinolone suspension 10 mg/mL (Kenalog)
◊ Using 27-30 gauge needle and a TB syringe (total dose 20-30 mg of triamcinolone). May inject 3 lesions at a time, using 10 mg/lesion.
◊ Advance needle while injecting in order to evenly distribute medication
◊ Early keloids are more responsive to this therapy than older lesions
◊ Reinject every 4 weeks until keloid shrinks to near skin surface
◊ If no response to 10 mg/mL triamcinolone suspension, may try 40 mg/mL suspension
◊ May mix dilute triamcinolone (5-10 mg/mL) with local anesthetic for excision of keloids. Postoperative steroid injections at 2-4 weeks and then monthly for 6 months helps prevent recurrences.
Contraindications: None absolute
Precautions:
• Systemic absorption with adrenal suppression (reversible)
• Local affects - skin atrophy, ulceration, depigmentation, telangiectasias
• Both types of side effects more common with 40 mg/mL triamcinolone suspension
Significant possible interactions: Rare interactions with very large doses of corticosteroids and systemic absorption

ALTERNATIVE DRUGS   None

FOLLOWUP

PATIENT MONITORING   Monthly visits for evaluation and possible steroid re-injections

PREVENTION/AVOIDANCE   Compressive pressure dressings may be useful in high risk (e.g., burn) patients. Local steroid injection postoperative in high risk patients is also effective.

POSSIBLE COMPLICATIONS   Skin atrophy, ulceration, depigmentation, telangiectasias can occur as a result of triamcinolone treatment

EXPECTED COURSE/PROGNOSIS
Lesions gradually diminish with therapy over a 6-12 month period, leaving a flat, shiny scar

MISCELLANEOUS

ASSOCIATED CONDITIONS   None

AGE-RELATED FACTORS   Keloid formation more common during adolescence
Pediatric: None
Geriatric: None
Others: N/A

PREGNANCY   Keloid formation more likely during pregnancy

SYNONYMS
• Razor bumps

ICD-9-CM
701.4

SEE ALSO   N/A

OTHER NOTES   N/A

ABBREVIATIONS   N/A

REFERENCES   Rook A, Wilkinson DS, Ebling FJG, et al: Textbook of Dermatology. 5th Ed. Oxford. Blackwell Scientific Publishing, 1992
Illustrations: 4 available on CD-ROM
Internet references: http://www.5mcc.com

Author(s)
Scott D. Miller, MD

Keratosis, actinic

BASICS

DESCRIPTION Common, usually multiple premalignant skin lesions of sun-exposed areas. They are the most common indicator of excessive cumulative ultraviolet light exposure. The risk of transformation to squamous carcinoma is quite low: 1/4% risk of malignant transformation per lesion per year.
Genetics: Relates to complexion
System(s) affected: Skin/Exocrine
Incidence/Prevalence in USA: Common in blondes and redheads; rare in blacks
Predominant age: 40+; progressive with age (if child, look for freckling and other stigmata of xeroderma pigmentosum)
Predominant sex: Male > Female (from occupational sun exposure)

SIGNS AND SYMPTOMS
• Lesions usually fairly flat, red, and rough to palpitation
• Mild hyperesthesia common over lesions
• Hypertrophic verrucous lesions (called "cutaneous horns" if extreme) may be impossible to differentiate from squamous cell carcinoma clinically
• A pigmented variant also exists
• Acute cheilitis usually involves lower lip only
• Only photo-exposed areas involved, often with other stigmata of chronic actinic damage: lentigines, actinic elastosis, atrophy

CAUSES
• Almost exclusively short-wave ultraviolet light (UVB)
• Role of long-wave ultraviolet (UVA) is unknown
• Bowen's disease can be caused by the carcinogenic types of human papilloma virus and arsenic exposure

RISK FACTORS
• Equatorial latitudes
• High elevations
• Outdoor occupation (farmers, sailors, ranchers)
• Outdoor athletics
• Sun worshippers
• Accompanying heat, wind, humidity augment carcinogenic effect
• Occupational exposure, i.e., petroleum products
• Immunosuppression, especially organ transplantation

DIAGNOSIS

DIFFERENTIAL DIAGNOSIS
• Squamous cell carcinoma (hypertrophic type)
• Verruca vulgaris (hypertrophic type)
• Seborrheic dermatitis or psoriasis (near hairline)
• Lentigo maligna (pigmented type)
• Lupus erythematosus

LABORATORY N/A
Drugs that may alter lab results: N/A
Disorders that may alter lab results: N/A

PATHOLOGICAL FINDINGS
Diagnosis usually made clinically except where there is a suspicion of carcinoma
• Hyperkeratosis
• Hypertrophic, atrophic, Bowenoid, acantholytic, and pigmented varieties show the corresponding epidermal findings
• Malignant cells sparse except in Bowenoid variety
• Usually a sparse lymphocytic and plasma cell infiltrate

SPECIAL TESTS N/A

IMAGING N/A

DIAGNOSTIC PROCEDURES Biopsy (shave)

TREATMENT

APPROPRIATE HEALTH CARE
Outpatient

GENERAL MEASURES Sun-protective techniques (See Patient Education)

SURGICAL MEASURES
• Cryosurgery for smaller number of lesions
• For extensive lesions (but medical treatment usually preferred)
  ◊ Skin peels, i.e., 35% trichloracetic acid
  ◊ CO_2 laser therapy
  ◊ Dermabrasion

ACTIVITY No restrictions

DIET No special diet

PATIENT EDUCATION
• Teach sun-protective techniques
• Transfer hobbies and other outdoor activities to early morning or late afternoon
• Wear protective clothing and hats
• Daily use of topically applied sunscreens with SPF greater than 15; preferably containing titanium dioxide or Parsol-1789 to afford protection in the UVA range also
• Teach self-examination for cutaneous carcinoma (melanoma, squamous cell, basal cell)

MEDICATIONS

DRUG(S) OF CHOICE
• Topical fluorouracil, destroys even subclinical lesions, also non-scarring; usually applied bid for 3-4 weeks (for larger number of lesions)
• Topical masoprocol (Actinex); usually applied bid for 4 weeks
Contraindications: N/A
Precautions: Continue treatment to involved skin
Significant possible interactions: N/A

ALTERNATIVE DRUGS
Topical tretinoin (Retin-A) every night for months (length of treatment is uncertain). It is not known if effects are permanent.

 FOLLOWUP

PATIENT MONITORING Dependent on associated malignancy and frequency with which new actinic keratoses appear

PREVENTION/AVOIDANCE Sun protective techniques (See Patient Education)

POSSIBLE COMPLICATIONS Actinic keratosis is a premalignant lesion and may undergo carcinomatous proliferation to become squamous cell carcinoma

EXPECTED COURSE/PROGNOSIS
Excellent, if prevention taken by patient

 MISCELLANEOUS

ASSOCIATED CONDITIONS
• Squamous cell carcinoma

AGE-RELATED FACTORS
Pediatric: Rare
Geriatric: Frequent problem
Others: N/A

PREGNANCY N/A

SYNONYMS N/A

ICD-9-CM 701.1 Keratoderma, acquired

SEE ALSO
• Dermatitis, seborrheic

OTHER NOTES N/A

ABBREVIATIONS N/A

REFERENCES
• Dodson JM, et al: Malignant potential of actinic keratoses and controversy over treatment. Archives of Dermatology 1991;127:1029
• Lever WF, Schaumburg-Lever G: Histopathology of the Skin. 7th Ed. Philadelphia, J.P. Lippincott, 1990
Illustrations: 5 available on CD-ROM
Internet references: http://www.5mcc.com

Author(s)
John R. Person, MD

Labyrinthitis

BASICS

DESCRIPTION Inflammation of the vestibular labyrinth (a system of intercommunicating cavities and canals in the inner ear). There are many possible causes (see Differential Diagnosis). The most constant and pervasive symptom is vertigo.
System(s) affected: Nervous
Genetics: No known genetic pattern
Incidence/Prevalence: Unknown
Predominant age: All ages beyond infancy
Predominant sex: Male = Female

SIGNS AND SYMPTOMS
• Vertigo
• Dizziness
• Hearing loss, fluctuating
• Nausea and vomiting
• Tinnitus
• Perspiration
• Increased salivation
• Generalized malaise
• Hypercapnia
• Nystagmus

CAUSES
• Physiological - mismatch of vestibular, visual and somatosensory systems triggered by an external stimulus, such as a stop after whirling turns, heights, motion sickness
• Pathological - imbalance in the vestibular system caused by a lesion within vestibular pathways (inner ear to cerebral cortex)
• Infections (especially viral)
• Tumors
• Vasculitis
• Infarction
• Ototoxic drugs, especially aminoglycosides
• Head injury
• Neuronitis

RISK FACTORS
• Trauma
• Stress
• Drug ingestion
• Predisposing virus infection
• Cardiovascular disease
• Cerebrovascular disease

DIAGNOSIS

DIFFERENTIAL DIAGNOSIS
• Acute viral labyrinthitis
• Benign positional vertigo
• Meniere's syndrome
• Postconcussion syndrome
• Chronic bacterial otomastoiditis
• Drug-induced damage to vestibular labyrinth
• Vascular insufficiency
• Cerebellopontine-angle tumors, such as acoustic neuroma
• Multiple sclerosis
• Para-infectious encephalomyelitis
• Para-infectious cranial polyneuritis
• Ramsay Hunt syndrome
• Cerebral or systemic vasculitis
• Temporal lobe epilepsy
• Benign positional vertigo

LABORATORY Routine laboratory studies not helpful
Drugs that may alter lab results: All drugs with potential ototoxicity
Disorders that may alter lab results: N/A

PATHOLOGICAL FINDINGS N/A

SPECIAL TESTS
• Electronystagmography
• Caloric test
• Doll's eye test
• Forced voluntary hyperventilation for 1 to 3 minutes to mimic symptoms if cause is physiologic or emotional

IMAGING CT or MRI for suspected lesions

DIAGNOSTIC PROCEDURES History and physical

TREATMENT

APPROPRIATE HEALTH CARE
Outpatient

GENERAL MEASURES
• Treat underlying disorder when possible
• Symptomatic treatment to accompany specific treatment

SURGICAL MEASURES N/A

ACTIVITY Lie still with eyes closed in darkened room during acute attacks. Otherwise, activity as tolerated.

DIET Reduced sodium

PATIENT EDUCATION Griffith, H.W.: Instructions for Patients, Philadelphia, W.B. Saunders Co.

Labyrinthitis

MEDICATIONS

DRUG(S) OF CHOICE
• Promethazine (Phenergan) 25 mg qid
or
• Diazepam 5 mg qid
or
• Prochlorperazine suppositories 25 mg, for vomiting
or
• Meclizine 25 mg qid
or
• Scopolamine, transdermal (where available)
Contraindications: Refer to manufacturer's literature
Precautions: All the listed medications have significant adverse reactions. Use with caution. Avoid scopolamine in the elderly.
Significant possible interactions: Refer to manufacturer's literature

ALTERNATIVE DRUGS N/A

FOLLOWUP

PATIENT MONITORING As needed

PREVENTION/AVOIDANCE No preventive measures

POSSIBLE COMPLICATIONS Permanent hearing loss

EXPECTED COURSE/PROGNOSIS
Depends on cause. Physiological labyrinthitis usually clears completely.

MISCELLANEOUS

ASSOCIATED CONDITIONS
• Meniere's syndrome
• Head injury

AGE-RELATED FACTORS
Pediatric: Unusual in this age group
Geriatric:
• Very common in this age group, especially benign positional vertigo
• Avoid scopolamine or use with extreme caution in this age group
Others: N/A

PREGNANCY Avoid medications

SYNONYMS
• Acute peripheral vestibulopathy
• Vestibular neuronitis

ICD-9-CM 386.30

SEE ALSO N/A

OTHER NOTES N/A

ABBREVIATIONS N/A

REFERENCES Baloh RW, Honrobia V: Clinical Neurology of the Vestibular System. 2nd Ed. Philadelphia, F.A. Davis Co, 1990
Illustrations: N/A
Internet references: http://www.5mcc.com

Author(s)
Marshall Godwin, MD

Lacrimal disorders

BASICS

DESCRIPTION Lacrimal disorders refer to diseases and abnormalities of tear production and tear film. The most common lacrimal disorder is "dry eye." Lacrimal duct disorders, seen in the pediatric age group, often result in "overflow" tearing.
System(s) affected: Skin/Exocrine
Genetics: None
Incidence/Prevalence in USA: Very common and more often seen in arid climates of the desert Southwest
Predominant age: Dry eye symptoms increase with age. Most common in the elderly.
Predominant sex: Female > Male

SIGNS AND SYMPTOMS
• Gritty sensation to the eyes
• Visual blurring
• Redness
• Excessive tearing and mucus production
• Inadequate tears on the ocular surface

CAUSES Poor tear production and/or rapid evaporation of the tears

RISK FACTORS Individuals who live in arid regions, are on diuretics or have a history of collagen vascular diseases such as rheumatoid arthritis, Sjögren's syndrome, Bell's palsy, eyelid abnormalities and thyroid disease, are most at risk.

DIAGNOSIS

DIFFERENTIAL DIAGNOSIS Lacrimal disorders need to be differentiated from ocular infections and allergy. Another important consideration is the variety of anticholinergic affecting drugs that decrease tear production.

LABORATORY Tear production can be measured using a Schirmer's filter strip after instillation of topical anesthetic. Wetting of less than 10 mm of the slip after 5 minutes is indicative of insufficient tear production.
Drugs that may alter lab results: N/A
Disorders that may alter lab results: N/A

PATHOLOGICAL FINDINGS In Sjögren's syndrome infiltration of the lacrimal gland with inflammatory cells may be evident

SPECIAL TESTS N/A

IMAGING None

DIAGNOSTIC PROCEDURES Staining of the ocular surface with fluorescein will show areas of abnormal uptake and patches of drying. Rose bengal will be taken up by dead or dying epithelial cells and may be a more sensitive test.

TREATMENT

APPROPRIATE HEALTH CARE
Outpatient

GENERAL MEASURES
• Those with systemic illnesses predisposed to dry eye should be informed and instructed in the appropriate use of artificial tear supplements
• Cool mist vaporizer and home humidification is helpful

SURGICAL MEASURES N/A

ACTIVITY No restrictions

DIET No special diet

PATIENT EDUCATION All individuals with systemic illnesses predisposed to dry eye, menopausal women, and those residing in arid climates or over the age of 60 should be instructed in the use of artificial tear supplements to combat dry eye symptoms

MEDICATIONS

DRUG(S) OF CHOICE
• Artificial tear drops excluding those that have preservatives. The dosage of the drop varies depending on the severity of the symptoms. Usually one drop in each eye several times throughout the day can prevent ocular discomfort.
• The use of a bland ophthalmic ointment at bedtime between the eyelid and the eye can help prevent drying of the eye at night
• Vitamin A supplements
Contraindications: N/A
Precautions: N/A
Significant possible interactions: N/A

ALTERNATIVE DRUGS N/A

 FOLLOWUP

PATIENT MONITORING Monitor early to determine the effectiveness of treatment. Occasionally the use of more viscous drops or increased frequency of tear supplements may be required.

PREVENTION/AVOIDANCE
• Prevent exposure to eye irritants from pollution, cigarette smoke, and sun exposure
• Ensure adequate vitamin A intake in the diet or as a supplement

POSSIBLE COMPLICATIONS Severe dry eye can lead to corneal break-down, secondary invasion by bacteria and eye infections

EXPECTED COURSE/PROGNOSIS
Lacrimal disorders can be adequately managed with artificial tear supplements. Blocked tear ducts can be managed with probing and punctal dilation and/or dacryocysto-rhinostomy procedures in more severe cases.

 MISCELLANEOUS

ASSOCIATED CONDITIONS Sjögren's syndrome and age-related factors more commonly seen in the elderly population

AGE-RELATED FACTORS
Pediatric: May find lacrimal duct blockage in infants
Geriatric: Most common in this age group
Others: N/A

PREGNANCY Dry eyes can frequently be associated with pregnancy in an otherwise healthy individual. Vitamin A intake should not exceed 6000 IU a day.

SYNONYMS Epiphoria (excessive tearing)

ICD-9-CM 375.15

SEE ALSO N/A

OTHER NOTES Symptoms of dry eye are most often overlooked by practitioners when considering conjunctivitis (pink eye) and allergic disorders

ABBREVIATIONS N/A

REFERENCES Orbit Eyelids And Lacrimal System, Basic and Clinical Course. San Francisco, American Academy of Ophthalmology
Illustrations: N/A
Internet references: http://www.5mcc.com

Author(s)
Robert M. Kershner, MD, FACS

Lactose intolerance

BASICS

DESCRIPTION Inability to digest lactose (the primary sugar in milk) into its constituents, glucose and galactose, due to low levels of lactase enzyme in the brush border of the duodenum
• Congenital lactose intolerance - very rare
• Primary lactose intolerance - common in adults in whom a low level of lactase has developed after childhood. Symptoms are experienced after consumption of milk. Intolerance varies with amount of lactose consumed.
• Secondary lactose intolerance - inability to digest lactose caused by any condition injuring the intestinal mucosa (e.g., diarrhea) or a reduction of available mucosal surface (e.g., resection). This is usually transient, with the duration of the intolerance determined by the nature and course of the primary condition.
• 50% or more of infants with acute or chronic diarrhea have lactose intolerance, especially with rotavirus disease. Also, fairly common with giardiasis and ascariasis, inflammatory bowel disease, and the AIDS malabsorption syndrome.
• Lactose malabsorption - inability to absorb lactose. This does not necessarily parallel lactose intolerance.
System(s) affected: Gastrointestinal, Endocrine/Metabolic
Genetics: Unknown
Incidence/Prevalence in USA:
• Primary lactose intolerance - varies according to race. 100% of American Indians, 80-90% of blacks, Asians, Mediterraneans and Jews, less than 5% of descendants of Northern and Central Europeans.
• Secondary lactose intolerance - 50% or more of infants with acute or chronic diarrheal disease have lactose intolerance, especially with rotavirus disease. Also fairly common with giardiasis and ascariasis, inflammatory bowel disease and the AIDS malabsorptive syndrome.
Predominant age:
• Primary - teenage and adult
• Secondary - depends on the underlying condition
Predominant sex: Male = Female. However, 44% of lactose intolerant women will regain the ability to digest lactose during pregnancy.

SIGNS AND SYMPTOMS
• Bloating
• Cramping
• Abdominal discomfort
• Diarrhea or loose stools
• Flatulence
• Rumbling (borborygmi)
• Only one-third to one-fifth of people with lactose malabsorption will develop symptoms. Degree of symptoms varies with lactose load and with other foods consumed at the same time.
• In children - vomiting is common; frothy, acid stools; malnutrition can occur

CAUSES
• Primary lactose intolerance - normal decline in the lactase activity in the intestinal mucosa after weaning which is genetically controlled and permanent
• Secondary lactose intolerance - associated with gastroenteritis in children
• Also nontropical and tropical sprue, regional enteritis, abetalipoproteinemia, cystic fibrosis, ulcerative colitis, immunoglobulin deficiencies in both adults and children

RISK FACTORS
• Race
• Age

DIAGNOSIS

DIFFERENTIAL DIAGNOSIS Sucrase deficiency, diseases listed under secondary lactose intolerance

LABORATORY Low fecal pH and reducing substances only valid when stools are collected fresh and assayed immediately. Fairly insensitive.
Drugs that may alter lab results: None
Disorders that may alter lab results: None

PATHOLOGICAL FINDINGS Lactase deficiency in intestinal mucosa - may be patchy or focal. Rarely used in clinical practice.

SPECIAL TESTS
• Lactose breath hydrogen test - especially in children
• Lactose absorption test - alternative to lactose breath hydrogen test in adults

IMAGING None

DIAGNOSTIC PROCEDURES Small bowel biopsy for assay of lactase activity - may be normal if deficiency is focal or patchy (not readily available and usually not necessary)

TREATMENT

APPROPRIATE HEALTH CARE
Outpatient except severe cases of malnutrition

GENERAL MEASURES No disease specific measures

SURGICAL MEASURES N/A

ACTIVITY Full activity

DIET
• Reduce or restrict dietary lactose to control symptoms
• Yogurt and fermented products such as hard cheeses are tolerated better than milk
• Supplement calcium in the form of calcium carbonate
• Commercially available "lactase" preparations (Lactaid or Lactrase) are effective in reducing symptoms in many people
• Prehydrolyzed milk (Lactaid) is available and effective

PATIENT EDUCATION
• Patients must read labels on commercial products since milk-sugar is used in many products and may cause symptoms
• Lactose intolerant patients may tolerate whole milk or chocolate milk better than skim
• Lactose consumed with other food products is better tolerated than when it is consumed alone
• Primary lactase deficiency is permanent; secondary lactose intolerance is usually temporary, though it may persist for several months after the inciting disease has been cured.

MEDICATIONS:

DRUG(S) OF CHOICE
• Lactase (Lactaid, Lactrase) tablets
◊ 1 to 2 capsules or tablets prior to ingesting milk products. These vary in effectiveness at preventing symptoms.
◊ Can add tablets or contents of capsules to milk before drinking
◊ Also available in milk in some areas
Contraindications: None
Precautions: Not effective for all people with lactose intolerance
Significant possible interactions: None

ALTERNATIVE DRUGS None

FOLLOWUP

PATIENT MONITORING N/A

PREVENTION/AVOIDANCE Avoidance of lactose in large quantities will relieve symptoms. Patients can learn what level of lactose is tolerable in their diet.

POSSIBLE COMPLICATIONS Calcium deficiency

EXPECTED COURSE/PROGNOSIS
• Normal life expectancy
• Symptoms can be controlled

MISCELLANEOUS:

ASSOCIATED CONDITIONS
• Tropical or nontropical sprue
• Giardiasis
• Immunoglobulin deficiencies
• Crohn's disease
• Cystic fibrosis

AGE-RELATED FACTORS
Pediatric:
• Primary lactose intolerance occurs after weaning - usually beginning in late childhood
• Breast milk contains a large quantity of lactose but does not seem to worsen diarrhea associated with viral or bacterial diseases
• Lactose free formulas are available
Geriatric: No increase in lactose intolerance in this age group
Others: Secondary lactose intolerance can begin at any age

PREGNANCY 44% of lactose intolerant women will be able to tolerate lactose while pregnant

SYNONYMS Lactase deficiency

ICD-9-CM 271.3 intolerance or malabsorption (congenital) of lactose

OTHER NOTES N/A

SEE ALSO N/A

ABBREVIATIONS N/A

REFERENCES
• Saavedra JM, Perman JA: Current Concepts in Lactose Malabsorption and Intolerance. Annu Rev Nutr 1989;9:475-502
• Hurst JW, ed: Medicine for the Practicing Physician. 2nd Ed. Boston, Butterworth, 1988
Illustrations: N/A
Internet references: http://www.5mcc.com

Author(s)
Kathryn Reilly, MD, MPH

Laryngeal cancer

 BASICS

DESCRIPTION Most common cancer representing less than 1% of all malignant lesions. Squamous cell carcinomas comprise 5-98% of all malignant neoplasms of the larynx.
• Less than 2% of all carcinomas
• At the time of diagnosis, 62% will have local disease, 26% regional disease and 8% distant disease in the lungs, liver and/or bone
• No racial predilection
System(s) affected: Pulmonary
Genetics: Unknown
Incidence/Prevalence in USA: 5/100,00 (12,500 new cases per year)
Predominant age:
• Median age of occurrence in the 6th and 7th decades
• Less than 1% of laryngeal cancers arise in patients under 30 years of age
Predominant sex: Male > Female (5:1). However, increasing incidence in women who smoke.

SIGNS AND SYMPTOMS
• Persistent hoarseness in an elderly or middle aged cigarette smoker
• Dyspnea and stridor
• Ipsilateral otalgia
• Dysphagia
• Odynophagia
• Chronic cough
• Hemoptysis
• Weight loss due to poor nutrition
• Halitosis due to tumor necrosis
• Mass in the neck from metastatic lymph node
• Laryngeal tenderness due to tumor necrosis or suppuration
• Lump in the neck
• Broadening of the larynx on palpation with loss of crepitation
• Tenderness of the larynx
• Fullness of the cricothyroid membrane

CAUSES
• Smoking
• Alcohol abuse

RISK FACTORS Included in Causes

 DIAGNOSIS

DIFFERENTIAL DIAGNOSIS
• Acute or chronic laryngitis
• Benign vocal cord lesions such as polyps, nodules, and papillomas
• Tuberculosis or fungal infection of the larynx

LABORATORY Liver function studies to rule out metastatic disease
Drugs that may alter lab results: N/A
Disorders that may alter lab results: N/A

PATHOLOGICAL FINDINGS N/A

SPECIAL TESTS
• Laryngoscopy - fungating, friable tumor with heaped up edges and granular appearance with multiple areas of central necrosis and exudate surrounding areas of hyperemia
• CT or MRI if chest and liver or brain metastasis suspected

IMAGING
• Bone scan if bone metastasis suspected
• Screening chest x-ray to rule out metastatic disease

DIAGNOSTIC PROCEDURES Indirect and/or direct laryngoscopy and biopsy to determine stage of disease as well as histologic confirmation

 TREATMENT

APPROPRIATE HEALTH CARE
Outpatient primarily

GENERAL MEASURES Tracheotomy care, when applicable

SURGICAL MEASURES
• Tracheotomy may be necessary if tumor is large enough to cause upper airway obstruction
• Early disease may be treatable by either radiation therapy or laser cordectomy on an outpatient basis. 90% cure rates are the rule.
• More advanced disease needs inpatient care necessitating partial or total laryngectomy, and post-operative radiation therapy 4-5 weeks after surgery depending on the stage of disease

ACTIVITY Fully active unless the patient is debilitated from more advanced disease and/or greater degree of surgery

DIET
• Nasogastric or gastrostomy feeding may be necessary if tumor involves esophageal inlet
• No special diet otherwise

PATIENT EDUCATION Material is available from local cancer society

MEDICATIONS

DRUG(S) OF CHOICE
• Narcotics may be necessary for pain control during treatment for mucositis secondary to radiation therapy
• Nystatin mouth rinses for oral thrush
Contraindications: N/A
Precautions: N/A
Significant possible interactions: N/A

ALTERNATIVE DRUGS N/A

FOLLOWUP

PATIENT MONITORING
• Repeat indirect laryngoscopy and complete head and neck examinations for at least five years after treatment to detect early recurrence or second primary
• Yearly chest x-ray and liver function tests
• Patients with dysphagia should undergo barium swallow and/or esophageal endoscopy to rule out second tumor in the esophagus
• Patients with unexplained pain should have appropriate radiological or nuclear medicine, bone scans
• Mental status change indicates CT scan of the brain to rule out brain metastases

PREVENTION/AVOIDANCE
• Indirect laryngoscopy for patients with persistent hoarseness lasting beyond one to two weeks
• Cessation of smoking and/or alcohol abuse

POSSIBLE COMPLICATIONS
• Temporary odynophagia or dysphagia secondary to mucositis and/or thrush during radiation therapy
• Persistent hoarseness despite adequate treatment necessitating further adjunctive procedures and/or speech therapy
• Tracheostomal stenosis requiring stenting with laryngectomy tubes or further surgery
• Dysphagia, secondary to upper esophageal stricture after total laryngectomy necessitating dilatation
• Aspiration, after partial laryngectomy necessitating completion laryngectomy or tracheotomy
• Inability to decannulate after partial laryngectomy due to laryngeal stenosis and/or aspiration
• Radiation induced chondronecrosis which mimics tumor recurrence
• Radiation edema necessitating emergent tracheotomy

EXPECTED COURSE/PROGNOSIS
• Early disease is expected to have greater than 90% cure

MISCELLANEOUS

ASSOCIATED CONDITIONS
• Less than 10% of patients may have a synchronous squamous cell carcinoma in the lower or upper aero-digestive tract; most notably in the esophagus or lungs

AGE-RELATED FACTORS
Pediatric: N/A
Geriatric: N/A
Others: N/A

PREGNANCY
• Very rare in young patients in general
• Natural history of disease and treatment side effects have to be weighed against the possibilities of continuing on to delivery

SYNONYMS Cancer of larynx

ICD-9-CM 161.0 Malignant neoplasm of larynx

SEE ALSO N/A

OTHER NOTES N/A

ABBREVIATIONS N/A

REFERENCES
• Suen JY, Myers EN: Cancer of the Head and Neck. 3rd Ed. Philadelphia, WB Saunders Co, 1996
• Ariyan S: Cancer of the Head and Neck. St. Louis, C.V. Mosby, 1987
Illustrations: N/A
Internet references: http://www.5mcc.com

Author(s)
Roy R. Casiano, MD

Laryngitis

BASICS

DESCRIPTION Inflammation of the mucosa of the larynx. Most common during peaks paralleling epidemics of individual viruses, late fall, winter, early spring. Course may be acute or chronic. Includes atrophic, hypertrophic, reflux, catarrhal, sicca, acute infectious, membranous, granulomatous.
System(s) affected: Pulmonary
Genetics: No known genetic pattern
Incidence/Prevalence in USA: Common
Predominant age: All ages
Predominant sex: Male = Female

SIGNS AND SYMPTOMS
• Hoarseness
• Abnormal sounding voice
• Aphonia or dysphasia
• Throat tickling
• Feeling of throat rawness
• Constant urge to clear the throat
• Fever
• Malaise
• Dysphagia
• Throat pain
• Cough
• Regional lymphadenopathy
• Stridor in children

CAUSES
• Virus infections - influenza A, B, parainfluenza, adenovirus, coronavirus, rhinovirus, HPV, CMV, HSV
• Bacterial infections - beta-hemolytic streptococcus, Streptococcus pneumoniae, H. influenza, tuberculosis, leprosy, Moraxella catarrhalis
• Excessive use of voice
• Inhaling irritating substances
• Aspiration of caustic chemical
• Aging changes - muscle atrophy, loss of moisture in larynx, bowing of vocal cords
• Esophageal reflux
• Fungal infections
• Parasites
• Spirochetes (syphilis)
• Allergic
• Autoimmune
• Idiopathic

RISK FACTORS
• Acute
  ◊ Upper respiratory tract infection
  ◊ Bronchitis
  ◊ Pneumonia
  ◊ Influenza
  ◊ Pertussis
  ◊ Measles
  ◊ Diphtheria
  ◊ Immunocompromised
• Chronic
  ◊ Allergy
  ◊ Chronic rhinitis
  ◊ Chronic sinusitis
  ◊ Voice abuse
  ◊ Reflux of gastric contents
  ◊ Smoking
  ◊ Alcohol abuse
  ◊ Constant exposure to dust or other irritants

DIAGNOSIS

DIFFERENTIAL DIAGNOSIS
• Croup
• Measles
• Diphtheria
• Vocal nodules
• Laryngeal malignancy
• Thyroid malignancy

LABORATORY WBC elevated in bacterial laryngitis
Drugs that may alter lab results: N/A
Disorders that may alter lab results: N/A

PATHOLOGICAL FINDINGS N/A

SPECIAL TESTS Virus culture (seldom necessary)

IMAGING Only if needed for differential diagnosis

DIAGNOSTIC PROCEDURES
• Fiberoptic or indirect laryngoscopy - red, inflamed and occasionally hemorrhagic vocal cords, with rounded edges, and exudate
• Consider biopsy - chronic laryngitis in adults with history of smoking or alcohol abuse
• Consider 24° pH probe - chronic laryngitis in adults with gastroesophageal reflux

TREATMENT

APPROPRIATE HEALTH CARE
Outpatient

GENERAL MEASURES
• Acute
  ◊ Usually a self-limited illness and not severe
  ◊ Voice rest
  ◊ Steam inhalations or cool-mist humidifier
  ◊ Increase fluid intake
  ◊ Analgesics
  ◊ Avoid smoking (or cigarette smoke from others) during acute phase
• Chronic
  ◊ Symptomatic treatment as above
  ◊ Voice therapy
  ◊ Stop smoking
  ◊ Reduce alcohol intake
  ◊ Occupational change or modification, if exposure
  ◊ For reflux laryngitis - elevate head of bed, other antireflux management

SURGICAL MEASURES
• Vocal cord stripping of hyperplastic mucosa and areas of leukoplakia (can be used for biopsy, may produce a more normal sounding voice)

ACTIVITY Rest until fever subsides then, no restrictions

DIET No special diet

PATIENT EDUCATION
• Provide assistance with smoking cessation
• Help patient with modification of other predisposing habits or occupational hazards

MEDICATIONS

DRUG(S) OF CHOICE
• Usually none
• Analgesics
• Antipyretics to reduce fever
• Cough suppressants
• Penicillin V 250 mg or erythromycin 250 mg - orally q6h for 10-12 days (for streptococcal or pneumococcal infections)
• Antacids or H2 blockers for GERD

Contraindications: Refer to manufacturer's literature
Precautions: Refer to manufacturer's literature
Significant possible interactions: Refer to manufacturer's literature

ALTERNATIVE DRUGS N/A

FOLLOWUP

PATIENT MONITORING None needed (usually)

PREVENTION/AVOIDANCE
• Avoid overuse of voice
• Prompt treatment of respiratory infections
• Influenza virus vaccine for high-risk individuals

POSSIBLE COMPLICATIONS Chronic hoarseness

EXPECTED COURSE/PROGNOSIS
Complete clearing of the inflammation without sequelae

MISCELLANEOUS

ASSOCIATED CONDITIONS
• Viral pharyngitis
• Croup
• Bronchitis
• Pneumonitis

AGE-RELATED FACTORS
Pediatric: Common in this age group
Geriatric: May be sicker and slower to heal
Others: N/A

PREGNANCY Use only safe antibiotics, if antibiotics are essential

SYNONYMS
• Acute laryngitis
• Chronic laryngitis

ICD-9-CM
• 464.0 Acute
• 476.0 Chronic

SEE ALSO N/A

OTHER NOTES N/A

ABBREVIATIONS N/A

REFERENCES
• Avila MM, Carballal G, Rovaletti H, et al: Viral etiology in acute respiratory infections. Am Rev Respir Dis 1989;140:634
• Adams GL, et al: Fundamentals of Otolaryngology. 6th Ed. Philadelphia, W.B. Saunders Co., 1989
• Ballenger JI, Snow JB, eds: Otorhinolaryngology Head and Neck Surgery. 15 Ed. Philadelphia, Williams & Wlkins, 1996
Illustrations: N/A
Internet references: http://www.5mcc.com

Author(s)
Bruce T. Vanderhoff, MD
Anna N Maxey, MD

Laryngotracheobronchitis

 BASICS

DESCRIPTION Subacute viral illness, characterized by barking cough, stridor and fever, often causing upper airway obstruction in children. Most common cause of stridor in children.
System(s) affected: Pulmonary
Genetics: Unknown, though 15% have family history
Incidence/Prevalence in USA: 15,000-40,000/100,000
Predominant age: Childhood
Predominant sex: Male = Female

SIGNS AND SYMPTOMS
- Barking, spasmodic cough
- Biphasic stridor
- Low-grade to moderate fever
- Upper respiratory infection prodrome lasting 1-7 days
- Hypoxia/cyanosis
- Fatigue
- Non-toxic appearing child
- Normal voice, no drooling
- No change in stridor with positioning
- Non-tender larynx
- Inflamed subglottic region
- Normal appearing supraglottic region

CAUSES
- Parainfluenza 1
- Paramyxovirus
- Influenza virus type A
- Other parainfluenza and influenza viruses
- Respiratory syncytial virus
- Other viruses - adenovirus, rhinovirus, enterovirus, coxsackievirus, ECHO virus, reovirus, measles virus

RISK FACTORS
- Past history of croup
- Recurrent upper respiratory infections

 DIAGNOSIS

DIFFERENTIAL DIAGNOSIS
- Epiglottitis
- Foreign body aspiration
- Subglottic stenosis (congenital or acquired)
- Bacterial tracheitis
- Simple upper respiratory infection
- Subglottic hemangioma
- Diphtheria

LABORATORY
- Leukopenia early
- Leukocytosis in severe later stage
Drugs that may alter lab results: N/A
Disorders that may alter lab results: N/A

PATHOLOGICAL FINDINGS
- Inflammatory reaction of respiratory mucosa
- Loss of epithelial cells
- Thick mucoid secretions

SPECIAL TESTS Rapid antigen tests are available in some centers

IMAGING
- PA and lateral neck films show funnel-shaped subglottic region with normal epiglottis - "steeple sign" or "pencil-point sign" (present in 40% of children with LTB)
- Patient should be monitored during imaging - progression of airway obstruction may be rapid

DIAGNOSTIC PROCEDURES
- Direct laryngoscopy - if child is not in acute distress
- Fiberoptic laryngoscopy - procedure of choice where available
- Bronchoscopy

 TREATMENT

APPROPRIATE HEALTH CARE
- Outpatient in mild cases only
- Intensive care unit for patients with tachypnea, tachycardia, hypoxia, cyanosis, reactions, pneumonia, or congestive heart failure

GENERAL MEASURES
- Humidification - "croup tent"
- Intravenous fluids
- Electrocardiographic monitoring and pulse oximetry

SURGICAL MEASURES
- Intubation required in 6-10% for 3-5 days; use smallest tube possible
- Tracheotomy - rarely

ACTIVITY Must keep patient quiet; crying may exacerbate symptoms

DIET
- NPO with IV fluids for severe cases
- Frequent small feedings with increased fluids for mild cases

PATIENT EDUCATION
- Educate parents about when to seek emergency care if mild cases progress
- Emotional support and reassurance for the patient

MEDICATIONS

DRUG(S) OF CHOICE
• Dexamethasone: 1-1.5 mg/kg up to 20 mg every 8-12 hours for 8 doses
• Racemic epinephrine (Vaponefrin): 0.2-0.5 mL of 2.25 percent racemic epinephrine delivered in 2-3 mL of normal saline - one dose per 30 minutes, monitoring for side effects and rebound
• Antibiotics controversial in this viral illness
• Oxygen as needed
Precautions: Avoid over sedation
Contraindications: Refer to manufacturer's literature
Significant possible interactions: Refer to manufacturer's literature

ALTERNATIVE DRUGS
• Budesonide 2 mg nebulized; a topical glucocorticoid
• Ribavirin for respiratory syncytial virus
• Amantadine for influenza A

FOLLOWUP

PATIENT MONITORING
Severe cases require ICU care with respiratory monitoring for hypoxemia and hypercapnia

PREVENTION/AVOIDANCE N/A

POSSIBLE COMPLICATIONS
• Subglottic stenosis in intubated patients
• Bacterial tracheitis
• Cardiopulmonary arrest
• Pneumonia

EXPECTED COURSE/PROGNOSIS
• Upper respiratory infection prodrome of 1-7 days
• If required, intubation is maintained for 3-5 days
• If required, tracheotomy is maintained for 3-7 days
• Recovery is usually full, without lasting effects

MISCELLANEOUS

ASSOCIATED CONDITIONS
If recurrent, search for underlying anatomic abnormality such as subglottic stenosis or consider foreign body

AGE-RELATED FACTORS
Pediatric: Common in children under the age of three
Geriatric: N/A
Others: N/A

PREGNANCY N/A

SYNONYMS
• Croup
• Infectious croup
• Viral croup
• LTB

ICD-9-CM
464.20 Acute
464.21 With obstruction
476.1 Catarrhal, chronic, atrophic

SEE ALSO
• Bronchiolitis
• Common cold
• Epiglottitis
• Tracheitis, bacterial

OTHER NOTES
Less severe " variant" form, spasmodic croup, consists of croupy cough which becomes worse at night, but has no fever or x-ray changes. Usually resolves with mist therapy at home.

ABBREVIATIONS
LTB = laryngotracheobronchitis

REFERENCES
• Ballenger JJ: Diseases of the Nose, Throat and Ear. Philadelphia, Lea & Febiger, 1991
• Gates GA: Current Therapy in Otolaryngology - Head and Neck Surgery. 4th Ed. Philadelphia, B.C. Decker, Inc., 1990
Illustrations: N/A
Internet references: http://www.5mcc.com

Author(s)
Laurene L. Howell, MD
Gregg W. Suits, MD

Laxative abuse

BASICS

DESCRIPTION Diarrhea caused by self-medication or by a patient simulating diarrhea by the addition of fluid (e.g., urine) to the stool.
System(s) affected: Gastrointestinal, Nervous
Genetics: N/A
Incidence/Prevalence in USA: N/A
Predominant age:
• 18 to 40 years with bulimia nervosa
• 40 to 60 years without bulimia.
Predominant sex: Female > Male
Predominant race: N/A

SIGNS AND SYMPTOMS
• Diarrhea
• Additional symptoms - abdominal pain, rectal pain, nausea, vomiting, weight loss, muscle weakness, bone pain
• Additional signs - hypokalemia, skin pigmentation, finger clubbing, cyclic edema, kidney stones, melanosis coli
• The signs and symptoms will persist in spite of years of investigation and re-evaluation

CAUSES
• Ingestion of any laxative agent
• Psychological factors
  ◊ Bulimia nervosa
  ◊ Secondary gain of attention
  ◊ Hysterical behavior
  ◊ Inappropriate perception of "normal" bowel habits
• Chronic constipation

RISK FACTORS See Causes

DIAGNOSIS

DIFFERENTIAL DIAGNOSIS Include any source of diarrhea of secretory or osmotic source

LABORATORY
• Serum test - hypokalemia, metabolic alkalosis
• Urinalysis may be abnormal
• Stool Na+, K+
• Stool pH (alkalinization suggests presence of phenolphthalein)
• Stool for laxative titers
• Urine volume and electrolytes
Drugs that may alter lab results: N/A
Disorders that may alter lab results: N/A

PATHOLOGICAL FINDINGS
• Melanosis coli
• "Cathartic colon" - refers to dilatation and ahaustral appearance on barium enema

SPECIAL TESTS Hospital room search

IMAGING Barium enema - cathartic colon

DIAGNOSTIC PROCEDURES
• Carefully selected when needed to rule out other diseases
• Try not to repeat prior evaluations
• Sigmoidoscopy

TREATMENT

APPROPRIATE HEALTH CARE
Hospitalization may be needed

GENERAL MEASURES
• Discontinue laxative use
• Psychological support is essential
• Long term laxative abuse requires weaning
• Confrontation of the patient, gently and with support and understanding
• Treat constipation

SURGICAL MEASURES N/A

ACTIVITY Physical exercise program

DIET
• Ensure good nutritional habits
  ◊ Increase fiber intake
  ◊ Adequate calories, especially with bulimia

PATIENT EDUCATION See General Measures

MEDICATIONS

DRUG(S) OF CHOICE
• Based on psychological assessment
• Non-stimulant laxatives if needed
  ◊ Senna best during pregnancy and lactation
  ◊ Lactulose
  ◊ Fiber
Contraindications: Dantron - hepatotoxic
Precautions: Patients will be manipulative in attempts to hide problem, and often large quantities of laxatives
Significant possible interactions:
• Increased rate of intestinal flow may affect rate of absorption of medications: antibiotics, hormones, etc.
• Docusate sodium may potentiate hepatotoxicity of other drugs

ALTERNATIVE DRUGS   N/A

FOLLOWUP

PATIENT MONITORING
• Careful psychological counseling
• Careful medical support. Show concern by frequent visits as needed.

PREVENTION/AVOIDANCE
• Suspicion in patients with unsolved chronic diarrhea
• Monitor "doctor hopping"
• Avoid exploratory surgery
• Avoid repeated testing

POSSIBLE COMPLICATIONS
• Risk of multiple tests and procedures and surgeries
• Malnutrition
• Electrolyte imbalances (hypokalemia)
• Renal failure
• Fatalities especially in children given laxatives by parents
• Renal calculi

EXPECTED COURSE/PROGNOSIS
• Protracted course
• Prognosis related to psychological response

MISCELLANEOUS

ASSOCIATED CONDITIONS   N/A

AGE-RELATED FACTORS
Pediatric:
• Death
• Life long laxative dependence
Geriatric:
• Unusual to start beyond age of 60 years
• Rectal incontinence
Others: N/A

PREGNANCY   N/A

SYNONYMS
• Factitious diarrhea
• Cathartic colon

ICD-9-CM   305.9 Other mixed, or unspecified drug abuse

SEE ALSO
• Bulimia nervosa
• Constipation
• Hypokalemia
• Renal failure, acute (ARF)
• Renal failure, chronic
• Renal calculi

OTHER NOTES   N/A

ABBREVIATIONS   N/A

REFERENCES
• Sleisenger MH, Fordtran JS., eds: Gastrointestinal Disease: Pathophysiology, Diagnosis, Management. 5th Ed. Philadelphia, W.B. Saunders Co., 1994
• Muller-Lisser SA: Adverse Effects of Laxatives: Fact and Fiction, Pharmacology 1993;47(supp1):138-145
Illustrations: N/A
Internet references: http://www.5mcc.com

Author(s)
Duane C. Roe, MD

Lead poisoning

BASICS

DESCRIPTION Consequence of a high body burden of lead, an element with no known physiologic value
System(s) affected: Endocrine/Metabolic, Nervous, Gastrointestinal
Genetics: N/A
Incidence/Prevalence in USA:
• 17% of preschoolers in the US have a blood lead greater than 15 µg/dL (0.72 µmol/L). Sporadic cases in adults.
• Estimated (1990's) in children 6 months to age 5 years (≥ 15 µg/dL [0.72 µmol/L]): 17,000/100,000
Predominant age: 1-5 years old; adult worker
Predominant sex: Male = Female

SIGNS AND SYMPTOMS
• Often asymptomatic
• Mild to moderate toxicity
  ◊ May cause myalgia or paresthesia, fatigue, irritability, lethargy
  ◊ Abdominal discomfort, arthralgia, difficulty concentrating, headache, tremor, vomiting, weight loss, muscular exhaustibility
• Severe toxicity - leads to 3 major clinical syndromes
  ◊ Alimentary type - anorexia, metallic taste, constipation, severe abdominal cramps due to intestinal spasm and sometimes associated with rigidity of the abdominal wall
  ◊ Neuromuscular type (characteristic of adult plumbism) - peripheral neuritis usually painless and limited to extensor muscles
  ◊ Cerebral type or lead encephalopathy (more common in children) - seizures, coma, long-term sequelae including neurologic defects, retarded mental development, chronic hyperactivity
  ◊ Chronic exposure may cause renal failure

CAUSES
Inhalation of lead dust or fumes, or ingestion of lead

RISK FACTORS
• Children with pica
• Children with iron deficiency anemia
• Residence or frequent visitor in deteriorating, pre-1960 housing with leaded-paint surfaces
• Children with seizures
• Children with hyperkinetic or autistic behavior
• Sibling or playmate with lead poisoning
• Dust from clothing of lead worker
• Lead dissolved in water from lead or lead-soldered plumbing
• Lead glazed ceramics, especially with acidic food or drink
• Food stored in inverted plastic bread bags printed with colored ink
• Colored comics
• Soil/dust near lead industries and roads
• Folk remedies (Mexican - azarcon, greta; Asian - chuifong tokuwan, pay-loo-ah, ghasard, bali goli, kandu; Middle Eastern - alkohl, surma, saoott, cebagin)

• Hobbies - glazed pottery making; target shooting at firing ranges; lead soldering; painting; preparing lead shot, fishing sinkers; stained-glass making; car or boat repair; home remodeling
• Occupational exposure - plumbers, pipe fitters, lead miners, auto repairers, glass manufacturers, shipbuilders, printers, plastic manufacturers, lead smelters and refiners, policemen, steel welders or cutters, construction workers, rubber product manufacturers, gas station attendants, battery manufacturers, bridge reconstruction workers
• Dietary - zinc or calcium deficiency

DIAGNOSIS

DIFFERENTIAL DIAGNOSIS
• Elevated erythrocyte protoporphyrin may be due to iron deficiency anemia, less commonly hemolytic anemia. Erythropoietic protoporphyria produces a very high erythrocyte protoporphyrin.
• Alimentary type may be confused with acute abdomen
• Neuromuscular type may be confused with other polyneuropathies
• Cerebral type may be confused with attention deficit disorder, mental retardation, autism, dementia, other causes of seizures

LABORATORY
• Blood lead (Pb) greater than 10 µg/dL (0.48 µmol/L), collected with lead-free container
```
CDC classification:
------------------------------
Class  Lead (µg/dL)
I      < 10      (< 0.48 µmol/L)
II     10-19     (0.48-0.92 µmol/L)
III    20-44     (0.97-2.12 µmol/L)
IV     45-69     (2.17-3.33 µmol/L)
V      > 70      (> 3.38 µmol/L)
------------------------------
```
• Asymptomatic patient screening with erythrocyte protoporphyrin level (EP) greater than 35 µg/dL (0.62 µmol/L) indicates need for testing blood Pb
• Hgb and Hct slightly low. Eosinophilia or basophilic stippling on peripheral smear may be seen, but are not diagnostic of lead toxicity.
• Renal function decreased in late stages
Drugs that may alter lab results: N/A
Disorders that may alter lab results: N/A

PATHOLOGICAL FINDINGS N/A

SPECIAL TESTS Calcium ethylenediaminetetraacetic acid (Ca EDTA) mobilization test if blood Pb 25-44 µg/dL (1.21-2.12 µmol/L). This test is not widely used because it is technically difficult to perform and may delay diagnosis and treatment.

IMAGING Abdominal radiograph for lead particles in gut. X-ray of long bones for lines of increased density in the metaphyseal plate resulting from growth arrest.

DIAGNOSTIC PROCEDURES N/A

TREATMENT

APPROPRIATE HEALTH CARE
Outpatient unless parenteral chelation required

GENERAL MEASURES
• Case report to local health department for Class III-V. Complete inspection of home or work-place to determine source of lead. Screen all family members.
• Consider oral chelation for Class III or IV. Chelation (preferably parenteral) for Class V or symptomatic Class III or IV
• Remove from potential source of lead for Class IV or V, until complete inspection is performed

SURGICAL MEASURES N/A

ACTIVITY
• Avoid activity at any site of potential contamination

DIET
• If symptomatic, avoid excessive fluids
• Avoidance of pica
• Consume adequate calcium and iron
• Eat a low fat diet to reduce absorption and retention of lead

PATIENT EDUCATION
• The Inside Story: A Guide to Indoor Air Quality, EPA/400/1-88/004. EPA and Consumer Product Safety Commission, 1988. Lead and Your Drinking Water. EPA, 1988, OPA-87-006
• Raising Children Toxic Free: How to keep your child safe from lead, asbestos, pesticides, and other environmental hazards. HL Needleman, PJ Landrigan. New York, Avon Books, 1994
• National Lead Information Center, 1025 Connecticut Ave, NW, Suite 1200, Washington DC 20036, (203)833-1071; http://www.nsc.org/ehc/lead.htm

MEDICATIONS

DRUG(S) OF CHOICE
• Oral chelation:
◊ Succimer (Chemet, dimercaptosuccinic acid, DMSA) 10 mg/kg q8h x 5 days, then 10 mg/kg q12h x 2 weeks. May be repeated after 2 weeks off if lead levels are not stabilized below < 15 µg/dL (< 0.72 µmol/L).
• Parenteral chelation (begin after establishment of adequate urine output):
◊ Class V or symptomatic: dimercaprol (British anti-Lewisite, BAL) 75 mg/m2 given deep IM, then BAL 450 mg/m2/d divided q4h x 5 days + Ca EDTA (edetate calcium disodium) 1500 mg/m2/d continuous IV infusion x 5 days. If rebound lead level ≥ 45 µg/dL (≥ 2.17 µmol/L), chelation may be repeated after 2 day interval if symptomatic, after 5 day interval if symptomatic.
◊ Class IV asymptomatic: Ca EDTA 1000 mg/m2/d x 5 days. May be repeated after 5-7 days.
• Diazepam for initial control of seizures, further control maintained with paraldehyde

Contraindications:
• BAL should not be given to persons allergic to peanuts (the drug solution contains peanut oil)

Precautions:
• Succimer: Gastrointestinal upset, rash, nasal congestion, muscle pains, elevated liver function tests
• Ca EDTA: Renal failure, increased excretion of zinc, copper and iron
• BAL: Nausea, vomiting, fever, headache, transient hypertension, hepatocellular damage

Significant possible interactions:
• Vitamins should not be given concurrently with oral chelation
• BAL may precipitate hemolytic crisis in a patient with G6PD deficiency

ALTERNATIVE DRUGS
• Oral chelation with penicillamine (d-penicillamine, Depen, Cuprimine)
◊ Penicillin allergic patient should not receive D-penicillamine (cross-sensitivity is common)
◊ 10-20 mg/kg bid mixed in apple juice/sauce on empty stomach (not FDA approved)
◊ D-penicillamine may cause gastrointestinal upset, renal failure, granulocytopenia, liver dysfunction, iron deficiency, drug induced lupus-like syndrome

FOLLOWUP

PATIENT MONITORING
• After chelation, check for rebound Pb level in 7-10 days. Follow with regular monitoring, initially biweekly or monthly.
• Correct iron deficiency or any other nutritional deficiencies present
• For Class II or higher, repeat testing every 3 months until Class I level achieved

PREVENTION/AVOIDANCE
• Family should receive counseling on potential sources of lead and methods to decrease lead exposure. Wet mopping and dusting with a high phosphate solution (e.g., powdered automatic dishwasher detergent with 1/4 cup per gallon of water) will help control lead-bearing dust.
• If the source is in the home, the patient must reside elsewhere until the abatement process is completed

POSSIBLE COMPLICATIONS
• CNS toxicity may be long lasting or permanent
• Long-term lead exposure may cause chronic renal failure (Fanconi-like syndrome); gout; lead line (blue-black) on gingival tissue

EXPECTED COURSE/PROGNOSIS
• Symptomatic lead poisoning without encephalopathy generally improves with chelation, but subtle CNS toxicity may be long lasting or permanent
• If encephalopathy occurs, permanent sequelae (mental retardation, seizure disorder, blindness, hemiparesis) in 25-50%

MISCELLANEOUS

ASSOCIATED CONDITIONS Iron deficiency anemia

AGE-RELATED FACTORS
Pediatric:
• Increasing evidence that low lead level exposure (as low as 10 µg/dL [0.48 µmol/L]) may produce neurotoxicity in children
• Children are at increased risk because of incomplete development of the blood-brain barrier before age 3 years allowing more lead into the central nervous system; ingested lead has 40% bioavailability in children compared with 10% in adults
• Common childhood behaviors such as frequent hand-to-mouth activity and pica (repeated ingestion of nonfood products) greatly increase the risk of ingesting lead
Geriatric: N/A
Others: N/A

PREGNANCY
• Lead exposure in pregnancy is associated with reduced birth weight and premature birth
• Lead is an animal teratogen

SYNONYMS Lead poisoning, inorganic

ICD-9-CM 984.9; when symptomatic, or a specific lead compound is the source, other codes may apply

SEE ALSO
• Iron deficiency anemia

OTHER NOTES Screening of all asymptomatic children during their first 6 years of life has been recommended. Screening EP is not sensitive for blood Pb less than 25 µg/dL (1.20 µmol/L).

ABBREVIATIONS
• Pb = lead
• EP = erythrocyte protoporphyrin
• BAL = British anti-Lewisite

REFERENCES
• Royce S: Case studies in environmental medicine: lead toxicity. US Dept. HHS, PHS, TSDR, 1990
• Centers for Disease Control: Preventing lead poisoning in young children. US Dept. HHS, PHS, CDC, Atlanta, 1991
Illustrations: 1 available on CD-ROM
Internet references: http://www.5mcc.com

Author(s)
Jason Chao, MD, MS

Légg-Calvé-Pérthes disease

BASICS

DESCRIPTION Idiopathic osteonecrosis of capital femoral epiphysis of the femoral head. 10-20% of cases are bilateral.
System(s) affected: Musculoskeletal
Genetics: No known genetic pattern
Incidence/Prevalence in USA: Incidence 15/100,000; prevalence 75/100,000
Predominant age: Susceptible age 2-12 years. However, 80% occur between 4-9 years
Predominant sex: Males > Females (4:1)

SIGNS AND SYMPTOMS
• Hip or groin pain with referral to knee and thigh not uncommon
• Range of motion limited, especially in internal rotation and abduction
• Atrophy of thigh musculature due to disease
• Leg length inequality

CAUSES
• Etiology remains unclear
• Felt to be related to interruption of blood flow to femoral epiphysis
• Role of trauma, hormonal and metabolic factors remains to be established

RISK FACTORS
• No genetic factors
• Increased incidence in children with low birth weight and delayed physical maturation

DIAGNOSIS

DIFFERENTIAL DIAGNOSIS
• Unilateral case - septic hip, toxic synovitis, juvenile rheumatoid arthritis, tuberculosis, lymphoma
• Bilateral cases - hypothyroidism, spondyloepiphyseal dysplasia

LABORATORY
• CBC
• Sedimentation rate (elevated in infection)
Drugs that may alter lab results: N/A
Disorders that may alter lab results: N/A

PATHOLOGICAL FINDINGS
• Early (necrotic, resorption) stage - necrosis of bone with subchondral bone fracture and subsequent collapse of subchondral bone
• Late (healing) stage - revascularization by creeping substitution of necrotic bone

SPECIAL TESTS
• Technetium 99 bone scan - helpful in delineating extent of avascular changes before they are evident on plain radiographs (sensitivity 98%, specificity 95%)
• Arthrography

IMAGING
• MRI - very sensitive test; facilitates early diagnosis of necrosis and visualization of articular surface
• Serial radiographs, AP and frog lateral, are crucial determinant of extent of involvement and progression of healing. Initial findings.
• Full extent of involvement may not be evident for several months
• Classification and prognosis based on radiographic extent of involvement; Herring and Catterall classification

DIAGNOSTIC PROCEDURES Hip aspiration when septic joint is suspected

TREATMENT

APPROPRIATE HEALTH CARE
• When necessary, a pediatric orthopedic surgeon should be consulted
• Ambulatory treatment is usual
• On occasion, inpatient traction or surgical procedure necessary

GENERAL MEASURES
• Goals of treatment are:
  ◊ Obtain and maintain range-of-motion
  ◊ Relieve weight bearing on affected, irritable hip as necessary
  ◊ Containment of femoral epiphysis within the confines of the acetabulum in order to encourage maximal normal growth and development of the femoral head
• Traction:
  ◊ Should be used to relieve pain and spasm of the hip and restore range-of-motion
  ◊ Home traction can be used, if available, as an alternative to inpatient traction

SURGICAL MEASURES N/A

ACTIVITY
• Bedrest and traction as necessary to relieve irritation of joint
• Ambulatory status depends on extent/stage of disease

DIET No special diet

PATIENT EDUCATION
• Patient and family should realize that Légg-Calvé-Pérthes disease (LCP) is a self-limited disease with revascularization occurring within 3 years
• Treatment is directed at maintaining an appropriate range-of-motion and maximizing the containment of the femoral head

MEDICATIONS

DRUG(S) OF CHOICE Ibuprofen 20-30 mg/kg/24 hours
Contraindications: Allergy to ibuprofen
Precautions: GI irritation
Significant possible interactions: N/A

ALTERNATIVE DRUGS N/A

FOLLOWUP

PATIENT MONITORING
• Initially, close followup needed to determine extent of necrosis and monitor clinical course
• Once healing phase entered, followup can be every 6 months
• Long-term followup necessary to determine final outcome

POSSIBLE COMPLICATIONS
• Permanent distortion of the femoral head
• Distorted joint susceptiable to early degenerative joint disease

PREVENTION/AVOIDANCE Since etiology is not clearly understood, prevention is not possible

EXPECTED COURSE/PROGNOSIS
• Most patients (60%) have a favorable outcome
• Outcome is dependent on the age at the time of the diagnosis (the younger the better)
• Prognosis is also proportional to the degree of radiologic involvement

MISCELLANEOUS

ASSOCIATED CONDITIONS N/A

AGE-RELATED FACTORS
Pediatric:
• Physical maturation is delayed
• The younger the patient at the time of diagnosis, the greater the chance for remodelling
Geriatric: N/A
Others: N/A

PREGNANCY N/A

SYNONYMS N/A

ICD-9-CM 732.1 Juvenile osteochondrosis of hip and pelvis

SEE ALSO N/A

OTHER NOTES N/A

ABBREVIATIONS N/A

REFERENCES
• Catterall A, Chir M: Perthes Disease. In: Steinberg ME, ed. The Hip and its Disorders. Philadelphia, W.B. Saunders Co., 1991:419-439
• Tachdjian M: Pediatric Orthopedics. 2nd Ed. Philadelphia, W.B. Saunders Co., 1990:933-1003
• Wenger DR, Ward TW, Herring JA: Légg Pérthes Disease: Current Concepts Review. Journal of Bone and Joint Surgery 1991;73A:778-788
Illustrations: N/A
Internet references: http://www.5mcc.com

Author(s)
Francisco G. Valencia, MD

Legionnaires' disease

BASICS

DESCRIPTION Legionnaires' disease was coined for an epidemic of lower respiratory tract disease occurring in Philadelphia in 1976 in war veterans. The causative bacterium was identified and named Legionella pneumophila and may cause pneumonia or flu-like illness.
System(s) affected: Pulmonary, Gastrointestinal
Genetics: None known
Incidence/Prevalence in USA: 2-4/100,000/year; 1-4% of commonly acquired pneumonias; up to 20% of nosocomial pneumonias; thought to be under reported
Predominant Age: 15 months-84 years, increased after age 50
Predominant sex: Male > Female

SIGNS AND SYMPTOMS
• Range of illness from asymptomatic seroconversion, mild febrile illness, to severe pneumonia
• Incubation 2-10 days
• Fever, chills
• Malaise, weakness, lethargy
• Anorexia
• Myalgia
• Headache
• Watery diarrhea in up to 50%
• Nausea and vomiting in 10-20%
• Dry cough which may become productive
• Pleuritic chest pain in up to 33%
• Relative bradycardia in up to 67% of patients
• Neuropsychiatric symptoms of confusion, disorientation, obtundation, depression, hallucinations, insomnia, seizures in up to 25%
• Blood streaked sputum; gross hemoptysis rare
• Hyponatremia
• Hypophosphatemia
• Elevated serum transaminases
• Hypotension (17%)

CAUSES Legionella pneumophila, a weakly gram negative organism widely distributed in soil and water, acquired by inhalation of infected aerosols

RISK FACTORS
• Smoking
• Alcohol abuse
• Immunosuppression/HIV
• Chronic cardiopulmonary disease
• Surgery
• Advanced age
• Renal failure

DIAGNOSIS

DIFFERENTIAL DIAGNOSIS Other bacterial pneumonias, atypical pneumonias with mycoplasma and chlamydia, viral pneumonias

LABORATORY
• Sputum:
◊ Gram stain many neutrophils, few organisms
◊ Direct immunofluorescence 25-80% sensitive
◊ DNA probe 70% sensitive
◊ Cultures 50-90% sensitive
• Urine radioimmunoassay (RIA):
◊ > 90% sensitivity + specificity
◊ Intended for detection of L. pneumophila serogroup 1 (which accounts for 70-80% of isolates)
• Blood:
◊ Indirect immunofluorescence 56% sensitive in three weeks and 90% sensitive after 6 weeks (acute and convalescent titers/seroconversion)
◊ Cultures 20% sensitive. Buffered charcoal yeast extract (BCYE) medium required.
• Polymerase chain reaction
◊ Experimental
Drugs that may alter lab results: N/A
Disorders that may alter lab results: Direct immunofluorescence can cross react with Pseudomonas and Bacteroides species, E. coli, Haemophilus

PATHOLOGICAL FINDINGS Multifocal pneumonia with alveolitis and bronchiolitis, with fibrinous pleuritis, and may have serous or serosanguinous pleural effusion. Abscess formation in up to 20%.

SPECIAL TESTS Silver and Gimenez stains for lung tissue/specimens

IMAGING
• Chest x-ray
◊ Not specific for Legionella
◊ Commonly with lower lobe patchy alveolar infiltrate with consolidation
◊ Cavitation or abscess, especially in immunocompromised
◊ Pleural effusion in up to 50%
◊ May take from 1-4 months for the x-ray to return to normal. Progression of infiltrate may be seen despite antibiotic therapy.

DIAGNOSTIC PROCEDURES
Transtracheal aspiration or bronchoscopy for sputum/lung samples

TREATMENT

APPROPRIATE HEALTH CARE Severity of illness and support available in the outpatient setting will dictate the appropriate site for care

GENERAL MEASURES
• Supportive care
• Maintaining oxygenation, hydration, and electrolyte balance while providing antibiotic therapy

SURGICAL MEASURES N/A

ACTIVITY As tolerated

DIET As tolerated

PATIENT EDUCATION Can educate patients regarding prevention/avoidance measures, lowering their risk status, and if infected already, about the expected course of the disease

Legionnaires' disease

MEDICATIONS

DRUG(S) OF CHOICE
• Erythromycin 30-60 mg/kg/day po or IV divided into four doses for 10-21 days
• Addition of rifampin 600 mg q 12 hours po or IV should be provided along with erythromycin in very ill patients
Contraindications: Hypersensitivity reactions
Precautions: Liver disease
Significant possible interactions:
• Erythromycin can increase theophylline, carbamazepine, and digoxin levels and can increase activity of oral anticoagulants
• Rifampin may decrease the effectiveness of oral anticoagulants, steroids, digoxin, quinidine, oral contraceptives and hypoglycemic agents

ALTERNATIVE DRUGS
• Tetracyclines may be used along with rifampin
  ◊ Doxycycline IV 200 mg every 12 hours x 2 doses, then 100 mg bid or po 200 mg x 1 dose, then 100 mg bid
• Trimethoprim-sulfamethoxazole, imipenem, and quinolones may also be effective
  ◊ Trimethoprim-sulfamethoxazole IV or po 5 mg/kg TMP every 8 hours
  ◊ Ofloxacin IV or po, 400 mg every 12 hours
  ◊ Ciprofloxacin IV 400 mg every 8 hours or po 750 mg every 12 hours
• Other macrolides (clarithromycin) or azalides (azithromycin)
  ◊ Clarithromycin 500 mg po bid
  ◊ Azithromycin 500 mg po qd

FOLLOWUP

PATIENT MONITORING
• Respiratory status, hydration and electrolyte status should be monitored closely
• Chest x-ray not useful to monitor clinical response

PREVENTION/AVOIDANCE
Heating water to 60-70 degrees centigrade may help prevent water contamination. UV light or copper-silver ionization are bactericidal.

POSSIBLE COMPLICATIONS
• Dehydration
• Hyponatremia
• Respiratory insufficiency requiring ventilator support
• Endocarditis
• Disseminated intravascular coagulation
• Renal failure
• Multiple organ dysfunction syndrome (MODS)
• Coma
• Death in 10% of treated non-immunocompromised patients, and in up to 80% of untreated immunocompromised patients
• Bacteremia or abscess formation in immunocompromised

EXPECTED COURSE/PROGNOSIS
• Recovery is variable, some patients experience rapid improvement with defervescence in 3-5 days and recovery in 6-10 days, while others may have a much more protracted course despite treatment
• Mortality rate can approach 50% with nosocomial infections

MISCELLANEOUS

ASSOCIATED CONDITIONS N/A

AGE-RELATED FACTORS
Pediatric: Less common
Geriatric: Increased incidence in those over age 50
Others: N/A

PREGNANCY N/A

SYNONYMS
• Legionella pneumonia
• Pontiac fever
• Legionellosis

ICD-9-CM
482.83 Pneumonia due to other gram negative bacteria

SEE ALSO
• Pneumonia, bacterial

OTHER NOTES
• Extrapulmonary disease can occur in the form of:
  ◊ Encephalitis
  ◊ Cellulitis
  ◊ Sinusitis
  ◊ Pancreatitis
  ◊ Pyelonephritis
  ◊ Endocarditis
  ◊ Pericarditis
  ◊ Perirectal abscess

ABBREVIATIONS N/A

REFERENCES
• Hoeprich P, Jordan MC: Infectious Diseases. 5th Ed. J.B. Lippincott, 1994
• Mandell GL, ed: Principles and Practice of Infectious Diseases. 4th Ed. New York, Churchill Livingstone, 1995
• Rubenstein E, Federman DD: Scientific American Medicine, 1995
• Edelstein PH: Legionnaire's disease. Clinical Infectious Diseases 1993;16:741-749
Illustrations: N/A
Internet references: http://www.5mcc.com

Author(s)
Carolyn Nine, MD
Mitchell S. King, MD

Leishmaniasis

BASICS

DESCRIPTION An infective condition caused by several species of the protozoan Leishmania. Four major clinical syndromes are recognized.
• Visceral leishmaniasis (Kala-azar, Black fever) may be endemic, epidemic or sporadic. Different forms are:
◊ African Kala-azar: Found in the eastern half of Africa from the Sahara in the North to the Equator. Disease of older children and young adults (10-25 years) Males > females.
◊ Mediterranean or infantile Kala-azar: Seen primarily in the Mediterranean area, China and Latin America. Dogs, jackals, foxes and rats are potential reservoirs. The strains responsible for the Mediterranean and American disease are sometimes referred to as L. infantum and L. chagasi respectively.
◊ Indian Kala-azar: Age and sex distribution similar to African Kala-azar. Humans are the only known reservoir and transmission is by anthropophilic sandflies.
• Cutaneous leishmaniasis of the old and new worlds. Characterized by one or more localized lesions on exposed areas. These ulcerate centrally and spread centrifugally. Spontaneous healing less common in new world disease. Satellite lesions and lymphadenopathy may or may not occur.
• Mucocutaneous leishmaniasis (espundia). One or more lesions on the legs which may ulcerate. In 2-5% of patients, metastatic lesions appear in the nasopharynx after months or years, and may result in painful mutilating erosions of soft tissue. Lesions may occur rarely in perineum.
• Diffuse cutaneous leishmaniasis. Extensive skin lesions, but no visceral lesions. Clinical picture may be similar to lepromatous leprosy.
System(s) affected: Gastrointestinal, Pulmonary, Hemic/Lymphatic/Immunologic, Skin/Exocrine
Genetics: N/A
Incidence/Prevalence in USA: Rare, but reported in states bordering Mexico.
Predominant age: Children and young adults. (10-25 years). Mediterranean or infantile Kala-azar - usually < 4 years age.
Predominant sex: African Kala-azar, Indian Kala-azar: Male > female

SIGNS AND SYMPTOMS
• Incubation period - about 3 months for the visceral form and 2-24 months for others
• Onset - insidious/abrupt
• Malabsorption; failure to thrive in infants and children
• Fever - nocturnal, no signs of toxemia
• Cough
• Diarrhea, GI bleeding
• Lymphadenopathy
• Splenomegaly
• Moderate hepatomegaly
• Cirrhosis, portal hypertension (in 10% of patients)
• Anemia, pancytopenia
• Cutaneous lesions, may ulcerate and heal spontaneously
• Nasal stuffiness

• Epistaxis
• Edema, cachexia and hyperpigmentation in late stages
• Hypoalbuminuria
• Hypergammaglobulinemia

CAUSES
Several species of Leishmania including L. donovani (Kala-azar), L.infantum, L.chagasi (Mediterranean and American forms), L. tropica (cutaneous form), L. major (in Middle East, Afghanistan and India), L. mexicana, L. braziliensis and others. The organisms are transmitted by female sandflies of the genus phlebotomus in the old world and Lutzomyia in the new world.

RISK FACTORS
• Children > young adults in endemic areas
• Malnutrition
• AIDS
• Incomplete therapy of initial disease

DIAGNOSIS

DIFFERENTIAL DIAGNOSIS
• Malaria
• Brucellosis
• Tuberculosis
• Typhoid
• Hepatic abscess
• Lepromatous leprosy for diffuse leishmaniasis
Post Kala-azar dermal lesion (PKDL) must be differentiated from leprosy, syphilis and yaws

LABORATORY
• Demonstration of parasites in
◊ Bone marrow aspirate
◊ Splenic aspirate
◊ Lymph node aspirate or biopsy
◊ Biopsy material from suspicious skin lesions after cleaning with alcohol to reduce bacterial contamination
◊ The intracellular amastigote form in the macrophages, formerly known as the Leishman-Donovan (LD) body, has a characteristic pear-shaped body with a dark circular nucleus and short rod-shaped kinetoplasts
• Hypergammaglobulinemia
• Direct agglutination test detects IgM antibody which indicates acute disease
Drugs that may alter lab results: N/A
Disorders that may alter lab results: N/A

PATHOLOGICAL FINDINGS
• Marked lymphocytic infiltration
• Ulcerating lesions in the skin and mucosa of nasopharynx

SPECIAL TESTS
• Leishmanin skin test is positive 6-8 weeks after recovery in cutaneous forms, but not in diffuse leishmaniasis. It is negative in visceral leishmaniasis.
• Monoclonal antibodies or hybridization of tissue touch blots with labelled kinetoplast DNA probes used for identification of different strains of Leishmania
• ELISA highly sensitive and specific in visceral disease
• Montenegro skin test is nonstandardized and used only in epidemiological studies. It is negative in visceral leishmaniasis.

IMAGING N/A

DIAGNOSTIC PROCEDURES
• Demonstration of the organism by smear or culture from aspirate or biopsy material. Novy-MacNeal-Nicolle medium or other liquid media used for cultures are maintained at 22-28°C for 21 days. Motile promastigotes can be observed microscopically.
• Speciation using monoclonal Ab or labelled DNA probes

TREATMENT

APPROPRIATE HEALTH CARE
Inpatient for blood transfusions and complicating superinfections. Outpatient care once the condition stabilizes.

GENERAL MEASURES
• Bed rest, oral hygiene, and good nutrition are important.
• Transfusions for anemia and antibacterial chemotherapy for bacterial complications must supplement specific therapy.
• Periodic ECG monitoring during prolonged therapy with pentavalent antimonials.

SURGICAL MEASURES
• Adjunctive splenectomy
• Reconstructive surgery for tissue damage

ACTIVITY
Bed rest during acute stages. Level of activity dependent on severity of disease and organ systems involved

DIET
Rich nutritious diet

PATIENT EDUCATION
Explain prevention measures

Leishmaniasis

MEDICATIONS

DRUG(S) OF CHOICE
• Sodium antimony gluconate (Pentostam) 100 mg Sb5+/mL IV/IM: single daily dose of 20 mg/kg/day for 20-30 days
• Meglumine antimoniate (Glucantime) 85 mg Sb5+/mL, same dose and duration of treatment as above, can also be used
Note: In the U.S., these drugs are available only from the CDC, Atlanta, GA 30333; emergency telephone 404-639-2888 (http://www.cdc.gov)
• Relapses and incomplete responses should be treated with the same regimen for 40-60 days. Addition of oral allopurinol (Zyloprim) 20-30 mg/kg/day in three divided doses has been effective.
Contraindications: Refer to manufacturer's profile of each drug
Precautions: Refer to manufacturer's profile of each drug. Periodic ECG monitoring is recommended during prolonged therapy.
Significant possible interactions: Refer to manufacturer's profile of each drug

ALTERNATIVE DRUGS
Relapses with drug resistant organisms are usually treated with:
• Amphotericin B (Fungizone)IV: 0.5-1 mg/kg on alternate days
OR
• Pentamidine (Pentam): 3-4 mg/kg, 3 times a week for 5-25 weeks; investigational only
• Recombinant human interferon gamma: an adjunct to pentavalent antimony in treatment failures

FOLLOWUP

PATIENT MONITORING
• Follow-up at 3 and 12 months to detect relapses
• PKDL should be treated in the same fashion as the initial illness
• Periodic monitoring of ECG, liver function and renal function during prolonged therapy

PREVENTION/AVOIDANCE
• Use of pesticides (e.g., DDT) against sandflies
• Insect repellants - for travelers
• Permethrin - coated fine netting for travelers
• Early treatment of human cases
• Elimination of diseased dogs

POSSIBLE COMPLICATIONS
• Edema, cachexia, hyperpigmentation in late stages
• Superinfections and gastrointestinal bleeding may cause death in untreated patients with visceral disease (Kala-azar)
• 3-10% of the treated cases develop PKDL characterized by depigmented macules and wart-like nodules over the face and extensor surfaces of limbs
• Metastatic lesions in nasopharynx with tissue destruction in patients with mucocutaneous leishmaniasis

EXPECTED COURSE/PROGNOSIS
With early treatment, cure rate is over 90%, though in advanced cases, mortality remains at 15-25%. In untreated cases, death occurs in 3-20 months in up to 95% of adults and 85% of children.

MISCELLANEOUS

ASSOCIATED CONDITIONS Fulminant Kala-azar has been described in association with AIDS and malnutrition

AGE-RELATED FACTORS
Pediatric:
• Pediatric Mediterranean or infantile Kala-azar usually a disease of children under 4 years
• African or Indian Kala-azar: usually a disease of children and young adults (10-25 years)
Geriatric: N/A
Others: N/A

PREGNANCY N/A

SYNONYMS
• Visceral leishmaniasis
• Kala-azar
• Black fever
• Dumdum fever

ICD-9-CM
085.0 Kala-azar

SEE ALSO N/A

OTHER NOTES N/A

ABBREVIATIONS
PKDL = Post Kala-azar Dermal Leishmaniasis
LD bodies = Leishman-Donovani bodies

REFERENCES
• Isselbacher KJ, et al, eds: Harrison's Principles of Internal Medicine. 13th Ed. New York, McGraw-Hill, 1994
• Berkow R, et al, eds: Merck Manual. 15th Ed. Rahway, NJ, Merck Sharp & Dohme, 1987
• Dhanda V: Classics in Indian Medicine. The National Medical Journal of India 1994;7(4):201
• Tracy JW, Webster LT Jr: In: Hardman JG, Limbird LE, eds. The Pharmacological Basis of Therapeutics. 9th Ed. New York, Mcgraw-Hill, 1996:987-1008
Illustrations: N/A
Internet references: http://www.5mcc.com

Author(s)
V. Vasudeviah, BSc, MBBS

Leprosy

BASICS

DESCRIPTION
A chronic granulomatous infection caused by Mycobacterium leprae, an organism which has a high predilection for cooler regions - skin, mucous membrane and peripheral nerves. The organism can be propagated in armadillos and in the foot pads of mice. The mouse model has been used for the study of anti-leprosy drugs and the armadillo model for immunologic and genetic studies. Leprosy is classified on a spectrum reflecting degrees of lost immunity (Ridley-Jopling classification)
• Indeterminate leprosy
Early cutaneous lesions; Findings are very subtle most commonly diagnosed in contacts of known leprosy cases. The lesions tend to heal spontaneously, but may progress to any of the other leprosy types.
• Tuberculoid leprosy (TT)
Characterized by early localized skin lesions and/or nerve lesions. Bacilli are few and difficult to find. Resistance to infection is high, and spontaneous recovery may occur; however peripheral nerves can be destroyed.
• Lepromatous leprosy (LL)
A generalized infection involving skin, oral, nasal, and upper respiratory mucous membrane, the anterior eye, cutaneous and peripheral nerve trunks, the RE system, adrenals, and testes. Numerous bacilli are easily found in tissue specimens. Patient's resistance to infection is low, and untreated disease is progressive
• Borderline (dimorphous) leprosy
This has features of both TT and LL poles in various combinations. Usually sub-divided into borderline tuberculoid (BT), mid-borderline (BB) and borderline lepromatous (BL). Borderline forms are unstable and may regress (reversal reaction) toward TT form or progress (Downgrading reaction) toward the LL form, depending on the effects of treatment and shifts in immune status
System(s) affected: Skin/Exocrine, Musculoskeletal, Nervous, Endocrine, Reproductive, Pulmonary, Hemic/Lymphatic/Immunologic
Genetics: Specific HLA-associated genes may be linked to different classes of disease, HLA-DR2 with TT and HLA-MT1 with LL
Incidence/Prevalence in USA: Extremely low; about 140 cases in 1992, mostly in immigrants from leprosy-endemic areas
Predominant age: Leprosy can present at any age, although cases in infants under 1 year are extremely rare
Predominant sex:
• Childhood: Male = Female
• Adults: Male > Female (2:1)

SIGNS AND SYMPTOMS
• Indeterminate leprosy
  ◊ One or more hypopigmented or hyperpigmented macules or plaques
  ◊ Anesthetic patches, though sensation is preserved in early stages
• TT
  ◊ Initial hypopigmented, hypesthetic macules with sharp demarcations
  ◊ Fully developed lesions are asymmetric and densely anesthetic with depressed atrophic central areas and elevated margins; loss of sweat glands and hair follicles near the lesion
  ◊ Nerve involvement occurs early
    - Ulnar, peroneal, and greater auricular nerves may be palpably and visibly enlarged
    - Neuritic pain
    - Muscle atrophy - small muscles of the hand
    - Facial nerve involvement leads to lagophthalmos, keratitis and corneal ulceration
  ◊ Hand and foot contracture
  ◊ Hand infection and plantar ulcers secondary to trauma
  ◊ Resorption and loss of phalanges may supervene
• LL
  ◊ Extensive cutaneous involvement, usually bilaterally symmetrical
  ◊ Highly variable cutaneous lesions macules, nodules, papules or plaques
  ◊ Sites of predilection are face, ears, wrists, elbows, buttocks and knees
  ◊ Loss of lateral eye brows
  ◊ Leonine facies
  ◊ Nasal stuffiness, epistaxis, septal perforation
  ◊ Nasal obstruction, laryngitis, hoarseness
  ◊ Saddle nose
  ◊ Keratitis, iridocyclitis
  ◊ Painless inguinal and axillary lymphadenopathy
  ◊ Testicular infiltrate and scarring - sterility
  ◊ Gynecomastia
• Borderline leprosy
Increasing variability in the appearance of skin lesions
  ◊ Papules and plaques may co-exist with macular lesions
  ◊ Anesthesia is less prominent than in TT
  ◊ Ear lobes slightly thickened, but eye brows and nasal region spared
  ◊ Skin lesions become even more numerous in BL type but without the symmetry typical of polar LL
  ◊ Skin lesions of BT generally resemble those of TT but are greater in number and have less well defined margins

CAUSES
Mycobacterium leprae: an acid fast rod is the causal agent. Incubation period is frequently 3-5 yrs although a range of 6 months to several decades has been seen

RISK FACTORS
• Close family contacts of untreated leprosy patients have 8 fold increased risk
• Compromised immunological status
• Poor socioeconomic status

DIAGNOSIS

DIFFERENTIAL DIAGNOSIS
• Lupus erythematosus
• Lupus vulgaris
• Sarcoidosis
• Yaws
• Dermal leishmaniasis
• Other skin conditions
• Peripheral neuropathy
• Syringomyelia

LABORATORY
• Demonstration of acid-fast bacilli in skin smears made by scraped-incision method is strong evidence of leprosy
• Skin biopsy specimen
• Histologic Involvement of peripheral nerves pathognomonic
• Mild anemia, elevated ESR and hyperglobulinemia
• Lepromin test: Usually positive in TT and negative in LL poles. It has no diagnostic value since it gives biological false positives in nearly all normal adults
• Sero-diagnostic assay: Based on the detection of antibody to phenolic glycolipid 1, this assay has a sensitivity of over 95% in LL and about 30% in TT
Drugs that may alter lab results: N/A
Disorders that may alter lab results: N/A

PATHOLOGICAL FINDINGS
• TT
Histologically, noncaseating granulomas containing lymphocytes, epithelioid cells, and perhaps giant cells; bacilli are difficult to demonstrate
• LL
Histologically, granulomas comprising macrophages, large foam (virchow or lepra) cells, and many intracellular bacilli, frequently in spheroidal masses
• Borderline leprosy
Histopathology of the granulomas changes from an epithelioid cell predominance in BT to a macrophage predominance as the lepromatous pole is approached

SPECIAL TESTS
Sero diagnostic assay

IMAGING N/A

DIAGNOSTIC PROCEDURES
• History and physical examination
• See details under Laboratory

TREATMENT

APPROPRIATE HEALTH CARE
Outpatient usually, except in reactional states where inpatient care is called for

GENERAL MEASURES
• Management involves a multi-disciplinary approach, including consultative services such as orthopedic surgery, ophthalmology and physical therapy in addition to specific drugs
• Plantar ulcers may be prevented by rigid soled foot wear or walking plaster casts
• Hand contractures can be prevented by physical therapy and casts
• Vocational retraining and rehabilitation along with psychological support should be instituted
• Immediate recognition of eye problems and prompt treatment are essential
• Mild reactional states such as reversal reaction and erythema nodosum leprosum (ENL) are best managed with bed rest, analgesics and sedatives. Severe reactions require treatment with corticosteroids, thalidomide or clofazimine. Specific therapy must be continued without any interruption.

SURGICAL MEASURES
Reconstructive surgery - nerve and tendon transplants, release of contractures and other cosmetic procedures can give more functional mobility and social acceptance

ACTIVITY
Dependent on severity of disease

DIET
Nutritious balanced diet

PATIENT EDUCATION
• Educate about the indolent course of the disease and importance of therapeutic course completion
• Information pamphlets and awareness to remove the psychological trauma and stigma associated with this malady
• Encourage case reporting

MEDICATIONS

DRUG(S) OF CHOICE
• Standard drug therapy for leprosy
◊ Dapsone 100 mg/day and rifampin 600 mg/day. Duration of treatment is prolonged and increases towards the LL pole.
◊ In patients with BB, BL and LL, clofazimine 50-100 mg/day and/or ethionamide 250-500 mg/day may be added
◊ The WHO recommends rifampin 600 mg per month for varying periods, but this is not approved in the U.S.
• Thalidomide is the most effective drug for ENL; initial dose is 200 mg bid tapering to 50-100 mg/day in chronic patients

The table displays the treatment duration given as minimum period beyond negativity except for rifampin.

```
Duration of treatment
Type/of
leprosy    D     R    C     E
-----------------------------------
Indeter-
minate TT 3y    6m   3y    -
BT        5y    6m   5y    -
BB        10y   2y   10y   10y
BL/LL     life  2y   life  life
-----------------------------------
D = Dapsone
R = Rifampin
C = Clofazimine
E = Ethionamide
y = years
m = months
Note: Dapsone-resistant cases,
 clofazimine 50-100 mg/day is
 used along with rifampin
```

Contraindications:
Clofazimine - pregnancy
Precautions:
• Hemolysis and methemoglobinemia are common untoward reactions to dapsone
• Patients should be screened for G6-PD deficiency to prevent drug-induced hemolysis
• Reactionary states should be anticipated during therapy, recognized early and treated aggressively
• Adverse effects to dapsone include GI upset, headaches, pruritus, agranulocytosis, fever and rash
• Clofazimine - GI upset and skin pigmentation, unacceptable to many light-skinned patients
Significant possible interactions: Refer to manufacturer's literature for each drug

ALTERNATIVE DRUGS N/A

FOLLOWUP

PATIENT MONITORING
• Frequent follow-up visits until therapy course is stabilized, then monthly supervision
• Periodic CBC, renal and hepatic function tests

PREVENTION/AVOIDANCE
• Early case finding and chemotherapy to suppress infectiousness and control spread
• Family and other close contacts need to be examined regularly for leprosy
• Vaccine trials with BCG have yielded conflicting results. At least four new experimental vaccines are currently in field trials in India and South America.

POSSIBLE COMPLICATIONS
• Crippling of the hand and foot
• Trauma and secondary infection leading to loss of digits and extremities
• Blindness
• Lucio phenomenon - arteritis
• Secondary amyloidosis
• Erythema nodosum leprosum (ENL)

EXPECTED COURSE/PROGNOSIS
The general course of leprosy is indolent, but may be interrupted by ENL and type I lepra reaction. Prognosis is good with early detection and prompt therapy.

MISCELLANEOUS

ASSOCIATED CONDITIONS
HIV-positive patients with early or subclinical leprosy are more likely to develop overt disease. Concurrent leprosy may accelerate HIV-disease course.

AGE-RELATED FACTORS
Pediatric: Rare in infants under one year
Geriatric: N/A
Others: N/A

PREGNANCY Clofazimine contraindicated during pregnancy; dapsone may be used

SYNONYMS
• Hansen's disease

ICD-9-CM
030.9 Leprosy

SEE ALSO N/A

OTHER NOTES Indeterminate, TT and perhaps BT are classified under paucibacillary leprosy whereas BB, BL or LL are classified under multibacillary leprosy. The National Hansen's Disease Center, Carville, LA 70721 (504-642-4722) can provide consultation for physicians if required. Thalidomide is available only from this center.

ABBREVIATIONS
TT = Tuberculoid type leprosy
LL = Lepromatous leprosy
BT = Borderline tuberculoid
BL = Borderline lepromatous
BB = Mid-borderline type
ENL = Erythema nodosum leprosum

REFERENCES
• Isselbacher KJ, et al, eds: Harrison's Principles of Internal Medicine. 13th Ed. New York, McGraw-Hill, 1994
• Berkow R, et al, eds: Merck Manual. 15th Ed. Rahway, NJ, Merck Sharp & Dohme, 1987
• Mandell GL, Petri WA Jr: In: Goodman, Gilman, eds. The Pharmacological Basis of Therapeutics. 9th Ed. New York, McGraw-Hill, 1996:1169-1172
Illustrations: N/A
Internet references: http://www.5mcc.com

Author(s)
V. Vasudeviah, BSc, MBBS

Leukemia

BASICS:

DESCRIPTION Proliferation and accumulation of abnormal immature blood cell progenitors (blasts) in the bone marrow and other tissues. The outstanding characteristic is the development of marrow failure. Intracerebral leukostasis may develop if the blood blast count becomes greatly elevated. Leukemia is classified according to the type of blast and according to the course, if untreated:
• Acute lymphoblastic leukemia (ALL)
• Acute nonlymphoblastic leukemia (ANLL)
• Chronic myelocytic leukemia (CML)
• Chronic lymphocytic leukemia (CLL)
System(s) affected:
Hemic/Lymphatic/Immunologic
Genetics: Unknown, some are familial
Incidence/Prevalence in USA: The yearly incidence is 13.2:100,000 in males and 7.7:100,000 in females
Predominant age:
• 70% occurs in adults, mostly CLL and ANLL. 30% in children, mostly ALL.
• With the current cure rate especially good for childhood ALL, it is estimated that by the year 2010, one in 1,000 young adults (15-45 years of age) in the USA will be a childhood ALL survivor
Predominant sex: Males > Females

SIGNS AND SYMPTOMS
• Mostly nonspecific and related to marrow failure or infiltration
• Fever
• Bleeding (e.g., petechiae, purpura, easy bruising, or oozing)
• Bone pain, pallor, fatigue
• Splenomegaly
• Hepatosplenomegaly
• Lymphadenopathy
• If CNS is involved, symptoms of increased intracranial pressure can be present
• Gingival swelling

CAUSES   Precise causes unknown

RISK FACTORS
• Genetic and chromosomal abnormalities (e.g., trisomy 21, breakage and translocation)
• Radiation exposure
• Immunodeficiency states
• Chemical and drug exposure (nitrogen mustard and benzene)
• Preleukemia
• Cigarette smoking

DIAGNOSIS

DIFFERENTIAL DIAGNOSIS
• Viral induced cytopenia, lymphadenopathy and organomegaly
• Immune cytopenias
• Drug induced cytopenias

• Other marrow failure and infiltrative diseases: aplastic, hypoblastic and refractory anemias; paroxysmal nocturnal hemoglobinuria; myelodysplastic syndromes, Gaucher's disease, etc.

LABORATORY
• CBC, differential, platelets show subnormal RBC, neutrophils, and possibly subnormal platelets
• In some types, no circulating leukemic blasts are necessary to be present to establish the diagnosis. If 2 of the 3 above parameters are affected, or only one profoundly decreased, bone marrow failure should be ruled out.
• Reticulocyte count < 0.5
• Sedimentation rate usually elevated
• Chemistries LDH, and uric acid can be elevated
• Immunoglobulins IgG can be low or rarely elevated
• Coagulation profile can be normal or prolonged especially in promyelocytic leukemia (ANLL subtype)
Drugs that may alter lab results:
Chemotherapy agents, especially corticosteroids. Don't prescribe these before finalizing the bone marrow studies. Some leukemic blasts are very sensitive and can have massive cell kill from as little as one dose of corticosteroids.
Disorders that may alter lab results: N/A

PATHOLOGICAL FINDINGS
• The marrow will be hypercellular and the normal architecture effaced
• The percentage of leukemic cells compared to the remainder of the cell population is usually more than 30%
• Liver, spleen, and kidneys can be enlarged and infiltrated with leukemic cells

SPECIAL TESTS   Spinal tap may reveal fluid with leukemic cells

IMAGING
• Chest x-ray may reveal a large mediastinal mass
• Ultrasonography or CT scan of the abdomen may discover organomegaly

DIAGNOSTIC PROCEDURES
• Bone marrow studies are necessary to make the final diagnosis
• Aspirates are stained with a buffered Wright's stain and provide good resolution for cell morphology
• Biopsies are demineralized, sectioned and stained with hematoxylin-eosin (H&E) stain. They provide valuable information for cellularity, architecture, and megakaryocytic series.
• Marrow cell suspension used for:
  ◊ Cytochemistries (e.g., myeloperoxidase and Sudan black are positive in myeloblasts)
  ◊ Immunophenotyping especially useful for lymphoid leukemia and can indicate whether it is monoclonal or polyclonal, B lymphocytes or T lymphocytes, early or late, etc.
  ◊ Chromosome studies will show the ploidy and/or the presence of a translocation which is of prognostic value

◊ Immunofluorescent stain for terminal deoxyribonucleotidyl transferase (TdT), another marker that differentiates between myeloid and lymphoid blasts

TREATMENT

APPROPRIATE HEALTH CARE
• Consult with a chemotherapist
• Induction for acute leukemia treatment requires inpatient care

GENERAL MEASURES
• Assessment of liver, heart, and kidney functions and performance status
• In acute leukemia induction, establish good hydration and urine flow (especially in ALL patients)
• Give platelet transfusion if platelet count is < 20,000 or if patient is having bleeding symptoms
• Avoid aspirin products
• Give packed red cells transfusion if patient is symptomatic from the anemia (e.g., orthostatic hypotension, dizziness, fatigue, hyperactive precordium) or if a cerebral or a cardiopulmonary problem is present
• If the absolute neutrophil count (ANC) < 1000, exert close temperature monitoring. (ANC = WBC x (Percentage of Polys + Bands) ÷ 100). If patient becomes febrile (even low grade fever), appropriate cultures should be taken and patient placed on broad spectrum IV antibiotics covering pseudomonas and gram positive bacteria.
• Isolation (when the ANC is low) has no value because majority of the infecting agents in this situation are the patient's own normal flora of the skin, mouth, or gut
• In promyelocytic leukemia (ANLL subtype), patients are especially at risk for DIC when treatment is started. Heparinization is indicated with close followup of coagulation parameters.

SURGICAL MEASURES
• Bone marrow transplant
  ◊ Allogenic bone marrow transplantation in first remission for ANLL is advocated if a matched sibling is available. Autologous bone marrow transplant is also acceptable in first remission.
  ◊ Allogenic or autologous bone marrow transplant is acceptable in first remission in high risk ALL, especially in adults. They are acceptable in second remission for childhood ALL.
  ◊ Early studies using an allogenic non-related match donor seem to be promising and might replace the autologous route when a full sibling match is not available

ACTIVITY   Ambulatory as tolerated

DIET
• Special attention should be given to ensure adequately balanced calorie and vitamin intake
• Weight should be followed closely because patients usually have decreased appetite.

PATIENT EDUCATION
• Particularly regarding prognosis and treatment toxicity.
• Leukemia Society of America has pamphlets and coloring books for children. 33 Third Ave. New York, NY 10017, (212)573-8484
• NCI (Bethesda, Maryland) has pamphlets: "Chemotherapy and You," "Young People with Cancer" and about "ALL" and "ANLL." NCI has a telephone number for over-the-telephone education and recent updates of treatment options.
• "You and Leukemia, A Day At A Time" by Dr. Lynn S. Baker, W. B. Saunders Co., Philadelphia

MEDICATIONS

DRUG(S) OF CHOICE
Change frequently as result of research
• ALL
◊ Induction: vincristine plus prednisone plus asparaginase with or without doxorubicin or daunorubicin. CNS prophylaxis, intrathecal methotrexate with or without cranial irradiation.
◊ Maintenance: mercaptopurine (6-mercaptopurine) daily and methotrexate weekly for 2-3 years
• ANLL
◊ Induction: cytarabine plus daunorubicin or cytarabine plus idarubicin. Idarubicin seems to be superior to daunorubicin in the treatment of ANLL. Yeast derived granulocyte-macrophage colony stimulating factor (GM-CSF) and granulocyte colony stimulating factor(G-CSF) do not stimulate leukemia cell growth; but help in the resolution of marrow hypoplasia associated with chemotherapy.
◊ Maintenance: combined agents and high dose cytarabine
• Promyelocytic leukemia:
◊ All-trans-retinoic acid (ATRA) promotes maturation to normal granulocyte and provide remissions with lower toxicity
• CLL. An anti-CD33 monoclonal antibody has the potential for eradicating minimal residual disease in promyelocytic leukemia.
◊ Chlorambucil with or without prednisone used only if symptomatic or cytopenic. Fludarabine and cladribine (2-CDA), recently FDA approved, are showing great promise in refractory CLL. New agents such as somatostatin analog, cyclosporine, theophylline have significant activity in CLL.
• Hairy cell leukemia
◊ Interferon
• CML
◊ Chronic phase, allogenic bone marrow transplantation. If not possible, busulfan, hydroxyurea, or interferon alpha can prolong survival.
◊ Acute phase - daunorubicin plus cytarabine plus vincristine plus prednisone with or without thioguanine, or
• High dose cytarabine with or without daunorubicin

Contraindications:
No absolute contraindication is present due to the variety of protocol options
Precautions:
• Administration of chemotherapy agents should be by skilled and specifically trained individuals. IV vincristine, daunorubicin, and doxorubicin may lead to chemical burns in the event of extravasation.
• If liver injury is present, the toxicity of vincristine, anthracyclines and antimetabolites can be pronounced. If liver injury is advanced and hyperbilirubinemia is present, avoid those medications or reduce dosage.
• Anthracyclines can cause cardiomyopathy. Avoid them if patient has a pre-existing cardiac problem.
• Close monitoring of the WBC's, polys, RBC and platelets is required especially in CML (chronic phase or ALL maintenance in order not to induce profound myelotoxicity
• Patients will be immunosuppressed during treatment. Avoid live vaccines. Administer varicella-zoster, or measles immunoglobulin as soon as exposure of a patient at risk becomes known.
Significant possible interactions:
Allopurinol accentuates the toxicity of 6-mercaptopurine

ALTERNATIVE DRUGS N/A

FOLLOWUP

PATIENT MONITORING
• Repeat bone marrow studies every week or every other week during induction of acute leukemia. Less frequently later. Also perform if a relapse is suspected.
• Follow uric acid level and urinary function closely
• Physical evaluation, including weight and blood pressure, should be done with every treatment and as frequently as once a week

PREVENTION/AVOIDANCE No intense or contact sports and no aspirin due to low platelets and RBC

POSSIBLE COMPLICATIONS
• Side effects of chemotherapy
• Rarely in lymphoid leukemia, acute tumor lysis syndrome may develop leading to hyperuricemia, hyperkalemia, hyperphosphatemia, hypocalcemia, and/or uric acid nephropathy
• Late onset cardiomyopathy has been described in children treated with standard dose anthracyclines

EXPECTED COURSE/PROGNOSIS
• ALL remission rate is very good. In children, long term survival is the rule.
• AML remission rate is 60-80%, with only 20-40% long term survival
• CML invariably transforms into the acute phase within 2 years (median of 45 months). Afterward, survival rate is poor.

• CLL usually is asymptomatic for several years especially Rai, stages 0-II. In Rai's series the mean interval (in stages 0-II) is 5.3 years from diagnosis until therapy was needed. Median overall survival in CLL is thought to be 9 years.

MISCELLANEOUS

ASSOCIATED CONDITIONS No specific condition is associated with leukemia. Leukemia can be the first manifestation of chromosomal abnormalities or an immunodeficiency.

AGE-RELATED FACTORS
Pediatric: Tolerate intense treatments better
Geriatric:
• Do not tolerate allogenic bone marrow transplant. Cut off age for transplant is usually 50 years.
• Autologous transplant may be tried in patients above 50 years, provided no organ failure is present and performance status is good
Others: N/A

PREGNANCY Chemotherapy is a viable option in the 2nd and 3rd trimesters. Refer patient to an oncologist.

SYNONYMS N/A

ICD-9-CM
204.0 ALL
202.4 Hairy cell leukemia
205.0 ANLL, AML or AGL
206.0 AMoL
204.1 CLL
205.1 CML or chronic granulocytic leukemia

SEE ALSO
• Leukemia, acute lymphoblastic in adults (ALL)

OTHER NOTES

ABBREVIATIONS
• ALL = acute lymphoblastic leukemia
• ANLL = acute nonlymphoblastic leukemia
• CML = chronic myelocytic leukemia
• CLL = chronic lymphocytic leukemia

REFERENCES
• Devita VT Jr, Helman S, Rosenberg SA, eds: Cancer: Principles & Practice of Oncology. 3rd Ed. Philadelphia, J.B. Lippincott, 1989
• The Medical Letter on Drugs and Therapeutics: Drugs of Choice for Cancer Chemotherapy. Vol. (33) (issue 840), March 22, 1991
• Yearbook of Hematology, 1997. St. Louis, C.V. Mosby and Co, 1997
Illustrations: 4 available on CD-ROM
Internet references: http://www.5mcc.com

Author(s)
Mustafa Barudi, MD

Leukemia, acute lymphoblastic in adults (ALL)

 BASICS

DESCRIPTION A malignant proliferation and accumulation of immature lymphocytes
System(s) affected:
Hemic/Lymphatic/Immunologic
Genetics: Increased incidence in children with Down syndrome or in rare familial diseases such as ataxia-telangiectasia, Bloom's syndrome, Fanconi's anemia, Klinefelter's syndrome, and neurofibromatosis. Can rarely occur in adult identical twins.
Incidence/Prevalence in USA: 1000 adult cases/year
Predominant age: Median age is 35-40 years but incidence increases with age
Predominant sex: Male > Female (slightly)

SIGNS AND SYMPTOMS
• Anemia - fatigue, shortness of breath, lightheadedness, angina, headache
• Thrombocytopenia - petechiae, ecchymoses, epistaxis, retinal hemorrhages
• Granulocytopenia - fever, infection
• Lymphocytosis - lymphadenopathy, hepato/splenomegaly, bone pain
• Immunosuppression
• Metabolic abnormalities - hyperuricemia, renal failure, increased lactic acid dehydrogenase (LDH)
• Central nervous system - cranial nerve palsies, confusion

CAUSES Unknown. Epstein-Barr virus is implicated in Burkitt's leukemia/lymphoma.

RISK FACTORS
• Age over 60
• Incidence appears increased following exposure to chemical agents such as benzene or to radiation (but acute myeloid leukemia [AML] is more common)
• May follow aplastic anemia

 DIAGNOSIS

DIFFERENTIAL DIAGNOSIS
• Malignant disorders - other leukemias, especially AML; prolymphocytic leukemia; malignant lymphomas; multiple myeloma; bone marrow metastases from solid tumors (breast, prostate, lung, renal); myelodysplastic syndromes
• Nonmalignant disorders - aplastic anemia; myelofibrosis; autoimmune diseases (Felty's syndrome, lupus); infectious mononucleosis; autoimmune thrombocytopenic purpura; leukemoid reaction to infection

LABORATORY
• Anemia - normochromic, normocytic
• Thrombocytopenia
• Peripheral blood lymphoblasts
• Elevated LDH
• Elevated uric acid
Drugs that may alter lab results: N/A
Disorders that may alter lab results: N/A

PATHOLOGICAL FINDINGS Diffuse replacement of marrow and lymph node architecture by sheets of malignant lymphoblasts

SPECIAL TESTS
• Immunophenotyping of marrow/blood lymphoblasts: B-lineage (CD19, CD20, CD24): T-lineage (CD2, CD5, CD7); CALLA ([common ALL antigen], CD10); human leukocyte antigen (HLA)-DR; terminal deoxynucleotidyl transferase (TdT); aberrant myeloid antigens; stem cell antigen (CD34)
• Cytochemical stains: Myeloperoxidase negative; Sudan black B usually negative; TdT positive; nonspecific esterase +/-; periodic acid Schiff (PAS) +/-
• Cytogenetics: Specific recurring chromosomal abnormalities have independent diagnostic and prognostic significance (hyperdiploidy > 50 chromosomes is favorable; the Philadelphia chromosome, t[9;22], the t[4;11], and the t[8;14] are unfavorable)
• Human leukocyte antigen (HLA) typing of patient and siblings for marrow transplantation

IMAGING
• Chest radiograph to evaluate for mediastinal mass or hilar adenopathy and for pulmonary infiltrates suggestive of infection
• Ultrasound exam to assess splenomegaly or renal enlargement suggestive of leukemic infiltration

DIAGNOSTIC PROCEDURES
• Bone marrow examination with aspiration, biopsy, immunophenotyping, cytochemistry, and cytogenetics
• Lymph node biopsy is rarely necessary but can be diagnostic
• Lumbar puncture should be done if neurological symptoms or signs are present. Repeat lumbar puncture after bone marrow remission is achieved to evaluate occult CNS involvement.

 TREATMENT

APPROPRIATE HEALTH CARE
• Inpatient care during remission induction chemotherapy
• Post-remission therapy is usually outpatient
• Access to the resources and expertise of a major oncology center is important for appropriate support

GENERAL MEASURES Protective isolation from infection

SURGICAL MEASURES Surgical placement of a percutaneous silastic double-lumen central venous catheter

ACTIVITY Ambulatory as tolerated

DIET
• Nutritional support including intravenous hyperalimentation, if necessary
• Avoid alcohol

PATIENT EDUCATION
• Risks of infection, transfusion, chemotherapy
• Stop smoking

MEDICATIONS

DRUG(S) OF CHOICE
Optimal therapy is not yet known. All treatment regimens are still investigational, although clearly effective for some fraction of patients. CALGB protocol 8811 is an example of therapy (from Blood 1995; 85:2025-2037):
- Remission induction
  ◊ Cyclophosphamide 1200 mg/square meter on day 1 (800 mg/m2 if > 60 years old)
  ◊ Daunorubicin 45 mg/m2 on days 1, 2, and 3 (30 mg/m2 if > 60 years old)
  ◊ Vincristine 2 mg on days 1, 8, 15, and 22
  ◊ Asparaginase (L-asparaginase) 6000 units/m2 on days 5, 8, 11, 15, 18, and 22
  ◊ Prednisone 60 mg/m2 on days 1-21 (days 1-7 if > 60 years old)
- Consolidation (repeat twice in 8 weeks
  ◊ Cyclophosphamide 1000 mg/m2 on day 1
  ◊ Intrathecal (IT) methotrexate 15 mg with hydrocortisone 50 mg on day 1
  ◊ Mercaptopurine (6-mercaptopurine) 60 mg/m2 on days 1-14
  ◊ Cytarabine 75 mg/m2 SC on days 1-4 and 8-11
  ◊ Vincristine 2 mg on days 15 and 22
  ◊ Asparaginase 6000 units/m2 on days 15, 18, 22, and 25
- CNS prophylaxis and interim maintenance - 2400 cGy cranial irradiation
  ◊ IT-methotrexate 15 mg with hydrocortisone 50 mg on days 1, 8, 15, 22, and 29
  ◊ Mercaptopurine (6-mercaptopurine) 60 mg/m2 on days 1-70
  ◊ Oral methotrexate 20 mg/m2 on days 36, 43, 50, 57, and 64
- Late intensification
  ◊ Doxorubicin 30 mg/m2 on days 1, 8, and 15
  ◊ Vincristine 2 mg on days 1, 8, and 15
  ◊ Dexamethasone 10 mg/m2 on days 1-14
  ◊ Cyclophosphamide 1000 mg/m2 on day 29
  ◊ Thioguanine (6-thioguanine) 60 mg/m2 on days 29-42
  ◊ Cytarabine 75 mg/m2 SC on days 29-32 and 36-39
- Prolonged maintenance
  ◊ Vincristine 2 mg/month for 16 months
  ◊ Prednisone 60 mg/m2 for 5 days with the vincristine
  ◊ Mercaptopurine (6-mercaptopurine) 60 mg/m2/day for 16 months
  ◊ Oral methotrexate 20 mg/m2/week for 16 months

Contraindications: Doses and schedule may need to be altered for older patients and for concurrent infection and organ toxicity

Precautions:
- Tumor lysis syndrome (elevated uric acid, potassium, and phosphate with decreased calcium leading to renal failure, disseminated intravascular coagulation, and cardiac arrhythmias) may be prevented by administering allopurinol 300 mg/day. Begin 2 days before chemotherapy begins. Reduce doses if used with mercaptopurine or azathioprine. Give increased fluids.
- Oral sulfamethoxazole-trimethoprim or aerosolized pentamidine is given for pneumocystis carinii prophylaxis
- Profound immunosuppression. Take appropriate precautions when patient is neutropenic
- High dose cyclophosphamide causes severe nausea and vomiting. Use appropriate antiemetic regimen to prevent.
- Neurotoxicity, ileus with vincristine
- Asparaginase may cause severe allergic reactions as well as impaired pancreatic and liver function. Monitor serum glucose concentrations frequently and carefully. Pancreatitis or thrombosis may occur.
Significant possible interactions: N/A

ALTERNATIVE DRUGS
Other anthracyclines, investigational chemotherapy agents

FOLLOWUP

PATIENT MONITORING
Daily during induction chemotherapy for metabolic and infectious complications. Weekly during remission consolidation chemotherapy. Monthly during maintenance therapy. Every 3 months thereafter.

PREVENTION/AVOIDANCE N/A

POSSIBLE COMPLICATIONS
- Infections (pneumocystis carinii pneumonia, bacterial pneumonia or sepsis, fungal pneumonia)
- Bleeding
- Need for transfusions
- Sterility from treatment
- Arachnoiditis and CNS effects from intrathecal chemotherapy and irradiation
- Pancreatitis and liver dysfunction from chemotherapy
- Relapse of ALL in marrow or extramedullary sites (CNS, testis)

EXPECTED COURSE/PROGNOSIS
- 80-95% of patients < 60 years old will achieve a complete remission, and 35-60% will remain free of disease at 5 years
- Patients with unfavorable cytogenetic subtypes (especially t[9;22]) should probably undergo allogeneic bone marrow transplantation in first remission if an HLA-identical donor were available

MISCELLANEOUS

ASSOCIATED CONDITIONS N/A

AGE-RELATED FACTORS
Pediatric: Bone growth and IQ development may be affected by treatment
Geriatric: N/A
Others: N/A

PREGNANCY Many chemotherapy drugs are teratogenic

SYNONYMS Acute lymphocytic leukemia

ICD-9-CM 204.0 Lymphoid leukemia

SEE ALSO N/A

OTHER NOTES N/A

ABBREVIATIONS HLA = human leukocyte antigen

REFERENCES
- Hoffman R, Benz EJ Jr, Shattil S, et al, eds: Hematology: Basic Principles and Practice. New York, Churchill Livingstone, 1995
- Laport GF, Larson RA: Treatment of adult acute lymphoblastic leukemia. Semin in Oncology 1997;24:70-82
Illustrations: N/A
Internet references: http://www.5mcc.com

Author(s)
Richard A. Larson, MD

Leukoplakia, oral

BASICS

DESCRIPTION A nonspecific clinical term used to describe a white patch in the oral mucosa which remains despite attempts to rub it off. It does not correlate with any specific microscopic findings and may be related to a variety of lesions, from benign hyperkeratosis to carcinoma.
System(s) affected: Gastrointestinal
Genetics: N/A
Incidence/Prevalence in USA: N/A
Predominant age: 90% of lesions found in patients over 40 years of age
Predominant sex:
• Males > Female
• Some studies show no preference

SIGNS AND SYMPTOMS
• Location
  ◊ 50% on tongue, mandibular alveolar ridge, and buccal mucosa
  ◊ Also seen on maxillary alveolar ridge, palate and lower lip
  ◊ Infrequently - floor of the mouth and retromolar areas
• Appearance
  ◊ Varies from nonpalpable, faintly translucent white areas to thick, fissured, papillomatous, indurated lesions
  ◊ May feel rough or leathery
  ◊ Color may be white, gray, yellowish-white, or brownish-gray
  ◊ Cannot be wiped off
  ◊ Macular or plaque-like

CAUSES
• Tobacco use
• Alcohol consumption
• Oral sepsis
• Oral snuff (smokeless tobacco)
• Human papillomavirus, types 11 and 15
• Actinic radiation
• Vitamin deficiency
• Syphilis
• Dental restorations
• Prosthetic dental appliances
• Alcoholism
• Estrogen therapy

RISK FACTORS
• Age over 40
• Tobacco or alcohol use
• Repeated or chronic trauma to oral regions

DIAGNOSIS

DIFFERENTIAL DIAGNOSIS
• White oral lesions that can be wiped away:
  ◊ Candida
  ◊ Aspirin burn
• White oral lesions that cannot be rubbed off:
  ◊ Traumatic or frictional keratosis
  ◊ Leukoedema
  ◊ Galvanic keratosis
  ◊ Lichen planus
  ◊ Verrucous carcinoma
  ◊ Lupus
  ◊ Squamous cell carcinoma
  ◊ Oral hairy leukoplakia
  ◊ Leukokeratosis nicotina palati

LABORATORY N/A
Drugs that may alter lab results: N/A
Disorders that may alter lab results: N/A

PATHOLOGICAL FINDINGS
• Biopsy specimens range from hyperkeratosis to invasive carcinoma
• 6% at initial biopsy are invasive carcinoma
• 4% subsequently undergo malignant transformation
• Location is important: 60% on floor of mouth are cancerous; rarely so on buccal mucosa

SPECIAL TESTS N/A

IMAGING N/A

DIAGNOSTIC PROCEDURES Biopsy necessary to rule out carcinoma

TREATMENT

APPROPRIATE HEALTH CARE
Outpatient biopsy, only if lesion persists despite elimination of possible etiologic factors

GENERAL MEASURES
• Eliminate habitual lip biting
• Correct ill fitting dental appliances
• Stop smoking and alcohol
• If dysplasia evident, remove lesion. Consider otolaryngologist referral.
• Some small lesions may respond to cryosurgery
• Beta-carotene may cause partial regression (experimental)

SURGICAL MEASURES N/A

ACTIVITY Full

DIET Regular

PATIENT EDUCATION
• If biopsy negative, stress importance of periodic and careful followup
• Aid the patient in discontinuing tobacco and/or alcohol use. Referral to support groups, recommendations for stop smoking programs, etc.

MEDICATIONS

DRUG(S) OF CHOICE N/A
Contraindications: N/A
Precautions: N/A
Significant possible interactions: N/A

ALTERNATIVE DRUGS N/A

FOLLOWUP

PATIENT MONITORING Regular, close followup, even after successful treatment. Biopsy as needed.

PREVENTION/AVOIDANCE
• Avoid tobacco, alcohol, habitual biting
• Provide well-fitting dentures

POSSIBLE COMPLICATIONS
• Carcinoma
• New lesions may develop after treatment

EXPECTED COURSE/PROGNOSIS
• Curable if detected early
• 4% of initially benign lesions subsequently develop cancer
• More likely cancerous if on floor of mouth

MISCELLANEOUS

ASSOCIATED CONDITIONS
Leukokeratosis nicotina palati is rarely malignant

AGE-RELATED FACTORS
Pediatric: N/A
Geriatric: More common in elderly
Others: Rare before age 40

PREGNANCY N/A

SYNONYMS N/A

ICD-9-CM 528.6

SEE ALSO N/A

OTHER NOTES Uncommonly - other mucosal surfaces (vaginal, anal, etc.)

ABBREVIATIONS N/A

REFERENCES
• Yeats D, Burn J: Common Oral Mucosal Lesions in Adults. Amer Fam Phys 1991;44:2043-50
• Fitzpatrick T, et al: Color Atlas and Synopsis of Clinical Dermatology. 2nd Ed. New York, McGraw-Hill, 1992
Illustrations: 1 available on CD-ROM
Internet references: http://www.5mcc.com

Author(s)
Paul Johnson, MD
Mark E. Sexton, MD

Lichen planus

 BASICS

DESCRIPTION A unique inflammatory disorder of the skin and mucous membranes. The disease is characterized by small flat, angular, violaceous, shiny, pruritic papules on the skin and white papules in the mouth. Onset abrupt or gradual. May be intermittent for years.
Genetics: N/A
System(s) affected: Skin/Exocrine
Incidence/Prevalence in USA: 450/100,000
Predominant age: 30-60 years, rare in children and the elderly
Predominant sex: Female > Male

SIGNS AND SYMPTOMS
• Skin
◊ Pruritus - often severe
◊ Papules - 1-10 mm, shiny, flat
◊ Color - violaceous, with white lace-like pattern (Wickham's striae) on papules. Wickham's striae best seen after topical application of mineral oil and if present, are almost pathognomonic for lichen planus.
◊ Shape - polygonal or oval shaped
◊ Arrangement - may be grouped, linear, annular, or scattered individual lesions.
◊ Koebner's phenomenon is often seen
◊ Distribution - ventral surface of wrists and forearms, glans penis, dorsa feet, groin, sacrum, shins and scalp. Hypertrophic (verrucous) lesions may occur on lower legs. An annular pattern may appear on trunk and mucous membranes. Linear arrangements of papules have been described.
• Mucous membranes
◊ Mucous membrane involvement is seen in 40-60% of patients with skin lesions. 20% of patients have mucous membrane lesions only.
◊ Milky-white papules with white lace-like pattern
◊ Usually seen on buccal mucosa, but may appear on tongue, gingiva, palate, and lips
◊ May be bullous or erosive
◊ Painful, especially if ulcers present
◊ Oral lesions may be precancerous (squamous cell carcinoma)
• Hair and nails
◊ Scalp - atrophic scalp skin and destruction of hair follicles. May result in permanent and total alopecia.
◊ Nails - (10%) may cause proximal to distal linear grooves and partial or complete destruction of nail bed with pterygium formation. Large toes most commonly affected.

CAUSES Etiology unknown. Possibly a disease of keratinization or an autoimmune disease. Emotional stress may antedate an attack.

RISK FACTORS Exposure to drugs or chemicals, graft versus host disease, or lupus erythematosus (LE-LP overlap syndrome)

 DIAGNOSIS

DIFFERENTIAL DIAGNOSIS
• Chemical exposure (chemicals used in color developing)
• Drug eruption (chloroquine, quinacrine, gold salts, methyldopa, penicillamine, arsenic, bismuth, ACE inhibitors)
• Lichen nitidus
• Leukoplakia
• Psoriasis
• Candidiasis
• Squamous cell carcinoma; basal cell carcinoma
• Aphthous ulcers
• Herpetic stomatitis
• Secondary syphilis
• Scabies

LABORATORY N/A
Drugs that may alter lab results: N/A
Disorders that may alter lab results: N/A

PATHOLOGICAL FINDINGS Inflammation with hyperkeratosis, increased granular layer, irregular acanthosis, basement-membrane thinning with "sawtoothing," hyaline bodies below the epidermis, band-like lymphocytic infiltrate of the upper dermis

SPECIAL TESTS N/A

IMAGING N/A

DIAGNOSTIC PROCEDURES Skin biopsy

 TREATMENT

APPROPRIATE HEALTH CARE
Outpatient

GENERAL MEASURES
• Goal is to relieve itching with topical and systemic antibiotics
• Psoralens and ultraviolet A (PUVA) photochemotherapy may be helpful for generalized or resistant cases
• Behavior modification for stress reduction may prevent recurrence

SURGICAL MEASURES N/A

ACTIVITY Fully active

DIET No special diet

PATIENT EDUCATION Help with stress reduction if appropriate

Lichen planus

 MEDICATIONS

DRUG(S) OF CHOICE
• Skin
◊ Topical steroids (e.g., 0.1% triamcinolone acetonide) with occlusion
◊ Intralesional corticosteroids, e.g., triamcinolone (Kenalog) 5-10 mg/mL) for hypertrophic lesions
◊ Antihistamine (e.g., hydroxyzine, dosage - 25 mg q6h) if needed for itching
• Mucous membranes
◊ Topical oral retinoids, e.g., 0.05% tretinoin (retinoic acid) in Orabase or topical oral corticosteroids (0.1% triamcinolone (Kenalog in Orabase) bid
◊ Intralesional corticosteroids for erosive, painful lichen planus, e.g., 0.5-1.0 mL methylprednisolone (Depo-Medrol) 40 mg/mL)
◊ Oral retinoids - isotretinoin (Accutane) or etretinate (Tegison)
Contraindications: Patients with history of hypersensitivity to corticosteroids or retinoids
Precautions:
• Systemic absorption of steroids may result in hypothalamic-pituitary-adrenal axis suppression, Cushing's syndrome, hyperglycemia, and glucosuria
• Increased risk with high potency - i.e., use over large surface area, prolonged use, occlusive dressings
• These medications are Category C teratogens. Avoid in pregnancy.
• Children may absorb a proportionally larger amount of topical steroid due to larger skin surface to weight ratio
Significant possible interactions: See manufacturer's profile of each drug

ALTERNATIVE DRUGS
• Oral prednisone - rarely used and only for a short course (e.g., prednisone 20 mg bid x 2-4 weeks)
• Cyclosporine may be used in severe cases, but cost and potential toxicity limits its use. Topical use for severe oral involvement refractory to other treatments.

 FOLLOWUP

PATIENT MONITORING Serial skin exams

PREVENTION/AVOIDANCE Reduce stress

POSSIBLE COMPLICATIONS
• Alopecia
• Nail destruction
• Squamous cell carcinoma of the mouth

EXPECTED COURSE/PROGNOSIS
• Spontaneous resolution in weeks is possible, but disease may persist for years - especially in the mouth and on shins
• There is a tendency toward relapse, especially with emotional stress
• Recurrence 12-20% especially in those with generalized involvement

 MISCELLANEOUS

ASSOCIATED CONDITIONS
• Lichen nitidus
• Bullous pemphigoid
• Alopecia
• Myasthenia gravis
• Lupus erythematosus
• Biliary cirrhosis
• Vitiligo
• Ulcerative colitis
• Graft-versus-host reaction
• Morphea and lichen sclerosus et atrophicus

AGE-RELATED FACTORS
Pediatric: N/A
Geriatric: N/A
Others: N/A

PREGNANCY Avoid corticosteroids, retinoids

SYNONYMS N/A

ICD-9-CM 697.0 Lichen planus

SEE ALSO N/A

OTHER NOTES Remember the 5 p's of lichen planus - purple, planar, polygonal, pruritic papules

ABBREVIATIONS N/A

REFERENCES
• Habif T: Clinical Dermatology. 3rd Ed. St. Louis, CV Mosby, 1996
• Fitzpatrick TB, et al: Color Atlas and Synopsis of Clinical Dermatology. New York, McGraw-Hill, 1983
• Fitzpatrick TB, et al: Dermatology in General Medicine. 4th Ed. New York, McGraw-Hill, 1993
• Arnold HL Jr, Odom RB, James WD, eds: Andrews' Diseases of the Skin: Clinical pharmacology. 8th Ed. Philadelphia, W.B. Saunders Co., 1990
Illustrations: 9 available on CD-ROM
Internet references: http://www.5mcc.com

Author(s)
Marc Darr, MD

Listeriosis

BASICS

DESCRIPTION Infection caused by the ubiquitous, weakly hemolytic, gram positive bacillus, Listeria monocytogenes, which is pathogenic to many animal species. Occurs most often in fetuses (disseminated infantile listeriosis), in neonates, and in immunosuppressed patients. Majority of adult patients have pre-existing disease (cirrhosis, lymphomas, solid tumors, AIDS, cancer therapy). Usual course - acute.
• In 1985 there was an epidemic affecting 142 persons in Southern California that resulted from eating contaminated Mexican cheese
System(s) affected: Pulmonary, Endocrine/Metabolic, Gastrointestinal, Renal/Urologic, Hemic/Lymphatic/Immunologic, Nervous
Genetics: No known genetic pattern
Incidence/Prevalence in USA: 1,850 cases a year (425 deaths). Rising incidence (due to AIDS) now estimated at 7.6/million.
Predominant age: Neonates, elderly
Predominant sex: Male > Female

SIGNS AND SYMPTOMS
• Asymptomatic
• Abdominal pain
• Adult respiratory distress syndrome
• Cervical lymphadenopathy
• Chills
• Conjunctivitis
• Decreased fetal movement
• Diarrhea
• Dysuria
• Fatigue
• Fever
• Hepatosplenomegaly
• Malaise
• Myalgia
• Nausea
• Pharyngitis
• Urinary frequency
• Vomiting
• Findings suggestive of meningitis - fever, headache, nausea and vomiting, stiff neck, delirium, coma
• Findings suggestive of sepsis - high fever and generalized severe illness without evidence of localized infection (in patients with alcoholism, malignancies, immunosuppression, AIDS)

CAUSES Listeria monocytogenes, a small gram-positive bacillus; infection with other species of Listeria are rare.

RISK FACTORS
• Age - fetus, neonates, elderly
• Metastatic malignant disease
• HIV infection
• Alcoholism
• Renal hemodialysis
• Pregnancy
• Immunosuppressed
• Exposure to infected animals (veterinarians, butchers, etc.). Animal-to-human transmission is rare.
• Ingesting contaminated food or drink (e.g., soft Mexican style cheese or feta cheese)

DIAGNOSIS

DIFFERENTIAL DIAGNOSIS
• Other infections - Staphylococcal, gram negative Klebsiella, Candida, cryptococcosis, viral
• Infantile listeriosis, E. coli, Group B streptococci
• Infectious mononucleosis

LABORATORY
• CSF
  ◊ Gram stain - may reveal small, gram-positive rods or coccobacillary forms with "tumbling" motility. (Sometimes difficult to identify since organisms are not present in large numbers and may be confused with diphtheroids and other bacteria.)
  ◊ Cell count - in most cases, the predominant cell type is the neutrophil; however, mononuclear cells may predominate. Counts range from 0-1200/mm3. RBC's frequently seen.
  ◊ Protein concentration - within normal limits to 735 mg/dL
  ◊ Glucose - within normal limits to undetectable
  ◊ CSF cultures - demonstrates beta-hemolysis (L. monocytogenes grows well on 5% sheep's blood or chocolate agar)
  ◊ Counterimmunoelectrophor (CIE) latex agglutination (LA) - possibly useful for differential diagnosis
• Other tests
  ◊ Blood cultures should be done
  ◊ CBC - peripheral WBC may show an elevated neutrophil count and/or left shift
  ◊ Other cultures in newborn - cervical vaginal secretions and lochia from the mother; cord blood; grossly abnormal portions of the placenta, meconium, and exudate expressed from an incised skin papule of the neonate
Drugs that may alter lab results: Antibiotics
Disorders that may alter lab results: Cultures may be confusing in patients with mixed infections

PATHOLOGICAL FINDINGS
• Gross - multi-organ miliary granulomatosis
• Micro - nodular focal abscess
• Micro - necrotic amorphous basophilic debris
• Micro - increased tissue macrophages
• Micro - gram-positive bacilli
• Motile bacilli
• Chinese-letter aggregates

SPECIAL TESTS Specimens for serologic testing should be submitted to the local public health laboratory. In outbreaks, serotyping may be desirable.

IMAGING MRI with any patient having central nervous system symptoms

DIAGNOSTIC PROCEDURES Lumbar puncture

TREATMENT

APPROPRIATE HEALTH CARE Inpatient during acute phase

GENERAL MEASURES
• Bedrest
• Isolation if immunosuppressed
• Secretion precautions
• Respiratory assistance (if apneic, or CNS depressed)

SURGICAL MEASURES N/A

ACTIVITY Bedrest

DIET
• Acute case, total parenteral nutrition, nasogastric tube, or softer diet if tolerated
• As a preventive, avoid eating raw or partially cooked foods and soft cheeses. Warm leftovers thoroughly and wash raw vegetables before cooking.

PATIENT EDUCATION Dietary guidelines for avoidance in high risk patients

Listeriosis

MEDICATIONS

DRUG(S) OF CHOICE
• Neonates:
◊ Meningitis - for infants older than one month: ampicillin 300-400 mg/kg/day IV
◊ Meningitis - neonate doses: < 2000 grams, less than 1 week old: ampicillin 50 mg/kg q12h. Older than 1 week: ampicillin 50 mg/kg every 8 hours. Plus gentamicin 7.5 mg/kg/day IV for 14 days. Discontinue gentamicin when cerebro-spinal fluid is sterile.
◊ Alternate therapy for neonates - penicillin G 100,000-200,000 units/kg/d IV x 14-21 days plus gentamicin as above
   - Bacteremia or pneumonia - ampicillin 100-150 mg/kg/day IV x 10 days (or penicillin G 200,000 units/kg/d IV x 10 days) plus gentamicin 5.0 mg/kg/day. Discontinue gentamicin when blood cultures become negative.
• Pregnant women:
◊ Ampicillin 2 gm IV q4h for 14 days plus gentamicin 120 mg IV q8h. Adjust for peak 5-6 mcg/mL.
• Immunocompromised/elderly patients:
◊ Ampicillin 200 mg/kg IV x 14 days. Note: Some experts recommend addition of gentamicin 3-5 mg/kg/d IV plus intrathecal doses of 4 mg q12h.
• For endocarditis and typhoidal listeriosis:
◊ Penicillin G 75,000-100,000 units/kg IV q4h and continue for 14 days after defervescence. plus tobramycin 2 mg/kg load, then adjust based on levels. Aim for peak at 5-6. Continue for 4 weeks after defervescence.
• For oculoglandular:
◊ Erythromycin 30 mg/kg/day as 4 equal doses q6h and continue for 1 week after defervescence
Contraindications: Allergy to penicillins
Precautions: Cephalosporins are not adequate treatment. Refer to manufacturer's literature.
Significant possible interactions: Refer to manufacturer's literature

ALTERNATIVE DRUGS
• In adult patients - trimethoprim-sulfamethoxazole. Base dose on trimethoprim component, 5 mg/kg IV q6h or erythromycin 10 mg/kg IV q6h, may not yield optimal results.
• Clarithromycin
• Ciprofloxacin

FOLLOWUP

PATIENT MONITORING
• Frequent arterial blood gases during acute phase
• Repeat lumbar puncture at 24-48 hours and at the end of treatment

PREVENTION/AVOIDANCE
• Avoid handling livestock during pregnancy
• Avoid contaminated silage
• Avoid contaminated sewage
• Avoid raw or contaminated milk products
• Avoid soft cheeses (Mexican and feta)
• Wash carefully all raw vegetables

EXPECTED COURSE/PROGNOSIS High mortality if symptomatic

POSSIBLE COMPLICATIONS
• Premature delivery
• Amnionitis
• Meningitis
• Septicemia
• Pulmonary abscess
• Hepatic abscess
• Placental abscess
• Splenic abscess
• Lymph node abscess
• Endocarditis
• Peritonitis
• Abortion
• Stillbirth
• Neonatal death

MISCELLANEOUS

ASSOCIATED CONDITIONS
• Cirrhosis
• Lymphomas
• Solid tumors
• Immunodeficiencies
• Pregnancy

AGE-RELATED FACTORS
Pediatric:
• Infected fetuses are usually stillborn or premature. More than half are infected with lethal listeriosis.
• 50% mortality in treated neonates
Geriatric: Greater morbidity and mortality
Others: N/A

PREGNANCY
• Pregnant women are more susceptible to infection with Listeria monocytogenes; transmission to the fetus and neonates occurs with high mortality.
• Requires prompt and vigorous treatment to prevent transfer of disease to fetus (pregnant patient's symptoms may begin as a flu-like illness or be absent)

SYNONYMS
• Listeria monocytogenes
• Listerial disease

ICD-9-CM 027.0 Listeriosis

SEE ALSO N/A

OTHER NOTES
• Notify laboratory at time of sending any specimen that listeriosis is a possibility
• Laboratory specimens must be sent to laboratory promptly (few organisms more difficult to culture)
• Need at least 10 cc of spinal fluid for culture

ABBREVIATIONS N/A

REFERENCES
• Linnan MJ, Mascola L, Lou X, May S, Salimen C, et al: Epidemic listeriosis associated with Mexican-style cheese. N Engl J Med 1988;319, 823:828
• Von Lichtenberg F: Pathology of Infectious Diseases. New York, Raven Press, 1988
• Haft RF, Kasper D: Group B Streptococcus Infection in Mother and Child. Hospital Practice 1991;26
• Foodborne and Diarrhea Diseases Branch, CDC Personal Communication, 1997
Illustrations: N/A
Internet references: http://www.5mcc.com

Author(s)
Susana May, MD, MPH

Low back pain

BASICS

DESCRIPTION
Mechanical low back pain is a diagnosis of exclusion. It is generally a self-limiting condition of the aging spine, responsive to conservative measures including rest and pain management. Patients typically present with pain at the posterior belt line with occasional referred pain to the buttocks and/or posterior thighs. These injuries often are the result of the mechanical stresses and functional demands placed on the low back area by everyday activities. The condition, for the vast majority of patients, is of short duration and complete recovery is the general rule. The primary goal of the clinician is to rule-out other more serious etiologies. It must be remembered that low back pain is a symptom, not a disease, and that the pathological basis of the pain frequently lies outside the spine.
System(s) affected: Musculoskeletal, Nervous
Genetics: N/A
Incidence/Prevalence in USA:
• 80% of Americans experience mechanical low back pain sometime in their lifetime
• One of the most common complaints for primary care visits
• Repetitive episodes are common
Predominant age: 25-45 years
Predominant sex: Male = Female

SIGNS AND SYMPTOMS
• History
  ◊ Onset of low back pain begins either suddenly after an injury or gradually over the next 24 hours
  ◊ Variable pain at posterior belt-line, typically bilateral
  ◊ Occasional radiation of pain to buttocks, and/or posterior thighs stopping at knees
  ◊ Pain pattern referred rather than radicular
  ◊ Back pain worse than leg pain
  ◊ Pain aggravated by back motion, sitting, standing, lifting, bending and twisting
  ◊ Pain relieved by rest (recumbency)
  ◊ Bowel and bladder function preserved
• Physical findings
  ◊ Normal motor, sensory, and reflex examinations
  ◊ Decreased lumbar range of motion, tenderness to palpation, paraspinous musculature spasm common
  ◊ Nerve root stretch tests are commonly negative
  ◊ Straight leg raise and other tests causing spinal motion may increase low back pain, but not leg pain

CAUSES
Normal aging process of musculoskeletal system aggravates an acute event

RISK FACTORS
• Age
• Activity
• Smoking
• Obesity
• Vibration, e.g., driving motor vehicles
• Sedentary lifestyle
• Psychosocial factors

DIAGNOSIS

DIFFERENTIAL DIAGNOSIS
• Structural
  ◊ Acute lumbar back pain
  ◊ Chronic lumbar back pain
  ◊ Low back strain/sprain
  ◊ Herniated lumbar intervertebral disc
  ◊ Degenerative disc disease
  ◊ Degenerative segmental instability
  ◊ Spinal stenosis
  ◊ Spondylolisthesis
  ◊ Fractures
• Inflammatory
  ◊ Ankylosing spondylitis and related inflammatory spondylopathies
  ◊ Infection: vertebral osteomyelitis, discitis
  ◊ Rheumatoid arthritis
• Neoplastic
  ◊ Primary tumors
  ◊ Metastases
• Referred pain
  ◊ Orthopaedic - osteoarthritis of hip
  ◊ Sacroiliac joint disease
  ◊ Gastrointestinal - duodenal ulcer, chronic pancreatitis, irritable bowel syndrome, diverticulitis
  ◊ Genitourinary - pyelonephritis, nephrolithiasis, prostatism
  ◊ Gynecological - pregnancy, endometriosis, ovarian cystic disease, pelvic inflammatory disease
  ◊ Cardiovascular - abdominal aortic aneurysm, vascular claudication

LABORATORY
• Generally negative and not typically indicated with initial presentation
• Indications
  ◊ Age > 50 years
  ◊ Nonmechanical nature of pain
  ◊ Atypical pain pattern or distribution
  ◊ Persistent symptomatology remittent to conservative treatment measures
• Screening laboratory studies
  ◊ CBC with differential
  ◊ Sedimentation rate
  ◊ Alkaline and acid phosphatase
  ◊ Serum calcium
  ◊ Serum protein electrophoresis
Drugs that may alter lab results: N/A
Disorders that may alter lab results: N/A

PATHOLOGICAL FINDINGS   N/A

SPECIAL TESTS   System directed investigation

IMAGING
• Plain radiographs
  ◊ Not indicated to initiate conservative management program
  ◊ Indicated for persistent symptoms > 1 week, patient age > 50 years, or suggestive history
  ◊ Radiographs utilized to rule-out tumor or identify other disease process
  ◊ Anteroposterior, lateral, spot lateral of L5-S1 and oblique x-rays are included in routine lumbo-sacral series
• Bone scan (scintigraphy)
  ◊ Technetium-99m labeled phosphorus indicates active mineralization of bone
  ◊ Rule-out tumor, trauma or infection

DIAGNOSTIC PROCEDURES   MRI, CT/myelography only indicated with persistent symptoms, sciatica or the development of neurologic abnormalities

TREATMENT

APPROPRIATE HEALTH CARE
Outpatient for majority

GENERAL MEASURES
• Initial short-term bedrest 2-3 days
• Short-term analgesics
• NSAID's 10 day course initially, then prn
• Muscle relaxants 10 day course
• Physical therapy
• Manipulation

SURGICAL MEASURES   N/A

ACTIVITY
• Restricted activities for 3-6 weeks
• Resume activities of daily living as tolerated

DIET   Weight reduction - if appropriate

PATIENT EDUCATION
• Home based exercise program
• Posture and body mechanics training
• "Back school" for chronic mechanical low back pain

MEDICATIONS

DRUG(S) OF CHOICE Nonsteroidal anti-inflammatory drugs - Ibuprofen, naproxen, salsalate. Less expensive, equally efficacious.
Contraindications: Refer to manufacturer's product information
Precautions:
• History of ulcer disease
• Elderly patients
• Renal disease
• Cardiac disease
Significant possible interactions: Refer to manufacturer's product information

ALTERNATIVE DRUGS N/A

FOLLOWUP

PATIENT MONITORING Estimated duration of care 1-6 weeks

PREVENTION/AVOIDANCE
• Smoking cessation
• Weight reduction
• General physical condition
• Avoid aggravating tasks, e.g., heavy lifting, bending, twisting, sudden unexpected movements or combination of above

POSSIBLE COMPLICATIONS
• Incorrect diagnosis
• Chronic low back pain
• Narcotic addiction
• Persistent psychosocial impairment

EXPECTED COURSE/PROGNOSIS
• Resumption of normal activity without residual symptoms in most cases
• May be hindered by secondary gain issues

MISCELLANEOUS

ASSOCIATED CONDITIONS
• Deconditioning
• Obesity
• Psychosocial disease

AGE-RELATED FACTORS
Pediatric: Thorough work-up imperative
Geriatric: Tumors, degenerative conditions, fractures and stenosis more common
Others: N/A

PREGNANCY Commonly associated with low back pain and/or sciatica. Treatment is conservative.

SYNONYMS
• Low back syndrome
• Lumbar strain/sprain
• Lumbago

ICD-9-CM
722 Intervertebral disc disorders
724.2 Lumbago
724.5 Backache, unspecified

SEE ALSO Lumbar (intervertebral) disk disorders

OTHER NOTES
• Adverse psychosocial factors to resolving back pain:
◊ Pending litigation or compensation
◊ Depressed or hostile patient
◊ Prolonged use of narcotics or alcohol

ABBREVIATIONS N/A

REFERENCES
• American Academy of Orthopedic Surgeons: Clinical Policy; Low back musculoligamentous injury (sprain/strain). AAOS Bulletin 3638, April, 1991
• Macnab I, McCulloch J: Backache. 2nd Ed. Baltimore, Williams & Wilkins, 1986
Illustrations: N/A
Internet references: http://www.5mcc.com

Author(s)
Michael J. Smith, MD
Robert A. Cheney, MD

Lumbar (intervertebral) disk disorders

BASICS

DESCRIPTION Many patients with low back pain have lumbar disc disease and involvement of surrounding spinal ligaments, muscles and skeleton. Over time may progress to disc degeneration, disc herniation, spinal narrowing and arthritic proliferation of the facet joint. Management is based on symptoms and disability, because the distinction between the normal aging of the spine and pathological findings are hard to distinguish.
• Non-radicular low back pain (acute and chronic) - low back pain remaining near belt-line caused by soft tissue or disc injury
• Radicular low back pain (acute and chronic) - neuropathic pain is to a greater degree in the buttocks, hips or legs rather than the back. There may or may not be signs of weakness, numbness, or loss of reflex. In younger patients, the source of the pain is likely to be mechanical compression or chemical irritation of a nerve root.
• Spinal stenosis is more likely to be the etiology of radicular pain in patients over 55 years
System(s) affected: Musculoskeletal, Nervous
Genetics: N/A
Incidence/Prevalence in USA:
• One of the most frequent complaints for which adults seek medical attention and second to the common cold for most time off work
• Lifetime prevalence of low back pain is 60-90%. The annual incidence is 5%. Among patients with acute back pain, 1% have nerve root symptoms.
• 95% of diseased disks are localized to L4-5 and L5-S1
• Less than 2% of patients with low back pain have infections, neoplasms, or inflammatory spondyloarthropathies
Predominant age: 25-45 years, first episode in 20's and 30's, infrequent before 20 years or after age 65
Predominant sex: Male = Female

SIGNS AND SYMPTOMS
• Variable pain; usually dull, originating in back, extending below knee
• Pain may or may not be followed by radiation (usually unilaterally) in nerve root distribution
• Back pain decreases at night. Bedrest usually improves symptoms at least temporarily.
• Pain increases with walking
• Constitutional symptoms absent
• Sciatica can occur without back pain
• Often sensory aberrations in extremities, paresthesia and numbness
• Occasionally muscle group weakness
• Most disc ruptures are postero-lateral and press upon lumbar nerve root with radiating pain
• Lumbar scoliosis possible, trunk tilted toward or away from affected side, depending on location of extrusion
• Paraspinal muscle spasm

CAUSES
• Trauma, major or minor
• Frequent lifting of objects weighing 25 pounds (11.3 kg) or more, especially if lifted with arms extended and knees straight, and body twisted
• Vibration; e.g., driving motor vehicles

RISK FACTORS
• Normal aging process after age 20 years
• Cigarette smoking
• Narrow lumbar vertebral canal (for prolapsed disk)
• Stress, muscle tension
• Obesity
• Osteoporosis

DIAGNOSIS

DIFFERENTIAL DIAGNOSIS Acute lumbosacral strain, chronic lumbosacral strain, spondylosis, spondylolisthesis, spinal arthritis, fibrositis, cauda equina syndrome, compression fracture, poor posture, bursitis, metastatic and primary tumors, vertebral infection, referred pain from hip, retroperitoneum, aneurysms, or pelvis, (geriatrics) neurogenic claudication

LABORATORY ESR - usually normal
Drugs that may alter lab results: N/A
Disorders that may alter lab results: N/A

PATHOLOGICAL FINDINGS Difficult to distinguish normal aging process of disc degeneration from specific lesions causing low back pain and sciatica

SPECIAL TESTS Electromyography - useful to exclude peripheral neuritis

IMAGING
• Lumbosacral plain films - rarely indicated just to initiate a conservative management program - indicated to rule out tumor or structural abnormality although presence of latter may not confirm source of pain
• Lumbosacral oblique views - controversial
• Myelography, CT scan, magnetic resonance - similar diagnostic accuracy for particular surgical candidate evaluation

DIAGNOSTIC PROCEDURES
• Sciatic stretch test - in supine position, elevation of affected leg (to 15-30% for severe, 30-60%, milder) elicits pain
• Laségue's sign - patient is supine, hip flexed, dorsiflexion of ankle accentuates sciatic pain or muscle spasm in posterior thigh
• Cross straight-leg-raising - elevating normal leg produces sciatica down other leg
• Doorbell sign - (insensitive) deep palpation of the spinous process over protruded disc reproduces sciatica
• Femoral stretch (for L2-3) in prone position, affected leg is extended reproducing pain along femoral nerve

• Faber's test - (positive only for hip pain) in supine position, flexion, abduction and external rotation produces pain
• Neurologic defects of lower extremities and perineum will usually locate level of lesion. Test gait, reflexes, motor strength, muscle atrophy; pulses and abdominal bruits; rectal sphincter.

TREATMENT

APPROPRIATE HEALTH CARE
Outpatient for majority. Inpatient for severe disability and/or surgery.

GENERAL MEASURES
• Initial: ordinary activities as tolerated, local heat, pelvic traction, sedation, physical therapy (90% response)
• Following bedrest: up and about with midline support. Wean from support over next several weeks.
• For chronic non-radicular pain: improve physical fitness with low impact aerobic exercise. Manipulation and physical therapy have shown benefit.
• Transcutaneous electrical nerve stimulation (TENS): very short term benefit

SURGICAL MEASURES
• Procedures available
  ◊ Standard discectomy - discectomy techniques all have comparable results
  ◊ Microsurgical discectomy
  ◊ Percutaneous discectomy - relatively new, contraindicated in spinal stenosis and sequestered disc fragments
  ◊ Chemonucleolysis - lower rate of benefit and occasional severe complications
  ◊ Spinal fusion (arthrodesis) - indicated for spinal instability
• Absolute indications for discectomy
  ◊ Cauda equina syndrome
  ◊ Progressive neurological deficit despite conservative treatment
• Relative indications for discectomy
  ◊ Intolerable pain
  ◊ Multiple episodes of radiculopathy
  ◊ Severe postural tilt
  ◊ Persistent dysfunctional pain - these patients have been reported to improve more rapidly postoperatively but long term results show no difference from nonoperative treatment
  ◊ Static neurological deficit - no reported difference between operative or nonoperative treatment for improvement in weakness or sensory disturbance

ACTIVITY
• After pain is controlled (7-10 days), begin progressive walking program. Short walks initially 4 times a day and lengthen as tolerated.
• Return to work as soon as possible with avoidance of high risk activities, e.g., heavy lifting, vibration, smoking

DIET
Weight reduction if appropriate

PATIENT EDUCATION
Good posture, proper body mechanics, physical fitness, physical therapy if appropriate

MEDICATIONS

DRUG(S) OF CHOICE
• Analgesics
• Nonsteroidal anti-inflammatory medication
• Muscle relaxants (controversial)
• Mild sedatives
Contraindications: Refer to manufacturer's profile of each drug
Precautions: Elderly, hypertension, prior peptic ulcer disease or bleeding, renal disease, liver disease, cardiac dysfunction
Significant possible interactions: Refer to manufacturer's profile of each drug

ALTERNATIVE DRUGS
N/A

FOLLOWUP

PATIENT MONITORING
Outpatient - return visit about 10 days following initial visit, should be improved. Follow pain history and neurological status. Thereafter monitor every 2 weeks until fully functional. Monitor exercise program.

PREVENTION/AVOIDANCE
• Modification of jobs to reduce exposure to known risk factors
• Selection of workers by such means as strength testing for certain jobs
• Avoid smoking

POSSIBLE COMPLICATIONS
• Foot drop with weakness of anterior tibial, posterior tibial and peroneal muscles
• Loss of ankle jerk
• Bladder and rectal sphincter weakness with retention or incontinence
• Limitation of movement and restricted activity
• Narcotic addiction

EXPECTED COURSE/PROGNOSIS
• Acute low back pain (90%) and/or radiculopathy (60-80%) can be expected to recover spontaneously with conservative therapy
• Chronic nonradicular low back pain - most patients respond to conservative management such as manipulation, fitness, weight reduction, and education regarding back care
• Chronic radicular pain - good selection of surgical candidates have found satisfactory results (80% in long-term studies)

MISCELLANEOUS

ASSOCIATED CONDITIONS
• Poor physical conditioning/posture
• Obesity
• Osteoarthritis
• Osteoporosis
• Depression, other psychiatric disorders

AGE-RELATED FACTORS
Pediatric: Scoliosis, onset age 10 years, rarely symptomatic until adulthood. Detect difference in leg length.
Geriatric: Usually multifactorial lesions of spine. Degenerative spondylolisthesis (especially in women), spinal stenosis, and neurogenic claudication are more likely.
Others: N/A

PREGNANCY
Commonly associated with low back pain and/or sciatica. Treatment is conservative.

SYNONYMS
• Degenerative disk disease
• Intervertebral disk dislocation

ICD-9-CM
722 Intervertebral disc disorders

SEE ALSO
• Low back pain

OTHER NOTES
• Features which predict best surgical outcome (90-95% improvement when all three exist)
  ◊ Definable neurological deficit
  ◊ Pathology in imaging which correlates with deficit
  ◊ Positive nerve root tension signs
• Adverse psychosocial factors to resolving back pain
  ◊ Sciatica with predominant back symptoms
  ◊ Pending litigation or compensation
  ◊ Depressed or hostile patient
  ◊ Low IQ or poorly educated may not be able to participate in assessment or decision
  ◊ Prolonged use of narcotics or alcohol

ABBREVIATIONS
N/A

REFERENCES
• Katz WA, ed: Diagnosis and Management of Rheumatic Diseases. 2nd ed. Philadelphia, Lippincott Co, 1988
• Eismont FJ, Currier B: Surgical Management of Lumbar Intervertebral-Disc Disease. J Bone & Joint Surg 1989:1266-1271
• Kent OL, Haynor DR, Longstreth WT, Larson EB: The clinical efficacy of magnetic resonance imaging in neuroimaging. Ann Int Med 1994:120;856-871
• Frost H, Moffett JAK, Moser JS, Fairbank JCT: Randomized controlled trial for evaluation of fitness programme for patients with chronic low back pain. Brit Med Jour 1995;310:151-159
• Malmivaara A, Hakkinen U, Aro T, Heinrichs MJ, et al: The Treatment of Acute Low Back pain - bed rest, exercises, or ordinary activity?. NEJM 1995:332; 351-355
Illustrations: N/A
Internet references: http://www.5mcc.com

Author(s)
Claudia A. Peters, MD

Lung abscess

BASICS

DESCRIPTION A localized cavity in the lung with pus resulting from necrosis of lung tissue surrounded by lung infection. May be caused by aerobic or anaerobic infection. Usual course is acute; progressive.
System(s) affected: Pulmonary
Genetics: No known genetic pattern
Incidence/Prevalence in USA: Unknown, relatively rare
Predominant age: Mainly 4th-6th decades
Predominant sex: Male > Female (4:1)

SIGNS AND SYMPTOMS
• Cough
• Sputum (purulent, foul-smelling)
• Fever
• Chest pain
• Dyspnea
• Chills, rigors
• Fatigue
• Malaise
• Weakness
• Weight loss
• Anorexia
• Night sweats
• Hemoptysis
• Decreased breath sounds
• Rales
• Wheezing
• Tachypnea
• Tachycardia
• Diaphoresis
• Dullness to percussion
• Consolidation by auscultation
• Cavernous breath sounds
• Asymmetric chest movement
• Clubbing

CAUSES
• Lung infection
• Aspiration pneumonia
• Necrotizing pneumonia
• Cavitary infarction
• Septic embolism
• Bacteremia
• Bronchial stenosis or obstruction
• Tumors
• Dental abscess in loose tooth

RISK FACTORS
• Periodontal disease
• Alcoholism
• Drug abuse
• Epilepsy
• Unconsciousness
• Lung neoplasia
• Immunosuppression/immunocompromised
• Diabetes mellitus
• Airway foreign body
• Gastroesophageal reflux with aspiration
• Sinusitis
• Gastric and esophageal surgery
• Dental and oropharyngeal surgery
• Cystic fibrosis

DIAGNOSIS

DIFFERENTIAL DIAGNOSIS
• Bronchogenic carcinoma
• Bronchiectasis
• Empyema with bronchopulmonary fistula
• Tuberculosis
• Mycotic lung infections
• Actinomycosis
• Nocardiosis
• Infected pulmonary bulla
• Wegener's granulomatosis
• Pulmonary sequestration
• Silicotic nodule
• Subphrenic or hepatic abscess with perforation into a bronchus
• Bronchogenic or parenchymal cyst (congenital)

LABORATORY
• Leukocytosis
• Anemia
• Hypoalbuminemia
• Sputum smear - mixed bacteria and neutrophils
• Sputum culture - mixed flora, anaerobes
• Gram-negative rods and cocci
• Transtracheal aspirate culture - anaerobes
• Pleural fluid - neutrophilia
• Bacteriology:
  ◊ Staphylococcus
  ◊ Klebsiella spp.
  ◊ Pseudomonas aeruginosa
  ◊ Anaerobes
  ◊ Other (uncommon)
Drugs that may alter lab results: Prior antibiotics
Disorders that may alter lab results: N/A

PATHOLOGICAL FINDINGS
• Gross - solitary abscess
• Multiple abscesses
• Micro - suppuration
• Cavitation

SPECIAL TESTS N/A

IMAGING
• Chest x-ray: consolidation with radiolucency
• Air-fluid level
• Pleural effusion
• CT: define location and extent

DIAGNOSTIC PROCEDURES
• Bronchoscopy if obstruction suspected
• Bronchoscopic protected brushing
• Bronchoalveolar lavage
• Transthoracic needle aspiration

TREATMENT

APPROPRIATE HEALTH CARE
• Inpatient if ill, otherwise outpatient
• Inpatient surgery

GENERAL MEASURES
• Postural drainage
• Pulmonary physiotherapy
• Treat underlying etiology (e.g., antibiotics)
• Bronchoscopy with selective therapeutic lavage

SURGICAL MEASURES
• Surgery for complications (pulmonary resection)
• Tracheostomy, if imperative

ACTIVITY Reduced activity until x-ray evidence of clearing

DIET No restrictions

PATIENT EDUCATION Pulmonary physiotherapy techniques

MEDICATIONS

DRUG(S) OF CHOICE Antibiotics according to culture and sensitivity results. For presumed anaerobes, data from prospective randomized trials have shown clindamycin 600 mg every 6-8 hours IV, followed by 300 mg every 6 hours orally for 4 weeks to result in fewer treatment failures than penicillin.
Contraindications: Refer to manufacturer's literature.
Precautions: Refer to manufacturer's literature
Significant possible interactions: Refer to manufacturer's literature

ALTERNATIVE DRUGS
• Anaerobes: standard therapy has been penicillin G 1-2 million units IV every 4 hours until improved, followed by 1.2 million units (750 mg) orally every 6 hours for 3-4 weeks. Metronidazole has not proven as effective as clindamycin.
• Bacteroides: cefoxitin, cefotetan, ticarcillin-clavulanate, chloramphenicol, imipenem
• Fusobacterium: first generation cephalosporin

FOLLOWUP

PATIENT MONITORING Continue treatment until cavity has disappeared or stabilized on serial x-rays (several weeks or months)

PREVENTION/AVOIDANCE Treat predisposing diseases

POSSIBLE COMPLICATIONS
• Extension
• Brain abscess
• Meningitis
• Empyema
• Pneumothorax
• Massive hemoptysis

EXPECTED COURSE/PROGNOSIS
Guardedly favorable. Increased sequelae with concomitant disease.

MISCELLANEOUS

ASSOCIATED CONDITIONS
• Pneumonia
• Alcoholism
• Epilepsy
• Empyema
• Periodontal disease
• Unconsciousness
• Neoplasia
• Bronchogenic carcinoma
• Tuberculosis
• Fungal diseases

AGE-RELATED FACTORS
Pediatric: Occurs in children, Staphylococcus most common organism
Geriatric: Mortality higher in this age group
Others: N/A

PREGNANCY N/A

SYNONYMS Pulmonary abscess

ICD-9-CM
513.0 abscess of lung

SEE ALSO
• Pneumonia, bacterial

OTHER NOTES N/A

ABBREVIATIONS N/A

REFERENCES
• Bartlett JG: Anaerobic bacterial infections of the lung and pleural space. Clinical Infectious Diseases 1993;16;Suppl4:s248-255
• Murray JF, Nadel JA, eds: Textbook of Respiratory Medicine. 2nd Ed. Philadelphia, W.B. Saunders Co., 1994
• Hagan JL, Hardy JD: Lung abscess revisited-a survey of 184 cases. Ann of Surg 1983;197:755-762
• Guidiol F, Manresa F, Pallares R, et al: Clindamycin vs penicillin for anerobic lung infections. Arch Int Med 1990;150:2525-2529
Illustrations: N/A
Internet references: http://www.5mcc.com

Author(s)
J. P. W. Cunnington, MD, FRCPC

Lung, primary malignancies

BASICS

DESCRIPTION
• The common lung cancers may be divided into two broad categories:
  ◊ Non-small cell cancer: includes squamous cell cancer, (most common); adenocarcinoma and large cell carcinoma
  ◊ Small cell cancer
• Other malignancies from the lung are numerous but uncommon (lymphoma, blastoma, sarcoma, etc.)
System(s) affected: Pulmonary
Genetics: N/A
Incidence/Prevalence in USA:
• 175,000 new cases per year
• 70/100,000 population
Predominant age: 50-70 years
Predominant sex: Male > Female

SIGNS AND SYMPTOMS
May be asymptomatic.
• Hypertrophic pulmonary osteoarthropathy
• Cough
• Shortness of breath
• Hemoptysis
• Exercise limitation
• Chest pain
• Hoarseness
• Wheezing
• Excess fatigue
• Dyspnea
• Shoulder/arm pain
• Dysphagia
• Bone pain
• Weight loss
• Superior vena cava syndrome
• Anemia

CAUSES
• Smoking (greater than 90%)
• Asbestos exposure
• Chronic interstitial pneumonitis
• Halogen ethers
• Inorganic arsenic
• Radioisotopes
• Atmospheric pollution
• Other metals

RISK FACTORS Listed under Causes

DIAGNOSIS

DIFFERENTIAL DIAGNOSIS
• Metastatic cancer
• Granuloma
• Hamartoma

LABORATORY
• CBC (look for anemia)
• SMA-18 (look for abnormalities of Na, K, Ca and liver enzymes)
• PT, PTT, platelet count
Drugs that may alter lab results: None likely
Disorders that may alter lab results: None likely

PATHOLOGICAL FINDINGS Cancer cell type from positive histology or cytology (see Description)

SPECIAL TESTS
• Electrocardiogram
• Pulmonary function studies
• Exercise treadmill
• Stress thallium or Persantine scans when applicable

IMAGING
• Chest x-ray, CT scan of chest, split perfusion lung scan:
  ◊ Pulmonary nodule, mass, or infiltrate
  ◊ Mediastinal widening
  ◊ Atelectasis
  ◊ Hilar enlargement
  ◊ Pleural effusion
• Other CT scans:
  ◊ Of brain - when applicable
  ◊ Of abdomen (may not be necessary if CT of chest includes screen for hepatic or adrenal metastasis)
• Bone scan:
  ◊ When applicable

DIAGNOSTIC PROCEDURES
• Fiberoptic bronchoscopy
• Mediastinoscopy, when applicable
• Fine needle aspiration biopsy
• Scalene node biopsy, when applicable

TREATMENT

APPROPRIATE HEALTH CARE
• Inpatient for surgery
• Outpatient chemotherapy or radiation therapy for small cell cancer

GENERAL MEASURES
• Radiotherapy
• Immunotherapy
• Pain relief when applicable

SURGICAL MEASURES Surgical resection for non-small cell cancer, when possible - stage I and II and some stage III

ACTIVITY Fully active

DIET No special diet

PATIENT EDUCATION
• General verbal information on lung cancer
• American Cancer Society for support groups and other information

MEDICATIONS

DRUG(S) OF CHOICE Pain medication
Contraindications: Refer to manufacturer's instructions
Precautions: Refer to manufacturer's instructions
Significant possible interactions: Refer to manufacturer's instructions

ALTERNATIVE DRUGS N/A

FOLLOWUP

PATIENT MONITORING
• Surgically resectable
  ◊ First year each 3 months
  ◊ Second year each 6 months
  ◊ Third though fifth year once a year
• Surgically unresectable
  ◊ As necessary for palliation

PREVENTION/AVOIDANCE
• Stop smoking
• Avoid asbestos
• Avoid occupational exposure to metals
• Consider prophylaxis with retinoid, such as beta-carotene

POSSIBLE COMPLICATIONS
• Development of metastatic disease
• Local recurrence

EXPECTED COURSE/PROGNOSIS
• Stage I, post-surgical resection of squamous/adeno/large cell is 50% survival
• Stage II, post-surgical is 33% for squamous (stage IIIa, post-surgical survival is 15% for squamous), and 20% for adeno/large cell
• Note: Pre-surgical staging is less accurate so survival figures are lower
• If nonresectable, prognosis is poor with mean survival rate of 8 to 14 months

MISCELLANEOUS

ASSOCIATED CONDITIONS N/A

AGE-RELATED FACTORS
Pediatric: N/A
Geriatric: More common in elderly (> 75 years)
Others: N/A

PREGNANCY N/A

SYNONYMS
• Lung cancer

ICD-9-CM
162.9 Malignant neoplasm of bronchus and lung, unspecified

SEE ALSO N/A

OTHER NOTES N/A

ABBREVIATIONS N/A

REFERENCES
• Shields TW, ed: General Thoracic Surgery. 3rd Ed. Philadelphia, Lea and Febiger, 1989
• Baue AE, ed: Glenn's Thoracic and Cardiovascular Surgery. 5th Ed. East Norwich, Appleton and Lange, 1990
• Sabiston DC, ed: Surgery of the Chest. 4th Ed. Philadelphia, W.B. Saunders Co., 1983
Illustrations: N/A
Internet references: http://www.5mcc.com

Author(s)
Joseph I. Miller, MD

Lupus erythematosus, discoid

 BASICS

DESCRIPTION Discoid lupus erythematosus (DLE) is a chronic skin disease characterized by sharply marginated dull, red macules with adherent scales extending into areas of atrophy, telangiectasias, or follicular plugging
• Localized DLE - more common form with lesions occurring on the face especially the malar areas, bridge of nose, lower lip, lower eyelids and ears
• Widespread DLE - lesions seen on upper extremities and thorax
System(s) affected: Skin
Genetics: N/A
Incidence/Prevalence in USA:
• 3/100,000 Caucasian females; 8/100,000 black females
• 100/100,000
Predominant age: 25 to 45
Predominant sex:
• Localized DLE - Female > Male (3:1)
• Widespread DLE - Female > Male (9:1)

SIGNS AND SYMPTOMS
• Red plaque-like lesions on face, thorax, or upper extremities
• Older lesions atrophy and appear as smooth white or hyperpigmented scars with telangiectasias
• Scarring alopecia with scalp lesions
• "Carpet tack" appearance of skin when scale removed
• Lesions occasionally slightly pruritic or stinging
• Oral ulceration in 15 percent of patients

CAUSES Unknown

RISK FACTORS Systemic lupus erythematosus (SLE)

 DIAGNOSIS

DIFFERENTIAL DIAGNOSIS
• Actinic keratoses
• Polymorphous light eruption
• Drug eruptions
• Sarcoid
• Cutaneous leishmaniasis
• Lupus vulgaris
• Seborrheic dermatitis
• Lichen planus
• Plaque psoriasis
• Rosacea
• Pemphigus erythematosus
• Tinea faciei
• Jessner-Kanof disease
• Granuloma faciale

LABORATORY
• Localized DLE - usually no lab abnormalities
• Widespread DLE (may occasionally find) - increased sedimentation rate, positive ANA, leukopenia, hematuria and albuminuria if concomitant SLE
Drugs that may alter lab results: N/A
Disorders that may alter lab results: Concomitant SLE

PATHOLOGICAL FINDINGS
• Hyperkeratosis
• Epidermal atrophy
• Liquefactive degeneration of basal cell layer
• Edema, mucin, and inflammation of dermis
• Follicular plugging
• Basement zone thickened with strong periodic acid-Schiff reaction staining

SPECIAL TESTS Immunofluorescent staining of skin biopsies (lupus band test)

IMAGING N/A

DIAGNOSTIC PROCEDURES Skin biopsy

 TREATMENT

APPROPRIATE HEALTH CARE Outpatient

GENERAL MEASURES Avoid sun exposure, avoid excessive heat, cold, or trauma

SURGICAL MEASURES N/A

ACTIVITY Full activity

DIET Regular

PATIENT EDUCATION
• Teach patients proper use of sunscreens and other measures to prevent sun exposure (e.g., wide-brimmed hats, long sleeves, etc.)
• Advise patient about symptoms of systemic lupus erythematosus (SLE) that should be watched for
• Griffiths: Instructions for Patients, Philadelphia, W.B. Saunders Co.

Lupus erythematosus, discoid

MEDICATIONS

DRUG(S) OF CHOICE
• Localized DLE:
◊ Mid to high potency topical corticosteroids applied tid (e.g., betamethasone, triamcinolone) to all active lesions
◊ Intralesional steroids for those resistant to topical treatment
• Widespread DLE:
◊ Hydroxychloroquine 200 mg or chloroquine 250 mg qd or bid and/or quinacrine 100 mg daily
◊ Short-term (1-2 weeks) of topical corticosteroids is helpful at the same time antimalarials are being started
Contraindications: Antimalarials such as hydroxychloroquine may have to be avoided in patients with preexisting retinal or hepatic disease. Do not give to individuals with G6PD deficiency. Quinacrine rarely causes hematologic cytopenia.
Precautions:
• Observe for skin atrophy with topical steroids especially with use on the face
• Patients on antimalarials should have an eye examination by an ophthalmologist at start of treatment and at 3-6 month intervals to monitor signs of retinal damage
Significant possible interactions: N/A

ALTERNATIVE DRUGS
• Localized DLE: Intralesional triamcinolone 2.5 mg/cc injected at monthly intervals. Prednisone 15 mg bid, then tapered after response.
• Widespread DLE: Quinacrine 100 mg qd, dapsone 100 mg qd, azathioprine 100 mg qd. Systemic retinoid, eg, etretinate 1 mg/kg; thalidomide is also effective

FOLLOWUP

PATIENT MONITORING
• Recheck patients once or twice per month
• Ophthalmology followup at 6 month intervals if patient on antimalarial
• If lesions subside, reduce dosage of antimalarials over 2-3 months, then discontinue

PREVENTION/AVOIDANCE Avoid sun exposure or excessive heat, cold, or skin trauma

POSSIBLE COMPLICATIONS
Hypertrophic scarring, hypopigmentation (especially in blacks)

EXPECTED COURSE/PROGNOSIS
• 40% remit completely; 1-5% may develop systemic lupus (these patients usually have widespread DLE)
• Not life-threatening unless it turns into systemic type

MISCELLANEOUS

ASSOCIATED CONDITIONS
• Systemic lupus erythematosus
• Mixed connective tissue disease (MCTD)
• Antiphospholipid syndrome

AGE-RELATED FACTORS
Pediatric: Neonatal lupus erythematosus is a syndrome of cutaneous lupus and/or congenital heart block. It is caused by transplacental passage of one of several maternal antibodies.
Geriatric: N/A
Others: N/A

PREGNANCY N/A

SYNONYMS Chronic cutaneous LE

ICD-9-CM 695.4 Lupus erythematosus

SEE ALSO
• Systemic lupus erythematosus (SLE)

OTHER NOTES N/A

ABBREVIATIONS N/A

REFERENCES
• Habif T: Clinical Dermatology. 3rd Ed. St Louis, Mosby, 1996
• Fitzpatrick TB, et al: Dermatology in General Medicine. 4th Ed. New York, McGraw-Hill, Inc., 1993
• Fitzpatrick TB, et al: Color Atlas and Synopsis of Clinical Dermatology. 3rd Ed. New York, McGraw-Hill, 1997
Illustrations: 8 available on CD-ROM
Internet references: http://www.5mcc.com

Author(s)
Gary J. Silko, MD

Lyme disease

BASICS

DESCRIPTION A multisystem infection caused by the spirochete Borrelia burgdorferi, which is transmitted primarily by Ixodid ticks
• Stage 1, early localized Lyme disease, includes a characteristic expanding skin rash (erythema migrans) and constitutional flu-like symptoms
• Stage 2, early disseminated Lyme disease, may present with involvement of one or more organ systems. Neurologic (15%) and cardiac (8%) disease are most common.
• Stage 3, chronic Lyme disease, involves arthritis (50%) and chronic neurological syndromes
System(s) affected: Skin, Musculoskeletal, Hemic/Lymphatic/Immunologic
Genetics: HLA - haplotype DR4 or DR2 may be more susceptible to prolonged arthritis
Incidence/Prevalence in USA: Overall incidence 4.4/100,000. Highest prevalence in Connecticut, Rhode Island, New York, New Jersey, Pennsylvania, Wisconsin, Maryland and Minnesota.
Predominant age: Can occur in all ages, but most common in children under 15 and in the 35-49 year age group
Predominant sex: Male = Female

SIGNS AND SYMPTOMS
• Stage 1:
 ◊ Erythema migrans (60-80%)
 ◊ Fever
 ◊ Headache
 ◊ Myalgias
 ◊ Arthralgias
 ◊ Some patients may be asymptomatic
• Stage 2: (involvement of one or more organ systems)
 ◊ Multiple erythema migrans
 ◊ Facial palsies, or other cranial neuropathies
 ◊ Aseptic meningitis
 ◊ Heart block
 ◊ Pericarditis
 ◊ Orchitis, hepatitis, or iritis
 ◊ Arthritis (usually large joint monarthritis)
• Stage 3:
 ◊ Recurrent synovitis
 ◊ Recurrent tendinitis and bursitis
 ◊ Neuropsychiatric symptoms, may include: Psychotic behavior, memory loss, dementia, depression, sleep disorders
 ◊ Encephalopathic symptoms: Headache, decreased memory, difficulty concentrating, confusion, fatigue
 ◊ Symptoms mimicking other CNS diseases: Multiple sclerosis-like syndromes, stroke-like symptoms, vestibular neuronitis, transverse myelitis, parkinsonian symptoms
 ◊ Peripheral neuropathic symptoms: Carpal tunnel syndrome, motor, sensory, or autonomic neuropathies
 ◊ Ophthalmic manifestations: Iritis, keratitis, retinal vasculitis, optic neuritis

CAUSES Infection with spirochete Borrelia burgdorferi, transmitted by the bite of Ixodid ticks

RISK FACTORS Exposure to tick infested area, most common from May to September

DIAGNOSIS

DIFFERENTIAL DIAGNOSIS
• Juvenile rheumatoid arthritis
• Viral syndromes
• Later stages may mimic many other diseases (see Signs and Symptoms)

LABORATORY
• ELISA for IgM and IgG B burgdorferi antibodies (frequently negative in stage 1 disease)
• Culture of CSF for B burgdorferi
Drugs that may alter lab results: Late stage disease with negative serology may be seen in patients who received early antibiotic treatment
Disorders that may alter lab results: False positive response has been seen with Rocky Mountain spotted fever, syphilis, systemic lupus erythematosus, and rheumatoid arthritis

PATHOLOGICAL FINDINGS Culture of B burgdorferi from blood or skin biopsy specimens has a very low yield

SPECIAL TESTS N/A

IMAGING N/A

DIAGNOSTIC PROCEDURES Lumbar puncture when neurologic findings are present, with ELISA of CSF for B burgdorferi antibodies

TREATMENT

APPROPRIATE HEALTH CARE
• Stage 1, clinical diagnosis, can be treated as an outpatient
• Stage 2 and 3 may require more intensive treatment, based on symptoms

GENERAL MEASURES Prevention of infection is possible by careful examination of skin for ticks after outdoor activities. Prompt removal of ticks may limit transmission. Clothing that covers the ankles should be worn in endemic areas, and the use of insect repellants is recommended.

SURGICAL MEASURES N/A

ACTIVITY No restriction

DIET No special diet

PATIENT EDUCATION
• In endemic areas, patients should be advised to protect themselves against tick exposure
• Information available from: American Lyme Disease Foundation, 293 Route 100, Suite 204, Somers NY 10589

MEDICATIONS

DRUG(S) OF CHOICE
• Stage 1:
◊ Doxycycline (Vibramycin) 100 mg po bid for 14-21 days (do not use in children under 12 or in pregnancy); or
◊ Amoxicillin 500 mg po tid for 14-21 days, (pediatric dose 25-100 mg/kg/day)
◊ Cefuroxime (Ceftin) axetil 500 mg bid for 14-21 days
• Stage 2:
◊ Normal CSF, treat for 28 days - doxycycline 100 mg po bid; or
◊ Amoxicillin 500 mg po tid
◊ Short course of corticosteroids (5-7 days) may be helpful
◊ With abnormal CSF, treat for 3-4 weeks - ceftriaxone (Rocephin) 2 g IV qd; or cefotaxime (Claforan) 2 g IV q 8 h; or penicillin G 20-24 million units/day IV
• Stage 3:
◊ Oral treatment for 28 days with doxycycline 100 mg bid; or
◊ Amoxicillin 500 mg tid
◊ If oral treatment fails, IV treatment for 2-3 weeks with ceftriaxone 2 g qd; or cefotaxime 2 g q 8 hr; or penicillin G 20-24 million units/day IV

Contraindications:
• Allergy to agent
• Doxycycline contraindicated in children and in women who are pregnant or breast feeding
Precautions: Refer to manufacturer's profile of each drug
Significant possible interactions:
• Oral anticoagulants may need reduced dose
• Oral contraceptives may be less effective

ALTERNATIVE DRUGS
• Cefuroxime (Ceftin) 500 mg bid for stage I disease, or tid for stage 2 or 3 disease

FOLLOWUP

PATIENT MONITORING
Stage 2 and 3 disease requires careful monitoring over a period of months to years, based on severity of symptoms

PREVENTION/AVOIDANCE
Awareness of the disease, protective clothing, and careful skin inspection with timely removal of ticks may reduce the incidence of disease

POSSIBLE COMPLICATIONS
• Recurrent synovitis, tendinitis, bursitis
• Chronic neurological symptoms
• Peripheral neuropathies
• See Signs and symptoms of Stage 3 disease

EXPECTED COURSE/PROGNOSIS
• Early treatment with antibiotics can shorten the duration of symptoms and prevent later disease
• Response of late stage disease is variable

MISCELLANEOUS

ASSOCIATED CONDITIONS N/A

AGE-RELATED FACTORS
Pediatric: Drug of choice in pediatrics is amoxicillin. Tetracyclines are contraindicated.
Geriatric: N/A
Others: Ixodid ticks are commonly found on deer. Hunters may be at increased risk.

PREGNANCY
Because B burgdorferi can cross the placenta, pregnant patients with active disease should receive parenteral antibiotics. Doxycycline should not be used in pregnancy.

SYNONYMS Lyme arthritis

ICD-9-CM
088.8 Other specified arthropod-borne diseases

SEE ALSO N/A

OTHER NOTES
Ixodid ticks require white footed mice to complete their life cycle. Investigators have had some success in eradicating the ticks by providing permethrin laced cotton in areas where the mice forage for bedding material.

ABBREVIATIONS N/A

REFERENCES
• The Medical Letter 1997; 39(1000);47-48
• MMWR 1996;45:481-484
• Rakel R, ed. Textbook of Family medicine. 5th Ed. Philadelphia, WB Saunders Co, 1995:337,1023
• Am J Med 1996;100;502-508
Illustrations: 3 available on CD-ROM
Internet references: http://www.5mcc.com

Author(s)
Barbara A. Majeroni, MD

Lymphogranuloma venereum

BASICS

DESCRIPTION Lymphogranuloma venereum (LGV) is a rare, systemic, sexually transmitted disease caused by the three most virulent strains or serovars of Chlamydia trachomatis, the same organism responsible for chlamydial urethritis
• Tender inguinal lymphadenopathy, especially unilateral, is the most common clinical manifestation. Painless vesicular or ulcerative lesions on the external genitalia may be seen in early disease and severe anogenital inflammation and scarring may result from untreated disease.
• Usually a disease of the tropics; especially Africa with a foci of endemicity also in the Caribbean (Haiti and Jamaica), South America, East Asia and Indonesia. Chlamydial infections now require reporting in most states.
System(s) affected: Reproductive, Hemic/Lymphatic/Immunologic
Genetics: N/A
Incidence/Prevalence in USA:
Approximately 300 cases reported to CDC each year. The prevalence of anorectal LGV is increasing in the USA in male homosexuals.
Predominant age: Third decade; corresponds with average age of peak sexual activity
Predominant sex: Male > Female (5:1)

SIGNS AND SYMPTOMS
Three stages:
Primary:
• Superficial lesions such as papules, vesicles, ulcers or erosions appear on the external genitalia 3 days to 3 weeks after exposure. Lesions are painless and disappear in a few days leaving no scar. This stage often escapes notice.
Secondary: the inguinal syndrome or bubonic stage
• Predominantly in men (Male:Female > 10:1)
• Fever, chills
• Regional lymphadenopathy occurring a week to months after the primary stage
• Buboes begin as a mass of firm, tender, enlarged, matted lymph nodes, often unilateral and eventually involve the overlying skin with erythema and adhesions. They may have a groove through them formed by the inguinal ligament.
• As the buboes enlarge:
  ◊ The patient experiences severe groin pain and often walks with a limp
  ◊ Within one to two weeks, the buboes may become fluctuant and rupture relieving the pain and leaving fistulas to drain, heal and scar. Sometimes buboes simply involute and form firm inguinal masses.
Tertiary: the anogenital stage
• Lymphatic obstruction or scarring
• Genitalia or anorectal canal inflammation
• Predominantly women and homosexual men. The rectal or vaginal mucosa can become involved after direct inoculation by receptive intercourse or may become involved through posterior lymphatic spread.

• Proctitis can occur producing fever, tenesmus, anal pruritus and mucinous rectal discharge
• Lymphatic obstruction can produce either unusual perianal growths of lymphoid tissue resembling hemorrhoids or genital elephantiasis
• Perirectal abscesses, ischiorectal and rectovaginal fistulas, anal fistulas, and rectal strictures or stenosis can occur

CAUSES Three of fifteen known strains of C. trachomatis described as serovars L1, L2, and L3 are responsible for LGV. These serovars are more invasive and virulent than the others and selectively infect lymphoid tissue rather than columnar epithelial cells.

RISK FACTORS
• Unprotected intercourse, especially outside of a mutually monogamous and disease-free sexual relationship
• Anal intercourse
• Residing in or visiting tropical or developing countries
• With the increasing incidence of anorectal LGV in male homosexuals in the USA, LGV should be kept in mind when a patient presents with symptoms of proctocolitis
• Prostitutes

DIAGNOSIS

DIFFERENTIAL DIAGNOSIS
• Inguinal adenitis - chancroid, genital herpes or syphilis. In the USA, one or more of these is much more likely than LGV, especially if the adenitis is associated with a prominent genital ulceration. Other causes of inguinal adenitis include cat-scratch disease, HIV or reactive adenopathy due to skin lesions on the lower extremities. Less common: lymphoproliferative disorders.
• Suppurative adenitis - chancroid, donovanosis, plague, tularemia, sporotrichosis, actinomycosis and tuberculosis
• Retroperitoneal adenitis - may present as lower abdominal pain with subsequent extensive differential diagnosis
• Proctitis - gonococcal and non-LGV chlamydial proctitis as well as antibiotic-induced and infectious, proctitis and inflammatory bowel disease
• Lymphatic obstruction - consider schistosomiasis along with malignancy if present

LABORATORY
• Mild leukocytosis with relative lymphocytosis or monocytosis
• Elevated erythrocyte sedimentation rate
• VDRL/RPR and HIV antibodies should be considered
Drugs that may alter lab results:
Antibiotics
Disorders that may alter lab results:
Chlamydial urethritis

PATHOLOGICAL FINDINGS N/A

SPECIAL TESTS
• Bubo pus, saline injected into a bubo and re-aspirated, infected tissue or primary lesion scrapings, preserved in proper transport media (ask your lab), can be studied with Giemsa stain or by immunofluorescence for inclusion bodies. They can also be cultured on McCoy cells. Yield is about 30% for all of these methods.
• Immunoglobulin M microimmuno-fluorescence (MIF) is a test used frequently to diagnose chlamydial pneumonia among infants, but can also be used for LVG
• Antibody levels to L1, L2, and L3 serovars of C. trachomatis can also be measured with complement fixation although cross-reactivity with other Chlamydial organisms is possible.
• A fourfold rise in MIF titer to LGV antigen or a complement fixation titer above 1:32, with the proper clinical scenario, is probably LGV. Complement levels above 1:128 confirm the LGV diagnosis. These levels are reached early in the disease. Acute and convalescent titers usually do not vary much at six weeks.
• MIF titers are more sensitive and specific than the complement fixation test
• Frei's intradermal test is obsolete

IMAGING
• Computerized tomography for retroperitoneal adenitis. Lymphography does not outline buboes, but may demonstrate the extent of lymph node involvement
• Barium enema may reveal the characteristic elongated stricture of rectal LGV

DIAGNOSTIC PROCEDURES Aspiration or incision and drainage of bubo for culture

TREATMENT

APPROPRIATE HEALTH CARE
Outpatient except for rare complications such as severe pain or for the surgical repair of complications. Surgery should only be attempted after antibiotic therapy.

GENERAL MEASURES Symptomatic treatment with nonsteroidal anti-inflammatories should be offered in those not contraindicated. Local heat may provide some analgesia.

SURGICAL MEASURES In the acute bubonic stage, fluctuant nodes should be aspirated before they burst and the occasional abscess should be incised and drained. Otherwise surgery should be avoided until antibiotics have been administered. Fever abates rapidly and bubo pain usually responds within a few days after starting antibiotics.

ACTIVITY Sexual abstention pending treatment, otherwise limited only by symptoms

DIET Avoid milk and milk products or any other agents that chelate tetracycline, such as iron supplements and antacids. Allow 2 hours for gastric emptying prior to medication administration if any of these agents are taken.

PATIENT EDUCATION
• LGV is a sexually transmitted disease. The patient should be counseled about other sexually transmitted diseases and safe sex practices
• Sexual partner(s) should be treated
• Offer HIV counseling and testing

MEDICATIONS

DRUG(S) OF CHOICE
• For acute cases: Doxycycline 100 mg po bid for 21 days
• For chronic or relapsing cases: Consider longer course of therapy
Contraindications: Tetracycline allergy or sensitivity
Precautions:
• For patients taking tetracyclines longer than 21 days, changes such as leukocytosis, atypical lymphocytes, toxic granulation of granulocytes, and thrombopenic purpura (rare) may be observed in the peripheral blood.
• Suprainfections such as antibiotic-induced diarrhea may ensue
• Tetracyclines may cause photosensitization. Advise patients to use sunscreen.
• Avoid tetracyclines in pregnancy and children under 8
Significant possible interactions:
• Avoid, when taking tetracyclines: milk and milk products, sodium bicarbonate, calcium and magnesium salts, silicate, iron preparations, and bismuth subsalicylate
• As opposed to the other tetracyclines, food does not otherwise interfere with absorption of doxycycline nor does doxycycline seem to have prolonged clearance in patients with impaired renal function
• Doxycycline's half-life is shortened from 20 to 7 hours in patients who are receiving chronic treatment with barbiturates or phenytoin and hence should be administered in the same dose three to four times a day in this group of patients

ALTERNATIVE DRUGS
• Tetracycline 500 mg po qid for 21 days or
• Sulfisoxazole 500 mg po qid for 21 days or equivalent sulfonamide course
• For pregnant women or patients allergic to tetracyclines and sulfas, erythromycin 500 mg po qid for 21 days

FOLLOWUP

PATIENT MONITORING
• Fever and bubo pain usually abate within 1 to 2 days after starting antibiotics. For persistent fever or malaise, monitor closely for complications such as abscesses or suprainfections.
• Treatment has no effect on preexisting scar tissue, therefore monitor for surgical complications
• Dual infections with other sexually transmitted diseases are common - appropriate monitoring should be performed, especially for syphilis and HIV

PREVENTION/AVOIDANCE
• Treat sexual contact(s)
• Abstinence or mutual monogamy in a proven disease-free sexual relationship is the only prevention. Condoms should be worn with sexual activity outside of such relationships.
• Condoms provide protection against genital-anogenital transmission but have no impact on transmission between other sites

POSSIBLE COMPLICATIONS
• Scarring - includes ureteral or bowel obstruction, persistent rectovaginal fistula or gross destruction of the anal canal, anal sphincter, or perineum. Repair of such complications as well as plastic repair of some of the complications of lymphatic obstruction such as genital elephantiasis are the more common surgical indications. Surgery should be performed only after antibiotic treatment.
• Mild rectal strictures can occasionally be dilated as an outpatient

EXPECTED COURSE/PROGNOSIS
• Early treatment improves the prognosis
• Complete resolution of symptoms is usual if treatment is undertaken before scarring
• Reinfection and/or inadequate treatment may result in relapse

MISCELLANEOUS

ASSOCIATED CONDITIONS Any of the sexually transmitted diseases. Screening should be done for syphilis and HIV.

AGE-RELATED FACTORS
Pediatric: N/A
Geriatric: N/A
Others: N/A

PREGNANCY
• Congenital transmission does not occur, but infection may be acquired during passage through an infected birth canal
• Pregnant and lactating women should be treated with erythromycin regimen

SYNONYMS
• Tropical bubo
• Climatic bubo
• Strumous bubo
• Poradenitis inguinalis
• Durand-Nicolas-Favre disease
• Lymphogranuloma inguinale
• Fourth and fifth and sixth venereal disease

ICD-9-CM
099.1 Lymphogranuloma venereum

SEE ALSO
• Chlamydial sexually transmitted diseases
• Chancroid
• Syphilis
• Herpes, genital

OTHER NOTES HIV infected patients with LGV should be treated with usual LGV regimen

ABBREVIATIONS
• HIV = human immunodeficiency virus
• CDC = Centers for Disease Control
• LGV = lymphogranuloma venereum
• RPR = Rapid plasma reagin test for syphilis
• VDRL = Venereal Disease Research Laboratories test for syphilis

REFERENCES
• Centers for Disease Control: 1993 sexually transmitted diseases treatment guidelines. MMWR 42(RR-14), 1993
• Woods GL: Update on laboratory diagnosis of sexually transmitted diseases. Clin Lab Med 1995;15(3):665-684
• Noble J, ed: Primary Care Medicine. 2nd Ed. St. Louis, Mosby, 1996:881
Illustrations: 2 available on CD-ROM
Internet references: http://www.5mcc.com

Author(s)
Grant C. Fowler, MD

Lymphoma, Burkitt's

BASICS

DESCRIPTION Highly undifferentiated B cell lymphoma. It may involve sites other than lymph nodes or reticuloendothelial system, particularly bone marrow and central nervous system. Endemic areas - Central Africa; New Guinea. Rare in USA.
System(s) affected:
Hemic/Lymphatic/Immunologic
Genetics: Translocation of chromosome 8 onto chromosome 14 (70%); c–myc activation
Incidence/Prevalence in USA: Rare
Predominant age: 3 months to 16 years
Predominant sex: Male > female

SIGNS AND SYMPTOMS
• African:
  ◊ Mouth pain
  ◊ Loose teeth
  ◊ Loose deciduous molars
  ◊ Jaw mass
  ◊ Anemia
• North American:
  ◊ Abdominal mass
  ◊ Abdominal pain

CAUSES Unknown; high association with Epstein-Barr virus

RISK FACTORS Living in endemic areas

DIAGNOSIS

DIFFERENTIAL DIAGNOSIS N/A

LABORATORY
• Anemia
• Serum uric acid often elevated
Drugs that may alter lab results: N/A
Disorders that may alter lab results: N/A

PATHOLOGICAL FINDINGS
• Stage AR - completely resected intra-abdominal tumor
• Stages A and B - indicate single or multiple extra-abdominal sites
• Stage C - intra-abdominal disease, including kidneys and/or gonads
• Stage D - stage C findings plus extra-abdominal sites including bone marrow, pleura and/or central nervous system
• High mitotic rate
• Starry sky pattern
• A sea of monotonous cells
• Round to oval nuclei
• 2-5 prominent nucleoli
• Pyroninophilic cytoplasm

SPECIAL TESTS
• Cytogenic studies - translocation between chromosomes 8 and 14
• Immunologic studies - presence of B cell markers (usually IgM) on cell surface

IMAGING CT scan

DIAGNOSTIC PROCEDURES
• Bone marrow aspiration
• Lumbar puncture
• Lymph node biopsy

TREATMENT

APPROPRIATE HEALTH CARE
• Inpatient - for staging surgery and chemotherapy (may require ICU for stages C and D)
• Outpatient - after definitive treatment

GENERAL MEASURES
• Symptomatic treatment for respiratory, gastrointestinal, or psychosocial problems that may follow chemotherapy
• Be alert to increased risk for renal failure and life-threatening metabolic abnormalities due to tumor lysis

SURGICAL MEASURES
• Staging surgery
• Surgery to excise the abdominal mass if present

ACTIVITY As tolerated

DIET
• May have difficulty in swallowing or chewing (jaw involvement). Suggest small meals of a soft diet (protein milk shakes) to help prevent malnutrition.
• Adequate fluid intake

PATIENT EDUCATION
Leukemia Society of America
733 3rd Avenue
New York, NY 10017
(212)573-8424

MEDICATIONS

DRUG(S) OF CHOICE Combination chemotherapy according to most recent protocols. Type and extent of therapy depends on stage of disease.
Contraindications: Refer to manufacturer's literature
Precautions: Myelosuppression, alopecia, mucositis, neurotoxicity with chemotherapy
Significant possible interactions: Refer to manufacturer's literature

ALTERNATIVE DRUGS Intensive chemotherapy with or without bone marrow transplantation for advanced cass

FOLLOWUP

PATIENT MONITORING
• For effects of chemotherapy
• Follow for detection of recurrence

PREVENTION/AVOIDANCE Avoid endemic areas

POSSIBLE COMPLICATIONS
• Tumor lysis syndrome with renal failure:
  ◊ Hyperkalemia
  ◊ Hyperphosphatemia
  ◊ Hyperuricemia
  ◊ Hypocalcemia
  ◊ Tetany

EXPECTED COURSE/PROGNOSIS
• 90% of patients with stage A and over 70% of patients with stages B and C experience long-term remission and possible cure
• With recent protocols, some patients with stage D have also been cured
• Without treatment, prognosis is grave

MISCELLANEOUS

ASSOCIATED CONDITIONS N/A

AGE-RELATED FACTORS
Pediatric: Common age group for this disorder
Geriatric: Unusual in this age group
Others: N/A

PREGNANCY N/A

SYNONYMS
• Monomorphic undifferentiated lymphoma
• African lymphoma
• Maxillary lymphosarcoma

ICD-9-CM 200.2

SEE ALSO N/A

OTHER NOTES N/A

ABBREVIATIONS N/A

REFERENCES
• Vietti T, Fernbach D, eds: Clinical Pediatric Oncology. 4th Ed. St. Louis, C.V. Mosby, 1992
• Williams WJ, et al: Hematology. 4th Ed. New York, McGraw-Hill, 1990
• Bennett JC, Plum F, eds: Cecil Textbook of Medicine. 20th Ed. Philadelphia, W.B. Saunders Co., 1996
Illustrations: N/A
Internet references: http://www.5mcc.com

Author(s)
John J. Hutter, Jr., MD

Macular degeneration, age-related (ARMD)

BASICS

DESCRIPTION One definition of ARMD is pigmentary changes in the macula or typical drusen associated with visual loss to the 20/30 level or worse, not caused by cataract or other eye disease in individuals over 50 years of age. Other definitions do not include age or visual acuity criteria. ARMD is the leading cause of irreversible severe visual loss in persons over 65 years of age.
• Stages:
  ◊ Atrophic/nonexudative: drusen and/or pigmentary changes in the macula
  ◊ Neovascular/exudative: growth of blood vessels underneath the retina
System(s) affected: Nervous
Genetics: N/A
Incidence/Prevalence in USA:
• In the Framingham Eye Study (FES) drusen were noted in 25% of all participants. Participants were 52 years of age or older. ARMD was noted in 5.7%.
• Prevalence increases with age. Over 75 years; one quarter of men and one third of women will have evidence of ARMD.
• The prevalence of severe visual loss from ARMD increases with age. 2.2% of patients over 65 years of age are blind in one or both eyes from ARMD.
• The atrophic/nonexudative stage accounts for 20% of cases of severe visual loss
• The neovascular/exudative stage accounts for 80% of cases of severe visual loss
Predominant age: FES prevalence rates:
• 1.6% of those individuals who were 52-64 years old
• 11% of those who were 65-74 years old
• 27.9% of those who were > 75 years
Predominant sex: Female > Male

SIGNS AND SYMPTOMS
• Atrophic/nonexudative Stage
  ◊ Drusen
    - Small yellowish-white lesions
    - Can be subdivided into types such as hard drusen and soft drusen
  ◊ Atrophy of the retinal pigment epithelium (RPE), a pigment layer underneath the retina
• Neovascular/exudative Stage
  ◊ Blood vessels can grow underneath the retina from the choroid. These blood vessels which grow from the choroid are called choroidal neovascular membranes (CNVMs) or subretinal neovascularization (SRN). The choroid is the vascular layer underneath the RPE.
    - Subretinal fluid
    - Exudates
    - Subretinal hemorrhage
    - Patients frequently notice distortion in their central vision. On Amsler grid testing the horizontal or vertical lines may become broken, distorted or missing. Patients may notice straight lines appear crooked, e.g., telephone poles.
  ◊ Disciform scar: An advanced stage resulting in a fibrovascular scar

CAUSES
• Visible light can result in the formation and accumulation of metabolic byproducts in the RPE which normally helps remove metabolic byproducts from the retina. The excess accumulation of these metabolic byproducts interferes with the normal metabolic activity of the RPE and can lead to the formation of drusen.
• The neovascular stage generally arises from the atrophic stage
• Most patients do not progress beyond the atrophic/nonexudative stage; however, those that do are at a greater risk to develop severe visual loss

RISK FACTORS
• Excess sunlight exposure
• Blue or light iris color
• Hyperopia
• History of cardiovascular disease (hypertension, circulatory problems)
• Short height
• History of lung infection
• Cigarette smoking

DIAGNOSIS

DIFFERENTIAL DIAGNOSIS
Idiopathic subretinal neovascularization, presumed ocular histoplasmosis syndrome, diabetic retinopathy, and hypertensive retinopathy

LABORATORY N/A
Drugs that may alter lab results: N/A
Disorders that may alter lab results: N/A

PATHOLOGICAL FINDINGS
• Drusen: deposits of hyaline material between the retinal pigment epithelium (RPE) and Bruch's membrane (the limiting membrane between the RPE and the choroid)
• Breaks in Bruch's membrane allows CNVM's to invade the RPE and grow into the subretinal space

SPECIAL TESTS
• Fluorescein angiography: Can detect CNVM's. This test helps to differentiate between atrophic and neovascular ARMD.
• Indocyanine green videoangiography: May be useful in identifying occult or hidden CNVM's

IMAGING N/A

DIAGNOSTIC PROCEDURES
• Daily Amsler grid testing
• Eye examination with detailed fundus examination
• Fluorescein angiography

TREATMENT

APPROPRIATE HEALTH CARE
Outpatient for laser treatment. Inpatient or outpatient for vitrectomy surgery.

GENERAL MEASURES
• Atrophic/nonexudative macular degeneration
  ◊ No specific treatment alters the course
  ◊ Free radical formation in the retina, induced by visible light may play a role in cellular damage that results in ARMD.
  ◊ Vitamin A, E, C and beta-carotene may be useful in preventing cellular damage
  ◊ Oral zinc may retard visual loss
  ◊ Laser photocoagulation to treat drusen is unwarranted
• Neovascular/exudative macular degeneration
  ◊ The Macular Photocoagulation Study (MPS) demonstrated a treatment benefit for laser treatment of CNVM's which were 200 microns (200 microns = 0.2 mm) or greater from the center of the macula.
    - The MPS showed that the benefits of argon laser photocoagulation were greatest one year after treatment. At that time the proportion of eyes with severe visual loss was reduced 51% by treatment, from 43% in untreated eyes to 21% in treated eyes. The deterioration in treatment effect in the MPS is primarily due to recurrent CNVMs growing towards the center of the macula.
    - Fluorescein angiogram usually can determine whether a CNVM is present, if it is well defined, and if it is in a treatable position.
    - Recurrent CNVM's, after laser treatment, were seen in 59% of patients with ARMD. Recurrent CNVMs develop early after treatment; 73% of the recurrences occurred within the first year of treatment, usually within the first 6 months.
• Treatment of CNVMs from 1 to 199 microns from the center of the macula has been studied by the Age-Related Macular Degeneration Study-Krypton Laser (ARMDS-K). The benefit of laser treatment was greatest among patients without evidence of hypertension. No benefit was observed among patients who had highly elevated blood pressure and/or used antihypertensive medication.
  ◊ Because patients in the ARMDS-K treatment group had CNVM's closer to the center of vision, the magnitude of treatment benefit after laser photocoagulation is smaller in the ARMDS-K treatment group than in the argon laser trial for CNVM's further away from the center of the macula.
  ◊ Laser treatment can be applied to CNVM's directly underneath the center of vision; however, this can result in immediate worsening of vision. The long term benefits of laser treatment for these lesions makes this form of laser treatment an option.

• Vitrectomy has been used to remove CNVM's, but the benefits are questionable
◊ CNVM's can bleed spontaneously leaving blood underneath the retina. The benefits of performing a vitrectomy to remove subretinal blood are questionable.
• Patients need to be monitored (usually with fluorescein angiography) after laser treatment to check for recurrent CNVM's. Changes in the Amsler grid or the patient's vision after treatment needs to be reported
• Low vision aids may be helpful
• Investigation/experimental treatments: transplanting of fetal RPE cells, photodynamic therapy using a light-activated drug and nonthermal light irridiation, laser treatment to drusen, low dose radiation therapy

SURGICAL MEASURES
See General Measures

ACTIVITY
Patients with the neovascular form of ARMD should avoid straining and anticoagulants if possible prior to laser treatment

DIET
• A diet high in vitamins A, E, C and beta-carotene along with zinc may be of benefit
• Eating dark green, leafy vegetables (spinach or collard greens) which are rich in carotinoids may decrease the risk of developing the neovascular/exudative stage

PATIENT EDUCATION
• Patient information is available from the American Academy of Ophthalmology, 655 Beach Street, San Francisco, CA 94109-1336
• Patients who are visually impaired should check with their local low vision center for low vision aids

MEDICATIONS

DRUG(S) OF CHOICE
Zinc and anti-oxidants may be of benefit. Zinc sulfate 100 mg twice daily with food has been recommended.
Contraindications: N/A
Precautions: Excess zinc ingestion can be associated with anemia and worsening of cardiovascular disease
Significant possible interactions: N/A

ALTERNATIVE DRUGS
• Interferon is currently undergoing investigation, but does not appear to be effective
• Thalidomide, investigational, is a potent inhibitor of angiogenesis and appears to be relatively safe in nonpregnant patients

FOLLOWUP

PATIENT MONITORING
• Laser treated patients should be re-examined promptly if new visual symptoms occur
• The Amsler grid can aid in discovering visual disturbances
• Patients with soft drusen or pigmentary changes in the macula are at an increased risk of visual loss. They should be instructed that it is important to monitor their vision, such as by Amsler grid testing and subjective measures of visual acuity, such as reading vision and image clarity. If there are no new symptoms, follow-up examination in 6-12 months.
• Follow-up examination for patients at increased risk of visual loss may permit early detection of treatable lesions with the laser

PREVENTION/AVOIDANCE
• Ultraviolet protection for eyes
• Well balanced diet which includes zinc, vitamins A, E, C, and beta-carotene
• Routine visits to an ophthalmologist
• Daily Amsler grid testing
• An eye exam should be performed every 2-4 years for patients between 40 and 64 years of age and every 1-2 years for patients >65

POSSIBLE COMPLICATIONS
Blindness

EXPECTED COURSE/PROGNOSIS
• Patients with bilateral soft drusen, and pigmentary changes in the macula, but no evidences of exudation, have an increased likelihood of developing CNVM's and subsequent visual loss
• Patients with bilateral drusen carry a cumulative risk of 14.7% over five years of suffering significant visual loss in one eye from the neovascular stage of ARMD.
• Patient's with neovascular stage in one eye and drusen in the opposite eye are at a risk of 5-14% annually of developing the neovascular stage in opposite eye with drusen
• There is a high incidence of recurrence after laser treatment for CNVM's

MISCELLANEOUS

ASSOCIATED CONDITIONS
• Presumed ocular histoplasmosis syndrome
• Exudative retinal detachment
• Vitreous hemorrhage
• Other causes of CNVM's

AGE-RELATED FACTORS
Pediatric: N/A
Geriatric: Prevalence will increase as population ages.
Others: N/A

PREGNANCY
N/A

SYNONYMS
• Senile macular degeneration
• Subretinal neovascularization

ICD-9-CM
362.51 Nonexudative senile macular degeneration
362.52 Exudative senile macular degeneration
362.57 Drusen (degenerative)

SEE ALSO
N/A

OTHER NOTES
N/A

ABBREVIATIONS
• ARMD = age-related macular degeneration
• SMD = senile macular degeneration
• SRN = subretinal neovascularization
• CNVM = choroidal neovascular membrane
• RPE = retinal pigment epithelium
• MPS = macular photocoagulation study
• ARMDS-K = Age-related macular degeneration study-Krypton Laser

REFERENCES
• Leibowitz H, Krueger DE, Maunder LR, et al: The Framingham Eye Study Monograph; an ophthalmological and epidemiological study of cataract, glaucoma, diabetic retinopathy, macular degeneration, and visual acuity in a general population of 2631 adults, 1973-1975. Surv Ophthalmol 1980;24(Suppl):335-610
• Bressler NM, Bressler SB, Fine SL: Age-related macular degeneration. Surv Ophthalmol 1988;32:375-413
• Macular Photocoagulation Study Group: Argon laser photocoagulation for neovascular maculopathy: Three year results from randomized clinical trials. Arch Ophthalmol 1986;104:694-701
• The Macular Photocoagulation Study Group: Recurrent choroidal neovascularization after argon laser photocoagulation for neovascular maculopathy. Arch Ophthalmol 1986;104:503-512
• Macular Photocoagulation Study Group: Krypton laser photocoagulation for neovascular lesions of age-related macular degeneration. Results of a randomized clinical trial. Arch Ophthalmol 1990;108:816-824
• Macular Photocoagulation Study Group: Subfoveal neovascular lesions in age-related macular degeneration. Guidelines for evaluation and treatment in the macular photocoagulation study. Arch Ophthalmol 1991;109:1242-1257
• Newsome, DA , Swatz M, Leone NC, et al: Oral zinc and macular degeneration. Arch. Ophthalmol 1988;106:192-198
• Smiddy WE, Fine SL: Prognosis of patients with bilateral macular drusen. Ophthalmology 1984;91:271-277
• Sedden JM, Ajani UA, Sperduto RD, et al: Dietary carotenoids, vitamins A, C, and E, and advanced age-related macular degeneration. JAMA 1994;272:1413-1420
Illustrations: 4 available on CD-ROM
Internet references: http://www.5mcc.com

Author(s)
Richard W. Allinson, MD

Malaria

BASICS

DESCRIPTION Malaria is an acute and chronic protozoan infection transmitted by Anopheles mosquitoes to humans. There are four species that cause human infection: Plasmodium falciparum, P. malariae, P. vivax, P. ovale.
System(s) affected:
Hemic/Lymphatic/Immunologic
Genetics: No known genetic pattern
Incidence/Prevalence in USA: Not endemic. Cases in the US are imported.
Predominant age: All ages
Predominant sex: Male = Female

SIGNS AND SYMPTOMS
• Chills
• Fever
• Hemolysis
• P. falciparum (also known as malignant tertian malaria) - does not have a specific periodicity in a non-immune individual. The patient may have persistent fever and in massive parasitemia may have serious complications including renal failure, central nervous system involvement, pulmonary edema, gastroenteritis, anemia, and thrombocytopenia. This is the only infection that is associated with fatal outcome.
• P. malariae (also known as quartan malaria) - patient will have attacks every 72 hours. This disease can become chronic. Nephrotic syndrome may be found in patients with chronic P. malariae infection.
• P. vivax (benign tertian) and P. ovale - patient will have attacks every 48 hours
• Splenomegaly is found in those with chronic infection

CAUSES Bites from infected Anopheles mosquitoes, or transfusion of infected blood

RISK FACTORS Traveling and/or living in endemic area

DIAGNOSIS

DIFFERENTIAL DIAGNOSIS
• Severe P. falciparum infection may present with signs and symptoms suggestive of acute hepatitis, acute hemolytic anemia, acute diarrheal illness, stroke, pneumonia, and acute viral infection
• Chronic infection may have to be differentiated from other causes of tropical splenomegaly and blood dyscrasias

LABORATORY
• Anemia
• Leukopenia
• Thrombocytopenia
• Elevated alanine aminotransferase (ALT), aspartate aminotransferase (AST)
• Direct and indirect bilirubin
• Depressed albumin
Drugs that may alter lab results:
Antimalarial agents may reduce parasitemia
Disorders that may alter lab results: N/A

PATHOLOGICAL FINDINGS
• Malaria causes hemolysis
• In the case of falciparum infection, the increased stickiness of the parasitized cells results in blocking of arterioles and capillaries
• Edema, localized hemorrhage, and the presence of malarial pigments are frequent findings

SPECIAL TESTS Malarial smear; indirect fluorescent antibody (IFA), ELISA, DNA probe

IMAGING Not contributory

DIAGNOSTIC PROCEDURES Malarial smear

TREATMENT

APPROPRIATE HEALTH CARE Inpatient for most cases of falciparum malaria in nonimmune patients. Outpatient for others, except during acute phase.

GENERAL MEASURES In severe cases watch for complications, such as severe anemia, and renal failure

SURGICAL MEASURES N/A

ACTIVITY May resume activity as soon as the fever is under control

DIET No restrictions in mild cases. In severe cases, give whatever the patient can tolerate.

PATIENT EDUCATION Prevention of future exposures. These measures include prevention of mosquito bites and malarial chemoprophylaxis.

MEDICATIONS

DRUG(S) OF CHOICE
For infection due to P. vivax, P. ovale, P. malariae, and chloroquine-sensitive P. falciparum:
- Oral therapy - chloroquine phosphate:
  ◊ Adult dose - 600 mg base (1 gm salt) followed by 300 mg in 6 h, then 300 mg daily for 2 days
  ◊ Pediatric dose - 10 mg/kg base (maximum of 600 mg) followed by half the dose in 6 h, then daily dose for 2 days
- Parenteral dose - quinidine or quinine IV (parenteral quinine is no longer available in the USA)
  ◊ Adult and pediatric dose - loading dose of 10 mg/kg over 1-2 hours followed by 0.02 mg/kg/min by continuous infusion or repeat initial dose every 8 h until oral therapy can be started
- Primaquine phosphate (to be given during or after the above anti-malarial therapy to eradicate the hepatic stage (hypnozoites) of P. vivax, and P. ovale)
  ◊ Adult dose - 15 mg base (26.3 mg salt) po daily for 14 days
  ◊ Pediatric dose - 0.3 mg base/kg/day for 14 days
- Caution - patients with glucose-6-phosphate dehydrogenase deficiency may develop hemolysis after given primaquine
For infection due to chloroquine-resistant P. falciparum
- Oral therapy - quinine sulfate plus tetracycline or clindamycin or sulfadoxine-pyrimethamine (Fansidar) - 25 mg p/500 mg s
  ◊ Adult dose - quinine sulfate 650 mg salt po tid for 3-7 days, plus tetracycline 250 mg qid for 7 days, or clindamycin 450 mg tid for 3 days
  ◊ Pediatric dose - quinine sulfate salt po tid for 3-7 days, plus sulfadoxine-pyrimethamine, < 4 years 1/2 tablet, 4-8 years 1 tablet, 8-12 years 2 tablets
  ◊ Pregnant women - quinine as above adult dose plus clindamycin 450 mg po every 8 hours for 3 days
- Alternate oral therapy - mefloquine hydrochloride or halofantrine
  ◊ Adult dose - mefloquine 15 mg/kg salt po, single dose (maximum 1250 mg); halofantrine 6 tabs (250 mg salt) po, 2 tabs 6 hours apart for 3 doses
- Parenteral therapy - quinidine gluconate
  ◊ Adult and pediatric dose - loading dose of 10 mg/kg over 1-2 hours followed by 0.02 mg/kg/min by continuous infusion or repeat initial dose every 8 hours until oral therapy can be started

Contraindications: Refer to manufacturer's literature
Precautions: Refer to manufacturer's literature
Significant possible interactions: Refer to manufacturer's literature

ALTERNATIVE DRUGS   See above

FOLLOWUP

PATIENT MONITORING   Watch for relapse of clinical symptoms

PREVENTION/AVOIDANCE
- Use of malarial prophylactic agents when visiting an endemic area
Chloroquine phosphate po (chemoprophylaxis of all species except chloroquine resistant P. falciparum)
  ◊ Adult dose - 300 mg base once weekly. Start 2 weeks before arrival (endemic area) and continue until 4-6 weeks after leaving the area.
  ◊ Pediatric dose - 5 mg/kg weekly; same as for adults. Maximum 300 mg dose.
Mefloquine po (chemoprophylaxis for chloroquine resistant P. falciparum)
  ◊ Adult dose - 250 mg (1 tablet) weekly. Begin 1 week before arrival and continue for 4 weeks after leaving the area.
  ◊ Pediatric dose - 15-19 kg 1/4 tablet; 20-30 kg 1/2 tablet; 31-45 kg 3/4 tablet; over 45 kg 1 tablet. Follow schedule as for adult.
- Patients with sickle cell disease, or trait, glucose-6-phosphate dehydrogenase deficiency, and hereditary ovalocytosis may have some protection against severe P. falciparum infection. Patients with Duffy-negative blood type are resistant to P. vivax infection.
For patients who cannot take mefloquine or chloroquine: For individuals > 8 years of age and not pregnant, doxycycline 100 mg po once daily. Start doxycycline 1-2 days before arrival, and up to 4 weeks after leaving endemic area. (Doxycycline may cause photosensitivity.)

POSSIBLE COMPLICATIONS
- P. falciparum - if not treated early, the patients may develop cerebral malaria, acute renal failure, acute gastroenteritis, pulmonary edema, massive hemolysis, and splenic rupture. Death from malaria is virtually limited to P. falciparum infection.
- P. malariae - nephrotic syndrome may develop in those with chronic infection
- Other complications - seizures, anuria, delirium, coma, dysentery, algid malaria, blackwater fever, hyperpyrexia

EXPECTED COURSE/PROGNOSIS   Only falciparum infection carries a poor prognosis with high mortality if untreated. However, if diagnosed early and treated appropriately the prognosis is excellent.

MISCELLANEOUS

ASSOCIATED CONDITIONS   N/A

AGE-RELATED FACTORS
Pediatric: N/A
Geriatric: More serious outcome in this age group
Others: N/A

PREGNANCY   Most antimalarial drugs contraindicated in pregnancy

SYNONYMS   N/A

ICD-9-CM
- Blackwater fever 084.8
- Cerebral malaria 084.9
- Congenital malaria 771.2
- Hepatitis 573.2
- Mixed malarial infection 084.5
- P. falciparum infection 084.0
- P. malariae infection 084.2
- P. ovale infection 084.3
- P. vivax infection 084.1
- Recurrent malaria 084.6
- Unspecified malaria 084.6

SEE ALSO   N/A

OTHER NOTES
- Most areas of the world now have chloroquine-resistant P. falciparum (the form of malaria most prevalent world-wide)
- Current information regarding malaria treatment and prophylaxis is always available from CDC, Atlanta, GA

ABBREVIATIONS   N/A

REFERENCES   Wyler DJ: Plasmodium Species (Malaria). In: Mandell GL, Douglas RG, Bennett JE, eds. Principles and Practice of Infectious Diseases. New York, Churchill Livingstone, 1990:2056-2066
Illustrations: N/A
Internet references: http://www.5mcc.com

Author(s)
James S. Tan, MD, FACP

Malnutrition, protein-calorie

BASICS

DESCRIPTION
Protein-calorie malnutrition (PCM) is present when sufficient energy and/or protein is not available to meet metabolic demands, leading to impairment in normal physiologic processes. PCM is classified according to degree of severity and by calculating the actual weight as a percentage of expected weight for height/length, using international standards (normal: 90-110%).
• 1st degree: mild form characterized by growth failure in children and wasting in adults. Weight as a percentage of expected weight: 85-90%
• 2nd degree: moderate form with additional biochemical changes, weight as a percentage of expected weight: 75-85%
• 3rd degree: severe PCM with the development of additional clinical signs, weight as a percentage of expected weight: < 75%
Kwashiorkor is a condition which develops when there is gross protein deficiency though nonprotein calorie intake may be adequate. Marasmus occurs with deficiency of both protein and calories.
System(s) affected: Gastrointestinal, Endocrine/Metabolic, Musculoskeletal, Nervous, Hemic/Lymphatic/Immunologic
Genetics: N/A
Incidence/Prevalence in USA: Institutionalized elderly, hospital patients and children of the poor have a significant prevalence
Predominant age: Infants and younger children (age 1-2) are more susceptible to PCM. However, PCM may occur at all ages.
Predominant sex: Male = Female

SIGNS AND SYMPTOMS
• Mild to moderate PCM
  ◊ Weight loss and reduction in subcutaneous fat in adults
  ◊ Stunted growth, wasted body habitus, delayed puberty and retarded cognitive and psychosocial development in children
  ◊ Decreased hand grip strength
  ◊ Impaired work capacity
  ◊ Risk of intrauterine growth retardation when pregnant women have PCM
  ◊ Reduced volume of breast milk with low fat content
• Severe PCM
  ◊ Severe alterations in the body habitus
  ◊ Muscle wasting in the extremities
  ◊ Associated micronutrient deficiency features
  ◊ Loss of subcutaneous fat
  ◊ Atrophy of interosseus hand muscles and temporalis
  ◊ Decreased skin elasticity
  ◊ Impaired immunity and susceptibility to infections
  ◊ Delayed wound healing and recovery
  ◊ Decubitus ulcers
  ◊ Dry, reddish-brown, sparse hair
  ◊ Lethargy, early satiety, vomiting and constipation
  ◊ Heart rate, BP and core body temperature may be subnormal
  ◊ Marasmic infants show gross weight loss, growth retardation and wasting of subcutaneous fat and muscle
  ◊ Kwashiorkor is characterized by generalized edema, flaky painful dermatoses, sparse and hair pigment changes, enlarged, fatty liver and petulant apathy

CAUSES
• Inadequate dietary intake
• Poor quality dietary protein
• Increased metabolic demands
• Increased nutrient losses

RISK FACTORS
• Nutritional
  ◊ Prolonged and severe reduction of intake
  ◊ Inadequate body reserves
  ◊ Concurrent deficiencies of the other nutrients
  ◊ Anorexia nervosa
• Underlying illnesses
  ◊ Fever, infection, trauma, burns and other hypercatabolic states
  ◊ Malabsorptive and maldigestive states
  ◊ Protein-losing enteropathy, nephrotic syndrome, enteric fistulas
  ◊ Metabolic disorders: Diabetes, hyperthyroidism
• Physiologic states in which requirements are increased
  ◊ Pregnancy and lactation
  ◊ Growth and development during infancy, childhood and adolescence

DIAGNOSIS

DIFFERENTIAL DIAGNOSIS
• Secondary growth failure due to malabsorption, congenital defects or deprivation
• Pellagra
• Nephritis or nephrosis
• Cardiac failure
• Disorders of glycogen metabolism
• Cystic fibrosis

LABORATORY
• Plasma albumin: Reduced
• Complete hemogram: Decreased lymphocyte count
• Serum chemistry
• Blood urea: Decreased
• Plasma transferrin: Decreased
• Plasma essential amino acids: Decreased
• Plasma betalipoprotein: Decreased
• Hypoglycemia with neuroglycopenia
• Plasma cortisol, GH: Increased, but insulin low
Drugs that may alter lab results: N/A
Disorders that may alter lab results: N/A

PATHOLOGICAL FINDINGS
• Marasmus
Muscle wasting and reduction in muscle mass due to gluconeogenesis. Mummified appearance. No edema. Fat depots reduced. Loss of subcutaneous fat.
• Kwashiorkor
Serum amino acid patterns distorted. Protein synthesis impaired. Hypoalbuminemia causes dependent edema. Impaired betalipoprotein synthesis causes fatty liver. Poor insulin response to glucose load. Growth, immune response, repair and production of enzymes and hormones are impaired in severe protein deficiency.

SPECIAL TESTS
• Triceps skin-fold thickness
• Mid-arm muscle area (MAMA)
• Protein index measurement
• Creatinine-height index
• Delayed-hypersensitivity index
• Prognostic-nutritional index (PNI)

IMAGING
Chest x-ray to rule out tuberculosis or other pulmonary infections

DIAGNOSTIC PROCEDURES
• History and physical examination
• MAMA = $[M - \pi(T)] \times [M - \pi(T)] \div 4\pi$
  M = mid-arm circumference (mm)
  T = triceps skin fold (mm)
  π = 3.1415
• Protein index = ratio of measured to predicted total body protein
• Creatinine-height index =
Actual 24 hr urinary creatinine excretion ÷ normative value for height and sex
• Delayed hypersensitivity index: This index quantitates the amount of induration elicited by skin testing with a common antigen such as Candida, Trichophyton or mumps.
Grading: 0 = < 0.5 cm; 1 = 0.5 cm; 2 = 1.0 cm
• Prognostic nutritional index is a weighted combination of 4 measures:
PNI% = 158 - [1.66 x A] - [0.78 x T] - [2.0 x F] - [5.8 x D]
where,
  A = serum albumin (g/L)
  T = triceps skin fold (mm)
  F = serum transferrin (g/L)
  D = delayed hypersensitivity index
All the above indices should be compared with the normative values in standard charts

Malnutrition, protein-calorie

TREATMENT

APPROPRIATE HEALTH CARE
Inpatient care for severe anemia, dehydration, electrolyte imbalance and superimposed infections. Outpatient care for stabilized cases.

GENERAL MEASURES
• Fluid and electrolyte balance should be restored and maintained
• In severe kwashiorkor, IV or SC infusion of amino acids
• Low-lactose formulas have been helpful in some cases with diarrhea due to disaccharidases deficiency
• Diarrhea due to other causes should be identified and treated
• Supplementary vitamins and micronutrients
• Mild anemia usually responds to oral protein, iron and folic acid supplements. Blood transfusion may be necessary in severe cases (Hb < 6 g/dL). Use oral iron with caution in kwashiorkor.

SURGICAL MEASURES   N/A

ACTIVITY   As tolerated

DIET
• Sufficient milk for infants and children to supply 2-5 g/kg/day protein. Lactic-acid fortified milk can be given.
• Adequate calories should be supplied by adding sugar and cereal to the milk diet (150-250 kcal/day)
• Gradual supplementation with high-energy foods such as candies, cake, puddings, meats, eggs and fruit juices
• Small, frequent feedings around the clock better tolerated in the early stages
• Prepared nutritional supplements available commercially are convenient

PATIENT EDUCATION
• Emphasis on nutrition education with the help of a dietician
• Need for a balanced food intake
• Educate about the composition of nutritional products to ensure balanced intake
• Awareness about risk factors and need for timely nutritional supplements

MEDICATIONS

DRUG(S) OF CHOICE
• Antibiotics may be indicated to treat infections
• Multivitamin-multimineral supplementation is required
Contraindications: N/A
Precautions: N/A
Significant possible interactions: N/A

ALTERNATIVE DRUGS   N/A

FOLLOWUP

PATIENT MONITORING
Initially periodic follow-up to ensure good nutritional status

PREVENTION/AVOIDANCE
• Emphasis on nutritional education and continuous nutritional care
• Routine record of height and weight
• Observe and record the patient's food intake
• Early recognition of increased nutritional needs during stress and infections
• Frequent interactions between physician, nurse and dietician to assess nutritional needs
• Avoidance of risk factors when possible

POSSIBLE COMPLICATIONS
Death in the first few days of treatment is usually due to electrolyte imbalance, infection, hypothermia or circulatory failure. Stupor, jaundice, petechiae and low serum sodium are ominous signs.

EXPECTED COURSE/PROGNOSIS
• Mortality varies between 15-40%
• Recovery is more rapid in kwashiorkor than in marasmus. Disappearance of apathy, edema and anorexia are favorable signs.
• In adequately treated cases, liver recovers fully without subsequent cirrhosis, but GI malabsorption and pancreatic deficiency may remain
• Compromised cell-mediated immunity returns to normalcy with recovery
• Behavioral and mental retardation is marked in the severely malnourished child. It is related to the duration of malnutrition and to the age of onset. Relatively mild degree of mental retardation persists into school age.

MISCELLANEOUS

ASSOCIATED CONDITIONS
• Malaria and other parasitic infections
• Multiple micronutrients deficiency
• Malabsorptive and maldigestive states

AGE-RELATED FACTORS
Pediatric:
Growth and development during infancy, childhood and adolescence increase nutritional requirements
Geriatric:
Institutionalized elderly are at special risk
Others: N/A

PREGNANCY
Pregnant women with mild to moderate PCM are at risk of delivering an infant with low weight/length for gestational age

SYNONYMS   N/A

ICD-9-CM
260 Kwashiorkor
261 Nutritional marasmus
263.9 Unspecified protein-calorie malnutrition

SEE ALSO   N/A

OTHER NOTES   N/A

ABBREVIATIONS
PCM = Protein - Calorie Malnutrition
PEM = Protein - Energy Malnutrition
MAMA = Mid - Arm Muscle Area
PNT = Protein Nutritional Index

REFERENCES
• Isselbacher KJ, et al, eds: Harrison's Principles of Internal Medicine. 13th Ed. New York, McGraw-Hill, 1994
• Berkow R, et al, eds: Merck Manual, 16th Ed. Rahway, NJ, Merck Sharp & Dohme, 1992
• Dempster WS, Sive AA, et al: Eur J Clin Nut 1995; 49: 202-210.
Illustrations: N/A
Internet references: http://www.5mcc.com

Author(s)
V. Vasudeviah, BSc, MBBS

Marfan's syndrome

 BASICS

DESCRIPTION A dominantly inherited disorder of connective tissue affecting primarily the musculoskeletal system, the cardiovascular system and the eye
System(s) affected: Musculoskeletal, Endocrine/Metabolic
Genetics: Autosomal dominant with high penetrance; 15% spontaneous mutation
Incidence/Prevalence in USA: 1 in 10,000 - 20,000 (estimated 1 in 15,000)
Predominant age: Congenital, so disorder is present from birth. However clinical manifestations do not usually become apparent until adolescence or young adulthood.
Predominant sex: No gender, ethnic or racial predilection

SIGNS AND SYMPTOMS
• Musculoskeletal
  ◊ Tall stature
  ◊ Thin, gangly body habitus (limb length out of proportion to trunk)
  ◊ Arachnodactyly i.e. long, thin fingers
  ◊ Pectus deformity
  ◊ High arched palate
  ◊ Hyperextensible joints
  ◊ Kyphoscoliosis
  ◊ Joint laxity
• Cardiovascular
  ◊ Aortic root dilatation
  ◊ Aortic regurgitation
  ◊ Aortic dissection
  ◊ Mitral valve prolapse
  ◊ Mitral regurgitation
• Ocular
  ◊ Subluxation of lens, usually upward
  ◊ Myopia
  ◊ Retinal detachment (uncommon)
• Other
  ◊ Easy bruising (uncommon)
  ◊ Excessive bleeding (uncommon)

CAUSES Genetic; at least 5% are obviously familial, the remainder arise from apparent spontaneous mutations

RISK FACTORS Advanced paternal age gives rise to a slightly increased risk only in those cases which are not clearly familial

 DIAGNOSIS

DIFFERENTIAL DIAGNOSIS
Homocystinuria, contractural arachnodactyly, Ehlers-Danlos syndrome, trisomy, all of which are rare conditions and all of which have clear cut distinguishing clinical features from the Marfan's syndrome

LABORATORY
• There are no specific laboratory abnormalities in the Marfan syndrome
• It is recommended that suspected patients have urinary homocystine measured to rule out homocystinuria
Drugs that may alter lab results: N/A
Disorders that may alter lab results: N/A

PATHOLOGICAL FINDINGS
• Cystic medial necrosis of the aorta
• Myxomatous degeneration of the cardiac valves
• FBN1 gene on chromosome 15 codes for fibrillin, a large glycoprotein constituent of microfibrils. Mutations in this gene have been found in over 90% of patients with the Marfan's syndrome, when tested.

SPECIAL TESTS Slit lamp examination is necessary to detect lens subluxation

IMAGING
• Plain x-rays of spine are necessary during growth years to detect and quantify scoliosis
• Annual screening echocardiograms are recommended beginning in adolescence in order to detect presymptomatic aortic root dilatation or valvular degeneration

DIAGNOSTIC PROCEDURES N/A

 TREATMENT

APPROPRIATE HEALTH CARE
Outpatient

GENERAL MEASURES Multidisciplinary approach including primary care physician, cardiologist, ophthalmologist and possibly orthopedic surgeon. A clinical geneticist if available, would be ideal as primary care physician.

SURGICAL MEASURES Many, if not most, of these patients will ultimately require reconstructive cardiovascular surgery

ACTIVITY
• Fully active unless limited by symptoms
• Several highly-trained athletes with the Marfan syndrome have suffered sudden death during competition leading to some concern that people with Marfan syndrome should be discouraged from participating in aerobically demanding sports

DIET No special diet

PATIENT EDUCATION Information available from the National Marfan Foundation, 382 Main St., Port Washington, NY 11959; 800-8MARFAN

Marfan's syndrome

MEDICATIONS

DRUG(S) OF CHOICE
• No specific medical therapy is available, however drugs are used to try to prevent certain complications
• Propranolol or other beta-adrenergic blocking drugs are used to decrease the force of cardiac contraction, in the hope of delaying the development or progression of aortic root dilatation. The dosage of these drugs are adjusted to target heart rate, i.e., resting rate of 60 per minute, with a rise to no more than 80 per minute after moderate exertion.
• Estrogen combined with progestogen has been used to induce puberty in pre-adolescent girls in an attempt to shorten the growth spurt thereby ameliorating scoliosis and preventing excessively tall stature. Do this only under the supervision of an endocrinologist.
Contraindications:
• Congestive heart failure, asthma, diabetes for the beta-adrenergic blocking drugs
• Thromboembolic disease for the estrogen/progestogen
Precautions: Refer to manufacturer's profile of each drug.
Significant possible interactions:
Amphetamines, antihistamines, anti-diabetics, oral contraceptives

ALTERNATIVE DRUGS N/A

FOLLOWUP

PATIENT MONITORING
• Frequent examinations (at least twice a year) while growing, with particular attention to cardiovascular system and scoliosis
• When cardiac symptoms develop or aortic root diameter becomes > 50 mm, surgical intervention must be considered
• When lens subluxation is detected, surgical correction is possible. However a high incidence of glaucoma results, so surgery should be offered only to those who cannot be treated with corrective lenses.

POSSIBLE COMPLICATIONS
• Bacterial endocarditis
• Aortic dissection
• Aortic or mitral valve insufficiency
• Dilated cardiomyopathy
• Retinal detachment

PREVENTION/AVOIDANCE
• No prenatal diagnosis yet available, but presymptomatic diagnosis may be possible at research centers using linkage analysis techniques
• Each child has a 50% chance of inheriting the disorder from an affected parent. Clinical manifestations are variable, however, so children may be more or less severely affected.
• Antibiotic prophylaxis for endocarditis should be prescribed for all Marfan syndrome patients with either a heart murmur or echocardiographic evidence of valvular or aortic root abnormalities

EXPECTED COURSE/PROGNOSIS
• Life-threatening complications are cardiovascular. Before routine corrective surgery was available most Marfan syndrome patients died before reaching the age of 35.
• With appropriate surgical intervention most patients can live a normal life span

MISCELLANEOUS

ASSOCIATED CONDITIONS N/A

AGE-RELATED FACTORS
Pediatric: Early medical or surgical intervention may reduce the degree of scoliosis
Geriatric: N/A
Others: N/A

PREGNANCY Pregnant women with the Marfan syndrome need to be managed as high-risk patients, preferably with involvement of a cardiologist. The outcome is usually excellent.

SYNONYMS N/A

ICD-9-CM 759.82 Marfan syndrome

SEE ALSO N/A

OTHER NOTES N/A

ABBREVIATIONS N/A

REFERENCES
• Pyeritz RE, McKusick VA: The Marfan Syndrome: Diagnosis and Management. New Engl J Med 1979;300:772-777
• Scriver RC, et al, eds: The Metabolic Basis of Inherited Disease. 7th Ed. New York, McGraw Hill, 1995
Illustrations: N/A
Internet references: http://www.5mcc.com

Author(s)
Robert J. Sliman, MD

Mastalgia

 BASICS

DESCRIPTION Chronic breast pain often occurring prior to menses. Breast pain could also be acute and caused by other problems such as breast abscess.
System(s) affected: Skin/Exocrine
Genetics: Familial tendency
Incidence/Prevalence in USA: Mild form is common; severe form is uncommon
Predominant Age: > age 20
Predominant Sex: Female only

SIGNS AND SYMPTOMS
• Breasts aching, heavy, or tender
• Enlarged breasts

CAUSES
• Associated with fibrocystic breast disease and premenstrual syndrome
• Hormonal influences; hormone replacement therapy

RISK FACTORS
• Caffeine consumption
• High fat diet

 DIAGNOSIS

DIFFERENTIAL DIAGNOSIS
• The major alternate disease to consider is breast cancer
• Manipulation or trauma can also make symptoms worse
• Chest-wall pain must also be differentiated from mastalgia
• Often concurrent with premenstrual syndrome
• Ductal ectasia of the breast

LABORATORY No relevant findings
Drugs that may alter lab results: N/A
Disorders that may alter lab results: N/A

PATHOLOGICAL FINDINGS Fibrocystic changes

SPECIAL TESTS
• Possibly TSH
• Prolactin if galactorrhea
• Pap test of other discharge, if present

IMAGING Mammography to differentiate from breast cancer

DIAGNOSTIC PROCEDURES
• Cysts may need to be aspirated for symptom relief and diagnostic verification
• Biopsies may be indicated based on exam or mammography

 TREATMENT

APPROPRIATE HEALTH CARE
Outpatient

GENERAL MEASURES
• Stop or modify current hormonal therapy
• Repeat examination within 30 days will help establish any cyclic nodularity pattern
• Well-fitting support bra (maybe fitted by a professional).
• Reassurance (this is sufficient for most women)
• Weight reduction, if obese

SURGICAL MEASURES N/A

ACTIVITY No restrictions

DIET
• Decreased caffeine
• Decreased fat intake to 20% of total calories

PATIENT EDUCATION
• Explain that breast pain does not mean the patient has cancer
• Explain relationship to menses

MEDICATIONS

DRUG(S) OF CHOICE
• No drugs are needed unless required by severity of symptoms. Reassurance, acetaminophen or ibuprofen may be all that is needed.
Contraindications: Refer to manufacturer's profile of each drug
Precautions: Refer to manufacturer's profile of each drug
Significant possible interactions: Refer to manufacturer's profile of each drug

ALTERNATIVE DRUGS
• Agents often used, whose value has been questioned:
◊ Diuretics (usually spironolactone) prior to menses
◊ Vitamin E 600 IU/day
◊ Evening primrose oil, includes high content of fatty acids
◊ Oral contraceptives may help some patients
• Other possibilities for refractory patients, used infrequently because of potential side effects:
◊ Danazol 100 mg bid (possibly lower doses) - this may be the most effective. Major side effects - menstrual irregularities, weight gain, acne, hirsutism and voice change.
◊ Bromocriptine 2.5-5.0 mg/day. Major side effects - nausea, dizziness, orthostatic hypotension.
◊ Tamoxifen 10 mg/day. Major side effects - cataracts, hepatocellular carcinoma, endometrial carcinoma.
◊ Gonadotropin-releasing hormone agonists

FOLLOWUP

PATIENT MONITORING
• As needed for patients not on prescription medications
• Time of followup will vary by type of prescription medication and patient problems

PREVENTION/AVOIDANCE See Risk Factors

POSSIBLE COMPLICATIONS N/A

EXPECTED COURSE/PROGNOSIS
• Premenstrual mastalgia increases with age, then generally stops at menopause unless on hormone replacement therapy
• Most patients will have control of symptoms without hormonal treatment
• Patients on hormonal treatment are likely to continue to need it for years

MISCELLANEOUS

ASSOCIATED CONDITIONS
Premenstrual syndrome

AGE-RELATED FACTORS
Pediatric: N/A
Geriatric: N/A
Others: N/A

PREGNANCY N/A

SYNONYMS
• Mastodynia
• Breast pain

ICD-9-CM 611.71 mastalgia

SEE ALSO
Premenstrual syndrome

OTHER NOTES
• Cyclic mastalgia responds better than noncyclic mastalgia to treatment
• Effects of long-term hormonal treatment are unknown
• If other treatment fails, a final possibility is subcutaneous mastectomy (used rarely)
• Oophorectomy also provides relief and may be drastic treatment for some patients

ABBREVIATIONS N/A

REFERENCES
• Holland PA, Gately CA: Drug therapy of mastalgia. Practical Therapeutics 1994;48:709-716
• BeLieu RM: Mastodynia. Obstetrics and Gynecology Clin of No Amer 1994;21:461-477
• Gateley CA, Miers M, Marisel RB, Hughes E: Drug treatment for mastalgia: 17 years experience in the Cardiff Mastalgia Clinic. J Royal Soc Med 1992;85:12-15
Illustrations: N/A
Internet references: http://www.5mcc.com

Author(s)
Marjorie A. Bowman, MD, MPA

Mastoiditis

BASICS

DESCRIPTION   Inflammatory process in the mastoid air cells
• Acute mastoiditis - acute suppurative inflammatory process, typically after acute otitis media
• Chronic mastoiditis - usually associated with cholesteatoma and chronic ear disease
System(s) affected: Pulmonary
Genetics: No known genetic pattern
Incidence/Prevalence in USA: Unknown
Predominant age: Children, middle age
Predominant sex: Male = Female

SIGNS AND SYMPTOMS
• Otalgia
• Bulging erythematous tympanic membrane
• Post-auricular edema/mass
• Post-auricular erythema
• Post-auricular tenderness
• Protrusion of auricle
• Fever
• Increased WBC
• Clouding of mastoid air cells on plain films
• Fluid density in middle ear/mastoid air cells with or without loss of bony architecture
• Possible otorrhea if perforated tympanic membrane
• Subperiostial abscess

CAUSES
• Acute otitis media
• Inadequately treated suppurative otitis media
• Cholesteatoma
• Blockage of outflow tract of mastoid air cells (additus ad antrum)

RISK FACTORS
• Cholesteatoma
• Recurrent acute otitis media
• Immunocompromised host

DIAGNOSIS

DIFFERENTIAL DIAGNOSIS
• Post-auricular inflammatory adenopathy
• Severe external otitis
• Post auricular cellulitis
• Benign neoplasm - aneurysmal bone cyst, fibrous dysplasia
• Malignant neoplasm - rhabdomyosarcoma

LABORATORY   CBC with differential - increased WBC
Drugs that may alter lab results: N/A
Disorders that may alter lab results: N/A

PATHOLOGICAL FINDINGS
• Inflammatory tissue in air cell system
• Granulation tissue
• Osteitis

SPECIAL TESTS   Consider audiogram

IMAGING
• Plain mastoid films - clouding of mastoid air cells
• CT scan if complication suspected. Cloud air cells - loss of bony septation of the air cell system.

DIAGNOSTIC PROCEDURES   N/A

TREATMENT

APPROPRIATE HEALTH CARE
Hospitalized during acute phase

GENERAL MEASURES
• Keep ear dry

SURGICAL MEASURES
• Myringotomy; placement of pressure equalization (PE) tube
• Culture material obtained at myringotomy
• Frequent cleaning of ear canal under microscope to assure PE tube patency and adequate drainage of middle ear
• IV antibiotics to cover the most common organisms
• Topical antibiotic drops are also usually used after insertion of PE tube
• If subperiosteal abscess present, it should be aspirated. If aspiration is not sufficient, incision and drainage should be performed.
• Mastoidectomy is reserved for those patients failing to respond to above measures within 18-72 hours or those with meningeal or intracranial complications

ACTIVITY   Fully active, water precautions

DIET   No special diet

PATIENT EDUCATION   Griffith: Instructions for Patients; Philadelphia, W.B. Saunders Co., 1994

Mastoiditis

MEDICATIONS

DRUG(S) OF CHOICE
• IV antibiotics:
◊ Directed against most common organisms - group A beta-hemolytic strep, S. pneumonia, Hemophilus influenza
◊ In patients with cholesteatoma, consider Proteus, Bacteroides and occasional S. aureus and Pseudomonas organisms
◊ IV antibiotics for adult - ampicillin, 1-2 gm q6h or ampicillin-sulbactam (Unasyn) or cefuroxime, 750 mg q8h, to ensure coverage of beta-lactamase producing organisms
◊ IV antibiotics for children - ampicillin, 100-200 mg/kg/day divided q6h or cefuroxime, 750 mg q8h
• Topical/oral antibiotics:
◊ Topical drops - neomycin-polymyxin B-hydrocortisone (Cortisporin) otic drops or gentamicin ophthalmic solution
◊ Oral antibiotic - amoxicillin-clavulanate (Augmentin)
Contraindications: Refer to manufacturer's literature
Precautions: Refer to manufacturer's literature
Significant possible interactions: Refer to manufacturer's literature

ALTERNATIVE DRUGS
Other antibiotics depending on pathogen sensitivity

FOLLOWUP

PATIENT MONITORING
• Postoperative - audiogram after acute process subsided
• Frequent cleansing of ear canal to keep PE tube patent

PREVENTION/AVOIDANCE
• Adequate antibiotic treatment for acute otitis media
• Treatment of chronic eustachian tube dysfunction (PE tubes)
• Early identification of cholesteatoma

POSSIBLE COMPLICATIONS
• Subperiosteal abscess
• Gradenigo's syndrome (sixth nerve palsy, draining ear and retro-orbital pain)
• Bezold's abscess
• Sigmoid sinus thrombosis
• Meningitis
• Intracranial abscess epidural/subdural/intraparenchymal

EXPECTED COURSE/PROGNOSIS
• Dependent on severity of disease
• Conductive hearing loss may require reconstructive surgery
• Expect to avoid complications with early treatment

MISCELLANEOUS

ASSOCIATED CONDITIONS N/A

AGE-RELATED FACTORS
Pediatric: N/A
Geriatric: N/A
Others: N/A

PREGNANCY N/A

SYNONYMS N/A

ICD-9-CM
• 383.9 Coalescent mastoiditis
• 383.00 Acute or subacute mastoiditis
• 383.02 Acute with Gradenigo's syndrome
• 383.02 Acute with petrositis
• 383.01 Acute with subperiosteal abscess

SEE ALSO N/A

OTHER NOTES N/A

ABBREVIATIONS PE = pressure equalization

REFERENCES Paparella MM, Shumrick DA, et al, eds: Otolaryngology. 4th Ed. Philadelphia, W.B. Saunders Co., 1991
Illustrations: N/A
Internet references: http://www.5mcc.com

Author(s)
Laurene L. Howell, MD
Sean O. McMenomey, MD

Measles, rubella

BASICS

DESCRIPTION An endemic and epidemic viral exanthematous infection of children and adults, worldwide in distribution. Many infections are subclinical, but this virus can potentially cause fetal infection with resultant birth defects.
System(s) affected: Nervous, Skin/Exocrine
Genetics: Children with congenital rubella syndrome and children with insulin dependent diabetes mellitus share a high frequency of HLA-DR3 histocompatibility antigen and a high prevalence of islet cell antibodies
Incidence/Prevalence in USA:
• Before rubella vaccine was introduced in 1969, epidemics occurred at 6-9 year intervals. Sporadic outbreaks continue to occur in hospitals, colleges, prisons, prenatal clinics and isolated religious communities.
• In 1996, the incidence of postnatal rubella was 0.08 cases per 100,000 population.
Predominant age: Children 5-9 years of age
Predominant sex: Male = Female

SIGNS AND SYMPTOMS
• Postnatal rubella
  ◊ Adenopathy - posterior auricular, posterior cervical, suboccipital
  ◊ Low-grade fever
  ◊ Exanthem - descending, maculopapular, may desquamate
  ◊ Enanthem - soft palate petechiae (Forschheimer's sign)
  ◊ Conjunctivitis
  ◊ Splenomegaly, rarely
  ◊ Coryza
  ◊ Malaise
  ◊ Headache
  ◊ Polyarthralgia/polyarthritis, especially in young women
  ◊ Asymptomatic (25%-50%)
• Congenital rubella: (T = Transient, P = Permanent, D = Developmental)
  ◊ Cataracts (P)
  ◊ Microphthalmia (P)
  ◊ Chorioretinitis (P)
  ◊ Patent ductus arteriosus (P)
  ◊ Pulmonic stenosis (P,D)
  ◊ Atrial and ventricular septal defects (P)
  ◊ Sensorineural deafness (P,D)
  ◊ Microcephaly (P)
  ◊ Meningoencephalitis (T)
  ◊ Mental retardation (P,D)
  ◊ Low birth weight (T)
  ◊ Purpuric ("blueberry muffin") skin lesions (T)
  ◊ Radiolucent bone disease (T)
  ◊ Hepatosplenomegaly (T)
  ◊ Large anterior fontanelle (T)
  ◊ Language and behavior disorders (P,D)
  ◊ Cryptorchidism (P)
  ◊ Inguinal hernia (P)

CAUSES Rubella virus is a single-stranded RNA virus in the togavirus family. Travelling via airborne droplets of nasopharyngeal secretions, the virus replicates in the nasopharynx and regional lymph nodes during a 16-18 day incubation period. After invading the bloodstream, it may spread to skin and other distal organs or, transplacentally, to the developing fetus. Fetal viremia may then produce disseminated fetal infection. Organogenesis occurs 2 to 6 weeks postconception, so that infection is a maximum hazard (40-80% risk) to heart and eyes at that time. During the second trimester, the fetus develops increasing immunologic competence, making it less susceptible (10% risk) to the effects of intrauterine infection.

RISK FACTORS
• Inadequate immunization
• Immunodeficiency states
• Immunosuppressive therapy
• Pregnancy
• Crowded living conditions
• School, day care
• Late winter, spring seasons

DIAGNOSIS

DIFFERENTIAL DIAGNOSIS
• Postnatal rubella
  ◊ Measles virus (rubeola)
  ◊ Scarlet fever
  ◊ Infectious mononucleosis
  ◊ Toxoplasmosis
  ◊ Roseola infantum (exanthem subitum)
  ◊ Erythema infectiosum (fifth disease)
  ◊ Drug eruptions
  ◊ Other exanthematous enteroviral infections
• Congenital rubella
  ◊ Cytomegalovirus
  ◊ Varicella-zoster virus
  ◊ Picornaviruses (coxsackievirus, echovirus)
  ◊ Poliovirus
  ◊ Herpes simplex virus
  ◊ Western equine virus
  ◊ Measles virus (rubeola)
  ◊ Hepatitis B virus
  ◊ Mumps virus
  ◊ Influenza virus
  ◊ Toxoplasmosis
  ◊ Congenital syphilis
  ◊ Malaria

LABORATORY
• Postnatal rubella
  ◊ Mild leukopenia with relative lymphocytosis
  ◊ Fourfold rise in serum levels of antibody to rubella virus
  ◊ Pharynx, nose and blood culture positivity to rubella virus
• Congenital rubella
  ◊ Presence of rubella-specific IgM antibody in serum up to one year of age, at which time, IgG becomes the dominant antibody
  ◊ Isolation of rubella virus from pharynx, blood, urine, cerebrospinal fluid
Drugs that may alter lab results: N/A
Disorders that may alter lab results: After re-exposure to rubella, a person with a low level of antibody from past infection or vaccination may experience an acute rise in antibody. This is not associated with a high incidence of contagion to others nor of fetal risk.

PATHOLOGICAL FINDINGS
• Inhibition of cellular growth after infection
• Fetal vasculitis
• Placental angiopathy
• Tissue necrosis

SPECIAL TESTS Cell-mediated immune responses (CMI) are impaired selectively in children with congenital rubella

IMAGING N/A

DIAGNOSTIC PROCEDURES Congenital rubella has been diagnosed by placental biopsy at 12 weeks

TREATMENT

APPROPRIATE HEALTH CARE
Outpatient usually

GENERAL MEASURES
• Postnatal rubella - mild and self-limited. Treat for symptomatic relief.
• Congenital rubella - supportive, unless neurologic or hemorrhagic complications develop

SURGICAL MEASURES N/A

ACTIVITY
• For postnatal rubella - contact isolation for 7 days after onset of rash, bedrest is not necessary
• Contact isolation of congenitally infected infants for one year, unless nasopharyngeal and urine cultures after 3 months of age are negative for rubella virus

DIET No special diet

PATIENT EDUCATION Make every effort to avoid exposing infected patient to pregnant women

MEDICATIONS

DRUG(S) OF CHOICE Acetaminophen for fever every 4 hours if needed - 10-15 mg/kg/dose
Contraindications: N/A
Precautions: N/A
Significant possible interactions: N/A

ALTERNATIVE DRUGS None

FOLLOWUP

PATIENT MONITORING
• Persons immune to rubella via natural infection or vaccine may be reinfected when re-exposed. This infection is usually asymptomatic and detectable only by serologic means.
• In congenital rubella, it is extremely important to detect auditory and visual impairment early, so that adequate education and counselling can begin

PREVENTION/AVOIDANCE
• Rubella vaccine
◊ A 2-dose schedule in combination with measles and mumps (MMR) is recommended for those born after 1956. The first dose is recommended at age 12-15 months; the second dose is recommended either at 4-6 years of age or at 11-12 years of age
◊ Recommended for susceptible individuals in the following groups: Prepubertal boys and girls, premarital or postpartum women, college students, day care personnel, health care workers, military personnel
◊ It is contraindicated in: Pregnancy, immunodeficiency or immunocompromised state (except HIV), receipt within the last 3 months of immunoglobulin (Ig) or blood, severe febrile illness, or hypersensitivity to vaccine components
◊ Persons who receive rubella vaccine do not transmit rubella to others, although the virus can be isolated from the pharynx

POSSIBLE COMPLICATIONS
• Postnatal rubella
◊ Postinfectious encephalitis (1/5,000 cases)
◊ Thrombocytopenic purpura (1/3,000 cases)
◊ Testicular pain
◊ Mild hepatitis
• Congenital rubella
◊ Spontaneous abortion
◊ Stillbirth
◊ Premature delivery
◊ Progressive rubella panencephalitis
◊ Endocrine disturbances (diabetes, thyrotoxicosis, hypothyroidism)
• Rubella vaccine
◊ Lymphadenopathy
◊ Fever
◊ Rash
◊ Arthritis/arthralgia (older girls, women)
◊ Polyneuropathy

EXPECTED COURSE/PROGNOSIS
• Postnatal rubella
◊ Fever, 1-2 days
◊ Rash, 3 days
◊ Coryza, 5 days
◊ Lymphadenopathy, 1 week
◊ Arthralgia (when present), 2 weeks
◊ Complete and full recovery without sequelae is the rule
• Congenital rubella
◊ Varied and unpredictable spectrum of consequences, ranging from stillbirth to completely normal infancy and childhood
◊ Disease characterized by chronic infection; infants may remain contagious for months after birth
◊ Detectable levels of hemagglutination-inhibiting antibody (IgG) persist for years, then may decline. By age 5, 20% have no detectable antibody.
◊ Overall mortality 10%; greatest during first 6 months
◊ 70% of those with encephalitis develop residual neuromotor defects, including an autistic syndrome
◊ Prognosis is excellent when only minor defects are present

MISCELLANEOUS

ASSOCIATED CONDITIONS N/A

AGE-RELATED FACTORS
Pediatric:
• Postnatal rubella is a milder disease in children than it is in adults
• Adolescents and young adults currently account for about 60% of all new cases
Geriatric: N/A
Others: N/A

PREGNANCY
• Women vaccinated against rubella are advised not to become pregnant for at least 3 months after receiving the vaccine
• The vaccine-type virus can cross the placenta. However, no case of congenital rubella has ever occurred in newborns of women who were inadvertently vaccinated while pregnant.
• The minimal fetal risk in women "accidentally" vaccinated while pregnant does not mandate automatic termination of a pregnancy
• If a pregnant woman is exposed to rubella (native disease, not vaccine associated), an immediate antibody titer should be obtained. Presence of antibody means that the woman is immune and not at risk. If antibody is not detectable, a second titer should be obtained 3 weeks later. If antibody is present in the second specimen, infection has occurred. If antibody is again negative, a third titer should be obtained in 3 more weeks (6 weeks after exposure). At this time, a negative test means that infection has not occurred; a positive test means that infection did occur, and that the fetus is at risk for congenital rubella.
• The use of commercially available human immunoglobulin (gamma globulin) in prophylaxis of rubella during pregnancy does not prevent rubella or the congenital rubella syndrome in a predictable or reliable fashion
• A reliable PCR-based method of detecting viral RNA may allow much more rapid prenatal diagnosis of rubella virus infection. Routine use is not yet available.

SYNONYMS
• German measles
• Three-day measles

ICD-9-CM
056.9 Uncomplicated postnatal rubella
056.XX Postnatal rubella with specific complications
771.0 Congenital rubella syndrome

SEE ALSO
• Measles, rubeola
• Immunizations

OTHER NOTES N/A

ABBREVIATIONS N/A

REFERENCES
• Committee on Infectious Diseases, Elk Grove, Illinois, AAP Red Book, ed. 23, 1994
• Mandell GL, ed: Principles and Practice of Infectious Diseases. 4th Ed. New York, Churchill Livingstone, 1995
• Rudolph AM, ed: Rudolph's Pediatrics. 20th Ed. Norwalk, CT, Appleton & Lange, 1996
• Revello MG, et al: Prenatal diagnosis of rubella virus infection by direct detection and semiquantitation of viral RNA in clinical samples by reverse transcription-PCR. J Clin Microbiol 1997;35:708-713
Illustrations: 1 available on CD-ROM
Internet references: http://www.5mcc.com

Author(s)
Richard Viken, MD

Measles, rubeola

BASICS

DESCRIPTION An acute epidemic viral exanthem which classically presents as a confluent erythematous maculopapular rash which begins over the head and spreads inferiorly to involve the trunk and extremities. The rash is preceded by the triad of cough, coryza, and conjunctivitis plus a pathognomonic enanthem (Koplik's spots).
System(s) affected: Skin/Exocrine
Genetics: N/A
Incidence/Prevalence in USA: Number of cases peaked during 1990, 27,786; followed by marked decline, 1995 total of 309 the lowest number ever recorded in the United States (1% of these secondary to imported cases)
Predominant Age: Increasing proportion of cases since 1991 have occurred among older age groups (1995, 39% of cases among persons age ≥ 20 years). Genomic sequencing of isolates from 1995 outbreaks were similar to viruses isolated in Europe and Japan suggesting interruption of indigenous measles transmission. Attack rate (# cases/100,000): 1991 - 3.82, 1992 - 0.87, 1993 - 0.12, 1994 - 0.37
Predominant sex: Male = Female

SIGNS AND SYMPTOMS
• Incubation period:
  ◊ 10+/-2 days from exposure to symptoms
  ◊ 14 days average to onset of rash (range 7-18 days)
  ◊ Patients contagious from 1-2 days before symptoms (3-5 days before rash) to 4 days after onset of rash, immunocompromised patients contagious for the duration of the illness
• Prodromal period:
  ◊ Lasts 3+/-1 days
  ◊ Classic triad (brassy cough, coryza, and conjunctivitis)
  ◊ Fever
  ◊ Malaise
  ◊ Photophobia
  ◊ Enanthem (Koplik's spots) - minute, whitish spots over buccal/labial mucosa; number rapidly increases and these coalesce. Underlying mucosa bright red and granular; spots appear 2 days before rash and resolve within 3 days after rash onset.
• Exanthem period:
  ◊ Begins behind ears and at hairline
  ◊ Spreads centrifugally from head to feet
  ◊ Red, morbilliform, blanching rash
  ◊ Discrete lesions become confluent
  ◊ Confluence more prominent over upper body
  ◊ Clearing begins after 3-4 days
  ◊ Rash becomes coppery and nonblanching
  ◊ Fever resolves 2-3 days after onset of rash
  ◊ Pharyngitis
  ◊ Lymphadenopathy
  ◊ Croup, vomiting, and diarrhea (in young children)
  ◊ Patients contagious from 2 days before symptoms to 4 days after onset of rash

• Modified illness:
  ◊ Attenuated measles in partially immune patient
  ◊ Secondary prior immune globulin, transplacental measles antibody, live vaccine failure
• Atypical measles:
  ◊ Most cases secondary to natural infection following vaccination with killed vaccine (available in U.S. 1963-68; Canada until 1975)
  ◊ Maculopapular rash begins distally and spreads centrally
  ◊ Rash frequently is petechial, purpuric, or urticarial
  ◊ Pulmonary involvement in all cases
  ◊ Frequency decreasing

CAUSES Single antigenic type of a RNA morbillivirus in the paramyxovirus family

RISK FACTORS Not being vaccinated

DIAGNOSIS

DIFFERENTIAL DIAGNOSIS
• Typical measles:
  ◊ Any erythematous maculopapular rash
• Exanthems secondary to:
  ◊ Drug eruptions
  ◊ Infectious mononucleosis
  ◊ Mycoplasma pneumoniae
  ◊ Rubella
  ◊ Erythema infectiosum
  ◊ Roseola
  ◊ Enteroviruses
• Atypical measles:
  ◊ Rocky Mountain spotted fever
  ◊ Drug eruptions
  ◊ Anaphylactoid purpura
  ◊ Mycoplasma pneumoniae infection

LABORATORY
• Viral isolation in tissue culture
• Detection of measles antigen in exfoliative cells by immunofluorescence
• Demonstration of measles specific IgM or substantial rise in IgG titers between acute and convalescent sera
Drugs that may alter lab results:
Immunosuppressive agents which may impair rise in specific antibody titers
Disorders that may alter lab results:
• Primary (severe combined immunodeficiency [SCID], etc.)
• Acquired immune deficiencies (HIV-1 infection, cancer chemotherapy)

PATHOLOGICAL FINDINGS
• Multinucleated giant cells
  ◊ Reticuloendothelial types (Warthin-Finkeldey) in lymphoid tissues
  ◊ Epithelial syncytial giant cells in skin, and respiratory mucosa
  ◊ Damaged respiratory ciliated epithelium

SPECIAL TESTS N/A

IMAGING N/A

DIAGNOSTIC PROCEDURES N/A

TREATMENT

APPROPRIATE HEALTH CARE
Outpatient except when complications develop (encephalitis, pneumonitis)

GENERAL MEASURES
• Symptomatic therapy (i.e., antipyretics, antitussives, humidification, encourage oral fluids)
• Control
  ◊ All cases should be placed in respiratory isolation until 4 days after the onset of the exanthem; immunocompromised patients should be isolated for the entire illness
  ◊ Notify public health officials of suspected cases
  ◊ Initiate preventive measures for all exposed susceptible persons or those at high risk for severe infection (i.e., symptomatic HIV infection, children less than 12 months)
  ◊ Live measles vaccine can provide protection to susceptible persons if given within 72 hours postexposure
  ◊ Immune globulin (Ig) given within 6 days postexposure can prevent or modify measles infection (0.25 mL/kg, maximum dose 15 mL; 0.5 mL/kg for immunocompromised patients)
  ◊ Patients with symptomatic HIV infection should receive Ig regardless of prior immunization
  ◊ Ig also indicated for susceptible household contacts of measles patient and pregnant women

SURGICAL MEASURES N/A

ACTIVITY Restricted during febrile phase

DIET As tolerated

PATIENT EDUCATION Avoid exposure to other children and potential secondary bacterial pathogens until respiratory symptoms resolve

MEDICATIONS

DRUG(S) OF CHOICE
• No proven specific antiviral agent is available
• Following the onset of infection, immune globulin has no significant effect on symptoms and duration of illness
• Antibiotics reserved for bacterial superinfection
Contraindications: Steroids contraindicated
Precautions: N/A
Significant possible interactions: N/A

ALTERNATIVE DRUGS
• Vitamin A
◊ 200,000 IU po per day for 2 days (100,000 IU between 6-12 months) has been shown to decrease the mortality and morbidity of severe measles in areas where vitamin A deficiency exists and mortality related to measles is ≥ 1%; efficacy in non-life-threatening infections not established
◊ Vitamin A currently recommended for the following patients:
1. Children 6-24 months hospitalized with complications of measles
2. Children over 6 months with immunodeficiency, malabsorption, moderate to severe malnutrition, ophthalmologic evidence of vitamin A deficiency, or recent immigration from areas with vitamin A deficiency
• Ribavirin
◊ Virus susceptible in vitro to ribavirin
◊ Immunosuppressed children with severe measles have been treated with IV or aerosolized ribavirin, but no controlled data and not approved by FDA

FOLLOWUP

PATIENT MONITORING   Not required unless complications develop

PREVENTION/AVOIDANCE
• Postexposure prophylaxis
◊ Vaccine use - protective if given within 72 hours postexposure
◊ Immune globulin (Ig) - prevents/modifies illness if given within 6 days postexposure. Dose - usually 0.25 mL/kg IM (for immunocompromised children 0.5 mL/kg IM) not to exceed 15 mL.
• Active immunization:
◊ Moraten strain vaccine - only currently licensed vaccine available as monovalent vaccine or in combination with mumps and rubella i.e., measles and rubella (MR); measles, mumps and rubella (MMR)
• Indications:
◊ Primary vaccination: Two doses of vaccine; 1st MMR at 12-15 months, 2nd at 11-12 years (2nd dose may be given at 4-6 years). Need for 2nd dose necessitated by recent outbreaks among adolescents and young adults. During outbreaks, monovalent measles vaccine may be given to infants > 6 months. These children must be vaccinated with MMR as above. For a comprehensive discussion of the complete use and control of measles outbreaks, the reader is referred to the first listing in References.
◊ HIV infected children should be vaccinated while asymptomatic
• Adverse events associated with vaccination (in 5-15% of susceptible vaccinees):
◊ Fever (7-12 days after)
◊ Transient rashes (in 5% of vaccinees)
◊ Convulsions (most likely febrile)

POSSIBLE COMPLICATIONS
• Otitis media (most common)
• Laryngotracheitis
• Bronchopneumonia - viral (Hecht's or giant cell pneumonitis) or bacterial in origin
• Encephalitis (incidence 1 per 1000)
• Hemorrhagic lesions ("black measles") of skin and bowel
• Thrombocytopenic purpura
• Myocarditis and pericarditis
• Subacute sclerosing panencephalitis - secondary to persistent infection following natural disease; disappearing as a result of mass vaccination

EXPECTED COURSE/PROGNOSIS
Self-limited; prognosis good

MISCELLANEOUS

ASSOCIATED CONDITIONS
• Primary measles in an immunosuppressed patient with leukemia or symptomatic HIV-1 infection may present with or without a rash and giant cell pneumonitis
• Giant cell pneumonitis
• Increased mortality with malnutrition
• Possible reactivation of latent tuberculosis secondary to measles

AGE-RELATED FACTORS
Pediatric: Infants have higher rate of complications than older children
Geriatric: N/A
Others: N/A

PREGNANCY   Increased fetal morbidity and mortality with infection during pregnancy

SYNONYMS   Rubeola

ICD-9-CM   055.9 Measles without mention of complication

SEE ALSO   Measles, rubella

OTHER NOTES   N/A

ABBREVIATIONS   N/A

REFERENCES
• Measles. In Report of the Committee on Infectious Diseases, 308-323, American Academy of Pediatrics, 1994
• Measles Prevention: Recommendations of the Immunization Practices Advisory Committee (ACIP). Morbidity and Mortality Weekly Report, Recommendations and Reports. 38 (S-9):1-13, 1989
• Cherry J: Measles. In: Feigin R, Cherry J, eds. Textbook of Pediatric Infectious Diseases. 3rd Ed. Philadelphia, W.B. Saunders Co., 1992
Illustrations: N/A
Internet references: http://www.5mcc.com

Author(s)
Charles D. Mitchell, MD

Melanoma

BASICS

DESCRIPTION Malignant degeneration of cells from the melanocytic system. The overwhelming majority of melanoma arises in the skin, but it may also present as a primary lesion in any tissue pigmentation. Metastatic spread may be to any region in the body.
• Lentigo maligna - a cutaneous lesion that is the slowest growing malignant melanoma and has the least tendency to metastasize. Occurs most often on the face, beginning as a circumscribed macular patch of mottled pigmentation showing shades of dark brown, tan, or black.
• Ocular - a malignant progressive lesion of the eye

System(s) affected: Skin/Exocrine

Genetics:
• The only genetic predisposition is in the familial dysplastic nevus syndrome. If the family history of a person with dysplastic nevus syndrome includes one relative with melanoma, then the risk of developing melanoma is 100%.
• Skin pigmentation is the only other risk factor transmitted genetically

Incidence/Prevalence in USA:
• 4.5/100,000 people in the USA
• Estimated year 1995, 38,000 cases, 6,700 deaths
• Estimated year 2000, 1 in 75 persons then living will eventually die of malignant melanoma

Predominant age:
• A median age is 53 with the highest annual incidence rate of any cancer in whites between the ages of 25-29 and in white males between 35-39
• Greater than 50% of all individuals with melanoma are between ages 20-40

Predominant sex: Male = Female

SIGNS AND SYMPTOMS Any change in a pigmented lesion including hypo- or hyperpigmentation, bleeding, scaling, size change, texture change

CAUSES Under investigation. Probably radiation in the ultraviolet A+B range.

RISK FACTORS
• Adulthood
• Previous pigmented lesions (especially dysplastic nevi)
• Fair complexioned, freckling, blue eyes and blond hair
• Twice the risk in persons with adolescent blistering sunburn, family history of previous melanoma, congenital nevi
• Intermittent UV exposure (seasonal)
• Those with increased numbers of nevi
• Family history of melanoma

DIAGNOSIS

DIFFERENTIAL DIAGNOSIS
• Dysplastic nevi
• Vascular skin tumors
• Pigmented squamous cell and basal cell carcinomas, seborrheic keratoses, other changing nevi. It follows the ABCDE mnemonic which stands for (1) asymmetry, (2) border irregularity, (3) color variegation, and (4) diameter great than 6 millimeters with the location on whites being primarily back and lower leg, and on African Americans being hands, feet, and nails, (5) elevation above skin surface.

LABORATORY N/A
Drugs that may alter lab results: N/A
Disorders that may alter lab results: N/A

PATHOLOGICAL FINDINGS
• Gross pathologic features include four clinical types:
  ◊ Superficial spreading melanoma - 70% of all cases
  ◊ Nodular - 15% of all cases
  ◊ Acral lentiginous - 2-8% of all cases
  ◊ Lentigo-maligna - 4-10% of all cases
  ◊ Note: Nodular melanoma is primarily vertical growth while the other three types are horizontal

SPECIAL TESTS The only special tests that exist for melanoma are those designed to follow metastatic disease

IMAGING Imaging studies are of benefit only in detecting metastatic disease which is usually to the brain, lymph nodes and lungs

DIAGNOSTIC PROCEDURES Surgical biopsy is the only form of appropriate diagnostic procedure

TREATMENT

APPROPRIATE HEALTH CARE
Outpatient or inpatient surgery

GENERAL MEASURES The key to the cure of melanoma is prevention: Avoidance of blistering solar radiation and the use of a sunscreen when exposure is unavoidable

SURGICAL MEASURES The appropriate health care for melanoma is surgical excision. Much debate exists as to the extent of the margins of excision once diagnosis has been made. The tendency now is toward margins of 1 cm if the lesion is less than 2 mm thick. If thicker, then margins can be extended to 3 cm. Regional lymph node dissection is of some benefit in a few studies.

ACTIVITY Avoid sun exposure

DIET No restrictions

PATIENT EDUCATION
• It is critical that a patient with melanoma or dysplastic nevi syndrome has frequent total body examinations for any abnormal appearing or changing nevi
• National Cancer Institute, Dept. of Health And Human Services, Public Inquiries Section, Office of Cancer Communications, Building 31, Room 101-18, 9000 Rockville Pike, Bethesda, MD 20892, (301)496-5583

Melanoma

MEDICATIONS

DRUG(S) OF CHOICE
• Adjuvant chemotherapy has included bacillus Calmette-Guérin (BCG) and levamisole
• Standard chemotherapy includes dacarbazine
• Adoptive immunotherapy with leukapheresis and IL-2 with LAK's (under investigation)
• Some benefit with vaccines containing melanoma associated antigens (MAAs) has occurred
Contraindications: Refer to manufacturer's literature
Precautions: Dacarbazine - myelosuppression, alopecia
Significant possible interactions: Refer to manufacturer's literature

ALTERNATIVE DRUGS Many have been tried; recent trials show some promise

FOLLOWUP

PATIENT MONITORING
• Current recommendations after diagnosis of malignant melanoma are skin exams every 3-6 months
• Only chest x-rays on an annual basis have been shown to be of any benefit at all in that 6% of recurrences were detected
• The patient should conduct his/her own skin examinations on a weekly basis. They must be thorough.

PREVENTION/AVOIDANCE Avoidance of burning solar exposures and the use of sunscreens is critical. Those at high risk should do all they can to avoid sunburn especially during the adolescent years.

POSSIBLE COMPLICATIONS
• Metastatic spread
• Unsatisfactory cosmetic results following the primary surgery

EXPECTED COURSE/PROGNOSIS
• Prognosis is entirely based on staging of the initial lesion
• Staging (falls into two categories)
  ◊ Breslow: This shows a 70% five-year survival of all patients who have no local or distant lymphatic spread.
  ◊ Clark's staging depends on depth of invasion by skin layer. The best prognosis is for those lesions which are less than .85 mm (especially if restricted to the stratum granulosum or higher) which carry 95-100% five-year survival. Spread to lymphatics or regional lymph nodes carries less than a 5% five-year survival.

MISCELLANEOUS

ASSOCIATED CONDITIONS As above

AGE-RELATED FACTORS
Pediatric: Rarely seen in pediatric age group
Geriatric: Lentigo maligna is most commonly seen in elderly patients who have had a slowly enlarging pigmented lesion, usually found on the face
Others: The most recent data on melanoma indicates that its highest incidence is between ages 30-50. However, it can occur at any age.

PREGNANCY
• Due to the facts that melanocyte-stimulating hormone (MSH) levels are markedly increased during pregnancy and that melanoma is one of the few carcinomas that can spread to the placenta, concern has been that pregnancy exacerbates melanoma. This has been neither proven nor disproven.
• If a person has had recent melanoma, many authors suggest waiting at least two years if further pregnancy is desired
• If invasion extends into the lymphatic structures, then further pregnancy is probably contraindicated
• If pregnancy occurs during metastatic melanoma, then there is clear risk to the fetus

SYNONYMS N/A

ICD-9-CM
172.9 Melanoma of skin, site unspecified

SEE ALSO N/A

OTHER NOTES It is imperative for the physician to realize that any nevus or pigmented lesion that is in any way suspect should be excised. A full thickness total excisional biopsy must be sent for pathologic specimen and never to be curetted, electrodesiccated, or shaved.

ABBREVIATIONS N/A

REFERENCES
• Koh HK: Cutaneous Melanoma. N Engl J Med 1991;325:171-182
• Malignant melanoma-CA. American Cancer Society. July/Aug 1996;46:4
• Johnson TM, et al: Current therapy for cutaneous melanoma. J Am Acad Dermatol 1995;32:689-707
Illustrations: 16 available on CD-ROM
Internet references: http://www.5mcc.com

Author(s)
David P. Sealy, MD

Ménière's disease

BASICS

DESCRIPTION An inner ear (labyrinthine) disorder in which there is an increase in volume and pressure of the inner-most fluid of the inner ear (endolymph), resulting in recurrent attacks of hearing loss, tinnitus, vertigo, and fullness
• Usually unilateral, but in 10-50% may later involve the second ear
• Severity and frequency may diminish over the years, but with increasing loss of hearing. It is not a synonym for dizziness.
System(s) affected: Nervous
Genetics: N/A
Incidence/Prevalence in USA:
• No reliable figures are available to provide comprehensive numbers for incidence and prevalence by age and sex, but using incidence figures from a Swedish study conducted in 1973, it is estimated that the incidence of Ménière's disease in the US is 46 (new cases/100,000/year). No figures for sex and age are available, but the disease is relatively equal in males and females, and is extremely rare in children.
• Using extrapolation, the estimated prevalence is 1,150 (cases/100,000 population)
Predominant age: Usual age of onset 20-60
Predominant sex: Male = Female

SIGNS AND SYMPTOMS
• Hearing loss - low frequency, fluctuating
• Vertigo - spontaneous attacks, duration 20 minutes to several hours
• Ear fullness
• Occurs as attacks, with intervening remission
• During severe attacks
  ◊ Pallor
  ◊ Sweating
  ◊ Nausea and vomiting
  ◊ Falling
  ◊ Prostration
  ◊ All symptoms aggravated by motion
  ◊ Between attacks may experience motion-related imbalance without vertigo

CAUSES
• Unknown. Best theory is inner ear response to variety of injuries (reduced middle ear pressure, allergy, endocrine disease, lipid disorders, vascular, viral, luetic).
• Recent theory is intracranial compression of balance nerve by blood vessel

RISK FACTORS
• Caucasian
• Stress
• Allergy
• Increased salt intake
• Noise

DIAGNOSIS

DIFFERENTIAL DIAGNOSIS
• Acoustic tumor
• Syphilis
• Perilymph fistula
• Multiple sclerosis
• Viral labyrinthitis
• Vertebro-basilar disease
• Other labyrinthine disorders producing same symptoms (Cogan's syndrome, benign positional vertigo, temporal bone trauma)

LABORATORY
• Lab studies done to rule out other conditions
• Serologic tests specific for Treponema pallidum - microhemagglutination (MHA), fluorescent treponemal antibody (FTA), Treponema immobilization test (TPI)
• Thyroid studies
• Lipid studies
Drugs that may alter lab results: Any medication that produces a significant degree of sedation is likely to affect vestibular testing and invalidate it
Disorders that may alter lab results: Many conditions may produce auditory and vestibular findings identical to those associated with Ménière's disease, making it a diagnosis of exclusion. A low frequency sensorineural hearing loss (nerve loss as opposed to conductive loss) is seen on audiometry, and a reduced caloric response on caloric testing is usual.

PATHOLOGICAL FINDINGS Autopsy only. Shows dilation of inner ear fluid system (endolymph).

SPECIAL TESTS
• Otoscopy with air pressure applied to the tympanic membrane
• Auditory
  ◊ Hearing test (audiometry using pure tone and speech) to show low frequency sensorineural [nerve] loss and impaired speech discrimination)
  ◊ Tuning fork test (Weber and Rinne) to confirm validity of audiometry
  ◊ Auditory Brainstem Response audiometry (ABR) to rule out acoustic neuroma
• Vestibular
  ◊ Spontaneous nystagmus (rapid rhythmic eye motion) seen visually. Must avoid eye fixation by having patient use 40 diopter glasses for test.
  ◊ Caloric testing - electronystagmography (ENG) may show reduced caloric response. Can obtain reasonably comparable information with use of 0.8 cc ice water instilled in ear canal, then noting duration and frequency of resulting nystagmus with 40 diopter lenses in place. Reduced activity on either side is consistent with Ménière's diagnosis, but is not diagnostic.

IMAGING MRI to rule out acoustic tumor, which can produce identical symptoms and findings

DIAGNOSTIC PROCEDURES N/A

TREATMENT

APPROPRIATE HEALTH CARE Can usually be managed in outpatient setting. Inpatient for surgery.

GENERAL MEASURES
• Medications are given primarily for symptomatic relief of vertigo and nausea. There is no medication available that influences the disease process.
• For attacks, bedrest with eyes closed and protection from falling. Attacks rarely last longer than four hours.
• Streptomycin therapy for bilateral Ménière's disease, when conventional management has failed. Streptomycin may be administered over a period of several days or weeks intentionally to damage the neuro-epithelium of the balance centers and reduce their function. Hearing must be carefully monitored during this time so that the treatment does not proceed to the point of damaging the hearing structures. This form of treatment should be administered only by an otolaryngologist and after careful patient education.

SURGICAL MEASURES
• Hearing good: Endolymphatic sac surgery, either (1) decompression or (2) drainage of endolymph into mastoid or subarachnoid space. Alternative procedure is to cut the vestibular nerve (intracranial procedure). A newer procedure involves placement of gentamycin through the tympanic membrane into the middle ear space.
• Hearing poor, but usable: Can do sac procedure, nerve section, or gentamycin instillation depending on quality of hearing. For poor hearing, can decompress cochlea (cochleocentesis), or perfuse cochlea with streptomycin.
• Hearing not useful: Destruction of inner ear (labyrinthectomy)

ACTIVITY
• Limit activity during attacks
• Between attacks patient may be fully active, but this may be limited by (1) fear of impending attack, (2) unsteadiness following attacks, (3) ear fullness or tinnitus, or (4) hearing loss in involved ear that may severely limit the patient's ability to perform work duties or to participate in social life

DIET Limit total intake during attacks because of nausea. Otherwise diet is usually not a factor unless attacks are brought on by certain foods. A restricted salt diet may be useful in some cases.

PATIENT EDUCATION Many otolaryngologists keep booklets on Ménière's disease as handouts. Ask your otolaryngology consultant for a supply.

MEDICATIONS

DRUG(S) OF CHOICE
• Acute attack. For severe episode, one of the following may be used. Adult doses are indicated
◊ Atropine 0.2-0.4 mg IV
◊ Diazepam (Valium) 5-10 mg IV slowly
◊ Transdermal scopolamine, 1 patch, or smaller segment of patch, applied to skin surface and not replaced sooner than 3 days
• Maintenance. Adult doses are indicated (frequently must be reduced to avoid sedating effects)
◊ Meclizine (Antivert, Bonine) 25-100 mg orally, either at bedtime or in divided doses
◊ Ergotamine-belladonna-phenobarbital (Bellergal Spacetabs), one q 12 hr
◊ Diazepam (Valium), 2 mg (or less) tid

Contraindications:
• Atropine - cardiac disease, especially supraventricular tachycardia and other arrhythmias
• Scopolamine - children and elderly

Precautions:
• Sedating drugs should be used with caution, particularly in elderly people. The need to reduce the dosage is common. Patients should be cautioned not to operate motor vehicles when they are sedated.
• Atropine, scopolamine, and Bellergal should be used with particular caution. If not prescribed frequently, refer to manufacturer's literature.

Significant possible interactions:
• Bellergal - oral anticoagulants, tricyclic antidepressants, phenothiazines, narcotics, beta blockers, estrogens, and others
• Transdermal scopolamine - anticholinergics, belladonna products, antihistamines, tricyclic antidepressants, and others

ALTERNATIVE DRUGS
• Acute attack
◊ Droperidol, 1.5-2.5 mg IV slowly (in hospital setting)
◊ Promethazine (Phenergan) 12.5-25 mg IV slowly
◊ Diphenhydramine (Benadryl) 50 mg IV slowly
◊ Carbogen (5% carbon dioxide and 95% oxygen) by mask from tank
• Maintenance
◊ Dimenhydrinate (Dramamine) 50 mg q4-6h po
◊ Promethazine (Phenergan) 12.5-25 mg q4-6h po
◊ Diphenidol (Vontrol) 25-50 mg tid po
◊ Diphenhydramine (Benadryl), 25-50 mg q6-8h po. Maximum, 100 mg/24 hours
◊ Chlorothiazide (Diuril) 500 mg daily po with potassium supplement

FOLLOWUP

PATIENT MONITORING
The most common complaint by Ménière's patients regarding prior treatment is that the primary care physician did not take the condition seriously and that he or she didn't seem interested in providing ongoing care. Because of the emotional impact alone, these patients need close followup care. It is important to monitor the status of their hearing, since it is at risk, and to continue to consider the possibility of a more serious underlying problem such as an acoustic tumor.

PREVENTION/AVOIDANCE
• Reduce stress
• Reduce salt intake
• Don't smoke
• Avoid significant noise exposure, or use ear protectors
• Avoid use of ototoxic medications (aspirin, quinine, kanamycin, and many others)

POSSIBLE COMPLICATIONS
• Failure to diagnose acoustic neuroma
• Loss of hearing
• Injury during attack
• Inability to work

EXPECTED COURSE/PROGNOSIS
• Alternating attacks and remission
• Over time the balance problem tends to resolve, but the hearing worsens
• The great majority of patients can be managed successfully with medication. About 5-10% of patients require surgery for incapacitating vertigo.
• Very important not to overlook acoustic tumor, which produces an identical clinical picture

MISCELLANEOUS

ASSOCIATED CONDITIONS
• Cochlear hydrops (hearing problem only)
• Vestibular hydrops (balance problem only)
• Drop attacks

AGE-RELATED FACTORS
Pediatric: Unusual, but occasional. Dizziness in children likely to be on basis of significant central nervous system disease.
Geriatric: Less likely to occur in elderly. Patients exposed to loud noise levels over many years are more susceptible.
Others: Usual onset age 20-60

PREGNANCY Not a common problem, but difficult to treat because of risk of producing fetal abnormalities with medication

SYNONYMS
• Ménière's syndrome
• Endolymphatic hydrops

ICD-9-CM 386.0 Meniere's disease

SEE ALSO N/A

OTHER NOTES N/A

ABBREVIATIONS N/A

REFERENCES
• Paparella MM, Shumrick DA, eds: Otolaryngology. 2nd Ed. Philadelphia, W.B. Saunders Co., 1980:1878-1889
• Schuknecht HF: Ménière's Disease. In: Britton BH, ed. Common Problems in Otology. St. Louis, Mosby Year Book, 1991:180-185
Illustrations: N/A
Internet references: http://www.5mcc.com

Author(s)
Gale Gardner, MD, FACS

Meningitis, bacterial

 BASICS

DESCRIPTION
Inflammation in response to bacterial infection of the pia-arachnoid and its fluid and the fluid of the ventricles. Meningitis is always cerebrospinal.
System(s) affected: Nervous
Genetics: Navajo Indian and American Eskimo may have genetic or acquired vulnerability to invasive disease
Incidence/Prevalence in USA: 3-10 cases per 100,000 population
Predominant age: Neonates, infants and geriatric aged
Predominant sex: Male = Female

SIGNS AND SYMPTOMS
• Antecedent URI
• Fever
• Headache
• Meningismus
• Signs of cerebral dysfunction
• Vomiting
• Photophobia
• Seizures
• Nausea
• Rigors
• Profuse sweats
• Weakness
• Altered mental status
• Focal neurologic deficits
• Elderly have subtle findings commonly including confusion
• Meningococcemia has rash - macular and erythematous at first, then petechial or purpuric

CAUSES
• Neonates: Group B or D Streptococcus, Escherichia coli, Listeria monocytogenes and non-group B Streptococcus
• Infants/children: H. influenzae (48%), Streptococcus pneumoniae (13%), and Neisseria meningitidis
• Adults: Streptococcus pneumoniae (30-50%), Haemophilus influenzae (1-3%), Neisseria meningitidis (10-35%), gram-negative bacilli (1-10%), Staphylococci (5-15%), Streptococci (5%) and Listeria species(5%)

RISK FACTORS
• Immunocompromised host
• Alcoholism
• Neurosurgical procedure or head injury
• Abdominal surgery for gram-negative

 DIAGNOSIS

DIFFERENTIAL DIAGNOSIS
• Bacteremia
• Sepsis
• Brain abscess
• Seizures
• Other non-bacterial meningitides

LABORATORY
• Turbid CSF
• Neonates
  ◊ > 10 WBC's in CSF
  ◊ CSF: blood glucose ratio < 0.6
  ◊ CSF protein >150 mg/dL (> 1500 mg/L)
• Infants/children
  ◊ > 5 WBC's in CSF
  ◊ CSF: blood glucose ratio < 0.6
  ◊ CSF protein > 50 mg/dL (> 500 mg/L)
• Adults
  ◊ 1000-100,000 WBC's in CSF (average 5000-20,000)
  ◊ CSF: blood glucose ratio < 0.4
  ◊ CSF protein > 45 mg/dL (> 450 mg/L) (usually 150-400 mg/dL [1500-4000 mg/L])
  ◊ Suspect ruptured brain abscess when WBC count is unusually high (±100,000)
• In all age groups:
  ◊ CSF opening pressure > 180 mm H2O (1.77 kPa)
  ◊ CSF Gram stain + in 75% of untreated patients
  ◊ CSF culture + 70-80% of the time
  ◊ Blood culture + 40-60% of the time
  ◊ CSF bacterial antigen test (sensitivity varies)
Drugs that may alter lab results: N/A
Disorders that may alter lab results: N/A

PATHOLOGICAL FINDINGS   N/A

SPECIAL TESTS   N/A

IMAGING
• CT scan of head if concern for increased intracranial pressure (ICP)
• Chest x-ray may reveal silent area of pneumonitis or abscess
• Sinus/skull x-rays may reveal cranial osteomyelitis, paranasal sinusitis or skull fracture
• Later in course, head CT scan, if hydrocephalus, brain abscess, subdural effusions or subdural empyema are considered

DIAGNOSTIC PROCEDURES   Lumbar puncture

 TREATMENT

APPROPRIATE HEALTH CARE
Inpatient often with ICU. If diagnosis is suspected, lumbar puncture should be done in office with antimicrobial therapy begun before transfer to hospital.

GENERAL MEASURES
• Appropriate antibiotic therapy
• Vigorous supportive care with constant nursing to ensure prompt recognition of seizures and prevention of aspiration
• Therapy for any coexisting conditions
• Measures to prevent hypothermia and dehydration

SURGICAL MEASURES   N/A

ACTIVITY
As tolerated in hospital and on discharge

DIET
Regular as tolerated, except when SIADH complicates course

PATIENT EDUCATION
For patient education materials on this topic, contact: American Academy of Pediatrics, 141 Northwest Point Blvd., P.O. Box 927, Elk Grove Village, IL 60009-0927, (800)433-9016

MEDICATIONS

DRUG(S) OF CHOICE Empiric therapy until culture results available (need to consider local patterns of bacterial sensitivity)
• 0 to 4 weeks: ampicillin 300-400 mg/kg/d plus a third-generation cephalosporin (cefotaxime 200 mg/kg/d q4-6h OR ceftriaxone 100 mg/kg/d q12-24h); or ampicillin plus an aminoglycoside (tobramycin 7.5 mg/kg/d q6-8h prematures or infants < 1 week, 2.5 mg/kg q12h. 14-21 days treatment.
• Age 4 to 12 weeks: ampicillin plus a third-generation cephalosporin. 10 days treatment (same doses as above).
• Age 3 months to 18 years: third generation cephalosporin; or ampicillin plus chloramphenicol 75-100 mg/kg/d. 10 days treatment.
• Age 18 to 50 years: penicillin G 18-24 million units q4-6h OR ampicillin 12-18 gm/d divided doses plus cefotaxime or ceftriaxone. 10 days treatment.
• Older than 50 years: ampicillin plus a third-generation cephalosporin (cefotaxime 2 gm q4h OR ceftriaxone 2 gm/d). 14-21 days treatment.
• For all ages > 1 month and < 50 years - evidence is convincing that corticosteroids decrease mortality and morbidity. Dexamethasone 0.15 mg/kg q6h, started 15-20 minutes before antibiotic x 4 days. (N Engl J Med 324:1525, 1991.)
Contraindications: Allergies to antibiotics
Precautions:
• Ototoxicity from aminoglycoside
• Hearing loss
• Developmental abnormalities related to meningitis
Significant Possible interactions: Refer to manufacturer's literature

ALTERNATIVE DRUGS
• Vancomycin
• Antipseudomonal penicillins
• Aztreonam
• Quinolones (e.g., ciprofloxacin)

FOLLOWUP

PATIENT MONITORING Brainstem auditory evoked response (BAER) test should be done with infants prior to hospital discharge. Further followup will depend on its results and course of meningitis while in hospital.

PREVENTION/AVOIDANCE
• Prompt medical treatment for infections
• Strict aseptic techniques when treating patients with head wounds or skull fractures
• Look for evidence of CSF fistula in patients with recurrent meningitis

POSSIBLE COMPLICATIONS
• Seizures (20-30% during course of illness)
• Focal neurologic deficit
• Cranial nerve palsies (III, VI, VII, VIII) 10-20% of cases, usually disappear within a few weeks
• Sensorineural hearing loss (10% in children)
• Neurodevelopmental sequelae (subtle learning deficits 30%)
• Obstructive hydrocephalus
• Subdural effusions

EXPECTED COURSE/PROGNOSIS
• Overall case fatality 14%
• H. influenza 6%
• Neisseria meningitidis 10.3%
• Streptococcus pneumoniae 26.3%

MISCELLANEOUS

ASSOCIATED CONDITIONS
Which worsen prognosis:
• Coma
• Seizures
• Alcoholism
• Old age
• Infancy
• Diabetes mellitus
• Multiple myeloma
• Head trauma

AGE-RELATED FACTORS
Pediatric: N/A
Geriatric: Several signs and symptoms may be less evident in elderly patients with other disorders (congestive heart failure, pneumonia)
Others: Different etiologic agents, antimicrobials and dosing, and CSF findings as listed above

PREGNANCY N/A

SYNONYMS N/A

ICD-9-CM
320 Bacterial meningitis

SEE ALSO
• Meningitis, viral
• Meningococcemia

OTHER NOTES N/A

ABBREVIATIONS N/A

REFERENCES
• Tunkel AR, Wispelwey B, Scheld WM: Bacterial meningitis: Recent advances in pathophysiology and treatment. Annals of Int Med 1990;112:610-623
• Shelton MM, Marks WA: Bacterial meningitis: An update. Neurologic Clinics of North America 1990;8:3:605-617
• Isselbacher KJ, et al, eds: Harrison's Principles of Internal Medicine. 13th Ed. New York, McGraw-Hill, 1994
Illustrations: N/A
Internet references: http://www.5mcc.com

Author(s)
Paul R. Gordon, MD

Meningitis, viral

 BASICS

DESCRIPTION Viral infection of the meninges and spinal fluid. The usual cause is acute and may be relapsing. Peak incidence occurs in summertime.
System(s) affected: Nervous
Genetics: N/A
Incidence/Prevalence in USA: Average of 10,000 reported cases per year. Probably many more unreported.
Predominant age: May affect all ages, but most common in young adults
Predominant sex: Male = Female

SIGNS AND SYMPTOMS
• Fever
• Headache, often severe
• Stiff neck
• Nausea and vomiting
• Photophobia
• Generalized aches and pains
• Occasional rash

CAUSES
• Coxsackie A, B
• ECHO virus (enteroviruses 70-75% of all cases)
• Poliovirus
• Lymphocytic choriomeningitis (LCM)
• Mumps
• Herpes (simplex and zoster)
• Epstein-Barr virus (EBV)
• Arthropod borne viruses
• Cytomegalovirus (CMV)
• Adenovirus

RISK FACTORS
• No specifics known
• Immunocompromised hosts may be more susceptible to CMV and adenovirus

 DIAGNOSIS

DIFFERENTIAL DIAGNOSIS
• Bacterial meningitis
• Encephalitis
• Acute encephalopathy
• Postinfectious encephalomyelitis
• Parameningeal infections (e.g., subdural empyema)
• Carcinomatous meningitis
• Meningeal leukemia
• Migraine headache
• Viral syndrome (e.g., influenza)
• Chemical meningitis
• Brain abscess
• Other infectious agents (TB, syphilis, ameba, leptospirosis)

LABORATORY
• CSF pleocytosis - usually predominantly mononuclear but may show more polys early on
• CSF cell count up to 3000-4000, but usually 50-200
• CSF - increased pressure
• CSF - serum antiviral antibody
• Elevated CSF protein, but usually < 150 mg/dL (< 1500 mg/L)
• CSF sugar usually normal (exceptions - herpes, mumps)
• Negative CSF Gram stain and culture for bacteria
• Negative CSF latex agglutination or CIEP for bacterial antigens
• Normal or mildly elevated WBC (blood)
• Viral cultures and/or antibody titers are seldom helpful
Drugs that may alter lab results:
Pretreatment with antibiotics may result in a "partially treated" bacterial meningitis, mimicking viral meningitis
Disorders that may alter lab results:
• Diabetes (alteration in spinal fluid sugar)
• Pre-existing neurologic diseases (e.g., brain tumor, demyelinating disease) could affect CSF findings

PATHOLOGICAL FINDINGS Lymphocyte infiltration of meninges and ventricles

SPECIAL TESTS EEG in some cases, especially if encephalitis is a consideration

IMAGING
• CT scan or MRI scan of the brain
• Usually CT or MRI performed prior to lumbar puncture

DIAGNOSTIC PROCEDURES Lumbar puncture

 TREATMENT

APPROPRIATE HEALTH CARE
• Usually inpatient, depending on severity of symptoms
• Private room indicated with moderate sterile precautions. Stress hand washing.

GENERAL MEASURES
• Fever control
• IV fluids if oral intake is poor or vomiting is present

SURGICAL MEASURES N/A

ACTIVITY Bedrest initially, then activity as tolerated

DIET Determined by symptoms; may need to NPO due to nausea or vomiting, advance to clear fluids and regular diet as tolerated

PATIENT EDUCATION
• Discuss possibility, but low probability, of transmission to contacts
• Expected duration of illness (2-7 days)
• For patient education materials favorably reviewed on this topic, contact: American Academy of Pediatrics, 141 Northwest Point Blvd., P.O. Box 927, Elk Grove Village, IL 60009-0927, (800)433-9016

MEDICATIONS

DRUG(S) OF CHOICE
• Analgesics (adult doses)
  ◊ Morphine 2-5mg IV q3h
  ◊ Nalbuphine (Nubain) 10mg IM
  ◊ acetaminophen-codeine or oxycodone-acetaminophen (Percocet), 1-2 q3h pm
• Anti-emetics
  ◊ Promethazine (Phenergan) 12.5-25 mg IV q4h
  ◊ Prochlorperazine (Compazine) 10 mg IM q4h, in adults
• Antipyretics
  ◊ Acetaminophen (Tylenol) 650 mg po or suppository q4h for adults. Approximately 60 mg per year of age in children or 10-15 mg/kg/dose.
• Antiviral agents are not indicated in the usual care of viral meningitis
• Antibiotics are not indicated for treatment of viral meningitis, but are often initiated until a diagnosis is firmly established. If all parameters suggest a viral etiology, it is usually prudent to treat symptomatically and follow the patient closely in the hospital setting. If in doubt, a broad spectrum antibiotic with good CSF penetration should be started intravenously. The choice may be dictated by local sensitivities, as well as a consideration of age related pathogens.
Contraindications: Refer to manufacturer's profile of each drug
Precautions:
• Aspirin should be avoided in children and adolescents due to a possible association with Reye's syndrome
• Phenothiazines may produce a dystonic reaction, especially in adolescents
Significant possible interactions: Refer to manufacturer's profile of each drug

ALTERNATIVE DRUGS
Symptomatic relief may be provided by a variety of anti-emetics and analgesics (e.g., nonsteroidal anti-inflammatory drugs)

FOLLOWUP

PATIENT MONITORING
• Once the acute illness begins resolving, follow at least once within 7-10 days
• Repeat of lumbar puncture is not necessary unless the clinical course is atypical

PREVENTION/AVOIDANCE N/A

POSSIBLE COMPLICATIONS
• Deafness
• Fatigue
• Irritability
• Muscle weakness
• Seizures (rare)

EXPECTED COURSE/PROGNOSIS
Complete recovery in 2-7 days; headaches and other uncomfortable symptoms may sometimes persist intermittently for 1-2 weeks

MISCELLANEOUS

ASSOCIATED CONDITIONS Encephalitis

AGE-RELATED FACTORS
Pediatric: N/A
Geriatric: Viral meningitis is rarely seen in the elderly, and suspicions should be raised about an alternative diagnosis, e.g., carcinomatous meningitis
Others: N/A

PREGNANCY N/A

SYNONYMS
• Abacterial meningitis
• Aseptic meningitis

ICD-9-CM 047.9 Unspecified viral meningitis

SEE ALSO
• Meningitis, bacterial
• Encephalitis, viral

OTHER NOTES
Enteroviruses and arthropod-borne viruses predominate in warm months; mumps usually occurs in the winter and spring, often in epidemics

ABBREVIATIONS
• CIEP - counterimmunoelectrophoresis
• CSF - cerebrospinal fluid

REFERENCES
• Mandell G, Douglas RG Jr, Bennett JE: Principles and Practice of Infectious Diseases. 4th Ed. New York, Churchill Livingstone, 1995
• Krugman S, Katz S, Gershon A, Wilfert C: Infectious Diseases of Children. 9th ed. New York, C.V. Mosby, 1990
• Rotbart HA: Enteroviral infections in the central nervous system. Clin Infect Dis 1995;20(4):971-81
Illustrations: N/A
Internet references: http://www.5mcc.com

Author(s)
Gary M. Miller, MD

Meningococcemia

BASICS

DESCRIPTION The presence of Neisseria meningitidis in the blood. This encompasses a broad spectrum of clinical manifestations.
• Bacteremia without sepsis: the patient has upper respiratory symptoms only and recovers spontaneously without antibiotic
• Bacteremia without meningitis: the patient is acutely ill, may have skin manifestations (rashes, petechiae, ecchymosis) and hypotension
• Bacteremia with meningitis: this clinical picture of meningitis predominates (headache, decreased sensorium, neck rigidity). Patient may also have skin manifestations and hypotension.
• Bacteremia with acute arthritis dermatitis syndrome: the patient may have tenosynovitis typical of gonococcal etiology
System(s) affected: Cardiovascular, Nervous, Skin/Exocrine, Musculoskeletal, Endocrine/Metabolic, Hemic/Lymphatic/Immunologic, Renal/Urologic
Genetics: N/A
Incidence/Prevalence in USA:
1-3/100,000 population
Predominant age: Highest attack rate in infants ages 3 months to 1 year and then decreases with age; it may affect all ages
Predominant sex: Male = Female

SIGNS AND SYMPTOMS
• Malaise
• Fever
• Chills, rigor
• Sore throat
• Cough
• Headache
• Changes in mental status - restlessness, agitation, confusion, delirium, lethargy, stupor, coma
• Myalgia
• Vomiting
• Convulsions
• Stiff neck
• Focal neurologic signs
• Tachycardia
• Tachypnea
• Hypotension
• Cyanosis
• Maculo-papular rash
• Petechiae
• Ecchymosis, purpura
• Arthritis
• Tenosynovitis

CAUSES
• Neisseria meningitidis, a gram-negative diplococcus
  ◊ At least 13 serotypes
  ◊ Major serogroups: A, B, C, Y, W -135
  ◊ Serogroup A may cause epidemics in many parts of developing world
  ◊ Serogroup C caused recent outbreaks in the U.S.

RISK FACTORS
• Age 3 months to 1 year
• Late complement component deficiency (C5, C6, C7, C8 or C9)
• Household contacts
• Contacts in nurseries, day care centers, dormitories and other close institutions

DIAGNOSIS

DIFFERENTIAL DIAGNOSIS
• Septicemia due to other microorganism
• Meningitis due to other pyogenic bacteria
• Gonococcemia
• Acute bacterial endocarditis
• Rocky Mountain spotted fever
• Hemolytic uremic syndrome
• Gonococcal arthritis dermatitis syndrome
• Influenza

LABORATORY
• Leukocytosis or leukopenia
• Left shift of leukocytes, toxic granulation
• Thrombocytopenia
• Lactic acidosis
• Prolonged prothrombin time
• Prolonged partial thromboplastin time
• Low fibrinogen
• Elevated fibrin degradation products
• Blood culture growing N. meningitidis
• Cerebrospinal fluid (CSF):
  ◊ Cloudy
  ◊ Increased WBC's with PMN's predominant
  ◊ Gram stain showing gram-negative diplococci
  ◊ Glucose to blood glucose ratio < 0.4
  ◊ Protein > 45 mg/dL (450 mg/L)
  ◊ Positive for N. meningitidis antigen
  ◊ Culture grew N. meningitidis
Drugs that may alter lab results: Prior antibiotic administration may make blood and/or CSF culture negative
Disorders that may alter lab results: N/A

PATHOLOGICAL FINDINGS
• Disseminated intravascular coagulation
• Exudates on meninges
• PMN infiltration of meninges
• Hemorrhage of adrenal glands

SPECIAL TESTS N/A

IMAGING CT scan of head if concern for space-occupying lesions

DIAGNOSTIC PROCEDURES
• Blood culture
• Lumbar puncture, done immediately after a brief history and physical examination, if meningitis suspected

TREATMENT

APPROPRIATE HEALTH CARE
• If meningitis suspected, immediate lumbar puncture
• If lumbar puncture is delayed, administer antibiotic immediately
• Admit patient to ICU, if severe sepsis or meningitis suspected
• Respiratory isolation, for 24 hours from the beginning of antibiotic therapy, is appropriate

GENERAL MEASURES
• Appropriate antibiotic
• Supportive care including IV fluids, oxygen when needed
• Close monitoring of patient for seizure activity
• Treat complications, e.g., DIC, ARDS, renal failure

SURGICAL MEASURES N/A

ACTIVITY As tolerated depending on clinical condition

DIET As tolerated depending on clinical condition

PATIENT EDUCATION
• Educate family and close contacts regarding risk of contracting meningococcal infections
• Educate healthcare personnel who are not at risk of contracting meningococcal infections

Meningococcemia

MEDICATIONS

DRUG(S) OF CHOICE
• In patients with severe mental changes, consider administering dexamethasone 0.15 mg/kg q 6h x 16 doses, starting 15 minutes before first dose of antibiotic
• For meningitis - penicillin G 4 million units IV q 4h (children 0.25 mU/kg IV q 4-6h) or ampicillin 2 g IV q 4h (children 200-300 mg/kg IV q 6h)
• For other infections - use half the dose for meningitis
• Duration of treatment 7-10 days
Contraindications: For patients with penicillin allergy, use alternate drugs
Precautions: Adjust dosage in patients with severe renal dysfunction
Significant possible interactions: Refer to manufacturer's literature

ALTERNATIVE DRUGS
• For meningitis - chloramphenicol 1 g IV q 6h (in children 75-100 mg/kg q 6h) or ceftriaxone 2 g IV q 12h (children 80-100 mg/kg q 12-24h)
  ◊ Ceftriaxone should not be used in patients with history of anaphylactic reactions to penicillin (hypotension, laryngeal edema, wheezing, hives, etc.)
  ◊ Chloramphenicol may cause aplastic anemia
• For other infections - ceftriaxone 1 g (children 40 mg/kg) IV q 24h

FOLLOWUP

PATIENT MONITORING
In patients with neurologic deficits, follow-up with neurologist may be needed

PREVENTION/AVOIDANCE
Before discharge, give patient rifampin 600 mg (children 10 mg/kg) po q 12h for 2 days to eradicate carriage or for adults only, one dose of ciprofloxacin 500-750 mg po

POSSIBLE COMPLICATIONS
• Disseminated intravascular coagulation
• Acute tubular necrosis
• Seizures
• Focal neurologic deficit
• Cranial nerve palsies
• Sensorineural hearing loss
• Obstructive hydrocephalus
• Subdural effusions

EXPECTED COURSE/PROGNOSIS
Overall mortality 10%

MISCELLANEOUS

ASSOCIATED CONDITIONS N/A

AGE-RELATED FACTORS
Pediatric: Age 3 months to 1 year - highest risk
Geriatric: Less common
Others: N/A

PREGNANCY N/A

SYNONYMS Spinal meningitis

ICD-9-CM
036.2 Meningococcemia
036.0 Meningococcal meningitis

SEE ALSO
• Septicemia
• Meningitis, bacterial

OTHER NOTES
• Chemoprophylaxis should be given to household contacts and contacts in nurseries, day care centers, nursing homes, dormitories and other closed institutions
• No chemoprophylaxis is needed for casual contacts, health care personnel (except persons giving mouth-to-mouth resuscitation), schoolmates, office co-workers
• Drug regimen - rifampin 600 mg (children 10 mg/kg) po q 12h for 2 days or for adults only, one dose of ciprofloxacin 500-750 mg po. Rifampin ingestion will cause orange-color urine.
• A vaccine containing polysaccharides of groups A, C, Y and W-135 is available for persons with late complement deficiency, anatomic or functional asplenia. Vaccination is also recommended for travelers to areas with epidemic meningococcal disease.

ABBREVIATIONS N/A

REFERENCES
• Apicella M: Neisseria meningitidis. In: Mandell GL, Bennett JR, Dolin R, eds. Principles and Practice of Infectious Diseases. 4th Ed. New York, Churchill Livingstone, 1995
• Marnejon T, Watanakunakorn C: Purpura fulminans and adrenal hemorrhage due to group Y meningococcemia in an elderly woman. South Med J 1991;84:527-529
• Rompalo AM, Hood EW, Roberts PL, et al: The acute arthritis dermatitis syndrome; The changing importance of Neisseria gonorrhea and Neisseria meningitidis. Arch Intern Med 1987;147:281-283
• Jackson LA, Schuchat A, Reeves MW, et al: Serogroup C meningococcal outbreaks in the United States. An emerging threat. JAMA 1995;273:383-389
Illustrations: N/A
Internet references: http://www.5mcc.com

Author(s)
Chatrchai Watanakunakorn, MD, FACP, FCCP

Meningomyelocele

BASICS

DESCRIPTION A defective closure of the vertebral column, in which the protruding sac contains meninges and spinal cord
• Meningomyelocele, anencephaly, and encephalocele belong to a group of disorders known as spina bifida, neural tube defects, or spinal dysraphism
• Meningomyelocele, anencephaly and encephalocele are serious congenital abnormalities of the nervous system, which develop in the first 4 weeks of gestation and represent faulty formation of the neural tube.
• Postneurulation defects:
  ◊ By 25 days of intrauterine life, neurulation is complete
  ◊ At this stage postneurulation defects of dysraphism develop
  ◊ Characterized by intact skin over the underlying lesion
  ◊ Lesions include simple meningocele, lipomyelomeningocele, diastematomyelia, myelocystocele, neurenteric cyst, intraspinal and pelvic meningoceles
System(s) affected: Nervous, Musculoskeletal, Skin/Exocrine
Genetics:
• Meningomyelocele, as well as the other forms of spina bifida (anencephaly and encephalocele) are a common example of multifactorial inheritance, i.e., they result from a number of genes and environmental factors acting together to determine the final result
• The parents of an affected infant have about a 1:30 chance of producing a 2nd affected offspring (this 3% risk has been calculated mathematically and confirmed by empiric data from population studies). Similarly, the patient with a neural tube defect, if able to have children, has a 3-4% chance of having an affected child. In the relatively rare instance where a couple has had 2 affected children, the risk for a 3rd rises further (7-8%). 2nd degree relatives of an affected individual (nieces, nephews) have about a 1:100 risk; for 1st cousins, the risk is about 1:200. There is little if any increased risk for other family members.
• Recent data have implicated vitamin deficiency as an environmental factor that plays a role in neural tube defects
Incidence/Prevalence in USA:
• Neural tube defects (also called spina bifida) incidence in Caucasians is about 1:700 live births
• Incidence among blacks is < 1:3000
Predominant age: Congenital abnormality which is usually apparent at birth
Predominant sex: Male = Female

SIGNS AND SYMPTOMS
• 75% of the lesions are situated in the lumbosacral spine
• The bony defect extends to the bottom of the vertebral column. Most are flat at birth but become cystic as time progresses.
• Infants are usually born with a single myelomeningocele
• Hydrocephalus - occurs in > 80% of infants with spina bifida and tends to arrest spontaneously over time
• Eventually only 1/2 of spina bifida patients are shunt-dependent
• Arnold-Chiari malformation (ACM)
  ◊ All spina bifida patients have an Arnold-Chiari malformation - overgrowth of cerebellar tissue into the spinal canal, elongated 4th ventricle and buckled medulla in the spinal canal
  ◊ ACM is symptomatic in only 20% of affected children
  ◊ If symptomatic - can impair nerve control of swallowing/breathing, can also lead to weakness of arms and legs
  ◊ In older children, ACM can lead to syringomyelia - cystic expansion of central spinal canal
  ◊ Syringomyelia causes weak legs/arms, cranial nerve dysfunction
  ◊ Decompression may reverse or arrest these problems

CAUSES
• Cause of spinal dysraphism is unclear
• General belief is that dysraphic malformations occur when environmental factors trigger an underlying hereditary predisposition that manifests itself in some form of spinal dysraphism

RISK FACTORS
• 1st trimester valproic acid and derivatives (Valproate Sodium) use
• High risk pregnancy - mother with one child with spina bifida
• High risk pregnancy - mother with close relative with spina bifida
• > 90% of spina bifida infants are from low-risk pregnancies

DIAGNOSIS

DIFFERENTIAL DIAGNOSIS N/A

LABORATORY
• Prenatal: Maternal serum alpha-fetoprotein (AFP) levels - if AFP level at 16-18 weeks is high, may suggest fetal neural defects. Amniocentesis is indicated.
• Newborn: No specific lab tests indicated
Drugs that may alter lab results: N/A
Disorders that may alter lab results: N/A

PATHOLOGICAL FINDINGS N/A

SPECIAL TESTS
• Prenatal
  ◊ Amniocentesis: Increased alpha-fetoprotein in amniotic fluid (by 14 weeks) indicates neural tube defects
  ◊ Ultrasound: Hydrocephalus usually easily diagnosable by ultrasonography > 80% of open neural tube defects have hydrocephalus. Banana sign - compression/anterior alignment of cerebellum. Banana sign on ultrasound may be sign of open spina bifida.
• Newborn
  ◊ Neurological testing to determine severity of functional defect
  ◊ Pinprick examination of trunk and legs shows level of sensory and motor involvement. Functional integrity is present if stimulus leads to limb movements, arousal, and crying.

IMAGING Newborn: MRI or CT scan of the brain may reveal an Arnold-Chiari malformation

DIAGNOSTIC PROCEDURES
• Newborn
  ◊ Usually, meningomyelocele is obvious on examination
  ◊ Defective innervation of the bladder is indicated by urinary dribbling

TREATMENT

APPROPRIATE HEALTH CARE Inpatient

GENERAL MEASURES
• A team approach is necessary for effective care (neurosurgeon, orthopedist, urologist, nurse, social worker, occupational and physical therapist)
• Most patients with myelomeningocele have neurogenic bladder. Intermittent catheterization prevents severe urologic disorders.

SURGICAL MEASURES
• Myelomeningocele repair - should be within 24-48 hours of birth. Orthopedist must address deformities of lower limbs and spine.
• ACM decompression - bony removal below level of herniated cerebellar tissue; dura opened and dural sac enlarged by sewing in a dural graft

ACTIVITY
• Guided by level of the lesion
• Activity assisted by physical therapy, braces, and wheelchair

DIET Liquid and food intake may need to be modified depending on bladder and bowel involvement

PATIENT EDUCATION
• Urologist instructs parents for protocol and techniques of catheterization
• Urologist instructs parents for prevention of urinary tract infections
• Neurosurgeon instructs parents about signs of shunt obstruction
• Genetic counseling
• Printed patient information available from: Spina Bifida Association of America, 1700 Rockville Pike, Suite 540, Rockville, MD, (800)621-3141

 MEDICATIONS

DRUG(S) OF CHOICE N/A
Contraindications: N/A
Precautions: N/A
Significant possible interactions: N/A

ALTERNATIVE DRUGS N/A

 FOLLOWUP

PATIENT MONITORING
• Physiotherapist looks for any deterioration in function
• Neurosurgeon follows patient's shunt function
• Urologist assesses urologic function
• Family physician provides general medical care/coordination

PREVENTION/AVOIDANCE Early recognition/decompression of ACM may reverse symptoms

POSSIBLE COMPLICATIONS
• Causes of late deterioration secondary to myelomeningocele repair
• Shunt obstruction - back pain and increasing neurologic deficit
• Shunt obstruction - can lead to hydrosyringomyelia
• Hydronephrosis - most occurs in 1st 5 years of life
• If operative procedures are not carried out, infants usually die within one year.

EXPECTED COURSE/PROGNOSIS
• > 80% of treated open neural tube defects have normal IQ
• Since 1970's, management techniques have improved tremendously
• Shunt infection and malfunction are now uncommon
• Early assessment in spina bifida may give misleading prognosis, i.e., a child with hydrocephalus and paraplegia may have normal IQ
• Small sacral lesion may result in severe physical/intellectual impairment from hydrocephalus or Arnold-Chiari malformation

 MISCELLANEOUS

ASSOCIATED CONDITIONS Infants with a simple meningocele may have an associated intraspinal abnormality that also requires treatment

AGE-RELATED FACTORS
Pediatric: Congenital defect
Geriatric: N/A
Others: N/A

PREGNANCY Diagnosable during pregnancy

SYNONYMS Myelomeningocele

ICD-9-CM
741.0 Spina bifida with hydrocephalus
741.9 Spina bifida without mention of hydrocephalus

SEE ALSO N/A

OTHER NOTES When an infant is severely affected, a decision about performing operative procedures or letting the disorder take its natural course presents serious ethical problems.

ABBREVIATIONS ACM = Arnold-Chiari malformation

REFERENCES
• Berklow R, et al, eds: Merck Manual. 16th Ed. Rahway, NJ, Merck Sharp & Dohme, 1992
• Hoffman HJ: Spinal Dysraphism. Amer Fam Phys 1987;36(6)
Illustrations: N/A
Internet references: http://www.5mcc.com

Author(s)
Mark R. Dambro, MD, FAAFP

Menopause

BASICS

DESCRIPTION The cessation of spontaneous menstrual cycles
• Climacteric: That period of time during which there is a decline in ovarian function. Although a woman may continue to have periodic uterine bleeding, such cycles may be anovulatory. During this time estrogen production diminishes and a woman may experience early signs of estrogen deficiency, such as vasomotor symptoms, even though she still has periodic bleeding.
• Postmenopause: The period after menopause usually accounting for more than a third of a women's total life.
System(s) affected: Reproductive, Endocrine/Metabolic, Skeletal
Genetics: N/A
Incidence/Prevalence in USA:
Increasingly common as life span increases - currently affects more than 30 million women
Predominant age:
• Average age is 51 and is unrelated to the age of the menarche. Virtually all women will be postmenopausal by age 58.
• If the menopause occurs before age 30, it is defined as premature menopause and may be associated with abnormalities of the sex chromosomes. A karyotype is indicated in such young women to rule out the presence of a Y chromosome.
Predominant sex: Female only

SIGNS AND SYMPTOMS
• Cessation of menses - either abruptly or preceded by a period of irregular cycles and/or diminished bleeding
• Vasomotor symptoms - hot flashes, sweating (85%)
• Psychologic symptoms - depression, nervousness, insomnia
• Vaginal atrophy - dyspareunia
• Urinary tract atrophy - stress or urge urinary incontinence
• Skin atrophy - wrinkles
• Osteoporosis - fractures (20% by age 85)
• Arteriosclerosis - coronary artery disease

CAUSES
• Physiologic - when due to depletion of oocytes
• Surgical - when due to removal of functioning ovaries because of disease or incidental to hysterectomy
• Medical - as a result of treatment of endometriosis (danazol [Danocrine] or GnRH analogues) or of breast cancer (antiestrogens). This etiology is reversible. May occur after cancer chemotherapy and be permanent or reversible.

RISK FACTORS
• Increasing age
• Pelvic surgery
• Sex chromosome abnormalities

DIAGNOSIS

DIFFERENTIAL DIAGNOSIS
• Pregnancy
• Polycystic ovarian disease
• Microadenoma of pituitary
• Hypothalamic dysfunction
• Asherman's syndrome
• Obstruction of uterine outflow tract

LABORATORY
• Usually none is required because patient's age and symptoms readily establish the diagnosis
• If the diagnosis is questionable in a young patient, an elevated serum FSH indicates ovarian failure (FSH greater than 100 mIU/mL [100 IU/L]). Measurement of LH is not necessary.
Drugs that may alter lab results:
• Estrogens
• Androgens
Disorders that may alter lab results:
Temporary, reversible cessation of ovarian function, e.g., during chemotherapy

PATHOLOGICAL FINDINGS
• Atrophy of endometrium - virtually 100% if untreated. The uterus may seem smaller on bimanual examination.
• Atrophy of vagina - loss of rugae, appearance of petechiae - virtually 100% after several years if untreated
• Atrophy of urinary tract
• Osteoporosis - approximately 2% loss of bone mass per year. This is most common in Caucasians and Orientals and least common in African-Americans.
• Arteriosclerosis
• Ovarian stroma only - or only a few inactive oocytes

SPECIAL TESTS Endometrial biopsy and/or D and C in patients who have intermenstrual or postmenopausal bleeding - may be accompanied by hysteroscopic examination of uterine cavity. Investigation for endometrial cancer is necessary even in the presence of an atrophic vagina (usually the cause of the bleeding).

IMAGING
• None for physiologic menopause
• MRI scan of head if pituitary tumor suspected
• Some physicians monitor bone density with photon beam absorptiometry - abnormal only after bone loss has occurred

DIAGNOSTIC PROCEDURES
• Serum FSH if diagnosis is questionable
• Peripheral blood karyotype if under age 30
• Endometrial sampling if intermenstrual or post menopausal bleeding occurs
• Pap smear
• Bimanual pelvic examination
• Mammography annually

TREATMENT

APPROPRIATE HEALTH CARE Periodic office visits

GENERAL MEASURES
• To retard development of osteoporosis - adequate calcium intake - at least 1500 mg elemental calcium per day obtained by diet or possibly by supplemental calcium; exercise; avoid smoking, excessive alcohol or caffeine intake
• Estrogen replacement therapy is indicated for long-term prophylaxis against osteoporosis and coronary artery disease as well as relief of vasomotor symptoms and urogenital atrophy. Exceptions are women with contraindications to therapy and obese women (who usually have sufficient endogenous estrogens produced by peripheral conversion of androgens by adipose tissue).
• Estrogen replacement has a favorable effect on lipoproteins, elevating the HDL levels, as well as retarding the development of osteoporosis, thereby reducing the incidence of fractures. It may also retard development of Alzheimer's disease.

SURGICAL MEASURES N/A

ACTIVITY Active exercise to the extent possible. Some type of weight-bearing exercise is recommended.

DIET Increased calcium intake

PATIENT EDUCATION
• American College of Obstetricians and Gynecologists (ACOG), 409 12th St. S.W., Washington, D.C. 20024, (800)673-8444
• For a listing of sources for patient education materials favorably reviewed on this topic, physicians may contact: American Academy of Family Physicians Foundation, P.O. Box 8418, Kansas City, MO 64114, (800)274-2237, ext. 4400

Menopause

MEDICATIONS

DRUG(S) OF CHOICE
• Estrogens - most commonly used are oral estrogen, conjugated (Premarin)
◊ Daily dose effective in retarding osteoporosis is 0.625 mg. Lesser doses are not effective.
◊ If vasomotor symptoms persist at 0.625 mg, a dose of 0.9 mg or 1.25 mg may be utilized, however, optimal cardioprotective effect is at 0.625mg
◊ Other forms of oral estrogen or the transdermal patch may be used and appear to be equally effective
• Progestogen
◊ Because estrogens are carcinogenic to the endometrium, a progestogen should be added for its protective effect against endometrial cancer. (If the uterus has been removed, a progestogen is not needed).
◊ Most often, medroxyprogesterone acetate (Provera) is used in a daily dose of 2.5 mg (for continuous use) or 5 mg (for cyclic use)
• Administration - estrogens and progestogens may be administered continuously or cyclically
◊ The advantage of continuous use is that withdrawal uterine bleeding is not expected
◊ With cyclic therapy, withdrawal bleeding may occur during the time that the patient is not on medication
◊ The most frequently used formulations are: Premarin 0.625 mg plus Provera 2.5 mg daily or Premarin 0.625 mg for 25 days per month - add Provera 5 mg during the last 14 days of estrogen therapy or Premarin 0.625 mg daily - add Provera 5 mg during 14 days of month. Some prescription packages contain both hormones (in same tablet) with days of week clearly marked, adding to convenience (Prempro, Premphase). Another option is Premarin and micronized progesterone.

Contraindications:
• Estrogen dependent malignancies
• Unexplained abnormal uterine bleeding
• History of thrombophlebitis
• Active liver disease

Precautions:
• Continuous combination therapy should not result in uterine bleeding
• Women on cyclic therapy may bleed normally only during those days when no therapy is given. Any bleeding other than that normally expected must be evaluated for the possibility of endometrial cancer.

Significant possible interactions: The estrogen dosage recommended is very low. It is unlikely that it will result in some of the complications that are associated with higher doses of estrogen, including hypercoagulability, breast tenderness, gall bladder disease and hypertension. The possible relationship to breast cancer is still controversial.

ALTERNATIVE DRUGS
• Oral - estropipate (Ogen) 0.625 mg, estradiol (Estrace) 1-2 mg
• Transdermal (patch) - estradiol (Estraderm; Vivelle; Alora; Climara) 0.05-0.1 mg/day applied twice weekly, or 0.05-0.1 mg/day applied weekly (Climara)
• Vaginal - conjugated estrogens (Premarin cream) - best for local therapy of atrophic vaginitis only. Systemic absorption occurs, but blood levels are unpredictable.
• Intramuscular - not recommended - may not be protective against coronary artery disease without first passing through the liver
• For women who cannot take estrogens - using progestogens (Depo-Provera) 150 mg IM every month is helpful in alleviating hot flashes. This may also retard the development of osteoporosis, but is not helpful in preventing coronary artery disease or urogenital atrophy.
• Clonidine (Catapres), oral or transdermal, may be used to treat vasomotor symptoms, but is not effective against other menopausal occurrences
• Vitamin D is not helpful as the sole treatment for preventing osteoporosis
• Calcitonin produces only a temporary increase in body calcium
• Sodium fluoride increases bone volume but has toxic side effects
• Alendronate (Fosamax) 10 mg/day (on empty stomach) used to treat postmenopausal osteoporosis

FOLLOWUP

PATIENT MONITORING
• Annual Pap smear and pelvic and breast examinations
• Annual mammography
• Endometrial sampling only in patients with abnormal bleeding

PREVENTION/AVOIDANCE
Menopause is a physiological process. It cannot be avoided, but the untoward effects can be moderated or eliminated by estrogen replacement therapy.

POSSIBLE COMPLICATIONS
• Vasomotor symptoms
• Uncomfortable psychologic symptoms
• Vaginal atrophy
• Skin wrinkles
• Osteoporosis
• Arteriosclerosis

EXPECTED COURSE/PROGNOSIS
• If untreated
◊ Ultimate disappearance of vasomotor symptoms - usually takes several years
◊ Urogenital atrophy
◊ Osteoporosis - possible fractures especially of the hip, vertebrae and wrists. Mortality associated with hip fractures is 15%.
◊ Coronary artery disease

• If treated
◊ Minimal effects of estrogen deprivation
◊ Slower development of significant bone loss and reduced incidence of coronary artery disease. Delayed appearance of Alzheimer's disease
◊ Therapy may be continued indefinitely if no contraindications appear since osteoporosis will rapidly occur after stopping therapy

MISCELLANEOUS

ASSOCIATED CONDITIONS Any medical problems that may occur with increasing age, especially osteoporosis

AGE-RELATED FACTORS
Pediatric: N/A
Geriatric: N/A
Others: N/A

PREGNANCY Mutually exclusive

SYNONYMS
• Climacteric
• Ovarian failure

ICD-9-CM
• 627.0 Premenopausal menorrhagia
• 627.2 Menopausal or female climacteric states
• 627.4 States associated with artificial menopause
• 716.3 Climacteric arthritis

SEE ALSO N/A

OTHER NOTES
• Estrogen replacement therapy is especially important in women having an early menopause, either spontaneous or surgical because of their long expected life without endogenous estrogens. Without such therapy, they may be at a significantly increased risk for osteoporosis and its life threatening or debilitating effects.
• Following surgical menopause, vasomotor symptoms often appear very rapidly. Estrogen replacement therapy may be started in the early postoperative period.
• In perimenopausal women bothered by severe vasomotor symptoms, cyclic estrogen and progestogen therapy may be started even though the patient is still having periodic uterine bleeding

ABBREVIATIONS N/A

REFERENCES Mishell DR Jr: Menopause. Physiology and Pharmacology. Chicago, Year Book Medical Publishers, 1987
Illustrations: N/A
Internet references: http://www.5mcc.com

Author(s)
Alvin Langer, MD

Menorrhagia

BASICS

DESCRIPTION Excessive amount or duration of menstrual flow, at more or less regular intervals
• Distinguish from, but may overlap with:
  ◊ Metrorrhagia - irregular or frequent flow, noncyclic
  ◊ Menometrorrhagia - frequent, excessive, irregular flow (menorrhagia plus metrorrhagia)
  ◊ Polymenorrhea - frequent flow, cycles of 21 days or less
  ◊ Intermenstrual bleeding - bleeding between regular menses
  ◊ Dysfunctional uterine bleeding (DUB) - abnormal endometrial bleeding of hormonal cause and related to anovulation
System(s) affected: Reproductive
Genetics: N/A
Incidence/Prevalence in USA: Abnormal bleeding is common; prevalence varies with definition (endometrial carcinoma: about 40,000 new cases per year)
Predominant age:
• Menarche to menopause; about 50% of cases occur after 40 years of age
• Dysfunctional bleeding is fairly common in adolescence and near menopause
Predominant sex: Female only

SIGNS AND SYMPTOMS
• "Excessive" menstrual flow defined subjectively varies greatly from woman to woman (average normal menstrual flow is about 30 mL per cycle)
• Useful historical features include:
  ◊ Bleeding substantially heavier than the patient's usual flow
  ◊ Bleeding lasting more than 7 days
  ◊ Flow associated with passage of significant clots
  ◊ Anemia
• The following symptoms tend to suggest that cycles are ovulatory:
  ◊ Regular menstrual interval
  ◊ Mid-cycle pain (mittelschmerz)
  ◊ Dysmenorrhea
  ◊ Premenstrual symptoms - breast soreness, mood changes, etc.
• Abdominal pain or cramps at other times of the cycle may be associated with structural causes:
  ◊ Myomas
  ◊ Polyps
  ◊ Ovarian tumors
• Hirsutism or acne
  ◊ May accompany Stein-Leventhal syndrome

CAUSES
• Hypothyroidism
• Endometrial proliferation/excess/hyperplasia:
  ◊ Anovulation, oligo-ovulation
  ◊ Polycystic ovarian disease (PCOD), Stein-Leventhal syndrome
  ◊ Ovarian tumor
  ◊ Obesity
  ◊ Hormone (estrogen) therapy

• Endometrial atrophy:
  ◊ Postmenopause
  ◊ Prolonged progestin or oral contraceptive administration
• Local factors:
  ◊ Endometrial polyps
  ◊ Endometrial neoplasia
  ◊ Adenomyosis/endometriosis
  ◊ Uterine myomata (fibroids)
  ◊ Intrauterine device (IUD)
  ◊ Uterine sarcoma
• Coagulation disorders:
  ◊ Thrombocytopenia, platelet disorders
  ◊ von Willebrand's disease
  ◊ Leukemia
  ◊ Ingestion of aspirin or anticoagulants
  ◊ Renal failure/dialysis

RISK FACTORS
• Obesity
• Anovulation
• Estrogen administration (without progestin)
• Prior treatment with progestational agents or oral contraceptives increases the risk of endometrial atrophy, but decreases the risk of endometrial hyperplasia or neoplasia

DIAGNOSIS

DIFFERENTIAL DIAGNOSIS
• Pregnancy complications:
  ◊ Threatened abortion
  ◊ Incomplete abortion
  ◊ Ectopic pregnancy
• Nonuterine bleeding:
  ◊ Cervical ectropion/erosion
  ◊ Cervical neoplasia/polyp
  ◊ Cervical or vaginal trauma
  ◊ Condylomata
  ◊ Atrophic vaginitis
  ◊ Foreign bodies
• Pelvic inflammatory disease (PID):
  ◊ Endometritis
  ◊ Tuberculosis

LABORATORY
• Pregnancy test
• CBC to assess severity of blood loss, exclude thrombocytopenia and leukemia
• In selected cases:
  ◊ TSH - elevated in hypothyroidism
  ◊ Platelet count, bleeding time, prothrombin time (PT), partial thromboplastin time (PTT) for coagulation screen
  ◊ Creatinine, BUN
  ◊ Serum progesterone - 5-20 ng/mL (15.9-63.6 nmol/L) in luteal phase, < 1 ng/mL (< 3.18 nmol/L) in follicular phase or anovulatory cycle
Drugs that may alter lab results: Progestins used prior to endometrial biopsy may cause decidualization and obscure true diagnosis
Disorders that may alter lab results: N/A

PATHOLOGICAL FINDINGS Vary with cause: see Causes

SPECIAL TESTS Endometrial biopsy detects hyperplasia, dysplasia, or atrophy. If done prior to expected menses, may also help make the diagnosis of anovulation or luteal phase defect.

IMAGING
• Ultrasonography to evaluate adnexal masses or fibroids suspected from pelvic exam
• Computerized tomography used in investigation of potentially malignant pelvic masses

DIAGNOSTIC PROCEDURES
• Pelvic and rectal examination
• Pap smear
• Endometrial biopsy
• Diagnostic dilatation and curettage
• Hysteroscopy

TREATMENT

APPROPRIATE HEALTH CARE
• Most cases can be managed as outpatients in office or emergency department
• Hospitalize for bleeding accompanied by orthostatic hypotension or hematocrit < 25%

GENERAL MEASURES
• Rule out pregnancy complications and non-uterine bleeding
• Treat severe or life-threatening bleeding acutely:
  ◊ Intravenous estrogen
  ◊ Curettage if necessary
  ◊ Hysterectomy in extreme case
• Proceed to identify underlying cause of bleeding and treat to prevent recurrence
  ◊ Hormonal therapy
  ◊ Dilatation and curettage for hormone-unresponsive cases
  ◊ Consider endometrial ablation or hysterectomy in persistent cases where fertility is not desired
  ◊ Specific treatment for neoplasia, polyps, systemic disease, etc.
  ◊ Patients who desire fertility may also need appropriate treatment for anovulation, endometriosis, myomata, etc.

SURGICAL MEASURES See general Measures

ACTIVITY As tolerated. Resting with feet elevated may be helpful.

DIET Iron supplementation may help correct for increased blood loss

PATIENT EDUCATION Information about side effects of medications

MEDICATIONS

DRUG(S) OF CHOICE
• For acute control of severe bleeding:
◊ Estrogen, conjugated (Premarin) 25 mg IV every 4 hours up to 6 doses until bleeding abates
• For less severe bleeding or after control of acute bleeding:
◊ Medroxyprogesterone acetate (Provera) 10-30 mg daily for 5-10 days
◊ Any combination oral contraceptive, (usually one of the "high dose" oral contraceptives) one tablet 4 times a day for 5-7 days
• To prevent heavy bleeding in subsequent cycles:
◊ Medroxyprogesterone acetate 10-20 mg daily for 10 days per month
◊ Usual cyclic dose of a combination oral contraceptive
• For endometrial atrophy in postmenopausal woman:
◊ Estrogen plus progesterone replacement therapy
Contraindications:
• To estrogen, oral contraceptives, or progestins:
◊ Pregnancy
◊ Breast or endometrial cancer
◊ Thromboembolic disease, past or present
◊ Impaired liver function
Precautions:
• Nausea and vomiting are common from IV estrogen; antiemetics are helpful
• Estrogen may precipitate acute intermittent porphyria or cholestatic jaundice in susceptible individuals
Significant possible interactions: Refer to manufacturer's profile of each drug

ALTERNATIVE DRUGS
• Norethindrone acetate (Norlutin, Norlutate) 2.5-10 mg daily for 10 days per month, during the assumed latter half of menstrual cycle
• Megestrol acetate (Megace) 40 mg daily for 10 days per month
• Megestrol acetate (Megace) 40 mg daily continuously to treat atypical hyperplasia
• Nonsteroidal prostaglandin-synthetase inhibitors (naproxen, mefenamic acid, ibuprofen, and others) can reduce blood loss with ovulatory cycles and reduce dysmenorrhea

FOLLOWUP

PATIENT MONITORING
• Varies with cause of bleeding
• Medical treatment of hyperplastic/dysplastic endometrium should be followed by repeat biopsy to confirm that histologic structure has returned to normal

PREVENTION/AVOIDANCE
Pap smear and pelvic examination annually

POSSIBLE COMPLICATIONS
Anemia

EXPECTED COURSE/PROGNOSIS
• Varies with cause of bleeding
• Most patients with hormonal causes will respond to hormonal manipulation

MISCELLANEOUS

ASSOCIATED CONDITIONS
Metrorrhagia; menometrorrhagia; androgenic disorders

AGE-RELATED FACTORS
Pediatric: Genital bleeding prior to puberty can result from trauma, foreign bodies, vaginal infection, or exogenous hormone administration
Geriatric: Genital atrophy may predispose to bleeding with minimal trauma. Neoplasm of ovary or endometrium must be ruled out.
Others:
• In adolescence, irregular bleeding due to anovulation and immaturity of the hypothalamic-pituitary-ovarian axis is common
• Beyond age 35-40, endometrial dysplasia and endometrial carcinoma are significant causes of bleeding. Obtain endometrial sampling before attempting hormonal treatment.

PREGNANCY
Bleeding in pregnancy is not menorrhagia. Complications of pregnancy or cervical/vaginal lesions should be considered.

SYNONYMS
N/A

ICD-9-CM
621.0 Endometrial polyp
621.3 Endometrial hyperplasia
621.8 Endometrial atrophy
626.2 Menorrhagia, menometrorrhagia, polymenorrhea
626.3 Pubertal menorrhagia
626.4 Irregular menses
626.6 Metrorrhagia
626.8 Dysfunctional uterine bleeding
627.0 Premenopausal (i.e., perimenopausal, climacteric) menorrhagia
627.1 Postmenopausal bleeding

SEE ALSO
• Amenorrhea
• Cervical dysplasia
• Cervical malignancy
• Cervical polyps
• Cervicitis
• Cervicitis, ectropion & true erosion
• Dysmenorrhea
• Uterine myomas
• Menopause
• Polycystic ovarian disease

OTHER NOTES
N/A

ABBREVIATIONS
N/A

REFERENCES
• Wentz AC: Abnormal Uterine Bleeding. In: Jones HW, ed. Novak's Textbook of Gynecology. 11th Ed. Baltimore, Williams & Wilkins, 1988
• Cowan BD, Morrison JC: Management of Abnormal Genital Bleeding in Girls and Women. N Engl J Med 1991;324(24):1710-1715
• Speroff L: Clinical Gynecologic Endocrinology and Infertility. 5th Ed. Baltimore, Williams & Wilkins, 1994
• Carlson JM: Menorrhagia and Metrorrhagia. In: Friedman EA, ed. Gynecologic Decision Making. 2nd Ed. Philadelphia, B.C. Decker, 1988
Illustrations: N/A
Internet references: http://www.5mcc.com

Author(s)
Donald A. F. Nelson, MD

Mental retardation

BASICS

DESCRIPTION Mental retardation (MR) is a symptom with multiple etiologies including chromosomal abnormalities, genetic defects, intrauterine, perinatal, neonatal, and postnatal causes. Mental retardation refers to substantial limitations in present functioning. It is characterized by significantly subaverage intellectual functioning, existing concurrently with related limitations in two or more of the following applicable adaptive skills areas: communication, self-care, home living, social skills, community use, self-direction, health and safety, functional academics, leisure and work. Cognitive and adaptive behavior deficits are manifested before age 18.
• Subgroups of mentally retarded:
  ◊ Mild: IQ 55-69 (85%)
  ◊ Moderate: IQ 40-54 (10%)
  ◊ Severe: IQ 25-39 (5%)
  ◊ Profound: IQ 0-24 (<1%)
System(s) affected: Nervous
Genetics:
• Autosomes: Trisomies and rearrangements - approximately 1500 variations are all associated with MR
• Sex chromosomes: 80 of 336 disorders cause MR
• Autosomal dominant: 180 of 3,000 disorders cause MR
• Autosomal recessive: 400 of 1,550 disorders cause MR
Incidence/Prevalence in USA: Incidence and prevalence are closely related to social, economic, and health conditions of the society. The general incidence of mental retardation in the United States has been estimated at 125,000 births per year by the American Association on Mental Retardation. This would correspond to approximately 3% of the population. The research on both incidence and prevalence of mental retardation in the US is exceedingly scant. A comprehensive Canadian study of the maritime Provinces found prevalences of 3.65 per 1000. Most professionals associated with the American Association on Mental Retardation accept a prevalence of 2.5% and they recognize that the prevalence varies with chronological age. Specifically, mildly retarded preschoolers are able to meet societies demands but are identified by the school system due to demands for cognitive processing. Conversely, once they leave the requirements of the educational system they may adapt to societies demands and the diagnosis need not apply.
Predominant age: By definition mental retardation occurs during the developmental period. Older adults who lose mental faculties are usually diagnosed as demented.
Predominant sex: Male > Female (1.5:1)

SIGNS AND SYMPTOMS
• Profoundly and severely retarded children are frequently diagnosed at the time of birth or during the newborn period. Children with dysmorphic features are more likely to be retarded
• Moderately retarded children may go undiagnosed until they fail to meet normal developmental milestones
• Mildly retarded children may go undiagnosed until well into the school years

CAUSES
• Chromosomal abnormalities
  ◊ Autosomal abnormalities
  ◊ Trisomy, e.g., Down syndrome
  ◊ Translocations
  ◊ Inversions
  ◊ Duplications
  ◊ Deletions, e.g., Prader-Willi
• Sex chromosome abnormalities
  ◊ Fragile X syndrome
  ◊ Turner syndrome
  ◊ Klinefelter's syndrome
  ◊ Various multiple X and/or Y conditions
• Autosomal dominant conditions
  ◊ Neurocutaneous syndromes, e.g., neurofibromatosis, tuberous sclerosis
• Autosomal recessive conditions
  ◊ Amino acid metabolism, e.g., phenylketonuria, Maple syrup urine disease
  ◊ Carbohydrate metabolism, e.g., galactosemia, fructosuria
  ◊ Lipid metabolism
  ◊ Tay-Sachs
  ◊ Gaucher's
  ◊ Niemann-Pick, e.g., mucopolysaccharidosis
  ◊ Purine metabolism, e.g., Lesch-Nyhan
  ◊ Other, e.g., Wilson's
• Multifactorial and sporadic conditions
  ◊ Cornelia de Lange's syndrome
  ◊ Spinal cord disorders (spina bifida, Arnold-Chiari malformation)
  ◊ Disorders of brain and skull
  ◊ Prenatal factors
  ◊ Rh incompatibility
  ◊ Maternal infections - all the TORCH viruses - rubella, toxoplasmosis, cytomegalic virus, and herpes simplex)
  ◊ Maternal diseases, e.g., diabetes mellitus, toxemia
  ◊ Maternal substance abuse, e.g., alcohol use/abuse. Fetal alcohol syndrome felt to be one of the leading causes of mental retardation.
  ◊ Prescription medications, such as Accutane or Dilantin
• Perinatal factors
  ◊ Prematurity
  ◊ Postmaturity
  ◊ Birth injuries
  ◊ High risk mothers
• Postnatal factors
  ◊ Childhood diseases, e.g., meningitis, encephalitis, general inflammatory disease with high fever, hypothyroidism
  ◊ Trauma, e.g., accidents, physical abuse, marked deprivation
  ◊ Poisoning, e.g., lead, carbon monoxide, household products

RISK FACTORS
Risk factors for future offspring of the parent couple must be calculated based upon the specific etiology of related retarded individuals

DIAGNOSIS

DIFFERENTIAL DIAGNOSIS
• Brain tumors
• Hearing and/or speech impairment
• Infantile autism
• Cerebral palsy
• Emotional disturbance
• Lack of environmental opportunities for appropriate development

LABORATORY
• Specific studies are available for those patients with identifiable genetic disease entities
• Chromosome studies
• Metabolic screens
• Amino acid
• Sugar substrates
• Molecular studies, e.g., DNA
Drugs that may alter lab results: N/A
Disorders that may alter lab results: N/A

PATHOLOGICAL FINDINGS N/A

SPECIAL TESTS
• Individually administered measure of intellectual abilities
  ◊ Measure utilized depends upon the age of the patient
  ◊ Birth through 42 months - Bayley's Scales of Infant Development
  ◊ 2 years of age through adulthood - Stanford Binet (form LM), Stanford Binet (4th edition), Wechsler Scales
    ◊ Preschool children - WIPPSI
    ◊ School age - WISC-III
    ◊ Adults- WAIS-R, and an adaptive behavior scale (Vineland Adaptive Scales)
    ◊ Other measures are available; however, these are the most widely recognized and utilized measures of individual ability and adaptive behavior

IMAGING N/A

DIAGNOSTIC PROCEDURES See Special tests

TREATMENT

APPROPRIATE HEALTH CARE
• Some specialized care may be necessary based upon the etiology of the retardation
• Care for the retarded is educational, not medical and should include early intervention

GENERAL MEASURES N/A

SURGICAL MEASURES N/A

ACTIVITY Full activity

DIET No research evidence supports the use of specific diets for mental retardation and/or Attention Deficit Hyperactivity Disorder (ADHD). Exception: Some metabolic and storage disorders, i.e., PKU.

PATIENT EDUCATION Parental education and consultation as to the development of appropriate behavioral and educational expectations are strongly advised. Families should be referred to the local Association for Retarded Citizens.

MEDICATIONS

DRUG(S) OF CHOICE None
Contraindications: N/A
Precautions: N/A
Significant possible interactions: N/A

ALTERNATIVE DRUGS N/A

FOLLOWUP

PATIENT MONITORING Regular pediatric care

PREVENTION/AVOIDANCE N/A

POSSIBLE COMPLICATIONS Learning inappropriate behaviors

EXPECTED COURSE/PROGNOSIS
• Mild retardation: Social and communication skills appropriate for community functioning, basic job skills, and functional literacy
• Moderate mental retardation: Speech deficits, social awareness, personal care skills, i.e., dressing, feeding, washing, sheltered employment, group home living
• Severe mental retardation: Limited speech and language, poor motor development, in need of supervision
• Profound mental retardation: Neurological defect, poor cognitive social ability, absent speech, possible self harm, extended care
• Specific etiologies, i.e., Down syndrome and fragile X patients show a decline in cognitive and adaptive behavior over time

MISCELLANEOUS

ASSOCIATED CONDITIONS
• Speech problems
• Seizures
• Maladaptive behaviors
• Attention deficit hyperactivity disorder (ADHD):
  ◊ Found with greater frequency among individuals with neuropsychological dysfunction
  ◊ Treatment for ADHD among the mentally retarded is not unlike that for the "normal" population
  ◊ Data indicates overuse of psychoactive substances to aid caretakers

AGE-RELATED FACTORS
Pediatric: N/A
Geriatric: N/A
Others: N/A

PREGNANCY Parents and first degree relatives could benefit from consultation with a genetic associate or counselor

SYNONYMS Mental deficiency

ICD-9-CM
• 317.00 Mild mental retardation
• 318.00 Moderate mental retardation
• 318.10 Severe mental retardation
• 318.20 Profound mental retardation
• 319.00 Unspecified mental retardation

SEE ALSO
• Cerebral palsy
• Down syndrome
• Fragile X syndrome
• Lead poisoning
• Attention deficit hyperactivity disorder

OTHER NOTES
• Extensive family history to aid in diagnosis is mandatory
• Genetic referral in cases without known etiology is appropriate

ABBREVIATIONS
MR = mental retardation

REFERENCES
• Holmes LB, et al: Mental Retardation: An Atlas of Diseases with Associated Physical Abnormalities. New York, The Macmillan Company, 1972
• Jones KL: Smith's Recognizable Patterns of Human Malformations. 4th Ed. Philadelphia, W. B. Saunders, 1988
Illustrations: N/A
Internet references: http://www.5mcc.com

Author(s)
Richard J. Simensen, PhD
Gene S. Fisch, PhD

Metatarsalgia

BASICS

DESCRIPTION   A catch-all term for pain in the forefoot, usually in the plantar aspect
• Pain and inflammation along the medial and transverse arches of the mid - and forefoot, involving the muscles, tendons and ligaments
System(s) affected: Musculoskeletal
Genetics: N/A
Incidence/Prevalence in USA: Common
Predominant age: 30's-80's
Predominant sex: Female > Male

SIGNS AND SYMPTOMS
• Predominantly located in the dorsal and plantar forefoot, especially distal half of metatarsal shaft
• Pain
• Swelling
• Tenderness
• Occasionally erythema

CAUSES
• Excess strain (anatomical variations)
  ◊ Hallux valgus and rigidus
  ◊ Plantar flexed metatarsals
  ◊ Hammer toe
  ◊ Obesity
• Repetitive and/or excessive and/or unaccustomed walking and running
  ◊ Long distance
  ◊ Hard surfaces
  ◊ Poor shoe construction
  ◊ Skeletal abnormalities
• Systemic disorder
  ◊ Gout
  ◊ Rheumatoid arthritis

RISK FACTORS
• Pes planus (flat foot)
• Old or poorly constructed shoes
• Poor physical condition

DIAGNOSIS

DIFFERENTIAL DIAGNOSIS
• Stress fracture
• Cellulitis or infection
• Neuroma (plantar or Morton's)
• Inflammatory arthritis
• Traumatic arthritis
• Foreign body
• Tumor (rare)

LABORATORY
• WBC - normal (elevated in infection)
• Sedimentation rate - normal (elevated in infection and inflammatory arthritis)
• Tests for gout, rheumatoid arthritis, or other systemic disorders if strongly suspect
Drugs that may alter lab results: N/A
Disorders that may alter lab results: N/A

PATHOLOGICAL FINDINGS   N/A

SPECIAL TESTS   N/A

IMAGING
• Routine anteroposterior and lateral foot x-ray - normal
• Bone scan if high index of suspicion of stress fracture
• MRI if suspect mass lesion

DIAGNOSTIC PROCEDURES   N/A

TREATMENT

APPROPRIATE HEALTH CARE
Outpatient

GENERAL MEASURES
• Ice initially
• Moist heat later
• Taping or Gelcast
• Walking cast - rarely
• Physical therapy - rarely
• Cane or crutch - temporary
• Arch support in a well-fitted, low-heel, air-soled shoe
• Energy-absorbing sole on shoe

SURGICAL MEASURES   N/A

ACTIVITY
• Rest during active, symptomatic phase
• Weight bearing as tolerated
• Progressive return to previous level of activities and sports - bike riding to jogging to running (with an arch support in running shoes)

DIET   No special diet

PATIENT EDUCATION   Instruct about proper shoes for specific activity and gradual return to usual activities

MEDICATIONS

DRUG(S) OF CHOICE
• Nonsteroidal anti-inflammatories such as:
◊ Oxaprozin (Daypro) 1200 mg once a day for 7-14 days
◊ Naproxen (e.g., Naprosyn) 500 mg bid 7-14 days
◊ Flurbiprofen (Ansaid) 100 mg bid 7-14 days
◊ Ibuprofen (Motrin) 800 mg tid 7-14 days
Contraindications:
• GI bleeding or ulcer history
• Liver diseases
Precautions:
• Renal disease
• Hepatic disease
• Fluid retention
• GI disorders, especially ulcers
• Coagulation disorders
• Anemia
Significant possible interactions:
• Anticoagulants
• Digoxin
• Lithium
• Methotrexate
• Cyclosporine

ALTERNATIVE DRUGS   N/A

FOLLOWUP

PATIENT MONITORING   Weekly for 2-4 weeks

PREVENTION/AVOIDANCE
• Appropriate shoes for appropriate activity
• Avoid overuse
• Treat systemic disorders

POSSIBLE COMPLICATIONS   Back and knee problems due to change in weight bearing dynamics

EXPECTED COURSE/PROGNOSIS
Expect complete healing with appropriate treatment

MISCELLANEOUS

ASSOCIATED CONDITIONS   See Causes

AGE-RELATED FACTORS
Pediatric: N/A
Geriatric:
• More frequent in older athletes and the aging
• Symptoms more pronounced
Others: N/A

PREGNANCY   N/A

SYNONYMS   N/A

ICD-9-CM   726.70 Metatarsalgia NOS

SEE ALSO   N/A

OTHER NOTES   N/A

ABBREVIATIONS   N/A

REFERENCES   Sullivan JA, Finberg L: The Pediatric Athlete. Park Ridge, Il, American Academy of Orthopedic Surgeons, 1990
Illustrations: N/A
Internet references: http://www.5mcc.com

Author(s)
Richard W. Cohen, MD

Migraine

BASICS

DESCRIPTION Paroxysmal headache lasting 4-72 hours. Episodes vary in frequency from more than once a week to less than one per year with symptoms abating completely between attacks. Prodromes consisting of non-specific symptoms occur frequently hours to days before headache. Most frequent sub-types are:
• Without aura - (common migraine) defining over 80% of attacks
• With aura - (classic migraine) characterized by focal disruption of neurological function begins and ends prior to headache onset
• Variants of migraine include:
  ◊ Transformed migraine - chronic headache pattern evolving from episodic migraine. Migraine-like attacks are superimposed on a daily or near-daily headache pattern, e.g., tension headache.
  ◊ Basilar migraine - occipital headache, with aura symptoms of dysarthria, vertigo, tinnitus, ataxia, and bilateral paresis or bilateral paresthesias
  ◊ Hemiplegic migraine - aura consisting of hemiplegia and/or hemiparesis
  ◊ Ophthalmoplegic - palsy of the ipsilateral third cranial nerve during the headache phase
  ◊ Retinal - symptoms of retinal vascular involvement during headache
  ◊ Childhood periodic syndromes - (migraine equivalents) recurrent often cyclic episodes of symptoms
  ◊ Status migrainous - persistent migraine which does not resolve spontaneously
  ◊ Migrainous stroke - persistent or permanent neurologic deficits persisting beyond migraine attack usually with neuro-imaging changes
System(s) affected: Nervous, Musculoskeletal, Cardiovascular, Gastrointestinal
Genetics: > 80% of patients have positive family history. Identification of a chromosomal abnormality has been confirmed in familial hemiplegic migraine.
Incidence/Prevalence in USA:
• Adults: 17.6% of females, 5.6% of males
• Childhood unknown; may be significant
Predominant age: Childhood; increase in early adolescence, through 30s and 40s; decreases with age, attacks may persist into mature adulthood
Predominant sex:
• Male ≥ Female in childhood
• Female > Male (3:1) after menarche to mid-adult life
• Female > Male (2:1) in postmenopausal female populations

SIGNS AND SYMPTOMS
Five phases of a migraine; symptoms vary from patient to patient or from attack to attack within the same individual
• Prodrome: A variety of "warnings" that precede migraine, frequently characterized by mood disruptions (e.g., euphoria, irritability, depression), fatigue, muscle tension, food craving, bloating, yawning, or subtle disruption of sensory processing

• Aura: Visual disruptions are most common, including scotoma, hemianopsia, fortification spectra, geometric visual patterns, and occasionally hallucinations. Somatosensory disruption in face or upper extremities is also common. Headache typically begins within 1 hour of aura resolution.
• Headache: Unilateral (30-40% bilateral), throbbing (40% non-throbbing) pain of 4-72 hours; intensified by movement; associated with systemic manifestations, e.g., nausea (87%), vomiting (56%), diarrhea (16%), photophobia (82%), phonophobia (78%), muscle tenderness (65%), lightheadedness (72%), vertigo (33%).
• Headache termination: Untreated, usually occurs with sleep; occasionally, vomiting or strong emotional experiences abort headache
• Postdrome: Headache pain resolved but another manifestation lingers on, such as, food intolerance, impaired concentration, fatigue, muscle soreness

CAUSES
• Exact etiology unknown; appears to be a genetically-linked, neuronal disease with vascular disruption as an epiphenomenon of underlying neurochemical disruption
• Serotonin and norepinephrine metabolism abnormalities may play a role
• Neurogenic inflammation and regional disruption of cerebral and/or extracranial blood flow may explain some clinical features

RISK FACTORS
• Specific foods, alcohol, missing meals, menstrual cycle, excessive sleep, fatigue, emotional stress, let down (relief of stress)
• Medications (estrogen replacement, BCP's, vasodilators)
• Family history of migraine
• Female gender
• Young age
• History of childhood cyclic vomiting, cyclic abdominal pain, motion sickness

DIAGNOSIS

DIFFERENTIAL DIAGNOSIS
• Other primary headache disorders
• Secondary headaches, such as tumor, infection, vascular pathology, or prescription or illicit drug, e.g., cocaine
• Drug seeking patients
• Psychiatric disease
• Rarely, migraine symptoms similar to certain forms of epilepsy

LABORATORY Only useful to rule out secondary causes of headache
Drugs that may alter lab results: N/A
Disorders that may alter lab results: N/A

PATHOLOGICAL FINDINGS
• Changes in blood serotonin levels and serotonin metabolites in the urine are reported
• Changes in regional blood flow
• Changes in sophisticated imaging studies

SPECIAL TESTS Only to rule out underlying pathology

IMAGING Occasionally required

DIAGNOSTIC PROCEDURES Based on careful history and physical findings

TREATMENT

APPROPRIATE HEALTH CARE
Outpatient. For status migrainous or cases complicated by concurrent medical problems or significant medication-withdrawal issues, hospitalization may be required.

GENERAL MEASURES
• Compression to ipsilateral temporal artery or tender areas of scalp or neck
• Cold compresses to area of pain
• Rest with pillows comfortably supporting head or neck in area devoid of sensory stimulation, including light, sound, and odors
• Withdrawal from stressful surroundings
• Sleep is desirable
• Biofeedback and early psychologic intervention in appropriate cases or when pain behaviors are first identified
• Most patients manage attacks with self-care

SURGICAL MEASURES N/A

ACTIVITY In bed in a dark quiet environment

DIET Maintain fluid intake. Avoid dietary precipitants of migraine.

PATIENT EDUCATION
• Emphasize migraine can not be cured, but symptoms can be managed
• Encourage use of diary and patient education
• Emphasize proper use of all medications
• Encourage lifestyle modifications

MEDICATIONS

DRUG(S) OF CHOICE
• 5-HT-1 agonists in moderate to severe migraine; a wide variety of vasoconstrictors, analgesics, anti-inflammatories, antiemetics, and sedatives used alone or in combination are prescribed based on symptoms and other factors. Except for parenteral 5-HT-1 agonists and antiemetics, drugs are most effective when taken early in migraine attacks.
5-HT-1 agonists
• Sumatriptan (Imitrex), most effective during headache phase of migraine
  ◊ Available as 6 mg self-administered injection with efficacy of 70-85% or 25 and 50 mg oral tablets with efficacy of 65%. 50 mg dose more effective than 25 mg.

◊ If initial injection fails to relieve migraine after 1 hour, don't repeat injection. Repeat injection or oral tablets, if headache returns.
  ◊ Oral tablet with slower onset (2-4 hrs)
  ◊ Restores normal function for most
  ◊ Appropriate patient selection important
Ergotamines
• Dihydroergotamine (DHE)
  ◊ Most effective ergotamine; available as IV, IM, or SC injection
  ◊ 0.5-1 mg dose with up to 3 mg IM or 2 mg IV in 24 hours. Maximum weekly doses of 4-6 mg. Many protocols utilize antiemetic, such as, metoclopramide or prochlorperazine 5-10 mg IM or IV prior to DHE administration.
  ◊ Drug of choice in status migraines
• Ergotamine tartrate
  ◊ Ergotamine-caffeine (Cafergot) suppositories 2 mg. Start with half and increase to 2 suppositories per attack. Avoid chronic use. Maximum 6 mg/attack; 10 mg/week.
  ◊ Oral preparations contain 1 mg of ergotamine and 100 mg of caffeine (Cafergot). Two tablets at onset of symptoms. Repeat after 30 minutes up to maximum dose of 6 mg per day. Cafergot PB contains 30 mg of pentobarbital and 0.25 mg of belladonna. Avoid chronic daily or near-daily use.
Nonsteroidal anti-inflammatories: No clear efficacy established for any particular agent; early administration improves efficacy.
Combination drugs
• Isometheptene - dichloralphenazone - acetaminophen (Midrin) 2 at onset then 1 q hr if needed up to 5 per 12 hour period
• Acetaminophen-butalbital (Phrenilin). 1 or 2 capsules at onset repeated q 4 hr prn up to 6/24 hours.
• Acetaminophen-butalbital (Fioricet) or acetaminophen-butalbital-codeine (Fiorinal #3, Fiorinal #4). 1 or 2 at onset q 4 hr prn up to 6/24 hours.

Contraindications:
• Avoid 5-HT-1 agonists in coronary heart disease, peripheral vascular disease, uncontrolled hypertension, and complex migraine, such as basilar or hemiplegic migraine. Avoid within 2 wks of MAO usage. Pregnancy category C.
• Avoid NSAIDs if danger of gastric erosion, renal, or hepatic disease
• Avoid acetaminophen in hepatic disease or with alcohol consumption
• Avoid drugs containing narcotics or butalbital in addiction prone patients
• Avoid vasoconstrictors in uncontrolled hypertension

Precautions:
• Administer ergotamines early
• Frequent use of acute treatment drugs may lead to changed migraine patterns
• Monitor use of aspirin and NSAID's for dyspepsia
• Monitor use of drugs with addictive potential
• Avoid concomitant sumatriptan and ergotamine

Significant possible interactions:
• Other sedatives, analgesics, alcohol, vasoconstrictors including decongestants
• Ergotamine and macrolide antibiotics

ALTERNATIVE DRUGS
• Any analgesic, antiemetic, or sedative
• Narcotics including butorphanol (Stadol) are reserved for rescue therapy
• In emergency department: sumatriptan, DHE, adequate analgesics, anti-emetic (chlorpromazine or prochlorperazine) and fluid replacement
• Other 5-HT-1 agonists

FOLLOWUP

PATIENT MONITORING
• Early intervention assist management
• Monitor frequency of attacks, pain behaviors. medication usage
• Encourage lifestyle modifications

PREVENTION/AVOIDANCE
• Avoid precipitants of attacks
• Prescribe biofeedback and psychologic intervention early if pain behavior evident
• Prophylactic therapy: If attacks significantly interfere with lifestyle or are not adequately controlled by appropriate acute interventions, daily prophylactic therapy may be appropriate. Regularly scheduled follow-up is mandatory.
  ◊ Propranolol (Inderal) 80-320 mg daily
  ◊ Atenolol (Tenormin) 50-100 mg daily
  ◊ Nadolol (Corgard) 40-80 mg daily
  ◊ Timolol (Blocadren) 10-20 mg daily
  ◊ Metoprolol (Lopressor) 100-450 mg daily
  ◊ Amitriptyline (Elavil) 10-150 mg daily
  ◊ Nortriptyline (Pamelor) 10-150 mg daily
  ◊ Verapamil (Calan, Isoptin) 80-120 mg daily
  ◊ Isradipine (DynaCirc) 2.5-10 mg bid
  ◊ Methysergide (Sansert) 5-8 mg daily
  ◊ Cyproheptadine (Periactin) 4-16 mg daily
  ◊ Valproic acid (Depakene) or divalproex (Depakote) 250-1500 mg daily
• Consultation/referral
  ◊ Obscure diagnosis, concomitant medical conditions, significant psychopathology
  ◊ Unresponsive to usual treatment
  ◊ Analgesic dependent headache patterns

POSSIBLE COMPLICATIONS
• Rare status migrainosis
• Rare cerebral ischemic events
• Iatrogenic effects of treatment

EXPECTED COURSE/PROGNOSIS
• With age - reduction in severity, frequency, and disability of attacks
• Most attacks subside within 72 hours

MISCELLANEOUS

ASSOCIATED CONDITIONS Depression, panic disorders, sleep disturbance, cerebral vascular disease, myocardial disease, peripheral vascular disease and seizure

AGE-RELATED FACTORS
Pediatric: Recurrent abdominal pain and cyclic vomiting may predominate; attacks may be of shorter duration. Headache description by younger children may appear atypical.
Geriatric: Rare onset of acephalgic migraine (aura without subsequent headache) after the age of 40. Possible relationship to transient global amnesia. Late onset of migraine requires diagnostic evaluation.
Others: Migraine affects all races, social classes, intelligence levels

PREGNANCY Attacks frequently diminish, esp. in 2nd/3rd trimester. No treatment drug has FDA approval in pregnancy; ergotamines are contraindicated.

SYNONYMS
• Hemicrania
• Sick headache

ICD-9-CM
346.0 Classical migraine
346.2 Variants of migraine (including cluster)
346.9 Migraine, unspecified
784.0 Headache

SEE ALSO
• Headache, cluster
• Headache, tension

OTHER NOTES N/A

ABBREVIATIONS N/A

REFERENCES
• Cady RK, Fox AW, eds: Treating the Headache Patient. New York, Marcel Dekker, 1995
• Sandler M, Collins GM, eds: Migraine: A Spectrum of Ideas. New York, Oxford University Press, 1990
• Raskin NH: Headache. 2nd Ed. New York, Churchill Livingstone, 1986
• Dalessio DJ, ed: Wolff's Headache. 5th Ed. New York, Oxford University Press, 1987
Illustrations: N/A
Internet references: http://www.5mcc.com

Author(s)
Roger Cady, MD

Miliaria rubra

BASICS

DESCRIPTION Miliaria rubra or prickly heat is a papulovesicular eruption
System(s) affected: Skin/Exocrine
Genetics: N/A
Incidence/Prevalence in USA: N/A
Predominant age: Common in infants, less common in adults
Predominant sex: Male = Female

SIGNS AND SYMPTOMS
• Fine papules and vesicles on an erythematous base
• May become inflamed pustules (miliaria pustulosa)
• Prevalent in areas of friction caused by clothing and in areas of flexure
• In infants - trunk, diaper area, neck, groin, axilla, face
• Pilosebaceous follicles, palms, soles spared
• Lesions appear after individual has been in a hot humid environment, resulting in sweating
• Pruritus or prickly, mildly stinging sensation in affected areas

CAUSES
• Keratinous plugging of the sweat ducts as a result of toxins produced by resident bacteria
• This leads to rupture of sweat duct producing sweat retention vesicle

RISK FACTORS
• Hot humid environment
• Occlusive bandages
• Plastic undersheets
• High fever

DIAGNOSIS

DIFFERENTIAL DIAGNOSIS
• Acne
• Folliculitis
• Viral exanthems
• Drug eruptions
• Erythema toxicum
• Yeast infections
• Pyogenic infections

LABORATORY N/A
Drugs that may alter lab results: N/A
Disorders that may alter lab results: N/A

PATHOLOGICAL FINDINGS
• Keratinous plugging of sweat ducts
• Sweat retention vesicle

SPECIAL TESTS N/A

IMAGING N/A

DIAGNOSTIC PROCEDURES N/A

TREATMENT

APPROPRIATE HEALTH CARE
Outpatient

GENERAL MEASURES
• Avoid wearing heavy, tight clothing or garments causing friction
• Avoid plastic or occlusive dressings/garments in hot environments
• Avoid excessive use of soap and contact with irritants
• Frequent cool baths with Aveeno colloidal, oatmeal or cornstarch
• Provide cool, dry environment for 8-10 hours a day

SURGICAL MEASURES N/A

ACTIVITY Avoid vigorous activity leading to sweating

DIET No special diet

PATIENT EDUCATION
• Cause of eruption/avoidance
• General measures for home care

Miliaria rubra

MEDICATIONS

DRUG(S) OF CHOICE
• Topical steroids to relieve pruritus - 0.1% betamethasone (Valisone) bid for 3 days
• Systemic antibiotics in cases of bacterial secondary infection - Staphylococcicidal antibiotic, e.g., dicloxacillin 250 mg qid for 10 days (unless resistance)
• If sweating due to fever, antipyretic drugs may be useful
Contraindications: N/A
Precautions: Care with fluorinated steroid application in children. They may cause systemic effects.
Significant possible interactions: N/A

ALTERNATIVE DRUGS Over-the-counter preparations with menthol, camphor for pruritus, e.g., hydrocortisone (Sarna) or pramoxine (Prax)

FOLLOWUP

PATIENT MONITORING As needed for persistence of symptoms

PREVENTION/AVOIDANCE
• See General measures
• Acclimatize slowly to hot weather

POSSIBLE COMPLICATIONS Secondary bacterial infections

EXPECTED COURSE/PROGNOSIS
• Benign - responds to cooling
• Avoidance of causative agents is key

MISCELLANEOUS

ASSOCIATED CONDITIONS N/A

AGE-RELATED FACTORS
Pediatric: More common
Geriatric:
• Less common
• Backs of hospitalized patients
Others: N/A

PREGNANCY N/A

SYNONYMS Prickly heat

ICD-9-CM
705.1 Prickly heat

SEE ALSO N/A

OTHER NOTES N/A

ABBREVIATIONS N/A

REFERENCES Bondi E, Jegasothy B, Lazarus G: Dermatology, Diagnosis and Therapy, 1991
Illustrations: 4 available on CD-ROM
Internet references: http://www.5mcc.com

Author(s)
Jeffrey A. Stearns, MD

Milk-alkali syndrome

BASICS

DESCRIPTION A condition resulting from ingestion of excessive amounts of calcium and absorbable alkali (e.g., sodium bicarbonate and calcium carbonate) usually during self-treatment for peptic ulcer or gastro-esophageal reflux
System(s) affected: Gastrointestinal, Renal/Urologic, Endocrine/Metabolic
Genetics: Unknown
Incidence/Prevalence in USA: Infrequent
Predominant age: 40-75 years
Predominant sex: Male = Female

SIGNS AND SYMPTOMS
- Anorexia
- Band keratopathy
- Constipation
- Dehydration
- Depression
- Dizziness
- Food distaste
- Headache
- Irritability
- Mental status changes
- Myalgias
- Nausea
- Periarticular calcinosis
- Polydipsia
- Polyuria
- Vomiting
- Weakness

CAUSES Excess intake of milk and alkali as therapy for gastrointestinal problems accompanied with gastric hyperacidity (e.g., peptic ulcer, esophageal reflux)

RISK FACTORS
- Peptic ulcer
- Hiatal hernia
- Malignancies

DIAGNOSIS

DIFFERENTIAL DIAGNOSIS Other causes of hypercalcemia, such as excessive osteolysis with malignant disease, vitamin intoxication, thyroid disease, sarcoidosis, thiazide diuretic treatment, hyperparathyroidism

LABORATORY
- Mild alkalosis
- Hypercalcemia
- Normocalciuria
- Decreased urine phosphate
- Increased BUN and serum creatinine
- Normal alkaline phosphatase
Drugs that may alter lab results: N/A
Disorders that may alter lab results: N/A

PATHOLOGICAL FINDINGS
Nephrocalcinosis, ectopic calcification

SPECIAL TESTS N/A

IMAGING N/A

DIAGNOSTIC PROCEDURES N/A

TREATMENT

APPROPRIATE HEALTH CARE Inpatient

GENERAL MEASURES
- Withdraw milk and alkali
- Treat the hypercalcemia
- Intravenous treatment to cause calcinosis (usually with sodium chloride solution)
- Goal of treatment: Maintain urine volume of 3 liters per day
- With significant renal insufficiency, employ renal dialysis

SURGICAL MEASURES N/A

ACTIVITY Bedrest during active treatment

DIET Increased fluid intake

PATIENT EDUCATION N/A

MEDICATIONS

DRUG(S) OF CHOICE
• To treat hypercalcemia: Isotonic sodium chloride 0.9% intravenously when serum calcium exceeds 15 mg/dL (3.75 mmol/L) (see Hypercalcemia), plus
• Furosemide 80-100 mgm IV q2 for 24 hours after volume depletion has been corrected
Contraindications: Refer to manufacturer's literature
Precautions: Replace sodium and potassium losses associated with furosemide use
Significant possible interactions: Refer to manufacturer's literature

ALTERNATIVE DRUGS
Disodium and monopotassium phosphate. (HAZARDOUS - should be used only by experienced nephrologist and only if dialysis is unavailable.)

FOLLOWUP

PATIENT MONITORING
• Kidney function
• Fluid intake and output
• Urine electrolytes

PREVENTION/AVOIDANCE
Avoid excess milk and/or absorbable antacids

POSSIBLE COMPLICATIONS
• Renal failure
• Nephrocalcinosis

EXPECTED COURSE/PROGNOSIS
Favorable with appropriate therapy

MISCELLANEOUS

ASSOCIATED CONDITIONS
• Peptic ulcer disease
• Hiatal hernia
• Gastroesophageal reflux
• Hyperparathyroidism
• Hypercalcemia of malignancy

AGE-RELATED FACTORS
Pediatric: N/A
Geriatric: Occurs predominantly in this age group
Others: N/A

PREGNANCY N/A

SYNONYMS
• Burnett's syndrome
• Milk poisoning
• Milk drinker syndrome

ICD-9-CM
999.9

SEE ALSO N/A

OTHER NOTES N/A

ABBREVIATIONS N/A

REFERENCES
• Wilson JD, Foster DW, eds: Williams' Textbook of Endocrinology. 8th ed. Philadelphia, Saunders, 1992
• Labhart A: Clinical Endocrinology: Theory & Practice. 2nd Ed. Springhouse, PA, Springer-Verlag, 1987
Illustrations: N/A
Internet references: http://www.5mcc.com

Author(s)
Stan G. Smith, MA, MB, FCFPC

Mitral stenosis

BASICS

DESCRIPTION Resistance to diastolic filling of the left ventricle due to valvular narrowing. In the adult, the most common etiology is rheumatic heart disease.
System(s) affected: Cardiovascular
Genetics: Congenital mitral stenosis is a rare congenital malformation, manifested in only 0.42% of children with congenital heart disease
Incidence/Prevalence in USA: The overall incidence of rheumatic heart disease is decreasing. The mitral valve is the valve most commonly affected with rheumatic heart disease.
Predominant age: Symptoms primarily occur in middle age (40-70 years)
Predominant sex: Female > Male

SIGNS AND SYMPTOMS
• History:
◊ History of murmur
◊ History of rheumatic fever
◊ History of pulmonary edema with pregnancy, exercise, infection or arrhythmia (commonly atrial fibrillation)
• Most common signs and symptoms:
◊ Effort induced dyspnea
◊ Palpitations
◊ Effort fatigue
◊ Hemoptysis (late)
◊ Apical early diastolic low-pitched rumble often with presystolic accentuation (listen with bell of stethoscope in left lateral decubitus position)
◊ Loud S1 (early in disease - as the valve becomes more stenotic and less mobile, this is less common)
◊ Opening snap after S2 (may also diminish in intensity with increasing stenosis)
◊ Right ventricle enlargement
• Other signs and symptoms:
◊ Paroxysmal nocturnal dyspnea
◊ Orthopnea
◊ Recumbent cough
◊ Hoarseness
◊ Digital clubbing
◊ Chest pain
◊ Peripheral edema
◊ Systemic embolization
◊ Rales, atrial fibrillation, malar rash (rare)
◊ Holosystolic murmur of mitral regurgitation may accompany the valvular deformity of mitral stenosis
◊ If pulmonary hypertension is present: right ventricular lift, increased pulmonic second sound, a high pitched decrescendo diastolic murmur of pulmonic insufficiency (Graham Steell's murmur)
◊ If right ventricular failure has developed: increased jugular venous distention, holosystolic murmur of tricuspid regurgitation at left sternal border, hepatomegaly and peripheral edema are often found
◊ May also find associated aortic, or less commonly, tricuspid murmurs (due to aortic or tricuspid valve involvement with rheumatic heart disease)

CAUSES In the adult, mitral stenosis is almost always secondary to rheumatic heart disease. Rarely, congenital in etiology.

RISK FACTORS History of rheumatic fever

DIAGNOSIS

DIFFERENTIAL DIAGNOSIS The major differential diagnosis to be considered in a patient with the relatively characteristic findings of mitral stenosis is the uncommon atrial myxoma or vegetation due to endocarditis obstructing left ventricle (LV) inflow. Diastolic flow murmurs can be also heard in the absence of true stenosis due to increased flow across a normal valve. These murmurs are generally limited to early diastole and may be associated with anemia, thyrotoxicosis, shunts as well as with significant mitral regurgitation.

LABORATORY N/A
Drugs that may alter lab results: N/A
Disorders that may alter lab results: N/A

PATHOLOGICAL FINDINGS
• Scarring of the leaflets with fibrosis restricting valve mobility
• Retraction then leads to further valvular narrowing, often with a funnel shaped deformity
• Chordal involvement leads to fusion of the chords and obliteration of the interchordal spaces, further limiting LV inflow
• Left atrial dilatation
• Left atrial thrombi may be found
• Right ventricular hypertrophy
• Pulmonary arterial thickening

SPECIAL TESTS
• ECG:
◊ Left atrial enlargement (manifested by broad, notched P waves in lead II with a negative terminal deflection of the P wave in lead V1)
◊ Atrial fibrillation is commonly noted
◊ With right ventricular hypertrophy, right axis deviation may be noted

IMAGING
• Chest x-ray:
◊ Left atrial enlargement with straightening of the left heart border, a "double density", and elevation of the left main stem bronchus
◊ Pulmonary venous patterns changes with redistribution of flow toward the apices
◊ Prominent pulmonary arteries at the hilum with rapid tapering
◊ Right ventricular enlargement
◊ Kerley's B lines
◊ Pulmonary edema pattern (late)

DIAGNOSTIC PROCEDURES
• Echocardiography: (2-D):
◊ Mitral valve thickening with decreased diastolic excursion and "doming" of the anterior leaflet in diastole
◊ Valvular calcification
◊ Decreased mitral orifice as directly measured by planimetry
◊ Enlarged left atrium
◊ Right ventricular enlargement
◊ Atrial thrombi
• Doppler:
◊ Transvalvular pressure gradients
◊ Calculated valve area
◊ Concomitant mitral regurgitation (MR), pulmonary insufficiency (PI), tricuspid regurgitation (TR)
• Cardiac catheterization:
◊ Increased left atrial or pulmonary capillary wedge pressure (PCWP)
◊ Increased left atrial or PCWP to left ventricular pressure gradient
◊ Calculated mitral valve orifice area
◊ Calcified mitral valve
◊ Concomitant mitral regurgitation
◊ Presence of coronary artery disease

TREATMENT

APPROPRIATE HEALTH CARE
Outpatient except for complications or surgery

GENERAL MEASURES
• Mitral stenosis is generally a progressive disease. The asymptomatic patient with non-critical mitral stenosis can be followed with appropriate evaluation.
• The patient should avoid unusual stresses (emotional and physical)
• All patients should receive endocarditis prophylaxis, prior to dental work or invasive procedures, regardless of age, etiology or severity of the stenosis (as recommended by the American Heart Association in Circulation, Vol 83, No 3, March, 1991)
• Patients who have mitral stenosis on the basis of rheumatic fever should also receive rheumatic fever prophylaxis (in addition to endocarditis prophylaxis) if under 35 years of age or continues to be in contact with young children
• If atrial fibrillation develops, it is important to slow the heart rate to allow more time for diastolic filling through the stenotic valve
• The development of pulmonary edema is often associated with atrial fibrillation and a rapid ventricular response. It is important to slow the heart rate. Cardioversion could be considered, particularly if the patient is chronically anticoagulated.
• Consider anticoagulation with warfarin (Coumadin) in all patients with mitral stenosis, particularly if a history of systemic embolism, or have atrial fibrillation or a large left atrium

SURGICAL MEASURES Surgical intervention: If the patient is eligible for a commissurotomy or balloon valvuloplasty, the onset of symptoms clearly referable to the mitral stenosis is generally considered an indication for early surgical intervention. If, however, the patient requires placement of a mitral valve prosthesis, often the timing of the surgical intervention is delayed until the symptoms are more severe.

ACTIVITY Adequate rest and reasonable physical activity

DIET Low salt

PATIENT EDUCATION Educate the patient about symptoms of mitral stenosis and report them should they occur

MEDICATIONS

DRUG(S) OF CHOICE
• Judicious addition of diuretics if symptoms indicate
• Atrial fibrillation - consider digoxin plus anticoagulation with warfarin (Coumadin). Beta or calcium channel blockers have been used in place of digoxin. Digoxin is used for rate control, not to convert to normal sinus rhythm. May require high levels (1.5-2.0 ng/mL) (1.9-2.6 nmol/L) to be effective. Monitor serum levels. The use of anti-arrhythmic therapy should be considered to maintain normal sinus rhythm.
• Rheumatic fever prophylaxis - preferably penicillin G benzathine, 1.2 million units IM every four weeks or penicillin V 250 mg twice daily
• Bacterial endocarditis prophylaxis - depends on procedure. For dental procedures - amoxicillin 3.0 g 1 hour prior to procedure and 1.5 g 6 hours after initial dose.
Contraindications: Penicillin allergy
Precautions: Refer to manufacturer's profile of each drug
Significant possible interactions: There are many when using the combination of warfarin and digoxin. Use caution when adding new medications. Refer to manufacturer's profile of each drug.

ALTERNATIVE DRUGS Erythromycin for prophylaxis

FOLLOWUP

PATIENT MONITORING Close regular visits for assessment of the gradually progressive symptoms

PREVENTION/AVOIDANCE
• Bacterial endocarditis prophylaxis for dental and invasive procedures continued for life
• Strep throat - treat appropriately when it occurs
• Rheumatic fever prophylaxis when indicated (See General Measures)

POSSIBLE COMPLICATIONS
• Thromboembolism from mitral stenosis is a major potential complication (anticoagulation therapy has lessened this risk substantially)
• Recurrent rheumatic fever
• Bacterial endocarditis
• Pulmonary hypertension
• Pulmonary edema

EXPECTED COURSE/PROGNOSIS
• Although a milder course is now seen in North America, the classic mitral stenosis history is 10 years from the episode of rheumatic fever to the development of a murmur, another 10 years until symptomatic and another 10 years for the patient to develop serious disability
• Operative mortality 1-2% for mitral commissurotomy; 2-5% for mitral valve replacement

MISCELLANEOUS

ASSOCIATED CONDITIONS Congestive heart failure

AGE-RELATED FACTORS
Pediatric: N/A
Geriatric:
• Atrial fibrillation and complicating arterial embolism more common
• Though there is an increased risk for bleeding, anticoagulation therapy recommended (unless specifically contraindicated) due to high risk of embolism and valve thrombosis (especially if atrial fibrillation present)
Others: N/A

PREGNANCY
• Can cause marked deterioration in cardiac function due to hemodynamic changes associated with increased intravascular volume and heart rate, with decreased diastolic filling time
• The associated pulmonary hypertension also poorly tolerated in pregnancy

SYNONYMS N/A

ICD-9-CM 394.0 Mitral stenosis

SEE ALSO N/A

OTHER NOTES N/A

ABBREVIATIONS N/A

REFERENCES
• Brandenburg RO, et al: Cardiology: Fundamentals and Practice, Chicago, Year Book Medical Publishers, 1987
• Dalen JE, Alpert JS: Valvular Heart Disease. 2nd Ed. New York, Little Brown, 1987
• Cotran RS, et al, eds: Robbins Pathological Basis of Disease. 4th Ed. Philadelphia, W.B. Saunders Co., 1989
• Hurst JW, et al: The Heart. 7th Ed. New York, McGraw-Hill, 1990
Illustrations: N/A
Internet references: http://www.5mcc.com

Author(s)
James M. Galloway, MD, FACP, FACC

Mitral valve prolapse

BASICS

DESCRIPTION Systolic bulging of mitral valve leaflets into left atrium. A subset of patient have mitral valve prolapse syndrome.
System(s) affected: Cardiovascular, Endocrine/Metabolic, Nervous
Genetics: Autosomal dominant with variable expression. Part of inherited connective tissue disorders such as Marfan syndrome and Ehlers-Danlos syndrome.
Incidence/Prevalence in USA:
Approximately 3% of the general population
Predominant age: Uncommon before adolescent growth spurt, usually detected in young adulthood
Predominant sex:
• Females > Males (under the age of 20)
• Females = Males (after age 20)
• Males more severely affected than females after age 50

SIGNS AND SYMPTOMS
• Usually asymptomatic, nonprogressive, and benign
• Subset of patients may have arrhythmias, emboli, endocarditis, severe mitral regurgitation, and sudden death.
• Characteristic systolic click (sound) and/or late systolic murmur, whose characteristics and timing change with body position and often fluctuate between exams.
• Chest pain: recurrent, located in left precordial and substernal areas, varies from instantaneous to hours in duration
• Fatigue
• Syncope/presyncope
• Dyspnea
• Body habitus: Thin, arm span greater than height, abnormal thoracic cage or spine including narrow AP chest and pectus excavatum, high arched palate
• "MVP" syndrome
  ◊ Low body weight
  ◊ Low blood pressure
  ◊ Minor skeletal abnormalities
  ◊ Orthostasis
  ◊ Palpitations
  ◊ Mitral regurgitation
  ◊ Autonomic dysfunction: chest pain, panic attacks, anxiety
  ◊ Neuroendocrine dysfunction

CAUSES
• Primary disorder: inherited; mitral valve and supportive structures disproportionately large for left ventricle
• Secondary disorder:
  ◊ Disorders of tissue structure: Marfan syndrome, Ehlers-Danlos, pseudoxanthoma elastica, osteogenesis imperfecta, myxomatous degeneration of connective tissue of the mitral valve
  ◊ Connective tissue diseases: rheumatic endocarditis, SLE
  ◊ Structural heart diseases: ruptured chordae tendineae, mitral stenosis
  ◊ Coronary artery disease
• Associated dysautonomia is cause of orthostasis and syncope, palpitations, anxiety, chest pain, fatigue, and dyspnea.

RISK FACTORS
• Positive family history
• Disorder of connective tissue/collagen
• Increased risk of complications
  ◊ Male sex and age over 50
  ◊ Posterior leaflet prolapse (associated with holo-systolic murmur)
  ◊ Mitral regurgitation (including exercise-induced MR)

DIAGNOSIS

DIFFERENTIAL DIAGNOSIS
• Click:
  ◊ Ejection clicks
  ◊ Opening snap (mitral/tricuspid stenosis)
  ◊ Split S2
  ◊ Ventricular aneurysm
  ◊ Constrictive pericarditis causing pericardial knock
• Late systolic murmur:
  ◊ Tricuspid valve prolapse
  ◊ Papillary muscle dysfunction
  ◊ Hypertrophic cardiomyopathy
  ◊ VSD

LABORATORY N/A
Drugs that may alter lab results: N/A
Disorders that may alter lab results: N/A

PATHOLOGICAL FINDINGS
• Myxomatous degeneration of the mitral valve
• Thickened, redundant mitral valve leaflets

SPECIAL TESTS
• ECG
  ◊ Usually normal
  ◊ Inferior ST-T wave changes
  ◊ Atrial arrhythmias, ventricular arrhythmias including complex arrhythmias, left atrial/ventricular enlargement secondary to mitral regurgitation
• Signal-averaged ECG helps predict PSVT and supraventricular arrhythmias

IMAGING Chest x-ray usually normal

DIAGNOSTIC PROCEDURES
• Echocardiogram (MVP be an incidental discovery):
  ◊ The most useful test for confirming and defining mitral valve prolapse.
  ◊ Should not be used to screen for mitral valve prolapse. Clinically significant mitral valve prolapse usually obvious on physical exam. Silent mitral valve prolapse common and clinically insignificant.
  ◊ Other valves may have myxomatous degeneration and prolapse. Echocardiogram evaluates other valves as well as the mitral valve.
  ◊ Doppler echocardiogram detects and quantitates mitral regurgitation
  ◊ Serial echocardiograms useful in following mitral regurgitation.
• Tilt table studies useful to diagnose autonomic dysfunction causing light-headedness and syncope
• Holter monitoring sometimes detects life-threatening arrhythmias. Atrial arrhythmias more common when mitral regurgitation present
• EKG stress test:
  ◊ Detects exercise-induced arrhythmias
  ◊ Detects exercise-induced mitral regurgitation which is associated with higher risk
  ◊ 50% false positive rate for ischemic changes
  ◊ Repeating the stress test after beta blockers improves specificity

TREATMENT

APPROPRIATE HEALTH CARE
Outpatient

GENERAL MEASURES
• 75% of cases have no increase in morbidity/mortality and no treatment required

SURGICAL MEASURES
• 25% of patients require valvular surgery after age 50, generally after long asymptomatic period
• Mitral valve and mitral annulus repair becoming preferred over mitral valve replacement

ACTIVITY
• Generally unrestricted
• Certain patients have arrhythmias precipitated by exercise which often respond to beta blockers
• Associated decreased intravascular volume may cause orthostasis and syncope with vigorous sports and/or dehydration
• Competitive sports should be avoided in patients with aortic root enlargement, unexplained syncope, uncontrolled tachyarrhythmias, etc.

DIET
• Adequate salt intake important: low baseline intravascular volume, abnormal renin-aldosterone response to volume depletion, and autonomic dysregulation limiting compensatory response.
• Caffeine, alcohol, and cigarettes should be avoided with palpitations

PATIENT EDUCATION
• Assurance of usually benign course
• Patient information can be obtained from: American Heart Association, 7320 Greenville Avenue, Dallas, TX 75231, (214)373-6300

MEDICATIONS

DRUG(S) OF CHOICE
• Usually none needed.
• Beta-blockers (e.g. atenolol) helpful if palpitations severe.
• Aspirin indicated for TIA
• When indicated (see Prevention/Avoidance):
  ◊ Antibiotics
  ◊ Warfarin (Coumadin)
Contraindications:
• Diuretics to be avoided (baseline low intravascular volume)
• Oral contraceptives to be avoided in patients with focal neurologic events
Precautions: Beta-blockers will increase fatigue and orthostasis/dizziness.
Significant possible interactions: Refer to manufacturer's literature

ALTERNATIVE DRUGS   None

FOLLOWUP

PATIENT MONITORING
• Serial echocardiograms in patients with posterior leaflet prolapse, mitral regurgitation (including exercise-induced), thickened or redundant leaflets, increased left ventricular size.

PREVENTION/AVOIDANCE
• Endocarditis prophylaxis for auscultatory murmur or redundant, thickened leaflets by echocardiogram. Prophylaxis not needed in MVP without a murmur.
• Good dental hygiene
• Anticoagulation in patients with atrial fibrillation and atrial enlargement

POSSIBLE COMPLICATIONS
Uncommon and related to advancing age, male sex, atrial/ventricular size rather than to presence/absence of valvular prolapse:
• Infective endocarditis
• TIA
• Stroke
• Congestive heart failure
• Cardiac dysrhythmias
• Heart block
• Sudden death
• Severe mitral regurgitation
• Syncope

EXPECTED COURSE/PROGNOSIS
• 75% excellent with same morbidity/mortality over age-matched controls
• 25% progressive mitral regurgitation with a long (25 year) asymptomatic phase followed by rapid deterioration requiring valvular repair within a year once symptoms occur

MISCELLANEOUS

ASSOCIATED CONDITIONS
< 5% of all mitral valve prolapse:
• Marfan syndrome
• Osteogenesis imperfecta
• Ehlers-Danlos syndrome
• Adult polycystic kidney disease
• Stickler syndrome
• Pseudoxanthoma elasticum
• Turner's syndrome
• Rheumatologic diseases including SLE, PSS, MCTD
• Primary cardiac disorders including rheumatic endocarditis, mitral stenosis, hypertrophic cardiomyopathy, LV aneurysm, coronary artery disease, and congenital abnormalities
• Duchenne's muscular dystrophy
• Inherited disorders of metabolism (Hunter's, Hurler's, & Sanfilippo's syndromes)

AGE-RELATED FACTORS
Pediatric:
Rarely detected before adolescent growth spurt
Geriatric: Complications occur mostly in men over 50
Others: N/A

PREGNANCY
• Mitral valve prolapse itself is not a contraindication to pregnancy.
• Connective tissue diseases (e.g., Marfan syndrome), especially with an enlarged aortic root, may be a contraindication to pregnancy
• Increased blood volume of pregnancy may improve symptoms of mitral valve prolapse

SYNONYMS
• Systolic murmur-click syndrome
• Mitral click murmur syndrome

ICD-9-CM
424.0 Mitral valve disorders
394.0 Mitral stenosis
394.1 Rheumatic mitral insufficiency
394.2 Mitral stenosis with insufficiency
394.9 Other and unspecified mitral valve diseases

SEE ALSO
• Mitral stenosis
• Mitral regurgitation due to papillary muscle dysfunction
• Mitral regurgitation due to rheumatic fever
• Marfan's syndrome
• Systemic lupus erythematosus (SLE)
• Polycystic kidney disease
• Turner's syndrome
• Muscular dystrophy

OTHER NOTES   N/A

ABBREVIATIONS
MVP = mitral valve prolapse

REFERENCES
• Hurst JW, et al: The Heart. 7th Ed. New York, McGraw-Hill, 1990
• Bennett JC, Plum F, eds: Cecil Textbook of Medicine. 20th Ed. Philadelphia, W.B. Saunders Co., 1996
• Stoddard MF, et al: Exercise-induced mitral regurgitation. Jrnl Am Coll Cardiol 1995; 25(3): 693-9
• Devereux RB: Recent developments in the diagnosis and treatment of MVP. Current Opinion Cardiol 1995; 10(2): 107-16
• Banasiak W, et al: P-wave signal-averaged ECG... Intl. Int. Cardiol 1995; 50(2): 175-80
• Kim S, et al: Relationship between severity of MR and prognosis of MVP... Am Ht Jnl 1996; 132(2(pt1)): 348-55
Illustrations: N/A
Internet references: http://www.5mcc.com

Author(s)
Hetty B. Hall, MD

Molluscum contagiosum

 BASICS

DESCRIPTION Common, benign viral skin disorder consisting of small umbilicated papules which tend to occur on the face, trunk and extremities in children and on the groin and genitalia in adults. Incubation period is 2 weeks to 2 months. In immunocompromised individuals (e.g., HIV infection), the lesions can be extensive and atypical. They are occasionally giant (up to 3 cm), involve face, neck and trunk, and are recalcitrant to treatment.
System(s) affected: Skin/Exocrine
Genetics: No known genetic pattern
Incidence/Prevalence in USA: Common
Predominant age: Children and young adults
Predominant sex: Male = Female

SIGNS AND SYMPTOMS
• Discrete pearly to flesh colored firm papules
• Diameter 2 to 6 mm (rarely giant nodules up to 3 cm occur)
• Usually grouped in one or two areas
• Centrally umbilicated with erythematous base
• Lesions can be pruritic or tender
• Beneath umbilicated center is white curd-like core
• Distribution: Anywhere. Predilection for face, trunk and extremities in children and groin and genitalia in adults.

CAUSES DNA virus of the poxvirus group. The virus cannot be grown in cell cultures. Incubation period is 2 weeks to 2 months after contact.

RISK FACTORS
• Close personal contact with infected persons
• In children, transmission can occur from swimming pools
• In adults, sexual transmission is common
• Immunocompromised individuals

 DIAGNOSIS

DIFFERENTIAL DIAGNOSIS
• Basal cell carcinoma
• Furunculosis
• Keratoacanthomas
• Warts
• Pyodermas (folliculitis, furunculosis
• Pyogenic granuloma
• Vesicular skin disorders
• Disseminated mycosis in AIDS patients

LABORATORY Virus particles cannot be cultured
Drugs that may alter lab results: N/A
Disorders that may alter lab results: N/A

PATHOLOGICAL FINDINGS
• Intracytoplasmic inclusion bodies in histological or cytological specimens
• Hypertrophied and hyperplastic epidermis

SPECIAL TESTS N/A

IMAGING N/A

DIAGNOSTIC PROCEDURES
• White, curd-like core easily expressed from beneath umbilication
• Biopsy

 TREATMENT

APPROPRIATE HEALTH CARE
Outpatient

GENERAL MEASURES Spontaneous resolution common in 6-12 months. Individual lesions resolve in 2 months.

SURGICAL MEASURES
• Removal by curettage alone, or curettage followed by trichloracetic acid or light electrodesiccation
• Cryotherapy is also effective

ACTIVITY No restrictions

DIET No special diet

PATIENT EDUCATION Instructions for Patients, W.B. Saunders Co., Philadelphia

MEDICATIONS

DRUG(S) OF CHOICE Curettage or cryotherapy are treatments of choice. Use of topical trichloroacetic acid, silver nitrate, phenol, tincture of iodine, podophyllin and tretinoin have all been reported. No clinical trials comparing efficacy or risk exist.
Contraindications: Refer to manufacturer's literature
Precautions: Refer to manufacturer's literature
Significant possible interactions: Refer to manufacturer's literature

ALTERNATIVE DRUGS N/A

FOLLOWUP

PATIENT MONITORING Recheck in 2 to 4 weeks after treatment for development of new lesions. Two to 4 visits are often required for complete course of treatment.

PREVENTION/AVOIDANCE In adults, avoid sexual contact with infected individuals

POSSIBLE COMPLICATIONS
• Autoinoculation is common
• Contagious to others
• Immunocompromised individuals may have extensive infections

EXPECTED COURSE/PROGNOSIS
• Untreated, the condition is usually self limited. Individual lesions spontaneously involute in 2 months. Total resolution usually takes 6 to 12 months.
• Recurrences are uncommon in immunocompetent individuals
• Lesions in HIV infected patients are more recalcitrant

MISCELLANEOUS

ASSOCIATED CONDITIONS Occurs in 5-18% of patients with HIV infection

AGE-RELATED FACTORS
Pediatric: Commonly seen on face, trunk and extremities. May be spread through swimming pools.
Geriatric: N/A
Others: In adults, is often a sexually transmitted disease.

PREGNANCY N/A

SYNONYMS N/A

ICD-9-CM
078.0 Molluscum contagiosum

SEE ALSO N/A

OTHER NOTES Spontaneous healing depends on triggering of a cell mediated immune response

ABBREVIATIONS N/A

REFERENCES
• Gottlieb SI, Myskowski PL: Molluscum contagiosum. Int'l J Dermatol 1994;33(7):453-461
• Epstein WL: Molluscum contagiosum. Seminars in Dermatol 1992;11(3):184-189
• Janniger CK, Swartz RA: Molluscum contagiosum in children. Cutis 1993;52:194-196
Illustrations: 2 available on CD-ROM
Internet references: http://www.5mcc.com

Author(s)
Nancy Elder, MD, MSPH

Mononucleosis

BASICS

DESCRIPTION Mononucleosis is a viral illness caused by the Epstein-Barr virus (EBV) of the herpes family. It causes 90% of the mono-like syndromes. EBV infection causes general involvement of the lymphoreticular system. The "mono" syndrome is characterized by fatigue, fever, splenomegaly, adenopathy and pharyngitis. Transmission is fecal-oral, often attributed to kissing. Incubation period is 20-50 days.
System(s) affected:
Hemic/Lymphatic/Immunologic
Genetics: N/A
Incidence/Prevalence in USA:
• Lower socioeconomic status: 50-85% seropositive by age 4
• Middle-upper socioeconomic status: 14-50% seropositive by college age
• By young adult life, 60-90% of persons are antibody positive
• Incidence is about 50/100,000 in general population to 5,000/100,000 in susceptible college students
Predominant age: High school and college predominate
Predominant sex: Male = Female

SIGNS AND SYMPTOMS
• Malaise (100%)
• Fatigue (100%)
• Headache (50%)
• Fever (85%)
• Adenopathy (85%)
• Tonsillitis (60%)
• Splenomegaly (45%)
• Hepatomegaly (35%)
• Petechiae (palate) (35%)
• Edema (periorbital) (35%)
• Rash (3-15%)

CAUSES Epstein-Barr virus - double-stranded DNA virus (herpes family)

RISK FACTORS
• College and high school students
• Kissing
• 70-90% shed virus 2-6 months after initial infection
• 20-30% individuals shed virus at any one time after 6 months

DIAGNOSIS

DIFFERENTIAL DIAGNOSIS
• Cytomegalovirus (CMV)
• Toxoplasmosis
• Rubella
• Adenovirus
• Herpes simplex
• Drug side effects
• Streptococcal pharyngitis
• Viral tonsillitis
• Vincent's angina
• Diphtheria
• Viral hepatitis A and B
• Lymphoma or leukemia
• Human herpesvirus -6

LABORATORY
• Positive EBV titers (IgG or IgM) (100%)
• Lymphocytosis (95%)
• Atypical monocytosis (95%)
• Elevated liver function tests (80%)
• Hypergammaglobulinemia (80%)
• Positive heterophil antibodies (70%)
• Thrombocytopenia (50%)
• Elevated bilirubin (40%)
• Cold agglutinins (30-80%)
• Monospot test useful as screen
Drugs that may alter lab results: N/A
Disorders that may alter lab results:
• CMV most frequently confused with EBV-induced mononucleosis
• Group A beta streptococcus often present (30%); does not rule out mononucleosis

PATHOLOGICAL FINDINGS
• B-cell lymphocytes infected
• Polyclonal proliferation of B-cells
• Strong T-cell response

SPECIAL TESTS
Positive results most likely during 2nd to 3rd week of clinical illness
• Heterophil antibody tests (Monospot or differential absorption). Tends to be negative in young children.
• Specific EBV titers (use in heterophil negative or complications)
   ◊ Viral capsid antigen (VCA): IgG and IgM - peak at 3-4 weeks. IgG then declines, but persists for life. IgM declines rapidly and is undetectable by 3 months. High persisting IgG suggests remote infection, systemic lupus, chronic renal failure, Burkitt's lymphoma, nasopharyngeal cancer, leukemia, sarcoidosis, cancer, AIDS, Hodgkin's lymphoma, rheumatoid arthritis, and immunodeficiency state.
   ◊ Early antigen (EA): Occur in 70-90%, persist 2-3 months. May persist in up to 20% of remote infections. High persisting titers might suggest: Pregnancy, immunodeficiency states, Hodgkin's lymphoma, lymphoma, leukemia, AIDS, Burkitt's, nasopharyngeal carcinoma.
   ◊ Epstein-Barr nuclear antigen (EBNA): Develop after 2 months and persist indefinitely. E antigen in mononucleosis primarily. K antigen in nasopharyngeal carcinoma primarily. Absence suggests immunodeficiency.

IMAGING Possible splenomegaly and/or hepatomegaly

DIAGNOSTIC PROCEDURES
• History and physical - fatigue, fever, splenomegaly, adenopathy, pharyngitis
• Heterophil antibodies - positive serology
• CBC/differential - abnormal white count
   ◊ Absolute lymphocytosis (> 4,000 cells/cc)
   ◊ Relative lymphocytosis (> 50%)
   ◊ Atypical lymphocytosis (10-20% or more)

TREATMENT

APPROPRIATE HEALTH CARE
Outpatient usually

GENERAL MEASURES
• No specific treatment
• Quarantine not indicated
• General supportive measures
• Gargles
• Avoid vigorous splenic palpation

SURGICAL MEASURES If splenic rupture, splenectomy (not always necessary) though probable mode of management for near future

ACTIVITY
• Rest (bedrest possibly during acute phase)
• Avoid contact sports, heavy lifting, strenuous athletics

DIET
• Healthy diet important
• To ease throat discomfort, patient may want to drink milk shakes, fruit juices and consume soft foods

PATIENT EDUCATION
• Convalescence may take several weeks
• Avoid stress
• Discuss feasibility of continuing with school or work
• Emphasize risk of splenic rupture from contact sports

Mononucleosis

 MEDICATIONS

DRUG(S) OF CHOICE
• Antibiotics for secondary infections only
• Analgesics
  ◊ acetaminophen (Tylenol)
  ◊ codeine
• Steroids may be indicated in certain complications only - prednisone, 40-80 mg/d then less over 5-7 days. Consider in threatened airway obstruction, hemolytic anemia, and thrombocytopenic purpura.
• Specific antiviral therapy is of no benefit
Contraindications: Aspirin (associated with Reye's syndrome)
Precautions: Refer to manufacturer's profile of each drug
Significant possible interactions: Refer to manufacturer's profile of each drug

ALTERNATIVE DRUGS N/A

 FOLLOWUP

PATIENT MONITORING
• Re-evaluate as needed based on clinical findings
• Preferable documentation of resolution of splenomegaly before resuming contact sports

PREVENTION/AVOIDANCE Most likely spread by saliva

POSSIBLE COMPLICATIONS
• Chronic EBV Infections (chronic fatigue syndrome- very controversial)
• Splenic rupture (rare, 0.1-0.5% of patients with proven mononucleosis)
• Hemolytic anemia (mild)
• Thrombocytopenic purpura
• Coagulopathy
• Aplastic anemia
• Hemolytic-uremic syndrome
• Seizures
• Cerebellar syndrome
• Nerve palsies
• Meningoencephalitis
• Optic neuritis
• Reye's syndrome
• Coma
• Transverse myelitis
• Guillain-Barré syndrome
• Psychosis
• Pericarditis
• Myocarditis
• ECG changes
• Airway obstruction
• Pneumonitis
• Pleural effusion
• Pulmonary hemorrhage
• Hepatitis/liver necrosis
• Malabsorption
• Dermatitis
• Urticaria
• Erythema multiforme
• Glomerulonephritis
• Nephrotic syndrome
• Mild hematuria/proteinuria
• Conjunctivitis
• Episcleritis
• Uveitis
• B-hemolytic streptococcal infections
• Staphylococcal infection
• Mycoplasma infection
• Bullous myringitis
• Orchitis
• Parotitis
• Monoarticular arthritis

EXPECTED COURSE/PROGNOSIS
• Fever subsides in about 10 days
• Adenopathy and splenomegaly subside in about 4 weeks
• Children should be able to return to school when signs of infection have decreased, appetite returns, and alertness, strength, and sense of well-being allow.
• Death is uncommon (splenic rupture, blood dyscrasias, hypersplenism, or encephalitis)
• Potential role in some malignancies, especially in context of immune suppression

 MISCELLANEOUS

ASSOCIATED CONDITIONS
Streptococcal pharyngitis

AGE-RELATED FACTORS
Pediatric:
• Children have subclinical or mild infections
• Most adolescents have clinically apparent infections
Geriatric: N/A
Others: N/A

PREGNANCY No other specific recommendations

SYNONYMS
• Mono
• Infectious mononucleosis (IM)

ICD-9-CM 075 Infectious mononucleosis

SEE ALSO Epstein-Barr virus infections

OTHER NOTES N/A

ABBREVIATIONS N/A

REFERENCES
• Neinstein L: Adolescent Health Care: A Practical Guide. 2nd Ed. Baltimore, Urban & Schwarzenberg, Inc., 1991
• Schroeder SA, Krupp MA, Tierney LM, McPhee SJ, eds: Current Medical Diagnosis and Treatment. Norwalk, CT, Appleton & Lange, 1989
• Isselbacher KJ, et al, eds: Harrison's Principles of Internal Medicine. 13th Ed. New York, McGraw-Hill, 1994
• Safran D, Bloom GP: Spontaneous Splenic Following Mononucleosis. American Surgeon 1990;56(10):601-605 (VI:91093752)
• Hanto DW: Clarification of EB virus associated posttransplant lymphoproliferative diseases. Ann Rev Med 1995:46:381-394
• Oren J, Sobel J: Human herpesvirus type 6. Review Clin Infectious Dis 1992;14:741-746
• Schuler J, Horst F: Spontaneous splenic rupture - the role of nonoperative management. Arch Surg 1995;130:662-665
• Goodman, Gilman: The Pharmacological Basis of Therapeutics. 9th Ed. New York, McGraw-Hill, 1996
Illustrations: 2 available on CD-ROM
Internet references: http://www.5mcc.com

Author(s)
Robert L. Weston, MD

Motion sickness

BASICS

DESCRIPTION Not a true sickness but a normal response to an abnormal situation in which there is a sensory conflict about body motion between the visual receptors, vestibular receptors and body proprioceptors. It can also be induced when patterns of motion differ from those previously experienced.
System(s) affected: Nervous
Genetics: N/A
Incidence/Prevalence in USA: N/A
Predominant age: N/A
Predominant sex: N/A

SIGNS AND SYMPTOMS
• Nausea
• Vomiting
• Diaphoresis
• Pallor
• Hypersalivation
• Yawning
• Hyperventilation
• Anxiety
• Panic
• Malaise
• Fatigue
• Weakness
• Confusion

CAUSES Motion (auto, plane, boat, amusement rides)

RISK FACTORS
• Travel
• Visual stimuli (i.e. moving horizon)
• Poor ventilation (fumes, smoke, carbon monoxide)
• Emotions (fear, anxiety)
• Zero gravity
• Other illness or poor health

DIAGNOSIS

DIFFERENTIAL DIAGNOSIS
• Mountain sickness
• Vestibular disease
• Gastroenteritis
• Metabolic disorders
• Toxin exposure

LABORATORY N/A
Drugs that may alter lab results: N/A
Disorders that may alter lab results: N/A

PATHOLOGICAL FINDINGS N/A

SPECIAL TESTS N/A

IMAGING N/A

DIAGNOSTIC PROCEDURES N/A

TREATMENT

APPROPRIATE HEALTH CARE Remove triggers or noxious stimuli

GENERAL MEASURES
• Minimize exposure (seat in middle of plane or boat)
• Improve ventilation

SURGICAL MEASURES N/A

ACTIVITY
• Semi-recumbent seating
• Fix vision at 45 degree angle above horizon
• Avoid fixation of vision on moving objects (i.e., waves)
• Avoid reading

DIET
• Decrease oral intake or take frequent small feedings
• Avoid alcohol

PATIENT EDUCATION N/A

Motion sickness

MEDICATIONS

DRUG(S) OF CHOICE
• Scopolamine (transdermal; where available) patch: Apply 6 hours before travel and replace every 3 days
or
• Dimenhydrinate (Dramamine) adults and adolescents 50-100 mg q4h, maximum 400 mg/day; children 6-12 years 25-50 mg q4h, maximum 150 mg/day

Contraindications: Glaucoma

Precautions:
• Young children
• Elderly
• Pregnancy
• Urinary obstruction
• Pyloric obstruction

Significant possible interactions:
• Sedatives (antihistamines, alcohol, antidepressants)
• Anticholinergics (belladonna alkaloids)

ALTERNATIVE DRUGS
• Antihistamines
  ◊ Meclizine (Antivert)
  ◊ Terfenadine (Seldane)

FOLLOWUP

PATIENT MONITORING N/A

PREVENTION/AVOIDANCE
• Minimize exposure (seat in middle of plane or boat)
• Improve ventilation
• Semi-recumbent seating
• Fix vision at 45 degree angle above horizon
• Avoid fixation of vision on moving objects (i.e., waves)
• Avoid reading
• Minimize food intake prior to travel

POSSIBLE COMPLICATIONS
• Hypotension
• Dehydration
• Depression
• Panic

EXPECTED COURSE/PROGNOSIS
• Symptoms should resolve when motion exposure ends
• Resistance to motion sickness seems to increase with age

MISCELLANEOUS

ASSOCIATED CONDITIONS N/A

AGE-RELATED FACTORS
Pediatric: Children more susceptible to motion sickness
Geriatric: Age confers some resistance to motion sickness
Others: N/A

PREGNANCY N/A

SYNONYMS
• Car sickness
• Sea sickness
• Air sickness
• Space sickness

ICD-9-CM
994.6 Motion sickness

SEE ALSO N/A

OTHER NOTES N/A

ABBREVIATIONS N/A

REFERENCES
• Dundee JW, McMillan C: Positive evidence for P6 acupuncture antiemesis. Postgrad Med 1991;67:417-422
• Bennett JC, Plum F, eds: Cecil Textbook of Medicine. 20th Ed. Philadelphia, W.B. Saunders Co., 1996
• Kohl RL, Calkins DS: Control of nausea & autonomic dysfunction with terfenadine, a peripherally acting antihistamine. Aviation, Space and Environmental Medicine 1991;62(5):392-396
Illustrations: N/A
Internet references: http://www.5mcc.com

Author(s)
Marshall Godwin, MD

Multiple myeloma

 BASICS

DESCRIPTION
Multiple myeloma (malignant tumor of plasma cells) is the most common primary malignancy of bone. It is the prototype of a monoclonal tumor cell proliferation that usually reveals monoclonal protein in the serum or urine of more than 90% of patients. The disease process encompasses a spectrum of localized and disseminated disease forms.

System(s) affected: Hemic/Lymphatic/Immunologic, Nervous, Musculoskeletal

Genetics: Occasional familial occurrence, indicating recessive heredity

Incidence/Prevalence in USA: Multiple myeloma accounts for approximately 1% of all types of malignant disease and slightly more than 10% of hematologic malignancies

Predominant age: Ages 40 to 80 (with a peak incidence in the 70's)

Predominant sex: Male = Female

SIGNS AND SYMPTOMS
• The majority of patients (65%) present with bone pain
• Pathologic fracture occurs in approximately one-third of these patients
• Weakness and fatigue are common
• Bleeding (nose, gums), often evidenced by purpura or epistaxis, may occur in the presence of thrombocytopenia or secondary amyloidosis
• Recurrent infections may occur
• Patients may also present with renal insufficiency or renal failure
• Swelling on ribs, skull, sternum, vertebrae, clavicles, shoulder, pelvis
• Weight loss
• Hyperviscosity syndrome

CAUSES
Unknown. There are tumor cells characteristic of plasma cells arising from bone marrow.

RISK FACTORS
Family history of myeloma

 DIAGNOSIS

DIFFERENTIAL DIAGNOSIS
Metastatic carcinoma, primary malignancy of bone (sarcoma, lymphoma), metabolic bone disease, monoclonal gammopathy of undetermined significance (MGUS)

LABORATORY
• Anemia is present in 70% of the patients at the time of diagnosis. Nearly all patients will develop anemia as the disease progresses.
• Peripheral blood smear - rouleaux formation
• Serum protein electrophoresis - usually shows a spike or a localized band (M spike in approximately 80% of patients). Of these, 50% are IgG protein, 20% IgA, and 17% free monoclonal light chains (Bence Jones protein).
• Urine electrophoresis - positive about 70% of the time for light chains, but inconsistencies hinder diagnosis
• Hypercalcemia
• Decreased platelets
• Elevated sedimentation rate
• Elevated creatinine and BUN

Drugs that may alter lab results: N/A
Disorders that may alter lab results: N/A

PATHOLOGICAL FINDINGS
• Secondary amyloidosis
• Myeloma kidney

SPECIAL TESTS   N/A

IMAGING
• Skeletal x-rays often show a radiolucent or a lytic lesion when the long bones are involved. The skull often shows punched-out lytic lesions with no sclerotic or reactive border. Periosteal reaction is uncommon. Vertebral compression fractures, with occasional extraosseous or extradural cord compression, are commonly seen.
• Although technetium-99 bone scans have often been described as cold, they will actually show some slight uptake increase in involved skeletal regions, particularly in the presence of fracture; however, the amount of uptake is far less than that demonstrated in other malignancies of bone
• MRI scans can be extremely valuable in determining the extent of marrow involvement as well as the difference between benign compression fractures and multiple myeloma lesions

DIAGNOSTIC PROCEDURES
The laboratory test most likely to yield a definitive diagnosis is a bone marrow biopsy. The bone marrow will contain increased numbers of plasma cells at various stages of maturation.

 TREATMENT

APPROPRIATE HEALTH CARE
Outpatient, except during intensive chemotherapy periods

GENERAL MEASURES
• Radiation therapy is limited to patients with intractable bone pain (failing chemotherapy)
• Patients with impending or pathologic fractures should have those fractures rigidly stabilized along with removal of the tumor, if possible. Patients with impending paraplegia secondary to spinal cord involvement should undergo immediate radiation therapy and bracing and/or surgical decompression and stabilization.

SURGICAL MEASURES   N/A

ACTIVITY   As tolerated

DIET   No special diet

PATIENT EDUCATION
American Cancer Society has literature available

MEDICATIONS

DRUG(S) OF CHOICE Chemotherapy is the primary treatment for symptomatic multiple myeloma, but the ideal chemotherapy is unknown. The most common initial protocol management includes the oral administration of melphalan (Alkeran) and prednisone. This protocol produces an objective response in 50-60% of the patients. This is usually given in oral doses of 0.25 mg/kg/day for four days, along with 50 mg of prednisone bid for the same period of time. The dosage should be repeated every six weeks with leukocyte and platelet counts evaluated at three-week intervals.

Contraindications: Refer to manufacturer's profile of each drug

Precautions:
• Melphalan - myelosuppression is the major dose-limiting toxicity of this drug (mainly leukopenia, thrombocytopenia). Monitor CBC, platelets every 3 weeks.
• Prednisone - usual hazards of long-term corticosteroid administration. Refer to manufacturer's literature.

Significant possible interactions: Refer to manufacturer's profile of each drug

ALTERNATIVE DRUGS In the event of failure of the above-mentioned regimen, alternate protocols include
◊ Cyclophosphamide, carmustine (BCNU), vincristine, and prednisone
◊ VAD - combination of vincristine, doxorubicin (Adriamycin), and dexamethasone

FOLLOWUP

PATIENT MONITORING CBC, platelets q 6 weeks

PREVENTION/AVOIDANCE N/A

POSSIBLE COMPLICATIONS
• Skeletal destruction
• Spontaneous fractures
• Secondary amyloidosis
• Renal insufficiency
• Recurrent infections (e.g., Streptococcus pneumoniae, Haemophilus influenzae)
• Hyperviscosity syndrome

EXPECTED COURSE/PROGNOSIS
• Average survival time varies considerably. The median survival of all patients is approximately 24 months. A significantly large number of patients survive for much longer periods of time with evidence of disease present.
• There are occasional temporary remissions with therapy
• Bone marrow transplantation should be considered in younger patients

MISCELLANEOUS

ASSOCIATED CONDITIONS Multiple myeloma has an association with systemic amyloidosis in which the amyloid is derived from immunoglobulin light chains. In one autopsy series, 15% of the patients had generalized amyloidosis with deposits in the kidneys, spleen, adrenal bodies, and liver. Kidney involvement often leads to azotemia and secondary renal failure.

AGE-RELATED FACTORS
Pediatric: N/A
Geriatric: More common in older adults
Others: N/A

PREGNANCY N/A

SYNONYMS Myeloma, plasma cell

ICD-9-CM 203.0 Multiple myeloma

SEE ALSO N/A

OTHER NOTES N/A

ABBREVIATIONS N/A

REFERENCES DeVita VT, Hellman S, Rosenberg SA: The Principles and Practices of Oncology. 4th Ed. Philadelphia, J.B. Lippincott, 1993
Illustrations: N/A
Internet references: http://www.5mcc.com

Author(s)
Mark C. Leeson, MD, FACS

Multiple sclerosis

BASICS

DESCRIPTION
Multiple sclerosis (MS) is a recurrent (occasionally progressive) inflammatory progressive demyelinization of the white matter of the brain and spinal cord resulting in multiple and varied neurologic symptoms and signs. Usual course - intermittent, progressive and relapsing. It may pursue an acute course or slowly progressive. It is a major cause of disability in young adults.
System(s) affected: Nervous
Genetics: Appears to be a strong genetic component in determining susceptibility to the disease.
Incidence/prevalence in USA: 25,000 new cases each year
Predominant age: Young adult (16-40 years)
Predominant sex: Female > Male

SIGNS AND SYMPTOMS
- Ataxia
- Babinski sign
- Blurred, double or loss of vision in a single eye; often triggered by retro-bulbar neuritis and its visual sequelae
- Clonus
- Clumsiness
- Dysarthria
- Emotional
- Lability
- Fatigue
- Genital anesthesia in women
- Hand paralysis
- Hemiparesis
- Hyperactive deep tendon reflexes
- Hyperesthesia
- Incoordination
- Loss of position sense
- Loss of vibration sense
- Monoparesis
- Ocular paralysis
- Paresthesias
- Sexual impotence in men
- Urinary frequency, hesitancy, incontinence
- Trigeminal neuralgia

CAUSES
- Unknown
- Autoimmune theory - supported by HLA linkage, hereditary pattern, immunocytes in plaques, changes in peripheral blood immunocytes
- Viral theory - supported by increasing incidence of disease at higher latitudes, clusters of cases with families, geographical clusters of cases, animal studies of infectious diseases of myelin
- Combined theory - autoimmune disorder triggered by environmental exposure to toxin or virus early in life

RISK FACTORS
- Living in temperate zone
- Northern European descent
- Family history of the disease

DIAGNOSIS

DIFFERENTIAL DIAGNOSIS
- Amyotrophic lateral sclerosis
- Behçet's disease
- Brain stem tumors
- Central nervous system infections
- Cerebellar tumors
- Friedreich's ataxia
- Hereditary ataxias
- Leukodystrophies
- Neurofibromatosis
- Pernicious anemia
- Progressive multifocal leukoencephalopathy
- Ruptured intervertebral disk
- Small cerebral infarcts
- Sarcoidosis
- Spinal cord tumors
- Syphilis
- Syringomyelia
- Systemic lupus erythematosus
- Vasculitides

LABORATORY
- Cerebrospinal fluid
  ◊ Abnormal colloidal gold curve
  ◊ Gamma globulin IgG elevated
  ◊ Mild mononuclear pleocytosis (less than 40 cells/mL)
  ◊ Myelin debris
  ◊ Negative serology for syphilis
  ◊ Protein normal or slightly elevated 50-100 mg/100 mL (50-100 mg/dL [500-1000 mg/L])
- Tests to exclude other disorders
  ◊ Fluorescent treponemal antibody absorption (FTA-ABS)
  ◊ Sedimentation rate
  ◊ Screens for clinically suspected vasculitic disorders
  ◊ Human T-lymphotropic virus-1 (HTLV-I) serology
Drugs that may alter lab results: N/A
Disorders that may alter lab results: N/A

PATHOLOGICAL FINDINGS
- Destruction of myelin sheaths of nerve fibers and axis cylinders, sparing axons, glia and other structures
- Atrophy of optic nerves and cerebral hemispheres
- T-cell lymphocytes about venules

SPECIAL TESTS
- Visual evoked response (VER) - abnormal in 75-97% of definite MS cases
- Somatosensory evoked potentials - abnormal in 72-96% of cases
- Brain stem auditory evoked responses - abnormal in 57-65% of cases
- CSF
  ◊ Oligoclonal bands
  ◊ Increased IgG

IMAGING N/A
- MRI (more sensitive than CT) - may show many plaques
- CT scan (double-dose, delayed) - plaques

DIAGNOSTIC PROCEDURES
- No test specific to diagnose MS
- History, physical, CSF analysis, MRI, evoked potential studies, repeated observations over a period of time

TREATMENT

APPROPRIATE HEALTH CARE
- Outpatient as long as possible
- Long-term care facility for physical therapy or complications such as pyelonephritis

GENERAL MEASURES
- No specific therapy. Remissions occur spontaneously and make treatment evaluations difficult.
- Emotional support, encouragement, and reassurances are necessary to help avoid a hopeless outlook
- Occupational therapy
- Urologic evaluation including any sexual dysfunction problems (impotence common in male patients)
- Self-catheterizations for inadequate bladder emptying (indwelling catheter may be necessary in a few patients)
- Custodial care, if patient cognitively impaired
- Physiotherapy to maintain range of movement and strength and to avoid contractures

SURGICAL MEASURES N/A

ACTIVITY
- Maintain activity, avoid overwork and fatigue
- Rest during periods of acute relapse

DIET If constipation a problem, high fluid intake, plus a high fiber diet

PATIENT EDUCATION For patient education materials favorably reviewed on this topic, contact: National Multiple Sclerosis Society, 205E 42nd Street, New York, NY 10017, (800)624-8236

MEDICATIONS

DRUG(S) OF CHOICE
Drug therapy directed toward relieving symptoms
• Methylprednisolone: IV 1000 mg for 5 days followed by tapered oral prednisone for acute attacks, especially retrobulbar neuritis (recommended by some clinicians)
• Spasticity: baclofen, low dosage to start, 5 mg 1-3 times a day, increase as needed, or diazepam 2-5 mg qhs
• Constipation: stool softeners, bulk producing agents, laxative suppositories
• Urinary problems: propantheline 7.5 mg every 3-4 hours to start, increase to 15 mg 3-4 times a day plus 15-30 mg at bedtime; or oxybutynin chloride 5 mg 3-4 times a day
• Prophylactic antibiotics: for urinary infections
• Incoordination or tremors: no ideal therapy; may try beta-blockers (if not contraindicated), primidone, or clonazepam.
• Depression and emotional lability: amitriptyline 10-25 mg at bedtime to start, increase as tolerated
• Paranoia or mania: haloperidol or lithium
• Musculoskeletal pain or discomfort: nonsteroidal anti-inflammatories
• Hemifacial and dysesthesias: carbamazepine 100-200 once or twice a day to start, increase to total daily dosage of 600-1600 mg 3-4 times a day. Must monitor serum levels.
• Immunosuppressive agents (e.g., azathioprine, ACTH (adrenocorticotropic hormone), methylprednisolone, cyclophosphamide, interferons, cyclosporine) still investigational
Contraindications: Refer to manufacturer's literature
Precautions: Refer to manufacturer's literature
Significant possible interactions: Refer to manufacturer's literature

ALTERNATIVE DRUGS
• Oral steroids: Poor evidence for use alone
• Chronic fatigue: amantadine 200-300 mg/day (no specific evidence that this works)
• Baclofen 40-80 mg/day in divided doses for reduction of spasticity
• Interferon beta approved for relapsing MS - 0.25 mg SC every other day
• Copolymer-1 and cladribine have shown promising results in clinical results

FOLLOWUP

PATIENT MONITORING Requires patient follow-up

PREVENTION/AVOIDANCE No known preventive measures. Avoid factors that may precipitate an attack, particularly stress from hot weather.

POSSIBLE COMPLICATIONS
• Coma
• Delirium
• Emotional lability
• Nystagmus
• Optic nerve atrophy
• Paraplegia
• Sexual impotence (men)
• Urinary tract infections

EXPECTED COURSE/PROGNOSIS
• Highly variable and unpredictable. Approximately 70% of patients lead active, productive lives with prolonged remissions.
• May disable the patient by early adulthood or cause death within months of onset
• Average duration exceeds 25 years
• 30% relapse in one year, 20% in 5-9 years, 10% in 10-30 years

MISCELLANEOUS

ASSOCIATED CONDITIONS N/A

AGE-RELATED FACTORS
Pediatric: Unlikely before puberty.
Geriatric: Remissions less frequent in this age group
Others: N/A

PREGNANCY A triggering factor for multiple sclerosis in some cases

SYNONYMS
• Disseminated sclerosis
• Insular sclerosis

ICD-9-CM 340 Multiple sclerosis

OTHER NOTES
• Since the course is highly variable and unpredictable, avoid a hopeless outlook
• 30-40% of patients with optic neuritis alone eventually develop other signs

ABBREVIATIONS N/A

REFERENCES
• Sibley WA: Therapeutic claims in multiple sclerosis. 2nd Ed. New York, Demos, 1988
• Matthews WB, et al: McAlpine's Multiple Sclerosis. 2nd Ed. New York, Churchill Livingstone, 1991
• Adams RD, Victor M: Principles of Neurology. 5th Ed. New York, McGraw-Hill, 1993
• Rowlan LP, ed: Merritt's Textbook of Neurology. 9th Ed. Philadelphia, Williams & Wilkins, 1995
• Beck RW, et al: The effect of corticosteroids for acute optic neuritis on the subsequent development of multiple sclerosis. New Engl J Med 1994;329;24:1764-1769
Illustrations: 1 available on CD-ROM
Internet references: http://www.5mcc.com

Author(s)
Stan G. Smith, MA, MB, FCFPC

Mumps

BASICS

DESCRIPTION Acute generalized paramyxovirus infection usually presenting with unilateral or bilateral parotitis. Epidemics occur in late winter and spring with transmission by respiratory secretions. Incubation is approximately 14 to 24 days.

System(s) affected: Reproductive, Hemic/Lymphatic/Immunologic, Skin/Exocrine

Genetics: N/A

Incidence/Prevalence in USA:
• 0.96/100,000 (2400 per year)
• 0 .0064/100,000
• 90% of adults are sero-positive even without history

Predominant age: 85% occur before age 15 years, but more severe in adults

Predominant sex: Male = Female

SIGNS AND SYMPTOMS
• Parotid pain and swelling in one or both glands
• Rare prodrome of fever, neck muscle ache, malaise
• Initial parotid swelling just behind jaw
• Swelling peaks in 1-3 days, lasts 3-7 days
• Obscures angle of mandible
• Elevates earlobe
• Redness at opening of Stensen's duct
• Sour foods cause pain in the parotid gland region
• Moderate fever, usually not above 104°F (40.0°C). High fever is frequently associated with complications.
• Meningeal signs in 15%, encephalitis in 0.5%
• Rarely arthritis, orchitis, thyroiditis, mastitis, pancreatitis
• Rare maculopapular erythematous rash
• Up to 50% of cases may be asymptomatic
• Swelling in the sternal area, rare, but pathognomonic of mumps

CAUSES
• Mumps paramyxovirus
• Other viruses, such as Coxsackie (rare)

RISK FACTORS
• Urban epidemics, non-vaccinated population
• Usual communicable period is 24 hours before to 72 hours after onset of parotitis
• Incubation period usually 18 days

DIAGNOSIS

DIFFERENTIAL DIAGNOSIS
• Parainfluenza parotitis, other viruses
• Suppurative parotitis - often associated with Staphylococcus aureus (presence of Wharton's duct pus nearly excludes diagnosis of mumps)
• Recurrent allergic parotitis
• Salivary calculus with intermittent swelling
• Lymphadenitis from any cause
• Cytomegalovirus parotitis in immunocompromised patients
• Mikulicz's syndrome (chronic, painless parotid and lacrimal gland swelling of unknown cause that occurs in tuberculosis, sarcoidosis, lupus, leukemia, and lymphosarcoma patients)
• Malignant or benign salivary gland tumors
• Drug-related parotid enlargement (iodides, guanethidine)
• Other causes of the complications of mumps (meningoencephalitis, orchitis, oophoritis, pancreatitis, polyarthritis, nephritis, myocarditis, prostatitis)
• Mumps orchitis must be differentiated from testicular torsion. (Testicular scan can be useful.)

LABORATORY
• Viral isolation from throat washings, urine, blood, or spinal fluid
• Serum amylase elevated
• Rise in paired antibodies: Anti-"S" antibodies peak early and may be seen at the time of presentation
• Cerebrospinal fluid (CSF) - leukocytosis
• Leukopenia

Drugs that may alter lab results: N/A
Disorders that may alter lab results: N/A

PATHOLOGICAL FINDINGS Periductal edema and lymphocytic infiltration

SPECIAL TESTS Rarely necessary

IMAGING Useful to differentiate mumps orchitis from testicular torsion

DIAGNOSTIC PROCEDURES N/A

TREATMENT

APPROPRIATE HEALTH CARE
Outpatient, if no complications

GENERAL MEASURES
• Supportive and symptomatic
• For patients with orchitis, ice packs to scrotum can help relieve pain
• Scrotal support with adhesive bridge while recumbent and/or athletic supporter while ambulatory
• Use IV fluids if severe nausea or vomiting accompanies pancreatitis

SURGICAL MEASURES N/A

ACTIVITY Mumps orchitis - bedrest and local supportive clothing, such as wearing 2 pairs of briefs, or adhesive-tape bridge

DIET Liquids if cannot chew

PATIENT EDUCATION
• Must be out of school until no longer contagious - about 9 days after onset of pain
• Orchitis is common in older children but rarely results in sterility
• Immunization of family may protect against later exposures but not the present one

MEDICATIONS

DRUG(S) OF CHOICE Corticosteroids or a nonsteroidal anti-inflammatory may diminish pain and swelling in acute orchitis and arthritis mumps, but usually not necessary. May use acetaminophen for fever and/or pain.
Contraindications: Refer to manufacturer's profile of each drug
Precautions: Avoid aspirin for pain in children. There may be an association of aspirin, virus infection, and Reye's syndrome in children.
Significant possible interactions: Refer to manufacturer's profile of each drug

ALTERNATIVE DRUGS Mumps arthritis may improve with corticosteroids or a nonsteroidal anti-inflammatory

FOLLOWUP

PATIENT MONITORING Most cases will be mild. Monitor hydration status.

PREVENTION/AVOIDANCE
• 2 doses of live mumps vaccine recommended for active immunization: At 15 months and at entry to middle school. (Postexposure vaccination does not protect from recent exposure).
• Isolate hospitalized patients until 9 days past onset

POSSIBLE COMPLICATIONS
• May precede, accompany, or follow salivary gland involvement and may occur (rarely) without primary involvement of the parotid gland
• Meningoencephalitis occurs clinically in approximately 10%. These symptoms may begin as late as 10 days following symptoms that signal onset of the illness.
• Cerebrospinal fluid (CSF) pleocytosis found in 65% of cases with parotitis
• Orchitis common (30%) in postpubertal boys, starts within 8 days after parotitis, fever, swollen testis of 4 day duration, fertility impaired in 13% but absolute sterility is rare
• Oophoritis in 7% of postpubertal females, no decreased fertility
• Pancreatitis, usually mild
• Nephritis, thyroiditis, or arthralgias are rare
• Myocarditis - usually mild, but may depress ST segment, may be linked to endocardial fibroelastosis
• Deafness - 1/15,000 unilateral nerve deafness, may not be permanent
• Inflammation about the eye (rare)
• Dacryoadenitis, optic neuritis

EXPECTED COURSE/PROGNOSIS
• Complete recovery is usual, immunity is permanent
• Sensorineural hearing loss in 4% of adults - transient
• Rare recurrence after 2 weeks may be recurrent nonepidemic parotitis

MISCELLANEOUS

ASSOCIATED CONDITIONS N/A

AGE-RELATED FACTORS
Pediatric:
• In adolescents - orchitis more common
• Most cases of acute epidemic mumps occur in children aged 5 to 15. Unusual in children less than 2 years. Most infants less than 1 year are immune.
• Less likely to develop complications
Geriatric: Most are immune
Others: Most complications occur in post-pubertal group

PREGNANCY
• No proven complications of vaccine, but theoretically should not vaccinate in pregnancy
• Disease may increase rate of spontaneous abortion in first trimester

SYNONYMS
• Epidemic parotitis
• Infectious parotitis

ICD-9-CM 072.9 Mumps without mention of complication

SEE ALSO N/A

OTHER NOTES A portion of people infected with mumps virus have no parotid swelling and a clinically inapparent infection

ABBREVIATIONS N/A

REFERENCES
• Behrman RE, ed: Nelson's Textbook of Pediatrics. Philadelphia, W.B. Saunders, 1996
• Report of the Committee on Infectious Diseases (Red Book). Elk Grove Village, Ill, American Academy of Pediatrics, 1994
Illustrations: N/A
Internet references: http://www.5mcc.com

Author(s)
Frances Wu, MD

Muscular dystrophy

BASICS

DESCRIPTION Inherited, progressive diseases of muscle with wide ranges of clinical expression. Included:
• Congenital muscular dystrophy
• Congenital myotonic dystrophy
• Duchenne's muscular dystrophy (DMD)
• Becker's muscular dystrophy (BMD)
• Myotonic dystrophy
• Fascioscapulohumeral dystrophy (FSH)
• Emery-Dreifuss muscular dystrophy (ED)
System(s) affected: Musculoskeletal, Nervous
Genetics: See Causes and Risk factors
Incidence/Prevalence in USA:
• Duchenne's muscular dystrophy (DMD): 1 per 3000 male births
• Myotonic dystrophy: 1 per 10,000 births
Predominant age:
• Birth to infancy: Congenital muscular dystrophy with or without cerebral involvement, congenital myotonic dystrophy
• Infancy to early childhood: Duchenne's muscular dystrophy (DMD), Becker's muscular dystrophy (BMD), fascioscapulohumeral dystrophy (FHS)
• Late childhood to adolescence: BMD, FSH, myotonic dystrophy
Predominant sex: Male > Female (DMD and BMD caused by defect in same gene)

SIGNS AND SYMPTOMS
• DMD and BMD:
  ◊ Leg pain may be an early complaint
  ◊ Normal motor milestones until child begins to walk
  ◊ Clumsiness - frequent falls, toe-walking, waddling gait
  ◊ Weakness - inability to jump or climb stairs, weak neck flexors, Gower's sign, lumbar lordosis
  ◊ Pseudohypertrophy of calf muscles and contractures of heel cords
  ◊ Kyphosis and scoliosis
• Myotonic dystrophy:
  ◊ Facial weakness - open, triangular mouth and droopy eyelids
  ◊ Sustained muscle contraction with percussion of thenar eminence
  ◊ High forehead with receding hairline
  ◊ Neonatal form - hypotonia, respiratory distress, hip dislocations
  ◊ Cataracts, gonadal dysfunction, cardiac conduction defects/arrhythmias
  ◊ Difficulty in letting go (myotonia) after handshake
• FSH:
  ◊ Facial weakness - inability to completely close eyes or whistle, pouting expression with transverse smile
  ◊ Shoulder and proximal arm weakness: inability to do push-ups, horizontal clavicles, exaggerated bicep muscles size ("Popeye" arms), winging of the scapula

• ED:
  ◊ Toe walking and small biceps
  ◊ Contractures of neck, biceps, Achilles tendons - even without significant weakness
  ◊ Cardiac conduction abnormalities with risk of sudden death

CAUSES
• X-linked: DMD and milder allelic form BMD have gene deletion at Xp21.2 for production of "dystrophin"; ED have abnormal gene at Xq 28
• Autosomal dominant: Myotonic dystrophy gene mapped to short arm of chromosome 19. FSH gene mapped to long arm of chromosome 4.

RISK FACTORS
• X-linked - affected male on maternal side of family (although female carriers may rarely be symptomatic)
• Autosomal dominant - affected parent. Myotonic dystrophy more severe if mother is affected parent.

DIAGNOSIS

DIFFERENTIAL DIAGNOSIS
• Onset from birth to early infancy: Encephalopathy, spinal muscular atrophy, infantile botulism, myasthenia gravis, congenital myopathies, metabolic myopathies, chromosomal disorders, paroxysmal disorders, neonatal spinal cord injury
• Onset from infancy to early childhood: Carnitine deficiency, acid maltase deficiency, spinal muscular atrophy, myotonia congenita
• Onset from childhood to adolescence: Other muscular dystrophies, spinal muscular atrophy, congenital myopathies, metabolic or inflammatory myopathies, myasthenia gravis, periodic paralysis

LABORATORY
• Creatine kinase:
  ◊ Marked elevation in DMD
  ◊ Moderate elevation in BMD, FSH
  ◊ Normal in congenital muscular dystrophy, late DMD
Drugs that may alter lab results:
• Opiates including codeine, heroin, meperidine, and morphine
• Dexamethasone
• Ethanol
• Digoxin
• Furosemide
• Aminocaproic acid
• Halothane
• Imipramine
• Phenobarbital
• Lithium
• Clofibrate
Disorders that may alter lab results:
• Polymyositis/dermatomyositis
• Muscle trauma - exercise, seizures, IM injections, needle EMG
• Hypothyroidism, hyperthyroidism
• Myocardial infarction, stroke, sepsis, shock

PATHOLOGICAL FINDINGS
Muscle biopsy in DMD - fiber splitting, necrosis, regeneration with interspersed fibrosis

SPECIAL TESTS EMG in myotonic dystrophy - high frequency repetitive discharges ("dive-bomber" effect)

IMAGING N/A

DIAGNOSTIC PROCEDURES
• Muscle biopsy of moderately weak muscle (vastus lateralis, triceps) not studied by needle electromyography
• Dystrophin level from muscle biopsy

TREATMENT

APPROPRIATE HEALTH CARE
Outpatient with team approach - neurologist, orthopedic surgeon, physical and occupational therapists, social worker, and orthotist

GENERAL MEASURES
• Physical therapy to maintain neuromuscular function
• Orthoses to sustain walking and delay development of scoliosis
• Respiratory care, ventilation during sleep for nocturnal hypoventilation syndrome

SURGICAL MEASURES Surgical release of contractures or fixation of joints

ACTIVITY Exercise as desired, but stop short of muscle pain or exhaustion

DIET Monitor nutrition and fat stores because of increased caloric requirements

PATIENT EDUCATION
• Family and individual counseling
• Genetic counseling
• Printed material and clinical services available through the Muscular Dystrophy Association, 3561 E. Sunrise Dr., Tucson, AZ 85718; (800)221-1142

MEDICATIONS

DRUG(S) OF CHOICE
• No drug treatment recommended at present
• Prednisone 0.15-0.75 mg/kg/day improves muscle strength in boys with DMD
Contraindications: N/A
Precautions: Careful monitoring for side effects of long-term steroid therapy is required; these include weight gain, hypertension, GI bleeding, immunosuppression
Significant possible interactions: N/A

ALTERNATIVE DRUGS   N/A

FOLLOWUP

PATIENT MONITORING
• Determined by interdisciplinary health care team
• In patients with ED, early detection of cardiac abnormalities may permit lifesaving pacemaker insertion

PREVENTION/AVOIDANCE
• Maternal carrier status evaluation in DMD (80% sensitive) and BMD (60% sensitive) by creatine kinase levels
• DNA probes for carrier status determination and antenatal diagnosis in DMD and BMD
• DNA linkage techniques in selected families for antenatal diagnosis of myotonic dystrophy

POSSIBLE COMPLICATIONS
• Cardiac arrhythmias or myopathy
  ◊ Especially in ED
  ◊ In DMD (< 80%)
  ◊ In BMD (< 40%)
• Hypertension - FSH
• Dysphagia or acute gastric dilation - DMD, myotonic dystrophy
• Malignant hyperthermia - DMD
• Respiratory failure and early death - congenital muscular dystrophy (15%), neonatal-onset myotonic dystrophy (> 50%)
• Endocrinopathies - myotonic dystrophy
• Cataracts - myotonic dystrophy
• Sensorineural hearing loss - FSH
• Seizures and cerebral dysplasia - congenital muscular dystrophy with cerebral involvement (> 50%)

EXPECTED COURSE/PROGNOSIS
• DMD and BMD:
  ◊ Progressive weakness, contractures, inability to walk
  ◊ Kyphoscoliosis and respiratory compromise
  ◊ Early death (Duchenne's 16 +/- 4 years; Becker's 42 +/- 16 years)
• Myotonic dystrophy (neonatal onset) and congenital muscular dystrophy with cerebral involvement:
  ◊ Progressive hypotonia and weakness
  ◊ Respiratory failure and early death
• Other types
  ◊ Slow progression and near normal life span

MISCELLANEOUS

ASSOCIATED CONDITIONS
• Mental retardation - DMD (25%), myotonic dystrophy with early onset
• Malignant hypothermia may be seen in patients with DMD

AGE-RELATED FACTORS
Pediatric: N/A
Geriatric: N/A
Others: N/A

PREGNANCY   Refer mother with myotonic dystrophy to perinatologist

SYNONYMS
• Pseudohypertrophic muscular dystrophy
• Steinert's disease
• Landouzy-Déjèrine dystrophy
• Fukuyama syndrome

ICD-9-CM
• 359.0 Congenital muscular dystrophy
• 359.1 DMD, BMD, FSH, ED and others
• 359.2 Myotonic dystrophy

SEE ALSO   N/A

OTHER NOTES   N/A

ABBREVIATIONS
• DMD = Duchenne's muscular dystrophy
• BMD = Becker's muscular dystrophy
• FSH = fascioscapulohumeral dystrophy

REFERENCES   Brooke MH: Clinician's View of Neuromuscular Diseases. 2nd Ed. Baltimore, Williams & Wilkins, 1986
Illustrations: N/A
Internet references: http://www.5mcc.com

Author(s)
David A. Griesemer, MD

Myasthenia gravis

BASICS

DESCRIPTION
A disorder of the neuromuscular junction resulting in a pure motor syndrome characterized by weakness and fatigue particularly of the extraocular, pharyngeal, facial, cervical, proximal limb and respiratory musculature. Typical and neonatal forms are immunologically mediated. A number of congenital forms of obscure pathogenesis exist. Onset may be sudden and severe (myasthenic crisis) but, more typically, is mild and intermittent over many years.

System(s) affected: Musculoskeletal, Hemic/Lymphatic/Immunologic

Genetics:
• 15% of infants born to myasthenic mothers have neonatal myasthenia gravis, due to the transplacental passage of acetylcholine receptor antibodies. The condition completely resolves in weeks to months. Neonatal myasthenia gravis is not a genetic disorder.
• Infants with congenital myasthenia gravis syndromes are born to normal mothers. The onset is at birth or in early childhood. Inheritance is typically autosomal recessive. The condition is persistent.
• Typical adult and juvenile myasthenia gravis do have a familial predisposition (5% of cases) and an increased frequency of HLA-B8 and DR3.

Incidence/Prevalence in USA:
2-5/year/million; 3/100,000

Predominant age: Ages 20-40, but occurs at any age (1-80). Incidence in females peaks in the 3rd decade, in males in the 5th and 6th decades.

Predominant sex:
• Adults - Female > Male (3:2)
• Children - Female > Male (3:2)
• Children with myasthenia plus associated disease - Female > Male (5:1)

SIGNS AND SYMPTOMS
• Ptosis
• Diplopia
• Facial weakness
• Fatigue on chewing
• Dysphagia
• Dysarthria
• Dysphonia
• Neck weakness
• Proximal limb weakness
• Respiratory weakness
• Generalized weakness

CAUSES
Humoral and cellular immune-mediated injury of the post-synaptic neuromuscular junction acetylcholine receptors

RISK FACTORS
• Female
• Age 20-40
• Familial myasthenia gravis
• D-penicillamine ingestion
• Other autoimmune diseases

DIAGNOSIS

DIFFERENTIAL DIAGNOSIS
• Chronic fatigue syndrome
• Oculopharyngeal muscular dystrophy
• Thyrotoxic ophthalmopathy
• Other disorders of neuromuscular transmission (myasthenic syndrome, botulism)
• Polymyositis
• Other myopathies
• Intracranial focal lesions involving cranial nerves
• Multiple sclerosis
• Depression

LABORATORY
• Acetylcholine receptor antibody - generalized myasthenia 80% positive; ocular myasthenia 50% positive; myasthenia + thymoma 100% positive; congenital myasthenia 0% positive; no clear correlation between antibody titer and disease severity
• Check thyroid function tests

Drugs that may alter lab results: N/A
Disorders that may alter lab results: N/A

PATHOLOGICAL FINDINGS
• Muscle electron microscopy - receptor infolding and the tips of the folds are lost, synaptic clefts are widened
• Immunofluorescence - IgG antibodies and complement on receptor membranes

SPECIAL TESTS
• Motor nerve conduction velocity - normal
• Sensory nerve conduction velocity - normal
• Concentric needle (conventional) electromyography- normal in mild cases; low amplitude, short duration, polyphasic motor unit potentials with a varying morphology (may be called "myopathic")
• Repetitive nerve stimulation - shows a decremental response at 3Hz which is seen more frequently in the proximal, cervical or facial muscles. The decrement is less pronounced 30 seconds after a 30 second maximal voluntary contraction (post-tetanic facilitation) and most pronounced 120 seconds after the contraction (post-tetanic depression).
• Single fiber EMG (SFEMG) - highly sensitive but less specific, technically difficult to perform, limited availability. SFEMG assesses the temporal variability between two muscle fibers within the same motor unit (jitter). Myasthenia is one condition that increases jitter.
• Edrophonium (Tensilon) test - initial dose is 2 mg IV, followed in 30 seconds by 3 mg, followed in 30 seconds by 5 mg to a maximum dose of 10 mg. A positive test is characterized by improvement of strength (of striated muscle) within 30 seconds of administration. False positives make a saline placebo control desirable. Atropine 0.4 mg IV may rarely be required as an antidote for severe bradycardia, but should always be available.

IMAGING
Chest CT scan - thymoma

DIAGNOSTIC PROCEDURES
• History and physical
• Electrodiagnostic studies; repetitive nerve stimulation (RNS)
• Edrophonium (Tensilon) test

TREATMENT

APPROPRIATE HEALTH CARE
• Typically outpatient
• Inpatient care for plasmapheresis, intravenous gamma globulin, management of pulmonary infections, myasthenic or cholinergic crises

GENERAL MEASURES
• Management of myasthenia gravis is difficult and should be carried out by a neurologist with experience in the field.
• Three basic approaches to treatment, 1) being symptomatic, 2) being immunosuppressive and 3) being supportive. No or few patients should receivesingle therapeutic modality.
• Symptomatic therapy consists of reversal of weakness with an acetylcholinesterase inhibitor (eg pyridostigmine bromide; also available as slow release oral preparation), or neostigmine methylsulfate which can be administered parenterally. Symptomatic therapy does nothing to stop the ongoing immunologically mediated damage to the muscle receptor. An overdose of these agents may induce severe weakness known as a cholinergic crisis. Suspect cholinergic crisis if there are other signs of cholinergic overactivity (excessive secretions, diarrhea, bradycardia).
• Immunosuppressive or immunomodulatory therapy in some form is necessary. This includes thymectomy, corticosteroids, plasmapheresis, immunosuppressive drugs (azathioprine, cyclophosphamide, cyclosporine) and/or intravenous human gamma globulin.
• Supportive therapy may be intermittently or occasionally eventually continually required; may include intubation, tracheostomy, artificial ventilation, respiratory therapy, administration of antibiotics, nasogastric tube and/or gastrostomy

SURGICAL MEASURES N/A

ACTIVITY
As tolerated. Heat and exercise both temporarily exacerbate symptoms.

DIET As tolerated

PATIENT EDUCATION
Printed materials, reference lists and other forms of patient and family support available from:
1. Myasthenia Gravis Foundation, 2225 Riverside Plaza, #1540, Chicago, IL 60606, (800)541-5454
2. Muscular Dystrophy Association, 3300 E. Sunrise Drive, Tucson, AZ 85718-3208, (800)572-1717, (520)529-2000

MEDICATIONS

DRUG(S) OF CHOICE
• Pyridostigmine bromide (Mestinon), 60 mg tablets and 180 mg sustained release tablets. Titrate dosage to clinical need. An average requirement would be 600 mg per day.
• Neostigmine methylsulfate (Prostigmin), 0.25, 0.5 and 1 mg/mL concentrations. Titrate dosage to clinical need. Starting dosages would be 0.5 mg SC or IM every 3 hours.
• Prednisone should be initiated with a daily, followed by a switch to an alternate day, regimen. Start with a 60-80 mg/day, taper the dosage every 3 days. Switch to an alternate day regimen within 2 weeks, continue to taper very slowly attempting to establish the minimum dosage necessary to maintain remission. A typical maintenance dosage would be 35 mg every other day.
• Azathioprine or cyclophosphamide 150-200 mg per day.
• Immune globulin
Contraindications: Refer to manufacturer's literature
Precautions: Numerous. Avoid aminoglycosides and other drugs with potential for neuromuscular blockade which may precipitate weakness. Refer to manufacturer's literature.
Significant possible interactions: Numerous. Refer to manufacturer's literature.

ALTERNATIVE DRUGS   Cyclosporine

FOLLOWUP

PATIENT MONITORING   Constant in an intensive care unit setting during myasthenic or cholinergic crises

PREVENTION/AVOIDANCE   Not possible

POSSIBLE COMPLICATIONS
• Acute respiratory arrest
• Chronic respiratory insufficiency
• Atelectasis, aspiration, pneumonia

EXPECTED COURSE/PROGNOSIS
Highly variable, ranging from remission to death. Mortality is probably less than 10%.

MISCELLANEOUS

ASSOCIATED CONDITIONS
• Thymoma
• Thymic hyperplasia
• Thyrotoxicosis
• Other autoimmune diseases

AGE-RELATED FACTORS
Pediatric: N/A
Geriatric: N/A
Others: Occurs in patients of all ages

PREGNANCY   N/A

SYNONYMS   N/A

ICD-9-CM   358.0 Myasthenia gravis

SEE ALSO   N/A

OTHER NOTES   N/A

ABBREVIATIONS
MG = myasthenia gravis

REFERENCES
• Rowland LP, ed: Merritt's textbook of Neurology. 9th Ed. Philadelphia, Williams & Wilkins, 1995
• Kimura J: Electrodiagnosis in diseases of nerve and muscle: principles and practice. 2nd Ed. Philadelphia, F.A. Davis, 1989
• Snead OC, Benton JW, Dwyer D, et al: Juvenile myasthenia gravis. Neurology 1980;30:732-739
• Soliven BC, Lang DJ, Penn AS, et al: Seronegative myasthenia gravis. Neurology 1988;38:514-517
Illustrations: N/A
Internet references: http://www.5mcc.com

Author(s)
Colin R. Bamford, MD

Myelodysplastic syndromes (MDS)

BASICS

DESCRIPTION A heterogeneous group of acquired hematopoietic stem cell disorders, characterized by cytologic dysplasia in the bone marrow and blood and by various combinations of anemia, neutropenia, and thrombocytopenia
• There is a natural progression of disease between categories as cellular maturation becomes more arrested and blast cells accumulate. There is a great deal of overlap between arbitrary diagnostic subgroups.
• Refractory anemia (RA) - < 5% blasts in marrow; < 1% blasts in blood
• Refractory anemia with ringed sideroblasts (RARS) - < 5% blasts in marrow; > 15% ringed sideroblasts; < 1% blasts in blood. Also known as acquired idiopathic sideroblastic anemia (AISA).
• Refractory anemia with excess of blasts (RAEB) - 5-20% blasts in marrow; < 5% blasts in blood
• Refractory anemia with excess of blasts in transformation (RAEBT) - 20-30% blasts in marrow; or > 5% blasts in blood; or Auer rods present
• Chronic myelomonocytic anemia (CMMOL) - 1-20% blasts in marrow; < 5% blasts in blood with > 1000 monocytes/μl
• Refractory cytopenia - same as RA but with leukopenia or thrombocytopenia without anemia
• Refractory anemia with dysplasia (RAD) - marked trilineage dysplasia but without excess of blasts
• Acute MDS with sclerosis - RAEB with marked myelosclerosis
• Refractory anemia with 5q minus syndrome - RA or RAEB with erythroid hyperplasia, mono- or bilobulated megakaryocyte nuclei and normal or increased platelets. Incidence is 2:1 female > male. Characteristic interstitial deletion on the long arm of chromosome 5.
• Therapy-related (t-MDS) - seen 3-7 years after treatment with alkylating agents and/or radiation therapy. Evolves to acute myeloid leukemia (AML) over about 6 months.
System(s) affected:
Hemic/Lymphatic/Immunologic
Genetics: Most are clearly clonal neoplasms by cytogenetics, G6PD isoenzyme analysis, or RFLP analysis. Mutations in RAS oncogene have been reported.
Incidence/Prevalence in USA: Apparent increased incidence (1-2/100,000/year) in recent years may be due to more accurate diagnosis
Predominant age: Median age is > 65 years; uncommon in children and young adults
Predominant sex: Male = Female

SIGNS AND SYMPTOMS
• Anemia - fatigue, shortness of breath, lightheadedness, angina
• Leukopenia - fever, infection
• Thrombocytopenia - ecchymoses, petechiae, epistaxis, purpura
• Splenomegaly - uncommon; mild to moderate enlargement may be encountered, particularly in CMMOL
• Skin infiltrates

CAUSES Unknown

RISK FACTORS
• Primary MDS is associated with occupational exposure to petroleum solvents (benzene, gasoline)
• Secondary (therapy-related) MDS is associated with prior treatment with alkylating agents or radiation therapy

DIAGNOSIS

DIFFERENTIAL DIAGNOSIS
• Other malignant disorders - evolving acute myeloid leukemia (AML) or erythroleukemia; chronic myeloproliferative disorders (chronic myelogenous leukemia (CML), polycythemia vera, myeloid metaplasia with myelofibrosis); malignant lymphoma; metastatic carcinoma
• Nonmalignant disorders - aplastic anemia; autoimmune disorders (Felty's syndrome, lupus); nutritional deficiencies (pyridoxine, vitamin B12, protein malnutrition); heavy metal intoxication; alcoholism; chronic liver disease; hypersplenism; chronic inflammation; recent cytotoxic therapy or irradiation; HIV infection.

LABORATORY
• Anemia - often macrocytic; occasional poikilocytosis, anisocytosis; variable reticulocytosis
• Granulocytopenia - hypogranular or agranular neutrophils with poorly condensed chromatin. Pelger-Huet anomaly with hyposegmented nuclei.
• Thrombocytopenia - occasionally giant platelets or hypogranular platelets
• Fetal hemoglobin - increased in 70%
• Sugar water (Ham's) test - increased RBC membrane sensitivity to complement lysis in some
• Direct antiglobulin (Coombs) test - positive in some
• Paraprotein - present in some
• Erythropoietin - usually normal or physiologically compensated levels unless renal failure is present
Drugs that may alter lab results: N/A
Disorders that may alter lab results: N/A

PATHOLOGICAL FINDINGS
• Ineffective hematopoiesis with dysplasia in one or more cell lineages dominates the bone marrow picture in MDS. Marrow cellularity is usually normal or increased for the patient's age but may be hypoplastic in about 10%.

• Reticulin fibrosis is usually minimal except in therapy-related MDS
• Myeloblasts may be clustered in the intertrabecular spaces, abnormal localization of immature precursors (ALIP)

SPECIAL TESTS
• Cytogenetics - at least half of patients with primary MDS and nearly all with therapy-related MDS have clonal chromosomal abnormalities (+8,-7,-5, del(5q), del(7q), del(20q), iso(17), and complex karyotypes). Detection of such a clonal abnormality establishes a diagnosis of neoplasm and rules out a nutritional, toxic, or autoimmune etiology.
• Granulocyte function tests - abnormal in half (decreased myeloperoxidase activity, phagocytosis, chemotaxis, and adhesion)
• Platelet function tests - impaired aggregation
• Marrow colony assays in vitro - results variable and correlate poorly with clinical course. Poor clonal growth may suggest more rapid evolution to AML.
• Immunophenotyping - nonspecific myeloid markers present. Occasionally evidence can be found for concomitant lymphoproliferative disorder.

IMAGING Liver/spleen scan or CT although rarely necessary may disclose occult splenomegaly or lymphadenopathy

DIAGNOSTIC PROCEDURES
• Bone marrow aspiration, biopsy, and cytogenetics
• Review peripheral blood smear

TREATMENT

APPROPRIATE HEALTH CARE Usually outpatient except when necessary to hospitalize for treatment of infection, blood transfusions, or intensive chemotherapy

GENERAL MEASURES
• Immunize for pneumococcal pneumonia and influenza
• RBC transfusions to alleviate symptoms
• Platelet transfusions only for bleeding or prior to surgery, in order to avoid alloimmunization
• Early use of antibiotics for fever, even while culture results are pending, due to quantitative and qualitative granulocyte disorder
• Iron chelation therapy to avoid iron overload from chronic transfusions

SURGICAL MEASURES N/A

ACTIVITY As tolerated

DIET Reduce alcohol use. Reduce iron intake.

PATIENT EDUCATION
• Stop smoking
• Seek early medical attention for fever, bleeding, or symptoms of anemia
• Advise about the risks of chronic transfusion therapy

MEDICATIONS

DRUG(S) OF CHOICE
• No medication has been proven more effective for these heterogeneous disorders than supportive care with antibiotics and transfusions as needed. Vitamins, iron, corticosteroids, androgens, or thyroid hormone are rarely helpful unless evidence of a specific deficiency exists.
• Intensive chemotherapy: younger patients with MDS may benefit from AML chemotherapy, especially if Auer rods are present, but toxicity may be severe for older patients. Remission durations are variable (median, about 1 year).
• Allogeneic bone marrow transplantation: recommended for younger patients with HLA-matched donors to eradicate the malignant clone and re-supply normal hematopoietic stem cells
• Aminocaproic acid (epsilon-aminocaproic acid, EACA) or tranexamic acid may benefit patients with chronic, severe thrombocytopenia and bleeding.
Contraindications: Cytotoxicity of chemotherapy may increase the risk of bleeding and infection and the need for transfusion support
Precautions: Aspirin, salicylates, and NSAID's should be avoided
Significant possible interactions: N/A

ALTERNATIVE DRUGS
• Possible differentiating agents such as all-trans-retinoic acid (ATRA) or homoharringtonine and other hematopoietic growth factors are under investigation
• Danazol or prednisone may benefit concomitant autoimmune thrombocytopenia
• Investigational agents: low doses of cytarabine or 5-azacitidine, 13-cis retinoic acid, interferon, cyclosporine, granulocyte-macrophage colony stimulating factor (GM-CSF) or granulocyte colony stimulating factor (G-CSF), interleukin-3 (IL-3)

FOLLOWUP

PATIENT MONITORING At least monthly during supportive care. More frequently if receiving treatment.

PREVENTION/AVOIDANCE N/A

POSSIBLE COMPLICATIONS Infection, bleeding, complications of anemia and transfusions

EXPECTED COURSE/PROGNOSIS
• Median survival for RA and RARS is 5 years but may extend much longer. Refractory anemia with 5q minus syndrome is quite favorable.
• Median survival for RAEB, RAEBT, and CMMOL is about 1 year with half of patients evolving to AML and the other half dying of infection or bleeding

MISCELLANEOUS

ASSOCIATED CONDITIONS N/A

AGE-RELATED FACTORS
Pediatric: Monosomy 7 syndrome; juvenile chronic myelogenous leukemia
Geriatric: N/A
Others: N/A

PREGNANCY N/A

SYNONYMS
• Dysmyelopoietic syndrome
• Hemopoietic dysplasia
• Preleukemia
• Smoldering or subacute myeloid leukemia
• CMMOL; Chronic myelomonocytic anemia
• CMML; Chronic myelomonocytic anemia

ICD-9-CM
238.7 Myelodysplastic syndrome

SEE ALSO N/A

OTHER NOTES N/A

ABBREVIATIONS N/A

REFERENCES Hoffman R, Benz EJ Jr, Shattil S, et al, eds: Hematology: Basic Principles and Practice. New York, Churchill Livingstone, 1995

Illustrations: N/A
Internet references: http://www.5mcc.com

Author(s)
Richard A. Larson, MD

Myeloproliferative disorders

 BASICS

DESCRIPTION The myeloproliferative disorders are neoplasms of the pluripotent hematopoietic stem cell. They include chronic myelogenous leukemia (CML), polycythemia vera (PV), agnogenic myeloid metaplasia with myelofibrosis (AMM/MF), and essential thrombocytosis (ET). PV is discussed in another chapter.
• With each disorder, the proliferation of one particular cell line tends to dominate. There is a variable tendency for reactive proliferation of the bone marrow fibroblast, which is not a part of the malignant clone, resulting in myelofibrosis, and for termination in an acute blastic leukemia.
• CML
  ◊ Characterized by marked splenomegaly and increased granulocytes, particularly neutrophils
  ◊ Runs a generally mild course until it transforms to a frankly leukemic (blastic) phase
• AMM/MF
  ◊ Characterized by the tendency of the neoplastic cells to lodge and grow in multiple sites outside the marrow
  ◊ Myelofibrosis appears to be a reaction to the presence of the abnormal, proliferating hematopoietic clone
• ET
  ◊ Dominated clinically by a markedly elevated platelet count
System(s) affected:
Hemic/Lymphatic/Immunologic
Genetics:
• CML - no genetic predisposition known
• AMM/MF - rare familial occurrence
• ET - may be familial
Incidence/Prevalence in USA:
• CML - annual incidence 1-2/100,000; 1/5 of all leukemia cases; incidence increases with age
• AMM/MF - annual incidence 0.5/100,000
• ET - annual incidence 0.1/100,000
Predominant age:
• CML - median age at diagnosis is 45-50
• AMM/MF; ET - median age at diagnosis is 60; distinct second peak incidence of ET occurs in younger patients
Predominant sex:
• CML - Male = Female
• AMM/MF - Male > Female (slightly)
• ET - Female > Male 1.3:1

SIGNS AND SYMPTOMS
• General
  ◊ Most are asymptomatic at the time of diagnosis
    ◊ Vague constitutional symptoms
    ◊ Hypermetabolic state (fever, sweating)
    ◊ Acute gouty arthritis
    ◊ Left-upper-quadrant abdominal pain or fullness from splenomegaly

• CML
  ◊ Marked splenomegaly (palpable in 90% of patients)
• AMM/MF
  ◊ Splenomegaly in virtually all patients, and can be massive
    ◊ Hepatomegaly in 50%
    ◊ Lymph node enlargement in 10%
    ◊ Jaundice, edema, and ascites in 10-20%
    ◊ Petechiae in up to 25%
• ET
  ◊ Easy bruiseability, unusual bleeding after minor dental procedures, large-vessel bleeding in the absence of trauma
  ◊ Transient ischemic attacks, or even frank strokes, may occur in patients with markedly elevated platelet counts

CAUSES Unknown. May be familial for some types.

RISK FACTORS
• Family history of myeloproliferative disorder (rare)
• CML - increased incidence in atomic bomb survivors and following radiation treatment of ankylosing spondylitis and cervical cancer

 DIAGNOSIS

DIFFERENTIAL DIAGNOSIS
• CML
  ◊ Low or absent leukocyte alkaline phosphatase (LAP) also seen in paroxysmal nocturnal hemoglobinuria, and occasional cases of myelodysplasia and AMM/MF
    ◊ Leukemoid reaction
• AMM/MF
  ◊ Hepatomegaly in the absence of splenomegaly is extremely rare in AMM/MF, and suggests secondary myeloid metaplasia
    ◊ Spent PV (late stage of PV)
    ◊ Secondary myelofibrosis
• ET
  ◊ Secondary thrombocytosis (including inflammation, iron deficiency, and neoplasia)

LABORATORY
• Basophilia
• Elevated serum vitamin B12 level
• Hyperuricemia
• CML
  ◊ Marked leukocytosis consisting of mature polymorphonuclear neutrophils and myelocytes or metamyelocytes
  ◊ Chronic phase typically with less than 5% myeloblasts in peripheral blood
  ◊ Blast crisis is defined when 30% or more blast cells are present in the bone marrow and/or peripheral blood
  ◊ Markedly decreased leukocyte alkaline phosphatase (absent in 5-10% of patients)
• AMM/MF
  ◊ Mild anemia - in more than 50% of patients at time of diagnosis, eventually in almost all patients, and is progressive
  ◊ Leukocytosis in 50% of patients (up to 50,000 leukocytes per mL, up to 10% blasts)
  ◊ Leukoerythroblastic blood picture
  ◊ Occasional RBC autoantibodies

• ET - the Polycythemia Vera Study group diagnostic criteria are:
  ◊ Thrombocytosis persistently greater than 600,000 per mL in the absence of an identifiable cause
  ◊ Normal total RBC mass
  ◊ Presence of iron in the bone marrow
  ◊ Absence of fibrosis in bone marrow biopsy
  ◊ Absence of the Philadelphia chromosome
Drugs that may alter lab results: N/A
Disorders that may alter lab results: In CML, LAP rises during infection, glucocorticoid use, or successful therapy

PATHOLOGICAL FINDINGS
• AMM/MF
  ◊ Foci of extramedullary hematopoiesis seen in kidneys, lymph nodes, adrenal glands, and lungs
  ◊ Special stains of the bone marrow reveal increased reticulin deposition, even in hypercellular areas

SPECIAL TESTS CML > 95% of patients are Philadelphia chromosome positive (shortened chromosome 22 due to a reciprocal translocation between chromosomes 22 and 9)

IMAGING AMM/MF - radiographic osteosclerosis in 50% of patients, particularly in the axial skeleton and proximal long bones

DIAGNOSTIC PROCEDURES
• Peripheral blood smear
• Bone marrow aspiration
• Cytogenetic studies

 TREATMENT

APPROPRIATE HEALTH CARE
Outpatient therapy. Inpatient for surgery when required.

GENERAL MEASURES
• Treatment to relieve symptoms and prevent infections
• Splenectomy has no impact on mortality, but is occasionally done for symptomatic relief. Extreme thrombocytosis, progressive and massive liver enlargement may ensue.
• CML
  ◊ Bone marrow transplantation is the only curative option, with disease-free survival in 50-70%, and should be offered to young patients with HLA matched donors
  ◊ Interferon alpha may produce hematologic remissions, and is appropriate for older patients and those without HLA-matched donors
  ◊ Hydroxyurea or an alkylating agent is used for controlling the excessive myelopoiesis in chronic phase disease
  ◊ Accelerated phase and blast crisis usually treated with regimens designed for the treatment of acute leukemia

- AMM/MF
  ◊ No definitive therapy
  ◊ Rule out other treatable causes for anemia
  ◊ Anemia is treated with transfusions as required
  ◊ Radiotherapy for localized bone pain, or symptomatic extramedullary hematopoietic tumors
  ◊ Successful bone marrow transplantation leads to the reversal of established fibrosis
- ET
  ◊ Young, asymptomatic patients generally not treated
  ◊ Lower the platelet count in those > 60, history of thrombosis, or with other cardiovascular risk factors

SURGICAL MEASURES See General Measures

ACTIVITY Restrictions will be dependent on symptoms and progression of the disorder

DIET
- Maintain good nutrition
- Small frequent meals, high-protein drinks
- Antacids as needed

PATIENT EDUCATION
- Explanations about the disorder, treatment protocols, lab studies, and prognosis
- Symptoms of recurrence to watch for
- Importance of followup examinations

 MEDICATIONS

DRUG(S) OF CHOICE
- Hydroxyurea 20-30 mg/kg/day as a single daily dose, generally favored over alkylating agents in the control of leukocytosis or thrombocytosis, as it has little to no known leukemogenic potential
- Allopurinol to control hyperuricemia - begin prior to hydroxyurea therapy
Contraindications: ET - because platelet function is often defective, drugs such as salicylates that impair platelet function are generally avoided
Precautions: ET - prolonged administration of platelet-antiaggregating agents may increase the risk of gastrointestinal hemorrhage
Significant possible interactions: Toxicity (bone marrow depression) of cyclophosphamide (Cytoxan) increased by allopurinol

ALTERNATIVE DRUGS
- Interferon controls leukocytosis and thrombocytosis
- AMM/MF
  ◊ Androgens and glucocorticoids may improve anemia
  ◊ Corticosteroids if autoimmune hemolysis present

- ET
  ◊ Aspirin, with or without dipyridamole, may prove useful in preventing thrombotic or ischemic symptoms in some patients
  ◊ Erythromelalgia (described below) responds to rapid reduction of the platelet count or to administration of nonsteroidal anti-inflammatory agents
  ◊ Ticlopidine, anagrelide, to inhibit platelet production

 FOLLOWUP

PATIENT MONITORING Individualized and dependent on therapy, ongoing studies, and stage of the illness

PREVENTION/AVOIDANCE N/A

POSSIBLE COMPLICATIONS
- Transformation to acute leukemia
- Gout due to hyperuricemia
- Uric acid nephropathy
- AMM/MF
  ◊ Portal hypertension
  ◊ Splenic infarcts
  ◊ Budd-Chiari syndrome
- ET
  ◊ Thrombohemorrhagic complications in one third
  ◊ Erythromelalgia (a vaso-occlusive syndrome with localized pain, burning, warmth of distal extremities - may progress to gangrene)

EXPECTED COURSE/PROGNOSIS
- CML
  ◊ In the 2 years following diagnosis, 10% of patients per year will develop into the accelerated phase or blast crisis. This rate then increases to 15-20% per year.
  ◊ Median survival > 5 years from the time of diagnosis, approximately 12-18 months after development of the accelerated phase, and 3 months after developing blast crisis
  ◊ Adverse prognostic factors include advanced age, large liver size, degree of splenomegaly, elevated platelet count, degree of leukocytosis, presence of blasts or of large numbers of eosinophils or basophils, percent of immature cells in the marrow, and clonal evolution
  ◊ 85% will die in blast crisis
- AMM/MF
  ◊ Progressive splenomegaly, anemia and thrombocytopenia
  ◊ Median survival is 5 years from the time of diagnosis, and 10 years from disease onset
  ◊ Usually die of hemorrhagic or thrombotic complications
  ◊ Adverse prognostic factors include platelet count less than 100,000 per mL, hemoglobin of less than 10 gm/dL, and hepatomegaly
- ET
  ◊ Overall life expectancy only slightly shortened

 MISCELLANEOUS

ASSOCIATED CONDITIONS AMM/MF - associations have been reported with systemic lupus erythematosus, periarteritis nodosa, scleroderma, and vasculitis

AGE-RELATED FACTORS
Pediatric: Rare in the young
Geriatric: These disorders more often found in middle and later years
Others: N/A

PREGNANCY
- CML
  ◊ Pregnancy does not affect the course of the disease
  ◊ Greater than 95% of mothers survive to delivery, with greater than 80% fetal survival rate through gestation
  ◊ Severe congenital defects have been reported with busulfan
- ET
  ◊ Increased risk of 1st trimester abortion. No need to treat if asymptomatic.

SYNONYMS N/A

ICD-9-CM
- 205.1 CML
- 289.8 AMM/MF
- 238.7 ET

SEE ALSO
- Leukemia
- Polycythemia vera

OTHER NOTES N/A

ABBREVIATIONS
- CML = chronic myelogenous leukemia, chronic myelocytic leukemia, chronic granulocytic leukemia
- PV = polycythemia vera
- AMM/MF = agnogenic myeloid metaplasia with myelofibrosis, idiopathic myelofibrosis
- ET = essential (primary) thrombocythemia, hemorrhagic thrombocythemia

REFERENCES Doll DC, et al, eds: Myeloproliferative disorders. Seminars in Oncology 1995;22(4):305-411
Illustrations: N/A
Internet references: http://www.5mcc.com

Author(s)
Robert Dolin, MD

Myocardial infarction

BASICS

DESCRIPTION Acute myocardial infarction (AMI) is the rapid development of myocardial necrosis resulting from a sustained and complete reduction of blood flow to a portion of the myocardium, produced by a superimposed thrombosis, generated by a ruptured atherosclerotic plaque
• Clinical consequences - dependent on the size and location of the infarction and the rapidity with which blood flow can be re-established by pharmacologic or mechanical modalities
• After total occlusion myocardial necrosis is complete in 4-6 hours. Flow to ischemic area must remain above 40% of pre-occlusion levels for that area to survive.
• Infarctions can be divided into Q-wave and non Q-wave, with the former being transmural and associated with totally obstructed infarct-related artery and the latter being non-transmural and associated with patent, but highly narrowed infarct-related artery
• Total occlusion of the left main coronary artery which usually supplies 70% of the LV mass is catastrophic and results in death in minutes
System(s) affected: Cardiovascular
Genetics: N/A
Incidence/Prevalence in USA: 600/100,000
Predominant age: Over 40
Predominant sex:
• Age 40-70: Male > Female
• Over age 70: Male = Female

SIGNS AND SYMPTOMS
• Pain - arm, back, jaw, epigastrium, neck, chest
• Anxiety
• Lightheadedness, pallor, weakness, syncope
• Nausea, vomiting, diaphoresis
• Chest heaviness, tightness
• Cough, diaphoresis, dyspnea, rales, wheezing
• S4 heart sound
• Arrhythmias
• Hypertension, hypotension
• Jugular venous distention
• Cannon jugular venous A waves (in presence of heart block or right ventricular failure)

CAUSES
• Coronary thrombosis - most common cause due to ruptured plaque inducing platelet aggregation and then thrombosis has been identified as the initiating factor in most cases
• Coronary artery spasm
• Arteritis
• Embolic infarction
• Congenital coronary anomalies
• Oxygen supply - demand imbalance; carbon monoxide poisoning
• In situ thrombosis - hematologic in origin (e.g., polycythemia rubra vera)
• Cocaine

RISK FACTORS
• Hypercholesterolemia (increased LDL; decreased HDL)
• Premature (<55) familial onset of coronary disease
• Smoking
• Diabetes mellitus
• Hypertension
• Sedentary life style
• Aging
• Hostile, frustrated personality
• Hypertriglyceridemia

DIAGNOSIS

DIFFERENTIAL DIAGNOSIS
• Unstable angina pectoris - serial ECG and enzymes to differentiate
• Aortic dissection
• Pulmonary embolism
• Pericarditis - differentiated by history of postural improvement of pain and pleuritic component, plus presence of a pericardial friction rub and upward concave diffuse ST segment elevation on ECG
• Esophageal spasm - no ECG or enzyme elevations
• Pancreatitis and biliary tract disease

LABORATORY
• Creatine kinase (CK): rises following infarction; beginning in 4-8 hours; peaking in 18-24 hours and subsiding over 3-4 days. Most specific indicator for myocardial necrosis, but has a 15% false positive rate.
• CK isoenzymes: MM, MB, and BB forms identified with skeletal muscle, BB in brain and kidney, and MB in cardiac. Elevation of CK-MB in serum is diagnostic of myocardial infarction. Rapid results forms now available.
• Troponin I has been shown to be a sensitive indicator of myocardial infarction
• LDH: rises above normal values within 24 hours of an acute MI and reaches a peak within 3-6 days and returns to baseline within 8-12 days. Can be used to date recent episode of acute MI well past the acute episode.
• ESR: rises above normal level within 3 days and may remain elevated for several weeks
• Leukocytes: rise within several hours after an MI, peak in 2-4 days, and are normal within 1 week
Drugs that may alter lab results: Refer to standard cardiology texts
Disorders that may alter lab results: Refer to standard cardiology texts

PATHOLOGICAL FINDINGS
• Myocardial necrosis
• Atherosclerosis, if etiologic
• Thrombosis; usually not seen because spontaneous thrombolysis occurs within 24 hours in most patients

SPECIAL TESTS
• Electrocardiography
◊ ST segment elevation in a regional pattern - typical of acute transmural ischemia
◊ ST segment depression with T-wave inversions - typical of subendocardial ischemia
◊ ST segment elevation and depression are early findings of myocardial ischemia. A significant percent of patients will have non-specific findings on presentation, such as peaked T-waves and ST-segment elevation less than 0.1 mv. A small percentage of patients, with transmural infarction, present with normal ECG.
◊ Q-waves representing transmural myocardial necrosis appear with 24-48 hours
• Echocardiography
◊ 2D and M-mode echocardiography useful in evaluating wall motion abnormalities in MI and overall left ventricular function
◊ Useful in delineating and assessing mechanical complications

IMAGING
• Chest x-ray
◊ Findings dependent on severity of MI
• Radionuclide studies
◊ Thallium scanning. Accumulates in viable myocardium.
◊ Technetium-99 gated blood pool scanning-noninvasive means of measuring ventricular function. Accumulates in recently infarcted myocardium.

DIAGNOSTIC PROCEDURES
Angiography prior to procedures to re-establish coronary perfusion

TREATMENT

APPROPRIATE HEALTH CARE Inpatient coronary care unit

GENERAL MEASURES
• General
Analgesia, prevention and treatment of electrical and mechanical complications, limitation of infarct size, and salvage of myocardium
• Arrhythmias
◊ Ventricular tachycardia: DC countershock, lidocaine, and/or procainamide (Pronestyl)
◊ Ventricular fibrillation: DC countershock and CPR
◊ Atrial flutter and fibrillation: digitalis or IV diltiazem (Cardizem) or verapamil. If hemodynamic compromise - DC countershock or rapid atrial pacing.
◊ Sinus bradycardia: no treatment unless accompanied by hypotension or hemodynamic compromise. Then treat with atropine and if ineffective, electrical pacing.
◊ Atrioventricular block: in inferior infarction requires transvenous pacing if patient hemodynamically compromised. In anterior infarction, pacing usually required as escape rhythm is unstable with ventricular asystole occurring quite suddenly.

Myocardial infarction

SURGICAL MEASURES
- Coronary reperfusion
  ◊ Emergency percutaneous transluminal angioplasty (PTCA) - mechanical form of coronary reperfusion. Recent studies suggest this technique may be superior to intravenous thrombolysis if initiated within first hour.
  ◊ Emergency surgical reperfusion - can be accomplished with low mortality. Must be carried out within 4 hours of beginning of the event. Many consider this treatment to be rarely indicated.
- Pump failure
  ◊ Intra-aortic balloon counter pulsation

ACTIVITY
- Bedrest for first 24 hours
- Medically supervised rehabilitation plan

DIET Nothing by mouth until stable; later, low fat, low salt diet

PATIENT EDUCATION Printed patient information available from: American Heart Association, 7320 Greenville Avenue, Dallas, TX 75231, (214)373-6300

MEDICATIONS

DRUG(S) OF CHOICE
- Coronary reperfusion
  ◊ Alteplase (tissue plasminogen activator, TPA, Activase). 15 mg IV bolus, 50 mg over 30 minutes, then 35 mg over 60 minutes.
  ◊ Heparin by standard or weight-adjusted protocol
  ◊ Aspirin 325 mg po acutely
- Acute MI, general
  ◊ Nitrates 5 μg/min IV, increase slowly. Do not lower arterial blood pressure beyond 20 mm Hg. Change to oral or topical when patient stable.
  ◊ Lidocaine 1-2 mg/kg once, then 1-4 mg/min. Use for arrhythmias only. Do not expect arrhythmia prophylaxis.
  ◊ IV heparin by standard or weight adjusted protocol
  ◊ Oxygen (2-4 L/minute)
  ◊ Oxazepam 10 mg po or lorazepam 0.5 mg IV, if needed for sedation every 4-6 hours
  ◊ Morphine 2-6 mg IV q2-4h prn pain
  ◊ Metoprolol (Lopressor) 5 mg IV x 3, 2 minutes apart followed by 50 mg po q6h starting 15 minutes after past IV dose
  ◊ Stool softeners - milk of magnesia, docusate sodium (dioctyl sodium sulfosuccinate) 100 mg bid, etc. to avoid straining and constipation secondary to immobility and narcotic use
- Post MI
  ◊ Beta-blockers reduce mortality
  ◊ Nitrates may be needed for angina
  ◊ ACE inhibitors prevent adverse remodeling, may improve longevity

Contraindications:
- Beta-blockers relatively contraindicated in CHF or incipient heart failure and bronchospasm
- IV thrombolysis (TPA/Streptokinase) contraindicated in patients with active internal hemorrhage; recent head trauma, intracranial neoplasm, hemorrhagic CVA; pregnancy; persistent hypertension (>200/120); prolonged (>10 minutes) or traumatic CPR; diabetic hemorrhagic retinopathy; severe trauma or major surgery within 2 weeks; calcium channel blockers, especially with LV dysfunction

Precautions:
- Use IV thrombolysis (TPA/Streptokinase) cautiously in patients with active peptic ulcer or heme positive stools; known bleeding disorders or current use of anticoagulants; uncontrolled hypertension; prior exposure to Streptokinase or Streptococcal infection in last 6 months; Trauma or major surgery within 2 months.

Significant possible interactions: N/A

ALTERNATIVE DRUGS
- Thrombolytics
  ◊ Streptokinase: produces systemic lytic effect in addition to local thrombolysis. Less costly then TPA. 1.5 million units in 50 cc D5W given over 60 minutes.
- Beta-blockers for acute arrhythmia
  ◊ Atenolol 5 mg IV over 5 minutes. Follow with a second dose 10 minutes later. Follow with 50 mg po in 10 minutes after the 2nd IV dose. Then q12h for at least 7 days.

FOLLOWUP

PATIENT MONITORING Determined by needs of patient

PREVENTION/AVOIDANCE
- Avoid risk factors
- Aspirin 81 mg/day may be helpful

POSSIBLE COMPLICATIONS
- Congestive heart failure
- Cardiogenic shock
- Myocardial rupture
- Left ventricular aneurysm
- Left ventricular thrombus and peripheral embolism
- Deep venous thrombosis and pulmonary embolism
- Pericarditis
- Dysrhythmias
- Mitral regurgitation
- Ventricular septal defect
- Dressler's syndrome
- Cardiac arrest
- Death

EXPECTED COURSE/PROGNOSIS
- Overall mortality rate is 10% during the hospital phase with an additional 10% mortality rate during the year after. More than 60% of the deaths occur within one hour of the onset of the event.
- Killip classification
  I - No CHF; mortality rate <5%
  II - Mild-Moderate CHF (bibasilar rales and/or S3 gallop); mortality rate 10%
  III - Severe CHF (rales over greater than 50% lung fields, S3 gallop, pulmonary edema); mortality rate 30%
  IV - Cardiogenic shock BP <90 mm Hg (<12 kPa) with hypoperfusion, e.g., oliguria, confusion, clammy skin; mortality rate >80%

MISCELLANEOUS

ASSOCIATED CONDITIONS
- Abdominal aortic aneurysm
- Extracranial cerebrovascular disease
- Atherosclerotic peripheral vascular disease

AGE-RELATED FACTORS
Pediatric: N/A
Geriatric: All incidences of complications are higher
Others: N/A

PREGNANCY N/A

SYNONYMS
- Coronary thrombosis
- Coronary occlusion
- Heart attack

ICD-9-CM
410.0 Acute myocardial infarction of anterolateral wall
410.9 Acute myocardial infarction, unspecified site

SEE ALSO
- Ventricular tachycardia (VT)
- Ventricular standstill
- Congestive heart failure

OTHER NOTES N/A

ABBREVIATIONS
CHF = congestive heart failure

REFERENCES
- Braunwald E: Heart Disease. 4th Ed. Philadelphia, W. B. Saunders Co., 1992
- Harvey AM: The Principles and Practice of Medicine. 22nd Ed. Norwalk, CT, Appleton & Lange, 1988
Illustrations: N/A
Internet references: http://www.5mcc.com

Author(s)
Phil Lobstein, MD

Narcolepsy

BASICS

DESCRIPTION A disorder of unknown etiology characterized by excessive sleepiness typically associated with cataplexy and other REM sleep phenomena, such as sleep paralysis and hypnogogic hallucinations. Commonly misconceived as representing low intelligence and/or poor motivation. The syndrome is frequently overlooked with an average of 15 years of symptoms prior to diagnosis. Onset is usually in teenage years.
System(s) affected: Nervous
Genetics:
• Inherited dominant with incomplete penetrance
• 60 fold increased incidence in families with positive history
• Incidence in first degree relative of index case is 30%
• Biologic marker HLA-DR2 allele on short arm of chromosome 6 in 100% of Caucasian patients; 1/3 normal subjects are also positive. 30% of black narcoleptic patients are non DR 2, but all with HLA-Dw1.
Incidence/Prevalence in USA: 1 in 3000
Predominant age: Mean age onset 18
Predominant sex: Male = Female

SIGNS AND SYMPTOMS
• Tetrad: 10-20% with all symptoms
• All with excessive daytime sleepiness (EDS)
• Sleep attacks - primary symptom, most severe form of EDS
  ◊ Instantaneous, irresistible REM sleep
  ◊ First and most disabling symptom
  ◊ Satisfied by naps lasting 5-10 minutes
  ◊ Lasts minutes to hours
  ◊ 1-8 naps per day, 24 hour duration of sleep normal
  ◊ Increased in monotonous environment, warm environment, after a large meal, or with strong emotions
  ◊ 20-25% of all patients with excessive somnolence
• Cataplexy (50%) auxiliary symptom, pathognomonic
  ◊ Momentary paralysis of voluntary muscles in association with sudden emotional reaction
  ◊ Can be limited to a particular muscle group, e.g., jaw droop with inability to speak; arm, neck or leg weakness
  ◊ Can be generalized causing patient to slump to floor while remaining fully conscious
  ◊ Can last seconds or minutes
• Sleep paralysis - auxiliary symptom (33%)
  ◊ When falling asleep or on awakening the patient wants to move but cannot
  ◊ The brain wakes from sleep while the body remains in REM sleep
  ◊ Lasts seconds to minutes
  ◊ Patients are aware of events around them, but cannot open eyes or move
  ◊ Can be preceded by hallucinatory phenomena
  ◊ 50% of normal population have at least one episode (nonspecific)

• Hypnagogic hallucinations - auxiliary symptom (33%)
  ◊ Vivid, frightening auditory or visual illusions or hallucinations at onset of sleep
  ◊ Dream-like experiences that occur during wakefulness or suddenly at sleep onset
  ◊ Characteristic hallucinations include seeing human or animal faces or feeling that someone else is in the room
• Disturbed nocturnal sleep (66%)
  ◊ Normal total sleep with decreased sleep efficiency
  ◊ More frequent transitions from wakefulness to sleep
  ◊ Retrograde amnesic and automatic behavior lasting minutes to hours
  ◊ Increased periodic leg movements (50%)

CAUSES
• Unknown
• Possible involvement of the immune system
• Widespread under-release of dopamine and a brainstem-specific proliferation of acetylcholine receptors and hypersensitivity to acetylcholine

RISK FACTORS
• Head trauma
• CNS infectious disease
• Anesthesia
• Family history

DIAGNOSIS

DIFFERENTIAL DIAGNOSIS
EDS present in 4% of population, most are not narcolepsy, causes include:
• Sleep apnea syndromes - 40-50% of those with excessive somnolence
• Epileptic seizures and syncope
• Idiopathic CNS hypersomnolence - 5-10% of those with excessive somnolence
• Nocturnal myoclonus
• Psychomotor seizures
• Abuse of sedative drugs
• Clinical diagnosis possible if cataplexy present

LABORATORY HLA-DR2
Drugs that may alter lab results: N/A
Disorders that may alter lab results: N/A

PATHOLOGICAL FINDINGS N/A

SPECIAL TESTS
• Nighttime polysomnography - monitoring of patients in a sleep laboratory will usually document fragmented sleep with a normal amount of REM sleep but a pattern of sleep onset REM. Polysomnography rules out other causes of excessive daytime sleepiness including sleep apnea syndromes and nocturnal myoclonus.
• Multiple sleep latency test (MSLT) - begins at least 90 minutes after nighttime test. Patient is monitored during 4-5 naps taken at two-hour intervals. The rapidity of sleep onset and type of sleep pattern are documented. A supportive test includes a mean sleep latency (time to fall asleep) of five minutes or less and at least two sleep-onset REM periods.
• HLA typing in ambiguous cases

IMAGING N/A

DIAGNOSTIC PROCEDURES
• Presence of excessive daytime sleepiness
• Documentation of at least two sleep-onset REM periods during MSLT

TREATMENT

APPROPRIATE HEALTH CARE Inpatient for sleep laboratory analysis, outpatient for followup

GENERAL MEASURES
• Usually managed with medication
• Regularly scheduled time for naps may help in mild cases

SURGICAL MEASURES N/A

ACTIVITY Exercise can sometimes decrease the number of sleep attacks. Seek to achieve optimal physical fitness.

DIET No special diet, avoid alcohol

PATIENT EDUCATION
• Symptoms can spontaneously improve or worsen
• The American Narcolepsy Association, P.O. Box 1187, San Carlos, CA 94070, (800)327-6085

Narcolepsy

MEDICATIONS

DRUG(S) OF CHOICE
• Recommended drugs either block norepinephrine uptake or cause central anticholinergic effects
• Excessive daytime sleepiness - stimulants that increase levels of daytime alertness:
  ◊ Methylphenidate (Ritalin) initial dose 30 mg/day divided 2-3/day; maximum dose 100 mg/day
  ◊ Pemoline (Cylert) - longer half life 8-10 hours; initial dose 37.5 mg/day divided AM and noon; maximum dose 150 mg/day. Monitor liver function studies 4 weeks after start and then once a year.
  ◊ Dextroamphetamine initial dose 15 mg/day divided 2-3/day; maximum dose 100 mg/day
  ◊ Combination of long and short acting - pemoline plus single or multiple doses of methylphenidate
• For auxiliary symptoms (cataplexy, hypnagogic hallucination, sleep paralysis) - tricyclic antidepressants suppress REM sleep. Imipramine 75-150 mg/day, protriptyline 10-40 mg/day, fluoxetine 20-60 mg/day.
Contraindications: Stimulants in hypertensive patients
Precautions:
• If patient develops tolerance to stimulants, switch drugs rather than increasing the dose - there is little cross-tolerance
• Patient may develop tolerance to the anticataplectic effect of tricyclic antidepressants and can get a rebound in cataplexy when withdrawn
• Stimulants - headaches, irritability, hypertension, psychosis, anorexia, habituation
• Pemoline - less cardiovascular side effects, longer acting, liver toxicity, little abuse potential
• Imipramine - dry mouth, sedation, urinary retention, impotence
Significant possible interactions:
Combination of tricyclic antidepressants and stimulants can lead to significant hypertension

ALTERNATIVE DRUGS
• Selegiline - selective MAO-B inhibitor
  ◊ 20-40 mg/day divided AM and noon
  ◊ Anticatapletic and effective for excessive daytime sleepiness
  ◊ Doses > 20 mg must be on low tyramine diet since it begins to lose selectivity
• Excessive daytime sleepiness:
  ◊ Propranolol 280-480 mg/day, good for patients during withdrawal from stimulants or patients with hypertension
  ◊ Dextroamphetamines 5-60 mg/day
  ◊ L-Tyrosine 64-120 mg/day
• Ancillary symptoms
  ◊ Gamma-hydroxybutyrate 5.25-6.75 g during sleep, has little effect on sleep architecture of REM sleep but increases slow-wave sleep. Also has mild effect on excessive daytime sleepiness without tolerance development. Gamma-hydroxybutyrate can increase sleep walking by increasing slow-wave sleep.
  ◊ Codeine 150 mg/day
  ◊ Triazolam 0.25 mg improves nocturnal sleep quality

FOLLOWUP

PATIENT MONITORING
• Frequent blood pressure checks
• Followup every 6 months

PREVENTION/AVOIDANCE   N/A

POSSIBLE COMPLICATIONS   N/A

EXPECTED COURSE/PROGNOSIS
• Life-long disease
• Symptoms can worsen with aging
• In women, symptoms can improve after menopause

MISCELLANEOUS

ASSOCIATED CONDITIONS   Obstructive sleep apnea

AGE-RELATED FACTORS
Pediatric: Uncommon syndrome of childhood
Geriatric: Symptoms worsen with aging
Others: N/A

PREGNANCY   N/A

SYNONYMS   N/A

ICD-9-CM
347 Cataplexy and narcolepsy

SEE ALSO
• Sleep apnea, obstructive

OTHER NOTES   N/A

ABBREVIATIONS
• REM = rapid eye movement
• MSLT = multiple sleep latency test

REFERENCES
• Mitler M, Hajdukovic R, et al: Narcolepsy. Journal of Clinical Neurophysiology 1990;7(1):93-118
• Scharf M, Fletcher K, et al: Current Pharmacologic Management of Narcolepsy. AFP 1988;38(1):143-148
• Nahmias J, Karetzky M: Current Concepts in Narcolepsy. New Jersey Medicine 1989;86:617-622
• Chaudhary B, Husain I: Narcolepsy. Jour Fam Prac 1993;36(2);207-213
• Standards of Practice Committee of the American Sleep Disorders Association: Practice parameters for the use of stimulants in the treatment of narcolepsy. Sleep 1994;17(4):348-351
• Parkes JD, Clift SJ, Dahlitz MJ: The narcoleptic syndrome. J of Psychiatry 1995;59(3):221-224
Illustrations: N/A
Internet references: http://www.5mcc.com

Author(s)
Jeffrey F. Minteer, MD

Near drowning

BASICS

DESCRIPTION Multisystem, potentially fatal disease, resulting from near suffocation secondary to submersion of a person's face or head. Approximately 10% of drowned patients die without actually aspirating. Most near drowning victims do not aspirate large volumes of fluid.
System(s) affected: Pulmonary, Nervous, Cardiovascular
Genetics: N/A
Incidence/Prevalence in USA:
• 8500 deaths yearly; 90,000 near-drowning victims
• Drowning is the 4th leading cause of accidental death in the United States
Predominant age: Teenagers and toddlers
Predominant sex: Male > Female

SIGNS AND SYMPTOMS
• Altered level of consciousness or comatose
• Absent or thready pulse
• Tachypnea or agonal respirations
• Cyanosis
• Wheezing
• Hypothermia
• Poorly reactive, dilated and fixed pupils
• Poor peripheral perfusion

CAUSES
• Swimming accidents
• Hyperventilation before underwater swimming
• Boating mishaps
• Motor vehicle accidents (i.e., auto submerged in water)
• Suicide
• Drug overdose (including alcohol)

RISK FACTORS
• Low socioeconomic class
• Alcohol
• Seizure disorder
• Inability to swim
• Improper pool fencing
• Inadequate adult supervision of children
• Cardiac arrhythmias
• Living in sunbelt states

DIAGNOSIS

DIFFERENTIAL DIAGNOSIS The submersion may have resulted from loss of consciousness and accidently falling into water because of another medical condition (i.e., head trauma, arrhythmia, seizure, etc.)

LABORATORY
• Salt water
  ◊ Hypoxemia
  ◊ Hypercarbia
  ◊ Hypokalemia
  ◊ Mixed acidosis
  ◊ Slight increase in serum sodium
  ◊ Normal or minimally increased Hb
  ◊ Rare albuminuria
  ◊ Rare oliguria
  ◊ Rare hemoglobinuria
  ◊ Hypovolemia possibly, or hypervolemia
• Fresh water
  ◊ Hypoxemia
  ◊ Hypercarbia
  ◊ Hypokalemia
  ◊ Mixed acidosis
  ◊ Slight decrease in serum sodium
  ◊ Normal or slightly decreased Hb
  ◊ Albuminuria rarely
  ◊ Oliguria rarely
  ◊ Rare hemoglobinuria
  ◊ Evidence of hemolysis
Drugs that may alter lab results: N/A
Disorders that may alter lab results:
Any underlying condition that may alter normal fluid and electrolyte balance (i.e., congestive heart failure) or alter normal pulmonary function (i.e., emphysema)

PATHOLOGICAL FINDINGS
• "Dry lungs" 10% of time
• Loss of normal pulmonary architecture (fresh water). Alveolar consolidations, collapse, hyaline membrane formation.
• Increased lung weight and intra-alveolar hemorrhages (salt water)
• Lung hyperexpansion
• Pneumonia, abscess and adult respiratory distress (ARDS) in those who survive only a few hours or days
• Renal - acute tubular necrosis
• Neurologic - cerebral edema

SPECIAL TESTS
• Lung compliance (reduced)
• Central venous pressure monitoring
• ECG
• EEG
• Calculation of V/Q mismatch, shunt, AaDO2

IMAGING Chest x-ray may show pulmonary edema, consolidation from aspiration, atelectasis or pneumothorax

DIAGNOSTIC PROCEDURES N/A

TREATMENT

APPROPRIATE HEALTH CARE
Hospitalize all patients initially. Monitor patients in an Intensive Care setting except for those few who present to the emergency room in an alert condition without evidence of respiratory compromise. The incidence of delayed drowning is 5%. Therefore all patients who have had a significant submersion accident should be hospitalized for 24-48 hours.

GENERAL MEASURES
• Begin resuscitation at the scene. Remove from water quickly and place in normal CPR position.
• Supplemental oxygen
• Positive airway pressure - positive end-expiratory pressure (PEEP) or continuous positive airway pressure (CPAP) for persistent hypoxia
• Avoid abdominal thrust unless airway obstruction is present
• Monitor pH and adjust bicarbonate administration accordingly
• Monitor arterial oxygenation
• Avoid steroids
• Avoid prophylactic antibiotics
• Hyperventilate patient (keep PaCO2 25-30 mm HG)

SURGICAL MEASURES N/A

ACTIVITY Bedrest for at least the initial 24 hours

DIET N/A

PATIENT EDUCATION Proper water safety techniques may help to avoid this problem

MEDICATIONS

FOLLOWUP

MISCELLANEOUS

DRUG(S) OF CHOICE
• All patients: Oxygen
• Unconscious patient without known pH: Sodium bicarbonate - 1.0 mEq/kg (1.0 mmol/kg)
• For bronchospasm: Aerosolized bronchodilator - albuterol (Proventil, Ventolin) 3cc of 0.083% solution OR 0.5mL of 0.5% solution diluted in 3cc saline
• Patients who develop pneumonia: Appropriate antibiotic based on sputum or endotracheal lavage culture
• Fresh water drowning patients with hemolysis: Transfusion may be necessary
• Prophylactic antibiotics and steroids are not helpful
Contraindications: Refer to manufacturer's profile of each drug
Precautions: Refer to manufacturer's profile of each drug
Significant possible interactions: Refer to manufacturer's profile of each drug

ALTERNATIVE DRUGS
• For bronchospasm
◊ Aerosolized bronchodilator - metaproterenol (Alupent) 0.3 mL in 3 mL normal saline
◊ Aminophylline

PATIENT MONITORING
• Frequent check of vital signs
• Arterial blood gas monitoring
• Pulmonary artery catheter may be needed for hemodynamic monitoring
• Pulse oximeter for oxygen saturation trending
• Intracranial pressure monitoring in selected patients
• Serial chest x-rays
• Serum electrolyte determinations

PREVENTION/AVOIDANCE
• Proper adult supervision of children
• Knowledge of water safety guidelines
• Mandatory pool fencing
• Avoidance of alcohol or recreational drugs around water
• Swimming instruction at an early age
• Boating safety knowledge
• Personal flotation device (life preserver if necessary)

POSSIBLE COMPLICATIONS
• Prolonged neurologic sequelae
• Fear of water
• Pneumonitis/lung abscess
• Secondary drowning
• Adult respiratory distress syndrome

EXPECTED COURSE/PROGNOSIS
• Patients who are alert or mildly obtunded at the time they present to the hospital have an excellent chance for a full recovery
• Patients who are comatose or receiving CPR at the time of presentation or who have dilated and fixed pupils and no spontaneous respiratory activity have a more guarded and often poor prognosis

ASSOCIATED CONDITIONS
• Cardiopulmonary arrest before the submersion
• Trauma, especially to the head causing altered mental status
• Seizure disorder
• Alcohol or drug overdose

AGE-RELATED FACTORS
Pediatric: Children frequently don't swim well
Geriatric: N/A
Others:
• Adolescents - may be intoxicated or using drugs
• Adults - most near-drownings are associated with boating accidents with or without alcohol

PREGNANCY N/A

SYNONYMS N/A

ICD-9-CM
• 994.1 Drowning and nonfatal submersion
• 518.5 Pulmonary insufficiency following trauma and surgery

SEE ALSO
• Respiratory distress syndrome, adult

OTHER NOTES
Accomplished swimmers may drown by hyperventilation before prolonged underwater swimming or by becoming fatigued following a particularly strenuous or long swim. Approximately 10% of victims drown without aspiration.

ABBREVIATIONS N/A

REFERENCES
• Wintemute G: Childhood Drowning and Near-Drowning in the United States. AJDC 1990;144:663
• Modell J, Graves S, Ketover A: Clinical Course of 91 Consecutive Near-Drowning Victims. Chest 1976;70:231
Illustrations: N/A
Internet references: http://www.5mcc.com

Author(s)
Alan J. Cropp, MD, FCCP

Nephropathy, urate

BASICS

DESCRIPTION Renal parenchymal damage and dysfunction associated with disordered uric acid metabolism. Several syndromes can present.
• Gout: Acute urate crystal-induced arthritis related to chronic hyperuricemia due to uric acid renal underexcretion in 80-90% and uric acid overproduction in 10-20%.
• Hyperuricemic acute renal failure: Precipitated by distal tubular obstruction resulting from acute massive overproduction of uric acid due to cell lysis. Serum uric acid usually greater than 15-20 mg/dL (0.88-1.18 mmol/L).
• Uric acid nephrolithiasis: Most commonly seen in gouty patients who are uric acid overproducers and have hyperuricosuria. Frequency of stone formation increases with increasing serum uric acid levels and urinary uric acid excretion rates. About 22% of gouty patients will form uric acid stones.
• Hyperuricemia of chronic renal failure: Occurs when creatinine clearance less than 15. Serum uric acid usually greater than 10 mg/dL. Secondary gout rare. Acute deterioration of renal function can be precipitated by an abrupt rise in serum uric acid.
• Chronic urate nephropathy: Renal insufficiency attributed to parenchymal damage secondary to medullary urate deposition. Bulk of evidence supports conclusion that typical gout or asymptomatic hyperuricemia are unlikely to lead to serious renal insufficiency. In patients with gout, renal insufficiency can usually be attributed to a complicating medical condition, most often hypertension, diabetes, renal vascular disease, obstructive uropathy, urinary tract infection or lead intoxication.
Incidence/Prevalence in USA: Gout 0.3%, Hyperuricemia 5-10%
System(s) affected: Renal/Urologic
Genetics: N/A
Predominant age: Adults
Predominant sex: Male > Female

SIGNS AND SYMPTOMS
• Hyperuricemic acute renal failure
  ◊ Precipitated by chemotherapy for leukemia or lymphoma
  ◊ Precipitated by heat stress and exercise
  ◊ Oliguria
  ◊ Anuria
  ◊ Anorexia, nausea, vomiting, encephalopathy and other manifestations of uremia
  ◊ Hypertension
  ◊ Anemia
  ◊ Dehydration
• Uric acid nephrolithiasis
  ◊ Flank pain
  ◊ Groin pain
  ◊ Micro or gross hematuria
  ◊ Anorexia
  ◊ Nausea
  ◊ Vomiting
  ◊ Dehydration

• Hyperuricemia of chronic renal failure
  ◊ Established chronic renal failure with glomerular filtration rate (GFR) less than 15-20
  ◊ Serum uric acid greater than 10 mg/dL chronically
  ◊ Intercurrent cause of abrupt increase in serum uric acid
  ◊ Acute decrease in GFR
  ◊ Acute onset of uremic symptoms

CAUSES
• Primary
  ◊ Congenital gout, hypertension and hyperuricemia (autosomal dominant)
  ◊ Congenital HGPRT deficiency (X-linked recessive)
  ◊ Congenital PRPP overactivity (X-linked recessive)
  ◊ Congenital glycogen storage disease, type I
• Secondary
  ◊ Lead intoxication
  ◊ Diuretics
  ◊ Cytotoxic chemotherapy in leukemia or lymphoma
  ◊ Heat stress and exercise
  ◊ Diabetic ketoacidosis
  ◊ Starvation ketosis
  ◊ Chronic myeloproliferative disease
  ◊ Psoriasis

RISK FACTORS
• Sudden increase in uric acid load
• Dehydration
• Urine pH less than 5
• Hypertension
• Diabetes mellitus
• Renal insufficiency
• Renal vascular disease

DIAGNOSIS

DIFFERENTIAL DIAGNOSIS Other causes of acute renal failure, other causes of nephrolithiasis, other causes of chronic renal failure

LABORATORY
• Gout and hyperuricemia
  ◊ Hyperuricemia
  ◊ Hyperuricosuria in 10-20%
  ◊ Decreased urinary ammonia production
• Hyperuricemic acute renal failure
  ◊ Serum uric acid greater than 15-20 mg/dL (0.88-1.18 mmol/L)
  ◊ Rising BUN and creatinine
  ◊ Urinary uric acid to creatinine ratio > 1
  ◊ Uric acid crystals in urine
• Uric acid nephrolithiasis
  ◊ Uric acid crystals in urine
  ◊ Urinary uric acid greater than 600-700 mg (3.54-4.13 mmol) per 24 hours (hyperuricosuria) on purine-free diet
  ◊ Hyperuricemia
  ◊ Microhematuria
  ◊ Pyuria
  ◊ Positive urine culture
  ◊ Stone composition uric acid or mixed uric acid and calcium oxalate or calcium phosphate

• Hyperuricemia of chronic renal failure
  ◊ Acute exacerbation of hyperuricemia with serum uric acid greater than 10 mg/dL (0.59 mmol/L)
  ◊ Acute on chronic BUN and creatinine elevations
Drugs that may alter lab results: N/A
Disorders that may alter lab results: N/A

PATHOLOGICAL FINDINGS
• Renal tophi-medullary monosodium urate deposits with inflammatory reaction and interstitial fibrosis
• Poor correlation between severity of renal pathology and severity of gout
• Tubulointerstitial nephritis with obstruction, recurrent infection or lead intoxication

SPECIAL TESTS Stone analysis

IMAGING
• IVP
• Renal ultrasound

DIAGNOSTIC PROCEDURES
• Cystoscopy and retrograde pyelography
• Renal biopsy

TREATMENT

APPROPRIATE HEALTH CARE
Outpatient except for complicated nephrolithiasis and hyperuricemic acute renal failure

GENERAL MEASURES
• Hydration to increase urine output
• Normalize serum uric acid
• Normalize renal uric acid excretion
• Decrease uric acid production
• Maintain urine pH greater than 6
• Antibiotic treatment of urinary tract infection
• Hyperuricemic acute renal failure:
  ◊ IV hydration
  ◊ Hemodialysis

SURGICAL MEASURES Uric acid nephrolithiasis: Cystoscopic or surgical stone removal for persistent ureteral obstruction

ACTIVITY Limited during attacks of acute gouty arthritis

DIET
• Purine restriction
• Protein restriction
• For nephrolithiasis, fluid intake adequate to produce urine output at least 2 L per day unless urine output is limited by acute or chronic renal failure
• In acute renal failure restrict sodium for hypertension and potassium for hyperkalemia

PATIENT EDUCATION Griffith, H.W.: Instructions for Patients. Philadelphia, W.B. Saunders Co., 1994

MEDICATIONS

DRUG(S) OF CHOICE
• Gout and hyperuricemia
◊ Uricosuric agent - probenecid (Benemid) starting with 250 mg bid and doubling 7-10 day intervals up to 500-1000 mg bid (maximum 3 gm/day)
◊ Xanthine oxidase inhibitor preferred for hyperuricosuria - allopurinol (Zyloprim) 200-300 mg/day.
◊ Treatment of symptomatic or asymptomatic hyperuricemia with uric acid-lowering drugs has no apparent favorable or adverse effect with respect to development of renal insufficiency
• Hyperuricemic acute renal failure
◊ Prevent by pretreating with allopurinol and hydrating patient prior to administration of chemotherapeutic agents for leukemia or lymphoma
◊ Loop diuretic
◊ IV alkalinizing solution
• Uric acid nephrolithiasis
◊ Allopurinol 200-300 mg/day
◊ Alkali to maintain urine pH 6.0-6.5 - sodium bicarbonate or potassium citrate-citric acid 0.5-1.5 mEq/kg in 5 or 6 divided doses
• Hyperuricemia of chronic renal failure
◊ Allopurinol in patients with prior history of gout
Contraindications: Avoid uricosuric agents in patients with hyperuricosuria, uric acid nephrolithiasis or chronic renal failure
Precautions:
• Avoid abrupt decreases or increases in serum uric acid, which may precipitate acute gouty arthritis
• Administer colchicine 0.5-0.65 mg/day 1-4 times/week concomitantly with allopurinol first 2-3 months to prevent precipitation of acute gouty arthritis
Significant possible interactions:
Phenylbutazone, diflunisal, aspirin (1-2 gm/day), radio-contrast agents, glyceryl guaiacolate, pyrazinamide, ethambutol, ethanol, diuretics, ascorbic acid (high dose), nicotinic acid

ALTERNATIVE DRUGS Sulfinpyrazone (Anturane)

FOLLOWUP

PATIENT MONITORING
• Serum uric acid, urinary uric acid excretion, BUN and/or serum creatinine at least twice a year
• Blood pressure screening at least once a year

PREVENTION/AVOIDANCE
• Appropriate pretreatment prior to chemotherapy of leukemia or lymphoma
• Avoid factors that can cause abrupt or persistent increases of serum uric acid or urinary uric acid excretion
• Prompt treatment of urinary obstruction or infection
• Control blood pressure in hypertensives

POSSIBLE COMPLICATIONS
• Gout and hyperuricemia
◊ No apparent renal complications
• Hyperuricemic acute renal failure
◊ Irreversible renal failure (end-stage renal disease)
◊ Residual renal insufficiency
◊ Persistent renal tubular functional defects
• Uric acid nephrolithiasis
◊ Urinary obstruction
◊ Urinary infection
◊ Renal insufficiency
• Hyperuricemia of chronic renal failure
◊ Progression to end-stage renal failure

EXPECTED COURSE/PROGNOSIS
• With effective drug therapy and general management prognosis is excellent in patients with gout, hyperuricemia, or nephrolithiasis
• Development or progression of renal insufficiency should not occur unless due to underlying renal disease or associated medical conditions with adverse renal effects

MISCELLANEOUS

ASSOCIATED CONDITIONS
• Hypertension
• Diabetes mellitus

AGE-RELATED FACTORS
Pediatric: Gout and uric acid nephrolithiasis may have onset in infancy or childhood with HGPRT deficiency or PRPP overactivity
Geriatric: Renal insufficiency more likely due to age and associated medical conditions
Others: N/A

PREGNANCY Women with nephrolithiasis have a slightly higher incidence of urinary tract infection, but no increase in stone formation rate

SYNONYMS N/A

ICD-9-CM
• 274.10 Gouty nephropathy
• 274.11 Uric acid nephrolithiasis

OTHER NOTES N/A

REFERENCES
• Jacobson HR, Striker GE, Klahr S, eds: The Principles and Practice of Nephrology. Philadelphia, B.C. Decker, Inc., 1995
• Brenner B, Rector F: The Kidney.5th Ed. Philadelphia, W.B. Saunders Co., 1995
• Puig JG, et al: Hereditary nephropathy associated with hyperuricemia and gout. Arch Int Med 1993;153:357
Illustrations: N/A
Internet references: http://www.5mcc.com

Author(s)
Donald F. Eipper, MD

Nephrotic syndrome

BASICS

DESCRIPTION
A syndrome comprising glomerular proteinuria (> 3 gm/day), hypoalbuminemia, lipiduria, hypercholesterolemia and edema as a result of a primary renal disease or secondary to another disease process.
Incidence/Prevalence in USA:
• Children - 2:100,000 new cases/year
• Adults - 3:100,000 new cases/year
System(s) affected: Renal/Urologic, Endocrine/Metabolic
Genetics: N/A
Predominant age:
• Children - 1.5-6 years (MCD)
• Adults - all ages (FGS, MGN more common USA; IgG-IgA worldwide)
Predominant sex: Male = Female

SIGNS AND SYMPTOMS
• Abdominal distention
• Anorexia
• Ascites
• Edema
• Hypertension
• Oliguria
• Orthostatic hypotension
• Puffy eyelids
• Retinal sheen
• Scrotal swelling
• Shortness of breath
• Skin striae
• Weight gain

CAUSES
• Primary renal disease
  ◊ Fibrillary glomerulopathy (primary)
  ◊ Focal glomerulonephritis
  ◊ Focal glomerulosclerosis (FGS)
  ◊ IgA nephropathy
  ◊ Membranoproliferative glomerulonephritis (MPGN)
  ◊ Membranous glomerulonephritis (MGN)
  ◊ Mesangial proliferative glomerulonephritis
  ◊ Minimal change disease (MCD)
  ◊ Rapidly progressive glomerulonephritis (RPGN)
  ◊ Congenital nephrotic syndrome
• Secondary renal disease
Associated primary renal disease are shown in brackets:
  ◊ Allergens (snake venoms, antitoxins, poison ivy, insect stings)
  ◊ Carcinoma (bronchogenic, breast, colon, stomach, kidney) (MGN)
  ◊ Diabetes mellitus
  ◊ Erythema multiforme
  ◊ Fibrillary glomerulopathy (secondary: amyloid, cryoglobulins, multiple myeloma, chronic lymphocytic leukemia (CLL)
  ◊ Schönlein-Henoch purpura
  ◊ Heredofamilial (Alport's syndrome, Fabry's disease)
  ◊ HIV infection
  ◊ Hodgkin's lymphoma (MCD)
  ◊ Infections: ventriculo atrial shunt infection, bacterial endocarditis [MPGN], viral (hepatitis B [MPGN, mesangial, MGN]) other viral (hepatitis C), protozoal and helminthic

  ◊ Leukemias
  ◊ Lymphomas (MGN)
  ◊ Non-Hodgkin's lymphoma
  ◊ Focal glomerulosclerosis (reflux nephropathy, heroin abuse, nephron ablation, extensive glomerular scarring in acute glomerulonephritis, chronic renal allograft rejection, end stage kidney, morbid obesity, a thromboembolism)
  ◊ Malignant hypertension
  ◊ Melanoma
  ◊ Nephrotoxins and drugs (gold penicillamine, mercury ([MGN])
  ◊ Nonsteroidal anti-inflammatory drug induced nephrotic syndrome (MCD) and interstitial nephritis.
  ◊ Polyarteritis nodosa
  ◊ Post streptococcal glomerulonephritis (PSGN) - 20% are nephrotic
  ◊ Sarcoid
  ◊ Serum sickness
  ◊ Sjögren's syndrome
  ◊ Systemic lupus erythematosus (SLE) (MGN, FGS, focal, mesangial, diffuse, proliferative)
  ◊ Toxemia of pregnancy

RISK FACTORS
• Drug addiction (e.g. heroin [FGS])
• Hepatitis B and C
• Immunosuppression
• Nephrotoxic drugs
• Infections
• HIV
• Vesicoureteral reflux [FGS]
• Cancer [MGN]

DIAGNOSIS

DIFFERENTIAL DIAGNOSIS   See Causes.
Is the disease predominantly nephrotic (protein without hematuria) such as MCD or MGN; or predominantly nephritic (protein plus blood) such as MPGN or FGS?

LABORATORY
• Hypoalbuminemia
• Hyperlipidemia
• Lipiduria
• Low complement in some diseases
• Azotemia
• Hypercholesterolemia
• Increased serum beta-globulin
• Increased serum IgG
• Urine
  ◊ Proteinuria (> 3 gm/24 hr)
  ◊ Glycosuria
  ◊ Hematuria
  ◊ Aminoaciduria
  ◊ RBC casts
  ◊ Granular casts
  ◊ Proteinuria
  ◊ Hyaline casts
  ◊ Fatty casts
  ◊ Foamy appearance
Drugs that may alter lab results: See description
Disorders that may alter lab results: Many

PATHOLOGICAL FINDINGS
• Light microscopy
  ◊ May see nothing (e.g., MCD)
  ◊ Disease specific: sclerosis (e.g., FGS in diabetes)
• Immunofluorescence: Mesangial IgA (Schönlein-Henoch, IgG-IgA nephropathy). Other specific for disease.
• Electron microscopy (specific for disease as in sub-epithelial deposits of IgG in MGN)

SPECIAL TESTS
• Complement levels
• Antinuclear antibody
• Serum protein electrophoresis
• Urine immune electrophoresis
• Blood cultures
• Renal venogram for thrombosis

IMAGING
• X-ray
• Ultrasound
• CT
• MRI or venography for renal vein thrombosis

DIAGNOSTIC PROCEDURES   History, physical, basic laboratory including electrolytes, renal biopsy with light, immunofluorescence, electron microscopy for definitive diagnosis

TREATMENT

APPROPRIATE HEALTH CARE
Outpatient

GENERAL MEASURES
• Treat infections vigorously (especially bacteriuria, endocarditis, peritonitis)
• Anticoagulant (heparin and warfarin) if thromboses occur
• Vaccines: Pneumococcal and flu
• Avoid excess sunlight
• Avoid nephrotoxic drugs
• Judicious use of diuretics
• Severe anemia may be treated with erythropoietin

SURGICAL MEASURES   N/A

ACTIVITY   Bedrest as tolerated

DIET
• Normal protein (1 g/kg/day)
• Low fat (cholesterol)
• Reduced sodium
• Liberal potassium (unless hyperkalemic)
• Supplemental multivitamins and minerals, especially D and iron
• Fluid restriction if hyponatremic
• Caloric restriction if obese or diabetic

PATIENT EDUCATION
• Printed material for patients: National Kidney Foundation, 30 E. 33rd Street, Suite 1100, NY, NY 10016, (800)622-9010
  ◊ "Childhood Nephrotic Syndrome" (Order #02-23NN)
  ◊ "Diabetes and Kidney Disease" (Order #02-09CP) and "Focal Glomerulosclerosis"

MEDICATIONS

DRUG(S) OF CHOICE
• Treat underlying disorder
• For steroid-responsive disease: MCD and FGS
◊ Adults-MCD: prednisone 1.0-1.5 mg/kg/day for 4-6 weeks. After response, continue steroid for 2 additional weeks, then shift to maintenance dose of 2-3 mg/kg q od for 4 weeks. Taper to zero during the next 4-6 months, or 120 mg po qod same duration, same period of taper. FGS all adults should receive 3-4 months of glucocorticoids and a cumulative dose of 6 gm of prednisolone.
◊ Children: prednisone 60 mg/m2 or 2 mg/kg/day orally for 4 weeks. After response, continue steroid for 2 additional weeks, then shift to maintenance dose of 2-3 mg/kg q od for 4 weeks. Taper to zero during the next four months.
• MGN patients with a poor prognosis: persistent, heavy proteinuria > 8 gm/day for > 6 months; elevated serum creatinine; hypertension; male sex; over age 50 or have a biopsy with sclerosis. Probably benefit from cytotoxic therapy (chlorambucil or cyclophosphamide [Cytoxan]). For hepatitis B virus glomular disease - interferon.
• For edema
◊ Most importantly salt restriction; then judicious thiazide, loop diuretics
◊ If resistant, a combination of loop and distal diluting segment diuretics, e.g., metolazone (Zaroxolyn) are synergistic
◊ It is possible that furosemide (Lasix) and albumin mixed and given IV may potentiate diuresis (eg, 150 mg furosemide plus 25 gm human serum albumin). Be wary of possible thromboses (especially renal vein thrombosis).
• Other nephrotic renal diseases: frequently relapsing MCD, RPGN, ?MGN, SLE
◊ Bolus steroids and/or immune suppression (cyclophosphamide, chlorambucil, cyclosporine)
◊ Consultation often required
• Hypercholesterolemia
◊ Diet and cholesterol lowering drugs (cholestyramine and/or HMG-CoA reductase inhibitors)
◊ Anticoagulants (heparin, followed by warfarin) for thrombotic events. There is data to suggest prophylactic oral anticoagulation in all cases of membranous GN (Kid Int. 1994;45:578-585).
◊ Hypocalcemia from vitamin D loss should be treated with oral vitamin D (dihydrotachysterol) 0.2 mg q day
Contraindications: See manufacturer's literature
Precautions: See manufacturer's literature
Significant possible interactions: See manufacturer's literature

ALTERNATIVE DRUGS N/A

FOLLOWUP

PATIENT MONITORING Frequent monitoring for azotemia, hypertension, edema, nephrotoxicity, serum cholesterol, weight

PREVENTION/AVOIDANCE
• Avoid causative factors whenever possible
• Detect and treat infections vigorously. Infections may involve the common (Pneumococcus) to the unusual (Strongyloides), especially with immunosuppression.

POSSIBLE COMPLICATIONS
• Low levels of: 25-hydroxycholecalciferol, serum calcium, adrenocortical hormones, thyroid hormones
• Hypercoagulability, thrombosis
• Pulmonary emboli
• Hyperlipidemia/accelerated cardiovascular disease
• Acute renal failure
• Progressive renal failure
• Renal vein thrombosis
• Protein malnutrition
• Infection
• Pleural effusion
• Ascites

EXPECTED COURSE/PROGNOSIS
Varies with specific causes. Complete remission expected if basic disease is treatable (infection, malignancy, drug-induced). Otherwise may progress to dialysis dependence (e.g., diabetic glomerulosclerosis).

MISCELLANEOUS

ASSOCIATED CONDITIONS
• Cancer
• Diabetes mellitus
• Connective tissue disease (e.g., SLE)
• Multiple myeloma

AGE-RELATED FACTORS
Pediatric: Relatively common in children aged 1.5-4 years (MCD)
Geriatric: Occurs in this age group. Prognosis is worse.
Others: N/A

PREGNANCY Toxemia of pregnancy may be nephrotic

SYNONYMS N/A

ICD-9-CM
581.9 Nephrotic syndrome with unspecified lesion in kidney

SEE ALSO
• Renal failure, acute
• Renal failure, chronic
• Diabetes mellitus, insulin-dependent (IDDM or Type I)
• Diabetes mellitus, non-insulin dependent (NIDDM)
• Multiple myeloma
• Systemic lupus erythematosus (SLE)
• Endocarditis, infective (part 1)
• Amyloidosis
• Breast cancer
• Colorectal malignancy
• HIV infection & AIDS
• Glomerulonephritis, acute

OTHER NOTES N/A

ABBREVIATIONS
• FGS = focal segmental glomerulosclerosis
• MGN = membranous nephropathy
• MPGN = chronic hypocomplementemic glomerulonephritis, chronic mesangiocapillary glomerulonephritis
• MCD = lipid nephrosis, four process disease, nil disease
• RPGN = crescentic glomerulonephritis

REFERENCES
• Harris RC, Ismail N: Extrarenal complications of the nephrotic syndrome. Am J Kidney Dis 1994;23:477-497
• Glassock RJ, Cohen AH: The primary glomerulopathies. Dis-A-Month 1996;42:329-383
• Cameron JS: Nephrotic syndrome in the elderly. Sem in Nephrol 1996;16:319-329
• Glassock RJ: Management of intractable edema in nephrotic syndrome. Kid Int Suppl 1997;58:S75-79
• Gansevoort RT, Vaziri NO, de Jong PE: Treatment of nephrotic syndrome with recombinant erythropoietin. Am J Kid Dis 1996;28:274-277
• Schnaper HW: Primary nephrotic syndrome of childhood. Curr Opin Pediatr 1996;8:141-147
Illustrations: N/A
Internet references: http://www.5mcc.com

Author(s)
Gregory W. Rutecki, MD

Neuroblastoma

BASICS

DESCRIPTION A neoplasm of neural crest origin which may arise anywhere along the sympathetic ganglion chain or in the adrenal medulla. The most common tumor in children less than 1 year of age in the USA.

Genetics:
• Familial cases reported
• Genetic abnormalities in 80%
• Deletions in short arm of chromosome 1p36
• Amplification of n-myc oncogene occurs on chromosome 2 (poor prognostic sign)

System(s) affected: Nervous, Endocrine

Incidence/Prevalence in USA: 27.8 cases/million children/year for 1st five years of life in USA; 8.7 cases/million in children/year for 1st 15 years of life in USA; Denmark: 1/12,000 - 14,000 live births; Japan: 1/15,000-18,749 infants

Predominant age:
• 90% occur in 1st 8 years of life
• 60% occur in < 2 years of age
• Most common intra-abdominal malignancy in the newborn

Predominant sex: Slightly more common in boys than girls(1.2:1)

SIGNS AND SYMPTOMS
• 50-60% present with metastatic disease
• Abdominal mass (50-75%)
• Weight loss
• Anemia
• Failure to thrive
• Abdominal pain and distension
• Bone pain
• Fever
• Diarrhea
• Hypertension (25%)
• Horner's syndrome (ptosis, miosis, enophthalmos, heterochromia of iris)
• Orbital ecchymosis (panda eyes)
• Respiratory distress
• Dysphagia
• Paraplegia
• Cauda equina syndrome
• Flushing, sweating, irritability
• Cerebellar ataxia (chaotic nystagmus): dancing eye syndrome

CAUSES
• Genetic abnormalities in 80% of cases

RISK FACTORS
• Beckwith-Wiedemann syndrome
• Pancreatic islet cell dysplasia
• Maternal phenytoin treatment
• Fetal alcohol syndrome
• Hirschsprung's disease

DIAGNOSIS

DIFFERENTIAL DIAGNOSIS
• Rhabdomyosarcoma
• Wilms' tumors
• Other tumors of neck, chest, abdomen and pelvis
• Hydronephrosis

LABORATORY
• CBC, platelet count
• Liver function studies
• Renal function studies
• Urinary catecholamines
• Uric acid
• Creatinine
• Magnesium, calcium
• LDH
• Electrolytes
• Bilirubin, SGOT, SGPT
• Gd2 monoclonal antibody levels
• Serum neuron-specific enolase
• Serum ferritin
• Bone marrow aspiration
• Assay for VIP

Drugs that may alter lab results: N/A
Disorders that may alter lab results: N/A

PATHOLOGICAL FINDINGS
• Small, dark, round cells
• Immature tumors tend to be large, red, lobular soft, friable
• Mature tumors are fibrous, contain calcification, hemorrhage, necrosis, cysts, rosettes, nerve filaments
• May be neuroblastoma, ganglioneuroblastoma, or benign neuroblastoma (depends on cell maturity)
• Favorable histology (Shimada): Stroma-rich, well-differentiated and intermixed tumors
• Unfavorable histology (Shimada): Stroma-rich nodular and stroma-poor, undifferentiated tumors
• Staging (Evans)
  ◊ I - confined to single organ, completely resected
  ◊ II - Extends beyond organ of origin but does not cross midline
  ◊ III - Extends across midline
  ◊ IV -Distant metastases
  ◊ IV-S - Infants under l year with metastases to liver, skin or bone marrow, sparing cortical bone
• Amplification of n-myc oncogene (poor prognosis)
• Normal DNA ploidy - worse prognosis than hyperploidy

SPECIAL TESTS N/A

IMAGING
• Chest x-ray
• Skeletal survey (including orbital views)
• Bone scan
• CT or MRI of neck, chest, abdomen or pelvis (depending on location of tumor)
• Myelogram for neurologic symptoms

DIAGNOSTIC PROCEDURES
• Myelogram if needed
• Bone marrow aspiration

TREATMENT

APPROPRIATE HEALTH CARE Inpatient workup and treatment until stable and induction chemotherapy completed

GENERAL MEASURES
• Radiation therapy in Stage III over 1 year of age
• Chemotherapy for stage II and greater

SURGICAL MEASURES
• Surgical resection may be complete, incomplete or biopsy only (for Stage I, excision only)
• If resection incomplete or biopsy, chemotherapy followed by 2nd look operation
• Dumbbell extension through vertebral foramina, chemotherapy alone vs. laminectomy and decompression
• Stage IV-S: resection of primary tumor and chemotherapy
• Bone marrow transplantation considered in stages III & IV

ACTIVITY As tolerated

DIET No special diet

PATIENT EDUCATION
• Patient and family teaching regarding long term outlook
• Possibility of second malignancy
• Side effects of treatment

MEDICATIONS

DRUG(S) OF CHOICE
• Cyclophosphamide
• Melphalan
• Vincristine
• Dacarbazine
• Teniposide
• Etoposide
• Doxorubicin (Adriamycin)
• Cisplatin
• Peptichemio
• Carboplatin
• Ifosfamide [with mesna to protect against hemorrhagic cystitis]
Contraindications: See manufacturer's information
Precautions: See manufacturer's information
Significant possible interactions: See manufacturers information

ALTERNATIVE DRUGS
• By protocol
• Ondansetron (Zofran), dronabinol (Marinol), metoclopramide (Reglan), and others for nausea control

FOLLOWUP

PATIENT MONITORING
• Multi-agent chemotherapy every 3-4 weeks for 4 courses then re-evaluate with bone marrow or second look operation
• Follow every 3 months for 1st year, every 4 months for 2nd year, every 6 months for 3rd year, then at least yearly
• Follow with CT or MRI every 3-6 months initially, then yearly

PREVENTION/AVOIDANCE N/A

POSSIBLE COMPLICATIONS
• Nausea, vomiting
• Alopecia
• Bone marrow depression
• Immunosuppression
• Hemorrhagic cystitis
• Azotemia
• Diarrhea
• ADH secretion
• Local tissue necrosis
• Myocardiopathy
• Renal toxicity
• Hearing loss
• Hypocalcemia, hypomagnesemia

EXPECTED COURSE/PROGNOSIS
• Overall survival 55%
• Stage I - expected survival approximates 100%
• Stage II - Survival 75%
• Stage III - Survival 43%
• Stage IV - Survival 15%
• Stage IV-S - Survival 70-80%
• Normal DNA ploidy, n-myc amplifications, unfavorable histology indicates worse than usual prognosis for same tumor
• Infants under 1 year of age have better outcome
• Patients with cervical, pelvic, and mediastinal tumors have better prognosis than those with retroperitoneal, paraspinal or adrenal tumors
• Survival for those presenting with opsoclonus and nystagmus is nearly 90% (seen especially in mediastinal tumors in infants under 1 year of age)

MISCELLANEOUS

ASSOCIATED CONDITIONS See Risk factors

AGE-RELATED FACTORS
Pediatric: Occurs only in children
Geriatric: N/A
Others: N/A

PREGNANCY N/A

SYNONYMS N/A

ICD-9-CM
194.0 Malignant neoplasm of adrenal medulla
171.8 Malignant pelvo-abdominal neoplasm
195.1 Thoracic neoplasm
173.4 Cervical neoplasm

SEE ALSO N/A

OTHER NOTES N/A

ABBREVIATIONS N/A

REFERENCES
• Ashcraft KW, Holder TM: Pediatric Surgery. 2nd Ed. Philadelphia, W.B. Saunders Co., 1993
• Grosfeld JL, Rscorla F, West KW, Goldman J: Neuroblastoma in the First Year of Life: Clinical and Biologic Factors Influencing Outcome. Seminars in Pediatric Surgery 1993;2(1):37-46
• Welch KJ, Randolph JG, Ravitch MM, O'Neill SA, Rowe MI: Pediatric Surgery. 4th Ed. Chicago, Year Book Medical Publishers, 1986
• Matthay KK: Neuroblastoma: A clinical challenge and biological puzzle. CA Cancer Jour Clin 1995;45:179-182
Illustrations: N/A
Internet references: http://www.5mcc.com

Author(s)
Timothy L. Black, MD, FACS, FAAP

Neurodermatitis

 BASICS

DESCRIPTION A chronic dermatitis resulting from continued, repeated rubbing or scratching part of the skin
System(s) affected: Skin/Exocrine
Genetics: None known
Incidence/Prevalence in USA: Common
Predominant Age: May occur in any age
Predominant sex: Female > Male

SIGNS AND SYMPTOMS
• Gradual onset
• Lichenified, pruritic, scaly patch on any part of the body
• Accentuation of normal skin lines
• Surface often excoriated
• Vesicles or weeping are rare
• Non-erythematous
• Postinflammatory hypopigmentation or hyperpigmentation may be present
• Scarring is rare except after serious secondary infections
• Most commonly involves nape of neck, lower legs, ankles, wrist, extensor surface of forearms, scalp, external ear or anogenital region
• Nuchal and suboccipital regions more commonly affected in women
• Perineal region more commonly affected in men

CAUSES
• Idiopathic in many instances
• Some causes of apparent idiopathic disease may be secondary to a previously unrecognized dermatosis
• Secondary forms may begin as another pruritic skin disease which evolves into neurodermatitis after resolution of the primary dermatitis
• Primary dermatoses from which neurodermatitis may develop include lichen planus, stasis dermatitis, atopic dermatitis, tinea corporis, seborrheic dermatitis, xerosis and eczema
• Social stress or obsessive-compulsive personality trait may play a role in development of this disease

RISK FACTORS
• Any pre-existing pruritic dermatosis as noted above
• Obsessive-compulsive personality/anxiety
• Exposure to irritants

 DIAGNOSIS

DIFFERENTIAL DIAGNOSIS
• Atopic dermatitis
• Contact dermatitis
• Cutaneous T-cell lymphoma
• Drug reaction
• Lichen planus
• Lichenified psoriasis
• Photodermatitis
• Stasis dermatitis
• Cutaneous amyloidosis
• Fungal infections
• Seborrheic dermatitis

LABORATORY None diagnostic
Drugs that may alter lab results: N/A
Disorders that may alter lab results: N/A

PATHOLOGICAL FINDINGS Thickening of all skin layers with minimal cellular infiltration is noted on skin biopsy

SPECIAL TESTS None

IMAGING N/A

DIAGNOSTIC PROCEDURES Skin biopsy

 TREATMENT

APPROPRIATE HEALTH CARE
Outpatient management

GENERAL MEASURES
• Treat pruritis to interrupt the scratch-itch cycle
• Occlusive dressings to prevent rubbing/scratching may be beneficial
• Nail trimming

SURGICAL MEASURES N/A

ACTIVITY As tolerated. Encourage exercise in those cases where stress may play a role.

DIET Regular

PATIENT EDUCATION
• Patients should understand the cause of this disease and their role in helping resolve the condition
• Various stress reduction techniques can also be used in those patients in whom stress plays a significant role

MEDICATIONS

DRUG(S) OF CHOICE
• Topical steroids
◊ High potency steroids alone, such as 0.05% betamethasone dipropionate cream or 0.05% clobetasol propionate cream can be used initially, but these should not be used on the face, anogenital region, or intertriginous areas. They should be used on small areas only , and for no longer than two weeks.
◊ An intermediate potency steroid such as 0.1% triamcinolone cream may be used initially under an occlusive dressing for one to two weeks instead
◊ Switch to intermediate or low potency steroids alone as response allows
◊ An intermediate potency steroid, such as 0.025% or 0.1% triamcinolone cream may be used for initial treatment of the face and intertriginous areas and for maintenance treatment of other areas. A low potency steroid, such as 1% hydrocortisone cream should be used for maintenance treatment of the face and intertriginous areas.
• Steroid tape (Cordran)
◊ Optimized penetration
◊ Provides some barrier to further trauma
Contraindications: High potency topical steroids are contraindicated for use on the face and intertriginous areas
Precautions: Topical and intralesional steroid therapy can cause epidermal and dermal atrophy as well as hypopigmentation
Significant possible interactions: N/A

ALTERNATIVE DRUGS
• Tar preparations are useful but cosmetically less appealing
• Menthol 0.25% solution can help relieve pruritis
• Oral antihistamines can be used for both their antipruritic and sedative effects
• In extreme cases, a short tapering course of oral prednisone could be considered
• Intralesional corticosteroids
• Capsaicin
• Anxiolytics or tricyclic antidepressants (e.g., lorazepam or amitriptyline)
• Topical doxepin cream
• Una boot as barrier protection
• Cold Burrow's solution compresses

FOLLOWUP

PATIENT MONITORING Patients should be followed closely and regularly for response to therapy and for development of complications from therapy

PREVENTION/AVOIDANCE Avoid known pruritic substances/exposure

POSSIBLE COMPLICATIONS
• Secondary infection
• Complications related to therapy, as mentioned

EXPECTED COURSE/PROGNOSIS
Often runs a chronic course, however, the prognosis is good for those patients in whom the scratch-itch cycle can be broken. After healing, the skin should have a normal appearance unless secondary infection has occurred.

MISCELLANEOUS

ASSOCIATED CONDITIONS Prurigo nodularis is a nodular variety of the same disease process

AGE-RELATED FACTORS
Pediatric: Rare in pre-adolescents
Geriatric: N/A
Others: N/A

PREGNANCY N/A

SYNONYMS
• Lichen simplex chronicus

ICD-9-CM
698.3 Neurodermatitis (circumscripta) (local)

SEE ALSO
• Pruritus ani
• Pruritus vulvae
• Dermatitis, contact
• Dermatitis, stasis
• Dermatitis, seborrheic

OTHER NOTES N/A

ABBREVIATIONS N/A

REFERENCES
• Orkin M, Maibach HI: 1st Ed. Dermatology. San Mateo, CA, Appleton & Lange, 1991
• Moschella SL, Hurley HJ: Dermatology. 3rd Ed. Philadelphia, W.B. Saunders, 1992
• Arnold HL, Odom RB, James WD: Andrews' Diseases of the Skin. 8th Ed. Philadelphia, W.B. Saunders Co., 1990
• Sauer GC: Manual of Skin Disease. 7th Ed. Philadelphia, J.B. Lippincott, 1996
• Sams WM, Lynch, PJ: Principles and Practice of Dermatology. 2nd Ed. New York, Churchill Livingstone, 1996
• Muramatsu T, et al: Localized cutaneous amyloidosis simulating lichen simplex chronicus. J of Derm 1995;22:759-763
Illustrations: 6 available on CD-ROM
Internet references: http://www.5mcc.com

Author(s)
Mitchell S. King, MD
Amy W. Waug, MD

Nocardiosis

BASICS

DESCRIPTION Nocardiosis is an acute, subacute, or chronic infection occurring in cutaneous, pulmonary, and disseminated forms. Nocardiosis produces suppurative necrosis and abscess formation at sites of infection.
• Primary cutaneous nocardiosis presents as cutaneous infection (cellulitis or abscess), lymphocutaneous infection (similar to sporotrichosis), or subcutaneous infection (actinomycetoma)
• Pulmonary infection presents as an acute, subacute, or chronic pneumonitis
• Disseminated nocardiosis may involve any organ (lesions in the brain or meninges most frequent)
System(s) affected: Pulmonary, Renal/Urologic, Nervous, Skin/Exocrine
Genetics: N/A
Incidence/Prevalence in USA:
0.4/100,000 (it is estimated that 500-1000 new cases occur per year)
Predominant age: All ages are susceptible, mean age at diagnosis is the fourth decade of life
Predominant sex: Males > Female (3:1)

SIGNS AND SYMPTOMS
• Pulmonary nocardiosis:
  ◊ Fever (70%)
  ◊ Cough (52%)
  ◊ Pleuritic chest pain (32%)
  ◊ Dyspnea (16%)
  ◊ Anorexia
  ◊ Weight loss
  ◊ Hemoptysis
  ◊ Tachypnea
  ◊ Rales
  ◊ Central nervous system dysfunction in those with CNS involvement
  ◊ Other focal infections in those with disseminated infection
• Cutaneous nocardiosis
  ◊ Abscesses
  ◊ Lymphadenopathy
• Disseminated nocardiosis
  ◊ Confusion
  ◊ Disorientation
  ◊ Dizziness
  ◊ Headache
  ◊ Nausea and/or vomiting
  ◊ Seizures

CAUSES Nocardiosis is caused by traumatic or inhalation inoculation of Nocardia species bacteria (predominantly Nocardia asteroides, but also N. brasiliensis, N. caviae, N. farcinica, N. transvalensis, N. otitidiscavarium, and N. nova) from soil

RISK FACTORS
• Most cases occur as opportunistic infection of immunocompromised hosts or hosts with predisposing pulmonary abnormalities
• Solid organ transplantation, chronic granulomatous disease of childhood, dysgammaglobulinemias, pemphigus, Cushing's disease, hemochromatosis, cirrhosis, bronchiectasis, tuberculosis, sarcoidosis, anthrosilicosis, pulmonary alveolar proteinosis, lymphoma, leukemia, glucocorticoid and cytotoxic therapy, solid malignancies, and AIDS.

DIAGNOSIS

DIFFERENTIAL DIAGNOSIS Includes other causes of acute, subacute, or chronic pneumonitis, particularly those occurring principally in immunocompromised hosts; tuberculosis, histoplasmosis, mixed bacterial lung abscess, and carcinoma

LABORATORY The diagnosis is established by observing the characteristic microscopical appearance of the organism in Gram stained and modified acid-fast stained preparations of sputum or pus or histopathologic samples. Confirmation is by culture of these same specimens.
Drugs that may alter lab results: N/A
Disorders that may alter lab results: N/A

PATHOLOGICAL FINDINGS
Histopathology reveals a suppurative lesion with acute necrosis and abscess formation and the microorganism

SPECIAL TESTS N/A

IMAGING
• X-ray - confluent bronchopneumonia with or without cavitation. Pleural effusion is common (up to 50%). Other chest x-ray presentations include masses, nodules, cavities, interstitial infiltrates.
• Imaging of the brain (brain scan, CT, or MRI) may reveal single or multiple intracranial abscesses, and is indicated in all patients with pulmonary nocardiosis. Other sites of focal infection may be identified by imaging in disseminated disease.

DIAGNOSTIC PROCEDURES If evaluation of sputum is nondiagnostic, bronchoscopy for bronchoalveolar lavage and transbronchial lung biopsy may prove valuable for diagnosis. Percutaneous aspiration of lung lesion is often useful.

TREATMENT

APPROPRIATE HEALTH CARE Patients with moderate or severe illness generally require hospitalization

GENERAL MEASURES Respiratory support is often necessary in such hospitalized patients

SURGICAL MEASURES Surgical drainage of abscesses other than intrapulmonary abscesses is generally indicated if technically feasible

ACTIVITY Acute phase usually requires bedrest. Increase activity as condition improves.

DIET No special diet

PATIENT EDUCATION
• Not a contagious disease
• Advise patients of the need for long-term antimicrobial therapy to reduce the likelihood of relapse

Nocardiosis

MEDICATIONS

DRUG(S) OF CHOICE
• Sulfonamides are the traditional mainstay of treatment for all forms of nocardiosis. Some prefer sulfadiazine because of possibly better CNS activity. Sulfadiazine should be given as 4-8 gm po per day in 4 divided doses. Dosage should be adjusted to maintain sulfonamide serum levels in the range of 8-16 mg/dL.
• Some prefer to use trimethoprim-sulfamethoxazole. This agent must be used if parenteral sulfonamide therapy is required. Initial dose based on trimethoprim component: 640 mg trimethoprim daily. Base subsequent doses on sulfamethoxazole level. Dosage should provide equivalent sulfonamide dosing and levels as when a sulfonamide is used alone.
Contraindications:
• Sulfonamides - in the last month of pregnancy (should only be used when the potential benefits outweigh the risks)
• All antimicrobial agents above are contraindicated in the presence of known hypersensitivity to the agent
Precautions: With the use of high dose sulfadiazine, high urine flow should be maintained to minimize risk of crystalluria. Generally, patient should be advised to drink 2-3 L/day.
Significant possible interactions:
• Sulfonamides can increase the therapeutic effects of oral anticoagulants, phenytoin, sulfonylurea hypoglycemic agents, methotrexate, and thiopental
• Decreased absorption of digoxin may be encountered

ALTERNATIVE DRUGS
Alternatives for sulfonamide allergic patients include doxycycline or minocycline, ampicillin plus erythromycin, amikacin, imipenem, ß-lactam/ß-lactamase inhibitor combinations, and cefotaxime or ceftriaxone. Clinical experience with these alternative regimens is limited.

FOLLOWUP

PATIENT MONITORING
Patients on high dose sulfonamide therapy should have a complete blood count and assessment of hepatic and renal function performed at least every other week

PREVENTION/AVOIDANCE N/A

POSSIBLE COMPLICATIONS
• Central nervous system infection (brain abscess or meningitis) (16%)
• Secondary cutaneous nocardiosis (13%)
• Septic arthritis (2%)
• Hematogenous osteomyelitis (1%)
• Other focal manifestations of disseminated infection (13%)

EXPECTED COURSE/PROGNOSIS
Overall modern mortality is 7-44%. In renal transplant recipients: overall mortality 25%, 0% mortality with isolated cutaneous involvement, 29% mortality with localized pleuropulmonary disease, 42% mortality with central nervous system involvement. In patients with the acquired immunodeficiency syndrome, mortality is 30%.

MISCELLANEOUS

ASSOCIATED CONDITIONS See Risk factors

AGE-RELATED FACTORS
Pediatric: Reported association between chronic granulomatous disease of childhood and nocardiosis
Geriatric: N/A
Others: N/A

PREGNANCY
Sulfonamides - in the last month of pregnancy should only be used when the potential benefits outweigh the risks

SYNONYMS N/A

ICD-9-CM 039.9 Nocardiosis, NOS

SEE ALSO N/A

OTHER NOTES
Unusual nocardial infections: keratoconjunctivitis associated with contact lenses, peritonitis in patients on continuous ambulatory peritoneal dialysis, upper respiratory and digestive tract infections, pericarditis, hematogenous endophthalmitis, prosthetic joint infections, natural or prosthetic valve endocarditis

ABBREVIATIONS N/A

REFERENCES
• Kalb RE, Kaplan MH, Grossman ME: Cutaneous nocardiosis. J Am Acad Derm 1985;13:125-133
• Wilson JP, Turner HR, Kirchner KA, Chapman SW: Nocardial infection in renal transplant recipients. Medicine 1989;68:38-57
• Kim J, Minamoto GY, Grieco MH: Nocardial infection as a complication of AIDS: Report of six cases & review. Rev Infect Dis 1991;13:624-629
• Mamelak AN, Obano WG, Flaherty JF, Rosenblum ML: Nocardial brain abscess: Treatment strategies and factors influencing outcome. Neurosurgery 1994;35:622-631
• Marrie TJ: Pneumonia caused by Nocardia Species. Sem Resp Infect 1994; 9:207
Illustrations: 2 available on CD-ROM
Internet references: http://www.5mcc.com

Author(s)
Ronald A. Greenfield, MD
Douglas P. Fine, MD

Obesity

BASICS

DESCRIPTION A condition of increased body weight (consisting of both lean and fat tissue) that leads to increased morbidity and mortality. Also defined as weight 20% greater than an individual's desirable weight as defined by the Metropolitan Life Insurance Company or BMI > 28.
• Android obesity (male pattern or abdominal obesity) is higher risk and gynecoid obesity (female pattern or gluteal obesity) is lower risk for long-term health problems.

```
Obesity threshold (BMI=28)
--------------------------
Height      Weight(lb)
 5'  0"       143
 5'  2"       153
 5'  4"       163
 5'  6"       173
 5'  8"       184
 5' 10"       195
 6'  0"       206
 6'  2"       218
 6'  4"       230
--------------------------
```

System(s) affected: Gastrointestinal, Endocrine/Metabolic
Genetics: 25-30% of the variance in body fat is genetically transmitted
Incidence/Prevalence in USA:
• Ages 35-44: 1600/100,000 males; 1400/100,000 females
• Ages 65-74: 500/100,000 males; 400/100,000 females
• 20-30% of adult men and 30-40% of adult women (according to an NIH panel)
Predominant age: All ages
Predominant sex: Female > Male

SIGNS AND SYMPTOMS Increased body weight and adipose tissue

CAUSES
• Multifactorial
• Rare genetic syndromes have been described
• Idiopathic obesity is assumed to be due to an imbalance between food intake and energy expenditure (physical activity and metabolic rate)
• Insulinoma
• Hypothalamic disorders
• Cushing's syndrome
• Corticosteroid drugs

RISK FACTORS
• Parental obesity
• Pregnancy
• Sedentary lifestyle
• High fat diet
• Low socioeconomic status

DIAGNOSIS

DIFFERENTIAL DIAGNOSIS N/A

LABORATORY
• Not needed for diagnosis
• Consider thyroid function tests
• Cardiac risk factors: serum cholesterol, triglycerides, glucose
Drugs that may alter lab results: N/A
Disorders that may alter lab results: Hypothyroidism

PATHOLOGICAL FINDINGS
• Hypertrophy and/or hyperplasia of adipocytes
• Cardiomegaly
• Hepatomegaly

SPECIAL TESTS
• Body mass index (BMI) = body weight (kg) divided by the square of body height (m). Obesity is BMI > 28 kg/m2.
• Determine fat distribution pattern by measuring waist and hips circumferences and calculating the waist to hips ratio (WHR)
• Android (male pattern, or abdominal obesity) has WHR greater than 0.85 for females; 0.95 for males
• Gynecoid (female pattern, or gluteal obesity) has WHR less than 0.85 for females; 0.95 for males

IMAGING N/A

DIAGNOSTIC PROCEDURES N/A

TREATMENT

APPROPRIATE HEALTH CARE
Outpatient

GENERAL MEASURES
• Appropriate functions for the primary care physician include: assessment of degree of health risk from BMI and WHR (see Diagnosis); assessment of motivation to lose weight; helping patients to set goals of therapy; office counselling or referral to a registered dietician or weight loss program for in depth counselling on diet, exercise, and behavior modification; and long term follow-up
• Many reputable commercial and community programs exist for obesity treatment. Desirable programs should include diets which meet the RDA for nutrients, exercise counselling, behavior modification, and provision for long term maintenance. Physicians can provide valuable additional monitoring and long term followup.

SURGICAL MEASURES Occasionally, patients with severe obesity (BMI > 40 kg/m2) are treated with a gastric bypass or stapling procedure. This involves complex pre-surgical evaluation, surgery and followup and should only be done in a center skilled in this treatment. Surgical treatment is the most effective long term weight loss treatment available for morbid obesity.

ACTIVITY Exercise alone rarely causes significant weight loss. It may improve long term results of weight loss treatment and should be an integral part of any weight loss program.

DIET
• Diet restriction is the cornerstone of obesity management (low-fat, high-complex carbohydrate and high-fiber)
• A 500 kcal (2.10 MJ) reduction in calorie intake will result in approximately 1 pound (.45 kg) weight loss per week
• Very low calorie diets (VLCD)
  ◊ 400-800 kcal (1.68-3.35 MJ) per day are usually based on liquid formulas and cause more rapid weight loss
  ◊ Complications of VLCD include: dehydration, orthostatic hypotension, fatigue, muscle cramps, constipation, headache, cold intolerance, and relapse after discontinuation
  ◊ Contraindications of VLCD include: recent myocardial infarction or cerebrovascular accident, renal or hepatic disease, cancer, pregnancy, insulin-dependent diabetes mellitus, some psychiatric disturbances
  ◊ Physician supervision is important for VLCD

PATIENT EDUCATION
• Educating the patient about the value of weight reduction is important
• Behavior modification can improve dietary adherence and long term results of weight loss and should be included in any weight loss program

MEDICATIONS

DRUG(S) OF CHOICE
Drug treatment is not usually recommended, although appetite suppressants may be indicated for short-term use (few weeks) in conjunction with a weight loss regimen
• Schedule IV drugs
  ◊ Diethylpropion
  ◊ Phentermine
  ◊ Fenfluramine
  ◊ Mazindol
  ◊ Dexfenfluramine (Redux) 15 mg bid with meals; has been approved by FDA without restrictions on length of use
  ◊ Combination therapy - usual starting dose: phentermine 15 mg qd plus fenfluramine 20 mg tid. Only FDA approved for short term use; clinical studies not available to assess efficacy and safety.
• Schedule III drugs
  ◊ Phendimetrazine
  ◊ Benzphetamine

Contraindications: Advanced atherosclerosis, symptomatic cardiovascular disease, hypertension, hyperthyroidism, glaucoma, history of drug abuse, agitated states, use of MAO inhibitors

Precautions:
• Abuse potential, especially for Schedule III
• Relapse after discontinuation of drug
• Phentermine + Fenfluramine (Phen-Fen) combination associated with pulmonary hypertension and cardiac valvular lesions; use only in patients with obesity causing significant comordid conditions.

Significant possible interactions:
Concurrent use with general anesthetics may cause arrhythmias

ALTERNATIVE DRUGS
Phenylpropanolamine is used in over-the counter-weight loss preparations

FOLLOWUP

PATIENT MONITORING Long term followup is crucial to prevent further weight gain or regain after weight loss

PREVENTION/AVOIDANCE Counselling in regular exercise and prudent diet with regular follow-up, especially in children and young adults and those with family history of obesity or diabetes mellitus

POSSIBLE COMPLICATIONS
• Increased mortality due largely to cardiovascular disease
• Diabetes mellitus
• Hypertension
• Hyperlipidemia
• Gall bladder disease with cholelithiasis
• Osteoarthritis
• Gout
• Thromboembolism
• Hypoventilation and sleep apnea syndromes
• Poor self-esteem
• Occupational discrimination

EXPECTED COURSE/PROGNOSIS
• Long term maintenance of weight loss is extremely difficult
• If patient is not motivated, successful weight loss is unlikely

MISCELLANEOUS

ASSOCIATED CONDITIONS See Possible complications

AGE-RELATED FACTORS
Pediatric: Prevalence of obesity is increasing. Among other factors, decreased physical activity and increased television viewing have been implicated.
Geriatric: Desirable weights (those associated with the lowest risk of mortality) increase with age
Others: Pre-puberty and young adulthood appear to be sensitive periods for development of obesity

PREGNANCY Pregnancy is a common time for onset of, or increase in obesity

SYNONYMS
• Overweight
• Adiposis
• Adiposity

ICD-9-CM 278.0 Obesity

SEE ALSO N/A

OTHER NOTES N/A

ABBREVIATIONS
RDA = recommended daily allowance
BMI = body mass index

REFERENCES
• Danford D, Fletcher JW, eds: Methods for voluntary weight loss and control. National Institutes of Health Technology Assessment Conference. Ann Intern Med 1993;119 (7 Part 2) S6:41-763
• Bray GA, ed: Obesity. Endocrinology and Metabolism Clinics of N Am 1996;25(4)
Illustrations: N/A
Internet references: http://www.5mcc.com

Author(s)
David S. Gray, MD

Obsessive compulsive disorder

BASICS

DESCRIPTION Psychiatric condition classified as an anxiety disorder in Diagnostic and Statistical Manual of Mental Disorders (DSM-IV-R) and characterized by recurrent, intrusive thoughts (obsessions) and ritualistic behaviors (compulsions)
• Obsessions and compulsions consume more than an hour per day and cause occupational/social impairment
• Patients know thoughts (obsessions) come from their own minds and are not imposed from outside (as in thought insertion). Thoughts are not associated with another disorder (for example, thought of food if an eating disorder is present).
• Compulsions are ritualistic behaviors designed to relieve the anxiety of obsessions
• Common obsessive themes:
  ◊ Violence, such as harming a beloved child
  ◊ Doubt, such as whether doors or windows locked or iron turned off
  ◊ Blasphemous thoughts, such as in a devoutly religious person
  ◊ Contamination, dirt or disease
  ◊ Symmetry or orderliness
• Common rituals or compulsions:
  ◊ Hand washing
  ◊ Checking
  ◊ Counting
  ◊ Hoarding
  ◊ Repeaters - such as dressing rituals
System(s) affected: Nervous
Genetics: Positive family history in about 20% of cases, no mode of transmission identified
Incidence/Prevalence in USA: 2.5% lifetime prevalence, 1.5-2.1% one year prevalence
Predominant age: Mean age 20. 1/3 cases present by age 15, new cases after age 50 rare.
Predominant sex: Male = Female (males tend to present at a younger age)

SIGNS AND SYMPTOMS
• Obsessions and/or compulsions that consume more than an hour a day and cause significant distress or impairment
• Obsessions (thoughts) are recurrent; patient attempts to ignore or neutralize thoughts with another thought or action
• Neither obsessions nor compulsions are related to another mental disorder
• Compulsions (actions) are repetitive, purposeful behaviors in response to thoughts in attempt to neutralize the thought - such as checking in response to doubt (locks, doors , windows or driving back over route to check for any possible damage inadvertently done while driving one's car)

• Repeated handwashing or ritualistic handwashing in response to fear of contamination
• 80-90% of patients have obsessions and compulsions
• 10-19% are pure obsessional
• 5% perform rituals until they "feel right" and may not have an identifiable obsession
• Hoarding and obsessional slowness comprise two other categories

CAUSES Dysregulation of neurotransmitter, serotonin

RISK FACTORS Greater concordance in monozygotic twins family history as above

DIAGNOSIS

DIFFERENTIAL DIAGNOSIS
• Impulse control disorders: Compulsive gambling, sex or substance abuse - the "compulsive" behavior is not in response to obsessive thought and patient derives pleasure from the activity, unlike OCD where obsessions and compulsions are ego dystonic
• Depression: Can see brooding, but ideas not perceived as senseless as in OCD
• Schizophrenia: Patient perceives thought to be true and from an external source
• Compulsive personality disorder: Not to be confused with OCD. In personality disorder, traits are ego-syntonic. Traits include perfectionism, preoccupation with detail, trivia or procedure and regulation. Patient tends to be rigid, moralistic and stingy. Often traits are rewarded in patient's job as desirable traits.

LABORATORY N/A
Drugs that may alter lab results: N/A
Disorders that may alter lab results: N/A

PATHOLOGICAL FINDINGS N/A

SPECIAL TESTS Yale Brown OCD checklist (Y-BOCS)

IMAGING PET scan - abnormal metabolism in frontal cortex and caudate nuclei (not generally available other than in research centers)

DIAGNOSTIC PROCEDURES Psychiatric interview

TREATMENT

APPROPRIATE HEALTH CARE Psychiatric referral for therapy (in vivo exposure)

GENERAL MEASURES In vivo exposure with response prevention (prevention or delay of ritual)

SURGICAL MEASURES Psychosurgery (last resort)

ACTIVITY No restriction

DIET With use of phenelzine must have tyramine-free diet to prevent precipitation of hypertensive crisis

PATIENT EDUCATION
• OCD Foundation, P.O. Box 9573, New Haven, CT 06535, (203) 772-0565
• Printed patient information available from: Obsessive-Compulsive Anonymous, P.O. Box 215, New Hyde Park, NY 11040, (516)741-4901

MEDICATIONS

DRUG(S) OF CHOICE
• Serotonin reuptake inhibitor, fluoxetine (Prozac)
◊ Adults: begin with 20 mg/day q morning and increase every 4-6 weeks to obtain maximal clinical response. Dose range: 20-60 mg/day. Doses >20 mg/day should be divided.
◊ Children: safety and efficacy has not been established
• Sertraline (Zoloft)
◊ Adults: begin with 50 mg per day and increase every week until clinical response. Dose range: 50-200 mg per day. Doses > 100 mg/day should be divided.
◊ Children: safety and efficacy have not been established

Contraindications:
• Absolute fluoxetine and sertraline contraindications
◊ Hypersensitivity to the selective serotonin re-uptake inhibitors
◊ Within 14 days of MAO inhibitor
• Relative fluoxetine and sertraline contraindications
◊ Severe liver impairment
◊ Seizure disorders (lowers seizure threshold)
• Clomipramine is of the tricyclic antidepressant class, so carries same contraindications as drugs in that class
• Absolute clomipramine contraindications:
◊ Within 6 months of myocardial infarction
◊ Narrow angle glaucoma
◊ 3rd degree AV block
◊ Within 14 days of MAO inhibitor
• Relative clomipramine contraindications:
◊ Prostatic hypertrophy (urinary retention)
◊ Seizure disorder (lower seizure threshold)
◊ 1st, 2nd degree AV block, bundle branch block and CHF (pro-arrhythmic effect)

Precautions:
• Drug should to be taken for a minimum of 8 weeks before considering it a treatment failure
• Because patients with OCD may have concomitant depression, suicide potential must be assessed
• Long half-life may be troublesome if patient has an adverse reaction
• May cause drowsiness and dizziness when therapy is initiated - warn patients about driving and heavy equipment hazards
• May alter glucose control by lowering blood glucose levels while on the medication and increase blood glucose after stopping the medication
• Tricyclic class of antidepressants dangerous in overdose

Significant possible interactions:
• Clomipramine
◊ Not yet fully elucidated
◊ May interfere with guanethidine, clonidine
◊ Serum level increased if used concomitantly with haloperidol
◊ Probable plasma increase if used with cimetidine, fluoxetine, methylphenidate
◊ Increases serum level of phenobarbital
• Fluoxetine and sertraline
◊ Causes increased concentrations of the following medications: warfarin, phenytoin, carbamazepine, diazepam, tricyclic antidepressants, and neuroleptics

ALTERNATIVE DRUGS
• Clomipramine
◊ Adults - beginning at 25 mg/day and increased gradually to 100 mg over first 2 weeks. Then to 250 mg over next several weeks, as tolerated.
◊ Children - beginning at 25 mg /day over first two weeks as in adults. Then titrated up to 3 mg/kg or 200 mg/day (which ever is smaller) over the next several weeks.

FOLLOWUP

PATIENT MONITORING Y-BOCS

PREVENTION/AVOIDANCE N/A

POSSIBLE COMPLICATIONS
• Depression
• Avoidant behavior (phobic avoidance)
• Anxiety and panic-like episodes associated with obsessions

EXPECTED COURSE/PROGNOSIS
• Chronic waxing and waning course in majority
• 24-33% fluctuating course
• 11-14% phasic with periods of remission
• 54-61% chronic progressive course

MISCELLANEOUS

ASSOCIATED CONDITIONS
• Depression
• Panic disorder
• Social phobia
• Phobia
• Tourette's
• Alcoholism
• Substance abuse

AGE-RELATED FACTORS
Pediatric: Adolescent onset in 15%. At this age males outnumber females 3:1.
Geriatric: Diagnosis not generally made after age 50
Others: N/A

PREGNANCY
• Onset of OCD has been noted after delivery
• Safety of fluoxetine and clomipramine has not been established in pregnancy nor lactation

SYNONYMS Obsessive compulsive neurosis

ICD-9-CM
300.3 Obsessive-compulsive disorders

SEE ALSO
• Anxiety
• Depression

OTHER NOTES Not to be confused with obsessive compulsive personality disorder (see Differential Diagnosis)

ABBREVIATIONS
• Y-BOCS = Yale Brown OCD checklist
• OCD = obsessive compulsive disorder

REFERENCES Diagnostic and Statistical Manual of Mental Disorders (DSM-IV-R). 4th Ed. American Psychiatric Association, Washington, D.C., 1994
Illustrations: N/A
Internet references: http://www.5mcc.com

Author(s)
Karl E. Miller, MD

Ocular chemical burns

 BASICS

DESCRIPTION Chemical exposure to the eye can result in rapid, devastating, and permanent damage and is one of the true emergencies in ophthalmology
• Separate alkaline from acid chemical exposure:
◊ Alkaline burns - more severe, alkali penetrates and saponifies tissues easily, may produce injury to lids, conjunctiva, cornea, sclera, iris, lens, and retina
◊ Acid burns - usually acid does not damage internal structures since protein coagulation limits acid penetration. Injury often limited to lids, conjunctiva, and cornea.
System(s) affected: Nervous, Skin/Exocrine
Genetics: N/A
Incidence/Prevalence in USA: Estimated 300/100,000/year
Predominant age: 18-65
Predominant sex: Male > Female

SIGNS AND SYMPTOMS
• Mild burns:
◊ Pain and blurred vision
◊ Eyelid skin erythema and edema
◊ Corneal epithelial defects or superficial punctate keratitis
◊ Conjunctival chemosis, hyperemia, and hemorrhages without perilimbal ischemia
◊ Mild anterior chamber reaction
• Moderate to severe burns:
◊ Severe pain and markedly reduced vision
◊ Second and third degree burns of eyelid skin
◊ Corneal edema and opacification
◊ Corneal epithelial defects
◊ Marked conjunctival chemosis and perilimbal blanching
◊ Moderate anterior chamber reaction
◊ Increased intraocular pressure
◊ Local necrotic retinopathy
◊ In alkaline burns, can have initial pain which later diminishes

CAUSES
• Alkali:
◊ Ammonia (NH3)
◊ Lye (NaOH)
◊ Magnesium hydroxide [Mg(OH)2]
◊ Potassium hydroxide (KOH)
◊ Lime [Ca(OH)2]
• Acids:
◊ Hydrochloric (HCl)
◊ Hydrofluoric (HF)
◊ Acetic (CH3COOH)
◊ Nitrous (HNO2)
◊ Sulfuric (H2SO4)

RISK FACTORS
• Construction work (plaster, cement, whitewash)
• Use of cleaning agents (drain cleaners, ammonia)
• Automobile battery explosions (sulfuric acid)
• Industrial work (many possible agents)
• Alcoholism

 DIAGNOSIS

DIFFERENTIAL DIAGNOSIS
• Thermal burns
• Ocular cicatricial pemphigoid
• Other causes of corneal opacification
• Ultraviolet radiation keratitis

LABORATORY None
Drugs that may alter lab results: N/A
Disorders that may alter lab results: None

PATHOLOGICAL FINDINGS
• Precipitation of glycosaminoglycans causes corneal opacification
• Saponification of cell membranes causes cell death
• Cation binding to collagen results in hydration, thickening, and shortening of collagen fibrils. This can mechanically elevate intraocular pressure.

SPECIAL TESTS Measure pH of tear film with litmus paper or electronic probe (irrigating fluid with non-neutral pH [e.g., normal saline has pH of 4.5] may alter results)

IMAGING Not necessary unless suspicion of intraocular or orbital foreign body is present

DIAGNOSTIC PROCEDURES
• Careful slit lamp examination, fundus ophthalmoscopy, tonometry, and measurement of visual acuity
• Full extent of damage from alkaline burns may not be apparent until 48-72 hours after exposure

 TREATMENT

APPROPRIATE HEALTH CARE
Emergency room with inpatient admission and ophthalmology consultation, depending on severity

GENERAL MEASURES Copious irrigation and removal of corneal or conjunctival foreign bodies are always the initial treatment. Continue irrigation until the tear film is of neutral pH and pH is stable. Sweep the conjunctival fornices every 12-24 hours to prevent adhesions.

SURGICAL MEASURES
• Punctal occlusion for tear film preservation and corneal epitheliopathy
• Tarsorrhaphy for persistent epithelial defects
• Tissue adhesive (e.g., isobutyl cyanoacrylate) for impending or actual corneal perforation
• Conjunctival or limbal autograft transplantation for epithelial stem cell restoration
• Lamellar or penetrating keratoplasty for tectonic stabilization or visual rehabilitation

ACTIVITY Ambulatory

DIET Usual for patient

PATIENT EDUCATION
• Safety glasses
• Need for immediate ocular irrigation with any available water following chemical exposure to the eyes

MEDICATIONS

DRUG(S) OF CHOICE
• Immediate treatment (any non-toxic irrigant):
◊ In hospital setting, sterile water, normal saline, lactated Ringer's solution are effective
◊ In the field, use what is available (tap water). Rapidity of irrigation is critical.
◊ Irrigation is continued until pH of superior/inferior cul-de-sac is neutral
◊ It is impossible to over-irrigate
• Further treatment: (depending on severity and associated conditions)
◊ Topical prophylactic antibiotics: Any broad spectrum agent, e.g., bacitracin-polymyxin B (Polysporin) ointment q2-4h, ciprofloxacin (Ciloxan) drops q 2-4h, chloramphenicol (Chloroptic) ointment q2-4h
◊ Tear substitutes: hydroxypropyl methylcellulose (Hypotears PF, Refresh Plus) drops q4h, carboxymethylcellulose (Refresh P.M.) ointment q hs
◊ Cycloplegics for photophobia and/or uveitis: Cyclopentolate 1% tid, or scopolamine 1/4% bid
◊ Anti-glaucoma for elevated intraocular pressure (IOP): Timolol (Timoptic) 0.5% bid or levobunolol (Betagan) 0.5% bid and/or acetazolamide (Diamox) 125-250 mg po q6h or methazolamide (Neptazane) 25-50 mg po bid and/or mannitol 20% 1-2 g/kg IV prn
◊ Corticosteroids for intraocular inflammation: Prednisolone (Pred-Forte) 1% or equivalent q1-4h for 10-14 days; if severe, prednisone 20-60 mg po qd for 5-7 days. Taper rapidly if epithelium intact by this time.
◊ Consider vitamin C (ascorbic acid) 500 mg po qid and/or acetylcysteine (Mucomyst) 10-20% top q4 h if corneal melting occurs
Contraindications: None
Precautions:
• For timolol and levobunolol - history of congestive heart failure or chronic obstructive pulmonary disease
• For acetazolamide and methazolamide - history of nephrolithiasis or metabolic acidosis
• For mannitol - history of congestive heart failure or renal failure
• For scopolamine - history of urinary retention
• Topical corticosteroids must be used with caution in the presence of damaged corneal epithelium as iatrogenic infection can occur. Daily follow-up or consultation with an ophthalmologist is recommended.
Significant possible interactions: Refer to manufacturer's literature

ALTERNATIVE DRUGS
Where available - topical fibronectin, epidermal growth factor, prokinase inhibitors

FOLLOWUP

PATIENT MONITORING
• Depending on severity of ocular injury, from daily to weekly visits initially
• May be inpatient
• If on mannitol or prednisone, consider frequent serum electrolytes

PREVENTION/AVOIDANCE
Safety glasses to safeguard uninvolved eye

POSSIBLE COMPLICATIONS
• Persistent epitheliopathy
• Fibrovascular pannus
• Corneal ulcer/perforation
• Progressive symblepharon and entropion
• Neurotrophic keratitis
• Glaucoma
• Cataract
• Hypotony
• Phthisis bulbi

EXPECTED COURSE/PROGNOSIS
• Depends on severity of initial injury
• Increasing amounts of limbal ischemia and corneal opacification correlate with poorer prognosis
• For severely injured eyes, permanent loss of vision is not uncommon
• Autologous cultivated corneal epithelium has been used for long term restoration of vision.
• Autologous nasal mucosal transplantation has also been successfully employed

MISCELLANEOUS

ASSOCIATED CONDITIONS
Facial cutaneous chemical or thermal burns

AGE-RELATED FACTORS
Pediatric: N/A
Geriatric:
• Compromised ocular surface from keratitis sicca or other disease associated with poorer prognosis
• Compromised corneal endothelium or pre-existing glaucoma may also complicate clinical management
Others: N/A

PREGNANCY N/A

SYNONYMS Chemical ocular injuries

ICD-9-CM
• 940.2 Alkali burn
• 940.3 Acid burn

SEE ALSO
• Burns
• Keratitis, superficial punctate

OTHER NOTES N/A

ABBREVIATIONS N/A

REFERENCES
• Fraunfelder FT, Roy FH: Current Ocular Therapy. 3rd Ed. Philadelphia, W.B. Saunders Co., 1990
• McCulley JP: Chemical Injuries. In: Smolin G, Thoft RA, eds. The Cornea: Scientific Foundations and Clinical Practice. New York, Little, Brown, 1987
• Shingleton BJ, Hersh PS, Kenyon KR: Eye Trauma. St. Louis, Mosby Year Book, 1991
• Ralph RA: Chemical Burns of the Eye. In: Tasman W, ed. Clinical Ophthalmology. Philadelphia, J.B. Lippincott, 1994
Illustrations: N/A
Internet references: http://www.5mcc.com

Author(s)
Robert G. Fante, MD

Onychomycosis

BASICS

DESCRIPTION Infection of nail by fungi
System(s) affected: Skin/Exocrine
Genetics: N/A
Incidence/Prevalence in USA: 22-130 cases/1000 population
Predominant age: Varies with type. Rare before puberty.
Predominant sex: Varies with type

SIGNS AND SYMPTOMS
Dermatophyte onychomycosis: Commonly preceded by dermatophyte infection at another site; most frequent form in adults; 80% involve toenails - especially hallux; simultaneous infection of finger and toe nails rare. Four clinical forms occur:
• Distal subungual onychomycosis
  ◊ Spreads from hyponychium to nailbed to nailplate
  ◊ Subungual hyperkeratosis: yellowish-gray mass which lifts off free border of nail
  ◊ Subungual paronychia: thickening of subungual region which lifts off nailplate
  ◊ Onycholysis (detachment of nailplate from nailbed)
  ◊ Dystrophic changes: thickening, deformation, crumbling
  ◊ Discoloration: yellow-brown
  ◊ Bois vermoulu: end stage nail, looks like worm-eaten wood
  ◊ Onychomadesis (shedding of nail) or traumatic avulsion may occur
  ◊ Subjective symptoms minimal except from secondary infection or deformity
  ◊ Rate of spread depends on pathogen
• Lateral onychomycosis (common)
  ◊ Yellowish discoloration lateral nail groove
  ◊ Progressive onycholysis, proximal or distal
  ◊ Very rarely will invade nailplate and spread to opposite lateral fold
• Proximal onychomycosis (rare)
  ◊ Hands or feet
  ◊ Leukonychia: yellowish-white spots begin under posterior nail groove, spreading to nail plate and lunula
• White superficial onychomycosis (rare)
  ◊ Hallux preferentially affected
  ◊ Infection of upper part of nailplate
  ◊ Opaque white spots on nail plate eventually merge to involve entire surface of the nail
  ◊ Trichophyton mentagrophytes most common pathogen
Candidal onychomycosis
• Predominantly adult women
• Hands 70% - especially dominant hand
• Middle finger most common
• Pain mild, unless secondarily infected
• Pain increases with frequent or prolonged contact with water
• Attacks the soft tissue surrounding the nail - penetrates keratin only secondarily
• Begins with detachment of cuticle from nailplate
• Dark yellowish to blackish-brown zone along lateral border of nail
• Secondary ungual changes - convex, irregular, striated nailplate with dull rough surface
• Onycholysis - frequent, especially on hands
• Distal subungual onychomycosis may occur
• Primary involvement of the nailplate uncommon (thin, crumbly, opaque, brownish nailplate deformed by transverse grooves)
• Periungual edema/erythema may occur (club-shaped, bulbous fingertips)
• Superficial white onychomycosis - young children
Mold onychomycosis
• More common over 60 years old
• More common in nails of hallux
• Resembles distal and lateral onychomycosis

CAUSES
• Dermatophytes
  ◊ Invade normal keratin
  ◊ Trichophyton rubrum - most common
  ◊ Trichophyton mentagrophytes var. interdigitale - 25% as common as T. rubrum
  ◊ Epidermophyton floccosum, T. violaceum and Microsporum less common
• Candida
  ◊ 70% Candida albicans
  ◊ C. parapsilosis, C. tropicalis, C. krusei (less common)
• Molds
  ◊ Invade altered keratin
  ◊ Found in following order of frequency: Scopulariopsis brevicaulis, Hendersonula toruloidea, Aspergillus species, Alternaria tenuis, Cephalosporium, Scytalidium hyalinium

RISK FACTORS
• Dermatophyte onychomycosis
  ◊ Warmth
  ◊ Moisture - hyperhidrosis, rubber shoes
  ◊ Cramped or tight fitting foot wear
  ◊ Peripheral vascular disease
  ◊ Depressed cell-mediated immunity
  ◊ Indirect contamination
• Candidal onychomycosis
  ◊ Direct contamination - ano-vulvar, perirectal pruritus
  ◊ Chemical or mechanical damage to cuticle
  ◊ Maceration
  ◊ Occlusion
  ◊ Contact with substances containing sugar
  ◊ Hyperhidrosis
  ◊ Chilblain
  ◊ Cold hands (Raynaud's phenomenon)
  ◊ Psoriatic onycholysis
  ◊ Diabetes mellitus
  ◊ Hyperparathyroidism
  ◊ Addison's disease
  ◊ Malnutrition
  ◊ Malabsorption
  ◊ Dyscrasias
  ◊ Malignant tumors
  ◊ Postoperative conditions
  ◊ Altered immune function
• Mold onychomycosis
  ◊ Soil contamination
  ◊ Peripheral vascular disease
  ◊ Overlapping toes
  ◊ Onychogryposis - deforming overgrowth of nails resulting in hooked or curved state

DIAGNOSIS

DIFFERENTIAL DIAGNOSIS
• Black nail paronychia
• Herpetic whitlow
• Eczema
• Pustular psoriasis
• Tumor
• Darier's disease
• Pityriasis rubra pilaris
• Trophic changes, peripheral vascular disease
• Endocrine disease
• Drugs; chemicals
• Trauma
• Alopecia areata
• Lichen planus
• Yellow-nail syndrome (icterus, carotenemia, amyloidosis)
• White acquired nail disease (trauma, acute infection, chronic disease, thallium or arsenic poisoning, hepatic cirrhosis, chronic albuminemia)
• Brown-black pigment (melanotic, hematoma)
• Green dyschromia (Pseudomonas aeruginosa)

LABORATORY
• Direct microscopy (KOH preparation) - clip or file away some of nailplate as needed, collect scales from stratum corneum of most proximal area (beneath nail or crumbling nail itself), 5% KOH + gentle heat, 100% sensitive if > 2 preps examined
• Cultures - negative in 30% (secondary to loss of dermatophyte viability)
• Histologic examination of keratin
• All are influenced by quality of sampling
Drugs that may alter lab results:
Discontinue all topical medication several days before obtaining sample
Disorders that may alter lab results: N/A

PATHOLOGICAL FINDINGS Pathogens within the nail keratin

SPECIAL TESTS N/A

IMAGING N/A

DIAGNOSTIC PROCEDURES
• Punch or scalpel biopsy - proximal lesions with PAS stain
• Nail scraping - KOH prep

TREATMENT

APPROPRIATE HEALTH CARE
Outpatient - unless secondary cellulitis/osteomyelitis

GENERAL MEASURES
• Avoid factors that promote fungal growth (heat, moisture)
• Treat underlying disease risk factors
• Treat associated fungal infections in other locations (40%)
• Treat secondary infection, if present

SURGICAL MEASURES
• Nail removal to remove infected keratin
  ◊ Mechanical: soften with occlusive dressing, detach from nailbed with tweezers or file with abrasive paper/grinding stone
  ◊ Chemical: protect peripheral tissue with adhesive strips, apply ointment of 30% salicylic acid, 40% urea or 50% potassium iodide under occlusive dressing
  ◊ Surgical avulsion: for involvement of a few nails

ACTIVITY
Restrictions based on promoting factors, underlying disease or secondary infection

DIET
No special diet

PATIENT EDUCATION
N/A

MEDICATIONS

DRUG(S) OF CHOICE
Dermatophytes - local: Less effective than systemic, apply under occlusive dressing, may mix with keratinolytic chemicals
• Most common agents
  ◊ Imidazoles: Clotrimazole (Lotrimin, Mycelex), miconazole (Monistat), butoconazole, tioconazole, econazole (Spectazole), ketoconazole (Nizoral), sulconazole (Exelderm), oxiconazole (Oxistat)
  ◊ Unsaturated fatty acid derivatives: Propionic acid, undecylenic acid; haloprogin (Halotex); tolnaftate (Tinactin)
• Other available agents: Ciclopirox (Loprox), naftifine (Naftin), cationic surfactants, e.g., benzalkonium chloride (Cetylcide), cetrimide, cetylpyridinium chloride (Ony-Clear, Fungoid)], Halogenated/chlorinated/iodinated derivatives [chloramine, tincture of iodine], Dyes [malachite green, crystal violet], Mercury derivatives [thimerosal], phenols, glutaraldehyde
Dermatophytes - systemic:
• Griseofulvin ultramicrosize (Fulvicin, Gris-PEG, Grisactin) usual adult dose 250-500 mg bid with meals
• Fluconazole 50-100 mg/d, overall better tolerated than ketoconazole; expensive; reserve for extreme cases (disseminated disease, immunocompromised)

• Itraconazole: 200 mg po qd for a week per month for 3 months for fingernails and 6-8 months for toenails
• New drugs: oral terbinafine (Lamisil); topical 5% amorolfine lacquer (Loceryl)
Candida:
• Treat with preparation effective against both Candida and bacteria - imidazole derivatives
• If bacterial infection present, treat with antibacterial plus agent effective against Candida e.g., nystatin (Mycostatin), topical amphotericin B (Fungizone), itraconazole (Sporanox) 200 mg po qd, or fluconazole 100 mg po qd
Mold:
• 1% iodinated alcohol, Whitfield's ointment, silver nitrate, glutaraldehyde, imidazole derivatives, itraconazole
Contraindications:
• Griseofulvin: porphyria, hepatocellular failure, serious side effects (leukopenia, persistent anemia), pregnancy
• Ketoconazole: prior sensitivity to drug, hepatocellular disease, pregnancy
• Fluconazole: hepatocellular failure, pregnancy
Precautions:
• Topical agents: use with caution on broken skin, vascular compromise, decreased sensation
• Griseofulvin: monitor for hepatic, renal, hematopoietic side effects; photo-sensitivity; lupus-like symptoms or exacerbation. Take with meals to enhance absorption.
• Ketoconazole: hepatotoxicity (may be severe or fatal), anaphylaxis may (rarely) occur with first dose, decreased testosterone levels
• Fluconazole: decrease dose in renal failure, hepatotoxicity
Significant possible interactions:
• Griseofulvin: warfarin, barbiturates, alcohol, oral contraceptives
• Ketoconazole: H2-blockers, antacids, warfarin, omeprazole, rifampin, cyclosporine, phenytoin, terfenadine
• Fluconazole: phenytoin (Dilantin), cyclosporine, oral hypoglycemics, oral anticoagulants, rifampin, hydrochlorothiazide

ALTERNATIVE DRUGS
N/A

FOLLOWUP

PATIENT MONITORING
• Topical agents: slow response expected; visits q 6-12 weeks, after initial followup to assess compliance
• Griseofulvin: CBC and liver function tests initially, then q 3 months
• Ketoconazole: liver function tests every 3 weeks for the first 3 months, then monthly
• Treatment duration: fingernails 6-9 months, toenails 9-12 months, great toenail 12-24 months

PREVENTION/AVOIDANCE
• Keep affected area clean and dry
• Avoid rubber or other occlusive footwear
• Avoid tight or ill-fitting footwear
• Wear absorbent cotton socks - avoid wool or synthetic fibers
• Change clothing and towels frequently and launder in hot water

POSSIBLE COMPLICATIONS
• Secondary infections with progression to cellulitis/osteomyelitis

EXPECTED COURSE/PROGNOSIS
• Relapse common; prognosis especially poor if one hand, 2 feet or multiple nails involved
• 20-40% of nails fail to respond
• 40-70% of patients show long term relapse

MISCELLANEOUS

ASSOCIATED CONDITIONS
Consider immunodeficiency or chronic metabolic disease in cases presenting with rapid spread

AGE-RELATED FACTORS
Pediatric:
• Dermatophyte onychomycosis rare before puberty
• Candidal infection presents more commonly as superficial white onychomycosis
• Drug dosing based on body mass and approved drugs more limited
Geriatric:
• Mold onychomycosis more common
• Predisposing diseases more common
• Hepatic/renal reserve limited
• Decreased ability for topical self-treatment
Others: N/A

PREGNANCY
Drug choices limited

SYNONYMS
• Tinea unguium
• Ringworm of the nail

ICD-9-CM
110.1 Dermatophytosis of nail
112.3 Candidiasis of skin and nails

SEE ALSO
• HIV infection & AIDS

OTHER NOTES
N/A

ABBREVIATIONS
N/A

REFERENCES
• Pariser DM: Superficial fungal infections. Postgraduate medicine 1990;87(5):205-214
• Baden HP: Diseases of the Hair and Nails. Chicago, Year Book Medical Publishers, 1987
Illustrations: 4 available on CD-ROM
Internet references: http://www.5mcc.com

Author(s)
Scott D. Miller, MD

Optic atrophy

BASICS

DESCRIPTION End result of loss of ganglion cells or axons of the optic nerve
System(s) affected: Nervous
Genetics: Inherited forms may be autosomally recessive, autosomally dominant or X-linked recessive
Incidence/Prevalence in USA: Unknown
Predominant age:
• Inherited forms occur shortly after birth to the third decade
• Acquired forms tend to occur later
Predominant sex: Male > Female (inherited forms)

SIGNS AND SYMPTOMS
• Loss of visual acuity
• Pallor of the optic disk
• Loss of pupillary reactions
• Visual field defects

CAUSES
• Glaucoma
• Post central retinal artery or vein occlusion
• Ischemic optic neuropathy
• Chronic optic neuritis
• Chronic papilledema
• Compression of the optic nerve or chiasm or tract by tumor or by aneurysm
• Trauma
• Syphilis
• Retinal degeneration (e.g., retinitis pigmentosa)
• Congenital optic atrophy
• Radiation neuropathy
• Drugs (amiodarone, chloroquine, ethambutol, oral contraceptives, streptomycin, vincristine)
• Thiamine deficiency

RISK FACTORS
• Hereditary
  ◊ Family history
• Acquired
  ◊ Diabetes mellitus
  ◊ Hypertension
  ◊ Radiation exposure
  ◊ Alcoholism
  ◊ Renal failure
  ◊ Arteriosclerosis

DIAGNOSIS

DIFFERENTIAL DIAGNOSIS
• Myopia
• S/p cataract extraction (no natural yellow color from the human lens)

LABORATORY
• CBC
• Antinuclear antibody (ANA)
• ESR
• Rapid plasma reagin (RPR)
• Fluorescent treponemal antibody absorption (FTA-ABS)
• Serological test for syphilis
• Heavy metal screen
Drugs that may alter lab results: N/A
Disorders that may alter lab results: N/A

PATHOLOGICAL FINDINGS N/A

SPECIAL TESTS
• Automated visual field test (i.e., Humphrey)
• Color vision testing

IMAGING CT or MRI of head

DIAGNOSTIC PROCEDURES
• Carotid Doppler (adult acquired optic atrophy)
• Complete ophthalmologic exam including dilated evaluation of retina

TREATMENT

APPROPRIATE HEALTH CARE
Outpatient

GENERAL MEASURES
• Treat underlying cause (rarely possible)
• Discontinue causative drug if possible
• If pressure against optic nerve is cause, neurosurgery to relieve it may help if done early

SURGICAL MEASURES N/A

ACTIVITY Fully active

DIET No special diet

PATIENT EDUCATION
• Low vision counseling if bilateral
• Genetic counseling if inherited
• For patient education materials favorably reviewed on this topic, contact: National Eye Institute, Information Officer, Dept. of Health and Human Services, 9000 Rockville Pike, Bethesda, MD 20892, (301)496-5248

MEDICATIONS

DRUG(S) OF CHOICE None
Contraindications: N/A
Precautions: N/A
Significant possible interactions: N/A

ALTERNATIVE DRUGS N/A

FOLLOWUP

PATIENT MONITORING Annual evaluations if stable

PREVENTION/AVOIDANCE N/A

POSSIBLE COMPLICATIONS N/A

EXPECTED COURSE/PROGNOSIS
• Rarely possible to treat the underlying cause effectively
• Visual loss occurs over weeks to months
• Optic atrophy secondary to vascular, trauma, degenerative changes and some toxic causes has a very bad prognosis

MISCELLANEOUS

ASSOCIATED CONDITIONS
• Inherited neurodegenerative conditions
   ◊ Hereditary ataxia
   ◊ Charcot-Marie-Tooth disease
   ◊ Storage diseases
   ◊ Leukodystrophies

AGE-RELATED FACTORS
Pediatric: Optic atrophy in small children is difficult to recognize because disks normally have a pale appearance
Geriatric: None
Others: None

PREGNANCY None

SYNONYMS N/A

ICD-9-CM 377.10 optic atrophy, unspecified

SEE ALSO N/A

OTHER NOTES American Council of the Blind (800)424-8666

ABBREVIATIONS N/A

REFERENCES
• Miller NR: Walsh and Hoyt's Clinical Neuro-Ophthalmology. 4th Ed. Baltimore, Williams & Wilkins, 1982
• Fraunfelder FT, Roy FH: Current Ocular Therapy. 3rd Ed. Philadelphia, W.B. Saunders Co., 1990
Illustrations: 1 available on CD-ROM
Internet references: http://www.5mcc.com

Author(s)
Robert Noecker, MD

Optic neuritis

 BASICS

 DIAGNOSIS

 TREATMENT

BASICS

DESCRIPTION Inflammation of the optic nerve
System(s) affected: Nervous
Genetics: N/A
Incidence/Prevalence in USA: N/A
Predominant age: Typically 18-50 years
Predominant sex: Female > Male

SIGNS AND SYMPTOMS
• Loss of vision, deteriorating from hours to days, usually reaching lowest level in one week
• Usually unilateral in adults, bilateral disease more common in children
• Tenderness of the globe, deep orbital pain or brow ache, especially with eye movement
• Central, cecocentral or arcuate visual field deficits
• Decreased color vision
• Apparent dimness of light intensities
• Impairment of depth perception
• Increase in visual symptoms with increased body temperature (Uhthoff's sign)
• May be either swollen optic disk (most commonly seen in children) or normal optic disc
• Relative afferent pupillary defect (Marcus Gunn pupil)

CAUSES
• Idiopathic
• Multiple sclerosis
• Viral infections of childhood (measles, mumps, chickenpox)
• Other viral infections (mononucleosis, herpes zoster, encephalitis)
• Contiguous inflammation of the meninges, orbit, or sinuses
• Granulomatous inflammations (syphilis, tuberculosis, cryptococcus, sarcoidosis)
• Intraocular inflammations
• Lead toxicity
• Chronic high doses chloramphenicol
• Posterior uveitis
• Vascular lesions of optic nerve
• Tumors
• Fungal infections

RISK FACTORS   N/A

DIAGNOSIS

DIFFERENTIAL DIAGNOSIS
• Acute papilledema
• Anterior ischemic optic neuropathy
• Severe systemic hypertension
• Toxic/nutritional optic neuropathy
• Orbital tumor compressing the optic nerve
• Intracranial tumor pressing on the afferent visual pathway
• Leber's congenital optic neuropathy

LABORATORY
• CBC
• Antinuclear antibody (ANA)
• ESR
• Rapid plasma reagin (RPR)
• Fluorescent treponemal antibody absorption (FTA-ABS)
• Serological test for syphilis
Drugs that may alter lab results: N/A
Disorders that may alter lab results: N/A

PATHOLOGICAL FINDINGS   N/A

SPECIAL TESTS
• Visual field test (preferably automated Humphrey or Octopus)
• Color vision testing

IMAGING
• Chest x-ray
• MRI head or CT head/orbits in atypical cases or when patient is not improving after 10-14 days and other tests are negative

DIAGNOSTIC PROCEDURES
• Check blood pressure
• Complete ophthalmologic exam including pupillary assessment, color vision evaluation with color plates, dilated retinal examination with optic nerve assessment
• Neurologic work-up

TREATMENT

APPROPRIATE HEALTH CARE
Outpatient observation

GENERAL MEASURES   No disease specific measures

SURGICAL MEASURES   N/A

ACTIVITY   Fully active

DIET   No special diet

PATIENT EDUCATION
• Reassurance about recovery of vision
• If felt to be secondary to demyelinating disease, patient should be informed of the risk of developing multiple sclerosis
• For patient education materials favorably reviewed on this topic, contact: National Eye Institute, Information Officer, Dept. of Health and Human Services, 9000 Rockville Pike, Bethesda, MD 20892, (301)496-5248

MEDICATIONS

DRUG(S) OF CHOICE None
Contraindications: N/A
Precautions: N/A
Significant possible interactions: N/A

ALTERNATIVE DRUGS
• Pulse steroids: methylprednisolone 250 mg IV q6h x 12 doses in the hospital followed by prednisone 1 mg/kg/day po for 11 days, taper over 1-2 weeks
• Anti-ulcer medication is given with steroids

FOLLOWUP

PATIENT MONITORING Monthly followup to monitor visual changes

PREVENTION/AVOIDANCE N/A

POSSIBLE COMPLICATIONS Permanent loss of vision

EXPECTED COURSE/PROGNOSIS
• Visual acuity begins to improve 2-3 weeks after onset
• Improvement continues over several months and vision often returns to normal or near normal levels
• Those patients with poor vision and who receive IV steroids often recover faster
• When baseline vision is good, IV steroids have no beneficial effect

MISCELLANEOUS

ASSOCIATED CONDITIONS Over 50% of adult optic neuritis patients will develop multiple sclerosis

AGE-RELATED FACTORS
Pediatric: N/A
Geriatric: N/A
Others: N/A

PREGNANCY N/A

SYNONYMS
• Papillitis
• Retrobulbar neuritis

ICD-9-CM 377.30 Optic neuritis

SEE ALSO Multiple sclerosis

OTHER NOTES N/A

ABBREVIATIONS N/A

REFERENCES
• Sergott R, Brown M: Current concepts of the pathogenesis of optic neuritis associated with multiple sclerosis. Surv Ophthalmol 1988;33:108-116
• Miller N: Walsh and Hoyt's Clinical Neuro-Ophthalmology. 4th Ed. Baltimore, Williams & Wilkins, 1982
• Fraunfelder FT, Roy FH: Current Ocular Therapy. 3rd Ed. Philadelphia, W.B. Saunders Co., 1990
Illustrations: 1 available on CD-ROM
Internet references: http://www.5mcc.com

Author(s)
Robert Noecker, MD

Oral cavity neoplasms

BASICS

DESCRIPTION Malignant tumors affecting the lip, tongue, floor of the mouth, salivary glands, inside of cheeks, gums, and palate. 90% of the neoplasms are squamous cell carcinomas and the remainder are lymphomas, melanomas, adenocarcinomas from minor salivary gland origin and sarcomas.
System(s) affected: Gastrointestinal
Genetics: N/A
Incidence/Prevalence in USA:
• 12/100,000 (30,300 new cases a year). 5000 persons die of this disease annually.
• Oral cavity neoplasms account for 4% of all cancers occurring in men and 2% in women
• High incidence in Asia, related to the habit of chewing betelnut, fresh betel leaf, and habitual reverse smoking in which the lighted end of the cigarette is held within the oral cavity
Predominant sex: Male > Female
Predominant age: 50 and over. However, increasingly being seen in younger age group with the use of smokeless tobacco.

SIGNS AND SYMPTOMS
• Dysphagia
• Odynophagia
• Problems articulating
• Regurgitation of liquids secondary to nasopharyngeal incompetence from the tumor
• Ipsilateral otalgia from referred pain
• Friable granular exophytic and/or infiltrative mass or ulcer which frequently is tender and confused with infection. Usually has hard indurated margins by palpation which extend beyond the confines of the ulcer itself.
• Hard neck mass suggesting metastatic disease in the nodal chain along the internal jugular vein

CAUSES
• Tobacco use (smokeless or smoked)
• Use of snuff
• Excess alcohol consumption
• Exposure to ultraviolet light in the instances of lip carcinoma
• Riboflavin or iron deficiency anemia, and Plummer-Vinson syndrome associated with oral cancers
• Betel nut or leaf chewing

RISK FACTORS N/A

DIAGNOSIS

DIFFERENTIAL DIAGNOSIS
• Exudative tonsillitis (usually bilateral involvement)
• Stomatitis or glossitis secondary to infectious etiology, most commonly candidiasis
• Benign tumors of the oral cavity (slow growing and usually not erosive or ulcerative)
• Kaposi's sarcoma
• Mycosis fungoides
• Premalignant lesions such as leukoplakia or erythroplasia
• Lichen planus

LABORATORY Liver function test to rule out metastasis to the liver
Drugs that may alter lab results: N/A
Disorders that may alter lab results:
• Alcoholism
• Hepatitis

PATHOLOGICAL FINDINGS Malignant changes characteristic of cell types

SPECIAL TESTS N/A

IMAGING
• Chest x-ray to rule out metastasis to the lungs
• Imaging bone scans if there is pain in the bones suggesting bone metastasis
• CT or MRI scan if clinical suggestion of intracranial or liver metastasis

DIAGNOSTIC PROCEDURES Transoral biopsy as an outpatient makes the definitive diagnosis

TREATMENT

APPROPRIATE HEALTH CARE
• Inpatient for surgery
• The treatment varies depending on location, i.e., tongue, buccal wall, pharynx, palate, lip

GENERAL MEASURES
• Unresectable lesions usually are treated with radiation therapy and/or chemotherapy for palliation
• Nutrition is of prime importance for normal wound healing should patient require surgery. Patients may need naso-gastric and/or gastrostomy feedings if orally disabled.

SURGICAL MEASURES
• Wide resection with or without radiation therapy and/or chemotherapy is the treatment of choice
• Tracheotomy may be necessary if the patient has problems handling secretions or difficulty breathing

ACTIVITY As tolerated by patient's nutritional and physical status

DIET
• Depends on the extent of disease and whether the patient is able to chew or swallow
• Usually early lesions can be managed with a regular diet. As disease progresses, a soft diet is necessary.

PATIENT EDUCATION Literature is available from American Cancer Society

MEDICATIONS

DRUG(S) OF CHOICE Narcotics for pain relief
Contraindications: N/A
Precautions: N/A
Significant possible interactions: N/A

ALTERNATIVE DRUGS N/A

FOLLOWUP

PATIENT MONITORING Routine periodic head and neck exams to detect possible second primary or recurrence in the upper respiratory and digestive tract

PREVENTION/AVOIDANCE
• Avoidance of smoking or the use of smokeless tobacco
• Avoid alcohol use

POSSIBLE COMPLICATIONS
• Functional and/or cosmetic disabilities proportional to the degree of surgery and stage of tumor
• Stomatitis with or without candidiasis secondary to radiation therapy or chemotherapy
• Persistent dysphagia secondary to surgery or radiation therapy
• Persistent problems with articulation or deglutition depending on the amount of tongue resection

EXPECTED COURSE/PROGNOSIS Early lesions with adequate treatment leads to a greater than 80% cure

MISCELLANEOUS

ASSOCIATED CONDITIONS Leukoplakia or erythroplasia should be biopsied, since they are considered premalignant and associated with carcinoma at least 10% of the time

AGE-RELATED FACTORS None
Pediatric: N/A
Geriatric: Greater incidence after 50
Others: N/A

PREGNANCY N/A

SYNONYMS N/A

ICD-9-CM
• 145.9 Malignant neoplasm of mouth, unspecified
• 198.89 Secondary malignant neoplasm, other specified sites, other
• 230.0 Carcinoma in situ lip, oral cavity and pharynx
• 210.4 Benign neoplasm other and unspecified parts of mouth
• 235.1 Neoplasm of uncertain behavior of lip, oral cavity and pharynx

SEE ALSO N/A

OTHER NOTES
• High incidence in Asia related to the habit of chewing the betel nut, fresh betel leaf, and habitual reverse smoking (lighted end is held within the oral cavity).

ABBREVIATIONS N/A

REFERENCES Cummings CW, Fredrickson JM, Harker LA, Crause CJ, Schuller DE: Otolaryngology: Head and Neck Surgery. Volume 2. New York, C.V. Mosby Company, 1986
Illustrations: 1 available on CD-ROM
Internet references: http://www.5mcc.com

Author(s)
Roy R. Casiano, MD

Oral rehydration

BASICS

DESCRIPTION
• Dehydration and ongoing fluid losses from infectious gastroenteritis (GE) can be effectively treated with oral rehydration solutions (ORS), except in the most severe cases where initial parenteral fluid resuscitation is required. This therapy takes advantage of the coupled transport of sodium and glucose in the small intestine even during course of GE. Water follows osmotically after sodium entry. Potassium is passively absorbed via solvent drag. A glucose concentration of 2% allows maximal sodium absorption.
• ORS for rehydration should have a sodium content of about 75 mEq/L (75 mmol/L). Maintenance ORS, with sodium content of 40-50 mEq/L (40-50 mmol/L), are useful for mild dehydration and treatment of ongoing losses with a relatively low sodium content (e.g., rotavirus). High sodium diarrheal losses as from cholera require higher sodium content ORS (WHO solution = 90 mEq/L Na).

System(s) affected: Gastrointestinal, Endocrine/Metabolic
Genetics: N/A
Incidence/Prevalence in USA: N/A
Predominant age: Primarily infants and children; effective for all ages
Predominant sex: Male = Female

SIGNS AND SYMPTOMS See
Dehydration

CAUSES N/A

RISK FACTORS N/A

DIAGNOSIS

DIFFERENTIAL DIAGNOSIS N/A

LABORATORY N/A

SPECIAL TESTS N/A
Drugs that may alter lab results: N/A
Disorders that may alter lab results: N/A

PATHOLOGICAL FINDINGS N/A

IMAGING N/A

DIAGNOSTIC PROCEDURES N/A

TREATMENT

APPROPRIATE HEALTH CARE Primarily outpatient. Designed to be administered by family members.

GENERAL MEASURES
• Estimate replacement at 60 mL/kg for mild- and 80-100 mL/kg for moderate dehydration over the first 4-8 hours. Very important to replace any ongoing losses and add maintenance fluids.
• Replace ongoing stool losses with ORS. In infant, estimate 5-10 mL/kg per stool or weigh diapers.
• Add maintenance requirements to replacement:
  ◊ Estimate:
    0-10 kg - 4 mL/kg/hr
    Plus 10-20 kg - 2 mL/kg/hr
    Plus > 20 kg - 1mL/kg/hr
  ◊ Use maintenance ORS. Traditional clear fluids (e.g., fruit juice, soda) are inappropriate for oral rehydration therapy.
• If the patient has hypertonic dehydration, oral rehydration should be planned for 12-24 hours
• If vomiting occurs, small amounts of ORS given frequently is usually effective
• If patient is not vomiting and is alert, patient's thirst is excellent indicator of fluid needs
• ORS is not to be diluted
• Maintenance oral rehydration therapy begins when the deficit is replaced and provides for ongoing losses. Maintenance ORS or a combination of ORS and water or other clear liquids can be used.
• Effective at all ages. If child refuses because of taste, flavor with a commercial artificially sweetened flavoring, such as, Nutrasweet-flavored Kool-Aid; use approximately 1/4 teaspoon to 4 oz ORS.

SURGICAL MEASURES N/A

ACTIVITY As tolerated

DIET
• For breast feeding infants - mother should continue nursing
• For bottle fed babies - early institution of lactose-free formulas. Delay using milk-based formula for several days.
• Age appropriate - easily digestible, carbohydrate rich, low lactose foods should be offered as soon as the dehydration deficit is replaced. Cow's milk can be added to diet after several days.

PATIENT EDUCATION
• Awareness and availability of ORS markedly diminishes morbidity from gastroenteritis
• Travelers concerned with severe diarrhea should carry ORS packets on trips

MEDICATIONS

DRUG(S) OF CHOICE
• The prototype ORS is the World Health Organization solution. In developed countries, when GE is unlikely to be caused by cholera, a lower sodium solution is advisable.
WHO ORS:
◊ 1 liter of clean water
◊ 1/2 tsp sodium chloride (salt)
◊ 1/2 tsp trisodium citrate
◊ 1/4 tsp potassium chloride (salt substitute)
◊ 2 tbsp glucose
• Notes:
◊ Glucose can be replaced by either sucrose (table sugar) or rice powder which are less expensive.
◊ Trisodium citrate can be replaced by sodium bicarbonate (baking soda). (Sodium bicarbonate was used in previous formulation.)

Comparison of ORS's

Solution	Type†	Na+	Storage form
WHO ORS	R	90	Powder
Rehydralyte	R	75	Liquid
Pedialyte	M	45	Liquid
Naolectro	M	52	Powder
Beech-nut- Ped. Electrolyte	M	50	Liquid

† R = rehydration
M = maintenance
Na+ = Sodium (mEq/L or mmol/L)

Contraindications:
• Conditions predisposing to risk of aspiration: Altered consciousness, seizure activity, severe hypotension, shock
• Persistent vomiting (as in pyloric stenosis)
• Absent bowel sounds

Precautions:
• The ingredients should be provided in pre-mixed packets in order to avoid iatrogenic errors in mixing
• If water safety is questionable, it should be boiled or treated for purification
• Discard the solution after 12 hours if held at room temperature, or 24 hours if refrigerated
• After rehydration is complete, ORS's should not be used as the only fluid intake because the high sodium content may lead to hypernatremia

Significant possible interactions: N/A

ALTERNATIVE DRUGS N/A

FOLLOWUP

PATIENT MONITORING
The patient needs to be frequently evaluated to ensure establishment of an improving clinical status and an adequate urine output

PREVENTION/AVOIDANCE N/A

POSSIBLE COMPLICATIONS
Change to IV hydration if the patient has increasing weight loss (fluid deficit), clinical deterioration, or intractable vomiting.

EXPECTED COURSE/PROGNOSIS
• Rapid clinical improvement despite continuing diarrhea is the usual course
• The overall complication rate for oral rehydration is the same as that for parenteral rehydration in cases of mild and moderate dehydration.

MISCELLANEOUS

ASSOCIATED CONDITIONS N/A

AGE-RELATED FACTORS N/A
Pediatric: See Diet
Geriatric: N/A
Others: N/A

PREGNANCY N/A

SYNONYMS N/A

ICD-9-CM N/A

SEE ALSO
• Dehydration
• Cholera
• Diarrhea, acute
• Gastroenteritis, viral
• Hypernatremia

OTHER NOTES
Advantages of oral rehydration include a much lower cost, minimal storage requirements (for powder forms) and no need for sterile conditions

ABBREVIATIONS
• GE = gastroenteritis
• ORS = oral rehydration solutions

REFERENCES
• The management of acute diarrhea in children: Oral rehydration, maintenance and nutritional therapy. MMWR 41:RR-16:10/16/92
• Goepp J, Santosham M: Oral rehydration therapy. In: Oski F, ed. Principles and Practice of Pediatrics. Philadelphia, J.B. Lippincott, 1992
• Meyers A: Modern management of acute diarrhea and dehydration in children. Am Fam Phys 1995;51:1103-18
• Santosham M, et al: A double-blind clinical trial comparing WHO ORS with a reduced osmolarity solution containing amounts of sodium and glucose. J Pediatr 1996;128:45-51
Illustrations: N/A
Internet references: http://www.5mcc.com

Author(s)
William A. Primack, MD
Charles N. Jacobs, MD

Osgood-Schlatter disease

BASICS

DESCRIPTION The syndrome associated with traction apophysitis in adolescent boys and girls consisting of pain of the tibial tubercle with swelling
System(s) affected: Musculoskeletal
Genetics: Unknown
Incidence/Prevalence in USA: Not known, but common (13% of athletes in one Finnish study)
Predominant age:
• Females 10-16
• Males 11-18
Predominant sex: Male > Female

SIGNS AND SYMPTOMS
• Unilateral or bilateral (30%) tibial tuberosity pain
• Pain exacerbated by exercise, especially jumping
• Tibial tuberosity swelling
• Pain increased with knee extension against resistance or kneeling
• Knee pain with squatting or crouching
• Absence of effusion or condyle tenderness
• Erythema of tibial tuberosity

CAUSES Basic etiology unknown, but clearly exacerbated by exercise - jumping and pivoting sports are the worst

RISK FACTORS
• Age between 11 and 18
• Male sex
• Rapid skeletal growth
• Involvement in repetitive jumping sports

DIAGNOSIS

DIFFERENTIAL DIAGNOSIS
• Stress fracture of the proximal tibia
• Pes anserinus bursitis
• Quadriceps tendon avulsion
• Patellofemoral stress syndrome
• Chondromalacia patellae
• Proximal tibial neoplasm
• Osteomyelitis of the proximal tibia
• Tibial plateau fracture

LABORATORY No blood tests indicated unless other diagnostic considerations are entertained
Drugs that may alter lab results: N/A
Disorders that may alter lab results: N/A

PATHOLOGICAL FINDINGS
• Osteochondritis of the tibial tubercle
• Heterotopic bone formation at insertion of the patellar tendon
• Bony fusion of the tibial metaphysis
• Inflammatory infiltrate of the epiphysis in severe cases
• Complete avulsion of the tibial tubercle with nonunion of the tubercle with the tibia - possible complication (extremely rare)

SPECIAL TESTS N/A

IMAGING
• X-ray imaging of the proximal tibia and knee may show heterotopic calcification in the patellar tendon
• Calcified thickening of the tibial tuberosity with irregular ossification at insertion of tendon to tibial tubercle
• Bone scan may show increased uptake in the area of the tibial tuberosity; will have increased uptake in apophysis in any child, but may be more than opposite side

DIAGNOSTIC PROCEDURES N/A

TREATMENT

APPROPRIATE HEALTH CARE
Outpatient

GENERAL MEASURES
• Frequent ice applications post exercise with pain
• Rest
• Knee immobilization in extension
• In more severe cases, avoidance of activities that increase pain or swelling
• Quadriceps isometric strengthening, hip extensions, adductor strengthening, hamstring and quadriceps stretching exercises

SURGICAL MEASURES Débridement of a thickened cosmetically unsatisfactory tibial tubercle (rare)

ACTIVITY Activity to be restricted to those activities not causing pain

DIET N/A

PATIENT EDUCATION
• Consider avoidance of jumping sports. Assure family that symptoms and findings will diminish with time and rest.
• OK to play sport with mild pain

MEDICATIONS

DRUG(S) OF CHOICE None in particular, but all analgesics may be considered. NSAID's are of minimal benefit.
Contraindications: N/A
Precautions: N/A
Significant possible interactions: N/A

ALTERNATIVE DRUGS More potent analgesics such as narcotics may be considered for short term use or in extreme situations

FOLLOWUP

PATIENT MONITORING Follow up on a prn basis for management of pain and disability

PREVENTION/AVOIDANCE
• Avoidance of those sports involving heavy quadriceps loading
• Patients may compete if the pain is minimal
• Increase hamstring and quadriceps flexibility

POSSIBLE COMPLICATIONS
• Nonunion of the tubercle to the tibia
• Upriding of the patella
• Patellar tendon avulsion
• Genu recurvatum
• Patellofemoral degenerative arthritis
• Patella alta
• Chondromalacia

EXPECTED COURSE/PROGNOSIS
Except in rare complicated cases, this is a self-limiting illness resolved within two years after full skeletal maturation

MISCELLANEOUS

ASSOCIATED CONDITIONS N/A

AGE-RELATED FACTORS
Pediatric: In skeletally mature boys and girls, with boys more frequent than girls
Geriatric: N/A
Others: Participants in sports involving heavy quadriceps activity

PREGNANCY N/A

SYNONYMS Osteochondritis of the tibial tubercle

ICD-9-CM 732.4 Juvenile osteochondrosis of lower extremity, excluding foot

SEE ALSO Tendinitis

OTHER NOTES N/A

ABBREVIATIONS N/A

REFERENCES
• Outerbridge AR, Micheli LJ: Overuse injuries in the young athlete. Sports Med 1995;14(3):503-516
• Peck DM: Apophyseal injuries in the young athlete. Am Fam Phys 1995;51(8):1891-1895
Illustrations: N/A
Internet references: http://www.5mcc.com

Author(s)
David P. Sealy, MD

Osteitis deformans

BASICS

DESCRIPTION Inflammatory focal (sometimes generalized) condition of the skeleton characterized by rapid, chaotic bone resorption followed by equally chaotic and excessive bone formation. Leads to enlarged but weakened and highly vascularized bone which is painful, easily deformed and subject to fractures with minimal trauma. Cranial and vertebral involvement can also cause neurologic deficits.
System(s) affected: Musculoskeletal
Genetics: 15-50% of patients have one or more involved first order relatives with osteitis deformans
Incidence/Prevalence in USA: 3% of Caucasian individuals above age 50 have at least one focus. Rare in African Americans and Asians.
Predominant age: Above age 50, occasional cases ages 20-50
Predominant sex: Male = Female

SIGNS AND SYMPTOMS
• Asymptomatic frequently
• Bone pain
• Skeletal deformities
• Bowing of extremities
• Acetabular protrusion
• Headaches
• Head enlargement
• Frequent fractures
• Secondary osteoarthritis
• Vertebral compression
• Neurologic deficits
• High output congestive heart failure (rare)
• Hypercalcemia (rare)
• Renal calculi (calcium, uric acid)
• Angioid streaks (rare)
• Mottled retinal degeneration (rare)
• Increased skin temperature over affected areas
• Bone sarcomas (rare)
• Peripheral neuropathies
• Carpal/tarsal tunnel syndromes
• Valvular/endocardial calcification
• Accelerated atherosclerosis
• Gouty diathesis
• Hyperparathyroidism
• Sensorineural hearing loss
• Conductive hearing loss

CAUSES Unknown; best evidence to date is for slow virus infection

RISK FACTORS None known

DIAGNOSIS

DIFFERENTIAL DIAGNOSIS
• Polyostotic fibrous dysplasia
• Osteitis fibrosis cystica (skeletal hyperparathyroidism)
• Primary bone neoplasms
• Osteolytic, osteoblastic metastases

LABORATORY
• Serum calcium - usually normal, occasionally increased
• Serum alkaline phosphatase (total or bone specific) - usually increased
• Serum GGT - normal
• Serum osteocalcin (BGP) - usually increased
• Urinary pyridinoline collagen crosslinks - usually increased
• N-telopeptide (collagen crosslinks) - usually increased
Drugs that may alter lab results:
• Vitamin D and its metabolites
• Hepatotoxic drugs
Disorders that may alter lab results:
• See Differential diagnosis
• Osteomalacia
• Liver disorders
• Traumatic fractures

PATHOLOGICAL FINDINGS
• Chaotic bone resorption at advancing edge of disease. Osteoclasts are large, contain 10-100 nuclei and have abnormal configuration.
• Electronphotomicroscopically, the nuclei and cytoplasm contain myriad of inclusion bodies resembling viral nucleocapsids
• Later, excessive osteoblastic bone formation predominates with sclerotic bone containing cement lines forming mosaic pattern

SPECIAL TESTS
• Neurologic examination
• Audiogram, if skull involvement
• Visual field study, if skull involvement

IMAGING
• X-rays show irregular pattern of alternating bone formation and resorption in enlarged deformed bones. Resorptive fronts at advancing edge.
• Bone scans show intense uptake in focal pattern
• CT/MRI show extra-bony extension if sarcomatous degeneration occurs

DIAGNOSTIC PROCEDURES Bone
biopsy needed only in confusing cases (rare)

TREATMENT

APPROPRIATE HEALTH CARE
Outpatient, except when intravenous treatment is used

GENERAL MEASURES
• Rarely, splints for severely resorbed areas with high risk of fracture
• Hearing aids for severe deafness; of some (but not great) value in sensorineural deafness

SURGICAL MEASURES N/A

ACTIVITY
• Full activity to maintain function
• Avoid excessive mechanical stress on involved bones

DIET No special diet

PATIENT EDUCATION Paget's Disease
Foundation, 200 Varick St., Suite 1004, New York, NY 10014-4810, (212)229-1582; fax (212)229-1502

MEDICATIONS

DRUG(S) OF CHOICE
• Synthetic injectable salmon calcitonin (Miacalcin, Calcimar, Osteocalcin): 50 IU three times weekly to 100 IU qd, courses 1.5 to 3 years
or
• Etidronate (Didronel), 5 mg/kg/day (approximately 400 mg) x 6 mos (taken on an empty stomach). Rarely, 20 mg/kg/day x 1 month. Courses may be repeated after a 3-6 month rest period
or
• Alendronate (Fosamax) 40 mg/day (taken on an empty stomach) for 6 mos
or
• Tiludronate (Skelid) 400 mg/day (taken on an empty stomach) for 3 months
or
• Pamidronate (Aredia) 60 mg/day by 4-6 hour infusions for 2-3 days. Alternately, 30 mg/day by 4-6 hour infusions once a week for 6 weeks. May be repeated several months later if effect wears off.
or
• Plicamycin (Mithracin), 25 mcg/kg/day or qod by 4-6 hr infusions x 9-10 infusions
• Add nonsteroidal anti-inflammatories (NSAID's) to above drugs for secondary osteoarthritis

Contraindications:
• Prior history of allergy or hypersensitivity
• For alendronate and tiludronate, esophageal dysfunction, severe upper GI symptoms, GERD, etc.
• For plicamycin, manifest hepatic or renal impairment or bone marrow depression

Precautions:
• Adverse side effects may require ameliorative measures or temporary dose reduction
• Salmon calcitonin - nausea, vomiting, anorexia, flushing, rash, including urticaria (rare)
• Etidronate disodium - nausea, vomiting, diarrhea, increased bone pain
• Alendronate and tiludronate - heartburn, epigastric pain, musculoskeletal pain. Take on an empty stomach with copious water. No food, beverages or other medications for 1 hour. Remain upright for 1 hour.
• Pamidronate disodium - transient fever, leukopenia, hypocalcemia, headache, malaise, loss of appetite
• Plicamycin - vomiting, anorexia, malaise, abnormal liver/renal function, thrombocytopenia with bleeding

Significant possible interactions: None

ALTERNATIVE DRUGS
NSAID's for mildly symptomatic disease in nonstrategic areas

FOLLOWUP

PATIENT MONITORING
• Followup visits every 2-4 months during drug therapy; yearly if drugs not being used. Alkaline phosphatase (total or bone specific) before each visit.
• Repeat x-rays and bone scan every 3-5 years

PREVENTION/AVOIDANCE
Avoid excessive mechanical stress on afflicted bones to reduce chance of fractures and other complications

POSSIBLE COMPLICATIONS
Fractures, severe deformities, head enlargement, acetabular protrusion, carpal/tarsal tunnel syndromes, neurologic deficits, deafness, visual impairment, congestive heart failure (high output), renal calculi, sarcomatous degeneration

EXPECTED COURSE/PROGNOSIS
• Depends on severity
• Slow progression if untreated
• Significant amelioration with treatment (85%)
• Poor prognosis if bone sarcoma develops

MISCELLANEOUS

ASSOCIATED CONDITIONS
• Hyperparathyroidism
• Gouty diathesis
• Secondary osteoarthritis
• Angioid streaks
• Mottled retinal degeneration
• Bone sarcoma (rare)

AGE-RELATED FACTORS
Pediatric: N/A
Geriatric: Common
Others: More prevalent if ancestry Caucasian, especially United Kingdom, Northern Europe (excluding Scandinavia), Italy, Australia and New Zealand. Rare in African Americans and Asians.

PREGNANCY N/A

SYNONYMS Paget's disease of bone

ICD-9-CM 731.0

SEE ALSO
• Hyperparathyroidism
• Arthritis, osteo
• Bone tumor, primary malignant

OTHER NOTES N/A

ABBREVIATIONS N/A

REFERENCES
• Hadjipavlou A, Lander P, Srolovitz H, Enker IP. Malignant transformation in Paget's disease of bone. Cancer. 1992;70:2802-2808
• Hamdy RC. Clinical features and pharmacologic treatment of Paget's disease. Endocrinol Metab Clin No Am. 1995;24(2):421-436
• Klein RM, Norman A. Diagnostic procedures for Paget's disease. Radiologic, pathologic and laboratory testing. Endocrinol Metab Clin No Am. 1995;24(2):437-450
• Morales-Piga AA, Rey-Rey JS, Corres-Gonzalez J, Garcia-Sagredo JM, Loopez-Abente G. Frequency and characteristics of familial aggregation of Paget's disease of bone. J Bone Miner Res. 1995;10:663-670
• Singer FR, Minoofer PN. Biphosphonates in the treatment of disorders of mineral metabolism. Adv Endocrinol Metab, 1995;6:259-288
• Delmas PD, Meunier PJ: The management of Paget's disease of bone. NEJM 1997;336:558-566
Illustrations: N/A
Internet references: http://www.5mcc.com

Author(s)
Stanley Wallach, MD

Osteochondritis dissecans

BASICS

DESCRIPTION Condition in which segment of articular and underlying subchondral bone becomes separated from surrounding bone.
System(s) affected: Musculoskeletal
Genetics: No distinct genetic pattern known
Incidence/Prevalence in USA: Unknown
Predominant Age: 2 main age groups; children under 12 years old and young adults
Predominant Sex: Male > Female (3:1)

SIGNS AND SYMPTOMS
• Intermittent joint pain, clicking, swelling, locking and stiffness
• May be asymptomatic until the fragment detaches, then experience locking of the joint or giving way in the knee
• Focal tenderness over involved part of joint
• May have effusion, atrophy of supporting musculature, crepitus, decreased range of motion

CAUSES
Most widely accepted theories are:
• Trauma (direct or indirect)
versus
• Ischemic theory due to focal insufficiency in end-arterial blood supply leading to necrosis
• Accessory growth centers that may have arterial supply disrupted leading to typical osteochondritis dissecans lesion (unlikely)

RISK FACTORS No apparent genetic predisposition

DIAGNOSIS

DIFFERENTIAL DIAGNOSIS
• Meniscal tear
• Osteochondral fractures
• Patellalgia
• Anomalous ossification center especially in lat condyle

LABORATORY No specific tests
Drugs that may alter lab results: N/A
Disorders that may alter lab results: N/A

PATHOLOGICAL FINDINGS
• Primary change in the bone
• Avascular necrosis occurs in a focal area
• Overlying cartilage changes are secondary to the bony changes
• Loss of subchondral bone support leads to degenerative. cartilage changes - softening, fibromatous, fissuring
• Fragment may detach and become loose body with traumatic event
• Healing occurs by revascularization and "creeping substitution"

SPECIAL TESTS N/A

IMAGING
• Plain radiographs - AP, lateral and "tunnel" view, first study to confirm diagnosis. Appears as a well demarcated fragment of bone surrounded by a radiolucent zone. If separated, the fragment may be seen elsewhere in the joint and a defect is present in the articular surface.
• Technetium 99 bone scan - now of historic value; was used to evaluate healing potential.
• CT scan - provides architectural description of lesion. Essentially replaced by MRI.
• MRI
  ◊ Very useful to delineate bony lesion
  ◊ Difficult to assess and identify the status of overlying articular cartilage. Healing progression difficult to follow.

DIAGNOSTIC PROCEDURES
• Arthroscopy - definitive procedure to assess the underlying cartilage and for definitive treatment

TREATMENT

APPROPRIATE HEALTH CARE
Outpatient usually; inpatient for surgery

GENERAL MEASURES
• Goals of treatment - maintain smooth congruous joint surface. Alleviate pain. Prevent degenerative joint disease. Promote revascularization of necrotic fragment.
• Splinting, crutches, non-weight bearing with active range of motion is the norm

SURGICAL MEASURES On occasion, early surgical intervention is needed. Orthopedic consultation recommended.

ACTIVITY
• Non-weight bearing, immobilization with intermittent maintenance of range of motion
• Follow closely for 12 weeks for healing; fragment displacement may occur, in which case arthroscopy is indicated.

DIET No specific diet recommended

PATIENT EDUCATION
• Compliance with immobilization and possibility of further trauma should be emphasized.
• Most lesions heal without surgical intervention.

MEDICATIONS

DRUG(S) OF CHOICE
• NSAIDs (e.g., ibuprofen 20-30 mg/kg/day)
Contraindications: N/A
Precautions: N/A
Significant possible interactions: N/A

ALTERNATIVE DRUGS N/A

FOLLOWUP

PATIENT MONITORING
Initially should be followed every 6-8 weeks with serial radiographs to check for healing and possible displacement. Expect healing in 3 months. In one year radiographs usually show no residual abnormality.

POSSIBLE COMPLICATIONS
• Failure to revascularize and heal
• Displacement of fragment becoming loose body within a joint

PREVENTION/AVOIDANCE No clear way to avoid its development.

EXPECTED COURSE/PROGNOSIS
• Most will heal without morbidity
• An incongruous joint surface may lead to degenerative changes if not managed adequately

MISCELLANEOUS

ASSOCIATED CONDITIONS N/A

AGE-RELATED FACTORS
Pediatric: N/A
Geriatric: N/A
Others: N/A

PREGNANCY N/A

SYNONYMS N/A

ICD-9-CM 732.7 Osteochondritis dissecans

SEE ALSO N/A

OTHER NOTES N/A

ABBREVIATIONS N/A

REFERENCES
• Federico DJ, et al: Osteochondritis Dissecans of the Knee: A historical review of etiology and treatment. Arthroscopy 1990;6(3):190-197
• Garrett JC: Clinics in Sports Med 1991;10(3):569-593
• Green WT, Banks HH: CORR; Osteochondritis Dissecans in Children 1990;(255):3-12
• Tachdjian MO: Pediatric Orthopedics 1990;2:1515-1534
Illustrations: N/A
Internet references: http://www.5mcc.com

Author(s)
Russell G. Cohen, MD
Francisco G. Valencia, MD

Osteomalacia & rickets

BASICS

DESCRIPTION Osteomalacia (referred to as rickets in children) is defined as an excess organic bone matrix secondary to defective or inadequate bone mineralization
System(s) affected: Musculoskeletal
Genetics: N/A
Incidence/Prevalence in USA: N/A
Predominant age: All ages. In adults, osteomalacia is usually a disease of the older population (50-80).
Predominant sex: Female > Male (slightly)

SIGNS AND SYMPTOMS
• Bone pain, tenderness, muscle weakness
• Bone pain is dull and tends to be poorly localized, usually affecting the ribs and upper thighs
• Muscle weakness is usually proximal
• Other symptoms of malnutrition or an underlying problem such as chronic renal disease may also be clinically evident
• Weight loss
• Anorexia
• Tetany
• In young children - restlessness, poor sleep patterns, craniotabes, costochondral beading, bowlegs, kyphoscoliosis

CAUSES
• Can be caused by a wide variety of pathogenic processes, including, but not limited to, vitamin D deficiency (reduced exposure to sunlight, poor nutrition, malabsorption syndromes)
• Defective metabolism of parent vitamin D to active metabolites (drug-induced, i.e., anticonvulsants— phenytoin (Dilantin), chronic renal failure), hypophosphatemia (renal tubular acidosis, hypophosphatemic syndrome), miscellaneous (long-term hemodialysis, malnutrition, vitamin D-dependent rickets)

RISK FACTORS
• Poverty
• Inadequate nutrition and sunlight exposure

DIAGNOSIS

DIFFERENTIAL DIAGNOSIS
• Osteoporosis
• Metastatic bone disease
• Primary bone malignancies (lymphoma, myeloma)

LABORATORY
• Alkaline phosphatase - increased
• Serum calcium is low or normal (never high)
• Hypophosphatemia
• Aminoaciduria
• Acidosis
• Glucosuria
• Hypouricemia
Drugs that may alter lab results: N/A
Disorders that may alter lab results: N/A

PATHOLOGICAL FINDINGS
• Defective calcification of growing bone
• Hypertrophy of epiphyseal cartilages

SPECIAL TESTS N/A

IMAGING Radiographic changes are non-specific. Earliest manifestations are thinning of cortical bone. In long-term osteomalacia: bone softening (protrusio acetabuli), looser lines, stress fractures, and pathologic fractures.

DIAGNOSTIC PROCEDURES Bone biopsy and subsequent histopathologic evaluation deliver the most accurate diagnosis of osteomalacia. The biopsy is usually taken from the iliac crest, and both calcified, and non-calcified studies, as well as special stains (including von Kossa's stain) are helpful.

TREATMENT

APPROPRIATE HEALTH CARE Can be managed on an outpatient basis, except for complicating emergencies/fractures

GENERAL MEASURES
• Treatment of osteomalacia depends upon the cause, i.e., gastrointestinal, renal, or nutritional.
• For nutritional osteomalacia, calcium and vitamin D have been shown to correct the disease process
• Treatment can be monitored by observing simple bone biochemistry
• Treatment results depend on identifying and correcting the cause

SURGICAL MEASURES N/A

ACTIVITY Full activity is encouraged, including a neuroconditioning program

DIET
• Ensure adequate vitamin D intake
• Provide instructions for a high calcium diet and information on calcium supplements, if appropriate

PATIENT EDUCATION Educate family and patient on nutrition

Osteomalacia & rickets

MEDICATIONS

DRUG(S) OF CHOICE For adults and uncomplicated rickets: vitamin D (ergocalciferol) 2000-4800 IU once a day for one month. Then reduce dose gradually.
Contraindications: N/A
Precautions: N/A
Significant possible interactions: N/A

ALTERNATIVE DRUGS
• IV calcium salts if tetany complicates. Single IM dose of 100,000 IU in adolescents each Fall.
• Alfacalcidol
• Calcitriol

FOLLOWUP

PATIENT MONITORING Office visits every 6 months

PREVENTION/AVOIDANCE
• Adequate dietary intake of vitamin D
• Adequate sunlight exposure
• Fortified cow's milk

POSSIBLE COMPLICATIONS
• Fractures
• Osteomyelitis
• Renal failure
• Renal tubular acidosis
• Seizures
• Growth deformity; bowing long bones in children

EXPECTED COURSE/PROGNOSIS
Variable

MISCELLANEOUS

ASSOCIATED CONDITIONS
• Chronic renal disease
• Epilepsy
• Malnutrition
• Previous gastric surgery
• Pregnancy-nutritional factors

AGE-RELATED FACTORS
Pediatric: N/A
Geriatric: Studies have suggested that vitamin D deficiency osteomalacia is a relatively common condition in the acutely ill elderly population, with an estimated prevalence of about 3-5%; however, it often goes undiagnosed
Others: N/A

PREGNANCY N/A

SYNONYMS Rickets

ICD-9-CM 268.2 Osteomalacia, unspecified

SEE ALSO N/A

OTHER NOTES N/A

ABBREVIATIONS N/A

REFERENCES Mare GM, McKenna MJ, Frame B: Osteomalacia. Bone Mineral Res 1986;4:335
Illustrations: N/A
Internet references: http://www.5mcc.com

Author(s)
Mark C. Leeson, MD, FACS

Osteomyelitis

BASICS

DESCRIPTION Osteomyelitis is an acute or chronic inflammation of the bone and its structures caused most commonly by bacteria and rarely by other microorganisms. This infection may be acquired either by hematogenous, contiguous, or direct inoculation.
System(s) affected: Musculoskeletal
Genetics: There is no genetic predisposition known in this disease
Incidence/Prevalence in USA:
Uncommon
Predominant age: This infection is commonly seen in older adults; hematogenous is bimodal, also seen in infants and children
Predominant sex: Males > Females

SIGNS AND SYMPTOMS
• Hematogenous long bone infection
(in children with hematogenous osteomyelitis)
◊ Abrupt onset of high fever
◊ Irritability
◊ Malaise
◊ Restriction of movement of the involved extremity
◊ Signs of localized inflammation
• Hematogenous vertebral infection
(in adults with vertebral osteomyelitis)
◊ Illness is insidious and behaves more like a chronic infection
◊ History of an acute bacteremic episode associated with infection of a specific organ may be found in some patients
• Contiguous and vascular insufficiency associated infection
◊ Acute constitutional manifestations are seldom seen
◊ Localized signs and symptoms of inflammation with or without drainage frequently found
• Chronic osteomyelitis
◊ Non-healing ulcer or draining sinus
◊ Constitutional symptoms, when present, indicate acute suppurative condition in the bone or surrounding tissues
• Prosthetic device associated infection
◊ Infection may be acquired either by hematogenous route, or by contiguous foci such as local infection, operative contamination, or postoperative infection
◊ Acute postoperative infection may present as fever, localized swelling, tenderness, and drainage
◊ Chronic infection is characterized by joint discomfort, swelling, erythema, and joint dysfunction

CAUSES
• Acute hematogenous osteomyelitis
◊ Staphylococcus aureus (most common)
◊ Streptococcus, coagulase negative Staphylococcus, Haemophilus influenzae, and gram negative organisms (less common)
• Vertebral osteomyelitis
◊ Staphylococcus aureus and gram negative enteric organisms (common)
◊ Other microorganisms to consider include Mycobacterium tuberculosis, and fungi
• Contiguous focus osteomyelitis and vascular insufficiency osteomyelitis
◊ Mixed aerobic/anaerobic microorganisms are frequently found
• Prosthetic device infection
◊ Coagulase negative Staphylococcus, and S. aureus (most common)
◊ Diphtheroids, and gram negative bacteria (less common)

RISK FACTORS
• Sickle cell disease
• Other conditions which predispose to bone infarcts
• IV drug use
• Hemodialysis
• Local trauma
• Open fractures
• Presence of prosthetic orthopedic implant
• Vascular insufficiency
• Neuropathy
• Diabetes mellitus

DIAGNOSIS

DIFFERENTIAL DIAGNOSIS
• Systemic infection from other source
• Aseptic bone infarction
• Other localized inflammation of skin and soft tissues
• Neuropathic joint disease
• Fractures
• Gout

LABORATORY
• Definitive diagnosis is made by needle aspiration or bone biopsy and demonstration of the microorganism by culture or histology
• Blood culture may be positive in about 50% of younger patients with acute hematogenous disease
• Leukocyte count is usually elevated in the acute cases, but not in the chronic cases
• Sedimentation rate is usually elevated, but non-specific
• Teichoic acid antibody may be elevated in a patient who has S. aureus infection for more than 2 weeks
Drugs that may alter lab results:
Antimicrobial agents given before bone culture
Disorders that may alter lab results:
Cultures from the sinus tract are unreliable because of frequent contamination

PATHOLOGICAL FINDINGS Inflammatory process of the bone with pyogenic bacteria

SPECIAL TESTS N/A

IMAGING
• Radiographic - routine x-ray (findings on plain x-ray often delayed for 10-14 days in acute infection), computed tomography, magnetic resonance imaging
• Radionuclide (technetium, indium, or gallium) are also useful

DIAGNOSTIC PROCEDURES Needle biopsy or open bone biopsy for bacterial culture

TREATMENT

APPROPRIATE HEALTH CARE
Hospitalize the patient with suspected acute osteomyelitis for diagnostic work-up and initial treatment

GENERAL MEASURES Symptomatic treatment of pain

SURGICAL MEASURES
• Surgical drainage and removal of necrotic tissues are of utmost importance to effect cure
• In patients with vascular insufficiency or severe gangrenous infection, amputation may be the only effective treatment

ACTIVITY Bedrest and immobilization of the involved bone and joint

DIET No restriction

PATIENT EDUCATION Stress need for long-term treatment and follow up

Osteomyelitis

MEDICATIONS

DRUG(S) OF CHOICE
Antimicrobial agent/agents based on susceptibility testing and known clinical efficacy. The duration of therapy for acute osteomyelitis should be at least 4-6 weeks. In chronic osteomyelitis, longer duration of therapy may be needed.
• Staphylococcus aureus and coagulase negative staphylococcus: nafcillin 2 g IV q4-6h. Vancomycin 1 g q12h for methicillin resistant Staph.
• Streptococcus spp.: penicillin G 2-4 million units q4h IV
• Enteric gram negative bacilli and Pseudomonas aeruginosa: piperacillin 4 g q4-6h IV, plus aminoglycoside
• Mixed aerobic/anaerobic infection (diabetic foot, bite wound): beta-lactamase inhibitor combination (ticarcillin-clavulanate 3.1 g q6h IV; ampicillin-sulbactam 3 g q6h IV); piperacillin-tazobactam 3.375 g q6h IV
Contraindications: Allergy
Precautions: In patients with renal or hepatic insufficiency, antimicrobial dose may need adjustment
Significant possible interactions: Refer to manufacturer's literature

ALTERNATIVE DRUGS
• Staphylococcus aureus and coagulase negative staphylococcus: clindamycin 600 mg IV q6h, nafcillin 2 g q4h, or cefazolin 1 g q8h IV, or vancomycin 1 g q12h
• Streptococcus spp.: penicillin G 2 million units q4h, cefazolin 1 g q8h IV, or clindamycin 600 mg q6h IV
• Enteric gram negative bacilli and Pseudomonas aeruginosa: ceftazidime 1 g q8h IV or ciprofloxacin [or other quinolone] 750 mg q12h orally.
• Mixed aerobic/anaerobic infection (diabetic foot, bite wound): clindamycin plus third generation cephalosporin or quinolone
• Home therapy often used - consider a simplified antibiotic regimen for outpatient use or oral therapy

FOLLOWUP

PATIENT MONITORING
Blood level of antimicrobial agents, serum antibacterial titers, sedimentation rate

PREVENTION/AVOIDANCE
Avoid further stress and weight bearing until healing

POSSIBLE COMPLICATIONS
• Abscess formation
• Bacteremia
• Fracture
• Loosening of the prosthetic implant
• Postoperative infection

EXPECTED COURSE/PROGNOSIS
• Cure of osteomyelitis with medical treatment is notoriously unpredictable especially when not accompanied by surgical debridement
• In patients with acute hematogenous osteomyelitis, the prognosis is usually good even without surgery. Cure takes about 6 weeks.
• The prognosis is improved if all infected bone has been removed

MISCELLANEOUS

ASSOCIATED CONDITIONS
Listed with Causes

AGE-RELATED FACTORS
Pediatric: Occurs most often in 5-14 age group and more frequently in boys
Geriatric:
• Vertebral osteomyelitis more common
• Contiguous focus of infection more common
• Vascular insufficiency is most common cause of osteomyelitis in 50-70 age group (usually due to presence of associated conditions)
Others: N/A

PREGNANCY N/A

SYNONYMS N/A

ICD-9-CM
• Acute osteomyelitis 730.0
• Chronic osteomyelitis 730.1
• Jaw osteomyelitis 526.4
• Orbital osteomyelitis 376.03
• For specific microbial etiology, see the ICD code of the specific organism, e.g., Salmonella - see Salmonella osteomyelitis 003.24. N.B.: 5th digit code required for site
0 - site unspecified
1 - shoulder
2 - upper arm
3 - forearm
4 - hand
5 - pelvis/thigh
6 - lower leg
7 - ankle/foot
8 - other, specified
9 - multiple sites

SEE ALSO N/A

OTHER NOTES N/A

ABBREVIATIONS N/A

REFERENCES Waldvogel FA: Osteomyelitis. In: Gorbach SI, Bartlett JG, Blacklow NR, eds. Infectious Diseases. Philadelphia, W.B. Saunders Co., 1992:1125-1129
Illustrations: 1 available on CD-ROM
Internet references: http://www.5mcc.com

Author(s)
James S. Tan, MD, FACP

Osteonecrosis

 BASICS

 DIAGNOSIS

 TREATMENT

DESCRIPTION Death of the cellular components of bony tissue
System(s) affected: Musculoskeletal
Genetics: The underlying condition of hemoglobinopathies, especially sickle cell disease, diabetes, and type II or IV hyperlipemia are inheritable and associated with a high incidence of osteonecrosis. Other forms have no proven genetic relationship.
Incidence/Prevalence in USA: Dependent upon the underlying condition
Predominant age: 3rd to 6th decade
Predominant sex: Male > Female

SIGNS AND SYMPTOMS
• The symptoms may be acute as in osteonecrosis of sickle cell disease or renal transplant. Usually insidious in other forms. Diagnosis may not be made for two years after onset of symptoms.
• Pain, the prominent symptom, is made worse with activity
• Loss of motion of the affected joint
• Stiffness (especially early morning)
• Swelling if the involved joint is superficial
• Locking may occur if a loose body has developed
• Proximal femur is the most common site and more prevalent in males in the 3rd-6th decade
• The distal femur, especially the medial femoral condyle, is the second most frequent site. This area is unique in that night pain is a prominent early symptom. Most common in females in the 6th-7th decade.
• Other sites in decreasing frequency are the proximal humerus, talus, carpal lunate (Kienböck's disease) and the humeral capitulum

CAUSES
• Idiopathic
• Fractures, especially the femoral neck
• Traumatic (fractures, dislocation)
• Dislocations
• Legg-Calvé-Perthes (seen in 6-12 year age group)
• Hemoglobinopathies (especially sickle cell disease)
• Metabolic (hemoglobinopathies, alcohol, steroids, renal failure/transplantation)

RISK FACTORS
• Gaucher's disease - especially likely as a postoperative infection
• Diabetes mellitus
• Alcoholism - the most frequent cause
• Type II or IV hyperlipemia
• Cortisone therapy (may be seen with Cushing's disease)
• Obesity
• Oral contraceptives
• Organ transplant, especially kidney
• Pregnancy
• Decompression sickness ("bends")

DIFFERENTIAL DIAGNOSIS Rheumatoid arthritis, septic necrosis and severe secondary parathyroidism. A crescent sign (a linear subchondral lucency indicates collapse of subchondral bone. Patchy lucencies reflect resorption; patchy sclerosis indicates growth of new bone over the scaffolding of dead trabeculae) in these conditions may occur because the bone may be so soft that it collapses producing a crescent sign.

LABORATORY N/A
Drugs that may alter lab results: N/A
Disorders that may alter lab results: N/A

PATHOLOGICAL FINDINGS The subchondral fracture occurs during bone repair as necrotic bone is resorbed. Later, a collapse of the bone occurs with subsequent irregularities at the joint surface. This will eventually produce osteoarthritic changes.

SPECIAL TESTS Bone scan shows decreased bone uptake (sometimes increased uptake depending on the stage). Later, the uptake increases as reparative processes begin within the bone.

IMAGING MRI will show a decreased signal intensity of the involved bone and is the most sensitive diagnostic exam.

DIAGNOSTIC PROCEDURES The presence of a crescent sign is practically diagnostic (see Differential Diagnosis of osteonecrosis). It is caused by a subchondral fracture.

APPROPRIATE HEALTH CARE Outpatient normally; inpatient if surgery indicated

GENERAL MEASURES
• Only four conditions can be treated to decrease the incidence of osteonecrosis
  ◊ Alcoholism - abstinence is obvious, but quite difficult to attain
  ◊ Dysbarism - new tables of decompression, if followed, will lower osteonecrosis incidence of divers
  ◊ Transplant patients - decreased doses of cortisone and regulation of calcium and phosphorous metabolism
  ◊ Sickle cell disease - treat a crisis vigorously with hydration, possible exchange transfusion and oxygenation, especially hyperbaric oxygen

SURGICAL MEASURES Bone grafts, arthroplasty, allografts and arthrodesis may be used, dependent upon the joint involved

ACTIVITY As tolerated

DIET No special diet

PATIENT EDUCATION The patient should be instructed in the use of crutches and/or canes when the lower extremity is involved. Proper use of a walking cane can decrease the pressure on the femoral head 20-30% when walking.

MEDICATIONS

DRUG(S) OF CHOICE
• NSAID's - consistent with the underlying disease may be used for painful episodes
• Acetaminophen - 500 mg qid can be quite helpful in alleviating symptoms
Contraindications: See manufacturer's profile of each drug
Precautions: NSAIDs - if history of peptic ulcer is present, the use of ranitidine (Zantac) 150 mg bid or 300 mg hs can be given. Misoprostol (Cytotec) 100 µg bid will usually prevent gastritis (not needed with acetaminophen).
Significant possible interactions: See manufacturer's profile of each drug

ALTERNATIVE DRUGS
Other H2-receptor antagonists in patients with a history of peptic ulcer disease

FOLLOWUP

PATIENT MONITORING
X-rays should be made every 12-18 months, more frequently if symptoms become more severe

PREVENTION/AVOIDANCE
Early diagnosis and treatment of underlying disease

POSSIBLE COMPLICATIONS
• Progression of disease
• The progression of osteonecrosis leads to osteoarthritis of the involved joint to a varying degree. Arthroplasty of the hip carries a much poorer prognosis than osteoarthritis alone. It should be postponed as long as possible.

EXPECTED COURSE/PROGNOSIS
Gaucher's disease is associated with a high risk of infection following surgery

MISCELLANEOUS

ASSOCIATED CONDITIONS
N/A

AGE-RELATED FACTORS
Pediatric: Legg-Calvé-Perthes occurs in the 6-12 year age group. Prognosis is better in younger patients.
Geriatric: N/A
Others: N/A

PREGNANCY
Is a risk factor

SYNONYMS
• Idiopathic osteonecrosis
• Avascular necrosis
• lunatomalacia, Kienböck's disease
• Subchondral fracture

ICD-9-CM
730.1 Osteonecrosis

SEE ALSO
• Arthritis, osteo
• Legg-Calvé-Perthes disease

OTHER NOTES
N/A

ABBREVIATIONS
N/A

REFERENCES
• Harris WH: Total Hip Replacement. American Academy of Orthopedic Surgeons, Institutional Course Lectures, Vol 23. St. Louis, C.V. Mosby Company, 1974
• Eftekhaur Khaur NS, Keirwam H: Systemic and Local Complications following low friction. Arthroplasty. In Archives of Surgery 1976;111:150
• Nicholson OR: Total Hip Replacement. In Clinical Orthopedics 1973;95:217
Illustrations: N/A
Internet references: http://www.5mcc.com

Author(s)
Furnie W. Johnston, MD
R. Bruce Hall, MD

Osteoporosis

BASICS

DESCRIPTION A multifactorial skeletal disease characterized by severe bone loss and disruption of skeletal micro-architecture sufficient to predispose to atraumatic fractures of the vertebral column, upper femur; distal radius, proximal humerus, pubic rami and ribs
• Postmenopausal osteoporosis (Type I): The most common form in Caucasian and Asian women. Due to excessive and prolonged acceleration of bone resorption following menopausal loss of estrogen secretion.
• Involutional osteoporosis (Type II): Occurs in both sexes above age 75. Due to a subtle, prolonged imbalance between rates of bone resorption and formation. A mixture of Types I and II is common.
• Idiopathic osteoporosis: A rare form of primary osteoporosis occurring in premenopausal women and in men below age 75. Not related to secondary causes or risk factors predisposing to bone loss. Causes unknown.
• Juvenile osteoporosis: A rare form of variable severity occurring in prepubertal children. Self-limited with cessation of fractures at puberty. Cause unknown. (Not covered in this topic.)
• Secondary osteoporosis: Severe bone loss sufficient to cause atraumatic fractures due to extrinsic factors such as corticosteroid excess, rheumatoid arthritis, chronic liver/kidney disease, malabsorption syndromes, systemic mastocytosis, hyperparathyroidism, hyperthyroidism, a variety of hypogonadal states, idiopathic hypercalciuria, and others
System(s) affected: Musculoskeletal
Genetics: Familial predisposition. More common in Caucasians and Orientals than in black and Latino ethnic groups.
Incidence/Prevalence in USA:
• 30-40% cumulatively in women, 5-15% in men
• Prevalence of idiopathic and juvenile types unknown
• Secondary osteoporosis cumulatively 5-10%, both sexes
Predominant age: Elderly
Predominant sex: Female > Male

SIGNS AND SYMPTOMS
• Back ache/pain; acute/chronic
• Kyphosis/scoliosis
• Atraumatic fractures
• No peripheral bone deformities
• Sclerae not blue/green/grey
• Loss of height

CAUSES
• Postmenopausal (Type I): Hypoestrogenemia
• Involutional (Type II): Unknown
• Idiopathic: Unknown
• Juvenile: Unknown
• Secondary: Various (see Description)
• Bone loss is a consequence of aging, however, osteoporosis occurs most frequently in individuals who fail to achieve optimal skeletal mass during development or lose bone rapidly thereafter. Such loses are due to excessive postmenopausal and/or involutional bone loss, or medical conditions/risk factors that increase bone loss.

RISK FACTORS
• Dietary - inadequate calcium, excessive phosphate/protein; inadequate vitamin D intake in the elderly
• Physical - immobilization, sedentary lifestyle
• Social - alcohol, cigarettes, caffeine
• Medical - chronic diseases, malabsorption, endocrinopathies, (see also secondary osteoporosis in Description)
• Iatrogenic - corticosteroids, excess thyroid hormone replacement, chronic heparin, chemotherapy, loop diuretics, anticonvulsants, radiation therapy
• Genetic/familial - suboptimal bone mass at maturity, "familial fast bone losers"

DIAGNOSIS

DIFFERENTIAL DIAGNOSIS
• Multiple myeloma
• Other neoplasia
• Osteomalacia
• Osteogenesis imperfecta tarda (Type I)
• Skeletal hyperparathyroidism (primary and secondary)
• Hyperthyroidism
• Mastocytosis (rare)

LABORATORY
• CBC, multipanel tests usually normal
• Alkaline phosphatase (bone specific and total) may be transiently increased following fractures
• Serum and/or urine protein electrophoresis normal
• Thyroid function tests and urinary free cortisol normal in primary types
• Serum osteocalcin, if high, indicates high turnover type
• Urine calcium normal (except if idiopathic hypercalciuria)
• Urinary pyridinoline and N-telopeptide collagen crosslinks, if high, indicates high turnover type
Drugs that may alter lab results:
• Hepatotoxins: changes in total alkaline phosphatase
• Estrogens: changes in thyroid function tests
Disorders that may alter lab results:
• Multiple myeloma or other neoplasia
• Osteomalacia
• Osteogenesis imperfecta
• Hyperparathyroidism
• Hyperthyroidism

PATHOLOGICAL FINDINGS
• Reduced skeletal mass, trabecular bone more so than cortical bone. Loss of trabecular connections.
• Osteoclast and osteoblast number variable
• No evidence of other metabolic bone diseases and no increase in unmineralized osteoid
• Marrow normal or atrophic

SPECIAL TESTS N/A

IMAGING
• X-rays - "early" changes of increased width of intervertebral spaces, relative accentuation of cortical plates, vertical striations of vertebral bodies
• "Late" changes of cortical plate fractures, vertebral compression, wedge and crush fractures, peripheral fractures at ends of long bones, rib fractures
• Bone scan may show increased uptake at previous fracture sites, otherwise negative
• Bone mineral density (BMD)
  ◊ DXA: Quantitates BMD of lumbar spine, forearm, and upper femur. Normal range: ± 1 standard deviation (SD) from mean (age and site specific).
  ◊ QCT: Special program and plastic phantom containing bone mass standards to quantitate either trabecular or cortical bone mass, or both (integral data) of lumbar spine. Normal range: ± 1 SD.

DIAGNOSTIC PROCEDURES Bone biopsy needed rarely, to rule out other metabolic bone diseases. Sometimes used to quantitate bone loss, utilizing quantitative histomorphometric technique.

TREATMENT

APPROPRIATE HEALTH CARE
• Usually outpatient
• Inpatient care for acute back pain, especially for new vertebral fractures and for acute treatment of upper femoral and pelvic fractures
• Nursing home or home care may be needed following peripheral fractures

GENERAL MEASURES As required by pain and disability, e.g., heat, analgesics, physical therapy. Decrease falls.

SURGICAL MEASURES N/A

ACTIVITY
• Maintain ambulation, walking 1 mile twice a day, if possible, swimming, tricycling
• Avoid exercises and maneuvers that increase compressive forces and mechanical stress on spine and peripheral bone sites
• Rehabilitation procedures for back muscle spasm, increase agility (e.g., decrease falls) and ambulation encouragement

DIET
• Reducing diet if overweight
• Calcium intake 1500 mg/day from all sources, if not hypercalciuric or with past medical history of calcium stones
• Avoid excess phosphate or protein intake, i.e., avoid phosphoric-acid-containing beverages and excess meat intake
• 600-1000 IU vitamin D daily from all sources

PATIENT EDUCATION Teaching
resources and patient literature available from National Osteoporosis Foundation, 2100 M St., Suite 602, Washington, DC 20037

MEDICATIONS

DRUG(S) OF CHOICE
• Hormone replacement therapy (HRT)
  ◊ estrogen-medroxyprogesterone (PremPro) q day
  ◊ estrogen (Premarin) 0.625mg q day, if post-hysterectomy
• Calcitonin (Miacalcin Nasal Spray) 200 IU intranasally; 1 puff per day, alternating nostrils
• Calcitonin (Osteocalcin, Calcimar, Miacalcin) 100 IU SC qd or qod preferred, 50 IU qd or 3 times a week may be effective in high turnover types. Should be used in conjunction with adequate calcium and vitamin D.
• Alendronate (Fosamax) 10 mg qd in the morning on an empty stomach

Contraindications:
• Calcitonins - none except allergy
• For alendronate, esophageal dysfunction, severe upper GI symptoms, GERD
• HRT absolute - past medical history of endometrial or breast cancer or premalignant breast conditions
• HRT relative - medical history uncontrolled hypertension, thromboembolic conditions, edematous conditions, endometriosis, migraine, severe hepatic dysfunction; family history of breast or uterine cancer

Precautions:
• Calcitonins - none
• HRT - annual gynecology exam, including Pap smear or endometrial biopsy, annual breast exam and mammography. Check blood pressure twice a week during initiation of HRT.
• Alendronate - must be taken on empty stomach in the morning with 1-2 glasses of water. No food, beverages or other medications for 1 hour and remain seated or standing for 1 hour.

Significant possible interactions: None

ALTERNATIVE DRUGS
• Other biphosphonates - etidronate, pamidronate, tiludronate - inhibitors of bone resorption (not FDA approved)
• Sodium fluoride - stimulates bone formation, but effects on cortical bone uncertain. Sustained release preparations may be better tolerated.
• Tamoxifen - has some estrogen effects on bone without potential for breast stimulation. May stimulate uterus and cause other side effects.
• Raloxifene and droloxifene - research drugs with estrogen effects on bone without potential for breast or uterine stimulation
• Androgens/anabolics - research drugs, may stimulate bone formation
• Parathyroid hormone analogues - research drugs, may stimulate trabecular bone formation

FOLLOWUP

PATIENT MONITORING
• Monthly during initiation, q 6 months thereafter
• Periodic multiphasic screening, annual gynecological exam, breast exam, and mammography
• Annual BMD using same technique as for baseline
• Repeat x-rays when indicated for acute pain, suspected fractures.

PREVENTION/AVOIDANCE
• General guidelines
  ◊ Diet, exercise, HRT at menopause
  ◊ Increased calcium intake; adequate vitamin D intake
• Prevention during the osteopenic phase (prolonged, usually asymptomatic phase prior to fracturing)
  ◊ Identification of osteopenia: BMD (regardless of method) between -1 and -2 SD
  ◊ Correction of treatable medical conditions and other risk factors (see Risk Factors); will also help achieve optimal skeletal mass during development
  ◊ HRT if postmenopausal and no absolute contraindications
  ◊ Low dose alendronate (5 mg qd) if HRT not usable and if no contraindications

POSSIBLE COMPLICATIONS
• Severe disabling pain
• Dorsal/lumbar neurologic deficits 2° to vertebral fracture (rare)
• Invalidism/death secondary to complications of upper femoral fractures

EXPECTED COURSE/PROGNOSIS
• With treatment, 70% of patients stabilize skeletal manifestations; increase bone mass, increase mobility, and have reduced pain
• 20-30% of upper femoral fractures lead to chronic care and/or premature death

MISCELLANEOUS

ASSOCIATED CONDITIONS
• Corticosteroid excess
• Rheumatoid arthritis
• Chronic liver/kidney disease
• Malabsorption syndromes
• Systemic mastocytosis
• Hyperparathyroidism
• Hyperthyroidism including iatrogenic
• Various hypogonadal states

AGE-RELATED FACTORS
Pediatric: Juvenile osteoporosis not discussed herein
Geriatric: Postmenopausal/involutional/mixed types
Others: Primary types rare in African Americans. Patients with British, North European, Scandinavian, and Oriental ancestry most susceptible.

PREGNANCY Rare acute osteoporosis of
pregnancy, not discussed herein

SYNONYMS N/A

ICD-9-CM 733.0 Osteoporosis

SEE ALSO N/A

OTHER NOTES N/A

ABBREVIATIONS
BMD = bone mineral density
SD = standard deviation
HRT = hormone replacement therapy

REFERENCES
• Ross PD: Osteoporosis: frequency, consequences and risk factors. Arch Int Med 1996;156:1399-1411
• Cummings SR, Nevitt MC, Browner WS, Stone K, Fox KM, Ensrud KE, et al: Risk factors for hip fractures in white women. NEJM 1995;332:767-773
• Miller PD, Bonnick, Rosen CJ: Consensus of an international panel on the clinical utility of bone mass measurements in the detection of low bone mass in the adult population. Calcif Tissue Int 1996;58:207-214
• Raisz LG: The osteoporosis revolution. Ann Int Med 1997;126(6):458-462
Illustrations: N/A
Internet references: http://www.5mcc.com

Author(s)
Stanley Wallach, MD

Otitis externa

BASICS

DESCRIPTION   Inflammation of the external auditory canal
• Acute diffuse otitis externa - the most common form, an infectious process usually bacterial, occasionally fungal
• Acute circumscribed otitis externa - synonymous with furuncle. Associated with infection of the hair follicle.
• Chronic otitis externa - same as acute diffuse, but of longer duration (greater than 6 weeks)
• Eczematous otitis externa - may accompany typical atopic eczema or other primary skin conditions
• Necrotizing "malignant" otitis externa - an infection which extends into the deeper tissues adjacent to the canal. May include osteomyelitis and cellulitis. Rare in children.
Incidence/Prevalence in USA:
• Unknown; incidence is higher in the summer months
• Acute, chronic and eczematous - common
• Necrotizing - uncommon
System(s) affected: Skin
Genetics: N/A
Predominant age: All ages
Predominant sex: Male = Female

SIGNS AND SYMPTOMS
• Itching
• Plugging of the ear
• Otalgia
• Periauricular adenitis
• Erythematous canal
• Purulent discharge
• Eczema of pinna
• Cranial nerve involvement (VII, IX-XII)

CAUSES
• Acute diffuse otitis externa
  ◊ Traumatized external canal
  ◊ Bacterial infection - pseudomonas (67% cases); staphylococcus; streptococcus; gram negative rods
  ◊ Fungal infection - aspergillus (90% cases); Phycomycetes; Rhizopus; actinomyces; Penicillium; yeast
• Chronic otitis externa
  ◊ Bacterial infection - pseudomonas
• Eczematous otitis externa (associated with primary skin disorder):
  ◊ Eczema
  ◊ Seborrhea
  ◊ Neurodermatitis
  ◊ Contact dermatitis
  ◊ Purulent otitis media
  ◊ Sensitivity to topical medications
• Necrotizing otitis externa
  ◊ Invasive bacterial infection - pseudomonas

RISK FACTORS
• Acute and chronic otitis externa
  ◊ Traumatization of external canal
  ◊ Swimming
  ◊ Hot humid weather
  ◊ Use of a hearing aid
• Eczematous
  ◊ Primary skin disorder
• Necrotizing otitis externa in adults
  ◊ Elderly
  ◊ Diabetes
  ◊ Debilitating disease
• Necrotizing otitis externa in children (rare)
  ◊ Leukopenia
  ◊ Malnutrition
  ◊ Diabetes mellitus
  ◊ Diabetes insipidus

DIAGNOSIS

DIFFERENTIAL DIAGNOSIS
• Ear pain
• Purulent ear discharge
• Hearing loss
• Cranial nerve palsy (VII, IX-XII) with necrotizing otitis externa
• Wisdom teeth eruption

LABORATORY   Gram stain and culture of canal discharge (occasionally helpful)
Drugs that may alter lab results:
Antibiotic pretreatment
Disorders that may alter lab results: N/A

PATHOLOGICAL FINDINGS
• Acute and chronic otitis externa - desquamation of superficial epithelium of external canal with infection
• Eczematous otitis externa - pathologic findings consistent with primary skin disorder, secondary infection on occasion
• Necrotizing otitis externa - vasculitis, thrombosis and necrosis of involved tissues; osteomyelitis

SPECIAL TESTS   N/A

IMAGING   Radiologic evaluation of deep tissues in necrotizing otitis externa

DIAGNOSTIC PROCEDURES   N/A

TREATMENT

APPROPRIATE HEALTH CARE
Outpatient, except for resistant cases and necrotizing otitis externa

GENERAL MEASURES
• Thorough cleansing of external canal
• Pain medications
• Antipruritic and antihistamines (eczematous form)

SURGICAL MEASURES   N/A

ACTIVITY   No restrictions

DIET   No restrictions

PATIENT EDUCATION   Methods for prevention

MEDICATIONS

DRUG(S) OF CHOICE
• Acute bacterial and chronic otitis externa
  ◊ Topical therapy for approximately 10 days
  ◊ 2% acetic acid
  ◊ Antibiotics
  ◊ Corticosteroids
• Fungal otitis externa
  ◊ Topical therapy anti-yeast for candida or yeast - nystatin
  ◊ Parenteral antifungal therapy - amphotericin B
• Eczematous otitis externa - topical therapy
  ◊ Aluminum acetate 8%
  ◊ Acetic acid 2% in aluminum acetate
  ◊ 5% aluminum acetate (Burrow's) solution
  ◊ Steroid cream, lotion, ointment
  ◊ Antibacterial, if superinfected
• Necrotizing otitis externa
  ◊ Parenteral antibiotics - antistaphylococcus and antipseudomonal
  ◊ 4-6 weeks of therapy

Contraindications:
• Hypersensitivity to topical or parenteral therapy
• Renal or hepatic failure when using amphotericin B

Precautions: Dosage adjustment for amphotericin B in patients with renal or hepatic dysfunction

Significant possible interactions:
• Hypokalemia associated with amphotericin B may lead to digitalis toxicity
• Concurrent administration of nonabsorbable anions, such as carbenicillin, may exacerbate hypokalemia

ALTERNATIVE DRUGS Azole antifungals for fungal otitis externa

FOLLOWUP

PATIENT MONITORING
• Acute otitis externa
  ◊ 48 hours after therapy instituted to assess improvement
  ◊ At the end of treatment
• Chronic otitis externa
  ◊ Every 2-3 weeks for repeated cleansing of canal
  ◊ May require alterations in topical medication, including antibiotics and steroids
• Necrotizing otitis externa
  ◊ Daily monitoring in hospital for extension of infection
  ◊ Baseline auditory and vestibular testing at beginning and end of therapy

PREVENTION/AVOIDANCE
• Avoid prolonged exposure to moisture
• Utilize preventive antiseptics
• Treat predisposing skin conditions
• Eliminate self-inflicted trauma to canal
• Diagnose and treat underlying systemic conditions

POSSIBLE COMPLICATIONS
• Mainly a problem with necrotizing otitis externa. May spread to infect contiguous bone and CNS structures.
• Acute otitis externa may spread to pinna causing a chondritis

EXPECTED COURSE/PROGNOSIS
• Acute otitis externa - rapid response to therapy with total resolution
• Chronic otitis externa - with repeated cleansing and antibiotic therapy the majority of cases will resolve. Occasionally, surgical intervention is required for resistant cases.
• Eczematous otitis externa - resolution will occur with control of the primary skin condition
• Necrotizing otitis externa - can usually be managed with debridement and prolonged parenteral antibiotics. Recurrence rate is 100% when treatment is inadequate. Surgical intervention may be necessary in resistant cases or if there is cranial nerve involvement. Mortality rate is significant, probably secondary to the underlying disease.

MISCELLANEOUS

ASSOCIATED CONDITIONS See Risk Factors

AGE-RELATED FACTORS N/A
Pediatric: N/A
Geriatric: N/A
Others: N/A

PREGNANCY N/A

SYNONYMS
• Swimmer's ear

ICD-9-CM
380.10 infective otitis externa, unspecified

SEE ALSO N/A

OTHER NOTES N/A

ABBREVIATIONS N/A

REFERENCES
• Marcy SM: Swimmer's Ear. Contemporary Pediatrics 1986;3:20
• Bluestone C, Stool S, eds: Pediatric Otolaryngology. 3rd Ed. Philadelphia, W.B. Saunders Co., 1996
Illustrations: N/A
Internet references: http://www.5mcc.com

Author(s)
James A. Nard, MD

Otitis media

BASICS

DESCRIPTION Inflammation of the middle ear
• Acute otitis media (AOM): Usually a bacterial infection accompanied by viral upper respiratory infection; rapid onset of signs and symptoms
• Recurrent AOM: 3 or more AOM in 6 months, or 4 or more AOM in 1 year
• Otitis media with effusion (OME): Persistent inflammation manifested as asymptomatic middle ear fluid that follows AOM or arises without prior AOM
System(s) affected: Nervous
Genetics: May be influenced by skull configuration or immunological defects
Incidence/Prevalence in USA: (Incidence) By age 7 years 93% of children have 1 or more AOM; 39% have 6 or more AOM; after AOM 10 to 20% still have OME 3 months later
Predominant age: Peak incidence age 6-18 months; declines after age 7 years; rare in adults
Predominant sex: Male > Female (for AOM and recurrent AOM)

SIGNS AND SYMPTOMS
• AOM:
  ◊ Earache
  ◊ Fever, although more often afebrile
  ◊ Accompanying URI symptoms
  ◊ Decreased hearing
  ◊ Otorrhea if eardrum perforated
  ◊ Eardrum mobility decreased (as observed by pneumatic otoscopy)
  ◊ Eardrum bulging, opaque, often yellowish or inflamed. Redness alone is not a reliable sign.
• AOM in infants:
  ◊ May cause no symptoms in the first few months of life
  ◊ Irritability is sometimes the only indication of earache
  ◊ Eardrum bulging, opaque, often yellowish or inflamed. Redness alone not a reliable sign.
• OME:
  ◊ Usually asymptomatic
  ◊ Decreased hearing probably universal, but not always measurable, and rarely appreciated by parents
  ◊ Eardrum often dull, but not bulging
  ◊ Eardrum mobility decreased (as observed by pneumatic otoscopy)

CAUSES
• AOM: A preceding viral upper respiratory infection produces eustachian tube dysfunction that is thought to promote bacterial infection via eustachian tube. Bacteriology:
  ◊ Pneumococci: 35%
  ◊ Haemophilus influenzae: 20-25%; 40% of these produce beta-lactamases that hydrolyze amoxicillin and some cephalosporins
  ◊ Moraxella (Branhamella) catarrhalis: 10-15%; 90% of these produce beta-lactamases that hydrolyze amoxicillin and some cephalosporins
  ◊ Group A streptococci: 3%
  ◊ Staphylococcus aureus: 1-2%
  ◊ Sterile/non-pathogens: 25-30%
• OME:
  ◊ 20-40% silent bacterial infection
  ◊ Eustachian tube dysfunction thought important
  ◊ Allergic causes rarely substantiated

RISK FACTORS
• Day care
• Formula feeding
• Smoking in household
• Male gender
• Family history of middle ear disease
• AOM in 1st year of life is a risk factor for recurrent AOM
• Sibling history of otitis media

DIAGNOSIS

DIFFERENTIAL DIAGNOSIS
• Tympanosclerosis
• Redness due to crying
• Earache with a normal ear exam may be caused by referred pain from the jaw or teeth

LABORATORY WBC higher in bacterial AOM than in sterile AOM
Drugs that may alter lab results: N/A
Disorders that may alter lab results: N/A

PATHOLOGICAL FINDINGS N/A

SPECIAL TESTS
• To document the presence of middle ear fluid - tympanometry, acoustic reflex measurement or acoustic reflectometry
• Hearing testing helpful to assess the need for early surgical intervention in OME
• Nasopharyngoscopy

IMAGING N/A

DIAGNOSTIC PROCEDURES
Tympanocentesis for microbiologic diagnosis recommended for treatment failures, may be followed by myringotomy

TREATMENT

APPROPRIATE HEALTH CARE
Outpatient except when surgery is indicated

GENERAL MEASURES
AOM: Outpatient except for febrile infants < 2 months

SURGICAL MEASURES
• OME: Referral for surgery if: > 4-6 months bilateral OME, and/or > 6 months unilateral OME, and/or hearing loss > 25 decibels
• Recurrent AOM: Referral for surgery if > 2 or 3 AOM while on chemoprophylaxis. Tympanostomy tubes and adenoidectomy effective surgical procedures for OME and recurrent AOM, but not in all cases.

ACTIVITY No restrictions

DIET No special diet

PATIENT EDUCATION N/A

MEDICATIONS

DRUG(S) OF CHOICE
• AOM: Amoxicillin 10-15 mg/kg tid for 10 days; probably the most effective of penicillins/cephalosporins against relatively resistant (but not highly resistant) pneumococci
• Recurrent AOM: Amoxicillin 20 mg/kg daily for 3-6 months or until summer
• OME: Antihistamines and decongestants ineffective, indications for steroids not defined, amoxicillin promotes resolution in 10-15% but effect is usually transitory - not recommended.
Contraindications: Allergy to penicillins
Precautions: Refer to manufacturer's profile of each drug
Significant possible interactions: Refer to manufacturer's profile of each drug

ALTERNATIVE DRUGS
• Alternative drugs are indicated for the following AOM patients:
  ◊ Patients with penicillin allergy
  ◊ Persistent symptoms after 48-72 hrs of amoxicillin
  ◊ AOM within 1 month of amoxicillin therapy
  ◊ AOM with severe earache
  ◊ Infants less than 6 months with high fever
  ◊ Immunocompromised hosts
  ◊ AOM due to Chlamydia trachomatis will respond to macrolides and sulfonamides
  ◊ AOM due to Mycoplasma pneumoniae will respond to macrolides
• AOM: Alternative drugs (treat for 10 days):
  ◊ Amoxicillin-clavulanate (Augmentin) 40 mg/kg/day of amoxicillin component tid - effective against resistant H. influenzae and M. catarrhalis, amoxicillin component effective against relatively resistant pneumococci
  ◊ Cefaclor (Ceclor) 40 mg/kg/day bid or tid is less effective than other alternatives
  ◊ Cefixime (Suprax) 8 mg/kg/day bid or single daily dose - effective against resistant H. influenzae and M. catarrhalis less effective than amoxicillin for pneumococci
  ◊ Cefpodoxime (Vantin) 10 mg/kg/day bid - less effective in vivo against H. influenzae than other drugs
  ◊ Ceftriaxone (Rocephin) 50 mg/kg IM single dose - effective against major pathogens, but expensive and painful so reserved for sick infants
  ◊ Clarithromycin (Biaxin) 15 mg/kg/day divided bid - not effective in vivo against H. influenzae
  ◊ Trimethoprim-sulfamethoxazole (Septra, Bactrim) 8 mg TMP/kg/day divided bid: up to 30% of pneumococci are resistant
  ◊ Erythromycin-sulfisoxazole (Pediazole) 40 mg erythromycin component/kg/day divided qid - some strains of pneumococci are resistant
• Recurrent AOM:
  ◊ Sulfisoxazole 75 mg/kg single daily dose for penicillin allergic patients
• Analgesics and antipyretics as needed

FOLLOWUP

PATIENT MONITORING
• AOM: Otoscopic examination 4 weeks after diagnosis
• OME: Monthly otoscopic or tympanometric exams as long as OME persists

PREVENTION/AVOIDANCE
• Breast-feeding decreases incidence of AOM
• Eliminate cigarette smoking in the household

POSSIBLE COMPLICATIONS
• AOM: Perforation/otorrhea, acute mastoiditis, facial nerve paralysis, otitic hydrocephalus, meningitis
• OME: Hearing loss. Extent and significance of impaired speech and language is controversial.
• Recurrent AOM and OME: Atrophy and scarring of eardrum, chronic perforation and otorrhea, cholesteatoma, permanent hearing loss, chronic mastoiditis, brain abscess and other intracranial suppurative complications

EXPECTED COURSE/PROGNOSIS
• AOM: Symptoms usually improve in 48-72 hrs; OME following AOM resolved in 90% by 3 months
• OME: Approximately 50% resolve after 8 weeks of observation
• Recurrent AOM and OME: Usually subside in school age children; only a small percentage have complications

MISCELLANEOUS

ASSOCIATED CONDITIONS
• Upper respiratory infection
• Bacteremia
• Meningitis
• Allergies

AGE-RELATED FACTORS
Pediatric: Primarily a pediatric disease
Geriatric: N/A
Others: N/A

PREGNANCY N/A

SYNONYMS
• Secretory otitis media
• Serous otitis media

ICD-9-CM
• 382.0 Acute otitis media
• 381.0 Acute suppurative otitis media

SEE ALSO N/A

OTHER NOTES In first few months of infancy, the eardrum is normally at an angle and less mobile in older adults

ABBREVIATIONS
AOM = acute otitis media
OM = otitis media
OME = otitis media with effusion

REFERENCES
• Bluestone CD, Klein JO: Otitis Media in Infants and Children. Philadelphia, W.B. Saunders Co., 1994
• Klein JO, Pediatr Inf Dis J 1993;12:973
• Nelson W, Behrman R, Kliegman R, Arvin A, eds: Nelson Textbook of Pediatrics. 15th Ed. Philadelphia, WB Saunders Co., 1996
Illustrations: N/A
Internet references: http://www.5mcc.com

Author(s)
Barbara J. Morant, MD
Marie A. Brister, MD
Janet M. Hahn, MD

Otosclerosis (otospongiosis)

BASICS

DESCRIPTION A primary bone dyscrasia involving the otic capsule. It is the leading cause of conductive hearing loss in adults.
• Histologic otosclerosis: Asymptomatic form in which abnormal bone spares vital structures of the ear
• Clinical otosclerosis: Abnormal spongy bone involves ossicular chain or other structures leading to altered physiology
System(s) affected: Nervous
Genetics:
• 60% of those affected give positive family history
• Appears to be transmitted by autosomal dominant gene with variable penetrance
Incidence/Prevalence in USA:
• 4-8% among Caucasians; 1% among African-Americans (histologic form)
• Caucasians 5000/100,000; Blacks 1000/100,000 (histologic form)
Predominant age: Clinical onset usually in early 20's. Peak incidence fourth and fifth decades.
Predominant sex: Female > Male (2:1)

SIGNS AND SYMPTOMS
• Progressive conductive hearing loss, usually with well preserved speech discrimination. May have sensorineural hearing loss with cochlear involvement.
• Carhart's notch: A dip in bone conductive threshold at 2000 Hz. on audiometric testing
• Schwartze's sign: Reddish hue on promontory upon otoscopic examination
• Patients often soft spoken and aware they seem to hear better in noisy environments

CAUSES Unknown; fluoride metabolism felt by some authorities to play a role in etiology

RISK FACTORS Unknown

DIAGNOSIS

DIFFERENTIAL DIAGNOSIS
• Chronic suppurative otitis media
• Serous otitis media
• External auditory canal occlusion
• Ossicular chain disruption
• Congenital fixation of stapes
• Presbycusis

LABORATORY N/A
Drugs that may alter lab results: N/A
Disorders that may alter lab results: N/A

PATHOLOGICAL FINDINGS
• Gross: Off-white to reddish bone formation, most often located anterior to the oval window and extending to involve the stapedial footplate. Sometimes covers entire oval window (obliterative). May be found anywhere in otic capsule. Bilateral in 75% of cases.
• Micro: "Spongy" appearing bone with increased vascular spaces. Osteoblasts and osteoclasts are plentiful.

SPECIAL TESTS Tuning fork and audiometric testing for conductive and/or sensorineural hearing loss. Will lateralize to more impaired ear with Weber's test.

IMAGING Coaxial or computerized tomography sometimes helpful

DIAGNOSTIC PROCEDURES N/A

TREATMENT

APPROPRIATE HEALTH CARE Inpatient for surgery. Outpatient if surgery not feasible.

GENERAL MEASURES Hearing aids

SURGICAL MEASURES
• Surgical correction (stapedectomy): Usually involves mobilization or removal of the stapedial foot plate with placement of a stapes prosthesis. Recent procedural innovations have involved use of lasers.
• Relative indications for surgery include: Negative Rinne's test (air-bone audiometric gap at least 20 dB); bilateral involvement

ACTIVITY No restrictions

DIET No special diet

PATIENT EDUCATION
• Because speech discrimination is usually preserved, patients should be advised of the possible benefit from hearing aids (as an alternative or adjunct to surgery)
• Mayo Foundation for Medical Education and Research, Section of Patient and Health Education, Sieber Subway, Rochester, MN 55905, (507)284-8140

MEDICATIONS

DRUG(S) OF CHOICE No specific drug therapy but sodium fluoride, vitamin D and calcium gluconate have been tried, especially in cases of predominantly sensorineural hearing loss
Contraindications: Refer to manufacturer's literature
Precautions: Refer to manufacturer's literature
Significant possible interactions: Refer to manufacturer's literature

ALTERNATIVE DRUGS N/A

FOLLOWUP

PATIENT MONITORING Interval audiometric testing

PREVENTION/AVOIDANCE N/A

POSSIBLE COMPLICATIONS Surgical risks include chorda tympani nerve injury, tympanic membrane laceration, ossicular chain disruption, otitis media and externa, labyrinthitis, granuloma formation, perilymph fistulae, and total deafness ("dead ear")

EXPECTED COURSE/PROGNOSIS
Progressive hearing loss if not treated. Surgery improves hearing by at least 15 dB in 90% of cases.

MISCELLANEOUS

ASSOCIATED CONDITIONS
• Van der Hoeve's syndrome (rare triad of osteogenesis imperfecta, blue sclera, and otospongiosis)
• Tinnitus
• Vertigo

AGE-RELATED FACTORS
Pediatric: N/A
Geriatric: Important differential diagnosis for presbycusis
Others: N/A

PREGNANCY Progression may accelerate during pregnancy. Some women first notice hearing loss at this time.

SYNONYMS N/A

ICD-9-CM
387.9

SEE ALSO Hearing loss

OTHER NOTES N/A

ABBREVIATIONS N/A

REFERENCES
• English GM: Otolaryngology: A Textbook. New York, Harper & Rowe, 1976
• Lee KJ: Essential Otolaryngology: Head & Neck Surgery. 4th Ed. New Hyde Park, NY, Medical Examination Pub. Co., 1987
Illustrations: N/A
Internet references: http://www.5mcc.com

Author(s)
Jeffrey D. Wolfrey, MD

Ovarian cancer

BASICS

DESCRIPTION A variety of malignancies that arise from the epithelium, sex cords, stromal cells, or germ cells or are metastatic to the ovary

System(s) affected: Reproductive, Endocrine/Metabolic

Genetics: Epithelial ovarian cancer may have a subset of inherited tendencies - two documented first degree relatives with epithelial ovarian cancer may give risk of 50%

Incidence/Prevalence in USA:
• 12,000 deaths/year
• 5th leading cause of cancer death in women

Predominant age:
• Epithelial: 40-75 years
• Germ cell malignancies: 12-40 years (although epithelial still the most common malignancy in this age)

Predominant sex: Female only

SIGNS AND SYMPTOMS
• Vague gastrointestinal symptoms
• Bloating and dyspepsia
• Abdominal swelling, pain, and distention
• Occasional vaginal discharge
• Irregular vaginal bleeding
• Ascites
• Cul-de-sac and/or pelvic nodularity
• Pelvic mass
• Dyspareunia
• Weight loss

CAUSES Etiology unknown

RISK FACTORS
• Low parity
• Late pregnancies (over 30)
• Family history

DIAGNOSIS

DIFFERENTIAL DIAGNOSIS
• Gastrointestinal or other gynecologic malignancies
• Irritable bowel syndrome
• Colitis
• Hepatic failure with ascites

LABORATORY
• Cancer antigen (CA) 125 (normal < 35 μ/mL)
• Liver function tests (LFT) to rule out hepatic involvement
• Carcinoembryonic antigen (CEA) if gastrointestinal primary suspected
• Chorionic gonadotropin (beta-hCG); alpha-FP for yolk-sac tumors

Drugs that may alter lab results: N/A

Disorders that may alter lab results: CA 125 may be elevated with benign disease (endometriosis, peritonitis, myomas) and with other malignancies

PATHOLOGICAL FINDINGS At surgery, most common type will be epithelial ovarian cancer and most common subtype will be serous cystadenocarcinoma

SPECIAL TESTS Pelvic ultrasound to differentiate other pelvic masses when ascites is not present

IMAGING If site of cancer is in question: Mammogram, barium enema (BE), upper gastrointestinal series (UGI), CT

DIAGNOSTIC PROCEDURES
• Surgery is definitive
• Occasionally paracentesis and thoracentesis for cytology may be helpful
• Guided needle aspiration of ovarian masses is not helpful

TREATMENT

APPROPRIATE HEALTH CARE
• Inpatient
• Surgical staging and primary debulking are critical. Chemotherapy and/or radiotherapy as recommended by oncologist.

GENERAL MEASURES N/A

SURGICAL MEASURES
• For epithelial malignancies:
  ◊ Total abdominal hysterectomy (TAH)/bilateral salpingo-oophorectomy (BSO)
  ◊ Omentectomy/debulking
  ◊ Staging biopsies including node sampling as indicated
• For germ cell cancers (which are less likely to be bilateral):
  ◊ Salpingo-oophorectomy (unilateral if only one ovary involved) in young patient
  ◊ Careful staging, including lymph node dissection, may be adequate

ACTIVITY As tolerated

DIET
• High protein diet
• Follow serum protein closely with significant ascites

PATIENT EDUCATION
• "What You Need to Know About Ovarian Cancer" - National Institutes of Health pamphlet
• "Chemotherapy and You: A Guide to Self-Help During Treatment" - National Institutes of Health pamphlet

Ovarian cancer

MEDICATIONS

DRUG(S) OF CHOICE
• Platinum-based regimen (cisplatin or carboplatin)
• Cyclophosphamide (Cytoxan)
• Paclitaxel (Taxol)
• Other drugs based on current protocol
Contraindications: Cisplatin - impaired renal function, hearing loss, neuropathy
Precautions: All regimens cause bone marrow suppression. Cisplatin associated with ototoxicity, renal toxicity, and peripheral neuropathy.
Significant possible interactions: All regimens may cause clinically significant bone marrow suppression

ALTERNATIVE DRUGS
• Etoposide
• 5-Fluorouracil
• Doxorubicin (Adriamycin)
• Other members of the alkylating agent family (melphalan, hexamethylmelamine, ifosfamide [with mesna to protect against hemorrhagic cystitis], thiotepa)
• Ondansetron (Zofran), dronabinol (Marinol), metoclopramide (Reglan), and others for nausea control

FOLLOWUP

PATIENT MONITORING
• A logarithmic or sevenfold fall in CA-125 suggests a good response, but normal value has only mild correlation with absence of disease
• A rise in CA-125 usually requires a change in therapy
• In germ cell cancers, markers should fall to normal range. Normal levels correlate closely with absence of disease.

PREVENTION/AVOIDANCE
• Prophylactic oophorectomy has been suggested for women with two first degree relatives with epithelial ovarian cancer
• Preventive role of oral contraceptive agents
• Mass screening for ovarian cancer by sonography and CA-125 is not cost-effective

POSSIBLE COMPLICATIONS
• Pleural effusion
• Pseudomyxoma
• Ascites
• Radiotherapy and chemotherapy adverse reactions
• Bowel obstruction

EXPECTED COURSE/PROGNOSIS
• Five year survival rate is dependent on cell type, stage and residual disease:
  ◊ Stage I, 80%
  ◊ Stage II, 60%
  ◊ Stage III (grade III epithelial cancer), 15-30%
  ◊ Stage IV, 10%

MISCELLANEOUS

ASSOCIATED CONDITIONS
• Ascites
• Pleural effusion
• Decrease of serum albumin
• Breast carcinoma

AGE-RELATED FACTORS
Pediatric: N/A
Geriatric: N/A
Others: Patients under 60 have a better prognosis

PREGNANCY   N/A

SYNONYMS   N/A

ICD-9-CM
183.0 Malignant neoplasm of ovary and other uterine adnexa

SEE ALSO   N/A

OTHER NOTES   N/A

ABBREVIATIONS   N/A

REFERENCES
• Bast RC, et al: A Radioimmunoassay Using a Monoclonal Antibody to Monitor the Course of Epithelial Ovarian Cancer. New Engl J of Med 1983;309:883-7
• Griffiths T, Parker L: Cancer of the Ovary. In: Knapp RC, Berkowitz RS, eds. Gynecologic Oncology. New York, Macmillan, 1986
• Classification and Staging of Gynecologic Malignancies. ACOG Technical Bulletin, 155, May 1991
Illustrations: N/A
Internet references: http://www.5mcc.com

Author(s)
Joanna M. Cain, MD

Ovarian tumor, benign

BASICS

DESCRIPTION The ovaries are a source of more varieties of tumors (benign and malignant) than any other part of the body. Benign tumors of the ovary create difficulties in differential diagnosis because of the need to identify malignancy. The tumors are often clinically silent until well developed; may be solid, cystic or mixed; may be functional (producing sex steroids) or nonfunctional.
System(s) affected: Reproductive, Endocrine/Metabolic
Genetics: N/A
Incidence/Prevalence in USA: Unknown due to asymptomatic character
Predominant age:
• All ages
• Concern for malignancy greater in postmenopausal women
Predominant sex: Female only

SIGNS AND SYMPTOMS
• Usually asymptomatic
• Pain related to torsion, endometriosis, or rupture
• Swelling in abdomen or bladder
• Bowel pressure or bladder pressure sensations

CAUSES
• Endometriosis with localized, repeated ovarian hemorrhage
• Physiologic cysts
• Etiology unknown

RISK FACTORS None known

DIAGNOSIS

DIFFERENTIAL DIAGNOSIS
• Malignancies
• Uterine myomas
• Appendicular cysts
• Diverticulitis and abscesses
• Pelvic inflammatory disease with tubo-ovarian abscess
• Distended urinary bladder

LABORATORY
• Serum tumor markers as indicated
  ◊ Cancer antigen (CA) 125
  ◊ Alpha fetoprotein (FP)
  ◊ Chorionic gonadotropin (beta-hCG)
Drugs that may alter lab results: N/A
Disorders that may alter lab results:
• CA 125
  ◊ Endometriosis
  ◊ Peritonitis
  ◊ Pelvic inflammatory disease (PID)
  ◊ Other cancers

PATHOLOGICAL FINDINGS
• Benign
  ◊ Simple cysts
  ◊ Physiologic cysts
  ◊ Endometrioma
  ◊ Epithelial cysts
  ◊ Granulosa cell/stromal tumors
  ◊ Fibroma
  ◊ Cystic teratoma

SPECIAL TESTS
• Pelvic exam is the most important
• Careful physical exam

IMAGING May differentiate tumors from other pelvic masses and identify features at high risk for malignancy, e.g., solid component, papillations, multiple septations

DIAGNOSTIC PROCEDURES N/A

TREATMENT

APPROPRIATE HEALTH CARE Inpatient if surgery necessary

GENERAL MEASURES N/A

SURGICAL MEASURES
• Surgical removal of tumor to establish diagnosis
  ◊ Premenopausal cysts greater than 5 cm or that persist
  ◊ Postmenopausal cysts
  ◊ Cysts with worrisome ultrasound features

ACTIVITY As tolerated

DIET No special diet

PATIENT EDUCATION Dependent on etiology, e.g., endometriosis vs. pelvic inflammatory disease vs. physiologic

MEDICATIONS

DRUG(S) OF CHOICE Oral contraceptives may be helpful in premenopausal patients to differentiate physiologic cysts. Suppression of formation of new cysts by this method and reexamination may resolve the issue.
Contraindications: Refer to manufacturer's profile of each drug
Precautions: Refer to manufacturer's profile of each drug
Significant possible interactions: Refer to manufacturer's profile of each drug

ALTERNATIVE DRUGS N/A

FOLLOWUP

PATIENT MONITORING
• Most require only yearly exams
• Varies by diagnosis

PREVENTION/AVOIDANCE Use of oral contraceptives may decrease risk

POSSIBLE COMPLICATIONS
Complications of untreated dermoid and mucinous cysts may include pseudomyxoma peritonei

EXPECTED COURSE/PROGNOSIS
Complete cure

MISCELLANEOUS

ASSOCIATED CONDITIONS N/A

AGE-RELATED FACTORS
Pediatric: N/A
Geriatric: Concern greater with postmenopausal emergence of ovarian masses
Others: N/A

PREGNANCY Rarely, tumors may be detected during pregnancy examinations

SYNONYMS N/A

ICD-9-CM 220 benign neoplasm of ovary

SEE ALSO N/A

OTHER NOTES N/A

ABBREVIATIONS N/A

REFERENCES
• Benacerrif BR, Finkler NJ, et al: Sonographic Accuracy in the Diagnosis of Ovarian Masses. Journal of Reproductive Medicine 1990;35:491-5
• Bird C, et al: Benign Neoplasms of the Ovary. In: Sciarra J, Droegmuller W, eds. Clinical Gynecology.Philadelphia, J.B. Lippincott, 1990
• Cain J: Pelvic Mass: Detection, Diagnosis and Management. In: Stenchever M, ed. Office Gynecology. St. Louis, Mosby Year Book, Inc., 1991
Illustrations: N/A
Internet references: http://www.5mcc.com

Author(s)
Joanna M. Cain, MD

Paget's disease of the breast

BASICS

DESCRIPTION Rare type of carcinoma that appears unilaterally as dermatitis of the nipple, representing an extension to the epidermis of an underlying carcinoma of a mammary duct.
System(s) affected: Skin/Exocrine
Genetics: No known genetic pattern
Incidence/Prevalence in USA:
• 1000-4000 new cases each year
• Approximately 1-2% of all cases of breast cancer
Predominant age: 40-75
Predominant sex: Female

SIGNS AND SYMPTOMS
• Nipple skin changes that do not respond to conservative treatment
• Nipple itching
• Nipple burning
• Nipple oozing
• Nipple bleeding
• Eczematoid nipple changes
• Breast mass
• Nipple fissures
• Nipple ulceration
• Local hyperemia
• Local edema

CAUSES Unknown

RISK FACTORS Same as for non-heritable breast carcinoma

DIAGNOSIS

DIFFERENTIAL DIAGNOSIS
• Eczema
• Psoriasis
• Skin tumors (e.g., Bowen's disease)
• Squamous cell carcinoma
• Basal cell carcinoma

LABORATORY N/A
Drugs that may alter lab results: N/A
Disorders that may alter lab results: N/A

PATHOLOGICAL FINDINGS
• Micro - malignant cell invasion of the epidermis with large pale staining sells
• Underlying ductal adenocarcinoma

SPECIAL TESTS N/A

IMAGING Mammography - useful, but cannot exclude malignancy without clinicopathological correlation

DIAGNOSTIC PROCEDURES Any chronic or nonhealing nipple lesion should be biopsied

TREATMENT

APPROPRIATE HEALTH CARE As determined by surgical consultant

GENERAL MEASURES
• Radiotherapy
• Chemotherapy
• Hormonal manipulation

SURGICAL MEASURES To be determined by surgeon

ACTIVITY Full activity

DIET No special diet

PATIENT EDUCATION National Cancer Institute, Dept. of Health And Human Services, Public Inquiries Section, Office of Cancer Communications, Building 31, Room 101-18, 9000 Rockville Pike, Bethesda, MD 20892, (301)496-5583

MEDICATIONS

DRUG(S) OF CHOICE According to protocols supervised by an oncologist
Contraindications: Refer to manufacturer's literature
Precautions: Refer to manufacturer's literature
Significant possible interactions: Refer to manufacturer's literature

ALTERNATIVE DRUGS N/A

FOLLOWUP

PATIENT MONITORING As dictated by needs of the various therapy modalities

PREVENTION/AVOIDANCE None known

POSSIBLE COMPLICATIONS
Metastases

EXPECTED COURSE/PROGNOSIS
• Dependent on stage of underlying breast carcinoma
• Stage and 10 year disease free survival
  ◊ 1 - 70-95%
  ◊ 2 - 40-45%%
  ◊ 3 - 10-15%
  ◊ 4 - < 5%

MISCELLANEOUS

ASSOCIATED CONDITIONS Underlying carcinoma

AGE-RELATED FACTORS
Pediatric: N/A
Geriatric: N/A
Others: N/A

PREGNANCY N/A

SYNONYMS N/A

ICD-9-CM
174.0 malignant neoplasm of breast and areola

SEE ALSO Breast cancer

OTHER NOTES Extramammary Paget's disease can also occur

ABBREVIATIONS N/A

REFERENCES
• Bland KI, Copeland EM, eds: The Breast. Philadelphia, W.B. Saunders Co., 1991
• Fitzpatrick TB, et al, eds: Dermatology In General Medicine. 4th Ed. New York, McGraw-Hill, 1993
• DeVita VT Jr, Hellman S, Rosenberg A, eds: Cancer: Principles and Practices of Oncology. 4th Ed. Philadelphia, J.B. Lippincott, 1993
Illustrations: N/A
Internet references: http://www.5mcc.com

Author(s)
Mark Horattas, MD, FACS

Pancreatic cancer, exocrine

BASICS

DESCRIPTION
Pancreatic exocrine malignancies (including adenocarcinoma, 90%; cystadenocarcinoma; and acinar cell carcinoma) represent 3% of all cancers but the fifth most common cause of cancer deaths in the United States.
These malignancies are divided into two broad categories:
• Periampullary lesions - most commonly adenocarcinoma of the head of the pancreas. Of lesser frequency are malignant lesions of the ampulla, duodenum and common bile duct. Lesions in these areas are characterized by jaundice, weight loss and abdominal pain.
• Lesions of body and tail - account for thirty percent of adenocarcinomas of the pancreas. Due to retroperitoneal location and distance from common bile duct, lesions tend to be much larger at diagnosis. Common symptoms are those of weight loss and pain.
System(s) affected: Gastrointestinal
Genetics: More common in blacks, diabetic patients
Incidence/Prevalence in USA:
• Approximately 28,000 new cases diagnosed per year
• Varies among ethnic groups, highest in Blacks and Hawaiians
Predominant age: Mean age in males = 63 years, females = 67 years
Predominant sex: Male > Female (1.5-2:1)

SIGNS AND SYMPTOMS
• Weight loss (90%)
• Pain (75%)
• Jaundice (65%)
• Anorexia (60%)
• Pruritus (40%)
• Diabetes mellitus (15%)
• Malnutrition (75%)
• Hepatomegaly (65%)
• Jaundice (70%)
• Palpable gallbladder (25%)
• Abdominal tenderness (20%)
• Mass (10%)
• Ascites (5%)

CAUSES
• No known etiology, though many associations
• Associations include race, diabetes mellitus, tobacco, environmental and occupational exposures, and dietary lipids
• Of interest, seemingly no association between pancreatitis, alcohol and coffee consumption when data adjusted for effect of tobacco use

RISK FACTORS
• Probable: Race, diabetes mellitus, tobacco
• Possible: Environmental/occupational exposures, dietary lipids

DIAGNOSIS

DIFFERENTIAL DIAGNOSIS
• Choledocholithiasis
• Pancreatitis
• Pancreatic pseudocyst
• Cholangiocarcinoma
• Carcinoma of the ampulla of Vater
• Duodenal neoplasms
• Endocrine tumors of pancreas
• Miscellaneous malignancies with extrinsic bile duct compression
• Biliary tract stricture
• Choledochal cyst

LABORATORY
• Bilirubin level mean of 15 mg/dL (256.5 μmol/L) in patients with jaundice due to pancreatic cancer; considerably higher than that in patients with benign diseases (choledocholithiasis, strictures)
• Patients with recent onset of jaundice with bilirubin greater than 10 mg/dL (171.0 μmol/L) should be considered to have neoplastic obstruction of common bile duct until proven otherwise
• Alkaline phosphatase elevated in most patients. Mean of 550 U/L not significantly different from level in patients with bile duct obstruction from benign disease
• Anemia present in approximately 60% of patients
• Stool occult blood present in approximately 90% of patients with periampullary tumors
• Elevated amylase found in less than 5% of patients
• Tumor markers:
  ◊ In general, useful for screening and assessment of extent of disease. Likely to have good specificity when multiple marker assays combined. Represent a dynamic area of research and discovery of new markers and development of sensitive and specific assays likely in the future.
  ◊ CA 19-9: Elevated in serum and pancreatic juice of patients with pancreatic cancer. Sensitivity/specificity in differentiating pancreatitis is undetermined.
  ◊ Carcinoembryonic antigen (CEA): Serum and pancreatic juice levels elevated beyond 10 ng/ml (10 μg/L) and 30 ng/mL (30 μg/L) respectively in patients with pancreatic cancer
  ◊ Pancreatic-oncofetal antigen: Sensitivity of 68% when used as screening test. Combining test with CEA and alpha-fetoprotein increases specificity.
Drugs that may alter lab results: N/A
Disorders that may alter lab results: N/A

PATHOLOGICAL FINDINGS
• Adenocarcinoma (90%)
• Acinar cell carcinoma (1.2%)
• Other (0.8%)
• Uncertain (9.2%)

SPECIAL TESTS
Pancreatic juice - for cytology and CEA, CA 19-9 assays

IMAGING
• Upper GI series - widening of duodenal sweep in large tumors
• CT scan - most useful imaging modality
• Ultrasound - limited by overlying bowel, less accuracy in staging
• MRI
• Endoscopic retrograde cholangiopancreatography (ERCP) - particularly useful in ampullary or duodenal lesions where biopsy may be performed, pancreatic juice sampled and pancreatic duct cytology
• PTC - delineates proximal biliary tree, important data in planning reconstruction following surgical procedure
• Angiography - role in preoperative staging, not in tumor localization

DIAGNOSTIC PROCEDURES
• Biopsy:
  ◊ CT-guided percutaneous needle aspiration has sensitivity of 85% with specificity of approximately 100% in pancreatic adenocarcinoma. Few complications and extremely low risk of tract seeding.
  ◊ Pseudocyst aspiration can differentiate benign pseudocysts from cystadenocarcinoma. Fluid in cystadenocarcinoma has low amylase, high CEA and lactate dehydrogenase (LDH) levels, and malignant cells are usually present.
  ◊ Liver biopsy may be useful in patients with hepatic metastases
  ◊ Laparoscopy with biopsy is becoming a popular technique and is likely to be more frequently used in the future for staging
• Esophagogastroduodenoscopy:
  ◊ Useful for evaluation of ampulla and duodenal regions in patients with periampullary and duodenal tumors

TREATMENT

APPROPRIATE HEALTH CARE Inpatient for testing, preliminary therapy, surgery or other protocols

GENERAL MEASURES
• Management highly variable and influenced by the overall health of the patient, presence of metastases, and location and size of tumor
• Analgesia
• Management of pruritus
• Control of diabetes (usually "brittle") if total pancreatectomy performed
• Non-operative procedures
  ◊ Biliary decompression by use of endoprostheses, transhepatic drainage catheters
  ◊ Celiac blockade and epidural catheter placement for analgesia
  ◊ Chemotherapy - multiple protocols
  ◊ Radiation therapy - external beam (intraoperative - largely investigational)

SURGICAL MEASURES
• Pancreaticoduodenectomy (Whipple's procedure)
• Total pancreatectomy
• Regional pancreatectomy - resection pancreas, portal vein, regional nodes, subtotal gastrectomy
• Biliary decompression for unresectable disease - T-tube, bilio-enteric anastomoses
• Gastrojejunostomy for gastric outlet obstruction in unresectable disease

ACTIVITY Ad lib

DIET As tolerated. Serve small frequent meals.

PATIENT EDUCATION Printed patient information available from: National Cancer Institute, Dept. of Health And Human Services, Public Inquiries Section, Office of Cancer Communications, Building 31, Room 101-18, 9000 Rockville Pike, Bethesda, MD 20892, (301)496-5583

MEDICATIONS

DRUG(S) OF CHOICE
• Analgesics
• Management of pruritus, e.g., phenothiazines or cholestyramine
• Chemotherapy - multiple protocols
• Antacids
• Pancreatic enzymes
• Diabetes control
Contraindications: N/A
Precautions: N/A
Significant possible interactions: N/A

ALTERNATIVE DRUGS N/A

FOLLOWUP

PATIENT MONITORING Variable

PREVENTION/AVOIDANCE Avoid tobacco

POSSIBLE COMPLICATIONS
• Pain
• Jaundice
• Malnutrition
• Diabetes - especially in patients undergoing total pancreatectomy
• Operative mortality - varies from 10-40%

EXPECTED COURSE/PROGNOSIS
• Three year survival - 2.5%
• Five year survival - 1%
• Following surgery for potentially curable disease, five year survival is about 4%. Reflects high likelihood of metastases at the time of diagnosis.

MISCELLANEOUS

ASSOCIATED CONDITIONS
• Diabetes
• Other findings associated with metastases, e.g., superior vena cava syndrome, Horner's syndrome

AGE-RELATED FACTORS
Pediatric: N/A
Geriatric: More common in this age group, particularly males
Others: N/A

PREGNANCY N/A

SYNONYMS N/A

ICD-9-CM
157.0 Malignant neoplasm of pancreas (site specified 157.x)

SEE ALSO N/A

OTHER NOTES N/A

ABBREVIATIONS
CEA = carcinoembryonic antigen
CA = cancer antigen

REFERENCES Howard JM, Jordan GL, Reber HA, eds: Surgical Diseases of the Pancreas. Philadelphia, Lea and Febiger, 1987
Illustrations: N/A
Internet references: http://www.5mcc.com

Author(s)
Leo C. Mercer, MD

Pancreatitis

 BASICS

DESCRIPTION
An inflammatory, auto-digestive process of the pancreas
- Acute pancreatitis
  ◊ Inflammatory episode with symptoms related to intrapancreatic activation of enzymes with pain, nausea and vomiting, and associated intestinal ileus
  ◊ It varies widely in severity, complications and prognosis
- Chronic pancreatitis
  ◊ Progressive functional destruction of the pancreas that may exist in the absence of an etiology
  ◊ Results in both exocrine and endocrine deficiencies
  ◊ Pain, maldigestion and diabetes mellitus are the major features

System(s) affected: Gastrointestinal
Genetics: Hereditary pancreatitis is a very rare condition with an autosomally dominant inheritance pattern
Incidence/Prevalence in USA: Urban - 22/100,00; rural - 10/100,000
Predominant age:
- Acute pancreatitis - none
- Chronic pancreatitis - 35-45 years (usually related to alcohol)

Predominant sex: Male = Female

SIGNS AND SYMPTOMS
- Abdominal pain - epigastric, may radiate straight through to back
- Nausea and/or vomiting
- Mild abdominal distention
- Fever (100-101°F [37.7-38.3°C])
- Hypotension/shock (40%)
- Mild jaundice
- Diminished or absent bowel sounds
- Flank discoloration (Grey Turner's sign)
- Umbilical discoloration (Cullen's sign)
- Pleural effusion

CAUSES
- Cholelithiasis/choledocholithiasis
- Alcoholism and acute intoxication
- Medications
- Metabolic hypercalcemia, hypertriglyceridemia
- Penetrating peptic ulcer (rare)
- Trauma/surgery
- Viral infections
- Endoscopic retrograde cholangiopancreatography (ERCP)
- Idiopathic
- Tumor
- Systemic lupus erythematosus
- Mumps
- Salmonella
- Cytomegalovirus
- Cystic fibrosis
- AIDS
- Insect/animal venom (certain scorpions, sea anemone)

RISK FACTORS
See Causes

 DIAGNOSIS

DIFFERENTIAL DIAGNOSIS
- Acute pancreatitis
  ◊ Penetrating or perforated peptic ulcer
  ◊ Acute cholecystitis
  ◊ Choledocholithiasis
  ◊ Macroamylasemia, macrolipasemia
  ◊ Mesenteric vascular obstruction and/or infarction
  ◊ Perforation of a viscus
  ◊ Intestinal obstruction
  ◊ Aortic aneurysm
- Chronic pancreatitis
  ◊ Pancreatic cancer
  ◊ Other malabsorptive processes
  ◊ Other cause of biliary obstruction

LABORATORY
- Acute pancreatitis
  ◊ Elevated serum amylase
  ◊ Elevated serum lipase
  ◊ Elevated (mild) alanine aminotransferase (ALT) and/or aspartate aminotransferase (AST) - when associated with alcoholic hepatitis or choledocholithiasis
  ◊ Elevated alkaline phosphatase (mild) - when associated with alcoholic hepatitis or choledocholithiasis
  ◊ Hyperbilirubinemia - when associated with alcoholic hepatitis or choledocholithiasis
  ◊ Glucose increased - in severe disease
  ◊ Calcium decreased - in severe disease
  ◊ WBC 10,000 - 25,000
- Chronic pancreatitis
  ◊ Sometimes none
  ◊ Hyperglycemia
  ◊ Steatorrhea
  ◊ Flare-ups may mimic acute pancreatitis
  ◊ Elevated alkaline phosphatase, bilirubin

Drugs that may alter lab results: Insulin and corticosteroids
Disorders that may alter lab results:
- Biliary tract disease
- Penetrating peptic ulcer
- Intestinal obstruction
- Intestinal ischemia/infarction
- Ruptured ectopic pregnancy
- Renal insufficiency
- Burns
- Macroamylasemia, macrolipasemia

PATHOLOGICAL FINDINGS
- Acute pancreatitis: autodigestion of the pancreas, interstitial edema, hemorrhage, cell and fat necrosis
- Chronic pancreatitis: calcification, fibrosis

SPECIAL TESTS
N/A

IMAGING
- Acute pancreatitis
  ◊ Plain film of abdomen - signs of ileus
  ◊ Chest x-ray - pleural effusion
  ◊ Ultrasound/CT scan of abdomen
  ◊ Endoscopic retrograde cholangiopancreatography (ERCP)
  ◊ Dynamic CT scan

- Chronic pancreatitis
  ◊ X-ray of abdomen - pancreatic calcification
  ◊ Ultrasound and/or CT scan of abdomen - pseudocyst formation/calcification
  ◊ Endoscopic retrograde cholangiopancreatography (ERCP) - ductal deformity, retained common bile duct (CBD) stone, pancreatic duct stones and strictures
  ◊ Endoscopic sphincterotomy - early CBD stone removal improves outcome in severe cases
  ◊ Endoscopic ultrasound

DIAGNOSTIC PROCEDURES
- Acute pancreatitis
  ◊ CT guided aspiration of necrotic areas
  ◊ ERCP for common duct stone removal
- Chronic pancreatitis
  ◊ Secretin stimulation test
  ◊ Para-aminobenzoic acid test (bentiromide [Chymex] test)
  ◊ Lunch test meal

 TREATMENT

APPROPRIATE HEALTH CARE
- Acute pancreatitis - hospitalization, unless very mild and able to maintain oral intake
- Chronic pancreatitis - outpatient except for complications

GENERAL MEASURES
- Acute pancreatitis
  ◊ P - pain control: meperidine
  ◊ A - arrest shock: IV fluids
  ◊ N - nasogastric tube for vomiting
  ◊ C - calcium monitoring
  ◊ R - renal evaluation
  ◊ E - ensure pulmonary function
  ◊ A - antibiotics
  ◊ S - surgery or special procedures in selected cases
- Chronic pancreatitis
  ◊ Pain - alcohol abstinence, analgesia (avoid narcotics if possible), celiac ganglion block, surgery, pancreatic enzyme preparations
  ◊ Maldigestion - pancreatic enzyme supplements, H2-blockers
  ◊ Diabetes mellitus - insulin

Pancreatitis

SURGICAL MEASURES
- Acute pancreatitis
  ◊ Infected necrosis
  ◊ Peritoneal lavage
- Chronic pancreatitis
  ◊ Pain
  ◊ Pseudocyst drainage

ACTIVITY
- Acute pancreatitis - usually bedrest although sitting in a chair may be more comfortable. Advance as able.
- Chronic pancreatitis - not restricted

DIET
- Acute pancreatitis: begin diet after pain, tenderness and ileus have resolved; small amounts of high carbohydrate, low fat and low protein foods. Advance as tolerated. NPO or nasogastric tube, if vomiting
- Chronic pancreatitis: small meals high in protein. Adjust if diabetes mellitus is present.

PATIENT EDUCATION
For patient education materials favorably reviewed on this topic, contact: National Digestive Diseases Information Clearinghouse, Box NDDIC, Bethesda, MD 20892, (301)468-6344

MEDICATIONS

DRUG(S) OF CHOICE
- Acute pancreatitis
  ◊ Meperidine (Demerol) 50-100 mg IM/IV every 3-4 hours
- Antibiotics
- Somatostatin
- Chronic pancreatitis
  ◊ Analgesics: acetaminophen (Tylenol), oxycodone-acetaminophen (Tylox), hydrocodone-acetaminophen (Vicodin), propoxyphene napsylate
  ◊ Pancreatic enzyme (Pancrease MT, Creon) supplements
  ◊ H2-blockers (reducing gastric acid increases availability of pancreatic enzymes)

Contraindications:
- Nor-meperidine, a metabolite of meperidine, may accumulate following several days of round-the-clock dosing. May cause mental status changes or seizures.
- Antibiotic allergy

Precautions: Narcotic addiction
Significant possible interactions: Refer to manufacturer's profile of each drug

ALTERNATIVE DRUGS N/A

FOLLOWUP

PATIENT MONITORING
- Assure alcohol abstinence
- Follow and correct any etiologic cause - hypertriglycerides, choledocholithiasis
- Persistent elevation of amylase weeks after acute pancreatitis suggests possibility of pseudocyst - should perform imaging study

PREVENTION/AVOIDANCE
- Avoid alcohol
- Correct underlying causes, i.e., lipids, drug use, ARDS

POSSIBLE COMPLICATIONS
- Acute pancreatitis - pseudocyst
- Chronic pancreatitis - pseudocyst, abscess, biliary/duodenal obstruction, portal/splenic vein thrombosis, diabetes mellitus

EXPECTED COURSE/PROGNOSIS
- Acute pancreatitis: 85-90% resolve spontaneously, 3-5% mortality
  ◊ Poor prognosis indicated by:
  - On admission: age > 55 years, WBC > 16,000/mm, blood glucose > 200 mg/dL (11.1 mmol/L), serum LDH > 2 x normal, serum SGOT > 6 x normal
  - Within 48 hours: hematocrit decrease > 10%, serum calcium < 8 mg/dL, BUN increase > 5 mg/dL, arterial pO2 < 60 mm Hg, base deficit > 4 mEq/L, fluid retention > 6L
- Chronic pancreatitis: may have recurrent episodes of "acute pancreatitis", slow progression, may "burn out" with resolution of symptoms. Narcotic addiction frequent.

MISCELLANEOUS

ASSOCIATED CONDITIONS N/A

AGE-RELATED FACTORS
Pediatric: Mumps, sometimes complicated by pancreatitis
Geriatric: Vascular disease
Others: N/A

PREGNANCY Acute fatty liver of pregnancy

SYNONYMS N/A

ICD-9-CM
577.0 Acute pancreatitis
577.1 Chronic pancreatitis

SEE ALSO
- Alcoholism
- Choledocholithiasis
- Peptic ulcer disease
- Systemic lupus erythematosus (SLE)

OTHER NOTES N/A

ABBREVIATIONS N/A

REFERENCES
- Silverman A, Roy CR: Pediatric Clinical Gastroenterology. St Louis, The C.V. Mosby Co., 1983
- Sleisenger MH, Fordtran JS, eds: Gastrointestinal Disease: Pathophysiology, Diagnosis, Management. 5th Ed. Philadelphia, W.B. Saunders Co., 1994
- Steinberg W, Tanner S: Acute pancreatitis. New Eng J Med 1994;330(17):1198
- Tran DD: Evaluation of severity in patients with acute pancreatitis. Am J Gastro 1992;87:607

Illustrations: N/A
Internet references: http://www.5mcc.com

Author(s)
Duane C. Roe, MD

Parkinson's disease

BASICS

DESCRIPTION An adult-onset neurodegenerative disorder of the extrapyramidal system characterized by a combination of tremor at rest, rigidity and bradykinesia. The diagnosis requires therapeutic response to levodopa which implies normal striatal neurons. This is the only neurodegenerative disease which is treatable long-term.

Genetics:
• 1/3-1/4 have family history
• Risk is higher if father (vs mother) has disease
• Subsequent generations develop disease earlier

System(s) affected: Neurologic, Musculoskeletal

Incidence/Prevalence in USA: 50,000 per year

Predominant age: Age 60 with 5% between the ages of 21 and 39

Predominant sex: Male > Female (1.4:1)

SIGNS AND SYMPTOMS
• Cardinal signs
  ◊ Tremor (48 Hz) in repose: Diagnostic, but not required; relieved with activity, concentration, and sleep; increases with stress; 10% of patients present with only tremor, 30% present without; most begin with unilateral tremor.
  ◊ Bradykinesia: required for diagnosis; most disabling symptom; movement initiation difficult, can be overcome with will; causes the gait and postural abnormalities
  ◊ Rigidity: lead pipe type; cogwheeling with tremor
• Other associated signs and symptoms
  ◊ Speech is poorly enunciated, low volume, clipped
  ◊ Ocular abnormalities: Decreased blinking, blepharospasm, impaired upward gaze
  ◊ Seborrhea
  ◊ Dysautonomia with constipation, incontinence, sexual dysfunction
  ◊ Depression in 2/3 of patients
  ◊ Dementia in 20% of patients; more common in patients whose disease onset was bilateral - mild to moderate, 90% with Folstein MMSE >15
  ◊ Gait disturbances including no arm swing, en mass turning, problems getting up from chair, festination, freezing
  ◊ Leaning posture
  ◊ Propulsion or retropulsion
  ◊ Micrographia
  ◊ Mask faces
  ◊ Neglect of swallowing with drooling

CAUSES
• Unknown
• Loss of dopaminergic neurons in the substantia nigra with rate of loss 1% per year in patients with Parkinson's versus 0.5% in normal aging.
• Probably not genetic rather toxic or infectious
• Known toxins: MPTP, pesticides. Other non-dopaminergic neurons can be affected.

RISK FACTORS Unknown in the idiopathic disease

DIAGNOSIS

DIFFERENTIAL DIAGNOSIS
• Parkinsonism: bradykinesia and occasionally tremor with little or no response to levodopa indicating that the striatal neurons are also degenerated
  ◊ Progressive supranuclear palsy
  ◊ Multisystem atrophy
  ◊ Alzheimer's disease with extrapyramidal features
  ◊ Side effects of neuroleptic medications
  ◊ Infectious - postencephalitic
  ◊ Vascular - lacunar state
  ◊ Toxins
  ◊ Metabolic - Wilson's disease: onset <40
• Benign essential tremor: positive family history and relief with alcohol

LABORATORY N/A
Drugs that may alter lab results: N/A
Disorders that may alter lab results: N/A

PATHOLOGICAL FINDINGS Typical changes that allow precise pathological diagnosis. Lewy bodies.

SPECIAL TESTS N/A

IMAGING
• CT or MRI help rule out other disorders
• PET scanning

DIAGNOSTIC PROCEDURES
Diagnostic criteria:
• Clinically possible - any one of:
  ◊ Rest tremor
  ◊ Rigidity
  ◊ Bradykinesia
• Clinically probable - any 2 of:
  ◊ Rest tremor
  ◊ Rigidity
  ◊ Bradykinesia
  ◊ Impaired postural reflexes
OR
One of first three displaying asymmetry
• Clinically definite - any 3 of:
  ◊ Rest tremor
  ◊ Rigidity
  ◊ Bradykinesia
  ◊ Impaired postural reflexes
OR
  ◊ Any 2 of above with one of first 3 displaying asymmetry

TREATMENT

APPROPRIATE HEALTH CARE
Outpatient

GENERAL MEASURES
• Drugs have therapeutic and toxic effects
• Acute worsening may indicate depression, non-compliance or supervening illness
• Course is progressive with or without drugs. Life-long therapy directed toward symptom control - treat disability
• Investigate for drug-induced cause; if found, discontinue drug. Symptom resolution may take weeks to months.
• Physical, occupational and speech therapy
• Physical limitations require adjustments in the home, e.g., special chairs, elevated toilet seat, eating utensils, dressing oneself

SURGICAL MEASURES
• Adrenal medullary transplants, fetal midbrain with substantia nigra neurons
• Thalamotomy
• Stereotactic pallidotomy

ACTIVITY Maintain activity to whatever degree possible; use cane for walking

DIET
• Small frequent meals if difficulty in eating
• High liquid intake important; high bulk foods
• Reduced protein diet is unnecessary

PATIENT EDUCATION
• Local support groups
• United Parkinson Foundation, 360 W. Superior St., Chicago, IL 60610, 312-664-2344
• Parkinson's Education Program - USA, 3900 Birch Street, #105, Newport Beach, CA 92660, 800-344-7872
• American Parkinson's Disease Foundation, 1250 Hyland Blvd., Staten Island, NY 10305, 800-223-2732

MEDICATIONS

DRUG(S) OF CHOICE
• Selegiline 5 mg in AM and noon: for patients with no limiting disability (neuroprotection unproven)
• Levodopa-carbidopa (Sinemet): for patients with manifested disability; although neuro-vegetative symptoms such as speech disorders and falls are resistant to levodopa
◊ Sinemet SR 50-200 (start with 1/2 tab) qid after food. Increase by 100 mg levodopa per day until desired effect or side effects occur. If early morning symptoms, add Sinemet 25-100 immediate release one half hour before arising
◊ If switching to the SR, increase daily dose by 25%
◊ Add agonist if "wear off" or dyskinesia appear or when 800-1000 mg levodopa SR per day being taken
• Dopamine agonists. Low potency; long half-life; reduces wearing-off effects of levodopa. Add when levodopa > 600 mg/day
◊ Bromocriptine - start with 1.25 mg qd or bid
◊ Pergolide - 0.05 mg/d for 2 days and increase by 0.1 mg/d q 3 days x 12 days. If higher doses needed, then increase by 0.25 mg q 3 days. Mean dose is 3 mg.
◊ Titrate the levodopa-carbidopa combination downward as these agents are added such that 1 mg of bromocriptine equals 10 mg of levodopa and 1 mg of pergolide equals 10 mg of bromocriptine
• MAO inhibitors. May prolong time prior to need for levodopa/carbidopa. Blocks metabolism of dopamine. May be neuro-protective.
◊ Selegiline 5 mg - start with 1/2 tab qAM and 1/2 q NOON; increase to 5mg bid. If add to levodopa-carbidopa, lower dosage 20%
• Anticholinergics. For tremor in early stages or as an adjunct (30% improvement in 50% of patients)
◊ Trihexyphenidyl (Artane): 1 mg/day, increase by 2 mg every 3 days until 6-10 mg/day
◊ Benztropine (Cogentin): 1-2 mg/day. Start with 0.5 mg/day and increase slowly by 0.5 mg every 6 days. Maximum 6 mg/day.
• Amantadine, mode of action unknown
◊ Similar to anticholinergics; improves bradykinesia and rigidity; rapid onset 48-72h
◊ Synergistic with L-dopa
◊ 100-200 mg/day
Contraindications: Refer to manufacturer's literature
Precautions:
• L-dopa/carbidopa - late effects
◊ Time related dosage problems occur in 50% of patients in 4-5 years
◊ Dyskinesias probably secondary to receptor hypersensitivity.
- Inter dose dyskinesia: occurs at peak level of drug 2 hours after immediate release form, limb choreoathetosis and grimacing; change to sustained release, reduce levodopa dose plus add agonist or clozapine 100-200 mg.

- Diphasic dyskinesia: mobile dystonia of limbs occurs as the dose is rising and falling; increase individual dose or subcutaneous apomorphine pulses.
- "Off" period dyskinesia: may begin as early morning dystonia (foot); reduce inter-dose interval or switch to sustained release or agonist
◊ Wear-off phenomena: usually occurs 3-4 hours after last dose. Usually first sign of drug-response problems caused by increased severity of nigral degeneration. Use sustained release form with an agonist or selegiline.
◊ On/off phenomena: 15-20% of patients develop severe fluctuation of response. Long-term high dose levodopa may be cause. Try low protein diet, slow release preparations, continuous subcutaneous infusions, or enteral infusion into duodenum. Also can decrease dose until on-off phenomena disappears and then restart drug.
◊ Hourly liquid preparation - 10 tablets 25-100 plus 2g abscorbic acid crystals in 1l of tap water; 75 mL in AM, then 35-50 mL/h
◊ Freezing: find a visual clue to "step over" or counting numbers in head
◊ Psychiatric side effects: confusion, hallucinations (well-formed visual or auditory) paranoia, nightmares. If mainly at night, reduce last evening dose or try clozapine.
• Agonists
◊ Nausea, nightmares, agitation, orthostatic hypertension, hallucinations
◊ Raynaud's phenomena in doses > 30 mg/day, edema, hypertension, worsening CHF
• MAO inhibitor: Anxiety/sleep disturbance
• Anticholinergics: Confusion, constipation, urinary retention, dry mouth and glaucoma
• Dopamine release stimulator: Confusion, hallucinations, edema, livedo reticularis, and worsening CHF
Significant possible interactions: Most have additive therapeutic and side effects

ALTERNATIVE DRUGS
• Tricyclic antidepressants for night time sedation and associated depression (50% of patients with Parkinson's)
• Antioxidants or vitamin E have shown no definite benefit
• Selective catechol-O-methyltransferase inhibitors
• Apomorphine as agonist or for "freezing" (use limited by adverse effects [vomiting] and need for parenteral administration)
• Clozapine: 70-200 mg/day can suppress frequency of dyskinesia and increase "on" time; also useful for hallucinations. Side effects include sedation and sialorrhea, and most serious, agranulocytosis.

FOLLOWUP

PATIENT MONITORING Life-long for medication adjustment and physical therapy

PREVENTION/AVOIDANCE Avoid drugs known to cause tardive dyskinesia, such as: Fluphenazine, perphenazine, prochlorperazine, thiopropazate, trifluoperazine, promazine, thioridazine, haloperidol, droperidol, benperidol, fluspirilene, pimozide, trifluperidol, chlorprothixene, clopenthixol, thiothixene

EXPECTED COURSE/PROGNOSIS
• More rapid progression: Older at disease onset; dementia
• Milder disease, the predominant feature is tremor

POSSIBLE COMPLICATIONS Dementia, depression, aspiration pneumonia, falls, freezing, dyskinesias; also associated with a twofold increase risk of death

MISCELLANEOUS

ASSOCIATED CONDITIONS Psychosis; depression

AGE-RELATED FACTORS
Pediatric: May occur as secondary parkinsonism in this age group
Geriatric: Common among elderly
Others: N/A

PREGNANCY N/A

SYNONYMS
• Paralysis agitans
• Shaking palsy

ICD-9-CM
332.0 paralysis agitans

SEE ALSO
• Depression
• Dementia
• Benign essential tremor syndrome

OTHER NOTES New approaches in treatment undergoing study

ABBREVIATIONS N/A

REFERENCES
• Sweeny PJ: Considerations in the diagnosis and management of Parkinson's disease. Fam Prac Recertification 1996;18(4)
• Poewe WH, Wenning GK: The natural history of Parkinson's disease. Neurology 1996;47(3):s146-s151
• Krauss JK, Jankovic J: Surgical treatment of Parkinson's disease. Am Fam Phys 1996;54(5):1621-1628
Illustrations: N/A
Internet references: http://www.5mcc.com

Author(s)
Jeffrey F. Minteer, MD

Paronychia

BASICS

DESCRIPTION Infectious inflammation of the folds of skin surrounding the fingernail or toenail. May be acute or chronic.
System(s) affected: Skin/Exocrine
Genetics: No known genetic pattern
Incidence/Prevalence in USA: Common
Predominant age: All ages
Predominant sex: Female > Male (3:1)

SIGNS AND SYMPTOMS
• Separation of nail fold from nail plate
• Red, painful swelling of skin around nail plate
• Purulent
• Secondary changes of nail plate
• Green changes in nail (pseudomonas)

CAUSES
• Acute - Staphylococcus aureus. Less frequently by Streptococci and Pseudomonas
• Chronic - Candida albicans. Less frequently by fungi - dermatophytes and occasionally, by molds (Scytalidium fusarium)

RISK FACTORS
• Acute - trauma to skin surrounding nail, ingrown nails
• Chronic - frequent immersion of hands in water, diabetes mellitus

DIAGNOSIS

DIFFERENTIAL DIAGNOSIS
• Herpetic whitlow
• Felon
• Reiter's disease
• Psoriasis

LABORATORY
• Gram stain
• Culture and sensitivity
• KOH preparation plus fungal culture
Drugs that may alter lab results: Use of over-the-counter antimicrobials or antifungals
Disorders that may alter lab results: N/A

PATHOLOGICAL FINDINGS N/A

SPECIAL TESTS None

IMAGING N/A

DIAGNOSTIC PROCEDURES N/A

TREATMENT

APPROPRIATE HEALTH CARE
Outpatient

GENERAL MEASURES
• Acute - warm compresses or soaks, elevation
• Chronic - keep fingers dry

SURGICAL MEASURES Incision and drainage (I&D) of abscess, if present. If there is a subungual abscess or ingrown nail present, will need partial or complete removal of nail.

ACTIVITY Full activity

DIET No special diet

PATIENT EDUCATION Chronic - keep fingers dry

MEDICATIONS

DRUG(S) OF CHOICE
• Acute (if diabetic, suppurative or more severe cases):
  ◊ Dicloxacillin 125-500 mg q6h
  ◊ Cloxacillin 250-500 mg q6h
  ◊ Erythromycin 500 mg q6h
  ◊ Cephalexin (Keflex) 250 mg q6h
• Chronic:
  ◊ Bacterial - mupirocin
  ◊ Yeast or dermatophyte - topical imidazoles (econazole, ketoconazole
• Systemic:
  ◊ Itraconazole 200 mg/day for 90 days (may have longer action because incorporated in nail plate)
  ◊ Fluconazole 150 mg/week for 4-6 months

Contraindications: Allergy to antibiotic
Precautions: Erythromycin may cause significant gastrointestinal upset
Significant possible interactions:
• Erythromycin affects levels of theophylline and effects of carbamazepine, digoxin and corticosteroids. Cardiac toxicity with terfenadine or astemizole.
• Ketoconazole, astemazole, itraconazole, fluconazole - terfenadine,

ALTERNATIVE DRUGS
Antipseudomonal drugs, e.g., third generation cephalosporin, aminoglycosides

FOLLOWUP

PATIENT MONITORING
Routine followup until healed

PREVENTION/AVOIDANCE
• Chronic - avoid frequent wetting of hands, wear rubber gloves with cloth liner
• Good diabetic control

POSSIBLE COMPLICATIONS
• Acute - subungual abscess
• Chronic - secondary ridging, thickening and discoloration of nail, nail loss

EXPECTED COURSE/PROGNOSIS
With adequate treatment and prevention, healing can be expected

MISCELLANEOUS

ASSOCIATED CONDITIONS
Diabetes mellitus

AGE-RELATED FACTORS
Pediatric: Anaerobes may be involved in cases with thumb/finger sucking
Geriatric: N/A
Others: N/A

PREGNANCY
N/A

SYNONYMS
• Eponychia
• Perionychia

ICD-9-CM
681.02 Onychia and paronychia of finger
112.3 Candidiasis of skin and nails

SEE ALSO
• Onychomycosis

OTHER NOTES
May be considered work-related in bartenders, waitresses, nurses and others who often wet their hands

ABBREVIATIONS
N/A

REFERENCES
• Fitzpatrick TB, et al, eds: Dermatology In General Medicine. 3rd Ed. New York, McGraw-Hill, 1987
• Moschella SC, Hurley HJ, eds: Dermatology. 3rd Ed. Philadelphia, W.B. Saunders Co., 1992
• Baran R, Dawber RPR, eds: Diseases of the Nail and Their Management. 2nd Ed. Boston, Blackwell Scientific, 1994
Illustrations: 2 available on CD-ROM
Internet references: http://www.5mcc.com

Author(s)
Larry Millikan, MD

Parvovirus B19 infection

BASICS

DESCRIPTION Human parvovirus B19 is the primary cause of erythema infectiosum (EI, or fifth disease). It also causes aplastic anemia in patients with increased RBC turnover (e.g., sickle cell anemia), chronic anemia in immunodeficient individuals, and arthritis and arthralgias in normal hosts. There is also the potential for intrauterine infection after maternal parvovirus B19 infection.
System(s) affected: Skin/Exocrine, Musculoskeletal, Hemic/Lymphatic/Immunologic
Genetics: Erythrocyte P antigen-negative individuals are resistant to infection
Incidence/Prevalence in USA: Extremely common; 50% of adults have evidence of prior infection. Most common as community epidemics in winter and spring in non-tropical regions.
Predominant age:
• Infection is common in childhood; approximately 2-11% of children under 11 years of age are parvovirus B19 seropositive
• Peak age for EI is 4-12 years
Predominant sex: Male = Female

SIGNS AND SYMPTOMS
• Erythema infectiosum (EI)
  ◊ Incubation period 4-14 days
  ◊ No preclinical symptoms most commonly. Fever is absent or low grade.
  ◊ Onset of rash noted first on the face ("slapped cheek appearance") with diffuse erythema of the face followed 1-4 days later by a second stage of a lacy reticular rash on the trunk and limbs
  ◊ A third stage of the rash is characterized by marked evanescence and recrudescence, sometimes associated with bathing, exercise, or sun exposure
  ◊ Pruritus and mild arthralgia may occur
  ◊ Headache, pharyngitis, coryza, myalgia, arthralgias, arthritis, and GI disturbances are more frequent and severe in adults
• Joint disease
  ◊ In adults, 80% of patients may manifest arthritis and/or arthralgia
  ◊ In children, joint symptoms are less common
  ◊ Knees, hands, and ankles (frequently symmetrical) are most commonly involved
  ◊ Joint symptoms usually subside in weeks but may persist for months. Joint destruction generally not seen.
• Transient aplastic crisis
  ◊ Seen in patients with chronic hemolysis, such as sickle cell anemia, spherocytosis, thalassemia, and pyruvate kinase deficiency
  ◊ Aplastic event is self-limited with reticulocytes reappearing in 7-10 days and full recovery in 2-3 weeks
• Chronic anemia
  ◊ Seen in immunodeficient individuals
  ◊ No manifestations of fever, rash, or joint symptoms usually

• Fetal/neonatal infection
  ◊ Risk of transplacental spread of virus approximately 33% in infected mothers
  ◊ Clinical manifestations range from asymptomatic seroconversion (most commonly), no seroconversion, second trimester fetal death, or stillbirth secondary to severe anemia and the development of fetal hydrops
  ◊ The principal organ involved in the fetus is the bone marrow: RBC survival is shortened and profound anemia can result from B19 induced erythroid bone marrow aplasia
  ◊ Risk of fetal loss in pregnancy is highest in first trimester B19 infection (9%)
  ◊ Anemia is the most common manifestation of later infection
  ◊ In one study, 84% of B19 infected pregnant women who carried to term delivered normal infants
  ◊ No known long-term developmental problems in infant survivors

CAUSES
• Small (20-25 mm), nonenveloped, single stranded DNA virus
• In EI, the period of viral shedding precedes the development of the rash, suggesting the pathogenesis of the rash is immune related
• In fetal infection, maternal viremia with transplacental passage is the source of infection. Respiratory secretions and rarely blood products are sources of human spread of virus.

RISK FACTORS
• Aplastic crisis - increased RBC turnover (e.g., sickle cell anemia)
• Chronic anemia - immunodeficient individuals
• Intrauterine infection - pregnant, non-immune woman

DIAGNOSIS

DIFFERENTIAL DIAGNOSIS
• Rubella
• Enteroviral disease
• Systemic lupus erythematosus
• Drug reaction
• Lyme disease
• Rheumatoid arthritis

LABORATORY
• Anemia with reticulocytopenia
• IgM antibody to B19 is usual method of confirming diagnosis. During acute infection B19 IgM persists for 1-2 months (less in neonates).
• To exclude congenital B19 in infants with negative B19 IgM, one must follow an infant's B19 IgG serology in the first year of life
• Maternal serum alpha-fetoprotein may be increased in fetuses with hydrops fetalis
Drugs that may alter lab results: N/A
Disorders that may alter lab results: N/A

PATHOLOGICAL FINDINGS
• Skin biopsy usually normal or mild inflammation, usually consisting of perivascular infiltrations of mononuclear cells
• In hydrops fetalis, may see intranuclear inclusions in nucleated red blood cells
• In stillbirths, virus can be detected in all tissues

SPECIAL TESTS
• Antigen detection in tissue or fluids by nucleic acid hybridization or polymerase chain reaction is available on an investigational basis in many academic centers
• B19 cannot be grown in traditional tissue culture systems, but can be isolated in special cell lines in research laboratories

IMAGING Maternal infection - fetal ultrasound

DIAGNOSTIC PROCEDURES Amniotic fluid and chorionic villus sampling may be useful diagnostically in investigation of some maternal infections

TREATMENT

APPROPRIATE HEALTH CARE
• Outpatient management for EI
• Inpatient for aplastic crisis, other severe manifestations

GENERAL MEASURES None

SURGICAL MEASURES N/A

ACTIVITY
• Unrestricted for EI
• Arthritis patients may require physical therapy/exercise program

DIET No special diet

PATIENT EDUCATION Patients with chronic hemolytic diseases should be aware of risks for aplastic crisis if exposed to EI

MEDICATIONS

DRUG(S) OF CHOICE
• No therapy needed usually
• Immune globulin, intravenous (IVIG) has been used for refractory anemias
• Red blood cell transfusions may be required for aplastic crisis
• Anti-inflammatory agents may alleviate arthritic symptoms
Contraindications: None
Precautions:
• Contact and respiratory isolation for patients hospitalized with aplastic crisis
• EI not contagious once rash has appeared
Significant possible interactions: None

ALTERNATIVE DRUGS   None

FOLLOWUP

PATIENT MONITORING   Periodic blood counts for anemic patients

PREVENTION/AVOIDANCE
• Standard hygienic practices can minimize spread
• Because EI is so common, it is not possible to avoid exposure completely. Also, period of contagion is before clinical illness (rash) appears.
• Pregnant health care workers should avoid caring for patients with aplastic crises
• Pregnant child care workers are at some increased risk; however, exclusion from the work place will not eliminate this risk, and therefore is not recommended

POSSIBLE COMPLICATIONS
Rare, but more commonly seen in adults than children
• Arthritis
• Persistent anemia
• Hemophagocytic syndrome
• Pneumonitis
• Encephalopathy
• Reports of congenital anomalies but no clear-cut association

EXPECTED COURSE/PROGNOSIS
• Usually self-limited
• Joint symptoms subside in weeks
• Full recovery from aplastic crisis in 2-3 weeks

MISCELLANEOUS

ASSOCIATED CONDITIONS   None

AGE-RELATED FACTORS
Pediatric: N/A
Geriatric: None known
Others:
• School-related epidemic and non-immune household contacts have a secondary attack rate of 50%
• Health care workers have a secondary attack rate of 35% with the highest rate being among nurses exposed to children with aplastic crises

PREGNANCY   See above

SYNONYMS
• Fifth disease
• Erythema infectiosum

ICD-9-CM
057.0 Erythema infectiosum (fifth disease)

SEE ALSO
• Abortion, spontaneous
• Anemia, sickle cell
• Schönlein-Henoch purpura
• Systemic lupus erythematosus (SLE)
• Arthritis, rheumatoid (RA)

OTHER NOTES   N/A

ABBREVIATIONS   EI = erythema Infectiosum

REFERENCES
• Kumar ML: Human parvovirus B19 and its associated diseases. Clin Perinatol 1991;18:209
• Adler SP: Risk of human parvovirus B19 infections among school and hospital employees during endemic periods. J Infect Dis 1993;168:361
• Harris JW: Parvovirus B19 for the hematologist. Am J Hematol 1992;39:119
Illustrations: 4 available on CD-ROM
Internet references: http://www.5mcc.com

Author(s)
Bernhard L. Wiedermann, MD
Elizabeth A. Frankel, MD

Patent ductus arteriosus

BASICS

DESCRIPTION Patent ductus arteriosus (PDA) is the failure of the ductus arteriosus to close after birth. 75% of time occurs as isolated defect.
System(s) affected: Cardiovascular
Genetics: No Mendelian inheritance. 1% chance of PDA in infant if one parent affected.
Incidence/Prevalence in USA: 8/1000 live births
Predominant age: Infancy
Predominant sex: Female > Male (2-3:1)

SIGNS AND SYMPTOMS
- Children
  ◊ Failure to grow
  ◊ Recurrent respiratory infections
  ◊ Easy fatigability
  ◊ Dyspnea on exertion
- Adult
  ◊ Leg fatigue
  ◊ Fatigue
  ◊ Shortness of breath
  ◊ Angina
  ◊ Syncope
- Signs (left-to-right shunt)
  ◊ Rough systolic murmur
  ◊ Continuous "machinery" murmur
  ◊ Thrill at left upper sternal border
  ◊ Bounding pulse with wide pulse pressure
  ◊ Prominent, displaced apical impulse
  ◊ Systolic ejection click
  ◊ Diastolic flow murmur (across mitral valve)
  ◊ Excessive sweating
  ◊ Tachypnea, tachycardia, rales if failure ensues
- Signs (right-to-left shunt)
  ◊ Cyanosis, especially lower extremities
  ◊ Clubbing
  ◊ Diastolic Graham-Steele murmur (pulmonic insufficiency)
  ◊ Right ventricular heave
  ◊ Polycythemia

CAUSES
- Prematurity
- Congenital
- Hypoxia
- Prostaglandins

RISK FACTORS
- Premature birth
- High altitudes
- Maternal rubella
- Coexisting cardiac anomalies
- Any condition resulting in hypoxia (pulmonary, hematologic, etc.)

DIAGNOSIS

DIFFERENTIAL DIAGNOSIS
- Venous hum
- Total anomalous pulmonary venous return
- Ruptured sinus of Valsalva
- Arteriovenous communications
- Anomalous origin of left coronary artery from pulmonary artery
- Absence or atresia of pulmonary valve
- Aortic insufficiency with ventricular septal defect
- Peripheral pulmonary stenosis (maternal rubella)
- Truncus arteriosus
- Aortopulmonary fenestration
- Coronary artery fistula

LABORATORY Arterial blood gas
Drugs that may alter lab results: None
Disorders that may alter lab results: None

PATHOLOGICAL FINDINGS
- Left ventricular and atrial enlargement
- Patent ductus may have abnormal intima (maternal rubella)

SPECIAL TESTS
- ECG in children and adults may show left ventricle and left atrial hypertrophy
- ECG in infants usually normal

IMAGING
- Echocardiography/Doppler
- Contrast echocardiography
- Radionuclide angiography
- Magnetic resonance imaging (MRI)
- Chest x-ray usually normal in infants
- Chest x-ray in children and adults (shunt vascularity, calcifications, left ventricle and left atrial enlargement, dilated ascending aorta, dilated pulmonary arteries)

DIAGNOSTIC PROCEDURES
- Cardiac catheterization and angiography - will demonstrate the shunt and determine the amount of shunt, pulmonary pressures, and other coexisting cardiac abnormalities
- Echocardiography - left atrial enlargement
- Doppler - displays direction of shunt and size of the patent ductus

TREATMENT

APPROPRIATE HEALTH CARE Inpatient surgery

GENERAL MEASURES
- Small, asymptomatic shunts may not need closure
- Pulmonary support
- Oxygen to correct hypoxia
- Sodium and fluid restriction
- Correction of anemia (hematocrit > 45)

SURGICAL MEASURES
- Surgical transection and ligation for moderate/large shunts
- Transfemoral catheter technique to occlude PDA with foam plastic plug or double umbrella

ACTIVITY As tolerated

DIET No special diet

PATIENT EDUCATION Discuss prematurity and explain different treatments of premature infants and full-term infants

MEDICATIONS

DRUG(S) OF CHOICE
• Indomethacin 0.2-0.25 mg/kg/dose IV preferred. Repeat every 12-24 hours x 3 doses. (Decreased efficacy in term infants; not effective in children or adults.)
• Oxygen
• Diuretics
• Antibiotic prophylaxis if not surgically repaired

Contraindications:
• To treatment with indomethacin
  ◊ Renal dysfunction
  ◊ Overt bleeding
  ◊ Shock
  ◊ Necrotizing enterocolitis
  ◊ Myocardial ischemia

Precautions: With indomethacin treatment - oliguria, hyponatremia

Significant possible interactions: Refer to manufacturer's profile of each drug

ALTERNATIVE DRUGS   Alprostadil

FOLLOWUP

PATIENT MONITORING
• Annual, routine followup after closure
• Shunts that have not been closed should be followed more closely

PREVENTION/AVOIDANCE   N/A

POSSIBLE COMPLICATIONS
• Left heart failure
• Pulmonary hypertension
• Right heart hypertrophy and failure
• Eisenmenger's physiology
• Bacterial endocarditis
• Myocardial ischemia
• Necrotizing enterocolitis

EXPECTED COURSE/PROGNOSIS
• Spontaneous closure after 3 months is rare
• Before 3 months, closure in premature infants is 75%
• Before 3 months, closure in term infants is 40%
• Best postoperative results if closed before age 3 years
• Increased pulmonary vascular resistance and pulmonary hypertension more common if closed after age 3 years
• No firm statistics but decreased survival for large shunts

MISCELLANEOUS

ASSOCIATED CONDITIONS
• Coarctation of the aorta
• Pulmonary valve stenosis or atresia
• Peripheral pulmonary stenosis (maternal rubella)
• Aortic stenosis
• Ventricular septal defect
• Necrotizing enterocolitis
• Club feet, cataracts, blindness, systemic arterial stenosis (associated with maternal rubella)

AGE-RELATED FACTORS   Moderate to large shunts usually diagnosed in infancy or childhood. Small shunts occasionally diagnosed in adults.
Pediatric:
• Symptoms and signs depend largely on size of shunt
• Some infants with coexisting cardiac anomalies benefit temporarily from a patent ductus to provide shunting to the lungs (right heart obstructions) or periphery (coarctation of the aorta). This benefit is short lived, so definitive treatment should proceed as soon as feasible
Geriatric: Good results expected with repair age 50-70 years
Others: N/A

PREGNANCY
• Women with small to moderate sized ductus and left-to-right shunt can expect an uncomplicated pregnancy
• High risk in those with high pulmonary resistance and right-to-left shunt

SYNONYMS
• Aorticopulmonary shunt
• Aorticopulmonary communication

ICD-9-CM
747.0

SEE ALSO   N/A

OTHER NOTES   No need for antibiotic prophylaxis after surgical repair

ABBREVIATIONS   N/A

REFERENCES
• Adams FH, Emmanouilides GC, Riemenschneider TA: Moss' Heart Disease in Infants, Children and Adolescents. 5th Ed. Baltimore, Williams & Wilkins, 1995
• Braunwald E: Heart Disease. 4th Ed. Philadelphia, W.B. Saunders Co., 1992
• Makowitz JS, et al: Transcatheter versus surgical closure of patent ductus arteriosus. New Engl J Med 1994;330(14);1014
Illustrations: N/A
Internet references: http://www.5mcc.com

Author(s)
Karil Bellah, MD

Pediculosis

BASICS

DESCRIPTION Pediculosis is an infestation by lice
• Characteristics of lice:
   ◊ Lice are ectoparasites that when removed from their human host die of starvation within ten days
   ◊ Lice feed solely on human blood by piercing the skin, injecting saliva, and then sucking blood
   ◊ Lice are mobile and can move quickly
   ◊ A mature adult female lays 3-6 eggs, or nits, a day. Nits are 0.8 mm long, white, and appear cemented to the base of the hair. They hatch in 8-10 days and reach maturity in 8-18 days.
   ◊ Nits may survive three weeks when removed from host
• Two species of lice infest humans:
   ◊ Pediculus humanus has two subspecies, the head louse (Pediculus humanus capitis), and the body louse (Pediculus humanus corporis). The head and body lice are anatomically identical, although the head louse is smaller. Both species are smaller than 2 mm, are flat, wingless, and have three pairs of legs that attach closely behind the head.
   ◊ Phthirus pubis (pubic or crab louse). The pubic louse resembles a sea crab and is shorter than the Pediculosis species with large, widespread claws on the 2nd and 3rd legs.
System(s) affected: Skin
Genetics: No genetic pattern
Incidence/Prevalence in USA: 10-40% in schools where accurate surveys have been conducted
Predominant age:
• Most common in adults - pubic lice
• Most common in children - Pediculosis capitis
Predominant sex: Female > Male

SIGNS AND SYMPTOMS
• Pediculosis capitis (head louse)
   ◊ Found most often on the back of the head and neck and behind the ears (warmer areas of the hair)
   ◊ Nits are white spheres found on the hair shaft. They cannot be moved.
   ◊ Itching common, mostly at night
   ◊ Scratching can cause inflammation and secondary bacterial infection, with pyoderma and posterior cervical lymphadenopathy
   ◊ Eyelashes may be involved
• Pediculosis corporis (body louse)
   ◊ Poor hygiene
   ◊ Adult lice and nits in the seams of clothing
   ◊ Pruritus
   ◊ Secondary infection

◊ Uninfected bites present as red papules, 2-4 mm in diameter, with an erythematous base
• Phthirus pubis (pubic louse)
   ◊ Anogenital pruritus
   ◊ May have no symptoms during 30-day incubation period
   ◊ Nits are present at the base of hair shafts
   ◊ Delay in treatment may lead to development of widespread groin inflammation, infection, and regional adenopathy
   ◊ Pubic hair most common site
   ◊ Lice may spread to hair around anus, abdomen, axillae, chest, beard, eyebrows, and eyelashes
   ◊ Infested adult patients may spread lice to eyelashes of children. This may induce blepharitis with localized pruritus and/or infection.

CAUSES
• Lice are transmitted by close personal contact and contact with objects such as combs, hats, clothing, and bed linen
• Infected sexual contacts

RISK FACTORS
• Pediculosis corporis - inability to change and launder clothing, overcrowded sleeping quarters
• Phthirus pubis - sexual contact with an infected person
• Immunosuppression
• Sharing combs, hats, etc.

DIAGNOSIS

DIFFERENTIAL DIAGNOSIS
• Scabies and other mite species that can cause cutaneous reactions in humans
• Dandruff for head lice

LABORATORY N/A
Drugs that may alter lab results: N/A
Disorders that may alter lab results: N/A

PATHOLOGICAL FINDINGS N/A

SPECIAL TESTS
• Scalp and pubic lice are apparent with careful examination of individual hairs
• Lice and nits can easily be seen under a microscope
• On Wood's lamp exam, live nits fluoresce white, empty nits fluoresce gray
• Examination of the seams of clothing reveals body lice and their eggs

IMAGING N/A

DIAGNOSTIC PROCEDURES History and physical exam

TREATMENT

APPROPRIATE HEALTH CARE
Outpatient

GENERAL MEASURES
• Nit removal:
   ◊ After treatment with shampoo or lotion, nits remain in scalp or pubic hair
   ◊ Nits are best removed with a very fine comb (nit comb). Removal may be made easier by soaking the hair in a solution of equal parts water and white vinegar and wrapping wet scalp in a towel for at least 15 minutes.
   ◊ Repeat treatment periodically as needed for stubborn nits
   ◊ All family contacts possibly infested with head lice should be treated concomitantly
   ◊ Discarding the clothes or washing them in hot water
   ◊ Evaluate for other sexually transmitted diseases (for pubic lice)

SURGICAL MEASURES N/A

ACTIVITY No restrictions

DIET No special diet

PATIENT EDUCATION
• Poor hygiene is not a risk factor in acquiring pediculosis capitis
• Printed patient information available from: Mayo Foundation for Medical Education and Research, Section of Patient and Health Education, Sieber Subway, Rochester, MN 55905, (507)284-8140

MEDICATIONS

DRUG(S) OF CHOICE
• Head lice - many topical preparations are effective. 1% lindane (Kwell) can be used but may have to be repeated in one week. 1% permethrin (Nix, Elimite) or pyrethrin (Rid) are also effective. They should be applied and washed off after 10 minutes.
• Pubic lice - treatments available include lindane, synergized pyrethrins, or permethrin. These can be used either as the shampoo left on for 10 minutes or the lotion which can be left on for several hours for best results.
• Body lice - best treated with lindane or synergized pyrethrins lotion applied once and left on for several hours
• Eyelash infestation - treated by careful manual removal of lice and nits, or by application of petroleum jelly (Vaseline) three or four times a day for 5 days
Contraindications: Avoid lindane in infants and pregnant women
Precautions:
• Pediculicides should never be used to treat eyelash infections
• Accidental ingestion and gross overuse of lindane may be associated with CNS toxicity
Significant possible interactions: N/A

ALTERNATIVE DRUGS
For resistant head lice, shaving the head or oral antibiotics may be indicated

FOLLOWUP

PATIENT MONITORING   As needed

PREVENTION/AVOIDANCE
• Ability to change and launder clothing eliminates risk of acquiring Pediculosis corporis
• Careful followup in schools by public health nurses may help prevent recurrence and spread of head lice
• Washing combs, brushes, hats, coats, collars, sheets, pillow cases, etc., will help to prevent reinfestation by head lice
• Safe sex (pubic lice)

POSSIBLE COMPLICATIONS
• Persistent itching may be caused by too-frequent use of the pediculicide
• Secondary bacterial infections

EXPECTED COURSE/PROGNOSIS
• With appropriate treatment over 90% cure rate
• Recurrence common, mainly from reinfection, failure to comply with treatment

MISCELLANEOUS

ASSOCIATED CONDITIONS
• Pubic lice are readily transmitted by sexual contact, with a 90% transmission rate. Up to 1/3 of patients have at least one concomitant sexually transmitted disease.
• Eyelash infestation on a child may be a sign of sexual abuse

AGE-RELATED FACTORS   N/A
Pediatric: N/A
Geriatric: N/A
Others: Typhus, relapsing fever, and trench fever are spread by body lice during wartime and in underdeveloped countries

PREGNANCY   N/A

SYNONYMS
• Lice
• Crabs

ICD-9-CM
132.9 Pediculosis, unspecified

SEE ALSO   N/A

OTHER NOTES   N/A

ABBREVIATIONS   N/A

REFERENCES
• Rakel RE (ed): Conn's Current Therapy. Philadelphia, WB Saunders Co, 1997
• Habif T: Clinical Dermatology. 3rd Ed. St. Louis, CV Mosby, 1996
Illustrations: N/A
Internet references: http://www.5mcc.com

Author(s)
George E. Kikano, MD

Pelvic inflammatory disease (PID)

BASICS

DESCRIPTION PID is a clinical syndrome caused by the ascent of microorganisms from the vagina and endocervix to the endometrium, fallopian tubes, ovaries, and contiguous structures. PID is a broad term that includes a variety of upper genital tract infections, unrelated to pregnancy or surgical procedures, such as salpingitis, salpingo-oophoritis, endometritis, tubo-ovarian inflammatory masses, and pelvic or diffuse peritonitis.
• Pathogenesis: The precise mechanism by which microorganisms ascend from the lower genital tract is not known. One possibility is that chlamydial or gonococcal endocervicitis alters the defense mechanisms of the cervix allowing ascent of the vaginal flora with or without the original pathogen. Other possibilities suggest that polymicrobial infection can occur without N. gonorrhoeae or C. trachomatis. Factors that predispose to the ascent of bacteria include the use of an intrauterine device (IUD) and the hormonal and physical changes associated with menstruation.
System(s) affected: Reproductive
Genetics: N/A
Incidence/Prevalence in USA: Estimated 1 million women are treated each year; 100-200/100,000
Predominant age: 16-40 years
Predominant sex: Female only

SIGNS AND SYMPTOMS
• May be asymptomatic
• Lower abdominal pain
• Fever and malaise
• Vaginal discharge
• Irregular bleeding
• Urinary discomfort, proctitis
• Nausea and vomiting
• Abdominal tenderness
• Tenderness with cervical motion
• Adnexal tenderness
• Unilateral or bilateral tender adnexal mass

CAUSES
Bacteriology - multiple organisms act as etiologic agents in PID and most cases are polymicrobial. Chlamydia trachomatis, Neisseria gonorrhoeae, and a wide variety of aerobic and anaerobic bacteria are recognized as etiologic agents. Mycoplasmas have also been implicated but their role is less clear. The proportion of cases infected with chlamydia or gonorrhea varies widely depending on the population studied. The most common anaerobes include Bacteroides, Peptostreptococcus, and Peptococcus species. The organisms involved in bacterial vaginosis are similar to the nongonococcal, nonchlamydial bacteria often found in the upper genital tract of women with PID, however, the relationship between these conditions is unclear.

RISK FACTORS
• Sexually active, reproductive age
• Most common in adolescents
• Multiple sexual partners
• Use of an IUD, greatest risk in first few months after insertion
• Previous history of PID; 20-25% will have a recurrence
• Chlamydial or gonococcal cervicitis; 8-10% will develop PID
• Gonococcal salpingitis occurs commonly within 7 days of onset of menses
• Condoms and vaginal spermicides lessen the risks of PID
• Oral contraceptives may reduce the risk of PID

DIAGNOSIS

DIFFERENTIAL DIAGNOSIS
• Appendicitis
• Ectopic pregnancy
• Ovarian torsion
• Hemorrhagic or ruptured ovarian cyst
• Endometriosis
• Irritable bowel syndrome
• Somatization disorder

LABORATORY
• Pregnancy test
• Leukocyte count greater than 10,000 cells per mm3
• Endocervical gram stain for gram-negative intracellular diplococci
• ESR of 15 mm/hour or higher
• Endocervical culture for gonorrhea
• Endocervical culture or antigen test for chlamydia
• Plasma cell endometritis on endometrial biopsy
Drugs that may alter lab results: N/A
Disorders that may alter lab results: N/A

PATHOLOGICAL FINDINGS N/A

SPECIAL TESTS
• Culdocentesis with culture of aspirated material
• Diagnostic laparoscopy with culture of fallopian tubes

IMAGING Pelvic ultrasound

DIAGNOSTIC PROCEDURES
• PID diagnosis is elusive and even asymptomatic patients are at risk for sequelae. Diagnosis incorrect in up to a third of women diagnosed. Laparoscopic diagnosis best but impractical as routine and generally reserved for problem situations. In general, wiser to over-treat lower tract genital infection than to miss an upper tract infection.

• Suggested criteria for diagnosis (sufficient for empiric treatment):
  ◊ Lower abdominal tenderness
  ◊ Cervical motion tenderness
  ◊ Adnexal tenderness
• Additional criteria:
  ◊ Temperature greater than or equal to 38°C
  ◊ WBC greater than or equal to 10,500/mm3
  ◊ Purulent material by culdocentesis
  ◊ Adnexal mass
  ◊ ESR > 15 mm/hour
  ◊ Laboratory evidence of gonorrhea or chlamydia
• Elaborate criteria:
  ◊ Histopathologic endometritis on biopsy
  ◊ Adnexal abscess on sonography
  ◊ Laparoscopic evidence of PID

TREATMENT

APPROPRIATE HEALTH CARE
• Outpatient, normally
• Hospitalization recommended in the following situations:
  ◊ Uncertain diagnosis
  ◊ Surgical emergencies cannot be excluded, e.g., appendicitis
  ◊ Suspected pelvic abscess
  ◊ Pregnancy
  ◊ Adolescent patient with uncertain compliance with therapy
  ◊ Severe illness
  ◊ Cannot tolerate outpatient regimen
  ◊ Failed to respond to outpatient therapy
  ◊ Clinical follow-up within 72 hours of starting antibiotics cannot be arranged
  ◊ HIV-infected

GENERAL MEASURES
• Avoidance of sex until treatment is completed
• Insure that sex partners are referred for appropriate evaluation and treatment. Partners should be treated, irrespective of evaluation, with regimens effective against chlamydia and gonorrhea.

SURGICAL MEASURES
• Reserved for failures of medical treatment and for suspected ruptured adnexal abscess with resulting acute surgical abdomen
• Conservative surgery preferred. This allows a 10-15% postoperative fertility rate.
• Hysterectomy and adnexectomy for older patients with completed childbirth
• Failure of medical therapy generally associated with adnexal abscess which may be amenable to transabdominal or transvaginal drainage under guidance by ultrasonography, computed tomography, or laparoscopy

ACTIVITY According to severity of illness

DIET According to severity of illness

PATIENT EDUCATION Information on written materials for patient distribution can be obtained from local and state health departments or from Information Services, CDC, E06, Atlanta, GA 30333, (404)639-1819

MEDICATIONS

DRUG(S) OF CHOICE
• Several antibiotic regimens are highly effective with no single regimen of choice
• Coverage must extend to include chlamydia, gonorrhea, anaerobes, gram-negative rods, and streptococci. The CDC regimens that follow are recommendations and the specific antibiotics named are examples.

Inpatient treatment
• Recommended regimen A
  ◊ Cefoxitin 2 g IV every 6 hours or cefotetan IV 2 g every 12 hours (or other cephalosporins such as ceftizoxime, cefotaxime, and ceftriaxone) plus doxycycline 100 mg orally or IV every 12 hours
  ◊ Therapy for 48 hours after clinical improvement and doxycycline continued after discharge for a total of 10-14 days
• Recommended regimen B
  ◊ Clindamycin 900 mg IV every 8 hours plus gentamicin loading dose IV or IM (2 mg/kg of body weight) followed by a maintenance dose (1.5 mg/kg) every 8 hours
  ◊ Therapy for 48 hours after clinical improvement with doxycycline after discharge as above, or clindamycin 450 mg orally qid for a total of 14 days

Outpatient treatment
• Recommended regimen A
  ◊ Cefoxitin 2 g IM plus probenecid, 1 g orally, concurrently or ceftriaxone 250 mg IM or equivalent cephalosporin plus doxycycline 100 mg orally bid for 10-14 days or tetracycline 500 mg orally qid for 10-14 days or erythromycin 500 mg orally qid for 10-14 days in patients who do not tolerate tetracyclines
• Recommended regimen B
  ◊ Ofloxacin 400 mg orally bid for 14 days plus either clindamycin 450 mg orally qid, or metronidazole 500 mg orally bid for 14 days

Contraindications: Refer to manufacturer's profile of each drug
Precautions: Refer to manufacturer's profile of each drug
Significant possible interactions: Refer to manufacturer's profile of each drug

ALTERNATIVE DRUGS
Many other antibiotic regimens have been proposed and used with success. For example, tobramycin in place of gentamicin, tetracycline in place of doxycycline.

FOLLOWUP

PATIENT MONITORING
• Close observation of clinical status, in particular for fever, symptoms, level of peritonism, white cell count
• Follow adnexal abscess size and position with ultrasonography

PREVENTION/AVOIDANCE
• Educational programs about safe sex practices
• Education, particularly for those who have had an episode of PID
• IUD contraindicated in women with history of PID or lifestyle associated with STD
• Oral contraceptive appears to decrease risk of PID in cases with cervicitis and the PID cases which do occur are generally less severe
• Barrier contraceptives, especially condoms, and spermicidal creams or sponges provide protection, the extent of which is not well documented
• Insure evaluation and treatment of sex partners
• Comply with management instructions
• Seek medical care early when genital lesions or discharge appear
• Seek routine check-ups for STD if in non-mutually monogamous relationship(s)

POSSIBLE COMPLICATIONS
• A tubo-ovarian abscess will develop in approximately 7-16% of patients
• Recurrent infection occurs in 20-25% of patients
• Risk of ectopic pregnancy increased by 7-10-fold to about 8% of women who have had PID
• Tubal infertility in 15, 35, and 55% of women after one, two, and three episodes of PID, respectively
• Chronic pelvic pain in 20% related to adhesion formation, chronic salpingitis, or recurrent infections

EXPECTED COURSE/PROGNOSIS
• Wide variation with good prognosis if early, effective therapy instituted and further infection avoided
• Poor prognosis related to late therapy and continued unsafe lifestyle

MISCELLANEOUS

ASSOCIATED CONDITIONS
• In PID patients with an IUD in situ, especially if an adnexal abscess is present, the possibility of actinomyces infection requiring penicillin treatment must be kept in mind
• The IUD is contraindicated in women with a previous episode of PID
• Rupture of an adnexal abscess is rare but life-threatening. Early surgical exploration is mandatory.
• Chlamydia or gonococcal perihepatitis may occur with PID. This combination is termed the Curtis-Fitz-Hugh Syndrome.

AGE-RELATED FACTORS
Pediatric:
• PID is rare before puberty
• Adolescents are highly vulnerable to sexually transmitted diseases (STD) including PID. Early vigorous therapy to prevent infertility is especially important in this age group.
Geriatric: PID is rare after menopause, although postmenopausal adnexal abscess is a well-documented entity
Others: N/A

PREGNANCY PID is rare during pregnancy but occurs occasionally and the possibility must be kept in mind

SYNONYMS
• Salpingitis
• Salpingo-oophoritis
• Adnexitis
• Pyosalpinx
• Tubo-ovarian abscess
• Pelvic peritonitis

ICD-9-CM
614.9 Unspecified inflammatory disease of female pelvic organs and tissue

SEE ALSO
• Chlamydial sexually transmitted diseases
• Gonococcal infections
• Syphilis

OTHER NOTES N/A

ABBREVIATIONS N/A

REFERENCES
• Pelvic inflammatory disease: Guidelines for prevention and management. MMWR. 40:1-25, 1991
• 1993 Sexually transmitted diseases treatment guidelines. MMWR. 42-RR-14
Illustrations: N/A
Internet references: http://www.5mcc.com

Author(s)
Michel E. Rivlin, MD

Pemphigoid, bullous

BASICS

DESCRIPTION Chronic benign bullous eruption considered to be an autoimmune disease. Confined to people over 60.
System(s) affected: Skin/Exocrine, Hemic/Lymphatic/Immunologic
Genetics: HLA typing does not reveal any typical pattern
Incidence/Prevalence in USA: Uncommon
Predominant age: Greater than 60 years
Predominant sex: Male = Female

SIGNS AND SYMPTOMS
• Large bullae 2 to 5 cm in diameter. Occasional tiny peripheral vesicles.
• Bullae that arise from normal-appearing skin (usually) or erythematous skin (sometimes)
• Bullae stay intact for many days
• Located on extremities at first, trunk later
• Occasionally located on the scalp, palms, soles, mucous membranes
• Intact blisters outnumber erosions (reverse is true with pemphigus)
• Clear fluid fills bullae (usually)
• Blood tinged fluid in bullae (sometimes)
• Itching (sometimes severe)
• Some patients are asymptomatic
• 10-20% of skin surface is continuously involved

CAUSES Autoimmune disorder

RISK FACTORS Male, age over 60

DIAGNOSIS

DIFFERENTIAL DIAGNOSIS
• Pemphigus
• Bullous erythema multiforme
• Dermatitis herpetiformis
• Drug eruptions

LABORATORY Circulating autoantibodies in 70% directed at the basement membrane (by immunofluorescence). These can be demonstrated in serum or skin.
Drugs that may alter lab results: N/A
Disorders that may alter lab results: N/A

PATHOLOGICAL FINDINGS Bullae located in a subepidermal location

SPECIAL TESTS
• Light microscopy reveals subepidermal blister with perilesional inflammation containing many eosinophils
• Immunofluorescent studies

IMAGING N/A

DIAGNOSTIC PROCEDURES
• History and physical
• Biopsy - essential for precise diagnosis

TREATMENT

APPROPRIATE HEALTH CARE
Outpatient, unless significant complications

GENERAL MEASURES
• Soak active lesions to debride and remove crusts
• Analgesic mouth washes (see Medications)

SURGICAL MEASURES N/A

ACTIVITY Depends on severity of disease and/or complications

DIET Liquid. Regular diet when tolerated.

PATIENT EDUCATION
• Use of oral analgesics
• Teach side effects and adverse reactions of steroids

MEDICATIONS

DRUG(S) OF CHOICE
• Prednisone 60 to 80 mg in single morning dose. Gradually taper in several weeks to maintenance level of 20 to 40 mg per day. Attempt switch to alternate day treatment.
• Consider adjunctive azathioprine if switch to alternate day treatment is not successful. Trial of cyclosporine for resistant disease.
• Topical intralesional corticosteroids may be sufficient for patients with localized disease
• Oral analgesics prn:
  ◊ Elixir of diphenhydramine (Benadryl) for oral ulcers
  ◊ lidocaine (Xylocaine) viscous
  ◊ Dyclonine solution
Contraindications: Refer to manufacturer's literature
Precautions: Some patients (who have only occasional lesions) can be managed without the need for internal medication
Significant possible interactions: Refer to manufacturer's literature

ALTERNATIVE DRUGS Dapsone

FOLLOWUP

PATIENT MONITORING Blood levels mandatory if prescribing cyclosporine

PREVENTION/AVOIDANCE N/A

POSSIBLE COMPLICATIONS
• Superimposed infection (may result in death in elderly debilitated patient)
• Complications of steroid therapy
• Associated malignancy
• Untreated severe disease can be fatal

EXPECTED COURSE/PROGNOSIS
• A chronic disease that lasts indefinitely
• Old lesions heal rapidly as new lesions appear
• Accompanying debilitation not as great as with pemphigus

MISCELLANEOUS

ASSOCIATED CONDITIONS May have an associated malignancy

AGE-RELATED FACTORS
Pediatric: Not a problem in pediatric age group
Geriatric: Older people with pemphigoid may have higher than expected rate of malignancy
Others: N/A

PREGNANCY N/A

SYNONYMS Pemphigoid

ICD-9-CM 694.5 pemphigoid

SEE ALSO N/A

OTHER NOTES N/A

ABBREVIATIONS N/A

REFERENCES
• Fitzpatrick TB, et al, eds: Dermatology in General Medicine. 3rd Ed. New York, McGraw-Hill, 1987
• Habif T: Clinical Dermatology. 3rd Ed. St. Louis, CV Mosby, 1996
Illustrations: 6 available on CD-ROM
Internet references: http://www.5mcc.com

Author(s)
Scott D. Miller, MD

Pemphigus vulgaris

BASICS

DESCRIPTION Uncommon, debilitating, potentially fatal skin disorder characterized by painful intraepidermal bullae that appear on normal appearing skin without surrounding inflammation, often starting in the mouth
System(s) affected: Skin/Exocrine, Gastrointestinal
Genetics: HLA-A10 and HLA-DR4 antigens; higher incidence among persons of Jewish or Mediterranean descent
Incidence/Prevalence in USA: Rare
Predominant age: 30-60 years of age
Predominant sex: Male = Female

SIGNS AND SYMPTOMS
• Oral mucous membrane lesions (particularly in the posterior mouth) often precede the cutaneous lesions (sometimes by several weeks or months)
• Lesion distribution - upper trunk or back initially. Gradual extension to face, groin, and axillae.
• Bullae arise from normal appearing skin
• Multiple shallow erosions which heal slowly
• Blisters are fragile
• Intact bullae are found only on the first day or two of their existence
• After blister roof breaks, a bright red or crusted shallow erosion follows which requires weeks or months to heal
• Outer layer of skin can easily be rubbed off (Nikolsky's sign)

CAUSES An autoimmune disorder with specific IgG antibodies and sometimes complement arising from bone marrow plasma cells which are deposited at sites of epidermal cell damage; a few cases from captopril and penicillamine

RISK FACTORS
• Genetic factors (more common in persons of Jewish or Mediterranean descent)
• Medications (particularly penicillamine)

DIAGNOSIS

DIFFERENTIAL DIAGNOSIS
• Eczematous disorders
• Herpes
• Tinea
• Varicella-zoster
• Erythema multiforme
• Bullous impetigo
• Pemphigoid
• Dermatitis herpetiformis
• Drug eruptions
• Transient acantholytic dermatosis

LABORATORY
• Autoantibody titers (by immunofluorescent studies)
• Titer corresponds to severity of the disease
Drugs that may alter lab results: N/A
Disorders that may alter lab results: N/A

PATHOLOGICAL FINDINGS
• Causative antigens are located on the exterior surface of the cytoplasmic membrane of epithelial cells
• Biopsy shows acantholytic intraepidermal bullae

SPECIAL TESTS N/A

IMAGING N/A

DIAGNOSTIC PROCEDURES
• Biopsy of lesions
• Light microscopy - suprabasal cleft formation and acantholysis

TREATMENT

APPROPRIATE HEALTH CARE Depends on severity of the disease and medical status of patient

GENERAL MEASURES
• May require reverse isolation procedures
• Topical treatment to prevent oozing skin from adhering to bed sheets
• Soak active lesions to debride and remove crusts
• Analgesic mouth washes (see Medications)
• Plasmapheresis, or cyclosporine, if patient fails to respond to an adequate trial of recommended regimens

SURGICAL MEASURES N/A

ACTIVITY As severity of disease and medical status of patient dictates

DIET Liquid or soft for patient with mouth lesions. Regular diet when tolerated.

PATIENT EDUCATION
• Use of oral analgesics
• Teach side effects and adverse reactions of steroids

MEDICATIONS

DRUG(S) OF CHOICE
• Prednisone: high doses 60-100 mg, higher if necessary. Start at 80 mg, increase by 50% every 7 days until no new blisters. Reduce to every other day dosage when possible. Taper over 6-8 months to every other day maintenance therapy, continued for life.
• Consider concomitant immunosuppressants, such as azathioprine 2-3 mg/kg/day, less effective than cyclophosphamide, but less toxic. Use with steroid, or cyclophosphamide 1-2 mg/kg/day - second best therapy, more toxic
• Severe cases require combination plasmapheresis, cyclophosphamide and prednisone
• Oral analgesics prn, choose one:
  ◊ Diphenhydramine (Benadryl) elixir
  ◊ Lidocaine (Xylocaine) viscous
  ◊ Dyclonine solution or lozenges
Contraindications: Refer to manufacturer's literature
Precautions: Refer to manufacturer's literature
Significant possible interactions: Refer to manufacturer's literature

ALTERNATIVE DRUGS
• Gold therapy (with or without concomitant corticosteroids)
• Dapsone controls some cases
• Methotrexate often helpful

FOLLOWUP

PATIENT MONITORING
• Frequent visits during acute phases
• If immunosuppressants prescribed, monitor blood levels frequently
• In elderly patients, chest x-ray to rule out reactivation of old tuberculosis, test urine daily for glycosuria

PREVENTION/AVOIDANCE N/A

POSSIBLE COMPLICATIONS
• Steroid complications that can lead to morbidity and mortality
• Inadequate nutrition and debilitation due to pain of oral lesions
• Sepsis/death for untreated or poorly controlled cases

EXPECTED COURSE/PROGNOSIS
• Chronic. Inevitably fatal if not treated.
• 10% fatality with vigorous treatment
• Ruptured bullae require weeks to heal

MISCELLANEOUS

ASSOCIATED CONDITIONS
• Thymomas
• Other internal malignancies
• Other autoimmune diseases

AGE-RELATED FACTORS
Pediatric: Unusual in this age group
Geriatric:
• This is the age group in which pemphigus is most likely to occur
• Close followup is needed for elderly patients on high doses of steroids
Others: N/A

PREGNANCY N/A

SYNONYMS Pemphigus

ICD-9-CM 694.4 Pemphigus

SEE ALSO N/A

OTHER NOTES
• Atypical presentation - pemphigus foliaceus has infrequent oral lesions and is not as debilitating
• In mild disease, gold salts alone can sometimes produce remission. This has the obvious advantage of avoiding immunosuppression, However, not uniformly beneficial and no controlled trials.

ABBREVIATIONS N/A

REFERENCES
• Fitzpatrick TB, et al, eds: Dermatology In General Medicine. 3rd Ed. New York, McGraw-Hill, 1987
• Habif T: Clinical Dermatology. 3rd Ed. St. Louis, CV Mosby, 1996
• Olson GL: Blistering disorders: which ones can be deadly? Postgrad Med 1994;46(1):53-64
Illustrations: 8 available on CD-ROM
Internet references: http://www.5mcc.com

Author(s)
Douglas M. Hoy, MD

Peptic ulcer disease

 BASICS

DESCRIPTION A chronic ulcer in the lining of the gastrointestinal tract.
• Duodenal ulcer (DU): Most located in the duodenal bulb. Multiple ulcers, and if distal to the bulb raise the possibility of Zollinger-Ellison syndrome.
• Gastric ulcer (GU): Much less common than DU (in the absence NSAID's). Most commonly located along the lesser curvature of the antrum near the incisura and in the pre-pyloric area.
• Esophageal ulcers: A peptic ulcer in the distal esophagus may be part of Barrett's epithelial change due to chronic reflux of gastroduodenal contents
• Ectopic gastric mucosal ulceration: May develop in patients with Meckel's diverticula or other sites of ectopic gastric mucosa
System(s) affected: Gastrointestinal
Genetics: Higher incidence with HLA-B12, B5, Bw35 phenotypes, identical twins
Incidence/Prevalence in USA:
• DU: 4 times more common than GU. Lifetime prevalence = 10% for men; 5% for women (gender gap is closing). 200,000-400,000 new DU cases/annually.
• GU: 87,500 new cases annually. Incidence of new GU in adults; 50/100,000
Predominant age:
• DU 25-75 years (rare before age 15)
• GU peak incidence age 55-65; rare < age 40
Predominant sex:
• DU: Male > Female (slightly)
• GU: Male = Female (female predominance among NSAID users)

SIGNS AND SYMPTOMS
• In adults (DU)
  ◊ Gnawing or burning epigastric pain 1-3 hours after meals, relieved by food, antacids, or antisecretory agents
  ◊ Nocturnal pain causing early morning awakening
  ◊ Epigastric pain in 60-90% (often vague discomfort, cramping, hunger pangs). Non-specific dyspeptic complaints (belching, bloating, abdominal distention, food intolerance) in 40-70%.
  ◊ Symptomatic periods occur in clusters lasting a few weeks followed by symptom-free periods for weeks to months. Some seasonal occurrence (spring and fall).
  ◊ Early satiety, anorexia, weight loss, abnormal saline load test, succussion splash, gastric retention of barium, nausea, vomiting suggest pyloric obstruction
  ◊ Heartburn (suggesting reflux disease)
  ◊ Sudden, severe mid-epigastric pain radiating to right shoulder, peritoneal signs and free peritoneal air may indicate perforation
  ◊ Dizziness, syncope, hematemesis or melena suggest hemorrhage

• In adults (GU)
  ◊ Symptom complex similar to DU
  ◊ NSAID-induced ulcers often silent; perforation or bleeding may be initial presentation
  ◊ Epigastric pain following a meal an uncommon finding; early satiety, nausea, vomiting suggest gastric outlet obstruction
  ◊ Weight loss can occur with either benign or malignant gastric ulcers
• In children (DU)
  ◊ Positive family history in 50% of early onset DU patients (under age 20)
  ◊ May account for chronic abdominal pain syndrome in young children
  ◊ Gastric outlet obstruction from ulcer must be distinguished from congenital infantile hypertrophic pyloric stenosis (seen within the first month after birth along with visible peristalses and a palpable pyloric mass)

CAUSES
Etiology of DU and GU is multifactorial. H. pylori gastritis is present in >80% of DU and >60% of GU.
• Imbalance between aggressive factors (e.g., gastric acid, pepsin, bile salts, pancreatic enzymes) and defensive factors maintaining mucosal integrity (e.g., mucus, bicarbonate, blood flow, prostaglandins, growth factors, cell turnover) which may relate to H. pylori infection
• Ulcerogenic drugs (e.g., NSAID's)
• Zollinger-Ellison syndrome
• Other hypersecretory syndromes

RISK FACTORS
• Strongly associated: Drugs (e.g., NSAID use), family history of ulcer, Zollinger-Ellison syndrome (gastrinoma), cigarettes (>1/2 pack/day)
• Possibly associated: Corticosteroids (high dose and/or prolonged therapy); blood group O; HLA-B12, B5, Bw35 phenotypes; stress; lower socioeconomic status; manual labor
• Poorly or not associated: Dietary spices, alcohol, caffeine, acetaminophen
• Annual risk of DU developing in H. pylori - positive individual ≤1%

 DIAGNOSIS

DIFFERENTIAL DIAGNOSIS
• Non-ulcer dyspepsia
• Gastric carcinoma
• H. pylori-associated gastritis (without ulcer)
• Gastroesophageal reflux (with or without esophagitis)
• Crohn's disease (gastroduodenal)
• Pancreatitis
• Variant angina pectoris
• Cholelithiasis syndrome
• Atrophic gastritis

LABORATORY
• Anemia uncommon in absence of hemorrhage. Fecal occult blood requires colonic evaluation before attributing positive test to ulcer alone (esp. in patients > 40 years).
• Elevated serum gastrin (to rule out Zollinger-Ellison syndrome)

• Gastric analysis (to rule out achlorhydria, acid hypersecretion)
• Secretin stimulation test (paradoxical rise seen in ZE)
• Serum pepsinogen
Drugs that may alter lab results:
Antisecretory medications may give falsely low gastric analysis or elevated gastrin
Disorders that may alter lab results: N/A

PATHOLOGICAL FINDINGS
• Helicobacter pylori gastritis
• Ulcer crater usually > 5 mm diameter; extends through the mucosa (in contrast to stress-related ulceration)

SPECIAL TESTS Serology or urea breath test for H. pylori

IMAGING
• Endoscopy more accurate than radiography
• Radiographic features of benign GU include ulcer projecting beyond the lumen, radiolucent band (Hampton line) paralleling ulcer base, radiating folds

DIAGNOSTIC PROCEDURES
• Endoscopy (accuracy > 95%)
• Barium meal (accuracy 70-90%)
• Mucosal biopsy, cytology (excludes malignancy in > 99%)
• Exploratory laparotomy
• Histology or urea breath test for H. pylori

 TREATMENT

APPROPRIATE HEALTH CARE
• Empiric treatment for young healthy patients with dyspepsia, otherwise endoscopy or barium meal for suspected complications, weight loss, persistent vomiting, etc., or symptom onset after age 50 years
• Emergency endoscopy and hospitalization for suspected ulcer bleeding
• ICU care for severe hemorrhage
• Surgical consult: suspected perforation/obstruction, uncontrolled bleeding

GENERAL MEASURES
• Reduce use of NSAID's and psychic stress
• Avoid or eliminate cigarette smoking

SURGICAL MEASURES For bleeding complication, obstruction or perforation

ACTIVITY Fully active for uncomplicated disease

DIET 3 regular meals daily with avoidance of dietary irritants

PATIENT EDUCATION National Digestive Diseases Information, Box NDDIC, Bethesda, MD 20892, (301)468-6344

MEDICATIONS

DRUG(S) OF CHOICE
Acute healing of DU and GU
• Acid suppression
◊ H2 blocker: ranitidine or nizatidine 150 bid or 300 mg hs; cimetidine 400 mg bid or 800 mg hs; famotidine 150 mg bid or 300 mg hs for 8-12 weeks
◊ Proton pump inhibitor, e.g., omeprazole 20 mg or lansoprazole 15 mg qd for 4 weeks
• Eradication of Helicobacter pylori (HP), single antibiotic regimens discouraged
◊ Classic "triple therapy": bismuth subsalicylate (Pepto-Bismol) 600 mg qid plus tetracycline 500 mg qid plus metronidazole 250 mg qid for 2 weeks; (amoxicillin 500 mg qid has been used in place of tetracycline)
• Currently optimal HP eradication regimens
◊ Omeprazole 20 mg or lansoprazole 30 mg bid plus 2 antibiotics (e.g., clarithromycin 500 mg bid and amoxicillin 1 gm bid for 2 weeks)
◊ Ranitidine bismuth citrate 400 mg bid plus clarithromycin 500 mg bid and amoxicillin 1 gm bid for 2 weeks
◊ Alternative antibiotics: Tetracycline and metronidazole
• Other:
◊ Treatment of H. pylori-negative ulcers: Most are due to NSAID's; treat acutely with H2-receptor antagonists or proton pump inhibitor for 4-12 weeks. Optimally, the NSAID should be discontinued.
◊ Unhealed refractory ulcers: higher doses of H2 blockers or proton pump inhibitors or surgery

Contraindications: Known hypersensitivity to the drug or another member of the class

Precautions:
• Renal insufficiency (GFR < 30 mL/min): reduce H2 blocker dose by 50%. Avoid magnesium-containing antacids
• Give sucralfate distant from meals to avoid binding with food proteins
• Bacterial resistance to metronidazole (50-60%) and clarithromycin (5-10%)
• Antibiotic-related side effects:
◊ Diarrhea (10%): change amoxicillin to tetracycline
◊ Nausea/vomiting (20%): avoid alcohol with metronidazole
◊ Unpleasant taste with metronidazole and clarithromycin
◊ Rash (5%): stop antimicrobial
◊ Pseudomembranous colitis (< 1%): treat with vancomycin
◊ Anaphylaxis, Stevens-Johnson syndrome (rare)

Significant possible interactions:
• Cimetidine interacts with many drugs (e.g., theophylline, warfarin, phenytoin, lidocaine) via inhibition of cytochrome P-450 isozymes, leading to reduced drug clearance; avoid cimetidine with interacting drugs.
• Ranitidine and famotidine have rarely been associated with increased theophylline levels
• Nizatidine has not been associated with drug interactions
• Omeprazole may prolong the elimination of diazepam, warfarin and phenytoin

• Sucralfate reduces absorption of tetracycline, norfloxacin, ciprofloxacin, and theophylline leading to subtherapeutic levels

ALTERNATIVE DRUGS
• Alternative ulcer healing drugs
◊ Sucralfate 1 gm qid or 2 gm bid for 4-8 wks
◊ Antacids, e.g., magnesium hydroxide, aluminum hydroxide 1 and 3 hours after meals (4-7 doses daily)

FOLLOWUP

PATIENT MONITORING
• Eradication of H. pylori: Expected in >90% (with 2 antibiotic regimen)
◊ Confirm eradication by CLOtest biopsy, urea breath test or serology in patients who remain symptomatic or relapse
◊ Treatment failure: use different antimicrobial regimen or test for sensitivity
• Acute DU: monitor clinical response. No need to repeat endoscopy or x-ray exam to document healing unless recurrence or complication suspected.
• Acute GU: confirm healing (endoscopy after 6-12 weeks for cytology and biopsy of poorly or unhealed ulcer to rule out malignancy)
• Symptomatic response to therapy does not preclude malignancy

PREVENTION/AVOIDANCE
• Eradication of HP: recurrence < 10% in the first year, off of all therapies
• Maintenance therapy (e.g., H2 blocker in 1/2 the acute healing dose at bedtime) suppresses ulcer relapse indefinitely while treatment is continued - however, relapses occur in most patients who remain HP positive
• Bleeding ulcers require continued maintenance therapy (e.g., H2 blocker or PPI if H. pylori not eradicated
• NSAID-related ulcers are best managed by avoiding salicylates and NSAID's. If NSAID's needed, add misoprostol (Cytotec), an H2 blocker or proton pump inhibitor.

POSSIBLE COMPLICATIONS
• Hemorrhage in up to 25% of cases (initial presentation in 10%)
• Perforation occurs in < 5%, usually related to NSAID use
• Gastric outlet obstruction occurs in up to 5% of patients with duodenal or pyloric channel ulcers. Men predominate.

EXPECTED COURSE/PROGNOSIS
• Ulcer relapse rates after H. pylori eradication low; suspect surreptitious NSAID use
• Reinfection rates < 1% per year
• The risk of rebleeding after H. pylori therapy alone remains less well defined
• NSAID-related ulcers may occur independently of H. pylori status
• Intractability now rare
• Cost effectiveness demonstrated for H. pylori eradication

MISCELLANEOUS

ASSOCIATED CONDITIONS
• Zollinger-Ellison syndrome (gastrinoma)
• Systemic mastocytosis
• MEN Type 1
• COPD, chronic renal failure, cirrhosis, hyperparathyroidism, carcinoid syndrome, polycythemia rubra vera, basophilic leukemia, porphyria cutanea tarda

AGE-RELATED FACTORS
Pediatric: Uncommon before puberty; hemorrhage and perforation more common
Geriatric: N/A
Others: N/A

PREGNANCY Unusual in gestation; safety of H2 blockers not established in first 16 wks, but considered reasonably safe later; sucralfate and antacids preferred as initial therapy

SYNONYMS
• Duodenal ulcer
• Gastric ulcer
• Helicobacter ulcer

ICD-9-CM DU 532.9, GU 531.9

SEE ALSO
• Zollinger-Ellison syndrome
• Pyloric stenosis

OTHER NOTES N/A

ABBREVIATIONS HP = Helicobacter pylori

REFERENCES
• Soll AH: Medical treatment of ulcer disease: Practice guidelines. JAMA 1996;275:622-629
• Hopkins RJ, Girardi LS, Turney EA: Relationship between Helicobacter pylori eradication and reduced duodenal and gastric ulcer recurrence: A Review. Gastroenterology 1996;110:1244-1252
• Silverstein MD, Petterson T, Talley NJ: Initial endoscopy or empirical therapy with or without testing for Helicobacter pylori for dyspepsia: A decision analysis. Gastroen 1996;110:72-83
• Ofman JJ, Etchason J, Fullerton s, et al: Management strategies for Helicobacter pylori-seropositive patients with dyspepsia: Clinical and economic consequences. Ann Int Med 1997:126:280-291
• Vakil N, Fennerty MB: Cost-effectiveness of treatment regimens for the eradication of Helicobacter pylori in duodenal ulcer. Am J Gastroenterology 1996;91:239-246
Illustrations: N/A
Internet references: http://www.5mcc.com

Author(s)
James H. Lewis, MD, FACP, FACG

Pericarditis

BASICS

DESCRIPTION The clinical manifestations of disease processes involving the pericardial sac surrounding the heart
• Acute pericarditis: an inflammatory process from a wide spectrum of etiologies of the pericardium with or without associated effusion. The most common etiology is idiopathic or nonspecific pericarditis.
• Pericardial tamponade: cardiac compression from pericardial effusion causing hemodynamic compromise and disruption of compensatory mechanisms
• Constrictive pericarditis: thickening and adherence of the pericardium to the heart after chronic inflammation
System(s) affected: Cardiovascular
Genetics: Unknown
Incidence/Prevalence in USA: N/A
Predominant age: Adolescents and young adults
Predominant sex: Male > Female

SIGNS AND SYMPTOMS
• Acute pericarditis
  ◊ Chest pain, typically sharp, retrosternal with radiation to the trapezial ridge
  ◊ Pain frequently sudden in onset
  ◊ Pain reduced by leaning forward and sitting up
  ◊ Splinted breathing
  ◊ Odynophagia
  ◊ Fever
  ◊ Myalgia
  ◊ Anorexia
  ◊ Anxiety
  ◊ Pericardial friction rub
  ◊ Cardiac arrhythmias often intermittent, supraventricular tachycardia (SVT)
  ◊ Tachypnea
  ◊ Localized rales
• Pericardial tamponade
  ◊ Dyspnea
  ◊ Tachycardia
  ◊ Distended jugular neck veins
  ◊ Cyanosis
  ◊ Relative or absolute hypotension
  ◊ Quiet precordium with little palpable cardiac activity
  ◊ Pericardial friction rub
  ◊ Lungs clear
  ◊ Ewart's sign - dullness and bronchial breathing between the tip of the left scapula and vertebral column
  ◊ Rapid thready pulse
  ◊ Varying degrees of consciousness
  ◊ Pulsus paradoxus: > 10 mm Hg (1.33 kPa) decrease in systolic pressure with inspiration

• Constrictive pericarditis
  ◊ Asymptomatic, early
  ◊ Dyspnea, pulmonary congestion
  ◊ Fatigue very common
  ◊ Peripheral edema
  ◊ Hepatomegaly
  ◊ Ascites
  ◊ Jugular venous distention - elevated, deep Y trough (not seen in tamponade)
  ◊ Kussmaul's sign - inspiratory increase in jugular venous pressure
  ◊ Pericardial "knock" - follows S2 by 0.06-0.12 sec, increases with squatting
  ◊ Hypovolemia may mask the signs of constriction

CAUSES
• Idiopathic
• Viral: Coxsackie, echo, adenovirus, Epstein-Barr, mumps
• Bacterial: Haemophilus (especially children), Staphylococcus, Pneumococcus, Salmonella, Meningococcus, Lyme disease, Legionella, Mycoplasma
• Fungal: Candida, Histoplasmosis, Aspergillus, Nocardia
• Mycobacterial: Mycobacterium tuberculosis
• Parasites, protozoa
• Neoplastic: Breast, lung, lymphoma, mesothelioma
• Drug-induced: Procainamide, hydralazine, bleomycin, phenytoin, minoxidil, mesalamine and perhaps others
• Connective tissue disease: Systemic lupus erythematosis, rheumatoid arthritis, scleroderma, acute rheumatic fever
• Radiation
• Myocardial infarction, Dressler's
• Postpericardiotomy
• Uremia
• Myxedema
• Cholesterol pericarditis
• Aortic dissection
• Sarcoidosis
• Pancreatitis
• Inflammatory bowel disease
• AIDS
• Chylopericardium

RISK FACTORS
• Chest trauma

DIAGNOSIS

DIFFERENTIAL DIAGNOSIS
• Acute myocardial infarction
• Pneumonia with pleurisy
• Pulmonary emboli
• Aortic dissection
• Pneumothorax
• Mediastinal emphysema
• Cholecystitis
• Pancreatitis

LABORATORY
• Leukocytosis and increased ESR
• May see elevated creatine kinase (CK), lactate dehydrogenase (LDH), serum glutamic-oxaloacetic (SGOT)
Drugs that may alter lab results: N/A
Disorders that may alter lab results: N/A

PATHOLOGICAL FINDINGS
Micro: acute inflammation

SPECIAL TESTS
• Electrocardiogram
• Echocardiogram
• Right heart catheterization

IMAGING
• Chest x-ray - small pleural effusion, transient infiltrates; "water bottle" silhouette in large associated pericardial effusion
• Chest CT or MRI in suspected constrictive pericarditis may reveal calcified or thickened pericardium; delineate effusions

DIAGNOSTIC PROCEDURES
• Pericardiocentesis
• Pericardial biopsy

TREATMENT

APPROPRIATE HEALTH CARE
• Outpatient unless signs of complications
• Inpatient with complications (hemodynamic compromise or effusion present)

GENERAL MEASURES N/A

SURGICAL MEASURES Pericardiectomy may be required if drugs are not effective

ACTIVITY No restrictions; limited by patients symptoms only

DIET No restriction. If patient overweight, suggest a weight loss program.

PATIENT EDUCATION Since 15% of patients have a recurrence, must educate for return of symptoms and followup

MEDICATIONS

DRUG(S) OF CHOICE
Uncomplicated: aspirin 650 mg q4h. If effective, continue for 2 weeks.
Contraindications: Hypersensitivity to aspirin, known coagulopathy
Precautions: Use with caution in patients with asthma, nasal polyps, severe carditis, pregnancy in the third trimester, history of GI disturbances or bleeding, bleeding disorders or diathesis, telangiectasis, anticoagulation, renal or hepatic dysfunction
Significant possible interactions:
Acetaminophen, acetazolamide, ammonium chloride, antacids, aurothioglucose, chlorpropamide, cimetidine, corticosteroids, diclofenac, dicumarol, diltiazem, dipyridamole, etodolac, flurbiprofen, ibuprofen, indomethacin, insulin, ketorolac, meclofenamate, mefenamic acid, methotrexate, metoclopramide, naproxen, nitroglycerin, nizatidine, penicillin G, phenprocoumon, phenylbutazone, phenytoin piroxicam, probenicid, protirelin, quinidine, spironolactone, sulfinpyrazone, sulfonylureas, sulindac, suprofen, tolmetin, valproic acid, warfarin

ALTERNATIVE DRUGS
• Ibuprofen 400-600 mg q6h for 2 weeks
• Indomethacin 25-50 mg q6-8h for 2 weeks
• Colchicine 1 mg q day
• Azathioprine, phenylbutazone, prednisone 60 mg q day x 2-3 days and quickly taper (last resort)

FOLLOWUP

PATIENT MONITORING
• Followup patients in office in 2 weeks and re-evaluate cardiac status and symptomatology
• Repeat chest x-ray and electrocardiogram should be considered at 4 weeks

PREVENTION/AVOIDANCE   N/A

POSSIBLE COMPLICATIONS
• Pericardial tamponade
• Recurrence of pericarditis
• Non-compressive effusion
• Chronic, constrictive pericarditis

EXPECTED COURSE/PROGNOSIS
• The majority of patients have complete resolution of pain and symptoms during the 2 weeks of therapy
• Fifteen per cent will have at least one recurrence in the first few months
• A rare patient may become refractory and require corticosteroids or pericardiectomy
• The hemodynamic effects of effusions depends on the volume and rapidity of development
• A very small percentage of patients can develop signs of right sided heart failure secondary to constriction. These patients are best treated with pericardiectomy.

MISCELLANEOUS

ASSOCIATED CONDITIONS Dependent on etiology

AGE-RELATED FACTORS
Pediatric: N/A
Geriatric: N/A
Others: N/A

PREGNANCY N/A

SYNONYMS Acute nonsuppurative pericarditis

ICD-9-CM
• 420.91
• 420.99 other acute pericarditis

SEE ALSO N/A

OTHER NOTES N/A

ABBREVIATIONS N/A

REFERENCES
• Rippe JM: Intensive Care Medicine. 1st Ed. Boston/Toronto, Little, Brown, 1985
• Bennett JC, Plum F, eds: Cecil Textbook of Medicine. 20th Ed. Philadelphia, W.B. Saunders Co., 1996
• Harvey AM: The Principles and Practice of Medicine. 22nd Ed. Norwalk, CT, Appleton & Lange, 1988
• Shabetai R: Diseases of the Pericardium. Cardio Clinics Nov;1990
Illustrations: N/A
Internet references: http://www.5mcc.com

Author(s)
Darell E. Heiselman, DO, FCCM, FACP, FACC, FCCP

Peritonitis, acute

BASICS

DESCRIPTION Acute inflammation of the visceral and parietal peritoneum
System(s) affected: Gastrointestinal, Endocrine/Metabolic, Cardiovascular
Genetics: No known genetic pattern
Incidence/Prevalence in USA: Common
Predominant age: None
Predominant sex: Male > Female

SIGNS AND SYMPTOMS
• Acute abdominal pain
• Fever
• Nausea
• Vomiting
• Constipation
• Abdominal pain exacerbated by motion
• Abdominal distention
• Dyspnea
• Diffuse abdominal rebound
• Generalized abdominal rigidity
• Decreased bowel sounds
• Abdominal hyper-resonance to percussion
• Hypotension
• Tachycardia
• Hippocratic facies
• Tachypnea
• Dehydration
• Ascites

CAUSES
• Primary - spontaneous bacterial peritonitis
  ◊ Ascites associated with cirrhosis,
nephrotic syndrome
• Secondary
  ◊ Following abdominal trauma
  ◊ Penetrating wounds
  ◊ Continuous ambulatory peritoneal dialysis
  ◊ Perforation
  ◊ Appendicitis
  ◊ Colitis - infectious, inflammatory
  ◊ Peptic ulcer perforation
  ◊ Gangrene of the bowel
  ◊ Diverticulitis
  ◊ Pancreatitis
  ◊ Postoperative
  ◊ Acute cholecystitis

RISK FACTORS
• Recent surgery
• Advanced liver disease
• Corticosteroid medication
• Nephrotic syndrome
• Continuous ambulatory peritoneal dialysis

DIAGNOSIS

DIFFERENTIAL DIAGNOSIS
• Abscess formation (subdiaphragmatic, subhepatic, peritoneal, pelvic)
• Other causes of ileus (volvulus, intussusception)
• Mesenteric adenitis
• Appendicitis
• Pancreatitis

LABORATORY
• Positive culture of peritoneal aspirate
• Leukocytosis
• Increased BUN
• Hemoconcentration
• Positive blood culture
• Metabolic acidosis
• Respiratory acidosis
• elevated amylase
• Ascitic fluid analysis
Drugs that may alter lab results:
Antibiotics prior to blood studies
Disorders that may alter lab results: N/A

PATHOLOGICAL FINDINGS
• Peritoneum - generalized fibrinopurulent exudate
• Peritoneum - polymorphonuclear infiltration

SPECIAL TESTS N/A

IMAGING
• Abdominal film - free air in peritoneal cavity, large bowel dilatation, small bowel dilatation, intestinal wall edema
• Chest x-ray - elevated diaphragm
• CT - intra-abdominal mass, ascites
• Sonography - intra-abdominal mass, ascites

DIAGNOSTIC PROCEDURES N/A

TREATMENT

APPROPRIATE HEALTH CARE Inpatient

GENERAL MEASURES
• Treat paralytic ileus (nasogastric decompression)
• Treat dehydration
• Antibiotics are started empirically to cover a broad spectrum of organisms. The choice of antibiotic may be altered after culture results are obtained.
• Respiratory support if needed
• IV fluids
• Blood transfusions (sometimes)

SURGICAL MEASURES Treat underlying condition(s) and infection (by surgery if necessary)

ACTIVITY Bedrest until infection is under control

DIET
• IV fluids and electrolytes
• Oral feedings only after return of bowel sounds, and passage of flatus and/or feces
• Total parenteral nutrition may be necessary

PATIENT EDUCATION N/A

MEDICATIONS

DRUG(S) OF CHOICE
- Monotherapy:
  ◊ Cefotaxime 2 g IV q8h
  or
  ◊ Ceftriaxone 2 g IV q24h
- Combination therapies:
  ◊ Ampicillin 1-2 g q6h plus gentamicin 1.5 mg/kg/dose plus clindamycin 600-900 mg q8h
  or
  ◊ Ampicillin plus gentamicin plus metronidazole 500 mg q6-8h
  or
  ◊ Gentamicin plus clindamycin
  or
  ◊ Imipenem 0.5-1.0 g q6-8h
- Continuous abdominal peritoneal dialysis:
  ◊ Intraperitoneal vancomycin 20 mg/L dialysate + 1 gm IV "load" plus gentamicin (6-8 mg/L dialysate)
  or
  ◊ Intraperitoneal ceftazidime
- Other:
  ◊ Morphine 2-10 mg IV or IM q3-4h, as needed, for pain
  ◊ Meperidine 50-100 mg IM

Contraindications: Refer to manufacturer's literature
Precautions: Refer to manufacturer's literature
Significant possible interactions: Refer to manufacturer's literature

ALTERNATIVE DRUGS
- Initial therapy with a third-generation cephalosporin (e.g., cefotaxime or ceftriaxone)
- Antibiotics, other than those mentioned, if indicated by culture of blood or peritoneal fluid

FOLLOWUP

PATIENT MONITORING
Inpatient and sometimes intensive care unit as indicated

PREVENTION/AVOIDANCE
Prophylactic antibiotics during abdominal surgery

POSSIBLE COMPLICATIONS
- Hypovolemic consequences
- Septicemia
- Septic shock
- Acute renal failure
- Acute respiratory insufficiency
- Liver failure
- Abscess formation

EXPECTED COURSE/PROGNOSIS
- Fully developed paralytic ileus requires 48 hours for recovery
- Mortality dependent on - age, duration, cause, and on pre-existing conditions

MISCELLANEOUS

ASSOCIATED CONDITIONS
- Abscesses: Subdiaphragmatic, subhepatic, peritoneal, pelvic
- Ileus

AGE-RELATED FACTORS
Pediatric: Get pediatric and surgical consultation, if available
Geriatric: Mortality greater in this age group. Symptoms may be muted.
Others: N/A

PREGNANCY Ruptured ectopic pregnancy may lead to peritonitis

SYNONYMS N/A

ICD-9-CM
567.2 acute generalized peritonitis

SEE ALSO N/A

OTHER NOTES N/A

ABBREVIATIONS N/A

REFERENCES
- Shands JW Jr: Empiric antibiotic therapy of abdominal sepsis and serious perioperative infections. Surg Clinics of North Amer 1993;73(2):291-306
- Isselbacher KJ, et al, eds: Harrison's Principles of Internal Medicine. 13th Ed. New York, McGraw-Hill, 1994
- Sleisenger MH, Fordtran JS, eds: Gastrointestinal Disease: Pathophysiology, Diagnosis, Management.5th Ed. Philadelphia, W.B. Saunders Co., 1994
- Bennett JC, Plum F, eds: Cecil Textbook of Medicine. 20th Ed. Philadelphia, W.B. Saunders Co., 1996
- Sabiston DC Jr, ed: Textbook of Surgery: The Biological Basis of Modern Surgical Practice. 14th Ed. Philadelphia, W.B. Saunders Co., 1991
- Ewald GA, McKenziem CR, eds: Manual of Medical Therapeutics. 28th Ed. Boston, Little-Brown & Co., 1995
- Sanford JP, Gilbert DN, Moellering RC, Sande MA. The Sanford Guide to Antimicrobial Therapy - 1997. Antimicrobial Therapy, Inc: Vienna, VA, 1997
Illustrations: N/A
Internet references: http://www.5mcc.com

Author(s)
Alan Adelman, MD, MS

Pertussis

BASICS

DESCRIPTION Pertussis or whooping cough is a highly communicable, respiratory bacterial infection. Characteristically, it produces a paroxysmal spasmodic cough, ending in prolonged high-pitched inspiratory whoop or crow. Transmission is by direct contact and patients are contagious for 3 weeks. Incubation period averages 7 to 14 days (maximum 3 weeks). Usual course - acute, but protracted (lasts 4-12 weeks after catarrhal period).
System(s) affected: Pulmonary
Genetics: N/A
Incidence/Prevalence in USA:
• 1.740 cases/100,000 people
• Annual average cases - 3,500, with 10 deaths
• Increasing as immunization rates decline.
Predominant age: 3 months-6 years (infants comprise about half of the cases)
Predominant sex: Female > Male

SIGNS AND SYMPTOMS
• Cough paroxysms
• Staccato cough
• Mild fever
• Rhinorrhea
• Anorexia
• "Whoop" cough
• Apnea, episodic
• Posttussive inspiratory gasp
• Posttussive emesis

CAUSES Bordetella pertussis. Bordetella parapertussis and Bordetella bronchiseptica produce a similar, but milder clinical illness.

RISK FACTORS
• Unimmunized children
• Contact with an infected person
• Epidemic exposure
• Pregnancy

DIAGNOSIS

DIFFERENTIAL DIAGNOSIS
• Common cold
• Adenoviral syndromes
• Bronchiolitis
• Influenza
• Bacterial pneumonias
• Cystic fibrosis
• Tuberculosis
• Interstitial pneumonitis
• Foreign body

LABORATORY
• ELISA: IgA against Bordetella pertussis
• WBC: elevated (15,000-60,000) with marked lymphocytosis
• Bordetella pertussis on Bordet-Gengou culture medium
Drugs that may alter lab results: N/A
Disorders that may alter lab results: N/A

PATHOLOGICAL FINDINGS
• Focal emphysema
• Mucopurulent exudate
• Patchy ulceration of respiratory epithelium

SPECIAL TESTS N/A

IMAGING Chest x-ray - focal atelectasis, peribronchial cuffing, emphysema

DIAGNOSTIC PROCEDURES N/A

TREATMENT

APPROPRIATE HEALTH CARE
Hospitalization for seriously ill infants. Outpatient for milder cases.

GENERAL MEASURES
• General supportive, skilled nursing care
• Isolation and quarantine for 4 weeks; 1 week after erythromycin started
• Parenteral fluid therapy if needed
• Oxygen
• Careful observation for apnea in young infants, and, to avoid stimuli that trigger paroxysms
• Mechanical ventilation
• Nutritional support - may require tube feedings in infants

SURGICAL MEASURES N/A

ACTIVITY Rest during active phase in quiet environment

DIET Encourage extra fluids. May need to provide small frequent meals to assure adequate nutrition.

PATIENT EDUCATION For patient education materials favorably reviewed on this topic, contact: American Academy of Pediatrics, 141 Northwest Point Blvd., P.O. Box 927, Elk Grove Village, IL 60009-0927, (800)433-9016

MEDICATIONS

DRUG(S) OF CHOICE
• Erythromycin, 30-40 mg/kg/day divided doses every 6 hours for 14 days
• Other antibiotics for bacterial complications such as bronchopneumonia or otitis media
• Antibiotics do not alter course of illness unless given very early. They prevent transmission.
Contraindications: Do not use cough suppressants
Precautions: N/A
Significant possible interactions: N/A

ALTERNATIVE DRUGS
• Steroids and/or theophylline have been suggested for treatment of severely ill patients (their effectiveness and potential hazards require further controlled studies)
• Beta-2 agonists may help with cough paroxysms.

 FOLLOWUP

PATIENT MONITORING
• Intensive care unit may be necessary for severely ill infants
• Older children and adults with mild cases do not need to be confined to bed

PREVENTION/AVOIDANCE
• Isolate infected persons
• Active immunization for all infants, usually combined with diphtheria and tetanus toxoids (DPT). Immunization or booster not recommended after age 6 years.
• Erythromycin - for susceptible children (under 2 months or unvaccinated) if they are exposed to an infected person during the contagious period

POSSIBLE COMPLICATIONS
• Can infect up to 90% of household members who are not immune
• Death in infants
• Pneumonia
• Hypoxic encephalopathy
• Coma
• Otitis media
• Tuberculosis activation
• Epistaxis
• Hernia
• Re-induction of paroxysmal coughing (for several months) especially with upper respiratory infections
• Convulsions
• Cerebral hemorrhage
• Neurologic disorders
• Weight loss
• Hemoptysis
• Atelectasis

EXPECTED COURSE/PROGNOSIS
Complete recovery

 MISCELLANEOUS

ASSOCIATED CONDITIONS
• Otitis media
• Bronchopneumonia
• Failure to thrive

AGE-RELATED FACTORS
Pediatric: Most serious and highest mortality in infants less than 6 months of age (death usually due to complications)
Geriatric: May be more serious in this age group
Others: N/A

PREGNANCY N/A

SYNONYMS
Whooping cough

ICD-9-CM
033 Whooping cough

SEE ALSO
• Immunizations
• Otitis media
• Failure to thrive (FTT)
• Common cold
• Adenovirus infections
• Bronchiolitis
• Influenza
• Pneumonia, bacterial
• Cystic fibrosis
• Tuberculosis

OTHER NOTES
• Do not use cough suppressants
• Reporting of selected adverse reactions with certain vaccines is now required by the National Childhood Vaccine Injury Act of 1986. Toll-free information number - (800)822-7967.

ABBREVIATIONS N/A

REFERENCES
• Mandell GL, ed: Principles and Practice of Infectious Diseases. 4th Ed. New York, Churchill Livingstone, 1995
• Centers for Disease Control: National Childhood Vaccine Injury Act: Requirements for permanent vaccination records and for reporting of selected events after vaccination. MMWR 1988;37:197-200
Illustrations: N/A
Internet references: http://www.5mcc.com

Author(s)
Nancy N. Dambro, MD

Pharyngitis

BASICS

DESCRIPTION Inflammation of the pharynx most commonly caused by acute infection. Group A streptococcus is a focus of diagnosis due to its potential for preventable rheumatic sequelae.
System(s) affected: Gastrointestinal
Genetics: Individuals with a positive family history of rheumatic fever have a higher risk of rheumatic sequelae following an untreated group A beta hemolytic streptococcal infection
Incidence/Prevalence in USA:
• Estimated 30 million cases diagnosed yearly
• 11% of all school age children visit a physician annually with pharyngitis
• 12-25% of sore throats seen by physicians
• Incidence of rheumatic fever is decreasing with estimate of 64 cases per 100,000
Predominant age:
• Pharyngitis occurs in all age groups
• Streptococcal infection has greatest incidence 5 to 18 years of age
Predominant sex: Male = Female

SIGNS AND SYMPTOMS
• Sore throat
• Enlarged tonsils
• Pharyngeal erythema
• Tonsillar exudates
• Soft palate petechiae
• Cervical adenopathy
• Absence of cough, hoarseness, or lower respiratory symptoms
• Fever (> 102.5°F [39.1°C] suggests Streptococcus)
• Scarlet fever rash: punctate erythematous macules with reddened flexor creases and circumoral pallor (Streptococcal pharyngitis)
• Gray pseudomembrane found in diphtheria and occasionally, mononucleosis
• Characteristic erythematous based clear vesicles in herpes stomatitis
• Anorexia
• Chills
• Malaise
• Headache
• Conjunctivitis, more commonly with adenovirus infections

CAUSES
• Acute - bacterial:
  ◊ Group A beta-hemolytic streptococci
  ◊ Neisseria gonorrhoeae
  ◊ Corynebacterium diphtheriae (diphtheria)
  ◊ Haemophilus influenzae
  ◊ Moraxella (Branhamella) catarrhalis
  ◊ Group C and G streptococcus, rarely
• Acute - virus:
  ◊ Rhinovirus
  ◊ Adenovirus
  ◊ Parainfluenza virus
  ◊ Coxsackievirus
  ◊ Coronavirus
  ◊ Echovirus
  ◊ Herpes simplex virus
  ◊ Epstein-Barr virus (mononucleosis)
  ◊ Cytomegalovirus

• Chronic
  ◊ More likely non-infectious
  ◊ Irritation from post-nasal discharge of chronic allergic rhinitis
    ◊ Chemical irritation
    ◊ Neoplasms and vasculitides

RISK FACTORS
• Group A beta hemolytic streptococcal epidemics occur
• Age (young are more susceptible)
• Family history
• Close quarters, such as in new military recruits
• Immunosuppression
• Fatigue
• Smoking
• Excess alcohol consumption
• Oral sex
• Diabetes mellitus
• Recent illness

DIAGNOSIS

DIFFERENTIAL DIAGNOSIS
• See causative factors
• Sore throat can be seen with leukopenia

LABORATORY
• Blood agar throat culture from swab. Bacitracin disc sensitivity of hemolytic colonies suggest group A streptococci.
• Rapid screening for streptococci can be done from throat swab with antigen agglutination kits. 5-10% false negatives lead some to suggest routine backup of all negatives with blood agar culture.
• Leukocytosis (if bacterial)
Drugs that may alter lab results: N/A
Disorders that may alter lab results: N/A

PATHOLOGICAL FINDINGS Culture of pathogens to identify causes

SPECIAL TESTS
• Special tests usually done only if history is suggestive
• Screening for gonococcal infection requires warm Thayer-Martin plate
• Viruses can be cultured in special media
• Mono spot test for Epstein-Barr virus
• Gram stain can be suggestive
• Streptococcal isolates can be immunologically typed

IMAGING N/A

DIAGNOSTIC PROCEDURES History and physical probably only 50% accurate. Laboratory required unless in epidemic setting.

TREATMENT

APPROPRIATE HEALTH CARE
Outpatient

GENERAL MEASURES
• Salt water gargles
• Acetaminophen
• Dyclonine lozenges
• Cool-mist humidifier

SURGICAL MEASURES N/A

ACTIVITY As tolerated

DIET No restrictions. Encourage extra fluids.

PATIENT EDUCATION
• Important to complete 10 day course of antibiotics regardless of symptom response
• Patients presumed to be non-infectious after 24 hours of antibiotic coverage

MEDICATIONS

DRUG(S) OF CHOICE
For streptococcal pharyngitis, penicillin is the standard. All choices should have complete 10 day course.
• Penicillin V 250 mg tid (25-50 mg/kg/day), or
• For penicillin allergic patients, erythromycin ethylsuccinate 300 to 400 mg tid (30 mg/kg/day), or
• Cephalexin 250 mg tid (30 mg/kg/day)
Contraindications: Allergy to specific antibiotic
Precautions: Refer to manufacturer's profile of each drug
Significant possible interactions: Refer to manufacturer's profile of each drug

ALTERNATIVE DRUGS
• Treatment of carrier state is difficult, usually requiring addition of rifampin to penicillin regimen
• Penicillin is the most documented treatment to prevent rheumatic sequelae but cephalosporins have lower rate of bacteriologic failure
• The newer macrolides, azithromycin and clarithromycin, are also effective against streptococcal pharyngitis, but more expensive. The chief advantage of azithromycin is its 5 day course with 10 day effective duration.
• Other cephalosporins are generally effective for streptococcal pharyngitis, but more expensive than cephalexin

FOLLOWUP

PATIENT MONITORING
• Routine followup cultures not necessary
• Telephone consult for duration of symptoms

PREVENTION/AVOIDANCE Avoid contact with infected people

POSSIBLE COMPLICATIONS
• Rheumatic fever
• Post-streptococcal glomerulonephritis
• Peritonsillar abscess
• Systemic infection
• Otitis media
• Mastoiditis
• Septicemia
• Rhinitis
• Sinusitis
• Pneumonia

EXPECTED COURSE/PROGNOSIS
• Streptococcal pharyngeal infection runs a 5-7 day course with peak of fever at 2-3 days
• Symptoms will resolve spontaneously without treatment, but rheumatic complications are still possible
• Suppurative complications such as peritonsillar abscess require surgical intervention

MISCELLANEOUS

ASSOCIATED CONDITIONS N/A

AGE-RELATED FACTORS
Pediatric: N/A
Geriatric: N/A
Others: N/A

PREGNANCY N/A

SYNONYMS
• Sore throat
• Tonsillitis
• Streptococcal throat

ICD-9-CM
• 462 Acute pharyngitis
• 463 Acute tonsillitis
• 472.1 Chronic pharyngitis
• 474.0 Chronic tonsillitis
• 034.0 Streptococcal sore throat
• 034.1 Scarlet fever

SEE ALSO
• Rheumatic fever
• Herpes simplex
• Mononucleosis

OTHER NOTES Unless clinical presentation is unusual, treatment is based on presence or absence of group A streptococci

ABBREVIATIONS N/A

REFERENCES
• Pichichero ME: Controversies in the treatment of streptococcal pharyngitis. Amer Fam Phys 1990;42(6):1558-1560
• Bennett JC, Plum F, eds: Cecil Textbook of Medicine. 20th Ed. Philadelphia, WB Saunders Co, 1996
Illustrations: N/A
Internet references: http://www.5mcc.com

Author(s)
David E. Burtner, MD

Pheochromocytoma

BASICS

DESCRIPTION Catecholamine-producing tumor. In 90% of cases, the tumors are found in the adrenal medulla, but may also be found in other tissues derived from neural crest cells.
System(s) affected: Endocrine/Metabolic
Genetics: N/A
Incidence/Prevalence in USA:
• 0.01% to 0.1% of the hypertensive population
Predominant age: Any age, peak incidence ages 30 to 60 years
Predominant sex: Male = Female

SIGNS AND SYMPTOMS
• Paroxysmal spells (the "5 P's")
  ◊ Pressure - sudden increase in blood pressure
  ◊ Pain - headache, chest and abdominal pain
  ◊ Perspiration
  ◊ Palpitation
  ◊ Pallor
• Additional symptoms
  ◊ Constipation
  ◊ Tremor
  ◊ Weight loss
  ◊ Anxiety
• Signs
  ◊ Hypertension - paroxysmal in half of the patients
  ◊ Orthostatic hypotension
  ◊ Grade II to IV retinopathy
  ◊ Fever
  ◊ Hyperglycemia
  ◊ Hypercalcemia
  ◊ Erythrocytosis

CAUSES
• Catecholamine-producing tumor - "Rule of 10:"
  ◊ 10% are extra-adrenal
  ◊ 10% are multiple or bilateral
  ◊ 10% are malignant
  ◊ 10% recur after surgical removal
  ◊ 10% occur in children
  ◊ 10% are familial

RISK FACTORS
• Familial pheochromocytoma
• Multiple endocrine neoplasia types II A and B
• Neurofibromatosis
• Von Hippel-Lindau syndrome

DIAGNOSIS

DIFFERENTIAL DIAGNOSIS
• Labile essential hypertension
• Anxiety and panic attacks
• Paroxysmal cardiac arrhythmia
• Thyrotoxicosis
• Menopausal syndrome
• Hypoglycemia
• Mastocytosis
• Withdrawal of adrenergic-inhibiting medications
• Angina
• Hyperventilation
• Migraine headache
• Amphetamine or cocaine use
• Sympathomimetic ingestion

LABORATORY
• Elevated 24-h urine metanephrine
• Elevated 24-h urine or plasma catecholamines measured by high performance liquid chromatography (HPLC)
• If results equivocal or normal, repeat 24-h urine collection with a spell
Drugs that may alter lab results:
• Increased by:
  ◊ Amphetamines
  ◊ Tricyclic antidepressants
  ◊ Clonidine or other drug withdrawal
  ◊ Labetalol
  ◊ Ethanol
  ◊ Methyldopa
  ◊ Sotalol
  ◊ Levodopa
• Decreased by:
  ◊ Central alpha-2 agonists
  ◊ Reserpine
Disorders that may alter lab results:
Major physical stress (e.g., surgery, stroke)

PATHOLOGICAL FINDINGS
Catecholamine-producing tumor in the adrenal medulla, para-aortic sympathetic chain, wall of the urinary bladder, sympathetic chain in the neck or mediastinum

SPECIAL TESTS Clonidine suppression test, suppression/provocative tests

IMAGING
• Computerized abdominal imaging (MRI preferred over CT)
• I-123: I-metaiodobenzylguanidine scan
• In-111: pentetreotide scan

DIAGNOSTIC PROCEDURES N/A

TREATMENT

APPROPRIATE HEALTH CARE Inpatient surgery

GENERAL MEASURES
• Combined alpha- and beta-adrenergic blockade
• Cardiovascular and hemodynamic variables must be monitored closely

SURGICAL MEASURES
• High risk surgical procedure
• Experienced surgeon/anesthesiologist team required

ACTIVITY No limitations

DIET High in salt content preoperatively

PATIENT EDUCATION N/A

MEDICATIONS

DRUG(S) OF CHOICE
• Combined alpha- and beta-adrenergic blockade required preoperatively
• Initiate alpha-blockade first - phenoxybenzamine (Dibenzyline) 10 mg daily and increase by 10-20 mg every 2 days as needed to control blood pressure and paroxysmal spells (average dose is 0.5-1.0 mg/kg daily)
• Beta-blockade after alpha-blockade is established - propranolol (Inderal) 10 mg q 6 hrs initially and increase as necessary to control tachycardia
• Acute hypertensive crises should be treated with phentolamine (Regitine) or nitroprusside administered intravenously
Contraindications: Beta-adrenergic blockade in patients with asthma, sinus bradycardia and greater than first degree block, or congestive heart failure. Avoid beta-blockers with intrinsic sympathomimetic activity
Precautions:
• Beta-adrenergic blockade alone may result in more severe hypertension due to the unopposed alpha-adrenergic stimulation; patients should be cautioned about postural hypotension
• Beta-adrenergic blockade is initiated at low doses of a short acting agent due to the possible side effect of pulmonary edema in the patient with catecholamine myocardiopathy
Significant possible interactions: For beta-adrenergic blockade - verapamil, phenytoin, phenobarbitone, rifampin, chlorpromazine, cimetidine

ALTERNATIVE DRUGS
• Alpha-adrenergic blocking agents - prazosin (Minipress), terazosin (Hytrin), doxazosin (Cardura)
• Beta-adrenergic blocking agents - nadolol (Corgard), atenolol (Tenormin), metoprolol (Lopressor)
• Combined beta- and alpha-adrenergic blocker - labetalol (Normodyne, TranDate)
• Catecholamine synthesis inhibitor - metyrosine (Demser)

FOLLOWUP

PATIENT MONITORING
• Daily blood pressure monitoring prior to surgery
• Intra-operative hemodynamic monitoring
• Two weeks postoperatively - 24-h urine for measurement of catecholamines and metanephrines; if normal, re-check annually for five years

PREVENTION/AVOIDANCE N/A

POSSIBLE COMPLICATIONS
• Postural hypotension with alpha-adrenergic blockade
• Pulmonary edema with beta-adrenergic blockade
• Intra-operative hypertensive crisis

EXPECTED COURSE/PROGNOSIS
• The survival rate after removal of a benign pheochromocytoma is nearly that of age- and sex-matched controls
• For malignant pheochromocytoma, the 5-year survival rate is less than 50%

MISCELLANEOUS

ASSOCIATED CONDITIONS
• Multiple endocrine neoplasia type IIA (medullary thyroid carcinoma and primary hyperparathyroidism)
• Multiple endocrine neoplasia type IIB (medullary thyroid carcinoma and mucosal neuromas)
• Neurofibromatosis
• Von Hippel-Lindau syndrome (retinal angiomatosis and cerebellar hemangioblastoma)
• Ataxia-telangiectasia
• Tuberous sclerosis
• Sturge-Weber syndrome
• Cholelithiasis
• Renal artery stenosis

AGE-RELATED FACTORS
Pediatric: N/A
Geriatric: N/A
Others: N/A

PREGNANCY
• First and second trimester - surgical resection
• Third trimester - cesarean section and removal of the pheochromocytoma in the same operation

SYNONYMS Paraganglioma

ICD-9-CM 194.0

SEE ALSO Hypertension

OTHER NOTES All patients with paroxysmal spells and hypertension or with difficult to control hypertension should be screened

ABBREVIATIONS HPLC = high performance liquid chromatography

REFERENCES
• Young WF Jr: Pheochromocytoma: 1926-1993: Trends in Endocrinology and Metabolism 1993;4:122
• Bravo EL, Gifford RW: Pheochromocytoma: Diagnosis, localization, and management. N Engl J Med 1984;311:1298
• Young WF Jr: Spells: In search of a cause. Mayo Clin Proc 1995;70:757-765
Illustrations: 2 available on CD-ROM
Internet references: http://www.5mcc.com

Author(s)
William F. Young, Jr., MD

Phimosis & paraphimosis

BASICS

DESCRIPTION
• Phimosis: tightness of the penile foreskin which prevents it from being drawn back from over the glans
• Paraphimosis: constriction of glans penis by proximally placed phimotic foreskin
System(s) affected: Renal/Urologic, Reproductive, Skin/Exocrine
Genetics: N/A
Incidence/Prevalence in USA: 1% of males over 16 years of age
Predominant age: Infancy and adolescence
Predominant sex: Male only

SIGNS AND SYMPTOMS
• Phimosis
  ◊ Unretractable foreskin
  ◊ Pain on erection
  ◊ Superimposed balanitis
• Paraphimosis
  ◊ Penile pain
  ◊ Drainage
  ◊ Ulceration
  ◊ Swelling

CAUSES
• Phimosis
  ◊ "Physiologic" - present at birth and resolves spontaneously during the first 2-3 years of life by nocturnal erections which slowly dilate the phimotic ring
  ◊ Congenital - unresolved physiologic phimosis
  ◊ Acquired - recurrent infection or irritation
• Paraphimosis
  ◊ Foreskin not pulled back over the glans after cleaning, cystoscopy or catheter insertion

RISK FACTORS
• Phimosis
  ◊ Poor hygiene
  ◊ Diabetes
  ◊ Frequent diaper rash in infant
• Paraphimosis
  ◊ Presence of foreskin
  ◊ "Inexperienced" health care provider, i.e., leaving foreskin retracted after catheter placement

DIAGNOSIS

DIFFERENTIAL DIAGNOSIS
Penile lymphedema which can be related to insect bites, trauma or allergic reactions

LABORATORY   N/A
Drugs that may alter lab results: N/A
Disorders that may alter lab results: N/A

PATHOLOGICAL FINDINGS   N/A

SPECIAL TESTS   N/A

IMAGING   N/A

DIAGNOSTIC PROCEDURES   N/A

TREATMENT

APPROPRIATE HEALTH CARE
Outpatient except for complications

GENERAL MEASURES
Paraphimosis: Reduction if possible (should be done with the patient sedated). Place the middle and index fingers of both hands on the engorged skin proximal to the glans. Place both thumbs on glans and with gentle pressure pushing on the glans and pulling on foreskin, attempt reduction. If unsuccessful, a dorsal slit will be necessary with eventual circumcision after the edema resolves.

SURGICAL MEASURES
• Phimosis: Circumcision
• Paraphimosis: Dorsal slit with subsequent circumcision

ACTIVITY   No sexual activity following circumcision until healing is complete

DIET   No limitations

PATIENT EDUCATION   If the patient is uncircumcised, appropriate hygiene and care of the foreskin is necessary to prevent phimosis and paraphimosis

MEDICATIONS

DRUG(S) OF CHOICE N/A
Contraindications: N/A
Precautions: N/A
Significant possible interactions: N/A

ALTERNATIVE DRUGS N/A

FOLLOWUP

PATIENT MONITORING 1 week after reduction of paraphimosis and 1 to 2 weeks after a circumcision

PREVENTION/AVOIDANCE Good patient and parental education

POSSIBLE COMPLICATIONS
• Unreduced paraphimosis can lead to gangrene of the glans
• Posthitis (inflammation of the prepuce)

EXPECTED COURSE/PROGNOSIS
Complete resolution if treatment is carried out effectively

MISCELLANEOUS

ASSOCIATED CONDITIONS N/A

AGE-RELATED FACTORS
Pediatric:
• Recurrent balanitis, either chemical or infectious, can lead to an acquired phimosis
• Forced reduction of a physiologic foreskin can lead to chronic scarring and acquired phimosis
Geriatric: Recurrent infection and irritations (condom catheters) can lead to phimosis
Others: N/A

PREGNANCY N/A

SYNONYMS N/A

ICD-9-CM
605 Phimosis
605 Paraphimosis

SEE ALSO N/A

OTHER NOTES N/A

ABBREVIATIONS N/A

REFERENCES Kelalis PP, King LR, Belman AB: Clinical Pediatric Urology. 3rd Ed. Philadelphia, W.B. Saunders Co., 1991
Illustrations: N/A
Internet references: http://www.5mcc.com

Author(s)
James P. Miller, MD, FACS, FAAP
Timothy L. Black, MD, FACS, FAAP

Phobias

BASICS

DESCRIPTION A persistent irrational fear of a specific object, activity or situation that results in a compelling desire to avoid the perceived fear. Psychiatric conditions classified in Diagnostic and Statistical Manual of Mental Disorders (DSM-IV-R) as anxiety disorders. When confronted with the phobic stimulus, patient reacts with intense anxiety, usually realizes the fear is excessive or exaggerated. When a fear causes significant distress and interferes with normal functions of life, then it is considered a psychiatric disorder.
• Agoraphobia: Fear of being trapped in a situation where escape is impossible or difficult. Fear centers on (1) fear of being alone, (2) fear of being away from home and (3) fear of being in a place from where escape is difficult - seen most often in association with panic disorder.
• Simple phobia: Fear of a discrete stimulus such as animals, insects, heights, flying, closed spaces (claustrophobia), blood-injury phobia
• Social phobia: Fear of humiliation or embarrassment in social situations where person may be under scrutiny by others, e.g., performance anxiety, speaking in public, or fear of using public toilets

Incidence/Prevalence in USA: 1 month prevalence of all phobic conditions: 6.2%; lifetime prevalence: 12.5%
System(s) affected: Nervous
Genetics: No consistent genetic pattern
Predominant age:
• Agoraphobia - onset 18-35 (mean 24)
• Simple phobia fear of animals - onset usually in childhood (mean 4.4 years)
• Simple phobia fear of heights, claustrophobia - 4th decade
• Other simple phobias - mean 22.7 years
• Social phobia - late childhood, adolescence (mean 19 years)
Predominant sex:
• Female > Male, overall phobias
• Male = Female, social phobia

SIGNS AND SYMPTOMS
• Extreme anxiety when exposed to phobic stimulus
• Tremors
• Palpitations
• Sweating
• Blushing
• Dyspnea
• Dizziness
• Associated nausea

CAUSES
• Persistence or exaggeration of learned response, learned initially as a protective mechanism (such as avoidance of large dogs by small children)
• Social - learned maladaptive anxiety response to social situation

RISK FACTORS
• For all phobias - presence of another psychiatric disorder
• Separation anxiety in childhood
• Introverted or dependent personality

DIAGNOSIS

DIFFERENTIAL DIAGNOSIS
• For agoraphobia:
  ◊ Paranoid and psychotic states
  ◊ PTSD (posttraumatic stress disorder)
  ◊ Depression - but do not see the other aspects of depression (anhedonia, loss of appetite and libido, sleep disturbance-early morning awakening, frequent night awakening, difficulty falling asleep)
• For simple phobia:
  ◊ Schizophrenia - avoidance can be seen but usually in response to a delusion and patient does not realize that fear is excessive. Schizophrenia is intimately intertwined with delusion.
  ◊ PTSD - phobic avoidance seen and is associated with the original trauma
  ◊ Obsessive compulsive disorder (OCD) - avoidance associated with obsessions (such as dirt avoidance)
• For social phobia:
  ◊ Avoidant personality disorder - central fear in avoidant personality disorder is that of rejection, not of humiliation or embarrassment as in social phobia
  ◊ Paranoid personality disorder
  ◊ Schizophrenia

LABORATORY None
Drugs that may alter lab results: N/A
Disorders that may alter lab results: N/A

PATHOLOGICAL FINDINGS N/A

SPECIAL TESTS None

IMAGING N/A

DIAGNOSTIC PROCEDURES
• Careful history and observation of the patient
• Description of the behavior by patient, family or friends
• Psychiatric examination

TREATMENT

APPROPRIATE HEALTH CARE
Outpatient

GENERAL MEASURES
• Agoraphobia:
  ◊ Behavioral treatment
  ◊ Graduated exposure
  ◊ Different treatment required when agoraphobia is associated with panic disorder
• Simple phobia:
  ◊ In vivo or graduated exposure
  ◊ Fear of flying specifically - benzodiazepine
• Social phobia:
  ◊ Social skills training
  ◊ Graduated exposure
  ◊ Performance anxiety or situations where patient in a circumscribed setting - beta blocker

SURGICAL MEASURES N/A

ACTIVITY No restriction

DIET Consider restriction of stimulants - such as caffeine, nicotine, xanthines, sympathomimetics, which can overdrive anxiety. Phenelzine - requires tyramine free diet.

PATIENT EDUCATION
• Cognitive therapy
• Phobia clinic or group therapy, if available

MEDICATIONS

DRUG(S) OF CHOICE
• Agoraphobia - none recommended
• Simple phobia - none recommended, except for fear of flying. A benzodiazepine, such as alprazolam, may help. Initial dose as low as 0.25 mg titrated upward as needed.
• Social phobia (acute) - beta-blocker, e.g., propranolol (Inderal) 20-40 mg, 45-60 minutes before anticipated performance, atenolol 50-100 mg/day for more generalized social phobia
• Social phobia (chronic) - phenelzine , a MAO inhibitor, up to 60 mg/day, if social phobia more generalized and requires more constant medication (as opposed to the sporadic treatment for performance anxiety)

Contraindications:
• Beta-blocker - asthma or bronchospasm, congestive heart failure, bradycardia
• Phenelzine - not with other antidepressants, tyramine in diet, decongestants, diet pills, meperidine (Demerol), dextromethorphan, L-dopa, and sympathomimetics

Precautions:
• Do not abruptly discontinue alprazolam due to potential for withdrawal seizures
• Monitor blood pressure in patients taking beta-blockers
• Consult drug information before using phenelzine

Significant possible interactions:
• Phenelzine - significant dietary restrictions due to potential for hypertensive crisis.
• Drugs to avoid include: Sympathomimetics, TCA's, fluoxetine, CNS depressants.
• Consult drug information sources before adding new medications in patients.

ALTERNATIVE DRUGS N/A

FOLLOWUP

PATIENT MONITORING Outpatient as needed

PREVENTION/AVOIDANCE N/A

POSSIBLE COMPLICATIONS
• Avoidance behavior
• Episodic alcohol, barbiturate and anxiolytic abuse/overuse and dependence as patients try to self-medicate to ameliorate symptoms
• Development of mild depression

EXPECTED COURSE/PROGNOSIS
• Agoraphobia - usually associated with panic disorder, chronic. Often patient becomes more and more home-bound as condition continues.
• Simple phobia - some spontaneously remit as person ages (as in some simple phobias of childhood), alternatively some become chronic. Impairment can be minimal if object can be avoided (such as snakes). Although improvement occurs with in vivo exposure, phobia can recur after successful treatment.
• Social phobia - chronic course

MISCELLANEOUS

ASSOCIATED CONDITIONS
• For all phobias - depression, substance abuse
• Social and agoraphobia - panic attacks or panic disorder

AGE-RELATED FACTORS
Pediatric: Animal phobia mean age of onset 4.4 years
Geriatric: N/A
Others: N/A

PREGNANCY No data

SYNONYMS N/A

ICD-9-CM
• 300.22 Agoraphobia
• 300.29 Simple phobia
• 300. 23 Social phobia

SEE ALSO
• Obsessive compulsive disorder
• Post-traumatic stress disorder
• Anxiety
• Depression
• Schizophrenia
• Dissociative disorders

OTHER NOTES N/A

ABBREVIATIONS
PTSD = posttraumatic stress disorder

REFERENCES
• Diagnostic and Statistical Manual of Mental Disorders (DSM-IV-R). 4th Ed. American Psychiatric Association, Washington, DC, 1994
• Hales RE, Yudofsky SC, eds: Synopsis of Psychiatry. 1st Ed. Washington, DC, American Psychology Press, 1996
Illustrations: N/A
Internet references: http://www.5mcc.com

Author(s)
Brian J. Murray, MD

Photodermatitis

BASICS

DESCRIPTION Light-induced eruptions seen in a pattern of photo-distribution
• Phototoxic reactions - result of the acute toxic effect on skin of ultraviolet light alone (sunburn) or together with a photosensitizing substance (non-allergic)
• Photoallergic eruptions - a form of allergic dermatitis resulting from combined effects of a photosensitizing substance (drugs or chemical) plus ultraviolet light (immunologic/delayed hypersensitivity)
• Polymorphous light eruption (PLE) - chronic, intermittent light-induced eruption with erythematous papules, urticaria, or vesicles on areas exposed to sunlight
System(s) affected: Skin
Genetics: Predisposition occurs in inbred populations (e.g., Pima Indians)
Incidence/Prevalence in USA: Unknown
Predominant age: All ages
Predominant sex: Male = Female

SIGNS AND SYMPTOMS
• Phototoxic
   ◊ Erythema
   ◊ With increasing severity - vesicles and bullae
   ◊ Classic example - sunburn
   ◊ Nails may exhibit onycholysis
   ◊ Chronic - epidermal thickening, elastosis, telangiectasia and pigmentary changes
   ◊ Sharp lines of demarcation between involved and uninvolved skin (sunlight exposure)
   ◊ Phototoxic eruption due to topicals - area of application
   ◊ Usually develops shortly after sun exposure
   ◊ Hyperpigmentation may follow resolution
   ◊ Pain
• Photoallergic
   ◊ Papules with erythema and occasionally vesicles
   ◊ Area exposed to light with less distinct borders
   ◊ Usually delayed - 24 hours or more after exposure
   ◊ May spread to unexposed areas
   ◊ Pruritus
• Polymorphous light eruption (PLE)
   ◊ Erythematous papules
   ◊ Occasionally urticaria or vesicles
   ◊ Scattered over sun exposed areas with normal skin in between
   ◊ Can spread to non-exposed areas
   ◊ Often flares in spring or early summer
   ◊ Desensitization affect (less over the course of the summer)
   ◊ Burning or pruritus may precede lesions

CAUSES
• Sunlight
• Phenothiazines
• Diuretics
• Tetracyclines
• Sulfonamides
• Oral contraceptives
• Topicals - psoralens, coal tars, photo-active dyes (eosin, acridine orange)

RISK FACTORS N/A

DIAGNOSIS

DIFFERENTIAL DIAGNOSIS Systemic lupus erythematosus

LABORATORY Antinuclear antibody (ANA) to rule out systemic lupus erythematosus
Drugs that may alter lab results: N/A
Disorders that may alter lab results: N/A

PATHOLOGICAL FINDINGS Nonspecific

SPECIAL TESTS
• Photo-testing
• Photopatch testing
• Skin biopsy - to rule out other disorders

IMAGING N/A

DIAGNOSTIC PROCEDURES Physical examination and medical history

TREATMENT

APPROPRIATE HEALTH CARE
Outpatient

GENERAL MEASURES
• Avoid sunlight/limit exposure
• Protective clothing/sunscreens
• Ice packs/cold water compresses

SURGICAL MEASURES N/A

ACTIVITY Avoid sunlight

DIET No special diet

PATIENT EDUCATION
• Avoidance of sunlight
• Avoidance of photosensitizing drugs
• Protective clothing
• Sunscreens

MEDICATIONS

DRUG(S) OF CHOICE
• Topical corticosteroids (betamethasone valerate 0.1% cream)
• NSAIDs (indomethacin 25 mg tid; aspirin; others)
• Prednisone for severe reactions (0.5-1 mg/kg/d) for 3-10 days
• Antihistamines for pruritus (hydroxyzine 25-50 mg qid)
• Sunscreens for prevention. Use broad-spectrum sunscreen to block both UVA and UVB. PABA may aggravate photodermatitis in sensitized patients (due to the sulfa moiety).
Contraindications: Refer to manufacturer's profile of each drug
Precautions: Refer to manufacturer's profile of each drug
Significant possible interactions: Refer to manufacturer's profile of each drug

ALTERNATIVE DRUGS N/A

FOLLOWUP

PATIENT MONITORING As necessary for persistence or recurrence

PREVENTION/AVOIDANCE
• Sunlight avoidance/protective clothing
• Identification and avoidance of causative drugs (see under Causes)
• Sunscreens - apply before exposure
  ◊ Zinc oxide - opaque, cosmetically less acceptable
  ◊ Chemical - use sun-protective factor > 15 for maximum protection; substantively resistant to sweat and swimming; cosmetically more acceptable

POSSIBLE COMPLICATIONS N/A

EXPECTED COURSE/PROGNOSIS
Good with avoidance/protection measures

MISCELLANEOUS

ASSOCIATED CONDITIONS
• Sunlight aggravation of systemic lupus
• Persistent light reactivity
• Actinic reticuloid

AGE-RELATED FACTORS N/A
Pediatric: N/A
Geriatric: More likely to experience adverse reactions to causative drugs
Others: N/A

PREGNANCY N/A

SYNONYMS
• Sun poisoning

ICD-9-CM
• 692.79 due to solar radiation, other
• 692.89 due to other specified agents, other

SEE ALSO N/A

OTHER NOTES N/A

ABBREVIATIONS
NSAID = nonsteroidal anti-inflammatory drugs

REFERENCES Bondi J, Jegasothy B, Lazarus G: Dermatology, Diagnosis and Therapy. Norwalk, CT, Appleton & Lange, 1991
Illustrations: N/A
Internet references: http://www.5mcc.com

Author(s)
Jeffrey A. Stearns, MD

Pinworms

BASICS

DESCRIPTION Intestinal infection with Enterobius vermicularis. Characterized by perianal itching, usually worse at night.
System(s) affected: Gastrointestinal, Skin
Genetics: N/A
Incidence/Prevalence in USA:
Approximately 20% of young children (ages 5-10)
Predominant age: 5 to 14
Predominant sex: Female > Male

SIGNS AND SYMPTOMS
• Perianal itching
• Perineal itching
• Vulvovaginitis
• Enuresis
• Abdominal pain
• Insomnia

CAUSES The intestinal nematode Enterobius (Oxyuris) vermicularis

RISK FACTORS
• Institutionalization (50-90% of institutionalized children have pinworms)
• Crowded living conditions
• Poor hygiene
• Warm climate

DIAGNOSIS

DIFFERENTIAL DIAGNOSIS
• Idiopathic pruritus ani
• Atopic dermatitis
• Contact dermatitis
• Psoriasis
• Lichen planus
• Infection with human papilloma virus
• Herpes simplex
• Fungal infections
• Erythrasma
• Scabies
• Vaginitis

LABORATORY N/A
Drugs that may alter lab results: N/A
Disorders that may alter lab results: N/A

PATHOLOGICAL FINDINGS Identification of ova on low power microscopy or direct visualization of the female worm (10 mm in length). Ova are asymmetric, flattened on one side, and measure 30 by 60 μm.

SPECIAL TESTS
• Transparent tape test - a piece of transparent cellophane tape is adhered to the perianal skin in the early morning and then affixed to a microscope slide. This procedure must be performed at least 3 times to achieve 90% sensitivity.
• Flashlight to perianal region at night for direct observation
• Digital rectal examination with saline slide preparation of stool on gloved finger

IMAGING N/A

DIAGNOSTIC PROCEDURES N/A

TREATMENT

APPROPRIATE HEALTH CARE
Outpatient

GENERAL MEASURES
• All symptomatic family members should be treated simultaneously
• Bedclothes and underwear of infected individuals should be washed in hot water at the time of treatment (ova can remain viable for 2-3 weeks in a moist environment)
• Strict hand washing can help prevent fecal-oral transmission
• Practice good hygiene (showers, nail cleaning)
• Topical use of antipruritic creams or ointments may help relive itching in the perianal region

SURGICAL MEASURES N/A

ACTIVITY No restrictions

DIET No restrictions

PATIENT EDUCATION For patient education materials on this topic: Centers for Disease Control, Dept. of Health and Human Services, Office of Public Affairs, Atlanta, GA 30333, (404)329-3534

MEDICATIONS

DRUG(S) OF CHOICE
Some clinicians recommend repeat treatment after 2 weeks.
• Mebendazole (Vermox) chewable tablet 100 mg as a single dose. Use with caution in children < age 2
or
• Pyrantel pamoate (Antiminth) oral suspension 11 mg/kg as a single dose. Maximum dose 1 gram. Use with caution in children < age 2
or
• Albendazole 400 mg orally as a single dose
Contraindications: Refer to manufacturer's profile of each drug
Precautions:
• All family members should be treated
• Take medicine on empty stomach
• May cause diarrhea and/or nausea
Significant possible interactions: Refer to manufacturer's profile of each drug

ALTERNATIVE DRUGS N/A

FOLLOWUP

PATIENT MONITORING Unnecessary unless symptoms do not abate following drug therapy

PREVENTION/AVOIDANCE
• Careful hand washing, keep nails short and clean
• Wash anus and genitals at least once a day, preferably in a shower
• Don't scratch anus or put fingers near nose or mouth

POSSIBLE COMPLICATIONS
• Perianal scratching may cause impetigo or excoriation
• Young girls - vulvovaginitis, urethritis, endometritis, salpingitis
• Urinary tract infections

EXPECTED COURSE/PROGNOSIS
• Asymptomatic carriers are common
• Symptomatic infections are cured > 90% of the time with drug therapy
• Reinfection is common

MISCELLANEOUS

ASSOCIATED CONDITIONS Pruritis ani

AGE-RELATED FACTORS
Pediatric: More common in children and more likely to get reinfected
Geriatric: N/A
Others: N/A

PREGNANCY Drug therapy is contraindicated in pregnancy

SYNONYMS Enterobiasis

ICD-9-CM 127.4 Enterobiasis

SEE ALSO N/A

OTHER NOTES N/A

ABBREVIATIONS N/A

REFERENCES
• Bennett JC, Plum F, eds: Cecil Textbook of Medicine. 20th Ed. Philadelphia, W.B. Saunders Co., 1996
• Berman RE, et al, eds: Nelson Textbook of Pediatrics. 14th Ed. Philadelphia, W.B. Saunders Co., 1992
• Sanford JP, et al: Guide to Antimicrobial Therapy. New York, Pfizer, 1997
Illustrations: N/A
Internet references: http://www.5mcc.com

Author(s)
Steven Eisenstein, MD

Pityriasis alba

BASICS

DESCRIPTION A chronic skin disorder characterized by one or more groups of poorly marginated, white patches and plaques that appear on the cheeks, neck and lateral arms of children and young adults
Genetics: Unknown, but is primarily seen in children with a genetic predisposition to atopic disease
System(s) affected: Skin/Exocrine
Incidence/Prevalence in USA: Common, exact incidence unknown. Common, especially in dark-skin individuals in sunnier climates (90% for ages 6-12).
Predominant age: 3-10 years. Rare after 25.
Predominant sex: Male = Female

SIGNS AND SYMPTOMS
• Description - small, ill-defined white patches
• Location - cheeks and lateral arms
• Number - 1-12 or more patches
• Palpation - smooth or slightly rough, and dry
• Appearance - pinpoint white papules (representing accentuation and keratinization of follicular orifices)
• Scale is either invisible or fine and light
• More common in dark skinned individuals
• Usually asymptomatic
• Pruritic (rare)
• More apparent in summertime in light skinned individuals
• Lesions do not tan in summer
• Even a small amount of sunlight exposure causes lesions to redden

CAUSES
• Unknown. Maybe part of an atopic diathesis.
• Possibly defects in melanin production or transfer

RISK FACTORS Children with a genetic predisposition to atopic disease

DIAGNOSIS

DIFFERENTIAL DIAGNOSIS
• Pityriasis versicolor
• Vitiligo
• Milia
• Keratosis pilaris
• Indeterminate or uncharacteristic leprosy

LABORATORY N/A
Drugs that may alter lab results: N/A
Disorders that may alter lab results: N/A

PATHOLOGICAL FINDINGS Irregular melanin pigmentation of basal layer, follicular plugging, follicular spongiosis, and atrophic sebaceous glands

SPECIAL TESTS N/A

IMAGING N/A

DIAGNOSTIC PROCEDURES History and physical exam. Atopic diathesis is of diagnostic significance.

TREATMENT

APPROPRIATE HEALTH CARE
Outpatient

GENERAL MEASURES No truly effective therapy available. Lubricating cream application may improve roughness and/or dryness.

SURGICAL MEASURES N/A

ACTIVITY No restrictions

DIET No special diet

PATIENT EDUCATION Stress long-term chronicity and permanent resolution in second or third decade of life

MEDICATIONS

DRUG(S) OF CHOICE
• Coal tar preparations - Alphosyl, Estar, Balnetar, applied topically once or twice a day. Treatment is not mandatory.
• Topical steroids if needed to reduce redness due to sunburn or spontaneous inflammation
• Note: Neither will change the pigmentation, but may improve pruritus, roughness and/or dryness, if the lubricating cream is not sufficient
• Phototherapy (e.g., UVB)
• Anecdotal evidence supports use of Lacticare HC 1% (Lac-Hydrin + 1% hydrocortisone lotion)
Contraindications: N/A
Precautions: Refer to manufacturer's literature
Significant possible interactions: N/A

ALTERNATIVE DRUGS N/A

FOLLOWUP

PATIENT MONITORING As needed only if lesions become symptomatic

PREVENTION/AVOIDANCE No known preventive measures

POSSIBLE COMPLICATIONS None expected

EXPECTED COURSE/PROGNOSIS
Permanent resolution during second or third decade of life

MISCELLANEOUS

ASSOCIATED CONDITIONS Atopic dermatitis

AGE-RELATED FACTORS
Pediatric: More common in children 3 to 10 years
Geriatric: Rare in this age group
Others: N/A

PREGNANCY N/A

SYNONYMS
• Pityriasis streptogenes
• Pityriasis simplex
• Pityriasis sicca faciei
• Erythema streptogenes
• Furfuraceous impetigo

ICD-9-CM 696.5

SEE ALSO
• Tinea versicolor
• Vitiligo
• Keratosis

OTHER NOTES N/A

ABBREVIATIONS N/A

REFERENCES
• Habif T: Clinical Dermatology. 3rd Ed. St. Louis, CV Mosby, 1996
• Sams WM, Lynch PJ, eds: Principles and Practices of Dermatology. 2nd Ed. New York, Churchill Livingstone, 1996
• Fitzpatrick TB, et al, eds: Dermatology in General Medicine. 4th Ed. New York, McGraw-Hill, 1993
• Arnold KL, Odom RB, James WD: Andrews' Diseases of the Skin. 8th Ed. Philadelphia, W.B. Saunders Co., 1990
• Vargas-Ocampo F: Pityriasis alba: a histologic study. Int J Dermatol 1993;32(12):870-3
Illustrations: 2 available on CD-ROM
Internet references: http://www.5mcc.com

Author(s)
Mitchell S. King, MD
Anne C. Reitz, MD

Pityriasis rosea

BASICS

DESCRIPTION An idiopathic self-limited skin eruption characterized by widespread papulosquamous lesions
System(s) affected: Skin/Exocrine
Genetics: Less than 5 percent of those affected give a positive family history
Incidence/Prevalence in USA: Relatively common but exact frequency unknown
Predominant age: 10-35, but occurs in all age groups
Predominant sex: Male = Female

SIGNS AND SYMPTOMS
• Salmon to light brown oval plaques with fine scales centrally and "collarette" of loose scales along borders
• Lesions average 1-2 cm in diameter and usually spare face, hands and feet in adults
• Lesions frequently oriented along skin cleavage lines in "Christmas tree" pattern
• Eruption often preceded by 2-6 cm "herald patch" of similar appearance days to weeks before generalized rash
• Mild pruritus, rarely severe
• Fever and malaise rare
• Variant forms include purpuric, urticarial, and vesicular lesions

CAUSES Unknown, may be a viral agent or an autoimmune disorder

RISK FACTORS Unknown

DIAGNOSIS

DIFFERENTIAL DIAGNOSIS
• Secondary syphilis
• Viral exanthems
• Drug rashes
• Psoriasis
• Parapsoriasis
• Eczema
• Lichen planus
• Tinea corporis

LABORATORY WBC normal. No specific lab markers. Serology to rule out syphilis.
Drugs that may alter lab results: N/A
Disorders that may alter lab results: N/A

PATHOLOGICAL FINDINGS Chronic inflammation with cytolytic degeneration of keratinocytes adjacent to Langerhans cells

SPECIAL TESTS KOH preparation to distinguish from tinea corporis

IMAGING N/A

DIAGNOSTIC PROCEDURES N/A

TREATMENT

APPROPRIATE HEALTH CARE
Outpatient

GENERAL MEASURES
• Symptomatic treatment
• Topical antipruritics as needed
• Ultraviolet therapy has been used but efficacy not proven
• Lukewarm oatmeal baths (not hot as it can intensify itching)

SURGICAL MEASURES N/A

ACTIVITY Full activity with good skin hygiene to prevent secondary infection

DIET N/A

PATIENT EDUCATION
• Reassurance as to self-limited nature of condition
• Printed patient information available from: American Academy of Dermatology (708) 330-0230.

MEDICATIONS

DRUG(S) OF CHOICE   Topical steroids to reduce itching, if needed
Contraindications: N/A
Precautions: N/A
Significant possible interactions: N/A

ALTERNATIVE DRUGS   N/A

FOLLOWUP

PATIENT MONITORING
• Check syphilis serology
• Return visit for reevaluation, if lesions persist longer than 8-10 weeks

PREVENTION/AVOIDANCE   N/A

POSSIBLE COMPLICATIONS   Secondary infection (e.g., impetigo)

EXPECTED COURSE/PROGNOSIS
Gradual resolution in 1-14 weeks (usually 2-6)

MISCELLANEOUS

ASSOCIATED CONDITIONS   N/A

AGE-RELATED FACTORS
Pediatric: Face, distal extremities more often involved in children and lesions may be more papular
Geriatric: N/A
Others: N/A

PREGNANCY   N/A

SYNONYMS   N/A

ICD-9-CM   696.3

SEE ALSO
• Pityriasis alba
• Dermatitis, exfoliative
• Tinea versicolor

OTHER NOTES   N/A

ABBREVIATIONS   N/A

REFERENCES
• Fitzpatrick TB, et al, eds: Dermatology In General Medicine. 3rd Ed. New York, McGraw-Hill, 1987
• Cheong WK, Wong KS: Pityriasis Rosea. Singapore Medical Jour 1989
Illustrations: 10 available on CD-ROM
Internet references: http://www.5mcc.com

Author(s)
Jeffrey D. Wolfrey, MD

Placenta previa

BASICS

DESCRIPTION Placental location near, partially, or completely over the cervical os
• Marginal previa: Placement near enough to cervical os to cause risk of hemorrhage during effacement and dilation of the cervix during labor
• Partial previa: Placement causing partial covering of the cervical os
• Total previa: Placement that causes entire os to be covered by placenta
System(s) affected: Reproductive, Cardiovascular
Genetics: N/A
Incidence/Prevalence in USA: 0.5% to 0.8% of all pregnancies; low lying placenta 4-8% in early pregnancy with < 10% persisting to term
Predominant age: Childbearing ages
Predominant sex: Female only

SIGNS AND SYMPTOMS
• Typically painless bright red bleeding 2nd or 3rd trimester
• Average time of first bleed, 27-32 weeks
• Contractions variably present
• First bleed usually self limited
• Maternal hemodynamic status consistent with clinical blood loss estimate
• Complete previas may bleed earlier and not "migrate"

CAUSES Prior uterine insult or injury or other uterine factors

RISK FACTORS
• Prior previa (4%-8%)
• First subsequent pregnancy following a cesarean section delivery
• Multiparity (5% in grand multiparous patient)
• Advanced maternal age
• Multiple gestation
• Prior induced abortions
• Smoking

DIAGNOSIS

DIFFERENTIAL DIAGNOSIS Abruptio placentae, vasa previa, vaginal and cervical causes including marked "bloody show" and infections

LABORATORY
• Maternal blood type and Rh
• Hemoglobin and hematocrit
• Platelet count
• PT, PTT, fibrinogen
• Type and cross match packed RBC (at least three units)
• Apt test: To determine fetal origin of blood (as in vasa previa). Mix vaginal blood with small amount tap water to cause hemolysis, centrifuge for several minutes, mix 1 cc of 1% NaOH with each 5 cc of the pink-hemoglobin-containing supernatant, observing pink fluid if fetal hemoglobin, and yellow-brown if adult origin.
• Wright's stain applied to a slide smear of vaginal blood looking for nucleated RBC's which are usually from cord blood and not adult blood
• L/S ratio for fetal maturity if needed
Drugs that may alter lab results: Drugs altering cell counts or clotting studies
Disorders that may alter lab results:
• Coagulopathies from other causes
• Red cell and hemoglobin disorders from other causes

PATHOLOGICAL FINDINGS
• Normocytic, normochromic anemia with acute bleed
• Coagulopathy rare, but may occur
• Positive Kleihauer-Betke if fetal/maternal transfusion

SPECIAL TESTS
• Kleihauer-Betke if concerned about fetal-maternal transfusion
• Bedside clot test: Draw red top tube from mother and observe for clot quality at 7-10 minutes. If there is no clot or if clot is friable may indicate disseminated intravascular coagulation (DIC).

IMAGING
• External sector sonography with moderately full and empty bladder
• Vaginal probe sonography may be done if not actively bleeding. Place the probe just inside os and use 5 or 6.5-mHz transducers.
• Magnetic resonance imaging (MRI) accurate, but more expensive, less available, and time consuming

DIAGNOSTIC PROCEDURES
• If placental location unknown and sonography not available, a double setup bimanual vaginal exam may be done in operating room with complete cesarean section readiness

• Careful vaginal speculum exam is not contraindicated and allows checking for cervical or vaginal source of bleeding, fern and nitrazine testing, cultures, and fluid for determining bleeding source
• Since fibrin degradation products rise in pregnancy, these levels are less helpful

TREATMENT

APPROPRIATE HEALTH CARE
• Inpatient observation at bedrest initially; once stable, and preterm, may be followed as outpatient
• May consider transfer to high risk center based on condition and local services

GENERAL MEASURES
• Optimizing maternal stability while delaying delivery, if possible, or if preterm to improve perinatal outcome
• Cesarean section indicated for partial or complete previa if fetus is mature or if the situation is urgent and the fetus is immature
• A trial of labor may be considered with anterior marginal previa, including oxytocin (Pitocin) augmentation IV
• Amniocentesis for L/S ratio for maturity as needed
• IV fluid support, oxygen, transfusions of packed RBC's, platelets and fresh frozen plasma if needed
• External fetal and labor monitoring
• Other intervention or observation based on maternal condition
• DIC risk low unless massive bleed. Follow coagulation studies and give fresh frozen plasma (FFP), platelets as needed, or cryoprecipitate if fibrinogen < 100-150 mg/dL (< 1.0-1.5 g/L).
• Transfuse platelets at < 20,000 or < 50,000 if surgery needed
• Low lying posterior marginal previa associated with dystocia and greater need for cesarean section
• Blood volume increased in pregnancy; can lose > 30% maternal blood volume before shock findings
• Central line placement only after checking coagulation studies
• May use sector probe with condom at introitus if vaginal probe unavailable

SURGICAL MEASURES N/A

ACTIVITY
• Bedrest
• Intercourse abstinence

DIET NPO initially, then based on delivery decisions

PATIENT EDUCATION
• First bleed rarely fatal
• Rebleed risk with activity or cervical stimulation
• Greatest cause of perinatal mortality is prematurity
• Risks and conditions associated with previa

MEDICATIONS

DRUG(S) OF CHOICE
• For IV fluids: Lactated Ringer's or saline
• Oxygen for all, since O2 consumption up 20% in pregnancy and fetus is more prone to hypoxia
• Fresh frozen plasma and platelets as needed
• Cryoprecipitate and fibrinogen if above unsuccessful
• Tocolytics may have role in certain preterm patients, but tachycardia of B-agonists (terbutaline) and risk of placental hypoperfusion with calcium channel blockers may make MgSO4 the drug of choice. For MgSO4, use 4 grams IV load and 1-4 grams/hour as indicated.

Contraindications:
Avoid tocolytics with term infant or unstable mother

Precautions:
• Beta-agonists and calcium channel blockers may complicate clinical picture
• Cryoprecipitate and fibrinogen may increase infection transmission risk

Significant possible interactions: Refer to manufacturer's profile of each drug

ALTERNATIVE DRUGS
• Ritodrine (Yutopar) IV may be an alternate beta-agonist, but carries same concerns as terbutaline
• Isoxsuprine may be used for tocolysis

FOLLOWUP

PATIENT MONITORING
• Inpatient followup
• Outpatient care with frequent visits

PREVENTION/AVOIDANCE
• Decrease activity to avoid rebleeding
• All vaginal exams, sexual intercourse, douching, or other vaginal manipulation may cause rebleeding

POSSIBLE COMPLICATIONS
• Maternal mortality is rare with cesarean section available. Greatest fetal risk is preterm delivery.
• Attempted tocolysis may compromise maternal status
• Rebleeding risk may be more risky than delivery and management
• If previa present after 30 weeks, there is greater risk of persisting previa

EXPECTED COURSE/PROGNOSIS
• If term and complete or partial: Cesarean delivery
• If term and anterior marginal: Trial of labor may be okay
• If preterm and maternal and fetal status stable: May observe and delay delivery

MISCELLANEOUS

ASSOCIATED CONDITIONS
• Abnormal presentations such as oblique and/or transverse lie
• Persistent high fetal station
• If previa present, then increased risk of intrauterine growth retardation (IUGR)
• Placenta accreta
• Postpartum hemorrhage
• Increased incidence of small for gestational age (SGA) babies with previas

AGE-RELATED FACTORS
Pediatric: N/A
Geriatric: N/A
Others: Advanced maternal age increases risk

PREGNANCY   As above

SYNONYMS   N/A

ICD-9-CM
• 641.0 Placenta previa without hemorrhage
• 641.1 Hemorrhage from placenta previa
• 641.2 Premature separation of placenta

SEE ALSO   Abruptio placentae

OTHER NOTES   N/A

ABBREVIATIONS
• DIC = disseminated intravascular coagulation
• L/S ratio = lecithin/sphingomyelin ratio
• PT = prothrombin time
• PTT = partial thromboplastin time

REFERENCES
• Pritchard JA, McDonald PC, Gant NF: Williams Obstetrics. Norwalk, CT, Appleton-Century-Crofts, 1985:407-411
• Lavery JP: Placenta Previa. Obstetrics and Gyn 1990;33(3)
Illustrations: N/A
Internet references: http://www.5mcc.com

Author(s)
Mark E. Sexton, MD

Plague

BASICS

DESCRIPTION
• Acute infection
• Sporadic world wide, especially Third World nations
• Epidemics associated with war, famine, and disaster
• Disease of rats and other small vertebrates
• Transmitted to humans by rat flea
• Occasional transmission to humans handling infected tissues
• Occasional human to human transmission by secretions or human flea
• Recently shown that infected cats may transmit disease to humans by bite, licking or scratch
System(s) affected: Hemic/Lymphatic/Immunologic, Skin/Exocrine, Pulmonary
Genetics: N/A
Incidence/Prevalence in USA: Few cases annually in Southwestern states, usually Spring, Summer, Fall
Predominant age: N/A
Predominant sex: Male = Female

SIGNS AND SYMPTOMS
• Bubonic plague
  ◊ Acute onset after 2-8 days incubation
  ◊ Fever
  ◊ Chills
  ◊ Weakness
  ◊ Headache
  ◊ Bubo - painful, very tender enlargement of regional lymph node(s) draining inoculation site. Overlying edema. Typically, absence of overlying skin lesion, ascending lymphangitis.
  ◊ Skin lesions - pustules, vesicles, eschars in area of flea bite(s), purpura
• Septicemic plague
  ◊ Features of bubonic plague
  ◊ Occasional occurrence without bubo
  ◊ Hypotension
  ◊ Hepatosplenomegaly
  ◊ Delirium
  ◊ Seizures in children
  ◊ Shock
• Secondary pneumonic plague
  ◊ Features of bubonic and septicemic plague
  ◊ Cough
  ◊ Chest pain
  ◊ Hemoptysis
• Primary pneumonic plague
  ◊ Acute onset within hours to one day after inhalation of bacteria
  ◊ Fever
  ◊ Chills
  ◊ Cough
  ◊ Chest pain
  ◊ Dyspnea
  ◊ Hemoptysis
  ◊ Lethargy
  ◊ Hypotension
  ◊ Shock

CAUSES
• Yersinia pestis, transmitted by bite of a flea from an infected rodent and by bite, lick or scratch by infected cat
• Untreated bubonic plague may progress to secondary pneumonic type which can be transmitted by contaminated respiratory droplets

RISK FACTORS
• Environmental exposure to rats and fleas
• Close contact with infected cat
• Close contact with pneumonic plague patient
• Plague bacillus in laboratory
• Hunters who skin wild animals

DIAGNOSIS

DIFFERENTIAL DIAGNOSIS
Other causes of fulminant bacteremia, pneumococcal pneumonia, lymphangitis

LABORATORY
• Elevated white cell count, predominantly mature and immature neutrophils. Leukemoid reaction sometimes.
• Stained smears of aspirate of bubo, sputum, peripheral blood reveal gram-negative coccobacilli with bipolar staining, "safety pin" appearance
• Aspirate, blood, sputum cultures (infusion broth, blood and MacConkey agar) grow typical bacteria. Public health authorities arrange definitive identification and serological followup.
Drugs that may alter lab results: Antibiotics
Disorders that may alter lab results: N/A

PATHOLOGICAL FINDINGS
Acute inflammation dominated by neutrophils, necrosis, masses of plague bacilli, seropurulent pericarditis

SPECIAL TESTS
Low platelet number; evidence of disseminated intravascular coagulation may be seen

IMAGING
Chest x-ray - patchy or confluent pulmonary consolidation in pneumonic plague

DIAGNOSTIC PROCEDURES   N/A

TREATMENT

APPROPRIATE HEALTH CARE
Hospitalization. For suspected pneumonic plague, respiratory isolation until 48 hours after initial effective therapy or after sputum negative.

GENERAL MEASURES
• Do not create aerosol
• Handle blood and bubo aspirate with gloves
• Notify laboratory to take precautions
• Intravenous fluids as required
• Hot, moist compresses for buboes

SURGICAL MEASURES   N/A

ACTIVITY   Bedrest until convalescent

DIET   As tolerated during recovery

PATIENT EDUCATION
• Avoid contact with wild animals
• Reduce rat and flea population in environment

Plague

MEDICATIONS

DRUG(S) OF CHOICE
• Streptomycin: 15 mg/kg IM bid for 10 days. If streptomycin not available, gentamicin.
• If streptomycin contraindicated or condition allows oral medication: tetracycline (Achromycin) 25-50 mg/kg/day, equally divided, every 6 hours for 10 days.
• For meningitis: chloramphenicol (Chloromycetin) 25 mg/kg followed by 60 mg/kg in 4 equally divided doses, daily for 10 days

Contraindications: None to antibiotic treatment of this often fatal infection

Precautions:
• Reduce dose of streptomycin for renal impairment, 20 mg/kg daily if mild and 8 mg/kg each 3 days if advanced
• Pregnant women and those with hearing disorders, shorten streptomycin to 3 days after afebrile
• Chloramphenicol associated with hematologic toxicity

Significant possible interactions: N/A

ALTERNATIVE DRUGS   None
demonstrated to be as effective or less toxic

FOLLOWUP

PATIENT MONITORING
• CBC for hematologic toxicity of chloramphenicol
• Streptomycin blood levels if available
• Hearing screening if streptomycin or gentamicin being used

PREVENTION/AVOIDANCE
• Avoid contact with vectors, infected tissue or aerosol, e.g., pneumonic plague case
• Killed vaccine for people at high risk to reduce risk and/or severity; tetracycline prophylaxis. Vaccine available from C.D.C., Atlanta.

POSSIBLE COMPLICATIONS
• Progression of bubonic form to septicemic and pneumonic forms
• Necrosis of bubo may require aspiration or incision and drainage
• Pericarditis
• Adult respiratory distress syndrome
• Meningitis

EXPECTED COURSE/PROGNOSIS
• Untreated plague mortality > 50%; 100% in primary pneumonic plague
• Plague may be fulminant, e.g., exposure, first symptoms and death in one day in primary pneumonic plague. Must not delay treatment of suspected cases until laboratory-confirmed diagnosis. Delay of initial therapy beyond 24 hours after onset of primary pneumonic plague regularly followed by death.

MISCELLANEOUS

ASSOCIATED CONDITIONS   N/A

AGE-RELATED FACTORS   N/A
Pediatric: N/A
Geriatric: N/A
Others: N/A

PREGNANCY   N/A

SYNONYMS   Black death

ICD-9-CM
• 020.0 Bubonic plague
• 020.2 Septicemic plague
• 020.5 Unspecified pneumonic plague
• 020.3 Primary pneumonic plague
• 020.4 Secondary pneumonic plague

SEE ALSO   N/A

OTHER NOTES   N/A

ABBREVIATIONS   N/A

REFERENCES   Mandell GL, Douglas RG, Bennett JE, eds: Principles and Practice of Infectious Diseases. 4th Ed. New York, Churchill Livingstone, 1995
Illustrations: N/A
Internet references: http://www.5mcc.com

Author(s)
William D. Sawyer, MD

Pleural effusion

BASICS

DESCRIPTION Excessive fluid collection in the pleural space, almost always caused by an underlying disease. Effusions may be from transudates (effusions due to imbalances in hydrostatic and oncotic pressures, such as those seen in congestive heart failure or hypoalbuminuria) or exudates (effusions that may be associated with many diseases - see Causes). Normal individuals will have a small amount of extracellular fluid that lubricates the pleural surfaces. Most patients with effusions will demonstrate symptoms relating to the underlying pathology.
System(s) affected: Pulmonary, Cardiovascular
Genetics: N/A
Incidence/Prevalence in USA: Not known
Predominant age: All ages
Predominant sex: Male = Female

SIGNS AND SYMPTOMS
• None in mild effusion
• Chest pain
• Cough
• Splint of chest wall
• Dyspnea
• Tachypnea
• Diminished chest wall excursion
• Reduced tactile fremitus
• Dullness to percussion
• Diminished or absent breath sounds over the effusion
• Displacement of trachea and the cardiac apex toward the contralateral side
• Friction rub in small effusion
• Weight loss
• Chills
• Hemoptysis
• Night sweats

CAUSES
• Parapneumonic effusion
• Empyema: Often associated with pneumonia exudate caused by pneumococcal or gram negative organisms in adult; pneumococcal, H. influenzae, Staphylococcus aureus, and mycoplasma organisms in children. Occasionally mycobacterial or fungal organism can be responsible in all age groups.
• Malignancy: Exudates, primary pleural malignancy vs. metastatic malignancy. Frequency scale - lung > breast > lymphoma > others.
• Congestive heart failure: Transudate often bilateral
• Renal: Nephrotic syndrome, renal failure. Transudates often bilateral.
• Cirrhosis: Transudate, usually right-sided
• Rheumatic disease: Exudate (small)
• Drug induced effusion: Exudate often with eosinophilia

• Dressler's syndrome (post cardiotomy or myocardial infarction syndrome): Exudate often associated with myocardial effusion
• Intra-abdominal abscess: Exudate, WBC, normal glucose, sterile
• Esophageal perforation: Exudate, air-fluid level, high amylase, unilateral, toxicity
• Pancreatitis: Exudate with high amylase, often left-sided

RISK FACTORS N/A

DIAGNOSIS

DIFFERENTIAL DIAGNOSIS See Causes

LABORATORY
• Leukocytosis
• Anemia
Drugs that may alter lab results: N/A
Disorders that may alter lab results: N/A

PATHOLOGICAL FINDINGS N/A

SPECIAL TESTS
• Examination of pleural fluid obtained by thoracentesis
  ◊ Cell count and differential
  ◊ Glucose, usually < 60 mg/dL (3.3 mmol/L) in empyema and rheumatoid arthritis. May also be this low in tuberculosis and parapneumonia effusions.
  ◊ Protein > 3 g/dL (> 30 g/L) with pleural serum ratio > 0.5 in exudate
  ◊ Pleural fluid lactic dehydrogenase (LDH) > 200 IU, with pleural/serum ratio > 0.6 in exudate
  ◊ pH < 7.2 in empyema
  ◊ Amylase, elevated in effusion secondary to pancreatitis or esophageal perforation
  ◊ RBC's in malignant, traumatic, or pulmonary embolism effusions. Large amounts of RBC (> 100,000) is termed hemorrhagic effusion and may also be seen in other causes.
  ◊ Cytology (tumor cells)
  ◊ Cultures, gram stain bacterial, fungal, mycobacterial.

IMAGING N/A
• Chest x-ray, anteroposterior (upright), lateral decubitus
• Chest ultrasounds: Echo-transmitting space due to encapsulated fluid
• CT scan

DIAGNOSTIC PROCEDURES
• Pleural biopsy in selective cases (useful in diagnosis of cancer or tuberculosis)
• Pleuroscopy in selective cases
• Thoracentesis

TREATMENT

APPROPRIATE HEALTH CARE Inpatient

GENERAL MEASURES
• Supportive, oxygen, hydration, chest physiotherapy
• Treat the primary disorder
• Empyema
  ◊ Antibiotics alone in selective cases (children)
  ◊ Chest tube drainage (initial therapy in adults)
  ◊ Pleurectomy (pleural stripping) in cases of "trapped lung"
  ◊ Thoracoscopy
  ◊ Fibrolytic agents
• Malignant pleural effusion
  ◊ Treatment of the primary malignancy
  ◊ Thoracentesis, chest tube drainage for symptomatic management
  ◊ Chemical pleurodesis in some patients
• Chylothorax
  ◊ Radiation therapy in some malignant chylothorax
  ◊ Surgical ligation of thoracic duct in traumatic chylothorax
• Hemothorax
  ◊ Fluid hematocrit equal to or similar to blood hematocrit - almost always caused only by trauma
  ◊ Thoracostomy tube drainage in traumatic hemothorax
• Hemorrhagic effusion
  ◊ Treatment of primary disease (usually malignancy)

SURGICAL MEASURES See General Measures

ACTIVITY As tolerated

DIET No special diet

PATIENT EDUCATION Patient instruction materials available from American Lung Association (local agency or 1740 Broadway, New York, NY 10038)

Pleural effusion

MEDICATIONS

DRUG(S) OF CHOICE
• Antimicrobial treatment according to pathogens and their sensitivities
• Chemical pleurodesis with doxycycline 500 mg or bleomycin 60 units in some patients
Contraindications: Refer to manufacturer's profile of each drug
Precautions: Refer to manufacturer's profile of each drug
Significant possible interactions: Refer to manufacturer s profile of each drug

ALTERNATIVE DRUGS N/A

FOLLOWUP

PATIENT MONITORING
• Chest x-ray every three months until return to normal
• Pulmonary function tests (PFT's) every three months until return to normal

PREVENTION/AVOIDANCE N/A

POSSIBLE COMPLICATIONS
• Chronic empyema
• Drainage through chest wall - pleurocutaneous fistula
• Bronchopleural fistula
• Toxic shock syndrome

EXPECTED COURSE/PROGNOSIS
Mortality rate around 20% for exudative effusions; worse for elderly patients or those with serious underlying conditions

MISCELLANEOUS

ASSOCIATED CONDITIONS N/A

AGE-RELATED FACTORS N/A
Pediatric: N/A
Geriatric: N/A
Others: N/A

PREGNANCY N/A

SYNONYMS N/A

ICD-9-CM
• 511.9 Unspecified pleural effusion
• 511.1 Pleurisy with effusion, with mention of a bacterial cause other than tuberculosis
• 197.2 Secondary malignant neoplasm of respiratory and digestive system, pleura

SEE ALSO N/A

OTHER NOTES N/A

ABBREVIATIONS N/A

REFERENCES
• Isselbacher KJ, et al, eds: Harrison's Principles of Internal Medicine. 13th Ed. New York, McGraw-Hill, 1994
• Kendig R, Chernick V: Disorders of the Respiratory Tracts in Children. 5th Ed. Philadelphia, W.B. Saunders Co., 1990
Illustrations: N/A
Internet references: http://www.5mcc.com

Author(s)
Sami K. W. Hadeed, MD

Pneumonia, bacterial

BASICS

DESCRIPTION An acute, bacterial infection of the lung parenchyma. Infection may be community-acquired or nosocomial (hospital acquired by an inpatient for at least 48 hours or inpatient in the previous 1-3 weeks). Most commonly, community-acquired disease is caused by Streptococcus pneumoniae or Mycoplasma pneumoniae. Hospital-acquired pneumonia is usually due to gram negative rods (60%) such as Pseudomonas, or if gram positive from Staphylococcus (14.5%).
System(s) affected: Pulmonary
Genetics: No known genetic pattern
Incidence/Prevalence in USA:
• Incidence - community-acquired: 1200 cases/100,000 population per year
• Incidence - nosocomial: 800 cases/100,000 admissions per year
Predominant age: Age extremes
Predominant sex: Male > Female

SIGNS AND SYMPTOMS
• Cardinal signs and symptoms
  ◊ Cough and fever
  ◊ Chest pain (pleuritic)
  ◊ Chill, with sudden onset
  ◊ Dark, thick or bloody (rusty) sputum
• Respiratory
  ◊ Signs of consolidation
    - Rales
    - Egophony
  ◊ Signs of pleural involvement
    - Decreased breath sounds
    - Dullness to percussion
    - Friction rub
• Signs of respiratory distress
  ◊ Tachypnea/tachycardia (or bradycardia)
  ◊ Cyanosis
  ◊ Mental status changes
• Central nervous system
  ◊ Mentation changes to include anxiety, confusion, restlessness, and meningeal signs
• Gastrointestinal
  ◊ Abdominal pain
  ◊ Anorexia
• Generalized
  ◊ Volume depletion
  ◊ Diaphoresis
  ◊ Malaise/myalgias
  ◊ Petechiae

CAUSES
• Sources
  ◊ Aspiration from the oropharynx
  ◊ Inhalation
  ◊ Hematogenous spread
• Bacterial pathogens
  ◊ Streptococcus pneumoniae (pneumococcus)
  ◊ Haemophilus influenzae
  ◊ Mycoplasma pneumoniae
  ◊ Staphylococcus aureus
  ◊ Legionella pneumophila
  ◊ Chlamydia pneumoniae, C. psittaci
  ◊ Moraxella catarrhalis (Branhamella catarrhalis)
  ◊ Pseudomonas aeruginosa
  ◊ Escherichia coli
  ◊ Anaerobes

RISK FACTORS
• Recent/concurrent viral infections
• Hospitalization to include mechanical ventilation, antecedent antibiotics, NG tubes
• Age extremes
• Alcoholism
• AIDS or other immunosuppression
• Tobacco smoking
• Renal failure
• Cardiovascular disease
• Functional asplenia
• Chronic obstructive pulmonary disease
• Diabetes mellitus
• Malnutrition
• Malignancy
• General anesthesia
• Altered level of consciousness or gag (e.g., seizures, stroke, neuromuscular disease, etc.)
• Occupational exposure
• Poorly implemented infection control practices

DIAGNOSIS

DIFFERENTIAL DIAGNOSIS Other causes of infectious pneumonitis: Viruses (respiratory syncytial, adenovirus, parainfluenza, influenzae A and B, varicella, measles, rubella, enterovirus, Epstein-Barr); Nocardia; Fungi (Blastomyces, Cryptococcus, Aspergillus, Histoplasma, Coccidioides, Pneumocystis carinii); Protozoans (Toxoplasma); Rickettsia (Coxiella burnetii - Q fever). Also tuberculosis, pulmonary embolism with infarction, bronchiolitis obliterans with organizing pneumonia (BOOP), pulmonary contusion, pulmonary vasculitis, acute sarcoid, hypersensitivity pneumonitis, ARDS, pneumothorax, and other causes.

LABORATORY
• Leukocytosis with left shift on differential
• Hyponatremia (SIADH)
• Hypoxemia
• Hypocapnia initially, then hypercapnia
• Blood culture - positive in 20-30% of patients with community-acquired pneumonia, 8-20/nosocomial pneumonia
• Bronchoscopic protected telescoping catheter brushing culture - significant at greater than or equal to 1000 microorganisms/mL
• Bronchoscopic bronchoalveolar lavage culture - significant at greater than or equal to 10,000 organisms/mL
Drugs that may alter lab results:
Antecedent antibiotics
Disorders that may alter lab results:
Refer to lab test reference

PATHOLOGICAL FINDINGS
• Lung:
  ◊ Segmental, lobar, or multifocal peribronchial consolidation
    ◊ Positive gram stain for bacteria

SPECIAL TESTS
• Decubitus chest roentgenograms to investigate for empyema or parapneumonic effusion
• Culture of pleural fluid
• pH of pleural fluid (iced, airless sample sent to blood gas laboratory)

IMAGING
• Chest roentgenogram (with lateral decubitus views if pleural effusion present)
  ◊ Lobar or segmental consolidation (air bronchogram)
    ◊ Bronchopneumonia
    ◊ Interstitial infiltrate
    ◊ Pleural effusion (free-flowing or loculated)

DIAGNOSTIC PROCEDURES
• Gram stain and culture of sputum (induced, if necessary)
• Nasotracheal suctioning for culture
• Transtracheal aspirate for culture
• Bronchoscopy with bronchoalveolar lavage or protected telescoping catheter brushing for culture
• Thoracentesis for pleural fluid studies
• Transthoracic fine needle aspiration for culture
• Blood culture, especially if hospitalized - prior to antibiotics

TREATMENT

APPROPRIATE HEALTH CARE
• Community-acquired - outpatient for mild case, inpatient for moderate to severe case such as multilobar presentation, hypoxemia, hypotension, significant co-morbid illness, and age extremes.
• Nosocomial - patients already hospitalized

GENERAL MEASURES
• Empiric antimicrobial therapy for most likely pathogen(s)
• Consider oxygen for patients with cyanosis, hypoxia, dyspnea, circulatory disturbances or delirium
• Mechanical ventilation for respiratory failure
• Chest physiotherapy
• Hydration
• Nasotracheal suction
• Analgesia for pain
• Electrolyte correction
• Respiratory isolation if TB is a possibility

SURGICAL MEASURES N/A

ACTIVITY Bedrest and/or reduced activity during acute phase

DIET
• Nothing by mouth if there is incipient respiratory failure
• Consider soft, easy-to-eat foods

Pneumonia, bacterial

MEDICATIONS

DRUG(S) OF CHOICE
• Initial therapy
  ◊ Usually empiric for most likely pathogens given clinical scenario (if specific etiology is identified, adjust antimicrobial therapy)
  ◊ Otherwise healthy young adult with community-acquired pneumonia: erythromycin 500 po q6h (the new macrolides should be considered in those intolerant of erythromycin and in smokers [to treat H. influenzae])
  ◊ Older patients or patients with preexistent illnesses, with mild community-acquired pneumonia: trimethoprim-sulfamethoxazole or 2nd generation cephalosporin or amoxicillin-clavulanate with or without erythromycin or other macrolide
  ◊ Patients with community-acquired pneumonia requiring hospitalization: second or third generation cephalosporin or beta-lactam/beta-lactamase inhibitor plus macrolide - if Pseudomonas aeruginosa is a concern, use ceftazidime plus an aminoglycoside
  ◊ For nosocomial pneumonia: either ceftazidime or an antipseudomonal penicillin (piperacillin, mezlocillin, or ticarcillin) plus an aminoglycoside. Vancomycin should be considered if strong suspicion of Staphylococcus aureus.
• Therapy for specific organisms
  ◊ S. pneumoniae: penicillin G or oral penicillin V. If high incidence of penicillin resistant S. pneumoniae in the area, consider either cefotaxime or ceftriaxone
  ◊ H. influenzae: trimethoprim-sulfamethoxazole. For severe infections - cefotaxime or ceftriaxone.
  ◊ S. aureus: nafcillin; vancomycin (if high incidence of methicillin resistant S. aureus)
  ◊ Klebsiella species: aminoglycoside plus cephalosporin
  ◊ E. coli: aminoglycoside plus cephalosporin
  ◊ Pseudomonas: aminoglycoside plus antipseudomonal penicillin or ceftazidime
  ◊ Moraxella catarrhalis: 2nd generation cephalosporin (cefuroxime axetil)
  ◊ Chlamydia pneumoniae: doxycycline
  ◊ Mycoplasma pneumoniae: erythromycin
  ◊ Legionella pneumophila: erythromycin (add rifampin for documented disease)
  ◊ Anaerobes: clindamycin

Contraindications: Allergy or likely cross-allergy to the prescribed antibiotic
Precautions: Possible significant sodium overload with antipseudomonal penicillins
Significant possible interactions: Refer to manufacturer's literature

ALTERNATIVE DRUGS
• S. pneumoniae: erythromycin; cephalosporin (if high level of resistance, vancomycin)
• H. influenzae: cefuroxime; fluoroquinolones; chloramphenicol; extended macrolides; beta-lactam/beta-lactamase inhibitor
• S. aureus: a first generation cephalosporin; vancomycin; clindamycin
• Klebsiella: chloramphenicol; fluoroquinolone
• E. coli: ampicillin; cephalosporin; fluoroquinolone; chloramphenicol
• Pseudomonas: aminoglycoside plus ceftazidime; ciprofloxacin; imipenem
• Moraxella catarrhalis: amoxicillin-clavulanate; trimethoprim-sulfamethoxazole; fluoroquinolone; clarithromycin; cefixime
• Chlamydia pneumoniae: clarithromycin; azithromycin; fluoroquinolone
• Mycoplasma pneumoniae: clarithromycin; doxycycline; azithromycin; fluoroquinolone
• Legionella pneumophila: clarithromycin; azithromycin; fluoroquinolone; doxycycline
• Anaerobes: beta-lactam/beta-lactamase

FOLLOWUP

PATIENT MONITORING
• If outpatient therapy, daily assessment of the patient's progress and reassessment of therapy if clinical worsening or no improvement in 48-72 hours
• Chest roentgenograms take time to clear and may not show clearing, even though patient is improving. Repeat study about 6 weeks after recovery to verify the pneumonia was not caused by an obstructing endobronchial lesion.
• Repeating the cultures after treatment has been started is unnecessary unless there has been treatment failure

PREVENTION/AVOIDANCE
• Reduce risk factors where possible
• Bedridden and postoperative patients - deep breathing and coughing exercises; prevent aspiration during nasogastric tube feedings
• Avoid indiscriminate use of antibiotics during minor viral infections
• Annual influenza vaccine for high risk individuals
• Polyvalent pneumococcal vaccine

POSSIBLE COMPLICATIONS
• Empyema
• Pulmonary abscess
• Superinfections
• Multiple organ dysfunction syndrome (MODS)
• Adult respiratory distress syndrome (ARDS)

EXPECTED COURSE/PROGNOSIS
• Usual course - acute. In otherwise healthy individual, improvement seen and fever resolved in 1-3 days.
• Overall mortality is about 5% in community acquired; 30-50% in nosocomial
• Poorest prognosis - age extremes, positive blood cultures, low WBC, presence of associated disease, immunosuppression respiratory failure, inappropriate antecedent antibiotics

MISCELLANEOUS

ASSOCIATED CONDITIONS
• Alcoholism
• Tobacco smoking
• Upper respiratory infection

AGE-RELATED FACTORS
Pediatric: Morbidity and mortality high in children under age 1
Geriatric: Morbidity and mortality high if > 70, especially if associated disease or risk factor
Others: N/A

PREGNANCY N/A

SYNONYMS
• Lobar pneumonia
• Classic pneumococcal pneumonia

ICD-9-CM 481 Pneumococcal pneumonia

SEE ALSO
• Pneumonia, viral
• Pneumonia, mycoplasma

OTHER NOTES Pneumococcal vaccine for all adults over age 65 and children over 2 years (and adults) with risk (cardio, pulmonary or metabolic disorders)

ABBREVIATIONS N/A

REFERENCES
• Bartlett JD, Mundy LM: Community-acquired pneumonia. N Engl J Med 1995;333:1618-1624
• Neiderman MS: Empirical therapy of community-acquird pneumonia. Sem Resp Inf 1994;9:192-198
• Laforce FM: Antibacterial therapy for lower respiratory tract infections in adults - A review. Clin Infect Dis 1992;14(S2):S233-237
• Barnes P: The pathology of community-acquired pneumonia. Sem Resp Inf 1994;9:130-139
• American Thoracic Society: Guidelines for the initial management of adults with community-acquired pneumonia. Am Rev Respir Dis 1993;148:1418-1426
• American Thoracic Society: Hospital acquired pneumonia in adults: diagnossis, assessment of severity, initial antimicrobial therapy, and preventive strategies. Am J Res Crit Care 1996;153:1711-1725
Illustrations: N/A
Internet references: http://www.5mcc.com

Author(s)
James K. Radike, MD
Ronald A. Greenfield, MD

PATIENT EDUCATION Printed patient information available from: American Lung Association, 1740 Broadway, New York, NY 100019 (212)315-8700; web site http://www.lungusa.org

Pneumonia, mycoplasma

 BASICS

DESCRIPTION Interstitial pneumonia caused by extensive infection of the lungs and bronchi, particularly the lower lobes of the lungs, by Mycoplasma pneumoniae. Usual course - acute. Incubation period is about 18-21 days and includes prodromal symptoms.
• Little seasonal variation of incidence, therefore a greater percentage of pneumonia in summer and fall are from Mycoplasma. Epidemics in communities tend to be prolonged (over many months) and occur every 4-5 years.
System(s) affected: Pulmonary
Genetics: None
Incidence/Prevalence in USA:
• 130 cases/100,000 people
• Estimated to be most common cause of pneumonia in school children and young adults (without chronic underlying condition)
Predominant age: Ages 5-15, but occurs at any age
Predominant sex: Male > Female

SIGNS AND SYMPTOMS
• Gradual onset with upper respiratory infection symptoms that progress
• Most will develop fever, cough, headache, sore throat, rales, and wheeze
• Many will develop myalgias, nasal congestion, chest pain
• Some will develop pleural effusion, pleural friction rub, cervical adenopathy, bullous myringitis, skin rash

CAUSES Mycoplasma pneumoniae infection

RISK FACTORS
• Close community living (e.g., hospitals, prisons, military bases, fraternity houses). Some of largest outbreaks have been in army recruits.
• Family exposure
• Immunocompromised patients

 DIAGNOSIS

DIFFERENTIAL DIAGNOSIS
• Viral pneumonia
• Bacterial pneumonia (including plague and tularemia in severe cases)
• Fungal pneumonias
• Pneumocystis carinii pneumonia
• Chlamydia pneumonia, TWAR or psittaci
• Legionella pneumonia

LABORATORY
• Increased sedimentation rate
• Increased complement fixation
• Positive cold agglutinins (titer of 1:258 or greater; or rising fourfold) in 50% of infections
• False-positive VDRL
• M. pneumoniae culture (requires 7-10 days)
• Peripheral white blood cell count - normal
• Complement fixation serologic assay shows fourfold rise in titer at 2-4 weeks after symptom onset
• IgM antibody to M. pneumoniae
Drugs that may alter lab results: N/A
Disorders that may alter lab results: N/A

PATHOLOGICAL FINDINGS Absence of bacterial pathogens on Gram stain and culture of sputum or transtracheal aspirate. Mycoplasma is a fastidious and slow-growing organism.

SPECIAL TESTS Radiolabeled DNA probe which detects M. pneumoniae ribosomal RNA in respiratory secretions, 90% sensitive

IMAGING Chest x-ray - diffuse interstitial infiltrates; small bilateral pleural effusion

DIAGNOSTIC PROCEDURES N/A

 TREATMENT

APPROPRIATE HEALTH CARE
Outpatient usually; inpatient if symptoms severe

GENERAL MEASURES N/A

SURGICAL MEASURES N/A

ACTIVITY Rest during acute phase

DIET Drink plenty of fluids

PATIENT EDUCATION Printed patient information available from American Lung Association, 1740 Broadway, New York, NY 10019, (212)315-8700

MEDICATIONS

DRUG(S) OF CHOICE
• Erythromycin - children 30-50 mg/kg/day for 10-14 days; adults 500 mg every 6 hours for 10-14 days
• Clarithromycin - children 15 mg/kg/d for 10-14 days; adults 500 mg bid for 10-14 days or azithromycin - children 10 mg/kg po first day, 5 mg/kg po for days 2-5; adults 500 mg first day, then 250 mg every day for 5 days. These newer macrolides might be used first if H. influenza is also suspected.
• Antibiotics such as penicillins are ineffective against M. pneumoniae
Contraindications: Refer to manufacturer's literature
Precautions: Refer to manufacturer's literature
Significant possible interactions:
Erythromycin and other macrolides inhibit the cytochrome P-450 microsomal enzyme system and can reduce elimination of other drugs such as carbamazepine, phenytoin, lovastatin, and theophylline. Prolongation of the QT interval and ventricular tachycardia has occurred in some patients receiving astemizide or terfenadine concomitantly with erythromycin.

ALTERNATIVE DRUGS
• Quinolones show moderate activity against Mycoplasma
• Adjunctive drugs - albuterol inhaler, 2 puffs qid for wheezing
• Children 9 yr and older - doxycycline 100 mg po bid

FOLLOWUP

PATIENT MONITORING
• Phone or in person followup
• Clearing of chest x-ray should be documented if the patient is older than 50. In smokers, document a clear x-ray in 6-8 weeks.

PREVENTION/AVOIDANCE
Isolation of active cases. Antibiotic prophylaxis of contacts is not indicated.

POSSIBLE COMPLICATIONS
Note: All complications are rare except reactive airway disease, hemolytic anemia, and erythema multiforme.
• Reactive airway disease
• Hemolytic anemia
• Erythema multiforme
• Meningoencephalitis
• Polyneuritis
• Polyarthritis
• Stevens-Johnson syndrome
• Pericarditis
• Myocarditis
• Respiratory distress syndrome
• Cerebral ataxia
• Thromboembolic phenomena
• Pleural effusion

EXPECTED COURSE/PROGNOSIS
• Mycoplasma infection symptoms usually resolve in about 2 weeks
• Some constitutional symptoms may persist for several weeks
• With correct therapy, even most severe cases can expect complete recovery

MISCELLANEOUS

ASSOCIATED CONDITIONS N/A

AGE-RELATED FACTORS
Pediatric:
• Unusual in infants
• M. pneumoniae is associated with an increased incidence of asthma attacks in older children
Geriatric: Unusual in this age group
Others: N/A

PREGNANCY Tetracycline contraindicated in pregnancy

SYNONYMS
• Primary atypical pneumonia (PAP)
• Eaton agent pneumonia
• Cold agglutinin-positive pneumonia

ICD-9-CM 483 Mycoplasma pneumonia

SEE ALSO
• Pneumonia, bacterial
• Pneumonia, viral
• Pneumonia, pneumocystis carinii (PCP)

OTHER NOTES N/A

ABBREVIATIONS N/A

REFERENCES
• Mandell GL, ed: Principles and Practice of Infectious Diseases. 4th Ed. New York, Churchill Livingstone, 1995
• Luby JP: Pneumonia caused by Mycoplasma pneumonia infection. Clinics in Chest Medicine 1991;12:237-99
• Luthan-Sadler BA, Morell VW: Viral and atypical pneumonias. Primary Care 1996;23:837-848
• Block S, Hedrick J, et al: Mycoplasma pneumonia and chlamydia pneumonia in pediatric community acquired pneumonia. Ped Infect Dis 1995;14:471-477
Illustrations: N/A
Internet references: http://www.5mcc.com

Author(s)
George R. Bergus, MD
Steven J. Havener, MD

Pneumonia, Pneumocystis carinii (PCP)

BASICS

DESCRIPTION A pneumonia arising in immunosuppressed persons caused by Pneumocystis carinii (PCP). This is one of the most common opportunistic infections occurring in patients with human immunodeficiency virus (HIV) infections. Pneumocystis infection can cause organ involvement and disseminated disease as well as pneumonia.
System(s) affected: Pulmonary
Genetics: N/A
Incidence/Prevalence in USA: Causes 43% of all opportunistic infections in AIDS patients
Predominant age:
• In HIV infected children, not taking prophylaxis, median age of onset is 5 months of age
• In HIV infected adults, PCP may occur at any age
Predominant sex: Male > Female

SIGNS AND SYMPTOMS
• Usually insidious but occasionally abrupt in onset
• Dyspnea on exertion progressing to continuous dyspnea
• Weakness, fatigue, malaise
• Fever, chills
• Cough - non-productive or productive of scant white or clear sputum
• Tachypnea

CAUSES The ubiquitous Pneumocystis carinii may cause infection in normal hosts (65-100% of young children have positive serology) but will rarely cause symptoms in immunocompetent individuals

RISK FACTORS Immunodeficiency (premature infants, neoplasia, congenital, acquired or drug-induced immunodeficiency states)

DIAGNOSIS

DIFFERENTIAL DIAGNOSIS
• Tuberculosis
• Mycobacterium avium intracellulare
• Viral pneumonias
• Fungal pneumonias
• Lymphoid interstitial pneumonitis (in children)
• Bacterial pneumonia

LABORATORY
• Serum LDH frequently elevated (mean elevation of 340 IU)
• Arterial blood gases reveal hypoxemia and increased alveolar-arterial gradient (varies with severity of disease)
• Sputum induced with inhaled 3-5% hypertonic saline may reveal pneumocystis on cytologic evaluation using Pap and Gomori methenamine-silver (GMS) stains. An IF (immunofluorescence) technique is also available. (Sensitivity may be as high as 78% in labs with experienced personnel.)
• CD4 cell count generally below 200 in HIV infected patients with PCP.
Drugs that may alter lab results: Inhaled pentamidine used to prevent PCP may change radiographic picture to infiltrates in predominantly upper-lobe distribution
Disorders that may alter lab results: N/A

PATHOLOGICAL FINDINGS Pneumonitis caused by presence of organism and inflammatory response

SPECIAL TESTS Gallium scanning of the lungs is highly sensitive for PCP but is not very specific. May be useful when sputum studies are inconclusive and bronchoscopy is not available.

IMAGING
• Chest x-ray
  ◊ Shows bilateral interstitial or perihilar infiltrate in 75% of cases
  ◊ May also show a normal chest x-ray, unilateral disease, pleural effusions, abscesses or cavitations, pneumothorax, and lobar consolidations

DIAGNOSTIC PROCEDURES
• Fiberoptic bronchoscopy with bronchoalveolar lavage or transbronchial biopsy is the preferred method of diagnosis when sputums are negative
• Open lung biopsy is rarely required
• A serum PCR test for pneumocystis may be useful in the future

TREATMENT

APPROPRIATE HEALTH CARE
Outpatient in mild cases, otherwise inpatient

GENERAL MEASURES Oxygen therapy often necessary

SURGICAL MEASURES N/A

ACTIVITY As tolerated

DIET No special diet

PATIENT EDUCATION For patient education materials on this topic, contact: American Lung Association, 1740 Broadway, New York, NY 10019, (212)315-8700

Pneumonia, Pneumocystis carinii (PCP)

MEDICATIONS

DRUG(S) OF CHOICE
• Trimethoprim-sulfamethoxazole (Bactrim, Septra) 15 mg/kg/day of trimethoprim component po in 3 divided doses or IV for 21 days. Reduce dose of trimethoprim-sulfamethoxazole in patients with renal failure.
• Adjunctive corticosteroid (prednisone or methyl prednisolone) therapy begun within 72 hours of diagnosis decreases mortality in AIDS patients (adults and children) with moderate to severe PCP (those with pO2<70 mmHg)

Contraindications: Use with care in pregnant patient and infants less than 2 months

Precautions:
• History of sulfa allergy
• A high percentage of patients with AIDS will develop intolerance to trimethoprim/ sulfamethoxazole. Especially common are dermatologic reactions, hematologic toxicity, or fever.
• Avoid sunlight

Significant possible interactions: Phenytoin, oral anti-coagulants, oral sulfonylureas, digitalis

ALTERNATIVE DRUGS
• Pentamidine 4 mg/kg/day IV for 21 days
• Dapsone 100 mg po daily plus trimethoprim 15 mg/kg/day po in 3 divided doses. Check G6PD level before beginning dapsone as hemolysis may result.
• Clindamycin 600 mg (450-650 mg) po tid plus primaquine 30 mg po daily for 21 days
• Trimetrexate glucuronate 45 mg/m2 IV qd over 60-90 minutes with leucovorin 20 mg/m2 IV or po q6h - continue for 72 hours after last dose of trimetrexate. Recommended course of therapy is 21 days of trimetrexate and 24 days of leucovorin. Doses may need to be adjusted for hematologic toxicity - monitor CBC/differential and platelets.
• Atovaquone 750 mg po bid-tid plus pyrimethamine 50-75 mg po q day for 21 days

FOLLOWUP

PATIENT MONITORING Serum LDH, pulmonary function tests and arterial blood gases generally normalize with treatment

PREVENTION/AVOIDANCE
• All AIDS patients with a history of PCP (or CD4 cells < 200 or evidence of immunodeficiency) require life-long prophylaxis with daily or thrice-weekly trimethoprim-sulfamethoxazole (double-strength), daily dapsone (100 mg/day) or monthly aerosolized pentamidine (300 mg). In patients intolerant of TMP-SMX, consider a rechallenge or desensitization with TMP-SMX - various protocols exist.
• All babies born to HIV infected mothers need to be on prophylaxis after the first month of life. Drug of choice is TMP-SMX; 150 mg/m2/day (TMP component) 3 times weekly. This should be continued until the baby is proven HIV negative or for the first year of life, after which CD4 cell count may be used to guide prophylaxis.

POSSIBLE COMPLICATIONS
• Respiratory failure
• Pneumothorax (even after successful treatment)
• Extrapulmonary pneumocystis (especially in patients on inhaled pentamidine prophylaxis)

EXPECTED COURSE/PROGNOSIS
• Previously, mortality from first episode PCP was 30-40%. Has declined to 10-15%. With prophylactic therapy, mean survival has increased.
• Approximately 11% of patients with PCP develop respiratory failure and 86% of these die

MISCELLANEOUS

ASSOCIATED CONDITIONS
• AIDS
• HIV infection

AGE-RELATED FACTORS
Pediatric:
• Early onset (5 months of age) and high mortality (median survival 1 month)
• Important to distinguish from lymphoid interstitial pneumonitis (LIP) as treatment and prognosis differ
• PCP prophylaxis with TMP-SMX, dapsone or pentamidine for all HIV positive children less than 1 year old is recommended. For older HIV positive children, prophylaxis individualized based on CD4 counts (see Prevention/Avoidance section).
Geriatric: N/A
Others: N/A

PREGNANCY
Trimethoprim-sulfamethoxazole has been used for treatment and prophylaxis. Avoid pentamidine.

SYNONYMS
• Pneumocystosis
• Pulmonary pneumocystosis
• Interstitial plasma cell pneumonia

ICD-9-CM   136.3 Pneumocystosis

SEE ALSO
• HIV infection & AIDS

OTHER NOTES   N/A

ABBREVIATIONS
• LDH = lactic acid dehydrogenase
• G6PD = glucose 6-phosphate dehydrogenase

REFERENCES
• Moe AA, Hardy WD: Pneumocystis carinii infection in the HIV-seropositive patient. Infect Dis Clin N Amer 1994;8(2):331-364
• Sistek CJ, et al: Adjuvant corticostroid therapy for Pneumocystis carinii pneumonia in AIDS patients. Ann Pharmacother 1992;9:1127-1133
• Recommendations of prophylaxis against PCP for adults and adolescents with Human Immunodeficiency Virus. MMWR, Recommendations and Reports, 41 RR-4 (April 10, 1992)
• Gluckstein D, Ruskin J: Rapid oral desensitization to trimethoprim-sulfamethoxazole: use in prophylaxis for pneumocystis carinii pneumonia in patients with AIDS who were previously intolerant of TMP/SMX. Clin Infect Dis 1995;20:849-53
Illustrations: N/A
Internet references: http://www.5mcc.com

Author(s)
Cynthia Gail Carmichael, MD

Pheumonia, viral

BASICS

DESCRIPTION Inflammatory disease of the lungs. Most viral pneumonia results from exposure of a non-immune individual to infected aerosolized secretions.
System(s) affected: Pulmonary
Genetics: No known genetic pattern
Incidence/Prevalence in USA:
• Approximately 90% of childhood pneumonia is viral
• 4-39% of pneumonia in adults has been attributed to viral etiologies in different series
• Prevalence is unknown and variable due to seasonal variation, though more common in winter months
• Mixed infections with bacterial pathogens common
Predominant age:
• More common in children than in adults
Predominant sex: Male = Female

SIGNS AND SYMPTOMS
• Fever
• Chills
• Cough (with or without purulent sputum production)
• Dyspnea
• Pulmonary rales and rhonchi
• Altered breath sounds
• Pleurisy
• Friction rub
• Headache
• Myalgias
• Malaise
• Gastrointestinal symptoms

CAUSES
• Influenza A, B and C
• Parainfluenza 1, 2, 3, and 4
• Respiratory syncytial virus (RSV, especially in young children)
• Adenovirus
• Cytomegalovirus (CMV), particularly in immunocompromised patients)
• Varicella (chickenpox)
• Herpes simplex
• Enterovirus
• Coronavirus
• Rubeola (measles)
• Epstein-Barr virus
• Hanta virus

RISK FACTORS
• Immunocompromised
• Living in close quarters
• Seasonal - epidemic upper respiratory illness
• Elderly
• Cardiac disease
• Chronic pulmonary disease
• Recent upper respiratory infection

DIAGNOSIS

DIFFERENTIAL DIAGNOSIS
• Bacterial pneumonia (especially atypical etiologies - Chlamydia pneumoniae and psittaci, Mycoplasma pneumoniae, Legionella pneumophila)
• Pulmonary edema
• Pneumocystis carinii pneumonia (PCP)
• Aspiration pneumonia
• Hypersensitivity pneumonitis
• Bronchial carcinoma with lymphangitic spread
• Bronchiolitis obliterans with organizing pneumonia (BOOP)
• Pulmonary embolus/infarction
• Cystic fibrosis (in infants)

LABORATORY
• Sputum gram stain and culture to identify bacterial co-pathogens if present
• Appropriate direct fluorescent antibody from throat swab, tracheal aspirate, or bronchoalveolar lavage specimens (HSV, VZV, Influenza A and B, RSV, adenovirus)
• Viral culture
• Cytopathology (CMV, HSV, Rubeola)
• Normal or near normal granulocyte count, occasionally leukopenic with increased lymphocyte percentage
• Hypoxemia with severe disease
• Hemoconcentration (Hanta virus)
• Serology (4-fold rise in acute vs convalescent titers)
• Polymerase chain reaction (PCR) detection if available
Drugs that may alter lab results: N/A
Disorders that may alter lab results: N/A

PATHOLOGICAL FINDINGS
• Heavy lungs
• Enlarged regional lymph nodes
• Cytoplasmic inclusion bodies (CMV)
• Intranuclear inclusion bodies (adenovirus, CMV, herpes virus, varicella)
• Intense inflammatory reaction with mononuclear cells
• Multinucleated giant cells (parainfluenza virus, Rubeola, HSV, varicella)

SPECIAL TESTS N/A

IMAGING
• Chest roentgenogram - interstitial or alveolar infiltrates, peribronchial thickening, pleural effusion

DIAGNOSTIC PROCEDURES
• Nasopharyngeal throat swab
• Tracheal aspiration (seldom needed)
• Bronchoscopy with bronchoalveolar lavage (BAL)

TREATMENT

APPROPRIATE HEALTH CARE
Outpatient for most cases. Inpatient for infants under 4 months of age or elderly, or for any patient with diffuse, severe infection (hypoxemia, hypercarbia, hypotension or shock, adult respiratory distress syndrome) or significant comorbidity (CHF, CAD, COPD, etc.)

GENERAL MEASURES
• Encourage coughing and deep breathing exercises to clear secretions
• Careful disposal of secretions/universal precautions
• Hydration
• Respiratory isolation for varicella which is highly contagious (i.e., negative pressure)

SURGICAL MEASURES N/A

ACTIVITY
• Rest

DIET
• Increase fluids, high calorie, high protein, soft diet

PATIENT EDUCATION
For patient education materials on this topic, contact: American Lung Association, 1740 Broadway, New York, NY 100919, (212)315-8700

MEDICATIONS

DRUG(S) OF CHOICE
• Amantadine (Symmetrel): Influenza A (not effective for influenza B)
  ◊ Age < 10: 4-8 mg/kg/day in 2 divided doses. Not to exceed 150 mg/day.
  ◊ Age 10-65: 100 mg orally q12 h (adults may be given a loading dose of 200 mg initially)
  ◊ Age > 65: 100 mg orally once a day
• Acyclovir (Zovirax): Pulmonary infections involving herpes simplex, herpes zoster or varicella
  ◊ Adults 5 mg/kg IV q8h for HSV pneumonia and 10 mg/kg IV q8h for varicella pneumonia
  ◊ Children 250 mg/square meter body surface area IV q8h
• Ganciclovir (Cytovene): CMV infection, HSV infection
  ◊ 5 mg/kg IV 12h
• Ribavirin (Virazole): RSV, possibly Hanta and Influenza B virus
(20 mg/mL via continuous aerosol administration for 12-18 hours/day for 3-7 days). Indicated only in severe RSV infections, given via small particle aerosol generator (SPAG).
Contraindications: Refer to manufacturer's literature
Precautions:
• Amantadine should be used cautiously in patients with liver disease, epilepsy, renal disease, eczematoid rash, and those with a history of psychotic illness
• Ribavirin is teratogenic and should not be administered by pregnant health-care personnel
Significant possible interactions: Refer to manufacturer's literature

ALTERNATIVE DRUGS
• Rimantadine (Flumadine), an amantadine analog, is equally effective as amantadine and has fewer CNS adverse effects. Useful for Influenza A.
• Antibiotics for superimposed bacterial infections.
• Foscarnet (Foscavir) for CMV, HSV, varicella infections, 60 mg/kg IV q8h
• Immune globulin, intravenous (IVIG) may increase response in non-AIDS, immunosuppressed patients with CMV pneumonia. Dose and dosage regimen not well established, but 500 mg/kg IV qod x 10 doses may be beneficial.

FOLLOWUP

PATIENT MONITORING
• Physical examinations and/or chest roentgenograms
• Oxygenation if illness severe enough for hospitalization

PREVENTION/AVOIDANCE
• Influenza A and B vaccine: Use for patients with chronic cardiovascular lung disease, residents of chronic care facilities, medical personnel with extensive contact with high risk patients, people over 65 years of age or those with chronic diseases, immunosuppressed patients
• For those patients unable to receive influenza vaccine (egg allergy or other) and are at high risk because of age, co-morbid illness, or other risk factor, amantadine or rimantadine can be given throughout the infectious season if tolerated
• For those who did not receive the vaccine and have been exposed to influenza, or there is an influenza A outbreak, amantadine or rimantadine may also be taken for 2 weeks until vaccination has produced immunity
• Health care workers who are pregnant need to take proper precautions to avoid infectious patients
• Measles vaccine
• Varicella vaccine

POSSIBLE COMPLICATIONS
• Superimposed bacterial infections such as S. pneumoniae, S. aureus, H. influenzae and others
• Respiratory failure requiring mechanical ventilation
• Adult respiratory distress syndrome (ARDS)
• Reye's syndrome after influenza in children

EXPECTED COURSE/PROGNOSIS
Usually favorable prognosis with illness lasting several days to a week. Post-viral fatigue is common. However, death can occur, especially in pediatric or bone-marrow transplant adenovirus infections or in elderly influenza infections.

MISCELLANEOUS

ASSOCIATED CONDITIONS
• Bacterial pneumonias
• Fungi, Pneumocystis carinii in immunosuppressed patients

AGE-RELATED FACTORS
Pediatric: Adenovirus infections in children are serious. More serious RSV infections are almost always seen in infants and immunocompromised patients.
Geriatric: Greatest morbidity and mortality
Others: N/A

PREGNANCY Should avoid contact with persons who may have viral infections

SYNONYMS N/A

ICD-9-CM
480.9

SEE ALSO N/A

OTHER NOTES N/A

ABBREVIATIONS
• RSV = respiratory syncytial virus
• PCP = Pneumocystis carinii pneumonia
• ARDS = adult respiratory distress syndrome
• BOOP = bronchiolitis obliterans with organizing pneumonia
• CMV = cytomegalovirus
• PCR = Polymerase chain reaction

REFERENCES
• Mandell GL, ed: Principles and Practice of Infectious Diseases. 4th Ed. New York, Churchill Livingstone, 1995
• Fields BN, ed: Virology. 2nd Ed. New York, Raven Press, 1990
• Greenburg SB: Viral Pneumonia. Infectious Disease Clinics of North America. vol. 5 (3), September 1991
• Gorbach SL, ed: Infectious Diseases. Philadelphia, W.B. Saunders Company, 1992
Illustrations: N/A
Internet references: http://www.5mcc.com

Author(s)
Gene W. Voskuhl, MD
Ronald A. Greenfield, MD

Pneumothorax

 BASICS

DESCRIPTION Accumulation of air or gas between the parietal and visceral pleurae. The amount trapped determines the degree of lung collapse.
• Spontaneous pneumothorax - may be primary or secondary
• Traumatic pneumothorax - may coexist with hemothorax
• Tension pneumothorax - the air in the pleural space is under higher pressure than air in adjacent lung and vascular structures
System(s) affected: Pulmonary, Cardiovascular
Genetics: No known genetic pattern, possible congenital predisposition in young men
Incidence/Prevalence in USA: 9/100,000
Predominant age: Adults 20-40 years
Predominant sex: Male > Female

SIGNS AND SYMPTOMS
• Chest pain, sudden, sharp, made worse by breathing, coughing or moving the chest
• Chest movements - asymmetrical
• Dyspnea
• Cyanosis (sometimes)
• Moderate to severe - profound respiratory distress
• Tension pneumothorax - weak, rapid pulse, pallor, neck vein distension, anxiety, tracheal deviation
• Shock
• Circulatory collapse
• Diminished breath sounds and voice sounds

CAUSES
• Perforation of the visceral pleura and entry of gas from the lung
• Gas generated by microorganisms in an empyema
• Penetration of the chest wall, diaphragm, mediastinum, or esophagus

RISK FACTORS
• Trauma (broken rib, ruptured bronchus, perforated esophagus)
• Rupture of superficial lung bulla following cough or blowing a musical instrument
• Vigorous or stretching exercises
• Flying (high altitude)
• Pneumoconioses
• Tuberculosis
• Bronchial obstruction
• COPD (particularly emphysema)
• Diving (at ascension or rapid decompression)
• Asthma
• Neoplasms
• Endometriosis (during menstruation)
• Rare diseases (Marfan's, Ehlers-Danlos)
• Rupture of an infected abscess
• Lymphangioleiomyomatosis
• Cystic fibrosis
• Subpleural Pneumocystis carinii pneumonia (PCP) (in AIDS patients on PCP prophylaxis via pentamidine aerosol)
• Cigarette smoking
• Broad swings in atmospheric pressure
• Intubation ventilation

 DIAGNOSIS

DIFFERENTIAL DIAGNOSIS
• Pleurisy
• Pericarditis
• Myocardial infarction
• Pulmonary embolism
• Diaphragmatic hernia
• Stomach herniation through diaphragm
• Dissecting aneurysm

LABORATORY
• Arterial blood gases in significant pneumothorax
  ◊ pH < 7.35
  ◊ pO2 < 80 mm Hg (10.6 kPa)
  ◊ pCO2 > 45 mm Hg (6.0 kPa)
Drugs that may alter lab results: N/A
Disorders that may alter lab results: N/A

PATHOLOGICAL FINDINGS N/A

SPECIAL TESTS N/A

IMAGING
• Chest x-ray:
  ◊ Air without lung markings peripherally, mediastinal shift to contralateral side
  ◊ Small pneumothorax may be evident only with expiratory or lateral decubitus film

DIAGNOSTIC PROCEDURES Careful history and physical. The physical findings depend on size of pneumothorax.

 TREATMENT

APPROPRIATE HEALTH CARE
• Outpatient - lung collapse less than 30%, no dyspnea, no signs of tension pneumothorax, no underlying lung disease
• Inpatient - if more than 30% collapse, tension or underlying lung disease

GENERAL MEASURES
• Outpatient
  ◊ Bed rest
  ◊ Monitoring blood pressure, pulse rate, respirations
  ◊ Oxygen at high concentration will accelerate rate of absorption by 4 times
  ◊ Treatment of any underlying condition
• Inpatient - see Surgical Measures
• Recurrent pneumothorax - see Surgical Measures

SURGICAL MEASURES
• Inpatient
  ◊ Simple aspiration - insert 16 gauge cannula into 2nd anterior intercostal space at midclavicular line and attach to three-way stopcock and 60 mL syringe. Withdraw air manually until no more can be aspirated.
  ◊ Thoracotomy tube - inserted in 4th, 5th or 6th intercostal space at midaxillary line and connect underwater seal
  ◊ Tension pneumothorax - insert 19-gauge or larger needle into the chest followed by using a 3-way stopcock attached to a large syringe to withdraw air. Follow with tube insertion
• Recurrent pneumothorax
  ◊ Can cause severe disability
  ◊ Consider thoracoscopy or thoracotomy following 2 or more spontaneous pneumothoraces, if lungs not expanded after 7 days therapy or persistent bronchopleural fistula
  ◊ Consider pleurodesis

ACTIVITY
• Bed rest until re-expanded
• No air travel until x-ray normal

DIET No special diet

PATIENT EDUCATION Stop smoking

MEDICATIONS

DRUG(S) OF CHOICE
• Pleurodesis for recurrent pneumothorax:
  ◊ Intrapleural doxycycline, 5 mg/kg in a total volume of 50 mL. Intrapleural doxycycline is painful so premedicate with short-acting benzodiazepine and give 4 mg/kg lidocaine in a total volume of 50 mL intrapleurally before doxycycline is injected.
  ◊ Intrapleural talc, 5g in 250 mL isotonic saline
Contraindications: If patient a possible candidate for future lung transplant, do not do sclerosing pleurodesis (sclerosing agents increase risk of bleeding at surgery so patients are not eligible for transplant)
Precautions:
• Talc procedure precipitated respiratory distress syndrome in 2 reports
• Pain at time of intrapleural instillation and postprocedure are most common side effects
Significant possible interactions: Refer to manufacturer's literature

ALTERNATIVE DRUGS   None

FOLLOWUP

PATIENT MONITORING
• Blood pressure, respiratory rate, arterial blood gases, for hospitalized patients
• After simple aspiration - clamp chest tube for 24 hours, then remove if no recurrence on x-ray. If lung not fully re-expanded after 7 days, consider persistent air leak/bronchopleural fistula.

PREVENTION/AVOIDANCE   No preventive measures known, but patients may avoid some risk factors, e.g., exposure to high altitudes, flying in unpressurized aircraft, scuba diving, smoking

POSSIBLE COMPLICATIONS
• Re-expansion pulmonary edema following suction
• Bronchopleural fistulae requiring surgical repair
• Surgery indicated following 2 spontaneous pneumothoraces on the same side

EXPECTED COURSE/PROGNOSIS
• Air reabsorbed from small spontaneous pneumothorax in a few days
• Air reabsorbed from larger air space in 2-4 weeks
• Risk of recurrence is 30-50%

MISCELLANEOUS

ASSOCIATED CONDITIONS   Listed with Causes

AGE-RELATED FACTORS
Pediatric: Unusual in this age group except following trauma
Geriatric: Higher morbidity and mortality
Others: N/A

PREGNANCY   A known, but unusual complication of labor and delivery. It should be suspected in the pregnant patient with dyspnea and chest pain.

SYNONYMS   N/A

ICD-9-CM
512.0 Spontaneous tension pneumothorax
512.1 Iatrogenic pneumothorax
512.8 Other spontaneous pneumothorax

SEE ALSO   N/A

OTHER NOTES   Chest pain may simulate an acute coronary occlusion or acute abdomen

ABBREVIATIONS   N/A

REFERENCES
• Light RW: Management of spontaneous pneumothorax. Ann rev Respir Dis 1993;148:245
• Miller AC, Harvey JE: Guidelines for the management of spontaneous pneumothorax. Br Med J 1993;307:114
Illustrations: N/A
Internet references: http://www.5mcc.com

Author(s)
Cheryl Zagozeski, MD, CCFP

Poliomyelitis

BASICS

DESCRIPTION Acute illness, symptomatic cases present as aseptic meningitis. Only a small number of cases with residual neurologic disease. Most symptomatic cases have nonspecific manifestations of infection. Illness is biphasic, paralysis occurs in second phase. Paralytic disease occurs with rapid onset.
Spread by direct contact - fecal/oral. More common in warm months. Virus secreted for weeks in stool.
• Three types
  ◊ Encephalitic - coma
  ◊ Bulbar - cranial nerve paralysis
  ◊ Spinal - arm(s) and leg(s) weakness
System(s) affected: Nervous, Musculoskeletal
Genetics: N/A
Incidence/Prevalence in USA: Two new cases per year
Predominant age: 3 months-16 years; rarely adults
Predominant sex: Male = Female

SIGNS AND SYMPTOMS
• Nonspecific
• Meningitis
• Neurologic symptoms

CAUSES Poliovirus - most common types are Brunhilde, Lansing and Leon

RISK FACTORS
• Living in areas where sanitation and hygiene are poor
• Low socioeconomic status
• Increasing age, if not immunized
• Pregnancy
• Recent tonsillectomy
• Inoculation (e.g., DPT injection)

DIAGNOSIS

DIFFERENTIAL DIAGNOSIS
• Guillain-Barré syndrome
• Mumps, herpes, coxsackievirus infection
• Aseptic meningitis
• Tick paralysis

LABORATORY
• Pleocytosis
• Increased protein
• Normal glucose
• Serology
• Virus culture - should be done when suspected
Drugs that may alter lab results: N/A
Disorders that may alter lab results: N/A

PATHOLOGICAL FINDINGS
• Spinal cord - perivascular cuffing, abnormal motor nuclei, chromatolysis of motor neurons, intermediate column inflammation, posterior column inflammation
• Diffuse mononuclear infiltrate
• Abnormal anterior horn cells
• Hypothalamic lesion
• Thalamic lesion
• Brainstem lesion
• Vestibular nuclei lesions
• Cerebellar deep nuclei lesions
• Reticular formation lesions
• Cortical motor area lesions
• Cerebral edema
• Edematous cord

SPECIAL TESTS Spinal fluid virus isolation from throat (early in disease) and/or feces (early and late in the disease)

IMAGING N/A

DIAGNOSTIC PROCEDURES Viral culture of CSF, stool and throat

TREATMENT

APPROPRIATE HEALTH CARE Inpatient for acute phase. Outpatient or rehabilitation facility for therapy.

GENERAL MEASURES
• Provide bed that has firm mattress, footboard, foam rubber pads or sandbags. Change positions frequently. Give good skin care.
• Mechanical ventilation, if required
• Management of fecal impaction and urinary retention. Catheterization may be necessary.
• Non-narcotic analgesics
• Hot, moist packs
• Physical therapy
• Public health - all suspected cases, report immediately to public health department

SURGICAL MEASURES Tracheostomy is frequently required in respiratory paralysis

ACTIVITY
• Bedrest during active phase. With paralysis, may require an extended period.
• Long-term rehabilitation plan - using physical therapy, braces, special shoes, possibly orthopedic surgery. Team effort with doctors, physical and occupational therapists, and social worker or psychiatrist, if necessary.

DIET Be sure patient has adequate well-balanced diet. May require tube feedings.

PATIENT EDUCATION For patient education materials favorably reviewed on this topic, contact: International Polio Network, 4502 Maryland Avenue, St. Louis, MO 63108, (314)361-0475

Poliomyelitis

MEDICATIONS

DRUG(S) OF CHOICE
• Aspirin or other non-narcotic analgesics
• Antibiotics, if other infection develops
• Parasympathomimetic (bethanechol) may help patient with urinary retention, 10-50 mg po bid-qid. Up to 100 mg qid may be required.
Contraindications: Refer to manufacturer's literature
Precautions: Bethanechol - adverse affects are rare, but may occur if dose increased. Includes colicky feeling, urinary urgency, skin flushing.
Significant possible interactions: Refer to manufacturer's literature

ALTERNATIVE DRUGS N/A

FOLLOWUP

PATIENT MONITORING Individualized depending on severity and long-term physical therapy requirements

PREVENTION/AVOIDANCE
• Poliovirus vaccines; live oral and inactive. Vaccine recommendations shifting toward using inactive vaccine in order to prevent vaccine-associated paralytic poliomyelitis (VAPP)
(Note: Use of these vaccines has effectively eliminated the disease in the industrialized world.)

POSSIBLE COMPLICATIONS
• Urinary tract infection
• Atelectasis
• Pneumonia
• Myocarditis
• Postpoliomyelitis progressive muscular atrophy (PPMA) - characterized by progressive weakness beginning 30 years or more after an attack of poliomyelitis
• Postpoliomyelitis motor neuron disease - occurs many years after acute poliomyelitis, less common than PPMA

EXPECTED COURSE/PROGNOSIS
• Often irreversible paralysis; less than 5% mortality during acute disease
• Increased mortality over age 40
• Poor recovery for totally paralyzed muscle groups
• Good recovery for partially paralyzed muscle groups

MISCELLANEOUS

ASSOCIATED CONDITIONS N/A

AGE-RELATED FACTORS
Pediatric: Most common in this age group. Polio is an extremely rare infection in U.S. since introduction of effective vaccines. (See Immunizations topic).
Geriatric: Extremely rare. Primary vaccination not recommended (except when traveling to endemic areas).
Others: N/A

PREGNANCY A risk factor for developing polio

SYNONYMS
• Infantile paralysis
• Acute anterior poliomyelitis
• Acute lateral poliomyelitis

ICD-9-CM 045.1 Acute poliomyelitis with other paralysis

SEE ALSO Immunizations

OTHER NOTES
WHO goal: eliminate polio in Americas by 2001

ABBREVIATIONS
WHO = World Health Organization

REFERENCES
• Bennett JC, Plum F, eds: Cecil Textbook of Medicine. 20th Ed. Philadelphia, W.B. Saunders Co., 1996
• Mandell GL, ed: Principles and Practice of Infectious Diseases. 4th Ed. New York, Churchill Livingstone, 1995
Illustrations: N/A
Internet references: http://www.5mcc.com

Author(s)
Mark M. Shelton, MD

Polyarteritis nodosa

BASICS

DESCRIPTION Polyarteritis nodosa (PAN) presents pathologically as an ongoing segmental inflammatory response within the media of small and medium sized muscular arteries
• Organ involvement - kidney, GI tract, skin, muscles, joints, genitourinary tract, peripheral and central nervous system, heart, testes, epididymis and ovaries
• One of the vasculitic syndromes which vary in involvement from mild, self-limited skin lesions to severe systemic isolated and combined, multi-organ dysfunction and death
• Although heterogeneity and "overlap" manifestations abound, PAN is classified as a systemic necrotizing vasculitis
System(s) affected: Cardiovascular, Nervous, Skin/Exocrine, Renal/Urologic, Gastrointestinal, Musculoskeletal
Genetics: Unknown
Incidence/Prevalence in USA: No definite figures because of inclusive grouping of different types of vasculitic syndromes
Predominant age: Childhood to geriatric age groups. Mean is 45 years.
Predominant sex: Male > Female (2.5:1)

SIGNS AND SYMPTOMS
• General (often nonspecific)
  ◊ Fever
  ◊ Weakness
  ◊ Weight loss
  ◊ Malaise
  ◊ Myalgia
  ◊ Livido reticularis
  ◊ Headache
  ◊ Abdominal pain and vague discomfort
• Related to organ system involved (may dominate clinical picture and course)
  ◊ Renal - hypertension, hematuria (usually microscopic), proteinuria, progressive renal failure
  ◊ Musculoskeletal - myalgia, migratory arthralgia and arthritis
  ◊ Skin - purpura, urticaria, subcutaneous hemorrhages, polymorphic rashes, subcutaneous nodules (uncommon but characteristic), persistent livedo reticularis and Raynaud's phenomenon (rare)
  ◊ Gastrointestinal - recurrent and severe pain, hepatomegaly, nausea, vomiting and bleeding
  ◊ Lung - Hilar adenopathy, patchy infiltrates, reticular or nodular lesions, often fleeting
  ◊ CNS - seizures, CVA's, headache, papillitis, altered mental states
  ◊ Peripheral nervous system - mononeuritis multiplex
  ◊ Cardiac - pericarditis, CHF associated with hypertension and/or myocardial infarction
  ◊ Genitourinary - usually asymptomatic but may have testicular, epididymal, ovarian pain. Neurogenic bladder reported.

CAUSES
• Unclear. Suggestive evidence for immunological involvement.
  ◊ Tissue deposition of immune complexes
  ◊ Hepatitis B antigenemia in 30% of cases
  ◊ Hepatitis B antigen in circulating immune complexes
  ◊ Hepatitis B antigen, complement and IgM demonstrated in vascular walls

RISK FACTORS N/A

DIAGNOSIS

DIFFERENTIAL DIAGNOSIS
• Systemic lupus erythematosis
• Cryoglobulinemia
• Subacute endocarditis
• Trichinosis
• Some rickettsial diseases
• Microscopic polyarteritis
• The key differences from other necrotizing vasculitides are lack of granuloma formation, sparing of veins and pulmonary arteries

LABORATORY
• Non specific:
  ◊ Abnormal urine sediment
  ◊ High neutrophil count
  ◊ Eosinophilia rare. Suggests granulomatous involvement when present
  ◊ Anemia of chronic disease
  ◊ Elevated sedimentation rate
  ◊ Hypergammaglobulinemia
  ◊ Hepatitis B surface antigen positive in 30% of cases (strong circumstantial evidence)
• Specific
  ◊ Mainly based on pathological findings of biopsy material from involved organs
  ◊ Careful examinations of biopsies from "acute abdomens", especially in males between the second and fourth decade
  ◊ Negative anti-neutrophil cytoplasm antibodies
Drugs that may alter lab results:
• Corticosteroids
Disorders that may alter lab results:
Allergic reactions and other immunologic disorders

PATHOLOGICAL FINDINGS
• Necrotizing inflammation, in various stages, of small and medium muscular arteries. Segmental in distribution, often seen at bifurcations and branchings. Involvement of venules not seen in classic PAN.
• Acute lesions show infiltration of polymorphonuclear cells through vessel wall and perivascular area
• Subsequent proliferation, degeneration, appearance of monocytes, necrosis with thrombosis and infarction of the involved tissue. Aneurysmal dilatations characteristic.
• Aortic dissection reported attributed to necrotizing vasculitis of the vasa vasorum

SPECIAL TESTS Angiographic demonstration of aneurysmal changes of small and medium sized arteries involving renal hepatic and mesenteric arteries represents strong evidence supporting the diagnosis

IMAGING Angiography: Mesenteric artery aneurysm, renal aneurysm, hepatic aneurysm, intestinal aneurysm

DIAGNOSTIC PROCEDURES N/A

TREATMENT

APPROPRIATE HEALTH CARE Depends on extent and involvement of specific organs

GENERAL MEASURES The same as those needed for patients under treatment with steroids (high risk of infections), cytotoxic agents and plasmapheresis

SURGICAL MEASURES N/A

ACTIVITY As tolerated

DIET Low salt if hypertensive

PATIENT EDUCATION Arthritis Foundation, 1314 Spring Street N.W., Atlanta, GA 30309, (800)283-7800

Polyarteritis nodosa

MEDICATIONS

DRUG(S) OF CHOICE
• Favorable results reported with prednisone and cyclophosphamide. Reports differ as to the benefits of adding plasmaphoresis.
• Hepatitis B vaccine may be considered for the amelioration of any subsequent development of life-threatening complications of hepatitis B virus-associated polyarteritis nodosa

Contraindications: Refer to manufacturer's profile of each drug

Precautions: Refer to manufacturer's profile of each drug

Significant possible interactions: Refer to manufacturer's profile of each drug

ALTERNATIVE DRUGS   N/A

FOLLOWUP

PATIENT MONITORING
• Careful monitoring for infection
• Delayed appearance of neoplasms
• Angiographic changes may improve rapidly with combination steroid/cyclophosphamide therapy
• Acute phase reactants such as Interleukin-6 and C-reactive protein may be useful in diagnosis and monitoring activity level during treatment and followup

PREVENTION/AVOIDANCE   N/A

POSSIBLE COMPLICATIONS
• Glomerulonephritis
• Thrombosis
• Infarction
• Tissue/organ necrosis

EXPECTED COURSE/PROGNOSIS
• Expected course of untreated polyarteritis nodosa is poor
• 5 year survival rate 13%
• Steroid treatment may increase percentage survival rate to 50-60% (prospective studies in progress)
• Renal and GI signs most serious prognostic factors

MISCELLANEOUS

ASSOCIATED CONDITIONS
• Churg-Strauss syndrome
• Benign cutaneous periarteritis nodosa (bears watching and investigating because not necessarily benign)

AGE-RELATED FACTORS
Pediatric: N/A
Geriatric: N/A
Others: N/A

PREGNANCY   One case report suggests that if a patient attains remission before becoming pregnant, the chance of a successful delivery is reasonable

SYNONYMS
• Periarteritis
• Panarteritis
• Necrotizing arteritis

ICD-9-CM   446.0 Polyarteritis nodosa

SEE ALSO   N/A

OTHER NOTES   N/A

ABBREVIATIONS   N/A

REFERENCES
• Isselbacher KJ, et al, eds: Harrison's Principles of Internal Medicine. 13th Ed. New York, McGraw-Hill, 1994
• Bennett JC, Plum F, eds: Cecil Textbook of Medicine. 20th Ed. Philadelphia, W.B. Saunders Co., 1996
• Iino T, et al: Polyarteritis nodosa. J Rheumatol 1992;19(10):1632-36
• Nakayama H: Distinct response interleukin-6 and other laboratory parameters to treatment in a patient with polyarteritis nodosa. Angiology 1992;43(6):512-6
• Garanger TA, et al: Anti-neutrophil cytoplasmic antibodies in patient's with the Americal College of Rheumatology criteria for pain. Autoimmunity 1995;20(1):33-7
Illustrations: N/A
Internet references: http://www.5mcc.com

Author(s)
J. Harlan Dix, MD, FACP

Polycystic kidney disease

 BASICS

DESCRIPTION Inherited disorders characterized by the development and growth of cysts in the kidneys; lined by epithelium, filled with fluid or semi-solid debris; accounts for 5-10% of patients with end stage renal disease

System(s) affected: Renal/Urologic
Genetics: See Causes
Incidence/Prevalence in USA: 1/200-1/1000
Predominant age: Usually diagnosed by age 45
Predominant sex: Male = Female

SIGNS AND SYMPTOMS
• Hypertension
• Hematuria; microscopic or macroscopic
• Palpable kidneys
• Hepatomegaly
• Abdominal pain
• Flank pain (60%)
• Headache
• Nocturia
• Dysuria
• Urinary frequency
• Polyuria

CAUSES
• Inherited autosomal dominant abnormality linked to chromosome 16. 90% penetrance by age 90 in gene carriers. A second gene on chromosome 4 recently identified. Rare autosomal recessive form exists in neonates. Offspring of affected individuals with 50% chance of acquiring disease. Can be detected in amniocentesis.
• Acquired polycystic kidney disease – found in 50% of patients on dialysis > 3 years

RISK FACTORS Dialysis

 DIAGNOSIS

DIFFERENTIAL DIAGNOSIS
• Simple cysts
• Nephronophthisis-medullary cystic disease
• Medullary sponge kidney

LABORATORY
• Hematocrit - elevated in 5% of cases
• Urinalysis - may have hematuria and mild proteinuria
• Serum creatinine - may be elevated
Drugs that may alter lab results: N/A
Disorders that may alter lab results: N/A

PATHOLOGICAL FINDINGS N/A

SPECIAL TESTS
• Gene linkage analysis
  ◊ Helpful for suspected cases with nondiagnostic imaging
    ◊ Expensive
    ◊ Requires other family members

IMAGING
• Ultrasonography: > 5 cysts in the renal cortex or medulla of each kidney, in children, 2 or more cysts in either kidney
• CT scan more sensitive
• 85% of patients can be detected by age 25

DIAGNOSTIC PROCEDURES N/A

 TREATMENT

APPROPRIATE HEALTH CARE
Outpatient except for complicating emergencies (infected cysts require 2 weeks IV antibiotics then long-term oral antibiotics)

GENERAL MEASURES
• Pain – bed rest and analgesics
• Hematuria (due to ruptured cyst) – bed rest, sedation, IV hydration

SURGICAL MEASURES
Renal transplant, by age 6-8 years, for autosomal recessive form

ACTIVITY Avoid contact activities that may damage enlarged organs.

DIET Low protein diet may retard progression of renal disease.

PATIENT EDUCATION
• Genetic counseling is critical
• Avoidance of nephrotoxic drugs

MEDICATIONS

DRUG(S) OF CHOICE
• No drug therapy available for polycystic kidney disease
• Hypertension – ACE inhibitors; avoid diuretics (possible adverse effects with cyst formation)
Contraindications: N/A
Precautions: N/A
Significant possible interactions: N/A

ALTERNATIVE DRUGS   N/A

FOLLOWUP

PATIENT MONITORING   Serum creatinine and blood pressure monitoring twice a year; more frequently as disease progresses

PREVENTION/AVOIDANCE   Genetic counseling

POSSIBLE COMPLICATIONS
• Progression to renal failure
• Renal calculi in up to 30%
• Cyst infection
• Cyst rupture

EXPECTED COURSE/PROGNOSIS
• The disease is slowly progressive and has a variable outcome
• End stage renal disease occurs in 70% of patients by age 65
• Acquired disease with 5% adenocarcinoma, cysts regress after renal transplant, once nonazotemic

MISCELLANEOUS

ASSOCIATED CONDITIONS
• Cerebral aneurysms present in 10-40% of patients
• Colonic diverticuli in 80%
• Liver cysts in approximately 50%
• Pancreatic and ovarian cysts
• Mitral valve prolapse in 26%

AGE-RELATED FACTORS
Pediatric: N/A
Geriatric: Renal insufficiency in 50% of patients by age 70, accounts for 5-10% of dialysis patients.
Others: Hypertension is secondary to high renin. Responds to angiotensin converting enzyme (ACE) inhibitors.

PREGNANCY   Higher frequency of new onset hypertension than in women without polycystic kidney disease. No adverse effect on the course of the polycystic kidney disease in asymptomatic patients. Patients with hypertension, proteinuria or renal insufficiency are at increased risk of complications. Also an increase in hepatic cysts with pregnancy (rarely a problem).

SYNONYMS   N/A

ICD-9-CM
753.1 Polycystic kidney, unspecified type
753.13 Polycystic kidney, autosomal dominant
753.14 Polycystic kidney, autosomal recessive

SEE ALSO
• Renal failure, chronic
• Renal calculi

OTHER NOTES   N/A

ABBREVIATIONS   N/A

REFERENCES
• Welling LW, Granthem JJ: Cystic and developmental diseases of the kidney. In: Brenner BM, Rector FC, eds. The Kidney. Philadelphia, W.B. Saunders, 1991
• Chapman AB, Johnson A, Gabow PA, Schrier RW: The renin-angiotensin-aldosterone system and autosomal dominant polycystic kidney disease. N Engl J Med 1990;323:1091-1096
• Beebe DK: Autosomal dominant polycystic kidney disease. Amer Fam Phys 1996;53(3):925-931
Illustrations: N/A
Internet references: http://www.5mcc.com

Author(s)
Douglas M. Hoy, MD

Polycystic ovarian disease

BASICS

DESCRIPTION Polycystic ovarian disease (PCOD) is characterized by a state of chronic oligo-ovulation and/or anovulation culminating in oligomenorrhea and/or amenorrhea
System(s) affected: Reproductive, Endocrine/Metabolic, Skin/Exocrine
Genetics: N/A
Incidence/Prevalence in USA: Unknown, but is a common cause of oligomenorrhea and/or amenorrhea
Predominant age: Women of reproductive age
Predominant sex: Female only

SIGNS AND SYMPTOMS
• Amenorrhea
• Oligomenorrhea
• Obesity
• Hirsutism
• Acne
• Dysfunctional uterine bleeding
• Infertility
• Acanthosis nigricans
• Hypertension
• Virilism
• Enlarged ovaries
• Enlarged clitoris
• Deep voice

CAUSES Disruption of hypothalamic-pituitary-ovarian axis (high normal luteinizing hormone and low normal follicle stimulating hormone leading to ovarian hyperandrogenism and follicular atresia and anovulation)

RISK FACTORS
• Endometrial hyperplasia
• Endometrial carcinoma
• Obesity
• Hypertension
• Diabetes mellitus
• Breast cancer
• Infertility

DIAGNOSIS

DIFFERENTIAL DIAGNOSIS
• Cushing's syndrome
• Hairan syndrome (hyperandrogenism, insulin resistance, acanthosis nigricans)
• Testosterone-producing ovarian or adrenal tumor
• Prolactin-producing pituitary adenoma
• Hyperthecosis
• Adult-onset adrenal hyperplasia
• Partial congenital adrenal hyperplasia (21-hydroxylase deficiency)
• Other adrenal enzyme deficiencies
• Endometrial hyperplasia
• Endometrial carcinoma

LABORATORY
• Luteinizing hormone/follicle stimulating hormone (LH/FSH) ≥ 2.5-3.0/1
• Testosterone increased, but less than 200 ng/dL (6.94 nmol/L)
• Dehydroepiandrosterone sulfate (DHEA-S) increased, but less than 800 µg/dL (20.8 µmol/L)
• Dehydroepiandrosterone (DHEA) increased
• 17-OH progesterone increased
• Estrone increased
• Androstenedione increased
• Sex hormone binding globulin decreased
• Prolactin
Drugs that may alter lab results:
• Oral contraceptives
• Steroids
• Antidepressants
Disorders that may alter lab results: N/A

PATHOLOGICAL FINDINGS
• Ovary usually enlarged with a smooth white glistening capsule
• Ovarian cortex lined with follicles in all stages of development but most are atretic
• Theca cell proliferation with an increase in the stromal compartment

SPECIAL TESTS N/A

IMAGING Pelvis ultrasound revealing enlarged ovaries with multiple small follicular cysts

DIAGNOSTIC PROCEDURES
• History and physical examination
• Endometrial biopsy to rule out hyperplasia and or carcinoma

TREATMENT

APPROPRIATE HEALTH CARE
• Outpatient
• Inpatient, if surgery for wedge resection recommended

GENERAL MEASURES No ideal treatment exists. Treatment must be individualized according to the needs and desires of the patient.

SURGICAL MEASURES N/A

ACTIVITY Full activity

DIET Regular (weight loss recommended, if overweight)

PATIENT EDUCATION Counsel the patient regarding the risk of endometrial and breast carcinoma, insulin resistance and diabetes mellitus, obesity and infertility

MEDICATIONS

DRUG(S) OF CHOICE
• If pregnancy not desired:
◊ Cyclic withdrawal bleeding with medroxyprogesterone acetate (Provera) 10 mg po x 12-14 days/month
or
◊ Low dose oral contraceptives
• If pregnancy desired:
◊ Ovulation induction with clomiphene citrate (Clomid, Serophene)
or
◊ Human menopausal gonadotropins - menotropins (Pergonal)
or
◊ Pure follicle-stimulating hormone (Metrodin) with or without the addition of gonadotropin releasing hormone (GnRH) agonist (leuprolide acetate (Lupron) or nafarelin acetate (Synarel))

Contraindications: None, but if using oral contraceptive agents to prevent sequelae of anovulation, be aware of contraindications

Precautions:
• Risks of multiple fetuses with clomiphene citrate is 8%
• Risks of multiple fetuses with HMG, FSH is 25%
• Risk of severe ovarian hyperstimulation syndrome (OHS) is less than 1%

Significant possible interactions: Refer to manufacturer's profile of each drug

ALTERNATIVE DRUGS
Bromocriptine if prolactin is elevated

FOLLOWUP

PATIENT MONITORING Monitor patient frequently throughout the menstrual cycle depending upon which drug combination is utilized for ovulation induction

PREVENTION/AVOIDANCE Prevent endometrial and breast carcinoma

POSSIBLE COMPLICATIONS
• Multiple pregnancies
• Ovarian hyperstimulation syndrome (OHS)
• Oral contraceptives are not without risk

EXPECTED COURSE/PROGNOSIS
• Prognosis for fertility is excellent depending upon other fertility factors
• Proper treatment and followup of chronic anovulation, can prevent endometrial hyperplasia and/or carcinoma

MISCELLANEOUS

ASSOCIATED CONDITIONS
• Obesity
• Hypertension
• Endometrial hyperplasia and/or carcinoma
• Breast carcinoma
• Diabetes mellitus
• Hairan syndrome
• Infertility
• Hyperthecosis

AGE-RELATED FACTORS
Pediatric: N/A
Geriatric: N/A
Others: N/A

PREGNANCY Does not cure the syndrome

SYNONYMS
• Stein-Leventhal syndrome
• Polycystic ovary syndrome

ICD-9-CM
• 256.4
• 628.0

SEE ALSO
• Amenorrhea
• Forbes-Albright syndrome

OTHER NOTES
• Drug costs high
• Monitoring (ultrasounds, estradiols) costs high

ABBREVIATIONS
OHS = ovarian hyperstimulation syndrome
HMG = human menopausal gonadotropins
FSH = follicle stimulating hormone

REFERENCES Danforth DM, Scott JR, et al, eds: Obstetric and Gynecology. 6th Ed. Philadelphia, J.B. Lippincott, 1990
Illustrations: N/A
Internet references: http://www.5mcc.com

Author(s)
Nicholas J. Spirtos, DO

Polycythemia vera

 BASICS

DESCRIPTION A clonal cell hematologic malignant disorder with excessive erythroid, myeloid and megakaryocytic elements in the bone marrow. It is one of a group of myeloproliferative disorders.

System(s) affected:
Hemic/Lymphatic/Immunologic

Genetics: Unknown genetic pattern (some suggestion that a chromosomal abnormality may be involved)

Incidence/Prevalence in USA: 0.5 per 100,000

Predominant age: Middle to late years, mean is 60 years (range 15-90)

Predominant sex: Male > Female (slightly)

SIGNS AND SYMPTOMS
• Early stages may produce no symptoms
• Headaches
• Tinnitus
• Vertigo
• Blurred vision
• Epistaxis
• Increased blood viscosity
• Spontaneous bruising
• Upper GI bleeding
• Peptic ulcer disease
• Arterial and venous occlusive events
• Pruritus
• Sweating
• Weight loss
• Plethora (face, hands, feet)
• Splenomegaly
• Hepatomegaly
• Hyperhistaminemia
• Bone pain (ribs and sternum)
• Bone tenderness (ribs and sternum)

CAUSES Unknown, all three hematopoietic cell lines originate in a single clone

RISK FACTORS
• Jewish ancestry (may have increased frequency)
• Familial history (rare)

 DIAGNOSIS

DIFFERENTIAL DIAGNOSIS
• Secondary polycythemias
• Hemoglobinopathy
• Spurious polycythemia

LABORATORY
• Tests used for diagnosis of polycythemia vera
  ◊ A1: Increased RBC mass - female ≥ 32 mL/kg, male ≥ 36 mL/kg
  ◊ A2: Normal arterial oxygen saturation (≥ 92%)
  ◊ A3: Splenomegaly
  ◊ B1: Thrombocytosis platelet count > 400,000/μL
  ◊ B2: Leukocytosis > 12,000/μL
  ◊ B3: Leukocyte alkaline phosphatase increased
  ◊ B4: Increased serum B12 or increased unsaturated vitamin B12 binding capacity (UB12CB)
• Diagnosis acceptable with following combinations:
  ◊ A1 + A2 + A3
  ◊ A1 + A2 + any 2 from B category (splenomegaly absent in about 25% of patients)
• Other lab findings
  ◊ Hyperuricemia
  ◊ Hypercholesterolemia
  ◊ Elevated blood histamine level

Drugs that may alter lab results:
Diuretics may cause a spurious polycythemia

Disorders that may alter lab results:
Excessive use of alcohol or tobacco

PATHOLOGICAL FINDINGS
• Plethoric congestion in all organs and tissues
• Major vessels contain thick, viscous blood
• Sinuses of spleen packed with red blood cells

SPECIAL TESTS Bone marrow aspiration (red cell hyperplasia, absent iron stores) and biopsy (fibrosis during spent phase of the disease)

IMAGING CT - splenomegaly

DIAGNOSTIC PROCEDURES Bone marrow aspiration - hyperplastic and panmyelosis

 TREATMENT

APPROPRIATE HEALTH CARE
Outpatient

GENERAL MEASURES
Individualized management necessary. Dependent on many factors - age, disease duration, disease phenotype, complications, disease activity.
Currently, phlebotomy is mainstay of therapy. Beyond that, differences exist among authorities about use and effectiveness of myelosuppressives.
• Phlebotomy
  ◊ To reduce hematocrit to approximately 45%
  ◊ Performed as often as every 2 or 3 days until normal hematocrit reached. Phlebotomies of 250-500 m/L. Reduce to 250-350 m/L in elderly patients or patients with cardiovascular disease.
  ◊ Concomitant therapy possibilities, e.g., some form of myelosuppression, radioactive phosphorus (in elderly patients)
  ◊ Phlebotomy repeated as necessary for maintenance
  ◊ If patient cannot tolerate phlebotomy - chemotherapy (hydroxyurea is the least mutagenic agent) or radiation therapy
• Other therapy
  ◊ Maintain hydration
  ◊ Pruritus therapy
  ◊ Manage thrombotic or hemorrhagic complications the same as with nonpolycythemic patient
  ◊ Uric acid reduction therapy

SURGICAL MEASURES N/A

ACTIVITY No restrictions

DIET
• No special diet (iron replacement not necessary)
• Phlebotomy regimen will produce pica, resulting in craving for crisp green vegetables (lettuce, celery) and ice

PATIENT EDUCATION
• Lifelong maintenance
• Complications to watch for

Polycythemia vera

 MEDICATIONS

DRUG(S) OF CHOICE
• Adjunctive
◊ Allopurinol 300 mg/day for uric acid reduction
◊ Cyproheptadine for pruritus, 4-16 mg as needed
◊ H2-receptor blockers or antacids for GI hyperacidity
• Myelosuppression
◊ Radioactive phosphorous in selected cases
◊ Busulfan or alkylating agents (e.g., hydroxyurea)
◊ The use of low-dose aspirin is controversial in view of bleeding risk, but small doses may be given if required
◊ Note: Refer to hematologist/oncologist for dosages and instructions
Contraindications: Refer to manufacturer's literature
Precautions: Refer to manufacturer's literature
Significant possible interactions: Refer to manufacturer's literature

ALTERNATIVE DRUGS
• Myelosuppression: chlorambucil, some authors believe contraindicated
• Interferon is an emerging treatment

 FOLLOWUP

PATIENT MONITORING
• Frequent during early treatment until satisfactory hematocrit is reached
• Monitor hematocrit often and phlebotomize when needed

PREVENTION/AVOIDANCE   No known preventive measures

POSSIBLE COMPLICATIONS
• Uric acid stones
• Secondary gout
• Vascular thromboses (major cause of death)
• Transformation to leukemia
• Hemorrhage
• Peptic ulcer
• Increased risk for complications and mortality from surgery procedures. Assess risk-benefits and assure optimal control of disorder before any elective surgery.

EXPECTED COURSE/PROGNOSIS
• Median survival without treatment - 6 to 18 months following diagnosis
• Survival up to 10 years with treatment
• Some patients live, symptom-free, for 20 or more years

 MISCELLANEOUS

ASSOCIATED CONDITIONS
• Budd-Chiari syndrome
• Mesenteric artery thrombosis

AGE-RELATED FACTORS
Pediatric: Rare in this age group
Geriatric: Phlebotomies and other therapies need to be adjusted for patients over 70
Others: N/A

PREGNANCY   Treat with phlebotomy alone

SYNONYMS
• Primary polycythemia
• Vaquez disease
• Polycythemia, splenomegalic
• Vaquez-Osler disease

ICD-9-CM   238.4 polycythemia vera

SEE ALSO   Myeloproliferative disorders

OTHER NOTES   N/A

ABBREVIATIONS   N/A

REFERENCES
• Williams WJ, Beutler E, Erslev AJ, et al, eds: Hematology. 4th Ed. New York, McGraw-Hill, 1990
• Conley CL: Polycythemia vera, diagnosis and treatment. Hosp Practice 1987;22:107
Illustrations: N/A
Internet references: http://www.5mcc.com

Author(s)
Stan G. Smith, MA, MB, FCFPC

Polymyalgia rheumatica

BASICS

DESCRIPTION A clinical syndrome characterized by aching and stiffness of the shoulder and hip girdle muscles affecting older patients, associated with an elevated ESR, lasting over 1 month and responsive to low dose steroids
System(s) affected: Musculoskeletal, Hemic/Lymphatic/Immunologic
Genetics: Associated with HLA determinants
Incidence/Prevalence in USA:
Approximately 50/100,000 patients over age 50/year
Predominant age: 60 or older. Incidence increases with age (rare under 50 years old).
Predominant sex: Females > Male (2:1)

SIGNS AND SYMPTOMS
• Onset - abrupt or insidious
• Pain and stiffness shoulder and hip girdle
• Usually symmetrical
• Symptoms more common in the morning
• Gel phenomena (stiffness after prolonged inactivity)
• Constitutional symptoms - fatigue, malaise, depression, weight loss, low grade fever
• Arthralgias/arthritis (non inflammatory)
• No weakness (pain may limit strength)
• Muscle tenderness mild to moderate
• No muscle atrophy
• Decreased range-of-motion of joints on active motion usually due to pain
• May have signs and symptoms of giant cell arteritis (seen in approximately 15% of patients)

CAUSES Unknown

RISK FACTORS
• Age greater than 50
• Presence of giant cell arteritis

DIAGNOSIS

DIFFERENTIAL DIAGNOSIS
• Rheumatoid arthritis
• Other connective tissue disease
• Fibromyalgia
• Depression
• Polymyositis/dermatomyositis (check CPK, aldolase)
• Thyroid disease
• Viral myalgia
• Osteoarthritis
• Occult infection
• Occult malignancy (extensive search usually not necessary)
• Myopathy (steroid, alcohol, electrolyte depletion)

LABORATORY
• ESR (Westergren) elevation greater than 50
• Anemia - normochromic/normocytic
• Creatine phosphdkinase (CPK)- normal
• Rheumatoid factor (RF) - negative (5-10% patients over 60 will have positive RF without disease)
• Mild elevations in liver function tests
Drugs that may alter lab results:
Prednisone
Disorders that may alter lab results:
Disorders causing acute phase reactants can elevate ESR (e.g., infection, neoplasm, renal failure)

PATHOLOGICAL FINDINGS
• None in muscle biopsy
• Mild non-specific synovitis

SPECIAL TESTS N/A

IMAGING N/A

DIAGNOSTIC PROCEDURES
• None, although in patients with symtoms suggesting giant cell arteritis, a temporal artery biopsy may be indicated. (Although the temporal artery biopsy may be positive, if there are no symptoms of giant cell arteritis, there is no reason to treat with high dose steroids. Increased morbidity has not been shown.)

TREATMENT

APPROPRIATE HEALTH CARE
Outpatient unless needs temporal artery biopsy

GENERAL MEASURES Physical therapy
for range-of-motion exercises if necessary

SURGICAL MEASURES N/A

ACTIVITY Do not overexercise to cause
exertion

DIET
• Adequate calcium and electrolyte intake (1500 mg/day)
• Regular diet

PATIENT EDUCATION
• Precautions regarding steroid use
• Instruct the patient about symptoms of giant cell arteritis and to report them immediately
• For a listing of sources for patient education materials favorably reviewed on this topic, physicians may contact: American Academy of Family Physicians Foundation, P.O. Box 8418, Kansas City, MO 64114, (800)274-2237, ext. 4400
• Excellent materials also available from Arthritis Foundation, 1330 W. Peachtree St, NW, Atlanta, GA 30309, (800)475-4700

Polymyalgia rheumatica

 MEDICATIONS

DRUG(S) OF CHOICE
• Prednisone
◊ 10 mg/day initially (average initial affective dose 10-15 mg/d)
◊ Usually dramatic (diagnostic) response.
◊ May increase gradually to 20 mg if no response
◊ Begin slow taper at 4-6 weeks by only 1 mg every 1-4 weeks to a dose of 5-7.5 mg. Continue at this dose for approximately 18 months to 2 years, if no recurrence of symptoms.
◊ Then attempt to taper by 1 mg every 2-4 weeks until drug discontinued. Patient may, however, require steroids for 3 or more years.
◊ Increase prednisone for recurrence of symptoms (relapse common).
Contraindications: Use steroid s with caution in patients with chronic heart failure, diabetes mellitus, systemic fungal or bacterial infection. Must treat infections concurrently if steroids are absolutely necessary.
Precautions: Long term steroid use associated with several significant adverse effects including sodium and water retention, exacerbation of chronic heart failure, hypokalemia, increased susceptibility to infection, osteoporosis, cataracts, avascular necrosis.
Significant possible interactions: Refer to manufacturer's literature

ALTERNATIVE DRUGS NSAID's have been used, rarely successful

 FOLLOWUP

PATIENT MONITORING
• Follow monthly initially and during taper of medication, every 3 months otherwise
• Follow ESR as steroids tapered
• Followup with patient for symptoms of giant cell arteritis. Educate patient to report such symptoms immediately (headache, visual and neurologic symptoms).

PREVENTION/AVOIDANCE N/A

POSSIBLE COMPLICATIONS
• Medication - complications related to steroid use
• Disease - exacerbation of disease with taper of steroids; development of giant cell arteritis (may occur when PMR is being adequately treated)

EXPECTED COURSE/PROGNOSIS
• Average length disease is 3 years (range 1-5 years)
• Exacerbation if steroids tapered too fast
• Prognosis very good if treated (may gradually remit even if no treatment)
• Relapse common

 MISCELLANEOUS

ASSOCIATED CONDITIONS
• Giant cell arteritis
• Temporal arteritis

AGE-RELATED FACTORS
Pediatric: Does not occur in this age group
Geriatric: Incidence increases with age
Others: N/A

PREGNANCY N/A

SYNONYMS
• Senile rheumatic gout
• Anarthritic syndrome
• Forestier-Certonciny syndrome
• Polymyalgia rheumatica syndrome
• Rhizomelic pseudoarthrosis

ICD-9-CM
725 polymyalgia rheumatica

SEE ALSO
• Giant cell arteritis
• Arthritis, rheumatoid (RA)
• Fibrositis
• Arthritis, osteo
• Polymyositis/dermatomyositis
• Depression

OTHER NOTES Westergren ESR is the preferred laboratory technique. If other types of ESR studies are used (e.g., Wintrobe, or zeta sedimentation rate [ZSR]), the guidelines listed in this chapter cannot be used for abnormal levels.

ABBREVIATIONS
PMR = polymyalgia rheumatica

REFERENCES
• Hunder GG: Giant Cell Arteritis and Polymyalgia Rheumatica. In: Kelly WN, Harris ED, Ruddy S, Sledge CB, eds. Textbook of Rheumatology. 3rd Ed. Philadelphia, W.B. Saunders Co., 1989
• Healey LA: Polymyalgia Rheumatica and Giant Cell Arteritis. In: McCarty DJ, ed. Arthritis and Allied Conditions: A Textbook of Rheumatology. Philadelphia, Lea and Febiger, 1989
• Wayland CM, Goronzy JJ: Polymyalgia rheumatica and giant cell arteritis. In:Koopman WJ, ed: Arthritis and Allied Disorders. 12th Ed. Philadelphia, Lea & Febiger, 1997
Illustrations: N/A
Internet references: http://www.5mcc.com

Author(s)
Bridget T. Walsh, DO
Eric P. Gall, MD

Polymyositis/dermatomyositis

 BASICS

DESCRIPTION
Systemic connective tissue disease characterized by inflammatory and degenerative changes in proximal muscles sometimes accompanied by characteristic skin rash.
• If skin manifestations are associated, it is designated as dermatomyositis
• Different types of myositis include:
  ◊ Idiopathic PM
  ◊ Idiopathic DM
  ◊ Childhood PM/DM
  ◊ PM/DM with malignancy
  ◊ PM/DM as an overlap
  ◊ Inclusion body myositis
  ◊ HIV associated myopathy

System(s) affected: Musculoskeletal, Pulmonary, Skin/Exocrine, Cardiovascular
Genetics: Mild association with HLA-DR3, HLA-DRw52
Incidence/Prevalence in USA: Estimated at 0.5-0.8 new cases/100,000; 1-2 patients/100,000
Predominant age: 5-15 years, 40-60 years
Predominant sex: Female > Male (2:1)

SIGNS AND SYMPTOMS
• Symmetrical proximal muscle weakness causing:
  ◊ Difficulty when arising from sitting or lying positions
  ◊ Difficulty kneeling
  ◊ Difficulty climbing stairs
  ◊ Difficulty descending stairs
  ◊ Difficulty raising arms
• Joint pain/swelling
• Dysphagia
• Respiratory impairment
• Decreased deep tendon reflexes of proximal muscle groups
• Muscle swelling, stiffness, induration
• Rash over face (eyelids, nasolabial folds), upper chest, dorsal hands, (especially knuckle pads)
• Periorbital edema
• Calcinosis cutis (childhood cases)
• Mesenteric arterial insufficiency/infarction (childhood cases)
• Cardiac impairment; arrhythmia, failure

CAUSES
• Unknown; potential factors:
  ◊ Inciting viral infection
  ◊ T cell activation
  ◊ Cytokine release
  ◊ Immune-mediate muscle destruction
  ◊ Genetic predisposition
  ◊ HTLV I

RISK FACTORS
Family history of autoimmune disease or vasculitis

 DIAGNOSIS

DIFFERENTIAL DIAGNOSIS
• Vasculitis
• Progressive systemic sclerosis
• Systemic lupus erythematosus
• Rheumatoid arthritis
• Muscular dystrophy
• Eaton-Lambert syndrome
• Sarcoidosis
• Amyotrophic lateral sclerosis
• Endocrine disorders
  ◊ Thyroid disease
  ◊ Cushing's syndrome
• Infectious myositis (viral, bacterial, parasitic)
• Drug-induced myopathies
  ◊ Cholesterol lowering agents
  ◊ Colchicine
  ◊ Corticosteroids
  ◊ Ethanol
  ◊ Chloroquine
  ◊ Zidovudine (AZT)
• Electrolyte disorders (magnesium, calcium, potassium)
• Heritable metabolic myopathies

LABORATORY
• Increased creatine kinase (CK)
• Increased aldolase
• Increased SGOT
• Increased LDH
• Myoglobinuria
• Increased ESR
• Positive rheumatoid factor (less than 50% of patients)
• Positive ANA (more than 50% of patients)
• Leukocytosis (less than 50% of patients)
• Anemia (less than 50% of patients)
• Hyperglobulinemia (less than 50% of patients)
• Increased creatinine (less than 50% of patients)
• Myositis specific antibodies have been described in a minority of patients - most are anti-synthetase antibodies, anti-Jo-1 is the most common and has been found in about 20% of patients; associated with an increased incidence of interstitial lung disease
Drugs that may alter lab results: N/A
Disorders that may alter lab results: N/A

PATHOLOGICAL FINDINGS
• Micro - muscle fiber degeneration
• Micro - phagocytosis of muscle debris
• Micro - perifascicular muscle fiber atrophy
• Micro - inflammatory cell infiltrates in adult form
• Micro (electron microscopy) - inclusion bodies (inclusion body myositis only)
• Sarcoplasmic basophilia
• Muscle fiber increased in size
• Vasculopathy (childhood PM/DM)

SPECIAL TESTS
• ECG - arrhythmias, conduction disturbances
• Electromyography (EMG) - muscle irritability, low amplitude potentials, polyphasic action potentials, fibrillations
• Muscle biopsy (deltoid or quadriceps femoris)

IMAGING
Chest x-ray: pulmonary interstitial disease

DIAGNOSTIC PROCEDURES
Diagnosis usually relies on 4 findings - weakness, CPK elevation, abnormal EMG, findings on muscle biopsy. Presence of skin rash of dermatomyositis also helpful.

 TREATMENT

APPROPRIATE HEALTH CARE
Outpatient

GENERAL MEASURES
• Search for malignancy in all adults
• Follow serum muscle enzymes carefully

SURGICAL MEASURES N/A

ACTIVITY
• Curtailed until after inflammation subsides
• Range-of-motion exercises to prevent contractures

DIET No special diet

PATIENT EDUCATION
Muscular Dystrophy Association, 3561 E. Sunrise Dr., Tucson, AZ 85718. Telephone (800)221-1142.

MEDICATIONS

DRUG(S) OF CHOICE
• Prednisone 40-60 mg/day initially in divided doses. Consolidate doses and reduce prednisone slowly when enzyme levels are normal. Probably need to continue 10-15 mg/day for maintenance.
• For steroid refractory cases:
◊ Azathioprine 1.0 mg/kg (arthritis dose) once or twice a day. Maintain at lowest possible dose.
◊ Methotrexate 10-25 mg weekly useful in some steroid-resistant cases
Contraindications: Refer to manufacturer's literature. Methotrexate contraindicated in patients with previous liver disease or current alcohol use.
Precautions:
• Prednisone - adverse effects associated with long-term steroid use include adrenal suppression, sodium, water retention, hypokalemia, osteoporosis, cataracts, increased susceptibility to infection
• Azathioprine - adverse effects include bone marrow suppression, increased LFT's, increased susceptibility to infection
• Methotrexate - adverse effects include stomatitis. bone marrow suppression, pneumonitis, and risk of liver fibrosis and cirrhosis with prolonged use
Significant possible interactions: Refer to manufacturer's literature

ALTERNATIVE DRUGS
Other immunosuppressant drugs such as cyclophosphamide, chlorambucil, cyclosporine can be added to steroids. Immune globulin, intravenous (IVIG) added to steroids being evaluated in resistant cases, also tacrolimus.

 FOLLOWUP

PATIENT MONITORING
• Serial testing for muscle enzyme activity in serum
• Any adult should be studied for malignancy
• Monitor for steroid-induced metabolic complications (hypokalemia, hypertension, hyperglycemia, etc.)
• If azathioprine, methotrexate or other immunosuppressant used, then appropriate laboratory monitoring should be done periodically. Refer to manufacturer's literature.

PREVENTION/AVOIDANCE N/A

POSSIBLE COMPLICATIONS
• Pneumonia
• Infection
• Myocardial infarction
• Carcinoma (especially breast, lung)
• Severe dysphagia
• Respiratory impairment due to muscle weakness, interstitial lung disease
• Aspiration pneumonitis
• Steroid myopathy
• Steroid induced diabetes, hypertension, hypokalemia, etc.

EXPECTED COURSE/PROGNOSIS
• 30% residual weakness
• 20% persistent active disease
• 75% 5-year survival
• Survival worse for women and African-Americans
• Most patients improve with therapy
• 50% have full recovery
• Possibly relapsing
• Inclusion body myositis tends to be more steroid-refractory and includes more distal weakness

 MISCELLANEOUS

ASSOCIATED CONDITIONS
• Malignancy
• Progressive systemic sclerosis
• Vasculitis
• Systemic lupus erythematosus
• Other connective tissue disorders

AGE-RELATED FACTORS
Pediatric:
• Childhood dermatomyositis occurs
• May be possible to discontinue prednisone gradually after a year or so
Geriatric:
• Rare after age 60
• Elderly male patient with polymyositis more likely to have underlying neoplasm
Others: N/A

PREGNANCY N/A

SYNONYMS
• Neuromyositis
• Wagner-Unverricht syndrome

ICD-9-CM
710.3 Dermatomyositis
710.4 Polymyositis

SEE ALSO N/A

OTHER NOTES
Classification of types of myositis: Childhood dermatomyositis, primary idiopathic dermatomyositis, dermatomyositis or polymyositis associated with malignancy, primary polymyositis, myositis associated with overlap syndrome. Inclusion-body myositis represents a variant with atypical presentation and variable response to therapy.

ABBREVIATIONS N/A

REFERENCES
• Kelley W, et al: Textbook of Rheumatology. 5th Ed. Philadelphia, W.B. Saunders Co., 1997
• Kagen LJ: Polymyositis/dermatomyositis. In: McCarty DJ, Koopman WJ, eds. Arthritis and Allied Conditions.12th Ed. Philadelphia, Lea & Febiger, 1993
• Kagen LJ, ed: Inflammatory disorders of muscle. Rheum Dis Clin of No Amer 1994;20:811-1057
• Plotz PH, et al: Myositis: Immunologic contributions to understanding cause, pathogenesis, and therapy. Ann Int Med 1995;122:715-724
Illustrations: 4 available on CD-ROM
Internet references: http://www.5mcc.com

Author(s)
Christopher M. Wise, MD

Porphyria

BASICS

DESCRIPTION Several heme synthesis pathway enzyme deficiencies with overproduction and accumulation of intermediate metabolic products and resultant neuropsychiatric-abdominal or dermatologic symptoms and syndromes. All more common in Caucasians than Blacks or Asians.
• Porphyria cutanea tarda (PCT) - dermatologic
• Acute intermittent porphyria (AIP) - pyrroloporphyria; neuropsychiatric-abdominal
• Protoporphyria (PP) - erythropoietic or hepatoerythropoietic; mild dermatologic
• Variegate porphyria (VP) - South African porphyria, prevalence in S. Africa is 1/400
• Hereditary coproporphyria (HCP) - neuropsychic, occasionally dermatologic
• Porphobilinogen synthetase deficiency (PBD) - delta-aminolevulinic aciduria; neuropsychiatric-abdominal
• Congenital erythropoietic porphyria (CEP) - Günther's disease; severe dermatologic
• Other rare genetic variants reported
System(s) affected: Gastrointestinal, Skin/Exocrine, Hemic/Lymphatic/Immunologic
Genetics:
• Autosomal dominant - PCT, AIP, PP, VP, HCP
• Autosomal recessive - PBD, CEP
• Latency common with variable expression, many asymptomatic or minimally symptomatic carriers
• PCT also sporadic and acquired
Incidence/Prevalence in USA:
• PCT - 1/10,000
• AIP, PP, VP - 1/10,000 to 1/100,000
• HCP - less than 1/100,000
• PBD, CEP - very rare
Predominant age:
• CEP - early childhood
• PP - older childhood
• AIP, VP, HCP, PBD - young adult
• PCT - middle age
Predominant sex:
• PP, CEP - male=female
• PCT - seen more commonly in male
• AIP, VP, HCP, PBD - seen more commonly in female

SIGNS AND SYMPTOMS
• All usually reversible, lasting days to weeks
• May be permanent
• Urine may turn dark red or brown on standing (word porphyria from Greek porphyra = purple)
• Abdominal:
  ◊ Rather severe abdominal pain, occasionally in back and extremities
  ◊ Generalized more often than localized
  ◊ Often colicky
  ◊ Can mimic acute abdomen
  ◊ No fever should be present
  ◊ Chronic constipation common
  ◊ Severity of symptoms often out of proportion to physical findings
• Neurologic:
  ◊ Essentially anything
  ◊ Includes sensory and motor systems
  ◊ Includes autonomic nervous system
  ◊ May include seizures
  ◊ May lead to quadriplegia and/or respiratory paralysis with death
• Psychiatric:
  ◊ Essentially anything
  ◊ Psychosis most common
  ◊ Visual hallucinations common
  ◊ Disorientation frequent
  ◊ Chronic depression frequent
• Dermatologic:
  ◊ Photosensitivity
  ◊ Scrapes, ulcerations, blisters with minimal trauma
  ◊ Hyperpigmentation, especially hands and face
  ◊ Scarring frequent
  ◊ CEP - mutilating, with hemolysis, erythrodontia, splenomegaly
  ◊ PP - occasional hepatic disease, including hepatic failure

CAUSES
• Genetic enzyme deficiencies
• PCT - uroporphyrinogen decarboxylase
• AIP - porphobilinogen deaminase
• PP - ferrochelatase
• VP - protoporphyrinogen oxidase
• HCP - coproporphyrinogen oxidase
• PBD - porphobilinogen synthetase
• CEP - uroporphyrinogen III synthetase (cosynthetase)
• Acquired PCT causes:
  ◊ Decreased enzyme associated with alcohol, steroids, hormones
  ◊ Specific exposure to polyhalogenated hydrocarbons (e.g., hexachlorobenzene)
  ◊ Lead poisoning may alter pathways
  ◊ HIV
  ◊ Hepatitis C virus

RISK FACTORS
• Multiple precipitating factors, especially AIP, VP, HCP
• Drugs (e.g., barbiturates and sulfas in AIP)
• Estrogens, especially oral contraceptives
• Steroids
• Liver disease
• Menstrual cycles
• Infection
• Fasting
• Heavy alcohol use

DIAGNOSIS

DIFFERENTIAL DIAGNOSIS Vast and protean

LABORATORY
• Urine for porphyrins during acute attack. Urine may be normal at other times.
• Individual enzyme activity in erythrocytes or other body cells/tissues
• Stool for porphyrins in PP, VP, HCP, CEP
• Bile for porphyrin in VP
• Plasma for fluorescence emission spectroscopy in VP
• Saliva for porphyria in PCT
• Erythrocyte uroporphyrin in CEP
• PP exception - urine unremarkable. Test erythrocyte protoporphyrin.
Drugs that may alter lab results:
Unknown
Disorders that may alter lab results:
• Numerous conditions may cause slight increase in porphyrinuria, but patients asymptomatic
• Acute liver disease
• Hepatoma
• Hodgkin's lymphoma
• Multiple neurologic diseases

PATHOLOGICAL FINDINGS N/A

SPECIAL TESTS Genetic studies when applicable

IMAGING N/A

DIAGNOSTIC PROCEDURES N/A

TREATMENT

APPROPRIATE HEALTH CARE
Outpatient, except for crises

GENERAL MEASURES
• Neuropsychiatric-abdominal - avoid drugs, alcohol, known toxins
• Dermatologic - shade, protective clothing; avoid skin trauma; PCT - phlebotomy weekly to monthly may help prevent
• CEP - consider bone marrow transplantation

SURGICAL MEASURES N/A

ACTIVITY Normal, except dermatologic avoid sun

DIET Neuropsychiatric - large quantities of carbohydrates have been reported to help

PATIENT EDUCATION American Porphyria Foundation, P.O. Box 22712, Houston, TX 77227, (713)266-9617

Porphyria

MEDICATIONS

DRUG(S) OF CHOICE
• Neuropsychiatric-abdominal
◊ Intravenous glucose 400 grams daily for one to two days
◊ Hematin (ferriprotoporphyrin IX, hemin [Panhematin]) IV 1-4 mg/kg/d over 10-15 minutes x 3-14 days
◊ Epilepsy - consider clonazepam or gabapentin
◊ Depression - consider selective serotonin re-uptake inhibitors
• Dermatologic:
◊ Oral carotenoids, e.g., beta-carotene (Solatene), 30 mg, 1-10 capsules per day
Contraindications: Known sensitivity to drug
Precautions: Hematin - phlebitis at IV site, reduced clotting ability
Significant possible interactions: None

ALTERNATIVE DRUGS
• PCT - chloroquine 125 mg twice weekly, or hydroxychloroquine 250 mg tid, in conjunction with phlebotomy
• Menstruating women - hematin premenstrual; cycle suppressors, e.g., luteinizing hormone releasing hormone (LHRH) analogues
• Autonomic manifestations - beta blockers
• Other symptoms - treat symptomatically

FOLLOWUP

PATIENT MONITORING Individualized

PREVENTION/AVOIDANCE
• Avoid precipitating drugs
◊ Alcohol
◊ Barbiturates
◊ Carbamazepine
◊ Chlorpropamide
◊ Danazol
◊ Ergots
◊ Estrogens and progestins
◊ Ethchlorvynol
◊ Glutethimide
◊ Griseofulvin
◊ Mephenytoin
◊ Meprobamate
◊ Methotrexate
◊ Methyprylon
◊ Phenytoin
◊ Pyrazolones
◊ Succinimides
◊ Sulfonamide antibiotics
◊ Valproic acid
• Eat an adequate diet with high carbohydrate intake

POSSIBLE COMPLICATIONS See list in Signs and Symptoms

EXPECTED COURSE/PROGNOSIS
• In all porphyrias:
◊ Patients who are asymptomatic or minimally symptomatic - unaffected longevity
◊ Patients who are more symptomatic - treatable and do well
◊ Neurologic complications (e.g., peripheral neuropathy, neurosis or hemiplegia), at times permanent
• In AIP
◊ Acute attacks have 25% mortality
◊ Increased risk of hepatocellular carcinoma
• Acquired PCT
◊ HIV
◊ Hepatitis C virus
◊ Hepatic malignancies

MISCELLANEOUS

ASSOCIATED CONDITIONS N/A

AGE-RELATED FACTORS
Pediatric: N/A
Geriatric: N/A
Others: N/A

PREGNANCY Unpredictable disease activity

SYNONYMS
• Delta-aminolevulinic aciduria
• Erythropoietic porphyria
• Günther's disease
• Hepatoerythropoietic porphyria
• Pyrroloporphyria
• South African porphyria

ICD-9-CM 277.1 disorders of porphyrin metabolism

SEE ALSO N/A

OTHER NOTES Some drugs considered safe - acetaminophen, aspirin, atropine, bromides, diazepam (in small doses), dicumarol, digoxin, diphenhydramine, ether, glucocorticoids, guanethidine, heparin, insulin, neostigmine, nitrous oxide, penicillin and derivatives, phenothiazines, narcotic analgesics, propranolol, streptomycin, succinylcholine, thiazides

ABBREVIATIONS
PCT = Porphyria cutanea tarda
AIP = Acute intermittent porphyria
PP = Protoporphyria
VP = Variegate porphyria
HCP = Hereditary coproporphyria
PBD = Porphobilinogen synthetase deficiency
CEP = Congenital erythropoietic porphyria

REFERENCES
• Isselbacher KJ, et al, eds: Harrison's Principles of Internal Medicine. 13th Ed. New York, McGraw-Hill, 1994
• Bennett JC, Plum F, eds: Cecil Textbook of Medicine. 20th Ed. Philadelphia, W.B. Saunders Co., 1996
Illustrations: 5 available on CD-ROM
Internet references: http://www.5mcc.com

Author(s)
Emil S Dickstein, MD, FACP

Portal hypertension

BASICS

DESCRIPTION Increased portal venous pressure (> 10 mm Hg.) that occurs in association with splanchnic vasodilatation, portosystemic collateral formation and a hyperdynamic circulation. Course is generally progressive and may produce one or more devastating clinical disorders.
System(s) affected: Gastrointestinal, Cardiovascular, Nervous
Genetics: No known genetic patterns except those associated with specific hepatic diseases that cause portal hypertension
Incidence/Prevalence in USA: Unknown. (Incidence of bleeding from gastroesophageal varices is approximately 120 episodes per 100,000 population per year.)
Predominant age: Adult
Predominant sex: Male > Female

SIGNS AND SYMPTOMS
May be general or related to specific complications
• General
  ◊ Splenomegaly
  ◊ Caput medusa
  ◊ Umbilical bruit
  ◊ Hemorrhoids
  ◊ Spider angiomata
  ◊ Gynecomastia
  ◊ Testicular atrophy
  ◊ Digital clubbing
  ◊ Palmar erythema
• Gastroesophageal varices
  ◊ Hematemesis
  ◊ Melena
  ◊ Anemia
  ◊ Hypotension
  ◊ Tachycardia
• Ascites
  ◊ Distended abdomen
  ◊ Fluid wave
  ◊ Shifting percussion dullness
• Hepatic encephalopathy
  ◊ Confusion
  ◊ Asterixis
  ◊ Hyperreflexia
• Hepatorenal syndrome
  ◊ Oliguria

CAUSES
May be intrahepatic or extrahepatic
• Cirrhosis present. Accounts for > 90% of cases.
  ◊ Alcoholic
  ◊ Viral (HBV, HCV, HGV)
  ◊ Wilson's disease
  ◊ Hemochromatosis
  ◊ Primary biliary cirrhosis
  ◊ Schistosomiasis
• Cirrhosis not present.
  ◊ Portal vein thrombosis
  ◊ Hepatic vein obstruction (Budd-Chiari syndrome)
  ◊ Right ventricular failure
  ◊ Myeloproliferative disorders

RISK FACTORS
Many different chronic liver diseases and hepatotoxins

DIAGNOSIS

DIFFERENTIAL DIAGNOSIS
Usually related to specific complications/presentations.
• Gastroesophageal varices with hemorrhage vs:
  ◊ Portal hypertensive gastropathy
  ◊ Hemorrhagic gastritis
  ◊ Peptic ulcer disease
  ◊ Mallory-Weiss tear
• Ascites vs:
  ◊ Spontaneous bacterial peritonitis
  ◊ Pancreatic ascites
  ◊ Peritoneal carcinomatosis
  ◊ Tuberculous peritonitis
  ◊ Nephrotic syndrome
  ◊ Cardiac ascites
• Hepatic encephalopathy vs:
  ◊ Delirium tremens
  ◊ Intracranial hemorrhage
  ◊ Sedative abuse
  ◊ Uremia
• Hepatorenal syndrome vs
  ◊ Drug nephrotoxicity
  ◊ Renal tubular necrosis

LABORATORY
Non-specific changes associated with underlying disease.
• Hypersplenism
  ◊ Anemia
  ◊ Leukopenia
  ◊ Thrombocytopenia
• Hepatic dysfunction
  ◊ Hypoalbuminemia
  ◊ Hyperbilirubinemia
  ◊ Elevated alkaline phosphatase
  ◊ Elevated liver enzymes
  ◊ Abnormal clotting factors (PT, PTT.)
• Gastrointestinal bleeding
  ◊ Iron deficiency anemia
  ◊ Elevated serum ammonia
• Hepatorenal syndrome
  ◊ Elevated serum creatinine, BUN
  ◊ Urine Na < 20 mEq/L.
Drugs that may alter lab results: N/A
Disorders that may alter lab results: N/A

PATHOLOGICAL FINDINGS Specific for underlying disease

SPECIAL TESTS Specific for underlying disease

IMAGING
• UGI series. May outline varices in esophagus and stomach.
• CT scan and ultrasound. May detect cirrhosis, splenomegaly, ascites and varices.
• Duplex-Doppler (ultrasound.) Can determine presence and direction of flow in portal and hepatic veins. Useful in diagnosing portal vein and/or shunt thrombosis.
• Angiography. Demonstrates cork-screwing of intrahepatic vessels (cirrhosis); can identify varices and vascular anomalies.

DIAGNOSTIC PROCEDURES
• Endoscopy. Can diagnose esophageal and gastric varices and portal hypertensive gastropathy or can directly visualize other bleeding sites (peptic ulcers, gastritis, Mallory-Weiss tears.)
• Hepatic venous wedge pressure. Correlates with portal pressure; risk of variceal bleeding is increased if HVWP > 12 mm./Hg.

TREATMENT

APPROPRIATE HEALTH CARE Inpatient

GENERAL MEASURES
• Treat underlying disease and support metabolic/nutritional needs.
• Avoid sedatives; may precipitate encephalopathy
• Transfuse packed RBCs as needed. Use caution; circulation is already hyperdynamic.
• Correct coagulopathy. Administer vitamin K and/or fresh-frozen plasma.
• Limit sodium administration; cirrhotic patients avidly retain sodium

SURGICAL MEASURES Liver transplantation may be recommended for selected patients with far-advanced hepatic disease. Other less aggressive approaches are available for specific complications of portal hypertension.

ACTIVITY Bed rest for acute complications (bleeding, encephalopathy or hepatorenal syndrome)

DIET Restrict sodium and protein

PATIENT EDUCATION N/A

Portal hypertension

MEDICATIONS

DRUG(S) OF CHOICE
• Therapy for variceal hemorrhage:
  ◊ For acute control: intravenous somatostatin or octreotide (synthetic analogue)
  ◊ Alternative: vasopressin; but, has more complications (decreased by addition of nitroglycerin)
  ◊ For prevention of recurrence: propranolol
• Therapy for encephalopathy:
  ◊ Lactulose. Induces diarrhea and traps intracolonic ammonia.
  ◊ Neomycin. Reduces bacterial production of nitrogenous substances in colon.
• Therapy for ascites:
  ◊ Furosemide (Lasix)
  ◊ Spironolactone.
Contraindications: Vasopressin is a systemic vasodilator and may cause hypotension, bradycardia and cardiac and peripheral ischemia. Cardiac monitoring is advisable.
Precautions: Vasopressin may cause hypertension, bradycardia, arrhythmias. Patient must be on a cardiac monitor while receiving this drug. Co-administration of nitroprusside may reduce cardiotoxicity.
Significant possible interactions: Refer to manufacturer's literature

ALTERNATIVE DRUGS
Glypressin and terlipressin are more selective splanchnic vasoconstrictors and may be associated with fewer complications. Studies are continuing.

FOLLOWUP

PATIENT MONITORING
Acute complications of portal hypertension require intensive monitoring of vital signs and organ function. Long-term management includes regular follow-up of all affected organ systems.

PREVENTION/AVOIDANCE
Abstinence from alcohol. Adequate and appropriate nutrition.

POSSIBLE COMPLICATIONS
As described above

EXPECTED COURSE/PROGNOSIS
• Variceal bleeding: 50% re-bleed, usually within 2 years unless portal pressure is reduced by shunt or TIPS procedure
• Ascites: Generally recurs. Frequency and severity can be reduced if salt restriction is observed.
• Hepatic encephalopathy. Often recurs especially if re-bleeding develops. Low protein diet advised.

MISCELLANEOUS

ASSOCIATED CONDITIONS
As described above

AGE-RELATED FACTORS
Pediatric: Uncommon. Generally different etiology than in adults.
• Intrahepatic
  ◊ Biliary atresia
  ◊ Viral hepatitis
  ◊ Metabolic liver disease.
• Extrahepatic
  ◊ Congenital anomalies of portal vein
  ◊ Neonatal omphalitis (umbilical vein catheterization, sepsis, abdominal trauma)
Geriatric: Mortality and complication rate are increased
Others: N/A

PREGNANCY N/A

SYNONYMS N/A

ICD-9-CM 572.3 Portal hypertension

SEE ALSO
• Cirrhosis of the liver
• Hepatitis, viral

OTHER NOTES
• Other treatment approaches (inadequately studied with non-control protocols)
  ◊ Transhepatic obliteration of varices
  ◊ Concomitant treatment with non-selective beta-adrenergic blockers

ABBREVIATIONS N/A

REFERENCES
• Sleisenger MH, Fortran JS, eds: Gastrointestinal Disease: Pathophysiology, Diagnosis, Management. 5th Ed. Philadelphia, WB Saunders Co., 1994
• Jaffe DL, Chung RT, Friedman LS: Management of portal hypertension and its complications. Med Clin N Am 1996;80:1021-1034
• Pagliaro L, D'Amico G, Luca A, et al: Portal hypertension: diagnosis and treatment. J. Hepatol. 1995: 23 (Suppl 1):36-44
Illustrations: N/A
Internet references: http://www.5mcc.com

Author(s)
Wayne H. Schwesinger, MD

Post-traumatic stress disorder (PTSD)

BASICS

DESCRIPTION A condition seen in people who experienced an event that would be extremely distressing to most human beings, e.g., serious threat to one's life, physical or psychological integrity; serious threat or harm to one's children, spouse, siblings, parents or other close relatives or friends; sudden destruction of one's home or community; seeing another person who has recently been (or is being) injured or killed as a result of a man-made violent act or natural disaster.
• The person's response involved intense fear, helplessness, or horror. Note: In children, this may be expressed instead by disorganized or agitated behavior.
• Symptoms of this condition did not exist prior to the trauma, and symptoms persist for at least one month following the trauma
• There is a subtype of post-traumatic stress disorder (PTSD) with a delayed onset of the symptoms which starts at least six months after the trauma
• The acute form of PTSD is defined as the duration being less than 3 months
• Chronic form is defined when the duration of symptoms is more than 3 months
System(s) affected: Nervous
Genetics: N/A
Incidence/Prevalence in USA: Up to 30% of victims of disasters develop PTSD. Lifelong prevalence in general population ranges from 1-14%.
Predominant age: The elderly and the very young are more vulnerable
Predominant sex: Adult women are more inclined to ask for help. Young boys may be more vulnerable to trauma than girls. Most men with PTSD have experienced combat or exposure to trauma on the job. Most women with PTSD have a history of rape or being physically assaulted.

SIGNS AND SYMPTOMS
• The traumatic event is persistently re-experienced in one or more of the following ways:
◊ Recurrent and intrusive distressing recollections of the event, including images, thoughts or perceptions. Note: In young children repetitive play may occur in which themes or aspects of the trauma are expressed.
◊ Recurrent distressing dreams of the event. Note: In children, there may be frightening dreams without recognizable content.
◊ Acting or feeling as if the traumatic event were recurring (includes a sense of reliving the experience, illusions, hallucinations, and dissociative flashback episodes, including those that occur on awakening or when intoxicated). Note: In young children, trauma-specific reenactment may occur.
◊ Intense psychological distress at exposure to internal or external cues that symbolize or resemble an aspect of the traumatic event
◊ Physiological reactivity on exposure to internal or external cues that symbolize or resemble an aspect of the traumatic event,

such as increased heart rate, changes in blood pressure, discoloration of the skin, blurred vision, hyperperistalsis in smooth muscle, nausea, vomiting, diarrhea, urinary urgency, etc.
• Persistent avoidance of the stimuli associated with the trauma, or numbing of general responsiveness (not present before the trauma) as indicated by three (or more) of the following:
◊ Efforts to avoid thoughts, feelings or conversations associated with the trauma
◊ Efforts to avoid activities, places or people that arouse recollections of the trauma
◊ Inability to recall an important aspect of the trauma (psychogenic amnesia)
◊ Markedly diminished interest or participation in significant activities (in young children, loss of recently acquired developmental skills such as toilet training or language skills)
◊ Feelings of detachment or estrangement from others
◊ Restricted range of affect (e.g., unable to have loving feelings)
◊ Sense of a foreshortened future (e.g., does not expect to have a career, marriage, or a normal life span)
• Persistent symptoms of increased arousal (not present before the trauma), as indicated by two or more of the following:
◊ Difficulty falling or staying asleep (insomnia)
◊ Irritability or outbursts of anger
◊ Difficulty in concentrating
◊ Hypervigilance
◊ Exaggerated startle response
• Others:
◊ Duration of the disturbance is more than 1 month
◊ The disturbance causes clinically significant distress or impairment in social, occupational, or other important areas of functioning

CAUSES Events which are insults to one's personal integrity, self-esteem and security are psychologically traumatic and may lead to PTSD

RISK FACTORS Individuals with a history of childhood neglect or dysfunctional families, children of alcoholic parents, or childhood abuse, are predisposed and more susceptible to developing PTSD in response to trauma

DIAGNOSIS

DIFFERENTIAL DIAGNOSIS
• Organic mental disorders
• Generalized anxiety disorder
• Phobic disorders
• Depressive disorder
• Panic disorder
• Conversion disorder
• Somatization disorder
• Personality disorders
• Substance and chemical dependency

LABORATORY N/A
Drugs that may alter lab results: N/A
Disorders that may alter lab results: N/A

PATHOLOGICAL FINDINGS Character pathology as shown on the Minnesota multiple personality inventory (MMPI)

SPECIAL TESTS
• Neuropsychological testing is helpful in cases of dementia and more subtle cognitive dysfunction
• EEG to rule out any brain damage (results may be altered by any drug affecting EEG patterns such as - sleeping pills, antidepressants, neuroleptics and other psychotropic medications)
• Psychological testing and a thorough mental status examination are valuable in a complete, thorough assessment of the patient
• Sleep lab studies of 8 hour EEG help in diagnosis of sleep disorders
• Through an examination and interview, assisted by sodium amytal (given intravenously) or similar substances, one may uncover traumatic material in patients with amnesia. Similarly, an examination assisted by hypnosis may help in the diagnosis.
• Tests may be affected by withdrawal or intoxication from drugs and alcohol; any organic brain syndromes such as multiple infarct dementia, other forms of dementia, and forms of epilepsy

IMAGING CT scan of the head and MRI of the brain are valuable to rule out any brain damage

DIAGNOSTIC PROCEDURES
• Psychiatric examination
• Psychological testing
• Note: The American Psychiatry Association has implemented in 1994, a new diagnostic manual for psychiatric disorders. This includes a new diagnostic category entitled Acute Stress Disorder. The signs and symptoms are essentially the same as those described for PTSD, except for the fact that in acute stress disorder, the disturbance lasts for a minimum of 2 days and the maximum of 4 weeks and occurs within 4 weeks of the traumatic event. If the symptoms last more than 4 weeks, or begin more than 30 days after the original trauma, the condition is diagnosed as PTSD.

TREATMENT

APPROPRIATE HEALTH CARE
• Most treatment is done on an outpatient basis
• In case of crisis such as a patient being suicidal or dysfunctional with activities of daily living, inpatient intensive treatment on a psychiatry unit is indicated

GENERAL MEASURES
• As indicated by the patient's general condition, treatment includes individual psychotherapy, group therapy, hypnotherapy, narcoanalysis and narcosynthesis, and behavior therapy
• Crisis intervention shortly after the traumatic event is very valuable for the immediate distress and may prevent the development of a chronic or delayed form of post-traumatic stress disorder
• Relaxation exercises to help reduce anxiety and improve sleep have been found helpful

SURGICAL MEASURES   N/A

ACTIVITY
• As indicated by patient's physical condition
• Restoration of regular sleep at night is essential in cases of insomnia

DIET   A healthy diet of complex carbohydrates, proteins, and multi-vitamins and minerals. Avoid fatty foods.

PATIENT EDUCATION   Lenore Terr: Too Scared to Cry. Harper & Row, NY, 1990

MEDICATIONS

DRUG(S) OF CHOICE
• Selective serotonin reuptake inhibitors (SSRI): (this group has recently been proven to be safe and effective for the control of many symptoms of PTSD)
  ◊ Fluoxetine 20-80 mg/day
  ◊ Sertraline 50-200 mg/day
  ◊ Paroxetine 20-60 mg/day
  ◊ Venlafaxine 75-325 mg/day
• Tricyclic antidepressants:
  ◊ Doxepin 50-150 mg/day
  ◊ Nortriptyline 30-100 mg/day
  ◊ Imipramine 50-300 mg/day
  ◊ Desipramine 50-300 mg/day
  ◊ Amitriptyline 50-300 mg/day
  ◊ Trimipramine 50-300 mg/day
  ◊ Protriptyline 15-60 mg/ day
  ◊ Amoxapine 50-300 mg/day
  ◊ Maprotiline 50-225 mg/day (increased risk of seizures with higher doses)
• Monoamine oxidase inhibitors:
  ◊ Phenelzine 45-75 mg/day is useful especially in PTSD patients with panic attacks
• Others:
  ◊ Trazodone 100-400 mg/day, given mostly at bedtime is helpful in patients with insomnia
  ◊ Nefazodone 200-600 mg/day in patients with insomnia improves REM sleep
  ◊ Small doses of neuroleptics are helpful in selective patients
  ◊ Bupropion 100-450 mg/day
  ◊ Neuroleptics - small doses are helpful in selective patients
  ◊ Benzodiazepines should be used selectively and with caution

Contraindications:
• Allergic reactions to specific drugs
• Use with caution in alcoholic patients with poor liver functions
Precautions:
• Do not mix tricyclic antidepressants with monoamine oxidase inhibitors
• Long-term use of benzodiazepines may lead to increased tolerance and drug dependency
Significant possible interactions:
Monoamine oxidase inhibitors may interact with other antidepressants, sympathomimetics such as pseudoephedrine and any foods with tyramine or its precursors

ALTERNATIVE DRUGS
• Clomipramine 75-250 mg/day or fluvoxamine 100-300 mg/day or fluoxetine 20-80 mg/day in patients with obsessive compulsive symptoms has been helpful in some cases
• Buspirone 30-80 mg/day has been found helpful in cases with severe anxiety
• Propranolol and clonidine have been used with limited results to control the psychophysiological hyperactivity during intense flashbacks

FOLLOWUP

PATIENT MONITORING   Psychotherapy for at least one hour per week is necessary in the first phase of treatment

PREVENTION/AVOIDANCE   Crisis intervention immediately after the traumatic event involving intensive support and treatment may prevent the development of chronic PTSD later

POSSIBLE COMPLICATIONS   Suicide; self-inflicted violence in reenactment of trauma

EXPECTED COURSE/PROGNOSIS
• The lack of crisis intervention immediately following the trauma may lead to the persistence of symptoms. If symptoms last less than 3 months, the patient is still in the acute form of PTSD. If symptoms persist over 3 months, patients may develop chronic PTSD which may lead to loss of job, marital conflicts, total disability and repeated and/or lengthy hospitalizations with severe morbidity.
• If the onset of symptoms is at least 6 months or more after the original traumatic event, the patient suffers from a delayed onset type
• The more chronic and delayed the onset, the worse the prognosis. Early treatment in acute phase associated with better prognosis.

MISCELLANEOUS

ASSOCIATED CONDITIONS   Personality disorders such as borderline personality disorder, depression, panic disorder, anxiety disorder, and dissociative disorders

AGE-RELATED FACTORS
Pediatric: Young children are susceptible to abuse and neglect; can develop chronic PTSD with failure to progress and grow in healthy way
Geriatric: Have fewer social support resources; adjustment to trauma less flexible; more sensitive to medication and need dose adjustment.
Others: N/A

PREGNANCY   Avoid psychotropics in the first trimester. Focus on non-pharmacologic treatment techniques such as psychotherapy, hypnotherapy, relaxation therapy, etc.

SYNONYMS
• Trauma syndrome
• Battle fatigue
• Shell shock
• Post-disaster syndrome
• Trauma survivor's syndrome
• Traumatic neurosis

ICD-9-CM   293.9

SEE ALSO   N/A

OTHER NOTES   N/A

ABBREVIATIONS   PTSD = post-traumatic stress disorder

REFERENCES
• Pynoos RS, ed: Posttraumatic stress disorder: A clinical review. Lutherville, MD, Sidran Press, 1994
• Rowan AB, Foy DW: Post-traumatic stress disorder in child sexual abuse. J of Traumatic Stress 1993;6:3-31
• Solomon SD, Gerrty DT, Muff AM: Efficacy of treatments for PTSD: an empirical review. JAMA 1992;268:633-638
• Terr L: Too Scared to Cry: Psychic Trauma in Childhood. New York, Harper & Row, 1990
• Williams MB, Sommer JF, eds: Handbook of post-traumatic therapy. Westport, CT, Greenwood Press, 1994
• Wilson JP, Raphael B, eds: The International Handbook of Traumatic Stress Syndromes. New York, Plenum Press, 1993
Illustrations: N/A
Internet references: http://www.5mcc.com

Author(s)
Moshe S. Torem, MD, FAPA

Preeclampsia

 BASICS

DESCRIPTION Hypertension associated with proteinuria, edema, and acute excessive weight gain developing during pregnancy after 20 weeks gestation
System(s) affected: Reproductive, Cardiovascular, Nervous
Genetics: N/A
Incidence/Prevalence in USA: 5-10% of all pregnancies
Predominant age:
• Young, primigravid women
• Women over 35 years of age
Predominant sex: Female only

SIGNS AND SYMPTOMS
• Elevated BP (> 140/90 [18.6/12 kPa] or increased 30 [4 kPa] systolic or increased 15 [2 kPa] diastolic) recorded on 2 BP readings 6 hours apart
• Proteinuria (> 300 mg/24 hours or > 1 gram/L)
• Edema
• Rapid excessive weight gain (> 5 lb/week) (2.3 kg/week)
• Epigastric pain
• Headache
• Hyperreflexia
• Visual disturbances
• Apprehension
• Retinal arteriolar spasm
• Papilledema
• Retinal cotton-wool exudate
• Amnesia
• Oliguria
• Anuria

CAUSES
• Altered cardiovascular reactivity
• Increased capillary permeability
• Widespread vasospasm
• Microthrombi
• Hypertension
• Improper implantation of placenta to uterine wall limiting blood and nutrients to fetus

RISK FACTORS
• Familial incidence
• Lower socio-economic
• Multiple fetuses
• Teenage
• Collagen disorders
• Females > 35 years old
• Primigravida
• First subsequent pregnancy with a different father
• Diabetes mellitus of pregnancy
• Chronic hypertension
• Hydatid mole
• Fetal hydrops
• History of renal disease

 DIAGNOSIS

DIFFERENTIAL DIAGNOSIS
• Chronic hypertension
• Pregnancy worsened hypertension
• Pregnancy induced hypertension

LABORATORY
• Proteinuria (> 300 mg/24 hrs or > 1 gram/L)
• Uric acid increased (mild increase > 5.5 mg/dL [0.32 mmol/L]);
(severe increase > 9.5 mg/dL [0.56 mmol/L])
• Thrombocytopenia
• CrCl < 90 mL/min/1.73m2 (0.87 mL/s/m2)
• Increased BUN (> 16 mg/dL [5.7 mmol/L])
• Increased creatinine (> 1.0 mg/dL [88 µmol/L])
• Abnormal increased liver function tests
• Increased fibrin degradation products
• Increased PT
• Decreased fibrinogen
• Granular casts in urine
• Red blood cell casts in urine
• Renal tubular cell casts in urine
• White blood cell casts in urine
• Increased urine specific gravity
• Increased T4
• Thrombocytopenia
• Decreased fibrinogen
• Disseminated intravascular coagulation
• Hyperbilirubinemia
Drugs that may alter lab results: N/A
Disorders that may alter lab results: Chronic renal disease

PATHOLOGICAL FINDINGS
• Fibrin deposits in kidneys
• Fibrin deposits in liver with necrosis and periportal hemorrhages
• Placental vascular abnormalities

SPECIAL TESTS N/A

IMAGING N/A

DIAGNOSTIC PROCEDURES 24 hour urine for protein

 TREATMENT

APPROPRIATE HEALTH CARE
• Outpatient care if mild
• Inpatient care if deterioration
• Delivery of fetus as soon as possible if severe
• Admit to hospital if blood pressure > 160/110 (21.3/14.6 kPa), proteinuria > 5 gm/24 hr, oliguria, cerebral or visual disturbances (scotoma, blurred vision), severe headache, altered consciousness, pulmonary edema, thrombocytopenia, impaired liver function tests, epigastric pain

GENERAL MEASURES
• If outpatient, keep a daily weight record; use a home test to check for proteinuria
• If outpatient, twice a week blood pressure tests

SURGICAL MEASURES N/A

ACTIVITY
• Bedrest on left side
• Ambulatory only to void

DIET
• Salt restriction is not good because the patient is in an intravascular contracted state
• Protein 80-100 gm/day

PATIENT EDUCATION Avoid excessive weight gain during pregnancy (> 25-30 lb [11.4-13.6 kg])

Preeclampsia

MEDICATIONS

DRUG(S) OF CHOICE For seizure prophylaxis - magnesium sulfate (MgSO4) loading dose 4 grams IV in 200 mL normal saline over 20-30 min. Maintenance dose - 1-2 grams/hr IV.
Contraindications: Refer to manufacturer's profile of each drug
Precautions:
• Therapeutic magnesium levels are 4-7 mEq/L (2-3.5 mmol/L)
• Toxicity (flushing, sweating, hyporeflexia, flaccid paralysis, CNS depression, oliguria, decreased cardiac function)
• Spinal/epidural anesthesia contraindicated
• Continue 24 hour postpartum
• Toxicity therapy with 10% calcium gluconate, 1 gram over 2-3 minutes plus oxygen
• Give oxytocin (Pitocin) postpartum to prevent bleeding (60 unit/L at 50 cc/hr)
• Keep urine flow > 25 cc/hr
• Recheck reflexes often. They may be hypoactive, but should be present.
Significant possible interactions: Refer to manufacturer's profile of each drug

ALTERNATIVE DRUGS
• Hypertension:
  ◊ Hydralazine (Apresoline) 5-10 mg IV q 20-30 minutes, or
  ◊ Diazoxide 30 mg minidose if refractory to hydralazine
  ◊ Avoid nitroprusside (decreased uterine blood flow plus possible lethal fetal cyanide levels)
• Seizures:
  ◊ MgSO4 - not as effective for treatment of seizures as it is for prophylaxis
  ◊ Diazepam (Valium) 10 mg IV followed by 10 mg IM q4h if MgSO4 unavailable or ineffective

FOLLOWUP

PATIENT MONITORING
• Keep urine output > 25 cc/hr
• Continue MgSO4 for 24 hr postpartum
• Give oxytocin (Pitocin) postpartum to prevent bleeding (60 unit/L at 50 cc/hr)

PREVENTION/AVOIDANCE
• Weight control
• Recent data indicates that low dose ASA may sometimes prevent preeclampsia

POSSIBLE COMPLICATIONS
• Eclampsia (seizures)
• Hypertensive crisis
• Acute pyelonephritis
• Acute fatty liver
• Acute pulmonary edema

EXPECTED COURSE/PROGNOSIS
• Prevention of seizures
• Delivery of viable fetus

MISCELLANEOUS

ASSOCIATED CONDITIONS Abruptio placenta

AGE-RELATED FACTORS
Pediatric: Increased incidence in teenagers
Geriatric: N/A
Others: Older pregnant females (> 35 years old) have increased incidence

PREGNANCY N/A

SYNONYMS
• Pregnancy-induced hypertension
• Toxemia of pregnancy

ICD-9-CM
642.4 Preeclampsia, mild
642.5 Preeclampsia, severe

SEE ALSO Eclampsia

OTHER NOTES N/A

ABBREVIATIONS
MgSO4 = magnesium sulfate
CrCl = creatinine clearance

REFERENCES
• Family Practice Recertification (Jan 88, Nov 1989)
• Cunningham FG, MacDonald PC, Gant NF, eds: Williams' Obstetrics. 19th Ed. Norwalk, CT, Appleton and Lange, 1993
• Fisher S: J of Clin Investigation 1997;5
Illustrations: N/A
Internet references: http://www.5mcc.com

Author(s)
Stoney A. Abercrombie, MD

Premature labor

 BASICS

DESCRIPTION
Labor occurring prior to the completion of 36 weeks' gestation
System(s) affected: Reproductive
Genetics: N/A
Incidence/Prevalence in USA: 8-12% of all births in the USA
Predominant age: Childbearing
Predominant sex: Female only

SIGNS AND SYMPTOMS
• Regular uterine contractions, with or without pain, continuing for 1 hour
• Dull, low backache, pressure, or pain
• Intermittent lower abdominal or thigh pain
• Intestinal cramping, with or without diarrhea or indigestion
• Change in vaginal discharge
• Palpable contractions on examination
• Dilatation of the cervix greater than 1 cm
• Effacement of the cervix more than 50%
• Signs of ruptured membranes (pH paper turns blue; fern positive)

CAUSES
• Infections (pyelonephritis)
• Subclinical chorioamnionitis (chlamydia or gonorrhea)
• Uterine abnormalities (incompetent cervix, leiomyomata; septa, diethylstilbestrol DES exposure)
• Over-distention (by multiple gestation or hydramnios)
• Premature rupture of membranes
• Unknown

RISK FACTORS
• Prior preterm delivery
• Multiple gestation
• Three or more first-trimester abortions
• Previous second-trimester abortion
• Cervical incompetence
• Abdominal surgery during pregnancy
• Uterine or cervical anomalies
• Placenta previa
• Premature placental separation (trauma or drug abuse - especially cocaine)
• Fetal abnormalities
• Hydramnios
• Serious maternal infection
• Second-trimester bleeding
• Prepregnancy weight less than 45 kg (100 lb)
• Single parent
• No prenatal care

 DIAGNOSIS

DIFFERENTIAL DIAGNOSIS
Dehydration, urinary tract infections, round ligament pain, viral gastroenteritis, lumbosacral muscular back pain, chlamydia vaginal infection, gonorrheal vaginal infection, yeast vaginitis, Braxton-Hicks contractions

LABORATORY
• Urinalysis and urine culture for evaluation of urinary tract infection
• Group B strep, gonorrhea, and chlamydial cultures for causes of chorioamnionitis
• Consider urine specific gravity and serum creatinine and BUN for dehydration
Drugs that may alter lab results: N/A
Disorders that may alter lab results: N/A

PATHOLOGICAL FINDINGS N/A

SPECIAL TESTS
Consider amniocentesis if 28-34 weeks' gestation for evaluation of lecithin/sphingomyelin (L/S) ratio and desaturated phosphatidylcholine (DSPC). If L/S ratio is greater than 2:1, and DSPC greater than 1000, hyaline membrane disease is unlikely.

IMAGING
Consider uterine ultrasound to quantitate gestational age, estimated fetal weight, multiple gestations, amount of amniotic fluid, and fetal growth

DIAGNOSTIC PROCEDURES
• Uterine monitoring for at least two hours
• Speculum vaginal examination for signs of infection and cultures
• pH and fern testing for ruptured membranes
• Digital cervical examination for effacement and dilatation

 TREATMENT

APPROPRIATE HEALTH CARE
Outpatient or inpatient depending on circumstances

GENERAL MEASURES
• Treat underlying risk factors with appropriate measures (antibiotics for infections, hydration for dehydration)
• If delivery is inevitable, but not immediate, consider transport to a tertiary care center or hospital equipped with a neonatal intensive care unit
• If mother is at 27-34 weeks' gestation, consider administering glucocorticoids to reduce incidence of neonatal respiratory distress
• No sexual intercourse

SURGICAL MEASURES N/A

ACTIVITY
• Bedrest. Discontinue work or other physical activities.
• Hospitalization may be necessary if on intravenous tocolysis or if bedrest is impossible at home

DIET
Liquids only, if delivery becomes imminent

PATIENT EDUCATION
Call physician or proceed to hospital whenever contractions last over an hour, low back pain, change in vaginal discharge, "menstrual cramping." or intestinal cramping

MEDICATIONS

DRUG(S) OF CHOICE
• Hydrate with 500 mL D5NS for first half hour
• For tocolysis, protocols include:
   ◊ Terbutaline 0.25-0.50 mg subcutaneously every 3h until contractions cease, or pulse is greater than 140. Change to oral terbutaline 2.5-5.0 mg every 3-6h if contractions have ceased.
   ◊ Ritodrine 150 mg per 500 mL of D5NS. Start at 100 µg/min, increase by 50 µg/min every 10 min. Stop for significant side effects or successful tocolysis. Decrease dose by 50 µg/min each hour to a minimum of 100 µg/min as long as tocolysis remains successful. Switch to po after 12-24h. Oral dose is 10 mg q2 for the first 24h, then 10-20 mg q4-6h. Total daily dose is 120 mg.
   ◊ Magnesium sulfate solution of 40 g per 1000 mL of D5NS. Bolus 4 g over 20 min, then begin infusion at 2 g/h, increasing by 0.5 g/h every 15-30 min; check serum magnesium levels (therapeutic is 6-8 mg/dL [2.47-3.29 mmol/L]). Stop for significant side effects or when tocolysis occurs. Decrease dose by 0.5 g/h each hour to a minimum of 2 g/h and then switch to oral therapy after 12h.
• Glucocorticoids to reduce incidence of neonatal respiratory distress, protocols include:
   ◊ Betamethasone 12 mg IM twice 24h apart
or
   ◊ Dexamethasone 5 mg IM bid x 4 doses
or
   ◊ Doses are repeated every 7-10 days as long as preterm delivery is likely; may not be helpful if fetus is older than 34 weeks or if delivery will occur in less than 24 hours
Contraindications:
• Severe preeclampsia, hemorrhage, chorioamnionitis, advanced labor, intrauterine growth retardation, or fetal heart decelerations
• Relative contraindications to terbutaline or ritodrine include maternal cardiac rhythm disturbance or poorly controlled diabetes or thyrotoxicosis
• Relative contraindications to magnesium sulfate are myasthenia gravis, hypocalcemia, or renal failure
Precautions:
• Palpitations, nausea, intractable vomiting, pulse greater than 140
• Long-term terbutaline may adversely affect glucose tolerance. Consider repeating glucose screen if using terbutaline for more than 1 week.
Significant possible interactions:
Pulmonary edema from rehydration fluids and tocolytic agents

ALTERNATIVE DRUGS   Nifedipine for tocolysis

FOLLOWUP

PATIENT MONITORING
• Weekly office visits and cervical checks for those at high risk for preterm labor
• Ambulatory external tocodynamometry has not yet been proven efficacious for prevention of preterm labor
• Treating bacterial vaginosis in second trimester with metronidazole 250 mg tid for 7 days and erythromycin base 333 mg tid for 14 days; alternatively, using clindamycin 300 mg bid for 7 days may reduce risk of premature delivery

PREVENTION/AVOIDANCE
• Patient education
• Consider cerclage placement before 20 week's gestation for those at high risk because of an incompetent cervix from DES or cone biopsy
• Controversy exists on whether maintenance tocolysis is useful

POSSIBLE COMPLICATIONS   Labor resistant to tocolysis

EXPECTED COURSE/PROGNOSIS   If membranes are ruptured, delivery generally occurs within 3-7 days. If membranes are intact, treat until 37 weeks, gestational age.

MISCELLANEOUS

ASSOCIATED CONDITIONS   See Risk Factors

AGE-RELATED FACTORS   N/A
Pediatric: N/A
Geriatric: N/A
Others: N/A

PREGNANCY   By definition, a problem of pregnancy

SYNONYMS   Preterm labor

ICD-9-CM   644.2 Premature labor

SEE ALSO   N/A

OTHER NOTES   N/A

ABBREVIATIONS   N/A

REFERENCES
• ACOG Technical Bulletin, No. 206, June, 1995
• Anon: Effect of corticosteroids for fetal maturation on perinatal outcomes. NIH Consensus Development Panel on the Effect of Corticosteroids for Fetal Maturation on Perinatal Outcomes. JAMA 1995;273(5):413-418
• Hauth JC, Goldenberg RY, Andrews WW, et al: Reduced incidence of preterm delivery with metronidazole and erythromycin in women with bacterial vaginosis. NEJM 1995;333(26):1732-1736
Illustrations: N/A
Internet references: http://www.5mcc.com

Author(s)
Cathryn Heath, MD

Premenstrual syndrome (PMS)

BASICS

DESCRIPTION Premenstrual syndrome is a constellation of symptoms that occurs prior to menstruation and is severe enough to interfere significantly with the patient's life
System(s) affected: Endocrine/Metabolic, Reproductive, Nervous
Genetics: Unknown, probably familial incidence
Incidence/Prevalence in USA: Almost all women have some symptoms prior to menses (this is not PMS). A low percentage have actual PMS.
Predominant age: Childbearing years, worse during late 20's and 30's
Predominant sex: Females only

SIGNS AND SYMPTOMS
Symptoms can involve any organ system but the following are more common:
• Depressed mood
• Mood swings
• Irritability
• Difficulty concentrating
• Fatigue
• Edema
• Breast tenderness
• Headaches
• Sleep disturbances

CAUSES Unknown, presumed hormonal; perhaps interacting with neurotransmitters

RISK FACTORS
• Premenstrual exacerbations can occur with other diseases (i.e., depression)
• Caffeine and high fluid intake exacerbate PMS symptoms
• Stress may precipitate
• PMS increases with age

DIAGNOSIS

DIFFERENTIAL DIAGNOSIS The major differentials are psychiatric syndromes, particularly depressive disorders and/or dysthymia. Other entities may be suggested by history or physical.

LABORATORY There are no laboratory tests which confirm or refute PMS. History and physical may disclose a need for specific laboratory tests.
Drugs that may alter lab results: N/A
Disorders that may alter lab results: N/A

PATHOLOGICAL FINDINGS N/A

SPECIAL TESTS N/A

IMAGING N/A

DIAGNOSTIC PROCEDURES Patients complete questionnaires over a minimum of two months to confirm premenstrual exacerbation of symptoms and lack of substantial symptoms in the follicular phase

TREATMENT

APPROPRIATE HEALTH CARE
Outpatient

GENERAL MEASURES
• Increase daily exercise
• Eat regular, balanced meals
• Stop smoking
• Get regular sleep
• Stress reduction techniques
• Individual or couples counseling
• Support groups

SURGICAL MEASURES N/A

ACTIVITY
• No restrictions
• Exercise is recommended

DIET Low-salt; low-caffeine; low-fat; frequent, small meals; high complex carbohydrates

PATIENT EDUCATION Explain PMS and treatment

MEDICATIONS

DRUG(S) OF CHOICE
• No single drug works for all women. Drugs that are used with varying degrees of success are listed.
• Diuretics (usually spironolactone) during luteal phase
• Symptomatic treatment of pain (ibuprofen or acetaminophen)
• Anti-depressants (fluoxetine, sertraline, clomipramine or nortriptyline), particularly for patients with depressive symptoms
• Alprazolam 0.25 mg tid-qid during symptoms
• Buspirone 5-10 mg tid during luteal phase
• Magnesium 300-500 mg/day
• Elemental calcium 1000 mg/day
• Vitamin B6 in modest doses (50 mg bid, may be toxic in higher doses)
• Vitamin E - up to 600 IU/day
• Evening primrose oil, high content of fatty acids, 500 mg qd to 1000 mg tid for breast tenderness
• Bromocriptine 2.5 mg tid at time of symptoms and danazol 100 mg bid may also work for breast tenderness, but have more side effects
• Danazol for the total PMS symptom complex
• Gonadotropin-releasing hormone agonists with or without concurrent estrogens/progestins

Contraindications: Refer to manufacturer's profile of each drug
Precautions: Refer to manufacturer's profile of each drug
Significant possible interactions: Refer to manufacturer's profile of each drug

ALTERNATIVE DRUGS
• Oral contraceptives may help
• Progesterone, during luteal phase, but recent research does not support much relief of symptoms

FOLLOWUP

PATIENT MONITORING See patient to provide general support and further patient education

PREVENTION/AVOIDANCE N/A

POSSIBLE COMPLICATIONS N/A

EXPECTED COURSE/PROGNOSIS
Many patients can have their symptoms adequately controlled

MISCELLANEOUS

ASSOCIATED CONDITIONS N/A

AGE-RELATED FACTORS
Pediatric: N/A
Geriatric: N/A
Others: N/A

PREGNANCY N/A

SYNONYMS N/A

ICD-9-CM 625.4 Premenstrual tension syndromes

SEE ALSO Mastalgia

OTHER NOTES Treatment may need to be continued for a long time. PMS sometimes continues after hysterectomy. Effects of long-term hormonal treatment unknown.

ABBREVIATIONS N/A

REFERENCES
• Parker PD: Premenstrual syndrome. Amer Fam Phys 1994;50:1309-1317
• Demonico SO, Brown CS, Ling F: Premenstrual syndrome. Current Opinion in Obstetrics and Gynecology 1994;6:499-502
• Carter T, Verhoef MJ: Efficacy of self-help and alternative treatments of premenstrual syndrome. Womens Health Issues 1994;4:130-137
• Barnhart KT, Freeman EW, Sandheimer SJ: A clinician's guide to premenstrual syndrome. Med Clin of NA 1995:70:1457-1472
Illustrations: N/A
Internet references: http://www.5mcc.com

Author(s)
Marjorie A. Bowman, MD, MPA

Pressure ulcer

BASICS

DESCRIPTION Skin breakdown is a common and serious complication affecting usually frail, disabled, acutely ill or immobile elderly patients, especially within long-term care settings. Most common sites are over bony prominences, such as elbows, hips, heels, outer ankles, and base of spine. Over 95% of ulcers develop on lower part of body. Median length of hospital stay to treat pressure sore is 46 days. Risk of death in elderly patient increases fourfold when sores heal and sixfold when sores do not heal.

System(s) affected: Skin/Exocrine
Genetics: N/A
Incidence/Prevalence in USA:
• 9% of all hospitalized and 23% of all nursing home patients
• 2 million patients develop these pressure sores each year
• Incidence is 43/100,000 population every year; 65% of elderly with femoral fractures; 33% of critical care patients, and a 60% prevalence among quadriplegic patients
• Estimated prevalence in nursing home residents ranges from 2.6-24%
Predominant age: 60-70% are elderly patients; age >85 at greatest risk
Predominant sex: Female > Male (due to survival differential); cost to heal pressure ulcer ranges from $5,000-$40,000

SIGNS AND SYMPTOMS
• Stage I - non-blanching erythema, warmth, tenderness
• Stage II - skin breakdown limited to dermis, excoriation, blistering, drainage, more sharply defined erythema, variable skin temperature, local swelling or edema
• Stage III - ulcer formation into subcutaneous tissues, crater formation, slough, eschar, and/or drainage
• Stage IV - ulcers extend beyond deep fascia into muscle or bone, decayed area may be larger than visibly apparent wound, osteomyelitis or sepsis may be present, granulation tissue and epithelialization may be present at wound margins

CAUSES
• Uneven application of pressure over a bony hard site; high pressure applied for two hours produces irreversible tissue ischemia and necrosis
• Shearing forces which develop when a seated person slides toward floor or toward foot of bed if supine
• Frictional forces which develop when pulling a patient across a bed sheet
• Moisture from incontinence or perspiration can increase the friction between two surfaces

RISK FACTORS
• Immobility (e.g., quadriplegia)
• Malnutrition and low body weight
• Hypoalbuminemia
• Fecal incontinence
• Urinary incontinence
• Bone fracture (especially femoral)
• Vitamin C deficiency
• Low diastolic blood pressure
• Age-related skin changes, such as diminished pain perception, thinning of epidermis, loss of dermal vessels, altered barrier properties, reduced immunity, and slowed wound healing
• Anemia
• Infections
• Peripheral vascular disease
• Dementia
• Malignancies
• Diabetes mellitus
• Cerebral vascular accidents
• Dry skin (low humidity, < 40%, and cold)
• Fractures
• Edema
• Assessment scale for evaluating risk factors include: Norton, Braden (Braden Q version for children), Waterlow and Walsall

DIAGNOSIS

DIFFERENTIAL DIAGNOSIS
• Stasis or ischemia ulcers
• Vasculitides
• Cancers
• Radiation injury
• Pyoderma gangrenosum and other dermatologic conditions

LABORATORY
• Culture of wound if there is evidence of infection (surrounding erythema, purulent drainage, foul odor)
• White blood cell count and differential if fever is present (greater than 37°C)
• Erythrocyte sedimentation rate
• If leucocytosis present, urinalysis to identify causative agents
• If above tests positive, blood and urine cultures
Drugs that may alter lab results: N/A
Disorders that may alter lab results: N/A

PATHOLOGICAL FINDINGS Extensive necrosis of affected part

SPECIAL TESTS N/A

IMAGING
• If leukocytosis present, chest radiograph
• Plain radiographs involved bone

DIAGNOSTIC PROCEDURES N/A

TREATMENT

APPROPRIATE HEALTH CARE
• An interdisciplinary approach usually indicated in nursing home, inpatient or home care settings if trained supervision available
• Complications will require inpatient setting to treat systemic infection, extensive debridement or skin grafting

GENERAL MEASURES
• Improve overall nutritional status (adequate protein intake)
• Clean wound each time dressing is changed to remove dead tissue, excess fluid and other debris
• Healing enhanced with body temperature maintained at 37°C (97.7°F) and an acidic pH
• Never use antiseptics and skin cleansers which harm the tissue
• Surgery for wounds not responding to treatment within 2-4 weeks
• Débridement of necrotic pressure ulcers using occlusive dressings, hydrotherapy, proteolytic enzymes, and surgical or laser débridement
• Pressure reduction products such as, specialized beds and repositioning every two hours to relieve pressure at site of ulceration (air-fluidized or low-air-loss beds); static-pressure and foam mattresses are less expensive. Water mattresses, sheepskins, and egg-crate mattresses are other less expensive devices.
• Avoid agents that delay wound healing, such as topical corticosteroids, hydrogen peroxide, povidone iodine solution, and hypochlorite solutions
• Control of fecal and/or urine incontinence Specific measures by stage as follows:
• Stage I: Nonblanchable erythema of intact skin
  ◊ Relieve pressure (floatation or airflow mattress/bed)
  ◊ Use moisture barrier lubricant, transparent bio-occlusive dressings (Opsite) or Granulex Spray on reddened areas
  ◊ Keep all skin areas clean and dry
  ◊ Assess skin every 8-12 hours
• Stage II: Partial thickness skin loss of epidermal and/or dermal layers
  ◊ Use saline soaked 4 x 4's to cleanse pressure sore followed by topical antibiotic
  ◊ Rinse with saline soaked 4 x 4's
  ◊ Pat dry with 4 x 4's
  ◊ Apply protective barrier film to unbroken skin surrounding pressure sore
  ◊ Apply occlusive hydrocolloid dressing (Duoderm)
  ◊ Repeat every three days
  ◊ Loosely pack wound
  ◊ Whirlpools useful for necrotic wounds
• Stage III: Full thickness skin loss through subcutaneous tissue to fascia
  ◊ Irrigate wound with saline solution
  ◊ Scrub and debride with dry gauze and gels for autolytic débridement
  ◊ Re-rinse wound
  ◊ Blot excess moisture with dry 4 x 4 gauze
  ◊ Apply protective barrier film
  ◊ Apply skin care product (occlusive hydrocolloid dressing, granules, or paste)
  ◊ If wound highly exudating, use absorption dressing (exudate absorbers) and change daily; consider wound culture

- **Stage IV:** Exposure or destruction of muscle, bone and other supportive structure
  - ◊ If eschar present, need to be debrided or sloughed
  - ◊ Irrigate wound with saline solution x 2
  - ◊ Blot excess moisture with 4 x 4 dry gauze
  - ◊ Apply protective barrier film to unbroken skin surrounding sore
  - ◊ Moisten packing gauze (Kerlix) in saline and pack wound
  - ◊ Apply outer dressing
  - ◊ Surgical intervention for definitive treatment of deep and complicated pressure ulcers, such as myocutaneous flaps, split-thickness skin grafts and primary closure

SURGICAL MEASURES
See under various stages in General Measures

ACTIVITY
- Any activity consistent with patient's ambulatory status and relief of pressure on wound
- Perform passive range-of-motion exercises for patient or encourage patient to do active exercises if possible

DIET
- Oral high-calorie and high-protein supplements
- Oral zinc sulfate, vitamin A and C, and iron

PATIENT EDUCATION
- Patient Care 1993; 27(7):65-66
- National Action Group for the Prevention and Treatment of Decubitus Ulcers, P.O. Box 1098, Union City, CT 06770
- AHCPR publication No. 92-0048, Preventing Pressure Ulcers: A Patient's Guide, May 1992.
- Patient information handout from: Findley D: Practical management of pressure ulcers. Amer Fam Phys 1996;54(3):1519-1536

MEDICATIONS

DRUG(S) OF CHOICE
- Clindamycin or gentamicin for complications such as cellulitis, osteomyelitis, or sepsis
- Supplements - vitamin C 500 mg twice a day, zinc sulfate
- Antibiotic prophylaxis for bacterial endocarditis if valvular lesions present
- Two week trial of topical antimicrobials (e.g., silver sulfadiazine or triple antibiotics) should be used only for a clean superficial ulcer not healing or producing moderate amount of exudate; cultures are necessary to determine whether antifungal (miconazole, clotrimazole, or haloprogin) or specific antibacterial agents (silver sulfadiazine, neomycin-polymyxin B-bacitracin, gentamicin, mupirocin 2%) are indicated
- Enzymatic debriding agents such as collagenase (Santyl), trypsin (Granulex), fibrinolysin-deoxyribonuclease (Elase), papain (Panafil) or sutilains (Travase) used with a moisture barrier to protect surrounding normal tissue

- Recommended dressings include polyurethane films (Op-site, Tegaderm), absorbent hydrocolloid dressings (Duoderm, Comfeel Ulcus)
Contraindications: Refer to manufacturer's literature
Precautions: Refer to manufacturer's literature
Significant possible interactions: Refer to manufacturer's literature

ALTERNATIVE DRUGS N/A

FOLLOWUP

PATIENT MONITORING
- Frequent evaluation of all patients with history of pressure sores, especially if limited mobility. Include nutritional status and dietary intervention.
- Early identification of areas of skin redness to prevent subsequent breakdown
- Skin cleansing as soon as soiled and at routine intervals

PREVENTION/AVOIDANCE
- Up to 95% of all pressure ulcers are preventable
- Pressure relief
- Early identification of at risk individuals and elimination of risk factors (risk assessment tools: Brader Scale for Predicting Pressure Sore Risk for nursing home patients and The Norton Scale for hospitalized patients)
- Underpads (non-cloth) to absorb moisture
- Quality nursing care
- Early interdisciplinary supportive care - include staff, patient, family/caregiver
- Nutritional assessment of patient, especially if cannot take food by mouth or has experienced involuntary change in weight. Additional protein and calories should be provided (vitamin C and zinc).
- Frequent patient repositioning if immobile - every hour if wheelchair bound and every 2 hours if bedridden
- Functional assessment of patient and treatment of incontinence
- Frequent physical examination of skin areas affected by pressure, moisture, shearing or friction sources
- Use mattress overlays, seat cushions or special mattresses and beds to reduce pressure on pressure points

POSSIBLE COMPLICATIONS
- Growth of resistant organisms if antibiotics used for local or systemic infection
- Gangrene

EXPECTED COURSE/PROGNOSIS
- Though pressure ulcers are associated with an increased rate of mortality, with good medical care, most can be expected to heal
- In a recent study among long-term care hospital patients, 79% of pressure sores improved and 40% completely healed during a six-week followup period using ordinary therapies

MISCELLANEOUS

ASSOCIATED CONDITIONS
- Malnutrition
- Fecal and/or urinary incontinence
- Immobility
- Impaired mental status
- Skin atrophy
- Low body weight
- Compromised immune states

AGE-RELATED FACTORS
Pediatric: N/A
Geriatric: Over 60% occur in elderly
Others: N/A

PREGNANCY N/A

SYNONYMS
- Decubitus ulcer
- Bedsore
- Trophic ulcer
- Pressure sore

ICD-9-CM 707.0 Decubitus ulcer

SEE ALSO N/A

OTHER NOTES N/A

ABBREVIATIONS N/A

REFERENCES
- Findley D: Practical management of pressure ulcers. Amer Fam Phys 1996;54(3):1519-1536
- Levine JM, Totolus E: Pressure ulcers; A strategic plan to prevent and heal them. Geriatrics 1995;50(1): 32-37
- Pressure Ulcer Guideline Panel: Pressure ulcer treatment. Amer Fam Phys 1995;51(5):1202-1222
- Panel for the Prediction and Prevention of Pressure Ulcers in Adults. Pressure Ulcers in Adults: Predicting and Prevention. Clinical Practice Guidelines, No. 3. AHCPR Publication No. 92-0047, May, 1992
Illustrations: N/A
Internet references: http://www.5mcc.com

Author(s)
Evan W. Kligman, MD

Priapism

BASICS

DESCRIPTION Painful and/or abnormally prolonged penile erection
System(s) affected: Reproductive
Genetics: N/A
Incidence/Prevalence in USA: Unknown
Predominant age: Young adult
Predominant sex: Male only

SIGNS AND SYMPTOMS
• Penile erection that is persistent, prolonged, painful, and tender
• Urination difficult during erection
• Loss of sexual function if treatment is not prompt and effective

CAUSES
• Intracavernosal injections of vasoactive drugs for erectile dysfunction; most common cause
• Pelvic vascular thrombosis
• Prolonged sexual activity
• Sickle cell anemia
• Leukemia
• Other blood dyscrasias
• Pelvic hematoma or neoplasia
• Cerebrospinal tumors
• Tertiary syphilis
• Bladder calculus
• Injury to penis
• Urinary tract infections, especially prostatitis, urethritis, cystitis
• Several drugs suspected as causing priapism, such as chlorpromazine, prazosin, trazodone, and certain corticosteroids, anticoagulants, antihypertensives
• Intracavenous fat emulsion

RISK FACTORS
• Erectile dysfunction (impotence)

DIAGNOSIS

DIFFERENTIAL DIAGNOSIS List with Causes

LABORATORY
• CBC
• Sickle prep and hgb electrophoresis
• Coagulation profile
• Platelet count
• Urinalysis
Drugs that may alter lab results: N/A
Disorders that may alter lab results: N/A

PATHOLOGICAL FINDINGS
• Pelvic vascular thrombosis
• Partial thrombosis of corpora cavernosa
• Corpus spongiosum, glans penis: No involvement

SPECIAL TESTS N/A

IMAGING N/A

DIAGNOSTIC PROCEDURES Physical examination

TREATMENT

APPROPRIATE HEALTH CARE Inpatient

GENERAL MEASURES
• Reassurance about outcome if warranted
• Continuous caudal or spinal anesthesia if etiology is neurogenic
• Treat any underlying cause
• In sickle cell anemia: Intravenous hydration; partial exchange or repeated transfusions to reduce percent of sickle cells below 50%
• Pian relief

SURGICAL MEASURES
• Introduction of 12 or 16 gauge needles into corpora cavernosa (best done by urologist if available)
  ◊ First: aspiration of 20-30 cc of blood from corpora cavernosum with 12-16 gauge needle
  ◊ Then: if caused by injected vasodilator, use intracavernous injection of 10-25 mg ephedrine sulfate or 5-10 µg epinephrine or 125-250 µg phenylephrine
  ◊ May repeat one time in 20-30 minutes if no response
• Create fistula between glans and corpus cavernosum (with biopsy needle by urologist)
• Semipermanent diversion by saphenous shunt from one or both corpora
• Caverноso-spongiosum shunt to permit reestablishment of pelvic circulation

ACTIVITY Bedrest until relieved

DIET N/A

PATIENT EDUCATION Information about long-term outlook, referral for counseling

MEDICATIONS

DRUG(S) OF CHOICE
• Narcotics for pain if needed
• Vasoconstrictors may be injected after dilution, e.g., metaraminol 1 mg into the penis
Contraindications: Refer to manufacturer's literature
Precautions: Refer to manufacturer's literature
Significant possible interactions: Refer to manufacturer's literature

ALTERNATIVE DRUGS N/A

FOLLOWUP

PATIENT MONITORING Close followup after surgery

PREVENTION/AVOIDANCE
• Avoid dehydration
• Avoid excessive sexual stimulation
• Avoid causative drugs (see Causes) when possible

POSSIBLE COMPLICATIONS Impotence

EXPECTED COURSE/PROGNOSIS
• Even with excellent treatment, detumescence may require several weeks
• Impotence is likely

MISCELLANEOUS

ASSOCIATED CONDITIONS Sickle cell anemia

AGE-RELATED FACTORS
Pediatric: > 85% likelihood of sickle cell in African American children
Geriatric: Treatment more difficult and less likely successful
Others: N/A

PREGNANCY N/A

SYNONYMS N/A

ICD-9-CM
607.3

SEE ALSO
• Anemia, sickle cell
• Erectile dysfunction

OTHER NOTES N/A

ABBREVIATIONS N/A

REFERENCES
• Smith DR: General Urology. 14th Ed. Los Altos, CA, Lange Medical Publications, 1995
• Tanagho EA, McAninch JW, eds: Smith's General Urology. 12th Ed. Norwalk, CT, Appleton & Lange, 1988
Illustrations: N/A
Internet references: http://www.5mcc.com

Author(s)
Bruce Block, MD

Primary pulmonary hypertension

BASICS

DESCRIPTION Pulmonary arterial hypertension of unknown cause, where secondary causes have been ruled out. Three pathologic subtypes have been identified: (1) thrombotic, (2) plexogenic, (3) veno-occlusive.
System(s) affected: Pulmonary, Cardiovascular
Genetics: 7% familial; autosomal dominant with variable expression and "genetic anticipation"
Incidence/Prevalence in USA: 1-2 cases/million. 1% of all causes of cor pulmonale at autopsy. 0.5-2% of patients with portal hypertension or HIV
Predominant age: Mean age 34-36 years; second incidence peak in males 50-59 years
Predominant sex: Female > Male (3:1)

SIGNS AND SYMPTOMS
• Loud P2 (> 80%)
• Right ventricular lift (> 80%)
• Dyspnea (> 75%)
• Murmur of tricuspid insufficiency (50-80%)
• Increased jugular venous pressure (50-80%)
• Right ventricular S4 (50-80%)
• Chest pain (> 50%)
• Fatigue (> 50%)
• Palpitations (< 50%)
• Syncope; dizziness (< 50%)
• Cough (< 50%)
• Raynaud's phenomenon (< 10%)
• Hepatomegaly (< 50%)
• Pulmonic ejection click (< 50%)
• Right ventricular S3 (< 50%)
• Murmur of pulmonic insufficiency (< 50%)
• Lower extremity edema (< 50%)
• Superficial thrombophlebitis (5%)

CAUSES
• Unknown; possible pulmonary arteriolar hyperactivity and vasoconstriction; occult thromboembolism; possible autoimmune (high frequency antinuclear antibodies)
• In Europe, reports of PPH associated with anorectic agent aminorex fumarate in late 1960's; tainted rapeseed oil
• HIV positive patients may have an increased incidence of primary pulmonary hypertension
• Anorectic agents (fenfluramine and dexfenfluramine)
• Amphetamines

RISK FACTORS Female sex

DIAGNOSIS

DIFFERENTIAL DIAGNOSIS
• Pulmonary parenchymal disease (COPD, asthma, pulmonary fibrosis, granulomatous disease, malignancy)
• Pulmonary vascular disease (pulmonary thromboembolism, collagen vascular disease, pulmonary arteritis, schistosomiasis, sickle cell disease)
• Cardiac disease (cardiomyopathy, valvular heart disease, congenital heart disease, persistent fetal circulation, pulmonary venous hypertension)
• Other disorders of respiratory function (sleep apnea syndromes, neuromuscular diseases, pleural diseases, thoracic cage abnormalities)
• IV drug abuse

LABORATORY
• ANA positive (1/3 of patients)
Drugs that may alter lab results: Hydralazine, procainamide, isoniazid, etc.
Disorders that may alter lab results: Many other diseases, e.g., lupus, scleroderma

PATHOLOGICAL FINDINGS
• Medial hypertrophy and arterial thrombosis are common in all subtypes
• Plexogenic pulmonary arteriopathy (30-70%): laminar "onion skin" intimal proliferation, focal medial disruption, aneurysmal dilatation
• Microthromboemboli (20-50%)
• Veno-occlusive disease (10-15%)

SPECIAL TESTS
• ECG - right ventricular hypertrophy and right axis deviation
• Pulmonary function testing - arterial hypoxemia, reduced diffusion capacity, hypocapnea
• V/Q scan - must rule out proximal pulmonary artery emboli
• Exercise test: reduced maximal O2 consumption, high minute ventilation, low anaerobic threshold, reduced maximal oxygen pulse, increased DO2A-a. Correlation to severity of disease with 6 minute walk test.

IMAGING
• Chest x-ray: enlarged central pulmonary arteries with pulmonary arterial branches attenuated. Right ventricular enlargement a late finding. If increased interstitial markings, consider lung parenchymal disease or veno-occlusive disease.
• Echo-Doppler: right ventricular enlargement and overload; important to rule out underlying cardiac disease such as atrial septal defect with secondary pulmonary hypertension or mitral stenosis

DIAGNOSTIC PROCEDURES
• Chest x-ray, pulmonary function tests, arterial blood gases, and V/Q scan should be done
• Cardiac catheterization - right heart catheterization is necessary to measure pulmonary artery pressures and hemodynamics; rule out underlying cardiac disease
• Pulmonary angiography - should be done if segmental or larger defect on V/Q scan. Caution in pulmonary hypertension as can lead to hemodynamic collapse; use low osmolar agents, subselective angiograms.
• Lung biopsy not recommended

TREATMENT

APPROPRIATE HEALTH CARE
• Medical therapy is first line and primarily palliative; health care is guided by clinical status
• Hospitalization with invasive monitoring is needed to screen vasodilator responsiveness and initiate vasodilator therapy
• There is a national registry established by the National Heart, Lung, and Blood Institute

GENERAL MEASURES
• Primary modalities are oxygen supplementation, vasodilators, anticoagulants, and treatment of heart failure (e.g., diuretics)
• Oxygen supplementation is indicated for rest, exercise, or nocturnal hypoxemia
• The acute response to vasodilators may improve survival

SURGICAL MEASURES
• Surgical procedures - patients with documented large vessel thromboembolic disease should be considered for pulmonary thrombectomy
• Heart-lung or lung transplantation is an option for appropriate patients when medical therapy has failed
• Blade-balloon atrial septostomy

ACTIVITY Restricted; exercise worsens pulmonary vascular resistance

DIET Low salt with heart failure

PATIENT EDUCATION
• Need to discuss prognosis; options such as transplantation
• Avoidance of pregnancy

MEDICATIONS

DRUG(S) OF CHOICE
• Medical therapy may be guided by suspected subtype:
◊ Plexogenic (clear lung fields, normal perfusion scan) - vasodilators potentially useful. Vasodilators - calcium channel blockers, first line, may be more effective in high doses. Other agents: ACE-inhibitors, alpha-antagonists, hydralazine - none shown to improve survival.
◊ Thrombotic (clear lung fields, patchy perfusion scan) - anticoagulants potentially useful. Anticoagulants - warfarin, heparin, antiplatelet agents.
◊ Veno-occlusive (pulmonary venous congestion, patchy perfusion scan) - vasodilators probably useless
All types: Heart failure may be treated with diuretics. Digoxin use controversial - not shown to be beneficial or detrimental. Digoxin may adversely affect exercise capacity due to increase in pulmonary vascular resistance.
• Chronic vasodilator therapy
◊ Nifedipine, diltiazem
◊ Prostacyclin
◊ Hydralazine
◊ Isoproterenol
◊ Terbutaline
◊ Prazosin
◊ Phentolamine
◊ Phenoxybenzamine
• Screening for responsiveness
◊ Prostacyclin
◊ Iloprost
◊ Acetylcholine
◊ Adenosine
◊ Nitrous oxide
◊ Nitroprusside
◊ Isoproterenol
◊ Hydralazine
◊ Phentolamine
• Anticoagulation: 2 small studies suggest prolonged survival. Warfarin with INR ~2.0.
Contraindications: Avoid warfarin in patients with syncope or hemoptysis
Precautions: Vasodilator therapy and response should be evaluated with invasive monitoring. Short acting agents such as prostacyclin, adenosine, or acetylcholine are useful for screening.
Significant possible interactions: Refer to manufacturer's literature

ALTERNATIVE DRUGS N/A

FOLLOWUP

PATIENT MONITORING Frequent

PREVENTION/AVOIDANCE None

POSSIBLE COMPLICATIONS
Thromboembolism, heart failure, sudden death

EXPECTED COURSE/PROGNOSIS
• Mean survival 2-3 years from time of diagnosis, 75% mortality at 5 years, although survival is quite variable as learned from the NIH registry.
• Mean age at diagnosis 34 years
• Mode of death:
◊ Right heart failure 63%
◊ Indeterminate 15%
◊ Pneumonia 7%
◊ Sudden death 7%
◊ Cardiac death 5%
• Poor prognostic factors:
◊ PaO2 < 63%
◊ RA pressure > 20 mm Hg
◊ Cardiac index < 2 L/min/m2
◊ Mean pulmonary arterial (PA) pressure > 85 mm Hg
◊ New York Heart Association (NYHA) class 3 or 4
◊ Raynaud's phenomenon

MISCELLANEOUS

ASSOCIATED CONDITIONS
• Portal hypertension
• Systemic lupus erythematosus
• HIV

AGE-RELATED FACTORS
Pediatric: N/A
Geriatric: N/A
Others: N/A

PREGNANCY Must be avoided; high mother and fetal wastage

SYNONYMS Primary pulmonary vascular disease

ICD-9-CM
416.0 Primary pulmonary hypertension

SEE ALSO
• Cor pulmonale
• Pulmonary embolism

OTHER NOTES N/A

ABBREVIATIONS
V/Q = ventilation/perfusion

REFERENCES
• Palevsky HE, Fishman AP: The management of primary pulmonary hypertension. JAMA 1991;265:1014-1020
• Hawkins JW, Dunn MI: Primary pulmonary hypertension in adults. Clinical Cardiology 1990;13:382-387
• Rich S: Primary pulmonary hypertension. In: Isselbacher KJ, et al, eds. Harrison's Principles of Internal Medicine. 13th Ed. McGraw-Hill, New York, 1994
• Cremona G, Higenbottom T: Role of prostacycline in the treatment of pulmonary hypertension. AF Cardio 1995;75(3):67A-71A
Illustrations: N/A
Internet references: http://www.5mcc.com

Author(s)
Darell E. Heiselman, DO, FCCM, FACP, FACC, FCCP

Proctitis

 BASICS

DESCRIPTION An acute or chronic inflammation of the rectal mucosa
System(s) affected: Gastrointestinal
Genetics: Higher incidence in Jews
Incidence/Prevalence in USA:
0.5-3/100,000 (ulcerative proctitis)/10-30/100,000 (ulcerative proctitis)
Predominant age: Adult
Predominant sex: Male > Female

SIGNS AND SYMPTOMS
• Rectal and/or perianal discomfort
• Rectal bleeding and/or mucous discharge
• Diarrhea
• Tenesmus
• Urgency
• Constipation
• Fever
• Weight loss

CAUSES
• Idiopathic
• Rectal gonorrhea
• Crohn's disease
• Syphilis (usually secondary)
• Nonspecific sexually transmitted infection
• Herpes simplex
• Chlamydia
• Papillomavirus
• Amebiasis
• Lymphogranuloma venereum
• Ischemia
• Radiation therapy
• Toxins (e.g., hydrogen peroxide enemas)
• Vasculitis

RISK FACTORS
• Rectal intercourse
• Radiation
• Rectal injury
• Rectal medications
• Jewish heritage

 DIAGNOSIS

DIFFERENTIAL DIAGNOSIS
• Traumatic proctitis
• Radiation proctitis
• Ulcerative colitis
• Crohn's disease
• Infections such as shigellosis or amebiasis

LABORATORY
• Serological tests for syphilis, ameba
• Smear, culture from rectal wall
• Stool cultures
Drugs that may alter lab results: N/A
Disorders that may alter lab results: N/A

PATHOLOGICAL FINDINGS
• Inflammation of rectal mucosa
• Ulceration
• Disruption of crypts

SPECIAL TESTS N/A

IMAGING N/A

DIAGNOSTIC PROCEDURES
• Flexible sigmoidoscopy
• Biopsy for histology, culture, viral studies, chlamydia culture
• Colonoscopy to exclude more proximal involvement

 TREATMENT

APPROPRIATE HEALTH CARE
Outpatient, unless severe and refractory to usual measures

GENERAL MEASURES
• Treatment depends upon the cause
• Rectal gram stains have significant false-negative rate and if clinician has strong suspicion of gonorrheal proctitis, empiric treatment warranted while culture results pending
• Avoidance of causative factors
• Sitz baths may provide some relief

SURGICAL MEASURES N/A

ACTIVITY No restrictions

DIET No special diet

PATIENT EDUCATION Counseling regarding HIV infection risk

Proctitis

MEDICATIONS

DRUG(S) OF CHOICE
• Ulcerative proctitis - topical steroids (enemas or foam), mesalamine (Rowasa, 5-ASA, 5-aminosalicylic acid) enemas or suppositories; oral mesalamine (Asacol, Pentasa), olsalazine (Dipentum), sulfasalazine; systemic steroids when refractory to above drugs
• Gonorrheal - IM ceftriaxone 250 mg in a single dose plus doxycycline 100 mg orally bid for 7 days
• Herpetic - oral acyclovir 200-400 mg 5 times a day for 10 days
• Chlamydial - oral tetracycline 500 mg tid or doxycycline 100 mg bid
Contraindications: Refer to manufacturer's literature
Precautions: Refer to manufacturer's literature
Significant possible interactions: Refer to manufacturer's literature

ALTERNATIVE DRUGS
For gonorrheal - in patients unable to take ceftriaxone - IM spectinomycin 2 g in a single dose or ciprofloxacin 500 mg orally in a single dose. Perform culture 4-7 days after treatment to verify efficacy of treatment.

FOLLOWUP

PATIENT MONITORING
Follow until completely healed and monthly thereafter for 6 months

PREVENTION/AVOIDANCE
Safe sex, if sexually transmitted

POSSIBLE COMPLICATIONS
• Chronic ulcerative colitis
• Fistulae/abscess formation
• Treatment failure (may be as much as 35% in gonorrhea proctitis)
• Perforation

EXPECTED COURSE/PROGNOSIS
Satisfactory cure or control with appropriate treatment

MISCELLANEOUS

ASSOCIATED CONDITIONS
• Syphilis
• Gonorrhea
• Other sexually transmitted disease
• Prostate cancer (radiation therapy)

AGE-RELATED FACTORS
Pediatric:
• Not common, but if found, is more apt to spread to full-blown disease in more proximal areas of the colon
• Consider sexual abuse, if gonorrheal infection
Geriatric: Slower to heal, consider ischemia
Others: N/A

PREGNANCY N/A

SYNONYMS N/A

ICD-9-CM 569.49 Proctitis nos

SEE ALSO
• Ulcerative colitis
• Crohn's disease of the colon
• Syphilis
• Gonococcal infections
• Lymphogranuloma venereum
• Herpes simplex

OTHER NOTES N/A

ABBREVIATIONS N/A

REFERENCES
• Wexner SD: Sexually transmitted diseases of the colon, rectum, and anus. The challenge of the nineties. Dis Colon Rectum 1990;33:1048-62
• Kirsner JB, Shorter G, eds: Diseases of the Colon, Rectum and Anal Canal. Baltimore, Williams & Wilkins, 1989
Illustrations: N/A
Internet references: http://www.5mcc.com

Author(s)
Philip E. Jaffe, MD

Prostatic cancer

 BASICS

DESCRIPTION The prostate is composed of acinar glands and their ducts arranged in a radial fashion with the stroma containing blood vessels, lymphatics and nerves. 95% of prostate cancers are acinar adenocarcinomas.
• Degree of malignancy based on grading various stages:
  ◊ A1, A2 and B1, B2 - confinement within the capsule
  ◊ C1 - extension beyond the capsule
  ◊ C2 - involving the seminal vesicles
  ◊ D1 - metastatic disease in regional lymph nodes
  ◊ D2 - metastatic disease in bone or other organs
System(s) affected: Reproductive
Genetics: Unknown
Incidence/Prevalence in USA: 69 per 100,000
Predominant Age: Sixth or seventh decade
Predominant sex: Male only

SIGNS AND SYMPTOMS
• May be asymptomatic early or late in the course of disease
• Induration of the prostate on digital rectal exam
• Hard prostate, localized or diffuse
• Bladder outlet symptoms
• Acute urinary retention
• Hematuria (rare)
• Urinary tract infection
• Bone pain
• Weight loss
• Anemia
• Shortness of breath
• Lymphedema
• Neurologic symptoms
• Lymphadenopathy

CAUSES Unknown

RISK FACTORS
• Genetic predisposition
• Endogenous hormonal influences
• Exposure to chemical carcinogens
• Sexually transmitted diseases
• Male over 60 years of age
• Increased risk with vasectomy has been newly proposed but is unsupported

 DIAGNOSIS

DIFFERENTIAL DIAGNOSIS
• Benign nodule prostate growth
• Prostate stones
• Nodular whorls of adenoma
• Seminal vesicle enlargement

LABORATORY
• Prostate specific antigen (PSA), elevated
• Free PSA - low in cancer (Catalana, et al: JAMA 1995;274:1213-1220)
• Alkaline phosphatase, elevated with metastasis
• Urine cytology, rarely helpful
Drugs that may alter lab results: None
Disorders that may alter lab results:
• Rectal manipulation will increase PSA
• Prior liver or bone disease

PATHOLOGICAL FINDINGS
• Size and shape of prostatic acini almost always altered
• Small closely packed interposed stroma
• Eosinophilic crystalloids present
• Architecture disrupted
• Cells invade perineural space

SPECIAL TESTS Prostate specific antigen

IMAGING
• Bone scan, positive with metastasis
• Skeletal survey, positive with metastasis
• Lymph node aspiration, positive with metastasis
• Computerized tomography of pelvic lymph nodes, positive with metastasis
• Prostatic ultrasound
• Lymphoscintigraphy
• Magnetic resonance imaging

DIAGNOSTIC PROCEDURES
• Biopsy, fine needle aspiration or core
• Ultrasound
• Bone marrow aspiration
• Bone biopsy
• Lymph node aspiration
• Lymph node biopsy
• Lymphoscopic lymph node dissection

 TREATMENT

APPROPRIATE HEALTH CARE Inpatient for surgery, outpatient for other treatment

GENERAL MEASURES
• Over age 70 conservative or palliative treatment
• Radiation, external beam or brachytherapy with implants
• Total androgen ablation

SURGICAL MEASURES
• Under age 70, aggressive surgery for cure
• Surgical for stages A-B and selected C under age 70
• Orchiectomy

ACTIVITY Full activity

DIET No special diet

PATIENT EDUCATION Printed material available from:
• American Cancer Society
• National Kidney & Urologic Diseases Information Clearinghouse, Box NKUDIC, Bethesda, MD 20893, (301)468-6345

Prostatic cancer

MEDICATIONS

DRUG(S) OF CHOICE
- None specific
- For androgen ablation:
  ◊ Flutamide (Eulexin) 250 mg tid
  ◊ Leuprolide (Lupron) 1 mg subcutaneously daily or 7.5 mg IM depot monthly or goserelin (Zoladex) 3.6 mg q 28 days

Contraindications: None

Precautions:
- Flare phenomenon with metastatic disease
- Fluid retention
- Nausea
- Vomiting
- Hot flashes
- Liver enzyme changes

Significant possible interactions: Refer to manufacturer's profile of each drug.

ALTERNATIVE DRUGS   None

FOLLOWUP

PATIENT MONITORING
- Routine clinical examination every 3 months for 1 year
- Routine clinical examination every 6 months for 1 year
- Annual examinations indefinitely
- PSA q 3 months for 1 year, q 6 months 1 year, then yearly
- Chest x-ray, bone scan, q 6 months for 1 year, then yearly

PREVENTION/AVOIDANCE   None

POSSIBLE COMPLICATIONS
- Cardiac failure
- Phlebitis
- Pathologic fracture

EXPECTED COURSE/PROGNOSIS
- Early diagnosis and treatment of lesions should be curable
- Advanced disease favorable prognosis if endocrine sensitive
- Advanced unresponsive disease progresses in 18 months average

MISCELLANEOUS

ASSOCIATED CONDITIONS   N/A

AGE-RELATED FACTORS
Pediatric: N/A
Geriatric: N/A
Others: N/A

PREGNANCY   N/A

SYNONYMS
Cancer of the prostate

ICD-9-CM
185 Malignant neoplasm of prostate

SEE ALSO   N/A

OTHER NOTES   N/A

ABBREVIATIONS   PSA = Prostate specific antigen

REFERENCES   Walsh PC, Gittes RF, Perlmutter AD: Campbell's Urology. 6th Ed. Philadelphia, W.B. Saunders Co., 1992
Illustrations: N/A
Internet references: http://www.5mcc.com

Author(s)
Jack L. Summers, MD, PhD

Prostatic hyperplasia, benign (BPH)

BASICS

DESCRIPTION Benign adenomatous growth of prostate which may result in bladder outlet obstruction
System(s) affected: Reproductive, Renal/Urologic
Genetics: Genetic factors may be involved
Incidence/Prevalence in USA:
• Universal pathologic phenomenon seen in older men
• No hard evidence suggesting racial predisposition
Predominant age:
• Rarely seen in men < 40
• Seen in 50% of men > 50; 80% of men > 70
Predominant sex: Male only

SIGNS AND SYMPTOMS
Prostate size correlates poorly with symptoms
• Obstructive symptoms: Due to mechanical obstruction and/or detrusor muscle decompensation
   ◊ Decrease force or caliber of stream
   ◊ Hesitancy
   ◊ Post-void dribbling
   ◊ Sensation of incomplete bladder emptying
   ◊ Overflow incontinence
   ◊ Inability to voluntarily stop stream
   ◊ Urinary retention
• Irritative symptoms: Due to incomplete bladder emptying and/or detrusor muscle instability
   ◊ Frequency
   ◊ Nocturia
   ◊ Urgency
   ◊ Urge incontinence
• Other symptoms and signs:
   ◊ Gross hematuria
   ◊ Observation of weak stream
   ◊ Distended bladder (> 150 cc in order to detect by percussion)
   ◊ Increased post-void residual (> 100 cc)
   ◊ Prostate enlarged (normal 20 gram prostate - size of horse chestnut)
   ◊ Clinical clues suggesting renal failure due to obstructive uropathy (edema, pallor, pruritus, ecchymoses, nutritional deficiencies, etc.)
   ◊ American Urological Association (AUA) symptom index score > 7

CAUSES Exact etiology unknown, but evidence suggests BPH arises from a systemic hormonal alteration which may or may not act in combination with growth factors stimulating stromal or glandular hyperplasia

RISK FACTORS
• Intact testes (BPH rare in eunuchs)
• Aging (thus, rare in men < 40 years old)
• No dietary, environmental, or sexual practices implicated yet

DIAGNOSIS

DIFFERENTIAL DIAGNOSIS
• Obstructive conditions:
   ◊ Prostate cancer
   ◊ Urethral stricture
   ◊ Bladder neck contracture (acquired or congenital)
      ◊ Anterior or posterior urethral valves
      ◊ Mullerian duct cysts
      ◊ Inability of bladder neck or external sphincter to relax appropriately during voiding
• Non-obstructive conditions:
   ◊ Neurogenic bladder (detrusor denervation)
   ◊ Myogenic cause (detrusor muscle failure)
   ◊ Medications (parasympatholytics, sympathomimetics, etc.)
   ◊ Psychogenic
• Irritative conditions:
   ◊ Neurogenic bladder
   ◊ Inflammatory disorders (prostatitis, urethritis, radiation cystitis, interstitial cystitis, etc.)
   ◊ Neoplasm (bladder carcinoma, especially carcinoma in situ)

LABORATORY
• BPH is a pathologic diagnosis - lab data is only suggestive
• Urinalysis: pyuria, pH changes due to chronic residual urine
• Elevated serum creatinine (if obstructive uropathy present)
• Urine culture positive (sometimes due to chronic residual urine)
• Prostate specific antigen (PSA) may be elevated but usually < 10 ng/mL (10 µg/L)
• Increased post-void residual (> 100 mL)
• Finasteride may lower the PSA
• Acute urinary retention, transurethral instrumentation may elevate the PSA
Drugs that may alter lab results:
• Finasteride (Proscar) may lower the PSA
Disorders that may alter lab results:
• Acute urinary retention, prostatitis, or prostatic infarction may elevate the PSA

PATHOLOGICAL FINDINGS Confirmation obtained by biopsy, resection or extirpation surgery. 5 types: Stromal (fibrous), fibromuscular, muscular ("leiomyoma"), fibroadenoma, fibromyoadenoma.

SPECIAL TESTS
• Transrectal prostate ultrasound gives volumetric estimate of gland
• Needle biopsy
• Have patient complete AUA test (see last column)
   ◊ Mild Symptoms (score 0-7): Offer watchful waiting only
   ◊ Moderate symptoms (score 8-19) to severe symptoms (score 20-35): Offer treatment options

IMAGING
• IVP - increased post-void residual, large prostatic impression on bladder, trabeculated bladder, bladder diverticula, upper tract dilation, bladder stones

• CT scan or MRI of pelvis - enlarged prostate
• Ultrasound - increase postvoid residual, prostate or hydronephrosis

DIAGNOSTIC PROCEDURES
• Uroflow - amount voided per unit time. Peak flow < 10 mL/sec suggests obstruction (accurate when voided volume is > 200 mL).
• Pressure-flow curve (urine flow versus voiding pressures) - decreased urine flow and increased pressure indicates obstruction
• Cystoscopy shows occlusive prostatic lobes, bladder trabeculation. Indicated if diagnosis is in doubt or helps guide the surgical approach (if surgery is an option)

TREATMENT

APPROPRIATE HEALTH CARE Inpatient or outpatient treatment required, either for surgery or medical treatment. Inpatient emergent treatment required to manage fluid and electrolyte abnormalities of obstructive uropathy.

GENERAL MEASURES
• Avoid large boluses of oral or IV fluids
• Avoid prolonged periods of not voiding
• Avoid sympathomimetic or anticholinergic medications (e.g., cold preparations)
• Urethral catheterization

SURGICAL MEASURES
• Surgery (indicators to determine necessity) One of the following:
   ◊ Urinary retention due to prostatic obstruction
   ◊ Intractable symptoms due to prostatic obstruction (gauged by AUA symptom index; score at least > 8)
   ◊ Obstructive uropathy
   ◊ Recurrent or persistent urinary tract infections due to prostatic obstruction
   ◊ Recurrent gross hematuria due to enlarged prostate
   ◊ Medical therapy indicated when surgery indicators not met.
• Surgical procedures
   ◊ Transurethral resection of prostate (TURP)
   ◊ Transurethral incision of prostate (TUIP), gland < 10 grams
   ◊ Open prostatectomy (glands > 40 grams)
   ◊ Transurethral (balloon) dilatation of prostate (TUDP)
   ◊ Transurethral microwave thermotherapy (TUMT)
   ◊ Transrectal prostatic hyperthermia
   ◊ Transurethral laser induced prostatectomy (TULIP)
   ◊ Visual laser assisted prostatectomy (VLAP)
   ◊ Prostatic urethral stenting
   ◊ Electrovaporization of prostate, transurethral (TVAP)
   ◊ Transurethral needle aspiration ablation of prostate (TUNA)

ACTIVITY No restriction

DIET Avoid caffeinated or alcoholic beverages, excessively spiced foods

PATIENT EDUCATION
• The Prostate Book, published by Krames Communications, 312 90th St, Daly City, CA 94015-1898
• National Kidney & Urologic Diseases Information Clearinghouse, Box NKUDIC, Bethesda, MD 20893, (301)468-6345

MEDICATIONS

DRUG(S) OF CHOICE
Indicated when no strong indications of surgery exist, patient refuses
• Alpha adrenergic antagonist: terazosin, doxazosin, tamsulosin
• Hormonal (anti-androgens) agents: finasteride (Proscar) works best for larger prostates; turosteride, flutamide and leuprolide are rarely used; sal pametto weak
Contraindications:
• Use alpha adrenergic antagonists with caution in patients with cardiac or cerebrovascular disease or those who operate machinery
• Hormones may cause impotence (except flutamide)
• The semen of men taking finasteride may cause effects on the fetus of pregnant sex partners
Precautions: Refer to manufacturer's profile of each drug
Significant possible interactions: Refer to manufacturer's profile of each drug

ALTERNATIVE DRUGS N/A

FOLLOWUP

PATIENT MONITORING
• Symptom index (AUA Symptom Index) monitored every 1-6 months
• Urodynamics every 3-12 months
• Digital rectal exam yearly
• PSA yearly

PREVENTION/AVOIDANCE Appears to be part of the aging process

POSSIBLE COMPLICATIONS
• Bladder stones
• Prostatitis
• Renal failure

EXPECTED COURSE/PROGNOSIS
• Symptoms improve or stabilize in 70-80% of patients; 20-30% require treatment because of worsening symptoms
• 11-33% men with BPH have occult prostate cancer

MISCELLANEOUS

ASSOCIATED CONDITIONS N/A

AGE-RELATED FACTORS
Pediatric: N/A
Geriatric: Much more prevalent in elderly men
Others: N/A

PREGNANCY N/A

SYNONYMS
• Prostatic hyperplasia
• Prostatic hypertrophy

ICD-9-CM 600 hyperplasia of prostate

SEE ALSO N/A

OTHER NOTES N/A

ABBREVIATIONS
• IVP = intravenous pyelogram
• AUA = American Urological Association

REFERENCES
• Grayhack JT: Benign prostatic hypertrophy. In: Gillenwater JY, Grayhack JT, Howard SS, Duckett JW, eds. Adult and Pediatric Urology. Chicago, Yearbook Medical Publishing, Inc., 1987
• Walsh PC: Benign prostatic hypertrophy. In: Walsh PC, Gittes RF, Perlmutter AD, et al, eds. Campbell's Urology. Philadelphia, W.B. Saunders Co., 1986
• Mebust WK: Surgical management of benign prostatic obstruction. Urology 1988;(Suppl)32(6):12
• Blaivas JG: Pathophysiology and differential diagnosis of benign prostatic hypertrophy., Urology 1988(Suppl)32(6):5
• Kapoor DA, Reddy PK: Surgical alternatives to TURP in the management of BPH. AUA Update Series 1993;3(12)
Illustrations: N/A
Internet references: http://www.5mcc.com

Author(s)
Charles Jennings, MD, FACS

Prostate Test (for urinary activities). Adapted from the American Urological Association (AUA) Symptom Index for BPH.

Circle the numerical score for each question below.

• 1. Over the last month or so, how many times did you most typically get up to urinate from the time you went to bed at night until the time you got up in the morning?
◊ None--------0
◊ 1 time-------1
◊ 2 times-----2
◊ 3 times-----3
◊ 4 times-----4
◊ 5 or more--5
• 2. Over the past month or so, how often have you had a sensation of not emptying your bladder completely after you finished urinating?
◊ Not at all------------------0
◊ Less than 1 time in 5---1
◊ Less than half the time---2
◊ About half the time---------3
◊ More than half the time---4
◊ Almost always---------------5
• 3. Over the past month or so, how often have you had to urinate again less than two hours after you finished urinating?
◊ Not at all------------------0
◊ Less than 1 time in 5------1
◊ Less than half the time---2
◊ About half the time---------3
◊ More than half the time---4
◊ Almost always---------------5
• 4. Over the past month or so, how often have you found that you stopped and started again several times when you urinate?
◊ Not at all------------------0
◊ Less than 1 time in 5------1
◊ Less than half the time---2
◊ About half the time---------3
◊ More than half the time---4
◊ Almost always---------------5
• 5. Over the past month or so, how often have you found it difficult to postpone urination?
◊ Not at all------------------0
◊ Less than 1 time in 5------1
◊ Less than half the time---2
◊ About half the time---------3
◊ More than half the time---4
◊ Almost always---------------5
• 6. Over the past month or so, how often have you had a weak urinary stream?
◊ Not at all------------------0
◊ Less than 1 time in 5------1
◊ Less than half the time---2
◊ About half the time---------3
◊ More than half the time---4
◊ Almost always---------------5
• 7. Over the past month or so, how often have you had to push or strain to begin urination?
◊ Not at all------------------0
◊ Less than 1 time in 5------1
◊ Less than half the time---2
◊ About half the time---------3
◊ More than half the time---4
◊ Almost always---------------5

• Total your score:_____
Total symptom score = sum of questions 1-7

Prostatitis

BASICS

DESCRIPTION
One of several inflammatory and/or painful conditions affecting the prostate gland
• Acute bacterial prostatitis – generally associated with urinary tract infection, has characteristically abrupt onset
• Chronic bacterial prostatitis –major cause of recurrent bacteriuria, less fulminant
• Nonbacterial prostatitis –findings similar to chronic bacterial, but no infection present
System(s) affected: Reproductive, Renal/Urologic
Genetics: No known genetic pattern
Incidence/Prevalence in USA: Common
Predominant age:
• Mostly ages 30-50, sexually active
• Chronic more common in ages over 50
Predominant sex: Male only

SIGNS AND SYMPTOMS
• Acute bacterial
  ◊ Fever; chills
  ◊ Tense, boggy, very tender and warm prostate
  ◊ Low back pain
  ◊ Perineal pain
  ◊ Frequency
  ◊ Urgency
  ◊ Dysuria
  ◊ Nocturia
  ◊ Bladder outlet obstruction
• Chronic bacterial
  ◊ Symptoms often absent
  ◊ Perineal pain
  ◊ Dysuria
  ◊ Irritative voiding
  ◊ Lower abdominal pain
  ◊ Low back pain
  ◊ Scrotal pain
  ◊ Penile pain
  ◊ Pain on ejaculation
  ◊ Hematospermia
• Nonbacterial
  ◊ Similar to chronic prostatitis

CAUSES
• Acute and chronic bacterial
  ◊ Ascending infection through urethra
  ◊ Refluxing urine into prostate ducts
  ◊ Direct extension or lymphatic spread from rectum
  ◊ Hematogenous spread
  ◊ Calculi serving as nidus for infection
  ◊ Aerobic gram negative bacteria (Escherichia coli, Pseudomonas, Klebsiella, Proteus), N. gonorrhea, Enterobacteriaceae
  ◊ Miscellaneous – Chlamydia trachomatis
  ◊ Gram positive bacteria (Streptococcus faecalis, Staphylococcus. aureus)
  ◊ Organisms suspected, but unproven (Staphylococcus epidermidis, Micrococci, non-group D streptococcus, Diphtheroids)
• Nonbacterial
  ◊ Currently unknown
  ◊ Ureaplasma, trichomonas vaginalis, and Chlamydia postulated, but not proven

RISK FACTORS
• Male sex
• Age over 50
• Prostatic calculi
• Urinary tract infection

DIAGNOSIS

DIFFERENTIAL DIAGNOSIS
• Cystitis
• Urethritis
• Pyelonephritis
• Malignancy
• Obstructive calculus
• Foreign body
• Acute urinary retention

LABORATORY
• Fractional urine examination (initial 10 mL from urethra for voided bladder 1 (VB1) test, next 200 mL discarded, then midstream from bladder for VB2 test, then expressed prostate secretion (EPS), lastly urine after prostate massage for VB3 test. Some feel vigorous massage may lead to bacteremia.
• Urinalysis, culture, sensitivities on all samples
• Over 10-15 white cells per high powered field or positive culture in EPS or VB3 but not VB1 or VB2 diagnostic of bacterial prostatitis
• Bacteria count generally less in chronic than acute
• Nonbacterial will show white blood cells with a negative culture
• No abnormal findings with prostatodynia
Drugs that may alter lab results: Antibiotics
Disorders that may alter lab results: N/A

PATHOLOGICAL FINDINGS
Inflammatory changes (except prostatodynia)

SPECIAL TESTS   N/A

IMAGING
• CT or ultrasound, if malignancy or abscess suspected
• Transrectal ultrasound (if prostatic calculi or abscess suspected)

DIAGNOSTIC PROCEDURES
• Needle biopsy or aspiration for culture
• Urodynamic testing (prostatodynia)
• Cystoscopy (in persistent nonbacterial prostatitis to rule out bladder cancer, interstitial cystitis)

TREATMENT

APPROPRIATE HEALTH CARE
• Inpatient (proven or suspected abscess, urosepsis, immunocompromised)
• Outpatient, if nontoxic

GENERAL MEASURES
• Analgesics
• Antipyretics
• Stool softeners
• Hydration
• Sitz baths to relieve pain and spasm
• Suprapubic catheter for severe urinary retention

SURGICAL MEASURES
Surgical resection for intractable chronic disease, or to drain an abscess; transurethral microwave thermotherapy for chronic nonbacterial prostatitis

ACTIVITY   Bedrest in severe cases

DIET
• Nonbacterial and prostatodynia – avoid spicy foods, excess caffeine and alcohol
• Acute and chronic bacterial – no special diet

PATIENT EDUCATION
• Printed patient information available from: National Kidney & Urologic Diseases Information Clearinghouse, Box NKUDIC, Bethesda, MD 20893, (301)468-6345

MEDICATIONS

DRUG(S) OF CHOICE
• Acute bacterial (outpatient): Trimethoprim-sulfamethoxazole (Septra), double strength, two tablets, twice daily for 30 days
• Acute bacterial (inpatient): Ampicillin 150-200 mg/kg/d IV divided q6h plus aminoglycoside – gentamicin 2.0 mg/kg loading dose; 1.7 mg/kg q8h maintenance
• Chronic bacterial: A fluoroquinolone (norfloxacin 400 mg bid, ciprofloxacin 500 mg bid) at standard dose for ≥ 3 months
• Nonbacterial: May benefit from erythromycin, doxycycline, trimethoprim-sulfamethoxazole
• Prostatodynia: Alpha-adrenergic blocking agents may be useful
• Analgesics
• Antipyretics
• Stool softeners

Contraindications: Drug allergies
Precautions:
• Renal disease
• Hepatic disease
• Elderly
• G6PD deficiency

Significant possible interactions:
Fluoroquinolones with magnesium/aluminum antacids, theophylline, probenecid, NSAID's, warfarin

ALTERNATIVE DRUGS
Carbenicillin with aminoglycoside, erythromycin, tetracycline, cephalexin, fluoroquinolones

FOLLOWUP

PATIENT MONITORING
• Acute bacterial - urinalysis and culture 30 days after initiating treatment
• Chronic bacterial - urinalysis and culture every 30 days (may take several months)

PREVENTION/AVOIDANCE
Suppression therapy may benefit patient with chronic bacterial prostatitis

POSSIBLE COMPLICATIONS
• Abscess
• Sepsis
• Urinary retention

EXPECTED COURSE/PROGNOSIS
Often prolonged and difficult to cure. Studies with 55-97% cure rate depending on population and drug used.

MISCELLANEOUS

ASSOCIATED CONDITIONS
• Prostatic hypertrophy
• Cystitis
• Urethritis

AGE-RELATED FACTORS
Pediatric: None
Geriatric: Consider prostatic hypertrophy and urinary retention more seriously
Others: N/A

PREGNANCY N/A

SYNONYMS N/A

ICD-9-CM
601.0 Prostatitis, acute
601.1 Prostatitis, chronic

SEE ALSO N/A

OTHER NOTES
• Prostatodynia: pain in the area of prostate. Sometimes inaccurately designated as a diagnosis.

ABBREVIATIONS
• VB = voided bladder
• EPS = expressed prostate secretion

REFERENCES
• Isselbacher KJ, et al, eds: Harrison's Principles of Internal Medicine. 13th Ed. New York, McGraw-Hill, 1994
• Moul JN: Prostatitis: Sorting out the different courses. Postgrad Med 1993;94-5:191-194
• Daneshgari F, Crawford ED: Benign prostatic disease: A growing challenge in the 1990's. Postgrad Med 1993;93(7):84-92
• Sable CA, Scheld WM: Fluoroquinolones: How to use (but not overuse) these antibiotica. Geriatrics 1993;48(6):41-51
• Nickel JC, Sorensen R: Transurethral microwave thermotherapy for nonbacterial prostatitis: a randomized double blind controlled study using new prostatitis specific assessment questionnaires. J Urol 1996;155(6):1950:1954
Illustrations: N/A
Internet references: http://www.5mcc.com

Author(s)
Gary A. Goforth, MD, MTMH

Pruritus ani

BASICS

DESCRIPTION Intense chronic itching in the anal and perianal skin. Usual course - acute. Chronic pruritus ani is a symptom, not a diagnosis or disease.
System(s) affected: Skin/Exocrine
Genetics: No known genetic pattern
Incidence/Prevalence in USA: Common
Predominant age: All ages
Predominant sex: Male > Female (4:1)

SIGNS AND SYMPTOMS
• Primary
  ◊ Rectal itching
  ◊ Anal erythema
• Secondary
Secondary infections with yeast, fungus, and/or bacteria are possible after prolonged scratching
  ◊ Anal itching
  ◊ Anal fissures
  ◊ Maceration
  ◊ Lichenification
  ◊ Excoriations

CAUSES
• Dermatologic disorders
  ◊ Allergies (soap, topical anesthetics, oral antibiotics)
  ◊ Fistulas
  ◊ Fissures
  ◊ Neoplasms
  ◊ Psoriasis
  ◊ Eczema
  ◊ Seborrheic dermatitis
  ◊ Contact dermatitis
• Infections
  ◊ Pinworms and other worms
  ◊ Scabies
  ◊ Pediculosis
  ◊ Candidiasis
  ◊ Tinea
• Other
  ◊ Poor hygiene (fecal material allowed to dry on the skin)
  ◊ Diabetes mellitus
  ◊ Chronic liver disease
  ◊ Diarrheic alkalotic irritation
  ◊ Trauma from scented toilet paper

RISK FACTORS
• Overweight
• Hairy, tendency to perspire a great deal
• Anxiety-itch-anxiety cycle

DIAGNOSIS

DIFFERENTIAL DIAGNOSIS
• Allergies
• Psoriasis
• Atopic dermatitis
• Fungus infection
• Bacterial infection
• Parasites
• Hyperhidrosis
• Diabetes mellitus
• Liver disease
• Neoplasia
• Anxiety

LABORATORY
• Glycosuria
• Hyperglycemia
• Skin scraping, yeast
• Fungi
• Parasites
• Stool - ova plus parasites
Drugs that may alter lab results: N/A
Disorders that may alter lab results: N/A

PATHOLOGICAL FINDINGS Excoriation of epithelial layer of skin

SPECIAL TESTS Blood sugar levels

IMAGING N/A

DIAGNOSTIC PROCEDURES
• Inspection
• Anoscopy biopsy (to exclude neoplasia)

TREATMENT

APPROPRIATE HEALTH CARE
Outpatient

GENERAL MEASURES
• Treat predisposing factors, such as parasites, diabetes, liver disease, cryptitis, scabies, pediculosis
• Resist overmeticulous use of soap and rubbing
• Avoid tight clothing and under clothing
• Cleanse anal area after bowel movements with moistened absorbent cotton and plain water; baby wipes may be a convenient alternative
• Dust anal area with non-medicated talcum powder
• If unable to completely empty rectum with defecation, use small plain water enema (infant bulb syringe) after each bowel movement. This may prevent postevacuation soilage and irritation.

SURGICAL MEASURES N/A

ACTIVITY Avoid getting overheated

DIET If suspicious of food allergy, eliminate as a trial: Coffee, beer, cola, vitamin C tablets in excessive doses, spices, citrus fruits

PATIENT EDUCATION See information in General Measures

MEDICATIONS

DRUG(S) OF CHOICE
• Specific treatment for allergies, micro-organisms, bacteria and worm infestation
• For symptomatic treatment - hydrocortisone cream 0.5-1% applied sparingly, usually at night. If severe, may need to apply several times a day. Discontinue once itching stops.
Contraindications: Refer to manufacturer's literature
Precautions: Refer to manufacturer's literature
Significant possible interactions: Refer to manufacturer's literature

ALTERNATIVE DRUGS
Albendazole for pinworms: 200 mg orally once for children <2 yrs, 400 mg for children over 2 and adults

FOLLOWUP

PATIENT MONITORING As needed

PREVENTION/AVOIDANCE
• Avoid topical agents
• Avoid laxatives
• Avoid tight underclothing made from synthetic material
• Practice good hygiene
• Use talcum powder
• Possibly lactobacillus acidophilus (tablets or in milk); possibly malt soup extract
• Eat yogurt when taking broad-spectrum antibiotics

POSSIBLE COMPLICATIONS
• Secondary bacterial infection
• Chronicity
• Excoriation
• Lichenification

EXPECTED COURSE/PROGNOSIS
• Depends upon etiology; usually good
• May be persistent and recurrent

MISCELLANEOUS

ASSOCIATED CONDITIONS
• Diabetes mellitus
• Psoriasis
• Hyperhidrosis
• Parasite infestations
• Hemorrhoids

AGE-RELATED FACTORS
Pediatric:
• Usually secondary to enterobiasis, anal fissures, other local inflammatory lesions, or coarse or moist undergarments. Nocturnal itching may be due to pinworms.
• Exposure to sunlight or dry heat may be helpful for infants with inflamed anal area
Geriatric: Common in this age group
Others: N/A

PREGNANCY N/A

SYNONYMS N/A

ICD-9-CM
698.0 Pruritus ani

SEE ALSO
• Pruritus vulvae
• Pinworms

OTHER NOTES N/A

ABBREVIATIONS N/A

REFERENCES
• Sleisenger MH, Fordtran JS, eds: Gastrointestinal Disease: Pathophysiology, Diagnosis, Management. 5th Ed. Philadelphia, W.B. Saunders Co., 1994
• Kirsner JB, Shortet G, eds: Diseases of the Colon, Rectum and Canal. Baltimore, Williams & Wilkins, 1988
Illustrations: N/A
Internet references: http://www.5mcc.com

Author(s)
Stan G. Smith, MA, MB, FCFPC

Pruritus vulvae

BASICS

DESCRIPTION Pruritus vulvae is both a symptom and a pathologic process affecting the vulva. It is a symptom of underlying disease in the vast majority of the patients. As a primary diagnosis, it consists of irritation and vulvar itching without an underlying pathologic etiology.
System(s) affected: Skin/Exocrine
Genetics: Unknown
Incidence/Prevalence in USA: The exact incidence is unknown, although most women will complain of vulvar pruritus at some time during their life
Predominant age:
• Any age can be affected
• In young girls, it is usually caused by an infection
• Frequent in postmenopausal women
Predominant sex: Female only

SIGNS AND SYMPTOMS
• Constant itching of the vulva
• Constant burning of the vulva

CAUSES
• Infectious causes - vaginal yeast infections, Gardnerella, other vaginal infections, and yeast dermatitis of the vulva itself
• Urinary tract infections will produce vulvar burning on occasion
• Vulvar vestibulitis (inflammation of the vestibular glands) produces a constant burning with pruritus and dyspareunia
• Human papillomavirus (HPV) has been associated with burning and itching of the vulva
• Vulvar tissues are estrogen sensitive. Estrogen deprivation can produce burning and itching.
• A search for underlying malignancy should be paramount. Carcinoma in situ (Bowen's disease) and invasive malignancy will often be associated with pruritus.
• Changes in the epidermis, such as lichen sclerosis et atrophicus (LSA) (thinning of the vulvar tissues and homogenization at the basement membrane) or hyperkeratosis of the vulva produce pruritus
• Anal incontinence with fecal soilage produces pruritus
• Excessive heat produces symptoms from sweat and irritation
• Environmental and dietary irritants such as nylon, soaps, perfumes, and over-zealous cleansing can produce symptoms
• Dietary irritants include methylxanthines (coffee, cola), tomatoes, peanuts

RISK FACTORS N/A

DIAGNOSIS

DIFFERENTIAL DIAGNOSIS
• The diagnosis of primary idiopathic vulvar pruritus must be made by exclusion
• A search for infectious causes should be undertaken with treatment of yeast and other vaginitis
• Biopsy of any abnormal-appearing epithelium on the vulva to insure that malignant changes are not present
• Only when all other factors have been ruled out can the diagnosis primary idiopathic vulvar pruritus be established

LABORATORY
• Vaginal secretions can be evaluated by wet mount (NaCl for trichomonas or Gardnerella, and KOH for yeast). Cultures seldom required.
• Gram stain of the vagina is non-diagnostic as multiple organisms are present in the normal flora
Drugs that may alter lab results: N/A
Disorders that may alter lab results: N/A

PATHOLOGICAL FINDINGS These are related to the underlying etiology. In primary vulvar pruritus, no changes will be noted. If HPV is present, these changes will be seen in the cornified layer of the squamous epithelium.

SPECIAL TESTS Whenever necessary, biopsy of the vulva should be used to establish the primary diagnosis

IMAGING N/A

DIAGNOSTIC PROCEDURES Biopsy when needed

TREATMENT

APPROPRIATE HEALTH CARE
Outpatient

GENERAL MEASURES
• Treatment of any underlying cause must be undertaken
• In cases of idiopathic primary vulvar pruritus, conservative measures include sitz baths, topical steroid creams, avoidance of chemical irritants and dietary changes
• When conservative measures fail, advanced cases can be treated with alcohol block or laser

SURGICAL MEASURES Bowen's disease and premalignant changes are treated with excision or laser vaporization

ACTIVITY Unlimited

DIET A trial of dietary alteration should be attempted for idiopathic pruritus. Coffee and caffeine-containing beverages should be avoided. Other foods to avoid include tomatoes, peanuts.

PATIENT EDUCATION See Prevention/Avoidance

MEDICATIONS

DRUG(S) OF CHOICE
• Infectious sources should be treated with appropriate antimicrobials or antifungals
• Lichen sclerosis is treated with 2% testosterone in petrolatum
• Hyperkeratotic lesions are treated with topical steroid
• Idiopathic primary vulvar pruritus can be treated with topical steroids such as triamcinolone (Kenalog) or desoximetasone (Topicort) cream
Contraindications: N/A
Precautions: N/A
Significant possible interactions: N/A

ALTERNATIVE DRUGS   N/A

FOLLOWUP

PATIENT MONITORING   These women should be followed closely for the development of premalignant or malignant changes within the area of pruritus

PREVENTION/AVOIDANCE
• Irritants to the vulva such as perfumes, soaps (use non-allergenic) or perfume douches must be avoided
• Only cotton underwear should be worn
• No tight fitting clothes or nylon pantyhose

POSSIBLE COMPLICATIONS   Chronic course

EXPECTED COURSE/PROGNOSIS
• Vulvar pruritus can be kept under control with conservative measures and topical steroids
• When it advances to uncontrollable symptoms, alcohol block or laser may be necessary

MISCELLANEOUS

ASSOCIATED CONDITIONS   N/A

AGE-RELATED FACTORS
Pediatric: N/A
Geriatric: More frequent
Others: N/A

PREGNANCY   N/A

SYNONYMS
• Vulvar pruritus
• Vulvodynia
• Burning vulva syndrome

ICD-9-CM   698.1 Pruritus of genital organs

SEE ALSO   N/A

OTHER NOTES   N/A

ABBREVIATIONS   N/A

REFERENCES
• McKay M: Vulvodynia vs. Pruritus vulvae. Clin Obstet Gynecol 1985;28:123-133
• Smith L, Henricks D, McCullah R: Prospective studies on the etiology and treatment of pruritus ani. Dis Colon Rectum 1982;25:258-363
• Hopkins MP: Anatomy and pathology of the vulva and vagina. In: Rebar R, Baker V, eds. Gynecology & Obstetrics, An Integrated Approach. New York, Churchill Livingstone, 1993
Illustrations: N/A
Internet references: http://www.5mcc.com

Author(s)
Michael P. Hopkins, MD

Pseudofolliculitis barbae

 BASICS

DESCRIPTION Foreign body inflammatory reaction surrounding an ingrown hair (usually in beard area, especially submandibular region, but can occur on scalp, axilla, or pubic area if these sites are shaved or plucked). Characterized by red papule/pustule at point of entry. A mechanical problem.
System(s) affected: Skin/Exocrine
Genetics: Curly haired people, especially Blacks
Incidence/Prevalence in USA: Widespread. Incidence of 45% in black soldiers who shave. Adult male blacks - 50,000/100,000; adult male Caucasians - 3000-5000/100,000.
Predominant age: Postpubertal, middle age (40-75)
Predominant sex: Male > Female

SIGNS AND SYMPTOMS
• Tender exudative, erythematous follicular papules or pustules in beard area (less commonly in scalp, axilla, pubic areas)
• Range from 2-4 mm in size
• Painful upon shaving
• Alopecia
• Lusterless brittle hair

CAUSES
• Reentry penetration of skin by external pointed tip of growing curved whisker, or sharped tipped whisker can grow into follicular wall if shaved too close
• Plucking of hair can cause abnormal hair growth in injured follicles

RISK FACTORS
• Curly hair
• Shaving too close with multiple razor strokes
• Plucking hairs
• Black race

 DIAGNOSIS

DIFFERENTIAL DIAGNOSIS
• Bacterial folliculitis
• Impetigo

LABORATORY N/A
Drugs that may alter lab results: N/A
Disorders that may alter lab results: N/A

PATHOLOGICAL FINDINGS
• Clinical pathology - follicular papules and pustules
• Histopathology - because of its curvature, the advancing hair's sharp-tipped free end causes an epidermal invagination as it approaches the skin. This is accompanied by inflammation and often an intra-epidermal abscess. As hair enters dermis, more severe inflammation occurs with downgrowth of epidermis in an attempt to ensheath hair. An abscess forms within the pseudofollicle and a foreign body reaction forms at the tip of invading hair.

SPECIAL TESTS
Culture of pustules - usually sterile. May show coagulase-negative micrococcus (normal skin flora).

IMAGING N/A

DIAGNOSTIC PROCEDURES Clinical diagnosis

 TREATMENT

APPROPRIATE HEALTH CARE
Outpatient

GENERAL MEASURES
• Acute treatment
  ◊ Dislodge embedded hair with sterile needle
  ◊ Discontinue shaving until red papules have resolved (minimum 3-4 weeks)
  ◊ Massage beard area with washcloths, coarse sponge or brush several times daily
  ◊ Systemic antibiotics if secondary infections present

SURGICAL MEASURES N/A

ACTIVITY Unlimited

DIET No restrictions

PATIENT EDUCATION
• Dunn 88, Pseudofolliculitis Barbae, pages 170-172
• American Family Physician (see References)

MEDICATIONS

DRUG(S) OF CHOICE
• Topical or systemic antibiotic for secondary infection
  ◊ Application of clindamycin (Cleocin-T) solution bid
  ◊ Low doses erythromycin or tetracycline 250 mg bid
  ◊ Administer until papule/pustule resolution
• Mild cases
  ◊ 5% benzoyl peroxide - apply after shaving
  ◊ 1% hydrocortisone cream - apply at bedtime
• Moderate disease - chemical depilatories
  ◊ Disrupt cross-linking of disulfide bonds of hair causing blunt hair tip
  ◊ Apply no more frequently than every 3rd day - 2% barium sulfide (Magic Shave) or calcium thioglycolate (Surgex)
• Moderate disease - adjunct treatment
  ◊ Tretinoin (Retin-A) liquid/cream, applied daily or every other day

Contraindications:
• Clindamycin - history of regional enteritis or ulcerative colitis; history of antibiotic associated colitis
• Erythromycin, tetracycline, tretinoin hypersensitivity only

Precautions:
• Clindamycin - colitis, eye burning and irritation, skin dryness, pregnancy category B
• Erythromycin - cautious use in patients with impaired hepatic function, GI side effects especially abdominal cramping, pregnancy category B
• Tetracycline - permanent discoloration of teeth if given during last half of pregnancy
• Tretinoin - severe skin irritation, pregnancy category C
• Benzoyl peroxide - skin irritation and dryness, allergic contact dermatitis
• Hydrocortisone cream - local skin irritation, skin atrophy with prolonged use

Significant possible interactions:
• Erythromycin - increases theophylline and carbamazepine levels, decreases clearance of warfarin; cardiac toxicity with terfenadine and astemizole
• Tetracycline - depresses plasma prothrombin activity (therefore need to decrease warfarin dosages)

ALTERNATIVE DRUGS
Topical application of glycolic acid lotion (8% buffered glycolic acid in a suitable carrier, either oil-in-water lotion or a non-lipid soap) twice daily. This treatment may allow shaving comfortably every day.

FOLLOWUP

PATIENT MONITORING
As needed. Educate patient on curative and preventive treatment.

PREVENTION/AVOIDANCE
• Mild cases
  ◊ Use tiny plastic hook for removing ingrown hairs before shaving
  ◊ Shave either with a manual adjustable razor at coarsest settings (avoids close shaves), a twin blade razor (Trac-II, The Bump-Fighter), a foil guarded razor (PFB razor), or electric triple "O" head razor
  ◊ Shave beard in direction of hair growth
  ◊ Do not stretch skin when shaving
  ◊ Use correct shaving cream/gel (Ef-Kay Shaving Gel, Edge Shaving Gel, Easy Shave Medicated Shaving Cream)
  ◊ Consider 5% benzoyl peroxide after shaving and application of 1% hydrocortisone cream at bedtime
• Moderate cases
  ◊ Chemical depilatories
  ◊ Consider 0.05% tretinoin (Retin-A) liquid or cream
• Severe cases
  ◊ Avoidance of shaving completely
  ◊ Electrolysis to destroy remaining hair follicles

POSSIBLE COMPLICATIONS
• Scarring (occasionally keloidal)
• Foreign body granuloma formation
• Disfiguring postinflammatory hyperpigmentation
• Impetiginization of inflamed skin

EXPECTED COURSE/PROGNOSIS
• Course is recurrent if preventative measures not followed
• Prognosis is poor in presence of progressive scarring and foreign body granuloma formation

MISCELLANEOUS

ASSOCIATED CONDITIONS
Keloidal folliculitis

AGE-RELATED FACTORS
Pediatric: N/A
Geriatric: N/A
Others: N/A

PREGNANCY
Do not use tretinoin (Retin-A), tetracycline, benzoyl peroxide

SYNONYMS
• Chronic sycosis barbae
• Pili incarnati
• Folliculitis barbae traumatica
• Razor bumps

ICD-9-CM
704.8 Other specified diseases of hair and follicles

SEE ALSO
• Folliculitis
• Impetigo
• Tinea barbae

OTHER NOTES
N/A

ABBREVIATIONS
N/A

REFERENCES
• Lever WF, Schaumburg-Lever G: Histopathology of the Skin. Philadelphia, J.B. Lippincott, 1990
• Dunn JF Jr: Pseudofolliculitis Barbae. Amer Fam Phys 1988;9
• Habif TP: Clinical Dermatology. St Louis, CV Mosby, 1995
• Sams W Jr, Lynch P: Principles and Practice of Dermatology. New York, Churchill Livingstone, 1990
• Perricone NV: Treatment of pseudofolliculitis barbae with topical glycolic acid: A report of two studies. Cutis 1993;52(4):232-235
Illustrations: N/A
Internet references: http://www.5mcc.com

Author(s)
W. Paul Slomiany, MD

Pseudogout (CPPD)

BASICS

DESCRIPTION An acute inflammatory arthritic disease usually involving large joints which primarily affects the elderly and is caused by calcium pyrophosphate dihydrate (CPPD) crystal deposition in joints. Associated with chondrocalcinosis.
• CPPD crystal deposition may cause a progressive degenerative arthritis in numerous joints
• CPPD crystal deposition may cause a more insidious, smoldering, symmetrical, polyarthritis which is similar to rheumatoid arthritis
System(s) affected: Musculoskeletal
Genetics:
• Uncommonly seen in familial pattern with autosomal dominant inheritance (< 1% of cases)
• Most cases sporadic
Incidence/Prevalence in USA: Unknown, primarily a disease of the elderly; chondrocalcinosis is present 1 in 10 in ages 60-75, over age 80 in 1 in 3. Only a small percentage develop pseudogout.
Predominant age: 80% of patients > than 60
Predominant sex: Male = Female

SIGNS AND SYMPTOMS
• Acute pain and swelling of one or more joints. Knee is involved in one-half of all attacks, ankle, wrist and shoulder also common.
◊ Inflammation, joint effusion, limitation of motion
◊ 50% associated with fever
◊ Any other synovial joint may be involved including first metatarsophalangeal
• Can present with a chronic progressive arthritis upon which acute inflammation attacks are superimposed
• Progressive degenerative arthritis in numerous joints including: wrists, metacarpophalangeal, hips, shoulders, elbows, and ankles without inflammatory attacks also seen
• Low grade inflammatory arthritis with multiple symmetrical joint involvement (mimics rheumatoid arthritis) < 5% of cases

CAUSES
• Acute inflammatory reaction to CPPD crystals shed into synovial cavity
• Physical and chemical changes in aging cartilage that favor crystal growth

RISK FACTORS
• Aging
• Trauma
• Pseudogout will often occur as a complication in patients hospitalized for other medical and surgical illnesses
• Metabolic diseases (10% or less of the cases)
◊ Hyperparathyroidism
◊ Hemochromatosis
◊ Gout
◊ Hypophosphatasia
◊ Hypothyroidism
◊ Ochronosis
◊ Wilson's disease
◊ Amyloidosis
◊ Hypomagnesemia

DIAGNOSIS

DIFFERENTIAL DIAGNOSIS
• Illness that may cause an acute inflammatory arthritis in a single or multiple joint(s): Gout, septic arthritis or trauma
• Other illnesses that may present with an acute inflammatory arthritis: Reiter's syndrome, Lyme disease, acute rheumatoid arthritis

LABORATORY
• Elevated sedimentation rate
• Leukocytosis with mild left shift
Drugs that may alter lab results: N/A
Disorders that may alter lab results: N/A

PATHOLOGICAL FINDINGS CPPD crystal deposition in articular cartilage, synovium, ligaments and tendons

SPECIAL TESTS
• Synovial fluid analysis consistent with an inflammatory effusion:
◊ Cell count from 2000 to 100,000 WBC/mL
◊ Differential predominantly neutrophils (80-90%)
◊ Wet prep with polarized microscopy demonstrates small numbers of weakly positively birefringent crystals in the fluid and within neutrophils
• Metabolic studies
◊ To exclude an underlying cause should always be obtained in patients under age 50 and considered in the elderly
◊ Serum calcium
◊ Serum phosphorus
◊ Serum alkaline phosphatase
◊ Serum parathormone
◊ Serum iron, total iron binding capacity, and serum ferritin
◊ Serum magnesium
◊ Serum thyroxine and thyroid stimulating hormone (TSH) level

IMAGING
• X-rays of joints
◊ May demonstrate punctate and linear calcification in articular hyaline or fibrocartilage: Knees, hips, symphysis pubis, and wrists most often affected, may also be found in asymptomatic individuals
◊ In the chronic destructive indolent form of the disease: Subchondral cyst formation, fragmentation with formation of intra-articular radiodense bodies in joints not typically affected by degenerative joint disease.

DIAGNOSTIC PROCEDURES Aspiration of joint fluid with synovial fluid analysis required for proper confirmation of pseudogout; aspiration may relieve symptoms and speed resolution of inflammatory process

TREATMENT

APPROPRIATE HEALTH CARE
• If septic arthritis is considered possible, inpatient care may be required for empiric antibiotic therapy pending culture results
• If patient does not have adequate support system inpatient care may be required until patient is able to walk

GENERAL MEASURES
• Rest and elevate affected joint(s)
• Apply moist warm compresses to affected joints

SURGICAL MEASURES N/A

ACTIVITY
• Non-weight bearing on affected joint while painful. Use crutches or walker.
• Perform isometric exercises to maintain muscle strength during the acute stage, i.e., quadriceps isometric contractions and leg lifts, if knee affected
• Begin range of motion of joint as inflammation and pain subside
• Resume weight bearing when pain subsides

DIET No special diet

PATIENT EDUCATION Specific instructions on exercise and activity

Pseudogout (CPPD)

MEDICATIONS

DRUG(S) OF CHOICE
• Nonsteroidal anti-inflammatory drugs (choose one of the following):
◊ Sulindac (Clinoril) 150-200 mg bid with food
◊ Ibuprofen (Motrin) 600-800 mg tid-qid with food. Maximum of 3.2 gm daily.
◊ Other NSAID's at anti-inflammatory doses are effective

Contraindications:
• History of hypersensitivity to NSAID's or aspirin
• Active peptic ulcer disease or history of recurrent upper gastrointestinal lesions
• Use with extreme caution when impaired renal function exists. Monitor serum creatinine.

Precautions:
• May interfere with platelet aggregation and prolong bleeding time. This effect is much shorter lived than with aspirin.
• May cause fluid retention and worsen congestive heart failure
• Abnormal liver function tests may develop in approximately 15% of patients. Discontinue if findings worsen or systemic manifestations occur.
• Serious gastrointestinal bleeding can occur without warning. Follow patient carefully for internal bleeding. Administer misoprostol 200 μg qid in patients with a history of peptic ulcer disease.

Significant possible interactions:
• May blunt the antihypertensive effects of angiotensin converting enzyme inhibitors
• May prolong the prothrombin time in patients taking oral anticoagulants
• Avoid concomitant usage of aspirin
• May blunt the diuretic effect of furosemide and hydrochlorothiazide
• May increase plasma lithium level in patients taking lithium carbonate
• May increase methotrexate levels

ALTERNATIVE DRUGS
• Intra-articular instillation of methylprednisolone acetate, 20-80 mg for large joints; 10-40 mg for medium joints. Available in 20, 40 and 80 mg/mL ampules.
• Intravenous colchicine 2 mg IV; may repeat 0.5 mg IV q6h; not to exceed 4 mg in 24 hours (oral colchicine ineffective). Contraindication: significant bone marrow dysfunction, renal insufficiency (creatinine clearance < 10 mL/min), biliary obstruction, sepsis.

FOLLOWUP

PATIENT MONITORING
Reevaluate patient for response to therapy 48-72 hours after treatment instituted. Reexamine 1 week later, then as needed.

PREVENTION/AVOIDANCE
None known

POSSIBLE COMPLICATIONS
• Erosive destructive arthritis in pattern of joints not usually affected by degenerative joint disease
• Recurrences may occur and a destructive arthritis may complicate CPPD

EXPECTED COURSE/PROGNOSIS
• Acute attack usually resolves in 10 days. Prognosis for resolution of acute attack is excellent.
• Some patients experience progressive joint damage with functional limitation

MISCELLANEOUS

ASSOCIATED CONDITIONS
Consider in patients with pseudogout - hyperparathyroidism, hemochromatosis, gout, hypophosphatasia, hypothyroidism, ochronosis, Wilson's disease, amyloidosis, hypomagnesemia

AGE-RELATED FACTORS
Pediatric: Not seen in children
Geriatric: Most cases are in patients over 60
Others: N/A

PREGNANCY N/A

SYNONYMS
• Calcium pyrophosphate deposition disease

ICD-9-CM
712.2 Chondrocalcinosis due to calcium phosphate crystals

SEE ALSO N/A

OTHER NOTES N/A

ABBREVIATIONS
CPPD = calcium pyrophosphate deposition disease

REFERENCES
• Beutler A, Schumacher H: Gout and pseudogout. Postgraduate Medicine 1994;95(2):103-116
• Jasmine J, McGrath H: Gout or 'pseudogout'? How to differentiate crystal induced arthropathies. Rheumatic Clin of NA 1995;21:151-161
• Rosenthal A, Ryan L: Treatment of refractory crystal-associated arthritis. Rheumatic Dis Clin of NA 1995;21:151-161
Illustrations: N/A
Internet references: http://www.5mcc.com

Author(s)
Paul T. Cullen, MD

Pseudomembranous colitis

 BASICS

DESCRIPTION Inflammatory bowel disorder associated with antibiotic use. May be mild diarrhea, or move through several stages to a severe colitis. Usual course - acute, relapsing.
System(s) affected: Gastrointestinal
Genetics: No known genetic factors
Incidence/Prevalence in USA:
• Epidemic or endemic in hospitals and nursing homes
  ◊ Nursing homes: 2-8%
  ◊ Hospitals: 7-15%
• Community: 6.7/100,000 patients treated with antibiotics
• Healthy adults: 5% colonized with C. difficile
• Hospitalized patients: 10-20% are colonized
• Neonates: 40% are colonized
Predominant age: 40-75 years
Predominant sex: Male = Female

SIGNS AND SYMPTOMS
• Diarrhea (classically watery, green, foul-smelling, bloody)
• Abdominal tenderness, pain, cramps
• Fever (up to 8% report fever only)
• Hypovolemia/dehydration
• Hypoalbuminemia

CAUSES Pathogenic Clostridium difficile toxins (A & B)

RISK FACTORS
• Antibiotic exposure (prior 6 weeks) particularly: clindamycin, lincomycin, ampicillin, cephalosporins. However, may also rarely occur with penicillins, erythromycin, sulfa-trimethoprim, chloramphenicol, tetracycline. In fact, nearly all antibiotics have been implicated.
• Cancer chemotherapy: fluorouracil, methotrexate, combination regimens.
• Recent surgery, especially bowel surgery
• Uremia or hemolytic-uremic syndrome
• Intestinal ischemia
• Shock
• Tube feedings
• Enemas
• GI stimulants
• Stool softener
• H2 blockers and antacids
• Immunocompromise (e.g., low CD4)
• Prolonged hospitalization
• Advancing age
• Hirschsprung's
• Inflammatory bowel disease

 DIAGNOSIS

DIFFERENTIAL DIAGNOSIS
• Other enteric pathogens
• Nonspecific inflammatory bowel diseases

LABORATORY
• Fecal leukocytosis
• Leukocytosis
• ELISA for C. difficile toxin, positive
• Culture
Drugs that may alter lab results: N/A
Disorders that may alter lab results: A high percentage of infants are normal carriers of C. difficile and are positive for toxin B

PATHOLOGICAL FINDINGS
• Mild, nonspecific colitis without plaques
• Gross - yellow-white plaques on colonic and small intestinal mucosa
• Micro - pseudomembrane arising from point of superficial ulceration
• Micro - fibrin
• Micro - thick confluent pseudomembrane
• Polymorphonuclear cells

SPECIAL TESTS
• Sigmoidoscopy - may be normal in 10-33%
• Colonoscopy may show involvement of the rectum and sigmoid colon and occasionally only right colon and/or distal ileum. Some patients do not have pseudomembrane.

IMAGING
• Abdominal film - distorted haustral markings, colonic distention
• CT - thickened or edematous colonic wall with pericolonic inflammation
• Note: Avoid barium enemas

DIAGNOSTIC PROCEDURES
Endoscopic visualization and sample collection

 TREATMENT

APPROPRIATE HEALTH CARE
• Outpatient for most patients
• Inpatient for severe or patients with co-morbidities

GENERAL MEASURES
• Fluid replacement
• Fluid plus electrolyte therapy
• Discontinue antimicrobial agent
• Successful in 25%

SURGICAL MEASURES Colectomy, not diversion, may be required

ACTIVITY Bedrest during acute phase

DIET Nothing by mouth during fulminant phase

PATIENT EDUCATION N/A

Pseudomembranous colitis

MEDICATIONS

DRUG(S) OF CHOICE
If drugs are not able to be taken orally, give via NG, enema, or direct instillation by colostomy/ileostomy or IV.
• Metronidazole (Flagyl) 250 mg po qid for 10 days
• Vancomycin 125 mg po qid (only for severe or resistant cases) for 10 days
• Teicoplanin 50 mg po qid for 3 days then 100 mg bid for 4 days
Contraindications: Refer to manufacturer's literature
Precautions: Avoid antiperistaltic drugs such as diphenoxylate, atropine, loperamide to reduce risk of toxic megacolon
Significant possible interactions: Alcohol and metronidazole. Refer to manufacturer's literature.

ALTERNATIVE DRUGS
• Bacitracin 500 mg qid
• For flora repletion: Lactobacilli capsules or saccharomyces bouldardii enema of mixed colonies
• For chronic recurrences, adjunct therapy with full colon irrigation with Golytely

FOLLOWUP

PATIENT MONITORING Careful monitoring through fulminant phase

PREVENTION/AVOIDANCE
• Judicious use of antimicrobial agents
• Keep courses of antibiotics as brief as possible
• Avoidance of recurrences
  ◊ Prolonged therapy
  ◊ Lactobacillus
  ◊ Repletion of other organisms which compete with C. Difficile
  ◊ In children, some success with IV gamma globulin

POSSIBLE COMPLICATIONS
• Reactive arthritis; Reiter's syndrome
• Hypoalbuminemia
• Ascites
• Dehydration, hypovolemia, shock
• Bowel perforation
• Toxic megacolon
• Death

EXPECTED COURSE/PROGNOSIS
• If treated, usual improvement in 3 days and virtually all patients recover
• Relapses do occur
• Untreated, 10-30% mortality
• In severely ill, colectomy sometimes required
• Significant morbidity and mortality in critical ill patients
• Poor prognostic factors: hypoalbuminemia, rapid fall in albumin, over 3 antibiotics, persistent C. difficile toxin after 7 days of treatment

MISCELLANEOUS

ASSOCIATED CONDITIONS
• Surgery
• Spinal fracture
• Intestinal obstruction
• Colon cancer

AGE-RELATED FACTORS
Pediatric:
• Unusual in children, but does occur
• Most infants are carriers; may become invasive in children with malignancy or Hirschsprung's disease
Geriatric: The elderly have a higher mortality rate from pseudomembranous colitis
Others: N/A

PREGNANCY Serious complication if it occurs during pregnancy

SYNONYMS
• Antibiotic associated colitis
• Pseudomembranous enterocolitis

ICD-9-CM 564.1

SEE ALSO N/A

OTHER NOTES N/A

ABBREVIATIONS N/A

REFERENCES
• Fekety R, Akshay S: Diagnosis and treatment of Clostridium difficile. JAMA 1993;269:71-75
• Leung D, et al: Treatment with intravenously administered gamma globulin of chronic relapsing colitis induced by Clostridium difficile toxin. Jour of Pediatr 1991;118:633-7
• Bartlett JG: Antibiotic-associated diarrhea. Clinical Infect Dis 1992;15:573-81
• Fualman S, et al: Clostridial difficile invasion & toxin circulation in fatal pediatric pseudomembranous colitis. Amer J Clin Pathol 1990;94:410-6
• McFarland L, Surawicz C, Stamm W: Risk factors for C. difficile carriage and C. difficile associated diarrhea in a cohort of hospitalized patients. J of Infect Dis 1990;162:678-84
• Ramaswamy R, et al: Prognostic criteria in Clostridium difficile colitis. Amer J Gastro 1996;91(3):460-4
• Hirschorn LR, et al: Epidemiology of community-acquired Clostridium difficile-associated diarrhea. J Infec Dis 1994;169:127-33
• Chatila W, Constantine M: Clostridium difficle causing sepsis and an acute abdomen in critically ill patients. Crit Care Med 1995;23(6):1146-1150
• Walker KJ, et al: Clostridium difficile colonization in residents in long-term care facilities: prevalence and risk factors. J Amer Geriatric Soc 41(9):940-6
• Simor AE, et al: Infection due to Clostridium difficile among elderly residents of a long term care facility. Clin Infec Dis 1993;17(4):672-8
• Reinke C, Messik CR: Update on Clostridium-difficile-induced colitis, Part 2. Amer J Hosp Pharm 1994;51(15):1892-901
• Tumbarello M, et al: Clostridium difficile-associated diarrhoea in patients with human immunodeficiency virus infection: a case control study. European J Gastro & Hepatol 1995;7(3):259-63
• Wenisch C, et al: Comparison of vancomycin, teicoplanin, metronidazole and fusidic acid for the treatment of Clostridium difficle associated diarrhea. Clin Infec Dis 1996;5:813-818
• Grundfest, et al: Clostridium difficile colitis in the critally ill. Dis of Colon Rectum 1996;6:619-623
• Liacouras CA, Piecol DA: Whole bowel irrigation as an adjunct to the treatment of chronic relapsing Clostridium difficle colitis. J Clin Gastroenterology 1996;22(3):186-189
Illustrations: N/A
Internet references: http://www.5mcc.com

Author(s)
Elizabeth McCord, MD, MS

Psittacosis

BASICS

DESCRIPTION Psittacosis is the clinical manifestation of a respiratory infection with the bacteria Chlamydia psittaci. The infection is virtually always contracted from an infected bird. Human to human transmission is rare.
• Pneumonia, bronchitis and fever of unknown origin (FUO) are most common diagnoses
• Can range from sub-clinical respiratory infection to severe systemic infection. Severity of illness may vary with strain of C. psittaci.
System(s) affected: Pulmonary
Genetics: No known genetic predisposition
Incidence/Prevalence in USA:
• .04-.08/100,000. 100-200 cases/year reported to Centers for Disease Control. True incidence probably greater.
• Outbreaks may occur, usually associated with occupational exposure to infected turkeys or ducks
Predominant age: Adults
Predominant sex: Male = Female

SIGNS AND SYMPTOMS
• Onset usually acute but may be insidious
• Fever (often > 39°C)
• Chills
• Cough (may develop later, usually non-productive)
• Headache (may be severe)
• Malaise
• Anorexia
• Myalgias
• Confusion
• Vomiting and/or diarrhea
• Abdominal pain
• Pleuritic chest pain
• Hemoptysis
• Dyspnea without wheezing
• Arthralgias
• Sore throat
• Hoarseness
• Epistaxis
• Photophobia
• Tachycardia
• Retractions
• Flaring
• Cyanosis
• Crepitations more common than signs of consolidation
• Auscultation may be normal even with pneumonia
• Relative bradycardia
• Tender hepatomegaly and splenomegaly
• Horder's spots (faint, reddish brown, blanching rash)
• Petechiae

CAUSES
Infection with Chlamydia psittaci (Arthus type immunologic reaction to inhaled avian antigen)

RISK FACTORS
Exposure to infected bird(s), usually a pet pigeon or parakeet, or occupational exposure at a turkey or duck processing plant. Infected birds may appear healthy.

DIAGNOSIS

DIFFERENTIAL DIAGNOSIS
• Consider other common bacterial respiratory pathogens including Streptococcus pneumoniae, Hemophilus influenzae, Klebsiella pneumoniae, Chlamydia pneumoniae, Mycoplasma pneumoniae, and Legionella species
• Early symptoms may suggest influenza, typhoid fever or mononucleosis

LABORATORY
• Leukocyte count often normal or low
• Erythrocyte sedimentation rate (ESR) usually elevated
• Sputum usually negative by gram stain and routine culture
• Proteinuria possible during febrile period
• Liver enzymes may be elevated
• Increased IgG, IgM, IgA
• Leukocytes with left shift
• Hypoxemia
• Hypocapnia
• Eosinophilia
Drugs that may alter lab results:
Serologic response may be blunted by early treatment with tetracycline
Disorders that may alter lab results: N/A

PATHOLOGICAL FINDINGS
• Alveolar phagocyte and lymphocyte infiltrate
• Granuloma formation
• Bronchial wall thickening
• Type III and IV immune complex deposition
• Diffuse miliary nodules

SPECIAL TESTS
• Culture requires special facilities and is rarely done
• Sera for serology should be collected 2 to 3 weeks apart (3-4 weeks for micro-immunofluorescence, and a second convalescent sera at 6-8 weeks if the pattern is uninterpretable)
• Complement fixation (CF) test most common serologic test for psittacosis, but is also positive with C. pneumoniae (a much more common respiratory pathogen) and C. trachomatis infections
• A fourfold rise in CF titer is diagnostic of an acute infection with Chlamydia
• A single or stable CF titer of > 1:64 suggests a recent infection
• The species specific micro-immunofluorescence test for C. psittaci is preferred, but not as widely available as the CF test

IMAGING
• Chest radiograph often shows patchy alveolar infiltrates of interstitial pneumonitis and small nodular densities
• Lobar consolidation less common
• Hilar adenopathy
• Pleural effusion possible but usually scanty
• Radiographic abnormalities may persist for several months after successful treatment

DIAGNOSTIC PROCEDURES N/A

TREATMENT

APPROPRIATE HEALTH CARE
• Outpatient
• Patients with dyspnea, hypoxia, confusion or other signs or severe disease should be hospitalized

GENERAL MEASURES
• History of avian exposure (particularly to a sick bird) is key to making early diagnosis
• Treatment depends primarily on severity of respiratory symptoms. Severely ill patients may require oxygen, intravenous fluids and antibiotics.
• While human to human transmission is rare, sputum and respiratory secretion precautions should be observed

SURGICAL MEASURES N/A

ACTIVITY
Based on disease severity. No disease-specific restrictions.

DIET No special diet

PATIENT EDUCATION
American Lung Association, 1740 Broadway, New York, NY 10019, (800)586-4872

MEDICATIONS

DRUG(S) OF CHOICE
• Azithromycin (Zithromax) 500 mg on first day; then 250 mg qd (length of treatment not established for psittacosis)
• Clarithromycin (Biaxin) 500 mg q12h (length of treatment not established for psittacosis)
• Doxycycline (Vibramycin) 100 mg po bid for 14-21 days or 100 mg IV q12h
• Tetracycline 500 mg po qid for 14-21 days
Contraindications: History of allergic reaction to the medication
Precautions: Tetracycline and doxycycline - avoid dairy products and sun exposure. Reduce dosage in renal failure. Avoid using in pregnancy or in children less than 8 years old (causes permanent discoloration of teeth).
Significant possible interactions: Refer to manufacturer's profile of each drug

ALTERNATIVE DRUGS
• Erythromycin also has in vitro activity and can be used at doses of 500 mg po qid for 14 to 21 days
• Rifampin (Rifadin, Rimactane) has in vitro activity and has been used in doses of 600 to 1200 mg po per day with erythromycin to treat endocarditis due to C. psittaci
• Beta-lactam (penicillin based) antibiotics not effective

FOLLOWUP

PATIENT MONITORING   Determined by severity of illness in the acute period. No disease-specific monitoring.

PREVENTION/AVOIDANCE
• Report to local health department
• Identify source of the infection if possible
• Public health surveillance of poultry flocks and pet shops
• Prophylactic antibiotic treatment with doxycycline (100 mg po qd for 10 days) has been advocated for people with known exposure

POSSIBLE COMPLICATIONS
• Meningitis and encephalitis
• Endocarditis, pericarditis and myocarditis
• Renal failure
• Erythema nodosum
• Sinusitis
• Respiratory failure
• Reactive arthritis (rare)
• Disseminated intravascular coagulation (rare)
• Valvular heart disease (rare)
• Spontaneous abortion (rare)
• Thyroiditis (rare)
• Pancreatitis (rare)
• Transverse myelitis (rare)

EXPECTED COURSE/PROGNOSIS
• Mortality rate less than 1% with appropriate treatment
• Patients usually respond within 24 to 48 hours following initiation of appropriate antibiotic therapy
• Full recovery may take weeks to months
• Relapse may occur necessitating second course of antibiotics
• Chest radiograph may not return to normal for up to 4 months

MISCELLANEOUS

ASSOCIATED CONDITIONS   None known

AGE-RELATED FACTORS
Pediatric: Uncommon in pediatric age group
Geriatric: Mortality rate may be higher in elderly or debilitated patients
Others: None

PREGNANCY   Spontaneous abortion has been reported with infection with some C. psittaci strains, primarily acquired from contact with sheep

SYNONYMS
• Ornithosis
• Bird breeder's disease
• Bird fancier's lung

ICD-9-CM
• 073.0 to 073.9 Ornithosis
• 495.8 - Other specified allergic alveolitis and pneumonitis

SEE ALSO
• Chlamydia pneumoniae
• Q fever

OTHER NOTES
• Incubation period ranges from 5 to 40 days; usually 7 to 15 days
• No persistent immunity to reinfection

ABBREVIATIONS   N/A

REFERENCES
• Macfarlane JT, Macrae A: Psittacosis. Br Med Bull 1983;39:163-167
• Schachter J, Dawson C: Human Chlamydial Infections. Littleton, Massachusetts, PSG Publishing Company, 1978
• Meyer KF: The ecology of psittacosis and ornithosis. Medicine 1942;21:175-206
Illustrations: N/A
Internet references: http://www.5mcc.com

Author(s)
David H. Thom, MD, PhD

Psoriasis

BASICS

DESCRIPTION Genetically determined (sporadic) common, chronic, epidermal proliferative disease. Clinically characterized by erythematous, dry scaling patches, recurring remissions and exacerbations. Flares may be related to systemic and environmental factors. Usual course - acute, chronic; unpredictable.
• Clinical forms:
◊ Discoid or plaque psoriasis - most common, patches appear on scalp, trunk and limbs, nails may be pitted and/or thickened
◊ Guttate psoriasis - occurs most frequently in children, numerous small papules over wide area of skin, but greatest on the trunk
◊ Pustular psoriasis - small pustules over the body or confined to one area (i.e., palms and soles) or arranged in annular patterns (especially children)
◊ Inverse flexural psoriasis - affects the flexural areas, lesions are moist and without scales (common in older people)
◊ Erythroderma (exfoliative psoriasis or red man syndrome) - patients skin turns red, may result from a flare of pre-existing dermatosis
◊ Ostraceous - grossly hyperkeratotic
Genetics:
• Genetic predisposition (probably polygenic)
• Type I psoriasis - young, strong family history = more aggressive disease
• Type 2 psoriasis - older, no family history = more stable disease
• Higher incidence in Caucasians and atopic families
• Increased incidence of human leukocyte antigens (HLA antigens)
System(s) affected: Skin/Exocrine
Incidence/Prevalence in USA:
1000-2000 cases/100,000 people in the U.S.
Predominant age: Two peaks of onset, age 16-22 and age 57-60; can develop in infants
Predominant sex: Male = Female

SIGNS AND SYMPTOMS
• Arthritis
• Pruritus
• Silvery scales on red plaques
• Knee-elbow-scalp distribution
• Stippled nails and pitting
• Positive Auspitz sign (underlying pinpoints of bleeding following scraping)
• Koebner's phenomenon (psoriatic response in previously unaffected area 1-2 weeks after skin injury)

CAUSES Possible genetic error in mitotic control. Activation of lymphocytes (antigen? autoimmune?).

RISK FACTORS
• Local trauma
• Local irritation
• Infection (streptococcal pharyngitis can stimulate acute guttate psoriasis, HIV)
• Endocrine changes
• Stress (physical and emotional)
• Sudden withdrawal of systemic and/or potent topical steroids
• Alcohol use

DIAGNOSIS

DIFFERENTIAL DIAGNOSIS
• Scalp - seborrheic dermatitis
• Body folds - intertrigo or candidiasis
• Diaper dermatitis
• Nails - onychomycosis
• Trunk - pityriasis rosea, pityriasis rubra pilaris, tinea corporis
• Squamous cell carcinoma
• Secondary and tertiary syphilis
• Cutaneous lupus erythematosus
• Eczema (nummular)
• Lichen planus
• Localized scratch dermatitis (lichen simplex chronicus)
• Mycosis fungoides
• Reiter's disease
• Subcorneal pustulosis
• Pustular eruptions

LABORATORY
• Negative rheumatoid factor
• Latex fixation test
• Leukocytosis and increased sedimentation rate often seen, especially in pustular psoriasis
• Fungal studies - may show a superimposed infection
• Uric acid increases in 10-20%
• In severe cases, anemia, B12, folate and iron deficiency can be present
Drugs that may alter lab results: N/A
Disorders that may alter lab results: N/A

PATHOLOGICAL FINDINGS
• Parakeratosis (focal), especially with neutrophils
• Hyperkeratosis
• Hypogranulosis
• Epidermal hyperplasia
• Elongation and thickening of rete ridges
• Thin epidermis above dermal papillae
• Spongiform pustule of Kogoj
• Munro's microabscess
• Abnormal mitoses
• Dilated tortuous capillary loops
• "Squirting" papillae

SPECIAL TESTS Biopsy

IMAGING N/A

DIAGNOSTIC PROCEDURES Usually diagnosis accomplished by inspection, occasionally biopsy required

TREATMENT

APPROPRIATE HEALTH CARE
• Outpatient usually
• May require inpatient for severe or resistant cases. Emergency: Severe and unstable forms like acute pustular psoriasis (Von Zumbusch's) or acute erythroderma.

GENERAL MEASURES
• Solar radiation
• Mild disease - ultraviolet radiation (UVA, UVB)
• Medication to soften scale, followed by soft brush while bathing
• Oatmeal baths for itching
• Tar shampoos
• Avoid excessive sun exposure
• Desert climates provide a favorable effect for some patients
• Wet dressings may help relieve pruritus
• For extensive, recalcitrant psoriasis, a referral to a specialist in psoriatic therapy is suggested

SURGICAL MEASURES N/A

ACTIVITY No restrictions

DIET No special diet

PATIENT EDUCATION
• Provide patient reassurance and anxiety relief to the extent possible
• Assurance to patient and family the condition is non-contagious
• For a listing of sources for patient education materials favorably reviewed on this topic, physicians may contact: American Academy of Family Physicians Foundation, P.O. Box 8418, Kansas City, MO 64114, (800)274-2237, ext. 4400
• National Psoriasis Foundation, Suite 300, 6600 S.W. 92nd Avenue, Portland, OR 97223, (503)244-7404; toll free (800)723-9166; fax (503)245-0626; E-mail 76135.2746@comserve.com

Psoriasis

MEDICATIONS

DRUG(S) OF CHOICE
• Mild disease:
◊ Emollients: to start treatment; bid soft yellow paraffin or aqueous cream; petrolatum or aquaphor cream greasier and more effective
◊ Topical, medium to high strength corticosteroids: tid-qid (overnight occlusion with plastic wrap will hasten resolution). Switching products prevents tachyphylaxis. Mid-potency topical corticosteroid mometasone furoate (non-fluorinated) is less atrophigenic. Limit use of potent steroids (halobetasol, betamethasone, clobetasol) to 2 weeks, avoid occlusive dressings, and taper to prevent rebound.
◊ Intralesional corticosteroid: 2-5 mg/mL triamcinolone acetonide
◊ Coal tar (Estar, PsoriGel) may be beneficial when alternated with topical steroids. Tar bath preparations for widespread involvement.
◊ Keratolytic agents: salicylic acid 6% gel (or 2-10% salicylate acid ointment) may be alternated with topical steroids
◊ Corticosteroid solutions and tar shampoos - scalp lesions
◊ Ultraviolet lamps and sun light effective. May be best treatment option during pregnancy or in young children.
◊ UVB + emollients in erythremogenic dose in fair-skinned patients - less toxic than PUVA
◊ Anthralin ointment 1% useful adjunctive treatment. Use prior to ultraviolet light (UVA, UVB). Indicated for quiescent or chronic psoriasis, contraindicated in acute or actively inflamed psoriatic eruptions. Start with 0.1% and gradually increase to 1%.
• Severe disease:
◊ Goeckerman's regimen - tar/UV light
◊ Methotrexate - single weekly dose (up to 25 mg) or 2.5-5 mg q12h for 3-4 days per week, but precautions necessary. Hydroxyurea for methotrexate failure. Azathioprine and intralesional cyclosporine, not common.
◊ Oral corticosteroids only for severe or life-threatening disease (risk of rebound)
◊ PUVA (psoralen plus ultraviolet light) - very effective, but causes skin-aging, cataracts and increases risk of skin cancers
◊ Etretinate, including RePUVA [PUVA and systemic retinoids] - for severe psoriasis (especially pustular and erythrodermic psoriasis) not responsive to standard treatments. Remains in body up to 2 years after treatment. Extremely fetotoxic. Do not use if pregnant or could become pregnant within 2 years of treatment.
◊ Isotretinoin: may work on some patients
◊ Triamcinolone, intralesional - mix with procaine or normal saline for concentrate of 4 mg/mL. Administer with syringe or dermajet. Effective in treating solitary resistant plaques and psoriasis involving the nails.
◊ Vitamin D analogs (calcipotriene ointment 0.005% for moderate plaque psoriasis). Results may not be maximal for 2 months. Too irritating for facial lesions.
◊ Cyclosporine or tacrolimus: only for recalcitrant psoriasis (possible nephrotoxicity)

Contraindications: Refer to manufacturer's literature
Precautions: Refer to manufacturer's literature
Significant possible interactions: Refer to manufacturer's literature

ALTERNATIVE DRUGS
• Cyclosporin: In recalcitrant disease for short-term use only, perhaps alternating with other agents

FOLLOWUP

PATIENT MONITORING
• Continuous supportive care
• Medications used in treatment require close followup. Certain lab studies may be necessary. Long-term use of topicals is not recommended.
• With methotrexate therapy check CBC, SGOT, albumin every month. Some recommend liver biopsy before treating or 3 months after treatment started and then regularly (usually every 2 years) based on a cumulative methotrexate dose of 1.5 grams.

PREVENTION/AVOIDANCE
• Avoid alcoholic beverages
• Avoid irritating drugs
• Avoid stimulating drugs (lithium, ACE inhibitors, beta-adrenergic blockers, tetracycline, NSAID's, amiodarone, morphine, procaine, potassium iodide, salicylates, sulfapyridine, sulfonamides and penicillin. Pustular flares may occur with steroids).
• Avoid antimalarial medications (aminoquinolone compounds)

POSSIBLE COMPLICATIONS
• Pustular psoriasis
• Exfoliative erythrodermatitis
• Rebound of the psoriatic process after corticosteroids are discontinued
• Topical corticosteroids may cause thinning of skin, striae, masking local infection, hypopigmentation and tachyphylaxis

EXPECTED COURSE/PROGNOSIS
• Usually benign
• Life-threatening forms do occur
• May be refractory to treatment

MISCELLANEOUS

ASSOCIATED CONDITIONS
• Extensive erythrodermic psoriasis may accompany AIDS
• Arthritis
• Psoriatic arthritis
• Myopathy
• Enteropathy
• Spondylitic heart disease
• Acute anterior uveitis

AGE-RELATED FACTORS
Pediatric:
• Onset common <10, rarely <3
• Disease may be atypical in its course
Geriatric:
• About 3% of psoriasis patients acquire the disease after age 65
• Detailed drug history important, since many drugs (e.g., beta-blockers) can exacerbate psoriasis
• If using cytotoxic medications for treatment of psoriasis, closely follow hepatic and renal functions, and creatinine clearance
• Elderly patients may have difficulty with application of topicals over all affected body parts
Others: N/A

PREGNANCY Unpredictable effect on disease. Avoid tars, topical corticosteroids, calcipotriene, and systemic therapies. Etretinate is fetotoxic.

SYNONYMS N/A

ICD-9-CM
696.1 Other psoriasis
696.2 Parapsoriasis

SEE ALSO N/A

OTHER NOTES N/A

ABBREVIATIONS N/A

REFERENCES
• Burrall B, Dijkstra J, Lowe N, Maibach H: Psoriasis therapies: Old, new and borrowed. Patient Care 1995;10:38-65
• Greaves MW, Weinstein GD: Treatment of psoriasis. NEJM 1995;332(9):581-588
• Habif T: Clinical Dermatology. 3rd Ed. St. Louis, CV Mosby, 1996
• Abel E: Diagnosis of drug induced psoriasis. Seminars in Dermatology 1992;11(4)
• Jegsothy B, et al: Tacrolimus (FK 506): A new therapeutic agent for severe recalcitrant psoriasis. Arc Dermatol 1992;128
• Ho C, Zioty D: Immunosuppressive Agents in Dermatology. Dermatology Clinics 1993;11(1)
• Moschella S, et al, eds: Dermatology. 3rd Ed. Philadelphia, W.B. Saunders Co., 1992
Illustrations: 15 available on CD-ROM
Internet references: http://www.5mcc.com

Author(s)
Paul J. Jaster, MD

Puerperal infection

BASICS

DESCRIPTION Bacterial infection of the genital tract following delivery. Includes perineal cellulitis, vaginal and cervical infections (all uncommon), necrotizing faciitis (rare), endomyometritis, pelvic cellulitis, septic pelvic thrombophlebitis, parametrial phlegmon.
System(s) affected: Reproductive
Genetics: N/A
Incidence/Prevalence in USA:
• Vaginal deliveries - 2% or 64,000 cases per year
• Cesarean sections - ≥13 % or 104,000 cases per year
Predominant age: Teens at higher risk
Predominant sex: Female only

SIGNS AND SYMPTOMS
• Fever > 38.6°C (101.4°F) in the first 24 hours, or > 38°C (100.4°F) on any of the first 10 days
• Localized pain and swelling
• Chills
• Abdominal pain
• Foul-smelling lochia
• Uterine tenderness on exam
• Peritonitis with severe pain, ileus
• Septic shock

CAUSES
• Puerperal infections often begin as wound infections following laceration of perineum, vagina, cervix, or the abdominal wound of C-section. Also, the entire endometrium is susceptible, especially at the site of placental attachment.
• Polymicrobial infections; primary pathogen often unclear
• Commonly found bacteria include:
  ◊ Aerobes/ facultative aerobes - Group A, B, and D Streptococci, Enterococcus, gram-negative bacteria (E. coli, Klebsiella and Proteus sp), Staphylococcus aureus, Staph. epidermidis, Gardnerella vaginalis, Hemophilus influenza
  ◊ Anaerobes - Peptococcus sp., Peptostreptococcus sp., Bacteroides bivius, B. fragilis, B. disiens, Clostridium sp., Fusobacterium sp.
  ◊ Other - Mycoplasma hominis, Chlamydia trachomatis, Urea urealyticum

RISK FACTORS
• Bacterial contamination (cervical exams, fetal monitoring devices, or operative manipulation)
• Blood loss
• C-section - risk increased following prolapse of umbilical cord or fetal extremity
• Diabetes
• Drug addiction
• History of sexually transmitted diseases
• Immune deficiency
• Poverty
• Bacterial vaginosis
• Urinary tract infection

• Malnutrition
• Obesity
• Pre-existing chorioamnionitis
• Pre-term labor
• Premature rupture of membranes
• Prolonged labor
• Trauma
• Group B Streptococcus vaginal colonization

DIAGNOSIS

DIFFERENTIAL DIAGNOSIS
• Fever from other sources:
  ◊ Urinary tract infection
  ◊ Respiratory infection
  ◊ Mastitis or breast engorgement
  ◊ Thrombophlebitis
  ◊ Wound infection

LABORATORY
• CBC
• Genital tract cultures and rapid test for group B streptococcus
• Amniotic fluid smear for WBC's and bacteria
• Blood cultures
Drugs that may alter lab results:
Previous antibiotics may alter culture results
Disorders that may alter lab results: N/A

PATHOLOGICAL FINDINGS
• Microscopic sections show a superficial layer of infected necrotic material
• Peritonitis (caused by lymphatic spread)
• Phlegmon may form in the leaves of the broad ligament, usually after C-section. Rarely this forms an abscess.
• Thrombosis may involve any of the pelvic veins, including the inferior vena cava

SPECIAL TESTS N/A

IMAGING
• CT or MRI for thrombophlebitis
• Ultrasound (sensitive for abscess)

DIAGNOSTIC PROCEDURES
Culdocentesis with culture

TREATMENT

APPROPRIATE HEALTH CARE Inpatient

GENERAL MEASURES
• IV antibiotics and close observation
• Infected wounds should be opened to establish drainage
• Peritonitis requires imaging to evaluate the cause
• Normalize fluid status

SURGICAL MEASURES
• Necrotizing fasciitis requires wide débridement
• Surgery may be needed to establish drainage or decompress the bowel
• Surgical drainage of a phlegmon is not advised unless suppurative

ACTIVITY As tolerated

DIET As tolerated, may be limited by ileus

PATIENT EDUCATION
• Avoidance of sexually transmitted diseases
• Prenatal discussion of premature rupture of membranes and preterm labor

Puerperal infection

MEDICATIONS

DRUG(S) OF CHOICE
• Preferred:
  ◊ Clindamycin 600-900 mg IV q8hr, plus
  ◊ Gentamicin 2 mg/kg IV q day
• If severe infection or poor response in first 48 hours, add ampicillin 1-2 gm IV q6hr
• There are several effective options
  ◊ Metronidazole 7.5 mg/kg IV q6h, plus gentamicin
  ◊ Ampicillin-sulbactam (Unasyn) - 2/1 gm IV q6hr
  ◊ Cefoxitin (Mefoxin) 2 gm IV q8hr. Add ampicillin if clinical failure in 48 hr.
Contraindications:
• Drug allergy
• Renal failure (aminoglycosides)
• Avoid chloramphenicol, sulfa, tetracyclines, fluoroquinolones before delivery or if breast-feeding
Precautions:
• Chloramphenicol rarely causes bone marrow suppression
• Clindamycin, others, occasionally cause pseudomembranous colitis
Significant possible interactions: Refer to manufacturer's literature

ALTERNATIVE DRUGS
• Piperacillin, mezlocillin, cefoperazone, cefotetan, cefotaxime
• Base therapy on cultures, sensitivities, and clinical response
• Heparin may be indicated for pelvic thrombophlebitis

FOLLOWUP

PATIENT MONITORING   Individualize according to severity

PREVENTION/AVOIDANCE
• Regular prenatal care
• Patient education regarding premature rupture of membranes and pre-term labor
• Minimize iatrogenic causes - cervical exams, fetal monitoring
• Prophylactic antibiotics for C-section if high risk
• Consider rapid test for group B strep for all patients during labor
• Consider antibiotics at the time of preterm premature rupture of membranes
• Amnioinfusion may decrease the incidence of puerperal infection in high risk labors

POSSIBLE COMPLICATIONS
• Infertility (uncommon)
• Need for surgery
• Wound infection
• Shock
• Death

EXPECTED COURSE/PROGNOSIS
• Depends on location and severity
• Most have dramatic response to therapy. If not, consider retained products of conception, abscess, hematoma, septic pelvic thrombophlebitis, or wound infection.
• Antibiotics can be stopped when afebrile for 24-48 hours. Oral antibiotics following this are not helpful.

MISCELLANEOUS

ASSOCIATED CONDITIONS   See Risk Factors

AGE-RELATED FACTORS   N/A
Pediatric: N/A
Geriatric: N/A
Others: Teen pregnancies at higher risk

PREGNANCY   A complication of pregnancy

SYNONYMS
• Endometritis
• Endoparametritis
• Endomyometritis
• Metritis with pelvic cellulitis

ICD-9-CM   670 Major puerperal infection

SEE ALSO   N/A

ABBREVIATIONS   N/A

OTHER NOTES   Interpret WBC with care; may be as high as 20,000 as physiologic leucocytosis

REFERENCES
• Cunningham FG, MacDonald PC, Gant NF, eds: Williams' Obstetrics. 19th Ed. Norwalk, CT, Appleton and Lange, 1993
• Watts DH, et al: Early postpartum endometritis: The role of bacteria, genital Mycoplasmas, and Chlamydia trachomatis. Obs and Gyn 1989;73(1):52-60
• Hamadeh G, et al: Postpartum fever. Amer Fam Phys 1995;52(2):531-538
Illustrations: N/A
Internet references: http://www.5mcc.com

Author(s)
Robert H. Scott, MD

Pulmonary edema

BASICS

DESCRIPTION Pulmonary interstitial and/or alveolar fluid accumulation that results when the forces moving fluid out of the pulmonary capillary exceed the forces restraining that fluid
System(s) affected: Cardiovascular, Pulmonary
Genetics: Multifactorial
Incidence/Prevalence in USA:
Approximately 150,000 persons per year in U.S. affected with non-cardiogenic pulmonary edema
Predominant age: Middle age and elderly
Predominant sex: Male = Female

SIGNS AND SYMPTOMS
• Respiratory
◊ Shortness of breath
◊ Dyspnea with exertion
◊ Orthopnea, paroxysmal nocturnal dyspnea
◊ Cough, often accompanied by pink or blood-tinged frothy sputum
◊ Wheezing, rhonchi, gurgles
◊ Moist, crepitant rales noted initially at bases and progressing to apices
◊ Breathlessness, air hunger
◊ Noisy respirations
◊ Tachypnea
◊ Dilated alae nasi
◊ Inspiratory retraction of the intercostal spaces and/or supraventricular fossae
◊ Cheyne-Stokes respirations
• Cardiovascular
◊ Tachycardia
◊ Elevated jugular venous pulse
◊ Increased P2
◊ S3
◊ S4
◊ Nocturnal angina
◊ Pulsus alternans or presence of valvular heart disease
• General
◊ Weakness, fatigue
◊ Other symptoms depending on etiology
◊ Anxiety
◊ Diaphoretic, cold, ashen, or cyanotic skin
◊ Lower extremity edema

CAUSES
• Cardiogenic
◊ Left heart failure
◊ Ischemic heart disease
◊ Acute myocardial infarction
◊ Aortic and mitral valvular disease
◊ Hypertensive heart disease
◊ Cardiomyopathy
◊ Volume overload
◊ Arrhythmias
◊ Endocarditis
◊ Myocarditis
◊ Congenital heart disease
◊ Acute rheumatic fever and rheumatic heart disease
◊ Septal defects
◊ Cardiac tamponade
◊ High cardiac output states (e.g., thyrotoxicosis, beriberi)

• Noncardiogenic
◊ Shock
◊ Multiple trauma
◊ Infection/sepsis (especially pneumonia)
◊ Liquid aspiration (e.g., drowning, gastric contents)
◊ Inhaled toxic gases
◊ Pulmonary lymphatic obstruction
◊ Drug overdose (especially narcotics)
◊ High-altitude illness
◊ Pancreatitis
◊ Embolism (thrombus, fat, air, amniotic fluid)
◊ Neurogenic
◊ Hematologic and immunologic disorders
◊ Disorders associated with high negative pleural pressure
◊ Radiation pneumonitis
◊ Disseminated intravascular coagulation
◊ Eclampsia
◊ Decreased plasma oncotic pressure (e.g., hypoalbuminemia)
◊ Postcardioversion, postanesthesia, postcardiopulmonary bypass
◊ Oxygen toxicity
◊ ARDS
◊ Renal failure

RISK FACTORS Dependent on etiology

DIAGNOSIS

DIFFERENTIAL DIAGNOSIS
Important to distinguish between cardiogenic and non-cardiogenic pulmonary edema
• Pneumonia
• Asthma
• COPD exacerbation
• Pulmonary embolism
• Hyperventilation syndrome

LABORATORY
• None specific for pulmonary edema; laboratory abnormalities (e.g., creatine kinase [CK], amylase, etc.) may point to underlying etiology
• Hypoxemia
• Hypocarbia
• Respiratory alkalosis
• Increased A-a gradient
• Leukocytosis
Drugs that may alter lab results:
Administered oxygen may complicate arterial blood gas interpretation
Disorders that may alter lab results:
Underlying pulmonary disease from an unrelated etiology may complicate arterial blood gas interpretation

PATHOLOGICAL FINDINGS
• Cardiogenic
◊ Heavy, wet, subcrepitant lungs
◊ Intra-alveolar granular pink precipitate
◊ Alveolar microhemorrhages and hemosiderin-laden macrophages
◊ "Brown induration," chronic passive congestion
◊ Hypostatic bronchopneumonia

• Noncardiogenic
◊ Heavy, firm, red, and boggy lungs
◊ Interstitial and intra-alveolar edema, inflammation, fibrin deposition, hemorrhage, and patchy atelectasis
◊ Hyaline membrane formation
◊ Interstitial and intra-alveolar fibrosis

SPECIAL TESTS
• Arterial blood gas
• Electrocardiogram
• Pulmonary function tests
• Mixed venous oxygen saturation

IMAGING
• Two-dimensional echocardiography with Doppler may be useful in some cases of cardiogenic pulmonary edema (e.g., valvular heart disease, systolic vs. diastolic dysfunction)
• Chest x-ray (may be difficult or impossible to differentiate cardiogenic from non-cardiogenic pulmonary edema)
◊ Cardiogenic chest x-ray; Interstitial edema, cardiomegaly, pulmonary venous redistribution, Kerley's B lines, alveolar edema (initially perihilar), pleural effusions (more common)
◊ Non-cardiogenic chest x-ray; alveolar edema, cardiomegaly absent, pulmonary venous redistribution absent, pleural effusions less common

DIAGNOSTIC PROCEDURES
• Swan-Ganz catheter may help differentiate cardiogenic from non-cardiogenic pulmonary edema
• Cardiac catheterization - occasionally beneficial

TREATMENT

APPROPRIATE HEALTH CARE
Generally inpatient or intensive care; outpatient for mildest forms

GENERAL MEASURES
• Treat underlying condition
• Patient sitting, with legs dangling
• Oxygen
• Rotating tourniquets or phlebotomy selectively
• Mechanical ventilation, often requiring positive end-expiratory pressure support
• Rapid reduction in altitude in cases of high altitude pulmonary edema

SURGICAL MEASURES   N/A

ACTIVITY   Bedrest in most cases

DIET   Low sodium diet

PATIENT EDUCATION
• Low sodium, fluid restriction
• Symptoms and signs of pulmonary edema
• Importance of medical compliance

MEDICATIONS

DRUG(S) OF CHOICE
• Acute cardiogenic pulmonary edema
◊ Morphine sulfate 2-5 mg IV
◊ Furosemide 20-80 mg IV
◊ Nitroglycerin paste 1-2 inches
◊ In selected cases: Nitroglycerin drip beginning at 5 µg/min and increasing by 5-10 µg/min every few minutes, titrating to blood pressure, etc. Nitroprusside IV drip beginning at 10 µg/min and increasing by 5-10 µg/min every few minutes, titrating to blood pressure, etc. Dobutamine 2 µg/kg/min IV titrating to blood pressure, cardiac output, pulmonary capillary wedge pressure, etc.
• Chronic management of cardiogenic pulmonary edema
◊ Furosemide 20-400 mg daily
◊ Angiotensin converting enzyme inhibitors (e.g., captopril 6.25-25 mg po tid, lisinopril 2.5-20 mg po qd, enalapril 2.5-15 mg po qd-bid)
◊ Digoxin 0.125-0.25 mg po qd
◊ Hydralazine 10-100 mg po qid
◊ Isosorbide dinitrate 10-60 mg po tid-qid
◊ Thiazide diuretics (e.g., hydrochlorothiazide [HCTZ] 25-50 mg po qd)
• Noncardiogenic pulmonary edema
◊ Oxygen
◊ Selected cardiovascular drugs to optimize tissue oxygen delivery
Contraindications: Refer to manufacturer's profile of each drug
Precautions:
• Avoid liberal intravenous fluids, especially normal saline or lactated Ringer's
• Avoid negative inotropic agents such as calcium channel blockers or beta-blockers in the setting of cardiogenic pulmonary edema
• Avoid high forced inspiratory O2 (FiO2) > 50% for prolonged periods of time if possible
• Avoid prolonged administration of nitroprusside due to risk of cyanide toxicity. If nitroprusside administered for > 72 hrs, obtain a thiocyanate level.
Significant possible interactions:
Additive hypotensive effects of nitrates, afterload reducers, diuretics, etc.

ALTERNATIVE DRUGS
• Chlorothiazide
• Metolazone
• Acetazolamide
• Bumetanide
• Potassium-sparing diuretics
• Other ACE inhibitors

FOLLOWUP

PATIENT MONITORING
• Inpatient
◊ Serial arterial blood gases or pulse oximetry, often in the intensive care unit with one-on-one nursing
◊ Strict measurement of intake and output
◊ Attention to optimal fluid management
◊ Attention to optimal ventilator settings
◊ Serial chest x-rays
• Outpatient
◊ Attention to clinical status
◊ Serial weights to assess fluid accumulation

PREVENTION/AVOIDANCE Compliance with medications and diet

POSSIBLE COMPLICATIONS
• Death
• Reversible or irreversible organ ischemia
• Pulmonary fibrosis, particularly with noncardiogenic pulmonary edema

EXPECTED COURSE/PROGNOSIS
• Dependent on underlying etiology
• Mortality approximately 50-60% for noncardiogenic pulmonary edema and up to 80% for cardiogenic shock

MISCELLANEOUS:

ASSOCIATED CONDITIONS (see Causes)

AGE-RELATED FACTORS
Pediatric: Usually secondary to lung immaturity, congenital heart disease, or associated with trauma
Geriatric: Higher mortality
Others: N/A

PREGNANCY An obstetrician and cardiologist or pulmonologist should be involved in care

SYNONYMS N/A

ICD-9-CM
• 428.1 Acute pulmonary edema with heart disease
• 518.4 Acute edema of lung, not otherwise specified

SEE ALSO
• Congestive heart failure
• Respiratory distress syndrome, adult
• Altitude illness

OTHER NOTES N/A

ABBREVIATIONS
ARDS = adult respiratory distress syndrome

REFERENCES
• Ingram RH, Braunwald E: Pulmonary edema. In: Braunwald E, ed. Heart disease - A Textbook of Cardiovascular Medicine. 4th Ed. Philadelphia, W.B. Saunders, Co., 1992
• Ingram RH, Braunwald E: Dyspnea and pulmonary edema. In: Braunwald E, ed. Harrison's Principles of Internal Medicine. 12th Ed. New York, McGraw-Hill, Inc., 1991
Illustrations: N/A
Internet references: http://www.5mcc.com

Author(s)
Peter Kozisek, MD

Pulmonary embolism

BASICS

DESCRIPTION Pulmonary embolism occurs when venous thrombi in the deep venous system of the legs dislodge and enter the pulmonary arterial circulation
• Pulmonary embolism presents as three different syndromes
◊ Acute cor pulmonale - due to massive pulmonary embolism, obstructing > 60-75% of the pulmonary circulation
◊ Pulmonary Infarction - occurs in patients with submassive pulmonary embolism with complete obstruction of a distal branch of the pulmonary circulation
◊ Acute unexplained dyspnea - occurs in patients who do not develop acute cor pulmonale or pulmonary infarction
System(s) affected: Pulmonary, Cardiovascular
Genetics: Hypercoagulability
Incidence/Prevalence in USA:
• 600,000-700,000 cases/year
• 100,000-200,000 deaths/year
Predominant age: Very rare in children, incidence increases with advancing age
Predominant sex: Male = Female

SIGNS AND SYMPTOMS
• Acute cor pulmonale
◊ Syncope
◊ Hypotension or cardiac arrest
◊ Dyspnea
◊ Anxiety
◊ Tachypnea
◊ Tachycardia
◊ Distended neck veins
◊ S3 gallop
◊ Clear lungs on auscultation
◊ ± Signs of deep venous thrombosis
◊ ECG - S1Q3T3 pattern or incomplete right bundle branch block
◊ Chest x-ray - usually normal
◊ Arterial blood gases (room air) decreased PO2, decreased PCO2
• Pulmonary infarction
◊ Pleuritic chest pain
◊ Dyspnea
◊ ± Hemoptysis
◊ Tachypnea
◊ Lungs - rales, wheezes and/or signs of pleural effusion
◊ ± Signs of deep venous thrombosis
◊ ECG - normal
◊ Chest x-ray - elevated hemidiaphragm, infiltrate or small pleural effusion
◊ Arterial blood gases (room air) - normal or decreased PO2, decreased PCO2, alkalosis
• Acute unexplained dyspnea
◊ Dyspnea
◊ ± Anxiety
◊ ± Tachycardia
◊ Tachypnea
◊ Clear lungs
◊ ± Signs of deep venous thrombosis
◊ ECG - usually normal
◊ Chest x-ray - normal

CAUSES
• Hypercoagulability (difficult to document)
• Deep vein thrombosis responsible for 95% of pulmonary embolism

RISK FACTORS
• Prolonged bed rest
• Advanced age
• Congestive heart failure
• Malignancy
• Stroke
• Pregnancy
• Oral contraceptives
• Postoperative
• Trauma to legs
• Obesity

DIAGNOSIS

DIFFERENTIAL DIAGNOSIS
• Pneumonia
• Myocardial infarction
• Congestive heart failure
• Viral pleuritis
• Pericarditis

LABORATORY N/A
Drugs that may alter lab results: N/A
Disorders that may alter lab results: N/A

PATHOLOGICAL FINDINGS Pulmonary infarction

SPECIAL TESTS N/A

IMAGING
• The diagnosis is confirmed by V/Q lung scan (multiple segmental or lobar perfusion defects with normal ventilation), or pulmonary angiogram (intraluminal filling defects and/or arterial cutoffs)
• Chest x-ray may reveal parachymal infiltrate, pleural effusion

DIAGNOSTIC PROCEDURES
• Lung scan
• Pulmonary angiogram
• Diagnosis suspected on basis of signs and symptoms consistent with one of the three syndromes in a patient with deep venous thrombosis (DVT) or with risk factors for DVT

TREATMENT

APPROPRIATE HEALTH CARE
Hospitalization, ICU if hemodynamically unstable

GENERAL MEASURES
• Designed to maintain adequate cardiovascular and pulmonary functions and to prevent recurrence of emboli
• Oxygen therapy as needed

SURGICAL MEASURES N/A

ACTIVITY
• Bed rest, move legs frequently
• Ambulation when patient stable

DIET No special diet, need to maintain adequate nutrition and fluids

PATIENT EDUCATION N/A

MEDICATIONS

DRUG(S) OF CHOICE
• Intravenous heparin by continuous infusion, at dose to prolong partial thromboplastin time to 1.5-2.0 times control for five to seven days. Usual regimen requires beginning with 80 units/kg load followed by 18 unit/kg/hr. Check PTT 6 hours after beginning infusion, then daily.
• Warfarin beginning day one or day two of hospitalization for at least three months. Warfarin dose adjusted to prolong prothrombin time to 2.0 to 3.0 INR.
• In event of hypotension requiring vasopressors in a patient with angiographically documented pulmonary embolism, pulmonary embolectomy or intravenous thrombolytic agents may be required

Contraindications: Refer to manufacturer's profile of each drug
Precautions:
• Refer to manufacturer's profile of each drug
• The major complication of heparin is the possibility of hemorrhage. If PTT is appropriately adjusted, the major hemorrhage rate should be low.
Significant possible interactions: Refer to manufacturer's profile of each drug

ALTERNATIVE DRUGS
Surgery to interrupt the inferior vena cava, if needed, in patients who have recurrent emboli, or can't take anticoagulants

FOLLOWUP

PATIENT MONITORING
After hospital discharge, prothrombin time should be prolonged to 2.0 to 3.0 (INR). Warfarin should be continued for at least three months. In patients with continuous predisposition to DVT, it should be continued indefinitely.

PREVENTION/AVOIDANCE
Recognition of hospitalized patients with multiple risk factors for deep venous thrombosis and implementation of prophylactic therapy including low dose heparin, warfarin or leg compression devices

POSSIBLE COMPLICATIONS
• Pulmonary infarction
• Acute cor pulmonale
• Recurrent deep venous thrombosis or pulmonary embolism, post phlebitic syndrome
• Treatment failure requiring surgical venous interruption

EXPECTED COURSE/PROGNOSIS
With appropriate therapy hospital mortality is less than 10%. Long-term prognosis determined by coexisting disease.

MISCELLANEOUS

ASSOCIATED CONDITIONS
• Deep vein thrombosis
• Occult cancer (lung, GI tract, breast, uterus, prostate)

AGE-RELATED FACTORS
Pediatric: Quite rare
Geriatric: More common, more often fatal.
Others: N/A

PREGNANCY
Higher risk of occurrence during pregnancy and puerperium

SYNONYMS
N/A

ICD-9-CM
415.1 Pulmonary embolism and infarction

SEE ALSO
• Thrombosis, deep vein (DVT)

OTHER NOTES
N/A

ABBREVIATIONS
N/A

REFERENCES
• Isselbacher KJ, et al, eds: Harrison's Principles of Internal Medicine. 13th Ed. New York, McGraw-Hill, 1994
• Rippe JM, et al, eds: Intensive Care Medicine. 2nd Ed. New York, Little, Brown, 1991:308-316
Illustrations: N/A
Internet references: http://www.5mcc.com

Author(s)
James E. Dalen, MD, MPH

Pulmonic valvular stenosis

 BASICS

DESCRIPTION
A congenital deformity consisting of obstruction to right ventricular outflow at the pulmonic valve level
System(s) affected: Cardiovascular
Genetics: N/A
Incidence/Prevalence in USA: 10% of congenital heart disease
Predominant age: Newborn, but often asymptomatic for years
Predominant sex: Male = Female

SIGNS AND SYMPTOMS
• History of heart murmur since birth
• Acyanotic
• Dyspnea and fatigue are the most frequent symptoms
• Occasionally dizziness or syncope occurs, particularly exertional, due to the low fixed cardiac output
• Chest pain can occur
• Myocardial infarction of the hypertrophied right ventricle has been noted
• Prominent A wave of the jugular venous pulse
• Right ventricular impulse
• Midsystolic murmur (increased duration and later peaking with increased severity)
• Pulmonic ejection sound
• Soft, delay in P2
• Occasional tricuspid regurgitation

CAUSES
• Congenital
• Rubella embryopathy

RISK FACTORS
Family history

 DIAGNOSIS

DIFFERENTIAL DIAGNOSIS
• Dysplastic pulmonic valve stenosis
• Discrete infundibular stenosis
• Subinfundibular obstruction
• Isolated pulmonary artery stenosis
• Supravalvar pulmonary stenosis
• Tetralogy of Fallot (Pink)

LABORATORY
N/A
Drugs that may alter lab results: N/A
Disorders that may alter lab results: N/A

PATHOLOGICAL FINDINGS
N/A

SPECIAL TESTS
ECG - generally sinus rhythm, occasional supraventricular arrhythmias, tall peaked P waves, rightward axis, severity correlates with R/S ratio in leads V1 and V6, right ventricular hypertrophy

IMAGING
• X-ray - post stenotic dilatation of the pulmonary trunk, prominence of right atrium and ventricle
• Echocardiogram - mobile dome, thickened pulmonic valve, post stenotic dilatation of the pulmonary trunk, small valve annulus; continuous wave Doppler provides an estimate of the transvalvular gradient
• Color-flow Doppler - delineates area of obstruction

DIAGNOSTIC PROCEDURES
• Cardiac catheterization
  ◊ Not indicated in mild pulmonic stenosis
  ◊ Essential in severe pulmonic stenosis
  ◊ Used to assess morphology of the right ventricle, pulmonary outflow tract and the pulmonary arteries
  ◊ Also used to rule out associated lesions e.g., atrial septal defect (ASD), though echocardiography may suffice.

 TREATMENT

APPROPRIATE HEALTH CARE
Usually outpatient. Inpatient, if surgery indicated.

GENERAL MEASURES
• Though infective endocarditis is rare, SBE prophylaxis is advisable
• Diagnostic treatment for critical pulmonary stenosis in newborns
• Intervention
  ◊ None required for mild pulmonic stenosis
  ◊ Intervention of asymptomatic patients with moderate PS is controversial. At minimum, regular assessment is advisable.

SURGICAL MEASURES
Percutaneous balloon valvotomy (preferred) or surgical pulmonic valvotomy required for patient with severe obstruction

ACTIVITY
No specific prescription. The lesion, if significant, will limit activity.

DIET
No specific regimen

PATIENT EDUCATION
American Heart Association, 7320 Greenville Avenue, Dallas, TX 75231, (214)373-6300

MEDICATIONS

DRUG(S) OF CHOICE
• No specific regimen in the absence of congestive heart failure
• Endocarditis prophylaxis
Contraindications: Refer to manufacturer's literature
Precautions: Refer to manufacturer's literature
Significant possible interactions: Refer to manufacturer's literature

ALTERNATIVE DRUGS N/A

FOLLOWUP

PATIENT MONITORING
• Postoperative (or post-balloon valvotomy) Doppler ultrasound suggested at approximately 1 year after procedure
• Post valvotomy SBE prophylaxis still required
• Regular followup assessment for patients not undergoing surgical correction

PREVENTION/AVOIDANCE N/A

POSSIBLE COMPLICATIONS
• Up to 10% late mortality following valvotomy in critical pulmonary stenosis in neonates
• Slower recovery in those with chronic severe right ventricular hypertrophy
• Post valvotomy pulmonic regurgitation reported in up to 50% (variable severity)
• Residual ASD or patent foramen ovale
• Persistent repolarization abnormalities on ECG associated with severe postoperative pulmonic regurgitation
• Late atrial arrhythmias

EXPECTED COURSE/PROGNOSIS
Outcome following either balloon or surgical valvotomy is excellent in general

MISCELLANEOUS

ASSOCIATED CONDITIONS Other cardiac abnormalities, e.g., ventricular and atrial septal defects

AGE-RELATED FACTORS
Pediatric: Congenital disorder
Geriatric: N/A
Others: N/A

PREGNANCY In asymptomatic young women with mild to moderate PS, pregnancy is generally well tolerated

SYNONYMS Pulmonic stenosis

ICD-9-CM
424.3 Pulmonary valve disorders
746.02 Stenosis, congenital

SEE ALSO Tetralogy of Fallot

OTHER NOTES N/A

ABBREVIATIONS
• SBE = subacute bacterial endocarditis
• PS = pulmonic stenosis

REFERENCES
• Braunwald E, ed: Heart Disease: A Textbook of Cardiovascular Medicine. 4th Ed. Philadelphia, W.B. Saunders Co., 1992
• Liberthson R: Congenital Heart Disease: Diagnosis & Management in Children and Adults. Boston, Little Brown & Co., 1989
• Perloff J: Clinical Recognition of Congenital Heart Disease. 4th Ed. Philadelphia, WB Saunders Co, 1994
Illustrations: N/A
Internet references: http://www.5mcc.com

Author(s)
Sylvia A. Mamby, MD

Pyelonephritis

BASICS

DESCRIPTION
• Acute pyelonephritis is a syndrome caused by an infection of the pyelo-calicial system, producing localized flank or back pain combined with systemic symptoms such as fever, chills and prostration. It is accompanied by bacteriuria, and often by bacteremia, which can progress to "septic shock" and death.
• Chronic pyelonephritis is the pathological result of progressive inflammation on the renal interstitium and tubules, and the radiologic diagnosis of the renal scarring and destructive changes in the caliceal system that are presumed to be caused by bacterial infection, vesicoureteral reflux, or both.
System(s) affected: Renal/Urologic
Genetics: N/A
Incidence/Prevalence:
• Community acquired acute pyelonephritis - 15.7 per 100,000/per year
• Hospital acquired acute pyelonephritis - 7.3 per 10,000 hospital persons
Predominant age: All ages, especially > 50
Predominant sex: Female > Male

SIGNS AND SYMPTOMS
• In adults
  ◊ Fever; above 38.5°C
  ◊ Chills
  ◊ Unilateral vs. bilateral pain in the lumbar flank area
  ◊ Malaise
  ◊ Myalgia
  ◊ Anorexia
  ◊ Nausea
  ◊ Vomiting
  ◊ Diarrhea
  ◊ Headache
  ◊ Dysuria
  ◊ Frequency
  ◊ Urgency
  ◊ Suprapubic discomfort
  ◊ Flank pain on palpation
  ◊ From no physical findings to septic shock
• In infants and children
  ◊ Sepsis
  ◊ Fever
  ◊ Irritability
  ◊ Poor skin perfusion
  ◊ Inadequate weight gain or weight loss
  ◊ Gastrointestinal symptoms
  ◊ Jaundice to gray skin color
  ◊ Flank mass
  ◊ Enuresis
  ◊ Vaginal discharge, vulval soreness or pruritus in girls

CAUSES
• E. coli (75%)
• Other gram-negative rods, Proteus mirabilis, klebsiella and Enterobacter account for 10-15%
• Enterococcus
• Staphylococcus - epidermis, saprophyticus and aureus
• Leptospira
• Salmonella typhi
• Mycoplasma
• Anaerobes

RISK FACTORS
• Underlying urinary tract abnormalities
• Indwelling catheter
• Nephrolithiasis
• Diabetes mellitus
• Immunocompromised conditions
• Elderly, institutionalized women
• Acute pyelonephritis within the prior year

DIAGNOSIS

DIFFERENTIAL DIAGNOSIS
• Renal infarction
• Acute renal vein thrombosis
• Acute renal artery dissection
• Obstructive uropathy
• Acute glomerulonephritis
• Acute bacterial pneumonia
• Myocardial infarction
• Acute hepatitis
• Cholecystitis
• Acute pancreatitis
• Appendicitis
• A perforated viscus
• Splenic infarct
• Aortic dissection
• Acute pelvic inflammatory disease
• Zona

LABORATORY
• Urine culture > 100,000 colony-forming units (CFU/mL)
• Pyuria
• The leukocyte esterase test in the urine
• Leukocyte casts
• Hematuria and mild proteinuria
• Leukocytosis
• Blood culture(s)
Drugs that may alter lab results:
Antibiotics
Disorders that may alter lab results: N/A

PATHOLOGICAL FINDINGS
• Acute:
  ◊ Abscess formation with neutrophils
  ◊ Glomeruli spared
  ◊ The area of the infection is wedge-shaped toward the medulla
• Chronic:
  ◊ Fibrosis
  ◊ Reduction in renal tissue
  ◊ Scarring
  ◊ Calyceal clubbing, dilatation and distortion

SPECIAL TESTS
• Bladder washout
• Antibody coated bacteria or ACB test

IMAGING 67gallium or 131I-Hippuran scanning

DIAGNOSTIC PROCEDURES
• Cystoscopy with ureteral catheterization
• Ultrasound
• Intravenous pyelogram (IVP)

TREATMENT

APPROPRIATE HEALTH CARE Inpatient, could be outpatient if toxic appearing with acute illness

GENERAL MEASURES
• Intravenous fluid when needed
• Treatment centers on antibiotic therapy according to culture and sensitivity studies

SURGICAL MEASURES N/A

ACTIVITY As tolerated

DIET Encourage fluid

PATIENT EDUCATION
• Griffith, H. W.: Instructions for Patients; Philadelphia, W.B. Saunders Co. 1994:211

MEDICATIONS

DRUG(S) OF CHOICE
• Gentamicin, tobramycin or netilmicin 1.5 mg/kg stat, then 1 mg/kg q8h if creatinine < 1.5 mg% and ampicillin 1 gm q4h IV or cefotaxime 1 gm q6h, cefoperazone 1 gm q12h, or piperacillin 2 gm q6h. (The cephalosporins and piperacillin are probably not needed for community-acquired infections. Piperacillin for suspected Pseudomonas aeruginosa.)
• Response within 48 hours (95% of patients); discharge on appropriate oral medication (one of: trimethoprim-sulfamethoxazole 160 mg/800 mg bid, cephalexin 500 mg qid, amoxicillin 500 mg qid; nalidixic acid 1 g qid) after patient is afebrile for 48 hours, continue treatment 2 weeks for women, 6 weeks for men.
• No response within 48 hours (5% of patients) - reevaluate, review cultures, consider ultrasound or IVP if no alternative diagnosis, continue therapy
• For outpatient treatment: trimethoprim-sulfamethoxazole, cephalexin, or amoxicillin-clavulanate
Contraindications:
• Allergies to penicillin-sulfa
• In impaired kidney function - nitrofurantoin, tetracyclines, sulfonamides
Precautions:
• Follow aminoglycoside levels and renal function
• In impaired kidney function use aminoglycosides for 1-2 days only or use aztreonam
Significant possible interactions: N/A

ALTERNATIVE DRUGS N/A

FOLLOWUP

PATIENT MONITORING At 2, 6, and 12 weeks with urine culture

PREVENTION/AVOIDANCE N/A

POSSIBLE COMPLICATIONS
• Metastatic infection: skeletal system, endocardium, eye, meningitis with subsequent seizures
• May complicate the pregnancy course and produce low weight babies
• Septic shock and death
• Chronic renal insufficiency
• Complications of antibiotics

EXPECTED COURSE/PROGNOSIS 95% respond in 48 hours

MISCELLANEOUS:

ASSOCIATED CONDITIONS N/A

AGE-RELATED FACTORS
Pediatric: Nonspecific systems, jaundice, enuresis, sepsis
Geriatric:
• May present as confusion
• Characteristics may change
Others: N/A

PREGNANCY The most common medical complications requiring hospitalization

SYNONYMS Acute upper urinary tract infection

ICD-9-CM
590.1 Acute pyelonephritis
590.10 Acute pyelonephritis without lesion of medullary necrosis
590.0 Chronic pyelonephritis

SEE ALSO
Urinary tract infection in men
Urinary tract infection in women

OTHER NOTES N/A

ABBREVIATIONS N/A

REFERENCES
• Schrier RW, Gottschalk CW: Diseases of the Kidney. 5th Ed. Boston, Little, Brown, 1993
• Kaye D: The Medical Clinics of N. America, Philadelphia, WB Saunders Co, March, 1991
Illustrations: N/A
Internet references: http://www.5mcc.com

Author(s)
Jehad Y. Asfoura, MD

Pyloric stenosis

BASICS

DESCRIPTION A progressive stenosis of the pyloric canal occurring in infancy
System(s) affected: Gastrointestinal
Genetics: Multifactorial inheritance risk; recurrence risk 3-9% if first degree relative affected
Incidence/Prevalence in USA:
1/300-1/1000 live births (male 1/150 live births; female 1/750 live births)
Predominant age: Infancy; onset usually at 3-4 weeks of age, rarely in the newborn period or as late as 5 months of age
Predominant sex: Male > Female (5:1)

SIGNS AND SYMPTOMS
• Intermittent, non-bilious, projectile vomiting of increasing frequency and severity
• Initially hunger, later weakness
• Epigastric distention
• Visible gastric peristalsis, sometimes retrograde
• Palpable tumor (olive) in right upper quadrant
• Jaundice, occasional
• Late signs: dehydration, weight loss
• Diminished stools

CAUSES
• Obscure, sometimes familial; 6% risk of recurrence if either parent had pyloric stenosis, much higher if the mother was affected

RISK FACTORS 2.5 times more common in Caucasians as in blacks

DIAGNOSIS

DIFFERENTIAL DIAGNOSIS
• Inexperienced or inappropriate feeding
• Gastroesophageal reflux
• Gastritis
• Congenital adrenal hyperplasia, salt-losing
• Pyloric diaphragm

LABORATORY
• Early - evidence hypochloremic alkalosis, with low serum chloride and high bicarbonate
• Later - may have acidosis with low bicarbonate and low potassium
• Elevated unconjugated bilirubin
Drugs that may alter lab results: N/A
Disorders that may alter lab results: N/A

PATHOLOGICAL FINDINGS Concentric hypertrophy of pyloric muscle

SPECIAL TESTS Abdominal ultrasound by experienced radiologist may outline the pyloric tumor

IMAGING
• Upright plain film of abdomen may reveal dilated stomach (filled with fluid and/or air) and relative lack of air in intestines
• Barium swallow (performed only when diagnosis is not clinically clear) reveals strong gastric contractions and elongated, narrow pyloric canal (string sign)
• Ultrasound (first choice if available)

DIAGNOSTIC PROCEDURES None

TREATMENT

APPROPRIATE HEALTH CARE
• Inpatient
• Surgery: Fredet-Ramstedt pyloromyotomy

GENERAL MEASURES N/A

SURGICAL MEASURES Surgery must be preceded by preoperative preparation, including: Empty stomach with nasogastric tube, fluid replacement, correction of electrolyte imbalance

ACTIVITY N/A

DIET
• No preoperative feeding
• No feeding for 8-16 hours postoperative
• Gradual increase in feedings thereafter
• Should reach full feedings 48-72 hours after surgery

PATIENT EDUCATION Instructions about preoperative and postoperative care

MEDICATIONS

DRUG(S) OF CHOICE N/A
Contraindications: N/A
Precautions: N/A
Significant possible interactions: N/A

ALTERNATIVE DRUGS N/A

FOLLOWUP

PATIENT MONITORING Routine pediatric health maintenance

PREVENTION/AVOIDANCE N/A

POSSIBLE COMPLICATIONS None; no long term morbidity

EXPECTED COURSE/PROGNOSIS
Complete recovery with catch-up growth and weight gain

MISCELLANEOUS

ASSOCIATED CONDITIONS Usually none; rarely hiatal hernia or esophageal atresia

AGE-RELATED FACTORS
Pediatric: N/A
Geriatric: N/A
Others: N/A

PREGNANCY N/A

SYNONYMS
• Infantile hypertrophic pyloric stenosis

ICD-9-CM
• 537.0 Acquired hypertrophic pyloric stenosis
• 750.5 Congenital hypertrophic pyloric stenosis

SEE ALSO N/A

OTHER NOTES N/A

ABBREVIATIONS N/A

REFERENCES
• Rudolph AM: Pediatrics. 18th Ed. Norwalk, CT, Appleton and Lange, 1987
• Garcia VF, Randolph TG: Pyloric Stenosis: Diagnosis and Management. Pediatrics in Review 1990;11:292-296
Illustrations: N/A
Internet references: http://www.5mcc.com

Author(s)
Kurt J. Wegner, MD

Rabies

BASICS

DESCRIPTION
A rapidly progressive infection of the central nervous system caused by an RNA virus and affecting mammals, including humans
• The disease is essentially 100% fatal once symptoms develop
• Infection can be prevented by prompt, postexposure treatment of persons bitten by, or otherwise exposed to, animals known, or suspected to be, carrying the disease
System(s) affected: Nervous
Genetics: N/A
Incidence/Prevalence in USA: 0-5 cases per year in humans; about 7000 cases per year in animals; about 30,000 postexposure treatments. In US citizens - rate of rabies < 0.001/100,000/year.
Predominant age: Any
Predominant sex: Male = Female

SIGNS AND SYMPTOMS
Usually proceed through four stages, although they may overlap
• Incubation
◊ The incubation period is the time between bite and first symptoms of disease. This time is between one and three months in 2/3 of the cases. Sometimes can be as short as 6 days or longer than 6 years. It is shortest in patients with extensive bites about the head and trunk.
◊ No symptoms except bite trauma
• Prodrome
◊ Lasts 2 to 10 days
◊ Pain or paresthesia at the bite site is the most specific symptom at this stage
◊ Symptoms are often extremely variable and nonspecific, including fever, headache
◊ May be referable to any of a number of organ systems
◊ May suggest any of a number of common infections
• Acute neurologic period
◊ Lasts 2 to 10 days
◊ Symptoms referable to central nervous system dominate clinical picture
◊ Generally takes one of two forms
◊ Furious rabies: Episodes of hyperactivity last about 5 minutes and include hydrophobia, aerophobia, hyperventilation, hypersalivation and autonomic instability interspersed with periods of normalcy
◊ Paralytic rabies: Paralysis dominates clinical picture, may be ascending (like Guillain-Barré syndrome) or affect one or more limbs differentially
• Coma
◊ Last hours to days; with intensive care, may rarely last months
◊ May evolve over a few days following acute neurologic period
◊ May be sudden, with respiratory arrest
• Death
◊ Usually occurs within three weeks of onset as result of complications
◊ Only 4 survivors reported in the world's literature

CAUSES
Rabies virus, a neurotropic virus present in saliva of infected animals

RISK FACTORS
For exposure to rabies:
• Professions or activities that may expose a person to wild or domestic animals, e.g., animal handlers, some lab workers, veterinarians, spelunkers (cave explorers)
• International travel to countries where canine rabies is endemic (most common risk factor)
• In the United States, most cases appear due to exposure to bats

DIAGNOSIS

DIFFERENTIAL DIAGNOSIS
• Any rapidly progressive encephalitis; important to exclude treatable causes of encephalitis, especially herpes
• Diagnosis should be considered if there is a bite by an animal capable of transmitting the disease; however, most patients in the U.S. do not recall exposure

LABORATORY
• WBC count in cerebrospinal fluid (CSF) exam may be normal or show moderate pleocytosis
• CSF protein may be normal or moderately elevated
• Viral isolation from saliva or CSF
• Serum CSF for rabies antibody
Drugs that may alter lab results: Immunosuppressive agents
Disorders that may alter lab results: None

PATHOLOGICAL FINDINGS
Encephalitis may be found in brain biopsy, but abnormal findings may be confined to parts (brainstem, midbrain, cerebellum) only examined postmortem

SPECIAL TESTS
• Only available in state and federal reference laboratories
• Rabies antibody titer should be obtained on serum and CSF
• Skin biopsy from nape of neck should be obtained for direct fluorescent antibody examination
• Saliva culture for rabies virus

IMAGING
Normal, or nonspecific findings consistent with encephalitis

DIAGNOSTIC PROCEDURES
• Spinal tap
• Skin biopsy to detect rabies antigen in hair follicles

TREATMENT

APPROPRIATE HEALTH CARE
• Suspect rabies encephalitis - inpatient with isolation
• Exposure to rabies - inpatient if wounds serious; outpatient for prophylactic treatment

GENERAL MEASURES
• Since there is no treatment for clinical rabies, this section is directed at prevention of disease following exposure to potentially rabid animals
• Physicians should evaluate each possible exposure to rabies and consult with local or state public health officials about the need for rabies prophylaxis. In the United States, raccoons, skunks, bats, foxes, coyotes are the animals most likely to be infected, but any carnivore can carry the disease. Outside the United States, dogs are a main reservoir in many developing countries.
• Before specific antirabies treatment is initiated, consider: Types of exposure (bite or nonbite), epidemiology of rabies in involved species, circumstances of biting incident and vaccination status of exposing animal

SURGICAL MEASURES N/A

ACTIVITY As tolerated

DIET No restrictions

PATIENT EDUCATION
• Avoid wild and unknown domestic animals
• Seek treatment promptly if bitten
• Careful wound cleansing is first line of treatment

Rabies

MEDICATIONS

DRUG(S) OF CHOICE
Postexposure prophylaxis regimen
• Essential components of rabies postexposure prophylaxis are local wound treatment and both passive and active vaccination
◊ Local wound treatment: Immediate and thorough washing of all bite wounds and scratches with soap and water
◊ Passive vaccination: rabies immune globulin, human (HRIG) is administered once, at the beginning of antirabies prophylaxis. Dose of HRIG is 20 IU/kg body weight (formula is applicable for all age groups, including children). If anatomically feasible, up to one-half the dose of HRIG should be thoroughly infiltrated in the area around the wound and the rest should be administered intramuscularly in the gluteal area. HRIG should never be administered in the same syringe or into the same anatomical site as vaccine.
◊ Active vaccination: rabies vaccine, human diploid cell (HDCV) or Rabies vaccine adsorbed (RVA) should be given intramuscularly in the deltoid. For children, the anterolateral aspect of the thigh is acceptable. Gluteal area should never be used for vaccine injections.
The first dose, 1 mL, should be given as soon as possible after exposure; one additional dose should be given on days 3, 7, 14, and 28 after the first vaccination.
For the previously vaccinated, two intramuscular doses (1 mL each) of vaccine should be administered, one immediately and one 3 days later. HRIG not necessary in these patients.
Preexposure vaccination
• Should be offered to persons in high risk groups, such as veterinarians, animal handlers, certain laboratory workers, and persons spending time (e.g., one month or more) in foreign countries where rabies is enzootic
◊ Primary preexposure: IM vaccination regimen consists of three 1.0 mL injections of HDCV or RVA given in deltoid area, one each on days 0, 7, and 28. HDCV may also be given in intradermal (ID) doses, administered with a special syringe developed for that purpose (Imovax Rabies I.D. Vaccine); the 0.1 mL ID dose is administered in the deltoid area, follow the same schedule as for IM doses.
◊ For persons at frequent risk of exposure to rabies, serum should be tested every 2 years. A preexposure booster should be administered if this is less than acceptable level. If titer cannot be obtained, a booster can be administered instead.

Contraindications: None for postexposure treatment
Precautions: About 6% of persons develop mild serum sickness reaction following HDCV boosters. Mild local and systemic reactions are very common following vaccination. Mild reactions should not be a cause for interruption of immunization.
Significant possible interactions: Antibody response may be suppressed by diseases that suppress immune system

ALTERNATIVE DRUGS None

FOLLOWUP

PATIENT MONITORING After primary vaccination, serologic testing only necessary if patient has disease or takes medications that may suppress immune system

PREVENTION/AVOIDANCE See Treatment

POSSIBLE COMPLICATIONS None

EXPECTED COURSE/PROGNOSIS No postexposure failures reported in the United States since the 1970's

MISCELLANEOUS

ASSOCIATED CONDITIONS N/A

AGE-RELATED FACTORS
Pediatric: N/A
Geriatric: N/A
Others: N/A

PREGNANCY N/A

SYNONYMS Hydrophobia

ICD-9-CM 071 (clinical rabies) or V01.5 (rabies exposure) or V04.5 (inoculation or prophylactic vaccination)

SEE ALSO Animal bites

OTHER NOTES N/A

ABBREVIATIONS
• HRIG = Human rabies immune globulin
• HDCV = Human Diploid Cell Rabies Vaccine
• RVA = Rabies Vaccine Adsorbed

REFERENCES
• Fishbein DB: Rabies in humans. In: Baer G, ed. Natural History of Rabies. 2nd Ed. Boca Raton, CRC Press, 1991:519-549
• Fishbein DB, Bernard KW: Rabies virus. In: Mandell GI, et al. Principles and Practice of Infectious Disease. 4th Ed. New York, Churchill Livingstone, 1995
• Rabies Prevention - United States, 1991. Morbidity and Mortality Weekly Reports 1991;40(RR-3):1-14
Illustrations: N/A
Internet references: http://www.5mcc.com

Author(s)
Daniel B. Fishbein, MD

Radiation sickness

BASICS

DESCRIPTION Any somatic or genetic disruption of function or form caused by electromagnetic waves or accelerated atomic particles
• Acute radiation sickness: Symptoms occurring within 24 hours of exposure
• Chronic radiation syndrome: Symptoms occurring greater than 24 hours after exposure, and generally over an extended time
• Radiation measures
◊ 1 rad is the absorption of 100 ergs of energy by 1 gram of tissue
◊ 100 rads = 1 gray (Gy)
◊ The REM (Radiation Equivalent Man) unit was developed because different tissues have different sensitivities to radiation. 1 REM (Radiation Equivalent Man) is radiation dose in rads multiplied by a relative biologic effectiveness factor for the tissue involved. 100 REM = 1 sievert (Sv).
• Radiation includes:
◊ Electromagnetic emissions. Energy (and hence penetration) is inversely proportional to wave length
◊ Particles. Alpha particles are the nuclei of helium atoms and beta particles are electrons. Both have low penetrance externally but are dangerous if ingested. Neutrons are damaging and penetrate well.
System(s) affected: Gastrointestinal, Endocrine/Metabolic, Skin/Exocrine, Reproductive, Hemic/Lymphatic/Immunologic, Pulmonary, Musculoskeletal
Genetics: Females tolerate better than males. The exception is pregnant females with risk of fetal injury at low dose.
Incidence/Prevalence in USA:
• Most acute radiation injury is related to accidents or radiation therapy
• 400,000 patients receive radiation therapy yearly for malignancies
• Accidents are sporadic and usually involve small numbers of individuals
• Historically:
◊ 120,000 individuals developed acute radiation syndrome in Japan as a result of nuclear explosions
◊ 7,266 natives of the Marshall Islands were exposed to radiation due to errors in judging winds after a nuclear test in the South Pacific
◊ Chernobyl accident in Russia in 1986 where an estimated 50,000 individuals received at least 0.5 Sv of exposure.
Predominant age: N/A
Predominant sex: N/A

SIGNS AND SYMPTOMS
• Acute radiation exposure is divided into several syndromes:
◊ Less than 200 rads = no disease. There may be some nausea more than 3 hours after the event. Nausea is not a reliable sign of exposure since most people involved in an accident of this type will complain of some nausea when questioned.
◊ 200-1000 rads = hematopoietic syndrome. Acute nausea and vomiting within 3 hours. Acute granulocyte elevation, then lymphopenia, then thrombocytopenia and neutropenia, then anemia. Peak lowering of platelets and granulocytes at 3 weeks (resolving in 12 weeks). Lymphopenia may last years. Survivors may get lung or kidney changes months after. Death rate 0-80% depending on dose received and treatment. Ld 50 for humans is 650 rads.
◊ 1000-5000 rads = gastrointestinal syndrome. Nausea and vomiting 30-60 minutes postexposure. Loss of the villus structure of small bowel. Severe GI bleeding, diarrhea and abdominal pain develop in 3 days and precede the hematopoietic syndrome. Death due to blood loss or gram negative sepsis. Survivors usually die late of bone marrow suppression. Death rate 80-100%.
◊ Over 5000 rads = neurovascular syndrome or "Spock syndrome". After a 15-30 minute asymptomatic period; tremors, ataxia, vomiting, hypotension, seizures and death. Death rate 100%.

CAUSES
• Nuclear weapons
• Industrial accidents
• Nuclear power accidents
• Radiation therapy

RISK FACTORS
• Young patients more susceptible than old
• Men more sensitive than women
• Debilitated more susceptible than healthy

DIAGNOSIS

DIFFERENTIAL DIAGNOSIS
Was the patient exposed to radiation?
• Acute viral illness or anxiety cause nausea and vomiting
• Blast or heat cause skin redness
• Chemical exposure causes blistering, pain

LABORATORY
• Lymphocyte count at 48 hours post event
◊ Over 1500 = trivial or no exposure
◊ Over 1000 = survival without treatment
◊ 500-1000 = survival with treatment
◊ 100-400 = death without bone marrow transplant
◊ Under 100 = certain death
Drugs that may alter lab results:
Chemotherapeutic agents cause bone marrow suppression identical to radiation exposure
Disorders that may alter lab results: N/A

PATHOLOGICAL FINDINGS
• Hypocellular marrow with the hematopoietic syndrome
• The GI syndrome with loss of villus margin and sloughing of villus structure
• Late cases with fibrosis of lung, liver and kidney tissues
• Loss of hair indicates exposure of 350 rads and is complete at 700 rads

SPECIAL TESTS Total body dosimetry may suggest dose of compound ingested. Most radioisotopes are not excreted well.

IMAGING N/A

DIAGNOSTIC PROCEDURES N/A

TREATMENT

APPROPRIATE HEALTH CARE Inpatient

GENERAL MEASURES
• Step 1 is decontamination to reduce external radiation and collateral exposure
• IV fluids, antinauseants and bedrest
• Platelet, RBC and WBC transfusion if needed
• Antibiotics for sepsis and neutropenia
• Treatment of collateral injuries such as burns and lacerations only after decontamination

SURGICAL MEASURES
• All wounds débrided to decontaminate
• All surgery within two days before loss of white cell and platelet function
• Bone marrow transplant for severe exposure

ACTIVITY Isolation techniques for immune system injury

DIET As tolerated. Hyperalimentation for severe GI syndromes.

PATIENT EDUCATION Recommend genetic counseling and screening to persons who have been exposed to significant amounts of radiation

MEDICATIONS

DRUG(S) OF CHOICE
• Supportive therapy
  ◊ Antibiotics for enteric organisms for GI syndrome, e.g., trimethoprim-sulfamethoxazole, ciprofloxacin
  ◊ Broad spectrum antibiotics for infections common with bone marrow suppression, e.g., neutropenia
  ◊ If radioactive iodine - potassium iodide (SSKI) in doses proportional to the exposure
  ◊ If radioactive phosphorus - use parenteral magnesium sulfate
  ◊ Nonspecific ingestions - use laxatives to increase GI transit rate
Contraindications: Refer to manufacturer's literature
Precautions: Refer to manufacturer's literature
Significant possible interactions: Refer to manufacturer's literature

ALTERNATIVE DRUGS N/A

FOLLOWUP

PATIENT MONITORING
• Daily CBC, platelet, granulocyte, lymphocyte counts
• Stools for blood
• Vital signs q4h looking for sepsis

PREVENTION/AVOIDANCE Follow safety procedures

POSSIBLE COMPLICATIONS
• Long-term fibrosis of kidneys, liver and lung. Occur within 6 months of acute exposure and with as little as 300 rads of exposure.
• Radiation exposure can induce malignancies
• Increased long-term risk of leukemia (acute lymphocytic or chronic myelogenous)
• Multiple myeloma and cancers of the breast, esophagus, stomach, colon, lung, ovary, bladder, thyroid
• Sterility

EXPECTED COURSE/PROGNOSIS
• Patients surviving 12 weeks have excellent prognosis but should be monitored for long-term complications
• Hair lost usually returns within 2 months

MISCELLANEOUS

ASSOCIATED CONDITIONS N/A

AGE-RELATED FACTORS
Pediatric: More sensitive to injury
Geriatric: Less sensitive to injury
Others: N/A

PREGNANCY Injury to fetus likely

SYNONYMS N/A

ICD-9-CM 990 radiation

SEE ALSO N/A

OTHER NOTES N/A

ABBREVIATIONS N/A

REFERENCES
• Bennett JC, Plum F, eds: Cecil Textbook of Medicine. 20th Ed. Philadelphia, W.B. Saunders Co., 1996
• Kissane JM, ed: Anderson's pathology. 9th Ed. St. Louis, Mosby, 1990
• Cotran RS, Ramzi S, et al, eds: Robbins Pathological Basis of Disease. 5th Ed. Philadelphia, Saunders 1994
Illustrations: 2 available on CD-ROM
Internet references: http://www.5mcc.com

Author(s)
Vicente J. Arano, MD

Rape crisis syndrome

 BASICS

DESCRIPTION
• Definitions (legal definitions may vary slightly from state to state)
◊ Sexual contact - intentional touching of a person's intimate parts (including thighs) or the clothing covering such areas, if it is construed as being for the purpose of sexual gratification
◊ Sexual conduct - vaginal intercourse between a male and female, or anal intercourse, fellatio, or cunnilingus between persons regardless of sex
◊ Rape - any sexual penetration, however slight, using force or coercion against the person's will
◊ Sexual imposition - similar to rape but without penetration or the use of force (i.e., non-consenting sexual contact)
◊ Gross sexual imposition - non-consenting sexual contact with the use of force
◊ Corruption of a minor - sexual conduct by an individual 18 years old or greater with an individual less than 15 years of age
System(s) affected: Nervous, Reproductive
Genetics: N/A
Incidence/Prevalence in USA:
• Over 100,000 cases of alleged rape reported in US every year
• Estimated that only 1 in 5 to 1 in 10 adult cases reported
• Estimated only 1 in 15 to 1 in 20 pediatric cases reported
• Estimated incidence of reported rape is 80/100,000 females (7% of violent crime)
Predominant age:
• Majority of adult victims are female in teens and 20's, (reported as high as 97 years)
• Pediatric victims may be either gender with predominance of females. Reported as young as 2 months.
• Increasing numbers of adult male victims presenting for treatment
Predominant sex: Female > Male

SIGNS AND SYMPTOMS
• In adults
◊ History of sexual penetration
◊ Sexual contact, or sexual conduct without consent and/or with the use of force
• In pediatrics
◊ Actual observation of, or suspicion of, sexual penetration, sexual contact, or sexual conduct
◊ Signs include evidence of the use of force and/or evidence of sexual contact (e.g., presence of semen and/or sperm)

CAUSES   Listed with Description

RISK FACTORS
• Numerous
• About 50% of rapes occur in the home, with 1/3 of these involving a male intruder

 DIAGNOSIS

DIFFERENTIAL DIAGNOSIS   Consenting sex among adults

LABORATORY
• Record results of wet mount noting the presence or absence of sperm and, if present, whether or not it is motile or immotile
• If indicated, a serum or urine pregnancy test should be obtained and the results recorded
Drugs that may alter lab results: N/A
Disorders that may alter lab results: N/A

PATHOLOGICAL FINDINGS   N/A

SPECIAL TESTS   N/A

IMAGING   N/A

DIAGNOSTIC PROCEDURES
• History:
◊ Record in patient's own words in so far as possible. Include date, approximate time, and general location as best possible. Document physical abuse other than sexual. Describe all types of sexual contact whether actual/or attempted. History of alcohol and/or drugs before or after alleged incident.
◊ Document time of last activity which could possibly alter specimens (e.g., bath, shower, or douche). Thorough gynecologic history is mandatory including last menstrual period (LMP), last consenting sexual contact, contraceptive practice, and prior gynecologic surgery.
• Physical examination:
◊ Use of drawings and/or photographs is encouraged. Use of UV light (Wood's lamp) to detect seminal stains on clothing or skin. Document all signs of trauma or unusual marks. Documentation of mental status/emotional state.
◊ Complete genital-rectal examination including evidence of trauma, secretions, or discharge. Use of a non-lubricated, water moistened speculum is mandatory since commonly used lubricants may destroy evidence.

 TREATMENT

APPROPRIATE HEALTH CARE
• Contact appropriate social services agency
• Majority of adult victims can be treated as outpatients unless associated trauma (physical or mental) requires admission
• Majority of pediatric sexual assault/abuse victims will require admission or outside placement until appropriate social agency can evaluate home environment

GENERAL MEASURES
• Providing health care to victims of sexual assault/abuse requires special sensitivity and privacy
• All such cases MUST be reported immediately to the appropriate law enforcement agency
• With the victim's permission, utilize personnel from local support agency(ies) (e.g., Rape Crisis Center). When available, use of in-house Social Services is extremely helpful to victim/family.
• Sedation and tetanus prophylaxis should be utilized when indicated
• Venereal disease prevention for gonorrhea/Chlamydia should be administered
• A discussion of possible pregnancy and pregnancy termination should be held with the victim. If hospital policy precludes such a discussion, then information about this option should be offered the victim via the followup mechanisms.
• Suspected HIV and hepatitis B exposure and testing should be discussed with the victim and be in keeping with hospital policies/protocols. The initial HIV test should be completed within seven days of the suspected exposure.

SURGICAL MEASURES   N/A

ACTIVITY   No restrictions

DIET   No restrictions

PATIENT EDUCATION
• Information and help available from local rape crisis support organizations
• National Institute of Mental Health, Public Inquiries Branch, Office of Scientific Information, Dept. of Health and Human Services, Parklawn Bldg., Room 15C-05, 5600 Fishers Lane, Rockville, MD 20857, (301)443-4513

Rape crisis syndrome

 MEDICATIONS

DRUG(S) OF CHOICE
• For gonorrhea - ceftriaxone 250 mg IM once or cefixime 400 mg po. Alternative medications would include spectinomycin, ciprofloxacin, norfloxacin, ampicillin/probenecid, or amoxicillin/probenecid.
• For chlamydia - azithromycin (Zithromax) 1.0 g po single dose; or doxycycline 100 mg po bid or tetracycline 250 mg qid for 10 days. If the patient is pregnant, erythromycin should be used, 500 mg every 6 hours.
• Specific treatment for vulvovaginitis if present
• Note - gonorrhea and chlamydia medications may be given concomitantly
Contraindications: Refer to manufacturer's literature
Precautions: Refer to manufacturer's literature
Significant possible interactions: Refer to manufacturer's literature

ALTERNATIVE DRUGS N/A

 FOLLOWUP

PATIENT MONITORING
• The patient should be seen in seven to ten days for followup care, including pregnancy testing, and counselling by a gynecologist or appropriate gynecologic clinic
• Close examination for vaginitis and treatment if necessary
• Followup test for syphilis and gonorrhea should occur in five to six weeks
• Followup testing for AIDS and hepatitis B should occur in six months
• Telephone numbers of counselling agency(ies) which can provide counselling/legal services to the patient should be provided
• Consider Sexual Assault Nurse Examiner (SANE) if available in area

PREVENTION/AVOIDANCE
• Scope of rape prevention is too complex and too broad to be discussed in these pages. True prevention will require many changes.
• Women may benefit from assertiveness training and self-defense training

POSSIBLE COMPLICATIONS
• Sexually transmitted disease and subsequent treatment
• Pregnancy (with the possibility of abortion)
• Trauma (physical and mental)

EXPECTED COURSE/PROGNOSIS
• Acute phase (usually 1-3 weeks following rape) - shaking, pain, wound healing, mood swings, appetite loss, crying. Also feelings of grief, shame, anger, fear, revenge or guilt.
• Late or chronic phase female victim may develop fear of intercourse, fear of men, nightmares, sleep disorders, daytime flashbacks, fear of being alone, loss of self-esteem, anxiety, depression, post-traumatic stress syndrome
• Recovery may be prolonged. Patients who are able to talk about their feelings seem to have a faster recovery.

 MISCELLANEOUS

ASSOCIATED CONDITIONS N/A

AGE-RELATED FACTORS
Pediatric: Assurance to the child that he or she is a good person and was not the cause of the incident
Geriatric: N/A
Others: N/A

PREGNANCY Baseline pregnancy test conducted. Pregnancy prevention discussed with patient.

SYNONYMS
• Sexual assault
• Rape trauma

ICD-9-CM V71.5

SEE ALSO N/A

OTHER NOTES
• Rape is a legal term and the examining physician is encouraged to use terminology such as "alleged rape" or "alleged sexual conduct".
• In majority of states, wife may now accuse husband of rape if they are estranged and living apart
• Since "consent defense" is common, documentation of evidence supporting the use of force or the administration of drugs/alcohol is imperative
• The use of a protocol is encouraged to assure every victim a uniform, comprehensive evaluation regardless of the expertise of the examining physician. The protocol must ensure that all evidence is properly collected and labeled, chain-of-custody is maintained, and the evidence is sent to the most appropriate forensic laboratory.
• All medical records must be well documented and legible
• All medical personnel must be willing and able to testify on behalf of the patient

ABBREVIATIONS N/A

REFERENCES
• Harwood-Nuss A, ed: The Clinical Practice of Emergency Medicine 2nd ed. Philadelphia, J.B. Lippincott-Raven, 1996
• Tintinalli JE, ed: Emergency Medicine: A Comprehensive Study Guide 4th ed. New York, McGraw-Hill, 1996
• Young WW, et al: Sexual Assault: Review of a National Model Protocol for Forensic and Medical Evaluation. Obs & Gyn 1992;80:5, 878-883
Illustrations: N/A
Internet references: http://www.5mcc.com

Author(s)
Daniel T. Schelble, MD, FACEP

Raynaud's phenomenon

 BASICS

 DIAGNOSIS

 TREATMENT

DESCRIPTION
Bilaterally occurring vasospastic disorder manifested by intermittent attacks of extreme pallor, then cyanosis of the fingers (rarely, of the toes) brought on by cold exposure. With warming, vasodilatation and intense redness develops, followed by swelling, throbbing, paresthesias. Resolves with warming. May accompany emotional upset. Thumbs rarely involved. 13% may progress to atrophy of digital fat pads, ischemic ulcers of fingertips. 50% idiopathic or primary Raynaud's disease, 50% secondary (Raynaud's phenomenon).
• Disease: progressive, symmetrical. Involves fingers; rarely toes. Ages 15 to 45. Spasm is more frequent, more severe with time. No gangrene; rarely ulcerates. Diagnose only after 2 years if no underlying associated disease. May be associated with coronary vasospasm or primary pulmonary hypertension. No histologic abnormality found in digital arteries.
• Phenomenon: may be unilateral, asymmetric; may affect only one or two fingers. Underlying condition usually identifiable with time. Usually has a worse morbidity and prognosis than primary disease.
System(s) affected: Skin/Exocrine, Musculoskeletal, Hemic/Lymphatic/Immunologic
Genetics: Little information available, but some suggest a dominant inheritance pattern. One study suggests there is a 5-fold increase in Raynaud's in family members of a Raynaud's patient. (Arthritis Rheum 1996; 39:1189-91)
Incidence/Prevalence in USA: 4 to 10% of population (based on reporting of characteristic color changes, cold intolerance)
Predominant age: After 40
Predominant sex:
• Female > Male (4:1 in primary form)
• Male = Female (secondary form)

SIGNS AND SYMPTOMS
• Pallor/whiteness of fingertips with cold exposure, followed by cyanosis, then redness and pain with warming
• Ulceration of finger pads, progressing to autoamputation in severe, prolonged cases (10-13% of cases)
• Normal physical exam in primary; may show signs of underlying vasospastic or autoimmune disease in secondary form

CAUSES
Unknown. May involve increased sensitivity of alpha-2-adrenergic receptors in digital vessels in primary type. Serotonin receptors (5-HT2 type) may be involved in secondary Raynaud's. Platelet and blood viscosity abnormalities also implicated.

RISK FACTORS
• Smoking
• Existing autoimmune or connective tissue disorder

DIFFERENTIAL DIAGNOSIS
• Thromboangiitis obliterans (Buerger's disease) - primarily affects men; involves legs and feet; less than 5% have hand involvement, 90% have Raynaud's; smoking related
• Rheumatoid arthritis
• Progressive systemic sclerosis (scleroderma) - 90% have Raynaud's; Raynaud's may precede other symptoms by years
• Systemic lupus
• Carpal tunnel syndrome
• Thoracic outlet syndrome
• CREST syndrome (calcinosis cutis, Raynaud's phenomenon, esophageal dysmotility, sclerodactyly and telangiectasia)
• Cryoglobulinemias
• Waldenström's macroglobulinemia
• Acrocyanosis
• Polycythemia
• Occupational injury (especially from vibrating tools, masonry work, etc.)
• Drugs (beta-blockers, clonidine, ergotamine, methysergide, amphetamines, bromocriptine, bleomycin, vinblastine, cisplatin, cyclosporine).

LABORATORY
Tests for underlying secondary causes (CBC, ESR, RA, ANA, immunoelectrophoresis, esophageal motility studies)
Drugs that may alter lab results: N/A
Disorders that may alter lab results: N/A

PATHOLOGICAL FINDINGS
Histology of skin biopsy correlates poorly with clinical presentation. May show edema, necrotizing or non-necrotizing vasculitis, and/or perivasculitis.

SPECIAL TESTS
• Cold challenge test to elicit characteristic color changes in hands
• Nailfold capillaroscopy to detect enlarged, irregular capillary loops of other connective tissue diseases (primary Raynaud's should show normal vasculature)

IMAGING
Rarely, cases may demonstrate osteolysis of distal metaphyseal portions of phalanges, tapering and calcification of soft tissues

DIAGNOSTIC PROCEDURES
Diagnosis largely determined by history, provocative exposure to cold

APPROPRIATE HEALTH CARE
Outpatient management usually sufficient

GENERAL MEASURES
• Dress warmly, wear gloves, avoid cold
• No smoking
• Avoid beta-blockers, amphetamines, ergot alkaloids, sumatriptan
• Biofeedback techniques to teach patients to increase hand temperature
• Finger guards over ulcerated fingertips

SURGICAL MEASURES
Cervical sympathectomy effect is transient - symptoms return in 1 to 2 years

ACTIVITY
Avoidance of situations in which exposure to cold is likely; avoid vibrating tools

DIET
No special diet

PATIENT EDUCATION
Emphasis on smoking cessation. Avoidance of aggravating factors (trauma, vibration, cold, etc.).

MEDICATIONS

DRUG(S) OF CHOICE
• Nifedipine 30-90 mg daily (sustained release form). (May only be needed during winter). Up to 75% experience improvement.
• Symptomatic responses do not correlate with objective evidence of improvement
Contraindications: Allergy to drug, pregnancy, congestive heart failure
Precautions: May cause headache, dizziness, lightheadedness, hypotension
Significant possible interactions:
• Increases serum level of digoxin - monitor digoxin levels closely after nifedipine added
• Cimetidine increases nifedipine level - may require dosage adjustment
• May increase prothrombin time in patients taking warfarin

ALTERNATIVE DRUGS
• Use of diltiazem, verapamil, reserpine, methyldopa, prazosin have equivocal support in literature
• Captopril studies suggest benefit, but need further evaluation (not FDA approved)
• Parenteral and oral prostacyclin have offered subjective improvement, but the effect is short-lived and not statistically significant
• Nitroglycerin patches may also be helpful, but limited by the incidence of severe headache

FOLLOWUP

PATIENT MONITORING
• Management of fingertip ulcers, including rapid treatment of infection
• Continue to observe for signs of associated illnesses, since Raynaud's may precede overt development of these conditions by an average of 11 years

PREVENTION/AVOIDANCE
• Avoid trauma to fingertips
• Avoid exposure to cold
• Smoking cessation

POSSIBLE COMPLICATIONS   Gangrene, autoamputation of fingertips

EXPECTED COURSE/PROGNOSIS
• Prolonged course with recurrent ischemia, ulceration
• In case of secondary phenomenon, may eventually develop hallmarks of underlying disease
• 50% of 64 patients with secondary Raynaud's developed a connective tissue disease within 8 years. (J Rheumatol 1995; 22:2226-32)

MISCELLANEOUS

ASSOCIATED CONDITIONS
• Lupus
• Rheumatoid arthritis
• Scleroderma
• Polymyositis
• Sjögren's
• Occlusive vascular disease
• Cryoglobulinemia
• Use of vibrating tools

AGE-RELATED FACTORS
Pediatric: Associated with systemic lupus erythematosus and scleroderma in children
Geriatric: Appearance of Raynaud's after 40 almost always indicates an underlying disease
Others: N/A

PREGNANCY   N/A

SYNONYMS   N/A

ICD-9-CM   443.0

SEE ALSO   N/A

OTHER NOTES   N/A

ABBREVIATIONS   N/A

REFERENCES
• Isselbacher KJ, et al, eds: Harrison's Principles of Internal Medicine. 13th Ed. New York, McGraw-Hill, 1994
• Maricq HR, et al: Prevalence of Raynaud phenomenon in the general population. A preliminary study by questionnaire. J Chronic Dis 1986;39:423
• Coffman JD: Raynaud's phenomenon: an update. Hypertension 1991;17:593
Illustrations: 2 available on CD-ROM
Internet references: http://www.5mcc.com

Author(s)
John E. Perchalski, MD, FAAFP

Rectal prolapse

 BASICS

 DIAGNOSIS

 TREATMENT

DESCRIPTION
Protrusion of the rectum through the anus
• Partial prolapse - involves only mucosa. This frequently follows anal operative procedures. (Radial rectal folds prolapsed through anus).
• Complete prolapse - involves the entire rectal wall (procidentia). This type occurs most commonly as a spontaneous event in children and complication of other disorders in the elderly. (Concentric rectal folds prolapsed through anus).
System(s) affected: Gastrointestinal
Genetics: Unknown
Incidence/Prevalence in USA: 4.2:1000 overall; 10:1000 after age 65 years
Predominant age: 2 years in children, 60-70 years in adults
Predominant sex: Male > Female (5:1 in adults, and a slight predominance in children)

SIGNS AND SYMPTOMS
• Children
  ◊ Sensation of anal mass
  ◊ Pain
  ◊ Rectal bleeding
  ◊ Protruding mass
• Adults
  ◊ Anorectal pain or discomfort during defecation
  ◊ Feeling of incomplete evacuation
  ◊ Rectal and urinary incontinence
  ◊ Rectal bleeding or discharge

CAUSES
• Children
  ◊ Idiopathic (most common)
  ◊ Abnormal innervation of levator ani muscle complex, puborectalis or anal sphincters or abnormal anatomic relationships of these muscle groups
• Adults
  ◊ Diastasis of levator ani
  ◊ Loose endopelvic fascia
  ◊ Loss of normal horizontal position of rectum
  ◊ Weak anal sphincter

RISK FACTORS
• Myelomeningocele
• Exstrophy of the bladder
• Cystic fibrosis
• Chronic constipation or diarrhea
• Imperforate anus
• Multiple sclerosis
• Stroke/paralysis
• Dementia

DIFFERENTIAL DIAGNOSIS
• Intussusception
• Rectal polyps
• Hemorrhoids

LABORATORY N/A
Drugs that may alter lab results: N/A
Disorders that may alter lab results: N/A

PATHOLOGICAL FINDINGS N/A

SPECIAL TESTS N/A

IMAGING
Barium enema is useful in selected cases of recurrent rectal prolapse

DIAGNOSTIC PROCEDURES
Sigmoidoscopy is useful in recurrent prolapse to rule out rectal lesions

APPROPRIATE HEALTH CARE
Outpatient, unless complications occur or surgical intervention required

GENERAL MEASURES
• Acute
  ◊ Prompt manual reduction of prolapse
  ◊ Treatment of diarrhea or constipation

SURGICAL MEASURES
• Recurrent
  ◊ Sub-mucosal injection of 5% phenol in glycerine in four quadrants under general anesthesia (outpatient)
  ◊ Linear electrocauterization (inpatient)
  ◊ Transabdominal Ripstein's procedure (suspension of rectum from sacrum by means of artificial material)
  ◊ Posterior sagittal rectal suspension and levator repair
  ◊ Ivalon sponge wrap procedure
  ◊ Anterior resection of rectum
  ◊ Transabdominal proctopexy (no artificial material used)
  ◊ Perineal rectosigmoidectomy
  ◊ Thiersch's wire (outpatient procedure; may be modified by using Marlex or Silastic strip instead of wire); used more commonly in children and elderly, poor-risk adults
  ◊ Gracilis Sling procedure

ACTIVITY Full activity, when able

DIET High fiber

PATIENT EDUCATION
• Particular reassurance to parents of infants with prolapse regarding benign nature of problem and high rate of spontaneous resolution
• Diet instructions
• Teach measures to avoid constipation

Rectal prolapse

 MEDICATIONS

DRUG(S) OF CHOICE
• Mineral oil
• Stool softeners
• Lactulose
Contraindications: N/A
Precautions: N/A
Significant possible interactions: N/A

ALTERNATIVE DRUGS N/A

 FOLLOWUP

PATIENT MONITORING Monthly visits until possible need for surgery has been determined or until prolapse has resolved

PREVENTION/AVOIDANCE Avoid constipation and diarrhea

POSSIBLE COMPLICATIONS
• Mucosal ulcerations
• Necrosis of rectal wall

EXPECTED COURSE/PROGNOSIS
• Spontaneous resolution expected in most children
• 5-10% recurrence rate for most procedures
• Good prognosis with treatment

 MISCELLANEOUS

ASSOCIATED CONDITIONS
• Cystic fibrosis
• Myelomeningocele
• Exstrophy of the bladder
• Chronic constipation or diarrhea
• Imperforate anus
• Paraplegia
• Stroke
• Incontinence

AGE-RELATED FACTORS
Pediatric: Idiopathic most common type of rectal prolapse in children
Geriatric: Common problem in the elderly
Others: N/A

PREGNANCY N/A

SYNONYMS N/A

ICD-9-CM 569.1

SEE ALSO
• Intussusception
• Hemorrhoids

OTHER NOTES N/A

ABBREVIATIONS N/A

REFERENCES
• Ashcraft KW, Garred JL, Holder TM, et al: Rectal prolapse: 17 year experience with the posterior repair and suspension. J Ped Surg 1990; 25(9): 992-995
• Holder TM, Ashcraft KW, eds: Pediatric Surgery. 2nd Ed. Philadelphia, W.B. Saunders Co., 1993
• Schwartz SI, Shires GT, Spencer FC, et al, eds: Principles of Surgery. 6th Ed. New York, McGraw-Hill Book Co., 1994
• Welch KG, Randolph JG, Ravitch MM, et al, eds: Pediatric Surgery. 4th Ed. Chicago, Year Book Medical Publishers, 1986
Illustrations: N/A
Internet references: http://www.5mcc.com

Author(s)
Timothy L. Black, MD, FACS, FAAP
James P. Miller, MD, FACS, FAAP

Refractive errors

 BASICS

DESCRIPTION
An inability of the eye to produce a focused image on the fovea or central part of the retina
- Emmetropia: When light rays are in perfect focus, the image being viewed is seen clearly
- Ametropia: Any refractive error of the eye which prevents normal focusing of the image
- Hyperopia: When the cornea of the eye is too flat or the eye is too short, light rays fall in focus behind the retina, and an individual is "farsighted"
- Myopia: When the cornea is too steep or the length of the eyeball is too long, light rays fall short of the retina, and the human eye is "nearsighted"
- Presbyopia: The natural tendency of the human crystalline lens to harden or become sclerotic, limiting the focusing of the eye on near objects (accommodation)
- Astigmatism: When the cornea is steeper in one meridian more than the other or the globe is not round (oval or almond-shaped), visual blurriness occurs

System(s) affected: Nervous
Genetics: Refractive errors are inherited
Incidence/Prevalence in USA: 70% of the general population have some form of ametropia
Predominant age: Refractive errors are present at birth, but not usually detected until puberty
Predominant sex: Male = Female

SIGNS AND SYMPTOMS
- Difficulty seeing objects at a distance
- Difficulty focusing on near objects
- Difficulty reading
- Squinting
- Headaches (from squinting)

CAUSES
- Developmental (most common)
- Ocular trauma
- Iatrogenic (e.g. post cataract removal)

RISK FACTORS N/A

 DIAGNOSIS

DIFFERENTIAL DIAGNOSIS
- Corneal disease
- Cataract
- Retinal abnormalities
- Diseases of the optic nerve

LABORATORY N/A
Drugs that may alter lab results: N/A
Disorders that may alter lab results: N/A

PATHOLOGICAL FINDINGS N/A

SPECIAL TESTS
- Pinhole vision test: To distinguish a refractive error from an organic cause of visual blurring, have the patient look through a pinhole in a card without a corrective lens. Patient's with a pure refractive error improve their vision since the pinhole blocks nonparallel and unfocusable rays of light.

IMAGING N/A

DIAGNOSTIC PROCEDURES
- Methods:
  ◊ Objective streak retinoscopy can be used to measure the degree of refractive error in spherocylinder correction for the proper spectacle or contact lens
  ◊ Antimuscarinic agents, e.g., clopentolate (Cyclogyl), tropicamide (Mydriacyl) applied topically paralyze the ciliary body, preventing accommodation. Cycloplegic refraction can then be performed.
- Age-related testing:
  ◊ Newborns should be examined for general eye health; ophthalmologic evaluation indicated for any discovered problems
  ◊ Vision screening should occur at each well child visit
  ◊ Visual acuity testing should be performed at approximately 3 1/2 years
  ◊ Visual acuity and motility testing should be performed at age 5
  ◊ Visual acuity should be retested prior to obtaining a driver's license, at age 40, and every 2-4 years until age 65, when evaluations are recommended every 1-2 years

 TREATMENT

APPROPRIATE HEALTH CARE
Outpatient

GENERAL MEASURES
- Spectacle lenses (glasses)
- Soft and hard contact lenses

SURGICAL MEASURES
- Radial keratotomy: With topical anesthesia, using a surgical diamond keratome, multiple (4-8) radial incisions are placed onto the surface of the peripheral cornea to flatten the central, optical zone. The length, depth and proximity of the incision to the central optical zone determines its effect, and degree of correction obtained. Radial keratotomy is safe and effective and corrects nearsightedness, astigmatism or a combination of both, after the age of 18 when the prescription has stabilized.
- Automated lamellar keratoplasty: A microsurgical dermatome removes a layer of the superficial cornea to induce flattening. It is presently available in the United States, though its use is still investigational.
- Excimer laser: The laser photoblates corneal tissue from the central visual axis, thus flattening it. Following the procedure, the cornea must re-epithelialize. Healing takes several months, during which there is a mild haze and blurring of vision. FDA approved Oct, 1995. Considered investigational.

ACTIVITY N/A

DIET N/A

PATIENT EDUCATION
- All patients should have their eyes examined when starting school, and periodically thereafter
- The options of eyeglasses, contact lenses and permanent surgical correction of refractive errors should be considered
- Aggressive control of diabetes mellitus should be encouraged

MEDICATIONS

DRUG(S) OF CHOICE N/A
Contraindications: N/A
Precautions: Antimuscarinic agents may induce acute glaucoma, via acute angle closure
Significant possible interactions: N/A

ALTERNATIVE DRUGS N/A

FOLLOWUP

PATIENT MONITORING
• Routine annual adult eye exams in individuals < age 40 are not indicated
• Individuals with risks will need ocular exams as indicated by their conditions

PREVENTION/AVOIDANCE N/A

POSSIBLE COMPLICATIONS
• Amblyopia
• Poor school performance

EXPECTED COURSE/PROGNOSIS
Good if discovered early and corrected appropriately.

MISCELLANEOUS

ASSOCIATED CONDITIONS Patients with diabetes mellitus have fluctuating myopia as a result of poorly controlled blood glucose and concomitant swelling of the crystalline lens

AGE-RELATED FACTORS
Pediatric: Refractive errors can be detected early in life
Geriatric: Presbyopia occurs in later life
Others: Individuals over the age of 40 are more likely to experience presbyopia or normal loss of accommodation which occurs with age, necessitating the use of reading glasses for close work

PREGNANCY It is not unusual for refractive errors to be temporarily worsened during pregnancy due to hormonal changes in tear function and corneal swelling

SYNONYMS N/A

ICD-9-CM
367.0 Hyperopia
367.1 Myopia
367.4 Presbyopia
367.21 Astigmatism, regular

SEE ALSO
• Amblyopia

OTHER NOTES Fax-On-Demand service of American Academy of Ophthalmology for policy statement and patient education materials (908)935-2761

ABBREVIATIONS N/A

REFERENCES
• Kershner RM: Lessons from the Practice: The Gift of Sight – A Guide to Understanding Your Eyes. Thorofare, NJ, Slack, Inc., 1994
• Infant and Children's Vision Screening. American Academy of Ophthalmology - Policy Statement (#812), June, 1991
• Frequency of Ocular exams. American Academy of Ophthalmology - Policy Statement (#808), Sept, 1990
Illustrations: N/A
Internet references: http://www.5mcc.com

Author(s)
Robert M. Kershner, MD, FACS

Reiter's syndrome

BASICS

DESCRIPTION   A triad of features including arthritis, conjunctivitis, and urethritis or cervicitis. Epidemiologically similar to other reactive arthritis syndromes characterized by sterile inflammation of joints from infections originating at non-articular sites. A fourth feature may be buccal ulceration or balanitis. (It is possible for only two features to be present.)
• Two forms:
  ◊ Sexually transmitted; symptoms usually begin 7-14 days after exposure
  ◊ Post-dysentery
System(s) affected: Musculoskeletal, Skin/Exocrine, Renal/Urologic
Genetics: HLA-B27 tissue antigen present in 60-80% of patients
Incidence/Prevalence in USA: 0.24-1.5% incidence after epidemics of bacterial dysentery; complicates 1-2% cases of non-gonococcal urethritis
Predominant age: 20-40 years
Predominant sex: Male > Female

SIGNS AND SYMPTOMS
• Musculoskeletal:
  ◊ Asymmetric arthritis (especially knees, ankles, MTP joints)
  ◊ Enthesopathy (inflammation at tendinous insertion into bone) such as plantar fasciitis, digital periostitis, Achilles tendinitis
  ◊ Spondyloarthropathy (spine and sacroiliac joint involvement)
• Urogenital tract:
  ◊ Urethritis
  ◊ Prostatitis
  ◊ Occasionally cystitis
  ◊ Balanitis
  ◊ Cervicitis - usually asymptomatic
• Eye:
  ◊ Conjunctivitis of one or both eyes
  ◊ Occasionally scleritis, keratitis, corneal ulceration
  ◊ Rarely uveitis and iritis
• Skin:
  ◊ Mucocutaneous lesions (small, painless, superficial ulcers on oral mucosa, tongue, glans penis)
  ◊ Keratoderma blennorrhagica (hyperkeratotic skin lesions of palms and soles and around nails)
• Cardiovascular:
  ◊ Occasionally pericarditis, murmur, conduction defects, aortic incompetence
• Nervous system:
  ◊ Rarely peripheral neuropathy, cranial neuropathy, meningoencephalitis, neuropsychiatric changes
• Constitutional:
  ◊ Fever, malaise, anorexia, weight loss
  ◊ Can appear seriously ill (fever, rigors, tachycardia, exquisitely tender joints)

CAUSES
• Chlamydia trachomatis the usual causative organism of postvenereal variety
• Dysenteric form following enteric bacterial infection due to Shigella, Salmonella, Yersinia, and Campylobacter organisms. This form more likely in women, children and the elderly.

RISK FACTORS
• Sexual intercourse 7-14 days prior to illness
• Food poisoning or bacterial dysenteric outbreak

DIAGNOSIS

DIFFERENTIAL DIAGNOSIS
• For specific diagnosis, arthritis associated with urethritis for longer than one month
• Rheumatoid arthritis
• Ankylosing spondylitis
• Arthritis associated with inflammatory bowel disease
• Psoriatic arthritis
• Juvenile rheumatoid arthritis
• Bacterial arthritis including gonococcal

LABORATORY
• Blood
  ◊ WBC 10,000-20,000
  ◊ Neutrophilic leukocytosis
  ◊ Elevated erythrocyte sedimentation rate
  ◊ Moderate normochromic anemia
  ◊ Hypergammaglobulinemia
• Synovial fluid
  ◊ WBC 1000-8000 cells/mm3
  ◊ Bacterial culture negative
• Collaborative tests
  ◊ Cultures or serology positive for Chlamydia trachomatis, or stools positive for Salmonella, Shigella, Yersinia or Campylobacter support the diagnosis
Drugs that may alter lab results: Antibiotics may affect isolation of the bacterial pathogens
Disorders that may alter lab results: N/A

PATHOLOGICAL FINDINGS
• A seronegative spondyloarthropathy (similar to ankylosing spondylitis, enteric arthritis and psoriatic arthritis)
• Villous formation in joints
• Joint hyperemia
• Joint inflammation
• Prostatitis
• Seminal vesiculitis
• Skin biopsy similar to psoriasis
• Non-specific conjunctivitis

SPECIAL TESTS   Histocompatibility antigen HLA-B27 positive in 60-80% of cases in non-HIV related Reiter's

IMAGING
• X-ray
  ◊ Periosteal proliferation, thickening
  ◊ Spurs
  ◊ Erosions at articular margins
  ◊ Residual joint destruction
  ◊ Syndesmophytes (spine)
  ◊ Sacroiliitis

DIAGNOSTIC PROCEDURES   N/A

TREATMENT

APPROPRIATE HEALTH CARE   Inpatient possibly, during acute phase

GENERAL MEASURES
• Treatment is symptomatic
• No treatment necessary for conjunctivitis. Iritis may require treatment.
• Treatment unnecessary for mucocutaneous lesions
• Physical therapy during recovery phase
• Arthritis may be prominent and disabling during the acute phase

SURGICAL MEASURES   N/A

ACTIVITY   Bedrest until joint inflammation subsides

DIET   No special diet

PATIENT EDUCATION
• Teach home physical therapy techniques
• For a listing of sources for patient education materials favorably reviewed on this topic, physicians may contact: American Academy of Family Physicians Foundation, P.O. Box 8418, Kansas City, MO 64114, (800)274-2237, ext. 4400
• Arthritis Foundation, 1314 Spring Street N.W., Atlanta, GA 30309, (404)872-7100

MEDICATIONS

DRUG(S) OF CHOICE
• Symptomatic management - NSAID's including indomethacin, naproxen; intraarticular or systemic corticosteroids for refractory arthritis and enthesitis
• Specific treatment of pathogenic microorganism should be attempted:
  ◊ C. trachomatis - doxycycline 100 mg po bid for 7-14 days
  ◊ Salmonella, Shigella, Yersinia Campylobacter infections - ciprofloxacin 500 mg po bid for 5 days (course may be extended to 14-28 days to eradicate chronic carrier state)
• For gastrointestinal upset - antacids
• For iritis - intraocular steroids
• For keratitis - topical steroids
Contraindications:
• Gastrointestinal bleeding
• Patients with peptic ulcer, gastritis, ulcerative colitis
• Renal insufficiency
Precautions: Refer to manufacturer's literature
Significant possible interactions: Refer to manufacturer's literature

ALTERNATIVE DRUGS
• Aspirin or other NSAID's
• Sulfasalazine is promising, but not yet approved
• Methotrexate or azathioprine in severe cases (still experimental and not approved or agreed to be effective. Contraindicated, if HIV related Reiter's).
• Consultation with specialist recommended when considering immunomodulatory agents such as sulfasalazine, methotrexate or azathioprine

FOLLOWUP

PATIENT MONITORING Monitor clinical response to medications. Surveillance for complications of therapy, sulfasalazine, immunosuppressives.

PREVENTION/AVOIDANCE N/A

POSSIBLE COMPLICATIONS
• Chronic or recurrent disease in 5-50%
• Ankylosing spondylitis develops in 30-50% of HLA-B27 positive patients
• Urethral strictures
• Cataracts and blindness
• Aortic root necrosis

EXPECTED COURSE/PROGNOSIS
• Urethritis within 1-15 days after sexual exposure
• Onset of Reiter's syndrome within 10-30 days of infection
• Mean duration 19 weeks
• Poor prognosis associated with local disease involving heel, eye or heart

MISCELLANEOUS

ASSOCIATED CONDITIONS
• Prior shigellosis
• Salmonellosis
• Yersinia infection
• Mycoplasma or ureaplasma infection
• Chlamydia urethritis
• HIV infection

AGE-RELATED FACTORS
Pediatric: Enteric etiology more likely than chlamydia
Geriatric: Enteric etiology more likely than sexually transmitted
Others: N/A

PREGNANCY No special considerations other than usual precautions regarding drugs

SYNONYMS
• Idiopathic blennorrheal arthritis
• Arthritis urethritica
• Urethro-oculo-articular syndrome
• Fiessinger-Leroy-Reiter disease

ICD-9-CM 099.3 Reiter's disease

SEE ALSO
• Behçet's syndrome
• Ankylosing spondylitis
• Arthritis, psoriatic

OTHER NOTES Effects of antibiotics on the development and long-term outcome of Reiter's syndrome not known

ABBREVIATIONS N/A

REFERENCES
• Kean WF, MacPherson DW: Reiter's syndrome. In: Bellamy N, ed. Prognosis in the Rheumatic Diseases. London, Kluwer Academic Publishers, 1991
• Rein MF: Urethritis. In: Mandell GL, Douglas RG, Bennett JE, eds. Principles and Practice of Infectious Diseases. 3rd Ed. New York, Churchill Livingstone, 1990
• Hughes RA, Keat AC: Reiter's syndrome and reactive arthritis: A current view. Sem in Arthritis and Rheumatism 1994;24(3):190-210
Illustrations: 3 available on CD-ROM
Internet references: http://www.5mcc.com

Author(s)
E. R. Jeans, MD, BSc, FRCPC
D. W. MacPherson, MD, MSc (CTM), FRCPC

Renal calculi

BASICS

DESCRIPTION Renal stones occur throughout the urinary tract and are common causes of pain, infection and obstruction. The pathogenesis is multifactorial. Stones are initially formed in the proximal urinary tract and pass distally. They usually become arrested at three points in the ureter - the ureteropelvic junction (UPJ), where the ureter crosses the iliac vessels, and the ureter-vesicular junction (UVJ). Renal stones consist of four basic types: (1) calcium stones - 80%, (2) uric acid stones - 5%, (3) cystine stones - 2%, (4) struvite stones.
System(s) affected: Renal/Urologic
Genetics: Genetic cause in production of cystine stones - inborn error in amino acid transport produces cystinuria
Incidence/Prevalence in USA:
• Of all renal calculi, roughly 1:1000 annual frequency of hospitalization
• Approximately 1% of autopsies
Predominant Age: 30-50 years, most common in third decade
Predominant sex:
• Varies depending upon type of stone
• Calcium stones - Male > Female (3:1)
• Struvite stones - Female > Male

SIGNS AND SYMPTOMS
• Back pain and "renal colic" - agonizing flank pain that waxes and wanes
• Pain may radiate to groin, testicles, suprapubic area or labia
• May be asymptomatic
• Hematuria, dysuria, urinary frequency
• Diaphoresis, tachycardia, tachypnea
• Chills and fever if associated with acute infection due to obstruction
• Hypertension due to pain
• Gastrointestinal symptoms - nausea, vomiting, diarrhea, abdominal distention with associated reflex ileus
• Costovertebral angle tenderness

CAUSES
• Increased supersaturation of urine with stone-forming salts
• Preformed crystals
• Abnormal crystal growth inhibitors
• Calcium stones - due to hypercalciuria, hyperparathyroidism, hyperoxaluria, hypocitruria
• Uric acid stones - due to low urinary volume, overproduction of uric acid, acidic urinary pH
• Cystine stones - inborn error in amino acid transport (cystinuria)
• Struvite stones - due to alkalotic pH usually secondary to infection with urea splitting organisms (i.e., Proteus mirabilis)

RISK FACTORS
• Intrinsic factors - renal tubular acidosis, cystinuria, genetic defects
• Extrinsic factors - geographical, climatic and seasonal factors, low water intake, high animal protein diet, sedentary lifestyle

DIAGNOSIS

DIFFERENTIAL DIAGNOSIS
• Acute peritonitis
• Gastroenteritis
• Acute appendicitis
• Colitis
• Diverticulitis
• Salpingitis
• Cholecystitis
• Peptic ulcer disease
• Pancreatitis

LABORATORY
• CBC with differential - look for signs of infection
• BUN/creatinine - evaluate renal function
• Urine culture and sensitivity if concerned about infection
• Ca+, PO4, uric acid if recurrent problem
• Urinalysis
  ◊ Microscopic or gross hematuria, pyuria
  ◊ Bacteriuria
  ◊ Crystals
  ◊ pH-acidic = uric acid or cystine stones
  ◊ Alkaline = struvite stones
Drugs that may alter lab results: None
Disorders that may alter lab results: Other underlying infections or renal abnormalities

PATHOLOGICAL FINDINGS Calcium, uric acid, cystine and struvite stones

SPECIAL TESTS 24 hour urine collections for Ca+, uric acid, Mg+, oxalate, citrate and creatinine

IMAGING
• Plain film x-ray of abdomen (may add oblique views) - 90% of stones are radiopaque. Ca+ phosphate stones most opaque followed by Ca+ oxalate, struvite and cystine stones. Uric acid stones radiolucent. Usually stones must be greater than 2 mm diameter to be seen on plain film.
• Intravenous urography - to evaluate the extent of obstruction and detect radiolucent stones
• Tomograms may reveal a stone obscured on plain film by gas or feces
• Retrograde urography - rarely needed, only if diagnosis is suspect or patient allergic to intravenous contrast medium
• Ultrasonography - if unable to obtain intravenous urography due to contrast allergy. Can assist in diagnosis of hydronephrosis.
• CT - useful if filling defect to help differentiate ureteral calculi from other causes such as malignancy. Also helpful if non-opaque stone or tumor suspected.
• MRI - not helpful

DIAGNOSTIC PROCEDURES Retrograde urography - rarely needed

TREATMENT

APPROPRIATE HEALTH CARE
Generally outpatient (90%) unless associated with infection, excessive nausea or vomiting, or when stones are greater than 6 mm in diameter

GENERAL MEASURES
• Pain relief
• Aggressive fluid management
• Strain urine for stone collection and analysis
• Treatment includes percutaneous chemolysis, systemic chemolysis, endo-urologic stone extraction, extracorporeal shock wave lithotripsy

SURGICAL MEASURES Rarely, open surgery

ACTIVITY As tolerated

DIET
• Low animal fat diet
• Increased fiber (especially bran)
• Increased fluid intake to keep urine output greater than 3 liters a day
• Other dietary restrictions depend upon specific type of stone formed

PATIENT EDUCATION
• Follow dietary and fluid intake recommendations
• Instruction on fitness

MEDICATIONS

DRUG(S) OF CHOICE
• First-line choice of drugs in outpatient setting:
 ◊ Oral NSAID's (e.g., ibuprofen 600-800 mg tid)
or
 ◊ Oral narcotics - hydrocodone-acetaminophen (Vicodin), acetaminophen-codeine (Tylenol #3), oxycodone-acetaminophen (Percocet)
• Second-line choice:
 ◊ IM ketorolac (Toradol), meperidine (Demerol) or morphine
 ◊ Analgesia: Demerol 50-100 mg IM q3-4h or morphine 10-15 mg IM q3-4 h
• For Ca+ stones due to hypercalciuria - hydrochlorothiazide 50 mg bid
• For Ca+ oxalate stones with hyperuricosuria - allopurinol 100 mg tid
Contraindications: Allergies to medications
Precautions: See manufacturer's profile of each drug
Significant possible interactions: See manufacturer's profile of each drug

ALTERNATIVE DRUGS
• Ketorolac tromethamine (Toradol) 30-60 mg IM, then 30 mg q6h prn (note: very costly, and may cause GI bleeding in some patients)
• Percocet, Tylenol 3, other oral narcotics

 ## FOLLOWUP

PATIENT MONITORING
• Consider urologic referral if evidence of obstruction and symptoms lasting more than 2 weeks
• Follow creatinine level at least weekly to evaluate kidney function
• Plain films of abdomen at 1-2 week intervals to monitor progress of stone in ureter
• Continue to strain urine until stone is passed
• Stone analysis required
• Usually resolved within 4 weeks
• Monitor K+ and blood pressure in patients taking hydrochlorothiazide

PREVENTION/AVOIDANCE Follow dietary restrictions and fluid management

POSSIBLE COMPLICATIONS
• Complete obstruction
• Hydronephrosis
• Kidney failure
• Infection, death

EXPECTED COURSE/PROGNOSIS
• Usually associated with complete return to previous baseline
• Recurrences common - up to 50% within 5 years

 ## MISCELLANEOUS

ASSOCIATED CONDITIONS
• Hyperparathyroidism
• Gout
• Cystinuria
• Hyperuricemia
• Sarcoidosis
• Infections
• Immobilization from trauma or chronic illness

AGE-RELATED FACTORS
Pediatric: Rare in this age group
Geriatric: Complications more likely
Others: N/A

PREGNANCY Approximately same prevalence

SYNONYMS
• Kidney stone
• Urologic stone
• Nephrolithiasis

ICD-9-CM 592.0 Calculus of kidney

SEE ALSO
• Urolithiasis

OTHER NOTES N/A

ABBREVIATIONS N/A

REFERENCES
• Stobo JD: The Principles and Practice of Medicine. 23rd Ed. Norwalk, CT, Appleton & Lange, 1996
• Rakel RE, ed: Conn's Current Therapy. Philadelphia, W.B. Saunders, Co., 1995
• Tanagho EA, McAninch JW, eds: Smith's General Urology. 14th Ed. Norwalk, CT, Appleton & Lange, 1995
Illustrations: N/A
Internet references: http://www.5mcc.com

Author(s)
Lee P. Ralph, MD

Renal cell adenocarcinoma

BASICS

DESCRIPTION The most common solid renal neoplasm, renal cell adenocarcinoma, represents 2-3% of all adult malignancies; 9th most common male malignant tumor, 13th most common female malignant tumor
System(s) affected: Renal/Urologic
Genetics:
• Oncogenes localized to the short arm of chromosome 3 may have etiologic implications. Chromosome 3p12-p26 are specific for clear cell RCC; 4% of RCC is familial.
• People with HLA antigen types Bw44 and DR8 are prone to develop renal cancer. These are rare familial renal carcinomas.
Incidence/Prevalence in USA:
• 30,000 new cases per year (1996); 12,000 deaths per year
• Men: 9.6/100,000
• Women: 4.2/100,000
Predominant age: 5th and 6th decades
Predominant sex: Male > Female (2:1)

SIGNS AND SYMPTOMS
• Solid renal masses, most 6-7 cm (incidentally discovered in asymptomatic patient due to increased use of CT and MRI)
• Hematuria 50-60%
• Elevated erythrocyte sedimentation rate 50-60%
• Abdominal mass 24-45%
• Anemia 21-41%
• Flank pain 35-40%
• Hypertension 22-38%
• Weight loss 28-36%
• Pyrexia 7-17%
• Hepatic dysfunction 10-15%
• Classic triad (hematuria, abdominal mass, flank pain) 7-10%
• Hypercalcemia 3-6%
• Erythrocytosis 3-4%
• Varicocele 2-3%
• Patients with vena caval thrombus present with lower extremity edema, new varicocele, dilated superficial abdominal veins, albuminuria, pulmonary emboli, right atrial mass or non-function of the involved kidney

CAUSES Unknown

RISK FACTORS
• Smoking
• Obesity
• Urban environment
• Cadmium
• Asbestos
• Petroleum by-products
• Herpes simplex virus exposure
• Phenacetin or analgesic abuse for transitional cell of the renal pelvis

DIAGNOSIS

DIFFERENTIAL DIAGNOSIS
• Hydronephrosis
• Polycystic kidneys
• Renal tuberculosis
• Renal calculi
• Renal infarction
• Benign renal cyst
• Transitional cell carcinoma (rare)

LABORATORY
• Anemia (21-41% of patients)
• Polycythemia
• Hematuria
• Alkaline phosphate may be elevated
• Increased erythrocyte sedimentation rate
• Urine - neoplastic cells
• Hypercalcemia
• Increased renin
• Transitional cell cancer (rare)
Drugs that may alter lab results: N/A
Disorders that may alter lab results: N/A

PATHOLOGICAL FINDINGS
• Renal cell tends to bulge out from the cortex producing a mass effect
• 48% of renal cell carcinomas measure < 5 cm and is grossly yellow to yellow/orange due to its high lipid content in the clear cell variety. Average renal cell size has been decreasing due to incidental discovery.
• The granuloma cell type more likely gray to white
• Small tumors are homogenous
• Large tumors may have areas of necrosis and hemorrhage
• A pseudocapsule covers some tumors
• Tumor thrombi into the vena cava generally do not invade the vena caval wall
• Microscopically there is a mixture of clear granular and occasionally sarcomatoid cells

SPECIAL TESTS
• Arteriography (rarely needed) - for tumors larger than 10 cm, it may identify parasitic capsular vessels for early control
• Cystoscopy - to rule out bladder cancer
• ECG as needed

IMAGING
• Intravenous pyelography with infusion nephrotomography remains the primary screening test for renal malignancy
• Ultrasonography - if there appears to be a mass on IVP, confirms the presence of a lesion and determines whether it is solid or cystic. Cystic lesions may either be observed or subjected to percutaneous cyst puncture.
• CT scan and, occasionally, arteriography - if solid or complex masses upon ultrasonography require further evaluation. 3% of RCC are bilateral by CT scan. The most common alteration with RCC is deletion of chromosome 3p. Recent evidence implicates gene p53 on chromosome 17p13.1 to be critical in renal cell carcinogenesis.

• Rapid sequence CT can demonstrate tumor enhancement
• MRI has not been shown to be superior to CT for tumors smaller than 8 cm, for larger tumors it may have advantage in delineating the vena cava
• Bone scans are indicated if the alkaline phosphatase is elevated or the patient has bone pain
• Brain CT is indicated if the patient has neurologic symptoms

DIAGNOSTIC PROCEDURES
• Simple cyst need not be aspirated unless painful
• Calcified cysts may contain renal cell cancer and therefore require open renal biopsy of the wall of the cyst or partial nephrectomy
• Hemorrhagic cyst - aspiration cytology may be helpful but needle biopsy of solid masses is to be discouraged, particularly if the patient has a normal contralateral kidney
• In solitary kidneys, open renal biopsy with wedge resection (not enucleation) can be performed if mass is ≤ 4 cm
• Doppler flow ultrasound of the renal veins or CT (thin cuts) that shows the renal vein entering the vena cava can be used to rule out tumor thrombus
• Venogram - when tumor thrombus is identified. The venogram can demonstrate when the thrombus goes above the hepatic veins or diaphragm (i.e., rarely cardiopulmonary bypass needed to remove the thrombus above the diaphragm at the time of nephrectomy).

TREATMENT

APPROPRIATE HEALTH CARE Inpatient

GENERAL MEASURES N/A

SURGICAL MEASURES
• Surgery is indicated. Drug therapy has been only erratically effective. Lesions are fairly radiation resistant.
• Maintain hydration during iodine injection diagnostic studies to prevent acute tubular necrosis
• Consider a mechanical bowel preparation to ease the nephrectomy
• Consider antibiotic bowel preparation for larger tumors (> 10 cm) where possible bowel injury or resection may be more likely
• Exploration wedge resection for solitary kidney or tumors less than 4 cm, otherwise radical nephrectomy in the face of a normal contralateral kidney is preferred
• Usual preoperative pulmonary toilet, pulmonary function tests if indicated
• Renal cell carcinoma (85% of renal parenchymal malignant tumors) - CT solid mass larger than 3 cm, radical nephrectomy if there is a normal contralateral kidney; smaller than 3 cm, wedge resection. Intraoperative Doppler ultrasound is undergoing study to determine the optimum partial nephrectomy approach to small tumors. Laparoscopy nephrectomy is still investigational.

- Angiomyolipoma (80% of tuberous sclerosis patients have these benign tumors) - classic CT findings, may be followed with CT
- Hemorrhage into a cyst - aspiration cytology
- Complex cyst (calcified cyst wall or irregular wall) - open cyst wall biopsy if cytology is inconclusive
- Transitional cell carcinoma of the renal pelvis or calyces - nephroureterectomy
- Oncocytoma - larger than 3 cm, radical nephrectomy
- Sarcoma - wide excision
- Adult Wilms' tumor - radical nephrectomy for unilateral disease
- Metastasis (lymphoma > lung > breast > stomach) - depends on prognosis of primary tumor; nephrectomy for uncontrolled bleeding
- Cortical adenoma smaller than 3 cm (7-22% at autopsy) - wedge resection

ACTIVITY
- No special preoperative activity
- Postoperatively - as tolerated; full activity in 8 weeks

DIET
Low protein diet for patients with proteinuria

PATIENT EDUCATION
- Preoperative nursing education is indicated for pulmonary toilet
- Pre-anesthesia education is needed if the patient is to have a patient controlled analgesia pump or epidural catheter for postoperative pain relief
- Printed patient information available from: National Kidney & Urologic Diseases Information Clearinghouse, Box NKUDIC, Bethesda, MD 20893, (301)468-6345

MEDICATIONS

DRUG(S) OF CHOICE None
Contraindications: N/A
Precautions: IUL monitoring for IL-2
Significant possible interactions: IL-2 associated with capillary leak syndrome (CLS)

ALTERNATIVE DRUGS
- For advanced renal cell carcinoma - interleukin-2 (IL-2) plus lymphokine-activated killer (LAK), or IL-2 alone, includes 4% complete responders and 11% partial responders
- Hormones - progesterone agents yield a 5-10% response rate
- Chemotherapy - vinblastine alone or with lomustine (CCNU) yields a 10-15% response rate

FOLLOWUP

PATIENT MONITORING
- One CT scan of the abdomen and renal fossa can be done 3-6 months later, particularly if the capsule or lymph nodes are positive, to monitor recurrences and repeat resection if needed for flank pain or mass
- For partial nephrectomy - renal ultrasound every 6 months for 3 years, then annually
- Chest x-rays to rule out pulmonary metastasis are performed quarterly for 2 years, then less often
- Skeletal x-rays and bone scan can be useful in detecting skeletal metastasis but should only be obtained if patient complains of bone pain or an alkaline phosphatase elevation
- Postoperative followup may be possible with plasma transcobalamin II or serum haptoglobin level to detect or monitor recurrences

PREVENTION/AVOIDANCE
- Do not smoke
- Eat a sensible diet
- Avoid stress, asbestos, cadmium, and petroleum distillates

POSSIBLE COMPLICATIONS
- Paraplegia can result with little warning from spinal vertebral metastasis
- CNS metastasis are not uncommon
- Approximately 30% of patients with RCC have metastatic disease when the diagnosis is established. The most common sites of metastasis are the lung (50-60%), bone (30-40%), regional nodes (15-30%), brain (10%) and adjacent organs (10%).

EXPECTED COURSE/PROGNOSIS

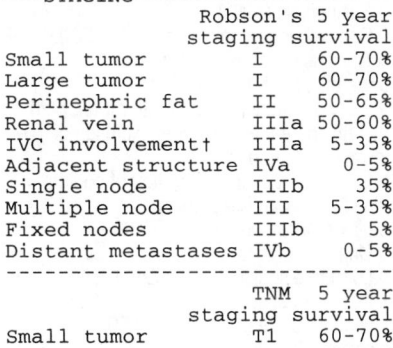

```
---STAGING-------------------
                        Robson's  5 year
                        staging   survival
Small tumor           I            60-70%
Large tumor           I            60-70%
Perinephric fat       II           50-65%
Renal vein            IIIa         50-60%
IVC involvement†      IIIa         5-35%
Adjacent structure    IVa          0-5%
Single node           IIIb         35%
Multiple node         III          5-35%
Fixed nodes           IIIb         5%
Distant metastases    IVb          0-5%
-----------------------------
                        TNM       5 year
                        staging   survival
Small tumor           T1           60-70%
Large tumor           T2           60-70%
Perinephric fat       T3           50-65%
Renal vein            T3b          50-60%
IVC involvement†      T3c          5-35%
Adjacent structure    T4a          0-5%
Single node           N1           35%
Multiple node         N2           5-35%
Fixed nodes           N3           5%
Distant metastases    M1           0-5%
-----------------------------
†Infradiaphragmatic vena caval
```

MISCELLANEOUS

ASSOCIATED CONDITIONS
- Von Hippel-Lindau disease (30-45% of these patients develop renal cell)
- Adult polycystic kidney disease
- Horseshoe kidney
- Acquired renal cystic disease from chronic renal failure

AGE-RELATED FACTORS
Pediatric: Extremely rare in children
Geriatric: Most commonly presents in the 5th and 6th decade
Others: N/A

PREGNANCY N/A

SYNONYMS
- Kidney cancer
- Hypernephroma
- Grawitz's tumor
- Hypernephroid cancer

ICD-9-CM 189.0 Malignant neoplasm of the kidney

SEE ALSO N/A

OTHER NOTES N/A

ABBREVIATIONS
- RCC = renal cell carcinoma
- IVC - inferior vena cava

REFERENCES
- Williams RD: Renal, perirenal and ureteral neoplasms, In: Gillenwater JY, ed. Adult and Pediatric Urology. Chicago, Year Book Medical Publishers, 1987
- Resnick MY: Current Therapy in Genitourinary Surgery. 2nd Ed. St. Louis, Mosby-Year Book Publishers, 1992
- Novick AC: Partial nephrectomy for renal carcinoma. Urol Clin N Am 198714:419
- Spencer W, Novick AC, et al: Conservative surgery for transitional cell carcinoma of the renal pelvis. J Urol 1988;139:507
- Montie J, Jackson C, Cosgrove D, Streem S, Novick AC: Resection of large inferior vena cava thrombi from renal cell carcinoma with the use of circulatory arrest. J Urol 1988;139:25
- Novick AC, Streem SB, et al: Conservative surgery for renal cell carcinoma; A single center experience with 100 patients. J Urol 1989;141:835
- Issac W: Molecular diagnosis of RCC. AUA Today, Dec, 1994
- Novick AC: Partial nephrectomy gaining wider acceptance as alternative treatment in surgery for RCC. The Kidney Cancer Jour 1994;1(2)
- Seminars in Urologic Oncology 1996;14(4):208-215/230-243
Illustrations: N/A
Internet references: http://www.5mcc.com

Author(s)
Mark D. Thomas, MD

Renal failure, acute (ARF)

BASICS

DESCRIPTION A syndrome of rapidly deteriorating kidney function with the accumulation of nitrogenous wastes
System(s) affected: Renal/Urologic, Cardiovascular
Genetics: No known genetic pattern
Incidence/Prevalence in USA: 5% of patients admitted to the hospital develop ARF; 10-15% of ICU patients develop ARF; 2-7% post open heart patients develop ARF; 50% of hospital ARF is iatrogenic.
Predominant age: All ages (average age increasing)
Predominant sex: Male = Female

SIGNS AND SYMPTOMS
• Anorexia
• Asterixis
• Back pain
• Coma
• Delirium
• Diarrhea
• Dyspnea
• Ecchymosis
• Edema
• Encephalopathy
• Epistaxis
• Fasciculation
• Fatigue
• GI hemorrhage
• Headache
• Hiccups
• Hyperpnea
• Hypertension
• Left ventricular failure
• Lethargy
• Muscle cramps
• Myoclonus
• Nausea
• Oliguria
• Pericarditis
• Petechiae
• Purpura (vasculitis)
• Rales
• Rash (acute interstitial nephritis)
• Retinopathy
• Seizure
• Somnolence
• Tachycardia
• Tachypnea
• Uriniferous odor
• Vomiting
• Weakness
• Xerostomia

CAUSES
• Pre-renal
  ◊ Hypovolemia
  ◊ Ineffective circulating volume: Congestive heart failure, cirrhosis, nephrotic syndrome and early sepsis
• Renal
  ◊ Tubular, interstitial: Acute interstitial nephritis (AIN) (drugs, infection); nephrotoxins; acute tubular necrosis; reflex anuria; contrast media
  ◊ Glomerular: Rapidly progressive (crescentic) glomerulonephritis (RPGN) (Immunofluorescence biopsy staining: linear,

immune complex or pauci-immune); pregnancy (2%); systemic lupus erythematosus
• Vascular
  ◊ Ischemic nephropathy (renal artery stenosis)
    ◊ Dissecting aortic aneurysm
    ◊ Ruptured abdominal aortic aneurysm
• Post-renal
  ◊ Obstruction (See topic for Hydronephrosis)

RISK FACTORS
• Surgery (especially with increased age, elevated creatinine, simultaneous cardiac valve and bypass surgery)
• Volume depletion (especially in diabetes)
• Aminoglycoside therapy, congestive heart failure, contrast exposure, septic shock
• Nephrotoxic drugs (e.g., ACE inhibitors in renal artery stenosis)
• Rhabdomyolysis
• Administration of contrast (parenteral) in susceptible individuals
• Dopamine and mannitol appear to increase the risk of acute renal failure in some groups; particularly patients with diabetes mellitus.

DIAGNOSIS

DIFFERENTIAL DIAGNOSIS See causes

LABORATORY
• Urinalysis
  ◊ Proteinuria
  ◊ Hematuria
  ◊ Brown granular urinary casts
  ◊ Urinary renal tubular epithelial cells
• Urine sediment
  ◊ Coarse granular casts
  ◊ Renal tubular epithelial cells
  ◊ Eosinophils (AIN?)
  ◊ Red cell or hemoglobin casts (RPGN)
  ◊ Crystals (lithiasis, obstruction)
• Urine electrolytes/osmolality
  ◊ Increased urine sodium (> 20 mEq/L [>20 mmol/L]), increased fractional excretion of sodium (> 3%) (e.g., renal).
Calculation: Fractional excretion of sodium = [(urine Na+/serum Na+) / (urine creatinine/serum creatinine)] X 100
  ◊ Urine isotonic to plasma
  ◊ Low urine sodium (< 10 mEq/L), low fractional excretion of sodium (≤ 1%), concentrate urine osmolality (≥ 500 mOsm/liter) (e.g., pre-renal)
• Other
  ◊ Azotemia
  ◊ Decreased creatinine clearance
  ◊ Hyperosmolarity
  ◊ Hyperphosphatemia
  ◊ Hyperkalemia
  ◊ Decreased serum bicarbonate
  ◊ Increased plasma volume
  ◊ Decreased hemoglobin
  ◊ Decreased hematocrit
  ◊ Hypocapnia
  ◊ Increased serum magnesium
  ◊ Acidemia (increased anion gap)
  ◊ Increased serum amylase/lipase
  ◊ Hyponatremia .
  ◊ Hypocalcemia

  ◊ Increased serum uric acid
  ◊ Increased bleeding time
  ◊ Impaired phagocytic function
Drugs that may alter lab results: Too many to list
Disorders that may alter lab results: Too many to list

PATHOLOGICAL FINDINGS Kidney biopsy: Not particularly helpful in acute tubular necrosis (ATN). Diagnostic in AIN and RPGN.

SPECIAL TESTS
• Angiogram (renal vascular disease)
• Cystoscopy - retrograde
• Bleeding time

IMAGING
• Obstruction - renal scan, CT scan
• Kidney ultrasound
  ◊ Renal cause: "Medical" renal disease (renal echogenicity = liver), normal size kidneys, kidney size disparity: ischemia
  ◊ Post renal cause - hydronephrosis

DIAGNOSTIC PROCEDURES Renal biopsy (ARF, unknown cause), diagnostic for AIN, RPGN

TREATMENT

APPROPRIATE HEALTH CARE Inpatient and intensive care

GENERAL MEASURES
• Correction of underlying hemodynamic abnormalities, especially volume
• Hemodialysis as soon as diagnosis of uremia is established (or continuous renal replacement therapy). The use of biocompatible membranes (e.g., polymethyl methylacrylate) as opposed to cuprophane results in a higher rate of recovery of renal function, more rapid recovery and better patient survival.
• Decrease catabolism
• Convert oliguria to nonoliguria
• Daily weight
• Correct reversible causes (volume and mannitol)
• Modify dosages of renal excreted drugs (see under Medications - Precautions)
• If drug induced, discontinue offending agent
• Meticulous aseptic technique
• Continuous arteriovenous hemofiltration
• Intravenous human immunoglobulin G
• Correct easy bleeding with DDAVP, estrogen and cryoprecipitate
• Question prednisone in AIN
• Hyperkalemia - severe (1 amp Ca gluconate IV); other IV insulin + glucose, if acidosis also present (1 amp NaHCO3) Kayexalate po 15-60 gm/day if gastrointestinal tract functions

SURGICAL MEASURES N/A

ACTIVITY As tolerated

DIET
• Restrict fluids to volume of urine output plus 500 mL/day
• Eliminate potassium if serum level increased
• Oral and IV amino acids
• Increase carbohydrates to decrease catabolism
• Alimentation to decrease catabolism

PATIENT EDUCATION
National Kidney & Urologic Diseases Information Clearinghouse, Box NKUDIC, Bethesda, MD 20893, (301)468-6345 and The National Kidney Foundation, Inc., 30 East 33rd Street, NY, NY 10016. "What Everyone Should Know About Kidneys and Kidney Disease" (Order #01-01BP - English), (Order #01-02BP -Spanish).

 MEDICATIONS

DRUG(S) OF CHOICE Prior to fixed renal failure: IV volume expansion with normal saline followed by mannitol, furosemide (Lasix), and calcium channel blockers. Dopamine has not been shown to be beneficial. Volume expansion alone is beneficial in contrast injury.
Contraindications: N/A
Precautions:
• Pharmacokinetics of all drugs used during renal failure should be reviewed for appropriate adjustment. For example, antiarrhythmic drugs:
◊ Quinidine: decrease dose, closely monitor drug level
◊ Procainamide: avoid in renal failure
◊ Disopyramide: reduction in maintenance dose
◊ Mexiletine: no dose adjustment-liver metabolized, etc.
Significant possible interactions:
Nonsteroidals plus other nephrotoxic drugs, male gender, increasing age, cardiovascular comorbidity and recent hospitalization are synergistic in causing ARF

ALTERNATIVE DRUGS N/A

 FOLLOWUP

PATIENT MONITORING As needed

PREVENTION/AVOIDANCE
• See risk factors
• Allopurinol prior to chemotherapy for hematologic malignancy
• Hydration most important, especially prior to contrast and chemotherapy
• Non biocompatible membranes
• Hypotension

POSSIBLE COMPLICATIONS
• Sepsis - infection (leading cause of mortality)
• Convulsions
• Edema
• Pulmonary edema
• Congestive heart failure
• Hyperkalemia
• Paralysis
• Arrhythmias
• Death (50%)
• Pericarditis/tamponade
• Uremia
• Bleeding
• Hypotension

EXPECTED COURSE/PROGNOSIS
Recover usually in days to 6 weeks. High mortality rate (5-80%) depending on cause/multi-organ involvement, and age.

 MISCELLANEOUS

ASSOCIATED CONDITIONS
• Hyperphosphatemia
• Hydronephrosis
• Muscle injury
• Congestive heart failure
• Cirrhosis
• Malignant hypertension
• Vasculitis
• Bacterial infections
• Drug reactions
• Hypercalcemia
• Hyperuricemia
• Sepsis
• Severe trauma
• Burns
• Transfusion reactions
• Internal bleeding

AGE-RELATED FACTORS
Pediatric: Congenital
Geriatric: Greater occurrence in this age group especially after surgery
Others: N/A

PREGNANCY
• Infected uterus (e.g., C. welchii [C. perfringens])
• Toxemia and a related obstetric complication
• Cortical necrosis
• Postpartum renal failure

SYNONYMS N/A

ICD-9-CM
584.9 acute renal failure unspecified

SEE ALSO
• Multiple myeloma
• Hepatorenal syndrome
• Reye's syndrome
• Rocky Mountain spotted fever
• Hydronephrosis
• Renal failure, chronic
• Rhabdomyolysis
• Glomerulonephritis, rapidly progressive

OTHER NOTES N/A

ABBREVIATIONS
• ATN = acute tubular necrosis
• AIN = acute interstitial nephritis
• RPGN = rapidly progressive glomerulonephritis
• ACE = angiotensin converting enzyme

REFERENCES
• Humes HD: Acute renal failure - the promise of new therapies. N Engl J Med 1997;336:870871
• Solomon R, Werner G, Mann D, et al: Effects of saline, mannitol & furosemide on acute decreases in renal function by radiocontrast agents. N Eng J Med 1994;331:1416-20
• Pascual J, Liano F, Ortuno J: The Elderly Patient with Acute Renal Failure. J Am Soc Nephrol 1995;6:144-53
• Abuel JG: Diagnosing Vascular Causes of Renal Failure. Ann Intern Med 1995;123:601-14
• Alkhunaizi AM, Schrier RW: Management of acute renal failure: new perspectives. Am J Kid Dis 1996;28:315-328
• Thadoni R, Pascual M, Bonventre JV: Acute renal failure. N Engl J Med 1996;334:1448-1460
• Gutthann SP, Rodriguez LAG, Raiford DS, et al: Nonsteroidal drugs and the risk of hospitalization. Arch Int Med 1996;156:2433-2439
Illustrations: N/A
Internet references: http://www.5mcc.com

Author(s)
Gregory W. Rutecki, MD

Renal failure, chronic

BASICS

DESCRIPTION The result of any renal injury that decreases renal excretory and regulatory function chronically. Characteristic findings: nitrogen retention, acidosis, and anemia.
System(s) affected: Renal/Urologic
Genetics:
• Compared to the general population, African Americans are 3.9 x more likely to have ESRD (irreversible, dialysis dependent renal failure) and 6.7 x more likely to have hypertensive ESRD
• Hereditary renal diseases can lead to chronic renal failure in children and some adults (Alport's syndrome, autosomal recessive polycystic kidney disease)
• Autosomal dominant polycystic kidney disease is a relatively common cause of chronic renal failure in adults affecting approximately 10% of dialysis population. Inherited in an autosomal dominant pattern with mutation on short arm chromosome 16.
Incidence/Prevalence in USA:
• Common (estimated that 160,000 persons per year are treated for end stage renal disease). Prevalence in the USA: 2.8/100,000 people in USA (estimate) with a chronic elevation of creatinine greater than 2.0 mg/dL (176.8 μmol/L). ESRD experienced an annual growth rate of 8.8% from 1982 to 1991.
• By the end of the decade, HIV-associated nephropathy will be the 3rd leading cause of ESRD in African Americans ages 20-64
Predominant age: All ages - much more common in adults. In children, chronic renal failure affects between 2 and 6 per 1 million population. The elderly represent 33,8% of new patients with ESRD from 1988-1991.
Predominant sex: Male = Female

SIGNS AND SYMPTOMS
• Anemia (normochromic, normocytic)
• Anorexia
• Confusion (late sign)
• Emotional lability
• Encephalopathy
• Endocrine dysfunction (thyroid, pituitary)
• Fatigue on slight exertion
• Hypertension
• Insomnia
• Intractable hiccups
• Lassitude
• Mental depression
• Metallic taste in mouth
• Muscle cramps
• Muscle twitching
• Nausea
• Neuropathy
• Nocturia
• Pallor
• Polyuria
• Pruritus
• Seizures (late sign)
• Serositis
• Skin dry
• Stomatitis
• Slight breathlessness
• Vomiting

CAUSES
• Renal parenchymal: Glomerular: membranous nephropathy, membrano-proliferative glomerulonephritis, systemic lupus erythematosus, focal glomerulosclerosis, diabetes mellitus, proliferative glomerulonephritis, amyloidosis, Alport's syndrome, connective tissue disease.
• Interstitial-tubular: Heavy metals, drugs, nephrotoxins, multiple myeloma, hypertension, gout(?), thrombotic microangiopathies, oxalate deposition, infection, renal artery stenosis or ischemic stenosis, connective tissue disease, autosomal dominant polycystic kidney disease, congenital.
• Post-renal: See hydronephrosis causes
• Pre-renal: Cirrhosis, cardiac, volume, nephrotic, drugs (e.g., NSAID's)

RISK FACTORS
• Contrast (diabetes, myeloma)
• Circulatory failure
• Urinary tract obstruction
• Analgesic abuse
• Untreated hypertension
• Diabetes mellitus
• The greater the proteinuria, the quicker the progression of CRF

DIAGNOSIS

DIFFERENTIAL DIAGNOSIS See causes

LABORATORY
• Blood:
◊ Smear - normochromic, normocytic anemia
◊ Decreased immune responsiveness
◊ Thrombocytopenia
◊ Decreased hematocrit
◊ Increased capillary fragility
◊ Increased bleeding time
• Chemistry:
◊ Azotemia
◊ Elevated ammonia
◊ Type IV hyperlipidemia
◊ Decreased active Vitamin D
◊ Increased parathyroid hormone
◊ Elevated glucose, insulin resistance
◊ Elevated phosphate
◊ Elevated potassium
◊ Elevated sulfate
◊ Elevated uric acid
◊ Reduced calcium
◊ Serum CO2 content - 15-20 mEq/L (15-20 mmol/L)
• Urine
◊ Proteinuria
◊ Casts

Drugs that may alter lab results:
• Cimetidine
• Trimethoprim
• Cefazolin: increase creatinine
Disorders that may alter lab results:
Ketosis may artificially raise creatinine

PATHOLOGICAL FINDINGS
• Kidney biopsy
• Glomerulonephritis
• Interstitial nephritis

SPECIAL TESTS
• 24 hour urine studies (protein, clearance)
• Glofil clearance
• Complement studies
• Antinuclear antibody
• Serum protein electrophoresis
• Urine immune electrophoresis
• Hepatitis B surface antigen

IMAGING
• Ultrasound - shows decreased kidney size, may show obstructed ureter and bladder outlet
• CT scan

DIAGNOSTIC PROCEDURES Kidney biopsy

TREATMENT

APPROPRIATE HEALTH CARE Inpatient or outpatient depending on severity

GENERAL MEASURES
• Treat any aggravating cause aggressively (salt and water depletion, nephrotoxins, congestive heart failure, infection, hypercalcemia, urinary obstruction)
• Drugs may exacerbate chronic renal failure
• Pay careful attention to dosing, and avoid use of nephrotoxic agents. When possible, treat anemia with erythropoietin.
• Dialysis: hemo, peritoneal, transplant
• Vitamin D (active) and calcium supplements (dihydrotachysterol 0.2-0.4 mg q day; calcium acetate tablets with meals tid
• Strict control of blood pressure. For patients with proteinuria > 1 gm/d ≤ 125/75; < 1 gm/d 130/80. ACE inhibitors in diabetes mellitus.

SURGICAL MEASURES N/A

ACTIVITY Restricted only by patient's condition

DIET
• Adequate caloric intake
• Restricted protein intake
• Restricted intake of phosphate
• Water intake limited to maintain serum sodium concentration of 135 to 145 mEq/L
• Sodium restriction if volume expanded
• Potassium restriction if hyperkalemic
• Vitamin supplementation (avoid extra-dietary intake of magnesium)
• Strict dietary restrictions in the elderly may not be necessary, since they often have a low protein and salt intake

PATIENT EDUCATION
• For patient education materials favorably reviewed on this topic, contact: National Kidney and Urologic Diseases Information Clearinghouse, Box NKUDIC, Bethesda MD 20893. (301)468-6345
• The National Kidney Foundation, Inc. 30 East 33rd Street, New York, New York 10016. "Bone Disease in Chronic Renal Failure" (Order #02-27CP), "Diabetes and Kidney Disease" (Order #02-09CP). "Drug Abuse Can Hurt Your Kidneys" (Order #02-22N) or "Nutrition and Changing Kidney Function" (Order #0401).

 MEDICATIONS

DRUG(S) OF CHOICE
• Multivitamin
• Lipid lowering agents appropriate for disorder (cholesterol lowering specifically for nephrotic syndrome); may use cholestyramine or HMG-CoA reductase inhibitor
• Erythropoietin for anemia, approximately 100-150 units/kg thrice weekly IV or subcutaneous
• Salt restriction and diuretics for edema. Thiazides do not work at glomerular filtration rate (GFR) < 30 cc/min (creatinine > 2.5 mg/dL).
• Calcium acetate and oral vitamin D for renal failure osteodystrophy (see information under General Measures)
• Hypertension: drugs to lower blood pressure. For diabetic CRF, angiotensin converting enzyme inhibitors slow progression to dialysis dependence (captopril 25-50 bid to decrease diastolic < 90).
• Muscle cramps: Vitamin E
• Pruritus: Skin moisturizes, diphenhydramine, activated charcoal
• Bleeding: DDAVP, cryoprecipitate, dialysis in uremia
Contraindications: Refer to manufacturer's literature
Precautions:
• Monitor serum electrolytes carefully
• Monitor loop diuretic use to avoid volume depletion
• Adjust the dose of all medications with a renal route of excretion
Significant possible interactions: Refer to manufacturer's literature

ALTERNATIVE DRUGS
• Multivitamin preparation excluding fat-soluble vitamins and magnesium containing products
• Angiotensin converting enzyme inhibitors may prevent or slow progression to end stage renal failure (non renal vascular) in some diseases; definitely in diabetic CRF

 FOLLOWUP

PATIENT MONITORING
• Blood, urine, chemistries and clinical status
• Blood pressure, volume monitored frequently

PREVENTION/AVOIDANCE
• Avoid nephrotoxic drugs when possible (especially iodinated contrast, NSAID's)
• Treat all disorders known to lead to chronic renal failure
• Many drugs require dosage reduction to prevent toxicity
• Avoid volume depletion

POSSIBLE COMPLICATIONS
• Anemia
• Changes in calcium and phosphorous metabolism
• Lipid disorders
• Pericarditis
• Serositis
• Pseudogout
• Hypothyroidism
• Infections
• Hyperkalemia
• Acidosis
• Hyponatremia
• Gout
• Accelerated hypertension
• Metabolic calcification
• Spontaneous abortion
• Infertility
• Impotence
• Bleeding
• GI mucosal ulcerations
• GI A-V malformations
• Seizures
• Fractures

EXPECTED COURSE/PROGNOSIS
Serious, chronic, mortality > 20% despite careful attention to fluid and electrolyte balance or other treatment

 MISCELLANEOUS

ASSOCIATED CONDITIONS
See conditions listed under Risk factors

AGE-RELATED FACTORS
Pediatric:
• Main causes in children include congenital renal and urinary tract malformations (signs appear before age 5), glomerular and hereditary renal diseases (signs appear between ages 5-15)
• Medical management much more difficult in children
• When it develops in infancy, growth impairment more profound than when disease develops in an otherwise healthy teenager
Geriatric:
• Highest incidence, highest morbidity, highest mortality. Renal disease is secondary to many age-dependent illnesses.
• Rule out such potentially reversible causes as urinary tract obstruction (particularly in men), renal arterial occlusion, hypercalcemia, use of nephrotoxic agents
• Older patients may tolerate dialysis quite well
Others: N/A

PREGNANCY
Pregnancy to term less common in CRF. Fertility and libido disturbed in CRF.

SYNONYMS
• Uremia
• CRF

ICD-9-CM
585 Chronic renal failure

SEE ALSO
• Renal failure, acute
• Hydronephrosis
• Nephrotic syndrome
• Polycystic kidney disease

OTHER NOTES
N/A

ABBREVIATIONS
N/A

REFERENCES
• Friedman AI: Etiology, pathophysiology, diagnosis and management of chronic renal failure in children. Curr Opin in Perdiatr 1996;8:148-151
• Jacobson HR, Striker GE: Report on a workshop to develop management recommendations for the prevention of progression in chronic renal disease. Am J Kid Dis 1995;25:103-106
• Bohle A, Muller GA, Wehrmann M, et al: Pathogenesis of chronic renal failure in the primary glomerulopathies, renal vasculopathies and chronic interstitial nephritides. Kid Int 1996;54:52-59
• Glassock RJ, Cohen AH: The primary glomerulopathies. Disease-A-Month;42:329-383
• Hood VL, Gennar FJ: End stage renal disease: measures to prevent it or slow its progression. Postgrad Med 1996;100:163-166
Illustrations: 3 available on CD-ROM
Internet references: http://www.5mcc.com

Author(s)
Gregory W. Rutecki, MD

Renal tubular acidosis (RTA)

BASICS

DESCRIPTION A group of disorders characterized by abnormal renal tubular acidification mechanisms, with glomerular function preserved, resulting in metabolic acidosis. These disorders are divided into three types:
• RTA-1: classic, distal, hypokalemic - due to inability to maintain H+ ion gradient
• RTA-2: proximal - due to decreased bicarbonate reabsorption. This is a limited acidosis because of the distal tubule resorptive capacity.
• RTA-3: no longer considered a distinct entity
• RTA-4: generalized, distal, hyperkalemic - due to primary or secondary aldosterone deficiency, or aldosterone resistance
Incidence/Prevalence in USA: N/A
System(s) affected: Renal/Urologic, Endocrine/Metabolic
Genetics: RTA-1 in children is autosomally dominant
Predominant age:
• RTA-1 and 2 mostly children
• RTA-4 mostly adults
Predominant sex: Male = Female

SIGNS AND SYMPTOMS
• Failure to thrive in RTA-1 and RTA-2
• Emesis
• Polyuria
• Dehydration
• Weakness due to potassium loss
• Respiratory distress, hyperventilation in attempt to compensate for acidosis
• Gait disturbance and bone pain from disturbed calcium metabolism in RTA-2

CAUSES
• RTA-1
  ◊ Drug induced - amphotericin B, toluene, lithium, NSAID's
  ◊ Hypergammaglobulinemic syndromes
  ◊ Cirrhosis of liver
  ◊ Pyelonephritis
• RTA-2
  ◊ Drug induced - deteriorated tetracycline, acetazolamide, sulfonamides, diachrome heavy metals
  ◊ Amyloidosis
  ◊ Multiple myeloma
• RTA-4
  ◊ Lupus nephropathy
  ◊ Diabetic nephropathy
  ◊ Nephrosclerosis due to hypertension
  ◊ Tubulo-interstitial nephropathies
  ◊ Addison's disease
  ◊ Acute adrenal insufficiency

RISK FACTORS
• Hyperparathyroidism
• Chronic renal failure (CRF)

DIAGNOSIS

DIFFERENTIAL DIAGNOSIS
• Metabolic acidosis of other causes - RTA has hyperchloremic non-anion gap acidosis
• Diarrhea with bicarbonate loss in stools
• CRF acidosis
• Respiratory acidosis

LABORATORY
• ABGs - metabolic acidosis picture
• Serum electrolytes - potassium is increased in RTA 4, and normal or decreased in RTA-1 and 2. Chloride is increased. Bicarbonate is decreased.
• Serum BUN and creatinine - to rule out renal failure
• Urine pH - not acidified with metabolic acidosis present in RTA-1
• Urine Ca++ elevated
• Urine culture - to rule out UTI with urea splitting organisms
• Renin and aldosterone levels - decreased in most types RTA-4 caused by aldosterone deficiency, aldosterone resistant type RTA-4 have high levels
• Anion gap - normal
Drugs that may alter lab results:
• Diuretics
• NaHCO3 (sodium bicarbonate)
Disorders that may alter lab results: N/A

PATHOLOGICAL FINDINGS Tubular transport dysfunction

SPECIAL TESTS
• Maximize metabolic acidosis and monitor for urine acidification. Give po NH4Cl (ammonium chloride), and monitor urine pH. Beware for problems associated with exacerbating metabolic acidosis.
• Bicarbonate titration curves

IMAGING
Necessary only if potential complications need to be ruled out
• Intravenous pyelogram (IVP) - nephrocalcinosis, nephrolithiasis, intrinsic renal disease
• Renal sonograms - to evaluate for renal size, cysts or stones
• Bone films - osteomalacia with pseudo-fractures

DIAGNOSTIC PROCEDURES N/A

TREATMENT

APPROPRIATE HEALTH CARE
Outpatient

GENERAL MEASURES
• Treatment with appropriate medications to correct acidosis
• May need respiratory support till acidosis corrected

SURGICAL MEASURES N/A

ACTIVITY As tolerated

DIET NaCl (sodium chloride) restriction

PATIENT EDUCATION For patient education materials on this topic, contact: National Kidney & Urologic Diseases Information Clearinghouse, Box NKUDIC, Bethesda, MD 20893, (301)468-6345

Renal tubular acidosis (RTA)

 MEDICATIONS

DRUG(S) OF CHOICE
• RTA-1

◊ Sodium bicarbonate - 1-4 mEq/kg/day (1-4 mmol/kg/day) starting and titrate up as needed. Bicarbonate wasting forms will need more. Dosing is 2 or 3 times daily.

◊ Potassium bicarbonate - if hypokalemia is a problem. Amount of HCO3 (the bicarbonate radical) given in this form depends on severity of hypokalemia.
• RTA-2

◊ Sodium bicarbonate - 5-20 mEq/kg/day (5-20 mmol/kg/day) titrated as necessary, with frequency of dosing 4-6 times a day
• RTA-4

◊ Sodium bicarbonate - 1-4 mEq/kg/day (1-4 mmol/kg/day) titrated as necessary with 2 or 3 times daily dosing

◊ Furosemide - to lower potassium levels, except if salt wasting is also occurring

◊ Sodium polystyrene sulfonate (Kayexalate) - initially to bring down very high potassium levels (via enemas)

◊ Fludrocortisone - 0.1-0.3 mg/day, if the patient is mineralocorticoid deficient, or in some cases of end organ resistance

Contraindications: Refer to manufacturer's literature
Precautions: Refer to manufacturer's literature
Significant possible interactions: N/A

ALTERNATIVE DRUGS
Hydrochlorothiazide (HCTZ) as an adjunct in RTA-2 after maximal NaHCO3. Shohl's solution (sodium citrate) can be used if large doses of bicarbonate are needed. Citrate is metabolized to bicarbonate in the liver, avoiding distention and flatulence caused by the gastric CO2 production.

 FOLLOWUP

PATIENT MONITORING Electrolytes, serum pH, urine pH, renal function studies

PREVENTION/AVOIDANCE Careful use or avoidance of causative agents listed above

POSSIBLE COMPLICATIONS
• Nephrocalcinosis
• RTA-1 - pyelonephritis
• Nephrolithiasis
• Rickets
• Hypercalciuria

EXPECTED COURSE/PROGNOSIS
• Permanent disorder, but prognosis is good with therapy if irreversible renal damage has not yet occurred
• Good, if not associated with any other autoimmune disease. Otherwise, prognosis dependent on the associated disease.

 MISCELLANEOUS

ASSOCIATED CONDITIONS
• RTA-1 in children - hypercalciuria leading to rickets, nephrocalcinosis, and nephrolithiasis
• RTA-1 in adults - autoimmune diseases such as Sjögren's disease
• RTA-2 - Fanconi's syndrome

AGE-RELATED FACTORS
Pediatric: N/A
Geriatric: N/A
Others: N/A

PREGNANCY N/A

SYNONYMS N/A

ICD-9-CM
• 588.8 Other specified disorder resulting from impaired renal function
• 270.0 Disorder of amino acid transport (Fanconi's syndrome)

SEE ALSO N/A

OTHER NOTES N/A

ABBREVIATIONS
• NaHCO3 = sodium bicarbonate
• RTA = renal tubular acidosis
• CRF = chronic renal failure

REFERENCES
• Isselbacher KJ, et al, eds: Harrison's Principles of Internal Medicine. 13th Ed. New York, McGraw-Hill, 1994
• Oski FA: Principles and Practice of Pediatrics. 3rd Ed. Philadelphia, J.B. Lippincott, 1990
Illustrations: N/A
Internet references: http://www.5mcc.com

Author(s)
Raghu Ram, MD

Respiratory distress syndrome, adult

BASICS

DESCRIPTION A patient with previously normal lungs who suffers a catastrophic pulmonary or nonpulmonary event followed by a cascade of events that occur at the alveolar-arteriolar capillary membrane. Reduction in functional residual capacity and lung compliance are hallmarks.
• Hypoxemia, decreased pulmonary compliance, and an increasing shunt forms as the proteinaceous material collects in the interstitium and alveoli. Hypoxemic respiratory failure secondary to noncardiogenic pulmonary edema almost always requires mechanical ventilation

System(s) affected: Pulmonary
Genetics: N/A
Incidence/Prevalence in USA: 150,000/year
Predominant age: All ages
Predominant sex: Male = Female

SIGNS AND SYMPTOMS Most patients demonstrate similar clinical and pathologic features regardless of the cause of the acute lung injury.
• There are 4 phases:
◊ Phase 1: Acute injury - normal physical exam, normal chest x-ray, tachypnea, tachycardia, and respiratory alkalosis
◊ Phase 2: Latent phase - 6-48 hours after injury: Hyperventilation, hypocapnia, increase in work of breathing, widening alveolar-arterial oxygen gradient
◊ Phase 3: Acute respiratory failure, tachypnea and dyspnea, decreased lung compliance, diffuse infiltrates on chest roentgenogram, high-pitched diffusely scattered crackles
◊ Phase 4: Severe abnormalities, severe hypoxemia unresponsive to therapy, increased intrapulmonary shunting, metabolic and respiratory acidosis
• Signs and symptoms common to all 4 phases:
◊ Tachypnea and tachycardia during the first 12 to 24 hours
◊ Moist and cyanotic skin
◊ Breathing difficulty with intercostal and accessory respiratory muscles
◊ Dramatic increase in work of breathing
◊ High-pitched end-expiratory crackles are heard throughout all lung fields
◊ Increased agitation
◊ Lethargy, then obtundation
◊ Hypoxemia may be present long before clinical signs

CAUSES
• Recent studies have revealed a number of mediators are involved in the initiation and perpetuation of ARDS
◊ Cytokines (tumor necrosis factor, interleukin 1, interleukin 6)
◊ Complement activation
◊ Coagulation activation
◊ Platelet - activating factor
◊ Oxygen radicals
◊ Lipoxygenase pathways (Leukotrienes C4, D4 and E4)
◊ Neutrophil proteases
◊ Nitric oxide - may be deleterious or advantageous
◊ Endotoxin
◊ Cyclooxygenase pathway products (thromboxane A2, prostacyclin)
• All of the following causes can initiate a systemic inflammatory response with activation of the previous mediators
◊ Aspiration
◊ Pulmonary and systemic infections (bacterial, fungal, viral and protozoan)
◊ Sepsis (gram negative, gram positive, fungi, tuberculous, pneumocystis pneumonia)
◊ Pulmonary contusion
◊ Near-drowning
◊ Multiple fractures, especially long bones (fat embolism)
◊ Multiple transfusions
◊ Pancreatitis, severe
◊ Head injury
◊ Inhalation of toxic gases (oxygen, smoke, NH3, chlorine, plastics, phosgene, cadmium)
◊ Burns
◊ Shock (hemorrhage, cardiogenic, septic, anaphylactic)
◊ Eclampsia
◊ Carcinomatosis
◊ Leukoagglutinin reaction
◊ Air or amniotic fluid emboli

RISK FACTORS
• Systemic sepsis
• Pulmonary contusion
• Aspiration
• Inhalation of toxic substances
• Diffuse pneumonia
• Multiple emergency blood transfusions

DIAGNOSIS

DIFFERENTIAL DIAGNOSIS Cardiogenic pulmonary edema

LABORATORY
• PaO2 < 50 mm Hg with FiO2 > 0.6
• Overall compliance < 50 mL/cm water (usually 20-30 mL/cm water)
• Increased shunt fraction Q's/Q't and dead space ventilation VD/VT
Drugs that may alter lab results: N/A
Disorders that may alter lab results:
• Multiple pulmonary embolism
• Cardiogenic pulmonary edema
• Severe chronic obstructive pulmonary disease
• Severe pneumonia

PATHOLOGICAL FINDINGS
• Lungs show exudative phase, early proliferative phase or late proliferative phase
• Interstitial and alveolar edema
• Inflammatory cells and erythrocytes spill into interstitium and the alveolus
• Type I cells are destroyed, leaving a denuded basement membrane
• Protein-rich fluid fills the alveoli
• Type II alveolar cells appear unaltered initially
• Type II cells begin to proliferate within 72 hours of initial insult
• The type II cells cover the denuded basement membrane
• Aggregates of plasma proteins, cellular debris, fibrin and surfactant remnants form hyaline membranes
• Over next 3-10 days, alveolar septum thickens by proliferating fibroblasts, leukocytes and plasma cells
• Capillary injury begins to occur
• Hyaline membranes begin to reorganize
• Fibrosis becomes apparent in respiratory ducts and bronchioles

SPECIAL TESTS
• Pulmonary artery catheter
• Measure pulmonary edema fluid content

IMAGING Chest roentgenogram

DIAGNOSTIC PROCEDURES
• Pulmonary artery catheterization to demonstrate:
◊ Normal pulmonary arterial occlusion pressure (PAOP)
◊ Note: The main point of this study is to determine if the PAOP is inconsistent with cardiogenic pulmonary edema. A low PAOP with low serum albumin may lead to cardiogenic etiology. The patient with chronic congestive heart failure may have high wedge, but still develop adult respiratory distress syndrome.

TREATMENT

APPROPRIATE HEALTH CARE
Intensive care unit

GENERAL MEASURES
• Treat underlying etiology as appropriate
• Corticosteroids have theoretical, but not proven, benefit. This is still controversial. Do not use if occult infection exists.
• Support ventilation mechanically as necessary
• Support oxygenation with positive end-expiratory pressure (PEEP) with an amount that allows adequate hemoglobin saturation (90-95%) with an FiO2 of ≤ 60%. PaO2 is less important than oxygen delivery.
• Maintain oxygen delivery:
    ◊ Increase O2 content with packed red blood cell transfusion as necessary
    ◊ Optimize cardiac output with fluid or inotropes. Measure CO with each PEEP change. If CO decreases, give fluids to regain adequate CO and allow additional PEEP adjustments if necessary.
• Avoid over-ventilation
• Avoid large tidal volumes (> 10 cc/kg) if peak airway pressures are high
• A pulmonary artery catheter may be helpful in assessing left ventricular function, CO, oxygen delivery and consumption. It is necessary if high levels of PEEP are used.
• Be aware of possible respiratory superinfection
• Deep vein thrombosis prophylaxis is essential
• Consider paralyzing agents (to improve compliance and decrease barotrauma) if patient is fighting ventilator. (Initiate anxiolytics when instituting treatment with paralytics.)
• Ulcer prophylaxis
• Extraordinary management
    ◊ 1. Extracorporeal membrane oxygenation (ECMO) is conceivable in children
    ◊ 2. High-frequency ventilation - it achieves adequate gas exchange; however, there is no improvement on outcome
    ◊ 3. Pressure controlled inverse ratio ventilation (PCIRV)
    ◊ 4 Extracorporeal CO2 removal with low frequency ventilation. (Used in Europe and Salt Lake City on NIH trial.)

SURGICAL MEASURES N/A

ACTIVITY Bedrest

DIET Nutritional support - avoid excess carbohydrates (could increase respiratory quotient)

PATIENT EDUCATION N/A

MEDICATIONS

DRUG(S) OF CHOICE
• Inotropic agents - dobutamine to maintain adequate cardiac output
• Vasodilators - nitroprusside, ACE inhibitors, hydralazine. (Only if BP is adequate.)
• Corticosteroids (controversial)
• Anxiolytics
• Heparin 5000 units q12h for deep-vein thrombosis prophylaxis
• Ulcer prophylaxis with H2 blockers or sucralfate
Contraindications: See manufacturer's profile of each drug
Precautions: See manufacturer's profile of each drug
Significant possible interactions: See manufacturer's profile of each drug

ALTERNATIVE DRUGS
• Specific mediator inhibitors: Are being evaluated in animal models and humans
    ◊ Xanthine oxidase inhibitors (early in burn patients)
    ◊ Monoclonal derived antibodies to released monokines, i.e., tumor necrosis factor
    ◊ NSAID's, i.e., ibuprofen
    ◊ High-dose corticosteroids are still being studied and reviewed
    ◊ Pentoxifylline - has shown to be of some benefit
    ◊ Maximizing gut barrier function by using early enteral feeds
    ◊ Surfactant replacement is being reviewed
    ◊ Ventilator management by using permissive hypercapnia with low tidal volumes to prevent extensive barotrauma from mechanical ventilation

FOLLOWUP

PATIENT MONITORING
• Vital capacity and static lung compliance are important measures of mechanics
• Daily labs until no longer critical
• Chest x-rays to assess - endotracheal tube placement; the possible development of barotrauma; the presence of infiltrates; PA cath migration
• Swan-Ganz catheter - to help assess 02 delivery and consumption; monitor cardiac output

PREVENTION/AVOIDANCE N/A

POSSIBLE COMPLICATIONS
• Multiple organ dysfunction syndrome (MODS)
• Death
• Permanent lung disease
• Oxygen toxicity
• Barotrauma
• Superinfection

EXPECTED COURSE/PROGNOSIS
• 50% mortality rate; the syndrome is heterogeneous and mortality runs from 15-90%, depending on multiple factors; mainly, underlying cause, age of patient, number of failed organs.
• There is a decrease in diffusing capacity due to fibrosis and restrictive lung disease. Many people will have abnormal pulmonary function tests up to 6 months after illness. Most who survive will reveal abnormalities only with sensitive function testing, such as pulmonary exercise tests.

MISCELLANEOUS

ASSOCIATED CONDITIONS See Causes

AGE-RELATED FACTORS N/A
Pediatric: N/A
Geriatric: Increasing mortality with increasing age
Others: N/A

PREGNANCY N/A

SYNONYMS
• Shock lung
• Wet lung
• Noncardiac pulmonary edema

ICD-9-CM
786.09 Dyspnea and respiratory abnormalities
518.5 Respiratory distress following surgery or trauma
518.82 Adult respiratory distress syndrome associated with other conditions

SEE ALSO N/A

OTHER NOTES N/A

ABBREVIATIONS
PEEP = positive end-expiratory pressure

REFERENCES
• Civetta JM: Critical Care. Philadelphia, J.B. Lippincott, 1988
• Matthay MA: Critical Care Medicines. JAMA 1991;265(23):3109-3110
• Murray JF, Matthay MA, et al: Amer Review Resp Disease 1988;138:720-723
• Bennett JC, Plum F, eds: Cecil Textbook of Medicine. 20th Ed. Philadelphia, W.B. Saunders Co., 1996
• Demling R: Adult respiratory distress syndrome: Current concepts. New Horizons 1993;1(3):388-401
Illustrations: N/A
Internet references: http://www.5mcc.com

Author(s)
Michael Ferrebee, MD
Darell E. Heiselman, DO, FCCM, FACP, FACC, FCCP

Respiratory distress syndrome, neonatal

 BASICS

DESCRIPTION
Serious disorder of prematurity, with clinical manifestation of respiratory distress. Pulmonary surfactants that are deficient at birth cause diffuse lung atelectasis. Must differentiate from pneumonia, sepsis.
System(s) affected: Pulmonary
Genetics: No known genetic pattern
Incidence/Prevalence in USA: Common
Predominant age: Neonatal
Predominant sex: Male = Female

SIGNS AND SYMPTOMS
• Onset within few hours after birth
• Delayed, weak cry
• Expiratory grunt
• Frothing at lips
• Intercostal, sternal retractions
• Nasal flaring
• Rapid respiratory rate
• Respiratory excursions decreased
• Rales
• Cyanosis
• Peripheral edema
• Oliguria

CAUSES
• Prematurity
• Deficient pulmonary surfactants in the neonatal period
• Possible pulmonary ischemia

RISK FACTORS
• Premature infants born prior to 37 weeks gestation
• Infants born of diabetic mothers
• More common and more severe with greater prematurity

 DIAGNOSIS

DIFFERENTIAL DIAGNOSIS
• Early group B streptococcal pneumonia
• Transient tachypnea of newborn
• Meconium aspiration pneumonia
• Sepsis with group B streptococcus pneumonia

LABORATORY
• Amniotic fluid:
  ◊ Lecithin:sphingomyelin ratio (L:S ratio < 2)
  ◊ Absence of phosphatidyl glycerol
  ◊ Surfactant production deficient
• Features of respiratory, metabolic acidosis
• Arterial blood gases - hypoxemia and hypercarbia
Drugs that may alter lab results:
Artificial or human surfactant; betamethasone
Disorders that may alter lab results: N/A

PATHOLOGICAL FINDINGS
• Voluminous, noncrepitant, purplish red lungs
• Dilatation right heart and vena cava
• Possible patent ductus
• Extensive resorptive atelectasis
• Hyaline membranes

SPECIAL TESTS
• Monitor arterial blood gases

IMAGING
• X-ray - reticulogranular appearance of lung fields demonstrating:
  ◊ Diffuse atelectasis
  ◊ Air bronchograms

DIAGNOSTIC PROCEDURES N/A

 TREATMENT

APPROPRIATE HEALTH CARE Inpatient - intensive care

GENERAL MEASURES
• Positive pressure ventilation
• CPAP
• Warm, humidified, oxygen enriched gases by hood
• Monitor respiratory and circulatory status carefully
• Umbilical artery catheter placed for monitoring blood pressure and sampling arterial blood gases
• Transcutaneous monitors to measure O2 and CO2 tension
• Pulse oximetry
• Radiant infant warmer
• Tube feedings or hyperalimentation
• High-frequency ventilation. Choices include conventional ventilation at faster-than-normal rates; high-frequency jet ventilation; high-frequency oscillation.
• Relationship between using surfactant and high-frequency ventilation still being studied
• Extracorporeal membrane oxygenation (ECMO) measure of last resort. Its use is still uncommon and there are risks associated. Not available for infants under 2 kg.

SURGICAL MEASURES N/A

ACTIVITY None; may require sedation or paralysis while on ventilator

DIET Special premature formula or parenteral alimentation

PATIENT EDUCATION For patient education materials favorably reviewed on this topic, contact: American Lung Association, 1740 Broadway, New York, NY 10019, (212)315-8700

MEDICATIONS

DRUG(S) OF CHOICE
• Beractant (Survanta): bovine surfactant.
Dose: 2.6-8.0 mL depending on patient's
weight (see Manufacturer's Dosing Table)
• Colfosceril (Exosurf): synthetic surfactant.
Dose: 67.5 mg/kg as soon as possible after
birth given by endotracheal tube adaptor
supplied by manufacturer.
Prophylaxis: as soon as possible after birth.
Therapeutic: when signs and symptoms of
RDS appear.
Contraindications: Refer to manufacturer's
literature
Precautions: Do not administer beractant
into a mainstem bronchus. Be prepared for
rapidly changing lung compliance; peak
ventilator pressures may need to be reduced
immediately.
Significant possible interactions: Refer
to manufacturer's literature

ALTERNATIVE DRUGS N/A

FOLLOWUP

PATIENT MONITORING Continuous
monitoring in an intensive care nursery

PREVENTION/AVOIDANCE
• Prevention of premature birth
• Systemic betamethasone given to mother
when fetal lung profile is immature; at least 24
hours before delivery

POSSIBLE COMPLICATIONS
• Intraventricular hemorrhage
• Intracranial pathology
• Tension pneumothorax
• Retinopathy of prematurity
• Apnea

EXPECTED COURSE/PROGNOSIS
• Course: acute, possibly fatal within 48 hours
in 20-30%, increasing with lower birth weights,
especially < 1,000 grams.
• Prognosis:
  ◊ Successful outcome expected in tertiary
care centers in children older than 28 weeks
gestation
  ◊ Chronic lung disease, bronchopulmonary
dysplasia (BPD), frequent in severe cases,
especially after prolonged artificial ventilation

MISCELLANEOUS

ASSOCIATED CONDITIONS N/A

AGE-RELATED FACTORS
Pediatric: A disorder of the neonatal period
Geriatric: N/A
Others: N/A

PREGNANCY N/A

SYNONYMS
• Hyaline membrane disease
• RDS

ICD-9-CM 770.8

SEE ALSO N/A

OTHER NOTES N/A

ABBREVIATIONS
CPAP = continuous positive airway pressure

REFERENCES
• Pons PT: Respiratory Emergencies.
Emergency Care Quarterly 1989;5(1)
• Freezer NJ, et al: Pulmonary mechanics of
neonates on ECMO. Pediatr Pulmonal
1991;11(2):108-12
• Bhutan VK, et al: Pulmonary mechanics and
energetics in preterm infants who had
respiratory distress syndrome treated with
synthetic surfactant. J Pediatr 1992;120:518-24
Illustrations: N/A
Internet references: http://www.5mcc.com

Author(s)
Kurt J. Wegner, MD

Respiratory syncytial virus (RSV) infection

 BASICS

DESCRIPTION
• RSV causes respiratory illness
  ◊ Adults: URI's
  ◊ Infants and children: bronchitis, bronchiolitis, pneumonia
  ◊ Leading cause of pediatric admissions for respiratory illness
System(s) affected: Pulmonary
Genetics: None known
Incidence/Prevalence in USA: Common in winter. Almost all persons infected one or more times during lifetime.
Predominant Age: Birth to age 2
Predominant Sex:
• Males = females as outpatients
• 2:1 males/females in hospital

SIGNS AND SYMPTOMS
• Cold signs and symptoms (mild disease)
  ◊ Fever
  ◊ Cough
  ◊ Coryza
  ◊ Congestion
  ◊ Otitis media
  ◊ Malaise
• Bronchitis/bronchiolitis/pneumonia
  ◊ Cough
  ◊ Chest congestion, rales/rhonchi
  ◊ Wheezing
  ◊ Dyspnea
  ◊ Hypoxia
  ◊ Cyanosis
• Vomiting

CAUSES Infection with RSV

RISK FACTORS
• Impaired immunity
  ◊ AIDS
  ◊ Chemotherapy
  ◊ Other types of impaired immunity
• Occupational exposure
  ◊ Day care workers
  ◊ Pediatric hospital staff
  ◊ School teachers
• Neonatal/congenital conditions
  ◊ Congenital cardiac anomalies
  ◊ Respiratory distress syndrome
• Low socio-economic status
• More common in urban vs. rural areas

 DIAGNOSIS

DIFFERENTIAL DIAGNOSIS
• Mild illness/upper respiratory tract
  ◊ Colds (non RSV)
  ◊ Allergic rhinitis
  ◊ Sinusitis
  ◊ Croup
• Severe illness/lower respiratory tract
  ◊ Asthma
  ◊ Bronchitis
  ◊ Bronchiolitis
  ◊ Pneumonia

LABORATORY
• WBC may be normal to elevated
• Positive RSV antigen test on nasal washings
Drugs that may alter lab results: None
Disorders that may alter lab results: None

PATHOLOGICAL FINDINGS Lymphocytic peribronchiole infiltrates (autopsy)

SPECIAL TESTS N/A

IMAGING
• Chest x-ray
  ◊ Hyperinflation - most common, characteristic finding
  ◊ Interstitial infiltrates - fairly common
  ◊ Segmental or lobar consolidation in pneumonia
  ◊ Pleural fluid

DIAGNOSTIC PROCEDURES None

 TREATMENT

APPROPRIATE HEALTH CARE
Outpatient for mild cases; inpatient for severe disease or for those with underlying disorders

GENERAL MEASURES
• Outpatient
  ◊ Rest/supportive care
  ◊ Bronchodilators - albuterol nebulizer/inhaler
  ◊ Monitor oxygenation-pulse oximeter
• Inpatient
  ◊ Oxygen
  ◊ Bronchodilators - albuterol nebulizer q4h
  ◊ Respiratory isolation
  ◊ Ribavirin
  ◊ Antibiotics for secondary bacterial pneumonia
  ◊ Monitor arterial blood gases/pulse oximeter
• Avoid exposing others
  ◊ Remove from day care/school until well
  ◊ Good hand washing practices
  ◊ Respiratory isolation in hospital

SURGICAL MEASURES N/A

ACTIVITY Decreased household activity/rest

DIET
• Maintain nutrition
• Avoid over-hydration (may increase lung congestion)

PATIENT EDUCATION Printed patient information available from: ICN Pharmaceuticals, Inc., ICN Plaza, 3300 Hyland Ave., Costa Mesa, CA 92626 "All about RSV: a guide for parents."

Respiratory syncytial virus (RSV) infection

MEDICATIONS

DRUG(S) OF CHOICE
• Ribavirin 20 mg/mL mist 12-18 hours/day for 3-7 days. (Can shorten duration and severity of illness.)
• Bronchodilators - albuterol nebulizer q4h (dose appropriate for age)
• Antibiotics for secondary bacterial infections/pneumonia
  ◊ Appropriate to particular pathogen
  ◊ Prophylactic use of antibiotics controversial
• Potential use of RSV immune globulin in high risk infants
Contraindications: See specific drug related information
Precautions: Avoid exposure of pregnant/potentially pregnant women to ribavirin
Significant possible interactions: See specific drug information

ALTERNATIVE DRUGS
• Antibiotic appropriate to identified or suspected bacterial pathogen
• Theophylline use all right, but not recommended

FOLLOWUP

PATIENT MONITORING
• Uneventful resolution is the norm
• No special monitoring is needed as illness resolves
• May want to educate parents about SIDS - avoid prone sleeping in infants

PREVENTION/AVOIDANCE
• Avoid exposure to those ill with RSV
• Good hand washing practices (since hand-nose and hand-eye transmission is common)
• Avoid rubbing the eyes (common RSV inoculation route)

POSSIBLE COMPLICATIONS
• Pneumonia
• Sudden infant death
• Death from severe lower respiratory tract infections
• Possible residual lung damage

EXPECTED COURSE/PROGNOSIS
• Usually resolves within two weeks without sequelae
• Hospitalization rate of children ill with RSV varies from 1:50 to 1:200 (children < 2 years old)

MISCELLANEOUS

ASSOCIATED CONDITIONS
• Asthma is worse with RSV and vice versa
• SIDS may be a sequelae of RSV

AGE-RELATED FACTORS
Pediatric: Most common under age 2
Geriatric: N/A
Others: Increasing immunity with subsequent infections by RSV usually results in less serious illness

PREGNANCY
Avoid ribavirin therapy in pregnancy

SYNONYMS N/A

ICD-9-CM
480.1 Pneumonia due to respiratory syncytial virus

SEE ALSO
• Bronchiolitis
• Pneumonia, bacterial
• Pneumonia, viral
• Bronchitis, acute

OTHER NOTES N/A

ABBREVIATIONS
• RSV = respiratory syncytial virus
• SIDS = sudden infant death syndrome
• URI = upper respiratory infection

REFERENCES
• Mandell GL, ed: Principles and Practice of Infectious Diseases. 4th Ed. New York, Churchill Livingstone, 1995
• Rudolph AM, ed: Rudolph's Pediatrics 19th Ed. Norwalk, CT, Appleton & Lange, 1991
• Gilchrist S, et al: National surveillance for RSV, U.S., 1985-1990. J Inf Dis 1994;170:986-990
• Levin MJ: Treatment & prevention options for RSV infections. J Pediatr 1994;124:322-325
• Groothuis J, et al: Prophylactic administration of RSV immune globulin to high risk infants and young children. New Engl J Med 1993;329:1524-1530
Illustrations: N/A
Internet references: http://www.5mcc.com

Author(s)
Joseph G. Ewing, MD

Retinal detachment

BASICS

DESCRIPTION Separation of the sensory retina from the underlying retinal pigment epithelium.
• Rhegmatogenous retinal detachment (RRD): Is the most common type. It occurs when the fluid vitreous gains access to the subretinal space through a break in the retina (Greek rhegma, rent).
• Exudative or serous detachment: Occurs in the absence of a retinal break, usually in association with inflammation and a tumor.
• Traction detachment: Vitreoretinal adhesions mechanically pull the retina from the retinal pigment epithelium. The most common cause is proliferative diabetic retinopathy.
System(s) affected: Nervous
Genetics: Most cases are sporadic
Incidence/Prevalence in USA:
• 1/10,000 per year in patients who have not had cataract surgery
• 1-3% of patients after cataract surgery will develop a retinal detachment
Predominant age: The incidence increases with age.
Predominant sex: Male>Female (3:2)

SIGNS AND SYMPTOMS
• Flashes (photopsia)
• Floaters
• Visual field loss
• Pigmented cells within the vitreous "tobacco dust"
• Central vision will be preserved if the macula is not detached
• Poor visual acuity (20/200 or worse) with loss of central vision when macula is detached.
• Elevation of retina associated with one or more retinal tears in RRD or elevation of the retina without tears in exudative detachment
• In 3-10% of patients with presumed RRD, no definite retinal break is found
• Tenting of the retina without retinal tears in traction detachment

CAUSES
• Traction from a posterior vitreous detachment (PVD) cause most retinal tears. With aging, vitreous gel liquefies leading to the separation of the vitreous from the retina. The vitreous gel remains attached at the vitreous base, in the retinal periphery, resulting in vitreous traction producing tears in the retinal periphery.
• PVD associated with vitreous hemorrhage has a high incidence of retinal tears
• Exudative detachment:
  ◊ Tumors
  ◊ Inflammatory diseases (Harada's, posterior scleritis)
  ◊ Miscellaneous (central serous retinopathy, uveal effusion, malignant hypertension)
• Traction detachment:
  ◊ Proliferative diabetic retinopathy
  ◊ Cicatricial retinopathy of prematurity
  ◊ Proliferative sickle cell retinopathy
  ◊ Penetrating trauma

RISK FACTORS
• Myopia (greater than 5 diopters)
• Aphakia or pseudophakia
• PVD and associated conditions (aphakia, inflammatory disease and trauma)
• Trauma
• Retinal detachment in fellow eye
• Lattice degeneration. Lattice degeneration is a vitreoretinal abnormality found in 6-10% of the general population
• Glaucoma. 4-7% of patients with retinal detachment have chronic open angle glaucoma
• Vitreoretinal tufts. Peripheral retinal tufts are caused by focal areas of vitreous tractions.
• Meridional folds. Redundant retina usually found in the supranasal quadrant

DIAGNOSIS

DIFFERENTIAL DIAGNOSIS
Retinoschisis (splitting of the retina). Vitreous cell or vitreous hemorrhage are rarely found in the vitreous with retinoschisis, whereas they are commonly seen in RRD. Retinoschisis usually has a smooth surface and is dome shaped; whereas, RRD often has a corrugated, irregular surface.

LABORATORY N/A
Drugs that may alter lab results: N/A
Disorders that may alter lab results: N/A

PATHOLOGICAL FINDINGS Elevation of the neurosensory retina from the underlying retinal pigment epithelium.

SPECIAL TESTS
• Visual field testing. Differentiate between a RRD and retinoschisis. An absolute scotoma is seen in retinoschisis whereas a RRD causes a relative scotoma.
• Ultrasonography can demonstrate a detached retina and may be helpful when the retina can not be visualized directly (cataracts, etc).

IMAGING Fluorescein dye leakage can be seen in exudative retinal detachment caused by central serous retinopathy

DIAGNOSTIC PROCEDURES
• Slit lamp examination
• Dilated fundus examination with binocular indirect ophthalmoscopy

TREATMENT

APPROPRIATE HEALTH CARE Referral to an ophthalmologist for examination and treatment, if indicated

GENERAL MEASURES
• Not all retinal tears or breaks need to be treated. Flap tears or horseshoe tears in symptomatic patients (that is patients with flashes or floaters) frequently are treated. Operculated holes in symptomatic patients are sometimes treated. Atrophic holes in symptomatic patients are rarely treated.
• Lattice degeneration with or without holes within the lattice in an asymptomatic patient with prior retinal detachment may be prophylactically treated.
• Flap retinal tears in asymptomatic patients are frequently treated prophylactically
• Exudative detachments are usually managed by treatment of the underlying disorder
• Traction detachments usually managed by observation. If the fovea is involved, then a vitrectomy is needed

SURGICAL MEASURES
• Timing of repairs
  ◊ Macula attached: within 24 hours. If the detachment is peripheral and does not have features suggestive for rapid progression (such as large and/or superior tears) then repair can be performed within a few days.
  ◊ Macula recently detached: within a couple of days
  ◊ Old macular detachment: elective repair within 2 weeks
• If a retinal break has lead to the development of a retinal detachment, then surgery will be needed. Surgical options (and combinations) include:
  ◊ Pneumatic retinopexy. Head positioning is required postoperatively.
  ◊ Scleral buckle.
  ◊ Vitrectomy.
  ◊ Perfluorocarbon liquids for giant tears (circumferential tears 90° or larger)
  ◊ Silicone oil for complex repairs
• Anesthesia. Usually with local anesthesia.
• RRD may have more than one break. If any retinal break is not closed at the time of surgery, the surgery will fail.
• Additional surgery may be required if the retina redetaches secondary to a new retinal break or due to proliferative vitreoretinopathy (PVR).

ACTIVITY Bedrest prior to surgery. Postoperatively, if an intraocular gas has been used, the patient may need specific head positioning and should not travel to high altitudes.

DIET NPO if surgery is imminent

PATIENT EDUCATION American Academy of Ophthalmology, 655 E. Beach Street, San Francisco, California 94109-1336

MEDICATIONS

DRUG(S) OF CHOICE
• Intraocular gases
◊ air
◊ perfluoropropane (C3F8)
◊ sulfur hexafluoride (SF6)
• Perfluorocarbon liquids
• Silicone oil
Contraindications: Patients with poorly controlled glaucoma.
Precautions: Expanding intraocular gas bubble increases intraocular pressure, therefore, avoid higher altitudes
Significant possible interactions: Nitrous oxide can expand an intraocular gas bubble

ALTERNATIVE DRUGS
Steroids can cause worsening of central serous retinopathy

FOLLOWUP

PATIENT MONITORING
• Alert ophthalmologist immediately:
◊ Symptoms of PVD and detachment (new onset of floaters or flashes, increase in floaters or flashes, sudden shower of floaters, curtain or shadow in the peripheral visual field, or reduced vision)
• Patients with an acute symptomatic PVD associated with mild vitreous hemorrhage should be reexamined in 3-4 weeks by the ophthalmologist. The development of a retinal detachment is unlikely if no retinal tears are present on reexamination in 3-4 weeks.
• A patient with an acute symptomatic PVD, even in the absence of vitreous hemorrhage, vitreous pigment or detectable retinal break, may need to be reexamined in 3-4 weeks by the ophthalmologist, depending on clinical circumstances such as aphakia or myopia, because retinal breaks may develop over time.
• If an acute symptomatic PVD is associated with gross vitreous hemorrhage which interferes with complete visualization of the retinal periphery by indirect ophthalmoscopy, then a patient should be reexamined at short intervals with indirect ophthalmoscopy until the entire retinal periphery can be observed.
• If the examiner is not certain that the retina is detached in the presence of opaque media, ultrasonography should be performed

PREVENTION/AVOIDANCE
• Patients at risk for a retinal detachment should have regular ophthalmologic examination

POSSIBLE COMPLICATIONS
• PVR is the most common cause of failed retinal detachment repair. 10-15% of patients, whose retinas reattach initially after retinal surgery, will subsequently re-detach; usually within 6 weeks due to cellular proliferation and contraction on the retinal surface.
• Partial or total loss of vision due to macular detachment and/or PVR
• Moderate to severe forms of PVR are usually treated with pars plana vitrectomy and fluid-gas exchange. If a segmental scleral buckle was placed at the initial procedure, then this will need to be revised.
• Scleral buckles may erode the overlying conjunctiva and lead to an infection

EXPECTED COURSE/PROGNOSIS
• RRD:
◊ 90% of retinal detachments can be reattached successfully after one or more surgical procedures. Postoperative visual acuity depends primarily on the status of the macula preoperatively. Also important is the length of time between the detachment and the repair (75% of macular detachments of less than one week will obtain a final visual acuity of 20/70 or better).
◊ 87% of eyes with a retinal detachment not involving the macula attain a visual acuity of 20/50 or better postoperatively. 37% of eyes with a detached macula preoperatively attain 20/50 or better vision postoperatively.
◊ In 10-15% of successfully repaired retinal detachments not involving the macula preoperatively, visual acuity does not return to the preoperative level. This decrease is secondary to complications such as macular edema or macular pucker.
• Tractional retinal detachment:
◊ When not involving the fovea, the patient can usually be observed since it is uncommon for these to extend into the fovea.
• Exudative retinal detachment:
◊ Management is usually nonsurgical
◊ The presence of shifting fluid is highly suggestive of an exudative retinal detachment. Fixed retinal folds which are indicative of PVR are rarely seen in exudative retinal detachment. If the underlying condition is treated the prognosis is generally good.

MISCELLANEOUS

ASSOCIATED CONDITIONS
• Lattice degeneration
• High myopia
• Cataract surgery
• Glaucoma
• History of retinal detachment in the fellow eye
• Trauma

AGE-RELATED FACTORS
Pediatric: Usually associated with underlying vitreoretinal disorders and/or retinopathy of prematurity
Geriatric:
• Posterior vitreous detachment
• Cataract surgery
Others: N/A

PREGNANCY Pre-eclampsia/eclampsia may be associated with exudative retinal detachment. No intervention is indicated, provided hypertension is controlled, prognosis is usually good.

SYNONYMS N/A

ICD-9-CM
361.00 Rhegmatogenous retinal detachment
379.21 Posterior vitreous detachment
361.2 Serous (nonrhegmatogenous) detachment
361.81 Tractional detachment
362.63 Lattice degeneration of retina
361.30 Retinal break without detachment

SEE ALSO
• Diabetic retinopathy

OTHER NOTES N/A

ABBREVIATIONS
RRD = rhegmatogenous retinal detachment
PVD = posterior vitreous detachment
PVR = proliferative vitreoretinopathy

REFERENCES
• Tani P, Robertson, DM, Langworthy A: Prognosis for Central Vision and Anatomic Reattachment in Rhegmatogenous Retinal Detachment with Macula Detached. Am J Ophthalmol 1981;92:611-620
• The American Academy of Ophthalmol. Ophthalmic Procedure Assessment: The Repair of Rhegmatogenous Retinal Detachments. Ophthalmology 1996;103:1313-1324
• The American Academy of Ophthalmol. Preferred Practice Pattern: Retinal Detachment 1990: 1-17
• The American Academy of Ophthalmology. Preferred Practice Pattern: Precursors of Rhegmatogenous Retinal Detachment in Adults 1994:1-19
• Benson WE: Retinal Detachment Diagnosis and Management. Second Edition. Philadelphia, J.B. Lippincott Co., 1988
• Vitrectomy with Silicone Oil or Perfluoropropane Gas in Eyes with Severe Proliferative Vitreoretinopathy: Results of a Randomized Clinical Trial. Silicone Study Report 2. Arch Ophthalmol 1992;110:780-792
Illustrations: 6 available on CD-ROM
Illustrations: 6 available on CD-ROM
Internet references: http://www.5mcc.com

Author(s)
Richard W. Allinson, MD

Retinitis pigmentosa

BASICS

DESCRIPTION Retinitis pigmentosa is characterized by poor night vision, constricted visual fields, bone spicule-like pigmentation of the fundus, and electroretinographic evidence of photoreceptor cell dysfunction.
System(s) affected: Nervous
Genetics:
• Autosomal dominant - 20%
• Autosomal recessive - 37%
• X-linked recessive - 4.5%
• Sporadic - 38.5%
Incidence/Prevalence in USA: RP affects approximately 1 in 4,000 people in the US
Predominant age:
• X-linked RP has the earliest onset of the major hereditary types and many X-linked patients are legally blind by the age 30
• Autosomal dominant RP has a later onset than autosomal recessive or X-linked recessive RP
• Leber's congenital amaurosis which is a variant of RP presents at birth
• Late onset RP typically is asymptomatic and unrecognized until age 40 or 50
Predominant sex: Male > female

SIGNS AND SYMPTOMS
• Night blindness (nyctalopia)
• Bone spicule pigmentation in the retina
• Retinal arteriolar narrowing
• Optic nerve head pallor, "waxy pallor"
• Progressive visual field loss
• Central visual acuity is usually preserved until the end stages of retinitis pigmentosa
• Most patients are myopic
• Posterior subcapsular cataracts are common in all forms of retinitis pigmentosa
• Cystoid macular edema
• Optic nerve head drusen
• Electroretinogram (ERG) changes
• Retinal neovascularization
• RP associated with an exudative retinal vasculopathy. Fundus findings would include serous retinal detachment, lipid deposition in the retina and telangiectatic vascular anomalies.
• Variants of RP exists with unusual or regional distribution including:
• Sectorial RP
• Pigmented paravenous atrophy
• Unilateral RP

CAUSES
• The genetic mutations responsible for RP have been identified in some families with RP, primarily those with the autosomal dominant form
• Mutations in the rhodopsin gene account for about 30% of cases with autosomal dominant RP
• Another 4-6% of autosomal dominant RP is due to a mutation in the gene for a photoreceptor protein, peripherin/RDS

RISK FACTORS Family history

DIAGNOSIS

DIFFERENTIAL DIAGNOSIS
Bone spicule-like retinal pigmentation and retinal atrophy are nonspecific findings and can result from conditions other than retinitis pigmentosa
• Infections
• Syphilis
• Rubella
• Inflammation (severe uveitis)
• Choroidal vascular occlusion
• Toxicity (chloroquine or thioridazine)
• Choroideremia
• Gyrate atrophy of choroid and retina (10 to 20 fold elevation of plasma ornithine levels)
• Systemic metabolic disorders such as Refsum's disease and abetalipoproteinemia
• Kearns-Sayre syndrome. Usually presents in adolescents. It is characterized by progressive external ophthalmoplegia, the first sign usually being ptosis, pigmentary degeneration of the retina and a cardiac conduction defect which may cause complete heart block.
• Cone-rod dystrophy. Characterized by bilateral and symmetric loss of cone function in the presence of reduced rod function.
• Cone dystrophy characterized by marked abnormality in cone function with some or no rod involvement.
• Congenital stationery night blindness
• Oguchi's disease
• Fundus albipunctatus
• Trauma

LABORATORY
• Elevated plasma levels of phytanic acid in Refsum's disease
• Acanthocytosis of red blood cells in peripheral blood smear in abetalipoproteinemia. This is an autosomal recessive disorder in which abetalipoprotein B is not synthesized, leading to fat malabsorption and deficiencies of fat soluble vitamins. Therapy with vitamin A and E can improve retinal function.
• Syphilic neuroretinitis can be diagnosed by performing a FTA-ABS or MHA-Tp
• Elevated plasma ornithine levels in gyrate atrophy of the choroid and retina. Usually a 10-20 fold elevation of plasma ornithine levels.
Drugs that may alter lab results: N/A
Disorders that may alter lab results: N/A

PATHOLOGICAL FINDINGS
• Disappearance of the rods, cones and outer nuclear layers in the retina.
• Bone spicule formation in the retina is secondary to the migration of retinal pigment epithelial cells into the anterior retina

SPECIAL TESTS
• Electroretinography (ERG). Photoreceptors generate reduced amplitude a- and b-waves in RP. Rod and cone responses may be undetectable in advanced RP.

• Visual field testing. A ring scotoma in the mid periphery may be identified. The ring scotomas generally starts as a group of isolated scotomas in the area 20-25° from fixation. Long after the entire peripheral field is gone, there remains a small island of intact central visual field.
• Fluorescein angiography can demonstrate cystoid macular edema.
• Fundus photography to document the status of the retina.
• Hearing tests in patients complaining of hearing loss such as patients with Usher's syndrome (RP with hearing loss).

IMAGING N/A

DIAGNOSTIC PROCEDURES N/A

TREATMENT

APPROPRIATE HEALTH CARE
Outpatient

GENERAL MEASURES
• Supportive
• Genetic counselling
• Low vision aids
• Educating the patient

SURGICAL MEASURES
• The efficacy of the "Cuban" therapy, which is electric stimulation, autotransfused ozonated blood, and ocular surgery has not been proven to be of benefit
• Macular grid laser photocoagulation may be of benefit for patients with cystoid macular edema secondary to RP

ACTIVITY Full activity. Caution should be exercised because of the reduced peripheral vision and poor night vision.

DIET No special diet

PATIENT EDUCATION
• Counsel patients to help them understand RP and its genetics
• RP is a slowly progressive, chronic disease; patients do not go blind rapidly and total blindness is not a frequent end-point of this disease
• RP Foundation Fighting Blindness, Executive Plaza One, Suite 800, 11350 McCormick Road, Hunt Valley, MD 21031-1014, (800)683-5555
• The American Academy of Ophthalmology, 655 E. Beach Street, San Francisco, CA 94109-1336, (415)561-8540

MEDICATIONS

DRUG(S) OF CHOICE
• Vitamin A 15,000 IU q day (retinal degeneration slowed as measured by ERG/visual fields). [Note: beta-carotene not a suitable substitute; not studied in patient under age 18]
• Vitamin E at 400mg q day results in faster retinal degeneration and is not recommended
• Acetazolamide 500 mg q day may be of benefit for cystoid macular edema occurring in RP.

Contraindications:
• Limit vitamin A to < 8,000 IU per day during pregnancy.

Precautions:
• Avoid vitamin A supplement dosages >15,000 IU per day

Significant possible interactions: N/A

ALTERNATIVE DRUGS   N/A

FOLLOWUP

PATIENT MONITORING
• Ophthalmic examinations every 1-2 years
• Check for complications (cataracts, etc.)

PREVENTION/AVOIDANCE
• Genetic counselling
• The amount of light does not modify the course of RP.
• Ultraviolet-absorbing sunglasses and brimmed hats are recommended when patients are at the beach or in the snow.

POSSIBLE COMPLICATIONS
• Cataract
• Cystoid macular edema
• Loss of visual field
• Poor night vision
• Blindness

EXPECTED COURSE/PROGNOSIS
• Reassurance about the slow course of RP
• Most of the deafness in Usher's syndrome is congenital. It is unlikely that an RP patient who is not born deaf will go deaf later in his life.
• RP severity varies with inheritance pattern
• Autosomal recessive form has an early age of onset and may have severely constricted visual fields by age 20. Tends toward more rapid progression as compared to autosomal dominant RP; also increased incidence of cataracts.
• X-linked RP is similar in clinical presentation to autosomal recessive RP
• Autosomal dominant RP generally has less severe findings initially than autosomal recessive RP; symptoms may not occur until 30 years of age
• Good central vision usually preserved. If the central visual field radius is >30°, >90% of patients will have visual acuities of 20/40 or better. If the central visual field radius is smaller than 10°, 30% of patients will have a visual acuity of 20/40 or better.

MISCELLANEOUS

ASSOCIATED CONDITIONS
• With systemic disorders:
◊ Usher's syndrome. RP and congenital sensorineural hearing impairment.
◊ Laurence-Moon-Biedl syndrome (also called the Bardet-Biedl syndrome) is an autosomal recessive disorder associated with retinal dystrophy, mental retardation, obesity, hypogonadism, and postaxial polydactyly.
◊ Cockayne syndrome. This is an autosomal recessive disorder in which children at the age of one or two years present with retinal dystrophy, sensorineural deafness, cerebellar dysfunction, dementia, and ultraviolet light photosensitivity.

AGE-RELATED FACTORS
Pediatric: Leber's congenital amaurosis is characterized by severely reduced vision from birth and impaired ERG responses from both cones and rods. Most cases are autosomal recessive.
Geriatric: Late onset RP is asymptomatic; generally unrecognized until age >40
Others: N/A

PREGNANCY   Remember risk of teratogenicity of high intake vitamin A during pregnancy

SYNONYMS
• Rod-cone dystrophy
• Retinal dystrophy

ICD-9-CM
362.74 Retinitis pigmentosa

SEE ALSO
• Laurence-Moon-Biedl syndrome
• Cataract

OTHER NOTES   N/A

ABBREVIATIONS
RP = Retinitis Pigmentosa
ERG = Electroretinogram

REFERENCES
• Berson EL, Remulla JFC, Rosner B, et al: Evaluation of patients with retinitis pigmentosa receiving electric stimulation, ozonated blood, and ocular surgery in Cuba. Arch Ophthalmol 1996;114:560-563
• Pagon RA: Retinitis pigmentosa. Surv Ophthalmol 1988;33:137-177
• Madreperla SA, et al: Visual acuity loss and retinitis pigmentosa. relationship to visual field loss. Arch Ophthalmol 1990;108:358-364
Illustrations: 1 available on CD-ROM
Internet references: http://www.5mcc.com

Author(s)
Richard W. Allinson, MD

Retinopathy of prematurity

 BASICS

DESCRIPTION Retinopathy of prematurity (ROP) is a proliferative disorder of the retinal blood vessels in premature infants. The normal retinal vascularization occurs nasally at approximately 36 weeks of gestation and temporally at approximately 40 weeks of gestation.
System(s) affected: Nervous
Genetics: Black infants appear less susceptible
Incidence/Prevalence in USA:
• Approximately one third of all infants weighing less than 1500 grams at birth may show evidence of retinopathy of prematurity
• 65.8% of infants weighing less than 1251 grams at birth, and 81.6% of those weighing less than 1000 grams
• Of babies born with a birth weight of 1001-1500 grams, 2.2% will develop cicatricial changes as a complication of ROP and 0.5% of them will be blind
Predominant age: Premature infants
Predominant sex: Male = Female

SIGNS AND SYMPTOMS
Acute ROP is classified as follows:
• Location:
  ◊ Zone I: posterior retina within a 60 degree circle centered on the optic nerve
  ◊ Zone II: extends from the edge of Zone I to the nasal ora anteriorly
  ◊ Zone III: is the residual temporal crescent of retina anterior to Zone II
• Extent: number of clock hours involved
• Degree of abnormal vascular response observed:
  ◊ Stage 1: the development of a demarcation line between the vascularized and nonvascularized retina
  ◊ Stage 2: the presence of a demarcation line that extends out of the plane of the retina (ridge)
  ◊ Stage 3: a ridge with extraretinal fibrovascular proliferation
  ◊ Stage 4: subtotal retinal detachment
  ◊ Stage 5: total retinal detachment
• "Plus" disease is characterized by the tortuosity of the retinal vasculature in the posterior fundus

CAUSES Oxidative processes, influenced by high levels of arterial oxygen, in immature retina, may be an important causative factor

RISK FACTORS
• Low birth weight
• Prematurity
• Supplemental oxygen. Once the retina becomes fully vascularized, oxygen will not affect the retina.

 DIAGNOSIS

DIFFERENTIAL DIAGNOSIS
• Retinoblastoma
• Congenital cataracts
• Norrie's disease
• Incontinentia pigmenti
• Familial exudative vitreoretinopathy
• Ocular toxocariasis
• Coat's disease
• Persistent hyperplastic primary vitreous
• X-linked retinoschisis

LABORATORY N/A
Drugs that may alter lab results: N/A
Disorders that may alter lab results: N/A

PATHOLOGICAL FINDINGS
• Peripheral retinal nonperfusion
• Retinal neovascularization
• Retinal hemorrhages
• Retinal detachment

SPECIAL TESTS N/A

IMAGING N/A

DIAGNOSTIC PROCEDURES
• An ophthalmologist skilled in the detection of this disorder should examine all infants who weigh less than 1,250 grams
• The initial eye exam should be performed at 4 to 6 weeks of age
• Follow-up exams are performed until the retina is noted to be fully vascularized

 TREATMENT

APPROPRIATE HEALTH CARE
Treatment usually is performed in the neonatal intensive care unit or as an outpatient or inpatient as the child grows older

GENERAL MEASURES
• The multicenter trial of cryotherapy demonstrated a favorable outcome for eyes treated at threshold (Stage 3+ retinopathy of prematurity) versus control eyes
• Stage 3 retinopathy defined as a ridge of extraretinal fibrovascular proliferation
• A plus sign is added to the ROP stage number when retinal vascular tortuosity is noted in the posterior fundus
• Threshold disease was defined as at least 5 contiguous or 8 cumulative clock hours of Stage 3 associated with retinal vascular tortuosity in the posterior segment of the eye ("plus" disease)

• Transscleral cryotherapy to the avascular retina when applied to high risk eyes can reduce the incidence of sight threatening complications. The multicenter trial of cryotherapy has shown that treatment of high risk eyes reduces the incidence of unfavorable outcomes by 46%.
• The multicenter trial of cryotherapy demonstrated an unfavorable outcome, defined as posterior retinal detachment, retinal fold involving the macula, or retrolental tissue, was significantly less frequent in eyes undergoing cryotherapy
• The results at one year from the multicenter trial of cryotherapy demonstrated an unfavorable outcome in 25.7% of eyes that received cryotherapy compared with 47.4% of the control eyes
• Using Teller Acuity Card assessment an unfavorable outcome was noted in 35.0% of the treated eyes compared with 56.3% of the control eyes, at one year in the multicenter trial of cryotherapy
• Laser treatment applied to the avascular retina in high risk eyes can reduce the incidence of sight-threatening complications; cataract formation is a possible complication
• Vitrectomy and/or scleral buckling can be used to treat retinal detachment associated with ROP
• The role of vitamin E administration for prophylaxis is controversial. It may reduce the severity, but not the incidence of ROP
• Extremely low birth weight infants receiving prophylactic treatment with calf lung surfactant extract demonstrated a lower incidence of any stage when compared with control infants

SURGICAL MEASURES See General Measures

ACTIVITY N/A

DIET N/A

PATIENT EDUCATION
• Expectant mothers should avoid behavioral and environmental risk factors associated with low birth weight. These include smoking, alcohol and other substance abuse, and poor nutrition.
• American Academy of Ophthalmology, 655 Beach St., San Francisco, CA 94109-1336

MEDICATIONS

DRUG(S) OF CHOICE None
Contraindications: N/A
Precautions: N/A
Significant possible interactions: N/A

ALTERNATIVE DRUGS N/A

FOLLOWUP

PATIENT MONITORING
• Close follow-up of patients with ROP is required
• Follow-up exams after the initial examination are performed every two weeks until the retina is fully vascularized or until the ROP regresses
• Follow-up exams are performed every week if "prethreshold" disease is present. Prethreshold disease is characterized by the following:
  ◊ Zone I, any stage
  ◊ Zone II, Stage 2 (ridge) with "plus" disease
  ◊ Zone II, Stage 3 (ridge) with extraretinal fibrovascular proliferation
• In some cases of regressed ROP, cicatrization can develop. This is associated with variable degrees of fibrosis. This can lead to vitreoretinal traction and subsequent retinal detachment from formation of a retinal hole.
• Retinal detachment secondary to cicatricial ROP can occur during the midteens, therefore, long term follow-up of cicatricial cases of ROP is indicated

PREVENTION/AVOIDANCE See Patient Education

POSSIBLE COMPLICATIONS
• Retinal detachment
• Retinal fold involving the macula
• Vitreous hemorrhage
• Angle closure glaucoma
• Amblyopia
• Strabismus
• Myopia

EXPECTED COURSE/PROGNOSIS
• Spontaneous regression occurs over a period of weeks or months in most cases. Spontaneous regression occurs in approximately 85% of eyes.
• The earliest sign of regression is the growth of blood vessels beyond the demarcation line into previously avascular retina
• Some cases of RLF do not regress spontaneously without sequela, but progress. A gradual transition then occurs from active RLF to cicatricial RLF. Cicatricial RLF is associated with varying degrees of fibrosis and vitreoretinal traction which can lead to retinal detachment.

MISCELLANEOUS

ASSOCIATED CONDITIONS Neonatal respiratory distress syndrome

AGE-RELATED FACTORS
Pediatric: N/A
Geriatric: N/A
Others: N/A

PREGNANCY N/A

SYNONYMS
• ROP
• Retrolental fibroplasia

ICD-9-CM
362.21 Retinopathy of prematurity

SEE ALSO N/A

OTHER NOTES N/A

ABBREVIATIONS
• ROP = retinopathy of prematurity
• RLF = retrolental fibroplasia

REFERENCES
• Cryotherapy for retinopathy of prematurity cooperative group. Multicenter trial of cryotherapy for retinopathy of prematurity: one year outcome - structure and function. Arch Ophthalmology. 108:1408-1416, 1990
• Ben-Sir I., Nissenkorn I, Kremer I: Retinopathy of Prematurity. Surv Ophthalmol 1988;33:1-16
• Cryotherapy for retinopathy of prematurity cooperative group. Multicenter trial of cryotherapy for retinopathy of prematurity. Preliminary results. Arch Ophthalmology 1988;106:471-479
• The committee for the classification of retinopathy of prematurity: An international classification of retinopathy of prematurity. Arch Ophthalmology 1984;102:1130-1134
Illustrations: N/A
Internet references: http://www.5mcc.com

Author(s)
Richard W. Allinson, MD

Retinopathy, diabetic

BASICS

DESCRIPTION Noninflammatory retinal disorder characterized by retinal capillary closure and microaneurysms. Retinal ischemia leads to release of a vasoproliferative factor stimulating neovascularization on the retina, optic nerve, or iris.
• Most patients with diabetes mellitus will develop diabetic retinopathy. It is the leading cause of new cases of legal blindness among Americans between the ages of 20-64.
• Diabetic retinopathy can be divided into three stages:
  ◊ Background diabetic retinopathy
  ◊ Preproliferative diabetic retinopathy
  ◊ Proliferative diabetic retinopathy
System(s) affected: Nervous
Genetics: N/A
Incidence/Prevalence in USA:
• Approximately 6.6% of the population between ages 20-74 has diabetes
• Approximately 25% of the diabetic population has some form of diabetic retinopathy
• Diabetic retinopathy accounts for approximately 10% of new cases of blindness each year
Predominant age:
• Peak incidence of Type I, juvenile onset diabetes mellitus, is between the ages of 12-15
• Peak incidence of Type II, adult onset, between the ages of 50-70
• The incidence of diabetic retinopathy is directly related to the duration of diabetes
• In children less than 10 years of age, it is unusual to see diabetic retinopathy, regardless of the duration of diabetes
• The risk of developing diabetic retinopathy increases after puberty
• Almost all diabetics will develop background retinopathy if they have had diabetes for at least 20 years
• Two-thirds of juvenile-onset diabetics who have had diabetes for at least 35 years will develop proliferative diabetic retinopathy, and one-third will develop macular edema. The proportions are reversed for adult-onset diabetes.
Predominant sex:
• Male = Female - juvenile onset diabetes mellitus
• Female > Male - non-insulin-dependent diabetes mellitus

SIGNS AND SYMPTOMS
• Background diabetic retinopathy
  ◊ Microaneurysms
  ◊ Intraretinal hemorrhage
  ◊ Macular edema
  ◊ Lipid deposits
• Preproliferative diabetic retinopathy
  ◊ Nerve fiber layer infarctions (cotton wool spots)
  ◊ Venous beading
  ◊ Venous dilation
  ◊ Intraretinal microvascular abnormalities (IRMA)
  ◊ Extensive retinal hemorrhage

• Proliferative diabetic retinopathy
  ◊ New blood vessel proliferation (neovascularization) on the retinal surface, optic nerve, and iris

CAUSES Related to the development of diabetic microaneurysms and microvascular abnormalities.

RISK FACTORS
• Duration of diabetes mellitus (usually over 10 years)
• Poor glycemic control
• Pregnancy
• Renal disease
• Systemic hypertension

DIAGNOSIS

DIFFERENTIAL DIAGNOSIS Other causes of retinopathy, e.g., radiation retinopathy, retinal venous obstruction, and hypertensive retinopathy.

LABORATORY N/A
Drugs that may alter lab results: N/A
Disorders that may alter lab results: N/A

PATHOLOGICAL FINDINGS
• Increased capillary permeability
• Microaneurysms
• Hemorrhages in retina
• Exudates in retina
• Capillary nonperfusion

SPECIAL TESTS Fluorescein angiography: Demonstrates retinal nonperfusion, retinal leakage, and proliferative diabetic retinopathy

IMAGING N/A

DIAGNOSTIC PROCEDURES
Eye examination: Measurement of visual acuity and documentation of the status of the iris, lens, vitreous and fundus

TREATMENT

APPROPRIATE HEALTH CARE Inpatient or outpatient surgery for vitrectomy; outpatient for laser treatment

GENERAL MEASURES
• The Early Treatment Diabetic Retinopathy Study demonstrated that systemic aspirin did not prevent the development of proliferative diabetic retinopathy, or reduce the risk of visual loss associated with diabetic retinopathy
• Microvascular complications, including proliferative diabetic retinopathy are significantly increased when blood-sugar levels are equal to or greater than 200 mg %
• Poor glycemic control is associated with an increases risk, both for developing diabetic retinopathy and with its progression, regardless of the type of diabetes, insulin-dependent or non-insulin dependent
• Cataracts are more common among diabetics. Try to delay cataract surgery in diabetics with retinopathy until the symptoms are more severe than in non-diabetics; cataract surgery can cause retinopathy to worsen

SURGICAL MEASURES
• Laser treatment: Recommended for patients with proliferative diabetic retinopathy and for patients with clinically significant macular edema
• The Diabetic Retinopathy Study demonstrated panretinal photocoagulation overall reduced the rate of severe visual loss from 15.9% in untreated eyes to 6.4% in treated eyes. In certain subgroups of eyes with proliferative diabetic retinopathy, the incidence of severe visual loss in untreated eyes was as high as 36.9% with a follow-up of 2 years.
• The Early Treatment Diabetic Retinopathy Study (ETDRS) demonstrated that eyes with clinically significant diabetic macular edema benefited from focal laser treatment. Clinical significant diabetic macular edema is defined as the following:
  ◊ 1. Thickening of the retina within 500 microns of the center of the macula
  ◊ 2. Hard exudates within 500 microns of the center of the macula associated with thickening of the adjacent retina
  ◊ 3. A zone of retinal thickening 1 disc area or larger within 1 disc diameter of the center of the macula
• Cryoretinopexy can be used instead of laser treatment in certain cases to decrease the neovascular stimulus and treat proliferative diabetic retinopathy
• Vitrectomy: Recommended for patients with severe proliferative diabetic retinopathy, traction retinal detachment involving the macula, and nonclearing vitreous hemorrhage. In eyes undergoing vitrectomy for severe proliferative diabetic retinopathy, the percentage of eyes with a visual acuity of 10/20 or better was greater in the group that underwent early vitrectomy versus conventional management.
• Vitrectomy can be considered after 1 month for a vitreous hemorrhage decreasing the vision to the 5/200 level or worse

ACTIVITY As tolerated

DIET Follow prescribed diabetic diet

PATIENT EDUCATION
• Patient information available from the American Diabetes Association - (800)232-3472 or local office
• American Academy of Ophthalmology, 655 Beach St., San Francisco, CA 94109-1336
• Stress importance of strict blood glucose control through diet, exercise, drugs/insulin and monitoring of blood glucose

MEDICATIONS

DRUG(S) OF CHOICE None are specific for retinopathy. See Other Notes. Lisinopril, an angiotensin-converting enzyme (ACE) inhibitor was found to slow the progression of retinopathy in insulin dependent diabetes.
Contraindications: N/A
Precautions: N/A
Significant possible interactions: N/A

ALTERNATIVE DRUGS N/A

FOLLOWUP

PATIENT MONITORING
• Scheduled eye examinations by an ophthalmologist:
 ◊ The diabetic patient with a normal exam should be followed yearly
 ◊ Patients with background diabetic retinopathy should be followed at least every six months
 ◊ Patients with preproliferative diabetic retinopathy should be followed at least every three to four months
 ◊ Patients with active proliferative diabetic retinopathy should be followed at least every two to three months

PREVENTION/AVOIDANCE
• Careful monitoring and control of blood glucose
• Routine visits to an ophthalmologist

POSSIBLE COMPLICATIONS Blindness

EXPECTED COURSE/PROGNOSIS If treated early, outlook good. If treatment delayed, blindness may result.

MISCELLANEOUS

ASSOCIATED CONDITIONS
• Glaucoma
• Cataracts
• Retinal detachment
• Vitreous hemorrhage
• Disc edema (diabetic papillopathy); can occur in type I or type II diabetes

AGE-RELATED FACTORS
Pediatric: N/A
Geriatric: Prevalence will increase as population ages and diabetic patients live longer
Others: N/A

PREGNANCY
• Pregnancy can exacerbate diabetic retinopathy
• Any woman with diabetes who becomes pregnant should be examined in the first trimester. She should be examined at least every three months until parturition.

SYNONYMS N/A

ICD-9-CM
• 362.01 Retinopathy, diabetic, background
• 362.02 Retinopathy, diabetic, proliferative

SEE ALSO
• Diabetes mellitus, insulin-dependent (IDDM or Type I)
• Diabetes mellitus, non-insulin dependent (NIDDM)

OTHER NOTES
• The Diabetes Control and Complications Trial (DCCT) recommends that for most patients with insulin-dependent diabetes mellitus, blood glucose levels should be as close to the nondiabetic range as is safe to do so, to reduce the risk and rate of progression of the diabetic retinopathy
• In the DCCT, insulin-dependent diabetics were randomly assigned into either conventional or intensive insulin treatment. Conventional treatment consisted of one or two daily insulin injections, with daily self-monitoring of urine or blood glucose. Intensive treatment consisted of insulin administered three or more times daily by injection or an external pump, with self-monitored blood glucose levels measured at least four times per day.
• The DCCT demonstrated intensive insulin therapy reduced the risk of macular edema and retinal neovascularization
• In the DCCT, intensive insulin therapy was more effective in reducing the risk of progression of diabetic retinopathy in the less advanced stages. However, advanced diabetic retinopathy also benefited from the intensive insulin.
• The DCCT demonstrated improvement in diabetic retinopathy was more likely to occur with intensive insulin therapy in insulin-dependent diabetes

ABBREVIATIONS
• BDR = background diabetic retinopathy
• PPDR = preproliferative diabetic retinopathy
• PDR = proliferative diabetic retinopathy

REFERENCES
• Diabetic Retinopathy Study Research Group: Indications for photocoagulation treatment of diabetic retinopathy. DRS Report No. 14. Int Ophthal Clin, 1987, 27:239-253
• Early Treatment Diabetic Retinopathy Study Research Group: Photocoagulation for Diabetic Macular Edema. ETDRS Report No. 1. Arch Ophthalmol, 1985; 103:1796-1806
• Early vitrectomy for severe proliferative diabetic retinopathy in eyes with useful vision: results of a randomized trial diabetic retinopathy vitrectomy study. Report No. 3. The Diabetic Retinopathy Vitrectomy Study Research Group. Ophthalmol 1988;95:1307-1320
• The Diabetes Control and Complications Trial Research Group: The effect of intensive diabetes treatment on the progression of diabetic retinopathy in insulin-dependent diabetes mellitus. Arch Ophthalmol 1995;113:36-51
• Diabetic Retinopathy Vitrectomy Study Research Group: Early vitrectomy for severe vitreous hemorrhage in diabetic retinopathy: Two year results of a randomized trial. Diabetic retinopathy Vitrectomy Study Report 2. Arch Ophthalmol 1985;103:1644-1651
• Regillo CD, Brown GC, Savino PJ, et al: Diabetic papillopathy: Patient characteristics and fundus findings. Arch Ophthamol 1995;113:889-895
Illustrations: 5 available on CD-ROM
Internet references: http://www.5mcc.com

Author(s)
Richard W. Allinson, MD

Reye's syndrome

 BASICS

DESCRIPTION Acute encephalopathy with cerebral edema and fatty infiltration of the liver. Occurs in previously healthy children, often associated with an antecedent viral infection such as varicella or influenza. Markedly decreased in incidence since late 1970's when association with aspirin use and Reye's syndrome made. Most cases currently seen are "Reye-like syndrome" (RLS) caused by inborn error of metabolism or toxin (see Differential Diagnosis).
System(s) affected: Nervous, Gastrointestinal
Genetics: No known genetic pattern
Incidence/Prevalence in USA: Currently very rare
Predominant age: Infants, children, adolescents. Peak incidence at 6 years of age. Most cases between 4-12 years of age.
Predominant Sex: Male = Female

SIGNS AND SYMPTOMS
• Symptoms reflected in clinical staging system
◊ I: Vomiting, sleepy, lethargic
◊ II: Confusion, delirium, hyperpnea, irritability, combative, hyperreflexia, altered muscle tone
◊ III: Obtunded, light coma and seizures, decorticate rigidity, loss of oculocephalic reflexes, intact pupillary reflex
◊ IV: Coma, decerebrate posturing spontaneously or in response to painful stimuli, seizures, fixed pupils
◊ V: Coma, flaccid paralysis, loss of deep tendon reflexes, seizures, respiratory arrest, isoelectric EEG

CAUSES Unknown - mitochondrion is major site of injury

RISK FACTORS
• Pediatric age group
• Viral illness, especially varicella, influenza A
• Use of preparations containing aspirin, salicylates, and/or salicylamides
• More common in rural and suburban areas

 DIAGNOSIS

DIFFERENTIAL DIAGNOSIS
• Acute encephalopathy without hepatic abnormalities
◊ Encephalitis, meningitis, diabetes mellitus, drug overdose, poisoning, psychiatric illness
• Acute toxic encephalopathy with hepatic abnormalities (Reye-like syndrome)
◊ Inherited metabolic disorders
- Organic acidurias with defects in hepatic fatty acid oxidation
- Fatty acid metabolism defects: Acyl-CoA dehydrogenase, carnitine deficiency
- Urea cycle defects: carbamyl phosphate synthetase, ornithine transcarbamylase
-Fructosemia
◊ Drug ingestions
-Valproate, aspirin
◊ Toxin ingestion (produce Reye-like syndrome)
-Margosa oil, hepantenate, aflatoxin, hypoglycin (akee fruit), Jamaican vomiting sickness

LABORATORY
• Usually severe elevations of AST (SGOT) and ALT (SGPT)
• Hypoglycemia
• Normal or slightly elevated bilirubin or alkaline phosphatase
• Elevated ammonia
• Prolonged prothrombin time - often not responsive to Vitamin K
• Increased CSF pressure without pleocytosis (< 8 leukocytes per cubic millimeter)
• Mixed respiratory alkalosis and metabolic acidosis
• Hyperaminoacidemia (glutamine, alanine, lysine)
Drugs that may alter lab results: N/A
Disorders that may alter lab results: N/A

PATHOLOGICAL FINDINGS
• Slightly enlarged, firm, yellow liver with fat droplets throughout
• Characteristic liver biopsy with foamy cytoplasm with microvesicular fat - may need special preparation
• Uniformly severe mitochondrial injury

SPECIAL TESTS EEG

IMAGING N/A

DIAGNOSTIC PROCEDURES
• Liver biopsy
• CSF pressure measurement

TREATMENT

APPROPRIATE HEALTH CARE Medical emergency requiring immediate hospitalization

GENERAL MEASURES
• Supportive depending on severity of illness
• IV glucose and close monitoring of blood or serum glucose (to prevent severe hypoglycemia)
• Hyperventilation, mannitol, barbiturates to reduce intracranial pressure
• Minimize noise and other CNS stimulation (to prevent increases in intracranial pressure)
• Vitamin K, fresh frozen plasma, platelets as needed
• Mechanical ventilation
• Dialysis to reduce high ammonia levels and/or residual salicylate

SURGICAL MEASURES
• Decompression craniotomy may be necessary

ACTIVITY Complete bedrest

DIET Nothing by mouth

PATIENT EDUCATION Printed material from the National Reye's Syndrome Foundation, (800)233-7393

MEDICATIONS

DRUG(S) OF CHOICE
All treatment is supportive.
• 10-15% glucose IV
• Vitamin K
• For increased intracranial pressure, for example:
  ◊ Mannitol 0.5-1.0 gm/kg IV, as long as there is urine output
  ◊ Dexamethasone 0.5 mg/kg/day
  ◊ Barbiturates

Contraindications: Mannitol - do not use if patient has no renal output
Precautions: Mannitol and poor renal output may result in vascular overload and pulmonary edema
Significant possible interactions: Refer to manufacturer's literature

ALTERNATIVE DRUGS   N/A

 FOLLOWUP

PATIENT MONITORING   Will depend on specific residual effects; may require care of physicians, nurses, psychologists, physical, occupational and/or speech therapists

PREVENTION/AVOIDANCE
• Avoidance of salicylates in children with viral illness
• Recognition of early symptoms of the disease

POSSIBLE COMPLICATIONS
See Signs and Symptoms also.
• Aspiration pneumonia
• Respiratory failure
• Cardiac dysrhythmia/arrest
• Inappropriate vasopressin excretion
• Diabetes insipidus
• Cerebral edema
• Seizures

EXPECTED COURSE/PROGNOSIS
• Majority will have mild illness without progression. Prognosis related to degree of cerebral edema and ammonia level on admission.
• Possible neurologic sequelae include problems with attention, concentration, speech, language, fine and gross motor skills - more common with higher stages

MISCELLANEOUS

ASSOCIATED CONDITIONS   N/A

AGE-RELATED FACTORS
Pediatric: Especially in infants under age 2, essential to make correct diagnosis; rule out other causes of Reye-like syndrome (see Differential Diagnosis section)
Geriatric: N/A
Others: N/A

PREGNANCY   N/A

SYNONYMS   White liver disease

ICD-9-CM
331.81

SEE ALSO
• Encephalitis, viral
• Hepatic encephalopathy

OTHER NOTES   N/A

ABBREVIATIONS   N/A

REFERENCES
• Balistreri W: Reye syndrome and "Reye-like" diseases in Behrman, RE, Kliegman RM, Arvin A, eds: Nelson Textbook of Pediatrics. Philadelphia, WB Saunders Co. 1996:1144-5
• Green A, Hall S: Investigation of Metabolic Disorders Resembling Reye's Syndrome. Arch Dis Child 1992;67:1313-7
• Salmona M, Tacconi MT: Reyes and Reye-like syndrome, Drug related diseases? Drug Met Rev 1995;27:517-39
• Hardie RM, Newton LH, Bruce JC, et al: The changing clinical pattern of Reye's syndrome 1982-1990. Arch Dis Child 1996;74:400-405
Illustrations: N/A
Internet references: http://www.5mcc.com

Author(s)
William A. Primack, MD

Rh incompatibility

 BASICS

DESCRIPTION Antibody-mediated destruction of red blood cells that bear Rh surface antigens by individuals who lack the antigens and have become isoimmunized ("sensitized") to them. Can occur with transfusion of incompatible blood. More commonly seen in the Rh-positive fetus or infant of an Rh-negative mother.

System(s) affected:
Hemic/Lymphatic/Immunologic

Genetics: Complex autosomal inheritance of polypeptide Rh antigens. At least three closely-linked loci on chromosome 2 carry an assortment of alleles: Dd, Cd, Ee. Individuals who express the D antigen antigen (also called Rho or Rho[D]) are considered Rh positive, as are those expressing the weak D (Du) variant. Individuals lacking the D antigen are Rh negative. Antibodies may be produced to C, c, D, E, or e in individuals lacking the specific antigen; only D is strongly immunogenic. Isoimmunization to Rh antigens is not inherited.

Incidence/Prevalence in USA:
• 15% of Caucasian population and smaller fractions of other races are Rh negative
• Risk of isoimmunization during or after an Rh-positive pregnancy is about 15%
• Only 1-2% of isoimmunizations occur antepartum
• With Rho(D) immune globulin prophylaxis, risk of sensitization is reduced to less than 1% of susceptible pregnancies

Predominant age: Childbearing
Predominant sex: Female only

SIGNS AND SYMPTOMS
• Hemolytic transfusion reaction in recipient of Rh-incompatible blood
• Jaundice of newborn
• Kernicterus
• Congenital or fetal anemia
• Fetal hydrops
• Fetal death in utero

CAUSES
• Transfusion of Rh-positive blood to Rh-negative recipient
• Maternal exposure to fetal Rh antigens, either antepartum or intrapartum

RISK FACTORS
• Any Rh-positive pregnancy in Rh-negative woman
• Induced abortion
• Spontaneous abortion
• Ectopic pregnancy
• Amniocentesis, chorionic villus sampling
• Fetomaternal hemorrhage (fetal death in utero)
• Fetal manipulation, external version
• Cesarean delivery
• Maternal trauma
• Placental abruption
• Placenta previa
• Manual placental removal

 DIAGNOSIS

DIFFERENTIAL DIAGNOSIS
• ABO incompatibility
• Other blood group (non-Rh) isoimmunization
• Nonimmune fetal hydrops
• Hereditary spherocytosis
• Red cell enzyme defects

LABORATORY Positive indirect Coombs' test (antibody screen) during pregnancy
Drugs that may alter lab results: Prior administration of D immune globulin may lead to weakly (false) positive indirect Coombs' test in mother and direct Coombs' test in infant
Disorders that may alter lab results: N/A

PATHOLOGICAL FINDINGS N/A

SPECIAL TESTS
• Paternal blood typing
• Kleihauer-Betke test to quantify an acute feto-maternal bleed

IMAGING N/A

DIAGNOSTIC PROCEDURES N/A

 TREATMENT

APPROPRIATE HEALTH CARE
Outpatient, ambulatory management in most cases. Because of the specialized, somewhat hazardous treatment measures involved, pregnancies usually managed at tertiary care level.

GENERAL MEASURES
• See Patient Monitoring also
• Depending on severity of involvement, treatment of newborn or fetus may include:
  ◊ Phototherapy
  ◊ Transfusion after delivery
  ◊ Exchange transfusion
  ◊ Diuretics and digoxin for hydrops
  ◊ Early delivery
  ◊ Intrauterine transfusion

SURGICAL MEASURES N/A

ACTIVITY N/A

DIET N/A

PATIENT EDUCATION Griffith: Instructions for Patients; Philadelphia, 1994 W.B. Saunders Co.

Rh incompatibility

MEDICATIONS

DRUG(S) OF CHOICE
• For prophylaxis:
Rho(D) immune globulin (RhIG, RhoGAM, Gamulin Rh) given to unsensitized, Rh-negative women following:
  ◊ Spontaneous abortion
  ◊ Induced abortion
  ◊ Ectopic pregnancy
  ◊ Antepartum hemorrhage
  ◊ Amniocentesis
  ◊ Chorionic villus sampling
  ◊ Routinely at 28 weeks
  ◊ Within 72 hours after delivery of Rh-positive infant
• Dose:
  ◊ 50 mcg dose for events up to 12 weeks gestation
  ◊ 300 mcg dose for events after 12 weeks
  ◊ Higher doses may be required in the event of a large fetal - maternal hemorrhage (> 30 mL whole blood)
Contraindications: Patient with known severe reaction to human globulin. Refer to manufacturer's profile.
Precautions: Refer to manufacturer's profile
Significant possible interactions: N/A

ALTERNATIVE DRUGS N/A

FOLLOWUP

PATIENT MONITORING
• Antibody titer measured every few weeks during pregnancy. A titer of 1:16 or greater indicates need for further testing.
• Amniocentesis for amniotic fluid bilirubin levels
• Umbilical blood sampling (cordocentesis) for fetal blood type, hematocrit, reticulocyte count, presence of erythroblasts
• Fetal heart rate testing/ultrasonography to assess fetal status
• Amniocentesis for fetal lung maturity

PREVENTION/AVOIDANCE
• Blood typing (ABO and Rh) on all pregnant women
• Antibody screening early in pregnancy
• Rh immune globulin prevents only sensitization to the D antigen
• Follow prophylaxis routine listed in Medications for unsensitized, Rh-negative women

POSSIBLE COMPLICATIONS
• Pregnancy loss from umbilical blood sampling
• Pregnancy loss from intrauterine transfusion
• Fetal distress requiring emergent delivery

EXPECTED COURSE/PROGNOSIS
• With appropriate monitoring and treatment, infants born of severely affected pregnancies have a survival rate of greater than 80%
• Hydropic fetuses have poor salvage rate
• Disease is likely to be more severe in affected subsequent pregnancies

MISCELLANEOUS

ASSOCIATED CONDITIONS
• Hemolytic disease of newborn
• Hydrops fetalis
• Neonatal jaundice
• Kernicterus

AGE-RELATED FACTORS
Pediatric: N/A
Geriatric: N/A
Others: N/A

PREGNANCY N/A

SYNONYMS
• Rh isoimmunization
• Rh alloimmunization
• Rh sensitization

ICD-9-CM
• 656.10-656.13 Rh isoimmunization in pregnancy
• 656.20-656.23 Other isoimmunization in pregnancy
• 773.0 Rh hemolytic disease in fetus or newborn
• 773.1 ABO hemolytic disease in fetus or newborn
• 773.2 Other hemolytic disease in fetus or newborn
• 773.3 Isoimmune hydrops fetalis
• 773.4 Isoimmune kernicterus
• 773.5 Isoimmune late anemia

SEE ALSO
• Jaundice
• Anemia, hemolytic
• Erythroblastosis fetalis

OTHER NOTES N/A

ABBREVIATIONS N/A

REFERENCES
• Perkins JT: Hemolytic Disease of the Newborn. In: Gleicher N, ed. Principles and Practice of Medical Therapy in Pregnancy. 2nd Ed. Norwalk, CT, Appleton & Lange, 1992
• Socol ML: Management of Blood Group Isoimmunization. In: Gleicher N, ed. Principles and Practice of Medical Therapy in Pregnancy. 2nd Ed. Norwalk, CT, Appleton & Lange, 1992
• Management of Isoimmunization in Pregnancy. ACOG Technical Bulletin, 148, Oct 1990
• Prevention of D Isoimmunization. ACOG Technical Bulletin, 147, Oct 1990
• Giblett ER: Blood Groups and Blood Transfusion. In: Braunwald E, et al, eds. Harrison's Principles of Internal Medicine. 12th Ed. New York, McGraw-Hill Inc., 1991
• Agre P, Cartron J: Molecular Biology of the Rh Antigens. Blood 1991;78(3):551-63
Illustrations: N/A
Internet references: http://www.5mcc.com

Author(s)
Donald A. F. Nelson, MD

Rhabdomyolysis

BASICS

DESCRIPTION A syndrome resulting from damage to skeletal muscle with the resultant appearance of free myoglobin in the circulation. Myoglobin is then filtered by the glomerulus and appears in the urine. Elevated urinary levels of myoglobin can lead to acute renal failure.

System(s) affected: Renal/Urologic, Musculoskeletal, Cardiovascular, Nervous, Gastrointestinal

Genetics: Certain inherited disorders of fatty acid metabolism (Carnitine Palmityltransferase deficiency - autosomal recessive) and glycogen storage diseases (phosphofructokinase deficiency autosomal recessive; phosphoglycerate kinase deficiency is the only of these categories which is X-linked recessive) are inherited and lead to muscle injury with exercise which may eventuate rhabdomyolysis and acute renal failure.

Incidence/Prevalence in USA: Unknown (estimate: at Harborview Medical Center, a Seattle municipal hospital, rhabdomyolysis accounts for approximately 10-15% of ARF cases, per Zager RA)

Predominant age: Depends on the etiology for rhabdomyolysis, i.e., inherited disorders lead to rhabdomyolysis at a younger age but other etiologies may occur at any time - trauma or rhabdomyolysis secondary to infection.

Predominant sex: M > F; because of greater incidence of trauma in males

SIGNS AND SYMPTOMS

Rhabdomyolysis may present with obvious muscle injury and swelling on examination, e.g., crush injury, compartment syndrome; or muscle exam may be completely negative despite severe rhabdomyolysis/myoglobinuria. The signs and symptoms with renal failure are the same as those for acute tubular necrosis (ATN) from other etiologies.

CAUSES
• Metabolic, electrolytes - hypokalemia, hypophosphatemia, myopathies, inherited disorders of fatty acid metabolism (i.e., acyl-CoA dehydrogenase deficiency), glycogen storage diseases (e.g., phosphorylase b-kinase deficiency) and others (lactate dehydrogenase A deficiency)
• Polymyositis
• Dermatomyositis
• Malignant hyperthermia
• Neuroleptic malignant syndrome (anesthesia, phenothiazines, MAO inhibitors)
• Muscle exertion (physical, secondary to convulsions or to heat injury)
• Trauma-crush syndromes and pseudo-crush syndrome
• Muscle ischemia secondary to arterial occlusion or insufficiency
• Burns
• Repetitive muscle injury (bongo drumming, torture)
• Status epilepticus
• Hyperosmolality
• Infections

◊ Viral (influenza A, Epstein-Barr virus, varicella, etc.)
◊ Bacterial
◊ Septicemia
• Toxic muscle injury
◊ Alcohol induced
◊ Tetanus
◊ Snake venom (viper bite) and rattlesnake
◊ Carbon monoxide exposure
• Drug induced
◊ Crack-cocaine, heroin, amphetamine abuse
• Drug overdoses
◊ Theophylline and INH
◊ Lipid lowering agents (clofibrate, gemfibrozil in combination with HMG CoA reductase inhibitors, HMG CoA reductase inhibitors and cyclosporine or itraconazole, possibly cyclosporine alone)
◊ Any drug that leads to neuroleptic malignant syndrome
• Carcinoma - acute necrotizing myopathy of carcinoma
• Diabetes mellitus; ketoacidosis
• Extreme lithotomy position for extended periods
• Extended periods of muscle pressure
◊ After allogenic bone marrow transplant
◊ Hyponatremia or correction thereof
◊ Hypothyroidism
◊ Water intoxication
◊ Hypokalemia

RISK FACTORS See Causes

DIAGNOSIS

DIFFERENTIAL DIAGNOSIS
• For acute renal failure with rhabdomyolysis - any disease that causes acute tubular necrosis can be confused with rhabdomyolysis
• Renal pigment injury from hemoglobin resembles pigment injury from myoglobin

LABORATORY
• Muscle enzyme elevations (creatinine kinase, aldolase, and lactic dehydrogenase)
• Marked elevations of potassium and phosphorus from muscle injury
• Hypocalcemia during oliguria with hypercalcemia occasionally during the recovery phase from acute tubular necrosis (in fact, hypercalcemia during recovery from ATN is almost diagnostic of rhabdomyolysis and myoglobulin tubular injury)
• Urinalysis - dipstick positive for blood without red cells in sediment is very suggestive of pigment injury from either hemoglobin or myoglobin; coarsely granular, pigmented casts
• Urine or serum myoglobin levels may be helpful, but normal levels do not rule out pigment injury
• Extreme hyperuricemia may be present and actually can cause acute uric acid nephropathy in the setting of rhabdomyolysis

• When measured, vitamin D levels are decreased in the oliguric phase of rhabdomyolysis
• Reversible hepatic dysfunction occurs

Drugs that may alter lab results: None
Disorders that may alter lab results: Hemoglobin may be confused with myoglobin on dipstick

PATHOLOGICAL FINDINGS Muscle
necrosis; kidney-myoglobin renal injury looks like ATN from other causes

SPECIAL TESTS
• Hypocalcemia during the oliguric phase helps but is not diagnostic of rhabdomyolysis
• Extreme hyperkalemia, hyperphosphatemia and hyperuricemia is very suggestive of rhabdomyolysis

IMAGING Any renal imaging is similar as for other etiologies of ATN

DIAGNOSTIC PROCEDURES A good
index of clinical suspicion with evidence of muscle damage on exam or by lab tests make the diagnosis likely

TREATMENT:

APPROPRIATE HEALTH CARE Inpatient

GENERAL MEASURES
(See also topic on acute renal failure)
• Dialysis will be necessary for severe renal failure
• Caution: Diagnose muscle entrapment syndromes (anterior compartment rhabdomyolysis may require surgical intervention and relief of pressure to stop rhabdomyolysis)
• Severe hypocalcemia with symptoms (Chvostek's and Trousseau's) during the oliguric phase would benefit from intravenous calcium gluconate and intravenous vitamin D (Calcijex)

SURGICAL MEASURES N/A

ACTIVITY Physical exertion can lead to
rhabdomyolysis and less exertion is tolerated in people with metabolic myopathies mentioned above. (See Genetics and Causes.)

DIET When acute renal failure occurs from
rhabdomyolysis, protein restriction to lower BUN, potassium restriction to lower potassium and volume restriction with anuria are essential

PATIENT EDUCATION Specific for
possible causes

MEDICATIONS

DRUG(S) OF CHOICE
• When rhabdomyolysis is identified, appropriate intervention may prevent renal failure
◊ Volume expansion attempt to increase urine output to approximately 150 cc/hr (3 mL/kg/hr), strong support for aggressive and early fluid replacement
◊ IV mannitol as a bolus - 12.5 to 25 grams (0.25-0.5 gm/kg); not to exceed approximately 50 grams in 24 hours; or as a constant infusion of 20% mannitol
◊ Alkalinization of the urine decreases myoglobin tubular injury (sodium bicarbonate to increase urine pH above 6.5)
• When renal failure supervenes from rhabdomyolysis, severe hyperkalemia may be life threatening. Treatment is based on EKG changes (tall, thin T waves; P-R prolongation; QRS widening; P wave flattening).
◊ Calcium gluconate IV 1-2 amps (0.5 mL of 10% calcium gluconate = 4 mg elemental calcium; give 4 mg/kg/hr x 4 hrs). Remember that bicarbonate administration may lead to alkalosis and worsening hypocalcemia.
◊ If acidosis is present 1-2 amps (2-3 mL/kg) sodium bicarbonate IV
◊ If tolerated oral sodium polystyrene sulfonate (Kayexalate) as much as 20 grams (1 gm/kg)
◊ insulin and glucose; tall peaked T waves-treatment resembles wide QRS.
◊ Dialysis may then become necessary to remove potassium.
• Vitamin D and calcium were mentioned above
Contraindications: See manufacturer's literature
Precautions: See Causes, especially drug combinations
Significant possible interactions: N/A

ALTERNATIVE DRUGS   N/A

 FOLLOWUP

PATIENT MONITORING
• Contingent on primary disease. Some cases (crush injury) are accidental and will not occur again.
• Contingent on disease - essential for metabolic myopathies

PREVENTION/AVOIDANCE
• Avoidance of situations leading to rhabdomyolysis (see Causes) prevent the injury
• Avoidance of metabolic states (hypokalemia) and drug combinations that lead to rhabdomyolysis (gemfibrozil and HMG CoA reductase inhibitors) are necessary

POSSIBLE COMPLICATIONS   Death
especially from hyperkalemia or renal failure. With dialysis and supportive care, prognosis much better.

EXPECTED COURSE/PROGNOSIS
Contingent on primary cause of rhabdomyolysis and contingent on recovery from acute renal failure without complications (infection, GI bleeding, cardiac standstill from hyperkalemia)

 MISCELLANEOUS

ASSOCIATED CONDITIONS See Causes

AGE-RELATED FACTORS
Pediatric: Inherited myopathies and trauma more common
Geriatric: N/A
Others: N/A

PREGNANCY   N/A

SYNONYMS   Myoglobinuria with renal failure

ICD-9-CM
728.89 Idiopathic rhabdomyolysis

SEE ALSO
• Renal failure, acute (ARF)
• Polymyositis/dermatomyositis

OTHER NOTES   N/A

ABBREVIATIONS
• ATN = acute tubular necrosis
• MAO = monoamine oxidase

REFERENCES
• Homis E: Prophylaxsis of acute renal failure in patients with rhabdomyolysis. Ren Fail 1997;19:283-285
• Lampley EC, Williams S, Myers SA: Cocaine-associated rhabdomyolysis causing renal failure in pregnancy. Obstet & Gynecol 1996;87:804-806
• Zager RA: Rhabdomyolysis and myohemoglobinuria acute renal failure. Kid Int 1996;49:314-326
• Daras M, Kakkouras L, Tuchman AJ, Koppel BS: Rhabdomyolysis & hyperthermia after cocaine abuse: A variant of the neuroleptic malignant syndrome? Acta Neurologica Scand 1995;92:161-165
• Singh U, Schels WM: Infectious etiologies of rhabdomyolysis: three case reports and review. CID 1996;22:642-649
Illustrations: N/A
Internet references: http://www.5mcc.com

Author(s)
Gregory W. Rutecki, MD

Rheumatic fever

BASICS

DESCRIPTION Rheumatic fever is an inflammatory disease, possibly autoimmune in nature. Rheumatic fever involves many tissues, including the heart, joints, skin, and central nervous system. Preceding infection of the upper tract with group A Streptococcus is a prerequisite to the development of acute rheumatic fever.
• Rheumatic fever can cause permanent cardiac valvular disease as well as acute cardiac decompensation.
• Recurrences are common if not prevented with "prophylactic" antibiotic treatment. In recent years there have been multiple reports of recurrences in adults as well as children.
System(s) affected: Cardiovascular, Hemic/Lymphatic/Immunologic, Nervous, Musculoskeletal, Skin/Exocrine
Genetics: A specific genetic marker that correlates with susceptibility to rheumatic fever has not been found, but the disease is known to occur in families
Incidence/Prevalence in USA:
• The incidence of rheumatic fever in the United States has been showing an overall decline for decades. In the 1970's it was a rare disease with an incidence of 0.5-1.88 cases per 100,000. However, since the mid-1980's there has been a resurgence of cases with multiple "outbreaks" having been reported in the U. S.
• The incidence calculated based on recent outbreaks has been as high as 18.1 per 100,000 in children aged 5-17 years
Predominant age: Most common in children ages 5-15. Recurrences can be seen in adulthood.
Predominant sex: Male = Female

SIGNS AND SYMPTOMS
• Joint symptoms ranging from arthralgias to frank arthritis (75%)
• Joints involved are medium to large, e.g., ankles, knees, wrists
• Joint involvement is classically migratory
• Joint symptoms usually disappear in 3-4 weeks without permanent deformities
• Carditis (65%), mild or severe with murmurs
• Cardiac involvement may include pericarditis, myocarditis, and/or valvular insufficiency. Appears within 2 weeks and lasts 6 weeks to 6 months.
• Valvular damage may be permanent
• P-R prolongation on ECG
• Erythema marginatum (classic rash) < 5%
• Subcutaneous nodules (painless, hard swellings overlying bony prominences) 5-10%
• Chorea is often a late finding but may be a presenting complaint. It occurs in 10-15% of patients, and its duration is not altered by treatment.
• Fever 101-104°F (38.3-40.0°C)
• Abdominal pain is common. It may be severe.
• Epistaxis (historically important, but rarely seen in acute rheumatic fever)
• Facial tics
• Facial grimace

CAUSES
• Autoimmune mechanisms
• A preceding upper respiratory infection with group A Streptococcus is a prerequisite

RISK FACTORS
• Crowded living, school or working conditions
• Tendency to upper respiratory infections

DIAGNOSIS

DIFFERENTIAL DIAGNOSIS Lupus, juvenile rheumatoid arthritis, infectious arthritis, viral myocarditis, innocent murmurs, Tourette's syndrome, Kawasaki syndrome

LABORATORY
• Increased acute phase reactants, including sedimentation rate (ESR) and C-reactive protein (CRP)
• Bacteriological or serological evidence of group A streptococcal infection, antistreptolysin O (ASO), Streptozyme, or anti-deoxyribonuclease B (DNase)
• Anemia
Drugs that may alter lab results: Prior treatment with aspirin or steroids
Disorders that may alter lab results: N/A

PATHOLOGICAL FINDINGS
• Subcutaneous nodules have a characteristic histological appearance
• Pericardial effusion
• Fibrinous pericardium

SPECIAL TESTS N/A

IMAGING
• Chest x-ray
• Echocardiogram (reveals pericardial effusion)

DIAGNOSTIC PROCEDURES
• Throat cultures for beta-hemolytic streptococci
• Diagnosis is dependent on fulfilling the modified Jones criteria of two major manifestations or one major and two minor manifestations. In either case, there must be evidence of preceding group A streptococcal infection. The five major criteria are carditis, arthritis, chorea, erythema marginatum, subcutaneous nodules. The minor criteria include fever, arthralgia (cannot use if arthritis was used as a major criteria), previous rheumatic fever, acute phase labs, prolonged P-R interval on EKG.

TREATMENT

APPROPRIATE HEALTH CARE
• Outpatient
• Initial hospitalization may be helpful to diagnose and establish stability of the patient

GENERAL MEASURES
• Mainstay of therapy is anti-inflammatory
• Patients with arthritis - therapy for relief of pain
• Patients with carditis - suppress inflammation
• Patients with arrhythmias - treat with appropriate agents

SURGICAL MEASURES N/A

ACTIVITY
• Initial bedrest with activity increasing gradually as tolerated
• Advance activity cautiously if there is evidence of carditis

DIET Regular; low sodium initially if the patient has carditis

PATIENT EDUCATION Information available from the American Heart Association

MEDICATIONS

DRUG(S) OF CHOICE
• If patient has carditis with cardiomegaly, start prednisone, 2 mg/kg/day (maximum 60 mg) for two weeks then taper over two weeks. Start aspirin at beginning of steroid taper. Continue aspirin for 6 weeks.
• If no cardiomegaly, start aspirin 60 mg/kg/day (to maintain salicylate level of 20-25μg/mL), 75-100 mg/kg/day for children, for 4-6 weeks
• Treat initially with penicillin as if active streptococcal infection is present, then begin prophylaxis. See Followup.
• Chorea may require treatment with haloperidol
Contraindications: Specific drug allergies
Precautions:
• Usual steroid side effects
• Extrapyramidal effects can occur with haloperidol
Significant possible interactions: Refer to manufacturer's profile of each drug

ALTERNATIVE DRUGS
Sulfadiazine may be used for prophylaxis in penicillin allergic patients. Patients who take sulfadiazine should take at least 2 liters of fluid daily to guard against sulfadiazine crystalluria.

FOLLOWUP

PATIENT MONITORING
Each week initially, then every 6 months

PREVENTION/AVOIDANCE
• Patients will need to be on prophylactic penicillin throughout childhood and possibly indefinitely during adulthood. Monthly injections of 1.2 million units of benzathine penicillin intramuscularly is the preferred treatment.
• Adults should be treated for a minimum of five years after an attack. Some treat adults indefinitely if there has been valvular disease. Oral penicillin V-K, 125 mg twice daily is an alternative to monthly injections. In the event of penicillin allergy, Sulfadiazine, 500 mg daily for children weighing less than 30 kg or 1 gr daily for all. Others may be used.
• If patients have valvular damage from acute rheumatic fever, they will require bacterial endocarditis prophylaxis for dental and other high risk procedures

POSSIBLE COMPLICATIONS
• Subsequent attacks of acute rheumatic fever secondary to streptococcal reinfection
• Carditis
• Mitral stenosis
• Congestive heart failure

EXPECTED COURSE/PROGNOSIS
Sequelae limited to the heart and dependent of severity of carditis during an acute attack

MISCELLANEOUS

ASSOCIATED CONDITIONS N/A

AGE-RELATED FACTORS
Pediatric: More common in children
Geriatric: N/A
Others: N/A

PREGNANCY
Residual valvular disease may be exacerbated by pregnancy. Refer pregnant patient to cardiologist for assistance in management.

SYNONYMS N/A

ICD-9-CM 390

SEE ALSO N/A

OTHER NOTES N/A

ABBREVIATIONS N/A

REFERENCES
• Vaughn VC, McKay RJ, eds: Nelson's Textbook of Pediatrics. Philadelphia, W.B. Saunders Co., 1992
• Ferrieri P: AJDC 1987;141 (7):125-7
• Quinn RW: Review Infect Dis 1989;11:128-153
Illustrations: N/A
Internet references: http://www.5mcc.com

Author(s)
H. Gratin Smith, MD, FAAP

Rhinitis, allergic

BASICS

DESCRIPTION Immediate and delayed reactions to airborne allergens, beginning with the generation and presence of specific antigen-responsive IgE antibody receptors on mast cells of the nasal mucosa
• An antigen-antibody chemical union initiates a cascade of events in the mast cell culminating in its degranulation and production of a melange of inflammatory mediators including histamine, heparin, leukotrienes, prostaglandins, proteases and platelet activating factor
• An immediate symptomatic response occurs followed by a more prolonged, persistent late phase reaction. This involves the infiltration into the reactive region of eosinophils, neutrophils, basophils and mononuclear cells
• May be seasonal or perennial depending on climate and individual response and the offending antigens
• Seasonal responses usually to grasses, trees and weeds
• Perennial responses exampled by house dust mites, mold antigens and animal body products
System(s) affected: Pulmonary, Skin/Exocrine, Hemic/Lymphatic/Immunologic
Genetics: Complex, but strong genetic determination present
Incidence/Prevalence in USA: 8-12% of the population affected
Predominant Age:
• Onset usually before the age of 30 with tendency to diminish with time
• Mean age onset approximately 10 years
Predominant sex: Male = Female

SIGNS AND SYMPTOMS
• Nasal stuffiness and congestion
• Pale, boggy mucous membranes
• Nasal polyps
• Sneezing, often paroxysmal
• Watery eyes
• Dark circles under eyes, "allergic shiners"
• Long eye lashes often associated
• Sensation of plugged ears
• Symptom associated sleeping difficulties
• Fatigue
• Mouth breathing
• Scratchy throat
• Voice change
• Irritating cough
• Postnasal drip
• Loss or alteration of smell
• Itchy nose, eyes, ears and palate
• Transverse nasal crease from rubbing nose upwards
• Dull facies

CAUSES
• Animal and plant proteins: Pollens, molds, mite dust, animal danders, dried saliva and urine
• Insect debris: Cockroach, locusts, fish food (thirps)

RISK FACTORS
• Family history
• Repeated exposure to offending antigen
• Exposure to multiple offending allergens
• Presence of other allergies, e.g., atopic dermatitis, asthma, urticaria
• Non-compliance to appropriate therapeutic measures

DIAGNOSIS

DIFFERENTIAL DIAGNOSIS
• Nonallergic rhinitis with eosinophilia syndrome (NARES)
• Vasomotor rhinitis
• Chronic sinusitis
• IgA deficiency with recurrent sinusitis
• Nasal polyps and tumor
• Reactive rhinitis of recumbency
• Cribriform plate defect with cerebrospinal fluid leakage (rule out by testing watery discharge for sugar)
• Foreign body
• Medications
  ◊ Rebound effect associated with continued use of topical decongestant drops and sprays
  ◊ Aldosterone converting enzyme inhibitors
  ◊ Chronic aspirin use
• Septal/anatomical obstruction
• Chronic rhinitis digitorum

LABORATORY
• CBC with differential. May have slight increase in eosinophils but often normal with uncomplicated rhinitis.
• Nasal probe smear with cytologic exam for eosinophils
• Increase IgE level. May do RAST determinations for specific suspected allergens.
Drugs that may alter lab results:
• Corticosteroids will ablate eosinophilia
Disorders that may alter lab results:
• Secondary infections may alter differential and decrease nasal eosinophils
• Parasitic infestations with more marked eosinophilia

PATHOLOGICAL FINDINGS
• Nasal washing/scraping
  ◊ Eosinophils predominate
  ◊ Basophils
  ◊ May see mast cells
• Nasal mucosa
  ◊ Submucosal edema but intact without evidence of destruction
  ◊ Eosinophilic infiltration
  ◊ Granulocytes to lesser extent
  ◊ Increased amount of tissue water with poor staining of ground substance
  ◊ Congested mucous glands and goblet cells

SPECIAL TESTS
• Skin tests using suspected antigens
Either technique manifests a positive reaction by inducing an expanding wheal and flare reaction. Special training recommended and available treatment for anaphylaxis mandatory
  ◊ Scratch or prick: a superficial injury to the epidermis with application of diluted test antigen
  ◊ Intradermal: Introduction of diluted material between layers of skin raising a 4 mm wheal using a 25 or 27 gauge needle
• Radioallergosorbent test (RAST)
  ◊ More expensive and used especially in cases where skin testing not practical, e.g., in atopic dermatitis and dermatographia
• Audiometry
  ◊ For deficits and base line evaluation
  ◊ Rhinoscopy (optional) - excellent visual advantages.

IMAGING Sinus film when indicated. Check for complete opacity, fluid level and mucosal thickening.

DIAGNOSTIC PROCEDURES See special lab tests. Appropriate diagnostic prick test kits available.

TREATMENT

APPROPRIATE HEALTH CARE
Outpatient

GENERAL MEASURES
• Patient education, assurance and understanding important
• Limit exposure to offending allergen
• Try to establish specific cause(s) - history and appropriate skin testing
• Intensity of treatment determined by severity of disease
• Immunotherapy:
  ◊ Usually reserved for seasonal allergies uncontrollable with drugs and not responding to environmental adjustment.
  ◊ Specific allergen extract is injected subcutaneously in increasing doses to patient tolerance as determined by local reaction
  ◊ Patient response should be evaluated each season or year

SURGICAL MEASURES Septoplasty when deviation significant enough to interfere with benefits of medication.

ACTIVITY No specific restrictions. Emphasize avoiding activity in areas of allergen exposure.

DIET No special diet unless concomitant food reactions suspected and evaluated

PATIENT EDUCATION Printed material available from many sources including: Asthma & Allergy Foundation of America. 1717 Massachusetts Ave., Suite 305, Washington, DC 20036, (800)7-ASTHMA

MEDICATIONS

DRUG(S) OF CHOICE
Most patients present because of inability to control symptoms and improve life style with avoidance of allergens or with over the counter medications.
• Antihistamines:
◊ Classification charts available. Five major classes:
   - Ethanolamines - diphenhydramine (Benadryl), clemastine (Tavist)
   - Alkylamine - chlorpheniramine, brompheniramine
   - Ethylenediamines - tripelennamine (PBZ)
   - Piperazines - hydroxyzine (Atarax)
   - Phenothiazines - promethazine (Phenergan), methdilazine (Tacaryl).
◊ Those with sedating side effects cheaper and often nonprescription. May start using at bedtime. Drowsiness often lessens with continued, regular dosage.
◊ Nonsedating type, e.g., terfenadine (Seldane) and astemizole (Hismanal) widely used. Emphasize that prescribed dosage not be exceeded. Be aware of drug interactions.
◊ Fexofenadine (Allegra)
• Decongestants
◊ Oral, e.g., pseudoephedrine
◊ Topical drops or sprays, e.g., phenylephrine
◊ Topical ophthalmic vasoconstrictors for annoying conjunctival itching
• Nasal sprays
◊ Physiologic saline solution
◊ Cromolyn sodium (Nasalcrom)
◊ Beclomethasone (Beconase AQ, Vancenase AQ), flunisolide (Nasalide, AeroBid), triamcinolone (Nasacort), budesonide (Rhinocort).
• Systemic steroids
◊ Only in urgent, selected cases and only for short-term use.
Contraindications:
• Antihistamines may precipitate urinary retention in males with prostatism and/or hypertrophy
• Decongestants if congestion is a "rebound" phenomenon
• Discourage decongestants if hypertension a problem
• Non-sedating antihistamines (Seldane and Hismanal) should not be used in patients with liver disease or in situations in which potassium channeling is a problem
Precautions: The elderly often require less aggressive treatment and will more frequently present with non-allergic rhinitis
Significant possible interactions:
• Refer carefully to manufacturer's literature for interactions
• Always mention antihistamine associated somnolence
• Terfenadine or astemizole
◊ Ketoconazole, macrolides, quinidine: may precipitate ventricular arrhythmias

ALTERNATIVE DRUGS Combinations with decongestants

 ## FOLLOWUP

PATIENT MONITORING
• Emphasize that you wish to do the most for, but the least to the patient
• Initiate patient education, supplementing with available videotapes and/or literature

PREVENTION/AVOIDANCE
• Avoidance - most patients with inhalant allergy have problems controlling their symptoms totally with allergen avoidance
• Air conditioning and limited outside exposure during season helpful
• Instructions as to the best housekeeping tactics and control for dust mites in patients sensitive to this allergen helpful
• Exposure to all animal contacts minimized. Discourage house pets.
• Avoid environmental irritants, e.g., smoke and fumes
• Air cleaners
• Use of allergy control covers especially on mattresses and pillows

POSSIBLE COMPLICATIONS
• Secondary infection
• Otitis media
• Sinusitis
• Epistaxis
• Nasopharyngeal lymphoid hyperplasia
• Decreased pulmonary function
• Continue to suspect effects of medications
• Facial changes (see Signs and Symptoms)

EXPECTED COURSE/PROGNOSIS
• Maximal, beneficially acceptable control of symptoms should be the goal
• Treatment tailored to each individual case.
• Immune system changes over time often associated with lessening of symptoms of allergic rhinitis. Therefore early, adequate control important.

 ## MISCELLANEOUS

ASSOCIATED CONDITIONS
• Other IgE mediated conditions, e.g., asthma and atopic dermatitis

AGE-RELATED FACTORS
Pediatric:
• Consider allergy as principle cause of persistent rhinitis
• Family understanding and involvement important
• Environmental control requires a cooperative effort and may include carpet and drape removal, removal of house plants, pet control, etc.
Geriatric:
• Increased medication side effects
• Number and specific types of allergens causing symptoms may change
• Symptoms may decrease by 4th-5th decade (not a hard rule)
Others: N/A

PREGNANCY Physiological changes of pregnancy may aggravate all types of rhinitis including allergic, vasomotor, nonallergic rhinitis with eosinophilia and chronic irritable airways

SYNONYMS
• Hay fever
• Pollinosis, seasonal and perennial
• IgE mediated rhinitis

ICD-9-CM 477 Allergic rhinitis

SEE ALSO Conjunctivitis

OTHER NOTES N/A

ABBREVIATIONS N/A

REFERENCES
• Middleton E Jr, Reed CE, Ellis EF: Allergy Principles and Practice. 4th Ed. St. Louis, C.V. Mosby Co, 1993
• JAMA. Primer on Allergic and Immunologic Diseases. 1992
• Baraniuk JA: Pathogenesis of allergic rhinitis. J of Allergy and Clinical Immunology 1997;99(2):S763-S772
Illustrations: N/A
Internet references: http://www.5mcc.com

Author(s)
J. Harlan Dix, MD, FACP

Rocky Mountain spotted fever

BASICS

DESCRIPTION Rocky Mountain spotted fever (RMSF) is an acute, potentially fatal febrile illness caused by Rickettsia rickettsii and transmitted by tick bite. The primary pathology is a vasculitis due to direct endothelial cell invasion by rickettsiae. The cardinal clinical features are headache, fever, and a centripetal rash which is often petechial.
System(s) affected: Cardiovascular, Skin/Exocrine, Musculoskeletal, Neurologic
Genetics: N/A
Incidence/Prevalence in USA: About 600 new cases are reported each year in the USA. There is considerable geographic variability; most cases are reported from south Atlantic and south central states. Peak incidence is in late spring and summer.
Predominant age: Highest incidences occur among children and young adults, primarily due to environmental exposure patterns. All ages are susceptible.
Predominant sex: Male > Female (due to greater male outdoor activity)

SIGNS AND SYMPTOMS
• Fever (100%)
• Rash (macular, maculopapular, petechial) (90-100%)
• Headache (65%)
• Rash (petechial) (50%)
• Headache, fever, rash (50-60%)
• Other neuropsychiatric symptoms (40-50%)
• Nausea, vomiting (30-50%)
• Headache, fever, petechial rash (33%)
• Abdominal pain (30%)
• Myalgias (30%)
• Hepatosplenomegaly (30%)
• Lymphadenopathy (25%)
• Arthralgias (10%)
• Cough (15%)
• Central nervous system dysfunction (stupor, confusion, coma, focal abnormalities) (10-30%)

CAUSES
RMSF is caused by Rickettsia rickettsii which is transmitted by the bite of ticks (Dermacentor andersoni, Dermacentor variabilis). Rarely by direct inoculation of tick blood into open wounds or conjunctivae.

RISK FACTORS
• Outdoor activity during warm months
• Contact with dogs

DIAGNOSIS

DIFFERENTIAL DIAGNOSIS
• Viral exanthems (measles, rubella, etc.)
• Meningoencephalitis (viral meningitis or encephalitis, bacterial meningitis)
• Typhus, rickettsialpox
• Ehrlichiosis
• Lyme disease
• Meningococcemia
• Leptospirosis

LABORATORY
• Nonspecific laboratory changes
  ◊ Thrombocytopenia
  ◊ WBC normal, increased, or decreased
  ◊ Anemia (mild)
  ◊ Hyponatremia (usually mild)
  ◊ CSF protein and WBC modestly elevated (lymphocytic predominance), glucose usually normal
  ◊ Prolonged PT, PTT; decreased fibrinogen; elevated fibrin degradation products (FDP) (uncommon)
• Specific laboratory diagnosis
  ◊ Serum Proteus Ox-19 antibody; fourfold increase (acute and convalescent) or solitary titer > 1:320 (relatively specific)
  ◊ Serum complement fixation (CF) antibody: fourfold increase or solitary titer > 1:16
  ◊ Serum indirect fluorescent antibody (IFA): fourfold increase or solitary titer > 1:64
  ◊ Direct fluorescent antibody (DFA) test on skin biopsy (not widely available)
Drugs that may alter lab results: N/A
Disorders that may alter lab results: Early treatment may blunt antibody response

PATHOLOGICAL FINDINGS
• The principal pathological abnormality is a systemic vasculitis
• Rickettsiae may be demonstrated within endothelial cells by DFA or electron microscopy
• Petechiae due to the vasculitis may be seen on various organ surfaces (e.g., liver, brain, epicardium)
• Secondary thromboses and tissue necrosis may be seen

SPECIAL TESTS N/A

IMAGING
Other than nonspecific pneumonic infiltrates which may be seen on routine chest x-ray, imaging procedures are rarely helpful

DIAGNOSTIC PROCEDURES
• Tissue (primarily skin) biopsy can be helpful if rapid DFA or electron microscopy are available
• Diagnosis is usually presumptive, based upon a compatible syndrome in a patient with exposure history in an endemic area; confirmation is obtained by subsequent serology
• Polymerase chain reaction currently unreliable

TREATMENT

APPROPRIATE HEALTH CARE
• Patients with the full clinical presentation or who are moderately ill should usually be hospitalized
• Patients with mild disease are treated presumptively as outpatients. Close followup is important in identifying complications.

GENERAL MEASURES
• Oxygen therapy and assisted ventilation for pulmonary complications, if necessary
• Good mouth care
• Blood transfusions for anemia
• Turning bed-confined patient frequently
• Watch patient closely for signs of renal failure

SURGICAL MEASURES N/A

ACTIVITY Bed rest until symptoms subside

DIET Critically ill patients may require IV nutrition. In others, small frequent meals may be necessary to maintain nutritional levels.

PATIENT EDUCATION See information in Prevention/Avoidance

MEDICATIONS

DRUG(S) OF CHOICE
• For adults (choose one of the following)
◊ Doxycycline (Vibramycin) 200 mg po initially, followed by 100 mg po bid for 7-10 days; same dosage IV; 100 mg q24h in renal failure
◊ Tetracycline 500 mg po q6h for 7-10 days; should not be used in renal failure
◊ Chloramphenicol 500-750 mg po q6h for 7-10 days; 20 mg per kg IV q6h (4 gm per day maximum); same dose in renal failure
• For children (choose one of the following)
◊ Chloramphenicol 20 mg per kg po q6h; same dosage IV
◊ Doxycycline (Vibramycin) 2.0-2.5 mg/kg po q12h for 7-10 days; 4.4 mg/kg IV initially, followed by 2.2 mg per kg IV q12h (see Contraindications)
◊ Tetracycline 10 mg per kg po q6h for 7-10 days (see Contraindications)

Contraindications:
• Children less than 9 years old - doxycycline and tetracyclines are generally not used because of the risk of tooth staining
• Pregnant women - doxycycline and tetracyclines are contraindicated because they may cause severe hepatic disease in the mother and retarded bone growth in the fetus

Precautions:
• Patients taking doxycycline or tetracyclines should minimize sun exposure to avoid photosensitization
• Infants or children with liver disease taking chloramphenicol should have serum drug levels monitored

Significant possible interactions:
Absorption of tetracyclines may be inhibited if they are ingested with milk products, iron preparations, or antacids containing aluminum or magnesium

ALTERNATIVE DRUGS
There are no currently available or adequately studied alternative drugs

FOLLOWUP

PATIENT MONITORING
• If patients are not hospitalized, they should be seen every 2-3 days until symptoms have fully resolved
• CBC, creatinine, electrolytes should be monitored

PREVENTION/AVOIDANCE
• People who go into tick-infested areas can take measures to prevent infection
◊ Occlusive clothing should be worn and insect repellants applied
◊ After possible exposure, all body areas should be carefully inspected for ticks, especially legs, groin, external genitalia, belt lines. Likelihood of infection increases with the duration of tick attachment.
◊ Ticks should be removed from humans or animals with caution; gloves should be worn or instruments used to minimize direct contact. Place a drop of oil, alcohol, gasoline or kerosine on the tick first. Hands should be washed thoroughly afterwards.

POSSIBLE COMPLICATIONS
• Encephalopathy, usually transient (30-40%)
• Seizures, focal neurologic signs (10%)
• Renal insufficiency (10%)
• Hepatitis (10%)
• Congestive heart failure (5%)
• Respiratory failure (5%)

EXPECTED COURSE/PROGNOSIS
• When treated promptly, the usual prognosis is excellent with resolution of symptoms over several days and no sequelae
• Mortality is rare with prompt institution of appropriate therapy
• If complications develop (see above), the course may be more severe and long-term sequelae may be present, particularly neurologic sequelae

MISCELLANEOUS

ASSOCIATED CONDITIONS N/A

AGE-RELATED FACTORS
Pediatric: N/A
Geriatric: Mortality risk higher
Others: N/A

PREGNANCY N/A

SYNONYMS Tick typhus

ICD-9-CM
082.0 Rocky Mountain spotted fever

SEE ALSO N/A

OTHER NOTES
Treatment should be initiated on the basis of clinical diagnosis or skin biopsy. Treatment should not be delayed for serologic confirmation.

ABBREVIATIONS N/A

REFERENCES
• Kirk JL, Fine DP, Sexton, DJ, Muchmore HG: Rocky Mountain spotted fever. A clinical review based on 48 confirmed cases, 1943-1986. Medicine 1990;69:35-45
• Melnick CG, Bernard KW, D'Angelo L: Rocky Mountain spotted fever: Clinical, laboratory, and epidemiological features of 262 cases. J Infect Dis 1984;150:480-488
• Archibald LK, Sexton DJ: Long-term sequelae of Rocky Mountain spotted fever. Clin Infect Dis 1995;20:1122-1125
Illustrations: N/A
Internet references: http://www.5mcc.com

Author(s)
Douglas P. Fine, MD
Ronald A. Greenfield, MD

Roseola

BASICS

DESCRIPTION An acute disease of infants or very young children with an incubation period of about 5-15 days. Characteristically, it causes first a high fever, followed by the appearance of an eruption (whose appearance is similar to that of measles) simultaneously with, or following defervescence. Both cause and transmission mode are unknown, but presumably it is a communicable virus.
System(s) affected: Endocrine/Metabolic, Skin/Exocrine
Genetics: No known genetic pattern
Incidence/Prevalence in USA:
• Estimated that 30% of all children
• More likely to occur in spring and fall
Predominant age: Infants and very young children (6 months to 3 years)
Predominant sex: Male = Female

SIGNS AND SYMPTOMS
• Abrupt fever without apparent cause (103-105°F [39.4-40.5°C]) for 3-5 days
• Sudden drop of fever. As fever disappears, skin rash begins (lasts hours to days).
• Anorexia
• Irritability
• Listlessness
• Does not appear seriously ill
• Maculopapular, nonpruritic rash, first appearing on the trunk, that blanches on pressure
• Rash appears as very slightly elevated, rose-pink papules that appear profusely on trunk, arms and neck; mild on face and legs
• Rash fades within a few hours to 2 days
• Febrile convulsions during height of fever (uncommon)
• Lymphadenopathy in cervical and posterior auricular regions
• Spleen enlarged (uncommon)

CAUSES
A communicable virus, human herpesvirus-6B (HHV-6B)

RISK FACTORS
• Day care center
• Exposure to infected infant

DIAGNOSIS

DIFFERENTIAL DIAGNOSIS
• Sepsis
• UTI
• Measles
• Rubella
• Fifth disease
• Enterovirus infection
• Otitis media
• Meningitis
• Bacterial pneumonia
• Drug eruption

LABORATORY
• Urinalysis
• CBC - leukopenia with relative lymphocytosis
• IgM, IgG for human herpesvirus-6 (HHV-6)
• PCR (serum) for HHV-6
Drugs that may alter lab results: N/A
Disorders that may alter lab results: N/A

PATHOLOGICAL FINDINGS   None

SPECIAL TESTS   N/A

IMAGING   Chest x-ray negative

DIAGNOSTIC PROCEDURES   Careful physical examination. Roseola should be suspected if it is known to be in the community and the child presents with a high temperature.

TREATMENT

APPROPRIATE HEALTH CARE
Outpatient

GENERAL MEASURES
• Symptomatic
• Tap water baths to cool excess temperature elevation
• Lightweight clothing
• Maintain normal room temperature

SURGICAL MEASURES   N/A

ACTIVITY   Rest until rash appears and fever breaks

DIET   Encourage fluids

PATIENT EDUCATION
• Infection is self-limiting
• If seizures occur, they will not cause brain damage and will cease after fever subsides

MEDICATIONS

DRUG(S) OF CHOICE
• Antipyretics for excessively high fever. Avoid aspirin. Instead use acetaminophen, 10-15 mg/kg/q4h to a maximum of 2.6 g/24h. (Aspirin may enhance the risk of Reye's syndrome.)
• Phenobarbital if needed for seizure
Contraindications: N/A
Precautions: N/A
Significant possible interactions: N/A

ALTERNATIVE DRUGS N/A

FOLLOWUP

PATIENT MONITORING   None after typical rash appears

PREVENTION/AVOIDANCE   None

POSSIBLE COMPLICATIONS
• Febrile seizures
• Encephalitis (rare)
• Meningitis

EXPECTED COURSE/PROGNOSIS
• Course - acute, benign, complete recovery without sequelae
• One attack confers permanent immunity

MISCELLANEOUS

ASSOCIATED CONDITIONS N/A

AGE-RELATED FACTORS
Pediatric: A disease of infants and very young children
Geriatric: N/A
Others: N/A

PREGNANCY N/A

SYNONYMS
• Exanthem subitum
• Pseudorubella
• Sixth disease

ICD-9-CM
• 056.9 Roseola
• 056.8 Roseola complicated

SEE ALSO N/A

OTHER NOTES N/A

ABBREVIATIONS N/A

REFERENCES
• Mandell GL, ed: Principles and Practice of Infectious Diseases. 4th Ed. New York, Churchill Livingstone, 1995
• Asano Y, Yoshikawa T, Suga S, Kobayashi I, et al: Clinical features of infants with primary human herpesvirus 6 (roseola infantum). Pediatrics 1994;93:104-108
• Donowitz LG: Infection Control in Child Care Center and Preschool. 2nd Ed. Baltimore, Williams & Wilkins, 1994
• Jenson HB, Baltimore RS, eds: Pediatric Infectious Diseases: Principles and Practices. 1st Ed. Norwalk CT, Appleton & Lange, 1995
Illustrations: N/A
Internet references: http://www.5mcc.com

Author(s)
Jeffery T. Kirchner, DO, FAAFP

Roundworms, intestinal

BASICS

DESCRIPTION Intestinal roundworms (nematodes) have adult stages infecting the intestinal tract of man. Larval stages may exist elsewhere in the body. Except for Trichinella spiralis, which is encysted in muscle; egg and/or larval stages can be isolated from the intestinal canal.
• Nematodes parasitizing the intestinal tract of man:
  ◊ Enterobius vermicularis (pinworm)
  ◊ Trichuris trichiura (whipworm)
  ◊ Ascaris lumbricoides (large roundworm of man)
  ◊ Necator americanus (hookworm)
  ◊ Ancylostoma duodenale (hookworm)
  ◊ Strongyloides stercoralis
  ◊ Trichostrongylus
  ◊ Trichinella spiralis (trichinosis)
System(s) affected: Gastrointestinal, Cardiovascular, Pulmonary, Nervous, Renal/Urologic, Musculoskeletal
Genetics: N/A
Incidence/Prevalence in USA:
• Up to 40% of children may have pinworms
• Trichinella 4-20%
• Others mostly in Southern regions
• Incidence of intestinal obstruction with ascaris is 2/1000
• Incidence of ascaris reportedly decreasing in the US, presumably due to improved sanitation
Predominant age: All ages; pinworm infestations more common in children
Predominant sex: Male = Female

SIGNS AND SYMPTOMS
• Lung Invasion:
  ◊ Fever
  ◊ Cough
  ◊ Blood-tinged sputum
  ◊ Wheezing
  ◊ Rales
  ◊ Dyspnea
  ◊ Substernal pain
  ◊ Pulmonary consolidations
  ◊ Eosinophilia
  ◊ Urticaria
  ◊ Asthma
  ◊ Angioneurotic edema
  ◊ Brain, kidney, eye, spinal cord, etc. (rare)
• Intestinal invasion:
  ◊ May be asymptomatic (small number)
  ◊ Abdominal pain (usually vague)
  ◊ Abdominal cramps/colic
  ◊ Diarrhea
  ◊ Rarely vomiting
  ◊ Occasionally constipation

• Muscle and other tissue invasion: (Trichinosis)
  ◊ Myalgias
  ◊ Fever
  ◊ Edema and spasm
  ◊ Periorbital and facial edema
  ◊ Photophobia
  ◊ Sweating
  ◊ Conjunctivitis
  ◊ Weakness or prostration
  ◊ Pain on swallowing
  ◊ Subconjunctival, retinal and nail hemorrhages
  ◊ Rashes and formication
  ◊ Encephalitis, myocarditis, nephritis
  ◊ Pneumonia, meningitis, neuropathy

CAUSES
• Ingestion of mature eggs in fecally contaminated food or drink
• Larval penetration of skin (hookworm)

RISK FACTORS
• Low standard of hygiene
• Poor sanitation
• Human feces fertilizer

DIAGNOSIS

DIFFERENTIAL DIAGNOSIS
• Pulmonary ascariasis with eosinophilia - consider asthma, Löffler's syndrome, eosinophilic pneumonia, systemic lupus erythematosus, Hodgkin's disease, and other parasitic causes (tropical pulmonary eosinophilia, toxocariasis, strongyloidiasis, hookworm, paragonimiasis)
• Worm-induced GI diseases - consider other causes of pancreatitis, appendicitis, diverticulitis, duodenitis, esophagitis, cholecystitis
• Anemia/hypoproteinemia (hookworm) - consider other etiology

LABORATORY
• Based on characteristics of eggs or larvae in stool or adult worm, if passed
• Cellophane-tape impression for pinworms
• Eosinophilia
• Larvae in sputum or adult worms seen on radiologic studies (uncommon)
Drugs that may alter lab results: N/A
Disorders that may alter lab results: N/A

PATHOLOGICAL FINDINGS
Characteristic eggs/worms

SPECIAL TESTS Serologic tests not useful

IMAGING Ultrasound is useful in the diagnosis of ascariasis as cause of biliary tract disease

DIAGNOSTIC PROCEDURES
• Stool exams
• Cellophane-tape impression

TREATMENT

APPROPRIATE HEALTH CARE
Outpatient

GENERAL MEASURES None other than medications to eradicate the worms

SURGICAL MEASURES N/A

ACTIVITY No restrictions

DIET No special diet

PATIENT EDUCATION Avoid fecally contaminated food, water, and soil

MEDICATIONS

DRUG(S) OF CHOICE
• Enterobius vermicularis (pinworm) - mebendazole 100 mg single dose, or albendazole 40 mg once, or pyrantel pamoate 11 mg/kg once (maximum of 1 g), repeat after 2 weeks (all dosages for adult and pediatrics)
• Trichuris trichiura (whipworm) - mebendazole 100 mg bid x 3 days or albendazole 400 mg once (all dosages for adult and pediatrics). Note - albendazole available in the US only from manufacturer.
• Ascaris lumbricoides (large roundworm of man), mebendazole 100 mg bid x 3 days or pyrantel pamoate 11 mg/kg once (maximum of 1 g) (all dosages for adult and pediatrics), or albendazole 40 mg once
• Necator americanus (hookworm), Ancylostoma duodenale (hookworm) - mebendazole 100 mg bid x 3 days or pyrantel pamoate 11 mg/kg (maximum of 1 g) x 3 days (all dosages for adult and pediatrics), or albendazole 40 mg once
• Trichostrongylus - pyrantel pamoate 11 mg/kg once (maximum of 1 g) or mebendazole 100 mg bid x 3 day (all dosages for adult and pediatrics)
• Trichinella spiralis - mebendazole 200-400 mg tid x 3 days, then 400-500 mg tid x 10 days (adult dosage) plus steroids if severe
• Strongyloides stercoralis - thiabendazole 50 mg/kg/d in 2 doses (maximum of 3 g a day) for 2 days (adult and pediatric), or albendazole 40 mg daily for 3 days (alternative), or ivermectin 200 mg as a single dose (also effective against co-existing ascaris, trichuris, enterobius). Superior to benzimidazoles for this indication.
• Note: FDA may consider certain uses of above drugs investigational, consult Medical Letter or appropriate drug reference
Contraindications: Refer to manufacturer's profile of each drug
Precautions: Refer to manufacturer's profile of each drug
Significant possible interactions: Refer to manufacturer's profile of each drug

ALTERNATIVE DRUGS N/A

FOLLOWUP

PATIENT MONITORING Followup stool studies at 2 weeks and retreat if necessary

PREVENTION/AVOIDANCE Good hygiene and sanitation

POSSIBLE COMPLICATIONS
• Vomiting worms
• Cholangitis - migration to common bile duct
• Pancreatitis - migration to pancreatic duct
• Appendicitis - migration to appendix
• Diverticulitis - migration to diverticuli
• Liver abscess
• Intestinal obstruction
• Volvulus
• Intussusception
• Bowel penetration
• Anemia (hookworm)
• Hypoproteinemia (hookworm)

EXPECTED COURSE/PROGNOSIS
Good for light to moderate infections. Ascariasis should always be treated due to the risk of migrating adult worms.

MISCELLANEOUS

ASSOCIATED CONDITIONS N/A

AGE-RELATED FACTORS Affects all ages
Pediatric: Children commonly infected
Geriatric: N/A
Others: N/A

PREGNANCY Benzimidazoles (mebendazole, albendazole, thiabendazole) should not be used; ivermectin has shown little teratogenic potential, and has provided an affective therapy though benefits should clearly outweigh risks

SYNONYMS Nematodes

ICD-9-CM 127 Other intestinal helminthiases

SEE ALSO
• Roundworms, tissue
• Intestinal parasites
• Pinworms

OTHER NOTES HIV infected patients have a higher risk of dissemination (e.g., strongyloides) and "standard" treatment failure

ABBREVIATIONS N/A

REFERENCES
• Markell EK, Voge M, John DT: Medical Parasitology. 6th Ed. Philadelphia, W.B. Saunders Co., 1986
• Schroeder SA, Krupp MA, Tierney LM, McPhee SJ, eds: Current Medical Diagnosis and Treatment. Norwalk, CT, Appleton & Lange, 1989
• Strickland GT: Hunter's Tropical Medicine. 6th Ed. Philadelphia, W.B. Saunders Co., 1984
• Drugs for Parasitic Infections. The Medical Letter. Vol 37 (issue 961) Nov 10, 1995
• Tietze PE, Tietze PH: Roundworms, Ascaris Lumbricoides. Primary Care; Clinics in Office Practice 1991;16(1):25-41
• Gomez NA, et al: Ultrasound in the diagnosis of roundworms in gallbladder and common bile duct. Surgical Endoscopy 1993;7(4):339-342
• Jensenius M: Hookworm disease: A differential diagnosis in iron deficiency anemia. Tidsskrift for den Norske Laegeforening 1995;115(3):367-369
• Lessnau KD, et al: Disseminated Strongyloides stercoralis in HIV infected patients. Chest 1993;104(1):119-122
• Goodman, Gilman: The Pharmacological Basis of Therapeutics. 9th Ed. New York, McGraw-Hill, 1996
Illustrations: N/A
Internet references: http://www.5mcc.com

Author(s)
Robert L. Weston, MD

Roundworms, tissue

BASICS

DESCRIPTION Tissue roundworms (nematodes) affect man when the adults or larval stages infect certain tissues. Infective larval stages are transmitted to man by arthropod vectors or from the soil. Once in human tissue, worms mature over 6-12 months and survive as long as 15 years. Symptoms depend on tissue infected.
- Filarial infections
  ◊ Wuchereria bancrofti (bancroftian filariasis)
  ◊ Brugia malayi (Malayan filariasis)
  ◊ Brugia timori (Timorian filariasis)
  ◊ Loa loa (eye worm)
  ◊ Onchocerca volvulus (river blindness, onchocerciasis)
  ◊ Mansonella perstans
  ◊ Mansonella ozzardi (Ozzard's filariasis)
  ◊ Mansonella streptocerca
- Other Tissue nematode infections
  ◊ Dracunculus medinensis (guinea worm, dracunculosis)
  ◊ Ancylostoma braziliense (cutaneous larva migrans, creeping eruption)
  ◊ Toxocara canis or cati (visceral larva migrans, toxocariasis)
- Distribution
  ◊ Over 300 million people are exposed to lymphatic filariasis in India and SE Asia; 30 million to onchocerciasis
  ◊ W. bancrofti: Tropics worldwide
  ◊ B. malayi: Southeast Asia
  ◊ B. timori: Indonesia
  ◊ L. loa: Africa
  ◊ O. volvulus: Africa, Central and South America
  ◊ M. perstans: Africa, South America
  ◊ M. ozzardi: Africa
  ◊ M. streptocerca: Central and South America
  ◊ D. medinensis: Africa, Asia
  ◊ A. braziliense: Tropics and Subtropics worldwide
  ◊ T. canis/cati: Over 50 countries worldwide, especially warmer tropical and subtropical regions

System(s) affected: Skin/Exocrine, Nervous, Gastrointestinal, Musculoskeletal, Hemic/Lymphatic/Immunologic, Cardiovascular, Renal/Urologic
Genetics: N/A
Incidence/Prevalence in USA:
- Visceral larva migrans - 4-30% seroprevalence has been reported, highest in southeastern United States
- Others - unknown
Predominant age: All ages, but children more commonly infected
Predominant sex: Male = Female

SIGNS AND SYMPTOMS
- Lymphatic filariasis (W. bancrofti, B. malayi, B. timori)
  ◊ Inflammatory signs - pain, tenderness, swelling, erythema
  ◊ Filarial adenolymphangitis
  ◊ Filarial orchitis
  ◊ Funiculitis and epididymitis
  ◊ "Filarial" and "Elephantoid" fever
  ◊ Filarial abscess
  ◊ Obstructive signs - lymph varices, lymph scrotum, hydrocele
  ◊ Lymphedema and elephantiasis
  ◊ Chyluria
  ◊ Filarial hypereosinophilia (tropical pulmonary eosinophilia)
- Loiasis (L. loa)
  ◊ Calabar swellings - recurrent subcutaneous inflammation/swelling
  ◊ Eye worm - adult or larvae migrate under conjunctiva
  ◊ Eosinophilia (may exceed 70%)
  ◊ Fever, irritability, urticaria and pruritus
- Onchocerciasis (O. volvulus)
  ◊ Dermatitis
  ◊ Nodules
  ◊ Lymphadenitis
  ◊ Ocular changes - intraocular microfilariae, punctate keratitis, sclerosing keratitis, anterior uveitis chorioretinitis, optic neuritis, optic atrophy, glaucoma, blindness (river blindness)
- Other filarial syndromes (M. ozzardi, M. perstans, M. streptocerca)
  ◊ Headaches, coldness, pruritus, and articular swelling/arthritis
  ◊ Eosinophilia and vague allergic signs
  ◊ Chronic dermatitis and macules can be confused with leprosy
  ◊ Lymphadenopathy
- Dracunculiasis (D. medinensis, guinea worm disease)
  ◊ Allergic manifestations - erythema, urticaria, pruritus, nausea, vomiting, giddiness, syncope, and occasional fever)
  ◊ Local lesions - papule, sterile blister, ulceration, abscesses
  ◊ Worm protrusion
- Toxocariasis (T. canis/cati, visceral or ocular larva migrans)
  ◊ Eosinophilia
  ◊ Visceral larva migrans
  ◊ Ocular larva migrans
- Cutaneous larva migrans (A. braziliense, creeping eruption)
  ◊ Itching and red papules
  ◊ Serpiginous track
  ◊ Edema and acute inflammation
  ◊ Scars
  ◊ Secondary infection

CAUSES Larvae introduced into human host by arthropod vector or infected soil

RISK FACTORS
- Geographic exposure to arthropod vectors
- Fishermen or women washing clothes have increased risk of 'river blindness'
- Contact with infected soil in cutaneous larva migrans (hence plumber's itch, sandworm, duckhunter's itch)

DIAGNOSIS

DIFFERENTIAL DIAGNOSIS
- Other causes of tissue inflammation (i.e., lymphangitis, epididymitis, dermatitis, conjunctivitis, blisters, pleuritis, peritonitis, pericarditis, encephalitis, nephropathy, cardiomyopathy, etc.)
- Nonfilarial causes of lymphangitis:
  ◊ Acute bacterial lymphangitis
  ◊ Phlebitis
  ◊ Unusual - plague, anthrax, TB, lymphogranuloma inguinale
- Nonfilarial causes of lymphedema, chyluria, and elephantiasis:
  ◊ Infiltrative or granulomatous process: Tumor, fungus, TB, leprosy
  ◊ Chronic venostasis or phlebitis
  ◊ Cardiac insufficiency
  ◊ Nutritional deficiencies
  ◊ Hereditary (Milroy's disease)
  ◊ Lateritious soil obstructing lymphatics

LABORATORY Examination of larvae or adult worms taken from the tissue; characteristic microfilariae on blood smear; eosinophilia. Distinction of species by larval exam is challenging and may require expert examination. Onchocerciasis is identified by skin snip/biopsy showing larval.
Drugs that may alter lab results: N/A
Disorders that may alter lab results: N/A

PATHOLOGICAL FINDINGS
Characteristic eggs/worms/larvae in tissue

SPECIAL TESTS Skin snip, nodulectomy, slit-lamp exam, and Mazzotti, test may be helpful in onchocerciasis

IMAGING Occasional worms seen on x-ray

DIAGNOSTIC PROCEDURES
Microfilariae on blood smear or other body fluids; clinical observations; serologies (e.g., ELISA)

TREATMENT

APPROPRIATE HEALTH CARE
Outpatient

GENERAL MEASURES
• Identify cause and treat accordingly
• Best treatment - direct removal of worm from tissue with caution not to break the worm
• Treat secondary infections

SURGICAL MEASURES
Long-standing lymphatic filariasis due to W. bancrofti and B. malayi may require surgical intervention to increase lymphatic drainage. This is unusual, and likely seen in long-term residents of endemic areas, subjected to extensive exposure to parasite.

ACTIVITY
No restrictions. If edema a problem, may want to elevate legs while sitting.

DIET
No special diet

PATIENT EDUCATION
• Avoid bites by arthropod vectors, insect repellants and other protective measures, e.g., proper clothing
• Avoid rivers and streams and soils known to be infected

MEDICATIONS

DRUG(S) OF CHOICE
• Visceral larva migrans (Toxocara): diethylcarbamazine (DEC) 6 mg/kg/d in 3 doses x7-10 days for adult and pediatric, or albendazole 400 mg bid x3-5 days for adult and pediatric or mebendazole 100-200 mg bid x5 days (adults only)
• Cutaneous larva migrans (Ancylostoma braziliense): thiabendazole topical and/or albendazole 200 mg bid x3 days for adult and pediatric. Topical 15% thiabendazole in a water soluble cream base is the treatment of choice given low toxicity and high cure rate (98%).
• Filariasis (Wuchereria, Bancrofti, Loa):
  ◊ Diethylcarbamazine: Adult: day 1) 50 mg po after meals; day 2) 50 mg tid; day 3) 100 mg tid; days 4-21) 6 mg/kg/d in 3 doses. Pediatric: day 1) 1 mg/kg po after meals; day 2) 1 mg/kg tid; day 3) 1-2 mg/kg tid; days 4-21) 6 mg/kg/d in 3 doses.
  ◊ Ivermectin 400 µg/kg as a single dose is highly effective (available from the CDC Drug Services 404-639-3670)
• Onchocerciasis: ivermectin 150 µg/kg po once, repeated every 6-12 months for adult and pediatric. Treatment with ivermectin only kills the larval worms, responsible for pathology, not the adult worms producing the larvae. Thus, treatment must be continued over a period of years until the adult worms die. DEC has been used for this purpose, but causes bad reactions, likely due to rapid killing of the larval worms with sudden release of large amounts of worm antigens. DEC is obsolete for this indication. Suramin, a drug used in the treatment of trypanosomiasis, is effective at killing the adult worms, but severe side effects prevent its use for onchocerciasis.
• Mansonella ozzardi: ivermectin 150 µg/kg in single dose may be effective. Diethycarbamazine has no effect.
• Mansonella perstans: mebendazole 100 mg bid x 30 days (approved drug, but considered investigational for this condition)
• Guinea worm (Dracunculus): metronidazole 250 mg tid x 10 days for adult; 25 mg/kg/d (max 750 mg/d) in 3 doses x 10 days for pediatric. Metronidazole does not cure the infection, but rather decreases the reaction to worm products. Cure is achieved only through physical removal of the adult worm.
• Note: FDA may consider certain uses of above drugs investigational and some may not be available in USA. Contact Parasitic Disease Drug Service, Parasitic Diseases Branch, Center for Disease Control, Atlanta 30333, (404)488-4240.

Contraindications: Refer to manufacturer's information
Precautions: Children, pregnancy, lactation
Significant possible interactions: Refer to manufacturer's profile of each drug

ALTERNATIVE DRUGS
Albendazole (available in USA only from the manufacturer)

FOLLOWUP

PATIENT MONITORING
N/A

PREVENTION/AVOIDANCE
• Avoid sources of infection (arthropod bites, rivers/streams, or contaminated soils)
• Diethylcarbamazine (DEC) once weekly has been used successfully in Peace Corps' workers for prophylaxis against L. loa
• Prophylaxis with ivermectin is under investigation
• Public health activities such as vector control

POSSIBLE COMPLICATIONS
• Depends upon type of worm
• Onchocerciasis - blindness
• Visceral worms - hepatitis, splenomegaly, pleuritis, peritonitis, eosinophilic granuloma or other organ damage as larvae migrate for up to 6 months
• Filariasis - lymphatic destruction leading to severe edema (elephantiasis)

EXPECTED COURSE/PROGNOSIS
• Good for light to moderate infections; depends on organ infected and extent of infection
• Long-term DEC treatment and immunomonitoring of filaria patients are essential in endemic areas to arrest and prevent pathology

MISCELLANEOUS

ASSOCIATED CONDITIONS
N/A

AGE-RELATED FACTORS
Pediatric: Children commonly infected
Geriatric: N/A
Others: Presence of onchocerciasis increases with age

PREGNANCY
N/A

SYNONYMS
• Creeping eruption
• Cutaneous larva migrans
• Dracunculosis
• Elephantiasis
• Filariasis
• Guinea worm
• Larva migrans
• Loiasis
• Nematodes
• River blindness
• Toxocariasis
• Visceral larva migrans

ICD-9-CM
127.0 Other intestinal helminthiases

SEE ALSO
Roundworms, intestinal

OTHER NOTES
N/A

ABBREVIATIONS
N/A

REFERENCES
• Markell EK, Voge M, John DT: Medical Parasitology. 6th Ed. Philadelphia, W.B. Saunders Co., 1986
• Schroeder SA, Krupp MA, Tierney LM, McPhee SJ, eds: Current Medical Diagnosis and Treatment. Norwalk, CT, Appleton & Lange, 1989
• Strickland GT: Hunter's Tropical Medicine. 7th Ed. Philadelphia, W.B. Saunders Co., 1991
• Warren KS, Mahmoud AAF: Tropical and Geographic Medicine. New York, McGraw-Hill, 1990
• Drugs for Parasitic Infections. Medical Letter. New Rochelle, NY, Medical Letter, Inc 1995;37:961
• Padrigel UM, et al: Immunomonitoring of filarial patients during DEC therapy in an endemic area: A seven year followup. Jour Tropical Med & Hygiene 1995;98(1):52-56
Illustrations: 1 available on CD-ROM
Internet references: http://www.5mcc.com

Author(s)
Robert L. Weston, MD

Salicylate poisoning

BASICS

DESCRIPTION A systemic disorder caused by acute and/or chronic intoxication from salicylate containing medications.
• Following accidental or intentional exposure, toxic actions of salicylates include:
  ◊ Stimulation of the CNS respiratory center
  ◊ Uncoupling of oxidative phosphorylation
  ◊ Inhibition of Krebs cycle dehydrogenases
  ◊ Stimulation of gluconeogenesis
  ◊ Increased lipolysis and lipid metabolism
  ◊ Inhibition of aminotransferases
  ◊ Cyclooxygenase inhibition and decreased production of clotting factors
  ◊ Irritation of the gastric mucosa and stimulation of the CNS chemoreceptor trigger zone.
• These actions cause sequential and progressively severe physiologic abnormalities with increasing doses of salicylates, time following exposure, duration of chronic exposure, extremes of age, and presence of concurrent medical conditions; abnormalities include:
  ◊ Respiratory alkalosis accompanied by progressive metabolic acidosis
  ◊ Hyperpyrexia
  ◊ Gastrointestinal, renal, pulmonary, and skin losses of body fluids and electrolytes
  ◊ Initial hyperglycemia followed by hypoglycemia, particularly CNS hypoglycemia
  ◊ Abnormal hemostasis and coagulation.
• The clinical presentation of patients with salicylate toxicity can range from minor symptoms to a syndrome initially indistinguishable from septic shock with multiple organ failure, including encephalopathy and adult respiratory distress syndrome (ARDS). The very young and elderly are particularly prone to develop severe toxicity, as are those with chronic intoxication. Also, conditions causing concurrent acidosis may increase tissue concentrations of salicylate and result in greater morbidity and mortality.
System(s) affected: Nervous, Hemic/Lymphatic/Immunologic, Gastrointestinal, Pulmonary, Renal/Urologic, Cardiovascular, Musculoskeletal, Skin/Exocrine, Endocrine/Metabolic
Genetics: N/A
Incidence/Prevalence in USA:
• > 18,000 ingestions of salicylate containing medications reported to poison control centers in 1995
• 52 deaths in 1995, 1 in children < 6
Predominant age: Occurs in children and adults at any age; over 70% of cases are in children > 6 and adults
Predominant sex: Male = Female

SIGNS AND SYMPTOMS
Acute intoxication
• Symptoms vary with the amount ingested, usually begin within 3-8 hours of ingestion, and progress more rapidly in children:
  ◊ < 150 mg/kg, minimal symptoms
  ◊ 150-300 mg/kg, moderate symptoms
  ◊ 300-500 mg/kg, severe symptoms
  ◊ > 500 mg/kg, potentially fatal
• Nausea and vomiting
• Hyperpnea
• Tachypnea
• Hyperpyrexia
• Tinnitus
• Disorientation
• Coma
• Convulsions
• Cardiac arrhythmias
• Hypotension
• Pulmonary edema
Chronic intoxication
• Signs and symptoms similar to acute intoxication may occur
• Onset of symptoms is usually gradual
• Signs and symptoms may be advanced at diagnosis and include severe hypotension and ARDS
• Neurologic symptoms often predominate, particularly in the elderly, and include agitation, confusion, stupor, hyperactivity, paranoia, bizarre behavior, dysarthria, restlessness

CAUSES
• Accidental or intentional ingestion of salicylates or salicylate containing medications
• Percutaneous absorption of dermatologic medications containing salicylate
• Breast feeding by mothers ingesting salicylate containing medications
• Teething gels containing salicylates

RISK FACTORS
• Dehydration
• Conditions causing metabolic or respiratory acidosis
• Extremes of age - the very young and elderly
• Psychiatric illness
• History of previous toxic ingestions or suicide attempts
• Concurrent oral poisoning with other substances
• Concurrent use of acetazolamide (Diamox)

DIAGNOSIS

DIFFERENTIAL DIAGNOSIS
• All ages: infection, sepsis, DKA, other causes of metabolic acidosis
• In the elderly: delirium, CVA, myocardial infarction, ethyl alcohol (ETOH) intoxication, congestive heart failure

LABORATORY
• Serum salicylate levels initially on all patients to confirm the diagnosis. Following acute ingestions, check levels 6 or more hours after ingestion and repeat q2h until levels are declining and the patient's condition has stabilized.
• Acid-base abnormalities common; usually respiratory alkalosis or mixed respiratory alkalosis and metabolic acidosis. Metabolic acidosis often predominates in chronic or severe acute poisonings and in poisonings in young children.
• Increased anion gap, esp. in acute poisonings and salicylate-only poisonings
• Initial hyperglycemia may be followed by hypoglycemia
• Electrolyte abnormalities such as hyper- or hyponatremia, and hypokalemia common
• Findings consistent with dehydration are common including an increased BUN/Cr ratio
• PT may be increased
• Liver function abnormalities may be present
• Proteinuria, renal function abnormalities may be present
• Stool hemocult testing may be positive
• Occasional hypouricemia
Drugs that may alter lab results:
• Diflunisal (Dolobid) may cross react with assay of salicylate concentration
• Medications affecting similar organ systems including oral anticoagulants and hypoglycemic agents
Disorders that may alter lab results:
Concurrent medical conditions involving similar organ systems

PATHOLOGICAL FINDINGS None specific for salicylate intoxication; associated findings include:
• Gastrointestinal = antral and prepyloric ulcers; small bowel ulcerations with enteric coated salicylates
• Renal = interstitial nephritis, acute tubular necrosis, minimal change nephrotic syndrome
• Pulmonary = noncardiogenic pulmonary edema

SPECIAL TESTS N/A

IMAGING
• Chest X-ray: noncardiogenic pulmonary edema; variable severity, from mild to ARDS
• Abdominal plain film: nonspecific bowel gas pattern with retained contrast in chronic bismuth subsalicylate ingestion

DIAGNOSTIC PROCEDURES None, other than correlating serum salicylate concentration with the clinical presentation.
• Following acute ingestions, the significance of the serum salicylate level can be estimated by using the Done nomogram. The nomogram may underestimate the severity of poisonings in patients with:
  ◊ Illnesses accompanied by dehydration and/or acidosis
  ◊ Chronic exposure to salicylates
  ◊ Ingestion of enteric coated or sustained release medications
  ◊ Unknown time of ingestion

TREATMENT

APPROPRIATE HEALTH CARE
Evaluate all patients at a healthcare facility; outpatient for non-toxic accidental ingestions; inpatient for toxic and intentional ingestions

GENERAL MEASURES
• Prevent further absorption:
◊ Gastric lavage, within 2-4 hours of ingestion. Ipecac if unable to be seen in a healthcare facility within 1 hour of ingestion.
◊ Activated charcoal after gastric emptying
• Fluid/electrolyte balance: IV fluids to restore intravascular volume and prevent hypoglycemia. With hypotension give isotonic fluid until orthostatic changes no longer present; the fluids should contain at least 5% dextrose unless hyperglycemia is a problem. Normal saline or a mixture of .45% NaCl with 1 ampule of sodium bicarbonate (50 mEq NaHCO3) may be administered at 10-15 mL/kg/hr for 1-2 hours, depending on the degree of acidosis. When blood pressure stable, fluid management is directed toward alkalinizing the urine to enhance salicylate excretion, preventing CNS hypoglycemia, and treating fluid and electrolyte abnormalities.
• Enhance elimination:
◊ Alkaline diuresis (urine pH 7-8) and prevention of hypoglycemia can usually be maintained with fluids containing approximately 40 mEq/L Na+, 35 mEq/L K+, 50 mEq/L Cl-, 20 mEq/L HCO3- and 5-10% dextrose, run at 4-8 mL/kg/hr until the salicylate level decreases into the therapeutic range. Additional bicarbonate may be needed for severe or persistent acidosis. Fluids should be run slower in patients with cardiovascular compromise. Thereafter, maintenance fluids with added bicarbonate as needed can be run at 2-3 mL/kg/hr until toxicity resolves.
◊ Hemodialysis should be considered in poisonings with markedly elevated salicylate levels (> 100 mg/dL in acute poisonings, > 40-60 mg/dL in chronic poisonings), acidosis unresponsive to alkalinization and diuresis, renal and/or hepatic dysfunction with impaired salicylate clearance, noncardiac pulmonary edema, and persistent, severe CNS symptoms.

SURGICAL MEASURES   N/A

ACTIVITY   Bedrest initially

DIET   No special diet

PATIENT EDUCATION
• Education of parents/caregivers during well child visits
• Education of patients on chronic salicylate therapy
• Anticipatory guidance for caregivers, family, and cohabitants of potentially suicidal patients
• Patient brochure: Child Safety: How to keep your home safe for your baby. American Academy of Family Physicians, 8880 Ward Parkway, Kansas City, MO 64114 2797

MEDICATIONS

DRUG(S) OF CHOICE
• Ipecac syrup
• Activated charcoal
• Bicarbonate
• Dextrose containing IV solution
At home
• Give ipecac syrup if patient is alert and unable to be evaluated at a health care facility within 1 hour. Dose: 6 months-1 year: 5 mL; 1-12 years: 15 mL; > 12 years: 30 mL. Give with 240 mL (8oz) of water when possible; may repeat in 30 min if emesis has not occurred.
Emergency facility/hospital:
• Patients evaluated within 4 hours of ingestion should have their stomachs evacuated. Gastric lavage is the preferred method
• Repeat activated charcoal every 4 hours (1 g/kg each dose) until passage of a charcoal stool
• Bicarbonate is used to alkalinize the urine (pH 7-8) and, when appropriate, to correct severe systemic acidosis (for pH < 7.1)
• Give dextrose-containing IV solution to prevent hypoglycemia; CNS hypoglycemia may be present despite a normal serum glucose

Contraindications:
• Ipecac syrup should not be given to patients with decreased responsiveness
• Medication allergies

Precautions:
• If ipecac has been given, activated charcoal should be given at least 30 minutes to 1 hour afterwards to avoid risks of decreased effectiveness and aspiration
• Intravascular overload may result from injudicious use of sodium bicarbonate, particularly in patients with cardiovascular compromise
• Dextrose should not be given to patients with severe hyperglycemia

Significant possible interactions: N/A

ALTERNATIVE DRUGS   N/A

FOLLOWUP

PATIENT MONITORING
• Fluid, acid base, blood glucose, and electrolyte status until stable; urine pH (to enhance elimination of salicylate)
• Psychiatric followup after intentional ingestions

PREVENTION/AVOIDANCE
• Patient and parent/caregiver education essential. See Patient Education.
• Ipecac syrup at home
• Emergency telephone numbers

POSSIBLE COMPLICATIONS
• Noncardiogenic pulmonary edema, including development of ARDS
• Rare following recovery from poisoning

EXPECTED COURSE/PROGNOSIS
• Complete recovery with early therapy
• Clinical course and prognosis are worse in the very young and elderly, chronic intoxications, and in patients with concurrent conditions which cause dehydration and/or acidosis

MISCELLANEOUS

ASSOCIATED CONDITIONS
Reye's syndrome with salicylate use and varicella or influenza viral infection

AGE-RELATED FACTORS
Pediatric: Acidosis is often more severe in the very young, particularly in chronic or repeated therapeutic dose poisonings
Geriatric:
• Increased risk for chronic toxicity because of decreased renal function
• Increased risk for bleeding or perforated gastric ulcers in patients over 70 years
Others: N/A

PREGNANCY
• No teratogenic effect in humans
• Salicylates may cause premature closure of ductus arteriosus in fetus
• Increased risk of ante and intrapartum hemorrhage

SYNONYMS   N/A

ICD-9-CM   965.1 Poisoning by salicylates (aspirin)

SEE ALSO   N/A

OTHER NOTES   N/A

ABBREVIATIONS   N/A

REFERENCES
• Yip L, Dart RC, Gabow A: Concepts and controversies in salicylate toxicity. Emerg Clin N Amer 1994;12:351-364
• Litovitz TL, Felberg L, White S, Klein-Schwartz W: 1995 Annual report of the American Association of Poison Control Centers Toxic Exposure Surveillance System. Am J Emerg Med 1996;14:487-537
Illustrations: N/A
Internet references: http://www.5mcc.com

Author(s)
Lars C. Larsen, MD

Salivary gland calculi

BASICS

DESCRIPTION The presence of stones within the ducts of any of the major salivary glands
System(s) affected: Gastrointestinal, Skin/Exocrine
Genetics: No known genetic pattern
Incidence/Prevalence in USA: Not uncommon
Predominant age: Middle to geriatric age groups. Uncommon in children.
Predominant sex: Male > Female (2:1)

SIGNS AND SYMPTOMS
• Mass palpable within the mouth or in the neck or face
• May be associated with sialadenitis
• Most stones are unilateral and tend to be recurrent

CAUSES
• Related to inflammation, trauma or factors that alter secretion
• Stones felt to be due to calcifications that occur around impacted food particles and organic debris. Increased with conditions that result in stasis of saliva. Examples include chronic parotitis, Sjögren's syndrome, cystic fibrosis, poor oral hygiene.

RISK FACTORS Existing chronic, debilitating illness

DIAGNOSIS

DIFFERENTIAL DIAGNOSIS
• Lymphadenitis
• Sialadenitis
• Oral or cervical carcinoma
• Foreign body
• Dental abscess
• Salivary carcinoma. Patients present with mass in the neck with or without intermittent swelling of the affected salivary gland.

LABORATORY Nonspecific except for factors altered by inflammation. If associated with sialadenitis there may be elevation of serum amylase.
Drugs that may alter lab results: N/A
Disorders that may alter lab results: N/A

PATHOLOGICAL FINDINGS
Submandibular glands are affected 90% of cases; parotid about 10%; other glands rarely

SPECIAL TESTS N/A

IMAGING
• Plain film of the head and neck
• Sialogram
• CT of head and neck
• 80% of stones are radiopaque and contain inorganic calcium and phosphate

DIAGNOSTIC PROCEDURES N/A

TREATMENT

APPROPRIATE HEALTH CARE Inpatient or outpatient surgery

GENERAL MEASURES
• Stone(s) within 2 cm of the end of the duct - the stone is removed intraorally by massage or by sectioning the duct
• Parotid stones are almost always removed intraorally
• Massage of the gland may cause expulsion of the stone if in the distal duct
• Look for primary diseases causing stasis such as Sjögren's syndrome
• Treat associated infections or conditions

SURGICAL MEASURES Stone(s) in the submandibular gland more than 2 cm from the orifice - treated by removal of the gland and the associated duct

ACTIVITY No restriction

DIET Avoid sour substances that may cause salivation

PATIENT EDUCATION Relate the general management and diet as listed above

MEDICATIONS

DRUG(S) OF CHOICE   If infection, use an antistaphylococcus antibiotic
Contraindications: Hypersensitivity to drug chosen
Precautions: Refer to manufacturer's literature
Significant possible interactions: Refer to manufacturer's literature

ALTERNATIVE DRUGS   N/A

FOLLOWUP

PATIENT MONITORING   Patients should be followed clinically approximately every 6 months for recurrence of the stone. Stones tend to be recurrent in the same gland in which the original stone was found.

PREVENTION/AVOIDANCE   Treat primary disease; good oral hygiene

POSSIBLE COMPLICATIONS
Postsurgery salivary fistula is possible. Sialadenitis may be caused by stones or they may cause stones and need separate treatment.

EXPECTED COURSE/PROGNOSIS
• Most patients have permanent recovery after the stone is removed
• Recurrence is possible

MISCELLANEOUS

ASSOCIATED CONDITIONS
• Sjögren's syndrome
• Cystic fibrosis
• Sialadenitis
• Oral trauma

AGE-RELATED FACTORS
Pediatric: N/A
Geriatric: N/A
Others: N/A

PREGNANCY   N/A

SYNONYMS   N/A

ICD-9-CM   527.5

SEE ALSO
• Sialadenitis

OTHER NOTES   Multiple calculi in 20% of cases. In past, stones were felt to be secondary to diseases of calcium metabolism but this has been disproven.

ABBREVIATIONS   N/A

REFERENCES
• Cotran RS, et al: Robbins Pathologic Basis of Disease. 4th Ed. Philadelphia, W.B. Saunders, Co., 1989
• Paparella MM, Shunrick DA: Otolaryngology. Philadelphia, W.B. Saunders Co., 1980
Illustrations: 1 available on CD-ROM
Internet references: http://www.5mcc.com

Author(s)
Michael Strange, MD

Salivary gland tumors

BASICS

DESCRIPTION Neoplasms benign or malignant of the major (parotid, submaxillary, sublingual) salivary glands or the minor (intra-oral, pharyngeal, nasal) salivary glands. Most tumors are discrete masses although some may manifest as diffuse enlargement of the gland or submucosal intraoral swelling. Malignant tumors are characterized by local recurrence and perineural spread (adenoid cystic), or local recurrence and lymph node metastases (mucoepidermoid, adenocarcinoma, squamous cell carcinoma).
• Types
  ◊ Pleomorphic adenoma (most common tumor) - 45% overall
  ◊ Monomorphic adenoma - 12% overall
  ◊ Mucoepidermoid carcinoma - 12% overall
  ◊ Adenoid cystic - 6% overall
  ◊ Less frequent lesions are - adenocarcinoma, squamous cell carcinoma, acinic cell carcinoma, oxyphilic adenomas, Warthin's tumor
• Distribution of neoplasms
  ◊ Parotid (80% benign, 20% malignant) - 70% are pleomorphic adenoma; 10% are monomorphic adenoma; 12% are mucoepidermoid carcinoma; 5% are adenoid cystic
  ◊ Submandibular (60% benign, 40% malignant) - 40% are pleomorphic adenoma; 10% are mucoepidermoid carcinoma; 20% are adenoid cystic carcinoma
  ◊ Minor salivary glands (40% benign, 60% malignant) - 40% are pleomorphic adenoma; 25% are mucoepidermoid carcinoma; 25% are adenoid cystic carcinoma
System(s) affected: Nervous, Digestive
Genetics: Increased incidence of adenocarcinoma of parotid in Eskimos, otherwise no known genetic pattern
Incidence/Prevalence in USA: 3% of new tumors; 6% of head and neck neoplasms
Predominant age: Malignant - age 55; benign - age 45
Predominant sex:
• Pleomorphic adenoma: Female > Male
• Other adenomas: Male = Female

SIGNS AND SYMPTOMS
• Discrete mass in anatomic area - 96% (malignant)
• Elevation of earlobe
• Pain 12-25% (malignant); 2.5% (benign)
• Trigeminal paresthesias
• Facial nerve palsy or dysfunction 8-26% (malignant)
• Fixation to masseter and pterygoids 17% (malignant)
• Skin ulceration 9% (malignant)
• Cervical lymph node metastases 20% (malignant)
• Pharyngeal mass (representing deep lobe tumors of the parotid gland)

CAUSES
• Unknown
• Possible ionizing radiation

RISK FACTORS None known

DIAGNOSIS

DIFFERENTIAL DIAGNOSIS
• Inflammatory masses
• Parotid and submandibular lymph nodes
• Mikulicz's syndrome
• Salivary gland stones
• Torus palatinus (minor)
• Necrotizing sialometaplasia (minor)
• Cervical lymph nodes
• Sjögren's syndrome
• Lymphadenopathy with AIDS

LABORATORY
• Autoimmune studies
• Fractionated amylase (inflammation)
Drugs that may alter lab results: None known
Disorders that may alter lab results: None known

PATHOLOGICAL FINDINGS Of 100 parotid masses, 70 will be non-neoplastic, 21 will be benign neoplasms, and 9 will be malignant neoplasms

SPECIAL TESTS
• Technetium-99 (Warthin's tumor)
• Ultrasound (inflammatory or malignant)
• Sialography (for calculi or chronic parotitis)

IMAGING
• CT/MRI. Both provide anatomic detail and diagnostic information.
• Chest x-ray - Sjögren's, metastases

DIAGNOSTIC PROCEDURES
• Fine needle aspiration (some authors would not utilize this procedure in fear of disseminating a malignant tumor)
• Superficial lobectomy

TREATMENT

APPROPRIATE HEALTH CARE Inpatient

GENERAL MEASURES
• Inpatient procedures with usual nursing care
• Drain parotid bed
• Usually 1-2 day hospitalization

SURGICAL MEASURES
• Benign tumors - superficial or total conservative (nerve-sparing) parotidectomy depending on site of tumor
• Malignant tumors - total parotidectomy, or sialadenectomy with adjuvant radiotherapy to parotid base of skull with/without neck depending on histology. Preservation of facial nerve unless involved by tumor.
• Cervical lymphadenectomy if palpable nodes or elective neck dissection in squamous cell carcinoma, high grade mucoepidermoid carcinoma or high grade adenocarcinoma
• Elevate head of bed postoperative
• Suction drainage x 1-2 days
• Suture line care with antibiotic ointment

ACTIVITY Moderate restriction for 1 day

DIET Non-stimulating liquid

PATIENT EDUCATION
• Basic cancer followup
• Recurrent masses
• Trigeminal nerve symptoms
• Frey's syndrome (gustatory sweating)
• Facial nerve symptoms (paresis)

Salivary gland tumors

MEDICATIONS

DRUG(S) OF CHOICE N/A
Contraindications: N/A
Precautions: N/A
Significant possible interactions: N/A

ALTERNATIVE DRUGS N/A

FOLLOWUP

PATIENT MONITORING
• For malignancy - once every 4 months the first year, once every six months subsequent 3 years, once per year subsequently
• For benign tumors - once per year for five years

PREVENTION/AVOIDANCE No known etiologic agents

POSSIBLE COMPLICATIONS
• Frey's syndrome (gustatory sweating) occurs symptomatically in about 20% of patients undergoing parotidectomy
• Facial neurapraxia from surgery should resolve within six months, even with use of adjuvant radiotherapy
• Cosmetic deformity of moderate facial flattening on side of parotidectomy
• Injury to hypoglossal or lingual nerve during submandibular resection
• Pleomorphic adenoma may recur, if inadequately excised, since it has pseudopods throughout the lobe

EXPECTED COURSE/PROGNOSIS
• Parotid pleomorphic adenoma untreated will demonstrate malignant degeneration in 2-10% over 20 years. Treated adequately, parotid pleomorphic adenoma has 1.5% recurrence rate. Malignancy prognosis depends on stage.
• Adenoid cystic - parotid 5 year survival 73%, 15 year 21%; submandibular 5 year 50%, 15 year 0%; palate 5 year 80%, 15 year 38%
• Adenocarcinoma - 5 year survival 78%, 20 year 41%
• Mucoepidermoid - low grade 5 year survival 81%, 15 year 48%, high grade 5 year survival 46%, 15 year 25%

MISCELLANEOUS

ASSOCIATED CONDITIONS None known

AGE-RELATED FACTORS
Pediatric: Hemangioma is the most common benign tumor in pediatric population followed by pleomorphic adenoma. Mucoepidermoid most common malignant.
Geriatric: N/A
Others: N/A

PREGNANCY Not affected

SYNONYMS N/A

ICD-9-CM 142-142.9 malignant neoplasm of major salivary glands

SEE ALSO N/A

OTHER NOTES N/A

ABBREVIATIONS N/A

REFERENCES
• Coleman JJ: Salivary gland disorders. In: Jurkiewicz MJ, Krizek TJ, Mathews SJ, Ariyan S, eds. Fundamentals of Plastic Surgery. St. Louis, C.V. Mosby Co., 1990
• Rankow RM, Polayes IM: Diseases of the Salivary Glands, Philadelphia, W.B. Saunders, 1976
• Batsakis JG: Tumors of the head and neck. Clinical and Pathological Considerations. 2nd Ed. Baltimore, Williams and Wilkins, 1979
Illustrations: 1 available on CD-ROM
Internet references: http://www.5mcc.com

Author(s)
John J. Coleman, MD

Salmonella infection

BASICS

DESCRIPTION Disease caused by any serotype of the genus Salmonella. Clinical syndromes include enterocolitis (75%), bacteremia (10%), enteric fever (10%) (see Typhoid fever), localized infection outside gastrointestinal tract (5%) and an asymptomatic carrier state (< 1%). Organisms invade gut mucosa, producing inflammatory, cytotoxic response. Organisms can then disseminate into systemic circulation via lymphatics. Infective dose and host defenses dictate extent of disease.

System(s) affected: Gastrointestinal

Genetics: A condition similar to Reiter's syndrome may follow Salmonella enterocolitis in patients with the HLA-B27 histocompatibility antigen

Incidence/Prevalence in USA:
• 800 cases/100,000 population/year. Peak frequency July-November. Salmonella isolations represent only 1-10% of actual yearly incidence. Second only to campylobacter as cause of bacterial diarrheal illness. Each year, an average of 55 outbreaks of salmonella infections are reported to CDC.
• Infants: 130/100,000
• Adults: 6/100,000

Predominant age:
• High prevalence in persons > 70 or < 20
• Highest in infants < 1 year

Predominant sex: Male = Female

SIGNS AND SYMPTOMS
• Acute uncomplicated illness
  ◊ Nausea, vomiting, diarrhea
  ◊ Abdominal cramps
  ◊ Headache, myalgias
  ◊ Fever to 102°F (39°C)
• Protracted disease
  ◊ Persistent fever
  ◊ Arthritis, reactive or septic
  ◊ Osteomyelitis
  ◊ Sacroiliitis
  ◊ Wound infection, soft tissue abscesses
  ◊ Meningitis
  ◊ Arteritis
  ◊ Endocarditis, pericarditis
  ◊ Pneumonia, lung abscess, empyema
  ◊ Hypovolemia
  ◊ Splenic (abscess)
  ◊ Hepatic (abscess)
  ◊ Urogenital tract infection

CAUSES
• Ingestion of contaminated food - (poultry, meat, eggs, dairy products) or water
• Person-to-person and/or fecal-oral spread
• Contact with animal reservoirs - poultry, cows, pigs, birds, sheep, seals, donkeys, lizards, snakes, pets (turtles, cats, dogs, mice, guinea pigs, hamsters)
• Iatrogenic contamination - blood transfusion, endoscopy
• Contact with asymptomatic chronic carrier
• Achlorhydria - gastroduodenal surgery, idiopathic
• Ulcerative colitis
• Systemic lupus erythematosus
• Schistosomiasis

• Cholelithiasis
• Nephrolithiasis
• Drugs - antibiotics, purgatives, opiates

RISK FACTORS
• Impaired gastric acidity—H2 blockers, antacids, gastrectomy, achlorhydria
• Hemolytic anemias - sickle-cell, malaria, bartonellosis
• Malignancy - lymphoma, leukemia, disseminated carcinoma
• Immunosuppression - AIDS, steroids, other immunosuppressants, chemotherapy, radiation
• Pets with high fecal carriage rates for salmonella, especially reptiles (snakes, iguanas)
  ◊ Antibiotic treatment of the animal is not recommended, due to temporary effect only

DIAGNOSIS

DIFFERENTIAL DIAGNOSIS
• Viral gastroenteritis
• Other bacterial enteritises (e.g., shigellosis, cholera)
• Other bacterial sources or systemic and localized sepsis (e.g., meningococci, staphylococci)
• Pseudomembranous colitis
• Inflammatory or granulomatous bowel disease
• Appendicitis
• Cholecystitis
• Perforated viscus

LABORATORY
• Enterocolitis
  ◊ Fecal leukocytes positive
  ◊ Stool culture positive for Salmonella species
  ◊ WBC normal or decreased
  ◊ Blood cultures negative
• Bacteremia
  ◊ Blood cultures positive
  ◊ Stool cultures negative
• Local infections
  ◊ Polymorphonuclear leukocytosis
  ◊ Tissue site culture positive
• Asymptomatic carrier state
  ◊ Stool culture positive for more than 1 year
  ◊ Urine culture may be positive with certain serotypes

Drugs that may alter lab results:
Antibiotics used early may lead to false-negative cultures and blunted immunologic response

Disorders that may alter lab results:
N/A

PATHOLOGICAL FINDINGS
• Mucosal ulceration, hemorrhage and necrosis
• Reticuloendothelial hyperplasia and hypertrophy
• Focal organ and soft tissues abscesses

SPECIAL TESTS Serologic tests identify particular clinical syndromes and serve as epidemiologic markers

IMAGING Angiography in patients over 50 with bacteremia. To rule out presence of infected aneurysm, particularly of aorto-iliac vessels.

DIAGNOSTIC PROCEDURES N/A

TREATMENT

APPROPRIATE HEALTH CARE
• Outpatient for uncomplicated enterocolitis and carrier state
• Inpatient for bacteremia and extra-intestinal infection (11% hospitalization rate)
• Do not wait for stool culture results before initiating important therapeutic decisions

GENERAL MEASURES
• Correct fluid and electrolyte deficits
• Control symptoms (pain, nausea, vomiting)

SURGICAL MEASURES Surgical drainage and vascular bypass procedures for infected tissue sites

ACTIVITY As tolerated

DIET Oral rehydration solution during diarrhea phase; advance to normal diet as tolerated

PATIENT EDUCATION Food Safety and Inspection Service, Office of Public Awareness, Dept. of Agriculture, Rm. 1165-S, Washington, DC 20205, (202)447-9351

Salmonella infection

MEDICATIONS

DRUG(S) OF CHOICE
• Enterocolitis uncomplicated:
◊ None recommended
• Enterocolitis complicated: (by age extremes, immunosuppression, underlying cardiovascular abnormalities, prosthetic orthopedic devices, hemolytic anemia)
◊ Ciprofloxacin (Cipro) po for 3-7 days--no pediatric dose; adult dose 500 mg q12h, or
◊ Ampicillin po for 10-14 days - pediatric dose 50-100 mg/kg/day in 4 divided doses; adult dose 500 mg qid, or
◊ Trimethoprim-sulfamethoxazole (Bactrim, Septra) po for 14 days - pediatric dose 10 mg/kg/day trimethoprim, 50 mg/kg/day sulfamethoxazole in 2 divided doses (maximum 320 mg/day trimethoprim; 1600 mg/day sulfamethoxazole); adult dose 1 double strength tablet q12h
• Bacteremia:
◊ Ampicillin IV for 10-14 days - pediatric dose 200-300 mg/kg/day in 4 divided doses; adult dose 1-2 gm q4h; or
◊ Cefotaxime (Claforan) IV for 14 days - pediatric dose 200 mg/kg/day q8h; adult dose 1-2 gm q8hr, maximum 12 gm/day; or ciprofloxacin (Cipro) 500 mg po or norfloxacin 400 mg po q12h for 7 days (adults only)
• Localized infection:
◊ Same as for bacteremia with additional option of chloramphenicol 25-75 mg/kg/day (maximum 4 gm/day) IV in 4 divided doses for 14 days
◊ In sustained bacteremia or prolonged local infection, antibiotics can be given po for 4-6 weeks (substitute trimethoprim-sulfamethoxazole for cefotaxime, using 2-4 double strength (DS) tablets given 3 times a day)
• Chronic carrier state:
◊ Ampicillin 2-4 gm/day plus probenecid 1-2 gm/day, both divided into 4 oral doses, for 6 weeks; or
◊ 40-160 mg/day trimethoprim and 200-800 mg/day sulfamethoxazole divided into 2 doses for 6 weeks
◊ Consider ciprofloxacin 500 mg po bid for 4 weeks, or norfloxacin (Noroxin) 400 mg po bid for 4 weeks, if gallstones are present
Contraindications: Known drug allergy
Precautions:
• Use bowel motility inhibitors (Lomotil, Imodium) with caution, if at all
• Monitor blood levels of chloramphenicol in neonates and infants
• Ampicillin-resistant strains increasing; now at 15-30% in US
Significant possible interactions:
Ampicillin failure rate is 75% in chronic carriers with gallbladder disease

ALTERNATIVE DRUGS Fluoroquinolones - ciprofloxacin (Cipro), ofloxacin (Floxin) gaining favor in management of gastroenteritis, osteomyelitis and carrier state. Use is restricted to nonpregnant adults only. For gastroenteritis in children > 1 year, consider furazolidone (Furoxone) 2.5 mg/kg po qid for 5 days.

FOLLOWUP

PATIENT MONITORING Repeat stool culture at 5 months (40% of children negative, 90% of adults negative) and at 1 year (> 99% of all patients negative)

PREVENTION/AVOIDANCE
• Proper hygiene in production, transport and storage of food
• Control of animal reservoir, especially by avoiding contact with animal feces
• Hand washing emphasized
• No vaccine available to oppose salmonellosis

POSSIBLE COMPLICATIONS
• Toxic megacolon
• Hypovolemic shock
• Metastatic abscess formation
• Acute or chronic hydrocephalus

EXPECTED COURSE/PROGNOSIS
• Prognosis for enterocolitis is excellent. Exceptions - in the very young (7.0% fatal), the very old (8.7% fatal) and the debilitated and/or institutionalized (2.3% fatal).
• Prognosis for meningitis or endocarditis is poor, unless effective treatment given early

MISCELLANEOUS

ASSOCIATED CONDITIONS N/A

AGE-RELATED FACTORS
Pediatric: Children, especially neonates, more likely to become chronic carriers
Geriatric: Patients over 60 also have high carrier rate presumably due to biliary sequestration of organisms
Others: Contaminated marijuana is important source of infection, particularly in young adults

PREGNANCY Consult obstetrician regarding antibiotics. Keep a low threshold for hospital admission.

SYNONYMS N/A

ICD-9-CM 003 Other salmonella infections

SEE ALSO
• Typhoid fever
• Gastroenteritis, viral
• Diarrhea, acute

OTHER NOTES If one member of a household becomes infected with salmonellosis, the chance of at least one other member becoming infected is 60%

ABBREVIATIONS N/A

REFERENCES
• Rubin RH: Infections due to gram-negative bacilli. Scientific American Medicine, 1995
• Sleisenger MH, Fordtran JS, eds: Gastrointestinal Disease: Pathophysiology, Diagnosis, Management. 5th Ed. Philadelphia, W.B. Saunders Co., 1994
• Mandell GL, ed: Principles and Practice of Infectious Diseases. 4th Ed. New York, Churchill Livingstone, 1995
• Sanford JP, Gilbert DN, Moellering RC, Sande MA: The Sanford Guide to Antimicrobial Therapy. 27th Ed. Dallas, Antimicrobial Therapy, inc., 1997
• Mermin J, Hoar B, Angulo FJ: Iguanas and Salmonella marina infection in children: a reflection of the increasing incidence of reptile-associated salmonellosis in the United States. Pediatrics 1997;99:399-402
Illustrations: N/A
Internet references: http://www.5mcc.com

Author(s)
Richard Viken, MD

Sarcoidosis

BASICS

DESCRIPTION Non-infectious multisystem disease of unknown cause, commonly affecting young and middle-age adults. Frequently presents with bilateral hilar adenopathy, pulmonary infiltrates, ocular and skin lesions. Other organs may be involved, including liver, spleen, lymph nodes, heart, and central nervous system.

System(s) affected:
Hemic/Lymphatic/Immunologic, Pulmonary, Cardiovascular, Gastrointestinal

Genetics: Although world-wide in distribution, increased prevalence found in Scandinavians, Japanese, Irish females, and African American women

Incidence/Prevalence in USA: 30-80 per 100,000

Predominant age: 20-60 years

Predominant sex: Female > Male

SIGNS AND SYMPTOMS
• Patients may be asymptomatic
• Cough
• Shortness of breath
• Skin (new lesions)
• Pain or irritation of eyes
• General fatigue, malaise
• Fever
• Night sweats
• Bell's palsy

CAUSES Unknown

RISK FACTORS None known

DIAGNOSIS

DIFFERENTIAL DIAGNOSIS
• Infectious granulomatous disease such as tuberculosis and fungal infections
• Foreign body reactions
• Lymphoma
• Other malignancies associated with lymphadenopathy
• Berylliosis

LABORATORY
• Lymphopenia, anemia, or leukopenia can be seen in over half of the patients
• Abnormal liver function, especially increased alkaline phosphatase is frequently encountered
• Hypercalciuria occurs in up to 10% of patients, with hypercalcemia less frequent

Drugs that may alter lab results:
Prednisone will lower serum-angiotensin converting enzyme and normalize Gallium scan

Disorders that may alter lab results:
Hyperthyroidism and diabetes will increase serum angiotensin converting enzyme level

PATHOLOGICAL FINDINGS
Noncaseating epithelioid granulomas without evidence of fungal or mycobacterial infection

SPECIAL TESTS
• Serum angiotensin converting enzyme (ACE) is elevated in over 60% of patients
• Gallium scan uptake in chest, lymph nodes, and parotids may be seen in active disease
• Characteristically in active disease, bronchoalveolar lavage (BAL) fluid has an increased percentage of lymphocytes, specifically CD4 positive (T-helper/inducer lymphocytes)
• Ophthalmologic exam

IMAGING
• Routine chest roentgenograms are staged using Scadding's classification:
    ◊ Stage 0 = normal
    ◊ Stage 1 = hilar adenopathy alone
    ◊ Stage 2 = hilar adenopathy plus parenchymal infiltrates
    ◊ Stage 3 = parenchymal infiltrates alone
    ◊ Stage 4 = pulmonary fibrosis
• Gallium scan will be positive in areas of acute disease
• Computerized tomography may enhance appreciation of lymph nodes and high resolution CT scan shows peribronchial disease

DIAGNOSTIC PROCEDURES
• Bronchoscopy with transbronchial biopsy and bronchoalveolar lavage is often performed to diagnose lung disease
• Mediastinoscopy, skin or lymph node biopsy (if needed to establish diagnosis)
• When available, Kveim-Siltzbach skin test can be performed. This test is fairly sensitive (approximately 80%) and highly specific (> 95%). Unfortunately, the antigen is not generally available.

TREATMENT

APPROPRIATE HEALTH CARE
Outpatient

GENERAL MEASURES
• The disease may require no specific therapy in the asymptomatic individual or may treat for specific indications, such as cardiac, central nervous system, ocular, or hypercalcemia
• Treatment of pulmonary and skin manifestations usually done on the basis of impairment

SURGICAL MEASURES N/A

ACTIVITY Generally no limitations

DIET
• Avoid high calcium diets
• In patients on corticosteroids, avoid high salt foods

PATIENT EDUCATION Generally stress the benign nature of the disease and the fact that it is not contagious to others and is not malignant

MEDICATIONS

DRUG(S) OF CHOICE
• Systemic corticosteroids in the symptomatic individual, usually prednisone initially 40 mg every day or every other day. Treatment with tapering doses of prednisone for at least one year.
• In patients with skin or ocular disease, topical steroids may be effective
Contraindications: Patients with known problems with corticosteroids
Precautions: Careful monitoring in patients with diabetes mellitus and/or hypertension
Significant possible interactions: Refer to manufacturer's profile of each drug

ALTERNATIVE DRUGS
Methotrexate 10 mg per week, hydroxychloroquine (Plaquenil) 100-200 mg per day, azathioprine 50-100 mg per day and chlorambucil 0.1-0.2 mg/kg. May increase risk of carcinogenicity. Use of immunosuppressants such as methotrexate, azathioprine or chlorambucil will require careful, regular monitoring of complete blood count.

FOLLOWUP

PATIENT MONITORING
• Patients on prednisone for symptoms should be seen every month or two while on therapy
• Patients not requiring therapy should be seen regularly (every three months) for at least the first two years after diagnosis
• Chest roentgenograms and pulmonary function tests are useful for monitoring for pulmonary changes
• Serum angiotensin converting enzyme level is used by some to follow disease activity. In patients with an initially elevated ACE level, it should fall towards normal while on therapy or when the disease resolves.

PREVENTION/AVOIDANCE None known

POSSIBLE COMPLICATIONS
• Patients may develop significant respiratory involvement including cor pulmonale
• Other organs, especially the heart (congestive heart failure, arrhythmias), eyes (rarely blindness) and central nervous system can be involved with serious consequences. Fortunately, cardiac, ocular, and CNS involvement usually manifests itself early on in patients with these manifestations of the disease.

EXPECTED COURSE/PROGNOSIS
• 80% of patients will have spontaneous resolution within two years
• 10% will have significant fibrosis but no further worsening of disease after two years
• 10% (higher in some populations, including African Americans) will have chronic disease

MISCELLANEOUS

ASSOCIATED CONDITIONS None known

AGE-RELATED FACTORS
Pediatric: Rare
Geriatric: Less than 5% of patients with active disease are 60 years or older
Others: Sarcoidosis is a disease of youth to middle age

PREGNANCY No increased incidence

SYNONYMS
• Loeffgren's syndrome (erythema nodosum, hilar adenopathy plus uveitis)
• Besnier-Boeck disease
• Boeck's sarcoid
• Schaumann's disease

ICD-9-CM 135 Sarcoidosis

SEE ALSO N/A

OTHER NOTES N/A

ABBREVIATIONS N/A

REFERENCES
• Thomas PD, Hunninghake GW: Current concepts of the pathogenesis of sarcoidosis. Am Rev Respir Dis 1987;135:747-760
• Sharma OP: Sarcoidosis. Dis Month 1990;36:469-535.3
• Baughman RP, Lower EE, Lynch JP: Treatment modalities for sarcoidosis. Clin Pulm Med 1995;1:223-231
• Lower LL, Baughman RP: Prolonged use of methotrexate for sarcoidosis. Arch Int Med 1995;155:846-851
Illustrations: 4 available on CD-ROM
Internet references: http://www.5mcc.com

Author(s)
Robert P. Baughman, MD
Elyse E. Lower, MD

Scabies

BASICS

DESCRIPTION A contagious disease caused by infestation of the skin by the mite Sarcoptes scabiei, var. hominis
System(s) affected: Skin/Exocrine
Genetics: N/A
Incidence/Prevalence in USA:
Common, although number of cases per year is declining as the epidemic, which began in 1971, passed its peak (1986). Worldwide incidence is 300 million cases per year.
Predominant age: Children and young adults
Predominant sex: Male = Female

SIGNS AND SYMPTOMS
• Generalized itching
• Nocturnal pruritus
• Burrows in finger webs, wrists, hands, feet, penis, scrotum, buttocks, waistline
• Vesicles and papules (discrete)
• Secondary erosions
• Pustules (if secondarily infected)
• Scaling
• Erythema
• Nodules in covered areas (buttocks, groin, axillae)
• Atypical infestations in immunosuppressed patients

CAUSES Skin infestation by the mite Sarcoptes scabiei, var. hominis

RISK FACTORS
• Personal skin-to-skin contact, e.g., sexual promiscuity, crowding, poverty, nosocomial infection
• Immunocompromised patients
• Atopic eczema

DIAGNOSIS

DIFFERENTIAL DIAGNOSIS
• Atopic dermatitis
• Dermatitis herpetiformis
• Eczema
• Insect bites
• Pityriasis rosea
• Prurigo
• Seborrheic dermatitis
• Syphilis

LABORATORY N/A
Drugs that may alter lab results: N/A
Disorders that may alter lab results: N/A

PATHOLOGICAL FINDINGS Skin biopsy of a nodule (although rarely performed) will reveal portions of the mite in the corneal layer

SPECIAL TESTS N/A

IMAGING N/A

DIAGNOSTIC PROCEDURES
• Examination of skin with magnifying lens - look for typical burrows in finger webs, on flexor aspects of the wrists, and penis. Look for a dark point at the end of the burrow (the mite). The mite can be extracted with a 25 gauge needle and examined microscopically.
• Mineral oil mounts - place a drop of mineral oil over a suspected lesion. Non-excoriated papules or vesicles may also be sampled. Scrape the lesion with a #15 surgical blade. Examine under a microscope for mites, eggs, egg casings or feces. Scraping from under fingernails may often be positive.
• Potassium hydroxide wet mount - transfer skin scrapings directly to a glass slide, add a drop of KOH (potassium hydroxide), and apply a cover slip. Examine the slide for diagnostic material. If none is evident, heat slide gently to separate squamous cells and reexamine.
• Burrow ink test - if burrows are not obvious, apply blue black ink to an area of rash. Wash off the ink with alcohol. A burrow should remain stained and become more evident. Then apply mineral oil, scrape and observe microscopically as previously noted.

TREATMENT

APPROPRIATE HEALTH CARE
Outpatient

GENERAL MEASURES
• Treat all intimate contacts and close household and family members
• Wash all clothing, bed linen, and towels in a normal wash cycle

SURGICAL MEASURES N/A

ACTIVITY Full activity

DIET No special diet

PATIENT EDUCATION
• Patient instruction sheet "Scabies" in Epstein: Common Skin Disorders (see References)
• Griffiths: Instructions for Patients, Philadelphia, W.B. Saunders Co.
• Schmitt: Instructions for Pediatric Patients, Philadelphia, W.B. Saunders Co.

MEDICATIONS

DRUG(S) OF CHOICE
• Permethrin (Elimite) cream: considered by many to be the drug of choice for scabies. Cream is applied into the skin from the head to the soles of the feet and left on for 8 to 14 hours, then thoroughly washed off. Thirty grams is usually adequate for an adult. A second application 48 hours later is sometimes recommended.
• Lindane (Kwell, Scabene): available in lotion, cream and shampoo. The cream or lotion should be applied to all skin surfaces from the neck down and washed off 8 to 12 hours later. Some dermatologists routinely retreat in 7 days.
• Crotamiton (Eurax): cream is applied into the skin from the head to the soles of the feet and left on for 8 to 14 hours, then thoroughly washed off. It is felt to be less toxic than lindane, but perhaps slightly less effective, therefore, application 2 nights in a row is advised.

Contraindications: Lindane should be avoided in children who are premature, malnourished or emaciated and those with severe underlying skin disease or a history of seizure disorders.

Precautions:
• Patients should be cautioned not to overuse the medication when applying it to the skin
• For medications other than permethrin, patients should use a second application only when specifically advised to do so by their physician

Significant possible interactions: N/A

ALTERNATIVE DRUGS
5% sulfur ointment: applied to the entire body from the neck down. It is malodorous and messy, but is thought to be safer than lindane, especially in infants under age 6 months

FOLLOWUP

PATIENT MONITORING Recheck patient at weekly intervals only if rash or itching persists. Rescrape new lesions and retreat if mite or products found.

PREVENTION/AVOIDANCE N/A

POSSIBLE COMPLICATIONS
• Eczema
• Pyoderma
• Postscabetic pruritus
• Nodular scabies

EXPECTED COURSE/PROGNOSIS
• Lesions begin to regress in 1 to 2 days along with the worst itching
• Some itching and dermatitis commonly persists for 10 to 14 days and can be treated with antihistamines and/or topical or oral corticosteroids
• Nodular lesions may persist for several weeks, perhaps necessitating intralesional or systemic steroids
• Some instances of lindane resistant scabies have now been reported. These do respond to permethrin.

MISCELLANEOUS

ASSOCIATED CONDITIONS N/A

AGE-RELATED FACTORS
Pediatric: Infants often have more widespread involvement. They are occasionally infested on the face and scalp (rare for adults). Vesicular lesions on the palms and soles are also more commonly seen. When treating infants with permethrin, the entire body should be treated.
Geriatric: The elderly often itch more severely, despite fewer cutaneous lesions. Elderly at risk for extensive infestations, perhaps related to a decline in cell-mediated immunity.
Others: N/A

PREGNANCY Lindane should be used cautiously and no more than twice during pregnancy due to its potential to cause neurotoxicity and convulsions

SYNONYMS N/A

ICD-9-CM 133.0 scabies

SEE ALSO N/A

OTHER NOTES N/A

ABBREVIATIONS N/A

REFERENCES
• Epstein E: Common Skin Disorders. 4th Ed., Montvale, NJ, Med. Econ. Books, 1994
• Hurwitz S: Clinical Pediatric Dermatology. 2nd Ed. Philadelphia, W.B. Saunders Co., 1993
• Habif T: Clinical Dermatology. 3rd Ed. St. Louis, CV Mosby, 1996
• Weston WL, et al: Color Textbook of Pediatric Dermatology. 2nd Ed. St Louis, CV Mosby, 1996
Illustrations: 5 available on CD-ROM
Internet references: http://www.5mcc.com

Author(s)
Gary J. Silko, MD

Scarlet fever

BASICS

DESCRIPTION "Streptococcal sore throat with a rash." A childhood disease characterized by high fever, vomiting, and rash caused by Group A beta-hemolytic streptococci (GAS) pyogenes that elaborate erythrogenic toxin. Incubation period 1-7 days, duration of illness 4-10 days.
System(s) affected: Gastrointestinal, Skin/Exocrine
Genetics: N/A
Incidence/Prevalence in USA: Up to 10% of GAS pharyngitis
Predominant age: 6-12 years
Predominant sex: Male = Female

SIGNS AND SYMPTOMS
• Prodrome 1-2 days
  ◊ Sore throat
  ◊ Headache
  ◊ Vomiting
  ◊ Abdominal pain (may mimic acute abdomen)
  ◊ Fever (up to 40°C or 103.6°F)
• Oral exam
  ◊ "Beefy red" tonsils and pharynx with or without exudate
  ◊ Petechiae on palate
  ◊ White coating on tongue "White strawberry tongue" appears on days 1-2. This sheds by day 4-5 leaving a "Red strawberry tongue" - shiny, red with prominent papillae.
• Exanthem (appears within 12-24 hours)
  ◊ Orange-red punctate skin eruption with sandpaper-like texture - "sunburn with goose pimples"
  ◊ Rash begins on chest and axillae and spreads to abdomen and extremities; prominent in skin folds (axillae, groin, buttocks)
  ◊ Flushed face with circumoral pallor
  ◊ Transverse red streaks in skin folds of abdomen, antecubital space, and axillae: "Pastia's lines"
  ◊ Desquamation begins on face after 7-10 days and proceeds over trunk to hands and feet; may persist for 6 weeks
  ◊ In severe cases, small vesicular lesions (miliary sudamina) may appear on abdomen, hands, feet

CAUSES
• Hypersensitivity to erythrogenic toxins produced by GAS
• Site of GAS infection: Usually tonsils, may occur with skin infection
• Erythrogenic toxin produced by Staphylococcus aureus can produce staphylococcal "scarlet fever" - may actually be a mild form of toxic shock syndrome or scalded skin syndrome

RISK FACTORS
• Age - most commonly affects school age children - by age 10, 80% have antibodies to erythrogenic toxin
• Contact with infected individual
• Crowded living conditions, eg, lower socioeconomic status, military, child care

DIAGNOSIS

DIFFERENTIAL DIAGNOSIS
• Measles
• Rubella
• Infectious mononucleosis
• Roseola
• Severe sunburn
• Secondary syphilis
• Arcanobacterium haemolyticum
• Toxic shock syndrome
• Staphylococcal scalded skin syndrome
• Kawasaki disease
• Drug hypersensitivity
• Mycoplasma pneumonia

LABORATORY
• Throat culture definitive diagnosis
• Rapid Strep antigen tests - diagnostic if positive, but sensitivity only 50-90%, so must do throat culture
• Serologic tests (includes anti-streptolysin O titer and streptozyme tests) - confirm recent GAS infection; not helpful for diagnosis of acute disease
Drugs that may alter lab results:
• Prior antibiotic therapy may result in negative throat culture
• Penicillin within 5 days of symptoms can delay/abolish anti-streptolysin O response
Disorders that may alter lab results: N/A

PATHOLOGICAL FINDINGS N/A

SPECIAL TESTS N/A

IMAGING N/A

DIAGNOSTIC PROCEDURES N/A

TREATMENT

APPROPRIATE HEALTH CARE
Outpatient except for severe suppurative complications

GENERAL MEASURES Supportive care

SURGICAL MEASURES N/A

ACTIVITY Fully active

DIET No special diet

PATIENT EDUCATION Must take antibiotics for full 10 days; brief delay in initiating treatment awaiting throat culture results does not increase the risk of rheumatic fever.

MEDICATIONS

DRUG(S) OF CHOICE
• Penicillin (oral; penicillin V and others)
◊ 125 mg po tid for under 60 lb/27 kg; 250 mg tid for others. If compliance good, many authorities believe bid dosing effective.
◊ If compliance questionable, use penicillin, benzathine (Bicillin LA): single IM dose 600,000 units for under 60 lb/27 kg; 1,200,000 million units for others
• Acetaminophen for fever and comfort
Contraindications: Penicillin allergy
Precautions: Refer to manufacturer's profile of each drug
Significant possible interactions: Refer to manufacturer's profile of each drug

ALTERNATIVE DRUGS
All are given for 10 days.
• Erythromycin estolate (20-40 mg/kg/day divided tid or qid or erythromycin ethyl succinate (40-50 mg/kg/day divided tid or qid). Maximum dose: 1 gm/day.
• Newer macrolides
◊ Azithromycin: 500 mg the first day, then 250 mg qd for 4 days (age ≥ 16 only)
◊ Clarithromycin: 250 mg bid
• Oral cephalosporins; many are effective, but first generation are less expensive.
◊ Cephalexin 40 mg/kg/day divided tid. Maximum: 250 mg tid.
◊ Cefadroxil 30 mg/kg/day divided bid. Maximum: 500 mg bid.
• Clindamycin 20 mg/kg/day divided tid.
• Tetracyclines and sulfonamides should not be used
• Sulfamethoxazole-trimethoprim is not effective against group A beta-hemolytic streptococci

FOLLOWUP

PATIENT MONITORING
• Routine follow-up throat cultures not needed unless patient is symptomatic.
• Since GAS uniformly susceptible to penicillin; bacteriologic treatment failures possibly due to:
◊ Poor compliance
◊ Beta-lactamase oral flora hydrolyzing penicillin
◊ GAS carrier state (requires no treatment) and concurrent viral rash

PREVENTION/AVOIDANCE
• GAS spread by contact with respiratory secretions. Avoid if possible.
• Children should not return to school or day care until after 24 hours of antibiotic therapy
• Prophylactic penicillin not recommended after exposure to scarlet fever

POSSIBLE COMPLICATIONS
• Suppurative
◊ Sinusitis
◊ Otitis media/mastoiditis
◊ Cervical adenitis
◊ Peritonsillar abscess/retropharyngeal abscess
◊ Pneumonia
◊ Septicemia/meningitis/osteomyelitis/septic arthritis
• Non-suppurative
◊ Rheumatic fever (penicillin prevents RF when started as long as 10 days after onset of acute GAS infection)
◊ Glomerulonephritis (prevention even after adequate treatment of GAS is less certain)
◊ "Streptococcal toxic shock syndrome": Fever, hypotension, disseminated intravascular coagulation (DIC); cardiac, liver, kidney dysfunction.

EXPECTED COURSE/PROGNOSIS
• With penicillin, defervescence in 24 hours
• Can have recurrent attacks

MISCELLANEOUS

ASSOCIATED CONDITIONS
• Pharyngitis
• Impetigo
• Puerperal sepsis

AGE-RELATED FACTORS
Pediatric: Rare in infancy
Geriatric: N/A
Others: N/A

PREGNANCY N/A

SYNONYMS Scarlatina

ICD-9-CM 034.1 Scarlet fever

SEE ALSO
• Pharyngitis

OTHER NOTES Asymptomatic carriers can spread disease

ABBREVIATIONS
GAS = Group A beta-hemolytic streptococci

REFERENCES
• Committee on Infectious Diseases of Amer Acad Ped. (Red Book). 483-94, 1997
• Krugman S, Katz S, Gershon A, Wilfert C: Infectious Diseases of Children. 9th ed. New York, C.V. Mosby, 1990
• Behrman R, Kliegman R, Arvin A: Nelson's Textbook of Pediatrics. 15th Ed. Philadelphia, WB Saunders Co., 1996
Illustrations: 1 available on CD-ROM
Internet references: http://www.5mcc.com

Author(s)
Mitchell S. King, MD
Mohammad Malik, MD
Carlo Niguidula, MD

Schizophrenia

 BASICS

DESCRIPTION Major psychiatric psychotic (out of touch with reality) disorder with prodromal, active and residual symptoms involving delusions, hallucinations, disturbed affect (emotion) and impaired thought processes, lasting at least six months
System(s) affected: Nervous
Genetics: Genetic predisposition necessary for development
Incidence/Prevalence in USA: Lifetime (1%). Highest prevalence in lower socioeconomic classes.
Predominant age: Onset before age 45
Predominant sex: Male = Female

SIGNS AND SYMPTOMS
• Withdrawal from reality
• Delusions (fixed false unreal beliefs - paranoid (people persecuting or after you)
• Reference (people or things have unusual significance)
• Others can hear your thoughts, put thoughts into you or control you; grandiose or religious delusions
• Hallucinations - usually auditory
• Affect - flat or inappropriate emotion
• Thought processes - loose associations (thoughts don't follow)
• Much speech but convey little information
• Extremes of gross overactivity to stupor with mutism

CAUSES Unknown - not initiated or maintained by an organic factor. Probably a complex interaction between inherited and environmental factors.

RISK FACTORS Biologic relative with schizophrenia

 DIAGNOSIS

DIFFERENTIAL DIAGNOSIS
• Organic mental disorder - characterized by JOMAC (a mnemonic that stands for impaired Judgment, Orientation, Memory, Affect and Concentration). Disorientation, in particular indicates organicity. Organic mental disorders may be due to trauma, infection, tumor, metabolic, endocrine, intoxication (psychoactive substance use), epilepsy, neurological disorders, etc.
• Organic delusional syndrome - secondary to substance use/abuse (e.g., amphetamines, LSD, or phencyclidine) may have identical symptoms
• Mood disorders - especially bipolar disorder (manic depressive disorder); schizoaffective disorder

LABORATORY
• No test available to indicate schizophrenia
• Laboratory tests needed to rule out organicity - may include CBC, blood chemistries, thyroid screen, urinalysis, vitamins (B12, folate, thiamine), blood and urine for drugs and alcohol
• Others for: heavy metals - ceruloplasmin, urine porphobilinogen
Drugs that may alter lab results: N/A
Disorders that may alter lab results: N/A

PATHOLOGICAL FINDINGS N/A

SPECIAL TESTS
• Psychological - Bender Gestalt, intelligence testing (WISC-R) thematic apperception test (TAT), and Rorschach
• EEG - to rule out seizure disorder, brain damage, etc.
• Glucose tolerance

IMAGING CT and MRI to rule out organicity

DIAGNOSTIC PROCEDURES Lumbar puncture

 TREATMENT

APPROPRIATE HEALTH CARE
• Usually hospitalize initially for organic workup and for treatment of psychotic symptoms
• Outpatient if not dangerous to self or others, able to cooperate with treatment, and supportive family

GENERAL MEASURES Ensure safety of patient and others - may act on delusional thinking

SURGICAL MEASURES N/A

ACTIVITY Establish safe hospital environment

DIET No special diet

PATIENT EDUCATION Education and support groups for patient and family available from National Alliance for the Mentally Ill (NAMI), 2101 Wilson Blvd., Suite 302, Arlington, VA 22201, (703)524-7600

Schizophrenia

MEDICATIONS

DRUG(S) OF CHOICE
• Benzodiazepines and/or neuroleptics
• While evaluating for organicity, may treat agitation with benzodiazepines - lorazepam (Ativan) 1, 2 or 4 mg po or IM every 2-6 hrs up to 10 mg/day
• If violent or severely disruptive - rapid neuroleptization - haloperidol 5 mg IM every 4-8 hrs up to 30 mg/day or chlorpromazine 10-25 mg IM test dose (check for hypotension in one hour) then 25 mg IM every 4 hr up to 150 mg day for low dose
• After stable - change to oral medicines and titrate dosage
• After 6 months in remission, may withdraw from neuroleptics. If relapse, reinstitute medications.
Contraindications: Refer to manufacturer's profile of each drug
Precautions:
• For acute side effects of neuroleptic - dystonic reaction (especially of head and neck) - diphenhydramine (Benadryl) 25-50 mg IM
• For pseudoparkinsonism reaction - trihexyphenidyl (Artane) 2 mg bid (may be increased to 15 mg/day if needed) or benztropine (Cogentin) 0.5 bid (range: 1-4 mg/day)
• Neuroleptic malignant syndrome-hyperthermia, severe extrapyramidal effect and autonomic dysfunction (hypertension, tachycardia, diaphoresis and incontinence)
Significant possible interactions: Refer to manufacturer's profile of each drug

ALTERNATIVE DRUGS
• Thioridazine (Mellaril) - only by mouth. Do not exceed 800 mg/day.
• Trifluoperazine (Stelazine) 4-30 mg/day for maintenance
• Thiothixene (Navane) 4-30 mg/day for maintenance
• Clozapine (Clozaril) 25 mg qd or bid. Increase slowly to dose of 300-400 mg given tid. Serious toxicity of agranulocytosis mandates weekly CBC; reserve for therapy resistant patients.
• Risperidone (Risperdal) - optimal dose 6 mg/day; possibly less extrapyramidal symptoms

FOLLOWUP

PATIENT MONITORING Continue neuroleptic as well as psychiatric therapies (individual, group, family), vocational rehabilitation, day hospital

PREVENTION/AVOIDANCE N/A

POSSIBLE COMPLICATIONS
• Side effects of neuroleptics especially risk of tardive dyskinesia with chronic use
• Self-inflicted trauma
• Combative behavior toward others

EXPECTED COURSE/PROGNOSIS
• Chronic course - remission and exacerbations
• Guarded prognosis, although 30% recover completely
• The negative symptoms (consisting of decreased ambition, energy and emotional responsiveness) are often most difficult to treat

MISCELLANEOUS

ASSOCIATED CONDITIONS N/A

AGE-RELATED FACTORS Onset in 30's - more paranoid type
Pediatric: Unusual before puberty
Geriatric: Those who survive enter into a chronic phase
Others: N/A

PREGNANCY Complications of being on neuroleptic medication

SYNONYMS N/A

ICD-9-CM 295 Schizophrenic disorders

SEE ALSO N/A

OTHER NOTES Schizophrenic patients occupy about half the beds in mental hospitals and 1/4 of all hospital beds

ABBREVIATIONS N/A

REFERENCES Schatzberg AF, Cole JO: Manual of Clinical Psychopharmacology. 2nd Ed. APA Press, Inc., Washington, DC, 1991
Illustrations: N/A
Internet references: http://www.5mcc.com

Author(s)
Steven L. Jaffe, MD

Schönlein-Henoch purpura

BASICS

DESCRIPTION A vasculitis of small vessels characterized by nonthrombocytopenic, usually dependent, palpable purpura, arthritis, abdominal pain and nephritis
System(s) affected: Skin/Exocrine, musculoskeletal, gastrointestinal, renal/urologic
Genetics: N/A
Incidence/Prevalence in USA: Incidence 14/100,000 in 2-14 year old age range. Seasonal variation - more common in winter.
Predominant age: Most occur between 2-8 years old, but can occur at any age
Predominant race: N/A
Predominant sex: Male > Female (2:1)

SIGNS AND SYMPTOMS
• Onset can be acute or gradual
• 50% of patients have malaise and low grade fever
• Skin lesions occur in all identified patients:
  ◊ Lesions appear on lower extremities and buttocks but may involve face, trunk and upper extremities
  ◊ Begin as small wheals or erythematous maculopapular
  ◊ Lesions blanch on pressure but later become petechial or purpuric
  ◊ Lesions appear in crops
  ◊ Angioedema of scalp, lips, eyelids, ears, dorsa of hands and feet, back, scrotum and perineum may be seen
• Two-thirds of patients experience arthritis:
  ◊ Large joints (knees and ankles) are most commonly involved
• One-half of patients experience GI symptoms:
  ◊ Colicky abdominal pain associated with vomiting is most common
  ◊ Occult or gross blood in stool
  ◊ Hematemesis
  ◊ Intussusception, obstruction or infarction rarely occurs
  ◊ Pancreatitis
• Renal involvement is less common
  ◊ Hematuria, with or without casts or proteinuria
• Other manifestations
  ◊ Seizures, neuropathies
  ◊ Hepatosplenomegaly
  ◊ Lymphadenopathy
  ◊ Cardiac involvement
  ◊ Pulmonary hemorrhage
  ◊ Rheumatoid-like nodules
• Infantile HSP
  ◊ Children < 2 years old
  ◊ Rare
  ◊ Edema and diffuse purpura of face and ears
  ◊ Fewer GI and renal symptoms

CAUSES Multiple infectious agents, drugs and toxins have been investigated, with no firm link found

RISK FACTORS N/A

DIAGNOSIS

DIFFERENTIAL DIAGNOSIS
• Hemorrhagic diathesis
• Septicemia
• Intussusception
• Acute appendicitis
• Acute glomerulonephritis
• Familial IgA nephropathy
• Polyarteritis nodosa
• Systemic lupus erythematosus
• Inflammatory bowel disease
• Subacute bacterial endocarditis
• Rocky Mountain spotted fever
• Thrombocytopenic purpura

LABORATORY
• Not diagnostic
• Sedimentation rate, white blood cell count may be elevated
• Coagulation studies, platelet count and complement determinations are normal
• Serum IgA elevated in 50%
• Urinalysis shows protein, red blood cells, white blood cells if renal involvement
Drugs that may alter lab results: N/A
Disorders that may alter lab results: N/A

PATHOLOGICAL FINDINGS
• Renal
  ◊ Focal and segmental increases in mesangial cells and matrix
  ◊ IgA deposition in glomerular basement membrane
  ◊ A minority show generalized mesangial changes
  ◊ Rarely, diffuse necrotizing glomerulonephritis with crescent formation
• Skin
  ◊ Small vessels are surrounded by an acute leukocytoclastic inflammatory reaction of neutrophils and round cells, with IgA deposition

SPECIAL TESTS N/A

IMAGING
• Abdominal x-rays may show ileus and segmental narrowing due to submucosal edema and hemorrhage
• Barium studies acutely may show large filling defects in the bowel wall, mimicking Crohn's disease or neoplasm

DIAGNOSTIC PROCEDURES
• Clinical diagnosis
• Renal biopsy rarely indicated except in cases of decreased renal function or development of nephrotic syndrome

TREATMENT

APPROPRIATE HEALTH CARE
• Outpatient
• Inpatient if hypertension, severe abdominal pain, renal insufficiency, or other major complication

GENERAL MEASURES N/A

SURGICAL MEASURES N/A

ACTIVITY No restrictions in uncomplicated cases

DIET Usually no restrictions; NPO for severe gastrointestinal disease

PATIENT EDUCATION N/A

MEDICATIONS

DRUG(S) OF CHOICE
• Anti-inflammatory agents may be used for arthritis and fever
• Corticosteroids (prednisone 1-2 mg/kg/day) for severe GI symptoms and/or painful angioedema. Corticosteroids do not alter the progression of the lesions.
Contraindications: N/A
Precautions: N/A
Significant possible interactions: N/A

ALTERNATIVE DRUGS
Azathioprine, cyclophosphamide, plasmapheresis, factor XIII have been used in severe cases

FOLLOWUP

PATIENT MONITORING
Urinalysis in follow-up, even if normal initially

PREVENTION/AVOIDANCE N/A

POSSIBLE COMPLICATIONS
• Hypertension
• Renal failure
• Intestinal hemorrhage
• Bowel obstruction or perforation
• Death very rare

EXPECTED COURSE/PROGNOSIS
• Disease may last for a few days with transient arthritis; however, in many cases, the average duration is 4-6 weeks
• Occasionally recurrent
• 25% of patients with initial renal involvement will have persistently abnormal urine sediment

MISCELLANEOUS

ASSOCIATED CONDITIONS N/A

AGE-RELATED FACTORS
Pediatric: More common in children
Geriatric: N/A
Others: N/A

PREGNANCY Rare reports only

SYNONYMS
• Henoch-Schönlein purpura
• Anaphylactoid purpura

ICD-9-CM
287.0 Allergic purpura

SEE ALSO N/A

OTHER NOTES N/A

ABBREVIATIONS
HSP = Henoch-Schönlein purpura

REFERENCES
• Amitai Y, et al: Henoch-Schonlein purpura in infants. Pediatrics 1993;92:865
• Tapson KMP: Henoch-Schonlein purpura. Amer Fam Phys 1993;47:633
• Martin SR, et al: Henoch-Schonlein syndrome. In: Oski FA, et al. Principles and Practice of Pediatrics. 2nd Ed. Philadelphia, J.B. Lippincott Co., 1994
Illustrations: N/A
Internet references: http://www.5mcc.com

Author(s)
Bernhard L. Wiedermann, MD
Elizabeth A. Frankel, MD

Scleritis

 BASICS

DESCRIPTION Scleritis is an inflammation of the scleral outer coat of the eye
System(s) affected: Nervous
Genetics: None
Incidence/Prevalence in USA: Scleritis is uncommon
Predominant age: None
Predominant sex: Male = Female

SIGNS AND SYMPTOMS
• Redness and inflammation of the sclera
• Pain ranging from mild discomfort to extreme localized tenderness

CAUSES The most common cause of scleritis is in association with collagen vascular diseases such as rheumatoid arthritis

RISK FACTORS Individuals with autoimmune disorders, and chronic rheumatoid arthritis are most at risk

 DIAGNOSIS

DIFFERENTIAL DIAGNOSIS
• Conjunctivitis
• Episcleritis
• "Pink eye"
• Iritis
• Trauma

LABORATORY
• Rheumatoid factor
• ANA, and HLA serotyping may help aid in the diagnosis
• Elevated sedimentation rate
Drugs that may alter lab results: None
Disorders that may alter lab results: None

PATHOLOGICAL FINDINGS
• Nodules can form on the sclera which demonstrate fibrinoid necrosis of the sclera
• There may or may not be adjacent inflammation
• The scleritis may be diffuse, nodular, or necrotizing
• If the posterior region of the globe is involved, adjacent swelling of orbital tissues may occur

SPECIAL TESTS N/A

IMAGING CT scan of the orbit may help differentiate the extensiveness and location of scleritis

DIAGNOSTIC PROCEDURES History and physical examination

 TREATMENT

APPROPRIATE HEALTH CARE
Outpatient

GENERAL MEASURES
• Treatment of the inflammation usually with systemic steroids is required
• All of the immunosuppressants and antimetabolites used for autoimmune and collagen vascular disorders may be of help in active scleritis

SURGICAL MEASURES N/A

ACTIVITY No restrictions

DIET No special diet

PATIENT EDUCATION N/A

MEDICATIONS

DRUG(S) OF CHOICE Prednisone is the mainstay of treatment including both topical, periocular, and systemic administration
Contraindications: None
Precautions: Scleritis can progress to ocular perforation which may be hastened with periocular steroid injection
Significant possible interactions: Refer to manufacturer's literature

ALTERNATIVE DRUGS Nonsteroidal anti-inflammatory medications

 ## FOLLOWUP

PATIENT MONITORING The patient should be followed very closely in the active stage of inflammation to assess the effectiveness of therapy

PREVENTION/AVOIDANCE None

POSSIBLE COMPLICATIONS
• Increased intraocular pressure
• Cataract and glaucoma can result as a result of treatment
• Ocular perforation can occur in severe stages

EXPECTED COURSE/PROGNOSIS
• Scleritis is indolent, chronic, and often times progressive
• Recurrent bouts of inflammation occur

 ## MISCELLANEOUS

ASSOCIATED CONDITIONS
• Sjögren's syndrome
• Pseudo tumor

AGE-RELATED FACTORS
Pediatric: N/A
Geriatric: N/A
Others: N/A

PREGNANCY N/A

SYNONYMS N/A

ICD-9-CM 379.0

SEE ALSO N/A

OTHER NOTES N/A

ABBREVIATIONS N/A

REFERENCES Merrill GM: Diseases of The Cornea. Boston, Little, Brown, 1990
Illustrations: N/A
Internet references: http://www.5mcc.com

Author(s)
Robert M. Kershner, MD, FACS

Scleroderma

BASICS

DESCRIPTION Scleroderma (systemic sclerosis [SSc]) is a chronic disease of unknown etiology, characterized by diffuse fibrosis, degenerative changes, and vascular abnormalities in the skin, articular structures and other organs (kidneys, lung, heart, gastrointestinal and skeletal muscles). The majority of manifestations have vascular features (e.g., Raynaud's phenomenon), but frank vasculitis is rarely seen. It can range from a mild disease, affecting the skin, to a systemic disease that can cause death in a few months.
Genetics: Familial clustering is rare, but has been seen
System(s) affected: Skin/Exocrine, Renal/Urologic, Cardiovascular, Gastrointestinal, Musculoskeletal, Pulmonary
Incidence/Prevalence in USA: 1/100,000
Predominant age:
• Young adult (16-40 years); middle age (40-75 years)
• Symptoms usually appear in the 3rd to 5th decade
Predominant sex: Female > Male (4:1)

SIGNS AND SYMPTOMS
• CREST syndrome (calcinosis, Raynaud's phenomenon, esophageal dysmobility, sclerodactyly, telangiectasia)
• Digital ulcerations
• Dry crackles at lung bases
• Dysphagia
• Dyspnea
• Finger tightness, swelling, thickening
• Flexion contractures
• Friction rub on tendon movement
• Hand swelling
• Hyperpigmentation, hypopigmentation
• Hypertension
• Joint stiffness
• Malapsorptive diarrhea
• Narrowed oral aperture
• Nausea and vomiting
• Peripheral neuropathy
• Polyarthralgia
• Proximal muscle weakness
• Pruritus
• Raynaud's phenomenon
• Scaling of skin
• Sclerodactyly
• Subcutaneous calcinosis
• Substernal fullness
• Telangiectasia
• Trigeminal neuropathy
• Weakness
• Weight loss
• Xerostomia

CAUSES
• Unknown
• Possible alterations in immune response
• Possibly some association with quartz mining, quarrying, vinyl chloride, hydrocarbons, toxin exposure, rape seed oil
• Treatment with bleomycin has caused a scleroderma-like syndrome

RISK FACTORS Unknown

DIAGNOSIS

DIFFERENTIAL DIAGNOSIS
• Sclerodermatomyositis
• Mixed connective tissue disease
• Toxic oil syndrome (Madrid, 1981, affecting 20,000 people)
• Eosinophilia-myalgia syndrome
• Diffuse fasciitis with eosinophilia
• Scleredema of Buschke's

LABORATORY
• Increased ESR
• Normocytic anemia
• Normochromic anemia
• Positive ANA
• Anti-centromere antibody
• Anti-Scl-70 (topoisomerase antibody)
• Positive nucleolar immunofluorescence
• Albuminuria
• Microscopic hematuria
• Eosinophilia
• Hemolysis
• Hypergammaglobulinemia
• Decreased maximum breathing capacity
• Increased residual volume
• Diffusion defect
• Positive rheumatoid factor test (33%)
Drugs that may alter lab results: N/A
Disorders that may alter lab results: N/A

PATHOLOGICAL FINDINGS
• Skin - edema
• Lymphocytic infiltrate around sweat glands
• Loss of capillaries
• Endothelial proliferation
• Hair follicle atrophy
• Subcutaneous tissue replaced by thick collagen bundles
• Synovium - pannus formation, fibrin deposits in tendons
• Kidney - small kidneys, intimal proliferation in interlobular arteries
• Heart - endocardial thickening, myocardial interstitial fibrosis
• Enlarged heart
• Cardiac hypertrophy
• Lung - interstitial pneumonitis, cyst formation
• Interstitial fibrosis
• Bronchiectasis
• Esophagus - esophageal atrophy, fibrosis

SPECIAL TESTS
• ECG - low voltage; possibly nonspecific abnormalities
• Lung function tests - decreased diffusion and vital capacity
• Skin biopsy - marked thickening of the dermis, occlusive vessel changes
• Nail fold capillary loop abnormalities

IMAGING
• Hand x-ray - absorption of tufts from terminal phalanges, soft tissue atrophy, subcutaneous calcinosis
• Upper GI - distal esophageal dilatation, atonic esophagus
• Barium enema - colonic diverticula, megacolon
• Chest x-ray - diffuse reticular pattern, bilateral basilar pulmonary fibrosis
• Gallium-67 lung scan - can be positive in early interstitial disease

DIAGNOSTIC PROCEDURES N/A

TREATMENT

APPROPRIATE HEALTH CARE
Outpatient. Inpatient possibly for some surgical procedures.

GENERAL MEASURES
• Treatment is symptomatic and supportive
• Esophageal dilatation
• Avoid cold, dress appropriately for the weather
• Avoid smoking (crucial)
• For chronic digital ulcerations - débridement after soaking in half-strength hydrogen peroxide solution, digital plaster to immobilize
• Physical therapy to maintain function and promote strength
• Avoid finger sticks (e.g., blood tests)
• Be wary of air conditioning
• Heat therapy to relieve joint stiffness
• Elevation of the head of the bed during sleep may help relieve gastrointestinal symptoms
• Skin - use softening lotions, ointments, bath oils to help prevent dryness and cracking
• Dialysis may be necessary as disease progresses

SURGICAL MEASURES Some success with gastroplasty for correction of gastroesophageal reflux

ACTIVITY Stay as active as possible, but avoid fatigue

DIET
• Soft, bland diet with frequent small meals
• Drink plenty of fluids with meals

PATIENT EDUCATION
• Printed patient information available from: Scleroderma Federation, 1725 York Avenue, No. 29F, New York, NY 10128, (212)427-7040
• Advise patient to report any abnormal bruising or non-healing abrasions
• Assist patient in smoking cessation, if needed

Scleroderma

MEDICATIONS

DRUG(S) OF CHOICE
• There are no drug therapies of proven value, except for ACE inhibitors for hypertensive renal crisis
• Corticosteroids - for disabling myositis, pulmonary disease or mixed connective tissue disease
• NSAID's - for joint or tendon symptoms
• Antibiotics - for secondary infections in bowel
• Antacids or cimetidine - for gastric reflux
• Dipyridamole (Persantine) or aspirin - antiplatelet therapy
• Hydrophilic skin ointments - skin therapy
• Topical clindamycin or erythromycin or silver sulfadiazine (Silvadene) cream - may prevent recurrent infectious cutaneous ulcers; use systemic antibiotic therapy for active infections
• Consider immunosuppressives - used alone or with plasmapheresis for treatment of life-threatening or potentially crippling scleroderma
• Vasoactive agents and antihypertensives - for Raynaud's phenomenon
• Penicillamine (d-penicillamine) - reduce skin thickening and delay the rate of new visceral involvement
• Angiotensin-converting enzyme (captopril) - for kidney disease
Contraindications: Refer to manufacturer's literature
Precautions: Refer to manufacturer's literature
Significant possible interactions: Refer to manufacturer's literature

ALTERNATIVE DRUGS
Many other drugs are currently under investigation, but no evidence of real benefits as yet

FOLLOWUP

PATIENT MONITORING
Frequent to monitor medications and offer encouragement

PREVENTION/AVOIDANCE
None

POSSIBLE COMPLICATIONS
• Renal failure
• Respiratory failure
• Flexion contractures
• Disability
• Esophageal dysmotility
• Reflux esophagitis
• Arrhythmia
• Megacolon
• Pneumatosis intestinalis
• Obstructive bowel
• Death

EXPECTED COURSE/PROGNOSIS
• Variable
• Possible improvement, but incurable
• Prognosis is poor if cardiac, pulmonary or renal manifestations present early

MISCELLANEOUS

ASSOCIATED CONDITIONS
• Rheumatoid arthritis
• Systemic lupus erythematosus
• Polymyositis

AGE-RELATED FACTORS
Pediatric: Rare in this age group
Geriatric: Not rare until after age 75
Others: N/A

PREGNANCY
N/A

SYNONYMS
• Progressive systemic sclerosis
• Morphea
• PSS

ICD-9-CM
710.1 Systemic sclerosis

SEE ALSO
N/A

OTHER NOTES
N/A

ABBREVIATIONS
N/A

REFERENCES
• Kelley WN, Harris ED, Ruddy S, Sledge CB, eds: Textbook of Rheumatology. 5th Ed. Philadelphia, W.B. Saunders, 1997
• Koopman WJ, eds: Arthritis and Allied Disorders. 13th Ed. Philadelphia, Lea & Febiger, 1997
• Kippel JH, Dippe PR, eds: Rheumatology, St. Louis, Mosby, 1994
Illustrations: 9 available on CD-ROM
Internet references: http://www.5mcc.com

Author(s)
John T. Boyer, MD

Seizure disorders

BASICS

DESCRIPTION A sudden alteration of behavior, characterized by a sensory perception or motor activity without or with change in awareness or consciousness, due to aberrant cortical electrical activity
• Classification of seizures
  ◊ I. Partial seizures (seizures begin locally) - (A) without impairment of consciousness, (B) with complex symptoms (with impairment of consciousness)
  ◊ II. Generalized seizures (bilaterally symmetrical and without local onset)
  ◊ III. Unclassified epileptic seizures
System(s) affected: Nervous
Genetics: Three times the prevalence of seizures in close relatives of seizure patients
Incidence/Prevalence in USA:
• 1.5 million for epilepsy
• Annual incidence is 1.2/1000 for all types of seizures and 0.54/1000 for recurrent seizures
• The age adjusted prevalence is 0.625% or 6.25/1000; isolated seizures may occur in 10% of the general population
• 10-20% of all patients have intractable epilepsy
Predominant age: All ages
Predominant sex: Male = Female

SIGNS AND SYMPTOMS
• General
  ◊ Fever - indicative of infectious etiology
  ◊ Focal neurologic finding - may indicate tumor or localized injury to the brain
  ◊ Papilledema - suggestive of increased intracranial pressure
  ◊ Hemorrhagic eye grounds - suggests underlying hypertension
  ◊ Meningismus - may be present with meningitis
  ◊ Headache - sometimes associated with infectious or hemorrhagic causes of seizures
• Generalized seizures
  ◊ Absence - loss of consciousness or posture
  ◊ Myoclonic - repetitive muscle contractions
  ◊ Tonic-clonic - sustained contraction followed by rhythmic contractions of all four extremities
• Partial seizures
  ◊ Simple - Focal seizures without alteration of awareness/consciousness
  ◊ Complex - Focal seizures with alteration of awareness/consciousness
• Febrile seizures (see separate chapter on febrile seizures)
  ◊ Occurs between three months and five years of age
  ◊ Fever without evidence of any other defined cause for seizures
  ◊ If febrile seizures occur in the first year, the recurrence rate is 51%
  ◊ If febrile seizures occur in the 2nd year, the recurrence rate is 25%.
  ◊ 88% of all recurrences of febrile seizures occur in the first 2 years
  ◊ The earlier the age of onset, the more likely repetitive febrile seizures will occur

  ◊ Recurrent febrile seizures probably do not increase the risk of epilepsy
• Status epilepticus (see separate chapter)
  ◊ Repetitive generalized seizures without return to consciousness between seizures
  ◊ Considered a neurological emergency

CAUSES
• Brain tumor
• Cerebral hypoxia (breath holding, carbon monoxide poisoning, anesthesia)
• Cerebrovascular accident (infarct or hemorrhage)
• Convulsive or toxic agents (lead, alcohol, picrotoxin, strychnine)
• Eclampsia
• Exogenous factors (sound, light, cutaneous stimulation)
• Fever (see chapter on febrile seizures)
• Head injury
• Heat stroke
• Infection
• Metabolic disturbances
• Withdrawal from, or hereditary intolerance of, alcohol

RISK FACTORS
• Susceptibility to seizures determined by a complex interplay between genetic factors and acquired brain disorders
• Children delivered breech have a prevalence rate of 3.8% compared with 2.2% in children delivered vertex

DIAGNOSIS

DIFFERENTIAL DIAGNOSIS
• Infancy (0-2)
  ◊ Perinatal hypoxia
  ◊ Birth injury
  ◊ Metabolic - hypoglycemia, hypocalcemia, hypomagnesemia, vitamin B6 deficiency, phenylketonuria
  ◊ Acute infection
• Childhood (2-10)
  ◊ Febrile seizure
  ◊ Idiopathic
  ◊ Acute infection
  ◊ Trauma
• Adolescent (10-18)
  ◊ Idiopathic
  ◊ Trauma
  ◊ Drug and alcohol withdrawal
  ◊ Arteriovenous malformations
• Early adulthood (18-25)
  ◊ Idiopathic
  ◊ Drug and alcohol withdrawal
  ◊ Trauma
• Middle age (25-60)
  ◊ Drug and alcohol withdrawal
  ◊ Trauma
  ◊ Tumor
  ◊ Vascular disease
• Late adulthood (over 60)
  ◊ Vascular disease
  ◊ Tumor
  ◊ Degenerative disease
  ◊ Metabolic - hypoglycemia, uremia, hepatic failure, electrolyte abnormality

LABORATORY
• Serum tests - glucose, sodium, potassium, calcium, phosphorus, magnesium, BUN, ammonia
• Anticonvulsant levels - inadequate level of anticonvulsant medication is the most common cause of recurrent seizures in children, and many adults
• Drug and toxic screens - include alcohol
• Complete blood count - helpful in evaluating infection
Drugs that may alter lab results:
• Anticonvulsant therapy may dramatically affect the EEG results
• Levels of anticonvulsants may be altered by a variety of common medications such as erythromycin, sulfonamides, warfarin, and cimetidine, as well as alcohol
Disorders that may alter lab results:
Pregnancy decreases serum concentration. Frequent monitoring and dosage adjustments are necessary.

PATHOLOGICAL FINDINGS None

SPECIAL TESTS
• Electroencephalogram (EEG). A negative EEG does not rule out a seizure disorder. Sensitivity, specificity and predictive value of the test depends on the underlying cause and anatomic location of the seizure focus.
• 24-hour ambulatory EEG - allows for continuous monitoring of cortical activity during regular activities
• Video-monitoring - useful in conjunction with simultaneous EEG monitoring in separating true events from pseudoseizures

IMAGING
• MRI of brain - superior in evaluation of the temporal lobes
• CT scan of brain - indicated routinely in work-up of tonic-clonic seizures

DIAGNOSTIC PROCEDURES None

TREATMENT

APPROPRIATE HEALTH CARE
Outpatient therapy except for status epilepticus

GENERAL MEASURES Protect the patient's airway

SURGICAL MEASURES N/A

ACTIVITY As tolerated

DIET Regular

PATIENT EDUCATION
• Stress the importance of compliance with anticonvulsant therapy
• Printed patient information available from: Epilepsy Foundation of America, 4351 Garden City Drive, Landover, MD 20785, (800)EFA-1000

MEDICATIONS

DRUG(S) OF CHOICE
• To avoid a particular side effect, one drug may be preferred within one of the seizure groups listed below
• Generalized seizures - tonic clonic
◊ Phenytoin (Dilantin) - 200-400 mg/day in 1-3 doses; therapeutic range: 10-20 µg/mL
◊ Phenobarbital - 100-200 mg/day in 1-2 doses; therapeutic range: 10-30 µg/mL
◊ Carbamazepine (Tegretol) - 600-1200 mg/day in 2-4 doses; therapeutic range: 4-12 µg/mL
◊ Valproic acid or divalproex sodium recommended - 750-3000 mg/day in 1-3 doses (begin at 15 mg/kg/day; increase in one week by 5-10 mg/kg/day; split at 250 mg; maximum 60 mg/kg/day); therapeutic range 50-150 µg/mL
• Generalized seizures - absence
◊ Ethosuximide (Zarontin) - 250-1500 mg/day in 1-2 doses; therapeutic range: 40-100 µg/mL
◊ Valproic acid (Depakene) - dose noted above; therapeutic range: 50-100 µg/mL
◊ Clonazepam (Klonopin) - 0.01-0.3 mg/kg/day in 2-3 doses (maximum 20 mg/day); therapeutic range: 20-80 ng/mL (63-254 nmol/L)
• Partial seizures
◊ Phenytoin (Dilantin)
◊ Carbamazepine (Tegretol)
◊ Phenobarbital
Contraindications: Refer to manufacturer's profile of each drug
Precautions: Doses should be individualized according to the patient's age and weight. Refer to manufacturer's profile of each drug.
Significant possible interactions: Refer to manufacturer's profile of each drug

ALTERNATIVE DRUGS
• Felbamate (Felbatol)
• Gabapentin (Neurontin)
• Lamotrigine (Lamictal)
• Primidone (Mysoline)
• Several additional drugs awaiting FDA approval

FOLLOWUP

PATIENT MONITORING
• Regular monitoring of anticonvulsant levels
• CBC as indicated
• Monitor medication side effects and adverse reactions

PREVENTION/AVOIDANCE   Maintain adequate epileptic drug therapy. Patient education on compliance.

POSSIBLE COMPLICATIONS   Drug toxicity

EXPECTED COURSE/PROGNOSIS
• Depends on the pathophysiology of seizure within particular patient
• Seizure activity may become quiescent. If a patient has been seizure-free for two years, withdrawal of therapy may be considered. Relapse rate after three years of being off medications is 33%.

MISCELLANEOUS

ASSOCIATED CONDITIONS
• Infections
• Tumors
• Drug abuse
• Metabolic disorders

AGE-RELATED FACTORS
Pediatric: Breastfeeding is not contraindicated in mothers receiving epileptic medication, although drug concentration in the infant may require monitoring if problems such as sedation occur
Geriatric: N/A
Others: N/A

PREGNANCY   There is a two-fold increased risk of congenital malformation in mothers taking anticonvulsant medication

SYNONYMS
• Convulsions
• Epilepsy
• Fits
• Spells

ICD-9-CM   780.3 Convulsions

SEE ALSO
• Seizures, febrile
• Status epilepticus

OTHER NOTES   Jacksonian epilepsy - characterized by unilateral clonic movements that start in one group of muscles and spread systematically to adjacent groups, reflecting the march of epileptic activity through the motor cortex. Usual course - chronic; recurrent; intermittent.

ABBREVIATIONS   N/A

REFERENCES
• Beignat JL: Getting a handle on an adult's first seizure. Emergency Med 1989;20:20-28,
• Schewer ML, Pedley TA: The evaluation and treatment of seizures. New Engl J Med 1990;323(21):1468-1474
• Applegate MS, Lo W: Febrile seizures: current concepts concerning prognosis and clinical management. Journal of Fam Prac 1989;299(4):422-428
• Freeman J, Vinny E: Decision making and the child with afebrile seizure. Pediatrics in Review 1992;13(8):305-310
Illustrations: N/A
Internet references: http://www.5mcc.com

Author(s)
William L. Toffler, MD
Scott A. Fields, MD

Seizures, febrile

BASICS

DESCRIPTION Seizure occurring with fever in infancy or childhood without evidence of other underlying cause. Seizures secondary to other CNS events like meningitis, tumor, or afebrile convulsive history excluded from this topic.
• Simple febrile seizure - single episode in 24 hours, lasting less than 15 minutes and generalized tonic-clonic activity. Accounts for 85% of febrile seizures.
• Complex febrile seizure - multiple episodes in 24 hours with focalizing findings and lasting more than 15 minutes. Accounts for 15% of febrile seizures.
System(s) affected: Neurologic
Genetics: Uncertain but may be autosomal dominant with variable expression and incomplete penetrance
Incidence/Prevalence in USA:
Approximately 2500/100,000. 2-5% of all children, comprising 30% of all childhood seizures.
Predominant age: 95% occur by 5 years; peak at 2 years
Predominant sex: Male > Female (slightly)

SIGNS AND SYMPTOMS
• Fever usually 39°C (102.2°F) or greater
• Tonic-clonic convulsive activity
  ◊ Generalized with simple seizure or focal with complex event
  ◊ Usually occurs within hours of fever onset
  ◊ The seizure is the initial sign of illness in 25% of patients
  ◊ Duration is less than 15 minutes with simple seizures; longer with complex episodes
  ◊ Average frequency is once in 24 hours with simple; more with complex

CAUSES
• Fever may lower seizure threshold in susceptible children
• Temperature usually greater than 39°C (102.2°F), but rate of change may be more important than temperature
• Viral illnesses: Upper respiratory infections, roseola infantum, influenza A, gastroenteritis
• Bacterial infections: Shigella, salmonella, otitis media
• Mumps, measles, rubella immunization (MMR) within prior 7-10 days or diphtheria, pertussis, tetanus immunization (DPT) within prior 48 hours

RISK FACTORS Febrile seizure in sibling raises risk 2-3 times

DIAGNOSIS

DIFFERENTIAL DIAGNOSIS
• Febrile delirium
• Febrile shivering with pallor and peri-oral cyanosis
• Breath holding spell during fever event
• Afebrile seizure occurring during fever event
• Acute meningitis presenting with seizure
• Head injury and fever
• Drug induced seizures
• Sudden discontinuance of anticonvulsants

LABORATORY
• First episode: CBC, calcium, glucose, magnesium, electrolytes (especially sodium), urinalysis, blood culture, BUN, creatinine
• A toxologic screen may be indicated in unclear cases
• First episode or under 1 year old, consider a lumbar puncture to rule out meningitis
Drugs that may alter lab results: N/A
Disorders that may alter lab results:
Infections

PATHOLOGICAL FINDINGS N/A

SPECIAL TESTS EEG may be indicated: If recurrent frequent febrile seizures, those with focal findings, complex type, underlying neurological disorder, family history of afebrile seizures, delayed awakening after event, or if this is first event after age 3. Perform EEG 2-4 weeks after event. EEG not indicated for simple febrile seizure when there is a ready explanation for fever and recovery is quick.

IMAGING CT scan of brain for complex types, focal findings, underlying neurological disorder, or prolonged recovery phase

DIAGNOSTIC PROCEDURES Lumbar puncture

TREATMENT

APPROPRIATE HEALTH CARE
Emergency room or extended observation based on clinical situation, seizure type and whether first or subsequent event

GENERAL MEASURES
• Supportive care
• If seizure ended and simple type with recovery progressing, determine fever source so underlying cause can be treated
• Tepid sponge bath to lower temperature
• If seizure less than 10 minutes, supportive measures with laying on side, protecting from injury, maintaining airway, low flow oxygen

SURGICAL MEASURES N/A

ACTIVITY Bedrest during observation interval

DIET Nothing by mouth until status clarified

PATIENT EDUCATION
• Parents need much support
• Febrile seizures do not cause developmental delay
• Febrile seizures do not cause retardation
• Febrile seizures do not cause behavioral abnormalities
• Febrile seizures do not cause death
• Recurrence risk 33%, with 95% occurring within next 1 year

MEDICATIONS

DRUG(S) OF CHOICE
• Rectal or oral acetaminophen for fever 10-15 mg/kg/dose or ibuprofen 10 mg/kg/dose
• Anticonvulsants rarely indicated. See topic Status epilepticus for treatment of prolonged seizures.
• Oxygen
Contraindications: Allergy to drug
Precautions: Respiratory compromise needing support or intubation
Significant possible interactions: N/A

ALTERNATIVE DRUGS
• Phenobarbital 10-15 mg/kg IV, slower onset of action and may cause respiratory depression and hypotension
• Phenytoin 10-15 mg/kg IV, slower onset of action and may cause cardiac arrhythmias and hypotension
• Valproic acid 40-60 mg/kg in equal parts water - 5 cm rectally is longer acting but may cause hepatotoxicity in under 2 year age group, slower onset of action
• Paraldehyde - 0.2 ml/kg up to 2 ml at one site IM, but slower onset of action, or paraldehyde in rectal dosage form - 0.3 cc (300 mg)/kg/dose in 1:1 dilution with cottonseed oil or olive oil (maximum dose 5 mL)

 FOLLOWUP

PATIENT MONITORING
Based on the site, severity, and origin of the fever.

PREVENTION/AVOIDANCE
• Acetaminophen 10 mg/kg orally or rectally or ibuprofen 10 mg/kg - temperature greater than 38°C (100.5°F) rectal
• May use intermittent prophylactic rectal diazepam for fever greater than 38.5°C (101.3°F); 5 mg if under 3 years or 7.5 mg 3 to 6 years or 0.5 mg/kg (up to 15 mg), repeated every 12 hours for 4 doses total
• Continuous prophylaxis is controversial; may consider for high risk child with strong family history, multiple recurrences, complex events, or underlying neurological abnormalities until 1 year after last seizure. Phenobarbital 3-5 mg/kg/day may be used but often causes behavioral problems; valproic acid 30-40 mg/kg/day may be tried but may cause severe hepatotoxicity

POSSIBLE COMPLICATIONS
• Febrile seizures do not cause death, retardation, behavioral problems nor developmental delays
• Children with febrile seizures are at greater than average risk to develop epilepsy later in life

EXPECTED COURSE/PROGNOSIS
• 33% develop recurrent febrile seizures, 50% if first episode before 12 months, 45% if two involved siblings
• 95% of recurrences occur within 1 year
• Epilepsy occurs in 0.5% of general population but 3-4% of population with prior febrile seizure
• Risks for epilepsy include: Complex initial event with risk climbing with each complex feature independently, age at first episode under 6 months, three or more recurrences, pre-seizure neurological abnormalities, and family history of epilepsy

MISCELLANEOUS

ASSOCIATED CONDITIONS
• Examine child for port wine stain over trigeminal nerve with Sturge-Weber syndrome, adenoma sebaceum and hypopigmented skin of tuberous sclerosis, and café-au-lait spots and subcutaneous nodules of neurofibromatosis
• 13-18% of meningitis cases present with seizures

AGE-RELATED FACTORS
Pediatric: Range 3 months to 5 years with 95% by age 5 and peak incidence at age 2 years
Geriatric: N/A
Others: N/A

PREGNANCY N/A

SYNONYMS
• Febrile convulsions
• Febrile fits

ICD-9-CM 780.3 Convulsions: febrile

SEE ALSO
• Seizure disorders
• Status epilepticus

OTHER NOTES
• Intermittent phenobarbital prophylaxis not recommended
• Phenytoin and carbamazepine are ineffective for prophylaxis
• No evidence that preventing recurrent febrile seizures prevents epilepsy
• Critical to distinguish between simple and complex events
• Post-ictal sleepiness is common; if marked may indicate underlying pathology

ABBREVIATIONS N/A

REFERENCES
• Leung AKC: Febrile Convulsions: How dangerous are they? Postgraduate Medicine 1991;89(5):217-224
• Applegate MS, Lo W: Febrile Seizures: Current Concepts Concerning Prognosis and Clinical Management. Journal of Family Practice 1989;29(4):422-428
• Sexton ME: Childhood Seizures. AAFP Home Study Audio Series, Sept. 1991
Illustrations: N/A
Internet references: http://www.5mcc.com

Author(s)
Mark E. Sexton, MD

Sepsis

BASICS

DESCRIPTION The systemic response to infection; it encompasses a broad array of clinical manifestations and overlaps with inflammatory reactions to other clinical insults (e.g., severe trauma or burn)
• Bacteremia: Bacteria in the blood; may have no accompanying symptoms
• Systemic inflammatory response syndrome (SIRS): inflammatory reaction to different clinical insults manifest by two of the following: (1) temperature >38°C or < 36°C, (2) heart rate > 90/min; (3) respiratory rate >20/min or PaCO2 < 32 mm Hg, and (4) WBC count > 12,000/mm3, < 4,000/mm3 or > 10% immature forms (bends)
• Sepsis: SIRS with documented infection (typically bacterial)
• Septic shock: Sepsis induced hypotension (systolic BP < 90 mmHg or ≥ 40 mmHg drop from baseline) despite adequate fluid resuscitation plus hypoperfusion abnormalities (oliguria, lactic acidosis, acute change in mental status)
• Multiple organ dysfunction syndrome (MODS): altered organ function in an acutely ill patient - requires intervention to maintain homeostasis
System(s) affected: Cardiovascular, Endocrine/Metabolic, Hemic, Renal, Neurologic, Pulmonary, Gastrointestinal
Genetics: N/A
Incidence/Prevalence in USA: 176/100,000 persons/year
Predominant age: All ages
Predominant sex: Male = Female

SIGNS AND SYMPTOMS
• Fever
• Chills, rigors
• Myalgias
• Changes in mental status - restlessness, agitation, confusion, delirium, lethargy, stupor, coma
• Tachycardia
• Tachypnea
• Hypotension
• Skin lesions - erythema, petechiae, ecthyma gangrenosum, embolic lesions
• Signs and symptoms related to site of primary infection:
  ◊ Respiratory tract - cough, sputum production, dyspnea, chest pain
  ◊ Urinary tract - dysuria, flank pain, frequency, urgency
  ◊ Intra-abdominal source - nausea, vomiting, diarrhea, constipation, abdominal pain
  ◊ Central nervous system - stiff neck, headache, photophobia, focal neurologic signs
• Signs and symptoms related to end organ failure:
  ◊ Pulmonary - cyanosis
  ◊ Renal - oliguria, anuria
  ◊ Hepatic - jaundice
  ◊ Cardiac - congestive heart failure

CAUSES
• Specific etiologic agents include:
  ◊ Gram positive organisms - most commonly Staphylococcus sp, Streptococcus sp, Enterococcus sp
  ◊ Gram negative organisms - most commonly Escherichia coli, Klebsiella sp, Proteus sp, Pseudomonas sp
  ◊ Fungi - most commonly Candida sp
  ◊ Other agents - anaerobes. Also, see Differential diagnosis.
• Common sources of septicemia include:
  ◊ Lungs
  ◊ Urinary tract
  ◊ Intra-abdominal focus - biliary tree, abscess, peritonitis
  ◊ Intravascular catheters
  ◊ Skin - cellulitis, decubitus ulcer, gangrene
  ◊ Heart valves

RISK FACTORS
• Age extremes (very old and very young)
• Impaired host (see associated conditions)
• Indwelling catheters - intravascular, urinary, biliary, etc.
• Complicated labor and delivery - premature and/or prolonged rupture of membranes, etc.
• Certain surgical procedures

DIAGNOSIS

DIFFERENTIAL DIAGNOSIS
• Viral diseases (influenza, dengue and other hemorrhagic viruses, Coxsackie B virus)
• Rickettsial diseases (Rocky Mountain spotted fever, endemic typhus)
• Spirochetal diseases (leptospirosis, relapsing fever [Borrelia sp], Jarisch-Herxheimer reaction in syphilis)
• Protozoal diseases (Toxoplasma gondii, Trypanosoma cruzi, Pneumocystis carinii, Plasmodium falciparum)
• Collagen vascular diseases, vasculitides, myocardial infarction, pulmonary embolus, thrombotic thrombocytopenic purpura/hemolytic-uremic syndrome, thyrotoxicosis, adrenal insufficiency (Addison's disease), dissecting aortic aneurysm, multiple trauma, third-degree burn

LABORATORY
• Positive blood cultures
• Positive cultures from other sites (sputum, urine, cerebrospinal fluid [CSF], etc.)
• Gram stain of clinical specimens (sputum, urine, CSF, etc.)
• Common:
  ◊ Leukocytosis
  ◊ Proteinuria
  ◊ Hypoxemia
  ◊ Eosinopenia
  ◊ Hypoferremia
  ◊ Hyperglycemia
  ◊ Hypocalcemia
  ◊ Mild hyperbilirubinemia
• Less common:
  ◊ Lactic acidosis
  ◊ Leukopenia
  ◊ Azotemia
  ◊ Thrombocytopenia

◊ Prolonged prothrombin time
◊ Anemia
◊ Hypoglycemia
Drugs that may alter lab results: Prior antibiotic use
Disorders that may alter lab results: N/A

PATHOLOGICAL FINDINGS
• Inflammation at primary site of infection
• Disseminated intravascular coagulation
• Noncardiogenic pulmonary edema

SPECIAL TESTS
• Antigen detection systems - counterimmune electrophoresis (CIE) and latex agglutination tests (pneumococcus, H. influenzae type B, group B streptococcus, meningococcus)
• Gram stain of buffy coat smears occasionally useful

IMAGING
• X-rays (e.g., chest)
• Ultrasound, CT scan, or MRI may be useful in delineating sites of infection

DIAGNOSTIC PROCEDURES
• Aspiration of potentially infected body fluids (pleural, peritoneal, CSF) when appropriate
• Biopsy, drainage of potentially infected tissues (abscess, biliary tree, etc.) when appropriate

TREATMENT

APPROPRIATE HEALTH CARE
• Hospitalization
• Intensive care treatment of patients with shock, respiratory failure

GENERAL MEASURES
• Removal or drainage of septic foci
• Correction of metabolic abnormalities (hypoxemia, hyperglycemia, hypoglycemia, severe acidemia [pH < 7.10])
• Mechanical ventilation for respiratory failure
• Transfusion of RBC, platelets, and/or fresh frozen plasma for bleeding
• Volume replacement followed by pressors for hypotension

SURGICAL MEASURES Drainage of infected sites, débridement of necrotic tissues

ACTIVITY Bedrest

DIET NPO initially; intravenous hyperalimentation appropriate in some severely malnourished patients and in patients who will be unable to receive enteral alimentation within the week

PATIENT EDUCATION N/A

MEDICATIONS

DRUG(S) OF CHOICE
• Antibiotic coverage should be broad initially and directed against organisms associated with identified septic foci. After culture results are available, treatment should be more organism-specific. Knowledge of the antibiotic susceptibility patterns of local pathogens extremely important.
• Neonatal (< 7 days old) sepsis - ampicillin 300 mg/kg/d in 3 divided doses and gentamicin (Garamycin) 5 mg/kg/d in 2 divided doses
• Non-immunocompromised child - cefotaxime (Claforan) 200 mg/kg/d in 4 divided doses
• Non-immunocompromised adult - cefotaxime (Claforan) 1-2 gm q8-12 or ticarcillin-clavulanate (Timentin) 3.1 g q6h plus gentamicin 5 mg/kg/day in 1-3 divided doses
• Neutropenic host - vancomycin (Vancocin) 1 gm q 12h, ceftazidime (Fortaz) 1-2 gm q8-12h, and gentamicin (Garamycin) or tobramycin 3-5 mg/kg/d in 2-3 divided doses
Contraindications: History of anaphylaxis or other allergic reaction to the antibiotic
Precautions: Dose adjustments required in renal failure
Significant possible interactions:
• Aminoglycosides - increased nephrotoxicity with enflurane, cisplatin and possibly vancomycin; increased ototoxicity with loop diuretics; increased paralysis with neuromuscular blocking agents
• Ampicillin - increased frequency of rash with allopurinol

ALTERNATIVE DRUGS
• Many other drug combinations are possible to get adequate coverage
• Antifungals
• Antimicrobials for anaerobic infections
• Antipseudomonals

FOLLOWUP

PATIENT MONITORING
• Depends upon source of infection, underlying disease(s)
• Peak and trough drug levels for aminoglycosides, vancomycin
• BUN, creatinine, electrolytes and complete blood counts at least twice weekly; more frequently if unstable

PREVENTION/AVOIDANCE
• Vaccination - pneumococcal (geriatric patients, patients with certain chronic diseases), Hemophilus influenzae type B (infants, young children)
• Gamma globulin (for hypo- or agammaglobulinemic patients)
• Hand washing by hospital personnel, appropriate catheter care, etc., for hospitalized patients

POSSIBLE COMPLICATIONS
• Death
• Adult respiratory distress syndrome (ARDS)
• Multi-organ failure (cardiac, pulmonary, renal, hepatic)
• Disseminated intravascular coagulation (DIC)
• Gastrointestinal hemorrhage

EXPECTED COURSE/PROGNOSIS Even with optimal care, mortality will be 10-50% overall; this is increased in patients with neutropenia, diabetes, alcoholism, renal failure, respiratory failure, hypogammaglobulinemia, certain etiologic agents (e.g., Pseudomonas aeruginosa), a delay in appropriate antimicrobial therapy, and those patients at the age extremes

MISCELLANEOUS

ASSOCIATED CONDITIONS
• Neutropenia
• Diabetes mellitus
• Alcoholism
• Leukemia, lymphoma, and solid tumors
• Cirrhosis
• Burns
• Multiple trauma
• Intravenous drug abuse
• Malnutrition
• Complement deficiencies
• Hypo- or agammaglobulinemia
• Splenectomy
• HIV infection

AGE-RELATED FACTORS
Pediatric: Screen newborns for infection due to prolonged rupture of membranes (> 24 h), maternal fever, prematurity
Geriatric:
• Often more difficult to diagnose clinically in the elderly
• Change in mental status/behavior may be only early manifestation
Others: N/A

PREGNANCY Beta lactam antibiotics, aminoglycosides, erythromycin are considered safe

SYNONYMS
• Septicemia
• Sepsis neonatorum

ICD-9-CM 038 Septicemia

SEE ALSO
• Pneumonia, bacterial
• Pyelonephritis
• Meningitis, bacterial
• Endocarditis, infective (part 1)
• Toxic shock syndrome
• Rocky Mountain spotted fever
• Candidiasis
• Listeriosis
• Tularemia

OTHER NOTES High dose steroids of no benefit

ABBREVIATIONS N/A

REFERENCES
• Bone RC, et al: Definitions for sepsis and organ failure and guidelines for the use of innovative therapies in sepsis. Chest 1992;101:1644-1655
• Harris RL, et al: Manifestations of sepsis. Arch Intern Med 1987;147:1895-1906
• Center for Disease Control: Increase in National Hospital Discharge Rates for Septicemia-United States. 1979-1987. MMWR 39:31-34, 1990
Illustrations: N/A
Internet references: http://www.5mcc.com

Author(s)
Robert L. Atmar, MD

Serum sickness

BASICS

DESCRIPTION   Allergic reaction to foreign serum or drugs, usually appearing 5-14 days after administration of the allergen. Characterized by fever, arthralgias, skin rash and lymphadenopathy.
System(s) affected: Musculoskeletal, Gastrointestinal, Skin/Exocrine, Hemic/Lymphatic/Immunologic, Cardiovascular
Genetics: N/A
Incidence/Prevalence in USA: Common
Predominant age: All ages
Predominant sex: Male = Female

SIGNS AND SYMPTOMS
• History of antibiotic therapy (especially penicillin and related drugs)
• History of injection of horse serum or other species serum
• Fever
• Arthralgias (particularly TM joint)
• Malaise
• Pruritus
• Nausea
• Vomiting
• Abdominal pain
• Splenomegaly
• Myalgias
• Extremity weakness
• Sneezing
• Coughing
• Dyspnea
• Melena
• Cutaneous eruptions
• Facial swelling
• Lymphadenopathy
• Urticaria
• Joint effusion
• Myocarditis (rare)

CAUSES
• IgG antibodies that form soluble complexes with the antigen to cause an immune complex (type III) reaction
• Drugs (penicillin, cephalosporins, sulfonamides, thiouracils, iodinated dyes, streptomycin)
• Tetanus toxoid
• Rabies antiserum
• Release of vasoactive substance
• Rabbit antiserum
• Crotalidae antivenin

RISK FACTORS   Previous exposure to injection of foreign protein (reaction usually occurs sooner than the expected 5-14 days)

DIAGNOSIS

DIFFERENTIAL DIAGNOSIS
• Periarteritis nodosa
• Anaphylaxis
• Drug hypersensitivity

LABORATORY
• Proteinuria
• Decreased C3
• Decreased C4
• Increased ESR
• Mixed IgG-IgM cryoprecipitates
Drugs that may alter lab results: N/A
Disorders that may alter lab results: N/A

PATHOLOGICAL FINDINGS   Nodular lesions in segments of arteries resembling periarteritis nodosa

SPECIAL TESTS   Test all persons prior to administering a foreign serum (see Prevention/avoidance)

IMAGING   N/A

DIAGNOSTIC PROCEDURES   N/A

TREATMENT

APPROPRIATE HEALTH CARE   Inpatient, if severe; outpatient for mild cases

GENERAL MEASURES   Treat symptomatically. Usually self-limited.

SURGICAL MEASURES   N/A

ACTIVITY   Bed rest during acute illness

DIET   No special diet

PATIENT EDUCATION   N/A

Serum sickness

MEDICATIONS

DRUG(S) OF CHOICE
• Antihistamine of choice for urticaria and generalized pruritus
• Aspirin 0.6-1.5 grams orally q 4h
Contraindications: Refer to manufacturer's literature
Precautions: Refer to manufacturer's literature
Significant possible interactions: Refer to manufacturer's literature

ALTERNATIVE DRUGS
Prednisone - 40 mg/day orally if simpler medicines do not bring symptomatic relief. Prednisone also used if peripheral neuritis or myocarditis (rare) develops.

FOLLOWUP

PATIENT MONITORING
During acute illness, monitor closely for signs of myocarditis or peripheral neuritis

PREVENTION/AVOIDANCE
• Special caution in patients who need foreign serum if they have history of asthma, hay fever, urticaria or other allergic symptoms
• Testing in patients with no previous exposure or allergic history: Before administering a foreign protein - prick test with 1:10 dilution. If this is negative, 0.02 mL of 1:10 dilution given intracutaneously.
• Testing in patients with previous exposure or allergic history: Test first with 1:1000 dilution
• If skin test is positive and serum treatment is essential, then desensitization is necessary

POSSIBLE COMPLICATIONS
• Vasculitis
• Neuropathy
• Glomerulonephritis (rare)
• Anaphylaxis
• Shock
• Death

EXPECTED COURSE/PROGNOSIS
Favorable; self-limiting with 2-3 weeks for recovery

MISCELLANEOUS

ASSOCIATED CONDITIONS
Drug hypersensitivity

AGE-RELATED FACTORS
Pediatric: N/A
Geriatric: N/A
Others: N/A

PREGNANCY
N/A

SYNONYMS
• Inoculation reaction
• Protein sickness

ICD-9-CM
999.5 Other serum reaction

SEE ALSO
N/A

OTHER NOTES
Horse antiserum still used in treatment of botulism, diphtheria, venomous snake bites, spider bites. Antilymphocyte or antilymphocyte serum is used to suppress immune reactions to transplanted organs.

ABBREVIATIONS
N/A

REFERENCES
• Isselbacker KJ, et al, eds: Harrison's Principles of Internal Medicine. 13th Ed. New York, McGraw-Hill Inc., 1994
• Virella G: Hypersensitivity reactions. Immunology Series 1993;58:329
Illustrations: N/A
Internet references: http://www.5mcc.com

Author(s)
Brian J. Murray, MD

Sexual dysfunction in women

BASICS

DESCRIPTION Difficulty getting or staying sexually aroused, reaching orgasm too quickly, difficulty or inability to reach orgasm, inability to relax, lack of interest in sex, distaste or revulsion with sex, too little foreplay, too little tenderness after intercourse.
• Most women who have orgasms do not do so invariably during intercourse, and some mistakenly think this is dysfunction
• Four major types:
 ◊ Disorder of desire - both hypo- and hyper-(initiation and response), global desire disorder, couple desire discrepancy, situational desire disorder - these must be evaluated in the context of the relationship overall
 ◊ Disorder of arousal
 ◊ Dyspareunia, vaginismus
 ◊ Orgasmic disorders - primary and secondary, during masturbation or coitus, situational or partner specific
System(s) affected: Reproductive, Nervous
Genetics: N/A
Incidence/Prevalence in USA:
• 1 in 5 women is sexually dissatisfied, and two thirds of women report some degree of sexual dysfunction. Only one third of anorgasmic women in general think it is a problem.
• Overall prevalence for dysfunction is 15-30% of all women. Desire disorders are complaint of 30-55% of individual patients presenting to clinics, and 31% of couples; arousal disorders present in about 14-48% in community studies. Orgasmic disorders probably the most common; about 10% primary, and up to 65-80% secondary in community studies.
• There are many barriers to seeking help, so data for prevalence incomplete; barriers include stigma of exposing sexual inadequacy, fear of unknown therapy, e.g., of having to perform before a therapist.
Predominant age: Can occur in post-pubertal age group; women's ability to experience orgasm increases gradually from puberty; in later teens nearly half have not had orgasm; by mid-thirties, about 10% have not
Predominant sex: Female (heterosexual, homosexual, and bisexual women)

SIGNS AND SYMPTOMS
• Complaint to health care provider (if the clinician inquires, over twice as many are revealed than if clinician waits for patient to mention)
• Infertility
• Marital conflict
• Family dysfunction

CAUSES
• Interrelational difficulties and conflict regarding intimacy
• Anxiety
• Survivor of sexual abuse, including incest
• Alcohol
• Drug use, including prescription medications (e.g., MAO inhibitors, tricyclic antidepressants, beta-blockers, especially SSRI antidepressants [Prozac, Paxil, Zoloft, etc.])
• Proximity of other people in household (mother-in-law)
• Anorgasmia can be due to diabetes
• Spinal cord damage
• Hormonal imbalance?
• Thyroid disease
• Sexual frequency myths
• Control issues in the relationships
• Dyspareunia, including vaginal dryness causing interference with lubrication, secondary to infection or endocrine
• There is little endocrine data on women with sexual dysfunction

RISK FACTORS Couple discrepancies in - expectations, cultural backgrounds, attitudes toward sexuality in family of origin, previous sexual trauma, low self-esteem

DIAGNOSIS

DIFFERENTIAL DIAGNOSIS
• Medications including psychotropics (monoamine oxidase inhibitors, tricyclic and other antidepressants)
• Marital dysfunction including domestic violence
• Decreased sensation secondary to back or nerve disease
• Multiple sclerosis
• Abdominal surgery (can interfere with pelvic innervation)
• Depression
• Vaginitis
• Decreased vaginal lubrication secondary to hormonal imbalance
• Pregnancy
• Anatomic or congenital abnormalities
• Pseudodyspareunia (use of complaint of pain to distance from partner)

LABORATORY As needed to identify infections and other medical causes
Drugs that may alter lab results: N/A
Disorders that may alter lab results: N/A

PATHOLOGICAL FINDINGS Varied if any

SPECIAL TESTS May need life experiences or some other psychological inventory to evaluate couple. (Alcohol, marijuana or other illicit drug use may make these evaluations unreliable.)

IMAGING N/A

DIAGNOSTIC PROCEDURES N/A

TREATMENT

APPROPRIATE HEALTH CARE
Outpatient

GENERAL MEASURES
• For childhood trauma - scripting, psychotherapy, cognitive restructuring
• For anorgasmia - directed masturbation and "homework" with partners
• For prescription drug causes - reduced dosages, or change to different medication
• Other - family therapy, sensate conditioning; referral to specialized sex therapy

SURGICAL MEASURES N/A

ACTIVITY Varies with couple

DIET Weight reduction if needed for either partner

PATIENT EDUCATION Information about normal sexual function and human reproductive anatomy and function and changes expected with aging

MEDICATIONS

DRUG(S) OF CHOICE These are usually multifactorial psychosocial conditions. Using medications doesn't address the cause of the problem and can make it worse.
Contraindications: N/A
Precautions: N/A
Significant possible interactions: N/A

ALTERNATIVE DRUGS N/A

FOLLOWUP

PATIENT MONITORING Varies with patient

PREVENTION/AVOIDANCE Sex education starting in elementary years, early intervention in dysfunctional family or incest

POSSIBLE COMPLICATIONS Marital or family stress, breakup and divorce

EXPECTED COURSE/PROGNOSIS Lack of desire is the most difficult to treat (less than 50% successful by patient report), and success is sometimes less optimal than patient's initial wish. Best predictors are desire to change and overall healthy relationship.

MISCELLANEOUS

ASSOCIATED CONDITIONS Marital stress

AGE-RELATED FACTORS
Pediatric: N/A
Geriatric:
• Societal expectations about geriatric sexuality, (especially the myth older women aren't sexually active) can cause distress if patient has sexual desires or sexual experience
• Normal physiologic changes in aging are misinterpreted as dysfunction
Others: Sex role stereotypes

PREGNANCY Often affects but the effect varies depending on the patient and couple's beliefs about pregnancy and the problem

SYNONYMS
• Hypoactive sexual desire disorder
• Sexual aversion disorder
• Female sexual arousal disorder
• Inhibited female orgasm

ICD-9-CM
302.70 Psychosexual dysfunction, unspecified
302.72 Psychosexual dysfunction with inhibited sexual excitement
302.73 Psychosexual dysfunction with inhibited female orgasm
302.76 Psychosexual dysfunction with inhibited functional dyspareunia

SEE ALSO
• Vaginismus
• Dyspareunia

OTHER NOTES
• Women must feel safe in order to let go and lose some control to experience orgasm
• Performance anxiety makes males ejaculate prematurely, while it inhibits orgasm in women
• Simple lack of knowledge about anatomy and physiology of sex can lead to problems

ABBREVIATIONS N/A

REFERENCES
• Leiblum SR, Rosen RC: Principles and Practice of Sex Therapy: Update for the 1990's. New York, The Guilford Press, 1989
• Wincze JP, Carey MP: Sexual Dysfunction: A Guide for Assessment and Treatment. New York, The Guilford Press, 1991
• Bancroft J: Human Sexuality and Its Problems. 2nd Ed. New York, Churchill Livingstone, 1989
Illustrations: N/A
Internet references: http://www.5mcc.com

Author(s)
S. Shevaun Duiker, MD
Julie Graves Moy, MD, MPH

Shock, circulatory

 BASICS

DESCRIPTION Inadequate perfusion (oxygen supply) of tissues which results in organ dysfunction, cellular and organ damage and, if not corrected quickly, death of the patient. Classification of shock:
• Hypovolemic shock - cardiac output is severely reduced due to loss of intravascular volume which results in reduced return of venous blood to the heart. Most often caused by blood loss.
• Cardiogenic shock - cardiac output is severely reduced due to a loss of myocardial muscle function, valvular dysfunction or arrhythmia. Most often caused by large myocardial infarctions.
• Obstructive shock - cardiac output is severely reduced by vascular obstruction to venous return to the heart (vena cava syndrome), compression of the heart, (pericardial tamponade, tension pneumothorax) or outflow from the heart (aortic dissection, pulmonary embolism)
• Distributive shock - maldistribution of blood flow
• Venous pooling (most often due to spinal shock or drug overdose) behaves much like hypovolemic shock, cardiac output severely reduced because blood is pooled in peripheral veins rather than being returned to the heart
• High output or vasodilating shock (most often due to sepsis or septic like states such as toxic shock) is unique in that cardiac output is normal or elevated, but not distributed appropriately, resulting in over perfusion of some tissues and underperfusion (to the point of critical ischemia) of other tissues.
System(s) affected: Cardiovascular
Genetics: Unknown
Incidence/Prevalence in USA: N/A
Predominant age: All ages. Determined by underlying diseases causing shock. More frequent and less well tolerated in the elderly.
Predominant sex: Male = Female

SIGNS AND SYMPTOMS
• Underlying disease:
◊ Upper gastrointestinal (UGI) bleeding (ulcer pain, hematemesis, melena)
◊ Sepsis (fever, chills, dysuria and/or costovertebral angle [CVA] tenderness with urinary tract infection)
◊ Myocardial infarction (chest pain, diaphoresis, nausea, vomiting, S4 or S3 gallop, new heart murmur, rales due to pulmonary edema)
• Underperfusion of organ systems:
◊ Brain: confusion, anxiety, agitation, coma only if severe
◊ Kidney: oliguria
◊ Skin: peripheral cyanosis, sluggish capillary refill, mottling, coolness, may be overperfused (flushed) in high output (septic) shock
◊ GI: absence of bowel sounds

◊ Circulation: thready pulses, tachycardia, hypotension (mean arterial pressure < 60 torr or systolic pressure < 90 torr or blood pressure > 40 torr less than usual blood pressure in chronic hypertension), secondary cardiac ischemia (ST depression) or heart failure may occur due to underperfusion of the heart during shock. Jugular-venous distention (JVD), pulsus paradoxus in pericardial tamponade.

CAUSES
• Hypovolemic shock
◊ Blood loss due to trauma or gastrointestinal bleeding
◊ Third space loss of plasma volume (pancreatitis, bowel obstruction, infarction, anaphylaxis)
◊ Diarrhea (e.g., in cholera like states)
◊ Burns
• Cardiogenic shock
◊ Acute myocardial infarction (> 40% of LV mass)
◊ Arrhythmia (heart block, ventricular tachycardia, atrial fibrillation with rapid ventricular response, etc.)
◊ Acute valvular dysfunction (mitral valve due to papillary muscle rupture following inferior MI's or chordal rupture) aortic or mitral valve due to bacterial endocarditis
◊ Ventricular septal rupture following anterior/septal MI's
• Obstructive shock
◊ Pericardial tamponade
◊ Inferior/superior vena caval obstruction usually due to neoplasms
◊ Aortic dissection
◊ Massive pulmonary embolism
• Distributive shock
◊ Venous pooling is due to a loss of venous tone caused by loss of sympathetic nervous system activity due to acute spinal injury, general or spinal anesthesia or overdose of sedative drugs
◊ High output shock is due to sepsis, toxic shock or anaphylaxis (once plasma volume normalized)

RISK FACTORS Included with Causes

 DIAGNOSIS

DIFFERENTIAL DIAGNOSIS N/A

LABORATORY
• Specific to shock
◊ Elevated lactate (> 2 mmol/L) indicates anaerobic metabolism due to underperfusion of tissues
◊ Reduced mixed venous P02 (< 28 mm Hg) (< 3.7 kPa) obtained from the pulmonary artery indicates vigorous extraction of oxygen from tissues due to underperfusion
• Underlying diseases responsible to shock
◊ ECG, CPK (serial)
◊ Chest x-ray
◊ Arterial blood gases
◊ Gram stain and culture of infected sites
◊ Blood cultures
◊ CBC (serial determination of Hgb/Hct in bleeding patients)

Drugs that may alter lab results: N/A
Disorders that may alter lab results: N/A

PATHOLOGICAL FINDINGS N/A

SPECIAL TESTS
• Certain tests are essential to making correct and prompt diagnosis in order to dictate specific therapy of disease states producing shock. For example:
• Endoscopy/Radioisotope bleeding scans enable localization of ongoing bleeding which may direct surgical intervention. The endoscopist may intervene directly via the endoscope. (e.g., injection of sclerosants into varices or ulcers).
• Echocardiograms may detect and/or quantify pericardial effusions in shock due to pericardial tamponade. Pericardiocentesis can then be performed under echocardiographic guidance. Also useful for detection of valvular failure.
• Lung scans and/or pulmonary arteriography for the detection of massive pulmonary embolism
• Pulmonary artery (Swan-Ganz) catheterization for serial measurement of cardiac output, central venous, pulmonary arterial and pulmonary arterial occlusion pressures (left atrial pressure) and vascular resistance. Mixed venous blood gases can be drawn from the catheter. Indicated when the etiology of shock is uncertain, in cardiogenic and septic shock, or when initial therapy of shock fails to provide for rapid correction of perfusion failure.

IMAGING See Special Tests

DIAGNOSTIC PROCEDURES
See Special Tests

 TREATMENT

APPROPRIATE HEALTH CARE
• Emergency room or intensive or coronary care unit
• Continuous electrocardiographic monitoring with frequent assessment of blood pressure, respiratory status, and urine output

GENERAL MEASURES
• Therapy must proceed quickly before extensive damage to vital organs occur. Therapy is directed simultaneously to correct both the deficit in tissue perfusion and the underlying disease causing shock (see Associated conditions).
• Maintain SaO2 > 95% with supplemental oxygen. Intubate and mechanically ventilate patient if patient cannot be oxygenated with 100% oxygen or has markedly increased breathing effort (excessive oxygen cost of breathing).
• Maintain pH above 7.3 (but less than 7.5) to preserve vascular responsiveness to endogenous or exogenous catecholamines.

• Correct plasma volume deficits rapidly by volume expanders consisting of isotonic saline (.9Ns or Ringer's lactate) with or without colloid (albumin 5% or hydroxyethyl starch 6%)
• Packed red blood cell transfusion to correct or prevent anemia. HB maintained at or above 10 grams/dl.
• Administer coagulation factors (fresh frozen plasma, cryoprecipitate) and platelets if coagulopathy (prolonged PT, PTT or platelet count < 50,000) is present in a patient who is bleeding
• Tachyrrhythmias (other than sinus tachycardia) should be promptly corrected by electrocardioversion. Transvenous pacemakers should be placed to correct bradyrhythmias.
• Vasopressors (see Medications) to correct hypotension or low cardiac output due to myocardial failure or hypotension due to low vascular resistance
• End points of resuscitation: adequate blood pressure (> 60 mm Hg [8.0 kPa] mean or > 90 mm Hg [12.0 kPa] systolic or within 40 mm Hg [5.32 kPa] of patient's normal blood pressure). Patient is awake/alert, urine output adequate, heart rate < 100, warm skin with brisk capillary refill, bowel sounds present. Lactate < 2 mmol/L, mixed venous PO2 > 30 mm Hg.

SURGICAL MEASURES N/A

ACTIVITY None

DIET N/A

PATIENT EDUCATION N/A

MEDICATIONS

DRUG(S) OF CHOICE
• Dopamine, low dose, 1-4 µg/kg/min augments contractility and cardiac output (beta-1) and increases heart rate. This provides increased blood flow to kidneys and gut. Also acts directly on dopaminergic receptors in the renal vasculature to enhance renal blood flow.
• Dopamine > 4 µg/kg/min: augments contractility, and cardiac output (beta-1) and increased heart rate. Increases blood pressure by a combination of increased cardiac output and vasoconstriction (alpha).
• Norepinephrine 2-12 µg/min: augments blood pressure by increased vascular resistance (alpha). Reduced blood flow to splanchnic bed can be reversed by low dose dopamine.
• Phenylephrine 20-200 µg/min: see norepinphrine
• Dobutamine 5-10 µg/kg/min augments contractility and cardiac output (beta-1). Has both vasoconstrictive (alpha) and vasodilator (beta-2) properties. These effects have a minimal effect on systemic vasculature.
Contraindications: Refer to manufacturer's profile of each drug

Precautions:
• Myocardial oxygen consumption is increased by increased heart rate, afterload, and contractility
• Pressors can increase myocardial ischemia if present
• May precipitate or worsen tachyarrhythmias
• Should be used in lowest possible dose for as limited period of time as possible
Significant possible interactions: Refer to manufacturer's profile of each drug

ALTERNATIVE DRUGS N/A

FOLLOWUP

PATIENT MONITORING Careful monitoring of all life functions in intensive care

PREVENTION/AVOIDANCE Shock is best avoided by prompt recognition and treatment of underlying diseases which cause shock (e.g., early antibiotic therapy for infections)

POSSIBLE COMPLICATIONS
• Multiple organs may be damaged by underperfusion during shock
• Acute tubular necrosis
• Ischemic hepatitis
• Ischemic bowel
• Disseminated intravascular coagulopathy
• Adult respiratory distress syndrome (ARDS)
• Encephalopathy and/or cerebrovascular accident

EXPECTED COURSE/PROGNOSIS
• Mortality is determined by a complex interaction of primary disease causing shock, age, coexisting chronic disease and shock severity as marked by the number of acute organ system failures that follow shock
• Best outcome (> 90% survival) in young patient with transient shock due to trauma or gastrointestinal blood loss without chronic irreversible illnesses
• Poor outcome (> 90% mortality) in elderly patient with septic shock, underlying chronic liver disease, who develops acute renal failure, ARDS, and coagulopathy

MISCELLANEOUS

ASSOCIATED CONDITIONS
• Gastrointestinal blood loss: may require endoscopic or surgical intervention if bleeding doesn't spontaneously cease, e.g., electrocoagulation or injecting sclerosant for bleeding peptic ulcers, sclerotherapy in esophageal varices

• Sepsis: empiric antibiotic therapy, based on the patient's underlying illnesses, age, site of infection, and hospital sensitivity patterns. After hemodynamic stabilization, surgical drainage of abscesses, if present. Antibodies directed against gram negative cell wall antigens (endotoxin) may reduce mortality in patients with gram negative bacteremia.
• Cardiogenic shock: therapy should help reduce cardiac ischemia (oxygen, nitrates) and accomplish rapid reperfusion of injured, but potentially viable, myocardium (thrombolysis with fibrinolytic agents, balloon angioplasty of stenotic vessels or surgical bypass grafting) A balloon pump may temporize by providing improved coronary blood flow during and following diagnostic testing and revascularization therapy. If shock is due to acute failure of the mitral or aortic valve, surgical valve replacement may be lifesaving.
• Pulmonary embolism: reduction in the obstruction to pulmonary outflow is accomplished by infusion of thrombolytics (streptokinase, urokinase, tissue plasminogen activator [TPA]). If fibrinolytic therapy is contraindicated (e.g., recent surgery, intracerebral lesion) then pulmonary embolectomy may be life saving although mortality may be 50% or higher.
• Pericardial tamponade: shock due to tamponade is best treated by prompt removal of pericardial fluid either by catheter or surgical drainage

AGE-RELATED FACTORS
Pediatric: N/A
Geriatric: N/A
Others: N/A

PREGNANCY N/A

SYNONYMS N/A

ICD-9-CM
785.50 Shock, unspecified
785.51 Cardiogenic shock
785.59 Other shock (endotoxic, septic, hypovolemic)

SEE ALSO
• Anaphylaxis
• Cardiac tamponade
• Myocardial infarction
• Pulmonary embolism
• Peptic ulcer with hemorrhage

OTHER NOTES N/A

ABBREVIATIONS N/A

REFERENCES
• Parillo JE: Shock. In: Braunwald E, et al. Harrison's Principles of Internal Medicine. 12th Ed. New York, McGraw-Hill, Inc, 1991
• Schuster DP, Lefrah SS: Shock. In: Civetta JF, et al. Critical Care. Philadelphia, J.B. Lippincott Corp, 1988:891-908
Illustrations: N/A
Internet references: http://www.5mcc.com

Author(s)
Sheldon M. Traeger, MD

Sialadenitis

BASICS

DESCRIPTION Inflammation of the salivary glands from nonspecific bacterial infection or inflammation most often arises in the excretory duct. The parotid is the most commonly affected gland with invasion of bacteria from the oral cavity. Inflammation may also follow trauma, spread of infection from adjoining tissues, and via hematogenous routes during bacteremia. Inflammation may lead to stone formation (sialolithiasis) or an obstructed duct may lead to inflammation of the gland. Stones are more commonly associated with the submaxillary glands. Recurrent infections or other chronic inflammatory processes can lead to decreased gland function with resulting xerostomia.
System(s) affected: Skin/Exocrine, Gastrointestinal
Genetics: Unknown
Incidence/Prevalence in USA: N/A
Predominant age: N/A
Predominant sex: N/A

SIGNS AND SYMPTOMS
• Enlarged, painful salivary gland
• Purulent discharge from duct orifice
• Red, painful duct orifice
• Fever
• Xerostomia
• Decreased salivary secretion (aptyalism)

CAUSES
• Bacteria from the oral cavity are the most common infectious cause of sialadenitis.
• The causative agents of the following diseases may also infect a salivary gland to cause sialadenitis:
  ◊ Mumps
  ◊ Actinomycosis
  ◊ Tuberculosis
  ◊ Syphilis
  ◊ CMV
  ◊ Cat-scratch disease

RISK FACTORS
• Dehydration
• Fever
• Hypercalcemia

DIAGNOSIS

DIFFERENTIAL DIAGNOSIS
Decreased salivary secretion is associated with:
• Drugs:
  ◊ Tricyclic antidepressants (amitriptyline, etc.)
  ◊ Phenothiazines (chlorpromazine, fluphenazine, thioridazine, prochlorperazine, etc.)
  ◊ Anticholinergics
• Myxedema
• Plummer-Vinson disease
• Pernicious anemia
• Febrile diseases
• Neuropsychiatric disorders
• Mikulicz's disease (benign lymphoepithelial lesion)
Enlarged glands may be the result of a variety of neoplasms including:
• Pleomorphic adenoma
• Mucoepidermoid carcinoma
• Other tumor types can also occur very rarely (lipoma, neurofibroma, fibrosarcoma, melanoma, lymphocytoma, Hodgkin's, etc.)
Also, obesity results in what appears to be enlarged parotids, but the bilateral nature and non-progressive course should help differentiate this from malignant neoplasms.

LABORATORY N/A
Drugs that may alter lab results: N/A
Disorders that may alter lab results: N/A

PATHOLOGICAL FINDINGS
With chronic infection of the gland:
• Enlarged gland
• Ductal dilatation with retention of saliva
• Acinar atrophy or dilated and filled with mucus
• Purulent/seropurulent exudate within the duct
• Glandular replacement by fibrotic tissue
• Infiltration with leukocytes

SPECIAL TESTS N/A

IMAGING Radiographs may reveal a stone in sialolithiasis

DIAGNOSTIC PROCEDURES
Digital manipulation of the duct may express pus from the ductal orifice

TREATMENT

APPROPRIATE HEALTH CARE
Outpatient

GENERAL MEASURES Heating pad and/or cool compresses may be comforting

SURGICAL MEASURES N/A

ACTIVITY Unrestricted

DIET Avoid pain-producing sialagogues (lemon, etc.) during an acute episode

PATIENT EDUCATION N/A

Sialadenitis

MEDICATIONS

DRUG(S) OF CHOICE
• Antibiotics
  ◊ Penicillin - penicillin V (Pen VK)
250-500mg QID or
  ◊ Erythromycin 250mg QID
  ◊ Amoxicillin-clavulanate (Augmentin)
  ◊ Cefuroxime (Ceftin)
• Analgesic: codeine, NSAID, etc
Contraindications: N/A
Precautions: N/A
Significant possible interactions: N/A

ALTERNATIVE DRUGS N/A

FOLLOWUP

PATIENT MONITORING N/A

PREVENTION/AVOIDANCE N/A

POSSIBLE COMPLICATIONS
Occasional loss of salivary function

EXPECTED COURSE/PROGNOSIS
Complete recovery and good prognosis

MISCELLANEOUS

ASSOCIATED CONDITIONS
• Rheumatoid arthritis (Sjögren's syndrome)
• Sarcoidosis (Herrfordt's syndrome)

AGE-RELATED FACTORS
Pediatric: Rare in children
Geriatric: N/A
Others: N/A

PREGNANCY N/A

SYNONYMS N/A

ICD-9-CM 527.2 sialadenitis

SEE ALSO N/A

OTHER NOTES N/A

ABBREVIATIONS
CMV = cytomegalovirus

REFERENCES Cotran RS, et al, eds:
Robbins Pathological Basis of Disease, 4th Ed.
Philadelphia, W.B. Saunders Co., 1989
Illustrations: N/A
Internet references: http://www.5mcc.com

Author(s)
Michael Strange, MD

Silicosis

 BASICS

DESCRIPTION
Pneumoconiosis (fibrogenic) caused by inhaling silica dust (in the form of quartz, cristobalite, or tridymite)
• Chronic (classical) silicosis can be simple or complicated
• Chronic simple silicosis (sim sil) is asymptomatic, non-progressive once exposure ends, and consists solely of small round radiographic pulmonary opacities
• Chronic complicated silicosis (comp sil) has progressively worsening symptoms and enlarging pulmonary opacities, even after exposure ends.
• Subacute silicosis (sub sil) develops after 3-6 years of high exposure, and resembles chronic complicated silicosis
• Acute silicosis (ac sil) develops within a couple years of massive exposure and is clinically distinct from the other forms

System(s) affected: Pulmonary
Genetics: No known genetic pattern
Incidence/Prevalence in USA: Unknown
Predominant age: 40-75
Predominant sex: Male > Female

SIGNS AND SYMPTOMS
• Sim sil
  ◊ Asymptomatic
  ◊ Cough and mild dyspnea typically accompany, and are due to smoking or occupational bronchitis
• Comp sil; sub sil
  ◊ Chest tightness
  ◊ Cough
  ◊ Dyspnea
  ◊ Expectoration
  ◊ Signs and symptoms of right heart failure as cor pulmonale develops
• Ac sil
  ◊ Dry cough
  ◊ Fever
  ◊ Severe dyspnea

CAUSES
• Sim sil: 10-12 years of exposure to silica dust
• Comp sil: > 20 years of exposure
• Sub sil: 3-6 years of heavy exposure
• Ac sil: < 2 years of massive exposure

RISK FACTORS
• Industrial activities that involve cutting, polishing, or shearing rock, or involve the use of sand, including:
  ◊ Metal mining (copper, silver, gold, lead, hard coal)
  ◊ Foundries
  ◊ Pottery making
  ◊ Sandstone cutting
  ◊ Granite cutting

DIAGNOSIS

DIFFERENTIAL DIAGNOSIS
• Sim sil
  ◊ Sarcoidosis
  ◊ Radiographic egg shell calcifications also seen in sarcoidosis and Hodgkin's disease
• Comp sil, sub sil
  ◊ Coal worker's pneumoconiosis
  ◊ Consider especially when consolidations are rapidly progressive, unilateral, or cavitating - tuberculosis, neoplasia, fungal pneumonia
• Ac sil
  ◊ Alveolar proteinosis

LABORATORY
• Hypoxemia
• Hypercarbia
Drugs that may alter lab results: N/A
Disorders that may alter lab results: N/A

PATHOLOGICAL FINDINGS
• Lung
  ◊ Pleural adhesions
  ◊ Pleural thickening
  ◊ Gray-black subpleural nodules
  ◊ Blackened lung
  ◊ Leathery lung
  ◊ Concentric layers of dense connective tissue
  ◊ Cellular infiltrate
  ◊ Ischemic degeneration of central nodule
  ◊ Metachromatic silica particles

SPECIAL TESTS
• Pulmonary function testing is normal in simple silicosis. Other forms show decreased pulmonary compliance, decreased lung volumes, decreased diffusing capacity.
• International Labor Office (ILO) classification system for quantification of chest radiograph abnormalities.
• Yearly PPD

IMAGING
Chest x-ray:
• Sim sil
  ◊ Egg shell calcification in hilar and mediastinal lymph nodes
  ◊ Small round opacities, initially in upper lobes
• Comp sil, sub sil
  ◊ Pulmonary opacities > 1 cm
  ◊ Opacities form bilateral conglomerate shadows (progressive massive fibrosis)
  ◊ Opacities initially peripheral, later migrate towards hilum.
  ◊ Opacities may cavitate (rule out tuberculosis!)

DIAGNOSTIC PROCEDURES
• Bronchoscopy
• Detailed occupational history
• Open lung biopsy

TREATMENT

APPROPRIATE HEALTH CARE
Prevention - respiratory protective devices for unavoidable short-term exposure

GENERAL MEASURES
• No known effective treatment
• Postural drainage
• Mist inhalation
• Chest physical therapy
• Breathing exercises
• Sequential whole lung lavage for acute silicosis

SURGICAL MEASURES
• Lung transplantation
• Whole lung lavage remains investigational

ACTIVITY
Maintain regular exercise program

DIET
• No special diet
• Increase fluid intake

PATIENT EDUCATION
Printed patient information available from: American Lung Association, 1740 Broadway, New York, NY 10019, (212)315-8700

MEDICATIONS

DRUG(S) OF CHOICE
• None specific for silicosis
• Isoniazid, 300 mg/d for one year, if tuberculin skin test is positive
• Silicotuberculosis requires at least 3 anti-tuberculous drugs initially, including rifampin
Contraindications: Avoid sedatives and hypnotics
Precautions: Refer to manufacturer's literature
Significant possible interactions: Refer to manufacturer's literature

ALTERNATIVE DRUGS
Antifibrinogenic agents remain investigational

FOLLOWUP

PATIENT MONITORING
• Monitor for heart failure and hypoxemia
• Treat intercurrent infections aggressively

PREVENTION/AVOIDANCE
Avoid dust exposure; substitute other materials for silica

POSSIBLE COMPLICATIONS
• Progressive massive fibrosis
• Respiratory infection
• Pneumothorax
• Emphysema
• Cor pulmonale
• Right heart failure
• Mycobacterial infections
• Fungal infections

EXPECTED COURSE/PROGNOSIS
• Sim sil - remains asymptomatic and does not progress if exposure ends
• Comp sil; sub sil - progressive pulmonary fibrosis with cor pulmonale and right heart failure, even after exposure ends.

MISCELLANEOUS

ASSOCIATED CONDITIONS
• Tuberculosis
• Caplan's syndrome

AGE-RELATED FACTORS
Pediatric: Unusual
Geriatric: Symptoms and complications more severe
Others: N/A

PREGNANCY N/A

SYNONYMS N/A

ICD-9-CM 502 Silicosis

SEE ALSO
• Tuberculosis
• Chronic obstructive pulmonary disease & emphysema
• Pneumothorax
• Cor pulmonale

OTHER NOTES
Silica - formula for calculating the threshold limit value (TLV) for respirable dust: TLV (threshold limit value) = (10 mg per cu meter/% SiO2) + 2

ABBREVIATIONS N/A

REFERENCES
• Silicosis and Silicate Disease Committee. Diseases associated with exposure to silica and non-fibrous silicate materials. Arch Pathol Lab Med 1988;112:673
• Banks DE, et al: Strategies for the treatment of pneumoniosis. Occ Med 1993;8(1):205-232
Illustrations: N/A
Internet references: http://www.5mcc.com

Author(s)
Robert Dolin, MD

Sinusitis

 BASICS

DESCRIPTION
Inflammation of the paranasal sinuses. Classified as acute or chronic depending on duration of infection. Occurs when an undrained collection of pus accumulates in the sinus.
System(s) affected: Pulmonary
Genetics: No known genetic pattern
Incidence/Prevalence in USA: Common
Predominant age: All ages
Predominant sex: Male = Female

SIGNS AND SYMPTOMS
• Nasal congestion (acute sinusitis)
• Gradual buildup of pressure feeling in sinus area with tenderness
• Nasal discharge - blood tinged, becoming purulent
• Malaise
• Sore throat (sometimes)
• Headache
• Fever
• Pain over cheeks and upper teeth (maxillary sinusitis) worse with bending
• Pain over eyebrows (frontal sinusitis)
• Pain over eyes (ethmoid sinusitis)
• Pain behind eyes (ethmoid)
• Cough (occasional)
• Postnasal discharge
• Periorbital edema
• Symptoms aggravated by air travel

CAUSES
• Bacterial infection (H. influenzae, pneumococci, streptococci, catarrhalis)
• Viral infections
• Fungal infections (Aspergillus, bipolaris, mucormycosis)
• Preceding upper respiratory infection
• Predisposing factors - chronic nasal edema, viscous mucous, polyps, nasal allergy, sudden temperature changes

RISK FACTORS
• Allergic diathesis
• Immunosuppression
• Continuous positive airway pressure
• Air travel during upper respiratory infection
• Tooth abscess
• Swimming in contaminated water

 DIAGNOSIS

DIFFERENTIAL DIAGNOSIS
• Viral rhinitis
• Allergic rhinitis
• Vasomotor rhinitis
• Tumors
• Cysts
• Foreign bodies
• Wegener's granulomatosis

LABORATORY
• Elevated WBC
• Culture for identification of infecting organism
Drugs that may alter lab results: N/A
Disorders that may alter lab results: N/A

PATHOLOGICAL FINDINGS
• Inflammation
• Edema
• Thickened mucosa
• Nasal polyps
• Ulcerations

SPECIAL TESTS
• Endoscopy - identify areas of persistent infection
• Maxillary sinuscopy - for biopsy and cyst removal
• Sphenoid sinuscopy - rarely needed

IMAGING
• Sinus x-rays - cloudiness, air-fluid levels, thick mucosa in affected sinuses
• CT scan - for ostiomeatal complex pathology; aids in diagnosing local underlying causes of chronic sinusitis
• MRI - not current choice for evaluation

DIAGNOSTIC PROCEDURES
Transillumination reveals opacity in affected sinus cavities

 TREATMENT

APPROPRIATE HEALTH CARE
Outpatient except for surgery (rarely indicated). Consider hospitalization for frontal or sphenoid sinusitis.

GENERAL MEASURES
• Early treatment is medical
• Steam inhalations can aid comfort and draining
• Avoid smoke and other environmental pollutants if possible
• Avoid smoking cigarettes
• If medical treatment fails, can perform irrigation to wash out the inspissated material

SURGICAL MEASURES
• Surgery for sinusitis that persists despite medical treatment
• Numerous techniques available for cleaning the different sinuses (nasal window procedure, Caldwell-Luc procedure, ethmoidectomy, external ethmoidectomy, fronto-ethmoidectomy, osteoplastic flap)

ACTIVITY
No restrictions. May need additional rest during acute phase.

DIET
No special diet. Drink plenty of fluids.

PATIENT EDUCATION
For patient education materials favorably reviewed on this topic, contact: Asthma & Allergy Foundation of America, 1717 Massachusetts Avenue, Suite 305, Washington, DC 20036, (800)7-Asthma

MEDICATIONS

DRUG(S) OF CHOICE
• Antibiotics - amoxicillin 500 mg tid for 14-21 days or trimethoprim-sulfamethoxazole. If no response, switch to antibiotics with activity against beta-lactamase producing bacteria.
• Analgesics
• Vasoconstrictors
• Antihistamines
Contraindications: Refer to manufacturer's literature
Precautions: Refer to manufacturer's literature
Significant possible interactions: Refer to manufacturer's literature

ALTERNATIVE DRUGS
Consider 3-5 days of topical decongestants at start of treatment. Chronic nasal steroid use indicated if sinusitis is secondary to allergic rhinitis.

FOLLOWUP

PATIENT MONITORING   Follow until clinically clear of disease

PREVENTION/AVOIDANCE   Treat nasal congestion prior to sinusitis

POSSIBLE COMPLICATIONS
• Meningitis
• Abscess (extradural, subdural, brain, retrobulbar)
• Osteomyelitis
• Orbital infection
• Septic cavernous thrombosis

EXPECTED COURSE/PROGNOSIS
• Acute - favorable prognosis with timely treatment and avoidance of complications
• Chronic - may improve if causative allergen is removed or drainage is feasible

MISCELLANEOUS

ASSOCIATED CONDITIONS
• Rhinitis
• Barosinusitis
• Pansinusitis

AGE-RELATED FACTORS
Pediatric:
• Incidence of both acute and chronic sinusitis increases in the latter part of childhood
• May be more prevalent in children who have had tonsils and adenoids removed
• Chronic sinusitis indicates a need to search for underlying cause, e.g., nasal deformities or infected and hypertrophied adenoids
Geriatric:
• Incidence increases up to age 75 and then decreases
• More difficult to heal when it occurs in this age group
Others: N/A

PREGNANCY   N/A

SYNONYMS   N/A

ICD-9-CM
• 461.9 Acute sinusitis, unspecified
• 473.9 Unspecified sinusitis (chronic)

SEE ALSO   N/A

OTHER NOTES   N/A

ABBREVIATIONS   N/A

REFERENCES
• Adams GL, et al: Fundamentals of Otolaryngology. 6th Ed. Philadelphia, W.B. Saunders Co., 1989
• Alberti PW, Ruben RJ, eds: Otologic Medicine and Surgery. New York, Churchill Livingstone, 1988
Illustrations: N/A
Internet references: http://www.5mcc.com

Author(s)
Michael Strange, MD

Sleep apnea, obstructive

 BASICS

DESCRIPTION
Repetitive episodes of upper airway occlusion during sleep, often with oxygen desaturation. Nearly always associated with snoring. Apneas often terminate with a snort or gasp. Repetitive apneas produce sleep disruption, leading to excessive daytime sleepiness (EDS). Usual course is chronic.

System(s) affected: Pulmonary, Nervous
Genetics: Hereditary factors unknown. Familial patterns sometimes seen.
Incidence/Prevalence in USA: 4% of middle-age and older males; 2% middle-age and older females
Predominant age: Middle-age
Predominant sex: Males > Females

SIGNS AND SYMPTOMS
• Cardinal symptom is excessive daytime sleepiness (EDS)
• Loud snoring
• Complaints of disrupted sleep
• Repetitive awakenings with transient sensation of shortness of breath or for unclear reasons
• Tired and unrefreshed upon A.M. awakening
• Witnessed apneas at night
• Complaints of poor concentration, memory problems, irritability
• Morning headaches
• Short-tempered
• Decreased libido is also common
• Depression
• Systemic and pulmonary hypertension

CAUSES
Upper airway narrowing may be due to obesity, enlarged tonsils or uvula, low soft palate, redundant tissue in soft palate or tonsillar pillars, large or posteriorly located tongue or craniofacial abnormalities. Anatomical narrowing superimposed upon a coexistent abnormality of neurological control of upper airway muscle tone or ventilatory control during sleep.

RISK FACTORS
• Obesity
• Nasal obstruction (due to polyps, rhinitis or deviated septum)
• Hypothyroidism
• Macroglossia
• Micrognathia (retrognathia)
• Acromegaly
• Persons with hypertension, cardiovascular or arteriovascular disease or alveolar hypoventilation have a much higher risk of obstructive sleep apnea (OSA)

 DIAGNOSIS

DIFFERENTIAL DIAGNOSIS
• Other causes of EDS such as narcolepsy, idiopathic daytime hypersomnolence, inadequate sleep, depressive episodes with EDS, periodic limb movements of sleep
• Respiratory disorders with nocturnal awakenings such as asthma, COPD, CHF
• Central sleep apnea may mimic OSA
• Sudden nocturnal awakenings due to panic attacks
• Sleep-related choking or laryngospasm
• Gastroesophageal reflux may also present with similar symptoms
• Sleep associated seizures (temporal lobe epilepsy)

LABORATORY
• Polycythemia (occasional) reflects the degree of nocturnal hypoxemia due to OSA
• Thyroid function should be evaluated to rule out concomitant hypothyroidism
• Daytime hypercapnia occasionally seen
Drugs that may alter lab results: Benzodiazepines or other sedatives can accentuate the severity of apnea seen on sleep study
Disorders that may alter lab results: N/A

PATHOLOGICAL FINDINGS
• Anatomically small upper airway common
• CNS abnormalities rare

SPECIAL TESTS
• Echocardiography may demonstrate right and/or left ventricular enlargement or pulmonary hypertension
• Polysomnogram (nighttime sleep study) including O2 saturation, CO2
• Multiple sleep latency testing (MSLT) provides an objective measurement of daytime sleepiness

IMAGING
• Cephalometric measurements from lateral head and neck x-rays are occasionally useful if surgery is contemplated
• MRI, CT scans or fiberoptic evaluation of upper airway occasionally helpful

DIAGNOSTIC PROCEDURES
• Nighttime sleep study (polysomnogram)
◊ Shows repetitive episodes of cessation or marked reduction in airflow despite continued respiratory efforts
◊ These apneic episodes must last at least 10 seconds and occur 10-15 times per hour to be considered clinically significant
◊ Polysomnogram demonstrates severity of hypoxemia, sleep disruption and cardiac arrhythmias associated with OSA and elevated end tidal CO2

 TREATMENT

APPROPRIATE HEALTH CARE
Outpatient for treatment or sleep study; inpatient for surgery

GENERAL MEASURES
• For patients with significant EDS and 15-20 apneas per hour or more, CPAP is probably the best treatment
• If OSA present only when supine - keep patient off the back (e.g., tennis ball sewn on nightshirt or fanny-pack with tennis balls worn at back)
• Mild to moderate OSA - surgery (tonsillectomy or uvulopalatopharyngoplasty [UPPP]), dental appliances or nasal continuous positive airway pressure (CPAP)
• Moderate to severe OSA - CPAP or BiPAP (biphasic positive airway pressure) is the standard therapy
• Avoid driving if EDS significant
• No alcohol within 6 hours of bedtime
• Avoid sedatives and sleeping pills

SURGICAL MEASURES
Severe OSA that is not controllable with nasal CPAP or UPPP - tracheostomy or craniofacial surgery (mandibular advancement)

ACTIVITY
Significantly sleepy patients should not drive motor vehicle or operate equipment with risk for injury until treated

DIET
Obese patients must lose weight. All patients must avoid weight gain and alcohol.

PATIENT EDUCATION
• Stress the fact that obesity can be the cause of OSA and weight loss may "cure" the condition
• Necessity to avoid alcohol and sedatives
• Stress the dangers of driving while suffering EDS

MEDICATIONS

DRUG(S) OF CHOICE Protriptyline 10-30 mg/d or fluoxetine 20-60 mg can occasionally be useful adjunct in the management of OSA (especially OSA in REM sleep) and to improve EDS
Contraindications: None
Precautions: May cause or exacerbate narrow angle glaucoma or urinary retention. Use with caution in patients with supraventricular tachycardia.
Significant possible interactions: See manufacturer's profile of each drug

ALTERNATIVE DRUGS
• Medroxyprogesterone is helpful in Pickwickian patients with both daytime alveolar hypoventilation and OSA
• Acetazolamide (Diamox) may increase central respiratory drive by acidifying blood/CSF. Used in central sleep apnea only.

FOLLOWUP

PATIENT MONITORING Physician followup improves compliance with CPAP therapy. Observe for return of snoring, EDS, or sleep disruption which may indicate inadequate control of apneas.

PREVENTION/AVOIDANCE See Patient Education

POSSIBLE COMPLICATIONS
• Untreated OSA can be associated with development of pulmonary hypertension, ventricular arrhythmias, cor pulmonale, CHF
• Significant morbidity and mortality due to accidents caused by EDS and inattentiveness
• Acute blood pressure elevations

EXPECTED COURSE/PROGNOSIS
• With appropriate control of apneas, EDS dramatically improves quickly
• All therapeutic measures other than surgery and aggressive weight loss in obese patients are methods of apnea control, rather than cure. Lifelong compliance with weight loss or nasal CPAP are necessary for therapy of OSA.
• Untreated, OSA appears to progress in severity
• Death due to OSA usually secondary to arrhythmias, cardiac ischemia or hypertensive complications, or motor vehicle accidents

MISCELLANEOUS

ASSOCIATED CONDITIONS
• Hypertension
• Arteriosclerotic vascular disease
• Coronary arterial disease
• Diabetes
• Obesity
• Nasal obstructive problems
• Acromegaly
• Hypothyroidism

AGE-RELATED FACTORS
Pediatric:
• OSA not as common in pediatric age group. If present, often due to tonsillar enlargement, craniofacial abnormalities. Response to tonsillectomy often good.
• Seen commonly in children with neuromuscular diseases, such as cerebral palsy, spinal muscular atrophy
Geriatric: OSA appears to increase in frequency after middle age and after the menopause in women. Often coexists with other health problems in the elderly.
Others: N/A

PREGNANCY Rare

SYNONYMS
• Pickwickian syndrome
• Sleep apnea syndrome
• Nocturnal upper airway occlusion

ICD-9-CM 306.1 Psychogenic apnea

OTHER NOTES OSA rare in premenopausal women unless there is coexistent morbid obesity or neurologic/craniofacial abnormalities

SEE ALSO N/A

OTHER NOTES N/A

ABBREVIATIONS
• CPAP = continuous positive airway pressure
• BiPAP = bilevel positive airway pressure
• UPPP = uvulopalatopharyngoplasty
• EDS = excessive daytime sleepiness
• OSA = obstructive sleep apnea

REFERENCES
• Kryger MH: Principles and Practice of Sleep Medicine. Philadelphia, W.B. Saunders Co., 1989
• Thorpy MJ: Handbook of Sleep Disorders. New York, Marcel Dekker Inc., 1990
Illustrations: N/A
Internet references: http://www.5mcc.com

Author(s)
Mary E. Klink, MD

Snake envenomations: Crotalidae

 BASICS

DESCRIPTION Symptom complex occurring following human envenomation by a snake of the family Crotalidae (pit vipers)
• These include those of the genus Crotalus (rattlesnakes), Agkistrodon (moccasins) and Sistrurus (pygmy rattlesnakes). Occurs most commonly in southeastern and southwestern US.
• These snakes characteristically have triangular-shaped heads, eyes with elliptical pupils, and small heat-sensing facial pits located between the nostril and the eye
System(s) affected: Cardiovascular, Skin/Exocrine, Nervous, Hemic/Lymphatic/Immunologic
Genetics: N/A
Incidence/Prevalence in USA:
3.2/100,000. 8,000 bites/year (20-25% of bites do not result in envenomation)
Predominant age: 19-30 years
Predominant sex: Male > Female

SIGNS AND SYMPTOMS
• These vary by species; prevalence as stated refers to family as whole
• Fang marks (may be two or only one) (>90%)
• Pain out of proportion to puncture wound (>50%)
• Edema of site, progressing proximally up extremity (>50%)
• Weakness, dizziness (>50%)
• Numbness/tingling in extremity, in mouth, tongue (>50%)
• Ecchymosis of skin, vesiculations around bite (>50%)
• Tachycardia (>50%)
• Nausea/vomiting (<50%)
• Hypo/Hypertension (<50%)
• Muscle fasciculations (<50%)
• Mental status changes including coma (<25%)
• Elevated creatine kinase (CK)

CAUSES Pit viper venom is a complex mixture which contains cytotoxins, hemotoxins, neurotoxins, and cardiotoxins

RISK FACTORS
• Risk taking behaviors
• Acute ethanol intoxication or intoxication with other drugs which impair judgment

 DIAGNOSIS

DIFFERENTIAL DIAGNOSIS Bite of non-venomous snake, bite of venomous species other than from Crotalidae family

LABORATORY
• CBC (Hgb/Hct decreased in < 50%)
• PT/PTT (prolonged in > 50%)
• Fibrinogen (decreased in < 50%), fibrin degradation products (increased in < 50%)
• Urinalysis - glycosuria (< 50%), proteinuria (< 25%), hematuria (< 25%)
• Decrease in blood platelets (< 50%)
• Type and crossmatch "to hold" in severe envenomations
• Electrolytes, blood urea nitrogen, creatinine
• Creatine kinase in severe envenomations
• Serum ethanol level if suspicious
Drugs that may alter lab results:
Anticoagulants
Disorders that may alter lab results: N/A

PATHOLOGICAL FINDINGS N/A

SPECIAL TESTS N/A

IMAGING N/A

DIAGNOSTIC PROCEDURES If suspicious of developing compartment syndrome, measure compartment pressures (rarely needed)

 TREATMENT

APPROPRIATE HEALTH CARE Patients with true envenomations and resulting signs/symptoms need emergency department evaluation with admission if necessary

GENERAL MEASURES
• Support vital signs
• Reassurance
• Remove rings and constrictive items proximal to site of envenomation
• Place affected injured part at level of heart
• Evaluate all pre-hospital care. If tourniquet has been placed in pre-hospital setting, sudden removal could "bolus" patient with venom.
• Obtain toxicology consultation by contacting American Association of Poison Centers (AAPCC) Regional Poison Information Center for your area
• Level 1:
  ◊ If local signs of edema are confined to area of bite without any other symptom of envenomation, place intravenous line of crystalloid at maintenance rates (if no history of renal or heart disease requiring fluid restriction) and draw laboratory studies
  ◊ Place reference marks for measuring circumference of extremity at 10 cm and 20 cm proximal to site of envenomation
  ◊ Measure every 15 minutes and trace leading edge of swelling
  ◊ Give tetanus toxoid
  ◊ Pain relief with opiate or acetaminophen (avoid aspirin)
  ◊ Repeat laboratory studies in six hours. If all remain normal and swelling does not progress, observe 8-12 hours then follow as outpatient.
  ◊ If swelling progresses or systemic signs and symptoms appear will need admission and further therapy (progresses to Level 2)
• Level 2:
  ◊ If edema, vesiculations, erythema progress beyond the immediate bite area and there are associated systemic signs/symptoms or laboratory abnormalities (as above), all therapy as in Level 1 above plus intravenous antivenom
  ◊ Intensive care monitoring may be necessary in most institutions
  ◊ Repeat laboratory evaluations every 6 hours initially until stable, then less frequently
  ◊ Continue to monitor vital signs and circumference of affected part

SURGICAL MEASURES N/A

ACTIVITY Bedrest with extremity elevated to level of atria

DIET Nothing by mouth initially

PATIENT EDUCATION Snake bite prevention and first aid

MEDICATIONS

DRUG(S) OF CHOICE
• Polyvalent Crotalidae antivenin
◊ First administer skin test according to product brochure. If negative, prepare five vials of antivenin in 250 mL normal saline IV fluid.
◊ Begin infusion at 3-5 mL/hr and, if no systemic reaction occurs, increase until a rate of 180-240 mL/hr is achieved (one vial every 15-20 minutes)
◊ Give by continuous infusion, not IV push
◊ If signs/symptoms continue to progress rapidly following the first 5 vials, repeat dose of 5 vials. Severe envenomations may require up to 30 vials.
Contraindications:
• History of allergy to horse serum product
• If skin test positive, and antivenin is necessary to save life or limb, contact Poison Information Center. Pretreatment with antihistamines, steroids, etc., in ICU setting may make antivenin administration possible.
Precautions:
• Have equipment and medications readily at hand to treat anaphylaxis
• Avoid aspirin or other anticoagulants
Significant possible interactions: N/A

ALTERNATIVE DRUGS
• Blood products only necessary for coagulopathies with clinical bleeding, not for treatment of laboratory abnormalities
• Steroid use is controversial.

FOLLOWUP

PATIENT MONITORING
• First return visit within 48 hours, then as clinically indicated
• Physical therapy referral should be made early for optimal outpatient intervention

PREVENTION/AVOIDANCE
• Use of preventive measures if handling snakes
• In snake-infested areas
◊ Wear protective shoes and clothing when walking
◊ Do not insert hands or feet into cracks or crevices or hollow logs
◊ Carry a flashlight if walking at night

POSSIBLE COMPLICATIONS
• Serum sickness from antivenom therapy (perhaps in > 50%)
• Local wound infection

EXPECTED COURSE/PROGNOSIS If
properly treated, mortality is very rare. Morbidity rare.

MISCELLANEOUS

ASSOCIATED CONDITIONS Underlying health of patient

AGE-RELATED FACTORS
Pediatric: Course may be more severe
Geriatric: Course may be more severe
Others: N/A

PREGNANCY N/A

SYNONYMS
• Snakebite
• Venomous snakebite
• Pit viper snake bite

ICD-9-CM 989.5 Venomous snake bite

SEE ALSO Snake envenomations: Elapidae

OTHER NOTES N/A

ABBREVIATIONS N/A

REFERENCES
• Ellenhorn MJ, Barceloux DG: Medical Toxicology: Diagnosis and Treatment of Human Poisoning. New York, Elsevier 1988;1113-1126
• Russell FE: Snake Venom Poisoning. Philadelphia, J.B. Lippincott, 1980
• Kurecki BA, Brownlee HJ: Venomous snakebites in the United States. J Fam Prac 1987;25(4):386-392
Illustrations: N/A
Internet references: http://www.5mcc.com

Author(s)
Gregory G. Gaar, MD, FAAP, FACEP

Snake envenomations: Elapidae

 BASICS

DESCRIPTION Symptom complex occurring following human envenomation by a snake of the family Elapidae
• In the US these include the genera Micrurus and Micruroides, commonly called "Coral Snakes." The Sonoran or Arizona coral snake is found mainly in Arizona (Micruroides euryxanthus), the Texas coral snake (Micrurus fulvius tenere) in Texas, Arkansas, and Louisiana, and the eastern coral snake (Micrurus fulvius fulvius) throughout the Southeastern US.
• The snakes have a characteristic rounded head with round pupils. Coloration is important in that in the U.S. broad rings of red and black are separated by narrow rings of yellow. ("Red on yellow, kill a fellow; red on black, venom lack.")
• Unlike Crotalidae envenomations, local signs and symptoms are mild in envenomation of Elapidae, even those which prove to be severe envenomations. Neurologic symptoms may be delayed; they have been reported to develop up to 12 or more hours after the envenomation.
System(s) affected: Nervous, Skin/Exocrine
Genetics: N/A
Incidence/Prevalence in USA: Unknown
Predominant age: 19-30 years
Predominant sex: Male > Female

SIGNS AND SYMPTOMS
• Fang marks; may be shallow or appear as scratch (> 75%)
• Local swelling (<50%)
• Numbness/change in sensation (< 50%)
• Nausea/vomiting (< 50%)
• Weakness (< 25%)
• Dizziness (< 15%)
• Diplopia (< 15%)
• Muscle fasciculations (< 15%)

CAUSES Venom is primarily a neurotoxin. Little or no cytotoxin to cause local tissue reaction.

RISK FACTORS Coral snakes are nocturnal and timid. Therefore they rarely bite humans. They must be deliberately provoked to bite.

 DIAGNOSIS

DIFFERENTIAL DIAGNOSIS
• Bite of other venomous snake (Crotalidae) without envenomation ("dry bite")
• Bite of a non-venomous snake

LABORATORY
• Creatine kinase (CPK) often elevated
• Blood ethanol level often elevated
• Laboratory not diagnostic
Drugs that may alter lab results: N/A
Disorders that may alter lab results: N/A

PATHOLOGICAL FINDINGS N/A

SPECIAL TESTS None

IMAGING N/A

DIAGNOSTIC PROCEDURES N/A

 TREATMENT

APPROPRIATE HEALTH CARE All patients with suspected coral snake envenomation need Emergency Department evaluation

GENERAL MEASURES
• All patients who have (1) confirmed bite by a snake identified as a coral snake, (2) history of the snake's having chewed on the person, and, (3) visible fang marks which pierce the epidermis, should be admitted to hospital for intensive care monitoring
• In this group of patients, perform a skin test for horse serum sensitivity. If negative, antivenom to Micrurus fulvius should be given early, even if there are no neurologic signs or symptoms present.
• If skin test is positive, and neurological symptoms are rapidly progressing, admission to ICU is indicated
• Pretreatment with IV diphenhydramine, steroids, and other antihistamines may allow for infusion of antivenom, although it is not clear from the literature if antivenom should be administered in light of a positive skin test. In this instance, obtain toxicology consultation from the American Association of Poison Control Centers (AAPCC) certified Poison Information Center for your area.
• Support vital signs, intubation may be necessary if respiratory compromise ensues
• Good supportive care with cardiac, respiratory, neurological monitoring
• Reassurance
• Immobilize extremity and keep at level of atria
• Contact AAPCC Regional Center for your area

SURGICAL MEASURES N/A

ACTIVITY Bedrest initially. May need physical therapy in severe cases of envenomation.

DIET Nothing by mouth initially

PATIENT EDUCATION N/A

MEDICATIONS

DRUG(S) OF CHOICE
• There is no antivenom available for Micruroides euryxanthus
• Tetanus booster if necessary
• Antivenom to the North American coral snake (Micrurus fulvius antivenin)
 ◊ Is available commercially. It is a horse serum product and is effective only for the envenomation of the Texas and eastern coral snakes (Micrurus fulvius tenere and Micrurus fulvius fulvius).
 ◊ If patients meet the criteria above (see General Measures), skin test should be performed according to directions taken from package insert. If negative, 4-6 vials of the antivenom should be reconstituted and diluted into 250 mL of normal saline. Begin infusion at 3-5 mL/hr and, if no systemic reaction occurs, increase until a rate of 1 diluted vial is being given every thirty minutes.
 ◊ Envenomations with more severe sequelae or prolonged sequelae may require larger doses of antivenom. Unfortunately it is impossible to specify dosage more specifically.
Contraindications: History of allergy to horse serum
Precautions: Have equipment and medications readily at hand to treat anaphylaxis
Significant possible interactions: N/A

ALTERNATIVE DRUGS
Steroid use is controversial.

FOLLOWUP

PATIENT MONITORING
First return visit within 48 hours, then as clinically indicated

PREVENTION/AVOIDANCE
• Use of preventive measures if handling snakes
• In snake-infested areas:
 ◊ Wear protective shoes and clothing when walking
 ◊ Do not insert hands or feet into cracks or crevices or hollow logs
 ◊ Carry a flashlight if walking at night

POSSIBLE COMPLICATIONS
• Serum sickness from antivenom therapy (perhaps in 10% or more)
• Local wound infection
• Aspiration pneumonia

EXPECTED COURSE/PROGNOSIS
• Neurologic deterioration may progress despite antivenom administration. Complete paralysis can occur.
• Early, elective intubation during progression of paralysis may help to prevent aspiration pneumonia
• Discharge should not occur until the patient has made neurologic recovery to the point that there is no concern of respiratory failure
• Muscle strength may not return to normal for 4-6 weeks
• Long-term morbidity rare
• Mortality does occur even with antivenom therapy

MISCELLANEOUS

ASSOCIATED CONDITIONS N/A

AGE-RELATED FACTORS
Pediatric: Not well described
Geriatric: Morbidity and danger of mortality is greater
Others: N/A

PREGNANCY N/A

SYNONYMS
• Neurotoxic snake bite
• Snakebite

ICD-9-CM 989.5 Venomous snake bite

SEE ALSO Snake envenomations: Crotalidae

OTHER NOTES N/A

ABBREVIATIONS N/A

REFERENCES
• Kitchens CS, Van Mierop LHS: Envenomation by the eastern coral snake (Micrurus fulvius fulvius). JAMA 1987;258(12):1615-1618
• Russell FE: Snake Venom Poisoning. Philadelphia, J.B. Lippincott, 1980
• Ellenhorn MJ, Barceloux DG: Medical Toxicology: Diagnosis and Treatment of Human Poisoning. New York, Elsevier, 1988:1127-1128
Illustrations: N/A
Internet references: http://www.5mcc.com

Author(s)
Gregory G. Gaar, MD, FAAP, FACEP

Sporotrichosis

 BASICS

DESCRIPTION Subacute or chronic fungal infection occurring in 4 forms: cutaneous or lymphocutaneous, pulmonary, osteo-articular, or disseminated; and rarely musculoskeletal (joint and tendon by puncture wounds). Most likely to occur in farmers, horticulturists, gardeners. Cutaneous lesions occur 20-90 days after cutaneous inoculation.
System(s) affected: Skin, Hemic/Lymphatic/Immunologic, Skeletal
Genetics: No known genetic pattern
Incidence/Prevalence in USA: N/A
Predominant age: Adults
Predominant sex: Male > Female (mostly due to occupational exposure)

SIGNS AND SYMPTOMS
• Cutaneous or lymphocutaneous:
  ◊ Characteristic skin lesions, beginning as an inoculation chancre, or erythematous plaque with satellite, small papule, painless, movable, subcutaneous nodules in a linear distribution. Lesions progress to larger nodules which may ulcerate and drain. Affects primarily upper extremities.
  ◊ Additional lesions spread proximally along lymphatics
• Pulmonary
  ◊ Cough, occasionally productive
  ◊ Cavitary lung disease
  ◊ Hilar adenopathy
  ◊ Signs and symptoms indistinguishable from other chronic pneumonias
• Osteo-articular
  ◊ Subacute or chronic inflammatory arthritis, often monoarticular, may persist for many years
  ◊ Signs and symptoms of osteomyelitis
  ◊ Generally afebrile
• Disseminated
  ◊ Multifocal skin lesions
  ◊ Polyarticular arthritis
  ◊ Weight loss
  ◊ Chronic lymphocytic meningitis

CAUSES Infection with Sporothrix schenckii, a fungus found in soil, sphagnum peat moss, and decaying vegetation. Infection acquired by direct inoculation (usual) or inhalation (rare).

RISK FACTORS
• Gardening - contact with mulch, sphagnum moss, hay, timber, thorny bushes
• Occupations handling gardening materials, such as nursery workers, landscapers, florists, carpenters
• Animal handlers (transmission from animals, especially cats, to humans has been documented)
• Immunocompromised (drugs or HIV infection)
• Alcoholism (pulmonary and disseminated)

 DIAGNOSIS

DIFFERENTIAL DIAGNOSIS
• Cutaneous or lymphocutaneous
  ◊ Sporotrichoid nocardiosis
  ◊ Leishmaniasis
  ◊ Chromomycosis
  ◊ Atypical mycobacterial infection (M. marinum, M. chelonei, M. kansasii)
  ◊ Tularemia
  ◊ Plague
• Pulmonary
  ◊ Tuberculosis
  ◊ Sarcoidosis
  ◊ Chronic fungal pneumonia
  ◊ Neoplasm
• Osteo-articular
  ◊ Rheumatoid arthritis
  ◊ Bacterial arthritis/osteomyelitis

LABORATORY
• Culture of S. schenckii in sputum, pus, synovial fluid or bone drainage
• Organism found with difficulty with PAS and Gomori stains of skin or other biopsied lesions
• Serum antibody tests may be useful for extracutaneous disease
Drugs that may alter lab results:
Antifungal drugs
Disorders that may alter lab results: N/A

PATHOLOGICAL FINDINGS Granulomas with central necrosis

SPECIAL TESTS Immunohistochemical staining of biopsy specimens

IMAGING Chest and skeletal x-rays

DIAGNOSTIC PROCEDURES
• Careful history and physical
• Culture of draining lesions
• Culture of inflammatory joint effusions or sputum
• Biopsy if diagnosis not confirmed

 TREATMENT

APPROPRIATE HEALTH CARE
• Many patients can be managed on outpatient basis
• Hospitalization for adjunctive surgical procedures or initiation of amphotericin B therapy

GENERAL MEASURES
• Local heat application useful for cutaneous and lymphocutaneous disease
• Keep cutaneous lesions clean
• Repeated drainage of infected joints may be indicated

SURGICAL MEASURES
• Synovectomy of infected joints may be indicated
• Surgical débridement of osteomyelitis usually indicated

ACTIVITY No restrictions

DIET No special diet

PATIENT EDUCATION Patients should be advised of the nature of the infection, the toxicities associated with therapy, and the need for sustained therapy

Sporotrichosis

MEDICATIONS

DRUG(S) OF CHOICE
• Cutaneous or lymphocutaneous disease:
◊ Itraconazole 200 mg per day orally for 3-12 months is a preferred treatment
◊ Potassium iodide saturated solution (SSKI) is an alternative treatment. Initially 10 drops orally tid increased by 1 drop each dose to maximum tolerated dose or 120 drops/day. Dilute in a beverage to disguise taste. Continue for 1-2 months after all lesions have healed.
• Extracutaneous disease:
◊ Itraconazole 400 mg per day orally is a preferred treatment. Therapy should be continued for 12-18 months.
◊ IV amphotericin B, 1.5-2.5 g total dose is alternative treatment
Contraindications: SSKI contraindicated in tuberculosis
Precautions:
• Amphotericin B can cause fever, chills, nausea and vomiting. Dosage varies for sex and age groups. Refer to manufacturer's literature for precautions, adverse effects and interactions.
• SSKI requires extra care if patient also has tuberculosis, kidney disease, renal dysfunction or hyperthyroidism. Can cause folliculitis and tender, swollen salivary glands.
Significant possible interactions: SSKI taken concurrently with amiloride, spironolactone or triamterene may result in hyperkalemia

ALTERNATIVE DRUGS
• Ketoconazole 400 mg orally daily may be effective alternative therapy in immunocompetent hosts
• Fluconazole 800 mg per day orally is an alternative therapy in patients unable to receive itraconazole therapy

FOLLOWUP

PATIENT MONITORING Check for compliance with long-term drugs (SSKI should be continued for 1-2 months after lesions heal)

PREVENTION/AVOIDANCE
• Avoid endemic areas
• Wear gloves when working in soil

POSSIBLE COMPLICATIONS
• Secondary bacterial infection
• Bone and joint deformities from osteo-articular disease

EXPECTED COURSE/PROGNOSIS
• Prognosis is excellent for complete recovery from cutaneous or lymphocutaneous infections
• Other disease forms demonstrate a chronic indolent course and are variably responsive to therapy

MISCELLANEOUS

ASSOCIATED CONDITIONS See Risk Factors

AGE-RELATED FACTORS
Pediatric: Rare
Geriatric: N/A
Others: N/A

PREGNANCY N/A

SYNONYMS
• Schenck's disease
• Beurmann's disease
• Rose gardener's disease

ICD-9-CM 117.1 Sporotrichosis

SEE ALSO N/A

OTHER NOTES Rare ocular disease due to direct inoculation

ABBREVIATIONS N/A

REFERENCES
• Winn RE: Sporotrichosis. Infect Dis Clinic North Am 1988;2:899
• Mandell GL, ed: Principles and Practice of Infectious Diseases. 4th Ed. New York, Churchill Livingstone, 1995
• Sharkey-Mathis PK, Kauffman CA, Graybill JR, Stevens DA, Hostetler JS, Cloud G, Dismukes WE & other members of the NIAID Mycoses Study Group: Treatment of sporotrichosis with itraconazole. Am J Med 1993;95:279
• Kauffman CA, Pappos PG, McKinsey DS, Greenfield RA, Perfect JR, Cloud GA, et al: Treatment of Lymphocutaneous and Visceral Sporotrichosis with Fluconazole. Clin Infect Dis 1996;22:46
Illustrations: N/A
Internet references: http://www.5mcc.com

Author(s)
E. Nan Scott, PhD
Ronald A. Greenfield, MD
Douglas P. Fine, MD

Sprains & strains

BASICS

DESCRIPTION
• Sprain: complete or partial ligamentous injury, either within the body of the ligament or at the site of attachment to bone. It may be classified as Grade I, II, or III. Grades I and II are incomplete tears and differ in severity; Grade III is complete dissolution of the ligamentous connection. Physical exam is key to the diagnosis. Usually secondary to trauma (falls, twisting injuries or motor vechicle accidents).
• Strain: partial or complete disruption of the muscle or tendon, usually associated with overuse injuries.
System(s) affected: Musculoskeletal
Genetics: N/A
Incidence/Prevalence in USA:
• Total incidence including spine, upper and lower extremities probably occurs in close to 80% of all athletes sometime in their career
• Prevalence - approximately 30,000
Predominant age:
• Sprains- any age where patient is physically active
• Strains - usually 15-40
Predominant sex: Male > Female

SIGNS AND SYMPTOMS
• Swelling
• Pain
• Erythema and/or ecchymosis
• Tenderness
• Gait disturbances if severe
• Decreased range of motion of joint and joint instability

CAUSES
• Falls
• Motor vehicle accident
• Trauma
• Excessive exercise or inadequate warm-up and stretching prior to activity
• Poor conditioning

RISK FACTORS
• Change in or improper shoe gear, protective gear, or environment (e.g., surface)
• Inappropriate increase in training schedule

DIAGNOSIS

DIFFERENTIAL DIAGNOSIS
• Sprains (ligament tears) must be differentiated from strains (muscle-tendon unit tears), although this is difficult and often the diagnosis is strain/sprain
• Tendonitis
• Bursitis
• Bony injuries
• Rarely, muscle hematomas account for some of the signs and symptoms of strains

LABORATORY   N/A
Drugs that may alter lab results: N/A
Disorders that may alter lab results: N/A

PATHOLOGICAL FINDINGS   N/A

SPECIAL TESTS
• Exam under anesthesia
• Arthroscopy in some cases
• For ankle, anterior drawer test, which tests the integrity of the anterior talofibular ligament

IMAGING
• Ankle films - only required if there is pain in malleolar zone and
1. Bone tenderness posterior edge or tip of lateral malleolus
or
2. Bone tenderness posterior edge or tip of medial malleolus
or
3. Unable to bear weight, both immediately and in emergency department
• Foot films - only required if there is midfoot zone pain and
1. Bone tenderness at base of 5th metatarsal
or
2. Bone tenderness at navicular
or
3. unable to bear weight, both immediately and in emergency department
• X-rays to rule out bony injury. Stress views may be helpful.
• CT scan of the affected area
• MRI
• Exam under anesthesia in difficult cases

DIAGNOSTIC PROCEDURES
• Sprains/strains
  ◊ Grade I - pain/tenderness without loss of motion
  ◊ Grade II - pain/tenderness; ecchymosis with some loss of range of motion
  ◊ Grade III - pain/tenderness; swelling and ecchymosis and complete loss of range of motion

TREATMENT

APPROPRIATE HEALTH CARE
Outpatient

GENERAL MEASURES
History and physical exam along with treatment of the worst possible suspected injury
• Acutely
  ◊ RICE therapy - Rest, Ice, Compression, Elevation
    - Elastic bandage wrap (Ace) is comfortable
    - Jone's dressing for more severe injuries
  ◊ Orthosis (splint) for pain relief and stability; "Air Cast" type devices provide effective stability and pain relief
  ◊ Crutches and crutch gait training

SURGICAL MEASURES
• Casting and surgery reserved for select Grade III injuries

ACTIVITY
• Bed rest for acute injuries
• Physical therapy for more severe injuries
• Elevate joint while sleeping

DIET   Weight loss if obesity etiologic

PATIENT EDUCATION
• Instructions on how to wrap with elastic bandage
• Prevention of injury

MEDICATIONS

DRUG(S) OF CHOICE Nonsteroidal anti-inflammatories (NSAID's)
Contraindications: Refer to manufacturer's profile of each drug
Precautions: Refer to manufacturer's profile of each drug
Significant possible interactions: Refer to manufacturer's profile of each drug

ALTERNATIVE DRUGS
• Painkillers acutely for severe pain (non-narcotics and/or narcotics as warranted)
• Analgesic balms
• Capsaicin cream

FOLLOWUP

PATIENT MONITORING After initial treatment, consider rehabilitation. Direct emphasis towards limiting swelling and providing a pain-free full range of motion.

PREVENTION/AVOIDANCE
• Maintaining a reasonable level of physical fitness
• Avoidance of excessive physical stresses and wearing of proper exercise gear (particularly shoes). Using proper equipment for the activity.
• Knowledge of the risks associated with the intended activity
• Appropriate conditioning, warm-up and cool-down exercises

POSSIBLE COMPLICATIONS
• Chronic joint instability
• Arthritis

EXPECTED COURSE/PROGNOSIS With appropriate treatment and rest, 6-8 weeks or longer for recovery, depending on severity of injury

MISCELLANEOUS

ASSOCIATED CONDITIONS
Hemarthrosis, stress, avulsion, or other fractures, syndesmotic injuries, contusions, wounds, dislocations

AGE-RELATED FACTORS
Pediatric: Sprains and strains accounted for 24% of injuries in an analysis of 1,124 sports injuries of children in a study done in West Germany, 1980-82
Geriatric: More likely to see associated bony injuries due to decreased joint flexibility and prevalence of osteoporosis and osteopenia
Others: N/A

PREGNANCY N/A

SYNONYMS N/A

ICD-9-CM 848.9

SEE ALSO
• Tendinitis

OTHER NOTES N/A

ABBREVIATIONS N/A

REFERENCES
• Kvist M, Kujala VM, Heinonen OJ, Vuori IV, Aho AJ, Pajulo O, Hintsa A, Parvinen T: Sports related injuries in children. IJSM 1989;10(2):81-86
• Strong WB, Stanitski EL, Smith RE, Wilmore JH: Diagnosis and treatment of ankle sprains. AJDC 1990;144:809-814
• Ruda S: Sports Nursing. In Nursing Clinics of North America. Philadelphia, W.B. Saunders Co., Mar, 1991
• Stiell I.G, McKnight D, Greenberg GH, et al: Implementation of the Ottawa ankle rules. JAMA 1994;271(11):827-832
Illustrations: N/A
Internet references: http://www.5mcc.com

Author(s)
Timothy Robinson, DO
Richard B. Birrer, MD

Status epilepticus

BASICS

DESCRIPTION Epileptic seizure which is more than 30 min long or absence of full recovery of consciousness between seizures. Tonic-clonic (grand mal) status epilepticus (SEp) is the most common and most serious form. SEp is a life-threatening emergency.
System(s) affected: Nervous
Genetics: Unknown
Incidence/Prevalence in USA: More than 60,000 cases per year; 1/3 as unprovoked first seizure, 1/6 in patients with known epilepsy, 1/2 secondary to acute CNS insult
Predominant age: > 50% of new cases of SEp occur in young children. Risk is also increased in those over age 60.
Predominant sex: Male = Female

SIGNS AND SYMPTOMS
• Depend on the duration and type of seizure
• Recurrent tonic-clonic convulsions: May be preceded by aura. Tonic phase (stiffening) for 30 to 45 seconds. Clonic phase (rhythmic jerking) for 2-5 minutes. No intervening consciousness before seizure recurs. (For additional seizure types see Other Notes).
• Associated autonomic phenomena: Excess catecholamine secretion resulting in glandular hypersecretion, piloerection, cyclic pupillary dilation, and prolonged apnea (may lead to cyanosis)
• Metabolic changes: Lactic acidosis, carbon dioxide narcosis, hyperkalemia, hyperglycemia - followed by hypoglycemia
• Cardiac changes: Hypertension (may be followed by hypotension), arrhythmias, high output failure
• Respiratory changes: Increased secretions, lax tongue, possible airway obstruction, pulmonary edema, aspiration
• Renal complications: Acute tubular necrosis from myoglobinuria after rhabdomyolysis
• Cerebrovascular changes: Loss of autoregulation, focal ischemia, cerebral edema
• Postictal findings: Fever, tachycardia, mydriasis, conjugate deviation of eyes, decreased corneal reflex, positive Babinski's sign, fecal and urinary incontinence and tongue, cheek, or lip lacerations

CAUSES
• Must search for the primary pathology
• Febrile convulsions (especially in children)
• Acute CNS injury - trauma, infection, mass/vascular lesion, metabolic disorder or anticonvulsant withdrawal/noncompliance
• Idiopathic
• Intoxication - multiple agents (especially cocaine, tricyclic antidepressants)
• Chronic CNS injury - previous trauma, stroke, infection, encephalopathy (hypoxic or other chronic or degenerative type)

RISK FACTORS
• Known seizure disorder plus any precipitating insult. Prior history of SEp (recurrence rate is 17% in children; 50% in those with neurologic abnormality).
• Porphyria

DIAGNOSIS

DIFFERENTIAL DIAGNOSIS
• Pseudostatus may occur with pseudoseizures; avoid dangerous therapy
• While tonic/clonic status is usually apparent, paralyzed patients and other forms of status require neurologic exam and EEG
• Primary diagnostic problem is identification of the underlying pathology

LABORATORY Glucose, electrolytes, CBC, calcium, magnesium and osmolarity; arterial blood gases; toxicology screen; anticonvulsants serum levels; liver/renal function.
Drugs that may alter lab results: N/A
Disorders that may alter lab results: N/A

PATHOLOGICAL FINDINGS Variable

SPECIAL TESTS EEG will differentiate pseudoseizures and prolonged seizures not classically recognized as status.

IMAGING CT scan, MRI

DIAGNOSTIC PROCEDURES Lumbar puncture. CAUTION - intra cranial pressure may be increased.

TREATMENT

APPROPRIATE HEALTH CARE
Tonic-clonic SEp is an emergency; treat if a seizure lasts >10 min. Requires continuous skilled care.

GENERAL MEASURES
• Manage airway, breathing and circulation (ABCs). Monitor pulse oximetry, end-tidal CO_2, blood pressure, ECG and temperature. Give oxygen. Ventilate and intubate if hypoventilation, hypoxia and/or hypercarbia occur or if aspiration is a concern.
• Observe and confirm the fit is SEp
• Pursue available drug history
• Establish IV (or intraosseous line for a child); obtain initial lab studies (above)
• Initiate anticonvulsant therapy to end seizure; then add maintenance therapy
• Use muscle relaxant if seizures impair ventilation or lactic acidosis develops

SURGICAL MEASURES N/A

ACTIVITY Protect the patient from injury. Place on side. Clear airway secretions. Prevent tongue laceration.

DIET NPO

PATIENT EDUCATION Epilepsy Foundation (800)EFA-1000

MEDICATIONS

DRUG(S) OF CHOICE Depend on the type of seizure. Tonic-clonic SEp is the most serious and may be approached as follows. (For other types, see Other Notes.)
Stabilization: Continue "ABC" assessment and monitoring. Intubate if treatment or seizures cause hypoventilation or loss of airway. Prevent hypotension with vasopressors if needed (e.g., dopamine).
• Thiamine: 100 mg IV or IM (adults only)
• 50% dextrose - if blood sugar is low or cannot be measured; give 50 mL IV (for child - use D25W; give 2 mL/kg IV slowly)
• Naloxone (Narcan): if pupils are myotic or drug overdose suspected; give 2 mg IV (for child - 0.1 mg/kg IV, up to 2 mg slowly)
To stop seizures (IV available):
Give BOTH a benzodiazepine and phenytoin. As each drug is added - watch for hypoventilation and hypotension.
• Lorazepam (Ativan): 0.05-0.1 mg/kg IV at 1 to 2 mg/min to maximum of 10 mg (for child 0.05-0.1 mg/kg IV at <2 mg/min to maximum of 4 mg). May repeat q 10 min/times 2 (some prefer diazepam [see below]).
PLUS
• Phenytoin (Dilantin): 15-20 mg/kg IV at < 50 mg/min with ECG monitoring (see Precautions). (In patients > 60 years old or with cardiac history, load with 15 mg/kg and slow to 0.4/kg/min.) May repeat 5 mg/kg q 30 min to total of 30 mg/kg, (for child < 50 kg, load with 20 mg/kg at 1 mg/kg/min and repeat as above). Fosphenytoin (Cerebyx) prodrug of phenytoin (FDA approved for SEp) has less local toxicity and cardiovascular depression. Follow package insert directions carefully.
To stop seizures (IV not available):
• Intraosseous infusion in small children for benzodiazepines, phenytoin and phenobarbital - doses are the same as IV
• Rectal diazepam: 0.5-1.0 mg/kg (child - 20 mg maximum) use the IV solution (less respiratory depression)
• Sublingual lorazepam: use IV dose
• Midazolam (Versed): 0.2 mg/kg IM or 0.5 mg/kg intranasal (onset 5-10 min, brief)
If seizures persist (refractory status):
• Induce drug coma (anesthesia) with a short acting barbiturate or benzodiazepine to obtain a burst suppression pattern EEG. Requires intubation, continuous respiratory support, cardiovascular monitoring, and (often) blood pressure support.
◊ Pentobarbital: induction dose 5 mg/kg IV or until EEG seizure activity is suppressed. Maintenance dose: 1-3 mg/kg/hr, adjusted according to the EEG response.
◊ Thiopental: induction dose 3-6 mg/kg IV, then add 50 mg IV q 2-5 min to produce EEG burst suppression. Maintenance dose: IV drip of 0.2% solution adjusted to keep EEG at burst suppression.
◊ Diazepam: 4-8 mg/hr IV drip
Contraindications:
• Review current package inserts
• Benzodiazepines (diazepam, lorazepam, midazolam) - in acute narrow-angle glaucoma
• Barbiturates - in acute intermittent porphyria

Precautions:
• Reduce dosage of depressants in patients with shock, coma or alcohol intoxication
• Benzodiazepines - apnea may occur with rapid IV injection, especially with barbiturates. Reduce dose in the chronic pulmonary patient, the elderly and hepatic insufficiency.
• Diazepam - venous thrombosis/phlebitis
• Phenobarbital - caution in pulmonary insufficiency, hepatic disease and pregnancy. Withdrawal seizures may occur following abrupt termination of high doses. Increase the dosing interval in renal failure. Reduce dose in severe liver disease.
• Phenytoin - monitor ECG for arrhythmias, prolonged QT interval, and hypotension. If these occur, decrease the rate of administration. Use with caution in pregnancy (increased risk of malformations), liver disease, hyperglycemia, and elderly patients. Abrupt withdrawal may precipitate status. Use in normal or half normal saline to prevent precipitation that occurs in dextrose solutions. Overdose may cause paradoxical inefficacy.

Significant possible interactions:
CNS depressants depression enhanced
• Phenobarbital: reduced efficacy of quinidine and warfarin; induces metabolism of phenytoin
• Phenytoin: increased serum levels and toxicity of warfarin, disulfiram, phenylbutazone, and isoniazid. Decrease dose with renal insufficiency; monitor free levels if possible.

ALTERNATIVE DRUGS
Alternate benzodiazepines:
• Medium acting/convenient: diazepam (Valium) 0.2-0.5 mg/kg IV at 5 mg/min up to a dose of 30 mg (for child 0.3 mg/kg at <2 mg/min up to 10 mg). Repeat q 5 min x 3.
• Faster/shorter acting: midazolam (Versed) 0.125-0.5 mg/kg IV (sedative to anesthetic dose) plus titrated infusion of 0.5-10 µg/kg/min
Second line drugs:
• Phenobarbital (Luminal): 10-20 mg/kg IV (in saline) at a rate of 25-50 mg/kg/min (use lower rate for old age or cardiac history); may repeat dose of 4-6 mg/kg IV until no seizures or total dose of 1-2 grams. (For child - 20 mg/kg IV at 1 mg/kg/min, maximum 30 mg/kg
• Lidocaine (Xylocaine): 1 to 3 mg/kg IV bolus; maintenance 3 to 10 mg/kg/hr
• Valproic acid: 500 mg via nasogastric tube or 500 mg with 300 mL water via rectal tube (clamp for 15 minutes)
• Paraldehyde: 0.3 mL(300 mg)/kg (usually 4-8 mL) via rectal (or gastric) tube diluted 1/1 in oil to prevent mucosal irritation (mix in a glass syringe). Rectal absorption is slow - peak levels in 2-4 hours. (No parenteral preparation is available in the US)
Investigational drugs:
Isoflurane, desflurane by inhalation; phenytoin prodrug (fosphenytoin) IV and IM; propofol by continuous IV and bolus; etomidate by continuous IV infusion; chlormethiazole by IV infusion; IV valproic acid; ketamine, NMDA antagonist–IV as neuroprotectants

FOLLOWUP

PATIENT MONITORING Therapeutic blood levels of anticonvulsants

PREVENTION/AVOIDANCE Establish maintenance regimen of anticonvulsants

POSSIBLE COMPLICATIONS
• Morbidity/mortality related to the acute CNS insult, stress, injury from repeated seizures
• Causes of death - cardiopulmonary arrest, renal failure, hyperthermia, aspiration pneumonia, the underlying pathology or the treatment instituted
• Anticonvulsants cause respiratory and cardiovascular depression

EXPECTED COURSE/PROGNOSIS
Mortality is 6-18% (3-6% in children) and is improving. Usually related to the underlying cause. Prolonged seizures (> 30 min) may cause neurologic injury or death. Seizure >4 hr, mortality = 50%; >12 hr = 80%.

MISCELLANEOUS

ASSOCIATED CONDITIONS Etiology or underlying pathology associated with SEp varies significantly by age group. In adults, usually related to a known condition, e.g., established epilepsy, alcohol withdrawal or acquired CNS lesion (especially frontal).

AGE-RELATED FACTORS
Pediatric: Lower mortality rate. More likely present in SEp as their first seizure due to febrile seizure; new onset epilepsy (idiopathic); CNS infection; metabolic derangement.
Geriatric: More likely to have SEp secondary to a change in drug therapy (noncompliance, drug interaction or toxicity); tend to have localized (often frontal lobe) CNS lesions.
Others: Neonatal status is most often related to meningitis or metabolic disorders (deficiencies of calcium, magnesium, or pyridoxine); needs careful workup for cause

PREGNANCY
• Phenytoin - use with caution (increased risk of malformations in first trimester)
• Phenobarbital - use with caution
• Valproate - increased risk of neural tube defects

SYNONYMS Status convulsivus

ICD-9-CM
345.3 grand mal status and status epilepticus
345.7 Epilepsia partialis continua, psychomotor status and temporal lobe status

SEE ALSO
• Seizure disorders
• Seizures, febrile

OTHER NOTES
Additional forms of status include:
• Focal motor status - starts distally with clonic jerking in ascending pattern; eyes and head deviate to side opposite the focus; may progress to generalized status; underlying CNS pathology is common. Treat like tonic-clonic SEp. May respond to carbamazepine.
• Epilepsia partialis continua - rapid focal jerking; no loss of consciousness; worsened by voluntary movements; may persist for hours to days; poor response to therapy; often associated with underlying pathology. Pentobarbital and diazepam recommended.
• Myoclonic status - sudden spasmodic contraction of limbs; usually secondary to widespread neurologic or metabolic dysfunction; consciousness usually maintained. Treat with diazepam.
• Complex partial status (psychomotor status) - short seizures with automatisms (e.g., lip smacking, random eye movements, chewing, staring); followed by post ictal confusion. With status, treat like tonic-clonic SEp.
• Absence status - varies from mild lethargy to severe confusion, 10 second duration, no aura, eyes flutter and turn upward, with irregular myoclonic jerks, automatisms, no post ictal confusion; may progress to generalized status. If so, treat as tonic-clonic status.
• Neonatal status epilepticus - subtle multifocal, clonic, tonic, and myoclonic features; risk of intracerebral hemorrhage; meningitis and metabolic disorders (deficiencies of calcium, magnesium, pyridoxine) more common. Begin with phenobarbital and diazepam.

ABBREVIATIONS SEp = status epilepticus

REFERENCES
• Working Group on Status Epilepticus: Treatment of status epilepticus: Recommendations of the Epilepsy Foundation of America Working Group on Status Epilepticus. JAMA 1993;270:854-859
• Sheperd SM: Management of status epilepticus. Emer Med Clin NA 1994;12:941-961
• Lowenstein SR: Status Epilepticus (Disease & Trauma Monographs for Acute Care). In: Honigman G, Rumack BH eds. EMERGINDEX® Information System. Denver, Micromedex, Inc., (Revised 3/96)
• Canadian Pediatric Society Statement: Management of the pediatric patient with generalized convulsive status epilepticus in the emergency department. Paediatrics & Child Health 1996;1(2):151-155
Illustrations: N/A
Internet references: http://www.5mcc.com

Author(s)
Jeff Ray Gibson, Jr., MD

Stevens-Johnson syndrome

BASICS

DESCRIPTION A severe variant of erythema multiforme. Acute, severe, generally self-limited hypersensitivity reaction involving the skin and mucous membranes. It may involve multiple organ systems as complications of the disease.
System(s) affected: Skin/Exocrine
Genetics: Possible association with HLA-B15
Incidence/Prevalence in USA: 0.1/100,000/year
Predominant Age: More common in children and young adults
Predominant sex: Males > Females (2:1)

SIGNS AND SYMPTOMS
• Variable and nonspecific prodrome, often with features of upper respiratory tract infection
• Sudden onset, rapidly progressive, pleomorphic rash, with vesicles and bullae
• Nikolsky's sign absent
• Mucous membrane with characteristic vesicles/ulcers
• Stomatitis
• Rash may have features of erythema multiforme
• Burning sensation to skin/mucous membranes, sometimes tenderness of skin also
• Pruritus usually absent
• Fever to 39-40°C (102-104°F)
• Headache
• Malaise
• Arthralgias
• Rhinitis
• Epistaxis
• Crusting of nares
• Conjunctivitis
• Corneal ulcerations
• Erosive vulvovaginitis, or balanitis
• Cough
• Thick mucopurulent sputum
• Tachypnea/respiratory distress
• Hematuria
• Albuminuria
• Arrhythmias
• Pericarditis
• Congestive heart failure
• Mental status changes
• Seizures
• Coma
• Sepsis
• Electrolyte disturbances

CAUSES
Idiopathic in up to 50% of cases. The remaining 50% may represent a hypersensitivity response to one of the following:
• Viral infections - particularly herpes simplex; also Epstein-Barr, Coxsackie, echovirus, varicella, mumps and poliovirus
• Bacterial infections - especially mycoplasma pneumoniae; also brucellosis, diphtheria, Yersinia, tuberculosis, tularemia, and gonorrhea
• Protozoan infections
• Collagen vascular disease

• Medications - especially sulfonamides, penicillins, anticonvulsants, salicylates
• Vaccines - diphtheria/typhoid, bacillus Calmette-Guérin (BCG), oral polio vaccine (OPV)
• Malignancy
• Pregnancy
• Premenstrual hormonal changes
• Consumption of beer
• Reiter's syndrome
• Sarcoidosis

RISK FACTORS
• Previous history of erythema multiforme/Stevens-Johnson syndrome
• Male sex

DIAGNOSIS

DIFFERENTIAL DIAGNOSIS
• Bullous impetigo
• Graft vs. host disease
• Pemphigus vulgaris
• Pemphigoid
• Septicemia
• Serum sickness
• Hand-foot-mouth disease
• Collagen vascular diseases
• Meningococcemia
• Behçet's syndrome
• Staphylococcal scalded skin syndrome

LABORATORY Culture for suspected sources of infection
Drugs that may alter lab results: N/A
Disorders that may alter lab results: N/A

PATHOLOGICAL FINDINGS Epidermal necrolysis is characteristic. Spongiosis, intracellular edema, vacuolar changes at the dermal-epidermal junction, edema and extravasated erythrocytes in the dermis may also be seen on biopsy specimen.

SPECIAL TESTS None

IMAGING N/A

DIAGNOSTIC PROCEDURES Skin biopsy

TREATMENT

APPROPRIATE HEALTH CARE Inpatient care, often in the intensive care setting

GENERAL MEASURES
• Withdrawal of any implicated medications or treatment of any identified underlying infection/disease
• Meticulous wound care - use Burow's solution or Domeboro solution dressings
• With extensive skin involvement - reverse isolation and treatment of skin (similar to burn care)
• Supportive care for maintenance of fluid, electrolyte and protein balance
• Empiric antibiotic use not recommended
• Oral lesions: To provide symptomatic relief, oral hygiene; to facilitate oral intake, treat with mouthwashes of warm saline, or a solution of diphenhydramine, Xylocaine, and Kaopectate
• Ophthalmological consultation for eye care

SURGICAL MEASURES N/A

ACTIVITY Bedrest, until clinically stabilized

DIET As tolerated. Increased fluid intake should be encouraged in those with more extensive skin involvement. Intravenous nutritional support may be required.

PATIENT EDUCATION
• Patients should be reassured that the disease is self-limited
• Recurrences are possible, and avoidance of any identified etiologic agent should be encouraged

Stevens-Johnson syndrome

MEDICATIONS

DRUG(S) OF CHOICE
• Systemic corticosteroids may provide benefit, particularly in rapidly evolving or more severe cases. Initial dosage equivalent to prednisone 1-2 mg/kg/day with subsequent tapering. Probably not beneficial after the first week of illness.
• Provide treatment to any underlying infection or disease
• Empiric antibiotic use not recommended
Contraindications: Any infectious process in which use of steroids would be contraindicated
Precautions: Refer to manufacturer's profile of each drug
Significant possible interactions: Refer to manufacturer's profile of each drug

ALTERNATIVE DRUGS
Acyclovir may be given to suppress recurrent herpetic disease if herpes is identified as the underlying cause.

FOLLOWUP

PATIENT MONITORING
The disease is generally self-limited. During the course of the disease, patients should be monitored for signs of secondary infections, dehydration, electrolyte imbalances, and malnutrition.

PREVENTION/AVOIDANCE
• Known or suspected etiologic agents should be avoided
• Acyclovir (used to treat viral infections) may help prevent herpes-related erythema multiforme
• Tamoxifen has been shown to prevent premenstrual related disease

POSSIBLE COMPLICATIONS
• Secondary infections
• Sepsis
• Pneumonia (10-20%)
• Dehydration/electrolyte disturbances
• Acute tubular necrosis
• Ophthalmic complications of corneal ulcerations or iritis
• Arrhythmias
• Death in up to 15% of untreated cases

EXPECTED COURSE/PROGNOSIS
• Disease may have a rapid onset or evolve over 1-2 weeks with subsequent resolution over 4-6 weeks
• Scarring may result from the skin involvement
• Blindness or corneal opacities may occur in 7-20% of patients
• The mortality rate for untreated cases is 5-15%
• Risk of recurrence may be as high as 37%

MISCELLANEOUS

ASSOCIATED CONDITIONS
• Any of the infections or diseases listed under Causes may be associated with Stevens-Johnson syndrome
• Toxic epidermal necrolysis
• Erythema multiforme (directly related, but a milder form of the disease)
• Mycoplasma pneumonia

AGE-RELATED FACTORS
Pediatric: More severe forms of the disease tend to occur in younger males. Rare under age 3 years.
Geriatric: Rare over age 50 years
Others: N/A

PREGNANCY
Reported as a possible etiologic condition

SYNONYMS
• Ectodermosis erosiva pluriorificialis
• Febrile mucocutaneous syndrome
• Herpes iris
• Erythema polymorphe

ICD-9-CM 695.1 Stevens-Johnson syndrome

SEE ALSO
• Erythema multiforme
• Pemphigus vulgaris
• Pemphigoid, bullous
• Serum sickness

OTHER NOTES
Because it is an immunologic reaction, drug related disease will not occur until 7-14 days after first exposure to the offending agent. Subsequent exposure may cause reaction to occur more quickly.

ABBREVIATIONS N/A

REFERENCES
• Fitzpatrick TB, et al, eds: Dermatology. In General Medicine. 3rd Ed. New York, McGraw-Hill, 1987
• Moschella SL, Hurley HJ: Dermatology. 3rd Ed. Philadelphia, W.B. Saunders Co., 1992
• Domonkos AN, Arnold HL, Odom RB: Andrews' Diseases of the Skin. 8th Ed. Philadelphia, W.B. Saunders Co., 1990
Illustrations: 2 available on CD-ROM
Internet references: http://www.5mcc.com

Author(s)
Marc LeDuc, MD
Mitchell S. King, MD

Stokes-Adams attacks

BASICS

DESCRIPTION Syncope due to transient complete heart block and resulting severe bradycardia or asystole with hypotension
System(s) affected: Cardiovascular, Nervous
Genetics: No known genetic pattern
Incidence/Prevalence in USA: Undocumented
Predominant age: Most commonly, greater than 40 years of age
Predominant sex: Male = Female

SIGNS AND SYMPTOMS
• Acute bradycardia
• Hypotension
• Paleness
• Altered sensorium or loss of consciousness, unrelated to position or exertion
• Acute onset of syncopal or near syncopal symptoms (with or without palpitations)

CAUSES
• Medications:
  ◊ Calcium channel blockers
  ◊ Beta blockers
  ◊ Sotolol
  ◊ Digoxin
  ◊ Clonidine
• Other causes:
  ◊ Myocardial ischemia involving the AV node
  ◊ Infiltrative or fibrosing diseases involving the heart and its conduction system
  ◊ Degeneration of the AV node secondary to aging
  ◊ Neuromuscular diseases (e.g., myotonic muscular dystrophy or Kearns-Sayre syndrome)

RISK FACTORS
• Use of the above mentioned medications
• Coronary artery disease
• History of previous AV nodal dysfunction
• Acute myocardial infarction (especially acute right coronary artery occlusion)
• Amyloidosis
• Chagas' disease
• Connective tissue diseases involving the heart (e.g., systemic lupus erythematosus, rheumatoid arthritis)

DIAGNOSIS

DIFFERENTIAL DIAGNOSIS
• Seizures
• Transient ischemia attacks
• Orthostatic hypotension
• Vasovagal attacks
• Neurocardiogenic syncope
• Cardiac arrhythmias
  ◊ Ventricular tachycardia
  ◊ Supraventricular tachycardia
  ◊ Re-entrant tachycardia
  ◊ Wolff-Parkinson-White syndrome
  ◊ Sinus arrest
  ◊ Sinus exit block
  ◊ "Sick-sinus syndrome"
  ◊ Transition from normal sinus rhythm to atrial fibrillation or from atrial fibrillation to normal sinus rhythm

LABORATORY
• Serum digoxin level
• Cardiac enzymes
Drugs that may alter lab results: None
Disorders that may alter lab results: Transient or long-standing renal failure may falsely elevate cardiac enzymes (creatine kinase)

PATHOLOGICAL FINDINGS N/A

SPECIAL TESTS N/A

IMAGING Transthoracic cardiac 2d-echo if infiltrative disease is suspected

DIAGNOSTIC PROCEDURES
• Cardiac coronary catheterization to rule out coronary ischemia
• Electrophysiologic testing to assess status of AV nodal conduction
• Myocardial biopsy if infiltrative disease is suspected
• ECG, event monitor or Holter monitor demonstrating (transient) complete heart block with slow or no ventricular escape

TREATMENT

APPROPRIATE HEALTH CARE
• Inpatient assessment in a monitored setting
• Continuing treatment - ambulatory

GENERAL MEASURES
• Cardiac monitoring
• Trans-thoracic pacer availability
• Atropine by the bedside

SURGICAL MEASURES
• Consider temporary pacemaker placement
• Permanent pacemaker placement, if etiology of transient complete heart block not reversible

ACTIVITY As tolerated after assessment

DIET Regular

PATIENT EDUCATION Once the diagnosis has been made and pacemaker has been implanted (if indicated) patient should be instructed in pacemaker guidelines

MEDICATIONS

DRUG(S) OF CHOICE
• For symptomatic bradyarrhythmias:
◊ For acute bradyarrhythmias - atropine, 1 mg IV push to be given during the complete heart block with hypotension; may be repeated once for a total dosage of 2 mg
◊ Epinephrine, 1 mg 1:10,000 IV push to be given during the complete heart block if associated with asystole; may be repeated every 5 minutes
◊ Isoproterenol drip,1 mg in 250 cc D5W or normal saline to be started at 5 micrograms per minute if patient maintains bradycardia and hypotensive after atropine given; may titrate drip as necessary
Contraindications: Use of epinephrine in bradycardia patient with a normal blood pressure may precipitate hypertensive crisis
Precautions: Possible tachycardiac response to the above mentioned medications
Significant possible interactions: None

ALTERNATIVE DRUGS   N/A

FOLLOWUP

PATIENT MONITORING
• Routine pacemaker checks, if permanent pacemaker implanted
• Followup Holter and/or event, monitor within two weeks after causal medications have been discontinued
• Discontinuation of driving, heavy machinery operation and being at unprotected heights pending normal followup

PREVENTION/AVOIDANCE   Avoidance of taking any drug similar to those causing the complete heart block

POSSIBLE COMPLICATIONS
• Protracted bradycardia with hypotension leading to end-organ damage or death
• Loss of consciousness while operating machinery or at unprotected heights

EXPECTED COURSE/PROGNOSIS
Once diagnosis is made and appropriate treatment is implemented (e.g., pacemaker insertion), prognosis is excellent and further difficulty not expected

MISCELLANEOUS

ASSOCIATED CONDITIONS
• Myocardial ischemia
• Acute myocardial infarction
• Systemic manifestations of connective tissue disease
• Unreliable self-administration of medications
• Neuromuscular disease

AGE-RELATED FACTORS
Pediatric: N/A
Geriatric: More common problem in this age group
Others: N/A

PREGNANCY   Rare during pregnancy

SYNONYMS   Drop attacks

ICD-9-CM
426.9 Stokes-Adams syndrome

SEE ALSO
• Seizure disorders
• Sinus bradycardia
• Complete heart block
• Myocardial infarction
• Amyloidosis

OTHER NOTES   N/A

ABBREVIATIONS   N/A

REFERENCES
• Brandenburg RO, Fuster V, Giuliani ER, McGoon DC: Cardiology: Fundamentals and Practice. Chicago, Year Book Medical Publishers, 1987
• Braunwald E, ed: Heart Disease: A Textbook of Cardiovascular Medicine. 4th Ed. Philadelphia, W.B. Saunders Co., 1992
Illustrations: N/A
Internet references: http://www.5mcc.com

Author(s)
David J. Framm, MD, FACC

Stomatitis

BASICS

DESCRIPTION Generalized inflammation of the oral mucosa of many possible etiologies
System(s) affected: Skin/Exocrine
Genetics: N/A
Incidence/Prevalence in USA:
• Herpetic stomatitis, hand-foot-and-mouth disease, and recurrent aphthous stomatitis are very common
• Herpangina is fairly common as are nicotinic and denture related stomatitis. The remaining causes are uncommon or rare.
Predominant age:
• Herpetic-primary infections - children
• Hand-foot-and-mouth disease - children
• Vincent's stomatitis - teenagers and young adults
• Behçet's disease - young adults
• Herpangina - children
• Others - N/A
Predominant sex: Male = Female

SIGNS AND SYMPTOMS
• General:
  ◊ Depends on etiology
  ◊ Varies from minimal to severe pain
  ◊ Many have multiple intraoral ulcers from 1 mm to several centimeters in diameter
  ◊ Some with constitutional symptoms - fever, malaise, headache
• Allergic stomatitis:
  ◊ Intense shiny erythema
  ◊ Slight swelling
  ◊ Itching
  ◊ Dryness
  ◊ Burning
• Vincent's infection:
  ◊ Necrotic ulceration of interdental papillae and mucous membrane
• Thrush (candidiasis):
  ◊ White patches, slightly raised (resembling milk curds)
  ◊ Distribution - tongue, buccal mucosa, palate, gums, tonsils, larynx, pharynx, GI tract, skin; commonly seen in infants, immunocompromised patients; patients on long-term antibiotics, corticosteroids, and anti-neoplastic treatment
• Pseudomembraneous stomatitis:
  ◊ Membrane-like exudate
• Mucous lesions accompanying systemic disease:
  ◊ Mucous patches (syphilis)
  ◊ Strawberry (measles)
  ◊ Koplik's spots (measles)
  ◊ Ulcers (erythema multiforme)
  ◊ Smooth, fire-red, painful (pellagra)

CAUSES
• Allergy - foods, drugs, contact (some erythema multiforme)
• Vitamin deficiency - riboflavin (angular stomatitis)
• Viral - herpes simplex I and II (herpetic stomatitis), Coxsackie A (herpangina and hand-foot-and-mouth disease)
• Smoking (nicotinic stomatitis)
• Hormonal (possibly recurrent ulcerative stomatitis)
• Uncertain (recurrent aphthous stomatitis, Vincent's stomatitis, recurrent scarifying stomatitis, Behçet's disease, angular stomatitis, gangrenous stomatitis, erythema multiforme)
• Bacterial (scarlatina)
• Uremic (uremic/nephritic)
• Dentures

RISK FACTORS Listed with Causes

DIAGNOSIS

DIFFERENTIAL DIAGNOSIS
• Herpetic stomatitis
• Hand-foot-and-mouth disease
• Recurrent aphthous stomatitis
• Vincent's stomatitis
• Nicotinic stomatitis
• Denture related stomatitis
• Erythema multiforme/Stevens-Johnson syndrome
• Recurrent ulcerative stomatitis
• Recurrent scarifying stomatitis
• Behçet's disease
• Angular stomatitis
• Noma (gangrenous stomatitis)
• Scarlatina (scarlet fever)
• Herpangina
• Uremic

LABORATORY
• Hematologic profile
• Tzanck test of historic interest only
• Serologic test for syphilis
Drugs that may alter lab results: N/A
Disorders that may alter lab results: N/A

PATHOLOGICAL FINDINGS Biopsy suspicious lesions or lesions that fail to heal or chronically recur to rule out cancer or vasculitis

SPECIAL TESTS N/A

IMAGING N/A

DIAGNOSTIC PROCEDURES Biopsy if persistent/recurrent/suspicious

TREATMENT

APPROPRIATE HEALTH CARE
Outpatient, unless severe

GENERAL MEASURES
• In most cases treatment is symptomatic only
• Severe cases may require parenteral fluids, particularly in children
• Topical anesthesia
• Analgesics
• Oral rinses such as 1/2 strength hydrogen peroxide
• Mycostatin, if superinfected with candida
• Stop smoking

SURGICAL MEASURES N/A

ACTIVITY As tolerated by patient

DIET May need to avoid spicy, sharp, hard, and dry foods

PATIENT EDUCATION Griffith: Instructions for Patients; Philadelphia, W.B. Saunders Co.

MEDICATIONS

DRUG(S) OF CHOICE
- Steroids and cytotoxic drugs for Behçet's disease
- 2% viscous lidocaine (Xylocaine) for local discomfort
- Liquid diphenhydramine (Benadryl) po, or swish and spit
- Antibiotics for gangrenous stomatitis
- Antifungal ointment, e.g., nystatin (Mycostatin) for candida complicating angular stomatitis
- For candidiasis - nystatin oral suspension 400,000 units (4 mL) qid for 10 days. Use as oral rinse, then swallow.

Contraindications: Allergy to specific medication

Precautions: Toxic dose of topical lidocaine uncertain, but likely only 25-33% of infiltration dose - may have significant absorption from open ulcers or mucous membrane

Significant possible interactions: Refer to manufacturer's literature

ALTERNATIVE DRUGS
Steroid oral rinses or topical preparations for aphthous ulcers

FOLLOWUP

PATIENT MONITORING Lesions need to be followed until resolved. If they fail to resolve, continuously recur, or appear suspicious, biopsy may be needed to establish a diagnosis.

PREVENTION/AVOIDANCE Avoid causative factors

POSSIBLE COMPLICATIONS
- Recurrent scarifying stomatitis may result in intraoral scarring with restriction of oral mobility
- Behçet's disease may result in visual loss, pneumonia, colitis, vasculitis, large artery aneurysms, thrombophlebitis, or encephalitis
- Gangrenous stomatitis may lead to death
- Scarlet fever may result in cardiac disease
- Herpetic stomatitis may be complicated by ocular or CNS involvement

EXPECTED COURSE/PROGNOSIS
- Herpetic - self-limited with resolution in 7-14 days
- Hand-foot-and-mouth disease - same as herpetic
- Recurrent aphthous - 7-14 day course per episode
- Vincent's - may progress to fascial space infection with airway compromise or sepsis
- Nicotinic - will resolve with cessation of smoking
- Denture - will resolve with careful oral hygiene and daytime denture wear only
- Erythema multiforme - resolution in 2-3 weeks
- Stevens-Johnson - resolution in about 6 weeks with adequate supportive care
- Recurrent ulcerative - as the name implies, these recur over time, but the overall prognosis is good
- Recurrent scarifying - occasional patients suffer continuous ulcers, others recur with eventual scarring. The prognosis is otherwise good.
- Behçet's disease - may recur for several years. Prognosis for vision is poor. Overall prognosis is related to other aspects of the disease.
- Angular - after correction of mechanical problems, allergic disorders, and nutritional deficiencies the prognosis is good
- Gangrenous - this is the most serious stomatitis, requiring aggressive treatment with IV antibiotics and débridement to avoid death
- Scarlatina - the prognosis is related to other manifestations of the disease
- Herpangina - 7-14 day course with total resolution
- Uremic - depends on the underlying renal disease

MISCELLANEOUS

ASSOCIATED CONDITIONS AIDS - associated with severe lesions

AGE-RELATED FACTORS
Pediatric: Certain etiologies more likely in the pediatric population: Herpetic-primary, hand-foot-and-mouth disease, herpangina
Geriatric: Certain etiologies more likely in the geriatric population, e.g., dentures
Others: N/A

PREGNANCY May bring on recurrent ulcerative stomatitis

SYNONYMS N/A

ICD-9-CM 528.0
- Herpetic - 054.2
- Hand-foot-and-mouth disease - 282.61
- Aphthous - 528.2
- Vincent's - 101
- Denture - 528.9
- Erythema multiforme/Stevens-Johnson syndrome - 695.1
- Ulcerative - 101
- Behçet's syndrome - 136.1
- Angular - 528.5
- Gangrenous - 528.1
- Scarlet Fever - 034.1
- Herpangina - 074.0
- Viral (epidemic) - 078.4
- Candidal - 112.0
- Secondary to vitamin or dietary deficiency - 266.0

SEE ALSO N/A

OTHER NOTES N/A

ABBREVIATIONS N/A

REFERENCES
- Moran WJ: Diseases of the mouth. In: Rakel E, ed. Conn's Current Therapy, Philadelphia, W.B. Saunders Co., 1990
- Teele DW: Inflammatory diseases of the mouth and pharynx. In: Paparella MM, Shumrick DA, eds. Otolaryngology. Philadelphia, W.B. Saunders Co., 1980:974-1017

Illustrations: 11 available on CD-ROM
Internet references: http://www.5mcc.com

Author(s)
Douglas M. Hoy, MD

Stroke (Brain attack)

BASICS

DESCRIPTION The sudden onset of a focal neurological deficit resulting from either infarction or hemorrhage within the brain
System(s) affected: Nervous, Cardiovascular
Genetics: Inheritance is polygenic with a tendency to clustering of risk factors within families
Incidence/Prevalence in USA: Overall incidence 160/100,000 (age 50-65, 1000/100,000; > 80, 3000/100,000). Prevalence 135/100,000.
Predominant age: Risk increases over age 45 and is highest in the seventh and eighth decades
Predominant sex: Male > Female (3:1)

SIGNS AND SYMPTOMS
• Carotid circulation (hemispheric): Hemiplegia, hemianesthesia, neglect, aphasia, visual field defects; less often headaches, seizures, amnesia, confusion
• Vertebrobasilar (brainstem or cerebellar): Diplopia, vertigo, ataxia, facial paresis, Horner's syndrome, dysphagia, dysarthria
• Impaired level of consciousness
• Cerebellar lesion in patients with headache, nausea, vomiting and ataxia

CAUSES
• Ischemic: Carotid atherosclerotic disease with artery-to-artery thromboembolism
• Cardiac: Cardioembolism secondary to valvular (mitral valve) pathology; mural hypokinesias or akinesias with thrombosis (acute anterior myocardial infarctions or congestive cardiomyopathies); cardiac arrhythmia (atrial fibrillation)
• Hypercoagulable states: Antiphospholipid antibodies, deficiency of protein S, protein C; presence of antithrombin 3, oral contraceptives
• Other causes: Spontaneous and post-traumatic (i.e., chiropractic manipulation) artery dissection, fibromuscular dysplasia, vasculitis, drugs (cocaine, amphetamines)
• Hemorrhagic
• Hypertension: may cause damage to putamen, internal capsule, cerebellum, brainstem, corona radiata
• Amyloid (congophylic) angiopathy: Lobar (cortical) hemorrhages in the elderly
• Vascular malformations: Arteriovenous malformation, cavernous angioma, venous angioma and capillary angioma

RISK FACTORS
• Age
• Hypertension
• Cardiac disease
• Smoking
• Diabetes
• Antiphospholipid antibodies
• Family history

DIAGNOSIS

DIFFERENTIAL DIAGNOSIS
• Migraine
• Focal seizure
• Tumor
• Subdural hematoma
• Hypoglycemia

LABORATORY N/A
Drugs that may alter lab results: N/A
Disorders that may alter lab results: N/A

PATHOLOGICAL FINDINGS N/A

SPECIAL TESTS
• Duplex carotid ultrasonography
• Cerebral angiography
• ECG
• Transthoracic echocardiogram (TTE); if normal and a cardiac source is suspected, followup with transesophageal echocardiogram
• Holter monitoring
• EEG for suspected seizure
• Prothrombin time (PT) and partial thromboplastin time (PTT). Coumadin prolongs PT.
• Antiphospholipid antibodies

IMAGING Acute phase: CT of head to rule out hemorrhage

DIAGNOSTIC PROCEDURES N/A

TREATMENT

APPROPRIATE HEALTH CARE
• Acute phase: Inpatient care
• Surgical therapy: In medically fit patients with non-disabling stroke, carotid endarterectomy is indicated for stenosis of > 70% on side ipsilateral to stroke; medical therapy for < 30% stenosis
• Best therapy for stenosis of 30-70% is unknown; consider a referral to a center involved in North American Symptomatic Carotid Endarterectomy Trial (NASCET)

GENERAL MEASURES
• Maintain oxygenation
• Monitor cardiac rhythm for 48 hours
• Control hyperglycemia (keep glucose < 220 mg/dL [12.1 mmol/L])
• Control of hypertension pressure if > 200/100 mm Hg (26.6/13.3 kPa)
• Prevent hyperthermia
• Early introduction of physiotherapy and ambulation
• Subcutaneous heparin 5,000 units subcutaneously every 12 hours

SURGICAL MEASURES N/A

ACTIVITY Ambulate as soon as possible

DIET
• Alert with no dysphagia: Diet as tolerated (no added salt if hypertensive)
• Alert with dysphagia: Pureed dysphagia diet or nasogastric feeding tube if indicated

PATIENT EDUCATION National Stroke Association, 300 East Hampden Ave., Suite 240, Englewood, CO 80110-2622

MEDICATIONS

DRUG(S) OF CHOICE
• Enteric coated aspirin (EC ASA) 325-1300 mg/day
or
• Ticlopidine (Ticlid) 250 mg po bid
Contraindications:
• EC ASA - active peptic ulcer disease, hypersensitivity to aspirin, patients who had bronchospastic reaction to ASA or other nonsteroidal anti-inflammatory drugs
• Ticlopidine - known hypersensitivity to the drug, presence of hematopoietic disorders, presence of a hemostatic disorder, conditions associated with active bleeding, severe liver dysfunction
Precautions:
• EC ASA - may aggravate pre-existing peptic ulcer disease, may worsen symptoms in some patients with asthma
• Ticlopidine - 2.4% of patients develop neutropenia (0.8% severe neutropenia) which is reversible with cessation of drug; monitor blood counts every 2 weeks for the first 3 months
Significant possible interactions:
• EC ASA - may potentiate effects of anticoagulants and sulfonylurea, hypoglycemic agents
• Ticlopidine - digoxin plasma levels decreased 15%, theophylline half-life increased from 8.6 to 12.2 hours

ALTERNATIVE DRUGS
• Dipyridamole (Persantine) of no proven benefit
• Sulfinpyrazone (Anturane) of no proven benefit
• Nimodipine and nicardipine have been useful when given early in some patients

FOLLOWUP

PATIENT MONITORING   Follow every 3 months for first year then yearly

PREVENTION/AVOIDANCE
• Stop smoking
• Control blood pressure, diabetes, hyperlipidemia
• EC ASA 650 mg bid or ticlopidine 250 mg po bid for patients with prior transient ischemic attack
• Use alcohol in moderation, if at all
• Regular exercise
• Maintain positive psychological outlook
• Maintain weight control

POSSIBLE COMPLICATIONS
• Shoulder subluxation
• Hyperextension knee injury
• Depression
• Sympathetic dystrophy

EXPECTED COURSE/PROGNOSIS
• Variable depending on severity of stroke
• Posterior circulation strokes have a higher acute mortality rate but generally make a better functional recovery than hemispheric strokes

MISCELLANEOUS

ASSOCIATED CONDITIONS   Major cause of death in first five years after a stroke is cardiac disease

AGE-RELATED FACTORS
Pediatric:
• Cardiac (especially developmental abnormalities)
• Metabolic: Homocystinuria, Fabry's disease
Geriatric: Amyloid (congophylic) angiopathy is most prevalent in elderly, especially if patient also has dementia
Others: Adults < 45 years old most likely to have a cardiac source of embolism

PREGNANCY
• Parturition may increase risk of rupture for aneurysm; amniotic fluid embolism may cause stroke at time of delivery
• Postpartum period associated with increased risk for cerebral venous thrombosis

SYNONYMS
• Cerebrovascular accident
• CVA
• Reversible ischemic neurological accident
• RIND

ICD-9-CM
436

SEE ALSO
• Transient ischemic attack (TIA)
• Stroke rehabilitation

OTHER NOTES   N/A

ABBREVIATIONS
EC ASA = enteric-coated aspirin

REFERENCES
• Hachinski V, Norris JW: The Acute Stroke. Philadelphia, F.A. Davis, 1985
• Barnett JHM, Mohr JP, Stein BM., Yatsu FM, eds: Stroke. New York, Churchill Livingstone, 1986
• Norris JW, Hachinski VC: Prevention of Stroke. Philadelphia, F.A. Davis, 1991
Illustrations: N/A
Internet references: http://www.5mcc.com

Author(s)
Carmelo Graffagnino, MD, FRCP
Vladimir Hachinski, MD, DSc, FRCP

Stroke rehabilitation

BASICS

DESCRIPTION Stroke rehabilitation involves restoration of function after medical and neurologic stability have been achieved
• Cerebrovascular diseases and/or disorders that affect central nervous system function by compromising delivery of blood or by hemorrhage resulting in ischemia, necrosis and gliosis
• Anterior lesions in the cerebrovascular system affect the arteries that supply the cerebral hemispheres and cause thrombotic strokes
• Posterior lesions affect arteries that supply the brain stem and yield crossed motor and/or sensory signs and symptoms
• Both anterior and posterior lesions can cause sudden death, but the lower in the central nervous system the lesion, or the more incomplete the lesion, or the more hemorrhagic the lesion, the higher the chance for neurologic return
System(s) affected: Nervous, Cardiovascular
Genetics: Similar to the probability of developing hypertension or coronary artery disease
Incidence/Prevalence in USA: 459/100,000
Predominant age: Over 45
Predominant sex: Male > Female

SIGNS AND SYMPTOMS
• Variable - depends upon the arterial system affected
• Hemiparesis
• Hemianesthesia
• Unilateral central facial palsy
• Homonymous hemianopsia
• Aphasia, apraxia (if the dominant cerebral hemisphere is involved)

CAUSES
• Coronary artery disease
• Hypertension
• Cerebral arteriosclerosis
• Cardiac thrombus embolus
• Foreign body embolus
• Frequently, the combination of gout, diabetes, hypertension has been untreated for some 5-10 years before the onset of the stroke disorder
• aneurysms and arteriovenous malformations

RISK FACTORS
• Many are lifestyle oriented and preventable. Factors include coffee ingestion, cigarette smoking, obesity, inactivity, hyperactivity to the point of exhaustion, emotional lability, sexual hyperactivity, starvation, antidepressant or diet reduction medication, alcohol or recreational drug habituation, unusual stress states.
• Ethnicity may be a risk factor but relationships to factors above first must be clarified

DIAGNOSIS

DIFFERENTIAL DIAGNOSIS
• Infection, tumor, bleeding disorders, endocrinologic, metabolic, gastrointestinal, toxic, etc.
• Different types of stroke disorders can occur in one patient

LABORATORY
• CBC
• Spinal fluid for routine studies (only if indicated)
• Urinalysis
• RPR
• ANA for collagen vascular disorders
• Consider quantitative immunoelectrophoresis with the combination of stroke disorders, anemia, hypertension
• Carotid flow studies
Drugs that may alter lab results: N/A
Disorders that may alter lab results: N/A

PATHOLOGICAL FINDINGS Thrombotic, hemorrhagic, mixed, combinations can be present

SPECIAL TESTS
• Somatosensory, auditory, and visual evoked potential technology can monitor neurologic recovery.
• EEG sometimes useful in evaluating seizure disorders

IMAGING
• Scanning - CT, MRI and PET scanning give good data about anatomy, blood flow, and metabolic activity
• Serial exams can delineate the course of this disease

DIAGNOSTIC PROCEDURES
• Spinal taps, myelography, pneumoencephalography, angiography all have special indications and contraindications at this time. None are routinely used.
• Electrodiagnosis for neuritis, radiculitis in specialized centers if available
• Endovascular procedures have great diagnostic implications.

TREATMENT

APPROPRIATE HEALTH CARE
Referral to a full service rehabilitation center - a rehabilitation medicine team can make the difference between independence and dependency. Refer when medically and neurologically stable.

GENERAL MEASURES
• Full service rehabilitation center characteristics: Comparison with national standards for admission, process, discharge, and followup care; closed units; regular team meetings to discuss long and short term objectives; quality assurance system in place; accreditation by Commission on Accreditation of Rehabilitation Facilities.
• Use heat with caution in patients with stroke or atherosclerotic vascular disease because of reduced sensation
• Use hydrotherapy and/or isometric exercise cautiously in patients with limited cardiopulmonary reserve
• In patients able to respond to the protocols after surgery, restorative, tendon transplant, or nerve transplants may be of value
• Cardiac precautions and a CPR team may be required during exercise programs since obese, hypertensive, or patients with coronary artery disease are at increased risk. Real-time monitoring might be required.
• Open units, especially in investor owned rehabilitation centers, need to be closely monitored for outcome and cost/benefit ratio type productivity quality
• Inpatient rehab in acute rehab units for 15-21 days after first uncomplicated strokes

SURGICAL MEASURES
• Microcatheter and microsurgical technology have been used to clip, embolize or reset aneurysms and other lesions.
• Applied cardioangiographic technology has generated new endovascular treatment procedures.

ACTIVITY
• Physical therapy, occupational therapy, speech pathology, psychology, nursing therapy should be delivered to the patient for at least three hours/day throughout the inpatient stay.
• The patient must be able to tolerate this vigorous activity level. If the patient becomes medically or neurologically unstable during the inpatient stay, a 48 hour leeway is usually built into the system. After that period, therapy must resume or the patient must be returned to an acute hospital bed. Most stroke rehabilitation units are usually able to deliver this type of functional return within one month of inpatient stay, although length of stay is individually determined.
• While most rehabilitative efforts take place within a very short time after ictus, successful rehabilitative efforts have taken place as long as five years later

DIET Depends upon other medical conditions

PATIENT EDUCATION
• Stroke is usually an unnecessary illness. Major risk factors are nearly all preventable. The difficulty that arises is that the patient's life style must be changed. Patients mount a great deal of active and passive resistance.
• The progressive physical and mental deterioration noted with hypertension and/or coronary artery disease is not inevitable
• Family pressure and support is helpful to interest the patient in his/her health in a consistent and sustained manner
• Disuse will add subsequent complications and sequelae
• Second complex strokes - patients with second ictus and/or renal failure, heart failure or cor pulmonale might require 20-30 days inpatient rehab in a skilled nursing facility before disposition

MEDICATIONS

DRUG(S) OF CHOICE
• Use only what is absolutely necessary. Sleeping medications, such as flurazepam, can accumulate over time in stroke patients.
• As needed for underlying disorders (e.g., hypertension, heart disease) or for complications (e.g., seizures, deep vein thrombosis, pneumonitis).
• Once neurological and medical stability have been achieved, depression can be treated with a serotonin inhibitor antidepressant, e.g., sertraline HCL 50 mg every morning.
Contraindications: Refer to manufacturer's profile of each drug
Precautions:
• Four or more medications will often have interactions; polypharmacy is frequent
• Antihypertensive medication can generate orthostatic hypotension
• Antidepressant medication can lower the seizure threshold and interact with antihypertensive medications
• Muscle relaxants, tranquilizers, major neuroleptic medication can confuse, delay return of memory and cognition, sedate, occasionally agitate, and obliterate spontaneous thought
• Unnecessary medications should be withdrawn
• Elderly patients regularly require lower dosages
Significant possible interactions: Refer to manufacturer's profile of each drug

ALTERNATIVE DRUGS
• Reflex sympathetic dystrophy (shoulder-hand syndrome) - can be treated with a series of seven stellate ganglion blocks
• Flexor spasms in spasticity - to help control, dantrolene sodium 25 mg po qid, diazepam 5 mg bid and/or baclofen 10 mg tid
• For spasticity in those not tolerating systemic medication: either intrathecal baclofen by pump or botulinum toxin IM administration

FOLLOWUP

PATIENT MONITORING
• Within the month following discharge, the patient and family should be seen in an outpatient group "alumni" day coordinated with an interdisciplinary outpatient clinic appointment
• If outpatient therapy is rendered, the team therapist(s) should meet with the physician regularly to rate progress and discuss long- and short-term objectives
• For first uncomplicated stroke patients - once the acute rehab is completed, the rest of the rehab can be accomplished as an outpatient or in a day care program

PREVENTION/AVOIDANCE See Risk factors and Patient education

POSSIBLE COMPLICATIONS
• Reflex sympathetic dystrophy syndromes - such as hand/shoulder syndrome - are nonspecific complications and last for 12 weeks before subsiding to adhesive capsulitis
• Tendonitis-bursitis-capsulitis may coexist with prolonged paralysis. Prolonged range-of-motion and neuromuscular re-education exercises help retard functional deterioration of the limb. Electrical stimulation and biofeedback for control and relaxation have also been used, but the treatment of choice is restoration of function.
• Diabetes, alcohol intake will add peripheral neuritis
• Many patients develop osteoporosis - especially on side of paresis. The normal side can develop osteoarthritis.

EXPECTED COURSE/PROGNOSIS
• Generally good, although pneumonia, respiratory failure, heart failure, and myocardial infarction occur more frequently after stroke
• Outcome studies have shown that acute rehab center programs generate 33% more functional improvement than comparable skilled nursing facilities, but tend to also cost more to health maintenance organizations

MISCELLANEOUS

ASSOCIATED CONDITIONS
• Hypertension
• Coronary artery disease
• Diabetes mellitus
• Gout
• Atherosclerosis
• Smoking
• Alcoholism

AGE-RELATED FACTORS
Pediatric: Aneurysms, hypertension, tumors, trauma
Geriatric: Heart disease, vascular disease, hypertension
Others: See Risk factors

PREGNANCY Hypertension in pregnancy can lead to stroke

SYNONYMS N/A

ICD-9-CM 438/(3429)/(7843) Late effects of cerebrovascular disease

SEE ALSO
• Stroke (Brain attack)

OTHER NOTES N/A

ABBREVIATIONS N/A

REFERENCES
• Clinchot DM, Kaplan PE, et al: Cerebral aneurysms and arteriovenous malformations. Arch Phys Med Rehabil 1994;75:1342-51
• Clinchot DM, Bogner JA, Kaplan PE: Cerebral aneurysms. Arch Phys Med Rehabil 1997;78:346-349
• Kaplan PE, Cerallo LJ, eds: Stroke Rehabilitation. Boston, Butterworth, 1986
Illustrations: N/A
Internet references: http://www.5mcc.com

Author(s)
Paul E. Kaplan, MD

Subarachnoid hemorrhage

 BASICS

DESCRIPTION Subarachnoid hemorrhage is the extravasation of blood into the subarachnoid space particularly of the basal cisterns and into the cerebral spinal fluid pathways.
• Traumatic: More common and it is related to head trauma
• Spontaneous: Rare. 50-60% of spontaneous subarachnoid hemorrhages are due to intracranial saccular aneurysms.
Incidence/Prevalence in USA:
Spontaneous: Incidence is 10.9/100,000 per year
System(s) affected: Nervous
Genetics: N/A
Predominant age:
• The majority of subarachnoid hemorrhages due to aneurysms occur in the fourth to seventh decades
• Subarachnoid hemorrhage due to arteriovenous (AV) malformation appears more commonly in the second, third, and fourth decades
Predominant Sex: Subarachnoid hemorrhage due to aneurysm occurs slightly more commonly in females (55%).

SIGNS AND SYMPTOMS
• Abrupt onset of headache associated with stiff neck and photophobia
• May or may not lose consciousness
• May develop focal neurological deficits such as hemiparesis or a dilated pupil
• Subhyaloid hemorrhages are more common in anterior communicating artery aneurysms

CAUSES
• Trauma
• Intracranial saccular aneurysm
• Intracranial A-V malformation
• Hypertension
• Rarely tumors and blood dyscrasias.

RISK FACTORS
• Intracranial aneurysms associated with coarctation of the aorta
• AV malformations
• Polycystic disease of the kidneys
• Fibromuscular dysplasia of the renal arteries
• Hypertension is not necessarily associated with saccular aneurysms, but is associated with rupture of an existing aneurysm

 DIAGNOSIS

DIFFERENTIAL DIAGNOSIS
• Intracerebral hematomas
• Meningitis
• Acute (usually first) migrainous attacks and thunderclap headaches

LABORATORY N/A
Drugs that may alter lab results: N/A
Disorders that may alter lab results: N/A

PATHOLOGICAL FINDINGS N/A

SPECIAL TESTS N/A

IMAGING
• CT scan:
◊ The diagnosis is established in more than 95% of the cases with a CT scan. This demonstrates blood in the basal cisterns and may help in localizing the source of hemorrhage.
◊ It also can rule out mass effect so that if this study is negative a spinal puncture can be safely performed
◊ A small percentage of subarachnoid hemorrhages will be missed on the CT scan
• Cerebral angiography
◊ Following the establishment of the diagnosis of subarachnoid hemorrhage, it is imperative to find out the source of bleeding, therefore, cerebral angiography is used to identify the source of hemorrhage such as a saccular aneurysm or AV malformation
• Other
◊ It must be remembered that occasional hemorrhage may occur from an AV malformation of the spinal cord or a vascular tumor in the spinal arachnoid space. Therefore, if no source of subarachnoid hemorrhage is found intracranially, consideration might be made for studies involving the subarachnoid space which would include MRI spinal scanning or myelography.

DIAGNOSTIC PROCEDURES See above

 TREATMENT

APPROPRIATE HEALTH CARE Initial therapy is carried out in the Intensive Care Unit

GENERAL MEASURES
• The treatment is directed to prevent complications of subarachnoid hemorrhage which include rebleeding, hydrocephalus, and cerebral vasospasm
• Vasospasm is treated with generous volume expansion and hypertension to promote cerebral perfusion after the aneurysm has been obliterated. This is not wise if an aneurysm is untreated.
• Once the patient has stabilized and recovered from the initial hemorrhage, then a vigorous rehabilitation program is indicated

SURGICAL MEASURES
• If the source of hemorrhage such as an aneurysm can be readily obliterated, this reduces the risk of rebleeding and allows more vigorous treatment with fluid and hypertensive therapy of cerebral vasospasm
• Hydrocephalus should be treated with cerebral spinal fluid drainage and may require permanent shunting procedures
• AV malformations may be obliterated with embolization and surgery
• Radiosurgery shows promise in the treatment of small deep AV malformations
• Endovascular obliteration of aneurysms is being performed in selected centers

ACTIVITY Strict bedrest until source of hemorrhage is eliminated

DIET N/A

PATIENT EDUCATION N/A

MEDICATIONS

DRUG(S) OF CHOICE
• Nimodipine
◊ Has been used at 60 mg q4h for the prevention of cerebral vasospasm
◊ Therapy should begin as soon as possible
◊ The capsule contents may be given via NG tube if patient can't swallow
Contraindications: Hypotension is contraindication in patients with vasospasm
Precautions:
• Quiet room
• Reduce stress
• Control blood pressure until source of hemorrhage eliminated
• Stool softeners to prevent straining
Significant possible interactions: Refer to manufacturer's profile

ALTERNATIVE DRUGS Nicardipine

FOLLOWUP

PATIENT MONITORING As needed

PREVENTION/AVOIDANCE Incidental aneurysms have a risk of hemorrhage of 2% per year so prophylactic surgery may be indicated

POSSIBLE COMPLICATIONS
• Death
• Paralysis

EXPECTED COURSE/PROGNOSIS
• Approximately 25-30% of the patients will die from a spontaneous subarachnoid hemorrhage due to an aneurysm. The highest morbidity is secondary to cerebral vasospasm.
• If the aneurysm can be successfully clipped and the vasospasm treated effectively, satisfactory outcome occurs in approximately 50-65% of patients
• Approximately 25-30% of aneurysms will be multiple. It is advisable to treat multiple aneurysms during the same operative procedure, but if this is not possible, surgery is directed at the aneurysm most likely to have hemorrhaged.
• Further surgical procedures may be necessary to obliterate additional aneurysms
• AV malformations do not have as high morbidity and mortality associated with the hemorrhage. Both untreated aneurysms and AV malformations are likely to bleed at about 2% per year. Therefore in the younger age groups, incidentally found A-V malformations and aneurysms may require aggressive treatment.

MISCELLANEOUS

ASSOCIATED CONDITIONS N/A

AGE-RELATED FACTORS
Pediatric: N/A
Geriatric: In the elderly patient, incidental aneurysms and AV malformations may best be followed since the chance of hemorrhage is only 2% per year
Others: In younger and middle-aged people, surgery is recommended

PREGNANCY
In the pregnant female, increased blood pressure and blood volume may predispose to hemorrhages. Under life-threatening situations, surgical procedures can be performed on a pregnant patient. However, with AV malformations, a less lethal lesion compared to aneurysms it may be worthwhile to allow the pregnancy go to term.

SYNONYMS N/A

ICD-9-CM
• 430 Subarachnoid hemorrhage
• 852 Subarachnoid, subdural, and extradural hemorrhage, following injury

OTHER NOTES N/A

ABBREVIATIONS
AV = arteriovenous

REFERENCES
• Weir B, ed: Aneurysm Affecting the Nervous System. Baltimore, Williams & Wilkins, 1987
• Sahs AL, Perret G, Nishioka H, eds: Intracranial and Subarachnoid Hemorrhage: A Cooperative Study. Philadelphia, J.B. Lippincott Co, 1969
• Youmans JR, ed: A Comprehensive Reference Guide to the Diagnosis and Management of Neurosurgical Problems. 3rd Ed. Philadelphia, W.B. Saunders Co., 1990
• Carter LP, Spetzler RF, eds: Neurovascular Surgery. New York, McGraw-Hill, 1995
Illustrations: N/A
Internet references: http://www.5mcc.com

Author(s)
L. Philip Carter, MD

Subclavian steal syndrome

 BASICS

DESCRIPTION Origin of the subclavian artery becomes compromised causing a reversal of flow in the branches of the first portion of the subclavian artery as a means of supplying blood to the upper extremity, especially during exercise. This may result in symptoms of vertebral-basilar insufficiency.
System(s) affected: Cardiovascular, Musculoskeletal, Nervous
Genetics: N/A
Incidence/Prevalence in USA: Unknown, not common; 70% of the time, the left subclavian artery is involved
Predominant age: > 55 years
Predominant sex: Male > Female (2:1)

SIGNS AND SYMPTOMS
• Most common - vertigo or presyncope following upper extremity exercise. The reversal of flow down the ipsilateral vertebral artery results in a relative vertebral-basilar insufficiency
• Less common: - weakness and clumsiness of an extremity, loss of vision, homonymous hemianopsia, ataxia and drop attacks
• Arm claudication following minimal exercise.
• Reduced blood pressure of > 20 mm Hg in involved arm
• Symptoms should be reproducible by exercising the arm

CAUSES
• Arteriosclerosis obliterans of the proximal subclavian artery in 95% of cases
• Less common causes of obstruction: dissecting aneurysm of aortic arch, embolus and Takayasu's arteritis

RISK FACTORS
• Smoking
• Hypertension
• Diabetes

 DIAGNOSIS

DIFFERENTIAL DIAGNOSIS
• Intracranial vascular disease
• Carotid artery disease
• Vertebral artery disease
• Brain tumor
• Subdural hematoma

LABORATORY
• Noninvasive measurement of blood pressure in upper extremities
• Arteriogram of arch vessels with delayed films of vertebral arteries
Drugs that may alter lab results: N/A
Disorders that may alter lab results: N/A

PATHOLOGICAL FINDINGS
• Absent or diminished pulses in ipsilateral arm
• Reduced blood flow (> 20 mm Hg) (> 2.7 kPa) in same arm

SPECIAL TESTS Pulse volume recording of upper extremities

IMAGING
• Duplex scanning of extracranial vessels
• Arteriography

DIAGNOSTIC PROCEDURES
Arteriography

 TREATMENT

APPROPRIATE HEALTH CARE Surgical correction of problem by carotid-subclavian bypass

GENERAL MEASURES None

SURGICAL MEASURES N/A

ACTIVITY Reduced exercise of arms

DIET None

PATIENT EDUCATION
• Prevent injury to arm
• Reduce exercise to arm

MEDICATIONS

DRUG(S) OF CHOICE None
Contraindications: N/A
Precautions: N/A
Significant possible interactions: N/A

ALTERNATIVE DRUGS N/A

FOLLOWUP

PATIENT MONITORING Annual physical to include blood pressure in both arms

PREVENTION/AVOIDANCE N/A

POSSIBLE COMPLICATIONS Completed stroke

EXPECTED COURSE/PROGNOSIS
Good

MISCELLANEOUS

ASSOCIATED CONDITIONS
• Carotid artery disease
• Heart disease
• Arteriosclerosis

AGE-RELATED FACTORS
Pediatric: N/A
Geriatric: Older patient more likely to have arteriosclerosis
Others: N/A

PREGNANCY N/A

SYNONYMS N/A

ICD-9-CM 435.2

SEE ALSO N/A

OTHER NOTES N/A

ABBREVIATIONS N/A

REFERENCES
• Rutherford RB: Vascular Surgery. Philadelphia, W.B. Saunders Co., 1984
• Sabiston DC Jr: Essentials of Surgery. Philadelphia, W.B. Saunders Co., 1987
Illustrations: N/A
Internet references: http://www.5mcc.com

Author(s)
William V. Sharp, MD

Subdural hematoma

BASICS

DESCRIPTION The accumulation of blood in the subdural space

Acute subdural hematoma: The most severe form, usually the result of trauma involving acceleration or deceleration head injury and commonly associated with parenchymal brain injury. Hematoma age is three days or less.

Chronic subdural hematoma: Often the result of trivial head injury in older patients, one-fourth to one-half have no history of head trauma. Hematoma is classically older than three weeks and is associated with an encapsulating membrane.

Subacute subdural hematoma: Appearing 4-21 days from maturation of acute subdural hematoma

System(s) affected: Nervous, Cardiovascular

Genetics: N/A

Incidence/Prevalence in USA:
• Acute subdural hematoma: 1-2/100,000
• Chronic subdural hematoma: 1-2/100,000
• Acute subdural hematoma in newborn infants and children are relatively infrequent, occurring approximately 25% as often as in adults. Chronic subdural hematomas occur in children of all ages. However, chronic subdural hematomas present a peak incidence at about 6 months and rarely, after 1 year of age.

Predominant age:
• Acute subdural hematoma - < age 60 years
• Chronic subdural hematoma - > age 50 years

Predominant sex: Male > Female

SIGNS AND SYMPTOMS
• Acute subdural hematoma:
 ◊ Altered level of consciousness 99%
 ◊ Pupillary irregularity (usually it is unilateral to hematoma) 47-53%
 ◊ Hemiparesis (usually contralateral to hematoma) 34-47%
 ◊ Decerebrate posturing or flaccid motor exam 47%
 ◊ Papilledema 16%
 ◊ Cranial nerve VI palsy 5%
• Chronic subdural hematoma:
 ◊ Impaired consciousness 53%
 ◊ Hemiparesis 45%
 ◊ Papilledema 24%
 ◊ Cranial nerve III abnormality 11%
 ◊ Hemianopsia 7%

CAUSES
• Acute subdural hematoma
 ◊ High velocity acceleration or deceleration head injury resulting in tearing of the bridging veins between cerebral cortex and the dural venous sinuses
 ◊ Bleeding from injured cortical vessels
• Chronic subdural hematoma
 ◊ Often from a trivial head injury in adults and birth trauma or abuse in children. A balance between recurrent bleeding from the hematoma membrane and resorption determines the ultimate size of the hematoma. The osmotic theory of fluid accumulation within the hematoma cavity has been discredited.

RISK FACTORS
• Acute subdural hematoma
 ◊ 0.5-1% of severe head trauma
 ◊ High velocity acceleration or deceleration head injury (motor vehicle accidents, falls, blunt head trauma)
 ◊ Suspected non-accidental trauma (SNAT) in infants
• Chronic subdural hematoma
 ◊ Chronic alcoholism
 ◊ Epilepsy
 ◊ Coagulopathy/anticoagulation therapy
 ◊ Cerebral spinal fluid shunt for hydrocephalus
 ◊ Rarely metastatic carcinoma to subdural space

DIAGNOSIS:

DIFFERENTIAL DIAGNOSIS
• Acute subdural hematoma and other forms of intracranial hematoma (epidural hematoma, cerebral contusion/hematoma)
• Chronic subdural hematoma
• Dementia
• Stroke
• Transient ischemic attack
• Brain tumor
• Subdural empyema
• Meningitis

LABORATORY
• Acute subdural hematoma - consumptive coagulopathy due to underlying parenchymal injury diagnosed with elevated PT and PTT, elevated fibrin degradation products, decreased fibrinogen, decreased platelet level, and extended bleeding time
• Chronic subdural hematoma - predisposing factors such as coagulopathy or anticoagulation therapy producing appropriate abnormalities in bleeding time or coagulation parameters. Subtherapeutic anticonvulsant levels in patients with epilepsy. Serum ethanol level in alcoholics.

Drugs that may alter lab results: Anticoagulants (e.g., warfarin)

Disorders that may alter lab results: DIC and other coagulopathies (e.g., hemophilia)

PATHOLOGICAL FINDINGS
• Acute subdural hematoma - this is a fresh hemorrhage
• Chronic subdural hematoma - there is a liquefied hematoma, an outer membrane beneath the dura after one week, and an inner membrane between the hematoma and arachnoid after three weeks. Cytology examination may reveal metastatic carcinoma cells on rare occasions to be associated with the hemorrhage.

SPECIAL TESTS EEG for seizures and intensive care consisting of continuous cardiac monitoring often in conjunction with continuous monitoring of intra-arterial pressure and intracranial pressure (ventriculostomy or intraparenchymal or subdural pressure monitoring probe)

IMAGING
• Acute subdural hematoma - the imaging study of choice is the CT head scan (with intravascular contrast if hemoglobin is less than or equal to 9 gm/dL)
• Chronic subdural hematoma - a CT head scan is also preferred. An MRI head scan is often necessary for hematomas isodense with brain due to the mixture of chronic hematoma with recurrent hemorrhage.

DIAGNOSTIC PROCEDURES N/A

TREATMENT

APPROPRIATE HEALTH CARE Inpatient

GENERAL MEASURES
• Acute subdural hematoma
 ◊ Medically, the management consists of controlling elevated intracranial pressure with osmotic and loop diuretics and hyperventilation to induce hypocapnia (PaCO2 of 22-28 mm Hg [2.9-3.7 kPa])
• Subacute subdural hematoma
 ◊ Maintenance of adequate airway and ventilation and support of cardiovascular system to promote normal cerebral perfusion
 ◊ Treatment of multi-system trauma and precautions for cervical and other spine injury

SURGICAL MEASURES
• Acute subdural hematoma
 ◊ Emergent craniotomy is indicated for evacuation of hematomas causing significant mass effect
• Subacute subdural hematoma
 ◊ If patient is neurologically stable, surgery may be delayed until hematoma matures and becomes chronic at which time a burr hole drainage can be performed
 ◊ Subacute hematomas causing significant mass effect and neurological deficit may require craniotomy for evacuation
• Chronic subdural hematoma - burr hole drainage of hematoma

ACTIVITY
• Acute subdural hematoma - the patient will need the head of the bed elevated to reduce intracranial pressure and flexion of lower body avoided until thoracic, lumbar, or sacral spine injuries are ruled out. The patient should be maintained in a rigid cervical collar until the cervical spine is cleared radiographically.
• Chronic subdural hematoma - the head of the bed is flat and appropriate precautions are taken if a spinal injury is present

Subdural hematoma

DIET
• Most patients with acute subdural hematoma require enteral or total parenteral nutrition initially
• Depending on level of consciousness, patients with chronic subdural hematoma can usually have the diet advanced to regular food as tolerated

PATIENT EDUCATION The National Institute of Neurological and Communicative Disorders and Stroke (NINDS), The National Institutes of Health, Bethesda, MD 20892

MEDICATIONS

DRUG(S) OF CHOICE
• Acute subdural hematoma:
◊ Prior to surgical therapy, management of cerebral edema and elevated intracranial pressure may require mannitol 20% solution 0.5-1.0 gm/kg followed by 0.25-0.75 gm/kg every 4-6 hours. If a loop diuretic is used in conjunction with mannitol, furosemide (Lasix) 0.5 mg/kg IV is administered. Check serum osmolality every 8 hours and serum electrolytes at least daily. A 5% or 25% albumin preparation (Plasmanate) may be used either as a continuous or an intermittent infusion to augment osmotherapy as needed.
◊ Seizure prophylaxis includes phenytoin (Dilantin) 1000 mg load (50 mg/min IV) with ECG monitoring followed by 100 mg IV every 8 hours or as needed to maintain therapeutic blood levels (10-20 µg/mL [40-79 µmol/L]). Dilantin therapy should be converted to the oral route as soon as possible to avoid cardiovascular complications of IV Dilantin administration.
◊ In the chronic subdural hematoma, medical management alone is frequently unsuccessful and entails risks of neurological deterioration. When small and asymptomatic, however, it may be appropriate to treat such patients conservatively with observation as some chronic subdural hematomas have been known to resolve spontaneously. Steroids may be helpful in some patients, if not otherwise contraindicated.
Contraindications: Refer to manufacturer's literature
Precautions: Refer to manufacturer's literature
Significant possible interactions: Refer to manufacturer's literature

ALTERNATIVE DRUGS N/A

FOLLOWUP

PATIENT MONITORING
• Anticonvulsant levels should be checked approximately every 3-6 months after initiation
• Consider discontinuing anticonvulsant if patient has no seizures for at least one year
• EEG may be complimentary in the decision making process for discontinuation of anticonvulsants

PREVENTION/AVOIDANCE
• Acute subdural hematoma
◊ Trauma prevention programs
• Chronic subdural hematoma
◊ Alcoholism prevention
◊ Medical and surgical management of epilepsy
◊ Conservative use of anticoagulation therapy
◊ Medium or high pressure ventriculoperitoneal shunt valves in at risk patients with hydrocephalus

POSSIBLE COMPLICATIONS
• Acute subdural hematoma - immediate postoperative complications include elevated intracranial pressure and brain edema, new or recurrent hematoma, infection, and seizures (in approximately one-third of cases)
• Chronic subdural hematoma - recurrent hematoma in up to 50% of cases (can be alleviated by the use of subdural drainage catheters), infection (subdural empyema, wound), and seizures in up to 10% of cases

EXPECTED COURSE/PROGNOSIS
• Acute subdural hematoma - mortality is greater then 50%. Significant neurological disability and impairment of function is seen in most surviving patients. Seizure prophylaxis is usually required for at least one year.
• Chronic subdural hematoma - mortality is less than 10%. Most patients resume preoperative functional status. Outcome highly dependent on pre-surgical neurological status.

MISCELLANEOUS

ASSOCIATED CONDITIONS
• Acute subdural hematoma
◊ Multi-system trauma
◊ Cervical spinal cord injury
◊ Injury to the thoracic, lumbar, or sacral spine
◊ Disseminated intravascular coagulation
◊ Epilepsy
• Chronic subdural hematoma
◊ Alcoholism
◊ Epilepsy
◊ Coagulopathy
◊ Cerebral spinal fluid shunt
◊ Birth trauma
◊ Child abuse
◊ Rarely metastatic carcinoma

AGE-RELATED FACTORS
Pediatric: N/A
Geriatric:
• Cerebral atrophy common
• Can be confused clinically with senile dementia
Others:
• Acute subdural hematoma - lower mortality in patients less than 40 years of age compared to those older then 40 years of age
• Chronic subdural hematoma - majority of patients are older than 50 years of age

PREGNANCY N/A

SYNONYMS Subdural hemorrhage

ICD-9-CM 852.30 Subdural hemorrhage following injury with open cranial wound

OTHER NOTES N/A

ABBREVIATIONS N/A

REFERENCES
• Cooper P: Traumatic intracranial hematomas. In: Wilkins R, Rengachary S, eds. Neurosurgery. New York, McGraw-Hill, 1985:1657-1666
• Fogelholm R, Waltimo O: Epidemiology of chronic subdural hematoma. Acta Neurochir 1975;32:247-250
• Seeling J, Becker D, Miller J, et al: Traumatic acute subdural hematoma. New Engl J Med 1981;304:1511-1518
• McLaurin R, Tobin R: Diagnosis and Treatment of Head Injury in Infants and Children. In: Youmans J, ed. Neurological Surgery. Philadelphia, W.B. Saunders, 1992
Illustrations: N/A
Internet references: http://www.5mcc.com

Author(s)
Martin E. Weinand, MD

Subphrenic abscess

BASICS

DESCRIPTION Any localized collection of pus below the diaphragm and in contact with the diaphragm
System(s) affected: Gastrointestinal, Pulmonary
Genetics: N/A
Incidence/Prevalence in USA: N/A
Predominant age: N/A
Predominant sex: N/A

SIGNS AND SYMPTOMS
• High spiking fever with chills and sweating
• Abdominal tenderness
• Ileus
• Anterior abdominal wall erythema
• Abdominal pain
• Tachycardia
• Chest pain
• Nausea
• Dyspnea
• Localized tenderness on palpation
• Pleural effusion
• Elevation of diaphragm
• Shoulder pain
• Hiccups
• Tenderness when compressing lower ribs
• Rales at lung base

CAUSES
• Complications of abdominal surgery cause 50%
• Penetrating trauma
• Gastrointestinal perforations - appendicitis, diverticulitis

RISK FACTORS
• Operative procedure with significant contamination
• Patients with chronic disease - cirrhosis, renal failure, malnutrition
• Patients on corticosteroids, chemotherapy, radiotherapy
• Myelosuppression

DIAGNOSIS

DIFFERENTIAL DIAGNOSIS
• Other intra-abdominal abscesses
• Empyema

LABORATORY
• White blood count
• Blood cultures
• Automated chemical profile
Drugs that may alter lab results: N/A
Disorders that may alter lab results: N/A

PATHOLOGICAL FINDINGS
• Pus under diaphragm
• Organisms: Escherichia, Streptococcus, Proteus, Klebsiella, Bacteroides fragilis, cocci, Clostridium

SPECIAL TESTS N/A

IMAGING
• CT scan
• Ultrasound
• Plain films of chest and abdomen display elevation and immobility of right diaphragm, fluid in right costophrenic sulcus; air-fluid level in subphrenic space
• Gallium scan

DIAGNOSTIC PROCEDURES CT or ultrasound directed aspiration

TREATMENT

APPROPRIATE HEALTH CARE Inpatient

GENERAL MEASURES
• Antibiotics
• Supportive care - nutrition, monitoring, oxygenation, hydration
• Swan-Ganz catheter if unstable
• Mechanical ventilation if necessary
• Vasopressors if indicated

SURGICAL MEASURES
• Adequate drainage of abscess - percutaneous and/or surgical
• Percutaneous drainage not advised if (1) abscess is multiloculated, (2) drainage route would traverse bowel, uncontaminated peritoneal or pleural space, (3) source of continued contamination still present, (4) fungal infection, (5) pus too viscous
• Surgical drainage mandated if patient fails to respond to percutaneous drainage in 24 to 48 hours

ACTIVITY As tolerated

DIET NPO until intestinal function returns

PATIENT EDUCATION N/A

MEDICATIONS

DRUG(S) OF CHOICE
• Broad spectrum antibiotics based on culture and sensitivity
• Aminoglycosides (tobramycin or gentamicin) 1.5-2.0 mg/kg loading dose
• Amikacin 5-7.5 mg/kg loading dose (very expensive)
• Plus clindamycin 600 mg IV q6h,
or
• Metronidazole (Flagyl) loading dose 15 mg/kg and maintenance dose 7.5 mg/kg q6h
Contraindications: Known allergy to antibiotics
Precautions:
• Aminoglycosides are ototoxic and nephrotoxic - follow BUN, creatinine and serum blood levels (peak and trough)
• Prolong dosing interval to achieve appropriate trough level; especially in renal failure
• Adjust dose for desired peak level
• Dosage adjustments in renal failure not needed for metronidazole since it is metabolized by the liver
Significant possible interactions: N/A

ALTERNATIVE DRUGS
• Cefoxitin 2 gm IV q4-6h
• Cefoperazone 1-2 gm IV q12h
• Cefotaxime 1 gm IV q6-8h
• Mezlocillin 3 gm IV q4h

FOLLOWUP

PATIENT MONITORING
• Frequent evaluation after discharge up to six weeks
• White blood counts regularly
• Chest x-rays until normal

PREVENTION/AVOIDANCE   N/A

POSSIBLE COMPLICATIONS
• Mortality - 10 to 90% if not adequately drained
• Multi-system organ failure
• Recurrent abscess
• Hemorrhage
• Bowel obstruction
• Wound dehiscence
• Continuing sepsis
• Pneumonia
• Pleural effusion
• Suppurative pylephlebitis

EXPECTED COURSE/PROGNOSIS
• Death if abscess is not adequately drained or patient vigorously supported

MISCELLANEOUS

ASSOCIATED CONDITIONS
• Multi-system organ failure
• Systemic sepsis
• Fistula

AGE-RELATED FACTORS
Pediatric: N/A
Geriatric: Worse prognosis
Others: N/A

PREGNANCY   N/A

SYNONYMS   Subdiaphragmatic abscess

SEE ALSO   N/A

ICD-9-CM   998.5 Postoperative infection

OTHER NOTES   N/A

ABBREVIATIONS   N/A

REFERENCES   Hau T, et al: Diagnosis and Treatment of Abdominal Abscesses, Current Problems in Surgery, Vol. XXI No. 7, Chicago, Year Book Medical Publishers, 1984
Illustrations: N/A
Internet references: http://www.5mcc.com

Author(s)
Gary B. Williams, MD

Substance abuse

BASICS

DESCRIPTION
• Substances of abuse include:
◊ Alcohol
◊ Amphetamines (e.g., methamphetamine, crystal, speed)
◊ Cocaine (eg, crack)
◊ Hallucinogens (e.g., LSD, peyote)
◊ Inhalants (e.g., glue, paint thinners)
◊ Marijuana or hashish
◊ Opioids (e.g., heroin, morphine, codeine)
◊ Phencyclidine (PCP)
◊ Polysubstances (i.e., abuse of multiple substances at the same time)
◊ Sedatives, hypnotics and anxiolytics
◊ Tobacco
◊ Others (anabolic steroids, nitrous oxide, OTC drugs, certain prescription drugs)
• Psychologists, psychiatrists, and addiction specialists debate the most appropriate definitions of "abuse" and "dependence", however DSM-IV provides a guideline:
Substance abuse: Criteria for diagnosis (adapted from the DSM-IV)
• A maladaptive pattern of substance use leading to clinically significant impairment or distress, as manifested by one (or more) of the following occurring within a 12 month period:
◊ Recurrent substance use resulting in a failure to fulfill major obligations at work, at school, or home
◊ Recurrent substance use in situations in which it is physically hazardous
◊ Recurrent substance-related legal problems
◊ Continued substance use despite having persistent or recurrent social or interpersonal problems caused or exacerbated by the effects of the substance
• The symptoms have never met the criteria for substance dependence for this class of substance
Substance dependence: Criteria for diagnosis (adapted from the DSM-IV):
• Maladaptive pattern of substance use leading to a significant impairment or distress, as manifested by 3 (or more) of the following occurring at any time in the same 12 month period:
◊ Tolerance as defined by either of the following:
- A need for markedly increased amounts of the substance to achieve intoxication or desired effect
- Markedly diminished effect with continued use of the same amount of the substance
◊ Withdrawal, as manifested by either of the following:
- The characteristic withdrawal syndrome for the substance
- The same (or closely related) substance is taken to relieve or avoid withdrawal symptoms
◊ The substance is often taken in larger amounts or over a longer period than was intended
◊ There is a persistent desire or unsuccessful efforts to cut down or control substance use
◊ A great deal of the time is spent in activities necessary to obtain the substance, use the substance, or recover from its effects
◊ Important social, occupational or recreational activities are given up or reduced because of substance use
◊ The substance use is continued despite knowledge of having a persistent or recurrent physical or psychological problem that is likely to have been caused or exacerbated by the substance
System(s) affected: Nervous, Endocrine/Metabolic
Genetics: Variants in the alleles of the dopamine D2 receptor may contribute to inter-individual differences in vulnerability to drug abuse
Incidence/Prevalence in USA:
• 74 million have used an illicit substance at least once
• 13 million use an illicit substance monthly
Predominant age: 18-25
Predominant sex: Male > Female

SIGNS AND SYMPTOMS
May result from the intoxication state, the withdrawal state, and of chronic use.
• History of infections, e.g., endocarditis, hepatitis B or C, tuberculosis, sexually transmitted diseases, or recurrent pneumonia
• Social or behavioral problems, including chaotic relationships and/or employment
• Frequent visits to emergency department
• Criminal incarceration
• History of blackouts or morning tremor, insomnia, mood swings, chronic pain, repetitive trauma
• Dilated or constricted pupils, reduced pupillary response to light
• Needle marks on skin
• Perforation of the nasal septum (with cocaine use)

CAUSES
Numerous factors have been identified as potential causes:
• Biomedical factors (genetic, physiological, biochemical, and prenatal)
• Psychological factors (emotional conflicts, personality traits, learned behavior, social and stress)

RISK FACTORS
• Family history of substance abuse
• Young adult
• Previous history of substance abuse
• Presence of other health-compromising behaviors
• Psychiatry disorders, especially depression
• Family and peer substance use

DIAGNOSIS

DIFFERENTIAL DIAGNOSIS
• If mental status acutely altered, consider metabolic derangements (hypoxia, hypothyroidism, hyperthyroidism, hypoglycemia, thiamine deficiency, etc.)
• Agitation
• Delirium
• Other altered mental states

LABORATORY
• Urine testing; positive test may be followed by more expensive confirmatory tests
• If mental status acutely altered, consider CXR, EKG, T4, TSH, CBC, chemical panel, UA, RPR
Drugs that may alter lab results: N/A
Disorders that may alter lab results: N/A

PATHOLOGICAL FINDINGS N/A

SPECIAL TESTS N/A

IMAGING N/A

DIAGNOSTIC PROCEDURES
• History (often unreliable) and physical; substance abuse screening tests
CAGE questionnaire (used for alcoholism)
• Have you ever felt you should cut down on your drinking?
• Have people annoyed you by criticizing your drinking?
• Have you ever felt bad or guilty about your drinking?
• Have you ever had a drink first thing in the morning to steady your nerves or to get rid of a hangover (eye-opener)?
Rost, et al screening:
• Have you misused one of these substances (see DESCRIPTION) more than 5 times in your life?
• Have you ever found that you needed to increase your use of a substance in order to get the same effect?
• Have you ever had emotional or psychological problems from using drugs - like feeling crazy or paranoid or uninterested in things?

TREATMENT

APPROPRIATE HEALTH CARE
• Outpatient usually. Some patients may benefit from inpatient rehabilitation units while others can be treated by individual physician or by outpatient substance abuse clinics.
• Severely ill patients or those with suicide ideation may require hospitalization

GENERAL MEASURES
• Behavioral therapies include drug counseling, behavioral and cognitive-behavior therapies, and psychodynamic strategies
• Family members should be involved in the recovery process (community reinforcement)
• Self-help groups:
◊ Can be important adjunct to treatment plan (Alcoholic Anonymous, Narcotics Anonymous, Cocaine Anonymous). Their twelve-step programs have been helpful for many patients.
◊ Encourage support groups for family members (Al-Anon and Alateen)
◊ Other support groups include the Rational Recovery and Secular Organizations for Sobriety. These are newer organizations and their success rate is still unclear.

SURGICAL MEASURES   N/A

ACTIVITY   No restrictions

DIET   Emphasize good nutrition

PATIENT EDUCATION
• Alcoholic Anonymous
• Narcotics Anonymous
• Cocaine Anonymous
• Rational Recovery
• Secular Organizations for Sobriety

MEDICATIONS

DRUG(S) OF CHOICE
• Methadone - 60 mg (or more) orally once a day; used for both detoxification of an opioid addict and for maintenance treatment to substitute for heroin and other injected opioids
• L-alpha-acetylmethadol (LAAM) - longer acting than methadone; given 3 times a week
• Naltrexone (ReVia) - given orally 3 times a week; blocks the euphoria produced by opiates; useful in conjunction with psychosocial and behavioral interventions in highly motivated patients
• Clonidine - used for managing symptoms of opioid withdrawal
Contraindications:
• Naltrexone - hepatic failure; acute hepatitis
Precautions:
• Clonidine may cause hypotension
Significant possible interactions:
• Naltrexone - opioid medications (naltrexone will precipitate or exacerbate withdrawal symptoms)

ALTERNATIVE DRUGS   None approved for cocaine or other stimulants

FOLLOWUP

PATIENT MONITORING
• Verify patient's compliance with the substance abuse treatment program
• Following treatment, follow-up on medical issues and provide support for continued abstinence

PREVENTION/AVOIDANCE
• Reduce risks through education
• Early identification and aggressive early intervention (mild substance abuse disorders respond better to treatment intervention)

POSSIBLE COMPLICATIONS
• Hepatitis, HIV, abscesses, pneumonia
• Malnutrition
• Social problems, including arrest
• Poor marital adjustment and violence
• Serious harm to self and others
• Overdoses resulting in seizures, arrhythmias, cardiac and respiratory arrest, coma, death
• Many other infectious diseases

EXPECTED COURSE/PROGNOSIS
• Success rates vary widely
• Patients who stay in treatment for longer periods of time (at least a year) have a higher success rate
• Counseling combined with drug therapy appears to be more successful than either one alone

---

Substance abuse

MISCELLANEOUS

ASSOCIATED CONDITIONS
• Depression
• Personality disorders
• Manic-depressive disorder

AGE-RELATED FACTORS
Pediatric: Levels of marijuana use among youth (12-17) have been steadily increasing since 1992. Between 1993 and 1994, rates of use of illicit drugs, alcohol and cigarettes has remained stable in persons age 18 and older.
Geriatric: Alcohol, prescription drugs
Others: N/A

PREGNANCY   Substance abuse may cause major problems that can lead to fetal abnormality, morbidity, and death of infant and mother

SYNONYMS
Drug abuse
Drug dependence

ICD-9-CM
304 Drug dependence
304.0 Opioid dependence
304.2 Cocaine dependence

SEE ALSO
• Alcoholism
• Depression

OTHER NOTES   N/A

ABBREVIATIONS
LSD = lysergic acid diethylamide
DSM-IV = Diagnostic and Statistical Manual of Mental Disorders, 4th ed.

REFERENCES
• Substance Abuse and Mental Health Services Administration, National Household Survey on Drug Abuse: Main findings 1994. Rockville, MD. SAMHSA, Office of Applied Sciences, Department of Health and Human Services, Public Health Service, 1994. DHHS Publication # (SMA)96-3085
• American Psychiatry Association Diagnostic and Statistical Manual of Mental Disorders. 4th Ed. Washington, DC, American Psychiatric Association, 1994
• Rost K, Burnam MA, Smith GR. Development of screeners for depressive disorders and substance disorder history. Med Care 1993;119:1017-28
• Haverkos HW, Stein MD: Identifying substance abuse in primary care. Amer Fam Phys 1995;52(7):2029-2035
Illustrations: 1 available on CD-ROM
Internet references: http://www.5mcc.com

Author(s)
Harry W. Haverkos, MD

Sudden infant death syndrome (SIDS)

BASICS

DESCRIPTION The sudden death of an infant under one year of age which remains unexplained after a thorough case investigation, including performance of a complete autopsy, examination of the death scene, and review of the clinical history. SIDS was first formally defined in 1969 and the definition was revised in 1989.
System(s) affected: Endocrine/Metabolic, Pulmonary, Nervous, Cardiovascular
Genetics: No genetic association has been identified
Incidence/Prevalence in USA: (for 1995)
• All races: 0.87/1000 live births (3,400 cases per year)
• White: 0.71/1000 live births (2,200 cases per year)
• Black: 1.79 live births (1,073 cases per year)
Predominant age: Rare in first month of life, peak occurs in infants between 2 and 4 months, 90% of deaths occur by 6 months
Predominant sex: Males > Females (52-60% of SIDS cases are males)

SIGNS AND SYMPTOMS These babies generally appear healthy, or may have had a minor upper respiratory or gastrointestinal infection in the last 2 weeks of life

CAUSES
• There are many theories about the cause of SIDS. There may be subtle developmental abnormalities resulting from pre- and/or perinatal brain injury.
• Possible causes:
 ◊ Abnormalities in respiratory control and arousal responsiveness
 ◊ Upper airway obstruction
 ◊ Bronchospasm
 ◊ Central and peripheral nervous system abnormalities
 ◊ Cardiac arrhythmias
 ◊ Carbon dioxide rebreathing in face down position on soft surface
 ◊ SIDS may occur when a combination of factors coincide; such triggers may include infectious agents, climatic changes, or environmental factors

RISK FACTORS
• Most SIDS deaths occur in children who are "low-risk." However, there are several risk factors associated with SIDS:
 ◊ Race: Native Americans and African Americans have highest incidence
 ◊ Season - late fall and winter months
 ◊ Time of day - between midnight and 6 AM
 ◊ Activity - during sleep
 ◊ Low birth weight; intrauterine growth retardation (IUGR)
 ◊ Poverty
• Maternal factors: Teenage mothers; maternal use of cigarettes or drugs (cocaine, opiates) during pregnancy; higher parity; maternal anemia during pregnancy

• Respiratory or gastrointestinal infection in recent past
• Sleep practices - prone and side sleep position, heavier clothing and bedding, soft bedding
• Lack of breast-feeding
• Passive cigarette smoke exposure after birth

DIAGNOSIS

DIFFERENTIAL DIAGNOSIS
• Suffocation
• Abnormalities of fatty acid metabolism (e.g., deficiency of medium-chain acyl-CoA dehydrogenase, or of carnitine)
• Homicide
• Dehydration/electrolyte disturbance
• Infant botulism

LABORATORY
• Pneumocardiograms have been abandoned in the workup
• Postmortem laboratory tests are done to rule out other cause of death (e.g., electrolytes to rule out dehydration and electrolyte imbalance). In SIDS, there are no consistently abnormal laboratory tests.
Drugs that may alter lab results: N/A
Disorders that may alter lab results: N/A

PATHOLOGICAL FINDINGS
• Characteristic findings on postmortem examination:
 ◊ Frothy discharge, sometimes blood-tinged, from nostrils and mouth in majority
 ◊ Petechiae on surface of lungs, heart and thymus gland in 50-85% (but not unique to SIDS)
 ◊ Pulmonary congestion and edema often present
 ◊ Morphologic markers of hypoxia: Increased gliosis in brain stem, retention of periadrenal brown fat, and hematopoiesis in the liver - present to varying degrees, not confirmed by all studies

SPECIAL TESTS N/A

IMAGING X-rays are taken to rule out possible child abuse

DIAGNOSTIC PROCEDURES N/A

OTHER Because the diagnosis of SIDS is often one of "exclusion," it is crucial to do a thorough death scene investigation and case review, in addition to the autopsy and lab tests

TREATMENT

APPROPRIATE HEALTH CARE
• Because a SIDS death is sudden and the cause is unknown, SIDS cannot be "treated." However, there are some measures that may be effective in preventing SIDS:
 ◊ Maternal avoidance of cigarette and illicit drug use during pregnancy
 ◊ Breast-feeding
 ◊ Avoidance of the prone and side sleep position, excessive bed clothing and soft bedding
 ◊ Avoidance of passive cigarette smoke exposure
• Recent studies from Europe, Australia and New Zealand suggest significant risk reduction with sleeping on back or side. U.S. data also indicate that rates are declining with reductions in prone sleep positions. Because infants placed on their side may turn during sleep to the prone position, it is now believed that back position is best.

GENERAL MEASURES N/A

SURGICAL MEASURES N/A

ACTIVITY N/A

DIET N/A

PATIENT EDUCATION
• Family counseling (see Expected Course/Prognosis))
• American Sudden Infant Death Syndrome Institute, (800)232-SIDS in Atlanta, Georgia
• SIDS Alliance, Baltimore, MD, (800)221-SIDS
• Back to Sleep Information Line, (800)505-CRIB (sponsored by the U.S. Public Health Service to provide information to parents and health providers about their recommendations to place infants on back, and general information about SIDS)
• National SIDS Resource Center, Vienna, VA, (703)902-1249

Sudden infant death syndrome (SIDS)

 MEDICATIONS

DRUG(S) OF CHOICE N/A
Contraindications: N/A
Precautions: N/A
Significant possible interactions: N/A

ALTERNATIVE DRUGS N/A

 FOLLOWUP

PATIENT MONITORING Some authorities recommend cardiopulmonary monitoring in siblings of prior SIDS victims

PREVENTION/AVOIDANCE N/A

POSSIBLE COMPLICATIONS N/A

EXPECTED COURSE/PROGNOSIS
• SIDS deaths have a powerful impact on families and their functioning. Physicians play an important role in providing immediate information about SIDS and sensitive counseling to limit parents' misinformation and feelings of guilt.
• Counseling needs of families vary from short-term to long-term; support groups are helpful to many couples. Physicians need to be familiar with resources available in their communities to help families mourning a SIDS death. Parents need to be counseled about subsequent pregnancies.
• Follow-up counseling, including review of the autopsy report with the family after some time has passed, will be important to help with understanding this condition and to clear the tremendous guilt these families experience.

 MISCELLANEOUS

ASSOCIATED CONDITIONS N/A

AGE-RELATED FACTORS N/A
Pediatric: Occurs in infants only
Geriatric: N/A
Others: N/A

PREGNANCY N/A

SYNONYMS
• Crib death
• Cot death

ICD-9-CM 798.0 Sudden infant death syndrome

SEE ALSO N/A

OTHER NOTES N/A

ABBREVIATIONS N/A

REFERENCES
• Corr CA, Fuller H, Barnickol CA & Corr DM.(eds.): Sudden Infant Death Syndrome. Who Can Help and How. New York, Springer Publishing Co., 1991
• Hoffman HJ, Damus K, Hillman L, Krongrad E: Risk factors for SIDS. Results of the National Institute of Child Health and Human Development SIDS Cooperative Epidemiological Study. Annals NY Acad Sciences 1988;533:13-30
• Dwyer T, Ponsonby AL: The decline of SIDS: A success story for epidemiology. Epidemiol 1996;7(3):323-25
• Willinger M, James LS, Catz C: Defining the Sudden Infant Death Syndrome (SIDS): Deliberations of an expert panel convened by the National Institute of Child Health and Human Development. Pediatr Pathol 1991;11:677-684
• AAP News Release, 4/15/92
• Willinger M, Hoffman HJ, Hartford RB: Infant sleep position and risk for sudden infant death syndrome: Report of meeting help January 13-14, 1994, National Institutes of Health, Bethesda, MD. Pediatrics 1994;93:814-819
Illustrations: N/A
Internet references: http://www.5mcc.com

Author(s)
Fern R. Hauck, MD, MS

Suicide

BASICS

DESCRIPTION Completed suicide refers to self-inflicted death. Attempted suicide refers to potentially lethal acts which do not result in death and non-lethal, attention-seeking gestures (e.g., superficial cuts on wrists).
System(s) affected:
Genetics: No known genetic pattern
Incidence/Prevalence in USA:
• 10-12 in 100,000. Ninth leading cause of death in US adults. Second leading cause of death among children and adolescents.
• Approximately 28,000 completed suicides yearly in US accounting for 2% of all deaths
• Attempted suicide is ten times more frequent than completed suicides
• Subpopulation incidence
  ◊ Ages 5-14 - 8/100,000
  ◊ Ages 15-24 - 13.1/100,000
Predominant age: Highest in elderly (> 65 years) and adolescent age period (15-24 years)
Predominant sex:
• Male > Female - complete suicide (3:1)
• Female > Male - attempted suicide (3:1)

SIGNS AND SYMPTOMS
• Hopelessness about future
• Suicidal thoughts with organized plan and intent
  ◊ Suicide note
  ◊ Giving away personal possessions
  ◊ Quitting a job
• Major depression (screen for symptoms)
  ◊ Change in sleep
  ◊ Loss of interest
  ◊ Loss of energy
  ◊ Loss of concentration
  ◊ Loss of appetite
  ◊ Diminished psychomotor activity
  ◊ Guilt
  ◊ Suicidal ideations
• Psychosis
  ◊ Ask about command auditory hallucinations to kill oneself

CAUSES
• Combination of psychiatric illness and social circumstances. Most patients have active psychiatric illness.
• Major depression and bipolar disorder account for 50% of completed suicides
• Alcoholism and drug abuse disorders account for 25% of completed suicides
• Schizophrenia and other psychotic disorders account for 10% of completed suicides

RISK FACTORS
• Psychiatric
  ◊ Mood disorders (major depression, bipolar), alcoholism, drug abuse, psychotic disorders, personality disorders
    ◊ Family history of suicide
    ◊ History of previous suicide attempt

• Medical diagnosis of terminal illness (cancer, AIDS), chronic intractable pain, chronic and disabling illness (renal dialysis patient)
  ◊ Hopelessness about future
• Epidemiologic
  ◊ Sex - males three times females
  ◊ Age - adolescent and geriatric population (males peaking at 75 years, females peaking at 55 years)
  ◊ Race - American Indian, Caucasian
  ◊ Marital status - single > divorced, widowed > married
• Psychologic
  ◊ History of recent loss (loved one, job, etc.)
  ◊ Loss of social supports
  ◊ Important dates (holidays, birthdays, anniversaries, etc.)
• Review mnemonic for risk factors = SAD PERSONS
  ◊ S = sex
  ◊ A = age
  ◊ D = depression
  ◊ P = previous attempt
  ◊ E = ethanol abuse
  ◊ R = rational thinking loss
  ◊ S = social support loss
  ◊ O = organized plan
  ◊ N = no spouse
  ◊ S = sickness
  ◊ If five risk factors present, consider very high suicidal risk

DIAGNOSIS

DIFFERENTIAL DIAGNOSIS
• Psychiatric
  ◊ Mood disorders (major depression, bipolar)
  ◊ Alcohol intoxication and other drug abuse
  ◊ Psychotic disorders (e.g., schizophrenia)
  ◊ Personality disorder (e.g., borderline)
  ◊ Organic mental disorders (e.g., dementia, delirium)
  ◊ Adjustment disorders
  ◊ Panic disorders
  ◊ Post-traumatic stress disorder
• Medical
  ◊ Hypothyroidism
  ◊ Cushing's disease/syndrome
  ◊ Addison's disease
  ◊ Hypopituitarism
• Other (medications associated with depression)
  ◊ Anti-hypertensives (methyldopa, reserpine, clonidine)
  ◊ Corticosteroids
  ◊ Opiates
  ◊ Anti-tuberculous agents (isoniazid, ethionamide, cycloserine)
  ◊ Anabolic steroid withdrawal
  ◊ Barbiturates
  ◊ Benzodiazepines
  ◊ Cocaine withdrawal
  ◊ Amphetamine withdrawal

LABORATORY There are no laboratory tests to determine who will commit suicide. Patients who have completed violent suicides were found to have low CSF levels of 5-Hydroxyindoleacetic acid (5-HIAA), a serotonin metabolite. Other findings have included: increased CSF methoxyhydroxyphenylglycol (MHPG), nonsuppression of dexamethasone suppression test (DST), low platelet MAO (mono amine oxidase), low platelet serotonin, high platelet serotonin-2 receptor responsivity.
Drugs that may alter lab results: N/A
Disorders that may alter lab results: N/A

PATHOLOGICAL FINDINGS Patients who have completed violent suicides were found to have low CSF levels of 5-Hydroxyindoleacetic acid (5-HIAA), a serotonin metabolite

SPECIAL TESTS N/A

IMAGING N/A

DIAGNOSTIC PROCEDURES N/A

TREATMENT

APPROPRIATE HEALTH CARE
• Admit to psychiatric ward (voluntarily/involuntarily) if patient is severely depressed, intoxicated, psychotic or status post serious suicide attempt
• Admit to general hospital for acute medical care with psychiatric consultation
• Consider outpatient treatment with scheduled followup appointment if patient has social support system and no evidence of severe depression, psychosis or intoxication
• If unsure or patient is high risk (i.e., five positive risk factors - SAD PERSONS), admit to hospital for further observation and evaluation

GENERAL MEASURES
• All patients with suicide threats, gestures or attempts should be screened for suicide risk factors and have a full mental status exam and psychiatric consultation
• Ensure patient safety by least restrictive method (i.e., remove potentially dangerous objects, provide one-to-one constant observation, medication, 2-4 point restraints)
• Diagnose and treat underlying psychiatric and medical disorder
• Electroconvulsive therapy provides rapid, safe, and effective treatment option for severely depressed, acutely suicidal patients

SURGICAL MEASURES N/A

ACTIVITY Suicide precautions; q 15 minute checks; one-to-one observation; 2-4 point restraints

DIET N/A

PATIENT EDUCATION
• For a listing of sources for patient education materials favorably reviewed on this topic, physicians may contact: American Academy of Family Physicians Foundation, P.O. Box 8418, Kansas City, MO 64114, (800)274-2237, ext. 4400

MEDICATIONS

DRUG(S) OF CHOICE
• Treat underlying psychiatric and medical illness
• Antidepressants, psychostimulants, carbamazepine, valproic acid, or lithium for mood disorders
• New generation antidepressants including selective serotonin reuptake inhibitors ([SSRIs], e.g., fluoxetine [Prozac], paroxetine [Paxil], sertraline [Zoloft]) and bupropion (Wellbutrin) and venlafaxine (Effexor) are less likely to be lethal with overdose attempts
• A minimum of two weeks required to obtain response from antidepressants
• Neuroleptic medications (e.g., haloperidol, chlorpromazine) for psychotic symptoms
• Benzodiazepines (e.g., lorazepam) for anxiety symptoms
• Agitated, combative and intoxicated patients in the emergency room:
◊ May require sedation with benzodiazepines (e.g., lorazepam 2 mg IM/IV) and/or neuroleptics (e.g., haloperidol 2-5 mg IM/IV)
◊ Clinical response typically seen within 20-30 minutes
◊ If no response, increase previous dose (e.g., 4-10 mg haloperidol)
Contraindications: Avoid tricyclic antidepressants in patient with evidence of 2°, 3° AV block or left bundle branch block ECG
Precautions: Use smaller doses in elderly patients
Significant possible interactions: Hypertensive crisis if MAO inhibitor antidepressants given in combination with medications containing sympathomimetic amines; tyramine-rich food; meperidine (Demerol); tricyclic antidepressants

ALTERNATIVE DRUGS N/A

FOLLOWUP

PATIENT MONITORING
• Weekly outpatient followup appointments
• Prescribe only a weekly supply of antidepressants or other psychotropic medications at each appointment

PREVENTION/AVOIDANCE
• Provide crisis hot-line phone number and nearest crisis emergency room location
• Mobilize social support system and inform family and friends of options if patient becomes more suicidal
• Instruct patient to avoid any alcohol consumption

POSSIBLE COMPLICATIONS Brief
period of increased suicide risk as depression resolves and patient's energy and initiative returns

EXPECTED COURSE/PROGNOSIS
• 15% of suicidal, depressed patients will ultimately complete suicide
• 82% of suicide victims have seen a doctor within the previous six months
• Approximately one-half of suicide victims have seen a doctor within one month of their death
• The key to a favorable course and prognosis is early recognition of risk factors, early diagnosis and treatment of a psychiatric disorder, and appropriate intervention and followup

MISCELLANEOUS

ASSOCIATED CONDITIONS Depression

AGE-RELATED FACTORS
Pediatric: Increasing suicide rate in adolescents. Suicide is second leading cause of death in adolescents.
Geriatric: Increasing rate with increasing age (women peak at 55 years, men peak at 75 years)
Others: N/A

PREGNANCY N/A

SYNONYMS N/A

ICD-9-CM N/A

SEE ALSO
• Alcoholism
• Depression
• Schizophrenia

OTHER NOTES
• Overdose is the most common method for suicide attempts
• Shooting is the most common method for completed suicides
• Men prone to more violent suicides (i.e., shooting, jumping, hanging)
• Jumping most common method of suicide among patients in a general medical/surgical hospital

ABBREVIATIONS N/A

REFERENCES
• Hackett TP, Cassem NH: MGH Handbook of General Hospital Psychiatry. 2nd Ed. New York, PSG Publishing Company, Inc., 1987
• Talbott JA, Hales RE, Yudofsky SC: Textbook of Psychiatry. Washington, DC, American Psychiatric Press, Inc., 1988
• Patterson WM, Dohn HH, et al: Evaluation of suicidal patients, THE SAD PERSONS Scale, Psychosomatics, 1983
Illustrations: N/A
Internet references: http://www.5mcc.com

Author(s)
M. Beatriz Currier, MD
Edwin J. Olsen, MD, MBA

Superior vena cava syndrome

BASICS

DESCRIPTION Partial or complete obstruction of the superior vena cava, 90% extrinsic, 70% from neoplasm (most frequently bronchogenic carcinoma), also thrombosis, fibrosis, invasion and aneurysm causing suffusion, varying degrees of airway obstruction and/or cyanosis of the face, neck, arms and occasionally chest and upper abdomen. Usual course - acute onset; chronic onset: often progressive.
System(s) affected: Cardiovascular, respiratory
Genetics: N/A
Incidence/Prevalence in USA: N/A
Predominant age: Young adult (16-40 years); middle age (40-60 years)
Predominant sex: Male > Female

SIGNS AND SYMPTOMS
• Dyspnea
• Facial swelling
• Truncal swelling
• Arm swelling
• Easy fatigability
• Orthopnea
• Chest pain
• Cough
• Headache
• Visual disturbances
• Altered consciousness
• Dysphagia
• Hoarseness
• Thoracic vein distention
• Neck vein distention
• Facial edema
• Chest vein distention
• Wheezing
• Tachypnea
• Facial plethora
• Cyanosis
• Arm edema
• Paralyzed vocal cord
• Conjunctival edema
• Proptosis
• Stridor
• Horner's syndrome
• Dilated retinal vessels
• Enlarged tongue
• Non-pitting edema of the neck (Stoke's collar)
• Fullness or stuffiness in ears/eyes
• Symptoms worse with lying down or leaning forward

CAUSES
• Obstruction of venous drainage of upper part of chest and neck. Sudden occlusion can cause rapid development of cerebral edema, intracranial thrombosis and death.
• Lung cancer, bronchogenic carcinoma/small cell
• Lymphoma
• Thymoma
• Fungus infections
• Breast cancer
• Other malignancies
• Iatrogenic
• Thyroid goiter
• Syphilitic aneurysm
• Tuberculous mediastinitis
• Primary superior vena caval thrombosis
• Pericardial constriction
• Idiopathic sclerosing mediastinitis

RISK FACTORS   HIV infection

DIAGNOSIS

DIFFERENTIAL DIAGNOSIS
• Aortic aneurysm
• Tuberculosis, Histoplasmosis
• Fungal infections

LABORATORY Sputum cytology-malignant cells
Drugs that may alter lab results: N/A
Disorders that may alter lab results: N/A

PATHOLOGICAL FINDINGS Sputum cytology, occasionally thoracentesis, bone marrow, lymph node biopsy, bronchoscopy or thoracotomy confirm - malignant cells.

SPECIAL TESTS Increased central venous pressure (CVP), usually 20-50 mm Hg.

IMAGING
• Tc 99m scan - block to flow of contrast material into right heart, large collateral veins
• Chest x-ray, MRI, CT scan, and/or tomography - mediastinal mass, superior mediastinal mass, pulmonary lesion, superior vena cava obstruction, hilar adenopathy, pleural effusion.
• Venography - superior vena cava obstruction

DIAGNOSTIC PROCEDURES
• Bronchoscopy
• Thoracentesis, thoracotomy, lymph node biopsy, as indicated

TREATMENT

APPROPRIATE HEALTH CARE Inpatient, intensive care

GENERAL MEASURES
• Radiotherapy
• Intravascular stenting

SURGICAL MEASURES Superior vena cava reconstruction for benign processes may be considered

ACTIVITY Bedrest (head of bed elevated)

DIET As tolerated, possibly salt restriction

PATIENT EDUCATION As appropriate

MEDICATIONS

DRUG(S) OF CHOICE
• Chemotherapy for cancer
• Steroids for some malignancies, esp. if cerebral or laryngeal edema
• Antifungal or antitubercular medications according to underlying cause
• Consider diuretics
• Anticoagulation role unclear
• Fibrinolytics (e.g., urokinase) for thrombosis
Contraindications: Refer to manufacturer's literature
Precautions: Refer to manufacturer's literature
Significant possible interactions: Refer to manufacturer's literature

ALTERNATIVE DRUGS
Streptokinase, tPA

FOLLOWUP

PATIENT MONITORING Linked to cause. If infection, monitor for evaluation of antimicrobial treatment. If malignant, monitor response to radiotherapy or chemotherapy.

PREVENTION/AVOIDANCE No preventive measures known

POSSIBLE COMPLICATIONS
Complications of underlying disease

EXPECTED COURSE/PROGNOSIS High probability of response; prognosis linked to cause; 20% 1-year survival for lung cancer; 50% 2-year survival for lymphoma. 85% neoplastic cases better in 3 weeks with radiation therapy, but symptoms usually recur.

MISCELLANEOUS

ASSOCIATED CONDITIONS
• Breast cancer
• Lung cancer
• HIV infection
• Hyperthyroidism
• Tuberculosis, histoplasmosis
• Lymphoma

AGE-RELATED FACTORS
Pediatric: N/A
Geriatric: Occurs in geriatric patients
Others: N/A

PREGNANCY Must treat underlying condition despite pregnancy

SYNONYMS
• Superior mediastinal syndrome
• Superior vena cava obstruction

ICD-9-CM
459.2 Compression of vein

SEE ALSO N/A

OTHER NOTES N/A

ABBREVIATIONS N/A

REFERENCES
• Sculier JP, Feld R: Superior Vena Cava Obstruction Syndrome: Recommendations for Management. In Cancer Treat Rev 1985;12:209
• DeVita VT Jr, Hellman S, Rosenberg SA, eds: Cancer: Principles and Practices of Oncology. 3rd Ed. Philadelphia, J.B. Lippincott, 1989
• Bennett JC, Plum F, eds: Cecil Textbook of Medicine. 20th Ed. Philadelphia, W.B. Saunders Co., 1996
• Schwartz SI, ed: Principles of Surgery. 4th Ed. New York, McGraw-Hill, 1984
• Wilkinson P, MacMahon J, Johnston L: Stenting and superior vena caval syndrome. Irish J Med Sci 1995;164(2):128-131
Illustrations: N/A
Internet references: http://www.5mcc.com

Author(s)
Paul J. Jaster, MD

Syncope

BASICS

DESCRIPTION Approximately 5-20% of adults will have one or more episodes of syncope by age 75. The disorder accounts for about 1% of hospital admissions and about 3% of emergency room visits. Its annual incidence in the institutionalized elderly is about 6%.
System(s) affected: Nervous, Cardiovascular
Genetics: N/A
Incidence/Prevalence in USA: 6% in persons over age 75 (incidence)
Predominant age: Elderly
Predominant sex: N/A

SIGNS AND SYMPTOMS
Transient loss of consciousness characterized by unresponsiveness, loss of postural tone, and spontaneous recovery

CAUSES
• Cardiac - obstruction to outflow:
  ◊ Aortic stenosis
  ◊ Hypertrophic cardiomyopathy
  ◊ Pulmonary embolus
• Cardiac - arrhythmias:
  ◊ Ventricular tachycardia
  ◊ Sick sinus syndrome
  ◊ 2nd and 3rd degree AV block
• Non-cardiac:
  ◊ Reflex mediated vasovagal, situational (micturition, defecation, cough)
    ◊ Orthostatic hypotension
    ◊ Drug induced
    ◊ Neurologic: Seizures, transient ischemic attack
    ◊ Carotid sinus
    ◊ Psychogenic

RISK FACTORS
• Patients with heart disease
• Patients taking following drugs:
  ◊ Antihypertensives
  ◊ Vasodilators (including calcium channel blockers, ACE inhibitors, and nitrates)
  ◊ Phenothiazines
  ◊ Antidepressants
  ◊ Antiarrhythmics
  ◊ Diuretics

DIAGNOSIS

DIFFERENTIAL DIAGNOSIS
• Drop attacks
• Coma
• A careful history, physical examination and an ECG are more important than other investigations in determining a diagnosis. Make sure that the patient or witness (if present) is not talking about vertigo, coma, or drop attacks. Prodromal manifestations of sudden weakness, nausea, and sweating, especially in circumstances provoking strong emotion, are diagnostic of vasovagal syncope. Syncope of sudden onset with no prodrome or brief premonitory symptoms suggest a cardiac cause. Vasovagal syncope does not occur when the patient is horizontal; cardiac syncope can occur in any position. Syncope with exertion suggestions a cardiac cause. Physical exam should be directed to blood pressure and pulse, both lying and standing. Check for a cardiac murmur or a focal neurologic abnormality.
After a careful evaluation, including diagnostic procedures and special tests, the cause of syncope will be found in only 50-60% of patients.

LABORATORY Rarely helpful. Less than 2% have hyponatremia, hypocalcemia, hypoglycemia or renal failure causing seizures.
Drugs that may alter lab results: N/A
Disorders that may alter lab results: N/A

PATHOLOGICAL FINDINGS N/A

SPECIAL TESTS
• If history and physical suggestive of ischemic, valvular or congenital heart disease - echocardiogram, cardiac catheterization
• If CNS disease suspected - EEG, head CT, head MRI. These tests should not be ordered unless there are hints of CNS disease on history or physical examination.

IMAGING Lung scan if history and physical examination suggestive of pulmonary embolism

DIAGNOSTIC PROCEDURES
• ECG monitoring, either in the hospital or ambulatory (Holter), is useful in 4-15% of patients. Arrhythmias are frequently documented, but rarely associated with syncope. Monitoring should be done in patients with heart disease, and in patients with recurrent syncope. Patient activated intermittent loop recorders, which the patient activates after regaining consciousness, can record 4-5 minutes of retrograde ECG rhythm. These have been helpful in patients with recurrent syncope with a diagnostic yield between 24-47%.
• Electrophysiologic studies (EPS) have been positive in 18-75% of patients. Induction of ventricular tachycardia and dysfunction of the His-Purkinje system are the two most common abnormalities. Although there is the problem of knowing whether the arrhythmia noted or induced during the study is the cause of syncope, EPS should be done in patients with heart disease or recurrent syncope.
• The following findings are probable causes of syncope:
  ◊ Sustained ventricular tachycardia
  ◊ Sinus node recovery time 3 seconds or more
  ◊ Pacing-induced infranodal block
  ◊ H-V interval greater than 100 msec
• Carotid hypersensitivity should be considered in patients with syncope on head turning, especially with head turning while wearing tight collar, and in patients with neck tumors and neck tissue scars. The technique is not standardized. One side should be massaged at a time for 20 seconds with constant monitoring of pulse and blood pressure. Atropine should be readily available.
• Tilt testing, with and without isoproterenol infusion, is a provocative test for vasovagal syncope which is not standardized, but has been reported positive (symptomatic hypotension and bradycardia) in 26-87% of patients. However, the test has been reported positive in 0-45% of control subjects. The role of this test in the workup of patients with syncope of unknown origin is not known, and should be done only in patients in which cardiac causes of syncope have been excluded. Patients with a positive tilt test often respond to beta-blocker treatment.
• Psychiatric evaluation should be considered in patients with multiple episodes of syncope (greater 5/year) who do not have heart disease. Anxiety, depression, alcohol and drug abuse can be associated with syncope.

TREATMENT

APPROPRIATE HEALTH CARE
• Patients with heart disease should be admitted to the hospital for evaluation
• Elderly patients without previously recognized heart disease should be admitted if the physician thinks that a cardiac cause of syncope is likely
• Patients without heart disease, especially young patients (less 60 years old), can be safely worked up as outpatients

GENERAL MEASURES
No specific measures

SURGICAL MEASURES   N/A

ACTIVITY
Fully active unless severe cardiac disease

DIET
No specific diet unless heart disease

PATIENT EDUCATION
• Reassure the patient that most cardiac causes of syncope can be treated, and that patients with non-cardiac causes do well, even if the cause of syncope is never discovered
• The physician and patient should carefully consider whether the patient should continue to drive while syncope is being evaluated. Physicians should be aware of the pertinent laws in their own state.

MEDICATIONS

DRUG(S) OF CHOICE
Antiarrhythmic drugs should be used to treat arrhythmias documented during monitoring which occur simultaneously with syncope or symptoms of presyncope. Asymptomatic arrhythmias found on monitoring usually do not require treatment.
The decision to treat patients on the basis of arrhythmias or conduction abnormalities provoked or detected during EPS is even more problematic. Does the arrhythmia or conduction abnormality have anything to do with the patient's symptoms? Most would treat a patient with provoked sustained ventricular tachycardiac with an antiarrhythmic drug that suppressed the arrhythmia during the study. Many recommend pacemaker implantation in patients with H-V intervals greater than 100 msec, pacing induced infranodal block, or sinus node recovery time of 3 sec or more. The rationale basis for such treatment is that recurrent syncope is less frequent in those patients with positive EPS who are treated than it is in those who have negative EPS.
Contraindications: N/A
Precautions: N/A
Significant possible interactions: N/A

ALTERNATIVE DRUGS   N/A

FOLLOWUP

PATIENT MONITORING
• Frequent followup visits for patients with cardiac causes of syncope, especially patients on antiarrhythmic drugs
• Patients with an unknown cause of syncope rarely (5%) have a diagnosis made during followup

PREVENTION/AVOIDANCE   Avoid Risk factors

POSSIBLE COMPLICATIONS
• Trauma from falling
• Death - see prognosis

EXPECTED COURSE/PROGNOSIS
• Cumulative mortality at 2 years:
◊ Low (2-5%) - young patients (< 60) with a non-cardiac cause or unknown cause of syncope.
◊ Intermediate (20%) - older patients (> 60) with a non-cardiac or unknown cause of syncope.
◊ High (32-38%) - patients with cardiac cause of syncope.

MISCELLANEOUS

ASSOCIATED CONDITIONS   See Causes

AGE-RELATED FACTORS
Pediatric: Rare in this age group
Geriatric: More common in this age group, prognosis worse in older patients
Others: N/A

PREGNANCY   N/A

SYNONYMS   N/A

ICD-9-CM
780.2 Syncope and collapse

SEE ALSO
• Aortic valvular stenosis
• Carotid sinus syndrome
• Stokes-Adams attacks
• Idiopathic hypertrophic subaortic stenosis
• Ventricular tachycardia
• Complete heart block
• Pulmonary embolism
• Seizure disorder
• Primary pulmonary hypertension
• Patent ductus arteriosus
• Atrial septal defect

ABBREVIATIONS   N/A

REFERENCES
• Linzer M, Gang EH, Estes NA, Wang P, Vonpenan V, Kapoor WN: Diagnosing syncope part 1: Value of history, physical examination and electrocardiography. The Clinical Efficacy of Assessment Project of the American College of Physicians. Ann Int Med 1997;126:989-996
• • Linzer M, Gang EH, Estes NA, Wang P, Vonpenan V, Kapoor WN: Diagnosing syncope part 2: Unexplained syncope. The Clinical Efficacy of Assessment Project of the American College of Physicians. Ann Int Med 1997;127:76-86
Illustrations: N/A
Internet references: http://www.5mcc.com

Author(s)
Jay W. Smith, MD

Synovitis, pigmented villonodular

BASICS

DESCRIPTION A proliferative disorder of unknown etiology affecting synovial lined joints, tendon sheaths or bursa. Occurs in diffuse or focal forms which have a quite different prognosis.
System(s) affected: Musculoskeletal
Genetics: N/A
Incidence/Prevalence in USA: Two occurrences per 1 million population
Predominant age:
• Diffuse form appears more commonly in the 3rd and 4th decades
• Focal is more common in the 5th and 6th decades
Predominant sex:
• Diffuse form: Male = Female
• Focal form: Female > Male

SIGNS AND SYMPTOMS
• Diffuse form:
  ◊ Unilateral and monoarticular with 80% occurring in the knee and affecting the hip, ankle and shoulder in decreasing order
  ◊ Mild and progressive pain in involved joint
  ◊ History of trauma (30% of cases)
  ◊ Recurrent swelling and tenderness to palpation of involved joint
  ◊ Increased skin temperatures over involved joint
• Focal form:
  ◊ More common in tendon than joints
  ◊ Involves the tendons of the hand and feet, usually, rarely the wrist and ankle or a major joint
  ◊ Presents as slow growing, painless mass
  ◊ Most common cause of tumor in hand, second to ganglion
• Chronic, inflammatory:
  ◊ Unusual monoarticular presentation

CAUSES Unknown, possibly repeated local hemorrhages

RISK FACTORS N/A

DIAGNOSIS

DIFFERENTIAL DIAGNOSIS
• Diffuse form (if soft tissue swelling is the main finding):
  ◊ Synovioma - frequently calcifies
  ◊ Synovial hemangioma - usually occurs in childhood and often associated with cutaneous hemangioma
  ◊ Lipoma - boggy fullness to palpation and absence of serosanguinous fluid on aspiration
  ◊ Unusual mono-articular presentation for other forms of chronic, inflammatory arthritis
• Diffuse form (if multiple subchondral cysts on x-ray are the main finding):
  ◊ Degenerative joint disease - cysts occur on weight bearing surfaces only, while cysts of PVNS may occur anywhere in joints. Osteophytes common in degenerative arthritis, absent in PVNS.
  ◊ Tuberculous arthritis is characterized by severe juxta-articular osteoporosis
  ◊ Amyloid arthropathy is usually symmetrical and more common in the upper extremities. The joint space is preserved.
  ◊ Synovial chondromatosis - presence of punctate calcifications along the margin. (Occurs 60-70% of time.)
• Focal form:
  ◊ Ganglion - contains jelly-like fluid on aspiration
  ◊ Dupuytren's nodules - not attached to tendon sheath and therefore does not move with tendon

LABORATORY Aspiration of a serosanguineous fluid from a joint in the absence of trauma is highly suggestive of diffuse pigmented villonodular synovitis (fluid can be clear, however). Aspirated joint fluid may contain high cholesterol.
Drugs that may alter lab results: N/A
Disorders that may alter lab results: N/A

PATHOLOGICAL FINDINGS The synovium shows proliferation into villi or nodules with subsynovial cellular infiltrate that includes fibroblasts, lymphocytes and lipid-laden macrophages (foam cells)

SPECIAL TESTS N/A

IMAGING
• The CT scan may be helpful, but MRI has the best potential for being diagnostic due to the presence of hemosiderin and fat within the abnormal tissue present in the joint
• X-ray shows soft tissue swelling of involved joints. Subchondral cysts and pressure erosions are limited mostly to the hip. The absence of osteophytes and juxta-articular osteoporosis is significant.

DIAGNOSTIC PROCEDURES
• Arthroscopy usually reveals characteristic synovial changes and allows definitive biopsy
• An arthrogram is not usually diagnostic
• Radioisotopes and ultrasound studies are also usually not definitive

TREATMENT

APPROPRIATE HEALTH CARE Inpatient or outpatient surgery

GENERAL MEASURES N/A

SURGICAL MEASURES
• Diffuse form - total synovectomy is the usual recommended treatment, but has a recurrence rate of 25-40%. X-ray therapy alone or combined with synovectomy has been tried, again with high recurrence rate. Recently, intra-articular injections of radioisotopes, in particular yttrium-90, has been tried and shows some early promise, but evaluation of this is incomplete.
• Focal form - local excision results in cure

ACTIVITY No restrictions

DIET No special diet

PATIENT EDUCATION N/A

MEDICATIONS

DRUG(S) OF CHOICE None
Contraindications: N/A
Precautions: N/A
Significant possible interactions: N/A

ALTERNATIVE DRUGS N/A

FOLLOWUP

PATIENT MONITORING Patients should be followed twice annually after treatment of the diffuse form by history and physical examination. X-rays yearly, especially if the hip is involved.

PREVENTION/AVOIDANCE N/A

POSSIBLE COMPLICATIONS
Osteoarthritis, especially in the hip joint

EXPECTED COURSE/PROGNOSIS
• Good in focal type
• Guarded in the diffuse form with recurrences of disease common as well as joint dysfunction

MISCELLANEOUS

ASSOCIATED CONDITIONS N/A

AGE-RELATED FACTORS
Pediatric: N/A
Geriatric: N/A
Others: N/A

PREGNANCY N/A

SYNONYMS
• Xanthoma
• Benign synovioma
• Giant cell tumor of tendon sheath
• Fibroxanthoma
• PVNS

ICD-9-CM 719.20 Villonodular synovitis

SEE ALSO Arthritis, rheumatoid (RA)

OTHER NOTES N/A

ABBREVIATIONS PVNS = pigmented villonodular synovitis

REFERENCES Flandry JB, Hughston JS: Pigmented Villonodular Synovitis. Current Concepts and Review, 1987
Illustrations: N/A
Internet references: http://www.5mcc.com

Author(s)
Furnie W. Johnston, MD
R. Bruce Hall, MD

Syplilis

BASICS

DESCRIPTION An infection, characterized by sequential stages (acute, subacute or chronic), with the spirochete, Treponema pallidum
• Infectious (primary or early syphilis) consists of a primary stage and a secondary stage. It may include neurosyphilis (central nervous system involvement). If the patient is untreated, the infectious stage may be followed by a latent stage.
• Latent stage syphilis (secondary) is an asymptomatic phase. If it occurs up to one year after the infectious stage, it is described as early latent. If it occurs 2 or more years after the infectious stage, it is termed late latent.
• Tertiary (or late syphilis) stage is late generalized syphilis
• Congenital is syphilis acquired in utero
System(s) affected: Reproductive, Skin/Exocrine, Nervous, Cardiovascular
Genetics: Unknown, however Caucasians more likely to develop CNS complications, African-Americans to develop cardiac problems
Incidence/Prevalence in USA:
• 1989 - nationally 18.4/100,000 new cases
• In urban African-American populations, as high as 124/100,000
• Cases reported are rapidly rising
Predominant age: Sexually active years
Predominant sex: Male > Female

SIGNS AND SYMPTOMS
• Infectious syphilis - primary
   ◊ Chancre begins as a papule which erodes to a 0.3 to 2 cm non-tender ulcer with a hard edge and clean, yellow base (unless secondarily infected) 9 to 90 days after exposure (median 3 weeks)
   ◊ Usually found on genitalia, frequently solitary, may be multiple, may have regional lymphadenopathy
   ◊ Heals with scarring in 3 to 6 weeks with 75% of patients having no further symptoms
• Infectious syphilis - secondary
   ◊ 25% of patients enter this stage 2-6 weeks after exposure, may overlap with chancre
   ◊ Resolves spontaneously in 2-6 weeks in most patients
   ◊ May wax and wane between secondary and latent stages
   ◊ Rash is bilaterally symmetric, polymorphic, palpable lesions with "fresh cut ham" color, non-pruritic, usually not bullous or vesicular, frequently on palms and soles
   ◊ Patchy alopecia of scalp, eyebrows and beard common
   ◊ Mucous patches - thin gray smears - and condyloma lata - moist, flat, pink, peripheral warty lesions - may be present on glans, perianal, vulva areas
   ◊ Generalized lymphadenopathy and flu-like symptoms occur early with rash
   ◊ Rarely may be accompanied by nephritis, meningitis, uveitis, hepatitis
   ◊ Mild hepatosplenomegaly often noticeable

• Latent syphilis
   ◊ Characterized by positive serology but no signs or symptoms
   ◊ Patient is not infectious after one year, but may relapse to infectious secondary stage if untreated (25% in first year, small percent second year, none after that)
• Tertiary syphilis
   ◊ Marked by cardiovascular (aortic valve disease or aneurysms)
   ◊ Neurological (meningitis, encephalitis, tabes dorsalis)
   ◊ Dementia (paresis)
   ◊ Deep cutaneous (gummas which are destructive granulomatous pockets)
   ◊ Orthopedic (Charcot's joints, osteomyelitis) complications (rare with antibiotics)
   ◊ Serologies often negative
• Congenital syphilis
   ◊ Failure to thrive
   ◊ Rhinitis
   ◊ Lymphadenopathy
   ◊ Jaundice
   ◊ Anemia
   ◊ Hepatosplenomegaly
   ◊ Nephrosis
   ◊ Meningitis
   ◊ Rash (the hallmark) similar to secondary syphilis in adults, but may be bullous or vesicular

CAUSES
• Exposure through sexual contact
• Exposure to infected body fluids
• Transplacentally
• Treponema pallidum

RISK FACTORS
• Multiple sexual partners
• IV drug use
• Male homosexuality

DIAGNOSIS

DIFFERENTIAL DIAGNOSIS
• Primary syphilis - chancroid, lymphogranuloma venereum, granuloma inguinale, herpes, Behçet's syndrome, trauma
• Secondary syphilis - pityriasis rosea, guttate psoriasis, drug eruption
• Positive serology and/or negative clinical signs and symptoms - previously treated syphilis, biological false positive, other spirochetal disease (yaws, pinta)

LABORATORY
• Requires either demonstration of organisms on microscopy or positive serology on blood or cerebrospinal fluid (CSF)
• Organism may not be cultured, but diagnosis is never made on clinical signs and symptoms alone

• Nonspecific treponemal tests: Venereal Disease Research Laboratory (VDRL) or rapid plasma reagin (RPR) are characterized as follows:
   ◊ Relatively inexpensive, primary screening test
   ◊ Positive within 7 days of exposure
   ◊ Titer decreases with time or treatment
   ◊ Used to monitor therapy: fourfold rise in titer indicates new infection while failure to decrease fourfold within one year is treatment failure
   ◊ False-positive common but positives are highly suggestive even without clinical signs and symptoms (confirm with fluorescent treponemal antibody absorption [FTA-ABS])
   ◊ Titer ≥ 1:64 even without confirming test is probably diagnostic of acute syphilis or other treponematoses
   ◊ Labs need to titer tests to final end point (not report as ">1:512" for example) to make best use of results in monitoring therapy response
   ◊ Beware of prozone phenomenon - negative results due to very high titers of antibody. Test diluted serum sample, as well, to declare a given specimen as negative.
• Specific treponemal tests: Fluorescent treponemal antibody absorption (FTA-ABS), microhemagglutination treponema pallidum (MHA-TP)
   ◊ More expensive, used to confirm diagnosis
   ◊ Usually positive for life after treatment
   ◊ Due to unusual nonspecific test results in HIV infected patients, these tests may be needed to absolutely rule out syphilis
• Lumbar puncture for CSF serologies should be done:
   ◊ In cases of latent syphilis where duration is unknown or non-penicillin therapy is planned
   ◊ Whenever neurological symptoms are present
   ◊ VDRL, not RPR is used on CSF, may be negative in neurosyphilis
   ◊ Negative FTA-ABS or MHA-TP on CSF excludes neurosyphilis
Drugs that may alter lab results: Many drugs reported to cause false-positive, but this is relatively uncommon with a good history
Disorders that may alter lab results:
• Rheumatoid disorders
• Acute febrile illness
• HIV infection
• Pregnancy

PATHOLOGICAL FINDINGS Aneurysm, osteomyelitis, gummas in late cases

SPECIAL TESTS
• Dark field microscopy
• Immunofluorescence
• Skin biopsy

IMAGING Only in late cases as indicated

DIAGNOSTIC PROCEDURES
Specialized test available from Center for Disease Control (CDC) to confirm false-positive if necessary

TREATMENT

APPROPRIATE HEALTH CARE
Outpatient, except for initiating IV penicillin or desensitization

GENERAL MEASURES
• Baseline serologies prior to treatment to monitor its success
• Symptomatic treatment of the chancres and rash of secondary syphilis (for patient's comfort only) prior to definitive antibiotic therapy

SURGICAL MEASURES N/A

ACTIVITY
• Full activity, but no sexual contacts until declared cured

DIET No special diet

PATIENT EDUCATION
• Need to trace and treat all sexual contacts of the patient
• Keep followup appointments to monitor success of therapy
• Advise patient to avoid intercourse until treatment is complete
• Local health department can provide literature and contact tracing

MEDICATIONS

DRUG(S) OF CHOICE
• Primary, secondary and latent less than one year - benzathine penicillin G, 2.4 million units IM for 1 dose
• Latent > 1 year - benzathine penicillin G, 2.4 million units IM weekly for 3 doses
• Neurosyphilis - aqueous procaine penicillin G (APPG) 2-4 million units IM daily for 10-14 days with probenecid 500 mg q6h, or 2-4 million units penicillin G IV every 4 hours for at least 10 days. Follow each therapy with benzathine penicillin G 2.4 million units IM weekly for 3 doses.
• Epidemiologic treatment for contacts without symptoms, treat as primary after baseline serologies are obtained
• Congenital - with abnormal CSF, 50,000 units/kg of aqueous procaine penicillin G (APPG) IM for at least 10 days. With negative CSF serologies, 50,000 units/kg benzathine penicillin G in one IM injection.
Contraindications: Allergy to penicillin
Precautions:
• HIV infected and pregnant patients may show poor response to recommended IM doses. Use IV therapy for all treatment failures in these patients.
• Do NOT give benzathine or procaine penicillins IV

Significant possible interactions: None, however, Jarisch-Herxheimer reaction, marked by fever, chills, headache, myalgias, new rash is common on starting treatment due to the lysis of treponemes and should not be confused with a reaction to antibiotics. It is managed with antihistamines and antipyretics.

ALTERNATIVE DRUGS
• Erythromycin, tetracyclines, ceftriaxone (Rocephin) may be used. However, in penicillin allergic patients, desensitization is easily accomplished and is recommended for HIV infected and pregnant patients so that penicillin can be used.
• Standard treatment with ceftriaxone and tetracycline used for gonorrhea is usually therapeutic for incubating syphilis

FOLLOWUP

PATIENT MONITORING Repeat serologies for 3 months, then yearly to confirm treatment. Do serological studies more frequently in HIV infected patients.

PREVENTION/AVOIDANCE
• Discuss safe sex
• Use of condoms

POSSIBLE COMPLICATIONS
• Cardiovascular disease
• Central nervous system disease
• Membranous glomerulonephritis
• Paroxysmal cold hemoglobinemia
• Organ damage that cannot be reversed
• Many other disorders

EXPECTED COURSE/PROGNOSIS
Excellent in all cases except late syphilis complications and a few HIV infected patients

MISCELLANEOUS

ASSOCIATED CONDITIONS
• Other sexually transmitted diseases
• HIV infection and hepatitis B (strongly urge patients treated for syphilis to obtain screenings for both)

AGE-RELATED FACTORS
Pediatric: In non-congenital cases, must consider possible child abuse
Geriatric: N/A
Others: N/A

PREGNANCY Early detection is imperative, all expectant mothers should have serologies as part of routine prenatal care

SYNONYMS
• Lues
• The Great Imitator

ICD-9-CM 090.0-097 Syphilis

SEE ALSO
• Chlamydial sexually transmitted diseases
• Pelvic inflammatory disease (PID)
• Gonococcal infections

OTHER NOTES Many experts urge more aggressive treatment than standard regimens in all patients and strongly advocate the use of penicillin rather than any alternative antibiotic

ABBREVIATIONS
• CSF = cerebrospinal fluid
• FTA-ABS = fluorescent treponemal antibody absorption
• MHA-TP = microhemagglutination treponema pallidum
• VDRL = Venereal Disease Research Laboratory
• RPR = rapid plasma reagin

REFERENCES
• Centers for Disease control: Sexually transmitted diseases: Treatment guidelines 1989. MMWR Morb Mortal Wkly Rep 1989;38 (Suppl 8):1
• Drugs for Sexually transmitted Diseases. Medical Letter, Vol. 36, Issue 913, Jan. 7, 1994
Illustrations: 3 available on CD-ROM
Internet references: http://www.5mcc.com

Author(s)
Kevin M. Hepler, MD, MBA

Systemic lupus erythematosus (SLE)

BASICS

DESCRIPTION A multi-system, autoimmune inflammatory condition characterized by a fluctuating, chronic course. Varies from mild to severe and may be lethal (CNS and renal forms).
System(s) affected: Hemic/Lymphatic/Immunologic, Nervous, Renal/Urologic, Endocrine/Metabolic, Skin/Exocrine, Gastrointestinal, Musculoskeletal
Genetics: Markers: HLA-B8; HLA-DR2; HLA-DR3
Incidence/Prevalence in USA: 20/100,000
Predominant age: All ages, but 30-50 are most common
Predominant sex: Female > Male (10:1)

SIGNS AND SYMPTOMS
• Arthritis
• Fever
• Anorexia
• Malaise
• Weight loss
• Skin lesions
• Oral ulcers
• Eye pain and/or redness
• Chest pain and/or shortness of breath
• Pallor
• Nausea, vomiting, diarrhea
• Muscles - tenderness, aching and stiffness
• Headaches and visual problems
• Psychosis/delirium

CAUSES
• Most cases are idiopathic
• Drugs - drug induced lupus is clinically different from idiopathic SLE

RISK FACTORS
• Race - blacks, Hispanics, Asians, and Native Americans have higher prevalence than whites.
• Genetic markers - HLA-B8, HLA-DR2, HLA-DR3.
• Hereditary complement deficiency especially C2 and C4

DIAGNOSIS

DIFFERENTIAL DIAGNOSIS
• SLE mimics numerous systemic conditions, especially those involving inflammation
• Many other disorders mimic SLE - rheumatoid arthritis, mixed connective tissue disease (MCTD), scleroderma, metastatic malignancy, fever of unknown origin, psychogenic rheumatism and many cutaneous rashes. No one test or biopsy is pathognomonic.

LABORATORY
• Positive antinuclear antibody (ANA)
• Anti-double standard DNA (dsDNA), anti-Sm, false-positive VDRL, or positive LE preparation. These tests have either high sensitivity (ANA, false-positive VDRL) or specificity (anti-dsDNA, anti-Sm and LE preparation) and are included as American Rheumatology Association (ARA) criteria for the diagnosis of SLE along with the clinical features.
• Sedimentation rate is nonspecific, but valuable in assessing activity of SLE
• Anemia
• Leukopenia
• Lymphopenia
• Abnormal urinary sediment
• Proteinuria
• Increased prothrombin time
• Positive anticardiolipin
• Hypoalbuminuria
• Thrombocytopenia
• Increased serum creatinine
• Positive Coombs test
Drugs that may alter lab results: N/A
Disorders that may alter lab results: N/A

PATHOLOGICAL FINDINGS Connective tissue disorders affecting skin, blood vessels, serous and synovial membranes
• Collagenous swelling
• Fibrinoid change
• Cellular necrosis
• Periarterial sclerosis
• Granulomatous reaction
• Infiltration of polymorphonuclear leukocytes, plasma cells, lymphocytes in walls of small vessels, arterioles of skin, spleen, glomeruli, endocardium pericardium, brain
• Hematoxylin bodies resembling those in LE cells
• Vegetation on heart valves

SPECIAL TESTS
• Complement levels, immune complex assays (cryoglobulins, Raji cell test, C1q precipitins)
• Coagulation studies (lupus anticoagulant)
• Biopsy of skin, kidney and peripheral nerves may reveal typical histopathology

IMAGING
• Cerebral angiography in CNS lupus
• Chest x-ray for pulmonary infiltration, pleural effusion
• MRI to detect CNS lupus
• Echocardiogram for pericardial effusion

DIAGNOSTIC PROCEDURES
American Rheumatology Association (ARA) criteria are a combination of any 4 manifestations of the 11 listed
1 Malar (butterfly) rash
2 Discoid rash
3 Photosensitivity
4 Oral/nasopharyngeal ulcers
5 Nonerosive arthritis
6 Pleuritis or pericarditis
7 Renal disorder - proteinuria or cylindruria
8 Neurologic disorder - psychosis or seizures
9 Hematologic disorder - hemolytic anemia, leukopenia (less than 4,000), lymphopenia (less than 1,500), thrombocytopenia (less than 100,000)
10 Immunologic disorder
11 Positive antinuclear antibody (ANA) in absence of drugs known to cause positive ANA
  Note: While the above criteria are required for proper epidemiologic classification of SLE, in practical situations, the combination of a multi-system inflammatory illness, positive antinuclear antibody (ANA) and absence of a better diagnosis often represents the most practical way to make a clinical diagnosis

TREATMENT

APPROPRIATE HEALTH CARE
Outpatient with regular monitoring

GENERAL MEASURES
• Avoidance of or protection from ultraviolet light by using sunscreens, hats, etc.
• Early intervention when infections occur
• Energy conservation
• Stress avoidance/management

SURGICAL MEASURES N/A

ACTIVITY
• As active as possible
• Those with arthritis may be limited by their pain, but active exercises are to be encouraged

DIET No special diet unless for complications such as renal failure

PATIENT EDUCATION Printed materials available on lupus from the Arthritis Foundation, 1314 Spring Street N.W., Atlanta, GA 30309, (404)872-7100; and from the Lupus Foundation of America, 1717 Massachusetts Avenue, NW, Suite 203, Washington, DC 20036, (800)558-0121

MEDICATIONS

DRUG(S) OF CHOICE
• No one drug of choice available. Treatment is symptomatic with certain exceptions. Use of local steroids for cutaneous manifestations, nonsteroidal anti-inflammatory drugs for minor arthritis symptoms, low dose steroids for minor discomfort and high dose steroids for major inflammatory disease.
• Use of immunosuppressants is indicated for renal disease and severe disease in other organs
• Minor arthritis - NSAID's
• More significant arthritis or dermal lupus - hydroxychloroquine 310 mg (400 mg of the sulfate salt) qd
• Major symptoms in any organ system or combination of organ systems - prednisone 30-60 mg qd
• Glomerulonephritis - cyclophosphamide 0.5 gm/m2 IV monthly together with prednisone 60 mg po qd tapering to 10 mg every other day after 4 months
• Methotrexate 5-25 mg oral or subcutaneous, weekly in 2 single doses has been effective as a "steroid sparer" for arthritis, rash, serositis or fever
• Immune globulin, intravenous (IVIG) pulse has been effective in the temporary treatment of SLE thrombocytopenia
Contraindications: Refer to manufacturer's profile of each drug
Precautions: Ensure good hydration when administering cyclophosphamide due to possibility of hemorrhagic cystitis
Significant possible interactions: Refer to manufacturer's profile of each drug

ALTERNATIVE DRUGS   Included in Drug(s) of Choice

 FOLLOWUP

PATIENT MONITORING
• Follow acute flares frequently, (weekly to monthly) for adjustment of medication based on clinical impression. Laboratory parameters are of limited value. CBC useful in hematologic lupus. Serum creatinine or renal clearance tests of value in renal lupus. Sedimentation rate often helps determine adequate suppression of symptoms or development of a remission.
• The confirming tests for lupus (ANA titers, anti-DNA titers, complement levels, etc.) are usually not helpful in follow-up assessment
• Use of continuing medication depends upon symptoms. Exception is in the case of renal lupus for which it has been shown that a defined course of monthly IV cyclophosphamide has been of value.

PREVENTION/AVOIDANCE
• Avoiding sun exposure is only necessary for approximately one sixth of SLE patients (those who self report such sensitivity)
• Routine vaccinations are safe and appropriate for SLE patients
• Drugs known to induce SLE in normal individuals are not necessarily contraindicated in patients who have idiopathic SLE

POSSIBLE COMPLICATIONS   Fever, vasculitis, panniculitis, myositis, avascular necrosis of bone, endocarditis, pulmonary fibrosis, renal failure, organic brain syndromes, peripheral neuropathy, stroke syndromes, pancreatitis and elevated liver enzymes, infertility, ascites, venous thrombosis, seizures

EXPECTED COURSE/PROGNOSIS
• Most patients with lupus follow a course of remissions and exacerbations. Many experience spontaneous permanent remission.
• Treatment of renal lupus (the most serious form) with immunosuppressors, renal dialysis, and renal transplantation, has increased the five year life expectancy to over 90%. For those patients surviving the first two years of disease, life expectancy is essentially normal.
• In patients with drug-induced lupus, symptoms should gradually decrease upon discontinuation of the suspected agent.

 MISCELLANEOUS

ASSOCIATED CONDITIONS   Other autoimmune diseases - rheumatoid arthritis, hypothyroidism, diabetes

AGE-RELATED FACTORS
Pediatric: Stroke syndromes frequently seen in children
Geriatric:
• Higher percentage of males involved among the elderly
• Since "false-positive ANA" reaches 15% in the elderly, caution in interpretation is required in this age group
Others: N/A

PREGNANCY
• Onset of lupus and lupus flares are more common during pregnancy
• Fetal loss is increased for mothers with lupus
• Newborns of mothers who have lupus are more likely to have cardiac arrhythmias
• Specialists' collaboration during pregnancy is indicated

SYNONYMS
• SLE
• Disseminated lupus erythematosus

ICD-9-CM   710.0 Systemic lupus erythematosus

SEE ALSO
• Anemia, autoimmune hemolytic
• Glomerulonephritis, membranous

OTHER NOTES   N/A

ABBREVIATIONS   N/A

REFERENCES
• Kelley WN, Harris ED, Ruddy S, Sledge CB: Textbook of Rheumatology. 4th Ed. Philadelphia, W.B. Saunders Co., 1993
• Kippel JH, Dippe PA, eds: Rheumatology, St. Louis, Mosby, 1994
Illustrations: 5 available on CD-ROM
Internet references: http://www.5mcc.com

Author(s)
John T. Boyer, MD

Tapeworm infestation

BASICS

DESCRIPTION Tapeworms, which can be parasitic in humans, are cestodes which in their adult phase are segmented flatworms that may reside in the gastrointestinal tract. Adult worms consist of a head (scolex), which is where it attaches to the host; the neck (germinal region); and a segmented body (strobila), with each individual segment (proglottid) containing sets of male and female reproductive organs that produce eggs. The life cycle of all but one tapeworm (Hymenolepis nana) requires an intermediate host, where they grow as larval forms in tissue that is then ingested by the final host such as humans, where it subsequently develops as an adult. Hymenolepis nana can complete all stages of development in humans, helping to make it the most common tapeworm in humans. Most tapeworm infections are confined to the gastrointestinal tract, however somatic disease can occur with Taenia Solium eggs being ingested (Cysticercosis), or Echinococcus infections, making these more serious. Tapeworms/their usual intermediate host/and type of infection in humans/description include:
• Taenia saginata/beef/intestinal worm/ Takes 2-4 months after ingestion to become adult tapeworm. 3-10 meters long. Usually single tapeworm. Proglottids are motile and can crawl out of anus.
• Taenia solium/pork/a.) intestinal worm, b.) Cysticercosis, a somatic infection/2-4 months to become adult worm. 3 meters long, occasionally multiple. Proglottids not motile. May live up to 25 years. Ingestion of encysted larvae (cysticerci) cause intestinal tapeworm. Ingestion of T.solium eggs causes Cysticercosis. Eggs look identical to T. saginata eggs.
• Diphyllobothrium latum and other species/fresh water fish/intestinal worm/longest adult tapeworm - up to 25 meters. Matures to adult in 3-5 weeks.
• Hymenolepis nana/rodent, insects, or even the human themselves/intestinal worm/ Mature to adult worms in 10-12 days. Seldom exceeds 40 mm long. Proglottids rarely seen in stool. Eggs can autoinfect individual, or occasionally insects (especially meal worms). Fecal oral transmission possible. Lifespan 4-10 weeks, but autoinfection can perpetuate infection. Usually self cleared by adolescence.
• Echinococcus a.) granulosis, b.)multilocularis/humans, sheep, cattle are intermediate hosts with dogs the definitive hosts for granulosis and rodents for multilocularis/Somatic infections: a.) hydatid disease of liver, spleen, etc., b.) alveolar hydatid disease/Adult worm lives in dogs (or rodents), human ingests eggs, larvae hatch and are carried through circulation to various organs such as liver and lungs where develop into hydatid cysts which enlarge causing symptoms perhaps 5-20 years later.

• Hymenolepis diminuta/rodents and insects/intestinal worm/90 cm long. Humans rare accidental host by swallowing contaminated mealworms or grain beetles in grain.
• Dipylidium caninum/dogs and cats and flea/intestinal worm/10-70 cm long. Motile proglottids, shape of cucumber seeds, can crawl out anus. Rare accidental infection of humans from ingesting infected flea that came from dogs or cats.

System(s) affected: Gastrointestinal, Nervous

Genetics: N/A

Incidence/Prevalence in USA: Occurs infrequently in USA. More often associated with immigrant population and ethnic groups with certain cultural eating habits. Can be endemic in other parts of the world, where fecal contamination can get into water or food source.

Predominant age: All ages affected. Hymenolepis nana and diminuta more common in children.

Predominant sex: Male = Female

SIGNS AND SYMPTOMS
• Taenia saginata (beef tapeworm): Generally asymptomatic. Often noted by passing eggs or proglottids, which can occasionally be felt crawling out of anus. Mild gastrointestinal symptoms may occur (one third) - nausea, abdominal pain, change in appetite, weakness, weight loss, allergic symptoms urticaria, pruritis.
• Taenia solium (pork tapeworm):
  ◊ Intestinal worm - generally asymptomatic, noted passing eggs or proglottids (which are not motile). Occasional minor abdominal complaints similar to T. saginata.
  ◊ Larval migration - Cysticercosis - most common to brain and skeletal muscle. Neurologic manifestations such as new onset of seizures, focal neurologic deficits, hydrocephalus, headache, vomiting, visual changes, dizziness.
• Diphyllobothrium latum (fish tapeworm): Generally asymptomatic, noted passing eggs, vomiting segment of worm, or occasionally passing proglottid segments. Occasionally mild abdominal discomfort, weight loss. Worm has marked affinity for vitamin B12, 40% decreased B12 levels, 2% megaloblastic anemia with glossitis, rare B12 associated neurologic symptoms.
• Hymenolepis nana (dwarf tapeworm): Usually asymptomatic. If heavy infection: anorexia, abdominal pain, and diarrhea.
• Echinococcosis (hydatid disease): Symptoms related to growth of cyst. Liver cysts - abdominal pain, RUQ mass, obstructive jaundice. Cyst rupture - fever, urticaria, pruritis, anaphylaxis. Pulmonary cyst, cough, chest pain, hemoptysis. Other organs possible - bone with pathologic fractures, CNS - space-occupying lesions, heart - conduction defects, pericarditis.
• Hymenolepis diminuta (rodent tapeworm): Most asymptomatic. Pass eggs in stool, proglottids disintegrate. Headache, mild GI symptoms - anorexia, nausea, cramps diarrhea.

• Dipylidium caninum (dog tapeworm): Most asymptomatic. Occasionally abdominal pain, diarrhea, anal pruritis, urticaria. May observe proglottid in diaper or stool.

CAUSES Eating the infective form of the parasite either by eating contaminated food such as undercooked beef, pork, fish, or infected insects that may be in cereals or grains, or through fecal-oral contamination.

RISK FACTORS
• Taenia's: Eating raw or undercooked beef or pork, particularly in Africa, Latin America, Middle East, Central Asia, India
• Cysticercosis: Presence of a tapeworm carrier in close environment
• Diphyllobothrium: Eating raw or undercooked fish, particularly in northern Europe
• Hymenolepis nana: More frequent in children, institutionalized, malnourished, immunodeficient
• Echinococcus: Keeping dogs around sheep and goats highest risk for hydatid cyst disease

DIAGNOSIS

DIFFERENTIAL DIAGNOSIS When diagnosed by passing egg or proglottid must differentiate from other parasitic diseases. Possible to present as gastroenteritis, irritable bowel syndrome, intestinal obstruction, cholecystitis, or biliary obstruction. Cysts disease, depending upon location of cysts, may resemble other mass lesions in similar locations. Diphyllobothrium may present as pernicious anemia.

LABORATORY
• May have mild to moderate eosinophilia, increased IgE
• Microscopic analysis of eggs or proglottids
Drugs that may alter lab results: N/A
Disorders that may alter lab results: N/A

PATHOLOGICAL FINDINGS
• Intestinal tapeworms generally no pathological findings
• Cysticercosis: Cysts, 5-10 mm in soft tissue. Calcified cysts in CNS, muscle
• Echinococcus: Hydatid cyst in liver, lung, other tissues
• Diphyllobothrium: Macrocytic megaloblastic anemia in 2%

SPECIAL TESTS
• Stool evaluation of O&P
• Microscopic evaluation of proglottid collected in water or saline
• Antibody testing by ELISA to differentiate T. saginata eggs from T. solium
• Immunoblot assay for certain parasites
• DNA probes for T. saginata or T. solium

IMAGING
• Intestinal tapeworms occasionally seen by small bowel enteroclysis
• Cysticercosis best diagnosed by CT or MRI. Possibly by plain films.
• Echinococcus cysts may be seen on CT, ultrasound, liver scan, plain films

DIAGNOSTIC PROCEDURES
• Occasional excisional biopsy of cysticercosis cyst.
• CT guided aspiration of hydatid cysts, with instillation of ethanol after aspiration and pretreatment for 1 month with albendazole.

TREATMENT

APPROPRIATE HEALTH CARE
Outpatient unless complications from cysts

GENERAL MEASURES
• Treatment of large percentage of population in endemic area can help
• General supportive care during treatment
• Good hygienic measures should be employed

SURGICAL MEASURES
Cysticercosis cysts and hydatid cysts have been removed surgically, with care not to leak fluid.

ACTIVITY As tolerated

DIET As tolerated

PATIENT EDUCATION
• Proper cooking of beef, pork, fish
• Proper freezing of meat or fish
• Fecal-oral precautions with good hand washing
• Treatment of infected dogs, and preventing fleas

MEDICATIONS

DRUG(S) OF CHOICE
• Praziquantel:
  ◊ Single dose of 5-10 mg/kg for taeniasis, diphyllobothriasis, and most other intestinal cestodes (cure rate > 95%)
  ◊ Single dose of 25 mg/kg for H. nana (cure rate >95%)
  ◊ 50 mg/kg/day divided tid x 14 days for children and adults for Cysticercosis
• Niclosamide: Single dose of 2 gm for adult or 1 gm for children (cure rate 90% for taeniasis and slightly less for Diphyllobothriasis)
• Albendazole: For Echinococcus hydatid cysts. Adults 400 mg bid x 28 days. May need several courses. Children > 2 years, use adult dose. Children 1-2 years, 200 mg/day.
• Steroids and anticonvulsants for neurocysticercosis
Contraindications: Prior sensitivity
Precautions:
• Niclosamide: Occasional nausea and abdominal pain, diarrhea, drowsiness, dizziness
• Praziquantel: Mild but frequent dizziness, myalgias, nausea, diarrhea, abdominal pain
• Albendazole: Occasional diarrhea and abdominal pain. Rare leukopenia, increased serum transaminase levels.
Significant possible interactions: None known

ALTERNATIVE DRUGS Niclosamide: 2 gm, then 1 gm qd X 5 more days for H. nana.

FOLLOWUP

PATIENT MONITORING Examine several stool specimens for O&P at sufficient interval to allow regrowth of worms: 3 months for Taenia species and 1 month for others

PREVENTION/AVOIDANCE
• Treatment of infected animals, populations and screening household contacts
• Improved sewage treatment
• See Patient Education

POSSIBLE COMPLICATIONS
• Larval form of T. solium can cause systemwide cysticercosis, including neurocysticercosis, which can be etiology of up to 25% of cases of new-onset seizures in indigenous areas
• Echinococcus hydatid cysts may occur causing abnormalities in the organ involved. Cyst rupture can cause spread of disease and anaphylaxis.
• B12 deficiency with D. latum
• Proglottid of T. saginata can rarely obstruct appendix, pancreatic and bile ducts
• D. latum can occasionally cause intestinal obstruction, cholangitis, cholecystitis

EXPECTED COURSE/PROGNOSIS
• Cure of > 95% of intestinal tapeworms with medications, occasionally requiring a second treatment
• H. nana often self cured by adolescence
• E. multilocularis often severe and even fatal
• Prognosis of systemic cysts influenced by their location

MISCELLANEOUS

ASSOCIATED CONDITIONS N/A

AGE-RELATED FACTORS
Pediatric: H. nana, highest among children with fecal-oral spread. H. diminuta, and Dipylidium caninum more common in children, as more likely to accidentally ingest insects.
Geriatric: N/A
Others: N/A

PREGNANCY N/A

SYNONYMS N/A

ICD-9-CM
• 122 Echinococcus (4th digit specifies location of disease)
• 123 Other cestode infection. (specific organisms coded separately)

SEE ALSO N/A

OTHER NOTES N/A

ABBREVIATIONS
O&P = Ova and Parasites

REFERENCES
• Isselbacher KJ, et al (eds): Harrison's Principles of Internal Medicine 13th Edition, New York, McGraw-Hill, 1994
• Miranda A: Neurocysticercosis. Amer Fam Phys 1993;47(5):1193-1197
• Schantz PM: Tapeworms (cestodiasis). Gastroenterology Clinics of North America 1996;25(3):637-653
• Wyngaarden JB, Smith LH, Bennett JC (eds): Cecil Textbook of Medicine. 19th Ed. Philadelphia, W.B. Saunders Co., 1992
Illustrations: N/A
Internet references: http://www.5mcc.com

Author(s)
Kenton Voorhees, MD

Teething

BASICS

DESCRIPTION Teething is the eruption of the deciduous teeth which most children experience without difficulty. It is a natural, gradual and predictable process but the timetable varies from baby to baby.
• Deciduous teeth
  ◊ Most deciduous teeth begin to erupt at 5-7 months of age and teething is completed by 2-3 years
  ◊ The mandibular central incisors erupt first, then the two or four maxillary incisors followed by the lower lateral incisors
  ◊ After a few months, the four molars appear (lower ones at 12 months, the upper ones at 14 months)
  ◊ After the cuspid teeth appear at 16-18 months of age the second molars erupt at 20-24 months
  ◊ About 25% normal babies may have delayed eruption of teeth until 4 or 6 teeth simultaneously appear after their first birthday
  ◊ Premature babies erupt teeth according to their gestational age rather than chronological age. If teething seems particularly delayed, refer patient to a pedodontist.
• Teeth in neonates
  ◊ One in 2000 neonates are born with a tooth (appears to be familial)
  ◊ These neonatal teeth may be loose but most are the normal deciduous lower central incisors and can persist
  ◊ Mild ulceration in the sublingual area has been reported in 18% of these babies
  ◊ Because of the potential for aspiration there is some controversy about elective removal of the loose teeth (most pediatric dentists would remove these teeth if they are loose)
System(s) affected: Gastrointestinal
Genetics: N/A
Incidence/Prevalence in USA: N/A
Predominant age: Birth to 2 years
Predominant sex: N/A

SIGNS AND SYMPTOMS
• A large percent of babies have no signs or symptoms of teething
• Excessive drooling and chewing on fingers begins at 3-4 months of age. This is also the time that normal hand-mouth stimulation increases salivation.
• A small red or white spot may appear over the swollen gum just prior to tooth eruption
• Local inflammation, swelling and occasional hemorrhage can be found on the involved gums
• Discomfort may be noted more with the eruption of the first tooth, the molars and/or with the simultaneous eruption of multiple teeth
• Restlessness, irritability, disturbed sleep, changes in feeding patterns, nasal discharge, mild cough, chin rash, fever, diarrhea, pulling of ear and rubbing of the cheeks have been reported by parents. It is impossible to document that these are caused by teething, so parents and health providers should consider other possible etiologies so as not to miss or delay diagnosing an illness.

CAUSES N/A

RISK FACTORS N/A

DIAGNOSIS

DIFFERENTIAL DIAGNOSIS
Herpetic gingivostomatitis - infants with fever, irritability, sleeplessness and difficulty feeding may have underlying infection caused by herpes simplex virus. Some of these infants with positive culture may not have evidence of inflammation or ulceration expected in gingivitis.

LABORATORY N/A
Drugs that may alter lab results: N/A
Disorders that may alter lab results: N/A

PATHOLOGICAL FINDINGS N/A

SPECIAL TESTS N/A

IMAGING N/A

DIAGNOSTIC PROCEDURES N/A

TREATMENT

APPROPRIATE HEALTH CARE
Outpatient

GENERAL MEASURES
• Treatment for teething include reassurance for the parents and symptomatic relief, if needed
• Provide the infant with a safe, one piece teething ring, clean cloth or pacifier for gumming
• Rub the involved swollen gums if the baby appears to be comforted
• Cool fluids may be offered but avoid frozen foods or objects. These could cause thermal damage to the tissues.
• Toast, cookies, bagels and crackers are offered by some parents for teething, but parents must observe carefully to prevent choking
• Avoid over-the-counter preparations for teething such as Xylocaine 2%, Baby Ora-Gel, Num-zit Gel, Num-zit Liquid, Ambesol. Misuse, overuse and sensitivity have been reported.
• Avoid the use of alcohol
• For the infant with low grade fever, irritability and/or inflamed gums (where other comforting measures have not been of help) - acetaminophen, in proper doses (10-15 mg/kg/dose every 4 hours prn), can be used intermittently
• Gum hematomas that erupt appear as a blue cyst. Most do not require medical intervention. Be sure there are no other signs of a bleeding disorder.
• Breast feeding babies may attempt to chew on the nipple at the end of sucking while teething but can be taught not to bite. Breast feeding can continue after teeth are present.
• Advise parents to avoid: Sugared pacifiers, painted furniture which may contain lead, tying teething ring with cord around the infant's neck, and imported fluid-filled teething rings

SURGICAL MEASURES N/A

ACTIVITY No restrictions

DIET No special diet

PATIENT EDUCATION
• Parents should be cautioned not to misinterpret teething as the cause of any systemic manifestation. The health provider should be consulted for any systemic complaints.
• The ABC's of Teething, Am Academy of Pediatric Dentistry, Public Relations Manual

MEDICATIONS

DRUG(S) OF CHOICE N/A
Contraindications: N/A
Precautions: N/A
Significant possible interactions: N/A

ALTERNATIVE DRUGS N/A

FOLLOWUP

PATIENT MONITORING N/A

PREVENTION/AVOIDANCE N/A

POSSIBLE COMPLICATIONS N/A

EXPECTED COURSE/PROGNOSIS
Normal progression through the teething
process without illness

MISCELLANEOUS

ASSOCIATED CONDITIONS N/A

AGE-RELATED FACTORS
Pediatric: N/A
Geriatric: N/A
Others: N/A

PREGNANCY N/A

SYNONYMS N/A

ICD-9-CM N/A

SEE ALSO N/A

OTHER NOTES N/A

ABBREVIATIONS N/A

REFERENCES
• King NM, Lee A: Prematurely erupted teeth in
the newborn infant. J Ped, 1989;114:807
• Gardiner J: Erupted teeth in the newborn. Proc
Roy Soc Med, 1961;4:504
• Falkner F: Deciduous tooth eruption. Archives
Disease of Childhood, 1957;32:386-391
• Seward M: General disturbances attributed to
the eruption of human primary dentition. J of
Dent for Children, 1972;39(3):178-183
• Golden N, Takieddine F, Hirsch V: Teething
age - prematurely born infants. Am J of Dis of
Child, 1981;135:903-904
• McDonald RE: Eruption of the teeth, local,
systematic and congenital factors that
influence the process. In: Dentistry for the Child
and Adolescent. 5th Ed. St. Louis, C.V. Mosby
Co., 1987:189-196
• King DL, Steinhauer W, Garcia-Godoy F,
Elkins CO: Herpetic gingivostomatitis and
teething difficulty in infants. Pediatric Denistry
1992;14:82-85
Illustrations: N/A
Internet references: http://www.5mcc.com

Author(s)
Nancy P. Fawcett, MD
Dina K. Varon, DDS, MS

Temporomandibular joint (TMJ) syndrome

 BASICS

DESCRIPTION Syndrome characterized by pain and tenderness in the jaw muscles, sound and/or pain over the temporomandibular joint (TMJ), with limitation of mandibular movement
System(s) affected: Musculoskeletal
Genetics: N/A
Incidence/Prevalence in USA:
Symptoms or signs of TMJ dysfunction are present in up to one half of the population but only 5-25% seek treatment
Predominant age: Symptoms more common age 30-50
Predominant sex: Female > Male (3:1)

SIGNS AND SYMPTOMS
• Facial and/or TMJ pain
• Locking or catching of the jaw
• TMJ noises - clicking, grinding, popping
• Headache
• Earache
• Neck pain

CAUSES
• TMJ synovitis
• TMJ disc derangement
• Hyper- or hypomobile TMJ
• Occluso-muscular dysfunction (bruxism)
• Masticatory muscle spasm
• Trauma
• Poorly fitting dentures

RISK FACTORS
• Chronic oral habits such as clenching or grinding of the teeth
• Osteoarthritis, rheumatoid arthritis
• Dental malocclusion
• Fibrositis
• Psychosocial stress

 DIAGNOSIS

DIFFERENTIAL DIAGNOSIS
• Condylar fracture/dislocation
• Trigeminal neuralgia
• Dental or periodontal conditions
• TMJ neoplasm

LABORATORY N/A
Drugs that may alter lab results: N/A
Disorders that may alter lab results: N/A

PATHOLOGICAL FINDINGS
• Condylar head displacement
• Anterior disc displacement
• Posterior capsulitis
• Loosening of disc and capsular attachments
• Chondroid metaplasia of disc leading to disc perforation and degeneration

SPECIAL TESTS Jaw range of motion (opening, closing, lateral, protrusive) and masticatory muscle strength

IMAGING
• Single-contrast videoarthrography demonstrates joint dynamics and disc movement
• Panoramic dental radiographs
• MRI - noninvasive study for disc position. Information gained helps in deciding conservative versus surgical management.

DIAGNOSTIC PROCEDURES
Arthroscopy

 TREATMENT

APPROPRIATE HEALTH CARE
Outpatient treatment

GENERAL MEASURES
• Jaw rest
• Local heat therapy
• Anti-inflammatory medications
• Muscle relaxants
• Analgesics
• Correction of malocclusion with orthodontic appliance
• Stress reduction
• Behavior modification to eliminate tension-relieving oral habits
• Buccal separator orthodontic appliance

SURGICAL MEASURES N/A

ACTIVITY Jaw rest

DIET Soft diet to reduce chewing

PATIENT EDUCATION
• Be aware of any teeth-clenching or grinding habits, and relax the jaw by disengaging the teeth
• Avoid wide uncontrolled opening such as yawning
• Management of stress. Behavioral modification counseling may be helpful.

MEDICATIONS

DRUG(S) OF CHOICE Nonsteroidal anti-inflammatory drugs (NSAID's) - no single drug more efficacious than another

Contraindications:
• History of anaphylaxis to aspirin
• Peptic ulcer disease
• Renal insufficiency

Precautions:
• Peptic ulcers, gastritis or GI bleeding may occur with chronic use
• May cause acute interstitial nephritis
• Drug accumulation with renal insufficiency
• Liver function abnormalities in up to 15% of patients

Significant possible interactions:
• Albumin-bound drugs - displacement of either drug
• Warfarin - increased prothrombin time
• Lithium - increased lithium plasma level
• Furosemide - decreased natriuretic effect
• Propranolol - decreased anti-hypertensive effect

ALTERNATIVE DRUGS Analgesic agents; muscle relaxants

FOLLOWUP

PATIENT MONITORING
• Ongoing assessment of clinical response to conservative therapies (NSAID's, behavior modification, occlusal splints) is necessary
• A surgical procedure to correct disc displacement or replace a damaged disc may be indicated only if the patient has not responded to conservative treatment

PREVENTION/AVOIDANCE Elimination of tension-relieving oral habits and reducing overall muscle tension

POSSIBLE COMPLICATIONS
• Secondary degenerative joint disease
• Chronic TMJ dislocation
• Loss of joint range of motion
• Depression and chronic pain syndromes

EXPECTED COURSE/PROGNOSIS
• With conservative therapy, symptoms resolve in 3/4 of the cases within three months
• Patients benefit the most from a comprehensive treatment approach including correction of occlusal discrepancies, restoration of normal muscle function, pain control, stress management and behavior modification

MISCELLANEOUS

ASSOCIATED CONDITIONS
Cranio-mandibular disorders

AGE-RELATED FACTORS
Pediatric: N/A
Geriatric: N/A
Others: N/A

PREGNANCY No association

SYNONYMS
• Myofascial pain-dysfunction (MPD) syndrome

ICD-9-CM 524.6

SEE ALSO
• Bruxism

OTHER NOTES N/A

ABBREVIATIONS N/A

REFERENCES
• Bronstein SL: Update on temporomandibular joint problems: Diagnosis and treatment. Res & Staff Phys 1988;34(1):71-87
• Dolwick MF, Dimitroulis G: Is there a role for temperomandibular joint surgery? British Jour of Oral and Maxillofacial Surg 1994;32(5): 307-313
• Wright EF, Schiffman EL: Treatment alternatives for patients with masticatory myofacial pain. J ADA 1995;126(7):1030-1039
• dosSantos J: Supportive conservative therapies for temporomandibular disorders. Dental Clin NA 1995;39(2):459-477
Illustrations: N/A
Internet references: http://www.5mcc.com

Author(s)
Scott A. Fields, MD

Tendinitis

BASICS

DESCRIPTION Inflammation of tendon occurring usually at its point of insertion into bone or at the point of muscular origin. The inflammation can extend to adjacent bursal tissue.
System(s) affected: Musculoskeletal
Genetics: N/A
Incidence/Prevalence in USA: Common
Predominant age: None
Predominant sex: Male > Female (slightly)

SIGNS AND SYMPTOMS
• Pain overlying the point of inflammation. This is usually worsened by active motion, but can be present at rest.
• Tenderness over the affected tendon
• Mild erythema and increased heat of overlying skin, especially if the tendon is superficial as in the case of the tendo Achilles

CAUSES Usually related to repetitive activity or trauma, but can be without obvious cause

RISK FACTORS Professional athletes and manual laborers are especially prone to tendinitis due to repetitive use

DIAGNOSIS

DIFFERENTIAL DIAGNOSIS
• Avulsion of the tendon - may occur with loss of function of the affected muscle. X-rays may show a portion of bone avulsed with the tendon, though this is not constant.
• Bursitis - can be impossible to differentiate, especially since the two conditions may coexist
• Infectious tenosynovitis - this occurs largely in the hand. The tenderness and swelling are located along the synovial lines proximally, instead of the insertion. Pain is more marked as is swelling and erythema. The sedimentation rate and white count will usually be elevated.
• Arthritis - the joint may be swollen. Tenderness and pain are in the joint proper in contrast to tendinitis which will be localized to the side of the joint where tendon insertion occurs.

LABORATORY Normal
Drugs that may alter lab results: N/A
Disorders that may alter lab results: N/A

PATHOLOGICAL FINDINGS Tendinitis is usually associated with some degenerative changes in the tendon under microscopic examinations with presence of fibrinoid, mucoid or hyaline degeneration of the connective tissue

SPECIAL TESTS Sonogram - this can be an accurate examination when done with real-time machines. Dynamics of the tendon during contraction may be obtained. Exert care that the ultrasound beam does not cross the tendon obliquely.

IMAGING The CT scan and MRI have replaced even arthrography of the shoulder in most instances. In case where diagnosis is in doubt, especially as regards tendon integrity, an MRI can be obtained and this will usually identify tears, partial tears, inflammation, or tumors. MRI cannot show irregularities of the tendon sheath itself however, and will not diagnose stenosing tenosynovitis or minimal tenosynovitis, unless fluid is present.

DIAGNOSTIC PROCEDURES N/A

TREATMENT

APPROPRIATE HEALTH CARE
Outpatient

GENERAL MEASURES Treatment goals are to relieve pain, reduce inflammation, rest the joint

SURGICAL MEASURES N/A

ACTIVITY
• In acute phases the involved muscle and tendon should be put at rest. Use slings and splints for the upper extremity. Use braces, canes and/or crutches for the lower limbs.
• Physical therapy, once patient is free of pain

DIET No special diet

PATIENT EDUCATION
• Explanation of the problem
• Instructions for use of supportive devices (e.g., crutches, slings)

MEDICATIONS

DRUG(S) OF CHOICE
• Anti-inflammatory drugs:
◊ NSAID's - all have about the same efficacy and the one which is most familiar to the prescriber can be used e.g., piroxicam (Feldene) 10 mg daily or indomethacin (Indocin) 25 or 50 mg tid after meals. Ibuprofen is a low-cost NSAID available over-the-counter.
◊ Corticosteroids - injectable, 40 mg of methylprednisolone (Depo-Medrol) accompanied by 4-6 cc of 1% or 2% lidocaine (Xylocaine) often results in dramatic relief. Never inject tendon, only into tendon sheath or surrounding bursa. (Careful preparation of the skin using Betadine or similar surgical prep is mandatory to prevent infection.)
Contraindications: A tendon should never be injected with a local anesthetic and/or cortisone to allow participation in an athletic event. This can result in complete rupture of the tendon.
Precautions: See manufacturer's profile of each drug
Significant possible interactions: See manufacturer's profile of each drug

ALTERNATIVE DRUGS N/A

FOLLOWUP

PATIENT MONITORING Symptoms will usually subside within a few days after treatment

PREVENTION/AVOIDANCE After adequate rest and treatment, prevention of recurrences is important. Splints such as circular bands for forearm extension tendinitis or patella tendinitis may be useful.

POSSIBLE COMPLICATIONS
• Tendon rupture or avulsion fractures may occur
• Repeated exacerbations of pain. This is probably the most common indication for MRI to confirm the diagnosis and determine the extent of attenuation of the tendon.

EXPECTED COURSE/PROGNOSIS The great majority subside without complications

MISCELLANEOUS

ASSOCIATED CONDITIONS Bursitis, arthritis - osteophytes may be a factor in traumatizing tendons if located adjacent to a tendon

AGE-RELATED FACTORS
Pediatric: A prevalent form of tendinitis is patellar tendinitis associated with inflammation of the tibial apophysis. Known as Osgood-Schlatter disease, it is seen in adolescents especially during a growth spurt. Splinting with a patella band and restricted activity usually alleviate symptoms. However, some are recalcitrant and may require steroid injections and even surgery with splitting of the patella tendon.
Geriatric: N/A
Others: N/A

PREGNANCY N/A

SYNONYMS N/A

ICD-9-CM 762.90

SEE ALSO Osgood-Schlatter disease

OTHER NOTES N/A

ABBREVIATIONS N/A

REFERENCES
• Fornage BD, Rifkin MD: Ultrasonic examinations of tendons. Radiologic Clinics of North America 1988;26(1):87-107
• Baker KS, Gilula LA: Current Role of tenography and bursoghraphy. American Journal of Roentgenography 1990;154(7):129-137
• Lawrence BD, et al: Recent advances in magnetic resonance imaging of the knee. Radiologic Clinics of North America 1990;28(1)
Illustrations: N/A
Internet references: http://www.5mcc.com

Author(s)
Furnie W. Johnston, MD
R. Bruce Hall, MD

Testicular malignancies

BASICS

DESCRIPTION Primary testicular neoplasms may arise from any testicular or adnexal cell component. They are divided into germinal (90-95%) and non-germinal tumors. The germinal tumors, discussed here, are further divided into seminomatous and non-seminomatous types (embryonal, teratoma, choriocarcinomas, yolk sac).
• Clinical staging - Memorial Sloan Kettering Cancer Center (MSKCC)
   ◊ A - tumor limited to testis and cord
   ◊ B - tumor of testis and retroperitoneal nodes
   ◊ B1 - nodes less than 5 cm
   ◊ B2 - positive retroperitoneal nodes > 5 cm in diameter (seen on imaging studies)
   ◊ B3 - positive retroperitoneal nodes > 10 cm in diameter (bulky)
   ◊ C - metastases above diaphragm or involving abdominal solid organs
System(s) affected: Reproductive
Genetics: Weak influence
Incidence/Prevalence in USA:
• 1-2% of all neoplasms in male
• 2.3-6.3 cases/year per 100,000 men (less common in African-Americans - 0.9 cases/year per 100,000)
• In adults, germ cell types comprise 90-95% of testicular cancers; in children, they represent only 60-75%
Predominant age: Peak incidence - age 20-40; smaller peaks between age 0-10 years and > 60
Predominant sex: Male only

SIGNS AND SYMPTOMS
• In adults
   ◊ Scrotal nodule or swelling most common
   ◊ Sensation of fullness or heaviness of scrotum, may be interpreted as "pain"
   ◊ Previously "small" testicle enlarging to size of "normal" contralateral one
   ◊ Firm, non-tender mass within confines of tunica albuginea usually palpably distinct from cord structures
   ◊ Acute or chronic epididymitis/epididymo-orchitis resulting in delay of diagnosis (10%)
   ◊ Manifestations due to metastasis e.g., neck mass (supraclavicular node), respiratory symptoms (lung metastasis), low back pain (nerve root or psoas irritation), uni- or bilateral lower extremity swelling (iliac or caval thrombosis or obstruction) palpable abdominal mass.
   ◊ Hydrocele (10-20%)
   ◊ Gynecomastia (may or may not be due to elevated hormones) (5%)
   ◊ Rapid tumor growth resulting in hemorrhage and necrosis
• In children
   ◊ Non-tender, non-painful scrotal mass
   ◊ Non-transilluminable, large, non-tender testicle
   ◊ Hydrocele (15-20%)
   ◊ With hormonally active tumors, the scrotal exam may be unrevealing

CAUSES No real clear cause and effect relations identified

RISK FACTORS
• Caucasian race; especially Scandinavian background
• Higher social status
• Unmarried
• Rural resident
• History of cryptorchism (even if previously repaired) - only undisputed risk factor
• Weak associations
   ◊ Maternal ingestion of hormones during 1st trimester
   ◊ Intersex disorders in genotypic male with dysgenetic gonad, trauma (no hard evidence of significant risk factor)
   ◊ Atrophy of any cause

DIAGNOSIS:

DIFFERENTIAL DIAGNOSIS
• Hernia
• Hydrocele
• Hematoma
• Spermatocele
• Syphilitic gumma
• Varicocele
• In children - epidermoid/dermoid cyst, para-testicular rhabdomyosarcoma, macro-orchidism, torsion

LABORATORY
• Alpha fetoprotein (AFP) - serum half life is 5-7 days; levels elevated by pure embryonal carcinoma, teratocarcinoma, yolk sac tumor or combinations of these three, but not by pure choriocarcinoma or seminoma
• Beta human chorionic gonadotropin (beta-HCG) - serum half life is 24-36 hours; elevated by all choriocarcinoma, 40-60% embryonal carcinoma; 5-10% pure seminomas have detectable levels of beta-HCG (usually < 500 ng/mL)
• Placental alkaline phosphatase (PLAP) - may be marker of choice for seminoma. 70-90% patients with recurrent or disseminated seminomas have elevated PLAP.
• Lactate dehydrogenase (LDH) - too ubiquitous to be specific. May be direct relationship between elevated LDH levels and tumor burden. Elevated LDH may be sole biochemical abnormality in 10% of patients with persistent or recurrent non-seminomatous tumors.

Drugs that may alter lab results: N/A
Disorders that may alter lab results:
• AFP alterations may be caused by - benign liver disease; telangiectasia and tyrosinemia; malignancies of the liver, pancreas, stomach and lung; heavy marijuana smoking
• PLAP may be elevated by heavy tobacco smoking
• Beta-HCG - pancreatic, stomach, kidney, breast and bladder cancers

PATHOLOGICAL FINDINGS Basically, two different groups based on germinal vs. non-germinal and seminomatous vs. non-seminomatous types

SPECIAL TESTS N/A

IMAGING
• Scrotal ultrasound - see mass clearly originating within testis with echotexture pattern (hypoechoic) distinct from surrounding normal testicular tissue. Echotexture may be mixed.
• For staging:
   ◊ Chest x-ray - good PA and lateral
   ◊ CT scan - very accurate; able to define pelvic retroperitoneal and mediastinal lymphadenopathy as well as to detect abdominal visceral and lung metastases
   ◊ Pedal lymphangiography (LAG) - is sensitive in picking up lymph node involvement intra-abdominally but not as accurate as CT scan in picking up upper para aortic nodes or visceral involvement
   ◊ MRI - still largely experimental

DIAGNOSTIC PROCEDURES
• Transinguinal scrotal exploration with biopsy and/or radical orchiectomy (testicle and spermatic cord excised) makes definite diagnosis
• Transscrotal open or percutaneous biopsy or transscrotal orchiectomy contraindicated secondary to anatomical trespassing into different lymph drainage system

TREATMENT

APPROPRIATE HEALTH CARE Inpatient and outpatient

GENERAL MEASURES
Adjuvent:
• Both seminomatous and non-seminomatous tumors are chemo-sensitive and have good chemotherapeutic response. Seminomas are extremely radiosensitive; more so than non-seminomas
• Treatment for seminomas stages:
◊ A - irradiation, 2500 R to ipsilateral inguinal, iliac chains and bilateral periaortic/pericaval nodes to level of diaphragm
◊ B2 - same as A, with irradiation using 600-1000 R to positive nodes
◊ B3 - chemotherapy - if post-chemotherapy lymph nodes persists more than 3 cm in diameter, then a retroperitoneal lymph node biopsy is added (43% of cases have viable tumor present) and further chemotherapy given if viable tumor found. If < 3 cm, observe.
◊ C - primary chemotherapy
• Treatment for non-seminomatous germ cell tumor stages
◊ A - nerve sparing staging and therapeutic retroperitoneal lymph node dissection (RPLND) alone
◊ B1 (microscopic metastasis in 1-6 nodes, < 2 cm) - observation
◊ B2 (microscopic metastases in more than 6 nodes or grossly positive nodes, 2-6 cm) - observation or two courses of chemotherapy
◊ B3 (nodes > 6 cm or tumor extension outside nodes) - initially 4 courses of chemotherapy. If complete response based on CT scan, serum markers, and no teratoma seen in original specimen, then observe. If partial response, do retroperitoneal lymph node dissection and tumor excision plus 2 more courses of chemotherapy. If tumor cannot all be excised, salvage chemotherapy.
• Children - radical orchiectomy plus initial AFP level
◊ If age ≤ 1 year and AFP rapidly normalizes, no metastases - then observe for 2 years with AFP and chest x-ray
◊ If AFP doesn't normalize or CT shows suspicious lymph nodes and chest x-ray negative - then do RPLND
◊ If lymph nodes are positive and chest x-ray negative - treat with chemotherapy; if chest x-ray positive for solitary lesion, add surgery
◊ If chest x-ray shows several lesions - give radiation
◊ If age > than 1 year - treat with chemotherapy

SURGICAL MEASURES
• All patients receive radical orchiectomy for diagnosis and excellent local control
• See General Measures

ACTIVITY As tolerated

DIET No special diet

PATIENT EDUCATION
• Discuss patient's concerns about sterility, impotence, testicular prostheses, hormone supplements
• Patient education material available from American Cancer Society

MEDICATIONS

DRUG(S) OF CHOICE
• Commonly used chemotherapeutic agents include cisplatin + etoposide ± bleomycin, taxol
• Salvage chemotherapy includes cyclophosphamide (Cytoxan), ifosfamide [with mesna to protect against hemorrhagic cystitis], carboplatin, chemo intensification with granulocyte colony stimulating factor (G-CSF) or autologous bone marrow transplant (BMT)
• In children - vincristine, dactinomycin (actinomycin-D), cyclophosphamide, doxorubicin (Adriamycin)
Contraindications: N/A
Precautions:
• Cisplatin - nephrotoxicity, ototoxicity, neurotoxicity
• Etoposide - marrow suppression, leukemia
• Cyclophosphamide/ifosfamide - hemorrhagic cystitis
• Bleomycin - pulmonary fibrosis
• Adriamycin - marrow suppression
• Vincristine - marrow suppression, neuromuscular toxicity
• Carboplatin - ototoxicity
• Taxol - neuropathy
Significant possible interactions: Refer to manufacturer's literature

ALTERNATIVE DRUGS
• Ondansetron (Zofran), dronabinol (Marinol), metoclopramide (Reglan), and others for nausea control

FOLLOWUP

PATIENT MONITORING
• First year - markers and chest x-ray every month, physical exam (emphasizing nodes) every 2 months
• After 1 year - markers and chest x-ray every 2 months and physical exam every 4 months
• After 2 years - markers and chest x-ray and physical exam every 6-12 months
• If patient had teratoma at diagnosis, need to followup for at least 5 years and get CT scan every year for 3 years

PREVENTION/AVOIDANCE N/A

POSSIBLE COMPLICATIONS
• RPLND treatment - loss of seminal emission (prevented by using nerve-sparing RPLND), atelectasis, hypoalbuminemia
• Radiation treatment - radiation nephritis, enteritis

• Non-seminomatous tumors are more likely to have metastatic disease than seminomas (50-70% vs. 25%, respectively)

EXPECTED COURSE/PROGNOSIS
Usually complete cure in patients with limited disease, 70-80% cure in patients with advanced disease

MISCELLANEOUS

ASSOCIATED CONDITIONS N/A

AGE-RELATED FACTORS
Pediatric: Rare in childhood (only 2% of all solid tumors in childhood)
Geriatric: N/A
Others: N/A

PREGNANCY N/A

SYNONYMS N/A

ICD-9-CM 186 Malignant neoplasm of testis

SEE ALSO N/A

OTHER NOTES N/A

ABBREVIATIONS
• AFP = alpha fetoprotein
• Beta-HCG = beta human chorionic gonadotropin
• LDH = lactate dehydrogenase
• PLAP = placental alkaline phosphatase
• RPLND = retroperitoneal lymph node dissection
• G-CSF = granulocyte cell stimulating factor
• BMT = bone marrow transplant

REFERENCES
• Rowland RG, Donohue JP: Scrotum and Testis. In: Gillenwater JY, Grayhack JT, Howards SS, Duckett JW, eds. Adult and Pediatric Urology. St. Louis, Mosby Yearbook, Inc., 1991
• Morse MJ, Whitmore WF: In: Walsh PC, Gittes RF, Perlmutter AD, et al, eds. Campbell's Urology. Philadelphia, W.B. Saunders Co., 1986
• Klein EA: Tumor Markers in Testis Cancer. The Urologic Clinics of North America 1993;20(1):67
• Motzer RJ, Bosl GJ: Role of adjuvant chemotherapy in patients with Stage II, non-seminomatiour germ cell tumors. The Urologic Clinics of North America 1993;20(1):111
Illustrations: N/A
Internet references: http://www.5mcc.com

Author(s)
Charles Jennings, MD, FACS

Testicular torsion

BASICS

DESCRIPTION Twisting of testis and spermatic cord resulting in acute ischemia.
• Intravaginal torsion: occurs within tunica vaginalis
• Extravaginal torsion: involves twisting of testis, cord and processus vaginalis (especially in newborns) and in undescended testes
System(s) affected: Reproductive
Genetics: Unknown
Incidence/Prevalence in USA: 1:160 males
Predominant age: Occurs from newborn period to 7th decade; 2/3 of cases occur in 2nd decade, with peak at age 14 years; 2nd peak in neonates
Predominant sex: Males only

SIGNS AND SYMPTOMS
• Scrotum is enlarged, red, and edematous
• First symptom is pain (sudden or gradual onset, increasing in severity)
• Nausea and vomiting are common
• Fever may occur
• Testicle exquisitely tender
• Testis may be high in scrotum with a transverse lie
• Absence of cremasteric reflex

CAUSES
• Torsion is usually spontaneous and idiopathic
• History of trauma in 20% of patients
• 1/3 have had prior episodic testicular pain
• Contraction of cremasteric muscle or dartos may play a role and is stimulated by trauma, exercise, cold, sexual stimulation
• Possible alterations in testosterone levels during nocturnal sex response cycle; possible elevated testosterone levels in neonates
• Testis must have inadequate, incomplete or absent fixation within scrotum

RISK FACTORS
• May be more common in winter
• Paraplegia

DIAGNOSIS

DIFFERENTIAL DIAGNOSIS
• Epididymo-orchitis
• Incarcerated/strangulated inguinal hernia
• Acute hydrocele
• Traumatic hematoma
• Idiopathic scrotal edema
• Torsion appendix testis
• Acute varicocele
• Testicular tumor
• Henoch-Schönlein purpura
• Scrotal abscess
• Leukemic infiltrate

LABORATORY Urinalysis may be helpful (usually not)
Drugs that may alter lab results: N/A
Disorders that may alter lab results: N/A

PATHOLOGICAL FINDINGS
• Venous thrombosis
• Tissue edema and necrosis
• Arterial thrombosis

SPECIAL TESTS N/A

IMAGING CT scan or ultrasound may confirm testicular swelling, but are rarely indicated

DIAGNOSTIC PROCEDURES
• Doppler ultrasonic flow detection demonstrates absent or reduced pulse with torsion, increased flow with inflammatory process (only reliable in 1st 12 hrs.)
• Radionuclide testicular scintigraphy with technetium 99m. pertechnetate demonstrates absent/decreased vascularity in torsion, increased vascularity with inflammatory processes (including torsion of appendix testes)

TREATMENT

APPROPRIATE HEALTH CARE
• Manual reduction - may be successful, facilitated by Lidocaine 1% (plain) injection at level of external ring. Must always be followed by orchidopexy.
• Surgical exploration via scrotal approach with detorsion, evaluation of testicular viability, orchidopexy of viable testicle, orchiectomy of non-viable testicle.

GENERAL MEASURES N/A

SURGICAL MEASURES
• Bilateral testicular fixation is recommended
• At least 3-4 point fixation with non-absorbable sutures
• Excision of window of tunica albuginea with suture to dartos fascia
• Any testis that is not clearly viable (and obvious) should be removed.

ACTIVITY As tolerated

DIET Regular

PATIENT EDUCATION Possibility of testicular atrophy in salvaged testis with depressed sperm counts

MEDICATIONS

DRUG(S) OF CHOICE N/A
Contraindications: N/A
Precautions: N/A
Significant possible interactions: N/A

ALTERNATIVE DRUGS N/A

FOLLOWUP

PATIENT MONITORING
• Postoperative visit at 1-2 weeks
• Yearly visits until puberty to evaluate for atrophy

PREVENTION/AVOIDANCE N/A

POSSIBLE COMPLICATIONS
• Possible testicular atrophy
• Abnormal spermatogenesis
• Infertility

EXPECTED COURSE/PROGNOSIS
• Testicular salvage directly related to duration of torsion (85-97% if less than 6 hours, less than 10% if greater than 24 hrs)
• 80-94% may have depressed spermatogenesis related to duration of ischemic injury (possibly related to autoimmune - mediated injury)
• As many as 2/3 of salvaged testicles may atrophy in first 2-3 years post torsion

MISCELLANEOUS

ASSOCIATED CONDITIONS N/A

AGE-RELATED FACTORS N/A
Pediatric: Most common at age 14
Geriatric: Rare in this age group
Others: N/A

PREGNANCY N/A

SYNONYMS N/A

ICD-9-CM
608.2 Torsion of testis

SEE ALSO N/A

OTHER NOTES N/A

ABBREVIATIONS N/A

REFERENCES
• Ashcraft KW: Pediatric Urology. Philadelphia, W.B. Saunders Co, 1990.
• Ashcraft KW, Holder TM: Pediatric Surgery. 2nd Ed. Philadelphia, W.B. Saunders Co., 1993.
• Kelalis PP, King LR, Belman AB: Clinical Pediatric Urology. 3rd Ed. Philadelphia, W.B. Saunders Co, 1992.
Illustrations: N/A
Internet references: http://www.5mcc.com

Author(s)
Timothy L. Black, MD, FACS, FAAP

Tetanus

 BASICS

DESCRIPTION Severe illness characterized by intermittent tonic spasms of voluntary muscles. Toxin enters the central nervous system along the peripheral nerves or is blood borne. Tetanospasmin binds at synapses and blocks inhibitors. Usual course is acute.

System(s) affected: Nervous
Genetics: N/A
Incidence/Prevalence in USA: Rare
Predominant age: Over 70% of cases in persons > 50 years of age
Predominant sex: Male = Female

SIGNS AND SYMPTOMS
• Arrhythmias
• Asphyxia
• Convulsions
• Cyanosis
• Drooling
• Dysphagia
• Fluctuating hypertension
• Hydrophobia
• Hyperhidrosis
• Hyperpyrexia
• Hyperreflexia
• Hypotension
• Irritability
• Low-grade fever
• Muscular rigidity
• Muscular spasticity
• Nuchal rigidity
• Opisthotonos
• Pain at wound site
• Painful tonic convulsions
• Risus sardonicus (fixed smile)
• Stiffness of the jaw
• Sudden bradycardia
• Sudden cardiac arrest
• Tachycardia
• Tingling at wound site
• Trismus
• Wound history (may be absent)

CAUSES
• Infection with Clostridium tetani
• Neurotoxin produced by Clostridium tetani
• Tetanospasmin (an exotoxin)

RISK FACTORS
• Burns
• Drug addiction (parenteral)
• Ear infection (with tympanic membrane perforation)
• Early postpartum with an infected uterus
• Exposure of open wounds to soil and animal feces
• Frostbite
• Newborn (umbilicus stump entry)
• Skin ulcers
• Surgical wounds
• Age > 50 years
• Traumatic wound

 DIAGNOSIS

DIFFERENTIAL DIAGNOSIS
• Dental abscess
• Subarachnoid hemorrhage
• Seizure disorder
• Meningoencephalitis
• Peritonsillar abscess
• Dystonic reaction to phenothiazines
• Hypocalcemic tetany
• Strychnine poisoning
• Alcohol withdrawal

LABORATORY
• Polymorphonuclear leukocytosis
• Culture of Clostridium tetani from wound (may not be positive even if tetanus is the problem)
Drugs that may alter lab results: N/A
Disorders that may alter lab results: N/A

PATHOLOGICAL FINDINGS N/A

SPECIAL TESTS
• ECG - supraventricular tachycardia
• Multifocal ventricular ectopia
• Bradycardia
• EEG sleeping pattern
• Culture of wound infrequently recover C. tetani

IMAGING N/A

DIAGNOSTIC PROCEDURES N/A

 TREATMENT

APPROPRIATE HEALTH CARE Intensive care

GENERAL MEASURES
• Wound excision
• Quiet observation
• Intubation
• IV hydration
• Catheterize the bladder
• Prevent jarring of bed or drafts

SURGICAL MEASURES Tracheostomy if needed

ACTIVITY Absolute bedrest with sedation

DIET Nothing by mouth until well

PATIENT EDUCATION Griffith: Instructions for Patients. Philadelphia, W.B. Saunders Co.,1994

MEDICATIONS

DRUG(S) OF CHOICE
• Anticonvulsants
• Diazepam for muscle rigidity
• Pancuronium bromide (administered by anesthesiologist) plus ventilation
• Tetanus toxoid in a previously immunized patient
• Tetanus immune globulin, human (TIG) 3000 units to 6000 units IM. May infiltrate the area around the wound with a portion of the dose.
• Penicillin G - 2 million units IV q6h. In a penicillin allergic patient, use doxycycline 100 mg q12h, or clindamycin 150-300 mg IV q6h.
Contraindications: Refer to manufacturer's literature
Precautions: Refer to manufacturer's literature. Do not use tetanus immune globulin intravenously.
Significant possible interactions: Refer to manufacturer's literature

ALTERNATIVE DRUGS
Equine tetanus antitoxin 50,000 units IM - only if tetanus immune globulin (human) is not available

FOLLOWUP

PATIENT MONITORING Careful observation in intensive care

PREVENTION/AVOIDANCE Active immunization with tetanus toxoid; wound débridement; passive immunization with tetanus immune globulin; benzathine penicillin; penicillin G; erythromycin

POSSIBLE COMPLICATIONS
• Respiratory arrest
• Cardiac failure
• Pulmonary emboli
• Bacterial infection
• Dehydration
• Vertebral fractures
• Airway obstruction
• Anoxia
• Urinary retention
• Constipation
• Pneumonia
• Rhabdomyolysis

EXPECTED COURSE/PROGNOSIS
• 25-50% mortality
• Poor prognostic factors:
  ◊ Form of tetanus
  ◊ Incubation period
  ◊ Onset period
  ◊ Patient's age
  ◊ Severity of symptoms
  ◊ Heart wound
• Recovery is complete if patient survives

MISCELLANEOUS

ASSOCIATED CONDITIONS N/A

AGE-RELATED FACTORS
Pediatric:
• Mortality high in young
• Infection may enter through umbilical cord
Geriatric: Mortality high in elderly
Others: N/A

PREGNANCY
• Must treat vigorously despite pregnancy
• Infection may enter uterus postpartum
• Tetanus toxoid probably safe, but few data available

SYNONYMS Lockjaw

ICD-9-CM 037 Tetanus

SEE ALSO
• Meningitis, bacterial
• Immunizations
• Anaerobic & necrotizing infections

OTHER NOTES N/A

ABBREVIATIONS N/A

REFERENCES
• Centers for Disease Control, Tetanus: United States 1981-1984. MMWR, 1985;34:602
• Mandell GL, ed: Principles and Practice of Infectious Diseases. 4th Ed. New York, Churchill Livingstone, 1995
Illustrations: N/A
Internet references: http://www.5mcc.com

Author(s)
Abdulrazak Abyad, MD, MPH, AGSF

Tetralogy of Fallot

BASICS

DESCRIPTION Large ventricular septal defect (VSD) associated with right ventricular outflow obstruction (infundibular and/or valvular pulmonic stenosis), right ventricular (RV) hypertrophy and an overriding aorta
• Pathophysiology dependent primarily on severity of right ventricular outflow tract obstruction
• Right and left ventricular pressures are generally equal (VSD is proximal to level of RV obstruction, therefore, RV pressures are elevated)
• Right to left shunting is typical
System(s) affected: Cardiovascular, Pulmonary
Genetics: Familial occurrence, components indicating dominant hereditary
Incidence/Prevalence in USA:
• 5-10% of all congenital heart disease. Most common cardiac cyanotic anomaly after age 1.
• 40 per 100,000 live births
Predominant age: Newborn
Predominant sex: Male > Female (slightly)

SIGNS AND SYMPTOMS
• With mild RV outflow tract obstruction a left to right shunt predominates, and the patient is acyanotic = ("Pink" tetralogy of Fallot)
• Cyanosis with severe RV outflow tract obstruction (generally recognized early)
• Exertional dyspnea, poor exercise tolerance
• Lower birth weight, retarded growth
• Clubbing and polycythemia commonly in children
• Squatting position, typical following exertion (allows increased systemic vascular resistance, lessening right to left shunting)
• No typical facies
• Scoliosis is common
• Normal arterial and jugular venous pulses
• Systolic thrill along the left sternal border
• Early systolic ejection sound (aortic)
• Single S2 (decreased P2)
• Systolic ejection murmur due to flow across narrowed RV outflow tract
• May auscultate the continuous diminished murmur of bronchial collateral vessels
• Right aortic arch in 30%
• Atrial septal defect (ASD) in 15%
• Anomalous coronary arteries in 2-10%
• Retinal engorgement
• Hemoptysis
• Aortic ejection click

CAUSES Unknown

RISK FACTORS
• Documented increased incidence with increased maternal age
• Occasional familial occurrence

DIAGNOSIS

DIFFERENTIAL DIAGNOSIS
• Fallot's tetralogy with absent pulmonic valve
• Fallot's tetralogy with absent pulmonary artery
• Pseudotruncus arteriosus

LABORATORY N/A
Drugs that may alter lab results: N/A
Disorders that may alter lab results: N/A

PATHOLOGICAL FINDINGS
• Anterior deviation of the infundibular septum, resulting in malalignment with the muscular septum, creating a ventricular septal defect
• Malposition of the infundibular septum, which encroaches on the right ventricular outflow tract, resulting in an increased aortic root size
• Aortic root rotated into overriding position

SPECIAL TESTS
• ECG
  ◊ Right axis deviation, right ventricular hypertrophy, subsequent right ventricular conduction abnormality
  ◊ Sinus rhythm in general, however, some may develop atrial fibrillation or flutter

IMAGING
• Chest x-ray
  ◊ In children, typically a small boot-shaped heart (coeur en sabot) with diminished pulmonary blood flow
  ◊ Prominent right ventricle
  ◊ Possibly a right sided aortic arch and knob
  ◊ Normal (or perhaps decreased) pulmonary vascularity in approximately 50% adults
• 2D echocardiogram/Doppler echocardiogram
  ◊ 2D images demonstrate the VSD, overriding aorta, extent and location of the infundibular obstruction, assessment of pulmonic valve, right ventricular hypertrophy, and coronary anatomy, additional ventricular septal defects, and peripheral branch pulmonic arteries
  ◊ Doppler echocardiogram allows quantification of the outflow gradient
  ◊ Colorflow Doppler provides assessment of the VSD
  ◊ Coronary anatomy

DIAGNOSTIC PROCEDURES
• Cardiac catheterization
  ◊ Assesses pulmonary annulus size and pulmonary arteries
  ◊ Assesses severity of right ventricular outflow obstruction
  ◊ Locates position of VSD and its size
  ◊ Rules out possible coronary artery anomalies

TREATMENT

APPROPRIATE HEALTH CARE Inpatient for diagnosis and surgery

GENERAL MEASURES
• Good dental hygiene
• Endocarditis prophylaxis

SURGICAL MEASURES
• Palliative surgical therapy
  ◊ It is important to emphasize that complete repair is the preferable modality of treatment
  ◊ Blalock-Taussig shunt or modified shunt (subclavian to pulmonary artery)
  ◊ Pott's procedure (descending aorta to pulmonary artery)
  ◊ Waterston's shunt (ascending aorta to pulmonary artery)
• Total correction surgical therapy
  ◊ Includes patch closure of VSD and relief of right ventricular outflow obstruction

ACTIVITY As tolerated

DIET Salt restriction

PATIENT EDUCATION American Heart Association, 7320 Greenville Avenue, Dallas, TX 75231, (214)373-6300

MEDICATIONS

DRUG(S) OF CHOICE No specific drug therapy in the absence of heart failure
Contraindications: N/A
Precautions: N/A
Significant possible interactions: N/A

ALTERNATIVE DRUGS N/A

FOLLOWUP

PATIENT MONITORING
• Postoperative (or post-balloon valvotomy) Doppler ultrasound suggested at approximately 1 year from procedure
• Post-valvotomy SBE prophylaxis still required
• Regular followup assessment for patients not undergoing surgical correction

POSSIBLE COMPLICATIONS
• Erythrocytosis may develop secondary to chronic hypoxemia (risk for thrombosis, thrombotic CVA and paradoxical emboli)
• Increased risk for brain abscess, acute gouty arthritis
• Infective endocarditis
• Cerebrovascular thrombosis
• Delayed puberty
• Postoperatively
  ◊ Residual right ventricular outflow obstruction
  ◊ Residual VSD
  ◊ Pulmonic regurgitation
  ◊ Ventricular arrhythmias
  ◊ Right bundle branch block quite common
  ◊ Left anterior hemiblock
  ◊ Infective bacterial endocarditis

PREVENTION/AVOIDANCE N/A

EXPECTED COURSE/PROGNOSIS Fatal if not surgically corrected

MISCELLANEOUS

ASSOCIATED CONDITIONS
• Stenotic pulmonary artery
• Patent ductus arteriosus
• Atrial septal defect
• Iron deficiency anemia

AGE-RELATED FACTORS
Pediatric: Congenital disorder
Geriatric: N/A
Others: N/A

PREGNANCY Well tolerated after total surgical correction

SYNONYMS N/A

ICD-9-CM 745.2

SEE ALSO N/A

OTHER NOTES N/A

ABBREVIATIONS
• VSD = ventricular septal defect
• RV = right ventricle

REFERENCES
• Braunwald E, ed: Heart Disease: A Textbook of Cardiovascular Medicine. 4th Ed. Philadelphia, W.B. Saunders Co., 1992
• Liberthson R: Congenital Heart Disease: Diagnosis & Management in Children and Adults. Boston, Little Brown, 1989
• Perloff J: Clinical Recognition of Congenital Heart Disease. 4th Ed. Philadelphia, W.B. Saunders Co., 1994
Illustrations: N/A
Internet references: http://www.5mcc.com

Author(s)
Sylvia A. Mamby, MD

Thalassemia

BASICS

DESCRIPTION A group of inherited disorders that affect the synthesis of hemoglobin. In beta-thalassemia, there is deficient synthesis of beta globin, while in alpha-thalassemia, there is deficient synthesis of alpha globin. This leads to deficient hemoglobin accumulation, resulting in hypochromic and microcytic red cells. Abnormality of the red cells is the most characteristic feature of the thalassemias. Thalassemia is prevalent in the Mediterranean region, Middle East and Southeast Asia, and among ethnic groups originating from these areas
• Types
◊ Beta-thalassemia major (Cooley's anemia) - severe anemia growth retardation, hepatosplenomegaly, bone marrow expansion and bone deformities. Transfusion therapy necessary to sustain life.
◊ Thalassemia intermedia - milder form. Transfusion therapy may not be needed.
◊ Thalassemia trait (alpha or beta) - mild anemia with microcytosis and hypochromia. No transfusion therapy needed.
• Varieties unique to Southeast Asians include hemoglobin H disease (a more severe form of alpha thalassemia) and hemoglobin E/beta thalassemia which often mimics Beta thalassemia major in its severity. Bother alpha and beta thalassemia trait (minor) are frequent in African-Americans but symptomatic thalassemia is very rare.
System(s) affected:
Hemic/Lymphatic/Immunologic
Genetics:
• Inherited in an autosomal recessive pattern
• Inheritance of one defective gene = milder type of thalassemia, two defective genes = severe type of thalassemia
Incidence/Prevalence in USA:
• Approximately 1000 patients with severe thalassemia
• The incidence of thalassemia trait within the ethnic groups involved ranges from 3-5%
Predominant age: Symptoms start to appear 3-6 months after birth
Predominant sex: Male = Female

SIGNS AND SYMPTOMS
(Thalassemia trait has no signs or symptoms)
• Pallor
• Poor growth
• Inadequate food intake
• Fatigue
• Shortness of breath
• Splenomegaly
• Jaundice
• Maxillary hyperplasia
• Dental malocclusion
• Cholelithiasis
• Pathologic fractures

CAUSES Genetic

RISK FACTORS Family history

DIAGNOSIS

DIFFERENTIAL DIAGNOSIS
• Iron deficiency
• Other hemoglobinopathies
• Other hemolytic anemias

LABORATORY
• Hemoglobin
◊ Elevated Hb A2 levels in beta-thalassemia trait
◊ Elevated Hb A2, elevated Hb F, reduced or absent Hb A1 in beta-thalassemia major or intermedia
• Peripheral blood
◊ Pronounced microcytosis
◊ Anisocytosis
◊ Hypochromia
◊ Punctate basophilic stippling
◊ High percentage of target cells
◊ Reticulocyte count elevated
• Hematocrit
◊ 28-40% in alpha-thalassemia trait and beta-thalassemia trait
◊ May fall to less than 10% in beta-thalassemia major
Drugs that may alter lab results: N/A
Disorders that may alter lab results: Parvovirus B19 infection may produce "aplastic crisis" and severe reticulocytopenia

PATHOLOGICAL FINDINGS
• Bone marrow hyperactivity
• Iron deposits in heart muscle
• Hepatic siderosis

SPECIAL TESTS
Bone marrow aspiration

IMAGING
Skull x-ray: thickened diploë of skull, osteoporosis

DIAGNOSTIC PROCEDURES
Family history

TREATMENT

APPROPRIATE HEALTH CARE
Outpatient for mild cases. Inpatient for transfusion therapy.

GENERAL MEASURES
• Mild cases require no therapy
• Thalassemia intermedia - normally no therapy necessary unless hemoglobin levels fall to a dangerous level, then may need transfusion therapy
• Patients with severe thalassemia
◊ Maintain the mean hemoglobin level of at least 9.3 g/dL (1.4 mmol/L) with a regular transfusion schedule (transfusions of about 15 mL per kg at 3-5 week intervals)
◊ Folate supplementation
◊ Treat infections promptly
• Iron overload
◊ Patients receiving transfusion therapy increase total body iron 4 times over the normal amount
◊ Therapy is iron chelation

SURGICAL MEASURES
• Splenectomy
◊ May be needed if hypersplenism causes a marked increase in the transfusion requirement
◊ Recommendation is to defer surgery until patient is 4-6 years of age (due to increased infection risk)
◊ Administer polyvalent pneumococcal vaccine one month prior to splenectomy
◊ Prophylaxis with a daily regimen of penicillin
• Bone marrow transplantation
◊ Available for selected patients with a matched sibling
◊ Cures the disease, but associated with significant mortality and morbidity

ACTIVITY
• Avoid strenuous activities (e.g., football, soccer)
• Acceptable activity levels will need to be determined on an individual basis depending on severity of disorder

DIET
• Avoid iron-rich foods (meats such as liver, and some cereals)
• Drinking tea may possibly help reduce iron

PATIENT EDUCATION
• Genetic counseling
• Teach parents signs of hepatitis, iron overload
• Printed patient information available from: Cooley's Anemia Foundation, 105 E. 22nd St., Suite 911, New York, NY 10010, (212)598-0911

MEDICATIONS

DRUG(S) OF CHOICE
• Antibiotics for infection
• Folic acid supplements
• Iron chelation with deferoxamine (Desferal). Continuous subcutaneous or intravenous infusion with a small infusion pump 40 mg per kg per day (about a 10 hour period). Usually started before 5-8 years of age.
Contraindications: Refer to manufacturer's literature
Precautions: Refer to manufacturer's literature
Significant possible interactions: Refer to manufacturer's literature

ALTERNATIVE DRUGS N/A

FOLLOWUP

PATIENT MONITORING Life-long monitoring necessary because both the therapy and disease progression have numerous possible complications

PREVENTION/AVOIDANCE
• Prenatal information
  ◊ Genetic counseling
  ◊ Prenatal diagnosis - study of beta globin genes performed on fetal cell DNA obtained by amniocentesis after 14 weeks
• Complication prevention
  ◊ Evaluation for thalassemia by 1 year of age for offspring of adult thalassemia patients
  ◊ Avoidance of infections
  ◊ Prompt treatment of infections (after splenectomy, patients should maintain a supply of ampicillin to take if symptoms of infection appear)
  ◊ Periodic dental checkups
  ◊ Avoidance of activities that could result in bone fractures

POSSIBLE COMPLICATIONS
• Chronic hemolysis
• Susceptibility to infections after splenectomy
• Infections from blood transfusion
• Intercurrent infections
• Worsening of anemia during infections
• Jaundice
• Leg ulcers
• Cholelithiasis
• Pathologic fractures
• Impaired growth rate
• Delayed or absent puberty
• Hepatic siderosis
• Hemolytic anemia
• Splenomegaly
• Cardiac disease from iron overload
• Aplastic and megaloblastic crises

EXPECTED COURSE/PROGNOSIS
• Outlook varies depending on type
• Thalassemia major patients live an average of 17 years, some into their mid-twenties.
• Thalassemia minor patients live a normal life span

MISCELLANEOUS

ASSOCIATED CONDITIONS See Possible complications

AGE-RELATED FACTORS
Pediatric: A disorder of childhood
Geriatric: N/A
Others: N/A

PREGNANCY Genetic counseling - advised for parents or other relatives of a child with thalassemia and for any individual with beta-thalassemia minor

SYNONYMS
• Mediterranean anemia
• Hereditary leptocytosis
• Thalassemia major and minor
• Cooley's anemia

ICD-9-CM 282.4

SEE ALSO N/A

OTHER NOTES N/A

ABBREVIATIONS N/A

REFERENCES
• Nathan DG, Oski F, eds: Hematology of Infancy and Childhood. Philadelphia, W.B. Saunders Co., 1991
• Fosburg MT, Nathan DG: Treatment of Cooley's anemia. Blood 1990;76:435
Illustrations: N/A
Internet references: http://www.5mcc.com

Author(s)
W. Paul Bowman, MD

Thoracic outlet syndrome

BASICS

DESCRIPTION A constellation of symptoms that affect the head, neck, shoulders and upper extremities caused by compression of the neurovascular structures (viz. cords of brachial plexus and subclavian artery and vein) at the thoracic outlet
• May be due to congenital bony muscular or tendonous anomalies; post traumatic, following clavicular or cervical spine injures; or idiopathic, without discernible cause
System(s) affected: Nervous, Musculoskeletal, Cardiovascular
Genetics: N/A
Incidence/Prevalence in USA: Unknown
Predominant age:
• Neurologic type (95%) - 20-60 years
• Venous type (4%) - 20-35 years
• Arterial type (1%) (atherosclerosis) - young adult or older than 50
Predominant sex:
• Neurologic type - Female > Male (3:1)
• Venous type - Male > Female
• Arterial type - Male = Female

SIGNS AND SYMPTOMS
• General symptoms
  ◊ Positive costoclavicular maneuver
  ◊ Positive hyperabduction maneuver
  ◊ Positive Adson's maneuver
  ◊ Positive elevated arm stress test
  ◊ Tenderness to percussion or palpation of supraclavicular area
  ◊ Worsening of symptoms with elevation of arm, overhead extension of arms, or with arms extended forward (e.g., driving a car, typing, carrying objects). Prompt disappearance of symptoms with arm returning to neutral position.
  ◊ Supraventricular bruit
• Neurologic type, upper plexus (C4-C7)
  ◊ Pain and paresthesias in head, neck, mandible, face, temporal area, upper back/chest, outer arm & hand in a radial nerve distribution
  ◊ Occipital headache
• Neurologic type, lower plexus (C8-T1)
  ◊ Pain and paresthesias in axilla, inner arm and hand in an ulnar nerve distribution
  ◊ Hypothenar and interosseous muscle atrophy
• Venous type
  ◊ Arm claudication
  ◊ Cyanosis
  ◊ Swelling
  ◊ Distended arm veins
• Arterial type
  ◊ Digital vasospasm
  ◊ Thrombosis/embolism
  ◊ Aneurysm
  ◊ Gangrene

CAUSES
• Upper thoracic neurovascular bundle compression
• Cervical rib
• Taut anomalous scalene muscles
• Elongated C7 transverse process
• Poor posture
• Pancoast's tumor
• Atherosclerotic plaques within vessels
• Subclavian muscle
• Costocoracoid tendon
• Callous bone formation from fractured clavicle or first rib
• Aberrant tissue

RISK FACTORS
• Exuberant callus after fracture of clavicle or first rib
• Exostosis of clavicle or first rib
• Postural abnormalities (e.g., drooping of shoulders, scoliosis)
• Body building, with increased muscular bulk in thoracic outlet area
• Rapid weight loss combined with vigorous physical exertion and/or exercise

DIAGNOSIS

DIFFERENTIAL DIAGNOSIS
• Cervical disk syndrome
• Carpal tunnel syndrome
• Orthopedic shoulder problems (shoulder strain, rotator cuff injury, tendinitis)
• Cervical spondylitis
• Ulnar nerve compression at the elbow
• Multiple sclerosis
• Spinal cord tumor or disease
• Angina pectoris
• Migraine

LABORATORY N/A
Drugs that may alter lab results: N/A
Disorders that may alter lab results: N/A

PATHOLOGICAL FINDINGS
• Bony abnormalities (cervical rib, anomalous first thoracic rib)
• Abnormal muscles
• Congenital fibromuscular bands

SPECIAL TESTS
• Plethysmography with previously mentioned maneuvers
• Doppler and duplex ultrasound if venous obstruct suspected
• Nerve conduction studies (< 70 m/sec is abnormal)

IMAGING
• X-ray (chest x-ray, oblique C-spine)
• Arteriogram - if arterial obstruction, aneurysm or emboli are suspected
• Phlebogram - if signs of venous obstruction
• CT scan - if cord compressive lesions (disc and/or tumor) are suspected

DIAGNOSTIC PROCEDURES Thoracic outlet syndrome (TOS) is a clinical diagnosis

TREATMENT

APPROPRIATE HEALTH CARE
• Outpatient for conservative treatment
• Inpatient if surgery required

GENERAL MEASURES
• Conservative
  ◊ If no vascular involvement is present and/or if no loss of function or lifestyle is present due to severity of symptoms, conservative therapy may be undertaken for 2-3 months
  ◊ Improvement can be expected in 60% of patients
  ◊ Exercise program to promote shoulder muscle function
  ◊ Physical therapy for postural faults
  ◊ Cervical collar, traction
  ◊ Weight loss if axillary folds are causing compression

SURGICAL MEASURES
• Operative - if vascular involvement is present and/or if there is loss of function or lifestyle secondary to severity of symptoms and if conservative therapy fails after 2-3 months
• Removal of first rib or cervical ribs (transaxillary, supraclavicular, posterior approaches)
• Removal of adhesive bands
• Anterior scalenectomy (not scalenotomy)

ACTIVITY
• Light activity with arm and hand encouraged
• No straining or heavy activity for 3 months

DIET N/A

PATIENT EDUCATION Physical therapy following surgery

MEDICATIONS

DRUG(S) OF CHOICE
• Analgesics
• Muscle relaxants
• Antispasmodics
Contraindications: Refer to manufacturer's profile of each drug
Precautions: Refer to manufacturer's profile of each drug
Significant possible interactions: Refer to manufacturer's profile of each drug

ALTERNATIVE DRUGS N/A

FOLLOWUP

PATIENT MONITORING Office follow-up visits e.g., q3 weeks x 2

PREVENTION/AVOIDANCE N/A

POSSIBLE COMPLICATIONS
• Postoperative shoulder, arm, hand pain and paresthesias in 10%, usually responds to physiotherapy
• 1.5-2% of patients will have symptomatic recurrences 1 month to 7 years postoperatively (usually within 3 months)
• 0.5-1% of patients have brachial plexus injury, probably due to intraoperative traction
• Re-operation indicated for symptomatic recurrence with long posterior remnant of first rib (posterior approach) or with disrupted fibrous adhesions (transaxillary approach)

EXPECTED COURSE/PROGNOSIS
• 60% improve with appropriate physiotherapy program
• 90% have excellent or good early results with surgery
• 70-80% have no recurrence at 5 years and 10 years

MISCELLANEOUS

ASSOCIATED CONDITIONS N/A

AGE-RELATED FACTORS N/A
Pediatric: N/A
Geriatric: N/A
Others: N/A

PREGNANCY Generalized tissue fluid accumulations and postural changes could aggravate symptoms

SYNONYMS
• Scalenus anticus syndrome
• Cervical rib syndrome
• Costoclavicular syndrome
• TOS

SEE ALSO N/A

ICD-9-CM 353.0 Thoracic outlet syndrome

OTHER NOTES 2-3 months trial of physiotherapy always indicated except in presence of obvious bony abnormality

ABBREVIATIONS N/A

REFERENCES
• Ursche HC, Rassuk MA: Thoracic Outlet Syndromes. In: Sabiston DC, Spencer FC, eds. Surgery of the Chest. 5th Ed. Philadelphia, W.B. Saunders Co.,1990
• Roos DB: Thoracic Outlet Nerve Compression. In: Ruthford RB, ed. Vascular Surgery. 3rd Ed. Philadelphia, W.B. Saunders Co.,1989
• Dale WQ: Thoracic outlet compression syndrome. Arch Surg 1982;117:1437
• Stallworth JM: Thoracic Outlet Compression Syndromes. In: Haimoviei H, ed. Vascular Surgery. 3rd Ed. Norwalk, Appleton & Lange,1989
Illustrations: N/A
Internet references: http://www.5mcc.com

Author(s)
Donald W. Moorman, MD
Michael A. Oddi, MD

Thromboangiitis obliterans (Buerger's disease)

 BASICS

DESCRIPTION Occlusion of small and medium sized arteries and veins caused by inflammatory changes in these vessels. It primarily occurs in men who smoke.
System(s) affected: Cardiovascular
Genetics: Greater prevalence of HLA-A9 and HLA-B5. Familial cases reported rarely.
Incidence/Prevalence in USA:
13/100,000
Predominant age: 20 to 40 years
Predominant sex: Male > Female (3:1). Increasing numbers of women are being diagnosed, presumably due to increased smoking.

SIGNS AND SYMPTOMS
Symptoms tend to wax and wane in early disease and are often asymmetric. Symptoms may be gradual or have a sudden onset related to impaired vasculature.
• Ulceration of digits; pain may be disabling
• Coldness in feet and/or fingers
• Cold sensitivity
• Paresthesias (numbness, tingling, burning, hypoesthesia) of feet and/or fingers
• Intermittent claudication in arch of foot or leg (rarely hand, forearm)
• Persistent extremity pain (may be worse at rest)
• Paroxysmal "electric shock" pain of ischemic neuropathy
• Raynaud's phenomenon
• Postural color changes (pallor on elevation; rubor on dependency)
• "Buerger's color" - cyanosis of hands and feet
• Migratory superficial phlebitis
• Tender skin nodules on extremities
• Impaired distal pulses; proximal pulses normal
• Foot edema
• Gangrene

CAUSES
(Postulated)
• Smoking
• Genetic factors
• Autoimmune disorder with cell mediated sensitivity to types I and III human collagens (both are constituents of blood vessels)

RISK FACTORS
• Smoking tobacco
• Incidence higher in Israel, Eastern Europe, Japan, India, Far East

 DIAGNOSIS

DIFFERENTIAL DIAGNOSIS
• Peripheral neuropathy
• Peripheral atherosclerotic disease
• Arterial embolus and thrombosis
• Idiopathic peripheral thrombosis
• Other causes of vasculitis
• Scleroderma
• Occupational trauma
• Cervical rib
• Livedo reticularis
• Raynaud's disease
• Acrocyanosis
• Ergotism
• Frostbite
• Neurotrophic ulcers
• Reflex sympathetic dystrophy
• Metatarsalgia
• Gout
• Periarteritis nodosa

LABORATORY Routine laboratory studies show no changes characteristic of this disorder. Auto-antibodies to collagen and circulating immune complexes may be present, but are considered a research tool only.
Drugs that may alter lab results: N/A
Disorders that may alter lab results: N/A

PATHOLOGICAL FINDINGS
• Segmental nonsuppurative panarteritis or panphlebitis with thrombosis
• Histologic findings may vary between acute, subacute, and chronic stages of the disease
• Histologic sine qua non - granulomas with collections of neutrophils in the organizing thrombus. Inflammation reaction permeates the entire thickness of the vessel wall.
• Chronic lesions show recanalized thrombus and perivascular fibrosis.

SPECIAL TESTS Doppler ultrasound (not specific)

IMAGING
• Arteriogram or digital-subtraction angiography (DSA)
  ◊ Multiple areas of segmental occlusion of small to medium arteries of arms and legs
  ◊ "Skip" areas may be demonstrated
  ◊ Numerous collateral vessels around occluded segments may give a characteristic "cork screw" appearance
  ◊ Larger arteries are spared

DIAGNOSTIC PROCEDURES
• History and physical examination
• Studies of nerve conduction velocity (to exclude neuropathy)

 TREATMENT

APPROPRIATE HEALTH CARE
• Outpatient
• Inpatient if surgery needed for gangrene
• Inpatient for dorsal or lumbar sympathectomy if indicated

GENERAL MEASURES
• Stop smoking (mandatory)
• Protect against trauma (poor fitting shoes)
• Protect against infections
• Protect against vasoconstriction from cold or drugs
• Eliminate exposure to thermal damage
• Eliminate exposure to chemical damage (iodine, carbolic acid, salicylic acid)
• Thrombolytic therapy of occlusive thrombus and angioplasty are experimental

SURGICAL MEASURES
• Amputation for non-healing ulcers, gangrene or intractable pain. Should preserve as much limb as possible. Rarely required.
• Omental autotransplantation has been successful in treating ulcers
• In severe disease, a lumbar sympathectomy to increase blood supply to the skin
• Direct revascularization of distal arteries is not practical unless coexistent atherosclerotic disease

ACTIVITY Restricted by symptoms. Use a bed cradle (non-heated) to prevent pressure from bed linens.

DIET No restrictions

PATIENT EDUCATION
• Must stop smoking
• Remove possibilities of exposure to others in the environment who smoke
• Use heel pads or foam rubber boots
• See General Measures

Thromboangiitis obliterans (Buerger's disease)

MEDICATIONS

DRUG(S) OF CHOICE
• Medications are not a substitute for discontinuance of smoking
• Antibiotics for infected digital ulcers and osteomyelitis
• Iloprost, a prostacyclin analogue, promotes ulcer healing
• No form of medical treatment has been shown to be effective (including steroids, calcium channel blockers, reserpine, pentoxifylline, vasodilators, antiplatelet drugs, anticoagulants)
Contraindications: Refer to manufacturer's literature
Precautions: Refer to manufacturer's literature
Significant possible interactions: Refer to manufacturer's literature

ALTERNATIVE DRUGS
Calcium channel blocking agents such as nifedipine may allow vasodilatation, but have not been proven effective.

FOLLOWUP

PATIENT MONITORING
Frequent history and physical examinations

PREVENTION/AVOIDANCE
Never smoke

POSSIBLE COMPLICATIONS
• Ulcerations
• Gangrene
• Need for amputation
• Rare involvement of cerebral, coronary, renal or mesenteric arteries

EXPECTED COURSE/PROGNOSIS
• Occasional remissions
• Unremitting progression if patient continues to smoke
• Death rare; normal survival curve

MISCELLANEOUS

ASSOCIATED CONDITIONS N/A

AGE-RELATED FACTORS
Pediatric: Not a problem in this age group
Geriatric: Not common in this age group, but diagnosis in the elderly is increasing
Others: N/A

PREGNANCY N/A

SYNONYMS
• Buerger's disease
• TAO

ICD-9-CM 443.1 Thromboangiitis obliterans (Buerger's disease)

SEE ALSO N/A

OTHER NOTES
May be difficult to differentiate from some types of atherosclerosis, systemic emboli or idiopathic peripheral thromboses

ABBREVIATIONS N/A

REFERENCES
• Hurst JW, et al: The Heart. 7th Ed. New York, McGraw-Hill, 1990
• Case records of the Mass. General Hospital. Weekly clinicopathological exercises. case 16-1989. A 36 year-old man with peripheral vascular disease. New Eng J Med 1989;20;320(16):1068-76
• Olin JW, et al: The changing clinical spectrum of thromboangiitis obliterans (Buerger's disease). Circulation Supplement IV 1990;82(5)
• Juergens JL: Thromboangiitis Obliterans (Buerger's disease, TAO). In: Juergens JL, ed. Peripheral Vascular Disease. Philadelphia, W.B. Saunders Co., 1980
Illustrations: N/A
Internet references: http://www.5mcc.com

Author(s)
Rick Kellerman, MD

Thrombophlebitis, superficial

BASICS

DESCRIPTION Superficial thrombophlebitis is an inflammatory condition of the veins with secondary thrombosis.
- Septic (suppurative) thrombophlebitis types:
  ◊ Iatrogenic
  ◊ Infectious, mainly syphilis and psittacosis
- Aseptic thrombophlebitis types:
  ◊ Primary hypercoagulable states - disorders with measurable defects in the proteins of the coagulation and/or fibrinolytic systems
  ◊ Secondary hypercoagulable states - clinical conditions with a risk of thrombosis

System(s) affected: Cardiovascular
Genetics:
- Septic - no known genetic pattern
- Antithrombin III deficiencies - autosomal dominant
- Proteins C and S deficiency - autosomal dominant with variable penetrance
- Disorders of fibrinolytic system - congenital defects inheritance variable
- Dysfibrinogenemia - autosomal dominant
- Factor XII deficiency - autosomal recessive

Incidence/Prevalence in USA:
- Septic
  ◊ Up to 10% of all nosocomial infections
  ◊ Incidence of catheter-related thrombophlebitis is 88/100,000
  ◊ Develops in 4-8% if cut down is performed
- Aseptic primary hypercoagulable state
  ◊ Antithrombin III and heparin cofactor II deficiency incidence is 50/100,000
- Aseptic secondary hypercoagulable state
  ◊ Trousseau incidence in malignancy 5-15%
  ◊ Trousseau in pancreatic carcinoma 50%
  ◊ In pregnancy 49-fold increased incidence of phlebitis
  ◊ Superficial migratory thrombophlebitis in 27% of patients with thromboangiitis obliterans

Predominant age:
- Septic
  ◊ More common in childhood
- Aseptic primary hypercoagulable state
  ◊ Antithrombin III and heparin cofactor II deficiency - neonatal period, but first episode usually at age 20-30 years
  ◊ Proteins C and S - before age 30
- Aseptic secondary hypercoagulable state
  ◊ Mondor's disease: women, ages 21-55 years
  ◊ Thromboangiitis obliterans onset: 20-50 years

Predominant sex:
- Suppurative:
  ◊ Male = Female
- Aseptic
  ◊ Mondor's - Female > Male (2:1)
  ◊ Thromboangiitis obliterans - Female > Male (1-19% of clinical cases)

SIGNS AND SYMPTOMS
- Swelling, tenderness, redness along the course of the veins
- May look like cellulitis or erythema nodosa
- Fever in 70% of patients
- Warmth, erythema, tenderness, or lymphangitis in 32%
- Sign of systemic sepsis in 84% in suppurative
- Red, tender cord
- Pain

CAUSES
- Septic
  ◊ Staphylococcus aureus in 65-78%
  ◊ Enterobacteriaceae, especially Klebsiella
  ◊ Multiple organisms in 14%
  ◊ Anaerobic isolate rare
  ◊ Candida spp.
  ◊ Cytomegalovirus in AIDS patients
- Aseptic primary hypercoagulable state
  ◊ Antithrombin III and heparin II deficiency
  ◊ Protein C and protein S deficiency
  ◊ Disorder of tissue plasminogen activator
  ◊ Abnormal plasminogen and co-plasminogen
  ◊ Dysfibrinogenemia
  ◊ Factor XII deficiency
  ◊ Lupus anticoagulant and anticardiolipin antibody syndrome
- Aseptic secondary hypercoagulable states
  ◊ Malignancy (Trousseau syndrome: Recurrent migratory thrombophlebitis). Most commonly seen in - metastatic mucin or adenocarcinomas of the GI tract (pancreas, stomach, colon and gall bladder); lung, prostate, ovary.
  ◊ Pregnancy
  ◊ Oral contraceptive
  ◊ Infusion of prothrombin complex concentrates
  ◊ Behçet's disease
  ◊ Buerger's disease
  ◊ Mondor's disease

RISK FACTORS
- Nonspecific
  ◊ Immobilization
  ◊ Obesity
  ◊ Advanced age
  ◊ Postoperative states
- Septic
  ◊ Intravenous catheter
  ◊ Duration of intravenous catheterization (68% of cannulae have been left in place for 2 days)
  ◊ Cutdowns
  ◊ Cancer, debilitating diseases
  ◊ Steroid
  ◊ Incidence is 40 times higher with plastic cannula (8%) than with steel or scalp cannulas (0.2%)
  ◊ Thrombosis
  ◊ Dermal infection
  ◊ Burned patients
  ◊ Lower extremities intravenous catheter
  ◊ Intravenous antibiotics
  ◊ AIDS
  ◊ Varicose veins
- Antithrombin II and heparin cofactor II deficiency
  ◊ Pregnancy
  ◊ Oral contraceptives
  ◊ Surgery; trauma; infection

- In pregnancy
  ◊ Increased age
  ◊ Hypertension
  ◊ Eclampsia
  ◊ Increased parity
- Thromboangiitis obliterans
  ◊ Persistent smoking
- Mondor's disease
  ◊ Breast abscess
  ◊ Antecedent breast surgery
  ◊ Breast augmentation
  ◊ Reduction mammoplasty

DIAGNOSIS

DIFFERENTIAL DIAGNOSIS
- Cellulitis
- Erythema nodosa
- Cutaneous polyarteritis nodosa
- Sarcoid
- Kaposi's sarcoma
- Hyperalgesic pseudothrombophlebitis

LABORATORY
- Septic
  ◊ Bacteremia in 80-90%
  ◊ Culture of IV fluid bag
  ◊ Leukocytosis
- Aseptic
  ◊ Acute phase reactant
  ◊ Factor levels
  ◊ Thrombin activity
  ◊ Platelet function test

Drugs that may alter lab results: In septic, broad spectrum antibiotics
Disorders that may alter lab results: N/A

PATHOLOGICAL FINDINGS
- The affected vein is enlarged, tortuous, and thickened
- Associated perivascular suppuration and/or hemorrhage
- Vein lumen may contain pus and thrombus
- Endothelial damage, fibrinoid necrosis and thickening of the vein wall

SPECIAL TESTS Leukocyte imaging

IMAGING
- Septic and aseptic
  ◊ Ultrasound of veins reveal an increase in the diameter of the lumen
  ◊ Chest x-ray - multiple peripheral densities or a pleural effusion consistent with pulmonary embolism, abscess, or empyema
  ◊ Bone and gallium scan - for associated subperiosteal abscess in septic thrombophlebitis
  ◊ Evaluation of complications (deep vein thrombosis and others)

DIAGNOSTIC PROCEDURES Skin biopsy

TREATMENT

APPROPRIATE HEALTH CARE
• Septic - inpatient
• Aseptic - outpatient

GENERAL MEASURES
• Heat application
• Extremity elevation

SURGICAL MEASURES
• Septic
  ◊ Excision of the involved vein segment and all involved tributaries
  ◊ Excision from ankle to groin may be required in some burn patients
  ◊ If systemic symptoms persist after vein excision, re-exploration is necessary with removal of all involved veins
  ◊ Drainage of contiguous abscesses
  ◊ Remove all cannulae
• Aseptic
  ◊ Mondor's disease, consider surgical transection of the phlebitic cord
  ◊ Management of underlying conditions

ACTIVITY Bedrest

DIET No restrictions

PATIENT EDUCATION
• Avoid trauma
• Be alert to change in skin color
• Be alert to tenderness over extremities

MEDICATIONS

DRUG(S) OF CHOICE
• Septic
  ◊ Initially: semisynthetic penicillin (e.g., nafcillin 2 g IV q6h) plus an aminoglycoside (e.g., gentamicin, 1.0-1.7 mg/kg IV)
  ◊ Duration of therapy is empiric
  ◊ If due to Candida albicans, consider a short course of amphotericin B, approximately 200 mg cumulative dose
  ◊ If osteomyelitis documented, antibiotic therapy for at least 6 weeks
• Aseptic general
  ◊ Nonsteroidal anti-inflammatories
  ◊ Oral anticoagulant warfarin
  ◊ Systemic anticoagulant heparin
• Antithrombin III and heparin cofactor II deficiency
  ◊ IV heparin
  ◊ Antithrombin III concentrate
  ◊ Prophylaxis: warfarin, oxymetholone
• Proteins C and S
  ◊ Long-term warfarin, lower dose, no loading
• Disorder of tissue plasminogen activator
  ◊ Phenformin and ethylestrenol
  ◊ Stanozolol and phenformin
  ◊ Stanozolol alone
  ◊ Ethylestrenol alone

• Dysfibrinogemia
  ◊ Acute attack - anticoagulation
  ◊ Prophylaxis - stanozolol
• Abnormal plasminogen and plasminogenemia
  ◊ Acute attack - anticoagulation
  ◊ Prophylaxis - warfarin
• Factor XII deficiency
  ◊ Standard therapy
• Lupus anticardiolipin
  ◊ Prophylaxis - warfarin
• Trousseau's syndrome
  ◊ Heparin
• For pregnancy
  ◊ Heparin
• Behçet's disease
  ◊ Phenformin
  ◊ Ethylestrenol
  ◊ Stanozolol
• Thromboangiitis obliterans
  ◊ Stop smoking
  ◊ Pentoxifylline
Contraindications: Refer to manufacturer's literature
Precautions: Refer to manufacturer's literature
Significant possible interactions: Refer to manufacturer's literature

ALTERNATIVE DRUGS
• Factor XII deficiency - streptokinase or alteplase (tissue plasminogen activator, TPA)
• Behcet's - oral anticoagulants plus cyclosporine
• Thromboangiitis obliterans - corticosteroid, antiplatelets and vasodilating drugs

FOLLOWUP

PATIENT MONITORING
• Septic
  ◊ Routine WBC and differential and culture
  ◊ Repeat culture from the phlebitic vein
• Aseptic
  ◊ Clinical followup to rule out secondary complications
  ◊ Repeat of blood studies for fibrinolytic system, platelets and factors

PREVENTION/AVOIDANCE
• Use of scalp vein cannulae
• Avoidance of lower extremity cannulations
• Insertion under aseptic conditions
• Secure anchoring of the cannulae
• Replacement of cannulae, connecting tubing, and IV fluid every 48-72 hrs
• Neomycin-polymyxin B-bacitracin ointment in cutdown

POSSIBLE COMPLICATIONS
• Septic: Systemic sepsis, bacteremia (84%); septic pulmonary emboli (44%); metastatic abscess formation; pneumonia (44%); subperiosteal abscess of adjacent long bones in children
• Aseptic: Deep vein thrombosis; thromboembolic phenomena

EXPECTED COURSE/PROGNOSIS
• Septic high mortality (50%), if untreated
• Aseptic
  ◊ Usually benign course; recovery 7-10 days
  ◊ Antithrombin III and heparin cofactor deficiency; recurrence rate is 60%
  ◊ Proteins C and S, recurrence rate 70%
  ◊ Prognosis depends on development of DVT and early detections of complications
  ◊ Aseptic thrombophlebitis can be isolated, recurrent or migratory

MISCELLANEOUS

ASSOCIATED CONDITIONS Varicose veins, manifestation of systemic disease, hypercoagulable states, surgery, trauma, burns, obesity, pregnancy

AGE-RELATED FACTORS
Pediatric: Subperiosteal abscesses of adjacent long bone may complicate
Geriatric: Septic thrombophlebitis is more common, prognosis poorer
Others: N/A

PREGNANCY
• Associated with increased risk of aseptic superficial thrombophlebitis
• Warfarin and NSAID's are contraindicated

SYNONYMS
• Phlebitis
• Phlebothrombosis

ICD-9-CM
451 Phlebitis and thrombophlebitis -
451.0 Phlebitis and thrombophlebitis of superficial vessels of lower extremities
451.1 Phlebitis and thrombophlebitis of deep vessels of lower extremities

SEE ALSO
• Thrombosis, deep vein (DVT)
• Cellulitis

OTHER NOTES N/A

ABBREVIATIONS DVT = deep vein thrombosis

REFERENCES
• Samlaskie CP, James WD: Superficial thrombophlebitis II. Secondary hypercoagulable states. J Am Acad Dermato 1990;23(1)1-18
• Samlaskie CP, James WD: Superficial thrombophlebitis I. Primary hypercoagulable states. J Am Acad Dermatol 1990;22:975-89
• Mandell GL, ed: Principles and Practice of Infectious Diseases. 4th Ed. New York, Churchill Livingstone, 1995
Illustrations: N/A
Internet references: http://www.5mcc.com

Author(s)
Abdulrazak Abyad, MD, MPH, AGSF

Thrombosis, deep vein (DVT)

BASICS

DESCRIPTION Development of single or multiple blood clots within the deep veins of the extremities or pelvis, usually accompanied by inflammation of the vessel wall. The major clinical consequence is embolization, usually to the lung, that is frequently life-threatening.
System(s) affected: Cardiovascular
Genetics: N/A
Incidence/Prevalence in USA: Common (approximately 2 million cases per year)
Predominant age: Usually over 40
Predominant sex: Female > Male (1.2:1)

SIGNS AND SYMPTOMS
• Many cases are completely asymptomatic, diagnosed retrospectively after embolization
• Limb pain (common)
• Limb swelling (common)
• Leg pain on dorsiflexion of the foot (Homan's sign; common)
• Palpable tender cord in affected limb (uncommon)
• Warmth of skin over area of thrombosis (uncommon)
• Redness of skin over area or thrombosis (uncommon)
• Fever (uncommon, except in septic thrombophlebitis)
• Non-tender swelling of collateral superficial veins (uncommon)
• Massive edema with cyanosis and ischemia (Phlegmasia cerulea dolens, rare)

CAUSES
• Venous stasis
• Injury to vessel wall
• Abnormalities of coagulation

RISK FACTORS
• Clinical risk factors:
  ◊ Trauma, especially long bone fractures or crush injuries
  ◊ Surgery, particularly hip and knee surgery
  ◊ Prolonged immobility
  ◊ Pregnancy, especially the puerperium
  ◊ Indwelling central venous catheters
  ◊ Oral contraceptive use (risk is confined to current usage and is proportional to estrogen content)
  ◊ Extreme high altitude (> 14,000 feet)
• Pathological risk factors:
  ◊ Carcinoma
  ◊ Deficiencies of protein C, protein S, antithrombin III, all endogenous anticoagulants
  ◊ Presence of anti-phospholipid antibodies (also known as lupus anticoagulant or anti-cardiolipin antibodies)
  ◊ Nephrotic syndrome
  ◊ Polycythemia vera
  ◊ Homocystinuria (rare)
  ◊ Campylobacter jejuni bacteremia (very rare)
  ◊ Mutation on Factor V conferring resistance to activated protein C (most common risk factor for idiopathic DVT)

DIAGNOSIS

DIFFERENTIAL DIAGNOSIS
• Cellulitis
• Ruptured synovial cyst (Baker's cyst)
• Lymphedema
• Extrinsic compression of vein by tumor or enlarged lymph nodes
• Pulled, strained, or torn muscle

LABORATORY
• No specific laboratory test is available for DVT
• Protein C, protein S, antithrombin III and anti-phospholipid antibodies can be measured in some laboratories. But as these are rare causes of DVT they are not routinely indicated and should be ordered only when the clinical circumstances suggest such a disorder.
Drugs that may alter lab results:
• Heparin, estrogens may lower antithrombin III levels
• Coumadin affects protein C and protein S function so may interfere with functional assays of these proteins
Disorders that may alter lab results:
• Thrombosis itself lowers antithrombin III levels so any workup for antithrombin III deficiency must be performed after patient has completed therapy
• Syphilis and systemic lupus erythematosus are associated with increased anti-phospholipid antibodies

PATHOLOGICAL FINDINGS
• Clot consisting predominantly of red blood cells, with some platelets and fibrin attached to vessel wall at one end with proximal end floating free in the lumen. Varying degrees of inflammation of the vessel wall are present.
• Biochemical abnormalities such as proteins S, C or antithrombin III deficiency, anti-phospholipid antibody or homocystinuria are found in only a small minority of cases
• Mutant Factor V conferring resistance to protein C ("Factor V Leiden") is a common abnormality, but routine clinical tests for the mutation are not yet in widespread use

SPECIAL TESTS N/A

IMAGING
• Imaging studies are necessary to diagnose or rule out suspected DVT
• Contrast venography is the gold standard test (i.e., most sensitive and specific). Disadvantages include discomfort, technical difficulty and small risk of morbidity.
• B-mode ultrasound combined with Doppler flow detection (duplex ultrasound); noninvasive, highly sensitive and specific for popliteal and femoral thrombi. Disadvantages include poor ability to detect calf vein thrombi; it is a highly operator-dependent technique; and its inability to reliably distinguish extrinsic compression of the vein from intrinsic clot.
• Impedance plethysmography (IPG); probably as accurate as duplex ultrasound, less operator dependency, but poor at detecting calf vein thrombi
• 125 I-fibrinogen scan; detects only active clot formation; very good at detecting ongoing calf thrombi. Major disadvantage is that it takes 4 hours for results. This test has generally been supplanted by duplex ultrasound and IPG.

DIAGNOSTIC PROCEDURES N/A

TREATMENT

APPROPRIATE HEALTH CARE Patients with DVT confined to the calf (i.e., distal to the popliteal system) can be managed conservatively as outpatients. All others should be admitted.

GENERAL MEASURES For hospitalized patient - intravenous anticoagulation, a brief period of bedrest, and close observation for embolic events

SURGICAL MEASURES Non-drug therapy - if anticoagulants and thrombolytics are contraindicated, filtering devices ("umbrellas") can he inserted into the vena cava to "trap" emboli before reaching the lungs

ACTIVITY Bedrest for 1-5 days, then gradual resumption of normal activity, with avoidance of prolonged immobility

DIET No special diet

PATIENT EDUCATION
• Advise women taking oral contraceptives of the risks, and the common symptoms of thromboembolic disease
• Discourage prolonged immobility

MEDICATIONS

DRUG(S) OF CHOICE
• Immediate therapy: Heparin 5,000-10,000 units intravenous bolus followed by continuous IV infusion at 1,000 units per hour. Weight-based heparin dosage may be used starting with a bolus of 80 units/kg , then an infusion starting at 18 units/kg/hr. Adjust dosage based on activated partial thromboplastin time (APTT) to achieve APTT of approximately 2 x control value.
• Maintenance therapy: warfarin (Coumadin) beginning 1-5 days after starting heparin, in a single daily dose starting at 5-10 mg daily and adjusting based on prothrombin time (PT) with a target value of PT of 1.3-1.5 x control value. Patient should remain on heparin until target PT level is achieved. Physicians should use international normalized ratio (INR), if available, to guide therapy. Aim for INR 2.0-3.0.
Contraindications:
• Absolute contraindications: Severe active bleeding, recent neurosurgical procedure (within 30 days), pregnancy (warfarin only), previous adverse reaction to the drug (other than bleeding, which is a known side effect)
• Relative contraindications: Recent severe hemorrhage, recent surgical procedure other than neurosurgery, history of significant peptic ulcer disease, recent non-embolic stroke
Precautions:
• Observe patient carefully for signs of embolization, further thrombosis or bleeding
• While on anticoagulant therapy avoid intramuscular injections. Periodically check stool and urine for occult blood, monitor complete blood counts including platelets.
• Heparin - other possible but rare adverse reactions include thrombocytopenia and/or paradoxical thrombosis with thrombocytopenia
• Warfarin - necrotic lesions of the skin (Warfarin necrosis) occasionally result from treatment
Significant possible interactions:
• Agents that may prolong or intensify the response to oral anticoagulants: Alcohol, allopurinol, amiodarone, anabolic steroids, androgens, many antimicrobials, cimetidine chloral hydrate, disulfiram, all nonsteroidal anti-inflammatory drugs (NSAID's), sulfinpyrazone, tamoxifen, thyroid hormone, vitamin E, ranitidine, salicylates
• Agents that may diminish the response to anticoagulants: Aminoglutethimide, antacids, barbiturates, carbamazepine, cholestyramine, diuretics, griseofulvin, rifampin, oral contraceptives

ALTERNATIVE DRUGS
• Thrombolytic agents (urokinase, streptokinase, alteplase [tissue plasminogen activator]) are effective in dissolving clots and are currently investigational for treatment of DVT. In current clinical practice they should he reserved for massive thromboembolic disease. The same contraindications apply as to anticoagulants.

• Low molecular weight heparin may be as effective as IV heparin in treatment of uncomplicated DVT
• If warfarin (Coumadin) is contraindicated, heparin can be given in the ambulatory setting by intermittent subcutaneous self-injection (see Pregnancy)

FOLLOWUP

PATIENT MONITORING
• APTT must be monitored several times a day while on IV heparin until dose stabilizes. Platelets should also be monitored and heparin discontinued if platelets fall below 75,000
• While on Coumadin, PT must be monitored daily until target achieved, then weekly for several weeks, then (if stable) monthly as long as patient is on the drug
• For first episode of DVT patients should be treated for 3-6 months. Subsequent episodes should be treated for at least a year.
• Significant bleeding such as hematuria or gastrointestinal hemorrhage should be thoroughly investigated since anticoagulant therapy frequently unmasks a pre-existing lesion such as cancer, peptic ulcer disease, or arteriovenous malformation

PREVENTION/AVOIDANCE
• General preventive measures such as avoiding prolonged immobility and using low-estrogen birth control pills when possible
• Surgical patients need active prophylaxis: Low dose subcutaneous heparin with dosage adjusted to slightly prolong the APTT, low dose Coumadin, enoxaparin (low molecular weight heparin) and intermittent mechanical compression of the legs have all been effective in reducing the risks of DVT following various types of surgery.

POSSIBLE COMPLICATIONS
• Pulmonary embolism (fatal in 10-20% of cases)
• Systemic embolism ("paradoxical embolization") in cases where there is arteriovenous shunting (rare)
• Chronic venous insufficiency
• Post-phlebitic syndrome, i.e., pain and swelling in affected limb without new clot formation
• Treatment induced hemorrhage
• Soft tissue ischemia associated with massive clot and very high venous pressures - phlegmasia cerulea dolens (very rare but should be considered a surgical emergency)

EXPECTED COURSE/PROGNOSIS
• About 20% of untreated proximal (i.e., above the calf) DVT's progress to pulmonary emboli and 10-20% of those are fatal. With aggressive anticoagulant therapy the mortality is decreased five to tenfold.
• DVT confined to the calf virtually never causes clinically significant emboli so does not require anticoagulation. However calf DVT's do sometimes propagate into the proximal system so known or suspected calf

DVT's should be followed with IPG or duplex ultrasound every 3-5 days for 10 days and treated aggressively if they propagate into the popliteal or femoral system.

MISCELLANEOUS

ASSOCIATED CONDITIONS
• Budd-Chiari syndrome (hepatic vein thrombosis)
• Renal vein thrombosis
• Homocystinuria
• Anti-phospholipid antibody syndrome

AGE-RELATED FACTORS
Pediatric: In this age group patients with DVT, in absence of preceding trauma, should be worked up for congenital coagulopathy
Geriatric: More common because predisposing conditions are more common
Others: N/A

PREGNANCY
• Warfarin (Coumadin) is a known teratogen so is contraindicated in pregnancy. Treat pregnant women with DVT with full dose heparin initially followed by subcutaneous heparin starting at 15,000 units twice daily with target APTT of 1.5-2 x control value.
• Septic thrombophlebitis, usually associated with childbirth, requires antibiotic therapy as well as anticoagulation

SYNONYMS Deep venous thrombophlebitis

SEE ALSO N/A

ICD-9-CM 451.19 Phlebitis and thrombophlebitis, of deep vessels of lower extremities, other

OTHER NOTES N/A

ABBREVIATIONS
• DVT = deep vein thrombophlebitis
• IPG = impedance plethysmography
• INR = international normalized ratio

REFERENCES
• Hirsh J: Venous thromboembolism. In: Rubenstein E, Federman DD, eds. Scientific American Medicine. New York, Scientific American, 1994
• Kontos HA: Vascular Diseases of the Limbs. In: Wyngaarden JB, Smith LH, eds. Cecil Textbook of Medicine. Philadelphia, W.B. Saunders Co., 1992
• Weinman EE, Salzman EW: Deep-vein thrombosis. New Engl J Med 1994;331:1630-1641
Illustrations: N/A
Internet references: http://www.5mcc.com

Author(s)
Robert J. Sliman, MD

Thyroglossal duct cyst

BASICS

DESCRIPTION Cystic remnant of thyroid descent in the neck
System(s) affected: Endocrine/Metabolic, Skin/Exocrine
Genetics: N/A
Incidence/Prevalence in USA: N/A
Predominant age: 50% less than 10 years, 65% less than 20 years of age
Predominant sex: Male = Female

SIGNS AND SYMPTOMS
• Midline neck mass
• Non-tender, unless infected
• Rises in the neck with tongue protrusion
• 80% juxtaposed to the hyoid bone

CAUSES
Failure of obliteration of the thyroglossal duct following descent of the thyroid in the 6th week of fetal life

RISK FACTORS
None

DIAGNOSIS

DIFFERENTIAL DIAGNOSIS
• Ectopic midline thyroid
• Dermoid cyst
• Thyroid adenoma of isthmus or pyramidal lobe
• Lymphadenitis

LABORATORY
None
Drugs that may alter lab results: N/A
Disorders that may alter lab results: N/A

PATHOLOGICAL FINDINGS
Cyst lined with stratified squamous or pseudostratified ciliated columnar epithelium. Thyroid tissue seen in 10-45% of cysts.

SPECIAL TESTS
N/A

IMAGING
• Ultrasound
• Thyroid scan if midline ectopic thyroid or thyroid nodule is suspected

DIAGNOSTIC PROCEDURES
N/A

TREATMENT

APPROPRIATE HEALTH CARE
Outpatient surgery

GENERAL MEASURES
N/A

SURGICAL MEASURES
• Once diagnosed, the excision can be done with Sistrunk procedure. This requires removal of the center portion of the hyoid bone to minimize recurrence.
• If the cyst is infected, it should be initially treated (antibiotics and local heat) or drained. After resolution of the inflammation, excision should be performed.

ACTIVITY
Unrestricted

DIET
Unrestricted

PATIENT EDUCATION
• Reassurance to family about absence of malignancy
• Patient may require thyroid medication for life, if ectopic, midline thyroid mistakenly removed

MEDICATIONS

DRUG(S) OF CHOICE None. All thyroglossal duct cysts should be surgically removed.
Contraindications: N/A
Precautions: N/A
Significant possible interactions: N/A

ALTERNATIVE DRUGS N/A

FOLLOWUP

PATIENT MONITORING 1-2 weeks after drainage or resection

PREVENTION/AVOIDANCE N/A

POSSIBLE COMPLICATIONS Infection and malignant degeneration if not excised

EXPECTED COURSE/PROGNOSIS Resolution with resection (less than 5% recurrence using the Sistrunk procedure)

MISCELLANEOUS

ASSOCIATED CONDITIONS None

AGE-RELATED FACTORS
Pediatric: N/A
Geriatric: N/A
Others: N/A

PREGNANCY N/A

SYNONYMS N/A

ICD-9-CM 759.2

SEE ALSO N/A

OTHER NOTES N/A

ABBREVIATIONS N/A

REFERENCES Welch KJ, Randolph JG, Ravitch MM, et al, eds: Pediatric Surgery. 4th Ed. New York, Year Book Medical Publishers, 1986
Illustrations: N/A
Internet references: http://www.5mcc.com

Author(s)
James P. Miller, MD, FACS, FAAP
Timothy L. Black, MD, FACS, FAAP

Thyroid malignant neoplasia

 BASICS

DESCRIPTION
Autologous growth of thyroid nodules with potential for metastases
- Papillary carcinoma - most common variety, 60-70% of thyroid tumors. May be associated with radiation exposure. Tumor contains psammoma bodies. Metastasizes by lymphatic route (30% at time of diagnosis).
- Follicular carcinoma - 10-20% of thyroid tumors. The incidence has been decreasing since the addition of dietary iodine. It occurs usually in females over 40 years of age. Metastasizes by the hematogenous route.
- Hürthle cell carcinoma - usually in patients over 60 years of age. Radioresistant. Composed of distinct large eosinophilic cells with abundant cytoplasmic mitochondria.
- Medullary carcinoma - arises from parafollicular cells, C-cells. 2-5% of all thyroid tumors. 25-35% are associated with multiple endocrine neoplasia (MEN) syndromes which can be familial or sporadic. Calcitonin is a chemical marker.
- Anaplastic carcinoma - 3% of thyroid tumors, usually in patients over 60 years of age
- Other - lymphoma, sarcoma, or metastatic (renal, breast or lung)

System(s) affected: Endocrine/Metabolic
Genetics:
- Medullary - autosomal dominant with MEN syndrome
- Others - none known

Incidence/Prevalence in USA:
0.0051/100,000 (16,100 new cases per year); < 1,200 deaths per year from thyroid cancer
Predominant age: Usually over 40 years of age
Predominant sex: Female > Male (2.6:1)

SIGNS AND SYMPTOMS
- Painless hard, fixed neck mass (in advanced cases; otherwise soft to hard masses)
- Hoarseness
- Dysphagia
- Cervical lymphadenopathy
- Dyspnea

CAUSES
Unknown

RISK FACTORS
- Family history
- Neck irradiation (6-2000 rads) - papillary carcinoma
- Iodine deficiency - follicular carcinoma
- MEN syndrome - medullary carcinoma
- Previous history of less than a total thyroidectomy for malignancy - anaplastic carcinoma

 DIAGNOSIS

DIFFERENTIAL DIAGNOSIS
- Multinodular goiter
- Thyroid adenoma
- Thyroglossal duct cyst
- Thyroiditis
- Thyroid cyst
- Ectopic thyroid

LABORATORY
Thyroid function tests usually normal
Drugs that may alter lab results: N/A
Disorders that may alter lab results: N/A

PATHOLOGICAL FINDINGS
- Papillary - psammoma bodies, anaplastic epithelial papillae
- Follicular - anaplastic epithelial cords with follicles
- Hürthle cell - large eosinophilic cells with granular cytoplasm
- Medullary - large amounts of amyloid stroma
- Anaplastic - small cell and giant cell undifferentiated tumors

SPECIAL TESTS
- Medullary carcinoma - calcitonin level (normal is less than 300 pg/mL [300 ng/L])
- Thyroglobulin level - post operative tumor marker
- DNA content of tumors from biopsy specimen. Diploid content has a better prognosis.

IMAGING
- Thyroid scan - cold nodules are more suspicious of malignancy
- Ultrasound - solid mass is more suspicious of malignancy
- CT and MRI can be useful to evaluate large substernal masses and recurrent soft tissue masses

DIAGNOSTIC PROCEDURES
- Fine needle aspiration
- Surgical biopsy/excision
- Laryngoscopy, if vocal cord paralysis is suspected

 TREATMENT

APPROPRIATE HEALTH CARE
Inpatient

GENERAL MEASURES
N/A

SURGICAL MEASURES
- Papillary carcinoma - lobectomy with isthmectomy (if lesion < 1.5 cm) or total thyroidectomy, and removal of suspicious lymph nodes
- Follicular carcinoma and Hurthle cell - total thyroidectomy and removal of suspicious lymph nodes
- Medullary carcinoma - total thyroidectomy with central node dissection. Unilateral or bilateral modified radical neck dissection if lateral nodes are histologically positive.
- Anaplastic carcinoma - aggressive en bloc thyroidectomy. Often times tracheostomy required.

ACTIVITY
As tolerated

DIET
Avoid iodine deficiency

PATIENT EDUCATION
National Cancer Institute
Building 31, Room 101-18
9000 Rockville Pike
Bethesda, MD 20892
(301)496-5583

Thyroid malignant neoplasia

MEDICATIONS

DRUG(S) OF CHOICE
• Post operatively will require thyroid replacement to suppress serum TSH level:
◊ Levothyroxine (T4, Synthroid) 100-200 μg/day or
◊ Liothyronine (T3, Cytomel) 50-100 μg/day

Contraindications: N/A

Precautions: N/A

Significant possible interactions:
• Amphetamines
• Anticoagulants
• Tricyclic antidepressants
• Antidiabetic medications
• Aspirin
• Barbiturates
• Beta adrenergic blockers
• Cholestyramine
• Colestipol
• Oral contraceptives
• Digitalis preparation
• Ephedrine
• Estrogens
• Methylphenidate
• Phenytoin

ALTERNATIVE DRUGS   N/A

FOLLOWUP

PATIENT MONITORING
• Thyroid scan at 6 weeks and administration of I131 for any visible uptake evidence of residual thyroid tissue (after total thyroidectomy) or lymph node disease is treated with radioactive iodine
• At 6 months and then yearly the patient should have a thyroid scan and chest x-ray
• Papillary and follicular - a thyroglobulin level should be done yearly
• Medullary - calcitonin level should be done yearly with pentagastrin stimulation
• The thyroid scan and thyroglobulin level should be done with the patient in the hypothyroid state induced by 6 week withdrawal of levothyroxine or 2-3 week withdrawal of liothyronine

PREVENTION/AVOIDANCE
• Physical exam in high risk group
• Calcium infusion or pentagastrin stimulation test in high risk MEN patients

POSSIBLE COMPLICATIONS
Recurrence of tumor

EXPECTED COURSE/PROGNOSIS
• Papillary carcinoma - overall mortality 3-8%
• Follicular carcinoma - overall 80% 5 year survival rate, 77% 10 year survival rate. Histologically microinvasive tumors parallel papillary tumor results while grossly invasive tumors do far worse.
• Hürthle cell carcinoma - 93% 5 year survival rate, and 83% survival rate overall. Grossly invasive tumors - survival is less than 25%.
• Medullary carcinoma - negative nodes 90% 5 year survival rate and 85% 10 year survival rate; with positive nodes 65% 5 year survival rate and 40% 10 year survival rate
• Anaplastic carcinoma - survival unexpected

MISCELLANEOUS

ASSOCIATED CONDITIONS Medullary carcinoma - pheochromocytoma, hyperparathyroidism, ganglioneuroma of the GI tract, neuromata of mucosal membranes

AGE-RELATED FACTORS
Pediatric: Over 60% of thyroid nodules are malignant
Geriatric: Risk of malignancy increases over age 60
Others: N/A

PREGNANCY   N/A

SYNONYMS
• Follicular carcinoma of the thyroid
• Papillary carcinoma of the thyroid
• Hürthle cell carcinoma of the thyroid
• Anaplastic cell carcinoma of the thyroid

ICD-9-CM
193 Malignant neoplasm of thyroid gland
198.89 Secondary malignant neoplasm of other specified sites, other

SEE ALSO   N/A

OTHER NOTES   N/A

ABBREVIATIONS   MEN = multiple endocrine neoplasia

REFERENCES
• Bell RM: Thyroid carcinoma. Surg Clin North Am 1986;66:13
• Lennquist S: The Thyroid Nodule, Surg Clin North Am 1987;66:213-232
• Gagel RF, Goepfert H, Callender RL: Changing Concepts in the Pathogenesis and Management of Thyroid carcinoma, CA Cancer J Clin 1996;46:261-283
Illustrations: N/A
Internet references: http://www.5mcc.com

Author(s)
James P. Miller, MD, FACS, FAAP
Timothy L. Black, MD, FACS, FAAP

Thyroiditis

BASICS

DESCRIPTION A variety of inflammatory thyroid disorders that can cause thyroid enlargement and thyroid atrophy. May lead to hypothyroidism or hyperthyroidism. Complete resolution can occur.
• Lymphocytic thyroiditis (Hashimoto's) - the most common form, an autoimmune disease, often presenting as an asymptomatic diffuse goiter. Often first detected after thyroid atrophy and hypothyroidism have occurred and occasionally as hyperthyroidism (Hashimoto's thyroiditis).
• Granulomatous thyroiditis ("subacute") - probably related to viral infection and usually presenting with thyroid pain (which may be severe), involving one or both thyroid lobes, accompanied by hyperthyroidism, going through a phase of mild hypothyroidism and then to permanent resolution to normal
• "Silent" thyroiditis - one form is characterized by spontaneously resolving hypothyroidism and/or hyperthyroidism often associated with pregnancy. Another form has the characteristics of granulomatous thyroiditis without the pain.
• Rare forms of thyroiditis - suppurative, due to bacterial infection and radiation due to ingested radionuclides or external irradiation
• One form is postpartum onset of goiter and/or hypothyroidism that may resolve spontaneously. Another is painless granulomatous thyroiditis.
• Riedel's thyroiditis - dense infiltration of thyroid and surrounding tissues of unknown cause
System(s) affected: Endocrine/Metabolic
Genetics: N/A
Incidence/Prevalence in USA:
• Not known definitively
• Lymphocytic thyroiditis increases with age, probably up to 10% over age 65
• Granulomatous thyroiditis much less common, has an epidemic pattern
Predominant age: All ages, postpuberty
Predominant sex: Female > Male

SIGNS AND SYMPTOMS
• Lymphocytic thyroiditis
  ◊ Insidious onset of goiter, often detected incidentally
  ◊ Slow onset of hypothyroidism
  ◊ Association with other autoimmune diseases
• Granulomatous thyroiditis
  ◊ Pain, tenderness and enlargement of one or both thyroid lobes
  ◊ Malaise, fever
  ◊ Mild to moderate symptoms of hyperthyroidism
  ◊ History of recent respiratory infection

CAUSES
• Lymphocytic thyroiditis
  ◊ Autoimmune response of thyroid tissue
  ◊ Genetic susceptibility
• Granulomatous thyroiditis
  ◊ Chronic inflammatory response of thyroid tissue
  ◊ Preceding infection with any of a variety of viruses

RISK FACTORS
• Lymphocytic thyroiditis
  ◊ Positive family history of thyroid disease
  ◊ Preceding autoimmune diseases including type I diabetes, primary adrenal insufficiency, rheumatoid arthritis, pregnancy/delivery
• Granulomatous thyroiditis
  ◊ Recent viral respiratory infection
  ◊ Other known cases in the community

DIAGNOSIS

DIFFERENTIAL DIAGNOSIS
• Lymphocytic thyroiditis
  ◊ Simple goiter
  ◊ Iodine-deficient goiter (especially in endemic areas)
  ◊ Early Graves' disease
  ◊ Lithium induced goiter
• Granulomatous thyroiditis
  ◊ Infections of oropharynx and trachea
  ◊ Hemorrhage into a thyroid cyst
  ◊ Subacute systemic illness
  ◊ Suppurative thyroiditis

LABORATORY
• Lymphocytic thyroiditis
  ◊ Elevated anti-thyroid antibodies (especially high titers of anti-microsomal [anti-TPO] antibodies)
  ◊ Free thyroxine index (FTI, normal 4.5-12) less than 5 with TSH greater than 5 mcg/dl (normal 0.5-5 mcg/dl)
  ◊ Thyroid radioactive iodine uptake (RAIU) variable with scintiscan showing patchy distribution of radioiodine
  ◊ Positive cytopathology of fine needle aspirate or positive formal biopsy
• Granulomatous thyroiditis
  ◊ Elevated erythrocyte sedimentation rate
  ◊ Normal or moderately elevated WBC without a granulocyte shift to band forms
  ◊ FTI greater than 12, TSH undetectable, RAIU less than 5% in 24 hours (often nil) early in course. FTI less than 4.5 with RAIU above normal (greater than 35% in 24 hours in USA) late in course
Drugs that may alter lab results:
• Thyroid
• Corticosteroids
• Iodine containing drugs and contrast media
• Lithium
Disorders that may alter lab results:
• Iodine-deficiency
• Non-thyroidal illness

PATHOLOGICAL FINDINGS
• Lymphocytic thyroiditis
  ◊ Lymphocytic infiltration
  ◊ Oxyphilic changes in follicular cells
  ◊ Fibrosis
  ◊ Atrophy
• Granulomatous thyroiditis
  ◊ Giant cells
  ◊ Mononuclear cell infiltrate

SPECIAL TESTS
• Radioimmunoassays
• Anti-thyroid antibody titers
• Complete blood count with differential count
• Erythrocyte sedimentation rate

IMAGING
• Thyroid radioiodine uptake and scan in granulomatous thyroiditis
• Ultrasonography if hemorrhage into thyroid cyst suspected

DIAGNOSTIC PROCEDURES Needle biopsy in confusing cases

TREATMENT

APPROPRIATE HEALTH CARE
Outpatient

GENERAL MEASURES
• Analgesics for pain
• Corticosteroids for severe granulomatous thyroiditis

SURGICAL MEASURES N/A

ACTIVITY Fully active

DIET No special diet

PATIENT EDUCATION N/A

MEDICATIONS

DRUG(S) OF CHOICE
• Lymphocytic thyroiditis:
◊ Levothyroxine if hypothyroid or goitrous. Generic levothyroxine may not be bioavailable. Carafate, iron preparations may decrease levothyroxine availability. Begin with 25 or 50 μg/day and titrate to TSH suppression to lower limit of assay normal range.
◊ Propylthiouracil and propranolol if thyrotoxic and symptomatic
• Granulomatous thyroiditis:
◊ Analgesics, e.g., codeine for pain
◊ Propranolol 40 mg q6h for symptomatic hyperthyroidism
◊ Levothyroxine 100 μg per 100 lbs (45.5 kg) body wt/day if hypothyroid phase is symptomatic
◊ Prednisone once daily in lowest effective dose, for severe symptoms
• Maintenance:
◊ Optimal dose can be established by measuring TSH at 6-8 week intervals until dosage level causes TSH to be at the lower level of normal for the assay used

Contraindications:
• Propylthiouracil - allergy or hypersensitivity to analgesics/narcotics
• Propranolol - insulin therapy, asthma
• Prednisone - adverse reactions
• Levothyroxine - none

Precautions: Reduce doses of corticosteroids, propranolol and narcotics as soon as feasible

Significant possible interactions:
Sucralfate (Carafate) and iron preparations may decrease levothyroxine availability

ALTERNATIVE DRUGS
Methimazole for propylthiouracil

FOLLOWUP

PATIENT MONITORING
• Repeat thyroid function tests every 3-12 months in lymphocytic thyroiditis
• Repeat thyroid function tests every 3-6 weeks in granulomatous thyroiditis until permanently euthyroid

PREVENTION/AVOIDANCE   N/A

POSSIBLE COMPLICATIONS   Treatment induced hypothyroidism or hyperthyroidism

EXPECTED COURSE/PROGNOSIS
• Lymphocytic thyroiditis - persistent goiter, eventual thyroid failure
• Granulomatous thyroiditis - eventual return to normal over weeks or months

MISCELLANEOUS

ASSOCIATED CONDITIONS
Other autoimmune diseases with lymphocytic thyroiditis including type I diabetes, primary adrenal insufficiency, premature ovarian failure

AGE-RELATED FACTORS
Pediatric: N/A
Geriatric: Remission of granulomatous thyroiditis may be slower in the elderly
Others: N/A

PREGNANCY
• Avoid radio-isotope scanning
• Avoid hypothyroidism
• Minimize use of antithyroid drugs

SYNONYMS
• Lymphocytic thyroiditis
• Granulomatous thyroiditis
• Silent thyroiditis
• Hashimoto's disease

ICD-9-CM   245 Acute thyroiditis

SEE ALSO
• Hypothyroidism, adult
• Hyperthyroidism

OTHER NOTES   N/A

ABBREVIATIONS
• RAIU = radioactive iodine uptake
• FTI = free thyroxine index
• TSH = thyroid stimulating hormone

REFERENCES
• Bardin CW, ed: Current Therapy In Endocrinology and Metabolism. 5th Ed. St. Louis, Mosby, 1994
• Braveman LE, Utiger RD, eds: The Thyroid. 6th Ed. Philadelphia, J.B. Lippincott, 1991
• DeGroot LW, Larsen PR, Hennemann G: The Thyroid and its Diseases. 6th Ed. Churchill, Livingston, 1996
Illustrations: N/A
Internet references: http://www.5mcc.com

Author(s)
Richard P. Levy, MD

Tinea capitis

BASICS

DESCRIPTION A fungal infection of the scalp often called "ringworm." The infection results from contact with infected persons or animals. It is contagious and may become epidemic. Affected areas of the scalp can show characteristic black dots resulting from broken hairs.
System(s) affected: Skin/Exocrine
Genetics: N/A
Incidence/Prevalence in USA: Although still common, the incidence and prevalence have markedly dropped over the past 30 years
Predominant age: Children particularly ages 3 to 9. Adult infection is rare.
Predominant sex: Male = Female

SIGNS AND SYMPTOMS
• Infection commonly begins with round patches of scale (alopecia less common)
• Frequently, infection will take on the patterns of chronic scaling with little inflammation or marked inflammation and alopecia. Less frequently, patients will present with multiple patches of alopecia and characteristic black dot pattern of broken hairs. Extreme inflammation results in kerion (exudative pustular nodulation).

CAUSES
• 90% Trichophyton tonsurans
• 10% Microsporum species (canis, audouinii, gypseum)

RISK FACTORS
• Day-care centers or schools
• Living in confined quarters
• Poor hygiene
• Immunosuppression

DIAGNOSIS

DIFFERENTIAL DIAGNOSIS
• Psoriasis and seborrhea dermatitis are most often confused with tinea capitis
• Pyoderma
• Alopecia areata and trichotillomania

LABORATORY
• Microscopy of a KOH preparation of hairs from affected area can show arthrospores that appear within hair shafts
• Fungal culture of hairs from affected areas allows the infection to be confirmed and the causative organism to be identified
Drugs that may alter lab results: N/A
Disorders that may alter lab results: N/A

PATHOLOGICAL FINDINGS
• Chronic inflammation
• Superficial infection producing lesions with follicular pustules, abscess
• Hyphae in follicles, keratin of skin

SPECIAL TESTS Viewed under a Wood's lamp, the 10% of infections caused by Microsporum species will fluoresce a light green. 90% of tinea capitis infections, those caused by Trichophyton, will NOT fluoresce.

IMAGING N/A

DIAGNOSTIC PROCEDURES N/A

TREATMENT

APPROPRIATE HEALTH CARE
Outpatient

GENERAL MEASURES
• Careful hand washing
• Launder towels, clothing, head wear of infected individual
• Check other family members

SURGICAL MEASURES N/A

ACTIVITY No restrictions

DIET No special diet except persons treated with griseofulvin should not be on a restricted fat diet

PATIENT EDUCATION See General Measures

MEDICATIONS

DRUG(S) OF CHOICE
• Griseofulvin - preferred treatment
  ◊ Microsized preparation
  ◊ Available in 125 mg, 250 mg and 500 mg tablets and 125 mg/5 mL suspension
  ◊ Dose at 10 mg/kg/day taken bid or as single daily dose up to 500 mg/day for 6 weeks
• Itraconazole
  ◊ Matches griseofulvin in treatment and is better tolerated
  ◊ 100 mg daily for 6 weeks

Contraindications:
• Griseofulvin contraindicated in patients with porphyria because of increased risk of hepatotoxicity

Precautions:
• Griseofulvin
  ◊ Headache in up to 10% of patients initially but generally resolves after first week of treatment
  ◊ Abdominal bloating, dyspepsia, and diarrhea also common
  ◊ Hypersensitivity and liver toxicity rare. The manufacturer recommends monitoring liver functions while on griseofulvin but due to rarity of hepatotoxicity many physicians choose to forgo any testing.
• Itraconazole
  ◊ Side effects - nausea, vomiting, diarrhea, headache, dizziness, abnormal hepatic function tests, rare significant liver toxicity (appears safer than ketoconazole)

Significant possible interactions:
Griseofulvin accentuates the effect of alcohol and increases the metabolism of warfarin and oral contraceptives.

ALTERNATIVE DRUGS
Oral terbinafine - adjunctive for severe kerion, prednisone 1 mg/kg/d for 1-2 weeks

FOLLOWUP

PATIENT MONITORING
Recheck after two weeks of therapy to document improvement and after the 6 week course of therapy. Patients might need liver function monitoring - see medication precautions.

PREVENTION/AVOIDANCE
• Good personal hygiene
• Don't share head wear
• Identification and treatment of infected individuals and household pets

POSSIBLE COMPLICATIONS
Permanent scarring and hair loss from kerion

EXPECTED COURSE/PROGNOSIS
Without treatment lesions will usually spontaneously heal in 6 months. Lesions with marked inflammation will spontaneously resolve much more rapidly but are more likely to leave scarring.

MISCELLANEOUS

ASSOCIATED CONDITIONS N/A

AGE-RELATED FACTORS
Pediatric: Highest incidence in this age group
Geriatric: N/A
Others: N/A

PREGNANCY
Oral antifungals are contraindicated in pregnancy

SYNONYMS Scalp ringworm

ICD-9-CM 110.0 Dermatophytosis of scalp and beard

SEE ALSO
• Tinea corporis
• Alopecia

OTHER NOTES N/A

ABBREVIATIONS N/A

REFERENCES
• Bergus GR, Johnson JS: Superficial fungal infections. Am Family Phys 1993;48:259-272
• Lopez-Gamez S, Del Palacio A, et al: Itraconazole versus griseofulvin in the treatment of tinea capitis. Int J Dermatol 1994;33(10):743-747
• Frieden IJ, Howard R: Tinea capitis: epidemiology, diagnosis, treatment and control. J Am Acad Dermatol 1994;31:542-546
• Greer DL: Treatment of tinea capitis with itraconazole. J Am Acad Dermatol 1996;35:637-638
Illustrations: 4 available on CD-ROM
Internet references: http://www.5mcc.com

Author(s)
George R. Bergus, MD

Tinea corporis

 BASICS

DESCRIPTION Scaling plaque characterized by a sharply defined annular pattern with peripheral activity and central clearing. Papules and occasionally pustules/vesicles present at border, and less commonly in center. Affects face, trunk, and extremities.
• Zoophilic infections (found in children and adults) are acquired from animals
• Anthropophilic infections (found only in adults) acquired from personal contact or fomites
System(s) affected: Skin/Exocrine
Genetics: There is evidence for genetic susceptibility in some people
Incidence/Prevalence in USA: Fairly common
Predominant age: All ages
Predominant sex: Male = Female

SIGNS AND SYMPTOMS
• Characteristic rash and mild pruritus
• Scaling plaques that are circular, bright red, sharply marginated, occur singly or in groups of 3-4
• Each plaque is less than 5 cm in diameter
• Plaques are solid, but annular forms occur
• Patient may experience intense itching
• Hyperpigmentation (occasionally)

CAUSES Fungal infection due to dermatophyte, e.g., Trichophyton rubrum (most common). Microsporum canis often results in multiple lesions.

RISK FACTORS
• Warm climates
• Direct contact with an active lesion on a human, an animal, or rarely from soil
• Working with animals
• Immunosuppression including prolonged use of topical steroids

 DIAGNOSIS

DIFFERENTIAL DIAGNOSIS
• Pityriasis rosea
• Eczema
• Contact dermatitis
• Syphilis
• Psoriasis
• Subacute lupus erythematosus
• Elastosis perforans serpiginosa
• Erythema annulare
• Gyrate erythemas, especially centrifugum

LABORATORY Potassium hydroxide preparation of skin scrapings. Fungal culture may be obtained, but is not generally necessary.
Drugs that may alter lab results: N/A
Disorders that may alter lab results: N/A

PATHOLOGICAL FINDINGS Branching hyphae with septa on potassium hydroxide preparation

SPECIAL TESTS
• Tinea corpora does not fluoresce with Wood's light
• Culture on Sabouraud's medium - sample by scraping or vigorous rubbing of a cotton swab on the lesion, then rolled/rubbed on the medium

IMAGING N/A

DIAGNOSTIC PROCEDURES
• Skin scraping:
  ◊ Use No.15 blade and place several small scrapings of the active border on glass slide with coverslip
  ◊ Apply 10-20% potassium hydroxide and heat gently without boiling
  ◊ Let stand for 5 minutes and examine for septate, branching hyphae. Use lowered condenser and dim light to enhance contrast. Hyphae may be accentuated with a commercial fungal stain or a drop of blue ink.

 TREATMENT

APPROPRIATE HEALTH CARE
Outpatient

GENERAL MEASURES Proper hygiene

SURGICAL MEASURES N/A

ACTIVITY Avoid contact sports, e.g., wrestling for 2 days while starting treatment

DIET Unrestricted diet

PATIENT EDUCATION Avoid contact with suspected lesions. Be careful with animal contacts.

Tinea corporis

MEDICATIONS

DRUG(S) OF CHOICE
• Topical antifungal creams - miconazole (Monistat-Derm) or clotrimazole (Lotrimin, Mycelex) applied bid for 2 weeks. Also ketoconazole (Nizoral) applied qd for 2 weeks. To prevent relapse should use for one week after resolution. Also econazole (Spectazole) and allylamines, e.g., naftifine (Naftin, Lamisil). For added benefit, wash with antifungal shampoo ketoconazole (Nizoral Shampoo) prior to use of cream.
• For resistant, extensive and/or invasive infections, oral agents are recommended for 4 weeks. Oral ultramicrosize griseofulvin (e.g., Gris-PEG) 7 mg/kg/day in children over 2 years; 375 mg/day in adults. Oral itraconazole, in lieu of ketoconazole - less toxic and less drug side effects. Although not indicated, itraconazole (Sporanox) is effective at 100-200 mg/day.
Contraindications: Known hypersensitivity to agent
Precautions: Ketoconazole contains a sulfite and should be avoided in sulfite sensitive people. There is a 1:10,000 reported incidence of hepatotoxicity with oral ketoconazole. Baseline liver function tests should be obtained prior to initiating oral ketoconazole and patients should be followed closely.
Significant possible interactions: Griseofulvin induces hepatic enzymes that metabolize warfarin and other drugs. H2 blockers and antacids reduce ketoconazole absorption. Ketoconazole is an enzyme inhibitor and may cause drug toxicity (case report of apparent terfenadine toxicity causing ventricular arrhythmia). Ketoconazole also significantly increases cyclosporine levels.

ALTERNATIVE DRUGS N/A

FOLLOWUP

PATIENT MONITORING Necessary for invasive disease or prolonged treatment with oral ketoconazole

PREVENTION/AVOIDANCE Avoid contact with suspicious lesions

POSSIBLE COMPLICATIONS
• Bacterial super-infection
• Generalized, invasive dermatophyte infection

EXPECTED COURSE/PROGNOSIS
Resolution without sequelae in 1-2 weeks of therapy

MISCELLANEOUS

ASSOCIATED CONDITIONS Other tineas - pedis, cruris, capitis, barbae, and manus

AGE-RELATED FACTORS
Pediatric: N/A
Geriatric: N/A
Others: N/A

PREGNANCY N/A

SYNONYMS
• Ringworm
• Tinea circinata

ICD-9-CM
110.5

SEE ALSO
• Tinea capitis
• Tinea cruris
• Tinea pedis

OTHER NOTES N/A

ABBREVIATIONS N/A

REFERENCES
• Habif T: Clinical Dermatology. 3rd Ed. St. Louis, CV Mosby, 1996
• Fitzpatrick TB et al: Color Atlas and Synopsis of Clinical Dermatology. 2nd Ed. New York, McGraw-Hill, 1992
Illustrations: 6 available on CD-ROM
Internet references: http://www.5mcc.com

Author(s)
Douglas M. Hoy, MD

Tinea cruris

BASICS

DESCRIPTION A superficial fungal infection of the groin area caused by a group of fungi known as dermatophytes, also called ringworm fungi. These dermatophyte infections may result from three genera of fungi: Microsporum, Trichophyton, and Epidermophyton.
• Tinea cruris is characterized by development of well marginated erythematous half-moon shaped plaques in the crural folds which spread to the upper thighs. The advancing border is well-defined often with fine scaling and sometimes includes vesicular eruptions. The skin within the border often heals to a red-brown with occasional red papules. The lesions are usually bilateral and do not include the scrotum or penis, but may migrate to the buttock and gluteal cleft area.
System(s) affected: Skin/Exocrine
Genetics: N/A
Incidence/Prevalence in USA: Common
Predominant age: Any age (rare prior to puberty)
Predominant sex: Males > Females

SIGNS AND SYMPTOMS
• Lesions may be asymptomatic but more frequently are quite pruritic
• Acute inflammation may result from wearing occlusive clothing
• Chronic scratching may result in an eczematous appearance
• Previous application of topical steroids may alter the appearance causing a more extensive eruption with irregular borders and erythematous papules. This modified form is called tinea incognito.

CAUSES
• Trichophyton rubrum
• Trichophyton interdigitale
• Trichophyton verrucosum
• Trichophyton tonsurans
• Trichophyton mentagrophytes
• Epidermophyton floccosum
• Microsporum canis

RISK FACTORS
• Summer months and/or increased sweating
• Wearing wet clothing
• Wearing multiple layers of clothing
• Depression of cell mediated immune response (atopic individuals, AIDS, etc.)
• Obesity

DIAGNOSIS

DIFFERENTIAL DIAGNOSIS
• Intertrigo - inflammatory process of moist opposed skin folds, often including infection with bacteria, yeast, and fungi. Painful longitudinal fissures occur in the creases of skin folds.
• Erythrasma - diffuse brown scaly noninflammatory plaque with irregular border often involving the groin. Caused by bacterial infection with Corynebacterium minutissimum. Fluoresces coral-red with Wood's lamp.
• Seborrheic dermatitis of the groin
• Psoriasis of the groin
• Candidiasis of the groin

LABORATORY
• Fungal culture using Sabouraud's dextrose agar or dermatophyte test medium (DTM)
• Potassium hydroxide preparation of skin scrapings from the dermatophyte leading border shows translucent branching, rod-shaped hyphae
Drugs that may alter lab results:
• Partial treatment with antifungal preparations
• Topical steroid treatment may confuse diagnosis by causing tinea incognito
Disorders that may alter lab results:
Pruritus with extensive itching

PATHOLOGICAL FINDINGS Skin biopsy showing fungal hyphae in the epidermis

SPECIAL TESTS Wood's lamp exam reveals no fluorescence

IMAGING N/A

DIAGNOSTIC PROCEDURES Potassium hydroxide, KOH preparation of skin scrapings form leading border

TREATMENT

APPROPRIATE HEALTH CARE
Outpatient

GENERAL MEASURES
• Avoid predisposing conditions, keep area as dry as possible
• Topical steroid preparations should not be used

SURGICAL MEASURES N/A

ACTIVITY Full activity

DIET No restrictions

PATIENT EDUCATION Explanation of the causative agents, predisposing factors, and prevention measures

MEDICATIONS

DRUG(S) OF CHOICE
• Topical antifungals including: naftifine, oxiconazole, clotrimazole (Lotrimin, Mycelex), ciclopirox (Loprox), econazole (Spectazole), haloprogin (Halotex), tolnaftate (Tinactin), miconazole (Monistat-Derm, Micatin) and undecylenic acid (Desenex). These should be applied bid for 14 days, up to 4 weeks.
• Terbinafine (Lamisil) - is a new topical antifungal with the advantage of being fungicidal, allowing for cure in as little as 7 days of therapy. It is approved for up to 4 weeks of treatment.
• If agents listed above are unsuccessful, a 14 day course of topical ketoconazole (Nizoral) applied once a day may be tried
• Absorbent powders may help to avoid excess moisture
Contraindications: Refer to manufacturer's literature
Precautions: Must continue therapy for at least 10 days even if symptoms resolve earlier
Significant possible interactions: N/A

ALTERNATIVE DRUGS
• Oral antifungal agents are effective, but not indicated in uncomplicated tinea cruris. If there is no response to topical therapy, or there is significant irritation, then griseofulvin, ultramicrosize, 500 mg daily with food for 3-4 weeks, or ketoconazole 200 mg qd for 2-3 months may be used and are FDA approved. Oral ketoconazole requires baseline laboratory evaluation of liver functions and a CBC, with LFT's repeated monthly. Concomitant use of oral ketoconazole and terfenadine or astemizole is contraindicated due to potential cardiac arrhythmia.
• Fluconazole (Diflucan) and itraconazole (Sporanox) are additional systemic antifungals which are being studied for treatment of cutaneous dermatophytoses. Their use is not FDA approved.

FOLLOWUP

PATIENT MONITORING
• Liver function testing prior to therapy and at regular intervals during the course of therapy for those patients requiring oral ketoconazole
• Monitor CBC, renal, and hepatic function of patients on griseofulvin.

PREVENTION/AVOIDANCE
Avoidance of risk factors

POSSIBLE COMPLICATIONS
Secondary bacterial infection

EXPECTED COURSE/PROGNOSIS
Excellent prognosis for cure with therapy

MISCELLANEOUS

ASSOCIATED CONDITIONS None

AGE-RELATED FACTORS
Pediatric: Rare in pediatric population prior to puberty
Geriatric: More common due to increase in risk factors
Others: N/A

PREGNANCY Rare

SYNONYMS
• Jock itch
• Ring worm

ICD-9-CM 110.3

SEE ALSO N/A

OTHER NOTES N/A

ABBREVIATIONS N/A

REFERENCES
• Fitzpatrick TB, et al: Color Atlas and Synopsis of Clinical Dermatology. 2nd Ed. New York, McGraw-Hill, Inc., 1992
• Habif T: Clinical Dermatology. 3rd Ed. St. Louis, CV Mosby, 1996
• Lynch PJ: Dermatology for the House Officer. 3rd Ed. Baltimore, Williams & Wilkins, 1994
• Clinical Courier CME Program. Superficial Fungal Infections: Diagnosis and Management 1994;12(7)
Illustrations: 2 available on CD-ROM
Internet references: http://www.5mcc.com

Author(s)
Michael Boespflug, MD

Tinea pedis

BASICS

DESCRIPTION Tinea pedis is a superficial infection of the feet caused by dermatophytes
System(s) affected: Skin/Exocrine
Genetics: No known genetic pattern
Incidence/Prevalence in USA: Extremely common
Predominant age: All ages, but most common in teens and young adults
Predominant sex: Male = Female

SIGNS AND SYMPTOMS
• Itching
• Scaling
• Maceration
• Vesicles/bullae
• Primarily in interdigital spaces
• May also involve sole and arch

CAUSES
• Trichophyton mentagrophytes
• Trichophyton rubrum
• Epidermophyton floccosum

RISK FACTORS
• Hot, humid weather
• Occlusive footwear
• Immunosuppressed patients
• Prolonged application of topical steroids

DIAGNOSIS

DIFFERENTIAL DIAGNOSIS
• Interdigital psoriasis
• Intertrigo
• Hyperkeratosis
• Contact dermatitis
• Eczema
• Dyshidrosis

LABORATORY
• Direct microscopic examination (KOH)
• Culture
Drugs that may alter lab results: N/A
Disorders that may alter lab results: N/A

PATHOLOGICAL FINDINGS
• Septate and branched mycelia on KOH
• Culture - dermatophyte

SPECIAL TESTS N/A

IMAGING N/A

DIAGNOSTIC PROCEDURES Culture

TREATMENT

APPROPRIATE HEALTH CARE
Outpatient

GENERAL MEASURES
• Treatment is generally with topical medications
• After soaking or bathing, patient should carefully remove or debride dead or thickened tissues

SURGICAL MEASURES N/A

ACTIVITY Avoid sweating feet

DIET No restrictions

PATIENT EDUCATION See Prevention/Avoidance

MEDICATIONS

DRUG(S) OF CHOICE
• Acute vesicular stage - Burow's wet dressings, followed by clotrimazole 1%
• Subacute (maceration, scaling) - clotrimazole cream or lotion bid for 4 weeks. Use antifungal powders between the toes and in the shoes.
• Chronic - same as treatment of subacute. Griseofulvin 375 mg orally bid for 4-8 weeks. If toenail involved, may need to treat at least 6 months.

Contraindications:
• Clotrimazole - do not use in any individual who has shown hypersensitivity to any of drugs' components
• Griseofulvin - patients with porphyria, hepatocellular failure, and in patients with a history of hypersensitivity to griseofulvin

Precautions:
• Clotrimazole - if irritation or sensitivity develop, treatment should be discontinued
• Griseofulvin - periodic monitoring of organ system functioning, including renal, hepatic, and hematopoietic. Possible photosensitivity reactions. Lupus erythematosus, lupus-like syndromes, or exacerbation of existing lupus erythematosus have been reported.
• Note: All systemic antifungal drugs have potential hepatotoxicity - ranging from low (griseofulvin), mid (itraconazole, to high (ketoconazole)

Significant possible interactions:
• Clotrimazole - none
• Griseofulvin - decreases the activity of warfarin-type anticoagulants. Barbiturates usually depress griseofulvin activity. The effect of alcohol may be potentiated, producing such effects as tachycardia and flush.

ALTERNATIVE DRUGS
• Topicals - imidazole, ketoconazole, sulconazole, miconazole, econazole, oxiconazole
• Allylamine topicals - naftifine, terbinafine
• Ketoconazole 200 mg daily by mouth, for griseofulvin-resistant dermatophytosis. Hepatotoxicity has been reported from its use. There is also a risk of cardiovascular events for patients taking terfenadine (Seldane) or astemizole (Hismanal) concomitantly with ketoconazole. Itraconazole is an alternative.

FOLLOWUP

PATIENT MONITORING   As needed

PREVENTION/AVOIDANCE
• Good personal hygiene
• Wearing rubber or wooden sandals in community showers or bathing places
• Careful drying between the toes after showering or bathing
• Changing socks frequently
• Applying drying or dusting powder

POSSIBLE COMPLICATIONS
• Secondary bacterial infections
• Eczematoid changes

EXPECTED COURSE/PROGNOSIS
Control, but not completely cured. Symptoms continue indefinitely with periods of relative quiescence.

MISCELLANEOUS

ASSOCIATED CONDITIONS
Hyperhidrosis

AGE-RELATED FACTORS
Pediatric: Rare in younger children (common in teens)
Geriatric: Elderly are more susceptible to outbreaks because of changes in the distal tissues resulting from peripheral vascular disease and the aging process
Others: N/A

PREGNANCY   N/A

SYNONYMS   Athlete's foot

ICD-9-CM   110.4 Dermatophytosis of foot

SEE ALSO
• Dyshidrosis
• Dermatitis, contact

OTHER NOTES   N/A

ABBREVIATIONS   N/A

REFERENCES
• Fitzpatrick TB, et al: Color Atlas and Synopsis of Clinical Dermatology. 2nd Ed. New York, McGraw-Hill, 1992
• Sober AJ, Fitzpatrick TB, eds: Year Book of Dermatology. St. Louis, C.V. Mosby, 1994
Illustrations: 6 available on CD-ROM
Internet references: http://www.5mcc.com

Author(s)
Robert B. Daigneault, MD, FAAP

Tinea versicolor

BASICS

DESCRIPTION Multiple patches on skin, generally asymptomatic. Ranges in color, usually white to brown. In blacks, lesions may be hyperpigmented. Probably the most common superficial mycosis.
System(s) affected: Skin/Exocrine
Genetics: No known genetic pattern
Incidence/Prevalence in USA: Common
Predominant age: Teenagers and young adults
Predominant sex: Male = Female

SIGNS AND SYMPTOMS
• Versicolor = various colors. Sun exposed areas - lesions usually white; on covered areas - they are often brown or red-brown.
• Distribution - (sebum-rich areas) chest, shoulders, back
• Appearance - sharply marginated 3 or 4 mm in diameter with centrifugal growth and coalescence
• Scale - fine, visible only with scraping
• Itching (rare)
• More prominent in summer
• Periodic recurrence

CAUSES
• Pityrosporon orbiculare (formerly Malassezia furfur)
• Variations in skin lipid formation

RISK FACTORS
• High heat
• High humidity
• Excessive sweating

DIAGNOSIS

DIFFERENTIAL DIAGNOSIS Other skin diseases with white patches and plaques including:
• Pityriasis alba
• Vitiligo
• Seborrheic dermatitis
• Nummular eczema

LABORATORY Routine lab not usually necessary
Drugs that may alter lab results: N/A
Disorders that may alter lab results: N/A

PATHOLOGICAL FINDINGS
• Short stubby fungal hyphae
• Y-shaped hyphae
• Small round spores in clusters on hyphae

SPECIAL TESTS KOH preparation to visualize budding yeast forms and club-shaped hyphae

IMAGING N/A

DIAGNOSTIC PROCEDURES Wood's lamp - golden fluorescence or pigment changes

TREATMENT

APPROPRIATE HEALTH CARE
Outpatient

GENERAL MEASURES
• Apply prescribed medications to affected parts with cotton balls
• Repeat treatment each spring prior to tanning

SURGICAL MEASURES N/A

ACTIVITY No restrictions

DIET No special diet

PATIENT EDUCATION For patient education materials favorably reviewed on this topic, contact: American Academy of Dermatology, 930 N. Meacham Rd., P.O. Box 4014, Schaumberg, IL 60168-4014, (708)330-0230

MEDICATIONS

DRUG(S) OF CHOICE
• Selenium sulfide shampoo (Excel and Selsun), allowed to dry for 40 minutes prior to showering daily for 1 week or allowed to remain on body for 12-24 hours before showering once a week for 4 weeks
or
• Clotrimazole topical (Lotrimin) bid for several weeks,
or
• Miconazole (Micatin, Monistat) bid for several weeks,
or
• Ketoconazole (Nizoral) cream bid for several weeks
Contraindications: Ketoconazole contraindicated in pregnancy
Precautions: N/A
Significant possible interactions: N/A

ALTERNATIVE DRUGS
• Ketoconazole (rarely needed and has significant adverse reactions): 400 mg in a single dose or 200 mg/day for a week
• Ketoconazole shampoo can be used weekly for maintenance
• Sulphur-salicylic acid (Sebulex) soap or shampoo can be used chronically for prophylaxis

FOLLOWUP

PATIENT MONITORING Recheck each spring

PREVENTION/AVOIDANCE N/A

POSSIBLE COMPLICATIONS None expected

EXPECTED COURSE/PROGNOSIS
Recurs almost routinely

MISCELLANEOUS

ASSOCIATED CONDITIONS N/A

AGE-RELATED FACTORS
Pediatric: Usually occurs after puberty
Geriatric: Not common in this age group
Others: N/A

PREGNANCY N/A

SYNONYMS Pityriasis versicolor

ICD-9-CM 111.0

SEE ALSO N/A

OTHER NOTES
• Warn patients that whiteness will remain for several months after treatment
• Treat again each spring prior to tanning season

ABBREVIATIONS N/A

REFERENCES
• Lynch PJ: Dermatology for the House Officer. 3rd Ed. Baltimore, Williams & Wilkins, 1994
• Rausch LJ, Jacobs PH: Tinea versicolor: treatment and prophylaxis. Cutis 1984;34:470
Illustrations: 4 available on CD-ROM
Internet references: http://www.5mcc.com

Author(s)
Kathryn Reilly, MD, MPH

Torticollis

BASICS

DESCRIPTION Rotation and tilting of head caused by primary pathology of the neck muscles or secondary to head and neck disorders. The condition may be congenital or acquired.
System(s) affected: Musculoskeletal, Nervous
Genetics: No known genetic pattern
Incidence/Prevalence in USA: Uncommon
Predominant age:
• Congenital - newborn
• Acquired - under age 10, and adults 30-60
Predominant sex: Male = Female

SIGNS AND SYMPTOMS
• Rotation and tilting of the head to the affected side, chin rotates to the opposite side
• Intermittent painful spasms of sternomastoid, trapezius and other neck muscles
• With congenital form, the first sign may be a firm, nontender, palpable enlargement of the sternocleidomastoid muscle that is visible at birth
• An early sign in acquired form is stiffness of neck muscles

CAUSES
• Congenital
 Injury to sternocleidomastoid muscle on one side at birth
  ◊ Possible malposition of head in utero
  ◊ Prenatal injury
  ◊ Fibroma
• Acquired
  ◊ Muscular damage from inflammatory disease (myositis, lymphadenitis, tuberculosis)
  ◊ Cervical spine injuries that produce scar tissue contracture
  ◊ Ocular muscle palsy
  ◊ Organic CNS disorder causing rhythmic muscle spasms
  ◊ Psychogenic inability to control neck muscles
  ◊ Tumor
  ◊ Cervical spondylosis
  ◊ Trauma
  ◊ Medications

RISK FACTORS
• Traumatic delivery, including breech
• Psychiatric illness, neurosis, stress, hypochondriasis
• Medications - phenothiazines and butyrophenones
• Acquired
  ◊ Inflammation
  ◊ Neurologic disorder
  ◊ Optical disorder
  ◊ Trauma

DIAGNOSIS

DIFFERENTIAL DIAGNOSIS
• Central nervous system infections
• Tumors of soft tissue or bone
• Basal ganglia disease
• Abscess of cervical glands
• Myositis of cervical muscles
• Cervical disk lesions

LABORATORY N/A
Drugs that may alter lab results: N/A
Disorders that may alter lab results: N/A

PATHOLOGICAL FINDINGS N/A

SPECIAL TESTS N/A

IMAGING
• X-ray to rule out skeletal abnormality (appearance may be subtle)
• CT or MRI of cervical spine to aid in differential diagnosis, especially for acquired cases

DIAGNOSTIC PROCEDURES History and physical examination

TREATMENT

APPROPRIATE HEALTH CARE
Outpatient

GENERAL MEASURES
• Physical therapy
• Sensory biofeedback
• Psychiatric treatment if there is an emotional disorder
• Acquired
  ◊ If less than 1 week in duration - soft collar and rest
  ◊ If less than 1 month duration - traction

SURGICAL MEASURES Congenital - operative division of involved muscle if physical therapy (i.e., passive stretching) is unsuccessful by one year of age

ACTIVITY No restrictions

DIET No special diet

PATIENT EDUCATION For congenital, training of parents to perform massage and range-of-motion exercises

The title is at top right.

MEDICATIONS

DRUG(S) OF CHOICE None indicated, other than analgesics for pain. If the torticollis has been drug induced, treatment can include diphenhydramine or diazepam.
Contraindications: N/A
Precautions: N/A
Significant possible interactions: N/A

ALTERNATIVE DRUGS Botulinum toxin (Ortholinum) injections are being studied for spastic form

FOLLOWUP

PATIENT MONITORING
• Periodic followup to assess progress
• In acquired cases, weekly followup required to assess progress

PREVENTION/AVOIDANCE No preventive measures known

POSSIBLE COMPLICATIONS
• Movement disorders
• Postural disorders
• May recur or persist throughout life
• Facial asymmetry in congenital cases

EXPECTED COURSE/PROGNOSIS
Good prognosis for correctable pathology

MISCELLANEOUS

ASSOCIATED CONDITIONS
• Difficult delivery in congenital cases

AGE-RELATED FACTORS
Pediatric: Congenital variety, associated with injury at time of birth that without treatment, becomes a fibrous cord
Geriatric: N/A
Others: N/A

PREGNANCY Associated with breech birth

SYNONYMS
• Spasmodic torticollis
• Wryneck

ICD-9-CM
• 333.83 Spasmodic torticollis
• 754.1 Certain congenital musculoskeletal deformities of sternocleidomastoid muscle
• 300.11 Hysterical

SEE ALSO N/A

OTHER NOTES Torticollis means "rotation", anterocollis means "tilting"

ABBREVIATIONS N/A

REFERENCE
• Tachdjian M: Pediatric Orthopedics. 2nd Ed. Philadelphia, W.B. Saunders Co., 1990
• Wenger DR, Rang M: Art and Practice of Childrens Orthopedics. New York, Raven Press, 1992
Illustrations: N/A
Internet references: http://www.5mcc.com

Author(s)
Francisco G. Valencia, MD

Tourette's syndrome

 BASICS

DESCRIPTION
Gilles de la Tourette's syndrome is a hereditary, chronic neuromuscular disorder consisting of various motor and vocal tics. Tics are sudden, involuntary, brief, repetitive, stereotypic motor movements. Symptoms begin in childhood and the location, number, frequency and complexity of tics change over time.

System(s) affected: Nervous
Genetics: Genetic predisposition, frequent familial history of tic disorders. Thought to be autosomal dominant with incomplete and sex-specific penetrances. Tourette's is concordant in identical twins and discordant in fraternal twins.
Incidence/Prevalence in USA: 0.1 to 0.5 cases per 1,000. It is estimated that there are one million sufferers of Tourette's in the U.S.
Predominant sex: Males 3 times more frequent than females
Predominant age: 2 to 15 years-old in 95% of cases, average age is 6-years-old

SIGNS AND SYMPTOMS
• Tics occur many times throughout the day and they change over time. May have only one tic at a time.
• Multiple motor tics such as: facial grimacing, blinking, head or neck twitching, tongue protruding, sniffing, touching
• Vocal tics such as grunts, snorts, throat clearing or barking and more complex vocal tics with echolalia (repeating the last words of someone else), palilalia (repeating one's own words), coprolalia (use of obscenities) copraxia, or copropraxia (use of obscene gestures)
• Tics usually worsen with stress and are most severe in the day and infrequent with sleep. When absorbed in a physical activity the tics are less severe or abate.
• Tics may persist for a few months and remiss then reoccur with a new motor tic

CAUSES
Possibly a gene defect that results in variable phenotypic expressions including Tourette's and chronic tic disorder, and obsessive-compulsive disorders. Possible pathology in the basal ganglia is suspected. Dopamine hypothesis suggests enhanced dopamine neurotransmitters within the striatum may be the cause.

RISK FACTORS
Increased prevalence in family members. Studies reveal 15 to 80% of patients have a family history of Tourette's, often undiagnosed.

 DIAGNOSIS

DIFFERENTIAL DIAGNOSIS
• Chronic-tic disorder (present for greater than 12 months and involves either motor or phonic tics)
• Huntington's disease
• Post-infectious encephalitis
• Drug intoxication
• Wilson's disease
• Cerebral palsy
• Sydenham's chorea
• Head trauma
• Hyperthyroidism

LABORATORY N/A
Drugs that may alter lab results: N/A
Disorders that may alter lab results: N/A

PATHOLOGICAL FINDINGS N/A

SPECIAL TESTS
• EEG studies may reveal nonspecific abnormalities in 50%
• EMG studies reveal short bursts of muscle activity

IMAGING N/A

DIAGNOSTIC PROCEDURES
A good history makes the diagnosis; no known biochemical abnormality and physical exam is typically normal. Most are diagnosed by parents, relatives or friends who are knowledgeable.

 TREATMENT

APPROPRIATE HEALTH CARE
Neurologic evaluation for therapy

GENERAL MEASURES
Patients are clinically heterogeneous and may have mild, moderate or very disturbing tics. Encourage a supportive environment, educate family and friends. The majority of patients require no medication. Adjustments may be required in work and school schedule to accommodate behaviors. Ignore outbursts and motor and vocal tics. Punishing the child rarely suppresses the present tic and classically provokes new tics which may be more problematic.

SURGICAL MEASURES N/A

ACTIVITY
No restrictions, encourage exercise

DIET N/A

PATIENT EDUCATION
Printed patient information available from:
Tourette's Syndrome Association (TSA)
42-40 Bell Blvd., Bayside, NY 11361-2861
National Hotline (800) 237-0717

MEDICATIONS

DRUG(S) OF CHOICE
• Haloperidol: The most frequently used; start at 0.25 mg at bedtime and slowly increase by 0.25 mg every week up to 2 mg a day. Side effects common, including lethargy and cognitive impairment.
• Clonidine: May help attention deficit disorders as well. Start at 0.05 mg/day and slowly increase by 0.05 mg every few weeks to 0.25 mg/day, given in divided doses. It may take many months to see an effect. Side effects common, such as sedation, will decrease with time.

Contraindications:
• Haloperidol
  ◊ CNS depression
  ◊ CNS disease
  ◊ Allergy
  ◊ Pregnancy
• Clonidine
  ◊ Allergy
  ◊ Pregnancy
  ◊ Hypotension

Precautions:
• Haloperidol
  ◊ Not recommended under age 3
  ◊ Not recommended during pregnancy
  ◊ Glaucoma
  ◊ Seizure disorders
  ◊ Thyrotoxicosis
• Clonidine
  ◊ Myocardial diseases
  ◊ Renal failure

Significant possible interactions:
• Haloperidol
  ◊ Possible increase toxicity with lithium
  ◊ Antagonized by anticholinergics
  ◊ May decrease anticoagulant effects
  ◊ May decrease guanethidine effects
  ◊ Potentiates CNS depression, especially if used with other CNS agents
• Clonidine
  ◊ Potentiates CNS depressants
  ◊ Antagonized by tricyclic antidepressants

ALTERNATIVE DRUGS
• Fluoxetine may alleviate the obsessive-compulsive symptoms. Naltrexone has been shown to be effective, but not recommended for long-term use due to its toxicity. A specific dopamine d2 antagonist, pimozide, has been shown to be effective in reducing tics, but its cardiotoxicity renders it a poor choice for routine clinical use.
• Other dopamine receptor antagonists that have been used include - thiothixene, trifluoperazine, fluphenazine
• Other agents used include - calcium channel blockers, benzodiazepines, alpha adrenergic receptor agonists (clonidine) and dopamine depletors

FOLLOWUP

PATIENT MONITORING Observe for associated attention deficit disorder or obsessive-compulsive disorders

PREVENTION/AVOIDANCE N/A

POSSIBLE COMPLICATIONS N/A

EXPECTED COURSE/PROGNOSIS
Clinically, symptoms wax and wane and new tics commonly develop. Up to 50% of patients show marked improvement during the teenage years. If tics abate, they do not usually reoccur in adulthood. If tics persist past age 15 then they tend to remain chronically.

MISCELLANEOUS

ASSOCIATED CONDITIONS
• Up to 50% develop attention deficit disorders and/or obsessive-compulsive disorders
• Phobias

AGE-RELATED FACTORS
Pediatric: Childhood onset, 90% by age 10
Geriatric: N/A
Others: None after age 21, by definition

PREGNANCY N/A

SYNONYMS N/A

ICD-9-CM 307.23

SEE ALSO N/A

OTHER NOTES N/A

ABBREVIATIONS N/A

REFERENCES
• American Psychiatric Association: Diagnostic and Statistical Manual of Mental Disorders (DSM-IV-R). 4th Ed. Washington, DC, 1994
• Dodick D, Adler CH: Tourette's syndrome. Postgraduate Medicine 1992;92:299
• Samuel MA, Feske S, eds. Office Practice of Neurology. 1st ed. New York, Churchill Livingstone Co., 1996
• Singer HS, Walkup JT: Tourette's syndrome and other tic disorders. Medicine (Baltimore) 1991;70:15-32
Illustrations: N/A
Internet references: http://www.5mcc.com

Author(s)
Brian J. Murray, MD

Toxic shock syndrome

BASICS

DESCRIPTION An acute multisystem illness associated with Staphylococcus aureus infections and characterized by the sudden onset of high fever, peculiar skin rash with desquamation, and shock
• Menstrual toxic shock: associated with menstruation and tampon use
• Nonmenstrual toxic shock: more common than the menstrual form; associated with postoperative wounds, barrier contraception, etc. Can occur in children, men, and women.
System(s) affected: Cardiovascular, Endocrine/Metabolic, Skin/Exocrine
Genetics: No specific mode of inheritance is recognized
Incidence/Prevalence in USA: 0.22 to 1.23 cases per 100,000
Predominant age: All ages, but especially 30-60 years
Predominant sex: Female > Male (3:2)

SIGNS AND SYMPTOMS
• Almost always present (> 80%)
  ◊ Temperature > 38.9°C (102°F)
  ◊ Erythroderma
  ◊ Diffuse macular rash
  ◊ Skin desquamation a few days after rash appears
  ◊ Shock, orthostatic hypotension or syncope
  ◊ Nausea or vomiting
• Commonly present (20-80%)
  ◊ Headache
  ◊ Confusion or agitation
  ◊ Acute respiratory distress syndrome
  ◊ Meningismus
  ◊ Pharyngeal erythema
  ◊ Vaginitis or vaginal discharge
  ◊ Conjunctivitis
  ◊ Periorbital edema
  ◊ Strawberry tongue
  ◊ Non-pitting edema
  ◊ Myalgia
  ◊ Oliguria
  ◊ Arthralgia
  ◊ Diarrhea
• Rarely present (< 20%)
  ◊ Arthritis
  ◊ Lymphadenopathy
  ◊ Hepatosplenomegaly
  ◊ Cardiomyopathy
  ◊ Pericarditis
  ◊ Photophobia
  ◊ Seizure

CAUSES Staphylococcus aureus exotoxins, especially toxic shock syndrome toxin-1 (TSST-1), and staphylococcal enterotoxins A, B and C (SEA, SEB, SEC)

RISK FACTORS
• High
  ◊ Absence of antibody to TSS toxin-1
  ◊ Infection with Staphylococcus aureus which produces TSST-1
  ◊ Continuous use of super absorbency tampons during menstruation
  ◊ Nasal surgery with packing
• Moderate
  ◊ Use of regular absorbency tampons during menstruation
  ◊ Use of contraceptive sponge
• Low
  ◊ Alternating use of tampons and pads during menstruation
  ◊ Intrauterine contraceptive device
  ◊ Surgical wound infections
  ◊ Early postpartum state

DIAGNOSIS

DIFFERENTIAL DIAGNOSIS
• Streptococcal scarlet fever
• Toxic strep syndrome
• Drug reactions
• Rocky Mountain spotted fever
• Leptospirosis
• Kawasaki disease
• Staphylococcal scalded skin syndrome
• Meningococcal or possibly gram negative sepsis
• Measles, rubeola

LABORATORY
• Microbiologic:
  ◊ Positive culture for Staphylococcus aureus from vagina or surgical wound (> 90%)
  ◊ Nasal or perineal carriage of Staphylococcus aureus
  ◊ Positive blood culture for Staphylococcus aureus (uncommon)
• Hematologic: (50-90%)
  ◊ Granulocytosis with increased band forms
  ◊ Lymphopenia
  ◊ Normocytic, normochromic anemia
  ◊ Thrombocytopenia
  ◊ Coagulopathy
• Biochemical: (50-90%)
  ◊ Hypoalbuminemia
  ◊ Abnormal electrolytes
  ◊ Hypocalcemia
  ◊ Hypomagnesemia
  ◊ Hypophosphatemia
  ◊ Increased SGOT
  ◊ Increased SGPT
  ◊ Increased CPK
  ◊ Increased BUN
  ◊ Increased serum creatinine
  ◊ Increased calcitonin
  ◊ Increased serum bilirubin
  ◊ Abnormal urine sediment
Drugs that may alter lab results: N/A
Disorders that may alter lab results: N/A

SPECIAL TESTS
• Absent serum antibodies to TSST-1, SEA, SEB or SEC
• Detection of TSST-1 or SEA-SEC in Staphylococcus aureus isolate

PATHOLOGICAL FINDINGS
• Subepidermic cleavage plane in the skin
• Minimal inflammatory reaction in tissues
• Lymphocyte depletion in lymph nodes
• Cervico-vaginal ulcerations

IMAGING No unusual or characteristic findings

DIAGNOSTIC PROCEDURES No specific diagnostic test is currently available

TREATMENT

APPROPRIATE HEALTH CARE Inpatient, admission to intensive care for monitoring

GENERAL MEASURES
• Removal of tampon or other vaginal foreign bodies
• Fluid resuscitation
• Management of renal or cardiac insufficiency
• Mechanical ventilation if necessary

SURGICAL MEASURES Surgical drainage of loculated infections

ACTIVITY Bed rest throughout acute illness

DIET As tolerated

PATIENT EDUCATION Advise patient regarding possible sequelae or recurrence

Toxic shock syndrome

 MEDICATIONS

DRUG(S) OF CHOICE
• Treatment of shock or hypotension
  ◊ Fluid replacement
  ◊ Dopamine
  ◊ Steroids or naloxone have not been proven to be of value
• Eradication of Staphylococcus aureus
  ◊ Oxacillin or nafcillin 100 mg/kg/day every 6 hours
Contraindications: Penicillin allergy
Precautions:
• Rash, diarrhea, seizures
• Reduce oxacillin dosage in patients with severe renal failure. Not necessary to reduce nafcillin dose for renal dysfunction.
Significant possible interactions: See manufacturer's profile of each drug

ALTERNATIVE DRUGS
• Clindamycin 25 mg/kg/day every 8 hours for patients allergic to penicillin
• Vancomycin 30 mg per kg per day every 6 hours
• Toxin neutralization. Benefit in humans is unproven, but animal and in vitro studies support this approach.
  ◊ Immune globulin, intravenous (IVIG) 0.4 g/kg over 6 hours

 FOLLOWUP

PATIENT MONITORING
• Admit to intensive care if in shock
• Daily vital signs until patient is afebrile and normotensive

PREVENTION/AVOIDANCE
• Avoidance of continuous tampon use during menstruation
• Avoidance of super absorbency tampons
• Encourage frequent tampon changes during the day
• Use sanitary napkins at night
• Early medical attention to infected wounds

POSSIBLE COMPLICATIONS
• Common (> 20%)
  ◊ Acute renal failure
  ◊ Adult respiratory distress syndrome
  ◊ Menorrhagia
  ◊ Alopecia
  ◊ Nail loss
• Rare (< 20%)
  ◊ Disseminated intravascular coagulation
  ◊ Ataxia, toxic encephalopathy
  ◊ Memory impairment
  ◊ Cardiomyopathy
  ◊ Protracted malaise

EXPECTED COURSE/PROGNOSIS
• Mortality 3-9%
• Recurrence 10-15%

 MISCELLANEOUS

ASSOCIATED CONDITIONS
Staphylococcal infections

AGE-RELATED FACTORS
Pediatric: May occur as a complication of chickenpox
Geriatric: Cellulitis or surgical wound infections
Others: None

PREGNANCY Postpartum infections, especially postcesarean section wound infection, or episiotomy infections

SYNONYMS Staphylococcal scarlet fever

ICD-9-CM
• 785.5 shock without mention of trauma
• 785.59 septic shock

SEE ALSO
• Scarlet fever
• Rocky Mountain spotted fever
• Measles, rubeola
• Pancreatitis

OTHER NOTES Streptococcal toxic shock syndrome or toxic strep syndrome may be clinically indistinguishable from staphylococcal toxic shock

ABBREVIATIONS N/A

REFERENCES
• Whiting JL, Chow AW: Toxic shock syndrome. In: Rakel RE, ed. Conn's Current Therapy. Philadelphia, W.B. Saunders Co., 1990:972-975
• See RH, Chow AW: Microbiology of TSS: overview. Rev Infect Dis 1989;11(suppl 1):S55-S60
• Reingold AL: Toxic shock syndrome: An update. Am J Obstet Gynecol 1991;165(suppl):1236-1239
• Barry W, et al: Intravenous immunoglobulin therapy for Toxic Shock Syndrome. JAMA 1992;267:3315-3316
• Kain KC, Schulzer M, Chow AW: Clinical spectrum of nonmenstrual toxic shock syndrome (TSS): Comparison with menstrual TSS by multivariate discriminant analyses. Clin Infect Dis 1993;16:100-106
Illustrations: 1 available on CD-ROM
Internet references: http://www.5mcc.com

Author(s)
Anthony W. Chow, MD, FRCPC, FACP

Toxoplasmosis

BASICS

DESCRIPTION Infection with the protozoan Toxoplasma gondii. Four types:
• Congenital toxoplasmosis: Acute infection of mother during gestation that is passed to fetus. Often asymptomatic, effects on fetus are more severe in first trimester infection.
• Ocular toxoplasmosis: Important cause of chorioretinitis, usually resulting from congenital infection but remaining asymptomatic until second or third decade of life
• Acute toxoplasmosis in immunocompetent host: Acute self-limiting asymptomatic or mildly symptomatic infection in normal host
• Acute toxoplasmosis in immunocompromised host: Primary or reactivation infection that can be a life-threatening disseminated infection involving many organ systems such as heart, lung, liver, but especially the central nervous system
System(s) affected: Nervous, Cardiovascular, Pulmonary, Gastrointestinal, Skin/Exocrine
Genetics: No known genetic pattern
Incidence/Prevalence in USA:
• Up to 70% of healthy adults are seropositive
• Seroconversion rate for women of childbearing age is 0.8% per year
• Affects more than 3500 newborns in U.S. each year
Predominant age: All ages
Predominant sex: Male = Female

SIGNS AND SYMPTOMS
• Congenital toxoplasmosis
  ◊ Most severe when maternal infection occurs early in pregnancy
  ◊ No signs or symptoms of infection (67%)
  ◊ Chorioretinitis (15%)
  ◊ Intracranial calcifications (10%)
  ◊ Cerebrospinal fluid pleocytosis and elevated protein (20%)
  ◊ Anemia, thrombocytopenia, jaundice at birth
  ◊ Microcephaly
  ◊ Affected survivors may have mental retardation, seizures, visual defects, spasticity, other severe neurologic sequelae
• Ocular toxoplasmosis
  ◊ Chorioretinitis - focal necrotizing retinitis
  ◊ Yellowish white elevated cotton patch with indistinct margins
  ◊ May be small clusters of lesions
  ◊ Congenital disease is usually bilateral
  ◊ Acquired disease is usually unilateral
  ◊ Symptoms include blurred vision, scotoma, pain, photophobia

• Acute toxoplasmosis in immunocompetent host
  ◊ 80-90% are asymptomatic
  ◊ Cervical lymphadenopathy with discrete, usually non-tender nodes, less than 3 cm in diameter
  ◊ Fever, malaise, night sweats, myalgias
  ◊ Sore throat
  ◊ Maculopapular rash
  ◊ Retroperitoneal and mesenteric lymphadenopathy with abdominal pain may occur
  ◊ Chorioretinitis
• Acute toxoplasmosis in immunocompromised host
  ◊ May be newly acquired or reactivation disease
  ◊ Central nervous system disease (50%)
  ◊ Encephalitis, meningoencephalitis or mass lesions
  ◊ Hemiparesis, seizures, mental status changes
  ◊ Visual changes
  ◊ May have signs and symptoms as seen in immunocompetent host
  ◊ Myocarditis, pneumonitis

CAUSES
• Etiologic agent for each of the clinical syndromes is Toxoplasma gondii
• Congenital disease is passed transplacentally from newly infected mother to fetus during pregnancy
• Other syndromes may result from newly acquired infection or reactivation of latent infection
• Ingestion of meats or foods containing cysts or oocysts present in cat feces
• Infection can be transmitted by blood transfusion or organ transplantation

RISK FACTORS
• Immunocompromised hosts especially those with defects in cellular immunity such as AIDS
• Risk of transplacental transmission is greatest during third trimester

DIAGNOSIS

DIFFERENTIAL DIAGNOSIS
• Congenital toxoplasmosis: Other members of TORCH syndrome (rubella, cytomegalovirus, herpes simple), syphilis, Listeria, other infectious encephalopathies, erythroblastosis fetalis, sepsis
• Ocular toxoplasmosis: Tuberculosis, syphilis, leprosy, ocular histoplasmosis
• Acute toxoplasmosis (normal and immunocompromised): Must consider lymphoma, infectious mononucleosis, cytomegalovirus, cat scratch disease, sarcoidosis, tuberculosis, tularemia, metastatic carcinoma, leukemia
• Toxoplasma encephalitis: Tuberculosis, fungal diseases, vasculitis, progressive multifocal leukoencephalopathy (PML), brain abscess, tumor, herpes encephalitis

LABORATORY
• Demonstration of Toxoplasma organism in blood, body fluids or tissue is evidence of infection
• Isolation of Toxoplasma from placenta is diagnostic of congenital infection
• Lymphocyte transformation to Toxoplasma antigens is indicator of previous Toxoplasma infection in adults
• Detection of Toxoplasma antigen in blood or body fluids by ELISA technique indicates acute infection
• Several serologic tests used in diagnosis, some measuring IgM and others IgG antibody
• Sabin-Feldman dye test is a sensitive and specific neutralization test, measures IgG antibody, is the standard reference test for toxoplasmosis, but requires live Toxoplasma organisms, so is not available in most labs. High titers suggest acute disease.
• Indirect fluorescent antibody test (IFA) measures same antibodies as dye test. Titers parallel dye test titers.
• IgM fluorescent antibody test detects IgM antibodies with first week of infection but titers fall within a few months
• Indirect hemagglutination test measures a different antibody than dye test. Titers tend to be higher and remain elevated longer.
• Double-sandwich IgM ELISA is more sensitive and specific than other IgM tests
• PCR on body fluids including CSF, amniotic fluid, BAL and blood may be useful in diagnosis
Drugs that may alter lab results: None
Disorders that may alter lab results:
• Antinuclear antibodies and rheumatoid factor may cause false positive serologic test
• Pregnancy may cause false negative hemagglutination test

PATHOLOGICAL FINDINGS
• Lymph node histology shows triad of:
  ◊ Reactive follicular hyperplasia
  ◊ Irregular clusters of epithelioid histiocytes encroaching on and blurring the margins of the germinal centers
  ◊ Focal distention of sinuses with monocytoid cells

SPECIAL TESTS
• Skin test showing delayed skin hypersensitivity to Toxoplasma antigens may be useful as a screening test
• Antibody levels in aqueous humor or cerebrospinal fluid may reflect local antibody production and infection at these sites
• Amniocentesis at 20-24 weeks in suspected congenital disease

IMAGING
• CT scan of head in cerebral toxoplasmosis
• Ultrasound of fetus at 20-24 weeks

DIAGNOSTIC PROCEDURES
• Lymph node biopsy showing characteristic pathologic triad
• Brain biopsy in CNS disease and demonstration of organisms by peroxidase-antiperoxidase technique

Toxoplasmosis

TREATMENT

APPROPRIATE HEALTH CARE
• Outpatient for acquired disease in immunocompetent host and ocular toxoplasmosis
• Inpatient initially for CNS toxoplasmosis and acute disease in immunocompromised host

GENERAL MEASURES
• Usually no treatment in asymptomatic hosts except in child under 5
• Symptomatic patients should be treated until immunity is assured

SURGICAL MEASURES N/A

ACTIVITY Level of activity dependent on severity of disease and organ systems involved

DIET No special diet

PATIENT EDUCATION
• Infected mother must be completely informed of potential consequences to fetus
• Explain prevention methods, e.g., protecting children's play area from cat litter
• Additional materials available from:
• National Institute of Allergy and Infectious Disease, Dept. of Health and Human Services, Bldg. 31, Rm 7A-32, 9000 Rockville Pike, Bethesda, MD 20892, (301)496-5717

MEDICATIONS

DRUG(S) OF CHOICE
• Acute toxoplasmosis in immunodeficient host:
◊ Sulfadiazine (Microsulfon) 100 mg/kg/day up to 8 grams/day plus pyrimethamine (Daraprim) 200 mg the first day, then 25-50 mg/day plus leucovorin (folinic acid) 10 mg/day for several weeks followed by maintenance therapy with the same drugs at lower dosage for several months
• Ocular toxoplasmosis: Above regimen for 1-2 months
• Acute toxoplasmosis in pregnant women: Above regimen may be used after the 16th week of pregnancy
• Congenital toxoplasmosis: Sulfadiazine 100 mg/kg/day plus pyrimethamine I mg/kg every 2 days plus leucovorin (folinic acid) 5 mg every 2 days

Contraindications:
• Pyrimethamine should not be used in first trimester of pregnancy
• Known hypersensitivity to pyrimethamine or sulfadiazine (Note: many HIV positive patients have a sulfa sensitivity)

Precautions:
• Bone marrow toxicity an important problem while treating toxoplasmosis
• Use with caution in patients with possible folate deficiency
• Use with caution in patients with renal or hepatic dysfunction
• Sulfonamides may increase anticoagulant effect of coumadin
• Sulfonamides may increase phenytoin (Dilantin) levels
• Sulfonamides may increase hypoglycemic effect of oral hypoglycemic agents
• Adequate hydration is essential since sulfadiazine is poorly soluble and may crystallize in the urine

Significant possible interactions:
Sulfonamides may interact with phenytoin, coumadin and oral hypoglycemic agents

ALTERNATIVE DRUGS
• In pregnancy - Spiramycin 3 g/day for 3 weeks, then 2 weeks off, then repeat 5 week cycles throughout pregnancy. Drug not yet FDA approved in U.S. Contact manufacturer - Rhone-Poulenc, Inc., CN5266, Princeton, NJ 08543-5266.
• Clindamycin 900-1200 mg tid IV has been used for ocular and CNS toxoplasmosis alone and in combination with pyrimethamine. May be as effective as the sulfa/pyrimethamine combination, but with fewer adverse effects.
• Corticosteroids (prednisone 1-2 mg/kg/day) may be added for macular chorioretinitis or CNS infection
• Atovaquone (Mepron), azithromycin (Zithromax) and clarithromycin (Biaxin) - promising new agents for CNS toxoplasmosis

FOLLOWUP

PATIENT MONITORING
• Followup visits every 2 weeks until stable, then monthly during therapy
• CBC weekly for first month, then every 2 weeks
• Renal and liver function tests monthly

PREVENTION/AVOIDANCE Prevention is important in seronegative pregnant women and immunodeficient patients. Avoid eating raw meat, unpasteurized milk, uncooked eggs and avoid contact with cat feces.

POSSIBLE COMPLICATIONS
• Seizure disorder or focal neurologic deficits in CNS toxoplasmosis
• Partial or complete blindness with ocular toxoplasmosis
• Multiple complications may occur with congenital toxoplasmosis including mental retardation, seizures, deafness and blindness

EXPECTED COURSE/PROGNOSIS
• Immunodeficient patients often relapse if treatment is stopped
• Treatment may prevent the development of untoward sequelae in both symptomatic and asymptomatic infants with congenital toxoplasmosis

MISCELLANEOUS

ASSOCIATED CONDITIONS Cellular immune compromised patients, especially those with AIDS, have a higher incidence of toxoplasmosis

AGE-RELATED FACTORS
Pediatric: With acute congenital toxoplasmosis, children often die in the first month of life. Subacute congenital disease may not be observed until some time after birth, when symptoms start to appear.
Geriatric: Acquired infection. Often reactivation disease more likely.
Others: None

PREGNANCY
• Have serum examined for Toxoplasma antibodies. Those with negative titers should take extra precautions to avoid contact with cats, not to eat raw meat and wash all fruits and vegetables carefully.
• For toxoplasmosis infection during pregnancy, refer patient to specialist

SYNONYMS N/A

ICD-9-CM
• 130.9 Toxoplasmosis, unspecified
• 771.2 Other congenital infections

SEE ALSO N/A

OTHER NOTES N/A

ABBREVIATIONS N/A

REFERENCES Mandell G, ed: Principles and Practice of Infectious Diseases. 4th Ed. New York, Churchill Livingstone, 1995
Illustrations: 2 available on CD-ROM
Internet references: http://www.5mcc.com

Author(s)
William G. Gardner, MD

Tracheitis, bacterial

 BASICS

DESCRIPTION
• Severe, potentially life-threatening infraglottic infection; relatively rare, caused by a secondary bacterial infection following a primary viral infection, usually H. parainfluenzae or H. influenzae
• Also called pseudomembranous croup or membranous tracheitis was described by C.L. Jackson as "an acute infection of the larynx, trachea, and bronchi characterized by toxemia, edema of the larynx and subglottic regions, and a thick, viscid, obstructive, often crusting exudate in the tracheobronchial tree."
System(s) affected: Pulmonary
Genetics: No known genetic predisposition
Incidence/prevalence in USA: True incidence is unknown; was a fairly common childhood illness in the pre-antibiotic era; a resurgence of cases has been noted since 1979; fall/winter predominance; in one series, 2% of all children hospitalized with "croup" had bacterial tracheitis
Predominant age: Mean age 54 months; range 3 weeks to 13 years; infections in adolescents have been reported
Predominant sex: Male > Female (1.8: 1); no gender predominance seen in other studies

SIGNS AND SYMPTOMS
• Barking, "brassy" cough
• Inspiratory stridor
• Variable degree of respiratory distress
• Child is usually lying flat
• Fever > 38°C (100.4°F)
• Toxic-appearing
• There is a gradual progression of mild upper airway symptoms over 1 hour to six days to an acute, febrile phase of rapid respiratory decompensation
• Voice and cry are usually normal
• Absence of drooling and dysphagia help distinguish it from epiglottitis
• Does not respond to aerosolized epinephrine (unlike patients with croup)
• Subglottic edema

CAUSES
• Staphylococcal aureus
• H. influenzae
• Streptococcus pneumoniae
• Moraxella catarrhalis
• Klebsiella
• Streptococci (group A)
• Neisseria

RISK FACTORS Periods of increased seasonal activity of respiratory viruses

 DIAGNOSIS

DIFFERENTIAL DIAGNOSIS
• Laryngotracheomalacia
• Epiglottitis
• Foreign body
• Retropharyngeal abscess
• Pneumonia
• Asthma
• Spasmodic croup
• Diphtheritic laryngitis

LABORATORY Elevated WBC count with predominance of PMN's and some bands present; blood cultures are usually negative
Drugs that may alter lab results: N/A
Disorders that may alter lab results: N/A

PATHOLOGICAL FINDINGS
• Mucosal destruction and/or local immunodeficiency caused by viral infection may predispose to bacterial infection
• Intense inflammation, sloughing of subglottic epithelium, and profuse mucopurulent secretions which compromise the airway and which make airway management very difficult

SPECIAL TESTS Rapid antigen tests are available for bacteria and viruses in some centers

IMAGING
• AP and lateral neck radiographs show subglottic and tracheal narrowing with haziness and radiopaque linear or particulate densities (crusts)
• In patients with risk of acute respiratory obstruction, either do not obtain radiographs or monitor carefully
• Often see pneumonic infiltrates

DIAGNOSTIC PROCEDURES
• Endoscopy is diagnostic and demonstrates severe inflammation of the subglottic region and trachea with copious mucopurulent secretions and sloughed epithelium that separates from the tracheal wall in sheets
• Obtain Gram stain and culture of tracheal secretions

 TREATMENT

APPROPRIATE HEALTH CARE ICU care

GENERAL MEASURES
• Constitutes a true pediatric emergency
• Maintain airway – this is often very difficult due to copious secretions
• Hydration, humidification, antibiotics
• Endotracheal or nasotracheal intubation
• Does not respond to epinephrine

SURGICAL MEASURES Tracheotomy may be necessary

ACTIVITY Complete bed rest

DIET Peripheral venous nutrition

PATIENT EDUCATION Usually requires 3-13 days intubation with complete recovery expected

MEDICATIONS

DRUG(S) OF CHOICE
• Nafcillin 150 mg/kg/day divided QID plus cefotaxime 150 mg/kg/day in 4-6 divided doses; maximum of 2 grams q6h
or
• Cefuroxime 75 mg/kg/day divided QID
• Does not respond to epinephrine
• Narrow the antibiotic regimen when pathogens and sensitivities available
Contraindications: Refer to manufacturer's literature
Precautions: Refer to manufacturer's literature
Significant possible interactions: See manufacturer's literature

ALTERNATIVE DRUGS
For patients with penicillin allergy: Clindamycin 40 mg/kg/day divided QID plus chloramphenicol 75 mg/kg/day divided QID

FOLLOWUP

PATIENT MONITORING   ICU care with cardiopulmonary monitoring

PREVENTION/AVOIDANCE   N/A

POSSIBLE COMPLICATIONS
• Postintubation subglottic stenosis
• Cardiopulmonary arrest
• Pneumonia
• Toxic shock syndrome secondary to enterotoxin-producing staphylococci

EXPECTED COURSE/PROGNOSIS
• With vigorous airway management and intubation for up to 13 days, complete recovery is expected
• Cardiopulmonary arrest and death have occurred.

MISCELLANEOUS

ASSOCIATED CONDITIONS   Consider anatomic abnormalities or foreign body

AGE-RELATED FACTORS
Pediatric: Typically affects children below the age of three
Geriatric: N/A
Others: N/A

PREGNANCY   No more contagious than the common cold; scrupulous handwashing is recommended

SYNONYMS
• Pseudomembranous croup
• Membranous tracheitis

ICD-9-CM
464.1 Acute tracheitis
464.2 Acute laryngotracheitis

SEE ALSO
• Common cold
• Epiglottitis
• Bronchiolitis
• Laryngotracheobronchitis

OTHER NOTES   N/A

ABBREVIATIONS
• ED = emergency department
• LTB = laryngotracheobronchitis

REFERENCES
• Cunningham MJ: The old and new of acute laryngotracheal infections. Clinical Pediatrics 1992;31(1): 56-64
• Donnelly BW, McMillan JA, Weiner LB: Bacterial tracheitis: report of eight new cases and review. Reviews of Infectious Diseases 1990;12(5):729-735
• Jackson CL: Acute infective laryngotracheobronchitis. In Mitchell-Nelson Textbook of Pediatrics. 4th Ed. Philadelphia, W.B. Saunders Co, 1945
• Kasian GF, Bingham WT, Steinberg, et al: Bacterial tracheitis in children. Canadian Medical Association Journal 1989;140(1):46-50
• Klassen TP, Feldman ME, et al: Nebulized budesonide for children with mild-to-moderate croup. New Engl J Med 1994;331:285-89
• Rabie I, McShane D, Warde D: Bacterial tracheitis. Journal of Laryngology & Otology 1989;103(11):1059-1062
• Walker P, Crysdale WS: Croup, epiglottitis, retropharyngeal abscess, and bacterial tracheitis: evolving patterns of occurrence and care. International Anesthesiology Clinics 1992;30(4):57-70
Illustrations: N/A
Internet references: http://www.5mcc.com

Author(s)
Barcey T. Levy, PhD, MD

Transfusion reaction, hemolytic

 BASICS

DESCRIPTION A cytotoxic, hemolytic reaction that occurs after administration of blood or blood components, resulting in hemolysis of donor's or recipient's RBC's (usually the latter). Reactions may be immune or nonimmune, and can vary from a mild to a fatal consequence. (Infection risks outweigh immune risks.)

System(s) affected:
Hemic/Lymphatic/Immunologic, Cardiovascular
Genetics: No known genetic pattern
Incidence/Prevalence in USA:
Uncommon
Predominant age: All ages
Predominant sex: Female > Male

SIGNS AND SYMPTOMS
• Immediate (intravascular) hemolytic transfusion reaction:
  ◊ Anxiety
  ◊ Flushing
  ◊ Tachycardia
  ◊ Hypotension
  ◊ Chest or back pain
  ◊ Dyspnea
  ◊ Fever
  ◊ Chills
  ◊ Note: symptoms are masked in anesthetized patient
• Delayed (extravascular) hemolytic transfusion reaction:
  ◊ Fever
  ◊ Anemia (2-14 days after transfusion)
  ◊ Jaundice

CAUSES
• Immune reactions - incompatibility within ABO system
• A nonhemolytic febrile reaction due to immune sensitivity to leukocytes, platelets, plasma constituents
• Hemolytic reactions:
  ◊ Transfusion of mismatched blood
  ◊ Destruction of donor erythrocytes by recipient incompatible isoantibodies
  ◊ Isosensitization by repeated transfusions
  ◊ Isosensitization by prior pregnancies
  ◊ Universal blood donor type considered dangerous unless thoroughly checked for agglutination titer
  ◊ Acquisition of B antigen by Group A individuals with colon cancer

RISK FACTORS
• Multiple blood transfusions
• Rh negative mother
• Multiple pregnancies

 DIAGNOSIS

DIFFERENTIAL DIAGNOSIS
• Other causes of acute hemolysis
  ◊ Autoimmune diseases
  ◊ Hemoglobinopathies
  ◊ Red blood cell enzyme defects
  ◊ Bacterial contamination of stored blood

LABORATORY
• Positive direct antiglobulin test (Coomb's)
• Plasma obtained 2-4 hours after lysis is red or pink, indicating free hemoglobin
• Increased BUN, creatinine
• Elevated serum bilirubin (mild)
• Wine-colored urine indicating hemoglobinuria
• Reduced serum haptoglobin
Drugs that may alter lab results: N/A
Disorders that may alter lab results: N/A

PATHOLOGICAL FINDINGS N/A

SPECIAL TESTS Blood bank evaluation for immune reactions

IMAGING N/A

DIAGNOSTIC PROCEDURES N/A

 TREATMENT

APPROPRIATE HEALTH CARE Inpatient

GENERAL MEASURES
• Stop transfusion immediately upon first sign of reaction
• Substitute infusion with normal saline at 150-300 mL per hour
• Check paperwork for any clerical error (usual cause of an ABO-incompatible transfusion)
• Monitor vital signs
• Maintain urine flow at 100 mL/hr for 6-8 hours or until hemoglobinuria clears
• Recognize and treat disseminated intravascular coagulation if it occurs
• Posttransfusion blood sample and discontinued blood to blood bank for investigation
• Maintain systolic blood pressure above 100 mm Hg

SURGICAL MEASURES N/A

ACTIVITY Bedrest

DIET As tolerated

PATIENT EDUCATION N/A

MEDICATIONS

DRUG(S) OF CHOICE
• Oxygen as needed
• Epinephrine for wheezing and/or dyspnea
• Corticosteroids to reduce inflammation
• Adequate colloid or crystalloid (may need 1000 mL/hr normal saline for 2-3 hours) to maintain systolic blood pressure above 100 mm Hg
• Mannitol not of proven value
• Dopamine effective against hypotension and impaired renal perfusion
• Heparinization, at moderate doses, is indicated if DIC present
• Diuretic: furosemide 80-120 mg IV or ethacrynic acid 50 mg IV
Contraindications: Refer to manufacturer's literature
Precautions: Refer to manufacturer's literature
Significant possible interactions: Refer to manufacturer's literature

ALTERNATIVE DRUGS
Diphenhydramine to combat cellular histamine release from mast cells

FOLLOWUP

PATIENT MONITORING   Until hemolytic signs are gone

PREVENTION/AVOIDANCE
• History of patient's responses to previous transfusions
• Risk/benefit of any transfusion needs to favor benefit
• Autologous transfusion
• Careful typing and crossmatch, double-check all data available
• Identity of unit of blood is carefully checked before administered
• Close observation of the patient during the transfusion
• Consider leukocyte depleted blood in people with history of recurrent febrile reactions
• Avoid prophylactic antipyretics
• Use of genotype specific RBCs in sickle cell anemia

POSSIBLE COMPLICATIONS
• Uremia, oliguria, anuria
• Right heart failure

EXPECTED COURSE/PROGNOSIS
• Usual course - acute
• Usually no harm if transfusion is stopped at onset of manifestations
• Severe - mortality 50%

MISCELLANEOUS

ASSOCIATED CONDITIONS
• Disseminated intravascular coagulation
• Acute renal failure

AGE-RELATED FACTORS
Pediatric: Reaction greater and outlook poorer in the very young
Geriatric: Outlook more grave in the elderly
Others: N/A

PREGNANCY   N/A

SYNONYMS   N/A

ICD-9-CM   999.8 Other transfusion reaction

SEE ALSO
• Renal failure, acute (ARF)
• Disseminated intravascular coagulation (DIC)
• Anemia, sickle cell
• Anemia, autoimmune hemolytic
• Anemia, hemolytic

OTHER NOTES   N/A

ABBREVIATIONS   N/A

REFERENCES
• Lee RG, Bithell TC, et al: Wintrobe's Clinical Hematology. 9th Ed. Philadelphia, Lea & Febiger, 1993
• Huestis DW, Bove JR, Case S: Practical Blood Transfusion. 4th Ed. Boston, Little, Brown and Co., 1988
Illustrations: N/A
Internet references: http://www.5mcc.com

Author(s)
Bruce G. Bellamy, MD

Transient ischemic attack (TIA)

BASICS

DESCRIPTION The sudden onset of a focal and transient (< 24 hours) neurological deficit due to brain ischemia
System(s) affected: Nervous
Genetics: Inheritance is polygenic with a tendency to clustering of risk factors within families
Incidence/Prevalence in USA: Incidence 160/100,000; prevalence 135 per 100,000
Predominant age: Risk increases over age 45 and is highest in the seventh and eighth decades
Predominant sex: Male > Female (3:1)

SIGNS AND SYMPTOMS
• Carotid circulation (hemispheric) - hemiplegia, hemianesthesia, neglect, aphasia, visual field defects; less often headaches, seizures, amnesia, confusion
• Vertebrobasilar (brainstem or cerebellar) - diplopia, vertigo, ataxia, facial paresis, Horner's syndrome, dysphagia, dysarthria
• Cerebellar or brainstem lesion in patients with headache, nausea, vomiting and ataxia

CAUSES
• Carotid atherosclerotic disease with artery to artery thromboembolism
• Small, deep, vessel disease associated with hypertension
• Cardiac - cardioembolism secondary to valvular (mitral valve) pathology; mural hypo- or akinesias with thrombosis (acute anterior myocardial infarctions or congestive cardiomyopathies); cardiac arrhythmia (atrial fibrillation)
• Hypercoagulable states - antiphospholipid antibodies, deficiency of protein S, protein C. Presence of antithrombin 3, oral contraceptives.
• Other causes - spontaneous and post-traumatic (i.e., chiropractic manipulation) arterial dissection, fibromuscular dysplasia

RISK FACTORS
• Age
• Hypertension
• Cardiac disease
• Smoking
• Diabetes
• Antiphospholipid antibodies
• Family History

DIAGNOSIS

DIFFERENTIAL DIAGNOSIS
• Migraine (hemiplegic)
• Focal seizure (Todd's paralysis)
• Hypoglycemia
• Todd's paralysis

LABORATORY N/A
Drugs that may alter lab results: N/A
Disorders that may alter lab results: N/A

PATHOLOGICAL FINDINGS N/A

SPECIAL TESTS
• Duplex carotid ultrasonography
• Cerebral angiography
• ECG
• Transthoracic echocardiogram (TTE); if normal and a cardiac source is suspected, follow with transesophageal echocardiogram
• Holter monitoring
• EEG for suspected seizure
• Prothrombin time (PT) and partial thromboplastin time (PTT) (Coumadin prolongs PT)
• Antiphospholipid antibodies

IMAGING
• Acute phase - CT of head to rule out hemorrhage
• Angiography - carotid arterial stenosis
• Digital substraction - stenosis

DIAGNOSTIC PROCEDURES N/A

TREATMENT

APPROPRIATE HEALTH CARE
• Acute phase: Outpatient for investigations; inpatient for surgery

GENERAL MEASURES
• Strict control of medical risk factors, e.g., diabetes, hypertension, hyperlipidemia, cardiac disease
• Counseling towards cessation of smoking

SURGICAL MEASURES In medically fit patients with non-disabling stroke, carotid endarterectomy is indicated for stenosis of >70% on side ipsilateral to stroke; medical therapy for <30% stenosis. Best therapy for stenosis of 30-70% is unknown, therefore it is best to refer the patient to a center involved in North American Symptomatic Carotid Endarterectomy Trial (NASCET).

ACTIVITY No restrictions

DIET As appropriate to underlying medical problems (diabetic diet, low fat diet, low salt diet etc.)

PATIENT EDUCATION National Stroke Association, 300 East Hampden Ave., Suite 240, Engle Wood, CO 80110-2622

MEDICATIONS

DRUG(S) OF CHOICE
• Enteric coated aspirin (EC ASA) 325-1300 mg/day,
or
• Ticlopidine 250 mg po bid
Contraindications:
• EC ASA - active peptic ulcer disease, hypersensitivity to aspirin, patients who had bronchospastic reaction to ASA or other nonsteroidal anti-inflammatory drugs
• Ticlopidine - known hypersensitivity to the drug, presence of hematopoietic disorders, presence of a hemostatic disorder, conditions associated with active bleeding, severe liver dysfunction
Precautions:
• EC ASA - may aggravate pre-existing peptic ulcer disease , may worsen symptoms in some patients with asthma
• Ticlopidine - 2.4% of patients develop neutropenia (0.8% severe neutropenia) which is reversible with cessation of drug. Monitor blood counts every 2 weeks for the first 3 months.
Significant possible interactions:
• EC ASA - may potentiate effects of anticoagulants and sulfonylurea, hypoglycemic agents
• Ticlopidine - digoxin plasma levels decreased 15%, theophylline half-life increased from 8.6 to 12.2 hours

ALTERNATIVE DRUGS
• Dipyridamole (Persantine) of no proven benefit
• Sulfinpyrazone (Anturane) of no proven benefit

FOLLOWUP

PATIENT MONITORING
Followup every 3 months for first year then yearly

PREVENTION/AVOIDANCE
• Stop smoking
• Control blood pressure, diabetes, hyperlipidemia
• EC ASA 650 mg bid or ticlopidine 250 mg po bid for patients with prior transient ischemic attack

POSSIBLE COMPLICATIONS
• Stroke
• Seizure
• Trauma if patient experiences sudden fall due to weakness

EXPECTED COURSE/PROGNOSIS
5-20% risk of stroke on ipsilateral side within one year and cumulative thereafter. Frequency increases with addition of multiple risk factors and severity of carotid stenosis.

MISCELLANEOUS

ASSOCIATED CONDITIONS
• Atrial fibrillation
• Major cause of death in first five years after a TIA is cardiac disease

AGE-RELATED FACTORS
Pediatric:
• Cardiac (especially developmental abnormalities)
• Metabolic - homocystinuria, Fabry's disease
Geriatric: Atrial fibrillation is a frequent cause of TIA among the elderly
Others: Adults < 45 years old most likely to have a cardiac source of embolism

PREGNANCY
A hypercoagulable state is associated with pregnancy and parturition

SYNONYMS
• Mini-stroke

ICD-9-CM
435.9

SEE ALSO
• Stroke (Brain attack)

OTHER NOTES N/A

ABBREVIATIONS
EC ASA = enteric coated aspirin

REFERENCES
• Hachinski VC, Norris JW: The Acute Stroke. Philadelphia, F.A. Davis, 1985
• Barnett JHM, Mohr JP, Stein BM, Yatsu FM, eds: Stroke. New York, Churchill Livingstone, 1986
• Norris JW, Hachinski V: Prevention of Stroke. Philadelphia, F.A. Davis, 1991
Illustrations: N/A
Internet references: http://www.5mcc.com

Author(s)
Carmelo Graffagnino, MD, FRCP
Vladimir Hachinski, MD, DSc, FRCP

Trichinosis

BASICS

DESCRIPTION
• Trichinosis is a parasitic disease that develops after ingesting infected pork or other meat containing viable cysts of Trichinella spiralis, a nematode, with rarer cases attributable to several different species of Trichinella. The cysts remain viable and can cause disease when the infected meat is undercooked. Most common outbreaks are attributable to undercooked pork, wild boar meat, homemade and commercial sausage, bear, walrus and other wild animal meats.
• Enteric phase, phase I: Cysts are broken down by digestive acid and pepsin in the stomach freeing larvae which develop into mature adult worms in the upper to middle small intestine, taking about one week after ingestion and may last 3 to 5 weeks
• Systemic phase, phase II: Female worms then release newborn larvae that migrate through blood vessels and lymphatics to multiple organ systems, occurring 2 to 3 weeks after ingestion and may last for 2 months
• Muscular encystment phase, phase III: Larvae become encysted in striated skeletal and sometimes cardiac muscle and can remain viable for years
System(s) affected: Gastrointestinal, and Musculoskeletal
Genetics: N/A
Incidence/Prevalence in USA: 50 to 100 cases are reported annually in the United States, but most mild cases probably are undiagnosed, based on autopsy studies.
Predominant age: Cases have been reported from all age groups. It occurs most frequently in ages 20-49.
Predominant sex: Male = Female

SIGNS AND SYMPTOMS
Signs and symptoms begin within one week of ingesting infected meat.
• Common symptoms:
  ◊ Diarrhea (mostly phase I)
  ◊ Abdominal Cramping (mostly phase I)
  ◊ Fever (mostly phase II and III)
  ◊ Myalgias (mostly phase II and III)
  ◊ Eosinophilia (mostly phase II and III)
  ◊ Periorbital edema (mostly phase II and III)
  ◊ Weakness (mostly phase II and III
• Clinical symptoms depend on the number of ingested infective larvae, and the phase of the parasitic invasion. Most light infections with <10 larvae per gram of muscle are asymptomatic. Skeletal muscle is the most frequent site of symptoms due to larval migration, however in severe cases there can be myocardial damage, pulmonary infiltration and focal neurologic damage. Most common muscles involved include the gastrocnemius, masseter, diaphragm, biceps, lower back, extraocular muscles, jaw and neck. Heavy infections with > 50 larvae per gram of muscle can be life threatening. Symptoms from the various phases can occur concurrently.

• Less common symptoms (mostly phase II and III):
  ◊ Conjunctivitis
  ◊ Subconjunctival hemorrhage
  ◊ Retinal hemorrhages
  ◊ Maculopapular rash
  ◊ Splinter hemorrhages
  ◊ Headache
  ◊ Photophobia
  ◊ Pneumonitis
  ◊ Tachycardia
  ◊ Heart failure

CAUSES
Eating undercooked meat that is infected with viable Trichinella cysts.

RISK FACTORS
• Access to wild game, homemade pork products, noncommercial sources of meat
• Eating pigs that were fed uncooked garbage
• Under cooking pork
• Eating wild game inadequately cooked or frozen
• Ethnic groups from Southeast Asia raising their own pork or favoring partially cooked pork products.
• Higher incidence in Alaska and northeastern United States.

DIAGNOSIS

DIFFERENTIAL DIAGNOSIS
• Acute rheumatic fever
• Arthritis, angioedema
• Botulism
• Collagen vascular disease
• Dermatomyositis
• Encephalitis
• Eosinophilia-myalgia syndrome
• Gastroenteritis
• Idiopathic hypereosinophilic syndrome
• Idiopathic polymyositis
• Influenza
• Meningitis
• Pneumonitis
• Polyarteritis nodosa
• Polymyositis
• Typhoid fever
• Tuberculosis

LABORATORY
• Eosinophilia (>600/cubic millimeter), with leukocytosis
• Increased creatine phosphate kinase (CPK)
• Increased lactate dehydrogenase (LDH)
• Hypergammaglobulinemia
• Elevated erythrocyte sedimentation rate (several weeks)
Drugs that may alter lab results: Rare increases in SGOT with thiabendazole
Disorders that may alter lab results: N/A

PATHOLOGICAL FINDINGS
Larvae on muscle biopsy (often gastrocnemius), however absence of larvae does not exclude diagnosis. Rarely find worm in stool.

SPECIAL TESTS
• Serologic tests for T. spiralis, IgM and IgG
• ELISA (enzyme linked immunosorbent assay) IgM and IgG
• Bentonite flocculation after 3rd week for parasite specific antibody
• Indirect immunoflourescence
• Complement fixation
• DNA testing [RAPD (random amplified polymorphic DNA), PCR (polymerase chain reaction)]

IMAGING
• CT may help see calcified muscle cysts
• MRI may help in evaluation of neurologic complications
• Chest x-ray may detect patchy infiltrates

DIAGNOSTIC PROCEDURES
Muscle biopsy of gastrocnemius or deltoid with at least 1 gram of muscle, including examination between compressed slides (higher detection rate)

TREATMENT

APPROPRIATE HEALTH CARE
• Outpatient unless complications such as cardiac, pulmonary, or neurological
• May call CDC for appropriate diagnostic tests (404-639-3311).

GENERAL MEASURES
Bedrest, antipyretics and analgesics.

SURGICAL MEASURES
Pacemaker has been required on occasion for severe myocarditis

ACTIVITY
As tolerated. Bedrest may help muscular pain.

DIET
As tolerated

PATIENT EDUCATION
• Manage complications as appropriate
• Measures at prevention
• Cook potentially contaminated meat such as pork to 170°F (77°C), no longer pink
• Freeze at -15°C for 21 days (longer if meat is >15 cm thick), however Trichinella larvae in wild game may be resistant to freezing
• Do not feed hogs uncooked garbage

Trichinosis

MEDICATIONS

DRUG(S) OF CHOICE
- For early intestinal phase (presenting in 1st 1 to 2 weeks), to treat adult worms:
  - ◊ Albendazole 400 mg bid x 15 days
  - ◊ Mebendazole may be used 200-400 mg tid x 3 days, then 400-500 mg tid for 10 days
- No drugs are very effective against larvae once encysted in muscle, however they may halt further dissemination
- Call CDC for current dosage and recommendation (404)639-3311
- Corticosteroids such as prednisone 40 to 60 mg/day for 3-5 days and then tapered as symptoms subside may be helpful in severe cases, particularly to help decrease inflammation when signs of myocarditis, neurologic disease, pulmonary insufficiency, or severe myositis

Contraindications: Corticosteroids have been reported to be contraindicated in the intestinal phase, as they could prolong this phase

Precautions: Minimal experience exists with the use of medications in small children and in pregnancy. Mebendazole should not be given in the first trimester, and any medications should only be used if felt absolutely necessary.

Significant possible interactions: Carbamazepine or alcohol may decrease the effect of mebendazole. Cimetidine may increase the level of mebendazole.

ALTERNATIVE DRUGS
Thiabendazole, which used to be the drug of choice at 25 mg/kg bid x 1 week, maximum dose 1.5 gm, has been replaced by the above drugs because they have fewer side effects, and are equally effective.

FOLLOWUP

PATIENT MONITORING
Monitor for signs and symptoms of complications such as cardiac, neurological and pulmonary

PREVENTION/AVOIDANCE
Avoid eating undercooked pork and game meat. Prolonged freezing may also be effective, but less so for wild game meat.

POSSIBLE COMPLICATIONS
- Meningitis
- Subcortical infarcts
- Encephalitis
- Myocarditis with congestive heart failure
- Nephritis
- Glomerulonephritis
- Sinusitis
- Pneumonitis

EXPECTED COURSE/PROGNOSIS
Most infections are asymptomatic, short-lived and generally have uneventful recovery without medication. Prognosis is good in most cases, although 5-10% of cases can be severe. There is no clear evidence that chronic trichinosis exists. Less than 1% of cases can be fatal, generally around the 4th-8th week, and a result of cardiac failure or pneumonia.

MISCELLANEOUS

ASSOCIATED CONDITIONS N/A

AGE-RELATED FACTORS
Pediatric: N/A
Geriatric: N/A
Others: N/A

PREGNANCY Although not much information, there is one case of a woman 16 weeks pregnant who delivered a normal child without complications or evidence of problems

SYNONYMS
Trichinellosis
Trichinelliasis

ICD-9-CM 124 Trichinosis

SEE ALSO N/A

OTHER NOTES N/A

ABBREVIATIONS N/A

REFERENCES
- Bailey T, Schantz P: Trends in the Incidence and Transmission Patterns of Trichinosis in Humans in the United States: Comparisons of the Periods 1975-1981 and 1982-1986. Reviews of Infectious Diseases 1990;12(1):5-11
- Clausen MR, et al: Trichinella infection and clinical disease. QJ Med 1996;89(8)631-636
- McAuley JB et al: Trichinosis surveillance, United States, 1987-1990. Morbidity and Mortality Weekly Report CDC Surveillance Summary 1992;40:35-42
- Stack PS: Trichinosis, Still a public health threat. Postgraduate Medicine 1995;97(6):137-139/143-144

Illustrations: N/A
Internet references: http://www.5mcc.com

Author(s)
Kenton Voorhees, MD

Trichomoniasis

BASICS

DESCRIPTION Trichomonas is a protozoan parasite found in men and women at genitourinary sites
System(s) affected: Reproductive, Renal/Urologic
Genetics: N/A
Incidence/Prevalence in USA:
• 300/100,000 women/year for first time diagnosis of trichomoniasis; 600/100,000 women/year for any diagnosis for trichomoniasis
• In sexually active adult women: 2,000/100,000 in a family planning clinic; 35,000/100,000 in a STD clinic
Predominant age:
• Young and middle aged adults
• Rare until onset of sexual activity
• Not uncommon in postmenopausal women
Predominant sex: Both affected, but women more commonly symptomatic

SIGNS AND SYMPTOMS
• Female
  ◊ 40% can be asymptomatic at time of diagnosis
  ◊ Symptoms typically begin or worsen at time of menstrual period
  ◊ Vaginal discharge (75%, usually copious and pooling, can be frothy)
  ◊ Vulvovaginal irritation (50%)
  ◊ Dysuria (50%)
  ◊ Vaginal odor (10%)
  ◊ A "strawberry cervix" from punctate hemorrhages (5% of cases)
  ◊ Vaginal hyperemia
  ◊ Dyspareunia
  ◊ Suprapubic discomfort
  ◊ Cervical erosion
• Male
  ◊ Many are asymptomatic
  ◊ Urethral discharge (50%)
  ◊ Dysuria
  ◊ Epididymitis (rare)

CAUSES
• Trichomonas vaginalis is a pear shaped protozoan which is a facultative anaerobe. It is usually sexually transmitted although a non-venereal route is possible as the organism survives for several hours in a moist environment.
• Transmission is rarely seen in female children of infected women
• Incubation period is 3-28 days

RISK FACTORS Multiple sexual partners

DIAGNOSIS

DIFFERENTIAL DIAGNOSIS
• Female - vaginal candidiasis, bacterial vaginosis. Cervical inflammation can lead to the mistaken diagnosis of cervicitis.
• Male - chlamydia urethritis

LABORATORY
• Female
  ◊ Wet prep is 60-70% sensitive and highly specific. Sensitivity is reduced with loss of motility due to cooling, low inoculum size and rapid scanning of the slide. Specificity is about 100%.
  ◊ Vaginal pH is > 4.5 in 90% of women
  ◊ Wet prep usually shows many more PMN's than epithelial cells
• Male
  ◊ A wet prep and culture of urethral discharge after prostatic exam is 50-80% sensitive
Drugs that may alter lab results: N/A
Disorders that may alter lab results: N/A

PATHOLOGICAL FINDINGS N/A

SPECIAL TESTS
• Culture has a sensitivity of greater than 95% but takes 4-7 days
• ELISA and direct fluorescent antibody tests are available and are 80-90% sensitive
• Pap smear has a 60% sensitivity and 99% specificity

IMAGING N/A

DIAGNOSTIC PROCEDURES N/A

TREATMENT

APPROPRIATE HEALTH CARE
Outpatient

GENERAL MEASURES Education about
the venereal aspect of the infection

SURGICAL MEASURES N/A

ACTIVITY Sexual activity should not be
resumed until patient and partner are both treated

DIET Should abstain from alcohol if
metronidazole used for therapy

PATIENT EDUCATION
• Vaginitis, Questions and Answers Planned Parenthood Federation of America, Inc., (212)541-7800
• Roses Have Thorns, RAJ Publications, P.O. Box 150720, Lakewood, CO 80215
• American College of Obstetricians & Gynecologists (ACOG), 409 12th St., SW, Washington, DC 20024-2188, (800)762-ACOG

Trichomoniasis

MEDICATIONS

DRUG(S) OF CHOICE
• Metronidazole: adult dose 2 grams at one time, or 250 mg tid for 7 days, or 500 mg bid for 7 days. The routines are effective in women but the one time dose has a higher failure rate in men. All sexual partners need treatment.
Contraindications: First trimester pregnancy or allergy to the antibiotic
Precautions: Avoid metronidazole or reduce the dosage in patients with liver failure
Significant possible interactions: Ethanol, warfarin, disulfiram, phenobarbital

ALTERNATIVE DRUGS
• Clotrimazole: 100 mg vaginal tablets qhs for 14 days. Cure rate is 20-25% but symptoms will be reduced in most women.
• Alternatively, saline or vinegar douching can be tried

FOLLOWUP

PATIENT MONITORING Monitor target symptoms. No followup is needed if symptoms resolve with treatment.

PREVENTION/AVOIDANCE Practice safe sex by using condoms

POSSIBLE COMPLICATIONS Recurrent infections

EXPECTED COURSE/PROGNOSIS
Prognosis is good but recurrent infection raises possibility of non-compliance with therapy, re-infection, or infection with a resistant organism. If resistance is suspected, try metronidazole 500 mg tid for 7 days along with vaginal 0.75% metronidazole gel.

MISCELLANEOUS

ASSOCIATED CONDITIONS Other sexually transmitted diseases

AGE-RELATED FACTORS
Pediatric: Very uncommon in prepuberty (confirmed diagnosis should raise concern of sexual abuse)
Geriatric: Older people remain at risk for Trichomonas
Others: N/A

PREGNANCY Do not use metronidazole in the first trimester

SYNONYMS
• Trick
• Trichomonal urethritis

ICD-9-CM
• 131.9 Trichomoniasis, unspecified
• 131.01 Vulva or vagina
• 131.00 Urogenitalis

SEE ALSO Vulvovaginitis, bacterial

OTHER NOTES N/A

ABBREVIATIONS N/A

REFERENCES
• Lossick JG, Kent H: Trichomoniasis: trends in diagnosis and management. Am J Obstet & Gyno 1991165;1217-22
• Krieger JN: Clinical manifestations of trichomoniasis in men. Ann Int Med 1993;118:844-849
• CDC: 1993 Sexually transmitted disease treatment guidelines. MMWR 1993;42:RR-14
• Heine P, McGregor JA: Trichmonas vaginalis: A reemerging pathogen. Clin OB Gyn 1993;36:137-142
• Schweke JR: Metronidazole utilization in the obstetric gynecologic patient. Sex Trans Dis 1995;22:370-376
Illustrations: N/A
Internet references: http://www.5mcc.com

Author(s)
George R. Bergus, MD

Trigeminal neuralgia

 BASICS

DESCRIPTION A disorder of the sensory nucleus of the 5th cranial nerve (trigeminal nerve), producing episodic, severe lancinating pain in the distribution of one or more of its divisions. Often precipitated by stimulation of well-defined, ipsilateral trigger paths, usually perioral, perinasal, occasionally intraoral.
System(s) affected: Nervous
Genetics: N/A
Incidence/Prevalence in USA:
16/100,000
Predominant age: Over age 50, peak age 60
Predominant sex: Male > Female (1.6:1)

SIGNS AND SYMPTOMS
• Unilateral (< 4% bilateral), symptoms rarely present at night
• Excruciating lip pain
• Excruciating gum pain
• Excruciating cheek pain
• Paroxysmal facial pain
• Wincing
• Pain elicited by tickle or touch
• Flushing
• Lacrimation
• Salivation
• Pain "bursts" several seconds with refractory period after
• Right > left side preference
• 2nd and/or 3rd division trigeminal nerve most commonly affected

CAUSES
• When present, most commonly compression of the trigeminal nerve by arteries or veins of the posterior fossa, usually the superior cerebral artery compressing the trigeminal root.
• Etiology classification
◊ Idiopathic
◊ Secondary - disseminated sclerosis; cerebellopontine angle tumors, e.g., meningioma; tumors of the 5th nerve, e.g., neuroma, vascular malformations

RISK FACTORS Unknown

 DIAGNOSIS

DIFFERENTIAL DIAGNOSIS
• Other forms of neuralgia usually have sensory loss. The presence of sensory loss nearly excludes the diagnosis of trigeminal neuralgia.
• Neoplasia in the cerebellopontine angle
• Vascular malformation of the brain stem
• Demyelinating lesion
• Vascular insult
• Migraine
• Chronic meningitis
• Acute polyneuropathy

LABORATORY N/A
Drugs that may alter lab results: N/A
Disorders that may alter lab results: N/A

PATHOLOGICAL FINDINGS
• Semilunar ganglion - inflammatory changes
• Degenerative changes

SPECIAL TESTS N/A

IMAGING N/A

DIAGNOSTIC PROCEDURES MRI or CT scan - neoplasm in cerebellopontine angle must be ruled out

 TREATMENT

APPROPRIATE HEALTH CARE
Outpatient

GENERAL MEASURES
• Drug treatment is first approach. Invasive procedures for patients who cannot tolerate, or fail to respond to, drug treatment.
• Alcohol, glycerol or radio-frequency gangliolysis
• Avoidance of stimulation (air, heat, cold) of trigger zones (lips, cheeks, gums)

SURGICAL MEASURES
• Microvascular decompression of the 5th cranial nerve at its entrance to (or exit from) the brainstem (73% relief)
• Partial sensory rhizotomy
• Peripheral block or section of 5th nerve proximal to the Gasserian ganglion
• Peripheral nerve ablation
◊ Alcohol block
◊ Neurectomy
◊ Cryotherapy
◊ Radiofrequency thermocoagulation

ACTIVITY Full activity

DIET No special diet

PATIENT EDUCATION Instruct regarding medication dosage and side effects

MEDICATIONS

DRUG(S) OF CHOICE Carbamazepine (Tegretol) 100-1200 mg/day (maximum)
Contraindications: MAO inhibitors taken concurrently
Precautions: Use with caution in presence of liver disease
Significant possible interactions: Macrolide antibiotics with Carbamazepine. Oral anticoagulants, anticonvulsants, tricyclics, oral contraceptives, steroids, digitalis, INH, MAO inhibitors, methyprylon nabilone, nizatidine, other H2 blockers, phenytoin, propoxyphene, benzodiazepines, calcium, channel blockers.

ALTERNATIVE DRUGS
• Phenytoin (Dilantin) 400 mg/day (synergistic with carbamazepine)
• Baclofen (Atrofen, Lioresal) 10-80 mg/day; start at 5-10 mg tid with food (as adjunct to phenytoin or carbamazepine)
• Clonazepam (Klonopin): frequently causes drowsiness and ataxia
• Valproic acid (Depakene) or divalproex (Depakote)

FOLLOWUP

PATIENT MONITORING
• Carbamazepine and/or phenytoin serum levels
• Liver and hematopoietic functions if carbamazepine is prescribed
• CBC as needed

PREVENTION/AVOIDANCE Reduce drugs after 4-6 weeks to determine if condition is in remission, resume at previous dose if pain recurs. Withdraw drugs slowly after several months again to check for remission or if lower dose of drugs can be tolerated.

POSSIBLE COMPLICATIONS Mental and physical sluggishness, dizziness with carbamazepine

EXPECTED COURSE/PROGNOSIS
Exacerbations in fall and spring; otherwise good

MISCELLANEOUS

ASSOCIATED CONDITIONS
• Sjogren's syndrome
• Rheumatoid arthritis
• Chronic meningitis
• Facial migraine
• Acute polyneuropathy
• Multiple sclerosis
• Hemifacial spasm
• Pretrigeminal neuralgia

AGE-RELATED FACTORS
Pediatric: Unusual in childhood
Geriatric: N/A
Others: N/A

PREGNANCY N/A

SYNONYMS
• Tic douloureux
• Fothergill's neuralgia
• Trifacial neuralgia

ICD-9-CM
350.1 Trigeminal neuralgia

SEE ALSO
• Migraine
• Headache, cluster

OTHER NOTES N/A

ABBREVIATIONS N/A

REFERENCES
• Bell WE: Orofacial Pain. 4th Ed. Chicago, Year Book Medical Publishers, 1989
• Adams RD, Victor M: Principles of Neurology. 5th Ed. New York, McGraw-Hill, 1993
• Sweet WH: The treatment of trigeminal neuralgia (tic douloureux). New Engl J Med 1986;174-177
• Moller AR: The cranial nerve vascular compression syndrome: A review of treatment. Acta Neurochirurgica 1991;113:18-23
• Merrill R, Graff-Radford SB: Trigeminal neuralgia: How to rule out the wrong treatment. JADA 1992;123:63-68
• Smith LH Jr, Bennett C: Trigeminal neuralgia. In: Wyngaarden JB, ed. Cecil Textbook of Medicine. Philadelphia, W.B. Saunders Co., 1992
• Fields HL: Treatment of trigeminal neuralgia (editorial). NEJM 1996;334(17):1125-1126
Illustrations: N/A
Internet references: http://www.5mcc.com

Author(s)
Paul J. Jaster, MD

Tropical sprue

 BASICS

DESCRIPTION Malabsorption syndrome of unknown etiology that occurs primarily in the tropics and subtropics. Characteristics include protein malnutrition and folic acid anemia. Usual course - relapsing without treatment. Symptoms may appear years after leaving an endemic area.
• Endemic areas - tropical regions only, Far East, India, Caribbean and the Middle East. Distribution is sporadic.
• The presence of normal jejunal biopsy nearly excludes this diagnosis
System(s) affected: Gastrointestinal, Hemic/Lymphatic/Immunologic
Genetics: N/A
Incidence/Prevalence in USA: Unknown
Predominant age: None
Predominant sex: Male = Female

SIGNS AND SYMPTOMS
• Fatigue
• Asthenia
• Weight loss, pallor
• Diarrhea
• Abdominal cramps
• Borborygmus
• Night blindness
• Stomatitis
• Glossitis
• Cheilosis
• Anorexia
• Steatorrhea
• Hyperkeratosis
• Edema
• Abdominal distension
• Hyperpigmentation
• Koilonychia

CAUSES
• Unknown
• Possible dietary deficiency
• Possible infectious agent
• Vitamin deficiency (folate), B12
• Food toxins (rancid fats)
• Toxigenic strains of coliform bacteria

RISK FACTORS Parasitic infestation

 DIAGNOSIS

DIFFERENTIAL DIAGNOSIS
• Other causes of megaloblastic anemia
• Other malabsorption syndromes
• Celiac disease
• Inflammatory bowel disease
• Giardiasis
• Strongylosis
• Other infectious causes:
  ◊ Coccidial isospora
  ◊ Capillaria philippinensis
  ◊ Cryptosporidium

LABORATORY
• Megaloblastic anemia in 60% of cases
• Steatorrhea
• Decreased D-xylose
• Decreased serum iron
• Decreased calcium
• Decreased folic acid
• Decreased serum vitamin B12
• Decreased serum carotene
• Decreased cholesterol, albumin
• Deficiency of magnesium
• Deficiency of alpha-tocopherol
Drugs that may alter lab results: N/A
Disorders that may alter lab results: N/A

PATHOLOGICAL FINDINGS Jejunal biopsy - mild villous atrophy, increased villous crypts, mononuclear cell infiltration

SPECIAL TESTS Serum vitamin B12

IMAGING
• Mild jejunal dilatation
• Jejunal fold coarsening
• Flocculation and segmentation of Barium meal

DIAGNOSTIC PROCEDURES
• Jejunal biopsy - not specific
• Malabsorption of at least two nutrients is considered essential for diagnosis
• D- Xylose, fat and radiolabeled vitamin B12 are used to test for absorptive capacity
• Stool microscopy
• Imaging - not specific

 TREATMENT

APPROPRIATE HEALTH CARE
Outpatient

GENERAL MEASURES
• Replace deficiencies, such as vitamin B12 and folic acid
• Control of diarrhea
• Fluid and blood replacement

SURGICAL MEASURES N/A

ACTIVITY No restrictions

DIET No special diet (gluten-free diets do not improve this disease)

PATIENT EDUCATION Written patient information available from:
National Digestive Diseases Information Clearinghouse
Box NDDIC
Bethesda, MD 20892
(301)654-3810

MEDICATIONS

DRUG(S) OF CHOICE
• Vitamin B12 1000 mcg SC for several days, then monthly thereafter for 6 months
• Folic acid 5 mg po daily
• Tetracycline 250 mg qid for 1-2 months, then half doses for up to 6 months. Occasionally, longer course is required.
• Combination folic acid and B12 plus tetracycline or sulfonamide
Contraindications: Allergy to tetracycline or oxytetracycline
Precautions:
• Use with caution in patients with lupus, myasthenia gravis, kidney or liver disease
• Don't take with milk, antacids or iron preparations
• Don't use during pregnancy
• Don't use in children under age 8
Significant possible interactions:
• Antacids, anticoagulants, bismuth subsalicylate
• Oral contraceptives
• Lithium

ALTERNATIVE DRUGS
• Oxytetracycline
• Nonabsorbable sulfonamides

FOLLOWUP

PATIENT MONITORING   As needed for symptoms

PREVENTION/AVOIDANCE   N/A

POSSIBLE COMPLICATIONS
• Malabsorption
• Relapse if medication regimen is stopped too soon

EXPECTED COURSE/PROGNOSIS
• Good with appropriate treatment
• Recurrences can happen in native residents treated in the tropics

MISCELLANEOUS

ASSOCIATED CONDITIONS   N/A

AGE-RELATED FACTORS
Pediatric: Don't treat with tetracycline
Geriatric: N/A
Others: N/A

PREGNANCY   Don't treat with tetracycline during pregnancy

SYNONYMS   N/A

ICD-9-CM   579.1

SEE ALSO
• Whipple's disease
• Diarrhea, chronic
• Celiac disease
• Anemia, pernicious

OTHER NOTES   N/A

ABBREVIATIONS   N/A

REFERENCES
• Sleisenger MH, Fordtran JS, eds: Gastrointestinal Disease: Pathophysiology, Diagnosis, Management. 5th Ed. Philadelphia, W.B. Saunders Co., 1994
• Mandell GL, ed: Principles and Practice of Infectious Diseases. 4th Ed. New York, Churchill Livingstone, 1995
Illustrations: N/A
Internet references: http://www.5mcc.com

Author(s)
Abdulrazak Abyad, MD, MPH, AGSF

Tuberculosis

BASICS

DESCRIPTION A common disease transmitted by inhaling airborne bacilli from a person with active tuberculosis (TB). The bacilli multiply in the aveolus and are carried by macrophages, lymphatics and blood to distant sites (eg., lung pleura, brain, kidney and bone). Tissue hypersensitivity usually halts infection within 10 weeks.
• Infected persons are those whose immunity has controlled the organism, they usually have a positive tuberculin skin test, but are asymptomatic and are not infectious
• TB refers to active disease which occurs in 10% of infected individuals without preventive therapy. Chance of disease increases with immunosuppression and is highest for all individuals within 2 years after infection - 85% of cases are pulmonary which is infectious.
• Primary TB refers to disease resulting from the initial pulmonary infection which the immune system is unable to control
• Recrudescent TB is active disease occurring after a period of latent asymptomatic infection
• Miliary TB refers to disseminated disease
System(s) affected: Pulmonary, Hemic/Lymphatic/Immunologic, Renal/Urologic, Gastrointestinal, Nervous, Endocrine/Metabolic, Musculoskeletal
Genetics: N/A
Incidence/Prevalence in USA: Overall 9/100,0000, but varies greatly, may be 32-100/100,000
Predominant age:
• Primary infection - any age, especially pediatric
• Recrudescent disease - adults and elderly
Predominant Sex: Male > Female

SIGNS AND SYMPTOMS
• Cough
• Hemoptysis
• Fever and night sweats
• Weight loss
• Malaise
• Adenopathy
• Pleuritic chest pain
• Hepatosplenomegaly
• Renal, bone or CNS disease are late findings

CAUSES
Mycobacterium tuberculosis, Mycobacterium bovis, and Mycobacterium africanum

RISK FACTORS
• For infection: Urban, homeless, minority, migrant workers; institutional (eg, prison, nursing home); close contact with infected individual; foreign born (Asia, Africa, Latin America); healthcare workers
• For disease: HIV; recent infection; IV drug abuse; lymphoma; diabetes mellitus; dhronic renal failure; malnutrition; steroids, immunosuppressive drugs; silicosis

DIAGNOSIS

DIFFERENTIAL DIAGNOSIS
• Other pneumonias
• Lymphomas
• Fungal infections, especially other atypical Mycobacteria or Nocardia

LABORATORY
• Tine test: not recommended for screening
• PPD:
  ◊ 5 units intermediate strength, 0.1 cc volar forearm
  ◊ Intradermal induration at 48 to 72 hrs
  ◊ > 5 mm - positive if HIV infection (or suspected), immunosuppressed, exposed household contact, clinical evidence of disease
  ◊ > 10 mm - positive if other risk factor or < 4 years old
  ◊ > 15 mm - positive if older than 4 years and no risk factors
  ◊ Two step testing if: no recent PPD, age > 55 years, nursing home, prison or healthcare worker
• Nonspecific laboratory includes anemia, monocytosis, thrombocytosis, hypergammaglobulinemia, syndrome of inappropriate antidiuretic hormone (SIADH) and sterile pyuria
Drugs that may alter lab results:
• BCG: false-positive skin test
• Inactive vaccine or improper placement: false-negative skin test
• Steroids: false-negative skin test
Disorders that may alter lab results:
Recent viral infections, new infection, < 10 weeks, severe malnutrition, HIV, anergy, age < 6 months. overwhelming TB: false-negative skin test

PATHOLOGICAL FINDINGS
• Granulomatous process with foci of caseating necrosis surrounded by epithelioid histiocytes and giant cells, in turn surrounded by lymphocytes
• AFB stains positive

SPECIAL TESTS
• Persons with TB should be tested for HIV
• Lumbar puncture, if meningitis suspected
• Bone marrow and liver biopsy for culture
• Polymerase chain reaction (PCR) - rapid diagnosis of TB, costly, false positives occur, does not replace standard tests

IMAGING
• CxR with primary disease: may show infiltrate with or without effusion atelectasis or adenopathy
• With recrudescent TB - cavitary lesions and upper lobe disease with hilar adenopathy common. Diffuse miliary pattern possible with appearance of "millet seeds."
• HIV - atypical findings with primary infection - right upper lobe atelectasis
• CxR useful to rule out TB in asymptomatic infected persons
• CT chest - good sensitivity

DIAGNOSTIC PROCEDURES
• AFB stain of infected specimens gives a presumptive diagnosis
• Culture confirms diagnosis, but takes 4-6 weeks on solid medium - can grow in 2 weeks on Bactec broth system
• For suspected pulmonary TB, obtain at least 3 morning sputum samples for AFB stain and culture - use aerosol induction, gastric aspirate (children) or bronchoalveolar lavage if needed
• Other specimens: bone marrow, urine, tissue, CSF, peritoneal/pleural fluids
• Culture and sensitivity guide treatment

TREATMENT

APPROPRIATE HEALTH CARE
• Prophylaxis for positive PPD at any age if: HIV, close contact, recent converter (< 2 years), IV drug use, abnormal CxR, high risk medical condition or if age < 35 in other high risk group
• Use INH (or rifampin if resistant) in usual daily dose for minimum 6 months, 12 months if HIV. Consider twice a week DOT if adherence not assured.
• For active disease, use minimum of 3 drugs for 2 months, then 2 drugs to complete 6 months - start with 4 drugs if resistance possible. Several regimen options available using DOT.
• If HIV infected, treat at least 6 months after culture negative

GENERAL MEASURES
Careful reevaluation required. Only change to twice weekly dosing if using DOT.

SURGICAL MEASURES
Indicated for extra pulmonary complications (spinal cord compression, constrictive pericarditis)

ACTIVITY
• As tolerated - respiratory isolation for infectious pulmonary TB
• Children without cough and negative sputum smears: no isolation required after treatment started

DIET
Regular. Consider pyridoxine (10-50 mg/day) supplement.

PATIENT EDUCATION
• Teach pathogenesis, emphasize importance of medical drug therapy, warn of effects and/or interactions, find contacts
• Inform local health department

MEDICATIONS

DRUG(S) OF CHOICE
• Isoniazid (INH) - scored tabs 100 mg, 300 mg or syrup 10 mg/mL
◊ Daily dose - adult 300 mg; pediatric 10-15 mg/kg (maximum 300 mg)
◊ Twice weekly - adult 15 mg/kg; pediatric 20-30 mg/kg (maximum 900 mg)
◊ Consider pyridoxine
• Rifampin (RIF) capsules (150/300 or syrup 10 mg/mL)
◊ Daily dose - adult 600 mg; pediatric dose 10-20 mg/kg (maximum 600 mg)
◊ Twice weekly - adult 600 mg; pediatric 10-20 mg/kg (maximum 600 mg)
• Pyrazinamide (PZA), scored 500 mg
◊ Daily dose - adult 20-35 mg/kg (maximum 1-3 gm); pediatric 20-40 mg/kg (maximum 2 gm)
◊ Twice weekly - adult 50-70 mg/kg; pediatric 50 mg/kg (maximum 4 gm)
• Streptomycin (SM) IM only, vials 1,4 gm
◊ Daily dose - 20-40 mg/kg (maximum 1 gm); pediatric 20-40 mg/kg (maximum 1 gm)
◊ Twice weekly - 25 mg/kg; pediatric 20-40 mg/kg (maximum 1.5 gm)
• Ethambutol (EMB) - tablets 100/400 mg bacteriostatic
◊ Daily dose 15-25 mg/kg, with maximum of 2.5 gm a week or twice weekly dose 50 mg/kg, with maximum of 2.5 gm

Contraindications:
• Streptomycin: avoid use longer than 12 weeks secondary to ototoxicity
• Ethambutol: because of optic neuritis, never use ethambutol unless patient old enough to cooperate for visual acuity and color testing.

Precautions:
• INH, RIF or PZA may cause hepatitis
• Follow liver function if the patient has history of liver dysfunction or develops new signs of liver disorder
• RIF - colors urine, tears and secretions orange. Can permanently stain contact lenses.
• INH - peripheral neuritis and hypersensitivity possible. Consider pyridoxine.
• PZA - may increase uric acid
• EMB - may cause optic neuritis; follow monthly vision and color tests
• SM - ototoxicity and nephrotoxic

Significant possible interactions: RIF alters the level of Dilantin and other drugs metabolized by the liver and may inactivate birth control pills (recommend a barrier method)

ALTERNATIVE DRUGS
• Steroids - use only with concurrent anti-TB therapy. Consider for meningitis, effusions, severe miliary disease or endobronchial disease.
• Other antituberculous drugs may be useful for multidrug resistant TB (MDRTB)
• Combination tablets to enhance adherence

FOLLOWUP

PATIENT MONITORING
• Every 2-3 months during treatment
• Follow chest x-ray at 2-3 month intervals and again if symptoms change
• During preventive therapy - monthly visits to assess adherence to regimen and monitor for hepatitis and neuropathy
• If age > 35, check liver enzymes, modify drugs if needed
• If culture positive after 2 months of therapy, reassess drug sensitivity and initiate DOT
• CxR at 3 months and at completion of therapy

PREVENTION/AVOIDANCE
• PPD screening
• Identify and treat contagious persons. Notify public health department and hospital infection control if admitted
• Inpatient - use personal sealed respirators, negative pressure ventilation, ultraviolet
• Ambulatory patients use mask and tissues
• Not infectious if: favorable clinical response after 2-3 weeks of therapy and 3 AFB smears are negative.

POSSIBLE COMPLICATIONS
• Cavitary lesions can be secondarily infected
• Spread to susceptible persons of all ages
• Drug resistance - suspect if immigrant, drug resistant source or noncompliant

EXPECTED COURSE/PROGNOSIS
Generally few complications and full resolution if drugs taken for full course as prescribed

MISCELLANEOUS

ASSOCIATED CONDITIONS HIV infection

AGE-RELATED FACTORS
Pediatric:
• Caution with ethambutol
• Children on medication may attend school
• Disseminated TB more common in infants; prompt treatment with 4 drugs if TB suspected
• Congenital infection may occur with miliary TB of maternal bacillemia, endometritis or amniotic aspiration. If suspected, get PPD, CxR, LP, culture placenta and infant, then start treatment promptly
• Protocol for newborn with mother/household member with infection or disease
◊ Member with positive PPD, but no disease: no special evaluation or treatment. Skin test all household members; prophylaxis if infected.
◊ Member has abnormal CxR: separate infant until infectious status known; if not contagious, monitor infant PPD
◊ Member with disease and possibly contagious: evaluate infant for congenital TB and test for HIV; separate newborn until member is noninfectious

◊ If congenital TB suspected, treat as above
◊ If no congenital disease, INH for 3-4 months, then repeat PPD: if positive, reassess for infant disease. If negative, finish 6 months INH. If repeat PPD negative and source not infectious, stop INH and monitor infant.
• Consider BCG
Geriatric:
• Symptoms may be more subtle and may be attributed to associated conditions or to aging
• Should have a PPD prior to entering a chronic-care facility using two step protocol
• Side effects of INH more pronounced
Others: N/A

PREGNANCY
• Treat pregnant woman with INH, rifampin (and ethambutol, if resistance suspected); add pyridoxine
• Avoid streptomycin and pyrazinamide
• Prophylaxis - postpone INH until delivery unless recent contact
• Breast feeding okay while taking TB drugs

SYNONYMS
• Consumption

ICD-9-CM
011.9 Pulmonary tuberculosis, unspecified

SEE ALSO N/A

OTHER NOTES
• BCG vaccine, live attenuated Mycobacterium bovis
◊ 50% efficacy for pediatric pulmonary TB
◊ In USA, consider BCG for children with negative PPD and HIV tests with unavoidable high risk and for health care workers at high risk for drug resistant infection
◊ Abscess, ulceration and regional lymphadenitis occur in 1-2%, osteitis and fatal infection can occur in immunosuppressed
◊ Used more commonly in developed countries to prevent complications of TB

ABBREVIATIONS
PPD = purified protein derivative
BCG = Bacillus Calmette-Guérin
DOT = directly observed treatment

REFERENCES
• Centers for Disease Control; Screening for tuberculosis and tuberculosis infection in high risk populations. MMWR, 39:1-12, 1990
• American Thoracic Society: Treatment of tuberculosis and tuberculosis infections in adults and children. AmJ Respir Crit Care Med 1994;149:1359-1374
• Report of the Committee on Infectious Diseases (Red Book). Elk Grove Village, Ill, American Academy of Pediatrics, 1997
• Centers for Disease Control: Core curriculum on tuberculosis-what the clinician should know, 1994
• Dutt AK: Tuberculosis. Part 1 and 2. Disease-A-Month 1997;43(3 & 4)
Illustrations: N/A
Internet references: http://www.5mcc.com

Author(s)
Gregory Snyder, MD

Tuberous sclerosis complex

BASICS

DESCRIPTION One of the neurocutaneous syndromes (phakomatoses). A genetic, developmental disorder with variable presentations, a broad clinical spectrum and multi-organ involvement. Organ systems may be few and subtle but can encompass multiple types of cutaneous lesions and tumor formation in the central nervous system and one or more areas including the skin, brain, retina, heart, lung, viscera, liver, kidney, bone, teeth, and nails. Other phakomatoses include neurofibromatosis, Sturge-Weber disease, von Hippel-Lindau syndrome and ataxia telangiectasia.
System(s) affected: Skin/Exocrine, Nervous, Cardiovascular, Pulmonary, Renal/Urologic, Musculoskeletal
Genetics:
• Inherited as an autosomal dominant trait with variable penetrance
• High rate of spontaneous mutation
• Two-thirds of cases sporadic and one-third familial
• Two chromosomal regions identified
Incidence/prevalence in USA:
• Reported to affect 1 in 9400 subjects in the population
• A detailed study in Olmsted County, Minnesota, reported the point prevalence on December 31, 1989, to be 6.9 per 100,000 persons, and the incidence at birth 6.0 per 100,000 live births
Predominant age: Clinical expression varies so that recognition and diagnosis may be delayed to well after birth
Predominant sex:
• If a parent has the gene, there is a 50- 50 chance that each child will have the gene
• Equal sex ratio among probands, but male probands with autism more than female

SIGNS AND SYMPTOMS
Most cases of tuberous sclerosis complex have more than one feature of the disorder
• Angiofibromata (labeled as adenoma sebaceum) ranging from 0.1-1.0 cm characteristic and often present as facial lesions in a "butterfly" distribution
• Hypopigmented areas mainly on trunk and extremities often the first sign (ash-leaf spots)
• Infantile spasms
• Seizure disorders (all types)
• Renal cysts
• Pulmonary lymphangiomatosis
• Multiple periventricular calcifications
• Retinal astrocytomas/hamartomas
• Cardiac rhabdomyomas associated with a variety of nonspecific clinical signs
• Mental retardation
• Autism
• Ungual fibromas, multiple
• Dental pits
• Liver hamartomas

CAUSES An inherited autosomal dominant genetic disorder

RISK FACTORS Family history

DIAGNOSIS

DIFFERENTIAL DIAGNOSIS
• Clinical diagnostic criteria are being periodically reviewed and updated
• Polycystic kidney disease
• Other causes for seizure disorders, mental retardation, autistic behavior, traumatic ungual fibromata
• Other neurocutaneous syndromes (see above)

LABORATORY
• Present day diagnostic criteria mainly confined to clinical evaluations
• Abnormal electroencephalogram
• Search for reliable molecular marker and gene appears fruitful
Drugs that may alter lab results: N/A
Disorders that may alter lab results: N/A

PATHOLOGICAL FINDINGS
• Nodular lesions made up largely of irregular groups of glial fibrils, ganglion cells and atypical cells seeming to result from faults in developing tissue combinations as in hamartomas
• Lesions may be sparse at birth
• Calcification of subependymal lesions may not occur until several months after birth
• Facial angiofibromas, ungual fibromas, renal angiomyolipomas are quite specific lesions which may develop months after birth
• 1% present with tuberous sclerosis and lymphangioleiomyomatosis and are almost always women of reproductive age
• Not practical to have age specific criteria. Periodic reassessment in at-risk families necessary.

SPECIAL TESTS
Must rely on clinical diagnostic criteria pending development of reliable molecular marker

IMAGING
• Magnetic resonance imaging (MRI) has become a major diagnostic technique
• With gadolinium enhancement, MRI provides more detailed imaging of characteristic subependymal nodules and cortical white matter tubers

DIAGNOSTIC PROCEDURES
• Biopsy and pathological evaluation often of highest importance. May not be necessary if lesions clinically obvious.
• Hypopigmented spots more clearly seen under ultraviolet light (Wood's lamp)

TREATMENT

APPROPRIATE HEALTH CARE
• Outpatient except for more severely involved cases and uncontrollable seizures

GENERAL MEASURES
• Team approach with neurological, orthopedic, dermatological, surgical and radiological involvement
• Physical, occupational and speech therapy
• Social worker, home care, support and genetic counseling important

SURGICAL MEASURES
Surgical excision of tumors where and when appropriate

ACTIVITY
Determined by degree and complexity of involvement

DIET
Balanced nutrition. A ketogenic diet has been used for seizure control.

PATIENT EDUCATION
• Swim alert for seizure prone children
• Seizure frequency changes with fever
• Updated information available from: National Tuberous Sclerosis Association, Inc., 8000 Corporate Drive, Suite 120, Landover, MD 20785

MEDICATIONS

DRUG(S) OF CHOICE
• Anticonvulsants to control seizures
• Surgeons choice of antibiotic prophylaxis if indicated
Contraindications: N/A
Precautions: See Patient Education
Significant possible interactions:
• Knowledge of anticonvulsant used is necessary to avoid drug interactions especially with antibiotics
• Refer to manufacturer's profile of each drug

ALTERNATIVE DRUGS   N/A

FOLLOWUP

PATIENT MONITORING
• Periodic reassessment of at-risk individuals very important in establishing clinical diagnosis
• Clinical features of patients periodically reviewed and updated

PREVENTION/AVOIDANCE   Genetic counseling

POSSIBLE COMPLICATIONS   See Signs and Symptoms

EXPECTED COURSE/PROGNOSIS
Variable. Decreased survival curves compared with general population.

MISCELLANEOUS

ASSOCIATED CONDITIONS   N/A

AGE-RELATED FACTORS
Pediatric: N/A
Geriatric: N/A
Others: Stigmata may be present at, or shortly after birth or may become apparent in late childhood or adulthood

PREGNANCY   Genetic counseling

SYNONYMS   Bourneville's disease

ICD-9-CM   759.5 Tuberous sclerosis

SEE ALSO
• Ataxia-telangectasia
• Von Hippel-Lindau disease
• Neurofibromatosis
• Sturge-Weber disease

OTHER NOTES   N/A

ABBREVIATIONS
• TS = tuberous sclerosis
• TSC = tuberous sclerosis complex

REFERENCES
• Shepherd CW, et al: Tuberous sclerosis complex in Olmsted County, Minnesota, 1950-1989 Department of Health Sciences Research, Mayo Clinic, Rochester, MN 55905. Arch Neurol 1991;48(4):400-1
• Isselbacher KJ, et al, eds: Harrison's Principles of Internal Medicine. 13th Ed. New York, McGraw-Hill, 1994
• Perspective Newsletter. National Tuberous Sclerosis Association, Inc. Spring/Summer, Fall, Winter publications
• Fuchs BD: Case records of the Massachusetts General Hospital - case 18-1994. New Engl J Med 1994;330
Illustrations: N/A
Internet references: http://www.5mcc.com

Author(s)
J. Harlan Dix, MD, FACP
Dorothy Lowder, RN

Tularemia

BASICS

DESCRIPTION Acute infection with Francisella tularensis. Incubation averages 3-4 days. May be ulceroglandular, glandular, typhoidal, oculoglandular, or oropharyngeal.
System(s) affected: Skin/Exocrine, Pulmonary, Cardiovascular, Hemic/Lymphatic/Immunologic
Genetics: N/A
Incidence/Prevalence in USA: (Incidence) 0.1 per 100,000
Predominant age: All ages
Predominant sex: Male > Female

SIGNS AND SYMPTOMS
- Nearly all cases have fever, chills, fatigue, malaise
- Ulceroglandular (3/4 of cases)
  ◊ Non-healing ulcer
  ◊ Regional adenopathy
  ◊ Failure of cephalosporin treatment
- Glandular
  ◊ Localized adenopathy
  ◊ No ulcer
- Typhoidal
  ◊ Systemic febrile illness
  ◊ Fulminating sepsis
  ◊ Pleuropulmonary disease
  ◊ No ulcer
- Oropharyngeal
  ◊ Exudative pharyngitis
  ◊ Membranous pharyngitis
  ◊ Cervical adenopathy
- Oculoglandular
  ◊ Purulent conjunctivitis
  ◊ Preauricular adenopathy
  ◊ Cervical adenopathy

CAUSES
- Inoculation of F. tularensis via:
  ◊ Tick bite
  ◊ Deer fly bite
  ◊ Cat bite
  ◊ Aerosol inhalation
  ◊ Contact with infected carcass (can penetrate unbroken skin)
  ◊ Ingestion

RISK FACTORS
- Location in endemic area (> 50% cases in AR, MO, OK, TN, TX)
- Outdoor work
- Rural residence
- Game handling
- Laboratory work

DIAGNOSIS

DIFFERENTIAL DIAGNOSIS
- Ulceroglandular/glandular
  ◊ Staphylococcal infections
  ◊ Streptococcal infections
  ◊ Cat-scratch disease
  ◊ Pasteurella infections
  ◊ Lymphogranuloma venereum
  ◊ Sporotrichosis
  ◊ Plague
  ◊ Toxoplasmosis
- Typhoidal
  ◊ Legionellosis
  ◊ Rocky Mountain spotted fever
  ◊ Ehrlichiosis
  ◊ Borreliosis (including Lyme disease)
  ◊ Infectious mononucleosis
  ◊ Non-typhoid salmonellosis
  ◊ Typhoid fever
  ◊ Brucellosis
  ◊ Q fever
  ◊ Psittacosis
  ◊ Tick-borne typhus
  ◊ Viral pneumonia
- Oropharyngeal
  ◊ Streptococcal pharyngitis
  ◊ Viral pharyngitis
  ◊ Diphtheric pharyngitis
  ◊ Infectious mononucleosis

LABORATORY
- Fourfold rise in antibody titer (peak in 4-8 weeks)
- Convalescent titer of 160 or greater
- Delayed growth on specific media or blood culture
- Elevated ESR
- Normal WBC, left shift
Drugs that may alter lab results: N/A
Disorders that may alter lab results: Brucella antibodies may cross-react

PATHOLOGICAL FINDINGS
- Necrotic areas in liver, spleen, other organs
- Caseating granulomata
- Microscopic foci with PMN's, macrophages, giant cells

SPECIAL TESTS
- Referral to specialized lab
- Pleomorphic Gram-negative coccobacilli
- Metabolic profile of isolate
- Specific immunofluorescent stain
- Culture ulcer

IMAGING
Chest x-ray may show ill-defined infiltrates, lobar consolidation, or pleural effusion

DIAGNOSTIC PROCEDURES
- Lymph node aspiration
- Thoracentesis
- Thorough history of patient's contact with wild rodents or exposure to arthropod vectors

TREATMENT

APPROPRIATE HEALTH CARE Inpatient during work-up and early treatment. Outpatient as soon as possible, depending on severity.

GENERAL MEASURES
- Isolation not needed for patient, but handle secretions carefully
- Hydration, fever control, antibiotics
- Wet saline dressings for skin lesions
- Recovery requires intact cell-mediated immunity

SURGICAL MEASURES Incision and drainage of abscesses

ACTIVITY As tolerated

DIET As tolerated, high caloric, easily digestible

PATIENT EDUCATION
- Person-to-person transmission not documented
- See Prevention/Avoidance
- Vaccine for high-risk persons; contact CDC

MEDICATIONS

DRUG(S) OF CHOICE
• Streptomycin 15-20 mg/kg IM per day, divided bid for 7-14 days
• Gentamicin
Contraindications: Known hypersensitivity, pregnancy
Precautions:
• Long-term therapy may produce eighth nerve damage
• Reduce dose in renal dysfunction
• Long-term therapy may produce renal dysfunction
• Use with care post-anesthesia (respiratory paralysis), and in patients with myasthenia gravis
Significant possible interactions: Other aminoglycosides, cephaloridine, polymyxin B, amphotericin B, colistin, muscle relaxants, paralyzing anesthetic agents

ALTERNATIVE DRUGS
• Ciprofloxacin - successful treatment reports increasing
• Chloramphenicol
• Tetracyclines - associated with higher relapse rate
• 3rd generation cephalosporins - high relapse rate or failure rate

FOLLOWUP

PATIENT MONITORING
• Monitor eighth nerve function in long-term therapy
• Monitor renal function in long-term therapy

PREVENTION/AVOIDANCE
• Tick repellents
• Remove tick by grasping near mouthparts
• Avoid squeezing body of embedded tick
• Wear gloves while dressing game
• Avoid contact if game appeared ill
• Lab workers - vaccine possibly protective. Wear protective hoods.
• Cook wild game thoroughly

POSSIBLE COMPLICATIONS
• Lung abscess
• Adult respiratory distress syndrome
• Hepatic dysfunction
• Rhabdomyolysis
• Renal failure
• Osteomyelitis, meningitis, endocarditis, pericarditis, peritonitis
• Mediastinitis

EXPECTED COURSE/PROGNOSIS
• Cure complete if treated early and vigorously
• Immunity is lifelong
• Mortality is 1-3%, higher in typhoidal-type disease

MISCELLANEOUS

ASSOCIATED CONDITIONS
• Other arthropod-borne diseases
• Tularemic conjunctivitis
• Bacteremia
• Atypical pneumonia

AGE-RELATED FACTORS
Pediatric: Often affected
Geriatric: Complications more likely, mortality rate higher
Others: More likely to occur in outdoor-type, young adult males

PREGNANCY
Streptomycin may cause fetal 8th nerve damage

SYNONYMS
• Rabbit fever
• Deer-fly fever
• Pasteurella tularensis
• Bacterium tularense
• Tick fever
• Ohara's disease
• Francis' disease
• Parvovirus B19 infection

ICD-9-CM 021.0-021.9 Tularemia

SEE ALSO N/A

OTHER NOTES Incidence higher in summer and fall

ABBREVIATIONS N/A

REFERENCES
• Mandell GL, Bennett JE, Dolin R, eds: Principles and Practice of Infectious Diseases. 4th Ed. New York, Churchill Livingstone, 1995
• Feigin RD, Cherry JD: Textbook of Pediatric Infectious Disease. 3rd Ed. Philadelphia, W.B. Saunders Co., 1992
Illustrations: N/A
Internet references: http://www.5mcc.com

Author(s)
Greg Elders, MD

Turner's syndrome

BASICS

DESCRIPTION Edema of hands and feet and excess skin of the neck (webbing) are presenting features during infancy. As children, girls are short and may have left sided heart or aortic abnormalities. Primary amenorrhea or delayed onset of puberty with short stature are important clues during adolescence.

System(s) affected: Nervous, Reproductive, Endocrine/Metabolic, Cardiovascular, Musculoskeletal, Renal/Urologic

Genetics: usually sporadic

Incidence/Prevalence in USA: 40 per 100,000 female births

Predominant age: All ages

Predominant sex: Female only

SIGNS AND SYMPTOMS
• Frequencies are for classic 45,X and vary somewhat with other chromosomal abnormalities associated with Turner's syndrome
• Short stature (98%)
• Gonadal dysgenesis (95%)
• Lymphedema (70%)
• Broad chest (75%)
• Hypoplastic, wide-spaced nipples (78%)
• Prominent, anomalous ears (70%)
• High palate (82%)
• Short neck (80%)
• Webbing of neck (65%)
• Low hairline (80%)
• Cubitus valgus (75%)
• Short fourth metacarpal (65%)
• Nail hypoplasia (75%)
• Excess nevi (70%)
• Renal anomalies (60%)
• Heart malformations (30%)
• Hearing impairment (70%)

CAUSES Monosomy for all or part of the X chromosome can result in symptoms consistent with Turner's syndrome

RISK FACTORS Familial chromosome translocations involving the X chromosome can increase the risk that an individual will conceive a child with Turner's syndrome

DIAGNOSIS

DIFFERENTIAL DIAGNOSIS
• Short stature
  ◊ Noonans syndrome
  ◊ Hypothyroidism
  ◊ Familial short stature
  ◊ Léri-Weil syndrome
  ◊ Brachydactyly E
  ◊ Growth hormone deficiency
  ◊ Glucocorticoid excess
  ◊ Klippel-Feil anomaly
  ◊ Short stature due to chronic disease
• Amenorrhea or delayed puberty
  ◊ Pure gonadal dysgenesis
  ◊ Stein-Leventhal syndrome
  ◊ Primary/secondary amenorrhea
• Lymphedema
  ◊ Hereditary congenital lymphedema
  ◊ Milroy's disease
  ◊ Lymphedema with recurrent cholestasis
  ◊ Lymphedema with intestinal lymphangiectasia
• Other
  ◊ Multiple pterygium syndrome
  ◊ Pseudohypoparathyroid

LABORATORY
• Chromosome analysis (a buccal smear is not an adequate test to rule out the diagnosis)
• At puberty FSH and LH levels may approach castration levels. FSH may be transiently high in infancy

Drugs that may alter lab results: N/A
Disorders that may alter lab results: N/A

PATHOLOGICAL FINDINGS
• Ovarian dysgenesis (> 90%)
• Renal - horseshoe kidney, double collecting system (60%)
• Cardiac - bicuspid aortic valve, coarctation of aorta, valvular aortic stenosis (70% with heart defects also have coarctation)
• Bone dysplasia (> 50%)
• Gonadoblastomas in X/XY mosaics

SPECIAL TESTS
• Upper/lower extremity blood pressures
• ECG

IMAGING
• Renal ultrasound
• Cardiac ultrasound

DIAGNOSTIC PROCEDURES   N/A

TREATMENT

APPROPRIATE HEALTH CARE
Outpatient

GENERAL MEASURES
Once diagnosis is confirmed by karyotype, the following measures are appropriate:
• Cardiology evaluation to include upper and lower extremity blood pressures, and echocardiography. If an abnormality exists, prophylactic antibiotics may be indicated (e.g., dental procedures).
• Renal ultrasound or intravenous pyelography
• Thyroid function test and antithyroid antibodies
• Routine hearing examination
• Therapy for gonadal failure is necessary for girls who do not enter puberty spontaneously to start at an age appropriate time. Replacement therapy usually begins with one to two years of low dose estrogen replacement followed by larger dose estrogens cycled with progesterone. Birth control pills can be used as maintenance therapy once menses and secondary sexual characteristics have been established. Therapy should continue into the late forties. Routine gynecologic evaluation is indicated. Infertility is the general rule, but alternatives such as in vitro fertilization and embryo transfer may be an option.
• Growth retardation has been managed with sex hormone replacement, anabolic agents, and most recently human recombinant growth hormone (hrGH). Current data shows that some Turner's syndrome patients increase final height attainment with hrGH treatment. Ideally, if hrGH therapy is provided, it is best started before significant growth deceleration occurs (between 3-10 years of age) and in a daily subcutaneous dose of approximately 0.05 mg/kg.
• Intelligence is usually normal. Problems may exist in non-verbal areas such as imagining objects in relationship to one another. If concerns about school performance arise, they should be appropriately evaluated and treated.
• Regular check-ups are recommended to detect problems early. Physicians and health care givers should be aware of the social problems and emotional problems associated with issues such as short stature and infertility.

SURGICAL MEASURES
• Removal of gonads in X/XY individuals
• Physical appearance may be enhanced by plastic surgery for inner canthal folds, protruding auricles and webbed neck.

ACTIVITY Normal other than limitations that may be placed on individuals with similar cardiac or renal abnormalities.

DIET Normal, but there is a tendency toward obesity

PATIENT EDUCATION
• Both families and patients need a thorough explanation of the condition and its management especially in regards to sexual development and growth. Jones/Smith suggest advising patient between age 8 and adolescence that she will probably not bear children.
• Excellent patient educational materials include:
  ◊ Plumridge D: Good things come in small packages: the whys and hows of Turner's Syndrome. Crippled Children's Division, University of Oregon Health Sciences Center, Portland, OR 97203.
  ◊ Rieser PA, Underwood LE: Turner's syndrome: a guide for families. Turner's Syndrome Society, York University, ASB 006, 4700 Keele St., Downsview, Ontario, Canada, M3J 1P3, (416)667-3773 or Turner's Syndrome Society, 3539 Tonkawood Rd., Minnetonka, MN 55345, (612)938-3118

MEDICATIONS

DRUG(S) OF CHOICE N/A
Contraindications: N/A
Precautions: N/A
Significant possible interactions: N/A

ALTERNATIVE DRUGS N/A

FOLLOWUP

PATIENT MONITORING
• Regular measurement of growth parameters
• Regular blood pressure checks
• Annual urine analysis if renal abnormality is present
• Monitor for signs of hypothyroidism
• Regular hearing testing
• Regular eye exams
• Monitor for blood in stool

PREVENTION/AVOIDANCE
Prenatal detection is available for couples who carry chromosomal translocations which would put them at high risk or for couples who have had an affected child. There is no in utero treatment, but pregnancy termination is an option if a fetus with Turner's syndrome is identified

POSSIBLE COMPLICATIONS
Complications are related to associated abnormalities

EXPECTED COURSE/PROGNOSIS
Most girls with Turner's syndrome can be expected to lead reasonably normal lives with appropriate medical management

MISCELLANEOUS

ASSOCIATED CONDITIONS
• Hashimoto's thyroiditis
• Hypothyroidism
• Alopecia
• Vitiligo
• Gastrointestinal disorders
• Carbohydrate intolerance

AGE-RELATED FACTORS
Pediatric: N/A
Geriatric: N/A
Others: N/A

PREGNANCY N/A

SYNONYMS
• Ullrich-Turner syndrome
• Bonnevie-Ullrich
• XO syndrome
• Monosomy X
• Short stature-sexual infantilism
• Gonadal dysgenesis

ICD-9-CM 758.6 Gonadal dysgenesis

SEE ALSO
• Amenorrhea
• Coarctation of the aorta
• Hypothyroidism, adult
• Thyroiditis

OTHER NOTES N/A

ABBREVIATIONS N/A

REFERENCES
• Buyse ML, ed: Birth Defects Encyclopedia. Cambridge, Massachusetts, Blackwell Scientific Publications, 1990
• Hall JG, Gilchrist DM: Turner's Syndrome and Its Variants. Pediatr Clinics NA 1990;37(6):1421-1440
• Jones KL: Smith's Recognizable Patterns of Human Malformation. Philadelphia, W.B. Saunders Co., 1988
• American Academy of Pediatrics Committee on Genetics. Health Supervision for Children with Turner Syndrome. Pediatrics 1995;96:1166-73
Illustrations: N/A
Internet references: http://www.5mcc.com

Author(s)
John R. Waterson, MD, PhD

Typhoid fever

BASICS

DESCRIPTION Typhoid fever is an acute systemic illness unique to humans caused by Salmonella typhi. It is a classic example of enteric fever caused by the Salmonella family of bacteria.
• It is endemic in Third World countries where sanitation is suboptimal. Majority of cases in North America are acquired after travel to endemic areas.
• Mode of transmission is fecal-oral through ingestion of contaminated food (commonly poultry), water and milk. Incubation period varies from 7 to 21 days.
System(s) affected: Gastrointestinal, Pulmonary, Skin/Exocrine
Genetics: N/A
Incidence/Prevalence in USA: 300-500 cases per year
Predominant age: All ages
Predominant sex: Male = Female

SIGNS AND SYMPTOMS
• Fever
• Headache
• Malaise
• Abdominal discomfort/bloating/constipation
• Diarrhea (less common)
• Dry cough
• Confusion/lethargy
• Rose spot (transient erythematous maculopapular rash in anterior thorax or upper abdomen)
• Splenomegaly
• Hepatomegaly
• Cervical adenopathy
• Relative bradycardia
• Conjunctivitis

CAUSES Salmonella typhi

RISK FACTORS Must be considered in any patient presenting with fever after tropical travel or exposed to chronic carrier

DIAGNOSIS

DIFFERENTIAL DIAGNOSIS
• Malaria
• "Enteric fever-like" syndrome caused by Yersinia enterocolitica, Yersinia pseudotuberculosis, and Campylobacter fetus
• Enteric fever caused by non-typhi Salmonella
• Infectious hepatitis
• Atypical pneumonia
• Infectious mononucleosis
• Subacute bacterial endocarditis
• Tuberculosis
• Brucellosis
• Q fever

LABORATORY
• Definitive diagnosis by isolation of S. typhi from blood. Isolation of S. typhi in sputum, urine or stool is presumptive diagnosis in typical clinical presentation.
• Serology is nonspecific and usually not useful
• If multiple blood cultures are negative or in patients with prior antibiotic therapy, diagnostic yield is better with bone marrow culture
• Anemia, leukopenia (neutropenia), thrombocytopenia or evidence of DIC (disseminated intravascular coagulopathy) are supportive evidence. Elevated liver enzymes are commonly seen.
Drugs that may alter lab results
• Prior antibiotic therapy
• Vaccination
Disorders that may alter lab results: N/A

PATHOLOGICAL FINDINGS Classically, mononuclear proliferation involving lymphoid tissue of intestinal tract especially Peyer's patch in terminal ileum

SPECIAL TESTS N/A

IMAGING Serial plain abdominal films for evidence of intestinal perforation

DIAGNOSTIC PROCEDURES Bone marrow aspirate for culture is rarely indicated

TREATMENT

APPROPRIATE HEALTH CARE
• Inpatient if acutely ill
• Outpatient for less ill patient or for carrier

GENERAL MEASURES
• Fluid and electrolyte support
• Strict isolation of patient's linen, stool and urine
• Monitor clinically with aid of serial plain abdominal films for evidence of perforation, usually in the third to fourth week of illness
• Indication for treatment must be determined on an individual basis. Factors to be considered are age, public health (food handler, chronic care facilities, medical personnel), intolerance to antibiotics, and evidence of biliary tract disease.
• For hemorrhage - need blood transfusion and shock management

SURGICAL MEASURES
Cholecystectomy may be warranted in carriers with cholelithiasis, relapse after therapy, or intolerance to antimicrobial therapy

ACTIVITY Bedrest initially, then as tolerated

DIET If abdominal symptoms severe, nothing by mouth. With improvement, normal low-residue diet, possibly enriched in calories.

PATIENT EDUCATION
• Discussion of chronic carrier state and its complications
• For family members, travelers or workers at risk, provide hygiene education, possibly vaccination

Typhoid fever

MEDICATIONS

DRUG(S) OF CHOICE
• Chloramphenicol: Children - 50 mg/kg/d po qid x 2 weeks; adult dose - 50 mg/kg per day, divided q6h x 2 weeks,
or
• Ampicillin: Children - 100 mg/kg/d qid po x 2 weeks; adults - 500 mg q6h x 2 weeks,
or
• Ciprofloxacin 500 mg po bid x 2 weeks, indicated in MDR-T, has been successfully and safely used in children
or
• Ceftriaxone 1-2 gm IV qd x 2 weeks,
or
• Furazolidone 7.5 mg/kg/d po x 10 days; in uncomplicated MDR-T; safe in children; efficacy > 85% cure
• Chronic carrier state
  ◊ Is treated with ampicillin 4-5 gram/day plus probenecid 2 grams/day qid x 6 weeks (for patients with normal functioning gallbladder without evidence of cholelithiasis)
  ◊ Ciprofloxacin 500 mg po bid x 4-6 weeks is also efficacious
Note: Chloramphenicol resistance - reported in Mexico, South America, Central America, Southeast Asia, India, Pakistan, Middle East and Africa
Contraindications: Refer to manufacturer's profile of each drug
Precautions: Rarely, Jarisch-Herxheimer reaction post antimicrobial therapy
Significant possible interactions: Refer to manufacturer's profile of each drug

ALTERNATIVE DRUGS
Trimethoprim-sulfamethoxazole

FOLLOWUP

PATIENT MONITORING See General Measures

PREVENTION/AVOIDANCE
• For travel to an endemic area, consider vaccination for typhoid, parenterally (phenol-killed or Vi vaccines) or live oral vaccine (Ty21a)
• Avoid tap water, salad/raw vegetables, unpeeled fruits, dairy products in tropical travel
• Avoid poultry or poultry products left unrefrigerated for prolonged period of time

POSSIBLE COMPLICATIONS
• Intestinal hemorrhage and perforation in distal ileum
• Patient may become chronic carrier state (up to 3%) defined as persistent stool excretor for longer than 1 year
• Predilection for seeding in the biliary tract exists and may become a focus for relapse of typhoid fever. Most common in female and the elderly (> 50 years old).
• Osteomyelitis especially in sickle cell anemia, systemic lupus erythematosus, hematologic neoplasms and immunosuppressed hosts
• Endovascular infection in the elderly and in patients with history of by-pass operation or aneurysm
• Rarely, endocarditis or meningitis

EXPECTED COURSE/PROGNOSIS
Overall prognosis good with therapy. < 2% mortality rate; 15% relapse rate with some antibiotic treatments; 3% bowel perforation

MISCELLANEOUS

ASSOCIATED CONDITIONS N/A

AGE-RELATED FACTORS
Pediatric: Disease more critical in infants, but may be milder in children
Geriatric: Disease more serious in elderly
Others: N/A

PREGNANCY Ciprofloxacin not recommended in pregnancy

SYNONYMS
• Typhoid
• Typhus abdominalis
• Enteric fever

ICD-9-CM 002.0 Typhoid and paratyphoid fevers

SEE ALSO N/A

OTHER NOTES N/A

ABBREVIATIONS N/A

REFERENCES Mandell GL, ed: Principles and Practice of Infectious Diseases. 4th Ed. New York, Churchill Livingstone, 1995
Illustrations: N/A
Internet references: http://www.5mcc.com

Author(s)
D. W. MacPherson, MD, MSc (CTM), FRCPC
T. C. Yang, MD, FRCPC

- 1107 -

Typhus fevers

BASICS

DESCRIPTION Acute infectious diseases caused by three species of rickettsiae
• Epidemic typhus - human to human transmission by body louse. Primarily in unclean circumstances such as refugee camps, war, famine and disaster. Recrudescent disease, occurring years after initial infection can be source of human outbreak. Flying squirrels also reservoir.
• Endemic (murine) typhus - infection of rodents. To humans by rat flea.
• Scrub typhus - infection of chiggers and of rodents. To humans by the chigger. Primarily in Asia and the Western Pacific.
System(s) affected: Endocrine/Metabolic, Pulmonary, Skin/Exocrine, Hemic/Lymphatic/Immunologic
Genetics: N/A
Incidence/Prevalence in USA:
• Epidemic typhus - rare
• Endemic typhus - fewer than 100 cases annually, primarily in gulf states, especially South Texas, under-reporting suspected
• Scrub typhus - none except for travelers returning from endemic areas
Predominant age: N/A
Predominant sex: N/A

SIGNS AND SYMPTOMS
• General
  ◊ Acute onset
  ◊ Fever
  ◊ Chills
  ◊ Headache
  ◊ Myalgia
  ◊ Malaise
  ◊ Diffuse organ involvement, e.g., intestine, liver, heart, kidneys, brain
• Epidemic typhus
  ◊ Incubation period about 1 week
  ◊ Macular or maculopapular rash beginning on trunk about fifth day of illness
  ◊ Nonproductive cough
  ◊ Pulmonary infiltrates
• Endemic typhus
  ◊ Incubation period 1-2 weeks
  ◊ Macular or maculopapular rash beginning on trunk third to fifth day of illness
• Scrub typhus
  ◊ Incubation period 1-3 weeks
  ◊ Eschar at bite site
  ◊ Regional lymphadenopathy
  ◊ Generalized lymphadenopathy
  ◊ Splenomegaly
  ◊ Macular or maculopapular rash beginning on trunk about the fifth day of illness
  ◊ Relative bradycardia early in disease
  ◊ Ocular pain
  ◊ Conjunctival injection

CAUSES
• Epidemic typhus by Rickettsia prowazekii
• Endemic typhus by R. typhi
• Scrub typhus by R. tsutsugamushi

RISK FACTORS
• Exposure to vectors, e.g., travel to certain countries
• Elderly may have more severe disease
• Laboratory worker

DIAGNOSIS

DIFFERENTIAL DIAGNOSIS
• Any acute febrile disease
• Rocky Mountain spotted fever
• Meningococcemia
• Bacterial meningitis
• Measles
• Rubella
• Toxoplasmosis
• Leptospirosis
• Typhoid fever
• Dengue
• Relapsing fever
• Secondary syphilis
• Infectious mononucleosis

LABORATORY
• WBC usually normal
• Abnormalities reflecting the particular organs affected
• Weil-Felix serological reaction may be positive; test limited to mid-illness or after, and by low sensitivity and non-specificity. Epidemic and endemic typhus, fourfold titer rise or titer > 1/320 to OX-19. Scrub typhus, fourfold rise in titer to OX-K.
• Hyponatremia in severe cases
• Hypoalbuminemia in severe cases
Drugs that may alter lab results:
Antibiotics
Disorders that may alter lab results: N/A

PATHOLOGICAL FINDINGS Diffuse vasculitis

SPECIAL TESTS Specific serological test showing a rising antibody titer. Isolation of rickettsia should be undertaken only in special laboratories to minimize risk of laboratory-acquired infection.

IMAGING N/A

DIAGNOSTIC PROCEDURES N/A

TREATMENT

APPROPRIATE HEALTH CARE
Outpatient unless severely ill

GENERAL MEASURES
• Protect agitated patient from injury
• Skin and mouth care
• Supportive care for the severely ill, directed to the complications

SURGICAL MEASURES N/A

ACTIVITY Bedrest during acute stages, otherwise as tolerated

DIET As tolerated

PATIENT EDUCATION
• Prevention information to travelers
• Vaccination information

MEDICATIONS

DRUG(S) OF CHOICE
• Treatment should begin when diagnosis is reasonably likely and continue until improved and afebrile for a minimum of 48 hours
• Children over 8 years and adults:
  ◊ Tetracycline (Achromycin), or a congener, orally 25 mg per kg initially, and then 25 mg per kg daily in equally divided doses every 6 hours
  ◊ If severely ill, may use doxycycline IV, adults 100 mg every 12 hours, children >8 years 5 mg per kg in 24 hours (maximum of 200 mg/24 hrs)
• Children under 8 years, pregnant women or if typhoid fever is possible cause of illness:
  ◊ Chloramphenicol (Chloromycetin) orally 50 mg per kg initially, and then 50 mg per kg daily in equally divided doses every 6 hours
  ◊ If severely ill, chloramphenicol (Chloromycetin) sodium succinate intravenously 20 mg per kg initially infused in 30-45 minutes, and then 50 mg per kg daily infused in equally divided doses every 6 hours until orally tolerable.
Contraindications: N/A
Precautions: Refer to manufacturer's profile of each drug
Significant possible interactions: Refer to manufacturer's profile of each drug

ALTERNATIVE DRUGS
• Doxycycline (Vibramycin) single oral dose of 100 or 200 mg in refugee camps, disasters or limited medical services
• Isolated reports indicate that erythromycin and ciprofloxacin are effective

FOLLOWUP

PATIENT MONITORING   Severely ill patients should be observed regularly in hospital. Outpatients checked periodically as improvement is evident.

PREVENTION/AVOIDANCE
• Avoid vectors for each disease, e.g., scrub typhus; wear protective clothing and use insect repellents, endemic typhus; practice ectoparasite and rodent control, and epidemic typhus; delousing
• Epidemic typhus vaccine considered for persons at high risk of exposure

POSSIBLE COMPLICATIONS
Consequences of specific organ system involvement in the second week, e.g., azotemia, meningoencephalitis, seizures, delirium, coma, myocardial failure, hyponatremia, hypoalbuminemia, hypovolemia, and shock

EXPECTED COURSE/PROGNOSIS
• Recovery expected if treatment is instituted before complications
• Relapses may follow treatment, especially if initiated within 48 hours of onset (this is not an indication to delay treatment). Relapses treated same as primary disease.
• Without treatment the mortality is 40-60% in epidemic, 1-2% in endemic, and up to 30% in scrub typhus. Mortality higher among the elderly.

MISCELLANEOUS

ASSOCIATED CONDITIONS   N/A

AGE-RELATED FACTORS
Pediatric: N/A
Geriatric: N/A
Others: N/A

PREGNANCY   N/A

SYNONYMS
• Louse-borne typhus
• Brill-Zinsser disease
• Murine typhus

ICD-9-CM
080 Louse-born [epidemic] typhus
081.0 Murine [endemic] typhus
081.1 Brill's disease

SEE ALSO   N/A

OTHER NOTES
• Severe headache often intractable and not eased by the usual drugs
• Report case to Health Department

ABBREVIATIONS   N/A

REFERENCES
• Mandell GL, Douglas RG, Bennett JE, eds: Principles and Practice of Infectious Diseases. 4th Ed. New York, Churchill Livingstone, 1995
• Dumlev JS, Taylor JP, Walker DH: Clinical and laboratory features of murine typhus in south Texas, 1980 through 1987. JAMA 1991;266:1365-1370
Illustrations: N/A
Internet references: http://www.5mcc.com

Author(s)
William D. Sawyer, MD

Ulcerative colitis

 BASICS

DESCRIPTION
One of a group of inflammatory bowel diseases of unknown etiology characterized by intermittent bouts of inflammation of all or portions of the colon. Manifested by recurrences of rectal bleeding and various constitutional symptoms.
System(s) affected: Gastrointestinal
Genetics: Family aggregates common, positive family history in 8-11%. More likely vertical than horizontal. More common in Jews.
Incidence/Prevalence in USA: 70-150 per 100,000. Incidence 6-8 new cases per 100,000 population.
Predominant age: Between ages of 15 and 35 years. There is a second and smaller peak in the 7th decade.
Predominant sex: Male = Female

SIGNS AND SYMPTOMS
• Bloody diarrhea
• Abdominal pain
• Fever
• Weight loss
• Arthralgias and arthritis (15-20%)
• Spondylitis (3-6%)
• Ocular complications (4-10%) includes episcleritis, uveitis, cataracts, keratopathy, marginal corneal ulceration, and central serous retinopathy
• Erythema nodosum
• Pyoderma gangrenosum
• Aphthous ulcers of mouth (5-10%)
• Asymptomatic fatty liver common - occasional hepatomegaly
• Pericholangitis (uncommon)
• Primary sclerosing cholangitis (1-4%)
• Cirrhosis of liver (1-5%)
• Bile duct carcinoma
• Thromboembolic disease (1-6%)
• Pericarditis (rare)
• Amyloidosis (rare)

CAUSES
Unknown (genetic, infectious, immunologic, and psychological factors have all been suggested)

RISK FACTORS
• None known
• Higher incidence in Jews and those with positive family history
• Negative association with smoking

 DIAGNOSIS

DIFFERENTIAL DIAGNOSIS
• Other sources of rectal bleeding including hemorrhoids, neoplasms, colonic diverticuli, A-V malformation, Crohn's disease
• Infectious causes of diarrhea including bacteria (Enterotoxigenic E. coli, E. coli 0157:H7, Salmonella, Shigella, Aeromonas, Plesiomonas), parasitic (Entamoeba histolytica)
• "Gay bowel" syndrome causes (herpes simplex, Chlamydia trachomatis, Cryptosporidium, Isospora belli, cytomegalovirus, and other infectious causes as listed above)
• Antibiotic associated diarrhea
• Radiation proctitis
• Ischemic proctitis

LABORATORY
• Nonspecific. Usually reflects the degree of severity of the bleeding and inflammation.
• Anemia may reflect chronic disease as well as iron deficiency from blood loss
• Leukocytosis during exacerbation
• Elevated sedimentation rate
• Electrolyte abnormalities, especially hypokalemia
• Hypoalbuminemia
• Elevated liver function tests (if there is associated hepatobiliary disease)
Drugs that may alter lab results: N/A
Disorders that may alter lab results: N/A

PATHOLOGICAL FINDINGS
Inflammation of the colonic mucosa with ulcerations. These appear hyperemic and hemorrhagic. Rectum involved 95% of time. The inflammation extends proximally in a continuous fashion, but for a variable distance. May affect terminal ileum - referred to as "backwash ileitis."

SPECIAL TESTS
None

IMAGING
Air contrast barium enema

DIAGNOSTIC PROCEDURES
• Sigmoidoscopy, may include biopsy
• Colonoscopy, may include biopsy for evaluation for premalignant features; also used to differentiate from Crohn's disease, and to investigate abnormalities that appear on radiography, such as stricture or mass lesions. Colonoscopy useful to define the extent of involvement and specific segments involved as this has bearing on therapy and prognosis.

 TREATMENT

APPROPRIATE HEALTH CARE
Outpatient, except for severe exacerbations which may require hospitalization

GENERAL MEASURES
Goal is to control inflammation, prevent complications, replace nutritional losses and blood volume

SURGICAL MEASURES
Complications or refractory disease may require surgical intervention

ACTIVITY
Full activity as tolerated

DIET
No specific diet; milk products not withheld unless an associated lactase deficiency exists

PATIENT EDUCATION
• Close doctor/patient relationship encouraged
• Self-help organizations such as:
National Foundation for Ileitis and Colitis
444 Park Avenue S., 11th Floor, New York, NY 10016-7374, (800)343-3637

MEDICATIONS

DRUG(S) OF CHOICE
• Sulfasalazine is treatment of choice both for mild flare-ups and for the chronic treatment used to decrease the frequency of relapses (dosage range 1-4 grams daily)
• Disease limited to the rectum (proctitis) or to the left side of the colon and rectum (proctosigmoiditis) may be treated topically with steroid enemas or mesalamine (5-aminosalicylic acid, 5-ASA) enemas and suppositories
• Oral or parenteral corticosteroids are used for more severe flare-ups (e.g., prednisone 40-60 mg qd, gradually tapered off over two months)
• Approximately 10% of patients have chronic disease activity and require continuous low - moderate steroid doses
• Newer agents include oral 5-ASA derivatives. Topical use of sodium cromoglycate and sucralfate being studied.
• Immunomodulators such as azathioprine, mercaptopurine (6-mercaptopurine), methotrexate, levamisole, and cyclosporine are controversial in a disease potentially curable by colectomy. However, have been shown to be effective in patients who either refuse surgery or are poor surgical candidates.
• Antimicrobial agents (anti-mycobacteriums and metronidazole) sometimes useful in Crohn's disease but not in ulcerative colitis
• Antidiarrheal agents, diphenoxylate-atropine and loperamide may be used to help control diarrhea, but require careful monitoring since they may precipitate toxic megacolon
Contraindications:
• Allergy to any of above agents
• Refer to manufacturer's profile of each drug
Precautions: Use of antidiarrheal agents in severe disease could precipitate toxic megacolon
Significant possible interactions: Refer to manufacturer's profile of each drug

ALTERNATIVE DRUGS   Included in Drug(s) of Choice

FOLLOWUP

PATIENT MONITORING   Regularly scheduled appointments are important to evaluate for disease activity, appearance of complications, and the psychological and social well being of the patient

PREVENTION/AVOIDANCE   Colonoscopic evaluation for cancer surveillance with biopsy evaluation of the mucosa for evidence of dysplasia must be performed every 1-2 years after the disease has been present for 7-8 years. This is particularly important in pancolitis. Low grade dysplasia warrants more frequent evaluation (e.g., every 3-6 months) and high grade dysplasia (or low grade dysplasia within a mass) warrant consideration of colectomy.
• Annual liver tests
• Cholangiography for cholestasis

POSSIBLE COMPLICATIONS
• Perforation
• Toxic megacolon
• Liver disease
• Stricture formation (less than Crohn's disease)
• Colon cancer (may occur in as many as 30% of those with pancolitis for 25 years). Incidence of cancer is cumulative and begins after 7-8 years of disease; risk may be considerably less in left sided disease.

EXPECTED COURSE/PROGNOSIS
• Course extremely variable; mortality for initial attack approximately 5%. Approximately 75-85% of patients experience relapse, and up to 20% in some studies eventually require colectomy.
• Colon cancer risk is the single most important risk factor affecting long-term prognosis
• Left-sided colitis and ulcerative proctitis have very favorable prognosis with probable normal life span

MISCELLANEOUS

ASSOCIATED CONDITIONS   Ankylosing spondylitis

AGE-RELATED FACTORS
Pediatric:
• Approximately 20% of patients are 21 years or younger
• Cancer surveillance is important since occurrence of cancer relates to the duration and extent of disease, whether frequently symptomatic or not
Geriatric: Increased mortality with initial attack in patients over 60
Others: N/A

PREGNANCY
• Outcome of pregnancy similar to general population. One study showed 30% of those with inactive disease at onset of pregnancy relapsed and 14% did so in first trimester.
• Treatment with sulfasalazine does not seem to affect outcome of pregnancy
• Recommend patient delay pregnancy until time when disease is inactive

SYNONYMS   Idiopathic proctocolitis

ICD-9-CM   556 Idiopathic proctocolitis

SEE ALSO
• Crohn's disease of the colon
• Diarrhea, acute
• Diarrhea, chronic
• Intestinal parasites

OTHER NOTES   N/A

ABBREVIATIONS   N/A

REFERENCES
• Isselbacher KJ, et al,eds: Harrison's Principles of Internal Medicine. 13th Ed. New York, McGraw-Hill, 1994
• Farmer RG: Inflammatory Bowel Disease. Medical Clinics Issue, Volume 74/number 1. Philadelphia, W.B. Saunders Co., January 1990
Illustrations: 3 available on CD-ROM
Internet references: http://www.5mcc.com

Author(s)
Mark Eric Worshtil, MD

Urethritis

BASICS

DESCRIPTION Syndrome of urethral inflammation marked by painful urination and discharge. Usually a sexually transmitted disease (STD); other causes not uncommon. Two types: Gonorrhea (GC) found usually in males, rarely in women, and nongonococcal urethritis (NGU).
• In males - gonorrhea marked by a yellow purulent discharge, abrupt onset of symptoms 3 to 5 days after exposure to Neisseria gonorrhea. Nongonococcal urethritis marked by clear to white scanty discharge developing gradually at least a week after exposure, waxing and waning in intensity from a variety of other organisms, most commonly Chlamydia trachomatis
• In females, classic urethral syndrome present when patient complains of dysuria, urinalysis is clear, urine cultures are negative and patient fails to respond to regimens for simple cystitis. However, females with GC or other infections which cause simple urethritis in males will often have symptoms besides dysuria, including vaginal discharge and suprapubic pain.
• Untreated cases will gradually resolve, but complications, especially urethral stricture in males or pelvic inflammatory disease (PID) in women, may then ensue
System(s) affected: Renal/Urologic
Genetics: N/A
Incidence/Prevalence in USA: Very common - annually 2 million cases of gonorrhea, probably many more cases of Chlamydia. Highest incidence in urban, non-white populations.
Predominant age: Sexually active, postpubertal
Predominant sex: Classic symptoms more commonly reported by males; incidence in females probably equal

SIGNS AND SYMPTOMS
• Both sexes may be asymptomatic carriers of the causative organisms
• Dysuria - pain throughout urination
• Urethral discharge - may be profuse and purulent in acute GC, or scanty, evident only with milking of the urethra in NGU
• Suprapubic discomfort
• Urethral itching or tenderness
• Tenderness, edema and inflammation of the urethral meatus, especially in women
• Dyspareunia
• Vaginitis, cystitis, cervicitis in women
• Proctitis, pharyngitis, conjunctivitis may also be present (sexual history is important)
• Lymphadenopathy or fever are not part of the syndrome and suggest another diagnosis
• Bloody discharge - rarely seen and suggests another diagnosis

CAUSES Sexual contact with carrier of causative organisms. Most common are N. gonorrhea, C. trachomatis, Ureaplasma urealyticum, Trichomonas vaginalis, viruses (including herpes, cytomegalovirus [CMV], human papilloma virus), many other bacteria, rarely fungi

RISK FACTORS
• Multiple sexual partners
• History of other STD's

DIAGNOSIS

DIFFERENTIAL DIAGNOSIS
• Postgonococcal urethritis (PGU) - following adequate treatment of acute GC, patient continues to have symptoms, due to a second organism resistant to original medication (see Treatment)
• Other urinary tract infections - cystitis, epididymitis, prostatitis, etc.
• Trauma - frequent milking of the urethra in males, caused by concern about possible infection may lead to dysuria and a clear discharge. Young girls may occasionally develop symptoms from external irritation.
• Atrophy, especially in postmenopausal women
• Intraurethral foreign bodies or growths, e.g., venereal warts, congenital polyps
• Allergic or sensitivity reactions - vaginal douches and lubricants, foods, other medications (rare)
• Substance abuse - frequent heavy users of amphetamines or other stimulants may develop a scant, clear discharge without white cells and mild dysuria
• Stevens-Johnson syndrome
• Reiter's syndrome - probably an immunological reaction to Chlamydial infection

LABORATORY
• Gram stain of discharge: Polymorphic neutrophils with intracellular gram-negative diplococci strongly indicates GC; sheets of polymorphonuclear leukocytes without organisms suggests NGU, few to no polymorphonuclear leukocytes suggests other etiologies
• Discharge cultures or slide reagins for GC: False-negatives can occur, so treatment should be directed by physical exam and Gram stain results and should not wait for culture results. Conjunctiva, pharynx, rectum cultured as indicated by history and symptoms. Labs should test positives for drug resistances.
• Cultures or reagin detection for Chlamydia: Negatives may be false results or indicate another infecting organism

• Urinalysis: If indicated, sample discharge before patient voids, usually normal in cases of simple urethritis
• Urine culture: Performed only if Gram stain of discharge is unremarkable or unobtainable
• Wet prep of discharge: may reveal Trichomonas, unusual to demonstrate trichomoniasis in infected males
• Syphilis, HIV serology as indicated to rule out concomitant STD's
Drugs that may alter lab results: Previous recent treatment with antibiotics may lead to false negative results
Disorders that may alter lab results: N/A

PATHOLOGICAL FINDINGS Urethral strictures (untreated GC), intraurethral lesions (venereal warts, congenital anomalies)

SPECIAL TESTS Viral cultures if typical lesions are present

IMAGING Urethrogram for persistent symptoms, rarely indicated

DIAGNOSTIC PROCEDURES
Urethrocystoscopy for persistent cases with suspected foreign body, intraurethral warts

TREATMENT

APPROPRIATE HEALTH CARE All cases can be treated as outpatients except females with severe symptoms of PID

GENERAL MEASURES Identification and treatment of sexual partners

SURGICAL MEASURES N/A

ACTIVITY Full activity, except no sexual intercourse until treatment is completed

DIET No special diet

PATIENT EDUCATION
• Many handouts available from local health departments on avoidance, causes and treatments
• Most important to emphasize need for compliance with therapy and treatment of sexual partners. Also, patients should be urged to undergoing screening for other STD's.

MEDICATIONS

DRUG(S) OF CHOICE
• Note: There is an ever-increasing incidence of multiple drug resistances
• Gonorrhea - ceftriaxone (Rocephin) 250 mg IM x 1 dose. All cases of GC need to be treated additionally with a regimen specific for Chlamydia due to the high incidence of mixed infections.
• Chlamydia - doxycycline 100 mg po bid for at least 7 days. Patients who continue with symptoms after treatment (and their sexual partners) should be retreated with erythromycin.
• NGU (especially U. urealyticum) - doxycycline 100 mg po bid for at least 7 days
• Trichomonas - 2 grams metronidazole (Flagyl) po for 1 dose or 250 mg tid for 7 days
Contraindications: Sensitivity to any of the indicated medications. Pregnant patients should not receive tetracyclines
Precautions: Patients taking tetracyclines need to be told of the possibility of increased sensitivity to sunlight
Significant possible interactions: Tetracyclines should not be taken with milk products or antacids. Oral contraceptives may be rendered ineffective by oral antibiotics. Patients and partners should use a back-up method of birth control for remainder of the cycle.

ALTERNATIVE DRUGS
• Gonorrhea
  ◊ Spectinomycin 2 grams IM once
  ◊ Ciprofloxacin (Cipro) 500 mg po once
  ◊ Ofloxacin (Floxin) 400 mg po once
  ◊ Amoxicillin 3 grams with 1 gram probenecid (Benemid) po once
• Chlamydia
  ◊ Erythromycin 500 mg po qid x 7 days
  ◊ Azithromycin (Zithromax)1 g po once
  ◊ Ofloxacin (Floxin) 300 mg po q12h x 7 days

FOLLOWUP

PATIENT MONITORING
• Patients with positive cultures should have cultures repeated several days after completing treatment as a test of cure
• Ensure that sexual partners were treated

PREVENTION/AVOIDANCE
Safer sex protection techniques, urinating immediately after intercourse, treatment of all sexual partners

POSSIBLE COMPLICATIONS
• Stricture formation in untreated patients, PID in women
• When urethritis is accompanied by suprapubic discomfort, consider prostatitis in males, PID in females

EXPECTED COURSE/PROGNOSIS
If diagnosis is firmly established, appropriate medications prescribed and patient is compliant with treatment, there will be relief of symptoms within 24 hours and the problem will resolve without sequelae

MISCELLANEOUS

ASSOCIATED CONDITIONS
Other STD's - patients should be strongly urged to undergo testing for syphilis and HIV

AGE-RELATED FACTORS
Pediatric: Proven cases of GC or Chlamydia, trichomoniasis should raise the question of sexual abuse
Geriatric: N/A
Others: None

PREGNANCY
Tetracyclines are contraindicated. Use erythromycin instead but not the estolate form because of an increased risk of cholestatic jaundice.

SYNONYMS N/A

ICD-9-CM
• 098.0 gonorrhea
• 099.4 nongonococcal urethritis
• 131.02 trichomonas infections
• 99.3 Reiter's syndrome

SEE ALSO
• Gonococcal infections
• Chlamydial sexually transmitted diseases
• Pelvic inflammatory disease (PID)
• Vulvovaginitis, bacterial
• Vulvovaginitis, candidal
• Urinary tract infection in men
• Urinary tract infection in women
• Prostatitis
• Epididymitis

OTHER NOTES
For patients who present without symptoms stating that a sexual partner was treated for this problem: Obtain specimens for lab tests, but treat this patient before the results are available (due to the high prevalence of the illness and the possibility of false-negative test results). Use any of the regimens discussed in Medications section.

ABBREVIATIONS
• STD = sexually transmitted disease
• GC = gonococcus infection
• NGU = nongonococcal urethritis
• PGU = postgonococcal urethritis

REFERENCES
• Centers for Disease control: Sexually transmitted diseases: Treatment guidelines 1989. MMWR Morb Mortal Wkly Rep 1989;38 (Suppl 8):1
• Drugs for Sexually transmitted Diseases. Medical Letter, Vol. 36, Issue 913, Jan. 7, 1994
Illustrations: N/A
Internet references: http://www.5mcc.com

Author(s)
Kevin M. Hepler, MD, MBA

Urinary incontinence

BASICS

DESCRIPTION Urinary incontinence is the involuntary loss of urine from the bladder. It can occur while asleep or awake. The amount of urine lost can vary greatly. The condition comes to medical attention when it is perceived to be a social and/or health problem by the patient or family.
System(s) affected: Renal/Urologic
Genetics: Unknown
Incidence/Prevalence in USA:
• 5-15% in community-dwelling elderly (over age 65)
• 10 million in U.S.
• Up to 50% in nursing home populations
Predominant age: Geriatric populations. Increases with age.
Predominant sex: Female > Male

SIGNS AND SYMPTOMS
• Involuntary loss of urine
• Urinary urgency
• Burning with urination
• Perineal irritation

CAUSES
• Pelvic floor muscle weakness
• Urethral sphincter weakness
• Bladder irritation (cystitis, tumors, stones, diverticula)
• Detrusor motor/sensory instability (stroke, dementia, parkinsonism)
• Anatomic obstruction (prostate, stricture, cystocele)
• Neurogenic bladder (diabetes, spinal cord injury, multiple sclerosis)
• Loss of central nervous system control (severe dementia)
• Fecal impaction
• Drugs (cyclophosphamide, caffeine, beta blockers, cholinergic agents)

RISK FACTORS
• Increasing age
• Female sex/estrogen deficiency
• Prostatic hypertrophy (males)
• Multiparity (females)
• Dementia
• Diabetes
• Spinal cord injury
• Multiple sclerosis
• General debilitated condition
• Stroke

DIAGNOSIS

DIFFERENTIAL DIAGNOSIS
• Urinary tract infection
• Vaginal discharge (women)
• Urethral discharge (men)
• Medication effect (diuretics)

LABORATORY
• Urinalysis - generally normal. May show glycosuria (diabetes), proteinuria (glomerular disease), white blood cells (infection), red blood cells (tumor), or bacteria (infection).
• Urine culture - will be positive in urinary tract infection
• IVP - may show renal pathology
Drugs that may alter lab results:
• Diuretics (low urine specific gravity)
• Antibiotics (negative urine culture)
Disorders that may alter lab results: Not applicable. Disorders producing abnormal lab results generally contribute to the problem of incontinence.

PATHOLOGICAL FINDINGS
• Relate to the primary cause of incontinence
• Urinary sphincter incompetence
• Prostatic hypertrophy
• Neurogenic bladder
• Bladder tumors
• Urinary tract infection
• Fecal impaction

SPECIAL TESTS
• Voiding cystourethrogram - may show bladder and/or urethral pathology
• Cystometrograms - may show abnormal sphincter pressure or bladder physiology
• Post-voiding residual measurement - may show increased residual urine

IMAGING
• Renal ultrasound - may show renal pathology
• Pelvic ultrasound - may show pelvic pathology
• Transrectal ultrasound - may show prostate pathology

DIAGNOSTIC PROCEDURES
• The diagnosis is generally made by history
• Physical examination of men should include palpation of abdomen (for distended bladder), digital rectal exam (for prostatic hypertrophy), and neurological exam
• Physical exam of women should include palpation of abdomen (for distended bladder), vaginal speculum and bimanual pelvic exam (for genitourinary pathology), and neurologic exam
• Both men and women should be examined for fecal impaction
• It is sometimes helpful to ask the patient to reproduce the activities (e.g., coughing, sneezing, laughing) which result in loss of urine
• Office cystometry - using a catheter and 60 cc Asepto syringe (without plunger)

TREATMENT

APPROPRIATE HEALTH CARE
Outpatient

GENERAL MEASURES
• All primary conditions relating to urinary incontinence should be identified and treated specifically (e.g., urinary tract infection, bladder tumors, prostatic hypertrophy)
• Good perineal hygiene
• Pelvic floor (Kegel) exercises
• Biofeedback/behavioral training
• Intermittent catheterization (selected patients)
• Incontinence pads
• Indwelling catheterization (selected patients)
• Condom catheters (male patients)
• Treatment for fecal impaction

SURGICAL MEASURES
• Some patients with overflow incontinence secondary to prostatic hypertrophy may benefit from transurethral resection of the prostate (TURP)
• Some patients with stress incontinence may benefit from bladder suspension procedures

ACTIVITY Full activities should be encouraged

DIET
• No special diet
• In situations where access to bathroom facilities is limited, may want to avoid high volume fluid intake and reduce intake of caffeine or alcohol-containing beverages

PATIENT EDUCATION
• Should be directed at the general problem, as well as any underlying diseases
• Should include instructions regarding good general nutrition and exercise practices
• Rational toileting schedule, based on the patient's pattern of incontinence
• Easy access to toilet facilities
• Pelvic floor (Kegel) exercises
• Bladder training - timed voiding, increasing slowly to 3 hours
• Examples of specific instructions can be found in Clinics in Geriatric Medicine, November, 1986, pages 841-855

MEDICATIONS

DRUG(S) OF CHOICE
• Detrusor instability
  ◊ Oxybutynin (Ditropan) 2.5-5 mg qid
  ◊ Propantheline (Pro-Banthine) 15-30 mg tid
  ◊ Dicyclomine (Bentyl) 10-20 mg qid
  ◊ Flavoxate (Urispas) 100-200 mg tid
  ◊ Imipramine (Tofranil) 25-50 mg tid
• Sphincter incompetence
  ◊ Pseudoephedrine (Sudafed) 30-60 mg tid
  ◊ Phenylpropanolamine (Ornade) 75 mg bid
  ◊ Imipramine (Tofranil) 25-50 mg tid
• Overflow/atonic bladder
  ◊ Bethanechol (Urecholine) 10-30 mg tid
• Overflow/prostatic enlargement
  ◊ Prazosin (Minipress) 1-2 mg tid
  ◊ Finasteride (Proscar) 5 mg q day

Contraindications:
• Should be reviewed for each specific medication prior to initiating
• Anticholinergic agents are contraindicated in patients with glaucoma or prostatic hypertrophy

Precautions:
• Use smallest dose possible in elderly patients
• Common side effects include: Dry mouth, blurred vision, constipation, postural hypotension, mental confusion

Significant possible interactions: Will vary for each of the drugs listed

ALTERNATIVE DRUGS
• Oral or topical estrogens for stress incontinence associated with atrophic vaginitis
• Prostaglandin inhibitors (investigational)
• Calcium antagonists (investigational)
• Desmopressin (DDAVP) nasal spray (nocturnal enuresis)

FOLLOWUP

PATIENT MONITORING
• Biweekly at first (while exercises are being learned and medication dosage is being adjusted)
• Quarterly, once incontinence is under control and medication doses are stable
• Ask about side effects of medication
• Check for orthostatic hypotension
• Consider measuring intraocular pressure in high risk patients
• Periodic urinalysis to detect early urinary tract infection

PREVENTION/AVOIDANCE
• Instruct women in routine use of Kegel exercises after birth of children
• Regular pelvic examination of female patients to detect pelvic pathology
• Regular rectal examination in male patients to pick up early prostatic pathology. Treatment for hypertrophy.

POSSIBLE COMPLICATIONS
• Urinary tract infection
• Hydronephrosis (with atonic bladder or outlet obstruction)
• Renal failure (with obstructive hydronephrosis)
• Adverse drug reactions

EXPECTED COURSE/PROGNOSIS
Prognosis is generally good. Most patients can achieve an increase in bladder control with appropriate medical management.

MISCELLANEOUS

ASSOCIATED CONDITIONS N/A

AGE-RELATED FACTORS
Pediatric: N/A
Geriatric: This problem is most commonly seen in the aging population
Others: N/A

PREGNANCY   Stress incontinence can occur during pregnancy

SYNONYMS
• Transient incontinence
• Urge incontinence
• Overflow incontinence
• Stress incontinence

ICD-9-CM   788.3 Incontinence of urine

SEE ALSO
• Urethritis
• Urinary tract infection in men
• Urinary tract infection in women
• Prostatic hyperplasia, benign (BPH)
• Vulvovaginitis, estrogen deficient

OTHER NOTES N/A

ABBREVIATIONS N/A

REFERENCES
• Hazard W, et al, eds: Principles of Geriatric Medicine and Gerontology. 2nd Ed. New York, McGraw-Hill Co, 1990
• Ouslander JG, ed: Clinics in Geriatric Medicine; 2:4. Philadelphia, W.B. Saunders Co., November, 1986
• Brocklehurs JC, ed: Gerontology; 36/52/90. Basel, Switzerland, S. Karger Publisher, September, 1990
• Houston KA: Clinics in Geriatric Medicine 1993;9(1):157-171
• Davila GW: Urinary incontinence in women: How to help patients regain bladder control. Postgrad Med 1994;96(2):103-109
• Fantl JA, et al: Estrogen therapy in the management of urinary incontinence in postmenopausal women; a meta-analysis. Obstet- Gynecol 1994;83:12-18
• Ramsey SD, et al: Estimated costs of treating stress urinary incontinence in elderly women according to the AHCPR Clinical Practice Guidelines. Am J Manag Care 1996;2(2):147-154
• Mold JW: Pharmacotherapy of urinary incontinence. Am Fam Phys 1996;54(2):673-680
Illustrations: N/A
Internet references: http://www.5mcc.com

Author(s)
Anthony J. Costa, MD

Urinary tract infection in men

BASICS

DESCRIPTION Cystitis is an infection of the lower urinary tract, usually resulting from a single gram-negative enteric bacteria. (See separate chapters for information on prostatitis, pyelonephritis, and non-gonococcal urethritis.)
System(s) affected: Renal/Urologic
Genetics: No specific genetic pattern
Incidence/Prevalence in USA: Not common
Predominant age: Increases with age. Uncommon in men under 50. 8 infections/10,000 men, ages 21-50.
Predominant sex: Male only (for this discussion)

SIGNS AND SYMPTOMS
• Urinary frequency
• Urinary urgency
• Dysuria
• Hesitancy
• Slow urinary stream
• Dribbling of urine
• Nocturia
• Suprapubic discomfort
• Low back pain
• Hematuria
• Systemic symptoms (chills, fever) present with concomitant pyelonephritis or prostatitis

CAUSES
• Escherichia coli (80% of infections)
• Klebsiella
• Enterobacter
• Proteus
• Pseudomonas
• Serratia
• Streptococcus faecalis and Staphylococcus

RISK FACTORS
• Benign prostatic hypertrophy
• Cognitive impairment
• Fecal incontinence
• Urinary incontinence
• Anal intercourse
• Recent urologic surgery, catheterization
• Infection of the prostate or kidney
• Urinary tract instrumentation
• Immunocompromised host
• Outlet obstruction

DIAGNOSIS

DIFFERENTIAL DIAGNOSIS
• Anatomic or functional pathology
• Urethritis
• Infections in other sites of the genitourinary tract (e.g., epididymis)

LABORATORY
• Pyuria
• Bacteriuria
• Urine dipstick leukocyte esterase (75-90%, sensitivity, 95% specificity), and nitrate (35-85% sensitivity, 70% specificity)
• Urine culture - 10/high power colonies of pathogens (or counts > 100,000 bacteria/mL of urine) confirms diagnosis (Escherichia coli, Klebsiella, Pseudomonas, other agents). Lower counts can also be indicative of infection, especially in presence of pyuria.
• Segmented bacteriologic localization cultures
  ◊ VB1 - collect 5-10 mL of urine of patient's initial voiding
  ◊ VB2 - then a sample of sterile midstream urine is obtained
  ◊ EPS - prostatic massage performed, and expressed prostatic secretion is collected from the meatus
  ◊ VB3 - patient completes voiding and 4th sample is collected
  ◊ Cultures and sensitivity collected from each specimen
Drugs that may alter lab results: Antibiotics prior to culture
Disorders that may alter lab results: N/A

PATHOLOGICAL FINDINGS Depends on site of infection

SPECIAL TESTS Urologic investigations necessary to rule out other disorders

IMAGING Intravenous pyelography, cystoscopy, ultrasound

DIAGNOSTIC PROCEDURES Careful history and physical

TREATMENT

APPROPRIATE HEALTH CARE
Outpatient, except for acute illness with toxicity or kidney failure

GENERAL MEASURES
• Hydration and analgesia if required
• Discontinue sexual activity until cured
• Patient with indwelling catheters
  ◊ If asymptomatic bacterial colonization - no need to treat (sterilization of urine not possible and resistant organisms can take up residence)
  ◊ If symptomatic of acute infection - institute treatment

SURGICAL MEASURES N/A

ACTIVITY Activity as tolerated.

DIET No special diet

PATIENT EDUCATION For patient education materials favorably reviewed on this topic, contact: National Kidney Foundation, 30 E. 33rd Street, Suite 1100, New York, NY 10016, (212)889-2210

MEDICATIONS

DRUG(S) OF CHOICE
• Acute UTI , first infection, no risk factors for treatment: 7-10 days of oral antibiotics either empirically or based on cultures and sensitivity results. For empiric therapy, trimethoprim-sulfamethoxazole (SMX-TMP) bid will usually treat the most likely pathogens.
• Complicated or recurrent UTI: 14-21 days of antibiotics based on antimicrobial sensitivities with repeat urine check after treatment
Contraindications: Refer to manufacturer's information
Precautions: Refer to manufacturer's information
Significant possible interactions: Refer to manufacturer's information

ALTERNATIVE DRUGS According to culture and sensitivity results and patient's history

FOLLOWUP

PATIENT MONITORING Close followup until clinically well and repeat urinalysis after treatment

PREVENTION/AVOIDANCE
• Prompt treatment of predisposing factors
• Catheter use only when necessary. If needed, use aseptic technique and closed system, with removal as soon as possible.

POSSIBLE COMPLICATIONS
• Pyelonephritis
• Ascending infection
• Recurrent infection

EXPECTED COURSE/PROGNOSIS
Clearing of infections with appropriate antibiotic treatment

MISCELLANEOUS

ASSOCIATED CONDITIONS
• Acute bacterial pyelonephritis
• Chronic bacterial pyelonephritis
• Urethritis
• Prostatitis
• Prostatic hypertrophy
• Prostate cancer

AGE-RELATED FACTORS
Pediatric: Usually associated with obstruction to normal flow of urine, such as vesicoureteral reflux
Geriatric: Bacteriuria is common in the elderly, appears related to functional status and is usually transient. If asymptomatic bacteriuria is noted, no treatment is needed.
Others: N/A

PREGNANCY N/A

SYNONYMS
• UTI
• Cystitis

ICD-9-CM
• 595 Cystitis
• 595.1 Acute cystitis
• 595.2 Chronic cystitis

SEE ALSO
• Prostatic cancer
• Prostatitis
• Prostatic hyperplasia, benign (BPH)
• Pyelonephritis
• Urethritis

OTHER NOTES N/A

ABBREVIATIONS N/A

REFERENCES
• Lipsky BA: Urinary tract infections in men. Epidemiology, pathophysiology, diagnosis, and treatment. Ann Intern Med 1989;110:138-150
• Finn SD: Urinary tract infections - diagnosis and treatment in women and men. Consultant 1992;10:43-58
• Hooton TM, Stamm WE: Management of acute uncomplicated urinary tract infection in adults. Med Clin of North Am 1991;75(2); 339-57
• Khan AJ, Schaffer HA, Evans H: Urinary tract infections in adolescent boys. J Nat Med A 1996;88(1):25-26
• Hutton J, Hughes M, Raymond CH: Management of bacterial urinary tract infections in adults. Ann Pharm 1994;28(11): 1264-1272
Illustrations: N/A
Internet references: http://www.5mcc.com

Author(s)
Scott A. Fields, MD

Urinary tract infection in women

BASICS

DESCRIPTION Inflammation of the bladder mucosa caused by bacterial infection. This topic refers primarily to infectious cyctitis. Other urinary tract infections are discussed elsewhere.
System(s) affected: Renal/Urologic
Genetics: N/A
Incidence/Prevalence in USA: 3-8% of women have bacteriuria at any given time. 43% of females aged 14-61 have had at least one UTI; 7 million doctor visits a year
Predominant age: Young adults and older
Predominant sex: Female

SIGNS AND SYMPTOMS
• Note: Any or all may be present
• Burning during urination
• Pain during urination
• Urgency (sensation of need to urinate frequently)
• Sensation of incomplete bladder emptying
• Blood in urine
• Lower abdominal pain or cramping

CAUSES Acute infection, usually with gram negative bacteria

RISK FACTORS
• Previous urinary tract infection
• Diabetes mellitus
• Pregnancy
• More frequent or vigorous sexual activity than usual
• Use of spermicides or diaphragm
• Underlying abnormalities of the urinary tract such as tumors, calculi, strictures, incomplete bladder emptying, etc.

DIAGNOSIS

DIFFERENTIAL DIAGNOSIS
• Vaginitis
• Sexually transmitted diseases causing urethritis or pyuria
• Hematuria from causes other than infection (e.g., neoplasia, calculi)
• Psychological dysfunction

LABORATORY
• Urinalysis demonstrating pyuria (more than 5-8 neutrophils per high power field on microscopic exam). Leukocyte esterase dipsticks also useful for detecting pyuria but fail to detect pyuria in up to 25% of patients, and false positives occur from vaginal leukocytes.
• Urinalysis demonstrating bacteriuria (any amount). Nitrate dipsticks also useful but fail to detect bacteriuria in 10-30 percent of patients.
• Urine culture demonstrating growth of single type of bacteria. Suspect contaminated specimen when culture shows multiple types of bacteria.
Drugs that may alter lab results: N/A
Disorders that may alter lab results: N/A

PATHOLOGICAL FINDINGS   N/A

SPECIAL TESTS   N/A

IMAGING
• For all infants and may be indicated for older patients with recurrent infections:
   ◊ Radiographic, ultrasound, and/or endoscopic imaging of upper and lower urinary tract
   ◊ Voiding cystourethrogram and ultrasound evaluation of the urinary tract

DIAGNOSTIC PROCEDURES
• Suprapubic bladder aspiration or urethral catheterization to obtain urine specimen from infants
• Urethral catheterization to obtain urine specimen from children and adults if voided urine suspected of being contaminated
• Classic symptoms in non-pregnant young adult female with first episode of UTI require no urine culture for diagnosis. Obtain urinalysis and culture in other age groups, if repeat episode, if pregnant, or if symptoms not classic.
• Some recent research suggests the most cost-effective approach is empiric treatment without lab tests in non-pregnant premenopausal women with symptoms of UTI

TREATMENT

APPROPRIATE HEALTH CARE
Outpatient, except for complicated or upper tract infections

GENERAL MEASURES
• Maintain good hydration
• One-fourth of women with simple UTI experience a second UTI within six months. Patients with multiple recurrent UTI and no underlying urinary tract abnormality may receive long-term prophylactic antibiotic treatment. Trimethoprim-sulfamethoxazole and nitrofurantoin commonly used.
• Patients with chronic indwelling urinary catheters always have infections that should not be treated unless symptomatic with fever, sepsis, or other systemic symptoms.

SURGICAL MEASURES   N/A

ACTIVITY   Avoid sexual intercourse when symptoms present

DIET   No special diet

PATIENT EDUCATION
• Take antibiotic as directed
• Return if symptoms not resolved or markedly improved within 48 hours
• Return if fever, chills, or flank pain develop

Urinary tract infection in women

MEDICATIONS

DRUG(S) OF CHOICE
• First UTI

In adolescents and adults who are non-pregnant, non-diabetic, afebrile, non-immunocompromised patients who have no abnormality of the urinary tract: 3 day treatment with trimethoprim-sulfamethoxazole (TMP-SMX) or fluoroquinolone

◊ Rare or infrequent uncomplicated UTI

In non-pregnant, non-diabetic, afebrile, non-immunocompromised patients who have no abnormality of the urinary tract: 3 days of TMP/SMX or fluoroquinolone

• Postcoital

Postcoital treatment with single-dose TMP/SMX or cephalexin may reduce frequency of UTI in sexually active women

• Pregnant patients

10-14 day treatment with pregnancy-safe antibiotic chosen based on culture/sensitivity results. May begin with cephalosporin, amoxicillin, or other antibiotic while awaiting culture/sensitivity results.

• All other patients

10-14 day treatment with antibiotic chosen based on culture/sensitivity results. May begin with fluoroquinolone, TMP/SMX, cephalosporin or other antibiotic while awaiting culture/sensitivity results.

Contraindications: Refer to manufacturer's literature. Fluoroquinolones not safe during pregnancy. TMP/SMX use in pregnancy not desirable, but appropriate is some circumstances.

Precautions: Refer to manufacturer's literature

Significant possible interactions: Refer to manufacturer's literature

ALTERNATIVE DRUGS
Change antibiotic if indicated by culture/sensitivity results

FOLLOWUP

PATIENT MONITORING
• First or rare UTI: In young or middle-age, non pregnant adult female requires no followup if patient cured after single dose therapy. If not resolved within two to three days after single dose therapy, obtain culture/sensitivity and change antibiotic accordingly.
• All other patients should have post-treatment urine culture to document eradication of infection

PREVENTION/AVOIDANCE
• Maintain good hydration
• Women with frequent or intercourse-related UTI should empty bladder immediately before and following intercourse and consider postcoital antibiotic treatment

POSSIBLE COMPLICATIONS
• Pyelonephritis
• Renal abscess

EXPECTED COURSE/PROGNOSIS
Symptoms resolve within 2-3 days after starting treatment in almost all patients

MISCELLANEOUS

ASSOCIATED CONDITIONS
Described under Risk Factors

AGE-RELATED FACTORS
Pediatric: Infants and young children at higher risk of pyelonephritis
Geriatric:
• Elderly may have bacteriuria without symptoms; generally does not require treatment if urinary tract otherwise normal
• Elderly more apt to have underlying urinary tract abnormality
• Acute UTI often associated with incontinence in the elderly
Others: N/A

PREGNANCY
UTI during pregnancy always requires culture/sensitivity and usually requires 10-14 day treatment. Limited data suggest that single dose or three-day treatment may be effective in some women. Following treatment of acute infection, pregnant women often receive prophylactic antibiotics for the remainder of pregnancy.

SYNONYMS
Cystitis

ICD-9-CM
• 595 Cystitis
• 595.1 Acute cystitis
• 595.2 Chronic cystitis

SEE ALSO
Pyelonephritis

OTHER NOTES
N/A

ABBREVIATIONS
TMP/SMX = trimethoprim-sulfamethoxazole

REFERENCES
• Stapleton MD, Latham RH, Johnson CJ, Stam W: Postcoital antimicrobial prophylaxis for recurrent urinary tract infection. JAMA 1990;264:703-706
• Stamm WE, Hooton T: Management of urinary tract infections in adults. New Eng J Med 1993;329:1328-1334
• Barry HG, Ebell MH, Hickner J: Evaluation of suspected urinary tract infection in ambulatory women: a cost-utility analysis of office-based strategies. J of Fam Prac 1997;44:49-60
Illustrations: N/A
Internet references: http://www.5mcc.com

Author(s)
Barry D. Weiss, MD

Urolithiasis

BASICS

DESCRIPTION The state describing the presence of calculi within the urinary system. Commonly known as kidney stones.
System(s) affected: Renal/Urologic
Genetics: Familial tendency
Incidence/Prevalence in USA: 70-210 in 100,000 population. 2%-5% of population in lifetime.
Predominant age: Peak 20-30. Range 20-60.
Predominant sex: Male > Female (4:1)

SIGNS AND SYMPTOMS
- Usually sudden onset
- Severe agonizing pain, costovertebral angle to groin depending on stone location
- Patient in constant motion, no comfort
- Nausea with or without vomiting
- Diaphoresis
- Tachycardia
- Intestinal ileus
- Abdominal guarding and rebound (rare)
- Tenderness to deep abdominal palpation, usually at CVA
- Lower tract stone with frequency, urgency, dysuria
- Fever, with infection
- Hematuria
- Pyuria, with infection
- May be asymptomatic if stone stays within kidney

CAUSES
- Calcium oxalate/calcium phosphate 65%-85%
  ◊ Supersaturation from any cause
  ◊ Dehydration
  ◊ Increased absorption
  ◊ Increased calcium excretion - familial
  ◊ Renal tubular acidosis
  ◊ Hyperparathyroidism
  ◊ Chronic bowel disease with absorptive disorders
  ◊ Poor GI citrate absorption
  ◊ Excessive oral vitamin D or C
  ◊ Alkaline urinary pH
  ◊ Chronic use of calcium antacids
  ◊ Diet high in calcium or oxalate
  ◊ Malignancy
- Struvite (staghorn calculus) 15%-20%
  ◊ Infection
  ◊ Alkaline urine
- Uric acid 5%
  ◊ Hereditary
  ◊ Gout
  ◊ Chronic bowel disease
  ◊ High purine diet
  ◊ Acidic urine, very low pH
  ◊ Malignancy with chemotherapy
- Cystine 1%-3%
  ◊ Hereditary homocystinuria

RISK FACTORS
- Family history
- Climate, hot
- Work in hot environment
- Poor fluid consumption
- Diet high in oxalate, purine, calcium
- Excessive vitamins
- Malignancy
- Sarcoidosis
- Gout
- Thiazide diuretics
- Bowel or kidney disease

DIAGNOSIS

DIFFERENTIAL DIAGNOSIS
- Pyelonephritis
- Clot or sloughed papillae (secondary to diabetes, infection, analgesic abuse)
- Drug-seeking addiction
- Acute abdomen
- Gynecological problems
- Diverticulitis

LABORATORY
- Urinalysis: Hematuria nearly 100%; if pH < 5.5 means uric acid, if pH > 7.5 means struvite
- Chemistries: Calcium, phosphorus, electrolytes, uric acid, creatinine
- Parathyroid hormone: If serum calcium high
- Urine cystine: If stone not visible on plain x-ray
- Urine culture: If pyuria or fever
Drugs that may alter lab results: Pyridium may alter urinalysis
Disorders that may alter lab results: See Causes and Risk Factors

PATHOLOGICAL FINDINGS Stone analysis: 60-80% calcium base, 15-20% struvite, 5% uric acid, 1-3% cystine

SPECIAL TESTS Stone analysis

IMAGING
- Plain kidney, ureter and bladder (KUB) x-ray: 80%-90% visible with some calcium
- Intravenous pyelogram (IVP): Primary study for urolithiasis
- Ultrasound: Technique varies, if good has equal sensitivity and specificity to IVP

DIAGNOSTIC PROCEDURES Retrograde pyelogram, if necessary

TREATMENT

APPROPRIATE HEALTH CARE 80% outpatient only, most will pass in 48 hours. 20% hospitalization and urology referral.

GENERAL MEASURES
- Reassurance
- Strain urine
- Hydration
- Pain control
- Refer to urologist for: Intractable pain, obstruction, size > 6 mm, infection, dehydration, failure to progress, stone growth, single kidney, persistent gross hematuria, pregnancy, severe renal disease

SURGICAL MEASURES
- Extracorporeal shock wave lithotripsy: Stone in renal pelvis or upper 2/3 ureter, size < 2 cm, noninfected, no coagulopathy
- Urethroscopy: Lower 1/3 ureter, normal anatomy present
- Percutaneous nephrolithotomy: Renal collecting system or upper 2/3 ureter, size > 2 cm, ureter stricture, cystine or uric acid stones, struvite, infection, obesity
- Open surgery: Less than 5% of patients, complex anatomy, obstruction, large infected struvite stone

ACTIVITY Bedrest, if necessary during acute phase. No restrictions after stone passes.

DIET
- Normal diet, 8 oz. water every 1 hour while awake, and if possible every 2 hours during sleep hours
- If uric acid stones, less protein in diet and take sodium bicarbonate to alkalinize urine

PATIENT EDUCATION
- Instructions on urine straining, dietary advice
- See Patient Care, August 15, 1990, p.42

MEDICATIONS

DRUG(S) OF CHOICE
• Acute therapy:
◊ Pain control (in office) - IM meperidine (Demerol) or morphine or buprenorphine (Buprenex), etc.
◊ 3 day supply pain control - oxycodone-acetaminophen (Percocet), pentazocine (Talwin), hydrocodone-acetaminophen (Vicodin), etc.
◊ Uric acid stone - potassium citrate (Urocit-K), 60-80 mEq/d (30-40 mmol/d) to keep urine pH 6.5-7.0. Check urine pH qid.
◊ Cystine stone - penicillamine (Cuprimine, Depen) 1-4 g/d, K-citrate (Urocit-K) 60 mEq/d (30 mmol/d)
◊ Infected stones - antibiotics for complicated pyelonephritis
• Maintenance therapy:
◊ Hypercalciuria - sodium cellulose phosphate 10-15 g/d (2.5-5.0 grams with each meal), hydrochlorothiazide (HCTZ) 50 mg bid, K-citrate 15-20 mEq (7.5-10 mmol) bid
◊ Uric acid - allopurinol (Zyloprim) 300 mg/d, K-citrate 20-30 mEq bid
◊ Cystine - K-citrate 30 mEq (15 mmol) bid, penicillamine 1-4 g/d
Contraindications: Penicillamine with pregnancy, renal failure, aplastic anemia, hypersensitivity reaction
Precautions: Penicillamine requires regular CBC with differential counts, urinalysis, liver function tests
Significant possible interactions: Refer to manufacturer's profile of each drug

ALTERNATIVE DRUGS
Individualize to any underlying metabolic etiology found

FOLLOWUP

PATIENT MONITORING
• Acute urolithiasis:
◊ Strain urine until stone or 72 hours after symptoms cease
◊ Repeat urinalysis 2-3 days
◊ Repeat KUB x-ray and or IVP/ultrasound if no stone passed
◊ Stone analysis
◊ KUB x-ray at 3-6 months and at 1 year, if no new stone, then no further followup needed
• Recurrent urolithiasis:
◊ 24 hour urine: volume, pH, calcium, phosphorus, sodium, uric acid, oxalate, citrate, creatinine clearance
◊ Measure parathyroid hormone (PTH)
◊ Calcium restricted diet test for urine calcium level

PREVENTION/AVOIDANCE
Hydration with urine > 2 liters a day (including nocturia once nightly). Dietary calcium < 1 g/d.

POSSIBLE COMPLICATIONS
• Hydronephrosis or kidney damage
• Infection and sepsis

EXPECTED COURSE/PROGNOSIS
80% will pass in 48-72 hours with outpatient therapy, 60% no recurrence at 10 years

MISCELLANEOUS

ASSOCIATED CONDITIONS
See Causes section

AGE-RELATED FACTORS
Pediatric: Homocystinuria or other hereditary disorder
Geriatric: N/A
Others: N/A

PREGNANCY
Urology referral

SYNONYMS
• Nephrolithiasis
• Kidney stone
• Renal colic

ICD-9-CM
592.9 Urinary calculus, unspecified

SEE ALSO
Renal calculi

OTHER NOTES
N/A

ABBREVIATIONS
KUB = kidney, ureter and bladder
IVP = intravenous pyelogram
HCTZ = hydrochlorothiazide

REFERENCES
• NIH Consensus Development Conference on Prevention and Treatment of Kidney Stones. J of Urology 1989;141;3(2):705-804
• O'Brien WM, Rotolo JE, Pahirz JJ: New Approaches in the Treatment of Renal Calculi. AFP 198736(5):181-194
• Coe FL, Parks JH, Asplin JR: The pathogenis and treatment of kidney stones. New Eng J Med 1992327(46):1141-1152
Illustrations: N/A
Internet references: http://www.5mcc.com

Author(s)
William H. Billica, MD

Urticaria

BASICS

DESCRIPTION Itchy rash. Single or multiple superficial raised pale macules with red halo. Subside rapidly; no scars or change in pigmentation. May be recurrent.
• Acute urticaria
◊ Response to many stimuli
◊ IgE-mediated histamine release from mast cells
◊ Sometimes idiosyncratic response to drug exposure
◊ Subsides over several hours
• Chronic urticaria: Persists > 6 weeks (30% of cases). Not mediated by IgE. Multiple types:
◊ Cold urticaria - from cooling, rewarming. Can be fatal (cold immersion with massive histamine release). Also a familial form with fever, chills, arthralgia, myalgia, headache, lymphocytosis.
◊ Cholinergic urticaria - heat urticaria. Small (5-10 mm) wheals on upper trunk from overheating, hot shower
◊ Exercise-induced urticaria - from extreme exercise; presents as cholinergic urticaria, angioedema, wheezing, hypotension. Often associated with eating food to which patient is allergic.
◊ Dermatographism - linear wheal and flare resulting from scratching the skin
◊ Solar urticaria - result of exposure to sunlight. Several types, by wavelength of light which induces reaction. Majority react to ultraviolet. Onset in minutes; subsides in 1-2 hours.
◊ Delayed pressure urticaria - occurs 4-6 hours after pressure to skin (elastic, shoes, etc.)
◊ Aquagenic urticaria - rare. Small wheals after contact with water at any temperature.
• Idiopathic urticaria
◊ Acute or chronic
System(s) affected: Skin/Exocrine
Genetics: No consistent genetic pattern known
Incidence/Prevalence in USA: 1 in 1000. Affects 15-20% of population at some time during life.
Predominant age: All ages. Acute form mainly in children, young adults.
Predominant sex: Male = Female (chronic forms more often in older women)

SIGNS AND SYMPTOMS
• Seen alone or with angioedema
• May occur with generalized anaphylactic reaction, potentially fatal
• Single or multiple raised, blanched, central wheals surrounded by red flare
• Intensely pruritic
• May occur anywhere on body
• Variably sized, 1-2 mm to 15-20 cm or larger; sometimes confluent
• Rapid onset, resolves spontaneously in less than 48 hours

CAUSES
• Allergic or non-allergic; massive histamine release from mast cells in superficial dermis
• Drug reaction (any drug) either from allergy or idiosyncrasy
• Aspirin, NSAID's seem to trigger by inhibiting cyclo-oxygenase, without IgE
• Food or food additive allergy
• Inhalant, contact, or ingestant allergy
• Transfusion reaction
• Insect bite, sting
• Infection - bacterial, viral (infectious mononucleosis, hepatitis), fungal, helminthic
• Collagen vascular disease (cutaneous vasculitis, serum sickness, lupus)
• Physical trauma (heat, cold, sunlight, etc.)
• Emotional stress (reported; little supporting evidence)
• Histamine-releasing autoantibodies have been identified in some cases of chronic idiopathic urticaria

RISK FACTORS Listed with Causes

DIAGNOSIS

DIFFERENTIAL DIAGNOSIS
• Insect bites
• Morbilliform drug eruptions
• Erythema multiforme
• Vasculitis and polyarteritis
• Systemic lupus erythematosus
• Urticaria pigmentosa (mastocytosis). Pink lesions urticate when scratched (Darier's sign).
• Bullous pemphigoid (urticarial stage)

LABORATORY
• Cause found in 10-25% of chronic cases
• Food and drug reactions - elimination diets, challenges with suspected agents
• Inhalant allergens - skin tests, radioallergosorbent (RAST)
• Idiopathic for > 6 weeks - CBC, skin biopsy, ESR, urinalysis, ANA
Drugs that may alter lab results:
Antihistamines, H2-blockers, tricyclic antidepressants
Disorders that may alter lab results: N/A

PATHOLOGICAL FINDINGS Edema, vasculitis and/or perivasculitis involving only superficial dermis

SPECIAL TESTS
• Cold urticaria - ice cube test (place ice cube on skin 5 minutes, observe 10-15 minutes)
• Cholinergic or exercise-induced: exercise challenge; methacholine skin test (local reaction to 0.01 mg in 0.05 ml saline intradermally. 50% false negatives).
• Dermatographism - scratch skin with piece of tongue blade, observe
• Solar - expose to defined wavelengths of light. Must rule out erythropoietic protoporphyria.
• Delayed pressure: apply 5-10 pound sandbag for 3 hours, observe
• Aquagenic - apply tap water at different temperatures
• Vibratory: apply vibration 4-5 minutes with a lab mixing device, observe
• Infection - pharyngeal culture, antistreptolysin (ASO) titer, rapid plasma reagin (RPR), parasitology, liver function tests, mononucleosis test
• Autoimmune - antinuclear antibody (ANA), rheumatoid arthritis (RA), complement, cryoglobulins, serum protein electrophoresis

IMAGING N/A

DIAGNOSTIC PROCEDURES Skin biopsy (correlates poorly with clinical picture)

TREATMENT

APPROPRIATE HEALTH CARE Don't work up acute cases (results usually inconclusive)

GENERAL MEASURES Cool moist compresses help to control itching

SURGICAL MEASURES N/A

ACTIVITY As desired. Avoid overheating.

DIET As desired. Avoid foods implicated as possible etiologic agents.

PATIENT EDUCATION Avoidance if etiology is apparent. Antihistamines if accidentally re-exposed.

MEDICATIONS

DRUG(S) OF CHOICE
• First generation antihistamines
  ◊ Older children and adults: hydroxyzine or diphenhydramine, 25-50 mg q6h
  ◊ Children under six: diphenhydramine 12.5 mg (elixir) q6-8h (5 mg/kg/day)
• Second generation H1 blockers are more expensive, about as effective as older antihistamines, but are less sedating (14% of patients, still less than 1st generation drugs), because they do not cross the blood-brain barrier.
  ◊ Terfenadine (Seldane) 60 mg bid or fexofenadine (Allegra) if Seldane not available
  ◊ Astemizole (Hismanal) 10 mg daily. Longest onset of action (3-4 days, so is not helpful for acute reactions), but has the longest duration of action; over 24 hours. This makes it good for chronic problems. Loading dose: 30mg on day 1, 20 mg on day 2, then 10 mg daily.
  ◊ Loratadine (Claritin) 10 mg daily
  ◊ Acrivastine (Semprex) 8 mg TID
  ◊ Cetirizine (Zyrtec)10 mg daily. More sedating than others in this class.
Contraindications: Danazol not for use in childhood, pregnancy.
Precautions:
• Drowsiness with first generation drugs
• Use caution when giving astemizole to patients in who metabolism may be delayed
• Second generation H1 blockers should be used with caution in pregnancy and the elderly
Significant possible interactions: Do not give astemizcle (Hismanal) or terfenadine (Seldane) to patients taking other inhibitors of the cytochrome P450 enzyme system (macrolides, ketoconazole, cimetidine, etc), because of a potential for cardiac arrhythmia induction (torsade de pointes)

ALTERNATIVE DRUGS
• Doxepin (Sinequan), tricyclic antidepressant with strong H1 and H2 blocking properties
• H2-blockers (cimetidine, ranitidine, etc.) may be helpful in chronic urticaria
• Corticosteroids for unresponsive cases (not acutely), e.g., prednisone 40 mg daily for 5-7 days, followed by taper

FOLLOWUP

PATIENT MONITORING
No followup for initial episode. Evaluate if symptoms persist or recur.

PREVENTION/AVOIDANCE
If etiology identified, avoidance is best solution

POSSIBLE COMPLICATIONS
Severe systemic allergic reaction (bronchospasm, anaphylaxis)

EXPECTED COURSE/PROGNOSIS
70% better in < 72 hours. 30% chronic. 20% have attacks for > 20 years. Becomes chronic in 75% of patients with both urticaria and angioedema.

MISCELLANEOUS

ASSOCIATED CONDITIONS
Angioedema, anaphylaxis

AGE-RELATED FACTORS
Pediatric: Acute isolated incidents are more frequent, chronic urticaria is rare
Geriatric: Less likely to occur in this age group
Others: N/A

PREGNANCY
Chronic urticaria

SYNONYMS
Hives

ICD-9-CM
708.8 Other specified urticaria

SEE ALSO
• Anaphylaxis
• Angioedema

OTHER NOTES
Same pathophysiology for urticaria and angioedema - localized anaphylaxis causes vasodilatation, vascular permeability of skin (urticaria) or subcutaneous tissue (angioedema)

ABBREVIATIONS
N/A

REFERENCES
• Lockey RF, Bukantz SC: Principles of Immunology and Allergy. Philadelphia, W.B. Saunders Co., 1987
• Cooper KD: Urticaria and angioedema: Diagnosis and evaluation. J Am Acad Dermatol 1991;25(1):166
• Monroe EW: Nonsedating H1 antihistamines in chronic urticaria. Ann Allergy 1993;71:585-91
• Woosley R, Darrow WR: Analysis of potential adverse drug reactions - a case of mistaken identity. Amer J Cardiol 1994;74:208-209
Illustrations: 8 available on CD-ROM
Internet references: http://www.5mcc.com

Author(s)
John E. Perchalski, MD, FAAFP

Uterine corpus malignancy

BASICS

DESCRIPTION
• Endometrial cancer: Malignancy of the endometrial lining of the uterus. Tumor grade - low, moderate, high. Cell types - adenocarcinoma, adenosquamous (benign or malignant squamous elements), clear cell, papillary serous.
• Sarcomas:
 ◊ Mixed müllerian sarcoma - heterologous elements not native to the müllerian systems, such as cartilage or bone; homologous elements native to the mullerian system
 ◊ Endometrial stromal sarcoma develops from the stromal component of the endometrium
 ◊ Leiomyosarcoma develops in the myometrium or in a myoma (fibroid)
System(s) affected: Reproductive
Genetics: Unknown
Incidence/Prevalence in USA: Most common gynecologic malignancy, 35,000 new cases per year
Predominant age:
• Endometrial cancer - postmenopausal (mid fifties to mid sixties). Also can occur in young women in their twenties and thirties with polycystic ovarian disease or chronic anovulation.
• Sarcomas - forties to sixties
Predominant sex: Female only

SIGNS AND SYMPTOMS
• Endometrial cancer:
 ◊ Postmenopausal bleeding is the most frequent sign. Any spotting should lead to evaluation.
 ◊ Pap smear is rarely positive
 ◊ Occasionally a patient will pass tissue that will render a diagnosis
• Sarcoma:
 ◊ Mixed müllerian sarcoma - bleeding and prolapsing tissue
 ◊ Leiomyosarcoma - increasing size of presumed uterine myomas
 ◊ D&C rarely diagnostic

CAUSES
• Unopposed estrogen due to:
 ◊ Polycystic ovarian disease
 ◊ Obesity
 ◊ Chronic anovulation
 ◊ Estrogen replacement therapy. (Estrogen replacement without concomitant progesterone increases the risk 70 times. When progesterone is added the risk does not decrease to zero but decreases to that of the population in general).
• Tamoxifen. Increases risk similar to that for unopposed estrogen.
• Sarcomas:
 ◊ Etiology unknown

RISK FACTORS
• Early menarche
• Late menopause
• Nulliparity
• Hypertension and diabetes are probably associated with underlying obesity

DIAGNOSIS

DIFFERENTIAL DIAGNOSIS
• Atypical complex hyperplasia (a premalignant lesion of the endometrium)
• Bleeding from cervical cancer
• Ovarian cancer invading the uterus
• Adenocarcinoma of the cervix
• Endometriosis

LABORATORY
• Liver function tests
• CA-125 can be elevated when intra-abdominal disease is present
Drugs that may alter lab results: N/A
Disorders that may alter lab results: A biopsy of a pregnant uterus can produce tissue which has a hyperplastic or premalignant appearance

PATHOLOGICAL FINDINGS
• Stage I
 ◊ A. Confined to endometrium
 ◊ B. Less than 50% myometrial invasion
 ◊ C. More than 50% myometrial invasion
• Stage II
 ◊ A. Endocervical involvement (microscopic)
 ◊ B. Cervical stromal invasion (macroscopic)
• Stage III
 ◊ A. Uterine serosal/adnexal involvement/positive peritoneal cytology
 ◊ B. Vaginal metastases
 ◊ C. Involved pelvic/para aortic lymph nodes
• Stage IV
 ◊ A. Extension to involve the mucosa of the bladder or rectum
 ◊ B. Distant metastatic disease or inguinal node involvement
• Stages are also subgrouped according to histologic grade:
 ◊ GI - Well differentiated
 ◊ G2 - Moderately differentiated
 ◊ G3 - Poorly differentiated

SPECIAL TESTS   Any that may be indicated preoperatively

IMAGING
• Chest x-ray - the most common site of metastases is the lungs. Rarely does this malignancy go to the bone or the liver except in advanced disease.
• CT scan, bone scan, liver spleen scan - not part of the routine evaluation, but may be needed occasionally
• Mammogram (endometrial cancer is associated with breast cancer)
• Barium enema (endometrial cancer is associated with colon cancer)
• MRI has been reported to accurately show the depth of myometrial penetration, but this is not always cost-effective
• Vaginal ultrasound can show increased endometrial echoes prior to D & C which will lead to the diagnosis

DIAGNOSTIC PROCEDURES
• Office endometrial biopsy (90% accurate). If this is negative, a D & C is necessary. Endometrial stromal sarcoma and leiomyosarcoma are rarely diagnosed preoperatively.
• D & C (99% accurate)

TREATMENT

APPROPRIATE HEALTH CARE   Inpatient surgery

GENERAL MEASURES
• Radiation is used to prevent the recurrence of tumor at the vaginal cuff
• When distant metastatic disease occurs, progesterone produces a 30% response rate. Active chemotherapeutic agents are cisplatin and Adriamycin.

SURGICAL MEASURES
• Surgical procedure is abdominal exploration with extrafascial total abdominal hysterectomy, bilateral salpingo-oophorectomy, cytology, pelvic and para-aortic node sampling
• Surgery is followed by radiation therapy in high-risk patients who have Stage 1B disease or greater, or for patients with poorly differentiated tumors regardless of stage. There is no adjuvant therapy that has been shown to be effective after surgery and radiation.

ACTIVITY   Patients are usually ambulatory and able to resume full activity by six weeks after surgery

DIET   Unrestricted unless they are undergoing radiation

PATIENT EDUCATION
• The American Cancer Society in the local community
• American College of Obstetricians & Gynecologists (ACOG), 409 12th St., SW, Washington, DC 20024-2188, (800)762-ACOG

MEDICATIONS

DRUG(S) OF CHOICE
• There are no drugs as adjuvant therapy
• Premalignant lesions in young women or in patients unsuitable for hysterectomy can be treated with megestrol (Megace), 160 mg qd x 3 months. This is followed by repeat D & C to ascertain whether the hyperplasia has resolved.
• Metastatic disease is treated with high dose progesterone, or doxorubicin (Adriamycin) or cisplatin

Contraindications:
• Progestational agents can cause significant fluid retention in 5-10% of patients
• Patients with congestive heart failure must be observed closely

Precautions: Usual precautions with chemotherapeutic agents. Refer to manufacturer's profile of each drug.

Significant possible interactions: Refer to manufacturer's profile of each drug

ALTERNATIVE DRUGS
• Ondansetron (Zofran), dronabinol (Marinol), metoclopramide (Reglan), and others for nausea control

FOLLOWUP

PATIENT MONITORING
• Pap smear every 3 months for two years, then every 6 months for 3 years
• Chest x-ray once a year

PREVENTION/AVOIDANCE
• In young women who are obese or anovulatory, endometrial cancer can be reduced by cyclic progesterone to prevent unopposed estrogen or by taking birth control pills
• Estrogen replacement therapy should always include progestational agents unless the woman has undergone hysterectomy

POSSIBLE COMPLICATIONS
Those attendant upon major abdominal surgery

EXPECTED COURSE/PROGNOSIS
Five year survival is based on stage and tumor grade

Grade	5 yr survival (%)
IAG1	98
IBG2	85
ICG3	60
IIA/B	60
III	40
IV	15

MISCELLANEOUS

ASSOCIATED CONDITIONS
• Obese patients with endometrial cancer should be screened annually because of increased risk of breast and colon cancer
• Patients who have breast or colon cancer are at increased risk for endometrial cancer. Granulosa cell tumors of the ovary produce estrogen and these patients will have an increased risk of endometrial cancer.

AGE-RELATED FACTORS
Pediatric: N/A
Geriatric: Older (especially obese) patients may be at high risk for surgery. Alternative radiation therapy can be considered.
Others: If preserving fertility is desired - young anovulatory women, polycystic ovarian patients with atypical complex hyperplasia, or patients with well differentiated endometrial cancer can be treated with progestational agents x 3 months followed by D&C

PREGNANCY This malignancy is not associated with pregnancy

SYNONYMS
• Uterine cancer
• Endometrial cancer
• Corpus cancer

ICD-9-CM
• 182.0 Malignant neoplasm of body of uterus, corpus uteri, except isthmus
• 182.8 Malignant neoplasm of body of uterus, other specified sites of body of uterus
• 182.1 Malignant neoplasm of body of uterus, isthmus
• 180.0 Malignant neoplasm of body of cervix uteri, endocervix

SEE ALSO
Cervical malignancy

OTHER NOTES N/A

ABBREVIATIONS N/A

REFERENCES
Hopkins MP: Benign and Malignant Diseases of the Uterus. In: Willson JR, ed. Obstetrics and Gynecology. St. Louis, Mosby Year Book, 1991
Illustrations: N/A
Internet references: http://www.5mcc.com

Author(s)
Michael P. Hopkins, MD
Eric L. Jenison, MD

Uterine myomas

BASICS

DESCRIPTION Uterine leiomyomas are well circumscribed, pseudo-encapsulated benign tumors composed mainly of smooth muscle but with varying amounts of fibrous connective tissue
• Three major types:
◊ Submucous: 5% of total, susceptible to abnormal uterine bleeding, infection and occasionally protrude from cervix
◊ Subserous: Common, may become pedunculated and rarely parasitic
◊ Intramural: Common, may cause marked uterine enlargement
System(s) affected: Reproductive
Genetics: N/A
Incidence/Prevalence in USA: 4-11% of all women, 20% of all women over 35 years of age and 40% of women over 50 years of age
Predominant age: Fourth and fifth decades
Predominant sex: Female only

SIGNS AND SYMPTOMS
• Majority are asymptomatic and are only suspected from pelvic examination
• Most common symptom is abnormal uterine bleeding. Hypermenorrhea most common. Secondary anemia with associated symptomatology may result.
• Pressure on bladder may result in suprapubic discomfort, urinary frequency
• Pressure on rectosigmoid may result in low back pain
• Edema and varicosities of the lower extremities may result from large tumors
• Pain may result from twisted, pedunculated myomas or degenerating, hemorrhagic or infected myomas
• Sterility may result from submucous myomas or with distortion of uterine cavity
• Rapid growth particularly in perimenopausal or postmenopausal may indicate sarcoma

CAUSES
• May arise from totipotential cells normally giving rise to muscle and connective tissue cells
• May arise from small immature smooth muscle cell nests
• Positive correlation with estrogen stimulation, i.e., not seen before menarche, may grow rapidly during pregnancy, with use of oral estrogen, and with estrogen producing tumors. Myomas regress following pregnancy and after menopause.

RISK FACTORS
• Later reproductive and perimenopausal age groups
• 3-9 times higher among African-Americans

DIAGNOSIS

DIFFERENTIAL DIAGNOSIS
• Intrauterine pregnancy
• Ovarian tumor
• Cecal or sigmoid tumor
• Appendiceal abscess
• Diverticulitis
• Pelvic kidney
• Urachal cyst

LABORATORY
• Pregnancy test
• CBC, differential count
• SED rate
• CA-125 - may be slightly elevated in some cases of uterine myomas, but generally is more useful in differentiating myomas from various gynecologic adenocarcinomas
Drugs that may alter lab results: N/A
Disorders that may alter lab results: N/A

PATHOLOGICAL FINDINGS
• Myomas are usually multiple and vary in size and location. Have been reported up to 100 pounds (45 kg).
• Gross pathology reveals firm tumors with characteristic whorl-like trabeculated appearance. A thin psuedocapsular layer is present.
• Microscopic appearance reveals bundles of smooth muscle mixed with varying amounts of connective tissue elements running in different directions
• Cellular variant has a preponderance of muscle cells. Mitoses are rare.
• May undergo various types of degeneration:
◊ I - Hyaline degeneration. Very common, eventually results in liquefaction and cyst formation.
◊ II - Calcification. Late result of circulatory impairment to myomas.
◊ III - Infection and suppuration. Submucous myomas most prone to infection and may lead to sepsis.
◊ IV - Necrosis. Pedunculated subserous fibroids most prone to necrosis secondary to torsion.
◊ V - Sarcomatous change. Incidence ranges from 1.0 to 0.1% of clinically apparent myomas.

SPECIAL TESTS N/A

IMAGING
• Ultrasonography shows characteristic hypoechoic appearance
• CT scan, MRI may help to differentiate complex cases
• Intravenous pyelogram (IVP)
• Barium enema

DIAGNOSTIC PROCEDURES
• Presumptive diagnosis by abdominal and pelvic examination: Firm, smooth nodules or masses arising from uterus. Masses are mobile without pain.
• Fractional D & C aids in ruling out cervical, uterine carcinomas
• Hysteroscopy may help diagnose submucous myomas
• Laparoscopy may be useful in complex cases and in ruling out other pelvic pathology

TREATMENT

APPROPRIATE HEALTH CARE
Outpatient usually; inpatient for some surgical procedures

GENERAL MEASURES
• Treatment must be individualized
• Patients with minimal symptoms may be managed with iron preparations and analgesics
• Conservative management: Asymptomatic myomas of less than 14 weeks' size gestation should be closely observed with pelvic examinations and ultrasonography at 3-6 month intervals, as long as size stable. Usually regress after menopause.
• Luteinizing hormone releasing hormone (LHRH) agonists induce an abrupt artificial menopause with cessation of bleeding and shrinkage of myomas. Not recommended for more than six months. May be useful in perimenopausal patients or as an adjunct in preparation for surgery.

SURGICAL MEASURES
• Surgical management is indicated in the following situations:
◊ Excessive uterine size (> 14 weeks gestation) or excessive rate of growth (except during pregnancy)
◊ Submucous location if associated with hypermenorrhea
◊ Pedunculated myomas may undergo torsion, pain, necrosis and hemorrhage
◊ Symptomatic from pressure on bladder or rectum
◊ If differentiation from ovarian mass is not possible
◊ If there is associated pelvic disease, i.e., endometriosis, pelvic inflammatory disease, etc.
◊ If infertility or habitual abortion is likely due to the anatomic location of the myoma
• Surgical procedures:
◊ Hysteroscopic or laparoscopic cautery or laser myoma resection can be performed in selected cases
◊ Myomectomies may be performed in younger women desiring to maintain fertility
◊ Hysterectomy, either vaginal or abdominal, is procedure of choice for symptomatic women no longer desiring fertility
◊ Preliminary Pap smear and endometrial sampling or D & C must be performed to rule out malignant or premalignant conditions

ACTIVITY
• Following hysteroscopic or laparoscopic myoma resection, bedrest 24 hours, no sexual intercourse for two weeks
• Following laparotomy for myomectomy or hysterectomy, 3-5 days hospital, followed by limited activity and no sexual intercourse for one month

DIET No restrictions

PATIENT EDUCATION ACOG (American College of Obstetricians and Gynecologists) pamphlet entitled "Uterine Fibroids," ACOG p-074

MEDICATIONS

DRUG(S) OF CHOICE
• Luteinizing hormone releasing hormone (LHRH) agonists (Synarel Nasal Spray, Zoladex Depot, Lupron Depot)
  ◊ Induce abrupt, artificial menopause and render patients asymptomatic
  ◊ Induce atrophy of myomas by 40-60% within 2-3 months
  ◊ May be valuable as a preoperative adjunct to myomectomy or hysterectomy by allowing recovery of anemia, donation of autologous blood and possibly converting abdominal to vaginal hysterectomy, thereby decreasing postoperative pain, hospitalization, and morbidity. Generally used two to three months prior to surgery.
  ◊ Not recommended for use longer than six months
  ◊ Following discontinuation, myomas return within 60 days to pretherapy size
• Patients with minimal symptoms
  ◊ May be managed conservatively with iron preparations and analgesics
  ◊ Progestins such as norethindrone, 10 mg daily, or medroxyprogesterone acetate (Depo-Provera) 200 mg IM, once monthly, may reduce the amount of blood flow. They do not reduce myoma size.
Contraindications:
• Progestins - history of thromboembolic phenomenon
• LHRH agonists - history of osteoporosis
Precautions: LHRH agonists induce acute menopausal symptoms: hot flashes, night sweats, insomnia, emotional lability, and osteoporosis
Significant possible interactions: Refer to manufacturer's profile of each drug

ALTERNATIVE DRUGS N/A

FOLLOWUP

PATIENT MONITORING
• Newly diagnosed uterine myoma, if symptomatic or excessive size, 2-3 months with pelvic exam and ultrasonography
• Consider CA-125 antigen
• Monitor hemoglobin and hematocrit, if uterine bleeding excessive
• If uterine size and symptoms stable, monitor every 6 months

PREVENTION/AVOIDANCE Excessive growth during estrogen stimulation, i.e., birth control pills, postmenopausal estrogen replacement therapy and pregnancy

POSSIBLE COMPLICATIONS
• Complications during pregnancy include abortion; premature labor; second trimester rapid myoma growth leading to degeneration and pain; third-trimester fetal dystocia during labor and delivery
• Previous myomectomy patients in labor may develop uterine rupture. C-section is recommended if entered endometrial cavity during myomectomy.
• May mask other gynecologic malignancies, i.e., uterine sarcoma, ovarian cancer

EXPECTED COURSE/PROGNOSIS
• Following myomectomy, 40% pregnancy rate in patients previously infertile
• At least 10% myomas recur following myomectomy

MISCELLANEOUS

ASSOCIATED CONDITIONS Endometrial carcinoma also associated with high unopposed estrogen stimulation

AGE-RELATED FACTORS
Pediatric: N/A
Geriatric: In postmenopausal patients with newly diagnosed uterine myoma or enlarging uterine myomas, highly suspect uterine sarcoma or other gynecologic malignancy
Others:
• Not seen in premenarchal females
• Incidence increases with each decade during reproductive years and is highest in perimenopausal age group

PREGNANCY See associations above

SYNONYMS
• Fibroids
• Myoma
• Fibromyoma
• Myofibroma
• Fibroleiomyoma

ICD-9-CM 218 (4th digit 0-9) Submucous leiomyoma of uterus

SEE ALSO N/A

OTHER NOTES N/A

ABBREVIATIONS N/A

REFERENCES
• Cunningham FG, MacDonald PC, Gant NF, eds: Williams' Obstetrics. 20th Ed. Norwalk, CT, Appleton and Lange, 1997
• Novak E, Woodruff JD: Novak's Gynecologic and Obstetric Pathology: With Clinical and Endocrine Relations. 8th Ed. Philadelphia, W.B. Saunders Co., 1979
• Ryan KJ, Berkowitz R, Barbieri RL: Kistners' Gynecology: Principles & Practice. 5th Ed. Chicago, Year Book Publishers, 1990
• Jones HW III, Wentz AC, Burnett LS: Novak's Textbook of Gynecology. 12th Ed. Baltimore, Williams and Wilkins, 1996
• ACOG (American College of Obstetricians and Gynecologists) pamphlet entitled "Uterine Fibroids," ACOG p-074
Illustrations: N/A
Internet references: http://www.5mcc.com

Author(s)
Eric L. Jenison, MD
Michael P. Hopkins, MD

Uterine prolapse

 BASICS

DESCRIPTION Uterine prolapse occurs when the integrity of supporting structures is lost. This allows the uterus to descend into the vagina. In advanced cases, complete protrusion with inversion of the vagina occurs.
• Prior to menopause, the degree and severity of prolapse is usually related to the number of children and the difficulty of childbirth. After menopause, atrophy and loss of tissue integrity further leads to prolapse.
System(s) affected: Reproductive, Renal/Urologic, Rectum, Gastrointestinal
Genetics:
• Common among Caucasian races
• Less common among Orientals and African Americans and particularly uncommon in South African Bantus and West Africans
Incidence/Prevalence in USA: Approximately 1 in 10 women will experience some degree of prolapse
Predominant age: Peri- and postmenopausal female
Predominant sex: Female only

SIGNS AND SYMPTOMS
• Pelvic pressure and low back pain
• As prolapse progresses, eventually a bulging is noticed as a result of protrusion
• Dyspareunia
• Difficulty with urination or defecation

CAUSES
• Advancing age and vaginal childbirth are the most important factors
• The incidence of prolapse increases with the frequency and difficulty of vaginal deliveries. Less than 2% of prolapse occurs in nulliparous women.
• Other causes of prolapse include connective tissue disorders with lax tissue, i.e., Marfan's syndrome and neurogenic disorders, i.e., multiple sclerosis, and the rare disorder of cloacal agenesis
• Patients who have undergone radical vulvectomy with loss of the external supporting structures have a higher rate of prolapse

RISK FACTORS
• Childbirth, particularly multiple parity
• Advancing age
• Caucasian race
• Various connective tissue and neurogenic disorders
• Conditions resulting in increased intra-abdominal pressure, such as obesity, abdominal or pelvic tumors, pulmonary disease with chronic coughing, chronic constipation
• Occupations requiring heavy lifting

 DIAGNOSIS

DIFFERENTIAL DIAGNOSIS Diagnosis is by physical and pelvic examination. With coughing and straining, the cervix will prolapse toward introitus or beyond. The patient may need to be examined in the standing as well as lying position for diagnosis. Herniations of the bladder (cystocele or urethrocele), rectum (rectocele) and small bowel (enterocele) are associated conditions that may be simultaneously diagnosed.

LABORATORY
• Evaluation of renal function to rule out ureteral obstruction
• Urinalysis to rule out urinary tract infection
Drugs that may alter lab results: N/A
Disorders that may alter lab results: N/A

PATHOLOGICAL FINDINGS
• Hyperkeratosis of the cervical and vaginal tissues occur with prolapse beyond the introitus due to chronic irritation and drying. As the irritation becomes more pronounced, bleeding and ulceration occur.
• Degrees of prolapse:
◊ First degree prolapse - to the ischial spine
◊ Second degree prolapse - to the introitus
◊ Third degree prolapse - just beyond the introitus
◊ Fourth degree prolapse - complete uterine and vaginal inversion involving bladder and bowel

SPECIAL TESTS N/A

IMAGING
• Intravenous pyelogram to rule out ureteral obstruction in complete uterine prolapse
• Pelvic ultrasound or CT scan to rule out other pelvic pathology, if suspected

DIAGNOSTIC PROCEDURES If ulceration or bleeding is present, Pap smears and appropriate cervical and endometrial biopsies should be done to rule out concomitant malignancies

 TREATMENT

APPROPRIATE HEALTH CARE
• Outpatient
• Inpatient when surgery is necessary

GENERAL MEASURES
• Treatment depends on multiple variables including the severity of prolapse, age, sexual activity, associated pelvic pathology and desire for future fertility
• Treatment of first and second degree prolapse is expectant unless patient is symptomatic
• Mildly symptomatic patients and poor surgical candidates - can be treated nonoperatively with perineal (Kegel) exercises, estrogen replacement and vaginal pessaries. Estrogen replacement restores healthy vaginal mucosa and promotes healing.

SURGICAL MEASURES
• Surgically able patients without additional pelvic pathology - vaginal hysterectomy with or without enterocele, cystocele, rectocele repair and vaginal vault suspension, provides excellent results
• Elderly, non-sexually active women - can be treated with a colpocleisis or vaginal obliteration procedure

ACTIVITY Heavy lifting or significant increases in intra-abdominal pressure will lead to worsening of prolapse or recurrence after surgical correction. Lifting should therefore be restricted.

DIET Unlimited. Avoid constipation.

PATIENT EDUCATION
• Kegel exercises when applicable
• American College of Obstetricians & Gynecologists (ACOG), 409 12th St., SW, Washington, DC 20024-2188, (800)762-ACOG

MEDICATIONS

DRUG(S) OF CHOICE Estrogen replacement therapy (oral or vaginal cream) can increase the blood supply to the vaginal tissues and in mild cases increase supporting tissue strength to a point where surgery or pessary use may be avoided
Contraindications: Those associated with the use of estrogen. Refer to manufacturer's literature.
Precautions: If estrogen therapy is utilized and the uterus is present, progesterone should be utilized to offset the potential of endometrial carcinoma
Significant possible interactions: Refer to manufacturer's literature

ALTERNATIVE DRUGS None

FOLLOWUP

PATIENT MONITORING
• Expectant management is appropriate with periodic follow-up examinations
• If a pessary is placed, it should be removed, cleaned and replaced each month or more often

PREVENTION/AVOIDANCE
• Kegel exercises will increase the strength of the pelvic diaphragm muscles and may provide some pelvic support
• Weight loss and proper management of conditions that would increase abdominal pressure help to prevent prolapse

POSSIBLE COMPLICATIONS
• Ureteral obstruction and renal failure
• Incarceration of bowel herniations
• Pessary use - may not always be effective, and may cause discomfort, ulcers, infection

EXPECTED COURSE/PROGNOSIS
• It is expected that as patients age, the incidence and severity of prolapse will increase
• Surgical correction usually successful

MISCELLANEOUS

ASSOCIATED CONDITIONS Cystocele, rectocele, enterocele and vaginal vault prolapse are often associated with uterine prolapse

AGE-RELATED FACTORS
Pediatric: Prolapse in newborn has been reported, but is rare and usually associated with congenital disorders and neuropathies
Geriatric: This is largely a disease of aging and will be much higher as the population ages
Others: N/A

PREGNANCY This disorder in large part results from vaginal childbirth and the distention and distortion of supporting tissues with childbirth

SYNONYMS
• Uterine prolapse
• Genital prolapse
• Genital relaxation
• Uterine descensus
• Total or partial procidentia
• Dropped uterus

SEE ALSO N/A

OTHER NOTES N/A

ICD-9-CM 618. Genital prolapse (fourth digits 1-9)

ABBREVIATIONS N/A

REFERENCES
• Nichols DH, Randall CL: Vaginal Surgery. 4th Ed. Baltimore, Williams & Wilkins, 1996
• Ryan KJ, Berkowitz R, Barbieri RL: Kistner's Gynecology: Principles and Practice. 6th Ed. Chicago, Year Book Medical Publishers, Inc., 1995
• Friedman EA, ed: Gynecologic Decision Making. 2nd Ed. St. Louis, C.V. Mosby Company, 1988
• American College of Obstetricians & Gynecologists (ACOG), 409 12th St., SW, Washington, DC 20024-2188, (800)762-ACOG
Illustrations: N/A
Internet references: http://www.5mcc.com

Author(s)
Eric L. Jenison, MD
Michael P. Hopkins, MD

Uveitis

BASICS

DESCRIPTION Uveitis is a nonspecific term used to describe any intraocular inflammatory disorder. Symptoms vary depending on depth of involvement and associated conditions.
• Anterior uveitis - refers to ocular inflammation limited to the iris (iritis) alone or iris and ciliary body (iridocyclitis)
• Intermediate uveitis - refers to inflammation of the structures just posterior to the lens (pars planitis or peripheral uveitis)
• Posterior uveitis - refers to inflammation of the choroid (choroiditis), retina (retinitis), or vitreous near the optic nerve and macula
System(s) affected: Nervous
Genetics: No specific pattern for uveitis in general; iritis: 50-70% of patients are HLA-B27 positive
Incidence/Prevalence in USA:
• Anterior uveitis most common (8.2 cases/100,000 annual incidence)
• Iritis is 4 times more prevalent than posterior uveitis
Predominant age: All ages
Predominant sex: Male = Female (except for HLA-B27 anterior uveitis male > female (2.5:1)

SIGNS AND SYMPTOMS
• Anterior uveitis (approximately 80% of patients with uveitis)
  ◊ Decreased visual acuity
  ◊ Generally acute in onset
  ◊ Deep eye pain
  ◊ Photophobia (consensual)
  ◊ Conjunctival vessel dilation
  ◊ Perilimbal (circumcorneal) dilation of episcleral and scleral vessels (ciliary flush)
  ◊ Small pupillary size of affected eye
  ◊ Frequently unilateral (95% of HLA-B27 associated cases)
  ◊ Bilateral involvement and systemic symptoms (fever, fatigue, abdominal pain) may be associated with interstitial nephritis
  ◊ Systemic disease is most likely to be associated with anterior uveitis (53% of patients found to have systemic disease in one study)
• Intermediate and posterior uveitis
  ◊ Decreased visual acuity
  ◊ Generally insidious in onset
  ◊ More commonly bilateral
  ◊ Posterior inflammation will generally cause minimal pain or redness unless associated with an iritis

CAUSES
• Infectious - may result from viral, bacterial, parasitic, or fungal etiologies
• Suspected immune-mediated - possible autoimmune or immune-complex mediated mechanism postulated in association with systemic (especially rheumatologic) disorders
• Isolated eye disease
• Idiopathic (approximately 25%)
• Masquerade syndromes - diseases such as malignancies that may be mistaken for inflammation of the eye

RISK FACTORS No specific risk factors. Higher incidence seen with specific associated conditions.

DIAGNOSIS

DIFFERENTIAL DIAGNOSIS
• Conjunctivitis
• Episcleritis
• Scleritis
• Keratitis
• Acute angle-closure glaucoma

LABORATORY
• No specific test for the diagnosis of uveitis. Tests for etiologic factors or associated conditions should be based on history and physical examination.
• CBC, BUN, creatinine (interstitial nephritis)
• HLA-B27 typing (ankylosing spondylitis, Reiter's syndrome)
• ANA, ESR (SLE, Sjögren's syndrome)
• VDRL, FTA (syphilis)
• PPD (tuberculosis)
• Lyme serology (Lyme disease)
Drugs that may alter lab results: N/A
Disorders that may alter lab results: Immune deficiency

PATHOLOGICAL FINDINGS Keratic precipitates, inflammatory cells in anterior chamber or vitreous, synechiae (fibrous tissue scarring between iris and lens), macular edema, perivasculitis of retinal vessels

SPECIAL TESTS Slit lamp examination and indirect ophthalmoscopy are necessary for precise diagnosis

IMAGING
• Chest x-ray (sarcoidosis, histoplasmosis, tuberculosis, lymphoma)
• Sacroiliac x-ray (ankylosing spondylitis)

DIAGNOSTIC PROCEDURES Slit lamp examination

TREATMENT

APPROPRIATE HEALTH CARE
Outpatient with urgent ophthalmologic consultation

GENERAL MEASURES
• Medical therapy best initiated following full ophthalmologic evaluation
• Treatment of underlying cause, if identified
• Cycloplegia
• Anti-inflammatory therapy

SURGICAL MEASURES N/A

ACTIVITY Full activity

DIET No special diet

PATIENT EDUCATION
• Instructions on proper method for instilling eye drops
• Wear dark glasses, if photophobia a problem
• Medication side effects to watch for and report

Uveitis

MEDICATIONS

DRUG(S) OF CHOICE
• Homatropine hydrobromide (Isopto) 2% ophthalmic solution - 2 gtts to the affected eye bid, or as often as every 3 hours if necessary, plus
• Prednisolone acetate 1% ophthalmic suspension - 2 gtts to the affected eye every 1 hour initially, tapering to qid with improvement

Contraindications:
• Hypersensitivity to the medication or component of the preparation
• Cycloplegia is contraindicated in patients known to have, or predisposed to, glaucoma
• Topical corticosteroid therapy is contraindicated in uveitis secondary to infectious etiologies

Precautions:
• Homatropine hydrobromide may produce adverse systemic antimuscarinic effects. Use extreme caution in infants and young children because of increased susceptibility to systemic effects.
• Topical corticosteroids may increase intraocular pressure. Prolonged use may cause cataract formation and exacerbate existing herpetic keratitis which may masquerade as iritis.

Significant possible interactions: Refer to manufacturer's profile of each drug

ALTERNATIVE DRUGS
• Cycloplegia - scopolamine hydrobromide 0.25% (Isopto Hyoscine) up to 3 times daily, or cyclopentolate hydrochloride 1% (Cyclogyl)
• Anti-inflammatory - prednisolone sodium phosphate 1% (Ocu-Pred Forte), dexamethasone sodium phosphate 0.1% (Ocu-Dex), and dexamethasone suspension
• Systemic nonsteroidal anti-inflammatory agents may provide some benefit

FOLLOWUP

PATIENT MONITORING
• Ophthalmologic followup as recommended by consultant
• Schedule for complete history and physical to evaluate for associated systemic disease

PREVENTION/AVOIDANCE   N/A

POSSIBLE COMPLICATIONS
Loss of vision as a result of the following:
 ◊ Keratic precipitate deposition on the corneal or lens surfaces
 ◊ Increased intraocular pressure, acute angle-closure glaucoma
 ◊ Formation of synechiae
 ◊ Cataract formation
 ◊ Vasculitis with vascular occlusion, retinal infarction
 ◊ Macular edema
 ◊ Optic nerve damage

EXPECTED COURSE/PROGNOSIS
• Dependent upon the presence of causal diseases, or associated conditions
• Uveitis resulting from infections (systemic or local) tend to resolve with eradication of the underlying infection
• Uveitis associated with seronegative arthropathies tend to be acute (lasting less than 3 months) and frequently recurrent

MISCELLANEOUS

ASSOCIATED CONDITIONS
• Viral infections: HIV, herpes simplex, herpes zoster, cytomegalovirus
• Bacterial infections: Tuberculosis, leprosy, Propionibacterium, syphilis, leptospirosis, brucellosis, Lyme disease, Whipple's disease
• Parasitic infections: Toxoplasmosis, acanthamebiasis, toxocariasis, cysticercosis, onchocerciasis
• Fungal infections: Histoplasmosis, coccidioidomycosis, candidiasis, aspergillosis, sporotrichosis, blastomycosis, cryptococcosis
• Suspected immune-mediated: Ankylosing spondylitis, Behçet's disease, Crohn's disease, drug or hypersensitivity reaction, interstitial nephritis, juvenile rheumatoid arthritis, Kawasaki disease, multiple sclerosis, psoriatic arthritis, Reiter's syndrome, relapsing polychondritis, sarcoidosis, Sjögren's syndrome, systemic lupus erythematosus, ulcerative colitis, vasculitis, vitiligo, Vogt-Koyanagi (Harada's) syndrome
• Isolated eye disease: Acute multifocal placoid pigmentary epitheliopathy, acute retinal necrosis, bird-shot choroidopathy, Fuch's heterochromatic cyclitis, glaucomatocyclitic crisis, lens-induced uveitis, multifocal choroiditis, pars planitis, serpiginous choroiditis, sympathetic ophthalmia, trauma

• Masquerade syndromes: Leukemia, lymphoma, retinitis pigmentosa, retinoblastoma

AGE-RELATED FACTORS
Pediatric: Infection should be the primary consideration. Allergies and psychological factors (depression, stress) may serve as a trigger factor.
Geriatric: The inflammatory response to systemic disease may be suppressed
Others: N/A

PREGNANCY   May be of importance in the selection of medications

SYNONYMS
• Iritis
• Iridocyclitis
• Choroiditis
• Retinochoroiditis
• Chorioretinitis
• Anterior uveitis
• Posterior uveitis
• Pars planitis
• Panuveitis

ICD-9-CM
364.3 Uveitis nos

SEE ALSO
• Conjunctivitis
• Scleritis
• Keratitis, superficial punctate
• Glaucoma, primary angle-closure

OTHER NOTES
• Synonyms are anatomic descriptions of the focus of the uveal inflammation
• Severe or unresponsive uveitis may require therapy including periocular injection of corticosteroids, systemic corticosteroids, cytotoxic agents (azathioprine, cyclophosphamide, chlorambucil and methotrexate), or immunosuppressive agents (cyclosporine)

ABBREVIATIONS
gtt = drop

REFERENCES
• Rosenbaum JT: Uveitis: an internist's view. Arch Intern Med 1989;149(5):1173-6
• Rosenbaum JT: An algorithm for the systemic evaluation of patients with uveitis: guidelines for the consultant. Semin Arthritis Rheum 1990;19(4):248-57
• Herman DC: Endogenous uveitis: current concepts of treatment. Mayo Clin Proc 1990;65(5):671-83
Illustrations: N/A
Internet references: http://www.5mcc.com

Author(s)
Dana W. Peterson, MD
William L. Toffler, MD

Vaginal adenosis

 BASICS

DESCRIPTION Adenosis is a term used to describe non-epithelialized columnar glandular epithelium in the vagina. At approximately the 15th week of embryological development, the müllerian system, which forms the upper two-thirds of the vagina, fuses with the invaginating cloaca, which forms the lower vagina. Squamous metaplasia from the cloacal region then produces a squamous epithelium through the vagina. Adenosis occurs when this squamous epithelium fails to completely epithelialize the vagina.
System(s) affected: Reproductive
Genetics: Unknown
Incidence/Prevalence in USA: Adenosis is relatively common, affecting 10-20% of young females studied. As maturation progresses with puberty, epithelialization occurs.
Predominant age:
• Teenage years. From puberty to approximately age twenty, epithelialization occurs.
• By age thirty, it is extremely rare to have adenosis present
Predominant sex: Female only

SIGNS AND SYMPTOMS A clear, watery vaginal discharge which is the glandular epithelium producing a small amount of mucus

CAUSES
• In the vast majority of young females, the etiology is incomplete squamous metaplasia. This occurs as a natural phenomenon and resolves with age.
• In diethylstilbestrol (DES) exposed females, the incidence of adenosis is higher and the etiology presumably is from the effect of the DES on the developing embryological system

RISK FACTORS Diethylstilbestrol (DES) exposed females

 DIAGNOSIS

DIFFERENTIAL DIAGNOSIS A thorough evaluation for adenocarcinoma of the vagina arising in adenosis should be done. A biopsy may be necessary to ensure that the process represents only benign adenosis. Colposcopy of the upper vagina aids in choosing the areas for biopsy. On visual inspection, adenosis appears as a fine, raised, reddened, granular type tissue.

LABORATORY
• When extensive adenosis is present
◊ Four-quadrant Pap smear of the vagina should be obtained
◊ Initial colposcopy performed
◊ Once squamous metaplasia is complete, four quadrant pap smear need not be performed
Drugs that may alter lab results: N/A
Disorders that may alter lab results: N/A

PATHOLOGICAL FINDINGS Biopsy will show benign glandular epithelium, which has not yet undergone squamous metaplasia. Biopsies in the areas of ongoing squamous metaplasia will be typical for this process.

SPECIAL TESTS N/A

IMAGING N/A

DIAGNOSTIC PROCEDURES
• Four quadrant Pap smear should be liberally utilized to isolate quadrants of the vagina which may contain abnormalities. This can be followed by colposcopy and biopsy.
• Colposcopy should be used to outline areas of adenosis and insure that no malignancy is present

 TREATMENT

APPROPRIATE HEALTH CARE
Outpatient

GENERAL MEASURES
• Unless malignancy is present, conservative treatment is indicated
• In the vast majority of young females with this condition, it will resolve with expectant management

SURGICAL MEASURES Aggressive therapy such as laser or surgical excision is only necessary if premalignant or malignant changes arise

ACTIVITY
• No limitations
• It is not necessary to avoid intercourse or placing objects in the vagina

DIET No special diet

PATIENT EDUCATION The patient should be educated that in the vast majority of situations this is benign and expectant management is all that is necessary
• American College of Obstetricians & Gynecologists (ACOG), 409 12th St., SW, Washington, DC 20024-2188, (800)762-ACOG

MEDICATIONS

DRUG(S) OF CHOICE N/A
Contraindications: N/A
Precautions: N/A
Significant possible interactions: N/A

ALTERNATIVE DRUGS N/A

FOLLOWUP

PATIENT MONITORING
• Initial evaluation consists of four-quadrant vaginal Pap smear, cervical Pap smear and colposcopy of the upper vagina and cervix
• If the initial colposcopy is normal, a yearly four-quadrant Pap smear of the vagina and Pap smear of the cervix is all that is necessary

PREVENTION/AVOIDANCE N/A

POSSIBLE COMPLICATIONS N/A

EXPECTED COURSE/PROGNOSIS
• It is expected that the vast majority of patients will have squamous metaplasia with complete resolution of the adenosis
• The rare patient, 1:1,000 to 1:10,000, may develop adenocarcinoma in the adenosis and will require definitive therapy as for vaginal cancer

MISCELLANEOUS

ASSOCIATED CONDITIONS
• DES exposure
◊ Adenosis from DES exposure should lead to an evaluation of other DES related abnormalities
◊ The greatest risk to the patient is from müllerian tract anomalies of the reproductive tract. These include cervical abnormalities with cervical hood, ridges, shortened cervix and incompetent cervix.
◊ Patients with a known DES exposure should have the reproductive tract evaluated prior to conception
◊ The vast majority of patients with adenosis have not been DES exposed and do not require evaluation of the reproductive system
◊ DES was last used to prevent spontaneous abortion in approximately 1970. This is a problem of decreasing importance.

AGE-RELATED FACTORS
Pediatric: N/A
Geriatric:
• Adenosis is a disorder of the young female. By the time of menopause the vagina and cervix should be completely epithelialized.
• The presence of glandular epithelium in the postmenopausal patient is an indication for excision and close evaluation for the possibility of a well-differentiated adenocarcinoma
Others: N/A

PREGNANCY Pregnancy produces a wide eversion of the transformation zone of the cervix. This will occasionally become so widely everted that it will extend onto the vaginal fornices leading to the impression of adenosis. This will resolve after the pregnancy is completed.

SYNONYMS N/A

ICD-9-CM 752.49 other anomalies of cervix, vagina, and external female genitalia

SEE ALSO N/A

OTHER NOTES N/A

ABBREVIATIONS N/A

REFERENCES
• Sandberg EC: The incidence and distribution of occult vaginal adenosis. Am J Obstet Gynecol 1968;101:322-34
• Hopkins MP: Vaginal Neoplasms. In: Copeland LJ, ed. Textbook of Gynecology. Philadelphia, W.B. Saunders Co., 1993
Illustrations: N/A
Internet references: http://www.5mcc.com

Author(s)
Michael P. Hopkins, MD
Eric L. Jenison, MD

Vaginal bleeding during pregnancy

 BASICS

DESCRIPTION Vaginal bleeding during pregnancy has many etiologies and ranges in severity from mild (with normal pregnancy outcome) to life-threatening for both infant and mother. The bleeding can vary from scant to excessive, from brown to bright red, and can be painless or painful. The different causes can be divided into vaginal, cervical and uterine factors. The differential diagnosis is guided by the gestational age of the pregnancy.
System(s) affected: Reproductive, Cardiovascular
Genetics: No known genetic pattern
Incidence/Prevalence in USA: Common
Predominant age: Childbearing
Predominant sex: Female only

SIGNS AND SYMPTOMS
• Bleeding can vary from scant to excessive
• Color of blood varies from brown to bright red
• May be painless or painful

CAUSES
• Vaginal infection or trauma
• Cervicitis
• Cervical polyp
• Cervical neoplasia
• Hyperemia of cervix
• Postcoital bleeding
• Ectopic pregnancy
• Molar pregnancy
• Implantation bleeding
• Spontaneous abortion
• Placenta previa
• Placental abruptio
• Bloody show
• Unknown - 50% of first trimester bleeding, no cause ever found

RISK FACTORS Varies, based on individual causes

 DIAGNOSIS

DIFFERENTIAL DIAGNOSIS
• Vaginal or cervical causes can occur throughout the pregnancy
• First trimester bleeding - ectopic pregnancy, molar pregnancy, or spontaneous abortion
• Second or third trimester bleeding - placenta previa, placental abruptio, or bloody show

LABORATORY
• CBC
• Quantitative beta human chorionic gonadotropin (HCG) - in early pregnancy bleeding; follow serially every couple of days. Levels fall in spontaneous abortion, are extremely high in molar pregnancy, and rise gradually in ectopic or intrauterine pregnancy.
• Blood type and screen - Rh negative patients need Rho(D) immune globulin (RhoGAM). If bleeding profuse, a transfusion may be required.
• Coagulation studies (fibrinogen, fibrin split products, platelets) - useful in late pregnancy bleeding and missed abortion
Drugs that may alter lab results: N/A
Disorders that may alter lab results: N/A

PATHOLOGICAL FINDINGS Depends on cause

SPECIAL TESTS N/A

IMAGING
• Ultrasound - gestational sac seen at 5-6 weeks, fetal heart tones at 8-9 weeks. Diagnostic of molar pregnancy with 98% accuracy, locates placenta, may show degree of placental separation in abruptio.
• Serial ultrasound may be required in early pregnancy to make diagnosis

DIAGNOSTIC PROCEDURES
• In first trimester bleeding - pelvic exam, culdocentesis, laparoscopy, laparotomy
• In second or third trimester bleeding - locate placenta by ultrasound prior to pelvic exam. If placenta previa, do not perform bimanual or speculum exam unless set up for immediate cesarean delivery.

 TREATMENT

APPROPRIATE HEALTH CARE
• In first trimester bleeding most patients can be managed as outpatient
• In late pregnancy bleeding, most patients need inpatient monitoring

GENERAL MEASURES
• In late pregnancy bleeding, the amount of bleeding and presence of maternal or fetal compromise indicates whether emergent cesarean section is performed or whether conservative measures are appropriate until greater fetal maturity can be obtained
• Threatened abortion: Bedrest and nothing per vagina. If bleeding is severe, hospitalization and close observation. Type and screen for possible transfusion

SURGICAL MEASURES
• If ectopic or molar pregnancy is diagnosed immediate surgical treatment is appropriate
• Inevitable or incomplete abortion: D&C (usually suction)
• If completeness of abortion is in doubt, then D&C and removal of retained products

ACTIVITY Bedrest, no coitus, no douching

DIET No restrictions

PATIENT EDUCATION
• Patient should be instructed to report any increase in the amount and frequency of bleeding and should seek immediate care if experiencing abdominal pain or sudden increased bleeding. She should bring for examination any tissue passed vaginally.
• Grief counseling is appropriate if pregnancy loss is inevitable
• American College of Obstetricians & Gynecologists (ACOG), 409 12th St., SW, Washington, DC 20024-2188, (800)762-ACOG

MEDICATIONS

DRUG(S) OF CHOICE None
Contraindications: N/A
Precautions: N/A
Significant possible interactions: N/A

ALTERNATIVE DRUGS
• Tocolytics in suspected premature labor

FOLLOWUP

PATIENT MONITORING Daily to weekly depending on diagnosis and severity of bleeding

PREVENTION/AVOIDANCE N/A

POSSIBLE COMPLICATIONS
• Anemia
• Shock
• Fetal or maternal death
• Infection
• Choriocarcinoma or invasive mole in the case of hydatidiform mole
• Premature delivery of infant with associated complications
• Coagulopathy

EXPECTED COURSE/PROGNOSIS
Depends on the cause of vaginal bleeding, the severity of bleeding and the rapidity of diagnosis. Maternal mortality is 1 in 826 of ectopic pregnancies.

MISCELLANEOUS

ASSOCIATED CONDITIONS Depends on cause of vaginal bleeding

AGE-RELATED FACTORS
Pediatric: N/A
Geriatric: N/A
Others: N/A

PREGNANCY A complication of pregnancy

SYNONYMS N/A

ICD-9-CM
• 630 Molar pregnancy
• 633.9 Ectopic pregnancy
• 634.9 Spontaneous abortion
• 641.1 Placenta previa
• 641.2 Placental abruptio

SEE ALSO
• Abortion, spontaneous
• Abruptio placenta
• Cervical malignancy
• Cervical dysplasia
• Cervical polyps
• Cervicitis
• Cervicitis, ectropion & true erosion
• Chlamydial sexually transmitted diseases
• Ectopic pregnancy
• Placenta previa
• Premature labor
• Vaginal malignancy
• Vulvovaginitis, bacterial
• Vulvovaginitis, candidal

OTHER NOTES N/A

ABBREVIATIONS N/A

REFERENCES
• Cunningham FG, MacDonald PC, Gant NF, eds: Williams' Obstetrics. 19th Ed. Norwalk, CT, Appleton and Lange, 1993
• Danforth DM, Scott JR., et al, eds: Obstetrics and Gynecology. 6th Ed. Philadelphia, J.B. Lippincott, 1990
Illustrations: N/A
Internet references: http://www.5mcc.com

Author(s)
Kimberle Vore, MD

Vaginal malignancy

BASICS

DESCRIPTION
• Vaginal intraepithelial neoplasia (carcinoma in situ): A premalignant phase with full thickness neoplastic changes in the superficial epithelium. However there is no invasion through the basement membrane.
• Invasive malignancies: Vaginal malignancies are squamous cell in 90% of the patients and the remaining 10% are adenocarcinomas, sarcomas and melanomas. The clear cell carcinoma is a subtype of adenocarcinoma.
• To be classified as a vaginal malignancy, only the vagina can be involved. If the cervix or the vulva is involved, then the tumor is classified as a primary cancer arising from the cervix or the vulva.
System(s) affected: Reproductive
Genetics: No known genetic pattern
Incidence/Prevalence in USA: This is the rarest of all gynecological malignancies
Predominant age:
• Carcinoma in situ - mid-forties to sixties
• Invasive squamous cell malignancy - mid-sixties to seventies
• Adenocarcinoma - any age range, fifties is mean age
• Mixed müllerian sarcomas and leiomyosarcomas in the adult population - mean age sixty
• Sarcoma botryoides and embryonal sarcomas - occur in the pediatric population
Predominant sex: Female only

SIGNS AND SYMPTOMS
• Abnormal bleeding is the most common symptom. This results from a fungating tumor present in the vagina.
• Dyspareunia
• Postcoital bleeding can result from direct trauma to the tumor
• Pain along with symptoms and signs of hydroureter are late findings when tumor has spread into the paravaginal tissues and extends to the pelvic side wall
• In the pediatric population, sarcomas can present either as a mass protruding from the vagina or as abnormal genital bleeding

CAUSES
• Women with a history of cervical malignancy have a higher probability of developing squamous cell malignancy in the vagina after hysterectomy
• The human papilloma virus (HPV) has been associated with vulvovaginal, cervical, adenocarcinoma and squamous cell carcinoma
• Smokers have a higher incidence
• Clear cell adenocarcinoma of the vagina in young women has been associated with diethylstilbestrol (DES) exposure. The incidence, however, is exceedingly rare estimated at 1:1,000 to 1:10,000 DES exposed females.
• Metastatic lesions can involve the vagina from the other gynecologic organs

• Renal cell carcinoma and breast cancer can metastasize to the vagina (rarely)

RISK FACTORS
• History of squamous cell cancer of the cervix or vulva
• Smoking
• Multiple sex partners

DIAGNOSIS

DIFFERENTIAL DIAGNOSIS
• Vaginal intraepithelial neoplasia (VAIN) involves premalignant changes that do not infiltrate beyond the basement membrane
• Adequate biopsies ensure that invasive lesions are not overlooked. Invasive lesions penetrate the basement membrane and cannot be treated conservatively. Other malignancies such as endometrial, cervix, bladder or colon cancer can invade directly into the vagina or metastasize to the vagina.
• In the childbearing age, female trophoblastic disease should be considered. The vagina is a common site of metastases. Biopsy will usually provide a clue to the primary site.

LABORATORY
Cytology will usually be positive when an obvious lesion is present
Drugs that may alter lab results: N/A
Disorders that may alter lab results: N/A

PATHOLOGICAL FINDINGS
• Stage 0 - carcinoma in situ
• Stage I - infiltrative tumor not involving the paravaginal tissues
• Stage II - paravaginal extension but not to the side wall
• Stage III - paravaginal extension to the side wall
• Stage IVA - tumor involving the bladder or the rectum
• Stage IVB - distant metastatic disease

SPECIAL TESTS   N/A

IMAGING
• Chest x-ray - lung metastases are a late finding.
• IVP - to evaluate for ureteral obstruction
• CAT scan to evaluate the retroperitoneum and especially the lymph nodes in the pelvic and periaortic area
• Lymphangiography is also useful for evaluation of the lymph node status
• Barium enema to rule out rectal invasion

DIAGNOSTIC PROCEDURES
• Colposcopy with directed biopsies for small lesions
• Wide excision under anesthesia of superficial disease may be necessary to insure that invasive cancer is not present
• Cystoscopy to rule out bladder invasion
• Sigmoidoscopy to rule out rectal invasion

TREATMENT

APPROPRIATE HEALTH CARE
Outpatient or inpatient depending on treatment

GENERAL MEASURES
• Carcinoma in situ can be treated by a variety of methods: Laser vaporization under microscopic guidance; fluorouracil (Efudex) intravaginal cream; partial vaginectomy
• There is no effective chemotherapy for squamous cell malignancy of the vagina
• In all tumor types, metastatic disease from the vagina to other sites is only minimally responsive to chemotherapy

SURGICAL MEASURES
• Whenever there is a doubt as to the presence or absence of invasive disease, vaginectomy must be performed
• Invasive lesions are usually treated by radiation therapy, however, stage I lesions can be treated with radical hysterectomy, radical vaginectomy with pelvic lymph node dissection
• If the lesion involves the lower vagina, inguinal node dissection must also be done as cancer involving the lower vagina can metastasize to the groin region
• Sarcomas are treated by radiation therapy followed by pelvic exenteration if persistent disease is present
• Childhood sarcomas are treated with chemotherapy followed by local resection. Childhood sarcomas are responsive to multiagent combination chemotherapies.

ACTIVITY
• The patients are usually ambulatory and able to resume full activity by six weeks after surgery
• Most patients are fully active while receiving radiation therapy

DIET   Unrestricted unless they are undergoing radiation

PATIENT EDUCATION
• This is a rare malignancy and these patients should be treated by a physician familiar and experienced with this malignancy
• Printed patient information available from: American College of Obstetricians & Gynecologists, 409 12th St., SW, Washington, DC 20024-2188, (800)762-ACOG

MEDICATIONS

DRUG(S) OF CHOICE
• With one exception, there are no chemotherapeutic agents to which this tumor is responsive. The exception is the childhood sarcomas, which have been treated with combinations of:
  ◊ Vincristine
  ◊ Dactinomycin (actinomycin-D)
  ◊ Cyclophosphamide (Cytoxan)
  ◊ Cisplatin
  ◊ Etoposide (VP-16)
• Adjuvant chemotherapy has no proven benefit in squamous cell or adenocarcinoma of the vagina
• Carcinoma in situ can be eradicated in 90% of patients with fluorouracil (Efudex) cream 5% applied bid x 2 hours x 7 days, then qd x 7 days, repeated in six weeks

Contraindications:
• Prior to treatment the diagnosis must be established with certainty
• If there is any doubt that a process beyond in situ disease exists, vaginectomy must be performed. Because these patients are often elderly, aggressive therapy is limited by the patient's performance status and ability to tolerate radical surgery, chemotherapy or radiation.

Precautions: Refer to manufacturer's literature
Significant possible interactions: Refer to manufacturer's literature

ALTERNATIVE DRUGS
• Ondansetron (Zofran), dronabinol (Marinol), metoclopramide (Reglan), and others for nausea control

FOLLOWUP

PATIENT MONITORING
• Pelvic examination and Pap smear every 3 months for 2 years and then every 6 months for subsequent 3 years
• Chest x-ray once a year

PREVENTION/AVOIDANCE
• A Pap smear should be performed for all women on a yearly basis, even after hysterectomy
• Premalignant changes discovered on Pap smear screening should be followed up with colposcopy, biopsy and treatment. This needs to be undertaken by a physician well trained in the diagnosis and treatment of vaginal disease.
• Patients with a history of in situ or invasive disease of the cervix and/or the vulva should be followed at close intervals for development of disease in the vagina

POSSIBLE COMPLICATIONS Those associated with major abdominal surgery or radiation therapy

EXPECTED COURSE/PROGNOSIS
• Stage and 5 year survival
  ◊ I - 60%
  ◊ II - 40%
  ◊ III - 20%
  ◊ IVA - 5%
  ◊ IVB - 0%

MISCELLANEOUS

ASSOCIATED CONDITIONS Due to the field effect, patients with vaginal cancer are more likely to develop malignancy in the cervix or vulva and should be followed closely

AGE-RELATED FACTORS
Pediatric: Childhood sarcomas can be treated in a conservative fashion with multi-modality therapy. This avoids the loss of the young child's bladder and/or rectum.
Geriatric: Older patients, many with a long smoking history are at a higher risk for surgery
Others:
• Younger patients, who have not completed their family, can occasionally be treated with limited resection and localized radiation to the area
• Premenopausal women, who desire to retain ovarian function, are better candidates for radical surgery for early stage disease

PREGNANCY This malignancy is not associated with pregnancy

SYNONYMS
• Bowen's disease
• Vaginal intraepithelial neoplasia (VAIN)

ICD-9-CM 184.0

SEE ALSO N/A

OTHER NOTES N/A

ABBREVIATIONS N/A

REFERENCES
• Hopkins MP: Vaginal Neoplasms. In: Copeland LJ, ed. Textbook of Gynecology. Philadelphia, W.B. Saunders Co., 1993
• Peters WA, Kumar NB, Morley GW: Carcinoma of the vagina: Factors influencing treatment outcome. Cancer 1985;55(4):892-97
Illustrations: N/A
Internet references: http://www.5mcc.com

Author(s)
Michael P. Hopkins, MD
Eric L. Jenison, MD

Vaginismus

BASICS

DESCRIPTION Involuntary painful contraction of perineal muscles prior to or during insertion of any object into vagina. The experience or even the anticipation of pain on vaginal entry causes these muscles to contract, occluding the vaginal opening and causing further pain when penetration is attempted.
System(s) affected: Reproductive
Genetics: N/A
Incidence/Prevalence in USA: Unknown
Predominant age: Postpubertal
Predominant sex: Female only

SIGNS AND SYMPTOMS
• Pain with vaginal sexual intercourse
• Reluctance or avoidance of pelvic examination
• Infertility
• Small and non-distensible vaginal opening
• Rigid hymen
• Anatomic or congenital abnormalities

CAUSES
• History of genital or psychic trauma, especially incest
• Previous traumatic gynecologic examination
• Vaginal infections
• Skin disorders involving vulva
• Bartholin's cysts or abscess
• Scarring following episiotomy or vaginal repair operations
• PID and endometriosis
• Vaginitis
• Decreased vaginal lubrication secondary to hormonal imbalance

RISK FACTORS
• Previous sexual trauma
• Incest
• Rape

DIAGNOSIS

DIFFERENTIAL DIAGNOSIS N/A

LABORATORY As needed to identify infections and other medical causes
Drugs that may alter lab results: N/A
Disorders that may alter lab results: N/A

PATHOLOGICAL FINDINGS Varied if any

SPECIAL TESTS Psychiatric consultation or psychologic tests. May be invalidated by any axis I from American Psychiatric Association's Diagnostic and Statistical Manual of Mental Disorders (DSM-IV-R).

IMAGING N/A

DIAGNOSTIC PROCEDURES
• Careful pelvic examination
• General and sexual history

TREATMENT

APPROPRIATE HEALTH CARE
Outpatient

GENERAL MEASURES
• Trusting and non-judgmental attitude on part of physician and all office staff
• Treatment of medical problems such as infections, cystocele, episiotomy scarring
• Referral to psychiatrist or counselor, if appropriate
• If patient has insufficient lubrication for intercourse, recommend use of lubricating creams or jellies

SURGICAL MEASURES N/A

ACTIVITY Simple techniques of gentle, progressive, patient-controlled vaginal dilation

DIET No special diet

PATIENT EDUCATION
• Education about reproductive biology, normal adult sexual function, link between past trauma and current symptoms
• Instruction in techniques for vaginal dilatation
• American College of Obstetricians & Gynecologists (ACOG), 409 12th St., SW, Washington, DC 20024-2188, (800)762-ACOG

MEDICATIONS

DRUG(S) OF CHOICE None
Contraindications: Anxiolytics, especially benzodiazepines
Precautions: Anxiolytics can disinhibit and lead to traumatic memories of incest, possible suicide
Significant Possible interactions: N/A

ALTERNATIVE DRUGS N/A

FOLLOWUP

PATIENT MONITORING When possible, initiate preventive health care such as Pap smear

PREVENTION/AVOIDANCE Societal action against incest, rape

POSSIBLE COMPLICATIONS
Precipitation of memory of incest prior to patient's readiness to deal with it

EXPECTED COURSE/PROGNOSIS
Some progress generally made if physician and therapist allow patient to proceed at her own pace

MISCELLANEOUS

ASSOCIATED CONDITIONS
• Marital stress, family dysfunction
• Dyspareunia

AGE-RELATED FACTORS Vaginismus is generally primary, e.g., happens with first attempt at intercourse (if previous incest, first attempt after puberty is time of onset)
Pediatric: N/A
Geriatric: N/A
Others: N/A

PREGNANCY Pregnancy can occur in patients with vaginismus via perineal ejaculation

SYNONYMS N/A

ICD-9-CM
306.51 Psychogenic vaginismus

SEE ALSO Sexual dysfunction in women

OTHER NOTES N/A

ABBREVIATIONS N/A

REFERENCES
• Leiblum SR, Rosen RC: Principles and Practice of Sex Therapy: Update for the 1990's. New York, The Guilford Press, 1989
• Wincze JP, Carey MP: Sexual Dysfunction: A Guide for Assessment and Treatment. New York, The Guilford Press, 1991
• Bancroft J: Human Sexuality and Its Problems. 2nd Ed. New York, Churchill Livingstone, 1989
Illustrations: N/A
Internet references: http://www.5mcc.com

Author(s)
Julie Graves Moy, MD, MPH
S. Shevaun Duiker, MD

Varicose veins

BASICS

DESCRIPTION Elongated, dilated, tortuous superficial veins with congenitally absent valves, or valves that have become incompetent. Affects legs where reverse flow occurs when dependent.
System(s) affected: Cardiovascular, Skin/Exocrine
Genetics: Familial, dominant, x-linked
Incidence/Prevalence in USA: About 20% of adults
Predominant age: Middle age
Predominant sex: Female > Male (5:1)

SIGNS AND SYMPTOMS
• Sometimes asymptomatic
• Leg muscular cramp
• Dilatation, tortuosity of superficial veins chiefly in the lower extremities
• Edema of affected limb
• Leg aching
• Fatigue
• Symptoms worse during menses
• Pain if varicose ulcer develops

CAUSES
• Faulty valves in one or more perforator veins in the lower leg causing secondary incompetence at the saphenofemoral junction
• Deep thrombophlebitis
• Increased venous pressure from any cause
• In many individuals, no cause or precipitating factor found

RISK FACTORS
• Pregnancy
• Occupations requiring prolonged standing, restrictive clothing (e.g., very tight girdles)

DIAGNOSIS

DIFFERENTIAL DIAGNOSIS
• Nerve root compression
• Arthritis
• Peripheral neuritis

LABORATORY None helpful
Drugs that may alter lab results: N/A
Disorders that may alter lab results: N/A

PATHOLOGICAL FINDINGS
• Elongation and tortuosity of veins
• Medial fibrosis of veins
• Disappearance or atrophy of valves

SPECIAL TESTS Trendelenburg's test

IMAGING N/A

DIAGNOSTIC PROCEDURES Clinical inspection

TREATMENT

APPROPRIATE HEALTH CARE
Outpatient

GENERAL MEASURES
• Conservative methods
  ◊ Frequent rest periods with legs elevated
  ◊ Lightweight, elastic compression hosiery. Best put on before getting out of bed.
  ◊ Avoid girdles and other restrictive clothing
  ◊ If stasis ulcers present, use warm, wet dressings
• Spider veins (idiopathic telangiectases)
  ◊ Fine intracutaneous angiectasis
  ◊ May be extensive/unsightly
  ◊ Eliminate with intracapillary injections of 1% solution of sodium tetradecyl sulfate (or hypertonic saline 23.4%) using a fine-bore needle
  ◊ Subsequent treatments may be required until optimal results attained

SURGICAL MEASURES
• Surgical and other methods
  ◊ If there is pain, recurrent phlebitis, skin changes, or for cosmetic improvement for severe cases
  ◊ Ligation and stripping of the saphenous vein
  ◊ Injection of sclerosing solution
  ◊ Stab evulsion phlebectomy - newer procedure with shorter recovery time
  ◊ For extensive fibrosis - excision of the entire area, followed by skin graft may be necessary

ACTIVITY
• Avoid long periods of standing
• Appropriate exercise routine as part of conservative treatment
• Walking regimen after sclerotherapy is important to help promote healing
• Apply elastic stockings before lowering legs from the bed
• Never sit with legs hanging down

DIET
• No special diet
• Weight loss diet recommended, if obesity a problem

PATIENT EDUCATION
• Inform patients that the surgery or sclerotherapy may not prevent development of varicosities and that the procedure may need to be repeated in later years
• For patient education materials favorably reviewed on this topic, contact: National Heart, Lung & Blood Institute, Communications & Public Information Branch, National Institutes of Health, Building 31, Room 41-21, 9000 Rockville Pike, Bethesda, MD 20892, (301)496-4236

Varicose veins

MEDICATIONS

DRUG(S) OF CHOICE Injection sclerotherapy with compression to totally obliterate the vein by fibrosis. Sclerosant is sodium tetradecyl sulfate 1-3% solution. Bandages remain 3 weeks or longer.
Contraindications: Refer to manufacturer's literature
Precautions: No oral contraceptives for at least 6 weeks prior to sclerotherapy because of their thrombogenic effect
Significant possible interactions: Refer to manufacturer's literature

ALTERNATIVE DRUGS Antibiotics for infected varicose ulcers

FOLLOWUP

PATIENT MONITORING Until surgery or conservative therapy brings maximal benefit

PREVENTION/AVOIDANCE N/A

POSSIBLE COMPLICATIONS
• Petechial hemorrhages
• Chronic edema
• Superimposed infection
• Varicose ulcers
• Pigmentation
• Eczema
• Recurrence after surgical treatment
• Scarring or nerve damage from stripping technique

EXPECTED COURSE/PROGNOSIS
• Usual course - chronic
• Prognosis - favorable with appropriate treatment

MISCELLANEOUS

ASSOCIATED CONDITIONS
• Stasis dermatitis
• Stasis ulcer

AGE-RELATED FACTORS
Pediatric: Unlikely in this age group
Geriatric:
• More common, usually valvular degeneration, but may be secondary to chronic venous deficiency
• Recommended therapy - elastic support hose and frequent rests with legs elevated rather than ligation and stripping
Others: N/A

PREGNANCY Frequent problem. Use of elastic stockings recommended for individuals who have a history of varicosities or when activities involve a great deal of standing.

SYNONYMS N/A

ICD-9-CM 454.1

SEE ALSO Dermatitis, stasis

OTHER NOTES N/A

ABBREVIATIONS N/A

REFERENCES Berkow R, et al, eds: Merck Manual. 16th Ed. Rahway, NJ, Merck Sharp & Dohme, 1992
Illustrations: N/A
Internet references: http://www.5mcc.com

Author(s)
Joseph A. Florence, MD

Ventricular septal defect (VSD)

BASICS

DESCRIPTION Congenital or acquired defect of the interventricular septum that allows communication of blood between the left and right ventricles. Other than bicuspid aortic valve, this is the most common congenital heart malformation reported in infants and children. It also occurs as a complication of acute myocardial infarctions (MI). Blood flow across the defect is typically left to right and depends on the size of the defect and the pulmonary vascular resistance (PVR). Prolonged shunting of blood can lead to pulmonary hypertension and eventually reversal of flow across the defect, and to cyanosis (Eisenmenger's complex).
System(s) affected: Cardiovascular
Genetics: Multifactorial etiology; autosomal dominant and recessive transmission have been reported
Incidence/Prevalence in USA:
• Congenital - 100-500 of 100,000 live births
• Acute myocardial infarctions - estimated to complicate 1-3%
Predominant age: Infants and children
Predominant sex: Male = Female (male > female if secondary to myocardial infarction)

SIGNS AND SYMPTOMS
• Depend on the degree of shunting across the defect
• Respiratory distress, tachypnea
• Forceful apical impulse
• Thrill along the left lower or midsternal borders
• High-frequency holosystolic murmur
• S3
• Increased intensity of P2
• Elevated jugular venous pressure
• Diastolic murmur of pulmonic insufficiency
• Diastolic rumble due to increased flow across the mitral valve
• If pulmonary hypertension exist: cyanosis with exertion
• If Eisenmenger's complex is present: cyanosis and clubbing

CAUSES
• Congenital
• In adults, secondary to myocardial infarction

RISK FACTORS
• Congenital
  ◊ 4.2% risk of sibling being affected
  ◊ 4.0% of offspring being affected
• Post-acute myocardial infarctions
  ◊ First MI
  ◊ Limited coronary artery disease
  ◊ Hypertension
  ◊ Most frequent within first week after myocardial infarction (MI)
  ◊ Occur in 1-2% of MI, most commonly after anterior MI

DIAGNOSIS

DIFFERENTIAL DIAGNOSIS
• Any disease with left-to-right shunt, such as large patent ductus arteriosus or atrial septal defect
• Children - Tetralogy of Fallot
• Adults - acute mitral regurgitation

LABORATORY None specific
Drugs that may alter lab results: N/A
Disorders that may alter lab results: N/A

PATHOLOGICAL FINDINGS
• Congenital VSD's (4 major anatomical types):
  ◊ Membranous (75%)
  ◊ Muscular (10%)
  ◊ Atrioventricular canal type (10%)
  ◊ Supracristal (5%; higher percent in Oriental population)
• Postmyocardial infarction VSD's
  ◊ Involve predominantly the muscular septum

SPECIAL TESTS
• ECG may suggest severity of VSD. Initially, left ventricular hypertrophy and left atrial enlargement may be evident. With pulmonary hypertension, right ventricular hypertrophy and right atrial enlargement may be seen.
• After surgical repair, right bundle branch block and left anterior hemi-block are common

IMAGING
• Chest x-ray may demonstrate increased pulmonary vascularity and/or cardiomegaly
• Two-dimensional echocardiogram for visualization
• Color-flow Doppler, for detection of ventricular septal defect jet

DIAGNOSTIC PROCEDURES
• Cardiac catheterization (left and right heart) can establish the diagnosis
• Demonstration of an oxygen saturation step-up (> 8 mm Hg) (1.1 kPa) from the right atrium to the distal pulmonary artery with Swan-Ganz catheter

TREATMENT

APPROPRIATE HEALTH CARE
• Outpatient, until surgical repair is indicated
• Inpatient in setting of acute MI
• Inpatient for treatment of severe congestive heart failure

GENERAL MEASURES N/A

SURGICAL MEASURES
• Surgical closure is indicated if the pulmonic to systemic flow is > 2:1
• Congenital VSD surgery is usually performed before the child enters school or earlier, if hemodynamically indicated
• In the post-MI setting, afterload reduction, inotropic support and intra-aortic balloon pump may be used to stabilize the patient prior to surgery

ACTIVITY As tolerated

DIET Low sodium

PATIENT EDUCATION
• Endocarditis prophylaxis
• Parents need support and instructions for prevention of complications until the child is ready for surgery

MEDICATIONS

DRUG(S) OF CHOICE
• Pediatric
◊ Nitroglycerin 0.5-5 μg/kg/min IV (max 60 μg/kg/min)
◊ Hydralazine 0.5 mg/kg/day po q6-8h (max 200 mg/day)
◊ Captopril 0.1-0.4 mg/kg/dose po given q6-24h. (max 6 mg/kg/24h)
◊ Nitroprusside 0.5-8 μg/kg/min IV
◊ Prazosin first dose 5 μg/kg po (max 25 μg/kg/dose q6h)
• Adult
◊ Nitroglycerin drip beginning at 5 μg/kg/min and increasing by 5 μg/kg/min every few minutes, then by up to 20 μg/kg/min and titrate effect blood pressure, cardiac output, etc.
◊ Nitroprusside beginning at 10 μg/min and increasing by 5-10 μg/min every few minutes, titrating to blood pressure, cardiac output, etc.
◊ Angiotensin converting enzyme (ACE) inhibitors (e.g., captopril 6.25-25 mg po tid or lisinopril 2.5-20 mg po qd or enalapril 2.5-15 mg po qd or bid)
◊ Hydralazine 10-100 mg po qid
◊ Dobutamine 2.5-10 μg/kg/min titrating to cardiac output and systemic resistance (SVR)
◊ Dopamine 5-10 μg/kg/min titrating to cardiac output and SVR
Contraindications: Drugs that increase peripheral vascular resistance may increase right-to-left shunting
Precautions: Hypotension
Significant possible interactions: Refer to manufacturer's profile of each drug

ALTERNATIVE DRUGS
Diuretics and digoxin may also be beneficial in certain circumstances

FOLLOWUP

PATIENT MONITORING Close followup (at least every 6 months) of a congenital VSD is necessary until primary intracardiac repair is performed to ensure that significant pulmonary hypertension does not develop

PREVENTION/AVOIDANCE For adults, avoiding risk factors for myocardial infarction

POSSIBLE COMPLICATIONS
• Congestive heart failure
• Infective endocarditis
• Sudden death
• Hemoptysis
• Chest pain
• Cerebral abscess
• Paradoxical emboli
• Cardiogenic shock
• Heart block may rarely accompany surgical closure

EXPECTED COURSE/PROGNOSIS
• Congenital
◊ 25-45% of VSD will close spontaneously by age 3
◊ Course is variable depending on the size of the VSD
◊ 4% of patients with VSD develop infective endocarditis by the third or fourth decade of life
◊ Progressive pulmonary vascular disease and pulmonary hypertension are the most feared complications of VSD caused by left-to-right shunting, and may eventually lead to reversal of the shunt (Eisenmenger's complex)
◊ Death usually occurs in the fourth decade of life if untreated
• Postmyocardial infarction
◊ 80-90% mortality in the first two weeks with medical management alone
◊ Prognosis worse with inferior MI compared to anterior MI

MISCELLANEOUS:

ASSOCIATED CONDITIONS
• Congenital
◊ Tetralogy of Fallot
◊ Aortic valvular deformities, especially aortic insufficiency
◊ Down's syndrome (Trisomy 21)
◊ Transposition of the great arteries
◊ Tricuspid atresia
◊ Truncus arteriosus
◊ Patent ductus arteriosus
◊ Atrial septal defect
◊ Pulmonic stenosis
◊ Subaortic stenosis
• Adult
◊ Coronary artery disease

AGE-RELATED FACTORS
Pediatric: Congenital
Geriatric: Almost entirely associated with myocardial infarction
Others: N/A

PREGNANCY
• May exacerbate symptoms and signs with a congenital VSD
• Tolerated during pregnancy if the septal defect is small

SYNONYMS N/A

ICD-9-CM 745.4

SEE ALSO
• Down's syndrome
• Myocardial infarction
• Tetralogy of Fallot

OTHER NOTES N/A

ABBREVIATIONS N/A

REFERENCES
• Friedman WF, Perloff JK: Congenital heart disease in infancy and childhood. In: Braunwald E, ed. Heart Disease. 4th Ed. Philadelphia, W.B. Saunders Co., 1992
• Hillis DL, Lange RA, Winniford MD, Page RL: Manual of Clinical Problems in Cardiology. New York, Little, Brown and Co., 1995
• Radford MJ, et al: Ventricular septal rupture: a review of clinical and physiologic features and an analysis of survival. Circulation 1981;64(3)
Illustrations: N/A
Internet references: http://www.5mcc.com

Author(s)
Robert Kowal, MD

Vitamin deficiency

BASICS

DESCRIPTION Vitamin deficiency syndromes develop slowly and are difficult to diagnose. Multiple deficiencies of vitamins occur more frequently than a deficiency in a single vitamin. Vitamin classification: follows:
- Fat-soluble
  ◊ Vitamin A (retinol)
  ◊ Vitamin D (vitamin D2 = ergocalciferol; vitamin D3 = cholecalciferol)
  ◊ Vitamin E
  ◊ Vitamin K (K1 = phytomenadione; K2 = menaquinone; K3 = menadione)
- Water-soluble
  ◊ Vitamin B1 (thiamine)
  ◊ Vitamin B2 (riboflavin)
  ◊ Vitamin B3 (niacin, nicotinic acid, niacinamide)
  ◊ Vitamin B6 (pyridoxine)
  ◊ Vitamin B12 (cobalamin)
  ◊ Vitamin C (ascorbic acid)

System(s) affected: Endocrine/Metabolic
Genetics:
- Hereditary vitamin D-dependent rickets - autosomal recessive syndrome
- Thiamine-dependent beriberi - rare hereditary metabolic disorder

Incidence/Prevalence in USA: Unknown
Predominant age: Elderly
Predominant sex: Male = Female

SIGNS AND SYMPTOMS
- Vitamin A (retinol)
  ◊ Night blindness
  ◊ Hyperkeratosis
  ◊ Xerophthalmia
  ◊ Growth retardation, loss of appetite, and anemia commonly found in children
  ◊ Bitot's spots (superficial foamy patches on exposed bulbar conjunctiva)
- Vitamin B1 (thiamine)
  ◊ Beriberi (peripheral neuropathy, muscular weakness, anorexia, congestive heart failure and generalized edema)
  ◊ Infantile beriberi (heart failure, aphonia, and absent deep tendon reflex; occurs in infants breast-fed by thiamine-deficient mothers
  ◊ Wernicke-Korsakoff syndrome (brain hemorrhage, mental confusion and aphonia are early symptoms followed by weakness of sixth nerve, total ophthalmoplegia, coma, and death)
- Vitamin B2 (riboflavin)
  ◊ Angular stomatitis
  ◊ Corneal vascularization
  ◊ Amblyopia
  ◊ Cheilosis
  ◊ Sebaceous dermatitis
  ◊ During pregnancy, deficiency leads to fetal skeletal abnormalities such as shortened bones and deformed growth
- Vitamin B3 (niacin [nicotinic acid], niacinamide)
  ◊ Pellagra (dermatosis, glossitis, GI dysfunction, CNS dysfunction, organic psychosis)
- Vitamin B6 (pyridoxine)
  ◊ Convulsions in infants
  ◊ Anemias
  ◊ Neuropathy
  ◊ Seborrhea-like skin lesions

- Vitamin B12 (cobalamin)
  ◊ Peripheral neuropathy
  ◊ Megaloblastic anemia
  ◊ Pernicious anemia
  ◊ Some psychiatric syndromes
- Vitamin C (ascorbic acid)
  ◊ Scurvy (loose teeth, gingivitis, hemorrhages)
- Vitamin D (vitamin D2 = ergocalciferol; vitamin D3 = cholecalciferol)
  ◊ Rickets
  ◊ Osteomalacia
- Vitamin E (alpha-tocopherol)
  ◊ RBC hemolysis
  ◊ Creatinuria
  ◊ Ceroid deposition in muscle
- Vitamin K (K1 = phytomenadione; K2 = menaquinone; K3 = menadione)
  ◊ Hemorrhage from deficient prothrombin

CAUSES
- Inadequate dietary intake
- Impaired absorption or storage

RISK FACTORS
- Alcoholism
- Parenteral nutrition
- Malabsorption
- Bile deficiency
- Dialysis
- Chronic protein-calorie undernutrition
- Deficiencies of other vitamins
- Interactions with medications
- Infants
- Elderly
- Lower socioeconomic status
- Laxative abuse
- Genetic disorder - abetalipoproteinemia (vitamin E)
- Prolonged lactation (vitamin C)
- Intestinal parasites
- Drug abuse
- Food faddism or bizarre nutritional practices
- Gastrointestinal surgery

DIAGNOSIS

DIFFERENTIAL DIAGNOSIS
- Vitamin A deficiency - retinitis pigmentosa
- Vitamin B1 deficiency - polyneuropathy
- Vitamin B2 deficiency - other causes of seborrheic dermatitis and ocular lesions
- Vitamin D - infantile scurvy; congenital syphilis; chondrodystrophy; readily distinguishable disorders (creatinism, hydrocephalus, poliomyelitis, etc.); convulsions due to other causes
- Vitamin K - liver damage, anticoagulant or salicylate therapy, other disorders that produce hemorrhagic symptoms (scurvy, allergic purpura, leukemia, thrombocytopenia)
- Niacin - other causes of stomatitis, glossitis, diarrhea, dementia

LABORATORY
- Vitamin A - serum levels below normal
- Vitamin B1 - elevated blood pyruvate, decreased urinary thiamine excretion
- Vitamin B2 - serum level < than 2 µg/dL (53 nmol/L), urinary excretion of < 30 µg of riboflavin/gm of creatinine
- Vitamin B3 - none
- Vitamin B6 - may be decreased serum levels or RBC transaminases (no generally accepted test to determine a deficiency)
- Vitamin B12 - serum levels < 150 pg/mL (111 pmol/L) (Schilling test)
- Vitamin C - serum levels < 0.4 mg/dL (23 µmol/L)
- Vitamin D - plasma calcium level < 7.5 mg/dL (1.88 mmol/L); low plasma vitamin D sterolsinorganic phosphate serum levels < 3 mg/dL (0.97 mmol/L); serum citrate levels, 2.5 mg/dL; alkaline phosphate < 4 Bodansky units/100 mL
- Vitamin E - serum levels < 0.8 mg/dL (18.5 µmol/L) (adults)
- Vitamin K - prothrombin time 25% longer than normal range (diagnostic for vitamin deficiency after ruling out other disorders), PIUKA II test

Drugs that may alter lab results: Refer to laboratory test reference
Disorders that may alter lab results: Refer to laboratory test reference

PATHOLOGICAL FINDINGS N/A

SPECIAL TESTS N/A

IMAGING N/A

DIAGNOSTIC PROCEDURES History and physical

TREATMENT

APPROPRIATE HEALTH CARE
Outpatient usually. Inpatient in severe cases.

GENERAL MEASURES
- Treatment of any underlying causes
- Oral or parenteral vitamin therapeutic replacement
- Maintenance vitamin supplement as required
- For vitamin D deficiency - adequate exposure to sunlight

SURGICAL MEASURES N/A

ACTIVITY As tolerated

DIET
- For dietary deficiencies - provide nutritional counseling with emphasis on appropriate foods and the proper methods for their preparation
- Abstain from alcohol

PATIENT EDUCATION
• Refer patients to appropriate social service agencies if socioeconomic factors contribute to deficient diet
• Emphasis on compliance with vitamin supplementation regimens
• Help with alcohol or smoking cessation

MEDICATIONS

DRUG(S) OF CHOICE
• Vitamin A: cod liver oil or halibut liver oil. Acute deficiencies require aqueous vitamin A solution IM.
• Vitamin B1: oral thiamine 5-30 mg tid depending on deficiency. Maintenance: supplemental B complex vitamin.
• Vitamin B2: oral riboflavin 10-30 mg/day in divided doses until patient response is evident, then decrease to 2-4 mg/day until recovered. May be given IM 5-20 mg/day.
• Vitamin B3: confirmed deficiencies require niacinamide 300-500 mg/day in divided doses by mouth or IV. Supplemental B complex vitamins and dietary increase in foods high in niacin.
• Vitamin B6: oral or parenteral replacement for confirmed deficiency. Prophylactic doses for epileptic children. Women on oral contraceptives may need supplement (2.5-10 mg po).
• Vitamin B12: for severe deficiency, parenteral cobalamin 30 mcg IM or subcutaneous for 5-10 days. Supplements as needed for maintenance.
• Vitamin C: daily doses of 100-200 mg in synthetic form or in orange juice for mild scurvy, doses up to 500 mg/day in severe disease
• Vitamin D: oral doses of vitamin D or cod liver oil. For rickets refractory to vitamin D, include 25-hydroxycholecalciferol (active form of vitamin D).
• Vitamin E: oral or parenteral replacement with a water soluble vitamin E supplement, 60-70 units/day for adult, 1 unit/kg/day for children
• Vitamin K: 10 mg (adult dose) vitamin K (phytomenadione) for hypoprothrombinemia given subcutaneously or IM. For nonemergency, give oral dose 5-20 mg.
Contraindications: Refer to manufacturer's literature
Precautions: Refer to manufacturer's literature
Significant possible interactions: Refer to manufacturer's literature

ALTERNATIVE DRUGS Calcitriol

FOLLOWUP

PATIENT MONITORING As needed depending on severity of problem

PREVENTION/AVOIDANCE
• Proper nutrition
• Supplemental vitamins if needed
• Reduce risk factors that lead to deficiency where possible
• Vitamin D deficiency - adequate exposure to sunlight (30 minutes several times a week)
• Postoperative vitamin K for patients who receive nothing by mouth
• Neonates - should receive vitamin K1 IM, subcutaneously or orally to prevent hemolytic disease of the newborn

POSSIBLE COMPLICATIONS
• Vitamin A deficiency - mortality high in advanced cases; eye lesions are a threat to vision
• Vitamin B1 (thiamine) deficiency - cardiac beriberi and Wernicke-Korsakoff syndrome may be fatal if left untreated
• Vitamin B6 chronic deficiency - may increase risk of kidney stone formation
• Vitamin D deficiency - skeletal deformities, greenstick fractures, bone pain
• Excessive synthetic vitamin K may lead to hemolytic anemia and kernicterus in infants

EXPECTED COURSE/PROGNOSIS With proper diagnosis and adequate therapy, expect full recovery without complications

MISCELLANEOUS

ASSOCIATED CONDITIONS N/A

AGE-RELATED FACTORS
Pediatric:
• Vitamin D deficiency rickets is now rare in the U.S., but may occur in breast-fed infants who do not receive a vitamin D supplement, or in infants fed a formula with a nonfortified milk base
• Vitamin E deficiency in infants usually results from formulas high in polyunsaturated fatty acids that are fortified with iron but not vitamin E
• Vitamin K deficiency - common among newborns
Geriatric: More likely to have multiple risk factors that can lead to vitamin deficiencies
Others: N/A

PREGNANCY Women should take a supplemental multivitamin tablet that contains at least 60 mg of elemental iron and 1.0 mg of folic acid

SYNONYMS N/A

ICD-9-CM
• Multiple deficiency 269.2
• Vitamin A deficiency 264.9
• Vitamin B complex 266.9
• Vitamin B1 265.1
• Vitamin B2 266.0
• Vitamin B6 266.1
• Vitamin B12 266.2
• Vitamin C 267
• Vitamin D 268.9
• Vitamin E 269.1
• Vitamin K 269.0
• Vitamin K newborn 776.0

SEE ALSO N/A

OTHER NOTES Alcohol withdrawal - initial therapy of alcohol withdrawal should include B vitamins, especially thiamine to avoid causing neurological complications

ABBREVIATIONS N/A

REFERENCES
• Machlin LJ, ed: Handbook of Vitamins. 2nd Ed. New York, Marcel Dekker, 1990
• Shils ME, Young VR, eds: Modern Nutrition in Health and Disease. 7th Ed. Philadelphia, Lea & Febiger, 1988
• Konis AB: Vitamin deficiency in the elderly. NY State Dent J;1991
Illustrations: N/A
Internet references: http://www.5mcc.com

Author(s)
Joseph A. Florence, MD

Vitiligo

BASICS

DESCRIPTION An acquired, slowly progressive depigmenting condition in small or large areas of the skin due to the disappearance of previously active melanocytes
• Type A is non-dermatomal and widespread. It represents 75% of cases
• Type B is dermatomal or segmental. It represents the remaining 25% of cases
System(s) affected: Skin/Exocrine
Genetics: Autosomal dominant with variable expression and incomplete penetrance. Positive family history in 30% of cases.
Incidence/Prevalence in USA: 1000-2000/100,000
Predominant age: All ages: 50% begin between ages 10 and 30
Predominant sex: Male = Female

SIGNS AND SYMPTOMS
• Loss of pigment
• Locally increased sunburning
• Pruritus (10%)
• Premature graying (35%)
• Koebner's phenomenon (aggravation by trauma)

CAUSES Etiology is unclear, but is thought to be an autoimmune reaction to preexisting melanocytes

RISK FACTORS
• Positive family history
• Autoimmune disorders

DIAGNOSIS

DIFFERENTIAL DIAGNOSIS Any condition that causes acquired hypomelanosis, including tinea versicolor, leprosy, lupus erythematosus, pityriasis alba, atopic dermatitis, albinism, alopecia areata, chemical exposure (phenols, arsenic, chloroquine, hydroquinone) steroid exposure, retinoic acid use, tuberous sclerosis, neurofibromatosis, melanocytic nevi (halo nevi), tumor regression of malignant melanoma, Addison's disease, hypopituitarism, hyperthyroidism

LABORATORY Routine blood and urine studies are usually normal in the absence of associated disease
Drugs that may alter lab results: N/A
Disorders that may alter lab results: N/A

PATHOLOGICAL FINDINGS Complete absence of melanocytes in skin biopsy. At the margins one may see a few lymphocytes and large melanocytes with abnormal melanosomes.

SPECIAL TESTS N/A

IMAGING N/A

DIAGNOSTIC PROCEDURES
• Examination under Wood's light accentuates the hypopigmented areas, especially in light-skinned individuals
• Skin scraping and a potassium hydroxide (KOH) preparation can be examined microscopically to rule out tinea versicolor

TREATMENT

APPROPRIATE HEALTH CARE Outpatient except in rare cases of surgical skin-grafting or transplantation

GENERAL MEASURES
• Sun exposure can accentuate the difference between normal and abnormal skin, so for cosmetic reasons patients may wish to avoid this
• Skin dyes and cosmetics may be used as cover-ups

SURGICAL MEASURES N/A

ACTIVITY Full activity

DIET No special diet

PATIENT EDUCATION Reassure patient that in absence of associated autoimmune illness the problem is purely cosmetic. Successful cosmetic cover-up is usually quite simple. Some areas offer vitiligo support groups.

MEDICATIONS

DRUG(S) OF CHOICE
• Localized vitiligo: Begin with a mid-potency steroid cream applied daily for 3-4 months. If no response, advance to high potency steroids. Clobetasol propionate (Temovate) cream applied qd for 2 months (qod on the face). Treatment may be resumed following a 1 to 4 month respite. Alternatively topical psoralens applied in a 1% solution followed in 90 minutes by ultraviolet exposure (UVA). Caution for subsequent exposure to light (sunburn).
• Widespread vitiligo: Oral systemic steroids, e.g., betamethasone 5 mg given 2 days in a row, then held the remainder of the week. This pattern continued for 2-4 months minimizes side effects and is effective in arresting the disease in many patients. Oral trimethylpsoralen or 8-methoxypsoralen (methoxsalen) (Oxsoralen-Ultra) and UVA over a 12-24 month period. Alternatively depigmenting the remaining normal skin with hydroquinone cream (Benoquin) may be elected.

Contraindications:
• Absolute contraindications to use of psoralen compounds: Idiosyncratic reaction to psoralens, photosensitive disease (e.g., systemic lupus erythematosus, albinism, porphyria), invasive squamous cell carcinoma, melanoma, aphakia
• Relative contraindications to use of psoralen compounds: Cardiac disease, hepatic dysfunction, multiple basal cell carcinomas, prior radiation therapy, prior arsenic therapy

Precautions:
• Watch for skin atrophy and telangiectasias when using topical steroids, especially on the face
• Watch for photosensitizers with UVA treatment
• Severe burns possible with topical psoralens. Partially avoided with - 1:10 or 1:50 dilution of psoralens.
• Psoralen plus UVA (PUVA) cannot be used for children less than 12 years of age due to immaturity of the ocular lens
• Patients undergoing PUVA therapy should have a screening ophthalmologic examination to rule out subclinical retinal pigmentary disease that is frequently associated with vitiligo

Significant possible interactions: Other photosensitizers, e.g., tetracyclines and retinoic acid

ALTERNATIVE DRUGS
Patients with unresponsive localized vitiligo may be candidates for minigrafting

FOLLOWUP

PATIENT MONITORING
If patient receives PUVA therapy, a complete blood count, liver and renal function tests, and an ANA should be repeated at 6 month intervals

PREVENTION/AVOIDANCE
While undergoing all therapies, excessive sun exposure should be avoided

POSSIBLE COMPLICATIONS
• Phototoxic reactions ranging from mild to severe with PUVA
• Skin atrophy and telangiectasias with topical steroids
• Contact dermatitis can occur with use of depigmenting agents and cosmetic covers

EXPECTED COURSE/PROGNOSIS
• Only 5% spontaneously repigment
• Best results are with PUVA therapy where 70% have repigmentation of head and neck area, less in other body areas. Lower percentages respond to topical therapy
• There is no response in at least 20% of cases, especially long-standing cases
• Once repigmentation occurs it usually persists.

MISCELLANEOUS

ASSOCIATED CONDITIONS
• Addison's disease
• Alopecia areata
• Chronic mucocutaneous candidiasis
• Diabetes mellitus
• Hypoparathyroidism
• Melanoma
• Pernicious anemia
• Polyglandular autoimmune syndrome
• Thyroid disorders (hyper- and hypothyroidism)
- 30% of patients with vitiligo
• Uveitis
• Halo nevi

AGE-RELATED FACTORS
Pediatric: Childhood vitiligo is a distinct subset of vitiligo. Higher incidence of Type B (segmental) vitiligo. Also higher incidence of autoimmune and endocrine disease. Response is poor to topical PUVA therapy, but can be tried, or topical steroids may be prescribed.
Geriatric: NA
Others: N/A

PREGNANCY
• Treatment with topical or oral psoralens is contraindicated

SYNONYMS
• Hypomelanosis
• Depigmentation

ICD-9-CM
709.0 Dyschromia

SEE ALSO
• Tinea versicolor
• Pityriasis alba
• Arsenic poisoning

OTHER NOTES
If PUVA therapy considered, dermatologic consultation should be considered

ABBREVIATIONS N/A

REFERENCES
• Hurwitz S: Clinical Pediatric Dermatology. 2nd Ed. Philadelphia, W.B. Saunders Co., 1993
• Habif T: Clinical Dermatology. 3rd Ed. St Louis, Mosby, 1996
• Fitzpatrick TB, et al: Color Atlas and Synopsis of Clinical Dermatology. 3rd Ed. New York, McGraw-Hill, 1997
Illustrations: 5 available on CD-ROM
Internet references: http://www.5mcc.com

Author(s)
Gary J. Silko, MD

Vulvar malignancy

BASICS

DESCRIPTION
• Carcinoma in situ (Bowen's disease). Premalignant changes involving the squamous epithelium of the vulva.
• Squamous cell carcinoma - invasive squamous cell carcinoma is the most common malignancy involving the vulva in 85% of the patients. The malignancy can be well, moderately or poorly differentiated.
• Other invasive cell types include melanoma, Paget's disease, adenocarcinoma, adenocystic carcinoma, small cell carcinoma and sarcomas. Sarcomas are usually leiomyosarcoma and probably arise at the insertion of the round ligament in the labium majus.
System(s) affected: Reproductive
Genetics: No known genetic pattern
Incidence/Prevalence in USA: Invasive vulvar malignancy is a rare gynecologic malignancy accounting for approximately 2,000 new cases per year in the USA
Predominant age:
• In situ disease - mean age, forties
• Invasive malignancy - mean age, sixties with a range of twenties to nineties
Predominant sex: Female only

SIGNS AND SYMPTOMS
• In situ disease - a small raised area associated with pruritus
• Invasive malignancy - an ulcerated, non-healing area; as lesions become large, bleeding occurs with associated pain and foul smelling discharge
• In far advanced diseases - the patients can develop rectal bleeding or urethral obstruction
• Large involved inguinal lymph nodes are also associated with advanced disease

CAUSES
• Patients with cervical cancer are more likely to develop vulvar cancer at a later date. This is due to the so-called field effect with a carcinogen involving the lower genital tract.
• Human papilloma virus (HPV) has been associated with squamous cell abnormalities of the cervix, vagina and the vulva but has not been proven to be the causative agent
• Smoking is associated with squamous cell disease of the vulva possibly from direct irritation of the vulva by the transfer of tars and nicotine on the patient's hands

RISK FACTORS
• Old age. Invasive disease is rarely seen before age forty and the majority of the patients are elderly.
• In situ disease can occur at any age but is rarely seen before the age of twenty-five

DIAGNOSIS

DIFFERENTIAL DIAGNOSIS
• The definitive diagnosis for vulvar lesions is made by biopsy. Infectious processes can present as ulcerative lesions and include syphilis, lymphogranuloma venereum and granuloma inguinale
• Crohn's disease can present as an ulcerative area on the vulva
• Rarely, lesions can metastasize to the vulva

LABORATORY
• Squamous cell antigen can be elevated with invasive disease
• Hypercalcemia can occur when metastatic disease is present
Drugs that may alter lab results: N/A
Disorders that may alter lab results: N/A

PATHOLOGICAL FINDINGS
• A surgical staging system is used for vulva cancer - TNM Classification = tumor, node, and metastases:
  ◊ T1 - tumor less than or equal to 2.0 cm
  ◊ T2 - tumor greater than 2.0 cm
  ◊ T3 - lower urethra or vagina involved
  ◊ T4 - upper urethra, bladder, or rectum involved
  ◊ N0 - nodes negative
  ◊ N1 - unilateral positive lymph nodes
  ◊ N2 - bilateral positive lymph nodes
  ◊ M0 - no metastatic disease
  ◊ M1 - distant metastatic disease, positive pelvic lymphs node
• International Federation of Obstetrics and Gynecology Classification using TNM:
  ◊ Stage I - T1, N0, M0
  ◊ Stage II - T2, N0, M0
  ◊ Stage III - T1-3, N1, M0; T3, N0-I, M0
  ◊ Stage IVA - T1-3, N2, M0
  ◊ Stage IVB - any T, any N, any M

SPECIAL TESTS N/A

IMAGING
• Chest x-ray to evaluate for metastatic disease to lungs
• CAT scan to evaluate pelvic lymph node status and periaortic lymph node status

DIAGNOSTIC PROCEDURES
• Office vulvar biopsy; vulvar punch biopsy should be done to establish the diagnosis
• Wide excision can be performed for carcinoma in situ and any lesion where there is doubt should be further excised for definitive diagnosis to insure that invasive disease is not coexistent with the carcinoma in situ
• Cystoscopy and sigmoidoscopy should be performed if there is a question of invasion into the urethra, bladder or rectum

TREATMENT

APPROPRIATE HEALTH CARE Inpatient for treatment

GENERAL MEASURES
• Radiation therapy is used as adjuvant therapy for patients with positive inguinal lymph nodes
• In advanced malignancy involving the urethra and rectum, concomitant cisplatin/5-FU chemotherapy with radiation produces significant decrease in size of the primary tumor, usually obviating the need for pelvic exenteration

SURGICAL MEASURES
• In situ disease can be treated with wide excision or laser vaporization of the affected area. Laser vaporization is preferable in the younger patient while wide excision is preferable in the elderly patient where the risk of invasive disease is also higher.
• Invasive disease is treated primarily by radical vulvectomy and bilateral groin node dissection
• In selected patients, pelvic lymphadenectomy can be performed. If the pelvic lymph nodes are negative, radiation therapy can be avoided.
• Pelvic exenteration provides effective therapy for advanced or recurrent malignancies involving the bladder or rectum after radiation
• Radical vulvectomy and bilateral groin node dissection can be performed through three separate incisions
• Unilateral lesions can be treated with radical hemivulvectomy and unilateral groin node dissection. These modified techniques provide fewer complications and better cosmetic results.

ACTIVITY The patients are usually ambulatory and able to resume full activities by six weeks after surgery unless wound breakdown occurs

DIET Unrestricted, unless undergoing radiation

PATIENT EDUCATION Two complications are common with radical vulvectomy and bilateral groin node dissection, which is the usual treatment of this disease. In the immediate postoperative period, approximately 50% of patients will experience breakdown of the wound. This requires aggressive wound care by visiting nurses approximately twice a day. The wounds usually will granulate and heal over a period of six to ten weeks. Approximately 15-20% of the patients experience some form of mild to moderate lymphedema after the groin node dissection. The patients should be instructed in use of leg elevation and support hose. Less than 1% of the patients will experience severe debilitating lymphedema.
• American College of Obstetricians & Gynecologists (ACOG), 409 12th St., SW, Washington, DC 20024-2188, (800)762-ACOG

MEDICATIONS

DRUG(S) OF CHOICE
• There are no curative drugs
• As an adjuvant therapy, fluorouracil (Efudex) cream for in situ disease can produce occasional results, but the regimen is not well tolerated because of the excoriation and irritation of the vulva. Adjuvant chemotherapy has not proven to be effective in this disease.
• Metastatic disease, especially in the subcutaneous tissues of the leg or abdomen will produce hypercalcemia, which is treated in the usual medical fashion for hypercalcemia
Contraindications: Elderly patients - if chemotherapeutic agents are used, pay close attention to the patient's performance status and ability to tolerate aggressive chemotherapy
Precautions: The usual precautions for chemotherapy agents. Refer to manufacturer's literature.
Significant possible interactions: Refer to manufacturer's literature

ALTERNATIVE DRUGS N/A

FOLLOWUP

PATIENT MONITORING
• Clinical examination of the groin nodes and vulvar area every 3 months for 2 years, then every 6 months for 3 years
• Chest x-ray should be obtained once a year

PREVENTION/AVOIDANCE
• Any woman complaining of symptoms related to the vulva should have a close examination and biopsies made of appropriate areas
• The vulva can be washed with 3% acetic acid to highlight areas. Areas of white raised epithelium should be biopsied.
• Patients with new onset of pruritus should be biopsied in the area of pruritus
• Liberal biopsy must be used to diagnose in situ disease prior to invasion and to diagnose early invasive disease
• The patient should not be treated for presumed benign conditions of the vulva without full examination and biopsy
• When symptoms persist, reexamination and rebiopsy should be undertaken
• The treatment of benign condyloma of the vulva has not been shown to decrease the eventual incidence of in situ or invasive disease of the vulva

POSSIBLE COMPLICATIONS The major complications from radical vulvectomy and groin node dissection are wound breakdown, lymphedema and urinary stress incontinence

EXPECTED COURSE/PROGNOSIS
• The five year survival is based on stage:
  ◊ Stage I 90%
  ◊ Stage II 85%
  ◊ Stage III 70%
  ◊ Stage IVA 25%
  ◊ Stage IVB 5%

MISCELLANEOUS

ASSOCIATED CONDITIONS
• The patients with invasive vulvar cancer are often times elderly and have associated medical conditions
• High rate of other gynecologic malignancies. Patients should be evaluated for these.

AGE-RELATED FACTORS
Pediatric: N/A
Geriatric:
• Older patients with associated medical problems are at high risk for radical surgery. The surgery, however, is external, usually well-tolerated and is the treatment of choice.
• In the very elderly, palliative vulvectomy provides relief of symptoms for ulcerating symptomatic advanced disease
Others:
• More limited surgery
  ◊ Has been undertaken for invasive lesions especially in young patients to preserve the clitoris and sexual function
  ◊ Radical vulvectomy with groin node dissection through separate incisions provides better cosmetic results than the en bloc technique
  ◊ Radical hemivulvectomy can also be utilized for smaller lesions

PREGNANCY This malignancy is not associated with pregnancy

SYNONYMS
• Bowen's disease
• Vulvar cancer

ICD-9-CM
184.4

SEE ALSO N/A

OTHER NOTES N/A

ABBREVIATIONS N/A

REFERENCES
• Hopkins MP: Disease of the vulva. In: Willson JR, ed. Obstetrics & Gynecology. St. Louis, C.V. Mosby Co., 1991
• Hopkins MP, Reid GC, Vettrano I, Morley GW: Squamous cell carcinoma of the vulva: Prognostic factors influencing survival. Gynecol Oncol 1991;43:113-7
Illustrations: N/A
Internet references: http://www.5mcc.com

Author(s)
Michael P. Hopkins, MD
Eric L. Jenison, MD

Vulvovaginitis, bacterial

BASICS

DESCRIPTION Infectious disease affecting the vagina, only rarely affecting the vulva
System(s) affected: Reproductive
Genetics: N/A
Incidence/Prevalence in USA: As low as 4% in unselected populations; up to 33% in STD clinics; up to 44% in patients with vaginitis
Predominant age: N/A
Predominant sex: Female

SIGNS AND SYMPTOMS
• Unpleasant vaginal odor, musty or fishy, exacerbated immediately after intercourse
• Thin gray-white vaginal discharge, mildly adherent to vaginal walls
• 10-30% with vaginal/vulvar irritation
• 10% with frothy discharge.

CAUSES
• Polymicrobial; Gardnerella vaginalis, Mobiluncus species, Mycoplasma hominis, Peptostreptococcus, other various anaerobes, including Prevotella, Bacteroides, and Fusobacterium
• There is a shift from a healthy lactobacilli based endogenous flora to an anaerobically based endogenous flora
• Rectal reservoir of organisms leading to autoinfection

RISK FACTORS
• Controversial regarding multiple sexual partners
• IUD

DIAGNOSIS

DIFFERENTIAL DIAGNOSIS
• N. gonorrhea
• Chlamydia
• Trichomonas
• E. coli
• Staphylococci
• Fungal
• Trophic

LABORATORY
• Affirm VP microprobe
• PH paper (pH > 4.5)
• Wet prep - clue cells in > 10-20% of epithelial cells, fewer WBC's than epithelial cells
• 10% KOH - "whiff test" transient amine or fishy odor
• Gram stain indicating absence of lactobacilli
• May be seen on cytology
• Culture difficult for mycoplasma, not useful
Drugs that may alter lab results: Recent douching
Disorders that may alter lab results: N/A

PATHOLOGICAL FINDINGS Biopsies demonstrate no histologic evidence of inflammation

SPECIAL TESTS N/A

IMAGING N/A

DIAGNOSTIC PROCEDURES N/A

TREATMENT

APPROPRIATE HEALTH CARE
Outpatient

GENERAL MEASURES Consider repletion of lactobacilli

SURGICAL MEASURES N/A

ACTIVITY No restrictions

DIET No restrictions

PATIENT EDUCATION N/A

MEDICATIONS

DRUG(S) OF CHOICE
• Metronidazole 500 mg bid for 7 days (95% cure)
• Clindamycin 450 mg q6h for 7 days, or topical 2% vaginal cream for 7 days, or metronidazole vaginal cream for bacterial vaginosis
Contraindications: Refer to manufacturer's literature
Precautions: Refer to manufacturer's literature
Significant possible interactions: Metronidazole and alcohol

ALTERNATIVE DRUGS
• Amoxicillin-clavulanate (Augmentin) 500 mg q8h for 7 days
• Cephradine 500 mg q6h for 7 days
• Less effective - ampicillin 500 mg q6h (66% cure rate)
• Consider treating partner, especially in recurrent cases
• Reported in vitro susceptibility to penicillin, erythromycin, chloramphenicol and trimethoprim

FOLLOWUP

PATIENT MONITORING   None indicated

PREVENTION/AVOIDANCE
• Good hygiene
• Use of condoms for sexual intercourse

POSSIBLE COMPLICATIONS
• Uncommon but include
  ◊ Adnexal tenderness
  ◊ PID
  ◊ Intrauterine infections
  ◊ Chorioamnionitis
  ◊ Post abortion PID
  ◊ Postpartum endometritis
  ◊ Pelvic abscesses
  ◊ Vaginitis emphysematous
  ◊ Rare extravaginal disease
  ◊ Pre-term labor
  ◊ Premature rupture of membranes
  ◊ Chorioamnionitis
  ◊ Rare newborn infections, including scalp electrode sites, abscesses, and 1 reported case of meningitis
  ◊ Fetal loss
• Post-hysterectomy infection, septicemia, gaseous crepitation in wound

EXPECTED COURSE/PROGNOSIS
Relapses fairly common, can be decreased by increased colonization of lactobacilli

MISCELLANEOUS

ASSOCIATED CONDITIONS   N/A

AGE-RELATED FACTORS
Pediatric: N/A
Geriatric: N/A
Others: N/A

PREGNANCY   N/A

SYNONYMS
• Gardnerella vaginosis
• Bacterial vaginosis
• Nonspecific vaginitis
• Haemophilus vaginitis
• Corynebacterium vaginitis

ICD-9-CM   616.0

SEE ALSO   N/A

ABBREVIATIONS   N/A

OTHER NOTES   N/A

REFERENCES
• Herbst A, Mishell D Jr, Stenchever A, Droegueller W: Comprehensive Gynecology. 2nd Ed. C.V. Mosby Yearbook, 1992
• Reed B, Eyler A: Vaginal infections: Diagnosis and management. Amer Fam Phys 1993;47(8)
• Holst E: Reservoir of four organisms associated with bacterial vaginosis suggests lack of sexual transmission. J of Clin Microbiolgy 1990;28(9)
• Ray A, et al: Non-specific vaginitis vis-a-vis Gardnerella vaginalis. J of Communicable Dis 1990;22(4)
• Livengood C, Thomason J, Hill G: Bacterial vaginosis: Diagnostic and pathogenetic findings during topical clindamycin therapy. Amer J of Obs and Gynecol 1990;163(2)
• Caitlin BW: Garderella vaginalis: Characteristics, clinical considerations and controversies. Clinical Microbiology Review 19925(3):213-217
• Kharsany AB, Hosen AA, Vanden Ende J: Antimicrobial susceptibility of Gardnerella vaginalis. Antimicrobial Agents and Chemotherapeutics 1993;37(12):2733-2735
• Briselden AM, Hillier SL: Evaluation of affirm VP microbial identification test for Gardnerella vaginalis and trichomonas vaginalis. J Clin Microbiology 1994;32(1):148-152
• Curry SL, Barclay: Benign disorders of the vulva-vagina. In: DeCherry & Perroll, eds. Current Obstetric & Gynecologic Diagnosis & Treatment. 8th Ed. Norwalk, Appleton & Lang, 1994
Illustrations: N/A
Internet references: http://www.5mcc.com

Author(s)
Elizabeth McCord, MD, MS

Vulvovaginitis, candidal

BASICS

DESCRIPTION Vulvar pruritus and/or burning, often with abnormal vaginal discharge
System(s) affected: Reproductive, Skin/Exocrine
Genetics: N/A
Incidence/Prevalence in USA:
• 40% of vulvovaginitis is caused by Candida
• 16% of non-pregnant premenopausal women are asymptomatic carriers
Predominant Age: Menarche to menopause
Predominant sex: Female only

SIGNS AND SYMPTOMS
• Intense vulvar itching
• Thick curd-like vaginal discharge
• Dyspareunia at times
• Erythema of vulva
• Erythema, pain and pruritus of crural and perineal area
• Thick white patches appear attached to vaginal mucosa
• Inflamed vulvar skin

CAUSES
Overgrowth of Candida species (C. albicans, C. glabrata, C. tropicalis) in vagina

RISK FACTORS
• Pregnancy
• Diabetes mellitus
• Antibiotic therapy
• Corticosteroid therapy
• Immunosuppressed states
• HIV infection
• Occlusive synthetic underpants and undergarments
• Hypothyroidism
• Oral contraceptive medications (low dose usually not a cause of increased infection risk)
• Anemia
• Zinc deficiency

DIAGNOSIS

DIFFERENTIAL DIAGNOSIS
• Trichomonas vaginitis
• Gonorrheal vaginitis - in prepubertal girls
• Pinworm vaginitis
• Contact dermatitis/vaginitis

LABORATORY
• Yeast, spores, and/or pseudohyphae on smear with 10% KOH solution
• Culture findings on Nickerson's or Sabouraud's media; usually only indicated for recurrent infections
• Vaginal pH < 4.5
Drugs that may alter lab results: N/A
Disorders that may alter lab results: N/A

PATHOLOGICAL FINDINGS N/A

SPECIAL TESTS N/A

IMAGING N/A

DIAGNOSTIC PROCEDURES
• Smear of discharge with 10% KOH solution
• Pap smear

TREATMENT

APPROPRIATE HEALTH CARE
Outpatient

GENERAL MEASURES
• Remove foreign body if one present
• Consider providone iodine douche 15 to 30 mL/L (2 tbsp/qt) of water for symptomatic relief until specific therapy is effective
• If urination causes burning, have the patient
  ◊ Urinate through a tubular device such as a toilet-paper roll or plastic cup with the end cut out
  ◊ Pour warm water over vaginal area while urinating
• Insist on strict diabetic control if patient is diabetic

SURGICAL MEASURES N/A

ACTIVITY
• Avoid overexertion, heat, and excessive sweating
• Delay sexual relations until symptoms clear

DIET Limit sweets (sucrose) and dairy products (lactose) in recurrent infections

PATIENT EDUCATION
• Keep the genital area clean. Use plain unscented soap.
• Take showers rather than tub baths
• Wear cotton underpants with a cotton crotch. Avoid clothing made from non-ventilating materials, including most synthetic underclothing. Avoid tight-fitting jeans or slacks
• Sleep in loose gown without underpants
• Don't sit around in wet clothing - especially a wet bathing suit
• Avoid frequent douches
• Avoid broad-spectrum antibiotics when possible
• After urinating or bowel movements, cleanse by wiping or washing from front to back (vagina toward anus)
• Lose weight, if obese
• American College of Obstetricians & Gynecologists (ACOG), 409 12th St., SW, Washington, DC 20024-2188, (800)762-ACOG

Vulvovaginitis, candidal

MEDICATIONS

DRUG(S) OF CHOICE
• Fluconazole (Diflucan): 150 mg po once
• Miconazole nitrate (Monistat): one suppository q night x 3, or miconazole vaginal cream q night x 7, or
• Butoconazole nitrate (Femstat): vaginal cream q night x 3, or
• Terconazole (Terazol): one suppository or vaginal cream q night x 3, or
• Clotrimazole (Gyne-Lotrimin): two 100 mg tablets intravaginally x 3 days or cream each night x 7 days
Contraindications: N/A
Precautions: Refer to manufacturer's profile of each drug
Significant possible interactions: Refer to manufacturer's profile of each drug

ALTERNATIVE DRUGS
• Retreat with different agent, if recurrence
• Course of oral nystatin; 100,000 units tid for 2 weeks
• Topical gentian violet 1% aqueous solution painted onto vagina weekly until infection resolves (usually 2-3 weeks)
• Boric acid 600 mg in gelatin capsule inserted vaginally daily for 2 weeks.

FOLLOWUP

PATIENT MONITORING Generally no specific followup needed. If symptoms persist, then repeat pelvic exam and culture.

PREVENTION/AVOIDANCE
• Follow instructions under patient education
• For recurrences consider re-infection from sexual partner(s). Examine and treat sex partner for Candida balanitis and oral Candida if vaginitis recurs.
• Review Risk Factors

POSSIBLE COMPLICATIONS Secondary bacterial infections of the vagina or vulva

EXPECTED COURSE/PROGNOSIS
• Complete cure with vigorous treatment
• Recurrences are common

MISCELLANEOUS

ASSOCIATED CONDITIONS Sexually transmitted diseases

AGE-RELATED FACTORS
Pediatric: Less common before puberty
Geriatric: N/A
Others: N/A

PREGNANCY Common

SYNONYMS
• Monilial vulvovaginitis

ICD-9-CM
112.1 Candidiasis of vulva and vagina

SEE ALSO N/A

OTHER NOTES N/A

ABBREVIATIONS N/A

REFERENCES
• Jones HW, Wentz-Colston A, eds: Novak's Textbook of Gynecology. 11th Ed. Baltimore, Williams & Wilkins Co., 1988
• Kaufman RH, Faro S, (eds: Benign Diseases of the Vulva and Vagina. 4th Ed. St. Louis, Mosby-Year Book, 1994
Illustrations: N/A
Internet references: http://www.5mcc.com

Author(s)
John Freeman, MD

- 1153 -

Vulvovaginitis, estrogen deficient

BASICS

DESCRIPTION   Decreased blood flow with a thinning and atrophy of the female genital tissue. Changes from estrogen deficiency occur throughout the body. The genital tissues are hormone responsive. Estrogen deficient vulvovaginitis is frequently associated with urinary incontinence.
System(s) affected: Reproductive
Genetics: No known genetic pattern
Incidence/Prevalence in USA: This disorder will affect all women, to some degree, unless estrogen replacement therapy is provided
Predominant age: This is predominantly a problem of the postmenopausal female. The average age of menopause in the United States is 52.5 years.
Predominant sex: Female only

SIGNS AND SYMPTOMS
• Vaginal dryness
• Decreased vaginal secretions
• Dyspareunia
• Vulva undergoes a thinning of the epidermis along with decreased integrity of the supporting structures. The thinning and atrophy often produces pruritus.

CAUSES
• Estrogen deficiency
  ◊ Menopause (surgical or natural)
  ◊ Ovariectomy
  ◊ Radiation of the pelvis

RISK FACTORS
• Estrogen deficient states accompanying metabolic disorders
• Vaginal infections with bacteria and fungi

DIAGNOSIS

DIFFERENTIAL DIAGNOSIS
• Malignancy
• Vulvar dystrophies

LABORATORY
• Cytology for maturation index will show a low maturation index, signifying a decreased turnover of the cells from the decreased estrogen effect
• In the perimenopausal or menopausal female, follicle stimulating hormone (FSH) will be elevated and estradiol will be decreased
Drugs that may alter lab results:
• Estrogen therapy will alter the maturation index
• Digoxin has estrogen-like properties
• Tamoxifen (Nolvadex) can produce menopausal type symptoms but also can act on genital tissues as a weak estrogen agonist. Symptoms can vary.
• Drugs used to treat endometriosis or uterine bleeding such as progestins, Danazol or gonadotropin releasing hormone (GnRH) agonists can produce a pseudomenopause which is reversible
Disorders that may alter lab results: N/A

PATHOLOGICAL FINDINGS   Thinning of the cornified squamous layer of both the vulva and the vagina

SPECIAL TESTS   N/A

IMAGING   N/A

DIAGNOSTIC PROCEDURES
• Examination of the vagina and the vulva for maturation index
• FSH level to confirm menopause
• Estradiol level to evaluate circulating estrogen level

TREATMENT

APPROPRIATE HEALTH CARE
Outpatient

GENERAL MEASURES
• Estrogen replacement therapy (ERT) will alleviate and reverse the symptoms and the thinning of the squamous epithelial layer. Replacement therapy leads to an increased blood supply to the genital tissues.
• Symptomatic relief, if needed, e.g., cool baths or compresses

SURGICAL MEASURES   N/A

ACTIVITY   No restriction

DIET   No special diet

PATIENT EDUCATION
• American College of Obstetricians & Gynecologists (ACOG), 409 12th St., SW, Washington, DC 20024-2188, (800)762-ACOG

MEDICATIONS

DRUG(S) OF CHOICE
• A wide variety of preparations are available:
  ◊ Estrogen, conjugated (Premarin) 0.625 mg daily
  ◊ Estradiol (Estrace) 1 mg daily
  ◊ Estradiol (Estraderm) patch 0.05 mg, changed twice weekly
  ◊ If the uterus is not removed, progesterone should be considered. This can be added as medroxyprogesterone (Provera) 2.5 mg daily or 10 mg for 10 days of each month.
  ◊ Conjugated estrogen vaginal cream (2-4 g/day intravaginally)
Contraindications:
• Estrogen therapy is contraindicated in patients with a history of breast cancer or estrogen positive tumor receptors
• A history of uterine malignancy is a relative contraindication
Precautions: Refer to manufacturer's literature
Significant possible interactions: Refer to manufacturer's literature

ALTERNATIVE DRUGS N/A

FOLLOWUP

PATIENT MONITORING The patient should be instructed that symptoms should resolve within 30-60 days. If they do not, reevaluation and reexamination for other causes should be undertaken.

PREVENTION/AVOIDANCE N/A

POSSIBLE COMPLICATIONS Those associated with estrogen replacement - postmenopausal bleeding, nausea, headache, libido changes, thrombophlebitis

EXPECTED COURSE/PROGNOSIS
Excellent. The vast majority of symptoms will be relieved with estrogen replacement therapy.

MISCELLANEOUS

ASSOCIATED CONDITIONS None

AGE-RELATED FACTORS
Pediatric: N/A
Geriatric: N/A
Others: N/A

PREGNANCY The lactating postpartum woman with high levels of prolactin are in a hypo-estrogenic state. These women should be instructed to use lubrication for symptoms of dyspareunia. The symptoms will resolve when breast-feeding is stopped.

SYNONYMS N/A

ICD-9-CM 616.10 Vaginitis and vulvovaginitis, unspecified

SEE ALSO N/A

OTHER NOTES The obese patient, especially those weighing more than 100 pounds (45 kg) over the ideal body weight, have higher levels of circulating estrogen and thus may have fewer symptoms. (Androstenedione is converted to estrone in peripheral adipose tissue and when there is an abundance of adipose, higher estrone levels are present.)

ABBREVIATIONS N/A

REFERENCES
• Cunningham FG, MacDonald PC, Gant NF, eds: Williams Obstetrics. 19th Ed. Norwalk CT, Appleton & Lange, 1993
• Novak ER, et al, eds: Novak's Textbook of Gynecology. 11th Ed. Baltimore, Williams & Wilkins, 1988
Illustrations: N/A
Internet references: http://www.5mcc.com

Author(s)
Michael P. Hopkins, MD
Eric L. Jenison, MD

Vulvovaginitis, prepubescent

 BASICS

DESCRIPTION Irritation and/or inflammation of the vulva and/or vagina frequently associated with vaginal discharge
System(s) affected: Reproductive, Skin/Exocrine
Genetics: Not well studied
Incidence/Prevalence in USA: Common
Predominant age: Toddlers to menarche
Predominant sex: Female only

SIGNS AND SYMPTOMS
• Irritation and erythema of vulva
• Vaginal discharge
• Offensive odor
• Itching
• Excoriation
• Bleeding

CAUSES
• Most often due to:
 ◊ Poor hygiene
 ◊ Secondary infection elsewhere, e.g., otitis media, pharyngitis
• Most common specific organisms:
 ◊ Group A beta-hemolytic streptococci; Streptococcus pyogenes, Streptococcus pneumoniae
 ◊ E. coli
 ◊ Staphylococcus aureus
 ◊ Hemophilus influenzae
 ◊ Pinworms
• Less common specific organisms:
 ◊ Neisseria meningitidis
 ◊ Candida sp.
 ◊ Shigella
 ◊ Neisseria gonorrhea
 ◊ Trichomonas vaginalis
 ◊ Chlamydia trachomatis
 ◊ Gardnerella vaginalis
 ◊ Herpes viruses
 ◊ Human papilloma virus
 ◊ Scabies
• Systemic illnesses:
 ◊ Measles
 ◊ Chickenpox
 ◊ Stevens-Johnson syndrome
• Localized vulvar disease:
 ◊ Seborrheic dermatitis
 ◊ Psoriasis
 ◊ Atopic dermatitis
 ◊ Contact dermatitis
 ◊ Lichen sclerosus et atrophicus
• Other:
 ◊ Sexual abuse
 ◊ Other trauma
 ◊ Foreign body
 ◊ Tumors or polyps
 ◊ Poor hygiene
 ◊ Masturbation
 ◊ Genital tract malformations

RISK FACTORS
• Co-existing pharyngitis or other systemic conditions
• Faulty hygiene
• Trauma or abuse
• Diabetes mellitus

 DIAGNOSIS

DIFFERENTIAL DIAGNOSIS
• Contact dermatitis
• Eczema
• Psoriasis

LABORATORY
• Gram stain
• Tape examination for pinworms
• Potassium hydroxide and saline smears
• Culture for bacteria, fungi or viruses
Drugs that may alter lab results: N/A
Disorders that may alter lab results: N/A

PATHOLOGICAL FINDINGS N/A

SPECIAL TESTS Exploration of vagina for foreign body may be necessary in long-standing vaginal discharge

IMAGING N/A

DIAGNOSTIC PROCEDURES
Visualization of the vagina may be necessary using a nasal speculum or infant laryngoscope. If blood or foul-smelling discharge is present, visualization is mandatory. Place child in knee-chest position for best result. Hold buttocks apart and slightly upward.

 TREATMENT

APPROPRIATE HEALTH CARE
Outpatient (except where systemic illness requires hospital care)

GENERAL MEASURES
• Hygiene:
 ◊ Wipe front-to-back after elimination
 ◊ Avoid bubble baths and other irritating products
 ◊ Clean daily with mild soap and water, drying thoroughly with soft towel
 ◊ Apply bland ointments for protection of the skin, if necessary

SURGICAL MEASURES N/A

ACTIVITY Normal

DIET N/A

PATIENT EDUCATION As noted above under General measures

MEDICATIONS

DRUG(S) OF CHOICE
• Group A beta-Streptococcus, Streptococcus pneumoniae - penicillin V (Pen Vee K) 25-50 mg/kg/day, maximum of 3 gm/day, divided qid x 10 days
• C. trachomatis - erythromycin 50 mg/kg/d po x 10 days
• N. gonorrhoea - ceftriaxone IM x 1, 125 mg if < 45 kg; 250 mg if > 45 kg
• Candida spp - topical nystatin (Mycostatin), miconazole, clotrimazole or terconazole
• Shigella - trimethoprim-sulfamethoxazole 8/40 mg/kg/day po x 7 days
• Staphylococcus aureus - cephalexin 25-50 mg/kg/day, divided qid x 7-10 days or dicloxacillin 12.5-25 mg/kg/day x 7-10 days
• H. influenzae - amoxicillin 20-40 mg/kg/day x 7 days; amoxicillin-clavulanate 20 mg/kg/day
• Trichomonas vaginalis - metronidazole 125 mg (15 mg/kg/day) tid x 7-10 days
• Estrogen deficiency with labial adhesion/agglutination - estrogen, conjugated cream to fused area nightly for two weeks
Contraindications: Allergy to proposed treatment
Precautions: Avoid potential allergens/topical sensitizers if possible
Significant possible interactions: See manufacturer's profile of each drug

ALTERNATIVE DRUGS Topical corticosteroids for pruritus

FOLLOWUP

PATIENT MONITORING Only if symptoms do not respond to treatment

PREVENTION/AVOIDANCE
• Perineal hygiene
• Avoidance of irritants and tight or occlusive, non-breathable clothing
• White, unscented toilet paper

POSSIBLE COMPLICATIONS Labial agglutination or adhesions

EXPECTED COURSE/PROGNOSIS
Usually clears with appropriate treatment with no permanent sequelae (if not due to underlying disease such as psoriasis, etc.)

MISCELLANEOUS

ASSOCIATED CONDITIONS N/A

AGE-RELATED FACTORS
Pediatric:
• Usual adult vulvitis/vaginitis organisms are rare in the prepubertal child
• Lack of estrogen causing thin vaginal mucosa which is more susceptible to trauma and infection
Geriatric: N/A
Others: N/A

PREGNANCY N/A

SYNONYMS Vaginitis, vulvitis

ICD-9-CM 616.1

SEE ALSO N/A

OTHER NOTES N/A

ABBREVIATIONS N/A

REFERENCES
• Dewhurst CJ: Practical Pediatric and Adolescent Gynecology. New York, Marcel Dekker Inc., 1980
• Vandeven AM, Emans SJ: Vulvovaginitis in the child and adolescent. Pediatric Rev 1993;14:141
• Pierce AM, Hart CA: Vulvovaginitis: causes and management. Arch Dis Child 1992;67:509-512
Illustrations: N/A
Internet references: http://www.5mcc.com

Author(s)
Janice E. Daugherty, MD

Warts

BASICS

DESCRIPTION Warts are painless, benign skin tumors characterized by an area of well circumscribed epithelial thickening. The DNA papillomavirus is causative and is passed by direct contact with an infected person or from recently shed virus kept intact in a moist, warm environment. Five types of warts are caused by specific genotypes of HPV:
• Common wart (verruca vulgaris)
• Plantar wart (verruca plantaris)
• Flat wart (verruca plana)
• Venereal wart (condyloma acuminatum)
• Epidermodysplasia verruciformis
System(s) affected: Skin/Exocrine
Genetics: N/A
Incidence/Prevalence in USA: 7-10% of the population
Predominant age: Young adults and children
Predominant sex: Female > Male

SIGNS AND SYMPTOMS
• Verruca vulgaris: Rough surfaced, raised, skin-colored papules 5-10 mm in diameter. They may coalesce into a mosaic 1-3 cm in diameter. Most frequently seen on hands.
• Verruca plantaris: Rough surfaced (although smoother than the common wart), flat, skin-colored papules not infrequently attaining 2-3 cm in diameter
• Verruca plana: Slightly elevated, flat-topped, skin-colored papules 1-3 mm in diameter sometimes in a linear arrangement often on hands and face
• Condyloma acuminatum: thin, flexible, tall, papules sometimes demonstrating a confluent growth resembling cauliflower. They do not have the visible or palpable keratin of the previous warts. In infants, laryngeal papillomatosis may occur if condyloma is transmitted during vaginal delivery.
• Epidermodysplasia verruciformis: Flat, reddish lesions on the hands and shoulders presenting in childhood with lifelong persistence

CAUSES Human papillomavirus (HPV)

RISK FACTORS
• AIDS and other immunosuppressive diseases (e.g., lymphomas)
• Immunosuppressive drug use
• Atopic dermatitis
• Locker room use
• Skin trauma

DIAGNOSIS

DIFFERENTIAL DIAGNOSIS
• Corns (on paring, a single "eye" of keratin is observed, whereas the wart shows hemorrhagic spots or "roots")
• Scar tissue
• Molluscum contagiosum (central umbilication and, after curettage, the characteristic pearl)
• Condyloma lata (flat warts of syphilis)
• Seborrheic keratoses

LABORATORY HPV cannot be cultured
Drugs that may alter lab results: N/A
Disorders that may alter lab results: N/A

PATHOLOGICAL FINDINGS
• Papillomavirus found in the nuclei and nucleoli of the stratum granulosum and keratin layers of the epidermis.
• Plantar warts have rete pegs (a downward proliferation of epidermal ridges).
• Thrombosed dermal capillaries

SPECIAL TESTS
Definitive diagnosis can be achieved with the following, but are not clinically relevant for most presentations:
• Electron microscopy
• Immunohistochemical study
• Nucleic acid hybridization

IMAGING N/A

DIAGNOSTIC PROCEDURES Paring or débridement and simple visualization will be diagnostic in most cases.

TREATMENT

APPROPRIATE HEALTH CARE
Outpatient

GENERAL MEASURES Spontaneous remissions are common, probably related to a host immune response. Conservative, non-scarring treatments are preferred. Each treatment is associated with a 60-70% cure rate. Cure is achieved when skin lines are restored to a normal pattern.

SURGICAL MEASURES
• Cryotherapy - often preferred because scar formation is minimized. Freezing periungual warts may result on nail deformation.
• Excision with electrocautery, laser ablation, curettage (the virus may be found in smoke so that masks should be worn)

ACTIVITY If plantar warts are on weight-bearing surface, they may cause significant discomfort requiring a decrease in activity

DIET N/A

PATIENT EDUCATION Infectious nature should be discussed; keep warts covered while under treatment to avoid auto-inoculation and transmission to others.

MEDICATIONS

DRUG(S) OF CHOICE
• Chemotherapy - all treatments begin by paring the wart, then soaking the area in warm water to moisten the wart
◊ Topical retinoids: tretinoin (retinoic acid, Retin-A) for flat warts, less scarring than cryotherapy or surgical approaches; may be best for warts on the face. Apply bid for 4-6 weeks.
◊ Lactic-salicylic acid (Duofilm): daily treatment for about 3 months
◊ Salicylic acid (Trans-Ver-Sal) in a transdermal delivery system : daily treatment for about 6 weeks
◊ Keralyt (salicylic acid in propylene glycol); rub into warts each night
◊ Occlusion - the easiest and least expensive; cover the wart with a waterproof tape and leave on for a week. Remove and leave open for 12 hours then re-tape if wart is still present. The environment under the tape does not foster viral growth. May be the best for periungual warts.
Contraindications: See specific treatments. Vascular insufficiency is a relative contraindication to some treatments.
Precautions: Avoid normal skin when using the topical chemicals
Significant possible interactions: N/A

ALTERNATIVE DRUGS
• Chemotherapy
◊ Benzoyl peroxide: apply bid for 4-6 weeks
◊ Bleomycin - intradermal injection, is expensive and causes severe pain, but has a 75% cure rate
◊ Cimetidine - 30-40 mg/kg divided tid for 3 months. 86% of patients will have partial or complete regression.
◊ 24% podophyllin applied weekly to anogenital warts, or 5% podofilox (Condylox) self-applied twice daily for 3 days each week for 1 month
◊ Others - dichloroacetic acid, trichloroacetic acid, podophyllin, 5-fluorouracil, silver nitrate, idoxuridine (Herplex Liquifilm)
• Immunotherapy
◊ Dinitrochlorobenzene (DNCB) - should be considered a last resort because of side effects and possible mutagenicity
◊ Interferon - intralesional for urogenital warts

FOLLOWUP

PATIENT MONITORING
One third of the warts of epidermodysplasia may become malignant

PREVENTION/AVOIDANCE
• Cover warts under treatment. Avoid the wound fluid after cryotherapy.
• Use personal footwear in locker room settings

POSSIBLE COMPLICATIONS
• Auto-inoculation
• Scar formation
• Chronic pain after plantar wart removal and scar formation
• Nail deformity after injury to nail matrix

EXPECTED COURSE/PROGNOSIS
Good; complete resolution with or without treatment

MISCELLANEOUS

ASSOCIATED CONDITIONS
• Acquired immunodeficiency syndrome
• Renal transplantation
• Other conditions with immunosuppression
• Lewandowsky-Lutz disease (associated with epidermodysplasia)

AGE-RELATED FACTORS
Pediatric: Generally more prevalent in children
Geriatric: Less common in non-immunocompromised adults
Others: N/A

PREGNANCY Podophyllin is contraindicated

SYNONYMS N/A

ICD-9-CM 078.1 viral warts

SEE ALSO
• Condyloma acuminata
• Warts, plantar

OTHER NOTES N/A

ABBREVIATIONS
HPV = Human papillomavirus

REFERENCES
• Bolton RA: Warts. Am Fam Phys 1991;43(6):2049-2056
• Lynch PJ: Dermatology for the House Officer. 3rd Ed. Baltimore, Williams & Wilkins, 1994
• Sams W, et al: Principles and Practices of Dermatology. 2nd Ed. New York, Churchill Livingston, 1996
• Ordoukhanian E: Warts and molluscum contagiosum; beware of treatments worse than the disease. Postgrad Med 1997;2:223-235
• Siegfried EC: Warts on children: an approach to therapy. Ped Annuals 1996;2:79-90
Illustrations: 12 available on CD-ROM
Internet references: http://www.5mcc.com

Author(s)
Barbara J. Morant, MD
Yates P. Lee, MD

Warts, plantar

BASICS

DESCRIPTION Discrete or grouped firm keratotic masses on the sole of the foot initiated by a viral infection of keratinocytes
System(s) affected: Skin/Exocrine
Genetics: Unknown
Incidence/Prevalence in USA:
Widespread; 2000/100,000
Predominant age: Any age, although more common in children and young adults
Predominant sex: Female > Male (slightly)

SIGNS AND SYMPTOMS
• Foot pain
• Discrete or grouped masses on sole of foot
• Rough, hyperkeratotic surface with brown-black dots (thrombised capillaries)
• Callus formation
• Leg or back pain (distortion of posture)

CAUSES Human papillomaviruses, types 1, 2 and 4

RISK FACTORS
• AIDS
• Atopic dermatitis
• Lymphomas
• Patient taking immunosuppressive drugs

DIAGNOSIS

DIFFERENTIAL DIAGNOSIS
• Corns (clavi)
• Calluses
• Black heel (ruptured capillaries)

LABORATORY N/A
Drugs that may alter lab results: N/A
Disorders that may alter lab results: N/A

PATHOLOGICAL FINDINGS Acanthotic epidermis with hyperkeratosis, papillomatosis, and parakeratosis

SPECIAL TESTS N/A

IMAGING N/A

DIAGNOSTIC PROCEDURES
• Inspection usually confirms the diagnosis
• If cannot distinguish between callus and wart, can examine with a magnifying lens. The wart should demonstrate a highly organized mosaic pattern.

TREATMENT

APPROPRIATE HEALTH CARE
• Outpatient cryotherapy at weekly intervals
• Repeated parings at weekly intervals with or without use of a keratolytic is also an option. Most successful appears to be curettage and chemical cautery (with phenol or trichloroacetic acid) or light electrocautery. (Note: extreme care must be exercised with this procedure because excessive cautery or curettage can cause a painful scar.)

GENERAL MEASURES
• If warts are asymptomatic, no treatment is necessary. However patient may be at risk for spread of warts.
• Warm soaks followed by patient's paring of the top layer of skin on repeated occasions may speed disappearance
• Patient may use pumice stone, emery board or a blade
• Over-the-counter keratolytics containing salicylic acid may help. The advised procedure is paring of skin followed by warm soaks, and finally application of a few drops of keratolytic.
• Other measures include use of a heel bar or appropriate padding to relieve pressure points where warts tend to aggregate

SURGICAL MEASURES
• Cryotherapy - application of liquid nitrogen is often effective. It usually requires at least 4 applications at weekly or biweekly intervals. Aggressive cryotherapy may cause blistering or even scarring, so light applications are preferred.
• Blunt dissection - a simple surgical procedure is effective and usually nonscarring. It requires inserting a blunt dissector between the wart and normal skin and separating the wart using short, firm stroke.
• CO2 laser surgery - used for recalcitrant warts

ACTIVITY Ambulatory unless warts or treatment is painful

DIET No special diet

PATIENT EDUCATION
• In Epsteln: Common Skin Disorders, patient instructions, pages 123 (see References)
• Griffith: Instructions for Patients, Philadelphia, W.B. Saunders Co.
• American Academy of Dermatology (708)330-0230

Warts, plantar

MEDICATIONS

DRUG(S) OF CHOICE
No effective antiviral wart medications currently exist. Keratolytics (over-the-counter or prescription) and a variety of chemotherapeutic acids may be used.
• Salicylic acid - see General Measures for instructions
• 40% salicylic acid plasters - available as Mediplast. It is supplied in 3 by 4 inch sheets which are cut to the size of the wart and the sticky surface applied to the wart. They are removed every 1 to 2 days, the white keratin peeled and a fresh plaster applied.
• Chemotherapy, dichloroacetic acid and trichloroacetic acid kits are available. Callus is pared and the surrounding skin is protected by a ring of petrolatum. The wart(s) are coated with acid which is then worked into the wart with a sharp toothpick. Procedure should be repeated at weekly intervals.
• Transdermal salicylates (Trans-Plantar)
• Vesicants containing cantharidin (Cantharone, Verrusol)
Contraindications: Infection, vascular insufficiency
Precautions:
• If the dermis is damaged with any of the above procedures, a scar may result which can be permanently painful
• Care should be taken to avoid excessive contact with normal skin when using keratolytics or chemotherapy
Significant possible interactions: N/A

ALTERNATIVE DRUGS N/A

FOLLOWUP

PATIENT MONITORING With any treatment modality, followup weekly

PREVENTION/AVOIDANCE Use rubber footwear in communal shower areas

POSSIBLE COMPLICATIONS Scarring with overly aggressive treatment

EXPECTED COURSE/PROGNOSIS The course of plantar warts is like that of other varieties of warts, i.e., highly variable. Most resolve spontaneously in weeks to months.

MISCELLANEOUS

ASSOCIATED CONDITIONS N/A

AGE-RELATED FACTORS
Pediatric: Duration of warts is generally shorter in children than in adults
Geriatric: N/A
Others: N/A

PREGNANCY N/A

SYNONYMS Verruca plantaris

ICD-9-CM 078.1

SEE ALSO
• Warts
• Condyloma acuminata

OTHER NOTES N/A

ABBREVIATIONS N/A

REFERENCES
• Epstein E: Common Skin Disorders. 4th Ed. Philadelphia, W.B. Saunders Co., 1994
• Hurwitz S: Clinical Pediatric Dermatology. 2nd Ed. Philadelphia, W.B. Saunders Co., 1993
• Habif T: Clinical Dermatology. 3rd Ed. St Louis, Mosby, 1996
Illustrations: 2 available on CD-ROM
Internet references: http://www.5mcc.com

Author(s)
Gary J. Silko, MD

Wegener's granulomatosis

BASICS

DESCRIPTION A multisystem disease characterized by granulomatous vasculitis involving multiple organs. The characteristic "triad" of involvement includes the upper airway (otitis, sinusitis, nasal mucosa), lung, and kidney. Other organ systems involved include skin, joints, nervous system (peripheral or central).
• As the condition progresses untreated, upper airway erosions, necrotic pulmonary nodules, and renal failure are common, and, without treatment, mortality rate is high
System(s) affected: Cardiovascular, Pulmonary, Renal/Urologic, Gastrointestinal, Nervous, Skin/Exocrine
Genetics:
• Increased presence in HLA-B8
• Increased presence in HLA-DR2
Incidence/Prevalence in USA: Incidence estimated at approximately 0.4/100,000; prevalence 3/100,000
Predominant age: Mean age of onset in mid-40's, but has been described in all age groups
Predominant sex: Male > Female (3:2)

SIGNS AND SYMPTOMS
• Pulmonary infiltrates (71%)
• Sinusitis (67%)
• Arthralgia/arthritis (44%)
• Fever (34%)
• Cough (34%)
• Otitis (25%)
• Rhinitis (22%)
• Hemoptysis (18%)
• Ocular inflammation (16%)
• Weight loss (16%)
• Skin rash (13%)
• Epistaxis (11%)
• Renal failure (11%)
• Chest pain, anorexia, proptosis, dyspnea, oral ulcers, hearing loss, headache (all < 10%)

CAUSES No known etiology. Autoimmune phenomena and immune complex deposition in arterial walls are implicated as pathogenetic factors. Triggering infectious agents, yet unidentified, may be involved.

RISK FACTORS None identified

DIAGNOSIS

DIFFERENTIAL DIAGNOSIS
• Infectious otitis and sinusitis (bacterial or fungal)
• Midline granuloma or other upper airway malignancy
• Relapsing polychondritis
• Fungal or tuberculous pulmonary infections, (Goodpasture's syndrome)
• Other vasculitic syndromes (including polyarteritis nodosa, lymphomatoid granulomatosis, Churg-Strauss vasculitis, and overlap vasculitis syndromes)
• Any disease associated with necrotizing and crescentic glomerulonephritis, sarcoidosis

LABORATORY
• Anemia, leukocytosis, and thrombocytosis common during active phases of disease
• Erythrocyte sedimentation rate (ESR) usually markedly elevated (75%)
• Rheumatoid factor present in low to moderate titer in up to 50%
• Hematuria and/or cellular casts with moderate range proteinuria
• Renal insufficiency, mild to moderate at first, but frequently progresses to end-stage renal disease
Drugs that may alter lab results: Corticosteroids and cytotoxic drugs, used to treat the disease, may cause normalization of most abnormal laboratory findings
Disorders that may alter lab results: See disorders listed under Differential Diagnosis

PATHOLOGICAL FINDINGS
• Upper airways: Granulomatous inflammation frequently seen, although not specific unless showing actual vasculitis
• Lung: Granulomatous arteritis involving vessels of all sizes, classically medium-sized arteries
• Kidney: Necrotizing and crescentic glomerulonephritis without immunofluorescent staining (pauci-immune) is common, granulomatous vasculitis rarely seen
• Skin: Vasculitic lesions, from leukocytoclastic vasculitis of small vessels; granulomatous arteritis seen occasionally

SPECIAL TESTS
Antibodies to neutrophilic cytoplasmic antigens with a cytoplasmic pattern of staining (c-ANCA) are detected in a majority (60-90%) of patients. Such pattern of staining is highly specific (90+%) for this diagnosis. A similar finding, with perinuclear staining (p-ANCA), is nonspecific, but frequently seen in patients with other vasculitic syndromes or isolated necrotizing glomerulonephritis.

IMAGING
• Upper airways: Chronic otitis and sinusitis, often with evidence of erosion into bony structures - seen on plain x-rays
• CT scans of sinuses useful in demonstrating mucosal and bony involvement
• Lungs: X-rays show nodular pulmonary densities, often with central necrosis and cavitation. Local infiltrates, or more diffuse interstitial involvement also described, as are radiographic findings of pulmonary hemorrhage.

DIAGNOSTIC PROCEDURES
• Renal biopsy may give findings consistent with diagnosis, although not always definitive
• Sinus or upper airway mucosal biopsy often helpful, although findings are often nonspecific
• Open lung biopsy most likely to confirm granulomatous arteritis
• Diagnosis best made by demonstration of granulomatous arteritis of involved organ, although compatible renal lesion in setting of chronic destructive sinusitis and/or pulmonary nodules can be used to make a presumptive diagnosis
• A positive serologic test for c-ANCA in proper clinical setting felt to be diagnostic by many

TREATMENT

APPROPRIATE HEALTH CARE
• Patients are usually ill enough with fever, sinus or pulmonary involvement, or renal disease to require hospitalization for diagnostic tests (to rule out infectious causes) and appropriate biopsies
• An occasional patient can be managed as an outpatient

GENERAL MEASURES Careful attention to upper airway drainage, and supportive measures for pulmonary, renal, or neurologic involvement

SURGICAL MEASURES N/A

ACTIVITY No specific restrictions. Fatigue, fever, and weight loss usually limit activity.

DIET Vigorous nutritional support may be needed early in illness

PATIENT EDUCATION Nutritional and drug counseling when patient is able to return home

Wegener's granulomatosis

MEDICATIONS

DRUG(S) OF CHOICE
• Prednisone - given initially in high doses (60-100 mg/day). After initial 2-4 weeks may be tapered to alternate-day regimen. Then gradually discontinued over 2-6 months in most patients, depending on clinical course.
• Cyclophosphamide - in critically ill patient, may be given initially at a dose of 4 mg/kg/day IV for 2-3 days, then continued at 2 mg/kg/day orally. In stable patient, may be started at 2 mg/kg/day orally. Dosage may need to be adjusted, based on patient response and toxicity (usually bone marrow suppression). Usually continued for 1-2 years after patient felt to be in remission, and tapered slowly, with careful monitoring for re-activation of disease.
Contraindications: No absolute contraindications, although diabetes, hypertension, metabolic bone disease are relative contraindications to prednisone
Precautions:
• Careful monitoring if taking corticosteroids
• Consider reducing dose of cyclophosphamide in patient with baseline leukopenia, renal insufficiency
Significant possible interactions:
• Prednisone may interfere with hypoglycemics, anti-hypertensives
• Cyclophosphamide may increase risk of other drugs with potential for bone marrow toxicity

ALTERNATIVE DRUGS
• Azathioprine: in patients with history of severe bone marrow toxicity or hemorrhagic cystitis from cyclophosphamide
• Trimethoprim-sulfamethoxazole (TMP-SMX) has been used alone with success in some patients with limited (usually upper airway) disease, and has some potential as adjunctive therapy with prednisone and cyclophosphamide
• Methotrexate: in some patients without renal involvement and may be useful in maintaining remission in patients with stable disease, as an alternative to chronic cyclophosphamide therapy

FOLLOWUP

PATIENT MONITORING
• Early, careful monitoring of upper airway, pulmonary, and renal manifestations for response to therapy
• Monitor blood pressure, glucose, potassium for steroid effects
• Frequent (every 2-4 weeks) CBC with differential to monitor for bone marrow toxicity from cyclophosphamide. Leukopenia most common. Dose needs to be reduced if peripheral WBC < 3000/ mm3.
• Monitor urinalysis for potential of hemorrhagic cystitis from cyclophosphamide. Consider cystoscopy for persistent or recurrent hematuria, especially later in course of treatment.

PREVENTION/AVOIDANCE
• Calorie and salt reduction in patients on prednisone
• High fluid intake to prevent hemorrhagic cystitis from cyclophosphamide
• Give cyclophosphamide dose in morning to decrease amount of drug present overnight in bladder.

POSSIBLE COMPLICATIONS
• Disease related
  ◊ Destructive nasal lesions with "saddle nose" deformity
  ◊ Deafness from refractory otitis
  ◊ Necrotic pulmonary nodules with hemoptysis
  ◊ Interstitial lung disease
  ◊ Renal failure
  ◊ Foot drop from peripheral nerve disease
  ◊ Skin ulcers, digital and limb gangrene from peripheral vascular involvement
• Drug related
  ◊ Prednisone - weight gain, hyperglycemia, hypertension, hypokalemia, skin thinning and bruising, infection, osteoporosis
  ◊ Cyclophosphamide - bone marrow suppression (especially leukopenia, neutropenia), alopecia, hemorrhagic cystitis, mucosal membrane irritation, sterility and premature gonadal failure, secondary malignancies (especially leukemias) with long term therapy. Risk of bladder cancer is 5% (10 years) and 16% (15 years) after first treatment, and is related to previous cystitis.

EXPECTED COURSE/PROGNOSIS
• Without treatment, almost uniformly fatal with 10% 2 year survival and mean survival of 5 months
• With aggressive treatment, survival improved to 75-90% at 5 years
• Treatment-related toxicity is significant, especially from long-term cyclophosphamide. After 1-2 years of disease-free interval, cyclophosphamide is usually tapered, although some patients demonstrate disease re-activation during this phase.

MISCELLANEOUS

ASSOCIATED CONDITIONS None

AGE-RELATED FACTORS
Pediatric: N/A
Geriatric: N/A
Others: N/A

PREGNANCY
• Rarely reported. Pregnancy should be considered only when patient is disease-free and off therapy.
• Cyclophosphamide often causes sterility and is potentially teratogenic

SYNONYMS N/A

ICD-9-CM 446.4 Wegener's granulomatosis

SEE ALSO
• Polyarteritis nodosa
• Goodpasture's syndrome, pulmonary component
• Goodpasture's syndrome, renal component

OTHER NOTES N/A

ABBREVIATIONS
• c-ANCA = antibodies to neutrophilic cytoplasmic antigens with cytoplasmic staining pattern
• p-ANCA = antibodies to neutrophilic cytoplasmic antigens with perinuclear staining pattern

REFERENCES
• Fauci AS, et al: Wegener's granulomatosis: Prospective clinical and therapeutic experience with 85 patients for 21 years. Ann Intern Med 1983;98:76-85
• Nolle B, et al: Anticytoplasmic autoantibodies: Their immunodiagnostic value in Wegener's granulomatosis. Ann Intern Med 1989;111:28
• Lieberman KV, Churg A: Wegner's granulomatosis. In: Churg A, Churg J, eds. Systemic Vasculitides. New York, Igaku-Shoin, 1991
• Roo JK, et al: The role of antineutrophil cytoplasmic antibody (c-ANCA) testing in the diagnosis of Wegner's granulomatosis. Ann Int Med 1995;123:925-932
Illustrations: 1 available on CD-ROM
Internet references: http://www.5mcc.com

Author(s)
Christopher M. Wise, MD

Wilms' tumor

BASICS

DESCRIPTION An embryonal renal neoplasm containing blastema, stromal or epithelial cell types usually affecting children before the 5th year.
Genetics: Several congenital anomalies are known to be associated with Wilms' tumor. A two stage mutational model has been proposed: occurrence in either hereditary form or sporadic form. Patients with aniridia have a deletion of the short arm of chromosome 11 (11p13).
System(s) affected: Renal/urologic
Incidence/Prevalence in USA:
0.69/100,000 people in the U.S. 8 cases/100,000 children under 15 year of age.
Predominant age: Median age of 36.5 months
Predominant sex: Female > Male (1.1 : 1)

SIGNS AND SYMPTOMS
• Usually asymptomatic
• Palpable upper abdominal mass
• Abdominal pain
• Fever
• Anemia
• Rarely, signs of acute abdomen with free intraperitoneal rupture
• Cardiac murmur
• Hepatosplenomegaly
• Ascites
• Prominent abdominal wall veins
• Varicocele
• Gonadal metastases

CAUSES
• Hereditary or sporadic forms of genetic mutation
• Familial form: autosomal dominant trait with incomplete penetrance (1%)
• Potential of paternal occupational exposure (machinists, welders, motor vehicle mechanics, autobody repairmen)

RISK FACTORS
• Aniridia (600 times greater than normal risk)
• Hemihypertrophy (100 times greater than normal risk)
• Cryptorchidism
• Hypospadias
• Duplicated renal collecting systems
• Wiedemann-Beckwith syndrome
• Drash's syndrome
• Klippel-Trenaunay syndrome
• Familial occurrence
• Paternal occupation (see Causes)

DIAGNOSIS

DIFFERENTIAL DIAGNOSIS
• Neuroblastoma
• Hepatic tumors
• Sarcoma
• Rhabdoid tumors

LABORATORY
• Urinalysis (occasional hematuria)
• CBC (anemia)
• LDH
• Plasma renin (rarely helpful)
• Urine catecholamines
Drugs that may alter lab results: N/A
Disorders that may alter lab results: N/A

PATHOLOGICAL FINDINGS
• Favorable findings (mortality of 7%)
  ◊ Bulky lesion, well-encapsulated
  ◊ Focal areas of hemorrhage and necrosis
  ◊ Absence of anaplasia and sarcomatous cell types
  ◊ Presence of blastema, stomal and epithelial elements
• Unfavorable histology (mortality rate of 57%)
  ◊ Anaplasia - markedly enlarged and multipolar mitotic figures 3-fold enlargement of nuclei in comparison with adjacent similar nuclei, hyperchromasia of enlarge nuclei. Anaplasia may be diffuse or focal.
  ◊ Sarcomatous changes - are now considered to be separate from Wilms, not subtypes. (Mortality of 64%)
• Nephroblastomatosis
  ◊ Considered premalignant

SPECIAL TESTS N/A

IMAGING
• Chest x-ray
• KUB (presence of linear calcifications)
• Abdominal ultrasound - gives best information about extension into IVC
• CT (with IV and oral contrast) of chest and abdomen
• IVP rarely helpful

DIAGNOSTIC PROCEDURES
Occasionally bone marrow aspiration necessary to distinguish from neuroblastoma

TREATMENT

APPROPRIATE HEALTH CARE
• In-patient work-up and treatment until stable postoperative and induction chemotherapy completed

GENERAL MEASURES
• Chemotherapy
• Radiation therapy in Stage II, unfavorable histology, Stage II and Stage IV

SURGICAL MEASURES
• Examination (visual and manual) of contralateral kidney
• Radical nephroureterectomy and biopsies as needed to provide precise staging information
• Sampling of any enlarged lymph nodes
• Identification of any retained tumor with titanium clips.
• Tumor should be given to pathologist fresh, not on formalin
• Vertical midline incision if tumor extension to right atrium present (possible use of cardiopulmonary bypass)
• With bilateral Wilms' tumors, biopsy, then chemotherapy and 2nd look operation 6 weeks to 6 month later for partial bilateral nephrectomy if possible

ACTIVITY As tolerated

DIET No special diet

PATIENT EDUCATION
• Patient and family teaching regarding long-term outlook
• Possibility of second malignancy
• Side effects of chemotherapy, radiation therapy

MEDICATIONS:

DRUG(S) OF CHOICE
• Dactinomycin (actinomycin-D)
• Vincristine
• Doxorubicin
• Cyclophosphamide (Cytoxan)
Contraindications: Refer to manufacturer's literature
Precautions: Refer to manufacturer's literature
Significant possible interactions: Refer to manufacturer's literature

ALTERNATIVE DRUGS
• Doxorubicin (Adriamycin)
• Cyclophosphamide

FOLLOWUP

PATIENT MONITORING
• Multidrug chemotherapy every 3-4 weeks for 16 weeks - 15 months depending on stage
• Every 4 months for 1 year, every 6 months for 2nd - 3rd year, yearly after that
• CBC, CT chest and abdomen with each visit

PREVENTION/AVOIDANCE N/A

POSSIBLE COMPLICATIONS
• 1-2% will develop second malignant neoplasms (leukemia, lymphoma, hepatocellular carcinoma, soft tissue sarcoma)
• High risk of low birth weight infants, perinatal mortality in offspring of female survivors of Wilms' tumor
• Chest is usual site of recurrence

EXPECTED COURSE/PROGNOSIS
• With favorable histology, 91% survival
• With diffuse anaplasia, 20% survival
• With focal anaplasia, 64% survival
• Staging
  ◊ I - tumor limited to kidney, completely excised
  ◊ II - Tumor extends beyond kidney, completely excised
  ◊ III - Residual non-hematogenous tumor confined to abdomen (lymph nodes positive, spillage of tumor, peritoneal implants, extension beyond resection region)
  ◊ IV - Hematogenous metastases
  ◊ V - Bilateral renal involvement

MISCELLANEOUS

ASSOCIATED CONDITIONS See risk factors

AGE-RELATED FACTORS Occurs only in children
Pediatric: N/A
Geriatric: N/A
Others: N/A

PREGNANCY N/A

SYNONYMS
• Nephroblastoma

ICD-9-CM
189.0 Malignant neoplasm of kidney

SEE ALSO N/A

OTHER NOTES
• Mesoblastic nephroma - distinguished only by histology. Age usually under 6 months. Essentially benign although metastases have been reported; tends to be locally invasive. Operative spillage may lead to recurrence. No chemotherapy or radiotherapy needed with complete excision.
• Nephroblastomatosis - considered premalignant; may present as nodularity as one or both kidneys; treated with biopsy and local excision (renal tissue sparing)

ABBREVIATIONS N/A

REFERENCES
• Ashcraft KW, Holder TM: Pediatric Surgery. 2nd Ed. Philadelphia, W.B. Saunders Co., 1993
• Shochat SJ: Wilms' Tumor: Diagnosis and Treatment in the 1990's. Seminars in Pediatric Surgery 1993;2(1):59-68
• Welch KJ, Randolph JG, Ravitch MM, O'Neill SA, Rowe MI: Pediatric Surgery. 4th Ed. Chicago, Year Book Medical Publishers, 1986
Illustrations: N/A
Internet references: http://www.5mcc.com

Author(s)
Timothy L. Black, MD, FACS, FAAP

Wiskott-Aldrich syndrome

 BASICS

DESCRIPTION A genetic disorder inherited as an x-linked recessive trait with clinical elements of eczema, thrombocytopenia with small platelets, proneness to infection. B and T cell functions are defective with inability to make antibodies to polysaccharide antigens. This syndrome may cause early death. Not all individuals have all features of the syndrome.
System(s) affected:
Hemic/Lymphatic/Immunologic, Skin/Exocrine
Genetics:
• X-linked recessive
• WASP gene located at Xp11.22; XLT maps to same site
• Familial history in 50% of individuals
Predominant age:
• Infants (symptoms develop as infants get older)
Predominant sex: Males (exclusively)
Incidence/Prevalence in USA: Rare; 4/million live male births in US

SIGNS AND SYMPTOMS
• Neonatal period:
  ◊ Bloody diarrhea
  ◊ Petechiae
  ◊ Purpura
• Childhood:
  ◊ Eczema (within the first year)
  ◊ Secondary skin infections
  ◊ Pneumonia
  ◊ Otitis media
  ◊ Chronic sinopulmonary infections
  ◊ Herpes infections (skin and eyes)
  ◊ Hepatosplenomegaly
• See Complications and Associated Conditions sections

CAUSES
• Inherited defect(s) in WAS gene affecting one or more hematopoietic cell lineages (other than red cells)
• Defective expression of cell surface protein CD43
• Abnormalities of glycosyl transferases
• Paucity of surface microvilli in T-cells
• Platelet storage pool defect
• Depletion of calcium dependent neutral protease calpain in platelets
  ◊ Primary cause of accelerated platelet destruction/TCP
  ◊ Platelets intrinsically abnormal
• Activation/expansion of B-cells/function
• Production of IgA may be 9x normal
• WASP defect may result in abnormal cytoskeleton of involved cells

RISK FACTORS Family history of congenital defects

 DIAGNOSIS:

DIFFERENTIAL DIAGNOSIS Diagnosis may be difficult in infancy if there are no definite immunological abnormalities present
• Restricted responsiveness of lymphoid cells
• Eczema
• Other causes of TCP
• Bronchitis
• Lymphoma
• Acute lymphoblastic anemia

LABORATORY
• Platelets often below 30,000/cubic millimeter and are small, MPV 2/3 normal; TCP and small platelets present at birth
• Low IgM in serum
• Absent/low isohemagglutinins
• IgE and IgA normal or elevated
• Normal IgG
• Low CD8+ count (61% of individuals); lymphopenia usually evident by age 6 years
Drugs that may alter lab results:
Antibiotics
Disorders that may alter lab results:
Infections

PATHOLOGICAL FINDINGS
• Multiple thromboses of small arterioles of kidneys, lungs, pancreas
• Hyperplasia of spleen, lymph nodes
• Inflammatory changes in skin

SPECIAL TESTS Lymphocyte proliferative response to periodate (impaired), response to other mitogens

IMAGING N/A

DIAGNOSTIC PROCEDURES Bone narrow aspiration. Although not diagnostic, it helps by excluding marrow aplasia and/or leukemia.

 TREATMENT:

APPROPRIATE HEALTH CARE Inpatient for acute problems

GENERAL MEASURES
• Crossmatched platelet transfusions
• Irradiated blood products for transfusions to prevent GVHD
• Corticosteroids and immunosuppressant drugs have no role in treatment of TCP in WAS
• Aggressive antibiotic therapy for any infection
• Bone marrow transplant (preferably with HLA-matched sibling; appears to correct all) problems except TCP

SURGICAL MEASURES Splenectomy, if there is special indication of severe TCP; TCP and small platelet size usually improve, but with increased risk of infection postsplenectomy

ACTIVITY
• Plan levels of activity to help in normal development, e.g., bike-riding (with acceptable protective gear) or swimming
• Avoid contact sports
• Avoid crowds

DIET No special diet

PATIENT EDUCATION
• Genetic counseling
• Patient/parent teaching for coping with disorder
and expected outcome

Wiskott-Aldrich syndrome

MEDICATIONS:

DRUG(S) OF CHOICE
• Immune globulin, intravenous (IVIG) infusions
• Topical corticosteroids
• Continuous antibiotics or as indicated by cultures and/or postsplenectomy (prophylactic penicillin)
• Immune-related complications respond variably to steroids (severe vasculitis, occasionally for autoimmune TCP), IVIG, vincristine or plasmapheresis
Contraindications: Refer to manufacturer's literature
Precautions: Corticosteroids in immunosuppressed patients. Refer to manufacturer's literature.
Significant possible interactions: Refer to manufacturer's literature

ALTERNATIVE DRUGS   N/A

FOLLOWUP:

PATIENT MONITORING   As needed for therapy, infection
treatment, progression of disorder, complications

PREVENTION/AVOIDANCE
• Genetic counseling
• Carriers may have mild TCP, but usually normal
• Carriers may sometimes be identified (G6PD alleles/other X-chromosomal markers useful); also by non-random patterns of x-chromosomal inactivation
• Prenatal diagnosis may also be possible in some instances

POSSIBLE COMPLICATIONS
• Severe infections - especially following splenectomy
• Hemorrhage; cerebral of particular concern
• Malignancies (lymphoreticular tumors, leukemia, Kaposi's sarcoma
• Nephropathy
• Autoimmune disorders including immune TCP and hemolytic anemia, glomerulopathy, leukocytoclastic or large vessel vasculitis, juvenile rheumatoid arthritis-like syndrome; sometimes aggressive autoimmune disease
• Malabsorption syndrome

EXPECTED COURSE/PROGNOSIS
Usual course - both acute and chronic. Cell mediated immunity becomes progressively dysfunctional with age. Broad range of disease severity even in patients with identical mutations. WAS has been fatal, as a rule before age 10, but prognosis improving. Some are surviving into twenties and thirties. Causes of death have been infection (50%), bleeding (27%), malignancies (12%). Splenectomy improves morbidity/mortality. Bone marrow transplant can restore all abnormalities to normal.

MISCELLANEOUS:

ASSOCIATED CONDITIONS
• Lyphomas, often involving brain (50%) - sometimes primary site
• Proneness to lymphoreticular tumors
• Nephropathy

AGE-RELATED FACTORS
Pediatric:
• Onset in male newborns/infants
• Within first year infections caused by pneumococcal and other bacteria with PS capsules; typically otitis media, pneumonia, meningitis or sepsis
• Later infection occurs with agents such as P. carinii, herpes more frequent
Geriatric: No patient has survived this long
Others: N/A

PREGNANCY   N/A

SYNONYMS
• Aldrich syndrome
• Eczema-thrombocytopenia-immunodeficiency syndrome
• Immunodeficiency-2; IMD2

ICD-9-CM   279.12 Wiskott-Aldrich syndrome

SEE ALSO
• Idiopathic thrombocytopenia
• Leukemia
• Immunodeficiency diseases

OTHER NOTES   N/A

ABBREVIATIONS
• WASP = Wiskott-Aldrich syndrome protein
• TCP = thrombocytopenia
• PS = Polysaccharide
• GVHD = graft versus host disease

REFERENCES
• Bennett JC, Plum F, eds: Cecil Textbook of Medicine. 20th Ed. Philadelphia, W.B. Saunders Co., 1996
• Online Mendelian Inheritance in Man, OMIM (TM). Johns Hopkins University, Baltimore, MD. MIM 301000. Updated 10/18/96. World Wide Web URL:http://www3.ncbi.nlm.nih.gov/omim/
• Sullivan KE, Mullen CA, Blaese RM, Winkelstein JA: A Multiinstitutional survey of Wiskott-Aldrich syndrome. J Pediat 1994;125:876-885
• Brochstein JA, Gillio AP, Ruggiero M, Kernan NA, Emanuel D, Laver J, Small T, O'Reilly RJ: Marrow transplantation from human leukocyte antigen-identical or haploidentical donors for correction of Wiskott-Aldrich syndrome. J Pediat 1991;119:907-912
• Ozsahin H, Le Deist F, Benkerrou M, Cavazzana-Calvo M, Gomez L, Griscelli C, Blanche S, Fischer A: Bone marrow transplantation in 26 patients with Wiskott-Aldrich syndrome from a single center. J Pediatr 1996;129:238-244
Illustrations: N/A
Internet references: http://www.5mcc.com

Author(s)
Douglas H. Sandberg, MD

Zinc deficiency

BASICS

DESCRIPTION Constellation of growth retardation, hypogonadism, cell mediated immune dysfunction, and skin changes related to decreased zinc
System(s) affected: Endocrine/Metabolic, Skin/Exocrine, Nervous
Genetics: Usually acquired, but rarely acrodermatitis enteropathica (autosomal recessive) and associated with sickle cell anemia (autosomal recessive)
Incidence/Prevalence in USA: Unknown
Predominant age: All ages, most often adolescent
Predominant sex: Male = Female

SIGNS AND SYMPTOMS
• Mild deficiency
  ◊ Hypogeusia
  ◊ Decreased dark adaptation
  ◊ Decreased lean body mass
• Moderate deficiency
  ◊ All of the above
  ◊ Diarrhea
  ◊ Growth retardation
  ◊ Hypogonadism (especially male)
  ◊ Mental lethargy
  ◊ Anergy
  ◊ Rough skin
  ◊ Delayed wound healing
  ◊ Glucose intolerance
  ◊ Impaired cell mediated immunity
• Severe deficiency
  ◊ All of the above
  ◊ Bullous pustular dermatitis
  ◊ Weight loss
  ◊ Dwarfism
  ◊ Emotional instability
  ◊ Tremors
  ◊ Ataxia
  ◊ Alopecia
  ◊ Death

CAUSES
• Increased requirements
  ◊ Pregnancy
  ◊ Lactation
  ◊ Rapid growth phase of childhood
  ◊ Burns
  ◊ Major trauma
• Increased losses
  ◊ Diabetes
  ◊ Cirrhosis
  ◊ Renal disease
  ◊ Malabsorption states, e.g., inflammatory bowel diseases
  ◊ Sickle cell anemia
• Decreased absorption
  ◊ Acrodermatitis enteropathica, an autosomal recessive deficiency in the enzyme required for intestinal absorption
  ◊ Geophagia
  ◊ Chelating agents
  ◊ Parasitism
  ◊ Diet high in phytates

• Insufficient dietary intake
  ◊ Vegetarianism
  ◊ Parenteral hyperalimentation without supplementation
  ◊ Breast feeding
  ◊ Suboptimal zinc conditions in diet (rare)
  ◊ Alcoholism

RISK FACTORS
• High milk consumption
• Low socioeconomic status

DIAGNOSIS

DIFFERENTIAL DIAGNOSIS
• Congenital dwarfism
• Failure to thrive in infants
• Primary hypogonadism
• Mental retardation

LABORATORY
• Plasma zinc levels decreased (in moderate to severe zinc deficiency)
• Erythrocyte or leukocyte zinc levels more adequately assess tissue stores, but these are more costly and not widely available
• Hair or fingernail zinc levels not useful
Drugs that may alter lab results: N/A
Disorders that may alter lab results: N/A

PATHOLOGICAL FINDINGS N/A

SPECIAL TESTS N/A

IMAGING N/A

DIAGNOSTIC PROCEDURES N/A

TREATMENT

APPROPRIATE HEALTH CARE
Outpatient

GENERAL MEASURES N/A

SURGICAL MEASURES N/A

ACTIVITY Full activity

DIET
• Balanced omnivorous diet
• Avoid excessive intake of foods with high phytate content, (e.g., cereals)

PATIENT EDUCATION Dietary consultation

Zinc deficiency

MEDICATIONS

DRUG(S) OF CHOICE
• Zinc gluconate or zinc sulfate 25-50 mg po qd for 6-9 months
• 4-6 mg of elemental zinc qd added to hyperalimentation in adult patient, may increase to 12 mg qd if suspect ongoing heavy zinc losses, e.g., burns or major trauma
• In pediatric patients, 0.02-0.04 mg zinc/kg/day in hyperalimentation
• Prenatal vitamins with minerals during pregnancy and lactation to prevent deficiency
Contraindications: None
Precautions: Avoid large (> 20 mg elemental zinc) parenteral doses
Significant possible interactions: N/A

ALTERNATIVE DRUGS N/A

FOLLOWUP

PATIENT MONITORING Clinical status such as improved outlook, weight gain, resolution of symptoms

PREVENTION/AVOIDANCE
• Adequate diet
• Supplementation when indicated (see Medications)

POSSIBLE COMPLICATIONS N/A

EXPECTED COURSE/PROGNOSIS
Immediate improvement in clinical status. Full resolution of signs and symptoms.

MISCELLANEOUS

ASSOCIATED CONDITIONS
• Sickle cell anemia
• Pregnancy and lactation
• Alcoholism
• Malabsorption
• Parenteral hyperalimentation
• In the older patient, diabetes, cirrhosis, those taking diuretics

AGE-RELATED FACTORS
Pediatric: Zinc deficiency may cause failure to thrive, impair growth and development of secondary sexual characteristics
Geriatric:
• Zinc deficiency may cause poor night vision leading to falls; poor wound healing or chronic skin ulcer; loss of taste which may cause worsening nutrition
• Elderly persons living in institutions may have low zinc intake
Others: N/A

PREGNANCY Requirements increase; deficiency may cause spontaneous abortion, inadequate weight gain

SYNONYMS N/A

ICD-9-CM
269.3

SEE ALSO
• Alcoholism
• Acrodermatitis enteropathica
• Failure to thrive (FTT)
• Anemia, sickle cell

OTHER NOTES N/A

ABBREVIATIONS N/A

REFERENCES
• Tasman-Jones C: Disturbances of trace mineral metabolism. In: Wyngaarden JB, et al, eds. Cecil Textbook of Medicine. 19th Ed. Philadelphia, W.B. Saunders Co., 1992
• Ronaghy H: World Review Nutr. Diet 1987:54
Illustrations: 3 available on CD-ROM
Internet references: http://www.5mcc.com

Author(s)
Clyde L. Harris, MD

Zollinger-Ellison syndrome

BASICS

DESCRIPTION
• A triad of
  ◊ Marked elevated gastric acid secretion
  ◊ Peptic ulcer disease
  ◊ A non-beta islet cell tumor of the pancreas (and sometimes other sites); frequently multifocal and small; one half are malignant with metastases into lymph nodes, liver and less frequently into the bone
• Gastrin producing tumor, single or multiple, large or small, benign or malignant: 80% sporadic, 20% associated with multiple endocrine neoplasia (MEN 1)
System(s) affected: Gastrointestinal, Endocrine/Metabolic
Genetics: 25-50% occur in association with the MEN 1 syndrome
Incidence/Prevalence in USA: 0.1% of patients with duodenal ulcer
Predominant age: Middle age (40-75)
Predominant sex: Male > Female (3:2)

SIGNS AND SYMPTOMS
• Abdominal pain
• Epigastric pain
• Reflux esophagitis
• Vomiting unresponsive to standard therapy
• 25% have diarrhea which persists with fasting
• Ulcer disease
• Complications of severe peptic ulcer disease (hemorrhage, perforation, obstruction)
• Signs related to MEN 1 (hyperparathyroidism, hypercalcemia)
• Weight loss
• Enlarged liver when metastasized
• Endoscopic (esophagitis, duodenal ulceration with multiple ulcers)
• Steatorrhea

CAUSES
Gastrinoma - found in the gastric triangle in 90%; 80% arise in the pancreatic islets and are located in the pancreatic head; 10-15% arise in the G cells of the duodenum

RISK FACTORS
• MEN 1
• Family history of ulcer disease
• Over age 60

DIAGNOSIS

DIFFERENTIAL DIAGNOSIS
• Elevated serum gastrin with hypochlorhydria/achlorhydria
  ◊ Atrophic gastritis
  ◊ Drug induced
  ◊ Gastric cancer
  ◊ Gastric ulcer
  ◊ Pernicious anemia
  ◊ Postvagotomy
  ◊ Vitiligo
• Elevated serum gastrin with normal or increased gastric acid
  ◊ Antral G-cell hyperfunction
  ◊ Chronic renal failure
  ◊ Gastric outlet obstruction
  ◊ Pheochromocytoma (rare)
  ◊ Retained gastric antrum
  ◊ Rheumatoid arthritis
  ◊ Small bowel resection
• Consider gastrinoma in all patients with:
  ◊ Recurrent or refractory ulcer disease
  ◊ Gastric hypertrophy and ulcers
  ◊ Duodenal and jejunal ulcers
  ◊ Ulcers and diarrhea
  ◊ Kidney stones
  ◊ Hypercalcemia
  ◊ Pituitary disease
  ◊ Family history of ulcer disease or endocrine tumors suggestive of MEN 1

LABORATORY
• Elevated serum gastrin - fasting
• Elevated basal gastric acid output >15 mEq/hr (> 15 mmol/hr)
• Elevated maximal acid output >150 mEq/hr (> 150 mmol/hr)
• Gastric pH < 2.0
• Increased pancreatic polypeptides
• Check serum calcium, phosphorus, cortisol and prolactin levels
Drugs that may alter lab results: N/A
Disorders that may alter lab results: N/A

PATHOLOGICAL FINDINGS
• Gastrinoma found in gastric triangle (60-70% in head of pancreas)
• 50% of tumors stain for VIP, ACTH, insulin, neurotensin
• In addition, 50% will have multiple metastases to liver, bone, lymph nodes, or with blood vessel invasion
• Duodenal ulcer
• Jejunal ulcer
• Gastric ulcer

SPECIAL TESTS
• Secretion stimulation test - gastrin level increases > 200 pg/mL (> 200 ng/L)
• Calcium infusion test

IMAGING
• Used to localize tumor
• Abdominal CT scan
• Abdominal ultrasound
• Abdominal angiography
• Selective venous sampling of gastrin from portal venous tributaries
• Sella turcica imaging

DIAGNOSTIC PROCEDURES
Endoscopy to look for tumors

TREATMENT

APPROPRIATE HEALTH CARE
Advise daily care based on symptoms

GENERAL MEASURES
Medical treatment alone in some cases; surgical correction if patient fails medical therapy

SURGICAL MEASURES
• Medical treatment plus laparotomy to search for resectable tumors
• Definitive therapy - removal of gastrinoma when found
• Total gastrectomy (is no longer used in most patients)
• Vagotomy in some patients to reduce acid secretion and add to inhibitory effect of medication
• In MEN I - parathyroidectomy; associated gastrinomas are generally benign and not amenable to surgery

ACTIVITY
As tolerated

DIET
Restrict only foods which aggravate symptoms

PATIENT EDUCATION
Inform as to nature of disease and prognosis

MEDICATIONS

DRUG(S) OF CHOICE
• Omeprazole first followed by H2 blockers. (Must correct hypercalcemia if caused by hyperparathyroidism.)
  ◊ Note: Dosages may exceed maximum recommended daily dose. Start at the recommended doses as listed below, and titrate up to maximum as listed.
  ◊ Omeprazole 60-120 mg/d
  ◊ Cimetidine start 300 mg q6h, up to maximum of 1.25-5.0 gm/day
  ◊ Ranitidine 150 mg q 12 hrs, up to maximum of 6 gm/day
  ◊ Famotidine 20 mg at bedtime, up to maximum of 800 mg/day

Contraindications:
• H2-receptor antagonists - anti-androgen effects; drug interactions due to hepatic oxides system
• Omeprazole - none

Precautions:
• Appropriate dose adjustment for renal and geriatric patients
• Gynecomastia reported with high doses of cimetidine (> 2.4 gm/day)

Significant possible interactions: Refer to manufacturer's literature

ALTERNATIVE DRUGS
• Chemotherapy regimens of streptozocin and fluorouracil have shown partial response
• Interferon

FOLLOWUP

PATIENT MONITORING
• Close followup necessary following any surgical procedure
• Careful dose titration required with medical therapy
• Gastric analysis to measure acid secretion rates for dose adjustment of H2-receptor antagonists

PREVENTION/AVOIDANCE
Must screen first degree relatives of patients with MEN 1

POSSIBLE COMPLICATIONS
• The complications of ulcer disease, e.g., bleeding or perforation
• Approximately two thirds of Zollinger-Ellison tumors are malignant with metastases
• Multiple hormone production and related syndromes such as Cushing's and others

EXPECTED COURSE/PROGNOSIS
• Survival rate - 5 year = 62-75%, 10 year = 47-53%
• Prognosis improves with complete resection
• If tumor inoperable due to metastases, 5 year = 43%, 10 year = 25%
• The presence of metastatic disease has decreased owing to the early detection

MISCELLANEOUS

ASSOCIATED CONDITIONS
• Hyperparathyroidism
• Prolactinoma
• Insulinoma
• Carcinoid tumors

AGE-RELATED FACTORS
Pediatric: N/A
Geriatric:
• One third of patients with Z-E are over age 50
• Consider this diagnosis for any patient with persistent or recurring peptic ulcer disease
Others: N/A

PREGNANCY   N/A

SYNONYMS
• Z-E syndrome
• Pancreatic ulcerogenic tumor syndrome
• Multiple endocrine neoplasia, partial
• Ulcerogenic islet cell tumor

ICD-9-CM
251.5 Zollinger-Ellison syndrome (other codes based on related diagnosis)

SEE ALSO   N/A

OTHER NOTES   N/A

ABBREVIATIONS
MEN = multiple endocrine neoplasia

REFERENCES
• McGuigan JE: Zollinger-Ellison Syndrome (Gastrinoma). In: Braunwald E, Isselbacher KJ, Petersdorf RG, et al. Harrison's Principles of Internal Medicine. 13th Ed. Vol.2. New York, McGraw-Hill, Inc., 1994:1375-1377
• Spiro HM: Ulcerogenic Tumor of the Pancreas (Zollinger-Ellison Syndrome). In: Spiro HM, ed. Clinical Gastroenterology. 4th Ed. New York, McGraw-Hill, Inc.,1993:313-327
• McGuigan JE: The Zollinger-Ellison Syndrome. In: Sleisenger MH, Fordtran JS, eds. Gastrointestinal Disease. 5th Ed. Philadelphia, W.B. Saunders Co.,1994:679-692
• Richardson CT: Zollinger-Ellison Syndrome. In: Wyngaarden JB, Smith LH, Bennett JC, eds. Cecil Textbook of Medicine. 19th Ed. Philadelphia, W.B. Saunders Co.,1992:665-667
Illustrations: N/A
Internet references: http://www.5mcc.com

Author(s)
Guy W. Neff, MD
Samuel Sim, MD
Ann Neff, MD

Short
Topics

Acanthosis nigricans

DESCRIPTION A circumscribed melanosis consisting of a brown pigmented velvety verrucosity or fine papillomatosis appearing in the axillae and other body folds. Occurs in association with endocrine disorders, underlying malignancy, administration of certain drugs, or as in inherited disorder. Usual course - chronic.

CAUSES
• congenital
• associated with malignant disease
• obesity
• idiopathic

TREATMENT
• treat underlying cause
• malignancy workup

ICD-9-CM
701.2 acquired acanthosis nigricans

Acquired adrenogenital syndrome

DESCRIPTION A condition of adults that is acquired or congenital in which excessive output of adrenal androgenic hormones causes virilization. The effects depend on age. Usual course - chronic; progressive.

CAUSES
• androgen producing tumors
• adrenal adenoma
• adrenal adenocarcinoma

TREATMENT
• surgery

ICD-9-CM
255.2 adrenogenital disorders

Acrodermatitis enteropathica

DESCRIPTION Previously fatal disorder resulting from malabsorption of zinc. Characteristics: psoriasiform dermatitis, hair loss, paronychia, diarrhea, and growth retardation. Symptoms begin in infants just after weaning.

SYNONYMS
• Danbolt-Closs syndrome
• Brandt syndrome

CAUSES
• zinc deficiency
• defective zinc absorption

TREATMENT
• oral elemental zinc

ICD-9-CM
686.8 acrodermatitis enteropathica

Acromegaly

DESCRIPTION A disorder due to excessive secretion of pituitary growth hormone, characterized by progressive enlargement of the head and face, hands and feet, and thorax. Usual course - progressive.

SYNONYMS
• Acromegalia
• Eosinophilic adenoma syndrome

CAUSES
• growth hormone excess from pituitary adenoma

TREATMENT
• transsphenoidal resection
• heavy particle irradiation
• radiotherapy
• bromocriptine

ICD-9-CM
253.0 acromegaly and gigantism

Actinomycosis of the kidney

DESCRIPTION Infectious bacterial disease that appears in 4 clinical forms - abdominal, cervicofacial, thoracic, and generalized. The generalized form can involve the kidneys as well as other organs. Characteristics - back pain, lethargy, weight loss, fever, hematuria. Usual course - acute.

CAUSES
• retrograde infection by actinomyces israelii

TREATMENT
• antibiotics
• drainage

ICD-9-CM
039.2 abdominal actinomycotic infection

Actinomycosis of the thorax

DESCRIPTION Infectious bacterial disease affecting the thorax and lungs. It also occurs in three other forms that include abdominal, cervicofacial and generalized. Usual course - progressive.

CAUSES
• actinomyces infection
• oral commensal
• aspiration of infected material
• impaired consciousness
• alcoholism

TREATMENT
• prolonged antibiotic therapy
• surgical drainage of suppurative lesions

ICD-9-CM
039.1 actinomycosis, thoracic

Adenocarcinoma of the bladder

DESCRIPTION Malignant growth in the bladder with characteristic hematuria, dysuria, urinary frequency, weight loss and suprapubic mass. Usual course - progressive.

CAUSES
• cystitis glandularis
• exstrophy of the bladder

TREATMENT
• segmental bladder resection
• total cystectomy

ICD-9-CM
188.9 malignant neoplasm of bladder, part unspecified

Adenocarcinoma of the colon

DESCRIPTION The colon and rectum account for more new cases of cancer each year than any other site, exclusive of the lung. The incidence increases with age and peaks at 60-75. Characteristics - melena, diarrhea, rectal mass, iron deficiency anemia. Usual course - progressive.

CAUSES
• familial polyposis
• chronic ulcerative colitis
• possibly low fiber, high fat diet
• granulomatous colitis

TREATMENT
• surgery
• radiotherapy
• palliative chemotherapy

ICD-9-CM
153.9 malignant neoplasm of colon, unspecified

Adenocarcinoma of the endometrium

DESCRIPTION Third rank in frequency of malignancies affecting women after breast and colon. Usually postmenopausal. Peak incidence between 50 and 60 years. Characteristics - positive Pap smear, menometrorrhagia, postmenopausal bleeding, perimenopausal bleeding. Usual course - progressive.

SYNONYMS
• Fundal carcinoma
• Corpus carcinoma
• Endometrial cancer

CAUSES
• irregular menses
• late menopause
• obesity
• diabetes mellitus
• hypertension
• infertility
• prolonged unopposed exogenous estrogen
• polycystic ovary disease

TREATMENT
• hysterectomy
• radiotherapy
• hormonal therapy with progesterone

ICD-9-CM
182.0 malignant neoplasm of corpus uteri, except isthmus

Adenocarcinoma of the gallbladder

DESCRIPTION The most frequent cause of extrabiliary obstruction. Characteristics - nausea, vomiting, abdominal pain, anorexia, jaundice, hepatomegaly, enlarged gallbladder.

CAUSES
• cholelithiasis
• calcified gallbladder

TREATMENT
• surgical resection
• palliative radiotherapy
• palliative chemotherapy

ICD-9-CM
156.0 malignant neoplasm of gallbladder

Adenocarcinoma of the rectum

DESCRIPTION A slow-growth rate malignancy that depends on routine examination to discover before symptom-producing size. Most common symptom is blood passage at the time of bowel movement. All rectal bleeding should raise suspicion of cancer until proven otherwise. Usual course - progressive; surgical cure.

CAUSES
• ulcerative colitis
• previous rectal cancer
• familial polyposis

TREATMENT
• surgery
• radiotherapy

ICD-9-CM
154.1 malignant neoplasm of the rectum

Adenoid hyperplasia

DESCRIPTION An enlargement of the adenoidal tissue of the nasopharynx. Normally small at birth (2-3 cm), adenoid tissue grows until child reaches adolescence, and then begins to atrophy slowly. With adenoid hyperplasia, however, this tissue continues to grow. Symptoms can include cough, earache, restlessness, headache, impaired taste or smell, mouth breathing, sleep apnea, snoring, chronic sinusitis, hyponasal voice, purulent rhinorrhea.

SYNONYMS
• adenoid hypertrophy

CAUSES
• unknown; factors that contribute: heredity, chronic infection, chronic nasal congestion, persistent allergy, insufficient areation, inefficient nasal breathing, and repeated infections

TREATMENT
• antibiotics
• adenoidectomy

ICD-9-CM
474.12 adenoids

Adrenoleukodystrophy

DESCRIPTION A sphingolipidosis which combines the features of leukodystrophy and Addison's disease. A rare, sex-linked recessive metabolic disorder that occurs in boys. Characteristics include - adrenal atrophy and widespread cerebral demyelinization. Usual course - progressive.

SYNONYMS
• sudanophilic leukodystrophy with adrenal atrophy
• Addison-Schilder disease
• Siemerling-Creutzfeldt disease
• diffuse cerebral sclerosis with adrenocortical atrophy
• Addison disease with cerebral sclerosis
• Sex-linked metachromatic leukodystrophy

CAUSES
• unknown biochemical enzyme defect

TREATMENT
• hormone replacement therapy
• dietary therapy

ICD-9-CM
330.0 leukodystrophy

Afibrinogenemia, congenital

DESCRIPTION Hereditary recessive disorder characterized by failure of synthesis of adequate amounts of fibrinogen causing blood to be incoagutable. Symptoms include bruising, epitaxis, easy posttraumatic bleeding.

CAUSES
• no fibrinogen
• no factor I

TREATMENT
• transfusion
• cryoprecipitate
• plasma
• whole blood

ICD-9-CM
286.3 afibrinogenemia, congenital

Agammaglobulinemia, acquired

DESCRIPTION Heterogenous disorder characterized by onset of recurrent bacterial infections in 2nd and 3rd decade, resulting from drastic decrease in Ig and antibody levels. It affects males and females equally and does not interfere with normal lifespan. Usual course - chronic.

SYNONYMS
• late-onset agammaglobulinemia
• common variable immunodeficiency

CAUSES
• Unknown, but most patients have defective synthesis or release of immunoglobulins.

TREATMENT
• maintenance gamma globulin
• fresh frozen plasma acutely

ICD-9-CM
279.06 common variable immunodeficiency

Agranulocytosis

DESCRIPTION Reduction of blood neutrophile (granulocyte) count, leading to increased susceptibility to bacterial and fungal infection. Acute, severe neutropenia due to impaired production is often life-threatening. Caracteristics - fever, fatigue, sore throat, buccal ulcers, dyspnea, tachycardia. Usual course - acute.

SYNONYMS
• malignant neutropenia
• primary granulocytopenia
• agranulocytic angina

CAUSES
• ionizing radiation, benzene, antimetabolites, nitrogen mustards, aminopyrine, phenothiazines, sulfonamides, chloramphenicol
• typhoid, paratyphoid, influenza, measles, rickettsia, cachexia, septicemia

TREATMENT
• eliminate etiological agent
• antibiotics
• supportive measures

ICD-9-CM
288.0 agranulocytosis

Agranulocytosis, infantile genetic

DESCRIPTION Rare, hereditary and congenital disease, including familial neutropenia, cyclic neutropenia, pancreatic insufficiency with neutropenia, and several other disorders combining impaired neutrophil production and severe immune deficiency. Characteristics include fever, recurrent skin and respiratory infections, cough. Usual course - progressive; chronic; spontaneous remission.

SYNONYMS
• Kostmann's syndrome

CAUSES
• defective bone marrow microenvironment
• progenitor defect

TREATMENT
• antibiotics
• bone marrow transplantation

ICD-9-CM
288.0 agranulocytosis

Ainhum

DESCRIPTION A condition occuring chiefly in Black people in tropical countries. Characteristics - linear constriction of a toe, especially the little toe, which by its contraction gradually amputates the toe. Usual course - progressive; leading to amputation. Endemic areas - tropics; Africa.

SYNONYMS
• dactylolysis spontanea
• dactylysis spontanea
• fibrous bands

CAUSES
• unknown

TREATMENT
• surgery
• Z-plasty
• relaxing incision
• amputation
• control infection

ICD-9-CM
136.0 ainhum

Albright's syndrome with precocious puberty

DESCRIPTION Fibrous dysplasia (cystic bone lesion) involving several bones plus cutaneous pigmentation and endocrine abnormalities. Characteristics - limb deformity, femoral fracture. Usual course - chronic; progressive.

SYNONYMS
• polyostotic fibrous dysplasia
• McCune-Albright syndrome
• osteitis fibrosa cystica

TREATMENT
• hyperthyroidism therapy
• adrenalectomy
• surgery

ICD-9-CM
756.54 polyostotic fibrous dysplasia of bone

Alcaptonuria

DESCRIPTION Inborn aminoacidopathy due to defective homogentisate 1,2-dioxygenase. The accumulation of homogentistic acid leads to homogentistic aciduria causing the urine to turn dark brown on standing or alkinization. Other characteristics include ochronosis and arthritis Usual course - asymptomatic until adulthood; progressive.

SYNONYMS
• homogentisicaciduria

CAUSES
• homogentisic acid oxidase activity
• increased homogentisic acid

TREATMENT
• supportive rehabilitation

ICD-9-CM
270.2 other disturbances of aromatic amino acid metabolism

Alveolar proteinosis of the lung

DESCRIPTION Rare disease of unknown etiology characterized by filling of alveolar spaces with granular, periodic acid-Schiff (PAS)- positive material consisting of phospholipids and proteins. Age predilection is 20 to 60 years. It predominantly occurs in previously healthy males or females. Usual course - progressive.

SYNONYMS
• pulmonary alveolar proteinosis

TREATMENT
• total lung lavage under general anesthesia
• steroids not indicated

ICD-9-CM
516.0 pulmonary alveolar proteinosis

Amaurosis fugax

DESCRIPTION Acute, transient episode of blindness or partial blindness, lasting ten minutes or less.

CAUSES
• retinal arteriolar emboli

TREATMENT
• medical:
  ◊ control hypertension
  ◊ antithrombotic medications
  ◊ aspirin
  ◊ dipyridamole
• surgical:
  ◊ carotid endarterectomy

ICD-9-CM
362.34 transient arterial occlusion

Amaurosis, congenital

DESCRIPTION A cone-rod abiotrophy causing blindness or amblyopia at birth; frequently found in Holland and Sweden. Usual course - stable; gradual deterioration.

SYNONYMS
• congenital retinal blindness
• amaurosis congenita of Leber
• heredoretinopathia congenita

CAUSES
• unknown

TREATMENT
• none

ICD-9-CM
362.76 dystrophies primarily involving the retinal pigment epitheluim

Amebic meningoencephalitis

DESCRIPTION A rare and often fatal, acute, febrile, purulent meningoencephalitis caused by usually free-living soil and water amebas of the genera Naegleria, Acanthamoeba, or Hartmannella. Generally seen in young persons who swim in contaminated fresh water. Also seen in a less fulminant form in older persons and in immunocompromised persons. Usual course -acute.

CAUSES
• naegleria
• acanthamoeba
• hartmanella

TREATMENT
• amphotericin B
• miconazole
• rifampin

ICD-9-CM
006.5 amebic brain abscess

Aminoaciduria

DESCRIPTION Impairment of renal tubular transport of amino acids.

SYNONYMS
• cystinuria
• dibasic aminoaciduria
• Hartnup disease
• iminoglycinuria
• dicarboxylate aminoaciduria

TREATMENT
• diet management
• high fluid intake
• lithotomy
• penicillamine
• nicotinamide

ICD-9-CM
270.9 unspecified disorder of amino-acid metabolism

Anemia due to chronic disease

DESCRIPTION The second most common anemia in the world. The major characteristic is that the marrow erythroid mass fails to expand appropriately in response to microcytic anemia from whatever cause. The defect, then, is one of decreased red blood cell production. The symptoms are primarily those of the underlying disease, such as rheumatoid arthritis, infections, or cancer. Usual course - chronic.

CAUSES
• chronic inflammation: iron metabolism abnormality
• defective RBC production
• inability to compensate for decreased red blood cell life span

TREATMENT
• treat underlying condition

ICD-9-CM
285 other and unspecified anemias

Anemia due to folate deficiency

DESCRIPTION Decreased red blood cells and hemoglobin content due to impaired production. This is one form of megaloblastic anemia charcterized by decreased red blood cells and decreased serum folate.

SYNONYMS
• nutritional macrocytic anemia
• tropical macrocytic anemia

CAUSES
• malnutrition
• inadequate folate intake
• malabsorption of folate
• increased demand for folate
• drugs

TREATMENT
• folic acid supplements
• avoid precipitating drug

ICD-9-CM
281.2 folate-deficiency anemia

Anemia, acquired sideroblastic

DESCRIPTION A microcytic (or normocytic), hypochromic anemia due to inadequate or abnormal utilization of intracellular iron for hemoglobin synthesis, despite adequate or increased amounts of iron within the mitochondria of the developing red blood cell precursors. Peripheral blood shows polychromatic, stippled, targeted red blood cells. Usual course - slowly progressive.

CAUSES
• idiopathic
• antituberculous drugs
• alcohol
• chloramphenicol

TREATMENT
• avoid precipitating drug
• avoid alcohol
• treat consequences

ICD-9-CM
285.0 sideroblastic anemia

Anemia, hemolytic

DESCRIPTION A general term covering a large group of anemias in which there is a shortened life span of the red blood cells (normal = 120 days). Most hemolysis occurs extravascularly in the spleen, liver, and bone marrow.
• Characteristics - signs and symptoms include chills, fever, pain in the back and abdomen, prostration, shock, jaundice, splenomegaly, hemoglobinuria, hemosiderinuria, reticulocytosis

CAUSES
• G6PD deficiency
• Intrinsic abnormalities of red blood cell contents (hemoglobin or enzymes) or membrane
• Serum antibodies, trauma in circulation, infectious agents
• Temporary failure of red blood cell production
• Autoantibodies against red cell antigens, idiopathic or secondary to autoimmune diseases
• Drug-induced (penicillin type or methyldopa type)

TREATMENT
• individualized to specific hemolytic disorders. Modalities may include splenectomy and iron replacement.

ICD-9-CM
282.9 Hemolytic anemias

Anemia, myelophthisic

DESCRIPTION Anemia characterized by appearance of immature myeloid and nucleated erythrocytes in the peripheral blood, resulting from infiltration of the bone marrow by foreign or abnormal tissue. Usual course - progressive.

SYNONYMS
• myelopathic anemia
• leukoerythroblastosis
• secondary myelofibrosis

CAUSES
• hematologic consequences of marrow infiltration
• lymphoma
• leukemias
• myelomas
• metastatic carcinoma
• tuberculosis
• lipid storage diseases
• fungus infection
• granulomatous disorders

TREATMENT
• treat underlying condition
• supportive measures
• splenectomy if hypersplenism

ICD-9-CM
285.8 other specified anemias

Anhidrosis

DESCRIPTION Abnormal deficiency of sweat. Other characteristics - malaise, easy fatiguability, headache, nausea, warmth, dry skin, tachycardia.

CAUSES
• senile skin
• radiodermatitis
• acrodermatitis chronica atrophica
• scleroderma
• lichen sclerosis et atrophica
• spinal cord lesions
• quinacrine toxicity
• miliaria
• sympathectomy
• peripheral neuropathy
• sympathetic ganglion antagonists
• hereditary anhidrotic ectodermal dysplasia
• acetylcholine antagonists
• hysteria
• brainstem, pontine or medulla tumors
• Franceschetti-Judassohn syndrome
• Fabry's disease

TREATMENT
• symptomatic

ICD-9-CM
705.0 anhidrosis

Anorectal fissure

DESCRIPTION An acute tear or chronic ulcer in the stratified squamous epithelium of the anal canal. Symptoms include rectal pain and bleeding with defecation.

SYNONYMS
• Anal fissure
• Fissure in ano
• Anal ulcer

CAUSES
• Unknown. Probably traumatic laceration from a hard or large stool with secondary infection.

TREATMENT
• Stool softeners
• psyllium seed laxatives
• glycerin suppositories
• warm sitz baths
• surgery if conservative measures fail

ICD-9-CM
565.0 anal fissure

Anthracosis

DESCRIPTION Usually asymptomatic form of pneumoconiosis caused by deposition of coal dust in the lungs. Usual course - progressive; chronic. Endemic areas - urban areas.

CAUSES
• inhalation of atmospheric particles
• inhalation of soot

TREATMENT
• none

ICD-9-CM
500 coal worker's pneumoconiosis

Anthrax of the intestine

DESCRIPTION Highly infectious disease of animals, (especially ruminants) that is rarely transmitted to man by contact with the animals or their products. Anthrax infection also occurs in a cutaneous form. Characteristics - fever, malaise, hematemesis, anorexia, abdominal pain, blody diarrhea. Usual course - acute.

CAUSES
• Bacillus anthracis
• ingestion of bacillus
• contaminated meat

TREATMENT
• penicillin
• tetracycline

ICD-9-CM
022.2 gastrointestinal anthrax

Anthrax of the lung

DESCRIPTION Highly infectious disease of animals (especially ruminants) that is rarely transmitted to man by contact with the animals or their products. Caracteristics - fever, malaise, cough, myalgia, dyspnea, headache. This infection can be severe enough to be fatal. Usual course - acute; 3-4 day incubation. (Rare in U.S.)

SYNONYMS
• woolsorter disease
• anthrax pneumonia

CAUSES
• bacillus anthracis
• inhalation

TREATMENT
• penicillin
• streptomycin
• hydration

ICD-9-CM
022.1 pulmonary anthrax

Anthrax of the skin

DESCRIPTION Highly infectious disease of animals, especially ruminants. Transmitted to man by contact with the animals or their products. Cutaneous form begins as a red-brown papule that enlarges with peripheral erythema, vesiculation, and induration, followed by ulceration and local lymphadenopathy. Usual course - acute.
Endemic areas - Haiti; South Africa; Asia.

SYNONYMS
• cutaneous anthrax
• charbon
• malignant pustule
• Siberian ulcer
• malignant edema
• splenic fever
• milzbrand
• ragpicker's disease

CAUSES
• bacillus anthracis
• skin contact

TREATMENT
• penicillin
• tetracycline
• erythromycin
• hydrocortisone

ICD-9-CM
022.0 cutaneous anthrax

Aortic regurgitation

DESCRIPTION Retrograde flow from the aorta into the left ventricle through incompetent aortic cusps. Symptoms include dyspnea, shortness of breath, palpitations, orthopnea. Usual course - acute; chronic.

SYNONYMS
• aortic valve insufficiency

CAUSES
• bacterial endocarditis, aortic dissection, ankylosing spondylitis, aortic stenosis, rheumatic fever, giant cell arteritis, syphilis, Marfan's syndrome, osteogenesis imperfection, Reiter's syndrome, rheumatoid arthritis, cystic medial necrosis, sinus of valsalva aneurysm, hypertension, arteriosclerosis, myxomatous degeneration of valve, dissection of aorta, bicuspid aortic valve

TREATMENT
• aortic valve replacement

ICD-9-CM
424.1 Aortic valve disorders

Apert's syndrome

DESCRIPTION Autosomal dominant mutation characterized by acrocephalosyndactyly and mental retardation. Usual course - chronic; progressive.

SYNONYMS
• acrocephalosyndactyly

CAUSES
• unknown
• probable early bridging of mesenchymal blastema
• probable early bridging of bone hypoplasia

TREATMENT
• supportive
• orthopedic surgery
• maxillofacial surgery
• neurosurgery

ICD-9-CM
755.55 acrocephalosyndactyly

Argininosuccinicaciduria

DESCRIPTION Presence in urine of argininosuccinic acid, characteristic of a condition resulting from an inborn error of metabolism (autosomal recessive) and accompanied by mental retardation, failure to thrive, ataxia, seizures. Usual course - progressive.

SYNONYMS
• arginosuccinicacidemia
• argininosuccinase deficiency

CAUSES
• argininosuccinase deficiency

TREATMENT
• decrease urea precursors
• decrease ureapoiesis
• decrease nitrogen waste production

ICD-9-CM
270.6 disorders of urea cycle metabolism

Arsenic poisoning

DESCRIPTION Toxic condition caused by exposure to arsenic. Characteristics - throat constriction, dysphagia, burning gastrointestinal pain, vomiting, diarrhea, dehydration, pulmonary edema, renal failure, liver failure. Usual course - acute; chronic.

CAUSES
• pentavalent arsenic salt
• trivalent arsenic salt
• arsine gas

TREATMENT
• dimercaprol
• induce vomiting
• gastric lavage
• milk
• penicillamine
• hemodialysis

ICD-9-CM
985.1 Toxic effect of arsenic and its compounds

Arteriosclerosis obliterans

DESCRIPTION Arteriosclerosis in which proliferation of the intima leads to occlusion of the lumen of the arteries. Usual course - progressive

CAUSES
• atherosclerosis

TREATMENT
• exercise
• pentoxifylline
• weight loss
• avoid tobacco smoking
• angioplasty
• surgery
• lumbar sympathectomy

ICD-9-CM
440.9 generalized and unspecified arteriosclerosis

Ascites, chylous

DESCRIPTION The presence of chyle in the peritoneal cavity as a result of anomalies, injuries, or obstruction of the thoracic duct. Characteristics - abdominal pain, fullness, discomfort, distention, shortness of breath, nausea, weight gain.

SYNONYMS
• chylous peritonitis

CAUSES
• abdominal neoplasm
• lymphoma
• abdominal lymphatic obstruction
• trauma
• intestinal obstruction
• chylous cyst rupture
• hodgkin's disease

TREATMENT
• paracentesis

ICD-9-CM
789.5 ascites

Astrocytoma

DESCRIPTION A tumor composed of astrocytes characterized by hemiparesis, cranial nerve palsy, personality changes, headache, seizures, and mentation change. Usual course - progressive.

SYNONYMS
• Astrocytic glioma
• Astroglioma

CAUSES
• tuberous sclerosis

TREATMENT
• grade I: surgery
• combined surgery plus radiotherapy
• grade II: combined surgery plus radiotherapy
• grade III: combined surgery plus radiotherapy

ICD-9-CM
191.9 astrocytoma, unspecified site

Ataxia-telangiectasia

DESCRIPTION Autosomal recessive progressive multisystem disorder characterized by cerebellar ataxia, skin and conjunctival teleangiectasia, recurrent infections of sinuses and lungs, and variable immunologic disease. Usual course - progressive.

SYNONYMS
• Louis-Bar syndrome
• cerebello-oculocutaneous telangiectasia

CAUSES
• immunoglobulin metabolic disorder
• defective mesodermal differentiation

TREATMENT
• treat complications

ICD-9-CM
334 spinocerebellar disease
334.8 other spinocerebellar ataxia

Atrial flutter

DESCRIPTION Atrial rate 240-400 beats per minute. QRS complexes uniform in shape, irregular in rate. P waves may have saw-toothed configuration.

CAUSES
• postoperative revascularization
• digitalis toxicity
• pulmonary embolism
• valvular heart disease
• congestive heart failure

TREATMENT
• Digoxin (except when due to digitalis toxicity), quinidine, propranolol
• Cardioversion
• Atrial pacemaker

ICD-9-CM
427.32 atrial flutter

Atrial myxoma

DESCRIPTION A benign tumor composed of primitive connective tissue cells forming a gelatinous growth, usually pedunculated. Symptoms include dyspnea of effort, weight loss, fatigue, low-grade fever, polyneuritis, nausea, syncopal attacks. Usual course: progressive.

CAUSES
• unknown

TREATMENT
• surgical excision of mass

ICD-9-CM
212.7 benign neoplasm of heart

 ## Atypical mycobacterial infection

DESCRIPTION Disease caused by mycobacteria other than the tubercle and lepra bacillus. The illnesses are similar both pathlogically and clinically to tuberculosis. Usual course - acute; progressive.
Endemic areas: Central USA; Texas; England; Wales; Southeastern USA

CAUSES
• Mycobacterium ulcerans
• Mycobacterium kansasii
• Mycobacterium avium intracellulare
• Mycobacterium xenopi
• Mycobacterium szulgai

TREATMENT
• rifampin
• ethambutol
• isoniazid
• surgery
• minocycline
• trimethoprim-sulfamethoxazole
• ethionamide
• pyrazinamide
• cycloserine

ICD-9-CM
031.9 unspecified diseases due to mycobacteria

 ## Babesiosis

DESCRIPTION A group of tick-borne diseases of cattle, sheep, goats, horses, swine, dogs and cats; caused by protozoans of the genus Babesia, which parasitize the red blood cells, producing hemolysis.
Usual course - acute
Endemic areas: Cape Cod; Nantucket Island; Martha's Vineyard; Fire Island; Shelter Island; Long Island

SYNONYMS
• piroplasmosis

CAUSES
• Babesia microti
• tick bite
• blood transfusion
• Ixodes dammini

TREATMENT
• quinine
• clindamycin
• pentamidine isethionate
• exchange transfusion

ICD-9-CM
088.82 babesiosis

 ## Balantidiasis

DESCRIPTION Infection by protozoan parasites of the genus Balantidium. B. coli may cause diarrhea and dysentery in man, with ulceration of the colon mucosa. Usual course - acute. Endemic areas - tropical areas.

CAUSES
• balantidium coli

TREATMENT
• tetracycline
• iodoquinol

ICD-9-CM
007.0 balantidiasis

 ## Balkan nephritis syndrome

DESCRIPTION A chronic progressive nephritis seen in a large percentage of the population living in the endemic areas of Yugoslavia, Romania, Bulgaria.

CAUSES
• unknown
• possible environmental toxin

TREATMENT
• treat renal failure
• avoid endemic areas

ICD-9-CM
582.89 nephritis, interstitial, chronic

 ## Bartter's syndrome

DESCRIPTION Hypertrophy and hyperplasia of the juxtaglomerular cells producing hypokalemic alkalosis and hyperaldosteronism. Characteristics - absence of hypertension in the presence of markedly increased plasma renin concentrations and insensitivity to the pressor effects of angiotensin. Usually affects children, is perhaps hereditary, and may be associated with other congenital anomalies, such as short stature and mental retardation.

CAUSES
• unknown
• primary renal potassium wasting
• defective renal tubular potassium transport
• defective renal tubular chloride transport

TREATMENT
• liberal dietary potassium and sodium chloride
• potassium supplementation
• spironolactone, indomethacin, ibuprofen, aspirin, captopril, propranolol

ICD-9-CM
255.1 Bartter's syndrome

 ## Beckwith-Wiedemann syndrome

DESCRIPTION A syndrome of multiple defects characterized primarily by umbilical hernia, macroglossia, and gigantism and secondarily by visceromegaly, hypoglycemia, ear abnormalities, etc. Usual course - acute.

SYNONYMS
• Beckwith syndrome
• Wiedemann II syndrome
• Exomphalos-macroglossia-gigantism syndrome

CAUSES
• unknown

TREATMENT
• steroids; feeding manipulations; non-ketogenic diet high in calories
• surgery

ICD-9-CM
759 other and unspecified congenital anomalies
759.8 other specified anomalies

 ## Benign essential tremor syndrome

DESCRIPTION A fine-to-coarse slow, rhythmic tremor, primarily affecting the hands, head and voice, with a frequency of 4-12 times per second. Affected body part may be in movement or held in one position. The tremor may begin at any age, most often affects upper extremities and can be aggravated by anxiety, stress, fatigue and cold. Tends to increase with age; generallyno disability; treatment often unnecessary.

SYNONYMS
• presenile tremor syndrome
• familial tremor

CAUSES
• exact cause is unknown
• inherited as an autosomal dominant trait in about 50% of cases

TREATMENT
• extra rest may help
• propranolol or primidone
• benzodiazepines
• ingestion of a small amount of alcohol provides short-term relief

ICD-9-CM
333.1 benign and other specified forms of tremor

 ## Beriberi heart disease

DESCRIPTION A form of beriberi caused by a deficiency of thiamine characterized by cardiac failure and edema, but without extensive nervous system involvement.

SYNONYMS
• vitamin B1 deficiency heart disease
• wet beriberi

CAUSES
• chronic alcoholism
• thiamine deficiency
• malnutrition

TREATMENT
• thiamine
• diuretics
• digoxin

ICD-9-CM
265.0 beriberi

Beriberi nervous system syndrome

DESCRIPTION Usual course - chronic; progressive; generally associated with beriberi heart disease; often progresses to cerebral beriberi

CAUSES
• thiamine deficiency
• malnutrition
• chronic alcoholism
• fever
• high carbohydrate intake
• thyrotoxicosis
• dialysis
• diuresis

TREATMENT
• intramuscular thiamine
• water-soluble vitamin repletion

ICD-9-CM
265.0 beriberi

Bezoar

DESCRIPTION Concretions of swallowed hair, fruit or vegetable fibers, or similar substances found in the alimentary canal. Usual course - acute.

CAUSES
• partial gastrectomy
• autonomic neuropathy
• accumulation of vegetable fibers
• accumulation of hairs

TREATMENT
• phytobezoars: cellulose digestion, papain digestion, lavage, surgery
• trichobezoars: lavage, surgery

ICD-9-CM
938 bezoar

Bezold abscess

DESCRIPTION Sore throat and nuchal rigidity caused by insufficiently treated otitis media. Named after Frederich Bezold, an otologist from Munich. Usual course - chronic.

SYNONYMS
• subperiosteal abscess of the temporal bone
• bezold mastoiditis

CAUSES
• insufficiently treated otitis media

TREATMENT
• antibiotics
• surgical drainage

ICD-9-CM
383.01 subperiosteal abscess of mastoid

Bladder tumors

DESCRIPTION
• The second most common site for tumors of the urinary tract. Most bladder tumors occur in men aged 50 and over. Common types include transitional cell carcinoma (the most common) type), epidermoid tumors, adenocarcinoma, and sarcoma with systemic disease.
• Characteristics - symptoms include hematuria, urinary frequency, urgency, dysuria, reduced force and size of the urinary stream, suprapubic pain, and sometimes a palpable suprapubic mass. Should rule out renal calculi, cystitis, nephritis. Measures to confirm diagnosis include cystoscopy, biopsy, CT scan, ultrasound.

CAUSES
• Unknown. Risk factors include alcoholism, tobacco smoking, radiation exposure.

TREATMENT
• tumor staging
• surgery
• radiation therapy
• hormone therapy
• immunotherapy
• chemotherapy

ICD-9-CM
188.9 neoplasm bladder primary

Bloom's syndrome

DESCRIPTION Autosomal recessive syndrome developing during infancy. Characteristics include erythema and telangiectasia (in a butterfly distribution the face), photosensitivity, and dwarfism. Usual course - chronic; onset in infancy; decreased infection rate with age. Information available - Bloom Syndrome Registry 212-570-3075.

SYNONYMS
• congenital telangiectatic erythema

CAUSES
• chromosomal breakage
• chromosomal instability
• sister chromatid exchanges
• chromosomal aberrations

TREATMENT
• sunscreens
• symptomatic
• cancer therapy as necessary

ICD-9-CM
757.39 Bloom's syndrome

Blue diaper syndrome

DESCRIPTION Defect in tryptophan absorption in which the urine contains abnormal indoles, giving it a blue color. This is similar to Hartnup's disease. Usual course - chronic.

SYNONYMS
• familial hypercalcemia; with nephrocalcinosis and indicanuria
• tryptophan malabsorption

CAUSES
• defective tryptophan absorption

TREATMENT
• low tryptophan diet
• definitive treatment unknown

ICD-9-CM
275.4 disorders of calcium metabolism

Boutonneuse fever

DESCRIPTION A febrile disease of the Mediterranean area, the Crimea, Africa and India, due to infection with Rickettsia conorii.
Usual course - acute; 5-7 day incubation period
Endemic areas: mediterranean littoral; africa; indian subcontinent

SYNONYMS
• African tick typhus
• African tick-borne fever

CAUSES
• Rickettsia conorii
• tick bite
• rodent reservoir
• dog reservoir

TREATMENT
• chloramphenicol
• tetracycline

ICD-9-CM
082.1 boutonneuse fever
087.1 tick-borne relapsing fever

Bowen's disease

DESCRIPTION An epidermal hyperplasia (often occurring in multiple primary sites), which may progress to squamous cell carcinoma

SYNONYMS
• precancerous dermatosis
• intradermal epidermoid carcinoma
• carcinoma in-situ
• intraepidermal squamous cell carcinoma

CAUSES
• sun damage
• arsenic

TREATMENT
• surgical excision
• topical 5-fluorouracil

ICD-9-CM
239.2 skin neoplasm, unspecified

Brill's disease

DESCRIPTION Recrudescence of epidemic typhus occurring years after the initial infection in which the etiologic agent Rickettsia prowazekii persists in body tissues in an inactive state (up to 70 years). Usual course - relapsing. Endemic areas - worldwide.

SYNONYMS
• Brill-Zinsser disease
• recrudescent typhus

CAUSES
• persistent rickettsia prowazekii in human reservoirs
• prior epidemic typhus fever

TREATMENT
• tetracycline
• chloramphenicol
• pediculocides

ICD-9-CM
081.1 Brill's disease

Broncholithiasis

DESCRIPTION Condition in which calculi (broncholiths) are present within the lumen of the tracheobronchial tree.

SYNONYMS
• calculi of bronchus
• bronchopulmonary lithiasis

CAUSES
• usually a late complication of a granulomatous disease

TREATMENT
• antibiotics
• endoscopic removal
• surgery

ICD-9-CM
518.8 broncholithiasis

Brown-Sequard syndrome

DESCRIPTION Syndrome due to damage of one half of the spinal cord, resulting in ipsilateral paralysis and loss of discriminatory and joint sensation, and contralateral loss of pain and temperature sensation.

SYNONYMS
• hemiparaplegic syndrome
• spastic spinal monoplegia syndrome

CAUSES
• spinal trauma
• unilateral spinal cord lesion
• spinal cord tumors
• spinal cord radiation
• spinal cord compression

TREATMENT
• surgery
• decompression

ICD-9-CM
344.8 Brown-Sequard syndrome

Bruxism

DESCRIPTION The grinding and clenching of teeth (usually performed during sleep) which may lead to occlusal trauma. It is common in persons of all ages (approximately 15% of children and as many as 96% of adults). Clinically, bruxism commonly accompanies the stress of marital strife, school examinations or work difficulties; it may resolve when these stresses lessen. A genetic predisposition may exist.

SYNONYMS
• tooth grinding

CAUSES
• unknown
• associated with stress, occlusal disorders, allergies and sleep position

TREATMENT
• biofeedback exercises
• changes in sleep position
• drug therapy, e.g., diazepam, methocarbamol, injections of botulinum toxin
• psychotherapy
• hypnotherapy
• physical therapy
• occlusal orthotics
• stress reduction
• coping techniques

ICD-9-CM
306.8 bruxism

Budd-Chiari's syndrome

DESCRIPTION Symptomatic occlusion or obstruction of the hepatic veins, causing hepatomegaly, abdominal pain and tenderness, intractable ascites, mild jaundice, portal hypertension and liver failure. The onset may be acute. In cases of complete occlusion, death may occur within days of onset. More often, there is a chronic course with survival for months or years.

SYNONYMS
• hepatic vein thrombosis

CAUSES
• trauma
• oral contraceptives
• polycythemia rubra vera
• paroxysmal nocturnal hemoglobinuria
• hypercoagulable state
• pyrrolizidine alkaloids

TREATMENT
• portacaval shunt

ICD-9-CM
453.0 Budd-Chiari syndrome

Byssinosis

DESCRIPTION An occupational airway disorder (in which bronchial constriction occurs); common to those who come in contact with crude cotton, hemp or flax. Characterized by chest tightness, wheezing, dyspnea that develop on the first day after a weekend or vacation away from the work environment; symptoms decrease during the week and by the end of the week, the individual is symptom-free.

CAUSES
• inhalation of substance; dust component not positively identified

TREATMENT
• discontinue exposure

ICD-9-CM
504 pneumonopathy due to inhalation of other dust

Campylobacter infections

DESCRIPTION Campylobacter species are small, gram-negative, curved or spiral bacilli associated with enteritis and systemic disease in humans. Outbreaks have been associated with day care centers, contaminated water supplies and raw milk. C. jejuni frequently causes acute enteritis (can be mild or severe), C. coli causes diarrhea and C. fetus causes bacteremia and meningitis in immunocompromised patients and may cause maternal fever, abortion, stillbirth, and severe neonatal infection. Helicobacter pylori (previously called Campylobacter pylori) has been associated with gastritis and peptic ulcer disease.

CAUSES
• contact with infected animals
• contaminated food and water
• improperly cooked poultry
• person-to-person spread via fecal-oral route

TREATMENT
• fluid and electrolyte replacement
• erythromycin (in children)
• tetracycline (in adults)
• note: trimethoprim-sulfamethoxazole and ampicillin are ineffective against Campylobacter

ICD-9-CM
008.43 intestinal infections due to other organisms, Campylobacter

Carcinoid syndrome

DESCRIPTION A symptom complex associated with carcinoid tumors (argentaffinoma). Characteristics - attacks of severe cyanotic flushing of the skin that lasts from minutes to days; watery stools; bronchoconstrictive attacks; sudden drop in blood pressure; edema; ascites. Symptoms are caused by the tumor secreting serotonin prostaglandins, and other biologically active substances.

SYNONYMS
• Thorson-Bioerck syndrome
• argentaffinoma syndrome
• flush syndrome
• Cassidy-Scholte syndrome

CAUSES
• tumor
• overproduction of serotonin

TREATMENT
• medical management of symptoms
• appropriate treatment of tumor

ICD-9-CM
259.2 carcinoid syndrome

Carcinoid tumor

DESCRIPTION Yellow, circumscribed tumor occurring in the small intestine, appendix, stomach or colon. Usually asymptomatic. Usual course - progressive.

SYNONYMS
• argentaffinoma
• carcinoid
• argentaffin carcinoid tumor

CAUSES
• multiple endocrine neoplasia, type 1
• regional enteritis
• Gardner syndrome

TREATMENT
• surgical excision
• antihormonal therapy as needed
• radiation therapy

ICD-9-CM
238.9 neoplasm of uncertain behavior, nos

Cardiospasm

DESCRIPTION Failure to relax the smooth muscle fibers of the esophagus. Usual course - chronic; progressive.

SYNONYMS
• achalasia
• megaesophagus
• esophageal dyssynergia

CAUSES
• unknown
• impairment of postganglionic innervation of esophagus

TREATMENT
• soft foods
• sedatives
• nitrates
• anticholinergics
• calcium channel blockers
• balloon dilatation
• myotomy

ICD-9-CM
530.0 achalasia and cardiospasm

Caroli's disease

DESCRIPTION Congenital dilatation of the intrahepatic bile ducts. Characteristics - abdominal pain, fever, intermittent jaundice, hepatomegaly. Usual course - chronic; progressive; relapsing.

CAUSES
• congenital dilatation of intrahepatic bile ducts
• intrahepatic stones
• biliary obstruction

TREATMENT
• antibiotics
• surgery not indicated

ICD-9-CM
751.69 other congenital anomalies of gallbladder, bile ducts, and liver

 Cauda equina syndrome

DESCRIPTION Dull aching pain of the perineum, bladder, and sacrum, generally radiating in a sciatic fashion, with associated paresthesias and paralysis, due to compression of the spinal nerve roots. Usual course - chronic.

SYNONYMS
• cauda equina pseudo-claudication

CAUSES
• lumbar spondylosis with cauda equina compression
• congenital narrowing of lumbar canal

TREATMENT
• decompressive laminectomy
• rest

ICD-9-CM
344.60 cauda equina syndrome without mention of neurogenic bladder
344.61 cauda equina syndrome with neurogenic bladder

 Cavernous sinus thrombosis

DESCRIPTION Infection of the venous channels that drain the orbit and face. Characteristics - symptoms include exophthalmos, papilledema, headache, convulsions, septic temperature curve. Prognosis is grave.

CAUSES Direct extension of infection from the orbit and face. Risk factors include diabetes mellitus and immunosuppression.

TREATMENT
• hospitalization, intensive care, IV fluids, and intense intravenous antibiotic treatment

ICD-9-CM
325 thrombosis, intracranial venous sinus

 Chagas' disease

DESCRIPTION An acute, subacute or chronic form of trypanosomiasis occurring widely in Central and South America, transmitted by bites of reduviid bugs. Usual course - acute; chronic; progressive.
Endemic areas: western hemisphere; Mexico to Central America; South America; identified mammalian reservoirs in USA

SYNONYMS
• Brazilian trypanosomiasis

CAUSES
• inoculation of trypanosoma cruzi
• congenital breast milk
• transfusion-related infection

TREATMENT
• no definitive treatment
• nifurtimox in acute phase
• metronidazole
• pacemaker
• esophageal dilatation
• gastrointestinal surgery

ICD-9-CM
086.2 Chagas' disease without mention of organ involvement

 Charcot joint

DESCRIPTION Neuropathic arthropathy associated with certain chronic disorders. Usual course - chronic; progressive.

SYNONYMS
• neuropathic arthropathy
• tabetic osteoarthropathy
• neuropathic joint disease

CAUSES
• peripheral neuropathy
• diabetes
• tertiary syphilis
• tabes dorsalis
• syringomyelia
• myelomeningocele

TREATMENT
• immobilization
• reduction of weight-bearing
• surgical arthrodesis

ICD-9-CM
094.0 tabes dorsalis
713.5 arthropathy associated with neurological disorders

 Charcot-Marie-Tooth disease

DESCRIPTION Progressive neuropathic (peroneal) muscular atrophy, usually autosomal dominant. Characteristics - cramps, paresthesias, leg and hand weakness, difficulty in walking. Usual course - chronic; progressive.

SYNONYMS peroneal muscular atrophy

CAUSES
• hereditary

TREATMENT
• leg braces

ICD-9-CM
356.1 Charcot-Marie-Tooth disease

 Cheese-worker's lung

DESCRIPTION A pathologic condition caused by inhalation of mold that grows on cheese. Usual course - acute; subacute; chronic.

SYNONYMS
• cheese-washer's lung

CAUSES
• antigens of aspergillus clavatus
• antigens of penicillium casei
• breathing cheese mold

TREATMENT
• avoid causative agents
• tapered steroids suppress alveolitis
• chronic disease: long-term steroids

ICD-9-CM
495.8 cheese washers' lung

 Chiari-Frommel syndrome

DESCRIPTION Persistent lactation and amenorrhea following pregnancy.
Usual course - chronic

SYNONYMS
• Frommel's Disease
• Persistent postpartum amenorrhea-galactorrhea syndrome
• Pregnancy-related A-G syndrome

CAUSES
• microadenoma of the pituitary

TREATMENT
• treat underlying disorder

ICD-9-CM
676.6 galactorrhea associated with childbirth

 Chikungunya

DESCRIPTION A self-limited dengue-like illness caused by an alphavirus transmitted by mosquitoes of the genus Aedes, principally occurring in Southeast Asia and Africa. Usual course - acute.

CAUSES
• group A arbovirus
• alphavirus
• arthropod-borne
• mosquito vector
• Aedes aegypti

TREATMENT
• supportive
• bed rest
• non-salicylate antipyretics
• analgesics
• anti-inflammatory agents
• physiotherapy
• anticonvulsants
• rehydration

ICD-9-CM
066.3 chikungunya fever

Chloasma

DESCRIPTION Sharply demarcated, blotchy, brown, macules found in a symmetric distribution over the cheeks and forehead and sometimes on the neck or upper lip. Frequently occurs during pregnancy, at menopause, and in patients taking oral contraceptives. Same type may be seen in patients with chronic liver disease. Usual course - variable; chronic; relapsing.

SYNONYMS
• melasma
• mask of pregnancy

CAUSES
• oral contraceptives plus ultraviolet light
• pregnancy plus ultraviolet light
• endocrine dysfunction
• cosmetics
• Mesantoin
• diphenylhydantoin

TREATMENT
• avoid sun exposure
• avoid oral contraceptives
• delivery
• discontinue implicated drug
• discontinue implicated cosmetic
• topical bleaching agents

ICD-9-CM
709.0 chloasma

Chondroma

DESCRIPTION Benign tumor of cartilage cells. Usual course - progressive; curable

SYNONYMS
• true chondroma
• enchondroma
• chondromyxoma

CAUSES
• cartilaginous exostoses

TREATMENT
• block excision of tumor
• combined surgery plus radiotherapy
• palliative radiotherapy for advanced disease

ICD-9-CM
213.9 neoplasm, cartilage, benign

Chromomycosis

DESCRIPTION Systemic infectious fungus disease caused by Hormodendrum pedrosoi, H. compactum, or Phialophora verrucosa. Characteristics - slowly develop into large papillomatous vegetations that frequently ulcerate. Usual course - chronic. Endemic areas - worldwide; most common in tropical and subtropical areas; Brazil; Costa Rica.

SYNONYMS
• dermatomycosis
• verrucous dermatitis
• phaeohyphomycosis
• cystic chromomycosis
• cerebral chromomycosis

CAUSES
• traumatic inoculation of saprophytic soil fungi
• phialophora fungi
• fonsecaea fungi
• cladosporium fungi

TREATMENT
• successful in inverse relation to duration and extent of infection
• antifungals: amphotericin B, flucytosine, ketaconazole
• anthelmintic: thiabendazole

ICD-9-CM
117.2 chromoblastomycosis

Chromophobe adenoma of the pituitary

DESCRIPTION Tumor of anterior lobe of the pituitary gland whose cells do not stain with either acid or base dyes. The tumor may be non- functioning or may be associated with hyperpituitarism including acromegaly or Cushing's syndrome. Usual course - progressive.

CAUSES
• increased incidence after bilateral adrenalectomy

TREATMENT
• radiotherapy for small tumors
• surgery with postoperative radiotherapy for large tumors

ICD-9-CM
227.3 benign neoplasms of pituitary gland and craniopharyngeal duct

Chronic pain disorder

DESCRIPTION Perceived pain that continues longer than 6 months without an accompanying injury or illness; or there is a medical problem, but it does not have a major role in causing the pain. Patients have often tried numerous medications and a variety of doctors in seeking a solution. Standard pain treatment brings only minimal relief. Characteristics include pain that is described as stinging, burning, aching. The pain may come and go, vary in intensity, duration, location and radiating pattern (moving from one body part to another); the pain may begin suddenly and increase in severity over days to weeks. Anxiety and depression are often present.

SYNONYMS
Somatoform pain disorder

CAUSES Unknown

TREATMENT
• Counseling, biofeedback, hypnosis
• Medications in some cases
• Group therapy

ICD-9-CM
306.9 unspecified psychophysiological malfunction

Cirrhosis, cardiac

DESCRIPTION Fibrosis of the liver following central hemorrhagic necrosis associated with congestive heart failure. Usual course - chronic.

SYNONYMS
• posthepatic cirrhosis

CAUSES
• right ventricular failure
• tricuspid stenosis
• rheumatic heart disease
• cardiomyopathy
• constrictive pericarditis

TREATMENT
• fluid restriction
• diuretics
• sodium restriction
• digitalis
• rest

ICD-9-CM
571.5 posthepatic cirrhosis

Cirrhosis, macronodal

DESCRIPTION Disorganization of liver structure by widespread fibrosis characterized by connective tissue bands of varying thickness and by nodules that vary in size and contain portal spaces and terminal hepatic veins. Characteristics - anorexia, fatigue, jaundice, right upper quadrant pain, ascites. Usual course - chronic; progressive.

SYNONYMS
• postnecrotic liver cirrhosis
• toxic cirrhosis
• posthepatic cirrhosis
• necrotic liver cirrhosis

CAUSES
• unknown
• possible sequela of viral hepatitis
• phosphorus intoxication
• poisons
• infection
• metabolic disorders

TREATMENT
• treat complications
• avoid drugs
• protein restriction

ICD-9-CM
571.5 postnecrotic cirrhosis

Cirrhosis, primary biliary

DESCRIPTION Fibrosis of the liver due to obstruction or infection of the major extra- or intrahepatic bile ducts. Characteristics include jaundice, abdominal pain, steatorrhea, and enlargement of the liver and spleen.

SYNONYMS
• Hypertrophic cirrhosis of Hanot
• Hanot syndrome
• Cholangiolitic biliary cirrhosis

CAUSES
• autoimmune

TREATMENT
• corticosteroids
• azathioprine
• penicillamine
• colchicine

ICD-9-CM
571.6 biliary cirrhosis

Colorado tick fever

DESCRIPTION A febrile illness characterized by chills, aches, vomiting, leucopenia, and sometimes encephalitis; caused by a retrovirus transmitted by the tick Dermacentor andersoni. Usual course - 3 to 7 day incubation period after tick bite; acute onset; brief symptom-free interval; second febrile illness. Endemic areas - Rocky Mountain area; western Canada.

SYNONYMS
• American mountain tick fever
• mountain tick fever

CAUSES
• arbovirus transmitted by bite of hard-shelled wood tick (dermacentor andersoni)

TREATMENT
• supportive therapy

ICD-9-CM
066.1 Colorado tick fever

Complete heart block

DESCRIPTION Characteristics - QRS interval normal (nodal pacemaker); wide and bizarre (ventricular pacemaker). No relationship between P waves and QRS complexes. No constant P-R interval.

CAUSES
• Myocardial infarction or ischemic heart disease, postsurgical valve replacement, hypoxia with syncope as with Stokes-Adams syndrome, digitalis toxicity

TREATMENT
• pacemaker

ICD-9-CM
426.0 complete heart block

Cor triloculare biatriatum

DESCRIPTION Three chambered heart

SYNONYMS
• single ventricle
• univentricular heart
• double inlet ventricle

CAUSES
• unknown

TREATMENT
• palliative surgery
• corrective surgery
• medical treatment of cardiac failure

ICD-9-CM
745.3 cor triloculare biatriatum

Cornelia de Lange's syndrome

DESCRIPTION A congenital syndrome in which severe mental retardation is associated with many abnormalities such as short stature, brachycephaly, low-set ears, webbed neck, bushy eyebrows and flat hands. Possible autosomal dominant; autosomal recessive; chromosomal mutation.

SYNONYMS
• typus degenerativus amstelodamensis
• Amsterdam dwarf syndrome of deLange
• Brachman de Lange syndrome

CAUSES
• genetic

TREATMENT
• dependent on congenital heart disease or respiratory failure

ICD-9-CM
759.8 Cornelia de Lange's syndrome

Cowden's syndrome

DESCRIPTION Autosomal dominant hereditary disease. Characteristics - ectodermal neoplasia, microstomia, trichilemmomas of the face, acral verrucous papules. Usual course - chronic; progressive.

SYNONYMS
• multiple hamartoma syndrome

CAUSES
• ectodermal neoplasia
• mesodermal neoplasia
• malignant transformation

TREATMENT
• surgical
• chemotherapy when applicable

ICD-9-CM
NA

Craniopharyngioma

DESCRIPTION A tumor arising from cell rests derived from the hypophyseal stalk, frequently associated with increased intracerebral pressure, and showing calcium deposits in the capsule or the tumor proper. Usual course - progressive.

SYNONYMS
• Rathke pouch tumor
• suprasellar cyst
• pituitary epidermoid tumor
• ameloblastoma
• pituitary adamantinoma

CAUSES
congenital in origin

TREATMENT
• surgery
• radiotherapy
• hormone replacement therapy

ICD-9-CM
237.0 craniopharyngioma

Creutzfeldt-Jakob disease

DESCRIPTION Rare, usually fatal, transmissible spongiform encephalopathy, occurring in middle life in which there is partial degeneration of the pyramidal and extrapyramidal systems accompanied by progressive dementia, tremor, muscle wasting, athetosis and spastic dysarthria. Usual course - progressive; 15-20 months incubation; 6 months average duration.

SYNONYMS
• spastic pseudosclerosis
• corticostriatal-spinal degeneration
• transmissible virus dementia

CAUSES
• risk factors:
  ◊ neurosurgery
  ◊ surgery
  ◊ trauma
  ◊ intraocular pressure testing
  ◊ ingestion of animal brains

TREATMENT
• effective treatment unknown
• experimentally amantadine
• experimentally vidarabine

ICD-9-CM
046.1 Jakob-Creutzfeldt disease

Crigler-Najjar syndrome

DESCRIPTION Two distinct, inherited, syndromes marked by deficiences of hepatic glucuronyl transferase. Both produce non-hemolytic unconjugated hyperbilirubinemia with jaundice.
• Type I is an autosomal recessive form. Kernicterus may develop at any age (homozygotes develop severe hperbilirebinemia in the first few days of life). Survival into childhood is possible with intensive therapy. Patients have no response to phenobarbital.
• Type II is an autosomal dominant form; one parent will have elevated bilirubin. Kernicterus has been reported in infants, but hyperbilirubinemia may be consistent with physiologic jaundice. Patients are reponsive to phenobarbital.

SYNONYMS
• congenital hyperbilirubinemia
• glucuronyl transferase deficiency type I
• familial unconjugated hyperbilirubinemia

CAUSES
• no uridine diphosphoglucuronic transferase

TREATMENT
• exchange transfusion
• phototherapy
• cholestyramine
• phenobarbital (in Type II)

ICD-9-CM
277.4 disorders of bilirubin excretion

Cryptosporidiosis

DESCRIPTION A gastrointestinal infection characterized by watery diarrhea and cramps, sometimes severe, produced by protozoa of the genus Cryptosporidium. Other characteristics include weight loss, nausea, vomiting and fever. Disease is self-limiting except in the immunocompromised, where it is typically chronic and may be fatal. The number of cases continues to rise.

CAUSES
• cryptosporidium spp

TREATMENT
• no known effetive therapy
• rehydration
• discontinuance of immunosuppressive drugs
• good hygiene

ICD-9-CM
136.9 unspecified infectious and parasitic diseases

Dehydration

DESCRIPTION Extracellular fluid volume depletion. Routes of loss are from the gastrointestinal tract, urinary tract, and skin.
• Characteristics - signs and symptoms include diminished skin turgor, diminished intraocular tension, dry shrunken tongue, low central venous pressure (measured from neck veins), postural hypotension, tachycardia, disorientation, shock, increased hematocrit.

CAUSES Excessive loss of fluid from the gastrointestinal tract, urinary tract and skin. Conditions favoring excess loss include vomiting, diarrhea, gastric suction, excessive sweating, dialysis, chronic renal failure, salt-wasting renal disease, interstitial nephritis, myeloma, acute real failure, diuretic therapy, diabetes mellitus with ketoacidosis or extreme glycosuria, Bartter's syndrome, adrenal disease (glucocorticoid deficiency), hypoaldosteronism.

TREATMENT
• fluid and electrolyte replacement
• discontinue diuretics

ICD-9-CM
276.5 dehydration

Delirium tremens

DESCRIPTION Severe alcohol withdrawal syndrome characterized by agitation, violence, anxiety, insomnia, muscle cramps, tremor, delusion, hallucinations, ataxia, fever, with clearing beginning in 12-24 hours up to 2-10 days. Usual course - acute; relapsing.

SYNONYMS
• alcohol withdrawal delirium

CAUSES
• cessation in alcohol consumption after heavy alcohol ingestion

TREATMENT
• benzodiazepines
• barbiturates
• beta-adrenergic blockers

ICD-9-CM
291.0 alcohol withdrawal delirium

Dengue fever

DESCRIPTION Acute, self-limited disease. Characteristics include fever, prostration, headache, myalgia, rash, lymphadenopathy, leukopenia, Caused by four antigenically related but distinct types of the dengue virus. Endemic areas are tropics and subtropics.

SYNONYMS
• breakbone fever

CAUSES
• Aedes aegypti mosquito vector
• group B arbovirus
• flavivirus

TREATMENT
• symptomatic
• supportive if hemorrhagic

ICD-9-CM
061 Dengue

Diffuse esophageal spasm

DESCRIPTION Retching, chest pain, dysphagia, and regurgitation associated to esophageal motor dysfunction. Usual course - progressive; intermittent.

CAUSES
• esophageal motor dysfunction

TREATMENT
• anticholinergics
• nitrates
• esophageal dilatation

ICD-9-CM
530.5 diffuse spasm of the esophagus

DiGeorge's syndrome

DESCRIPTION An embryonic fault in the derivation of the thymus and parathyroid glands. Also with defects in the aortic arch and heart, hypoplastic mandible, defective ears, and short philtrum. Marked variability occurs, but patient with this syndrome must have both parathyroid dysfunction (lack of PTH) and T-cell dysfunction.

SYNONYMS
N/A

CAUSES
• congenital

TREATMENT
• thymic transplantation

ICD-9-CM
279.11 DiGeorge's syndrome

Diphtheria of the skin

DESCRIPTION Occurs when any disruption of the skin becomes colonized by C. Diphtheriae. Poor personal and community hygiene are particular risk factors. Lesions are punched out ulcers and appear on extremities. Usual course - acute. Endemic areas - tropics; Pacific Northwest; Southwest USA.

SYNONYMS
• cutaneous diphtheria

CAUSES
• corynebacterium diphtheriae
• skin trauma
• poor hygiene

TREATMENT
• intramuscular diphtheria antitoxin
• penicillin
• erythromycin
• quarantine

ICD-9-CM
032.85 Cutaneous diphtheria

Dubin-Johnson syndrome

DESCRIPTION Rare autosomal recessive disorder characterized by various organic anions as well as bilirubin. The hyperbilirubinemia is conjugated and bile appears in the urine. Rotor syndrome is a variant differentiated by liver histology. Splenomegaly occurs in half of patients and jaundice may occur as early as age 5. Usual course - intermittent.

SYNONYMS
• chronic idiopathic jaundice
• Dubin-Sprinz disease

CAUSES
• impaired intrahepatic bilirubin secretion
• conjugated hyperbilirubinemia

TREATMENT
• decrease bilirubin with phenobarbital

ICD-9-CM
277.4 Dubin-Johnson syndrome

Dyslexia

DESCRIPTION Disparity between intellectual potential and achievement in reading and spelling. Characteristics - normal, intelligent child 2 years behind expected reading level for his grade. Affects children in all socioeconomic levels. Affects more boys than girls.
Signs and symptoms include:
◊ Confusion in orientation of letters
◊ Reading from right to left
◊ Letter and word reversals
◊ Omitting words
◊ Losing place on a page
◊ Images appear blurred
◊ Frustration symptoms - behavioral problems, delinquency, withdrawal
◊ Cognitive abilities may take over by age 7 or 8 years in some children

SYNONYMS
• congenital word blindness
• primary reading disability

CAUSES
• unknown

TREATMENT
• remedial, corrective, compensatory education. Balance child's academic difficulties with enjoyable successful activities.

ICD-9-CM
784.61 dyslexia

Echinococcosis of the lung

DESCRIPTION Infection of the lung with hydatid cysts of the larvae of small tapeworms of the family Taeniidae. Usual course - progressive; 5-20 year latency. Endemic areas - Middle East; Australia; South Africa; South America; Central Europe.

CAUSES
• larval echinococcus granulosus
• canine fecal contamination
• childhood ingestion of contaminated material

TREATMENT
• surgical cystectomy

ICD-9-CM
122.1 echinococcus granulosus infection of lung

Ecthyma

DESCRIPTION An ulcerative pyoderma usually caused by group A beta-hemolytic streptococcal infection at the site of minor trauma, predominantly of the shins and feet. Healing is with variable scar formation. Usual course - acute; progression of vesiculopustule to crusts to ulceration.

CAUSES
• bacterial infection (streptococcal, staphylococcal)
• poor hygiene
• minor injuries

TREATMENT
• antibiotics
• good hygiene
• proper nutrition

ICD-9-CM
686.8 ecthyma

Ectrodactyly, ectodermal dysplasia, clefting syndrome

DESCRIPTION A congenital ectodermal dysplasia. Characteristics - lobster claw deformity, cleft lip, cleft palate, decreased hair growth, photophobic ectrodactyly, syndactyly. Usual course - chronic; progressive.

SYNONYMS
• EEC syndrome

CAUSES
• unknown

TREATMENT
• oral surgery
• ophthalmologic surgery
• orthopedic surgery

ICD-9-CM
757.31 congenital ectodermal dysplasia

Ehlers-Danlos syndrome

DESCRIPTION A group of inherited disorders of the connective tissue occurring in many types based on clinical, genetic and biochemical evidence, varying in severity from mild to lethal. Transmitted as autosomal recessive, autosomal dominant, or X-linked recessive traits. The major manifestations include hyperextensibility of skin and joints, easy brusability, friability of tissues with bleeding and poor wound healing, calcified subcutaneous spheroids and pseudotumors, and cardiovascular, gastrointestinal, orthopedic, and ocular defects. Usual course: chronic; progressive.

CAUSES
• probable defective cross-linkage of collagen

TREATMENT
• symptomatic
• preventive
• prolonged wound fixation
• conservative surgical repair

ICD-9-CM
756.83 Ehlers-Danlos syndrome

Elephantiasis, filarial

DESCRIPTION A chronic disease of the tropics due to infection of the lymphatic channels characterized by inflammation and obstruction of the lymphatics and hypertrophy of the skin and subcutaneous tissues. Usual course - acute; chronic; progressive. Endemic areas - South America; Africa; Asia; tropics; subtropics.

SYNONYMS
• filariasis
• wuchereriasis
• lymphatic filariasis

CAUSES
• microfilariae
• Wuchereria bancrofti
• Brugia malayi
• mosquito vector

TREATMENT
• diethylcarbamazine citrate
• plastic surgery
• fulguration
• elastic stockings

ICD-9-CM
125.9 elephantiasis, filarial, nos
457.1 elephantiasis, scrotal

Empyema

DESCRIPTION Presence of pus in a hollow organ or body cavity, particularly the pleural cavity. Usual course - acute.

CAUSES
• purulent inflammatory exudate of pleural cavity
• pulmonary infection
• thoracic surgery
• esophageal perforation
• hematogenous spread from other sites
• idiopathic
• subphrenic abscess

TREATMENT
• drainage
• antimicrobial therapy

ICD-9-CM
510.9 empyema without mention of fistula

Encephalitis, Saint Louis

DESCRIPTION A viral disease first observed in Illinois in 1932, closely similar to western equine encephalomyelitis. It occurs in late summer and early fall. Transmitted usually by mosquitoes of the genus Culex. It ranges from an abortive type of infection to severe disease. Endemic areas - Eastern USA; Midwestern USA.

CAUSES
• group B arbovirus
• transmitted by culex mosquito

TREATMENT
• supportive

ICD-9-CM
062.3 St. Louis encephalitis

Endomyocardial fibrosis, eosinophilic

DESCRIPTION Idiopathic myocardiopathy occurring endemically in various regions of Africa, characterized by cardiomegaly, marked thickening of the endocardium with dense, white fibrous tissue that frequently extends to involve the inner third or half of the myocardium.

SYNONYMS
• loeffler endomyocardial fibrosis
• loeffler fibroplastic parietal endocarditis

CAUSES
• unknown
• possibly eosinophil disorder

TREATMENT
• inotropic support
• fluid restriction plus diuretics
• anticoagulants
• immunosuppression
• endomyocardiectomy
• valve replacement
• glenn shunt

ICD-9-CM
425.0 endomyocardial fibrosis

Eosinophilic adenoma of the pituitary

DESCRIPTION A tumor of the eosinophilic cells of the anterior lobe of the pituitary gland whose presence is associated with acromegaly and gigantism. Usual course - slowly progressive.

CAUSES
• unknown

TREATMENT
• transsphenoidal surgery
• frontal craniotomy
• radiotherapy
• bromocriptine
• combined therapy

ICD-9-CM
194.3 malignant neoplasms of pituitary gland

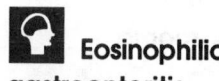

Eosinophilic fasciitis

DESCRIPTION Inflammation of the fascia of the extremities caused by unusual strenuous exercise. Usual course - acute; progressive; relapsing.

CAUSES
• unusual strenuous physical exercise
• inflammatory reaction due to chemotactic collagen breakdown products

TREATMENT
• corticosteroids
• nonsteroidal anti-inflammatory drugs

ICD-9-CM
729.4 fasciitis, unspecified

Eosinophilic gastroenteritis

DESCRIPTION A disorder characterized by infiltration of the mucosa of the small intestine by eosinophils, with edema but without vasculitis. Symptoms include diarrhea, abdominal pain, nausea, fever, malabsorption. The stomach is also frequently involved. This disorder is commonly associated with intolerance to specific foods. Usual course: -chronic; recurrent.

CAUSES
• food allergy
• idiopathic

TREATMENT
• exclusionary diets
• prednisone

ICD-9-CM
558.9 other noninfectious gastroenteritis and colitis

Epithelial mesothelioma

DESCRIPTION A malignant tumor derived from mesothelial tissue of the pleura, with some regions containing spindle-shaped, sarcoma-like cells and other regions showing adenomatous patterns. Usual course - progressive.

CAUSES
• asbestos
• tobacco smoking

TREATMENT
• surgical resection for solitary lesion
• palliative radiotherapy for advanced disease
• palliative chemotherapy for advanced disease
• pleurocentesis for pleural effusion

ICD-9-CM
163.9 malignant neoplasm of the pleura

Erythema marginatum

DESCRIPTION Superficial, often asymptomatic, form of gyrate erythema associated with some cases of rheumatic fever. Characterized by presence on the trunk and extensor surfaces of the extremities of a transient eruption of flat to slightly indurated, non-scaling multiple lesions. Usual course - acute.

CAUSES
• rheumatic fever

TREATMENT
• treat underlying disease

ICD-9-CM
695.0 erythema marginatum

Ewing's sarcoma

DESCRIPTION Malignant tumor of bone arising in medullary tissue, occurring more often in cylindrical bones. Prominent symptoms include pain, fever and leukocytosis. Usual course - acute; relapsing probable.

CAUSES
• enchondroma
• aneurysmal bone cyst

TREATMENT
• cyclophosphamide
• possibly surgery
• megavoltage radiotherapy
• vincristine
• actinomycin D
• adriamycin

ICD-9-CM
170.9 malignant neoplasms of the bone

Fabry's disease

DESCRIPTION An x-linked lysosomal storage disease of glycosphingolipid catabolism. Usual course - progressive.

SYNONYMS
• glycosphingolipidosis
• angiokeratoma corporis diffusum
• ceramide trihexoside lipoidosis

CAUSES
• alpha-galactosidase a deficiency
• ceramide trihexosidase deficiency

TREATMENT
• analgesic
• phenytoin
• carbamazepine
• corticosteroid

ICD-9-CM
272.7 Fabry's disease

Factor X deficiency

DESCRIPTION Deficiency of Factor X, a storage-stable factor essential to the clotting process that participates both in the intrinsic and extrinsic pathways of blood coagulation. Usually inherited as an autosomal recessive trait, though it can be acquired. It is characterized by defective activity in both the intrinsic and extrinsic pathways, impaired thromboplastin time, and impaired prothrombin consumption. Usual course - chronic; intermittent.

SYNONYMS
• Stuart-Prower factor deficiency

CAUSES
• inherited metabolic abnormality

TREATMENT
• fresh frozen plasma for hemorrhagic episodes

ICD-9-CM
286.3 congenital deficiency, factor X

Familial Mediterranean fever

DESCRIPTION Hereditary disease transmitted in an autosomal recessive manner, usually occurring in Armenians and Sephardic Jews. Characteristics include short, recurrent attacks of fever with pain in the abdomen, chest, or joints and erythema resembling that seeen in erysipelas. It is sometimes complicated by amyloidosis. Usual course - intermittent.

SYNONYMS
• paroxysmal polyserositis
• familial recurrent polyserositis
• periodic fever
• periodic disease

CAUSES Genetic

TREATMENT
• colchicine

ICD-9-CM
277.3 familial mediterranean fever

Familial neonatal hyperbilirubinemia

DESCRIPTION Transient familial form of hyperbilirubinemia with onset of jaundice within four days after birth. This form can lead to kernicterus.

SYNONYMS
• transient familial neonatal hyperbilirubinemia

CAUSES
• unknown

TREATMENT
• exchange transfusion

ICD-9-CM
774.6 unspecified fetal and neonatal jaundice

Fanconi's syndrome

DESCRIPTION A general term for a disorder marked by dysfunction of the proximal tubules of the kidney, with generalized hyperaminoaciduria, renal glycosuria, hyperphosphaturia, and water and bicarbonate loss. It occurs in genetic and acquired forms.

CAUSES
• multiple myeloma
• amyloidosis
• sjogren's syndrome
• nephrotic syndrome
• renal transplantation
• vitamin D deficiency
• lead
• mercury
• cadmium
• uranium
• strontium
• tetracycline
• maleic acid
• cystinosis
• wilson's disease
• galactosemia
• hereditary fructose intolerance
• tyrosinemia
• lowe's syndrome

TREATMENT
• no specific treatment
• Shohl's solution
• potassium replacement

ICD-9-CM
270.0 Fanconi syndrome

Fascioliasis

DESCRIPTION Infection with a trematode worm found in the small intestines of residents in many parts of Asia. Intermediate hosts are snails, Characteristics include nausea, diarrhea, and malabsorption. Usual course - acute; chronic; progressive; 3 month incubation.

CAUSES
• fasciola hepatica

TREATMENT
• praziquantel

ICD-9-CM
121.3 fascioliasis

Fasciolopsiasis

DESCRIPTION The state of being infected with flukes of the trematode worm genus Fasciolopsis. Characteristics - asymptomatic. Usual course - chronic; progressive. Endemic areas - Southern China; Southeast Asia; Indian subcontinent.

CAUSES
• fasciolopsis buski

TREATMENT
• praziquantel

ICD-9-CM
121.4 fasciolopsiasis

Fatigue

DESCRIPTION A state of discomfort and decreased efficiency resulting from prolonged or excessive exertion or loss of power (from any cause) to respond appropriately to stimulation.
• Characteristics - closely related to approximately equal terms: Lassitude, tiredness, lethargy, malaise, and ennui

CAUSES Drugs, overexertion, Addison's disease, alcohol, anemia, chronic fatigue syndrome (Epstein-Barr virus infection has unclear, possible association), diabetes mellitus, emotional problems (depression, somatization disorder), emphysema, endocarditis, environmental toxins, hepatitis, inadequate nutrition, inadequate rest, infectious mononucleosis, intestinal parasites, malignancies, myasthenia gravis, obesity, poor physical conditioning, rheumatoid arthritis, sedative-hypnotics, systemic lupus erythematosis, thyroid disease, tuberculosis, and others.

TREATMENT
• treat underlying disorder

ICD-9-CM
780.7 malaise and fatigue

Fatty liver due to pregnancy, acute

DESCRIPTION A serious complication of pregnancy that can lead to encephalopathy, bleeding and shock. Usual course - acute.

CAUSES
• unknown

TREATMENT
• delivery

ICD-9-CM
646.7 pregnancy complicated by fatty metamorphosis of liver

Favism

DESCRIPTION Hemolytic anemia due to the ingestion of fava beans or after inhalation of pollen from the Vicia fava plant by person with glucose-6-phosphate dehydrogenase deficient erythrocytes. Usual course - acute; chronic; intermittent; relapsing. Endemic areas - malarial endemic areas; worldwide.

CAUSES
• acute hemolysis
• fava bean ingestion
• vicia faba ingestion
• Mediterranean type glucose-6-phosphate dehydrogenase deficiency

TREATMENT
• supportive
• transfusion
• folic acid
• maintain adequate urine output
• alkalinize urine

ICD-9-CM
282.2 favism

Felty's syndrome

DESCRIPTION Chronic rheumatoid arthritis with leukopenia, splenomegaly, pigmented skin spots on the extremities, anemia, and thrombocytopenia. Usual course - chronic.

SYNONYMS
• rheumatoid arthritis-hypersplenism syndrome

CAUSES
• rheumatoid arthritis

TREATMENT
• splenectomy

ICD-9-CM
714.1 Felty's syndrome

Fetal alcohol syndrome

DESCRIPTION A syndrome found in infants whose mothers have consumed alcohol during pregnancy. Signs include microcephaly, short palpebral fissures, flat midface, underdeveloped philtrum and thin upper lip. Other, less common signs include low nasal bridge, epicanthal folds, minor ear anomalies, short nose, and micrognathia. Intrauterine or postnatal growth retardation, mental retardation or other neurologic abnormality and two or more of the facial features are needed for the diagnosis.

CAUSES
• Alcohol ingestion during pregnancy. All trimesters have been associated with abnormalities and no lower limit of alcohol dose is known. Therefore, alcohol consumption during pregnancy should be avoided entirely.

TREATMENT
• Counseling pregnant women
• Patient interventions include behavioral (special education, setting realistic family expectations), surgical (cardiac defects), dental (caries are common), ophthalmic (vision correction), and others as appropriate.

ICD-9-CM 760.71 Fetal alcohol syndrome

Filariasis

DESCRIPTION Infection with the filarial worm, Wuchereria bancrofti. The adult worms migrate to the lymphatic system producing recurrent lymphangitis with obstruction and fibrosis. Edema progresses to elephantiasis. Transmitted by mosquitoes, which harbor the larval forms. Usual course - chronic; relapsing; 8-12 month incubation. Endemic areas - Africa; Pacific islands; Southeast Asia; West Indies; Central America; eastern coastal plains of South America.

SYNONYMS
• bancroftian filariasis
• Malayan filariasis
• lymphatic filariasis
• Filarioidea infection

CAUSES
• adult filarial worms
• Wuchereria bancrofti
• Brugia malayi
• Brugia timori
• lymphatic obstruction

TREATMENT
• diethylcarbamazine
• treat hypersensitivity to dying parasite
• aspirin
• antihistamine
• steroids

ICD-9-CM
125.9 filariasis, nos

First degree AV block

DESCRIPTION P-R interval prolonged to greater than .20 seconds. Normal QRS complex. Usually asymptomatic.

CAUSES
• anterior or inferior myocardial infarction, hypothyroidism, digitalis toxicity, potassium imbalance

TREATMENT
• correct underlying cause
• use caution with use of digitalis

ICD-9-CM
426.11 first degree block

Floppy infant syndrome

DESCRIPTION Congenital myopathy marked by hypotonia and muscle weakness

CAUSES
• CNS diseases, atonic diplegia, congenital cerebellar ataxia, kernicterus, chromosomal defects, oculocerebrorenal syndrome, cerebral lipidoses, Prader-Willi syndrome, spinal cord diseases, spinal cord trauma, Werdnig-Hoffmann disease, peripheral nerve diseases, polyneuritis, familial dysautonomia, congenital sensory neuropathy, neuromuscular junction diseases, myasthenia gravis, infantile botulism, muscle diseases, congenital muscular dystrophy, myotonic dystrophy, glycogen storage disease of muscle and heart, central core disease, nemaline myopathy, mitochondrial myopathies

TREATMENT
• treat underlying disorder

ICD-9-CM
781.9 other symptoms involving nervous and musculoskeletal systems

Forbes-Albright syndrome

DESCRIPTION Galactorrhea-amenorrhea syndrome usually associated with a pituitary tumor. There is no relationship to pregnancy. Usual course - chronic; indolent.

SYNONYMS
• amenorrhea-galactorrhea syndrome
• nonpuerperal galactorrhea

CAUSES
• pituitary prolactinoma

TREATMENT
• bromocriptine
• surgery

ICD-9-CM
253.1 Forbes-Albright syndrome

 Formaldehyde poisoning

DESCRIPTION Unusual poisoning with formaldehyde due to occupational exposure. Toxic symptoms include gastrointestinal upsets, vascular collapse and coma. 60 mL of 40% formalin can cause fatality. Usual course - acute; chronic; progressive. Endemic areas - occupational exposure.

CAUSES
• cytotoxicity
• conversion to formic acid

TREATMENT
• activated charcoal
• supportive
• bicarbonate infusion
• avoid emetics
• avoid lavage

ICD-9-CM
989.8 formaldehyde poisoning

 Friedreich's ataxia

DESCRIPTION Antosomal recessive disease beginning in childhood or youth. Characteristics include sclerosis of the dorsal and lateral columns of the spinal cord. symptoms include ataxia, speech impairment, lateral curvature of the spinal column, peculiar swaying and irregular movements, and paralysis of the muscles of the lower extremities. Usual course - chronic; progressive.

SYNONYMS
• spinocerebellar ataxia
• familial ataxia
• hereditary ataxia of Friedreich
• hereditary spinal ataxia

CAUSES
• usually hereditary

TREATMENT
• surgery for scoliosis
• intervention for heart disease

ICD-9-CM
334.0 Friedreich's ataxia
334.2

 Gardner's syndrome

DESCRIPTION An autosomal dominant disorder characterized by familial polyposis of the large bowel, with supernumerary teeth, fibrous dysplasia of the skull, osteomas, fibromas and epithelial cysts. The polyps of the large bowel have malignant potential. Usual course - progressive.

SYNONYMS
• intestinal polyposis III
• polyposis-osteomatosis-epidermoid cyst

CAUSES
• genetic

TREATMENT
• total colectomy

ICD-9-CM
211.3 intestinal polyposis

 Gastroenteritis, viral

DESCRIPTION Acute inflammation of the lining of the stomach and intestines accompanied by fever and caused by any one of a number of viruses. Usual course - acute.

SYNONYMS
• epidemic diarrhea
• winter vomiting disease

CAUSES
• rotavirus
• adenovirus
• astrovirus
• Norwalk-like agents
• coxsackievirus
• echovirus

TREATMENT
• fluid replacement
• bismuth subsalicylate

ICD-9-CM
008.8 viral gastroenteritis

 Gaucher's disease

DESCRIPTION Hereditary disorder of glucocerebroside metabolism, usually occurring in infancy, and characterized by mental retardation, bulbar palsy, opisthotonus and enlargement of the spleen and liver. Usual course - acute; progressive.

SYNONYMS
• cerebroside lipoidosis

CAUSES
• beta-glucosidase deficiency
• glucocerebroside accumulation

TREATMENT
• splenectomy for hemorrhage
• orthopedic immobilization
• bone marrow transplantation
• analgesics

ICD-9-CM
272.7 Gaucher's disease

 Geotrichosis

DESCRIPTION An oral, bronchial, pulmonary or intestinal fungal infection. Symtoms include cough, mucopurulent gelatinous sputum (streaked with blood), mouth lesions resembling thrush, fever. Prognosis - uneventful.

CAUSES
• Geotrichum candidum

TREATMENT
• gentian violet
• oral potassium iodide for pulmonary infections

ICD-9-CM
117.9 geotrichosis

 Gestational trophoblastic neoplasm

DESCRIPTION A tumor usually arising in the uterus developing from hydatidiform mole,(50%), following abortion (24%), or during normal pregnancy (22%). Usual course - slow onset; curable. Endemic areas - Asia.

SYNONYMS
• choriocarcinoma
• chorioadenoma destruens
• hydatidiform mole

CAUSES
• increasing age

TREATMENT
• hydatidiform mole: removal of mole
• hysterectomy
• stage I: chemotherapy with optional hysterectomy
• stage II: chemotherapy with recommended hysterectomy
• stage III: combination chemotherapy with optional hysterectomy
• stage IV: combination chemotherapy with local radiotherapy plus optional surgery

ICD-9-CM
239.5 unspecified neoplasm of the placenta

 Giant hypertrophic gastritis

DESCRIPTION Excessive proliferation of the gastric mucosa, producing diffuse thickening of the stomach wall. Frequently associated with inflammatory changes. Usual course - chronic. The presence of diffuse carcinoma; diffuse lymphoma; Zollinger-Ellison syndrome nearly excludes this diagnosis.

SYNONYMS
• Menetrier's disease
• protein-losing gastroenteropathy

CAUSES
• idiopathic

TREATMENT
• observation
• H2-receptor blockers
• anticholinergic medications
• vagotomy
• antifibrinolytic medications
• partial gastrectomy

ICD-9-CM
535.2 hypertrophic gastritis

Glioblastoma multiforme

DESCRIPTION   Astrocytoma of grade III or IV. Characteristics include rapid growth, confinement to the cerebral hemispheres and cell types of a mixture of spongioblasts, astroblasts, and astrocytes. Headache, vomiting, and personality changes comprise prominent symptoms. Most likely in males ages 40-75 years. Usual course - progressive over months.

SYNONYMS
• grade 3 and 4 astrocytoma
• spongioblastoma multiforme

CAUSES   Unknown

TREATMENT
• surgical excision plus radiotherapy plus chemotherapy

ICD-9-CM
191.9 malignant neoplasm of the brain, unspecified

Globus hystericus

DESCRIPTION   A condition in which the patient has a sense of fullness or lump in the throat. However, no difficulty is encountered when actually swallowing (i.e., not true dysphagia).

CAUSES
• Anxiety disorders

TREATMENT
Antianxiety agents may be needed although simple reassurance is usually sufficient.

ICD-9-CM
300.11 Globus hystericus

Glomerulonephritis, membranous

DESCRIPTION   A disease of the glomerulus manifested clinically by proteinuria, and sometimes by other features of the nephrotic syndrome. Histologically characterized by deposits in the glomerular capillary wall between the epithelial cell and the basement membrane and a thickening of the membrane. Also characteristic are outward projections of the membrane between the epithelial deposits in the form of "spikes". There is some agreement that the deposits are antigen-antibody complexes. Usual course - progressive.

SYNONYMS
• membranous glomerulopathy
• membranous nephropathy
• extramembranous glomerulopathy
• idiopathic membranous glomerulonephritis
• idiopathic membranous nephropathy
• membranous glomerulonephropathy
• MGN

CAUSES
• idiopathic
• circulating antigen-antibody complexes

TREATMENT
• steroids
• cytotoxic drugs

ICD-9-CM
583.1 nephritis and nephropathy, not specified as acute or chronic, with lesion of membranous glomerulonephritis

Glomerulonephritis, rapidly progressive

DESCRIPTION   Acute glomerulonephritis marked by a rapid progression to end-stage renal failure and, histologically, by profuse epithelial proliferation. The principal signs are anuria, proteinuria, hematuria, and anemia. Usual course - progressive.

SYNONYMS
• extracapillary glomerulonephritis

CAUSES
• idiopathic

TREATMENT
• corticosteroids
• azathioprine
• cyclophosphamide
• anticoagulants
• plasmapheresis
• renal transplantation

ICD-9-CM
583.4 nephritis and nephropathy, not specified as acute or chronic, with lesion of rapidly progressive glomerulonephritis

Glomerulopathy, membranous

DESCRIPTION   A noninflammatory disease of the renal glomerulus. Characteristics - edema, hypertension, subendothelial immune deposits, thickened glomerular basement membrane.

SYNONYMS
• membranous nephropathy

CAUSES
• idiopathic
• drugs
• penicillamine
• gold
• captopril
• hepatitis B
• parasitic infestation
• SLE
• malignancy
• NSAID

TREATMENT
• corticosteroids
• anti-metabolites
• antiplatelet drugs
• anticoagulants

ICD-9-CM
583.1 nephritis and nephropathy, not specified as acute or chronic, with lesion of membranous glomerulonephritis

Glossopharyngeal neuralgia

DESCRIPTION   Rare disease of the 9th cranial nerve (glossopharyngeal). Characteristics - paroxysms of sharp, darting pain affecting the posterior pharynx, base of tongue, jaw.

CAUSES   Rare tumor (nasopharyngeal or other intracranial tumor), trauma, usually no known cause

TREATMENT
• carbamazepine with or without phenytoin
• surgery

ICD-9-CM
352.1 glossopharyngeal neuralgia

Glucagonoma

DESCRIPTION   Glucagon-secreting tumor of the pancreatic alpha cells characterized by a distinctive rash, weight loss, stomatitis, glossitis, diabetes, hypoaminoacidemia, and normochromic normocytic anemia. Usual course - progressive.

SYNONYMS
• alpha cell tumor
• alpha-cell adenoma

CAUSES
• unknown

TREATMENT
• surgical enucleation to partial pancreatectomy
• fluorouracil plus streptozotocin for unresectable tumor

ICD-9-CM
235.5 neoplasm of the pancreas

Goodpasture's syndrome, pulmonary component

DESCRIPTION   Glomerulonephritis associated with pulmonary hemorrhage and circulating antibodies against basement membrane antigens. This condition exists most frequently in young men. It has a course of rapidly progressive renal failure with hemoptysis, pulmonary infiltrates, and dyspnea. Usual course - chronic.

CAUSES   Unknown

TREATMENT
• corticosteroids
• cytotoxic agents
• plasmapheresis

ICD-9-CM
446.2 goodpasture's syndrome

Goodpasture's syndrome, renal component

DESCRIPTION   Glomerulonephritis occurring most often in young men accompanied by rapidly progressive renal failure. Other characteristics include hemotysis, dyspnea, and pulmonary infiltrates. Usual course - progressive.

CAUSES
• anti-glomerular basement membrane antibody

TREATMENT
• corticosteroids
• plasmapheresis
• cyclophosphamides
• renal transplantation

ICD-9-CM
446.2 Goodpasture's syndrome

Granuloma inguinale

DESCRIPTION Genital ulcers (not to be confused with lymphogranuloma inguinale) caused by Donovania granulomatis; also called donovanosis. Diagnosis is by demonstration of typical intracellular Donovan bodies in crushed-tissue smears. Usual course - acute; progressive; relapsing; indolent. Endemic areas - tropics; subtropics.

SYNONYMS
- donovanosis
- donovania
- granuloma venereum

CAUSES
- sexual transmission
- calymmatobacterium granulomatous
- fomites
- autoinoculation

TREATMENT
- antibiotics

ICD-9-CM
099.2 granuloma inguinale

Granulomatous disease of childhood, chronic

DESCRIPTION A group of immunodeficiency of X-linked or autosomal recessive inheritance, caused by failure of the respiratory or metabolic burst resulting in deficient microbacidal activity. Characteristics - patients sustain frequent, severe, and prolonged bacterial and fungal infections. Usual course - chronic.

SYNONYMS
- congenital dysphagocytosis
- familial chronic granulomatosis
- septic progressive granulomatosis

CAUSES
- bacterial infection
- fungal infection
- defective phagocytic cell microbicidal activity
- abnormal oxidative metabolism during phagocytosis

TREATMENT
- antibiotics

ICD-9-CM
686.1 granulomatosis

Halitosis

DESCRIPTION Unpleasant odor to the breath. Characteristics - gastrointestinal disorders do not generally cause halitosis, so breath odor does not reflect the state of digestive system or bowel function.

CAUSES
- inhaled substances
- ingested substances
- gingival disease
- dental disease
- food fermentation in mouth
- systemic disease (tonsillitis, pneumonia, bronchiectasis, lung abscess)
- hepatic encephalopathy
- diabetic acidosis
- infectious diseases
- neoplastic disease of the respiratory tract
- hypochondriasis

TREATMENT
- treat any discovered specific cause
- attentive listening
- assurance regarding benign nature (if appropriate)

ICD-9-CM
784.9 foul breath

Hallervorden-Spatz disease

DESCRIPTION Autosomal recessive hereditary disorder usually beginning in first or second decade. Characteristics include marked reduction in the number of myelin sheaths of the globus pallidus and substantia nigra, progressive rigidity in legs, dyarthria, choreoathetoid movements, and progressive mental degeneration. Usual course - chronic; progressive.

SYNONYMS
- pigmentary pallidal degeneration syndrome
- progressive pallidal degeneration syndrome
- late infantile neuroaxonal dystrophy

CAUSES
- genetic

TREATMENT
- L-dopa
- tryptophan
- megavitamins

ICD-9-CM
333.0 hallervorden-spatz disease or syndrome

Hand-foot-and-mouth disease

DESCRIPTION Usually mild and self-limited exanthematous eruption most often caused by Coxsackievirus. It occurs primary in preschool children. Characteristics include vesicles on the buccal mucosa, tongue, soft palate, gingivae, and hand and feet, including the palms and soles. Usual course - subacute; chronic; recurrent.

CAUSES
- coxsackie virus

TREATMENT
- symptomatic

ICD-9-CM
074.3 hand, foot, and mouth disease

Hand-Schueller-Christian syndrome

DESCRIPTION Disseminated, chronic form of Langerhans-cell histiocytosis. May exhibit the classic triad of exophthalmos, diabetes insipidus and bone destruction. Usual course - chronic; remission.

SYNONYMS
- craniohypophyseal xanthoma
- idiopathic chronic xanthomatosis
- multifocal eosinophilic granuloma
- histiocytosis x
- Schueller-Christian Disease

CAUSES
- eosinophilic infiltration

TREATMENT
- chemotherapy
- access to free water

ICD-9-CM
277.8 Hand-Schueller-Christian disease

Hantavirus

DESCRIPTION A genus of the Bunyaviridae family responsible for pneumonia and hemorrhagic fevers. Disease transmission is associated with infected rodents, who manifest no apparent symptoms, but shed virus in feces, urine and saliva. The hantavirus strain that causes disease in Europe and Asia is distinctly different from the hantavirus pulmonary syndrome occurring mainly in southwestern U.S. This syndrome, progressing from flulike symptoms to respiratory failure, and possibly death is known for its high mortality.

CAUSES
- human infection may occur from inhalation, ingestion (e.g., contaminated food or water), contact with rodent excrement or rodent bites; person-to-person spread or transmission by mosquitos, fleas or other arthropods has not been reported

TREATMENT
- supportive (oxygenation, vital signs monitoring, stabilization of heart rate and blood pressure)
- fluid volume replacement (with caution not to overhydrate)
- dopamine or epinephrine for hypotension
- ribavirin

ICD-9-CM
079.99 infection, viral, unspecified nature or site

Hartnup disease

DESCRIPTION Familial syndrome characterized clinically by a pellagrous rash, cerebellar ataxia, and mental retardation and biochemically by the loss of renal tubular and intestinal transport of neutral amino acids. Usual course - intermittent

CAUSES
- abnormal intestinal amino acid transport
- abnormal renal tubular amino acid transport

TREATMENT
- nicotinamide
- high protein diet

ICD-9-CM
270.0 Hartnup disease

Heat cramp

DESCRIPTION A form of heat exhaustion characterized by muscle spasm attended by pain, dilated pupils, and weak pulse. It occurs in people who lose much salt and water by working intensely in excessive heat. Usual course - acute; intermittent. Endemic areas: tropics; subtropics.

CAUSES
- electrolyte depletion

TREATMENT
- rest
- adequate salt replacement
- isotonic saline solution

ICD-9-CM
992.2 heat cramps

Hemangioma of the liver

DESCRIPTION Benign tumor made of newly formed blood vessels resulting from malformation of angioblastic tissue of fetal life. Usual course - stable; usually asymptomatic.

SYNONYMS
• cavernous hemangioma of the liver
• cavernoma of the liver

TREATMENT
• none for small asymptomatic lesions
• surgical excision
• radiotherapy has been used for massive hemangiomas

ICD-9-CM
228.04 hemangioma of intraabdominal structures

 ## Hemiplegia, acute infantile

DESCRIPTION Hemiparesis, weakness, seizures present at or before birth, due to cerebral thrombosis. Numerous causes for cerebral thrombosis. Usual course - acute.

CAUSES
• cerebral artery embolism
• cerebral artery thrombosis
• vasculitis
• tonsillar infection
• cervical adenitis
• trauma
• arteriosclerosis
• fibromuscular hyperplasia
• sickle cell disease
• lupus
• polyarteritis nodosa
• cyanotic heart disease

TREATMENT
• treat underlying condition
• control seizures
• treat increased intracranial pressure if present

ICD-9-CM
343.4 infantile hemiplegia

 ## Hemoglobin C disease

DESCRIPTION A disease characterized by compensated hemolysis with a normal hemoglobin level or a mild to moderate anemia. There may be intermittent abdominal discomfort, splenomegaly, and slight jaundice. Hereditary, autosomal recessive. Usual course - chronic.

CAUSES
• point mutation in hemoglobin beta gene

TREATMENT
• supportive
• transfusions
• folate therapy

ICD-9-CM
282.7 hemoglobin C disease

 ## Hemosiderosis, pulmonary

DESCRIPTION Rare disease of unknown etiology. Must be distinguished from Goodpasture's syndrome and from lung hemorrhage in systemic lupus erythematosus. • Characteristics - episodes of hemoptysis, hemorrhage into the lung, pulmonary infiltration, secondary iron deficiency anemia. Most common in children. Pathology shows diffuse infiltration with hemosiderin-containing macrophages. Death may occur from massive hemorrhage, although patients may live for several years with pulmonary fibrosis and insufficiency.

CAUSES
• unknown

TREATMENT
• symptomatic and supportive

ICD-9-CM
275.0 Hemosiderosis, pulmonary
516.1

 ## Hemothorax

DESCRIPTION A collection of blood in the pleural cavity. Characteristic signs and symptoms include chest pain, dyspnea, weakness, tachycardia, and asymmetrical chest movement. Usual course - acute.

CAUSES
• frank bleeding into pleural space
• penetrating chest trauma
• blunt chest trauma
• hematologic disorders

TREATMENT
• drainage by catheter
• thoracotomy if continuous serious bleeding

ICD-9-CM
511.8 hemothorax
860.2

 ## Hepatic artery aneurysm

DESCRIPTION Aneurysmal dilatation of a portion of the hepatic artery. Characteristics - right upper quadrant pain, bruit in right upper quadrant, jaundice. Usual course - progressive.

CAUSES
• weakening of vessel wall by stone eliciting aneurysmal dilatation

TREATMENT
• surgery

ICD-9-CM
442.84 hepatic artery aneurysm

 ## Hepatic fibrosis, congenital

DESCRIPTION Developmental disorder of the liver characterized by irregular broad bands of fibrous tissue containing multiple cysts formed by disordered terminal bile ducts, chiefly in the portal areas, which leads to portal hypertension. Symptoms include splenomegaly, hepatomegaly, and gastrointestinal bleeding.

CAUSES
• genetic

TREATMENT
• splenectomy
• splenorenal shunt

ICD-9-CM
571.5 cirrhosis of liver without mention of alcohol

 ## Hepatitis, alcoholic

DESCRIPTION An acute or chronic degenerative and inflammatory lesion of the liver in the alcoholic patient which is potentially progressive or reversible; it does not necessarily include steatosis, fibrosis, or cirrhosis of alcoholics, although it is frequently associated with these conditions. Usual course - acute; chronic.

SYNONYMS
• alcoholic steatonecrosis
• sclerosing hyaline necrosis

CAUSES
• alcoholism

TREATMENT
• well-balanced diet
• intravenous alimentation
• avoid alcohol

ICD-9-CM
571.1 acute alcoholic hepatitis

 ## Hereditary angioneurotic edema

DESCRIPTION Inherited C1 inhibitor deficiency. An autosomal dominant disorder characterized by recurrent episodes of edema of the skin, upper respiratory tract, and gastrointestinal tract. Frequently mediated by minor trauma, sudden changes in environmental temperature, and sudden emotional stress. Usual course - acute; intermittent; relapsing.

SYNONYMS
• hereditary angioedema

CAUSES
• No complement C1 esterase inhibitor

TREATMENT
• antifibrinolytic agent
• epsilon-aminocaproic acid

ICD-9-CM
277.6 hereditary angioneurotic edema

Hereditary anhidrotic ectodermal dysplasia

DESCRIPTION A congital ectodermal defect that is x-linked recessive; autosomal recessive. Only males fully express the condition; female carriers may have mild symptoms in x-linked recessive form; both sexes equally affected in autosomal recessive form. Symptoms: heat intolerance, facial anomalies, anhidrosis, hypotrichosis, short stature, dry skin, no mammary glands, mental retardation. Chronic course.

SYNONYMS
• Christ-Siemens-Touraine syndrome
• Siemens syndrome

CAUSES
• defective ectodermal structures
• inherited disease

TREATMENT
• dental reconstruction

ICD-9-CM
757.31 congenital ectodermal dysplasia

Hereditary hemorrhagic telangiectasia

DESCRIPTION Autosomal dominant vascular anomaly. Characteristics - multiple small telangiectases of the skin, mucous membranes, gastrointestinal tract and other organs; recurrent episodes of bleeding; gross or occult melena. Usual course - very slowly progressive.

SYNONYMS
• Osler-Weber-Rendu disease

CAUSES
• genetic

TREATMENT
• symptomatic

ICD-9-CM
448.0 hereditary hemorrhagic telangiectasia

Hernias, external

DESCRIPTION Abnormal protrusion of intra-abdominal tissue through a fascial defect in the abdominal wall. Most often, a hernial mass consists of covering tissues (skin, subcutaneous tissues, etc.), a peritoneal sac, and any contained viscera. Groin hernias (indirect inguinal, direct inguinal, femoral) are the most common (about 75% of cases), followed by incisional and ventral hernias (10%), umbilical (3%), and others (3%). Reducible hernia is one where the contents of the sac may spontaneously or with pressure return to the abdomen. Irreducible (incarcerated) hernia is one whose contents cannot be returned to the abdomen. A strangulated hernia is one where there is compromise to the blood supply of the contents of the sac. Signs and symptoms of a hernia include a heavy feeling in groin, a painful or painless inguinal swelling or lump (may or may not persist with recumbency).

CAUSES
• congenital defect
• postoperative complication (incisional hernia)
• abnormal muscular structures around umbilical cord (umbilical hernia); common in newborns
• weakness in in the fascial margin of the internal inguinal ring (indirect inguinal hernia)
• weakness in fascia floor of the inguinal canal (direct inguinal hernia)

TREATMENT
• herniorrhaphy; bowel resection (strangulated or necrotic hernia); elastic corset

ICD-9-CM
533.00 femoral (unilateral) hernia
550.9 inguinal (direct, indirect) hernia
553.1 umbilical hernia
553.21 incisional hernia

Histiocytosis, pulmonary

DESCRIPTION A disorder of the mononuclear phagocyte system caused by tobacco smoking. Characteristics - cough, dyspnea, chest pain, weight loss. No known treatment except to stop smoking. Usual course - chronic; progressive in some cases.

SYNONYMS
• histiocytosis X
• pulmonary eosinophilic granuloma

CAUSES
• disorder of the mononuclear phagocyte system
• tobacco smoking

TREATMENT
• unknown

ICD-9-CM
277.8 histiocytosis X

Hutchinson-Gilford syndrome

DESCRIPTION Premature old age. Characteristics - small stature; absence of facial and genital hair; wrinkled skin; gray hair; and appearance, manner, and attitude of old age. Usual course - progressive; fatal. Possibly autosomal recessive.

SYNONYMS
• childhood progeria
• premature senility syndrome

CAUSES
• unknown

TREATMENT
• none

ICD-9-CM
259.8 Hutchinson-Gilford syndrome

Hyperbilirubinemia, physiologic neonatal

DESCRIPTION A mild, transient physiological hyperbilirubinemia of unconjugated type occurring in the normal neotate.

SYNONYMS
• icterus neonatorum
• hyperbilirubinemia in the newborn

CAUSES
• fetal hemolysis
• inadequate bilirubin conjugation
• prematurity

TREATMENT
• phototherapy

ICD-9-CM
774.6 transient neonatal jaundice

Hyperhidrosis

DESCRIPTION Excessive perspiration due to over-activity of the sweat glands. Distribution - general or confined to palms, soles, axillas, inframammary region, groin. Symptoms include skin maceration, fissuring, scaling. A bad odor may be produced by decomposition of sweat and cellular debris resulting from yeast and bacteria infection.

CAUSES
• various skin diseases, such as pyogenic or fungal infections, contact dermatitis, fever, hyperthyroidism, central nervous system disorders, psychogenic

TREATMENT
• bromhidrosis (malodorous exudate). Treat with soap containing chlorhexidine. Apply aluminum chlorhydroxy complex after bathing.
• treat any uncovered underlying cause
• localized hyperhidrosis - treat with nighttime applications of aluminum chloride in absolute ethyl alcohol. Cover with polyethylene films if possible. Wash applications away next morning.

ICD-9-CM
780.8 hyperhidrosis

Hyperthermia, malignant

DESCRIPTION Autosomal inherited condition occurring in patients undergoing general anesthesia. Characteristics - sudden, rapid temperature rise, tachycardia, tachypnea, sweating, cyanosis, muscle rigidity. Usual course - acute.

SYNONYMS
• fulminating hyperpyrexia
• malignant hyperpyrexia

CAUSES
• general anesthesia
• sukamethonium
• succinylcholine
• halothane
• duchenne muscular dystrophy

TREATMENT
• cooling
• cessation of anesthesia
• correct acidosis
• dantrolene
• mannitol

ICD-9-CM
995.89 hyperpyrexia, malignant, due to anesthetic

Hyphema

DESCRIPTION Hemorrhage within the anterior chamber of the eye. Usual course - acute; recurrent.

CAUSES
• traumatized iris roof
• traumatized stromal vessels
• spontaneous bleeding

TREATMENT
• strict bed rest
• keep upright
• binocular patching
• mydriatics
• miotics
• antifibrinolytic agents
• surgery
• sedation
• ocular hypotensives

ICD-9-CM
364.41 hyphema of iris and ciliary body

Hypocalcemia

DESCRIPTION Calcium level of 8.5 mg/dL (2.13 mmol/L) or less (with a normal albumin)
• Characteristics - symptoms include neuromuscular irritability, weakness, weight loss, diarrhea, abdominal cramping, bone pain, paresthesias, headache, seizures, dry skin. Signs include Chvostek's sign and Trousseau's sign.

CAUSES
• Surgically induced hyperparathyroidism, Addison's disease, candidiasis, carcinoma of the thyroid, chronic liver disease, hyperphosphatemia, idiopathic, malabsorption, malnutrition, nephrosis, pancreatitis, pernicious anemia, pseudohypoparathyroidism, renal disease, rickets and osteomalacia

TREATMENT
• treat any discovered underlying disorder
• carefully replace calcium

ICD-9-CM
275.4 hypocalcemia

 Hypohidrotic ectodermal dysplasia syndrome

DESCRIPTION Inherited, ectodermal hypoplasia disorder characterized by decreased or no sweating, hairlessness, thin skin, anodontia, mental deficiency, hyperthermia. Usual course - chronic.

CAUSES
• ectodermal hypoplasia

TREATMENT
• cool climate
• water cooling
• dentures
• wig

ICD-9-CM
757.31 congenital ectodermal dysplasia

 Hypophosphatasia

DESCRIPTION Genetic metabolic disorder resulting from serum and bone alkaline phosphatase deficiency leading to ethanolamine phosphaturia and ethanolamine phosphatemia. Clinical characteristics include severe skeletal defects resembling rickets, failure of the calvarium to calcify, dyspnea, cyanosis, and gastrointestinal symptoms, renal calcinosis, failure to thrive. Usual course - chronic; progressive.

SYNONYMS
• juvenile Paget's disease
• hyperostosis corticalis juvenilis deformans
• Rathbun's syndrome

CAUSES
• unknown

TREATMENT
• symptomatic
• sodium fluoride
• calcitonin
• corticosteroids

ICD-9-CM
275.3 hypophosphatasia

 Hypoprothrombinemia

DESCRIPTION Deficiency of prothrombin (coagulation Factor II) in the blood. Characteristics - epistaxis, gingival bleeding, hematuria, melena, excessive bleeding with injury. Usual course - chronic.

SYNONYMS
• prothrombin deficiency
• factor II deficiency

CAUSES
• genetic deficiency
• vitamin K deficiency

TREATMENT
• fresh frozen plasma
• vitamin K

ICD-9-CM
286.3 hypoprothrombinemia

 Ichthyosis

DESCRIPTION A symptom in several rare hereditary syndromes - ichthyosis vulgaris; X-linked ichthyosis; lamellar ichthyosis (nonbullous congenital ichthyosiform erythroderma), epidermolytic hyperkeratosis (bullous congenital ichthyosiform erythroderma). Also occurs in several systemic disorders. Xeroderma, the mildest form is neither congenital nor associated with systemic disease. Characteristics - skin is dry, scaling, thick over widespread parts of the body.

SYNONYMS
• Xeroderma
• Dry skin
• Xerosis

CAUSES
• inherited, Refsum's syndrome (hereditary mental deficiency and spastic paralysis), Sjögren-Larrson syndrome, leprosy, hypothyroidism, AIDS

TREATMENT
• skin lubricants

ICD-9-CM 757.1 ichthyosis congenital

 Icterohemorrhagic leptospirosis

DESCRIPTION A severe form of leptospirosis. Characterized by jaundice usually accompanied by azotemia, hemorrhages, anemia, continued fever, and disturbances of consciousness. Usual course - acute; biphasic.
Endemic areas: worldwide

SYNONYMS
• Weil's syndrome
• leptospiral jaundice
• spirochetal jaundice
• spirochaetosis icterohemorrhagica

CAUSES
• spirochetes of genus leptospira
• systemic infectious disease
• zoonosis
• contact with infected animal tissues
• contact with infected animal urine

TREATMENT
• supportive therapy
• antibiotics

ICD-9-CM
100.0 leptospirosis icterohemorrhagica

 Idiopathic edema

DESCRIPTION Swellings of unknown cause affecting women, occurring intermittently over a period of years. Usually worse during premenstrual phase. Associated with increased aldosterone secretion. Usual course - intermittent; relapsing.

SYNONYMS
• cyclic edema
• periodic edema
• stress edema
• distress edema
• periodic swelling

CAUSES
• unknown
• abnormal albumin metabolism
• hormonal imbalance

TREATMENT
• DECR salt intake
• elastic stockings
• captopril
• bromocriptine
• diuretics

ICD-9-CM
782.3 edema

 IgG heavy chain disease

DESCRIPTION A rare malignant neoplasm of lymphoplasmacytic cells consisting of monoclonal immunoglobulin heavy chains. Usual course - progressive; fatal.

SYNONYMS
• gamma chain disease
• franklin disease

CAUSES
• secretion of free gamma immunoglobulin chains

TREATMENT
• unresponsive to chemotherapy

ICD-9-CM
273.2 heavy chain disease

 IgM heavy chain disease

DESCRIPTION Rarest heavy chain disease. Found in patients with chronic lymphocytic leukemia. Characteristics - hepatomegaly, splenomegaly. Usual course - slowly progressive.

SYNONYMS
• mu chain disease

CAUSES
• secretion of free mu chains

TREATMENT
• no specific therapy

ICD-9-CM
273.2 heavy chain disease

Interstitial keratitis

DESCRIPTION Chronic, non-ulcerative infiltration of the deep layers of the cornea, rare in the USA. Characteristics - signs and symptoms include photophobia, pain, lacrimation, gradual loss of vision.

CAUSES
• congenital or acquired syphilis; tuberculosis

TREATMENT
• refer to an ophthalmologist for treatment

ICD-9-CM
090.3 interstitial keratitis

 ## Intrahepatic cholestasis due to pregnancy

DESCRIPTION A benign disorder of pregnancy causing jaundice, pruritus, and hepatomegaly that clears upon delivery. Usual course - intermittent.

SYNONYMS
• cholestatic jaundice of pregnancy

CAUSES
• sensitivity to hormones normally produced in pregnancy

TREATMENT
• unnecessary
• cholestyramine for pruritus

ICD-9-CM
646.7 icterus gravis of pregnancy

 ## Jaundice

DESCRIPTION A descriptive term implying deposition of bile pigment in the skin and mucous membranes with resulting yellow appearance of the patient. Yellow skin and sclerae appear whenever bilirubin reaches 3 mg/mL. Characteristics - jaundice is usually brought about by hemolysis, virus infection, alcoholism, drugs, stones in the bile ducts, cancer of the pancreas or liver.

CAUSES
• preponderance of direct (conjugated) bilirubin:
  ◊ obstruction - gallstones, common duct stones, tumors, strictures
  ◊ hepatitis
  ◊ cirrhosis
  ◊ drugs
  ◊ pregnancy (idiopathic cholestatic jaundice of pregnancy)
  ◊ hereditary
• preponderance of indirect (unconjugated) bilirubin:
  ◊ hemolysis
  ◊ neonatal
  ◊ drugs
  ◊ Gilbert's syndrome
  ◊ congestive heart failure

TREATMENT
• according to cause

ICD-9-CM
782.4 jaundice

 ## Jaundice, breast milk

DESCRIPTION Self-limited hyperbilirubinemia in a healthy vigorous neonate. Cause unknown. Usual course - progressive; self-limiting.

CAUSES
• unknown
• possibly maternal estrogen isomer interference with infant bilirubin conjugation

TREATMENT
• interrupt nursing as diagnostic trial

ICD-9-CM
774.3 neonatal jaundice due to delayed conjugation from other causes

 ## Jet lag

DESCRIPTION The syndrome of jet lag results from transmeridian (east-west) travel between different time zones. (North-south travel does not cause jet lag.) It is a state of physiological desynchronization (e.g., clock shows that it is lunchtime, but the body says it is the middle of the night). The degree of severity depends on the number of time zones crossed and the direction traveled. Most people find traveling eastward and adapting to a shorter day is more difficult than traveling westward and adapting to a longer day. Resulting symptoms include: extreme fatigue, sleep disturbances, loss of concentration, malaise, disorientation, sluggishness, gastrointestinal upset and loss of appetite.

CAUSES
• disturbance in the body's physiological processes (circadian dysrhythmia) that control not only sleep and wakefulness, but also alertness, hunger, digestion, urine production, temperature and hormone secretion

TREATMENT
• no clear evidence that extensive and elaborate prevention programs to avoid jet lag are of value
• short-acting benzodiazepines (e.g., lorazepam) for sleep in transit
• plan destination activities to accommodate for time differences
• the hormone melatonin may be a promising remedy

ICD-9-CM
N/A

 ## Juvenile amaurotic familial idiocy

DESCRIPTION Neuronal ceroid lipofuscinosis. Characteristics - loss of vision, onset 5-10 years, death during late adolescence, atypical retinitis pigmentosa, cerebellar ataxia, dementia. Genetics - autosomal recessive. Usual course - progressive.

SYNONYMS
• Spielmayer-Sjogren chronic neuronal ceroid lipofuscinosis
• Spielmayer-Vogt disease
• Batten disease

CAUSES
• neuronal accumulation of ceroid
• neuronal accumulation of lipofuscin

TREATMENT
• rehabilitation as needed

ICD-9-CM
330.1 Spielmayer-Vogt disease

 ## Kartagener's syndrome

DESCRIPTION An inherited disorder involving a combination of situs inversus, bronchiectasis, and sinusitis. Genetics - familial; autosomal recessive; 1/70 persons of those involved are heterozygous. Usual course - chronic; variable onset.

SYNONYMS
• Kartagener triad

CAUSES
• defective mucociliary clearance

TREATMENT
• chest physiotherapy
• antibiotics
• bronchodilators

ICD-9-CM
759.3 Kartagener's syndrome

 ## Kearns-Sayre syndrome

DESCRIPTION Inherited disorder (autosomal dominant with onset before age 15). Characteristics - progressive ophthalmoplegia, pigmentary degeneration of the retina, ataxia, myopathy, cardiac conduction defect. Usual course - progressive; ophthalmic onset at ages 5-20; retinal onset at ages 8-40; cardiac onset at ages 10-40.

SYNONYMS
• oculocraniosomatic neuromuscular disease
• ragged red fiber disease
• ophthalmoplegia-plus
• hereditary external ophthalmoplegia

CAUSES
• unknown

TREATMENT
• folic acid
• coenzyme Q10
• pacemaker

ICD-9-CM
378.55 external ophthalmoplegia

 ## Keratitis, superficial punctate

DESCRIPTION Loss of epithelium from the corneal surface of one or both eyes. Often associated with trachoma, staphylococcus blepharitis, conjunctivitis, or a respiratory tract infection.
• Characteristics - symptoms include photophobia, pain, lacrimation, diminished vision, conjunctival injection

CAUSES ultraviolet light exposure, bacterial infection, viral infection

TREATMENT
• topical antibiotics after positive culture
• for gram-positive organisms: 10-30% sulfacetamide drops every 2 hours and 0.5% erythromycin or 500 u./gm bacitracin ointment tid
• gram-negative organisms: 0.3% gentamycin drops every 2 hours
• use dark glasses
• systemic analgesics for pain

ICD-9-CM
370.21 keratitis, superficial punctate

Keratoconus

DESCRIPTION Degenerative eye disorder characterized by thinning and anterior protrusion of the cornea, usually bilateral, beginning between ages 10 and 20. More frequent in females. Signs and symptoms: blurred vision, myopia, astigmatism.

CAUSES
• transmitted as an autosomal recessive trait

TREATMENT
• hard contact lenses
• glasses with high astigmatic correction
• corneal graft or transplantation

ICD-9-CM
371.60 keratoconus

Kernicterus

DESCRIPTION A condition characterized by high levels of nonconjugated bilirubin in the blood with biliary pigmentation of certain nuclei in the brain and spinal cord and frequently resulting in cerebral palsy, mental retardation, and hearing deficit. It is commonly a sequel to icterus gravis neonatorum. Usual course - acute; progressive; chronic.

SYNONYMS
• bilirubin encephalopathy
• nuclear jaundice

CAUSES
• isoimmunization
• erythrocyte biochemical defects
• erythrocyte structural abnormalities
• infection
• sequestered blood

TREATMENT
• physical therapy

ICD-9-CM
773.4 kernicterus due to isoimmunization
774.7 kernicterus not due to isoimmunization

Klinefelter's syndrome

DESCRIPTION Congenital disorder. Characteristics - small testes, azoospermia, infertility, increased urinary excretion of gonadotropin, tall long legs, gynecomastia. Associated with an abnormality of the sex chromosomes. Usual course - chronic; manifestations begin at puberty.

SYNONYMS
• seminiferous tubule dysgenesis
• XXY syndrome

CAUSES
• congenital
• supernumerary X chromosome
• mosaicism
• advanced maternal age predisposes

TREATMENT
• mastectomy for disfiguring gynecomastia
• supplemental androgens for delayed secondary sexual characteristics
• supplemental androgens for impotence

ICD-9-CM
758.7 Klinefelter's syndrome

Korsakoff's psychosis

DESCRIPTION Anterograde and retrograde amnesia with confabulation associated with alcoholic or nonalcoholic polyneuritis. Usual course - subacute; possibly acute; possibly chronic.

SYNONYMS
• alcohol amnestic syndrome

CAUSES
• alcoholism
• thiamine deficiency
• malnutrition

TREATMENT
• parenteral thiamine replacement
• vitamin supplementation

ICD-9-CM
291.1 Korsakoff's psychosis

Krabbe leukodystrophy, infantile form

DESCRIPTION Lysosomal storage disease. Characteristics - begins in infancy, fretfulness, rigidity, followed by tonic seizures, convulsions, quadriplegia, deafness, progressive mental deterioration. Usual course - progressive.

SYNONYMS
• globoid cell leukodystrophy; Krabbe's disease
• Krabbe's brain leukodystrophy
• globoid cell brain sclerosis

CAUSES
• galactocerebrosidase deficiency

TREATMENT
• none

ICD-9-CM
330.0 leukodystrophy

Kuru

DESCRIPTION Progressive nervous system disorder of melanesian tribes of central New Guinea thought to be associated with cannibalism. Usual course - progressive.

CAUSES
• unknown
• slow virus of central nervous system

TREATMENT
• none

ICD-9-CM
046.0 kuru

Kyasanur forest disease

DESCRIPTION Severe hemorrhagic fever. Tick-borne arbovirus infection occurring the in the Kyasanur Forest in India. Characteristics - fever, hemorrhagic manifestations and rash. Usual course - recurrent.

CAUSES
• ixodes
• haemaphysalis spinigera
• tick-borne flavivirus
• rodent hosts
• monkey hosts

TREATMENT
• symptomatic
• fluid replacement
• transfusion

ICD-9-CM
065.2 kyasanur forest disease

Lassa fever

DESCRIPTION Acute, possible fatal infectious disease occurring in West Africa. Characteristics - high fever, pharyngitis, vomiting, abdominal pain, dyspnea followed by hemorrhages and shock. Usual course - acute; gradual defervescence.

CAUSES
• lassa virus form of arenavirus found in excreta of wild rodents

TREATMENT
• supportive care
• fluid plus electrolyte therapy

ICD-9-CM
078.89 lassa fever

Lathyrism

DESCRIPTION A morbid condition resulting from eating leguminous plants (includes many kinds of peas). characteristics - spastic paraplegia, pain, hyperesthesia, paresthesia. Usual course - progressive. Endemic areas - Africa; Asia.

SYNONYMS
• neurolathyrism

CAUSES
• beta-aminopropionitrile ingestion
• sweet peas of species Lathyrus sativus

TREATMENT
• none

ICD-9-CM
988.2 lathyrism

Laurence-Moon-Biedl syndrome

DESCRIPTION A hereditary syndrome of childhood, transmitted as an autosomal recessive trait, with obesity, retinitis pigmentosa, mental retardation, polydactyly, and hypogonadism as the main features. Usual course - progressive.

SYNONYMS
• Laurence-Moon syndrome
• Bardet-Biedl syndrome

CAUSES
• genetic

TREATMENT
• supportive

ICD-9-CM
759.8 Laurence-Moon-Biedl syndrome

Left ventricular failure, acute

DESCRIPTION Left heart failure. Characteristics - dyspnea, cough, sense of suffocation, frothy sputum, cyanosis, rales, wheezing, tachycardia, Cheyne-Stokes respiration. Usual course - acute.

SYNONYMS
• ventricular failure
• left heart failure

CAUSES
• hypertension
• coronary artery disease
• incompetent mitral valve
• incompetent aortic valve
• myocardial infarction

TREATMENT
• diuretics
• vasodilators
• digitalis

ICD-9-CM
428.1 left heart failure

Leptospirosis

DESCRIPTION Infection by leptospira organisms transmitted to man from dogs, swine, and rodents or by contact with contaminated water. Characteristics - lymphocytic meningitis, hepatitis, nephritis. Weil's syndrome is severe leptospirosis with jaundice, bleeding and renal failure. Usual course - acute; abrupt; biphasic; relapsing. Endemic areas - Southern USA; tropics.

SYNONYMS
• autumnal fever
• Fort Bragg fever
• mud fever
• pea-picker's disease
• European swamp fever
• wycon fever
• Bushy Creek fever
• cane field fever
• swineherd disease

CAUSES
• leptospira interrogans
• spirochete
• contact with infected animal tissues
• contact with infected animal excrement

TREATMENT
• antibiotics, supportive care, fluid replacement, electrolyte therapy, possibly steroids if hepatic coma

ICD-9-CM
100.9 leptospirosis, unspecified

Lesch-Nyhan syndrome

DESCRIPTION An X-linked disease caused by a deficiency of an enzyme of purine metabolism, hypoxanthine-guanine phosphoribosyl transferase, and characterized by physical and mental retardation, hyperuricemia, self-mutilation, and choreoathetosis.

SYNONYMS
• hypoxanthine-guanine phosphoribosyltransferase deficiency syndrome
• HG-PRT deficiency syndrome

CAUSES
• hypoxanthine-guanine phosphoribosyltransferase deficiency

TREATMENT
• symptomatic and supportive
• protective restraint

ICD-9-CM
277.2 Lesch-Nyhan syndrome

Letterer-Siwe disease

DESCRIPTION Acute, disseminated, rapidly progressive form of Langerhans-cell histiocytosis. Genetics - Some familial predisposition. Characteristics include - hemorrhage tendency, eczematoid skin eruption, hepatosplenomegaly, progressive anemia, lymphadenopathy. Usual course - acute; fulminant; progressive; chronic.

SYNONYMS
• acute diffuse histiocytosis
• acute infantile reticuloendotheliosis
• acute reticulosis of infancy
• generalized histiocytosis
• non-lipid reticuloendotheliosis

CAUSES
• nonneoplastic proliferation of langerhans cells

TREATMENT
• irradiation, chemotherapy, steroids, vasopressin replacement, antibiotics

ICD-9-CM
202.50 Letterer-Siwe disease, unspecified site

Leukemia, acute monocytic

DESCRIPTION Leukemia in which the predominating leukocytes are identified as monocytes. Characteristics - fever, fatigue, bleeding, lymphadenopathy, hepatosplenomegaly, anemia. Usual course - acute; possibly relapsing.

SYNONYMS
• acute monocytoid leukemia
• monoblastic leukemia
• acute monoblastic leukemia

CAUSES
• chloramphenico, phenylbutazone, ionizing radiation, benzene, Down syndrome, alkylating agents

TREATMENT
• cytosine arabinoside
• daunorubicin
• 6-thioguanine

ICD-9-CM
206.0 monocytic leukemia, acute

Leukemia, acute myeloblastic

DESCRIPTION An acute nonlymphoblastic leukemia occurs at all ages and is the more common leukemia among adults. Usually associated with irradiation as a causative agent and occurring as a second malignancy following cancer chemotherapy. Characteristics - bleeding, pallor, fever, headaches, vomiting, weakness, lethargy, pallor, joint pain. Usual course - acute; progressive; relapsing.

SYNONYMS
• acute granulocytic leukemia
• acute myelocytic leukemia

CAUSES
• idiopathic
• retroviral infection
• ionizing radiation
• genetic defect
• chemical poisoning

TREATMENT
• chemotherapy
• immunotherapy
• bone marrow transplantation

ICD-9-CM
205.0 myeloid leukemia, acute

Leukemia, acute myelogenous

DESCRIPTION Leukemia arising from myeloid tissue in which the granular, polymorphonuclear leukocytes and their precursors predominate. Characteristics - fever, anorexia, bleeding, hepatosplenomegaly, anemia, lymphadenopathy. Usual course - acute; possibly relapsing.

CAUSES
• Bloom's syndrome
• Philadelphia chromosome
• chloramphenicol
• ionizing radiation
• benzene
• Down syndrome
• Fanconi's syndrome
• phenylbutazone
• alkylating agents

TREATMENT
• cytosine arabinoside, daunorubicin, 6-thioguanine, prednisone, vincristine, intrathecal methotrexate, cranial radiotherapy

ICD-9-CM
205.0 myeloid leukemia, acute

Leukemia, chronic myelogenous

DESCRIPTION Clonal myeloproliferation caused by malignant transformation of a pluripotent cell. Characteristics - extraordinary overproduction of granulocytes. Usual course - slowly progressive.

SYNONYMS
• chronic granulocytic leukemia

CAUSES
• unknown
• possibly ionizing radiation

TREATMENT
• busulfan, allopurinol, leukophoresis, localized radiotherapy, vincristine, prednisone, cytosine arabinoside, doxorubicin

ICD-9-CM
205.1 myeloid leukemia, chronic.

Leukemia, hairy cell

DESCRIPTION A neoplastic disease of the lymphoreticular cells which is considered to be a rare type of chronic leukemia. It is characterized by an insidious onset, splenomegaly, anemia, granulocytopenia, thrombocytopenia, little or no lymphadenopathy, and the presence of "hairy" or "flagellated" cells in the blood and bone marrow. Usual course - chronic; progressive.

SYNONYMS
• leukemic reticuloendotheliosis

CAUSES
• precise cause unknown

TREATMENT
• splenectomy
• interferon

ICD-9-CM
202.4 hairy-cell leukemia

Lichen sclerosis of the vulva

DESCRIPTION Thickened skin and accentuated markings affecting the vulva. Characteristics - external genital itching and pain. Usual course - chronic; progressive; may have spontaneous regression.

SYNONYMS
• lichen sclerosis et atrophicus
• lichen albus
• Csillag's disease
• white spot disease
• circumscribed scleroderma

TREATMENT
• vitamin A ointment
• intralesional corticosteroids
• topical corticosteroids
• oral estrogen

ICD-9-CM
701.0 circumscribed scleroderma

Lipoid nephrosis

DESCRIPTION Nephrosis characterized by edema, albuminuria, changes in lipids and proteins in the blood, accumulation of globules of cholesterol esters in the tubular epithelium of the kidney.

SYNONYMS
• minimal change disease
• foot process disease
• nil disease
• minimal change nephropathy
• minimal change glomerulopathy

CAUSES
• loss of negative charge in glomerular capillary wall

TREATMENT
• steroids
• antibiotics
• cyclophosphamide
• chlorambucil

ICD-9-CM
581.3 lipoid nephrosis

Loiasis

DESCRIPTION A parasitic infection caused by the nematode Loa loa. The vector in the transmission of this infection is the horsefly (Tabanus) or the deerfly or mango fly (Chrysops). The larvae may be seen just beneath the skin or passing through the conjunctiva. Eye lesions are not uncommon. The disease is generally mild and painless. Usual course - chronic; progressive; 10-15 year incubation period. Endemic areas - West Africa; Central Africa.

SYNONYMS
• calabar swellings

CAUSES
• Loa loa filaria

TREATMENT
• diethylcarbamazine

ICD-9-CM
125.2 loiasis

Ludwig's angina

DESCRIPTION Severe form of cellulitis affecting the submandibular, submental, and sublingual spaces. Characteristics - tongue elevation, difficult eating and swallowing, edema of the glottis, fever, tachypnea, and moderate leukocytosis. Usual course - acute.

CAUSES
• oral trauma
• aerobic infection of submandibular space
• anaerobic infection of submandibular space

TREATMENT
• broad-spectrum intravenous antibiotics
• maintain airway
• tracheostomy if necessary

ICD-9-CM
528.3 Ludwig's angina

Lupus nephritis

DESCRIPTION Glomerulonephritis associated with systemic lupus erythematosus. Characteristics - hematuria, a fulminant or chronic progressive course. Hypertension does not occur until late in the course of the disease. Usual course - relapsing; progressive.

SYNONYMS
• focal glomerulonephritis
• lupus glomerulonephritis

CAUSES
• SLE

TREATMENT
• steroids
• renal transplantation

ICD-9-CM
710.0 lupus nephritis

Lymphangitis

DESCRIPTION Inflammation of a lymphatic vessel or vessels. Characteristics - painful subcutaneous streaks along the course of the vessels. Usual course - acute; relapsing.

CAUSES
• beta-hemolytic streptococci
• staphylococcus

TREATMENT
• antibiotics
• drainage
• heat
• moisture

ICD-9-CM
457.2 lymphangitis

Lymphoma, non-Hodgkin's

DESCRIPTION Heterogenous group of malignant lymphomas with absence of giant Reed-Sternberg cells characteristic of Hodgkin's disease. Characteristics - widespread disease, painless enlargement of one or more peripheral lymph nodes. Usual course - progressive.

CAUSES
• malignant tumors of lymphoid tissues with the exception of hodgkin's disease

TREATMENT
• radiotherapy
• chemotherapy

ICD-9-CM
202.8 non-hodgkin's lymphoma, nos

Lymphoma, pulmonary

DESCRIPTION Malignant disease of the lung. Characteristics - cough, weight loss, chest pain. Usual course - progressive.

CAUSES
• tumor of the immune system
• Hodgkin's lymphoma
• lymphocytic lymphoma

TREATMENT
• radiotherapy
• chemotherapy

ICD-9-CM
202.8 malignant lymphoma, nos

Magnesium deficiency syndrome

DESCRIPTION Abnormally low magnesium content of the blood plasma. Characteristics - neuromuscular hyperirritability. Usual course - progressive; acute; relapsing.

SYNONYMS
• hypomagnesemia

CAUSES
• dietary deficiency
• decreased absorption
• increased excretion
• alcoholism
• uremia
• diuretics
• parathyroid disease
• eclampsia

TREATMENT
• magnesium

ICD-9-CM
275.2 magnesium deficiency

Mallory-Weiss syndrome

DESCRIPTION Mucosal tears usually linear and confined to the esophagogastric junction but may be located in the fundus of the stomach or in the distal esophagus. Upper gastrointestinal bleeding from these lacerations is often precipitated by retching or vomiting. Usual course - acute.

SYNONYMS
• gastroesophageal laceration-hemorrhage syndrome

CAUSES
• retching after alcoholic bout
• hiatus hernia
• atrophic gastritis
• esophagitis
• straining at stool

TREATMENT
• vasopressin
• gastrotomy with sutures

ICD-9-CM
530.7 Mallory-Weiss syndrome

Maple bark stripper's disease

DESCRIPTION Granulomatous, interstitial pneumonitis caused by a mold found under the bark of maple logs. Usual course - acute; relapsing.

CAUSES
• hypersensitivity reaction to spores of cryptostroma corticale

TREATMENT
• eliminate etiological agent

ICD-9-CM
495.6 maple bark-strippers' lung

Maple syrup urine disease

DESCRIPTION Familial cerebral degenerative disease caused by a defect in branched chain amino acid metabolism and characterized by severe mental and motor retardation and urine with a maple-syrup-like odor. Usual course - progressive.

SYNONYMS
• branched chain ketoaciduria

CAUSES
• deficiency of branched chain alpha-ketoacid decarboxylase

TREATMENT
• controlled intake of branched-chain amino acids
• peritoneal and/or hemodialysis

ICD-9-CM
270.3 maple syrup urine disease

Marburg virus disease

DESCRIPTION Severe, acute often fatal viral hemorrhagic fever. Characteristics - prostration, fever, pancreatitis, hepatitis. The Marburg virus first infected laboratory workers handling infected African green monkeys. Usual course - acute. Endemic areas: Germany; Yugoslavia; Africa.

SYNONYMS
• green monkey virus disease

CAUSES
• Marburg virus

TREATMENT
• isolation
• treat dehydration
• nasogastric suction
• heparin

ICD-9-CM
078.89 Marburg virus disease

Marchiafava-Bignami syndrome

DESCRIPTION Progressive degeneration of the corpus callosum. Characteristics - progressive intellectual degeneration, confusion, hallucinations, tremor, rigidity, and convulsions. Usual course - chronic; progressive.

SYNONYMS
• Marchiafava disease
• callosal demyelinating encephalopathy

CAUSES
• chronic alcoholism
• addiction to crude red wine

TREATMENT
• avoid alcohol

ICD-9-CM
341.8 Marchiafava-Bignami disease or syndrome

Mastocytosis

DESCRIPTION A rare disease characterized by an abnormal increase in mast cells in various body organs and tissues. It can occur in any age group and demonstrates a slight male predominance. Various forms are identified: mastocytoma (a benign cutaneous tumor); urticaria pigmentosa (multiple, small collections of mast cells, salmon or brown color, that may become vesicular or even bullous); and systemic mastocytosis (mast cell infiltrates in the bone marrow, liver, spleen, lymph nodes, gastrointestinal tract, skin and bones). Symptoms include arthralgias, bone pain and anaphylactoid symptoms. Mast cell leukemia is a form of mastocytosis.

SYNONYMS
• cutaneous mastocytosis
• systemic mast cell disease

CAUSES
• exact cause is unknown

TREATMENT
• cutaneous mastocytosis and urticaria pigmentosa seldom require treatment
• systemic mastocytosis:
  ◊ H1 and an H2 antihistamine
  ◊ aspirin therapy (use with caution)
  ◊ oral cromolyn sodium (if GI symptoms are inadequately controlled)
  ◊ surgical excision of mast cells (rare)

ICD-9-CM
757.33 urticaria pigmentosa
202.6 mastocytosis

Meckel's diverticulum

DESCRIPTION Sacculation or appendage of the ileum derived from an unobliterated yolk stalk. Symptoms of infection may resemble those of appendicitis. Usual course - acute; intermittent; chronic.

CAUSES
• vestigial remnant of omphalomesenteric duct

TREATMENT
• surgery

ICD-9-CM
751.0 Meckel's diverticulum

Meigs' syndrome

DESCRIPTION Ascites and hydrothorax associated with ovarian fibroma or other pelvic tumors. Usual course - acute; relapsing.

SYNONYMS
• ovarian ascites-pleural effusion syndrome
• Demons-Meigs syndrome
• Meigs-Coss syndrome

CAUSES
• benign fibroma
• ovarian tumor
• movement of the ascitic fluid across the diaphragm

TREATMENT
• tumor excision

ICD-9-CM
789.5 ascites

Melioidosis

DESCRIPTION A glanders-like infection of man and animals endemic in SE Asia, NE Queensland Australia, Central, West and Eastern Africa. Likely to be one of the infections seen in patients with AIDS. May be asymptomatic or symptoms can include chills; cough; bloody purulent sputum; abdominal pain; diarrhea.

SYNONYMS
• Stanton disease
• Whitmore disease
• pneumoenteritis
• pseudocholera

CAUSES
• pseudomonas pseudomallei; transmitted by direct contact with infected rodents or infected food, soil, water, excreta; person-to-person transmission possible through use of injection needle

TREATMENT
• trimethoprim-sulfamethoxazole
• ceftazidime

ICD-9-CM
025 melioidosis

Meningioma

DESCRIPTION Hard, slow growing, vascular tumor arising along the meningeal vessels and superior longitudinal sinus. It invades the dura and skull and leads to thinning and erosion of the skull. Usual course - progressive; surgical cure.

SYNONYMS
• arachnoidal fibroblastoma
• leptomeningioma
• dural endothelioma
• meningeal fibroblastoma

CAUSES
• unknown

TREATMENT
• surgical excision
• radiotherapy for incomplete removal
• radiotherapy for recurrence

ICD-9-CM
225.2; 225.4 benign neoplasm of meninges

Mesenteric adenitis, acute

DESCRIPTION Inflammation of lymph glands located in the mesentery. It causes a clinical picture at times that is difficult to differentiate from acute appendicitis.

SYNONYMS
• acute mesenteric lymphadenitis

CAUSES
• yersinia enterocolitica
• yersinia pseudotuberculosis
• streptococcus viridans
• giardia lamblia
• staphylococcus aureus

TREATMENT
• antibiotics

ICD-9-CM
289.2 acute mesenteric lymphadenitis

Metachromatic leukodystrophy, late infantile form

DESCRIPTION A form of leukoencephalopathy transmitted autosomal recessive. Characteristics - accumulation of sphingolipid in neural and non-neural tissues with a diffuse loss of myelin in the central nervous system. The infantile form begins in the second year of life with blindness, motor disturbances, mental deterioration. Usual course - progressive.

SYNONYMS
• metachromatic brain leukodystrophy
• metachromatic leukoencephalopathy
• sulfatidosis
• Greenfield disease
• arylsulfatase A deficiency

CAUSES
• arylsulfatase A deficiency

TREATMENT
• none

ICD-9-CM
330.0 leukodystrophy

Metastatic neoplasm of the liver

DESCRIPTION Progressive form of hepatic cancer that has metastasized from malignancies arising primarily from other locations. Usual course - progressive.

CAUSES
• colon metastases
• rectal metastases
• gastric metastases
• pancreatic metastases
• breast metastases

TREATMENT
• palliative chemotherapy
• palliative radiotherapy
• surgical resection in rare cases

ICD-9-CM
197.7 secondary malignant neoplasm to the liver

Milker's nodules

DESCRIPTION A disease caused by paravaccinia virus, transmitted to humans during milking. Characteristics - purple nodules on fingers or adjacent areas. Lesions break down and crust and heal without scarring. It can be retransmitted to uninfected cows. Usual course - acute; relapsing. Endemic areas - dairy farms.

SYNONYMS
• pseudocowpox
• paravaccinia

CAUSES
• paravaccinia virus of poxviridae family
• transmitted through direct contact
• cutaneous disease of cow teats
• oral lesions in suckling calves

TREATMENT
• none

ICD-9-CM
051.9 paravaccinia, nos

Millard-Gubler syndrome

DESCRIPTION Paralysis caused by infarction of the pons involving the 6th and 7th cranial nerves and fibers of the corticospinal tract. Characteristics - crossed paralysis affecting the limbs on one side of the body and the face on the opposite side. Additionally, paralysis of outward movement of the eye. Usual course - acute; chronic; progressive.

SYNONYMS
• alternating inferior hemiplegia
• Gubler paralysis
• abducens-facial syndrome

CAUSES
• basal pontine infarction
• basal pontine tumor

TREATMENT
• supportive plus rehabilitative
• treat underlying cause of infarction

ICD-9-CM
344.8 Millard-Gubler syndrome

Mitral regurgitation due to papillary muscle dysfunction

DESCRIPTION Retrograde blood flow from the left ventricle in the left atrium through an incompetent mitral valve. Characteristics - fatigue, orthopnea, systolic murmur, left ventricular hypertrophy, S3 gallop. Usual course: chronic; progressive; acute (after myocardial infarction).

CAUSES
• coronary artery disease
• infiltrative diseases
• cardiac tumors

TREATMENT
• dental endocarditis prophylaxis
• surgical endocarditis prophylaxis
• nitrates
• calcium channel blockers
• diuretics
• digitalis
• inotropic agents
• afterload reducing agents
• mitral valve replacement

ICD-9-CM
394.9 other and unspecified mitral valve diseases

Mitral regurgitation due to rheumatic fever

DESCRIPTION Retrograde blood flow from the left ventricle into the left atrium through an incompetent mitral valve. Characteristics - history of rheumatic fever, fatigue, dyspnea, holosystolic murmur, left ventricular hypertrophy. Usual course - chronic; progressive disability.

CAUSES
• autoimmune cross reaction between streptococcal antigens and heart tissue

TREATMENT
• medical endocarditis prophylaxis
• dental endocarditis prophylaxis
• surgical endocarditis prophylaxis
• afterload reducing agents
• nitrates
• calcium channel blockers
• digitalis
• diuretics
• mitral valve replacement

ICD-9-CM
394.1 rheumatic mitral insufficiency

Munchausen's syndrome

DESCRIPTION A chronic disorder characterized by habitual presentation for medical care. Often requires hospitalization. The patient gives a plausible and dramatic history, all of which is factitious.
Also, Munchausen's by proxy, in which a caregiver creates a history or illness requiring frequent medical care. The caregiver often has a medical background.

SYNONYMS
• chronic factitious disorder with physical symptoms
• hospital-addiction syndrome

CAUSES
• factitious
• external incentives

TREATMENT
• psychotherapy
• behavior modification techniques

ICD-9-CM
301.51 Munchausen syndrome

 Mushroom poisoning, Amanita phalloides

DESCRIPTION Characteristics include: nausea, vomiting, abdominal pain, diarrhea, followed by a period of improvement up to 48 hours. Then culminating in severe renal, hepatic, and central nervous system damage. Usual course - acute; progressive. Endemic areas - Western USA; Europe.

CAUSES
• cyclic octapeptide amatoxin
• hepatic cytotoxicity by interference with RNA polymerase
• renal cytotoxicity by interference with RNA polymerase

TREATMENT
• intragastric activated charcoal
• intensive supportive care
• charcoal hemoperfusion
• thiotic (alpha-lipoic acid)

ICD-9-CM
988.1 toxic effect of mushrooms eaten as food

 Mushroom-worker's disease

DESCRIPTION Allergic respiratory disease, resembling farmer's lung, developing in persons working with moldy compost prepared for growing mushrooms. Characteristics - fever, dyspnea, dry cough, chills, malaise, myalgia, tachypnea. Usual course - acute; chronic; intermittent; progressive; relapsing.

SYNONYMS
• pulmonary granulomatosis of mushroom pickers

CAUSES
• immunological reaction to inhaled antigens
• micropolyspora faeni
• thermoactinomyces vulgaris

TREATMENT
• corticosteroids
• eliminate etiological agent

ICD-9-CM
495.5 mushroom workers' lung

 Mussel poisoning

DESCRIPTION Food poisoning due to ingestion of toxin from dinoflagellate Gonyaulax. Characteristics - dysesthesias of tongue, lips, fingertips, dysphagia, abdominal cramps, ascending weakness, seizures. Usual course - acute; progressive. Endemic areas - Mid-Pacific coast from May to October; Northeastern seaboard; Western European coast.

SYNONYMS
• mytilotoxism
• paralytic shellfish poisoning

CAUSES
• alkaloid saxitoxin of dinoflagellate gonyaulax catanella
• alkaloid saxitoxin of dinoflagellate gonyaulax tamarensis
• neuromuscular blockade by preventing depolarization
• aerosolized ingestion has been reported

TREATMENT
• emergent gastrointestinal decontamination
• supportive
• mechanical ventilation

ICD-9-CM
988.0 toxic effect of fish and shellfish eaten as food

 Mycetoma

DESCRIPTION Infectious disease of the skin, subcutaneous tissues, and bone, usually affecting the lower extremities, especially the foot. Characterized by chronicity, tumefaction and multiple sinus formation. With early diagnosis, prognosis is good; if identified late in disease, treatment response is limited and amputation may be necessary.

SYNONYMS
• maduromycosis
• madura foot

CAUSES
• allescheria boydii or actinomycetales bacteria; more than 20 species of fungi and bacteria have been implicated

TREATMENT
• penicillin
• tetracycline
• sulfonamides
• streptomycin
• itraconazole
• dapsone
• surgery

ICD-9-CM
039.4 madura foot

 Myiasis

DESCRIPTION The invasion of living tissues of man and other mammals by dipterous larvae (fly maggots). Usual course - acute. Endemic areas - tropical America; Africa; South America; Mexico; California.

SYNONYMS
• maggot infestation

CAUSES
• ingestion of fly eggs
• eggs deposited in open wounds

TREATMENT
• surgery
• local anesthesia
• mineral oil
• ether bath

ICD-9-CM
134.0 myiasis

 Myringitis, infectious

DESCRIPTION Inflammation, hemorrhage and emission of fluid into the tissue at the end of the external ear canal and the tympanic membrane. Pain is typically sudden in onset and continues for 24 to 48 hours. Bacterial ottis media is suggested if hearing loss and fever are present.

SYNONYMS
bullous myringitis

CAUSES
• bacterial or viral infection

TREATMENT
• analgesics
• antibiotics for secondary infection
• rupture of vesicles with myringotomy knife

ICD-9-CM
384.00 myringitis

 Myxedema heart disease

DESCRIPTION Heart disease associated with primary hypothyroidism. Usual course - acute; progressive.

CAUSES
• decreased thyroid hormone
• congenital developmental defect
• idiopathic
• postablative
• postradiation
• iodine deficiency

TREATMENT
• thyroid hormone replacement

ICD-9-CM
244.9 myxedema

Necrobiosis lipoidica diabeticorum

DESCRIPTION Degenerative disease of dermal connective tissue. Characteristics - erythematous papules or nodules in the pretibial area that extend to form waxy, yellowish red plaques covered with telangiectatic vessels. The plaques have a red-violet border and depressed atrophic center. Usual course - chronic.

SYNONYMS
• Oppenheim-Urbach disease

CAUSES
• unknown

TREATMENT
• triamcinolone acetonide

ICD-9-CM
250.8 necrobiosis lipoidica diabeticorum
709.3

Nephropathy, analgesic

DESCRIPTION Kidney damage due to massive intake of analgesics, particularly phenacetin. Usual course - chronic.

CAUSES
- phenacetin
- aspirin
- acetaminophen

TREATMENT
- cessation of analgesic use

ICD-9-CM
965 poisoning by analgesics, antipyretics, and antirheumatics

 ## Nephropathy, chronic lead

DESCRIPTION Kidney damage due to lead poisoning. Particularly present in Queensland, Australia. Usual course - chronic.

SYNONYMS
- lead related hyperuricemia
- hyperuricemic nephropathy
- saturnine gout

CAUSES
- lead poisoning
- lead paint ingestion
- lead vapor inhalation
- moonshine alcohol

TREATMENT
- EDTA

ICD-9-CM
984 toxic effect of lead and its compounds (including fumes)

 ## Nephrosclerosis

DESCRIPTION Hardening of the kidney due to overgrowth and contraction of interstitial connective tissue. Characteristics - edema, headache, hypertension, retinal hemorrhages. Usual course - chronic; progressive.

CAUSES
- unknown
- essential hypertension
- diabetes

TREATMENT
- antihypertensive medication

ICD-9-CM
403.9 nephrosclerosis

 ## Neuritis/neuralgia

DESCRIPTION Degeneration of peripheral nerves
- Characteristics - insidious onset, muscle weakness with sensory loss, muscle atrophy, decreased tendon reflexes, paresthesias, hyperesthesias in hands and feet. Electromyography shows delayed action potential.

SYNONYMS
- Multiple neuritis
- Peripheral neuropathy
- Polyneuritis

CAUSES
- chronic intoxication (alcohol, arsenic, lead, other drugs)
- infections
- metabolic and inflammatory (diabetes) gout, rheumatoid arthritis, systemic lupus erythematosus
- nutritive (vitamin deficiencies, cachexia)

TREATMENT
- supportive
- physical therapy
- analgesics
- treat underlying specific disorders if possible
- drugs - amitriptyline, carbamazepine, phenytoin (uneven and unpredictable response, but helpful for some)

ICD-9-CM
729.2 neuritis/neuralgia

 ## Neutropenia, autoimmune

DESCRIPTION Decreased number of neutrophilic leukocytes in the blood due to an autoimmune mechanism. Usual course - acute; chronic; intermittent; progressive; relapsing.

CAUSES
- antineutrophil antibodies

TREATMENT
- antibiotics
- prednisone
- splenectomy
- supportive

ICD-9-CM
288.0 neutropenia

 ## Neutropenia, chronic idiopathic

DESCRIPTION An autosomal dominant, familial disorder with a chronic decrease in number of neutrophilic granulocytes. Characteristics - repeated non-life-threatening infections of skin, oral cavity, and sometimes upper respiratory tract. Usual course - chronic; relapsing.

SYNONYMS
- chronic benign neutropenia

CAUSES
- abnormal homeostasis of mitosis of granulocyte precursors

TREATMENT
- symptomatic

ICD-9-CM
288.0 neutropenia

 ## Neutropenia, cyclic

DESCRIPTION Autosomal dominant disorder of children and young adults characterized by cyclical neutropenia, producing fever, malaise, mouth ulcers and cervical lymphadenopathy. Usual course - relapsing; 21-day cycles.

SYNONYMS
- cyclic agranulocytosis
- periodic neutropenia
- cyclic leukopenia
- periodic myelocytic dysplasia

CAUSES
- defective regulation of hematopoietic cell proliferation

TREATMENT
- glucocorticoids
- androgens
- splenectomy
- antibiotics

ICD-9-CM
288.0 agranulocytosis

 ## Nevus of ota

DESCRIPTION A macular lesion on the side of the face (usually lifelong and unilateral), involving the conjunctiva and lids, as well as the adjacent facial skin, sclera, ocular muscles, and periosteum. Histological features vary from those of a mongolian spot to those of a blue nevus. Usual course - chronic.

SYNONYMS
- oculodermal melanocytosis
- nevus fusco-caeruleus ophthalmo-maxillaris

CAUSES
- unknown

TREATMENT
- cosmetic cover up

ICD-9-CM
224.3 nevus conjunctiva

 ## Niemann-Pick disease

DESCRIPTION Sphingolipidosis due to sphingomyelinase deficiency with sphingomyelin accumulation in the reticuloendothelial system. There are 5 types (A, B, C, D, and E) with differing ages of onset and differing amounts of CNS involvement and sphingomyelinase activity. Genetics - autosomal recessive. Usual course - acute; chronic; progressive.

SYNONYMS
- sphingomyelin lipidosis
- sphingomyelinase deficiency

CAUSES
- sphingomyelinase deficiency

TREATMENT
- supportive
- splenectomy
- bone marrow transplantation

ICD-9-CM
272.7 Niemann-Pick disease

Nitrobenzene poisoning

DESCRIPTION   Poisoning due to excessive exposure to nitrobenzene, a benzene derivative used in the manufacture of aniline. Complete recovery from pathologic changes can be expected if survival greater than 24 hours.

SYNONYMS
• nitrobenzol toxicity
• oil of mirbane toxicity

CAUSES
• direct mucous membrane irritation
• methemoglobin formation

TREATMENT
• cutaneous plus gastric decontamination
• oxygen
• 1% methylene blue
• exchange transfusion
• hemodialysis

ICD-9-CM
983.0 poisoning, nitrobenzene

Osteopetrosis

DESCRIPTION   Excessive formation of dense trabecular bone leading to pathological fractures, osteitis, splenomegaly with infarct, anemia and extramedullary hemopoiesis. Genetics: malignant form: autosomal recessive; benign form: autosomal dominant. Usual course - progressive; chronic.

SYNONYMS
• marble bone disease
• Albers-Schonberg disease
• osteosclerosis fragilis generalisata

CAUSES
• replacement of marrow space with bone
• no carbonic anhydrase II in erythrocytes
• defective osteoclast function

TREATMENT
• bone marrow transplantation
• calcitriol

ICD-9-CM
756.52 osteopetrosis

Ovarian mucinous cystadenocarcinoma

DESCRIPTION   Carcinoma and cystadenoma of the ovary. Characteristics — multilocular tumor produced by the epithelial cells of the ovary having mucin-filled cavities. Symptoms include abdominal pain and distention, menstrual disturbances, weight loss, dyspareunia, ascites. Clinical findings are the same as those with ovarian serous cystadenocarcinoma.

SYNONYMS
• pseudomucinous ovarian cystadenocarcinoma

CAUSES
• unknown

TREATMENT
• hysterectomy
• stage I: bilateral salpingo-oophorectomy plus omentectomy if high grade
• stage II: add radiotherapy or chemotherapy
• stage III: surgical debulking

ICD-9-CM
183.0 malignant neoplasm of ovary

Paralysis of the recurrent laryngeal nerve

DESCRIPTION   Paralysis may be unilateral or bilateral with many possible underlying causes. Characteristics — dysphagia, stridor, dyspnea, and aphonia. Usual course: acute; insidious.

CAUSES
• innominate artery aneurysm
• right subclavian artery aneurysm
• neck surgery
• thyroid goiter
• trauma
• aortic aneurysm
• left atrial enlargement
• laryngeal tuberculosis

TREATMENT
• treat underlying condition

ICD-9-CM
478.31 partial unilateral paralysis of vocal cords

Parapsoriasis

DESCRIPTION   A group of slowly evolving erythrodermas. common characteristics: chronicity, resistance to treatment. The group includes chronic and acute lichenoid pityriasis and large and small plaque parapsoriasis. Usual course - chronic; relapsing; benign forms; premalignant forms.

SYNONYMS
• maculopapular erythroderma

TREATMENT
• ultraviolet B light therapy

ICD-9-CM
696.2 parapsoriasis

Paratyphoid

DESCRIPTION   An infection due to any of the salmonella serotypes except S. typhi and salmonellosis. Characteristics — prolonged febrile illness less severe than typhoid fever, frequently follows an attack of salmonella food poisoning.

SYNONYMS
• paratyphoid fever
• enteric fever

CAUSES
• salmonella paratyphi A
• salmonella paratyphi B
• salmonella paratyphi C
• salmonella sendai
• enteric pathogens

TREATMENT
• fluid replacement
• antibiotics in elderly at greatest risk
• antibiotics in infants at greatest risk

ICD-9-CM
002.9 paratyphoid fever, nos

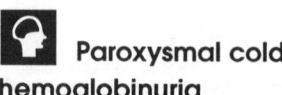

Paroxysmal atrial tachycardia

DESCRIPTION   Heart rate greater than 140 beats per minute. May increase up to 250. P waves regular but aberrant. Onset may be sudden. Symptoms include light-headedness and palpitations.

SYNONYMS
• Premature atrial tachycardia
• Paroxysmal supraventricular tachycardia

CAUSES
• abnormal AV conduction system
• physical or psychological stress
• hypokalemia, hypoxia, caffeine, marijuana, digitalis toxicity, sympathomimetics

ICD-9-CM
427.0 paroxysmal atrial tachycardia

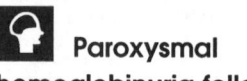

Paroxysmal cold hemoglobinuria

DESCRIPTION   A rare disease in which blood hemolyzes minutes to hours after exposure to cold (atmospheric, drinking cold water, handwashing in cold water). Usually occurs following a non-specific viral type illness. Usual course - acute; progressive; relapsing.

SYNONYMS
• Donath-Landsteiner hemolytic anemia
• Dressler syndrome
• Harley syndrome

CAUSES
• immune-mediated hemolysis upon rewarming after cold exposure

TREATMENT
• supportive
• transfusion
• oxygen
• maintain adequate urine output
• alkalinize urine
• steroids

ICD-9-CM
283.2 paroxysmal cold hemoglobinuria

Paroxysmal hemoglobinuria following exercise

DESCRIPTION   A benign disorder characterized by red urine, hemoglobinuria, myoglobinuria and abdominal pain. Usual course - acute.

SYNONYMS
• march hemoglobinuria

CAUSES
• strenuous exercise
• running on hard ground
• poorly cushioned shoes

TREATMENT
• unnecessary

ICD-9-CM
283.2 march hemoglobinuria

Paroxysmal nocturnal hemoglobinuria

DESCRIPTION Chronic acquired blood cell dysplasia with proliferation of a clone of stem cells producing erythrocytes, platelets, and granulocytes that are abnormally susceptible to lysis by complement. Characteristics — episodic intravascular hemolysis, particularly following infections, and by various thromboses, particularly of the hepatic veins. Usual course - chronic. Genetics - genetic mutation

SYNONYMS
• Marchiafava-Micheli syndrome

CAUSES
• intrinsic erythrocyte defect
• unusual complement sensitivity

TREATMENT
• transfusion
• androgens
• corticosteroids
• anticoagulants

ICD-9-CM
283.2 paroxysmal nocturnal hemoglobinuria

 ## Pellagra

DESCRIPTION Clinical deficiency syndrome. Characteristics — dermatitis, diarrhea, dementia, inflammation of mucus membranes. Skin lesions appear in area exposed to light and/or trauma. Mental symptoms include depression, irritability, anxiety, confusion, disorientation, delusions and hallucinations. Usual course - progressive. Endemic areas - Southern USA.

SYNONYMS
• niacin deficiency disease

CAUSES
• nicotinic acid deficiency
• tryptophan deficiency
• folic acid deficiency
• carcinoma
• isoniazid

TREATMENT
• nicotinic acid

ICD-9-CM
265.2 pellagra

Pemphigus, benign chronic familial

DESCRIPTION Benign, persistently recurrent bullous dermatitis (autosomal dominant; 66% positive family history). Characteristics — crops of lesions (may remain localized or become generalized), that rupture, undergo erosion and become thickly crusted. sites: sides of the neck, axillae, groin, and flexural and opposing surfaces of the body. Usual course - intermittent; spontaneous exacerbations with remissions.

SYNONYMS
• Hailey-Hailey disease

CAUSES
• defective intercellular cohesion
• defective tonofilament attachment to desmosomes
• precipitated by infection
• precipitated by trauma

TREATMENT
• antibiotics
• dapsone
• systemic steroids for severe cases
• topical steroids of limited value
• complete excision with split thickness skin graft

ICD-9-CM
694.4 pemphigus

 ## Pemphigus, Brazilian

DESCRIPTION Progressive and sometimes fatal variant of pemphigus foliaceous endemic in south central Brazil. Most frequently in children and adolescents. Characteristics — flaccid blisters that rupture easily, forming erosions with peripheral rolls of epidermis, associated with a burning sensation. Usual course - progressive; variable. Endemic areas - South Central Brazil.

SYNONYMS
• fogo selvagem

CAUSES
• unknown
• possibly infectious agent

TREATMENT
• topical corticosteroids for localized disease
• systemic corticosteroids for generalized disease

ICD-9-CM
694.4 pemphigus

 ## Pericholangitis

DESCRIPTION Inflammation of the tissues that surround the bile ducts. Characteristics — fever, mild icterus, hepatomegaly, mild pruritus. Usual course - progressive.

CAUSES
• unknown

TREATMENT
• none

ICD-9-CM
576.9 biliary tract disorder, nos

Perleche

DESCRIPTION Single or multiple fissures and cracks at corners of the mouth. In advanced stages may extend to lips and cheeks. Usual course - chronic; relapsing; acute.

SYNONYMS
• angulus infectiosus

CAUSES
• poorly fitting dentures
• monilia infection
• dietary deficiency

TREATMENT
• antimonilial drugs
• vitamins
• refit dentures

ICD-9-CM
686.8 perleche

 ## Personality disorders

DESCRIPTION A group of conditions that are not forms of illnesses, but ways of behaving. They are classified depending on the predominant symptoms and their severity. Characteristics include relatively fixed, inflexible and maladaptive patterns of behavior that cause trouble with relationships, work and the law. The individuals feel their behavior patterns are "normal" and "right."
• Paranoid: shows unwarranted suspiciousness and distrust of others, defensive, oversensitive.
• Schizoid and schizotypal: cold emotionally, difficulty in forming relationships, withdrawn, shy, superstitious, socially isolated.
• Compulsive: perfectionist, rigid in habits, indecisive, need for control.
• Histrionic: dependent, immature, excitable, vain, constantly crave stimulation.
• Narcissistic: exaggerated sense of own importance, exhibitionist, preoccupied with power, lack of interest in others, demands attention,
• Avoidant: fears and overreact to rejection, low self-esteem, socially withdrawn, dependent.
• Dependent: passive, overaccepting, unable to make decisions, lack of confidence.
• Passive-aggressive: stubborn, sulking, fear of authority, procrastinates, chronic lateness, argumentative, helpless, clinging.
• Antisocial: selfish, callous, promiscuous, impulsive, reckless, unable to learn from experience, failure at school and work.
• Borderline: impulsive, has unstable and intense inter-personal relationships, inappropriate anger, fear and guilt, lacks self-control, has identity problems, is suicidal.

CAUSES Exact cause is unknown

TREATMENT
• Long-term psychotherapy
• Antidepressants for depression or anxiety
• Clomipramine or fluoxetine for compulsive disorders
• Antipsychotic drugs for psychoses

ICD-9-CM
301.9 unspecified personality disorder

 ## Peutz-Jeghers syndrome

DESCRIPTION Multiple pigmented (melanin) macules of the skin and mouth mucosa and multiple polyposis of the small intestine. Usual course - chronic.

SYNONYMS
• intestinal polyposis II
• intestinal polyposis-cutaneous pigmentation syndrome
• periorificial lentiginosis syndrome

CAUSES
• hereditary

TREATMENT
• surgery

ICD-9-CM
759.6 Peutz-Jeghers syndrome

 ## Phlyctenular keratoconjunctivitis

DESCRIPTION Conjunctivitis and keratitis with discrete nodules of inflammation (phlyctenules).
• Characteristics - signs and symptoms include blepharospasm, severe lacrimation, photophobia, and pain

CAUSES
• atopic reaction of a hypersensitive conjunctiva to an unknown allergen, perhaps the protein of staphylococcal, tuberculous or other bacteria

TREATMENT
• topical corticosteroid and antibiotic combination. Ophthalmological referral or consultation.

ICD-9-CM
370.31
phlyctenular keratoconjunctivitis

Phosphine poisoning

DESCRIPTION Poisoning by hydrogen phosphide, PH3, a malodorous gas. Usual course - acute; progressive

CAUSES
• acid on phosphorus-contaminated metals
• water on phosphorus-contaminated metals
• acetylene to release phosphine gas
• phosphides to release phosphine gas

TREATMENT
• gastric decontamination
• irrigate eyes
• supportive
• excise sequestered jaw bone

ICD-9-CM
987.8 poisoning, phosphine

 Phosphorus poisoning

DESCRIPTION Condition resulting from inhalation or ingestion of phosphorous. Characteristics — garlic breath odor, mandibular necrosis, toothache, anemia, anorexia, weakness, luminescent vomitus. Usual course - acute; progressive.

SYNONYMS
• yellow phosphorous poisoning

CAUSES
• cytotoxicity

TREATMENT
• gastric decontamination
• irrigate eyes
• supportive
• bone excision

ICD-9-CM
983.9 poisoning, phosphorus

 Pick's disease

DESCRIPTION Rare progressive degenerative disease of the brain. Clinically similar to Alzheimer's with impaired reasoning, poor insight, memory loss, apathy, amnesia, aphasia, incontinence, and extrapyramidal signs. Pathologically, cortical atrophy is confined to frontal and temporal lobes. Usual course - chronic; progressive.

SYNONYMS
• lobar atrophy
• circumscribed brain atrophy
• presenile dementia

CAUSES
• degenerative disease

TREATMENT
• occupational therapy
• family counseling

ICD-9-CM
331.1 Pick's disease

 Pickwickian syndrome

DESCRIPTION Extreme obesity with polycythemia, somnolence, hypoventilation, arterial unsaturation and hypercapnia, and pulmonary hypertension. Usual course - chronic; intermittent.

SYNONYMS
• hypoventilation associated with extreme obesity

CAUSES
• marked obesity

TREATMENT
• caloric restriction
• progesterone
• tracheostomy

ICD-9-CM
278.8 pickwickian syndrome

 Pilonidal cyst

DESCRIPTION Hair-containing sacrococcygeal dermoid cyst or sinus that opens at a post anal dimple. Usual course - acute; chronic.

SYNONYMS
• pilonidal sinus
• jeep driver's disease
• coccygeal sinus
• pilliferous cyst

CAUSES
• ingrown broken hair
• stocky body build
• trauma

TREATMENT
• drainage
• excision

ICD-9-CM
685.1 pilonidal cyst without mention of abscess

 Pituitary basophilic adenoma

DESCRIPTION Small tumor of the anterior lobe whose cells stain with basic dyes and give rise to excessive secretion of ACTH resulting in Cushing's syndrome. Characteristics include truncal obesity, hypertension, visual disturbances, menstrual irregularity, impotence, muscle atrophy, osteoporosis, psychic disturbances. Usual course - chronic; progressive.

CAUSES
• unknown

TREATMENT
• transsphenoidal resection
• pituitary irradiation
• bromocriptine

ICD-9-CM
227.3 benign neoplasm of the pituitary

 Pituitary chromophobe adenoma

DESCRIPTION Anterior lobe of the pituitary gland tumor. Characteristics — hypopituitarism, headache, lassitude, visual disturbances, galactorrhea, hypogonadism. Usual course - chronic; progressive.

CAUSES
• unknown

TREATMENT
• transsphenoidal resection
• irradiation
• bromocriptine

ICD-9-CM
227.3 benign neoplasm of the pituitary

 Pituitary dwarfism

DESCRIPTION Dwarfism caused by hypofunction of the anterior pituitary gland with decreased secretion of growth hormone.

SYNONYMS
• ateliotic dwarfism
• panhypopituitary dwarfism
• hypopituitary dwarfism

CAUSES
• idiopathic
• pituitary tumor
• intrathecal methotrexate
• trauma
• CNS irradiation
• hemochromatosis
• sarcoidosis
• hypothalamic failure
• hypothalamic tumor
• CNS infection
• histiocytosis
• septo-optic dysplasia
• holoprosencephaly
• biologically inactive growth hormone
• growth hormone receptor insensitivity
• deficiency insulin-like growth factor I
• psychosocial dwarfism

TREATMENT
• exogenous growth hormone
• counseling

ICD-9-CM
253.3 pituitary dwarfism

Pituitary eosinophilic adenoma

DESCRIPTION A tumor of the anterior lobe of the pituitary associated with acromegaly and gigantism Usual course - chronic; progressive.

SYNONYMS
• pituitary acidophilic adenoma

CAUSES
• unknown

TREATMENT
• transsphenoidal resection
• pituitary irradiation
• bromocriptine

ICD-9-CM
227.3 benign neoplasm of the pituitary

Pituitary gigantism

DESCRIPTION Gigantism due to excessive pituitary secretion occurring before puberty and before epiphyses close. May be caused by eosinophilia or chromophobe adenoma. Usual course - insidious.

CAUSES
• somatotropic cell adenoma of the pituitary
• somatotropic cell adenoma of mixed cell
• somatotropic cell adenoma of stem cell
• bronchial adenoma
• pancreatic islet cell tumor
• carcinoid tumor
• ectopic growth hormone production

TREATMENT
• surgery
• irradiation
• bromocriptine

ICD-9-CM
253.0 pituitary gigantism

 Pituitary hypothyroidism

DESCRIPTION Hypothyroidism caused by deficiency of thyrotropin secretion. Usual course - chronic.

CAUSES
• pituitary irradiation
• pituitary ablative surgery
• failure of anterior pituitary due to infarction

TREATMENT
• thyroid hormone replacement

ICD-9-CM
244.9 pituitary hypothyroidism

 Placental insufficiency syndrome

DESCRIPTION Malnutrition and hypoxia of the fetus due to degenerative changes in the placenta.

CAUSES
• postterm fetus

TREATMENT
• good perinatal care

ICD-9-CM
762.2; 656.5 placental insufficiency

 Pleural malignant mesothelioma

DESCRIPTION Malignant tumor derived from mesothelial tissue. Characteristics — chest pain, dyspnea, weight loss, asthenia, cough, hemoptysis. Usual course - progressive; insidious onset.

CAUSES
• primary tumor of the pleura
• asbestos
• first exposure 20 to 60 years prior to diagnosis

TREATMENT
• surgery
• radiotherapy
• chemotherapy

ICD-9-CM
163.9 malignant neoplasm of the pleura

 Portal vein thrombosis

DESCRIPTION Clotting of the portal vein of the liver usually from unknown cause. Characteristics — hematemesis, melena splenomegaly, pancytopenia, encephalopathy, portal hypertension. It occurs in pregnancy (especially eclampsia) chronic heart failure, constrictive pericarditis, malignancies. Diagnosis established by angiography. Usual course - chronic; progressive.

CAUSES
• usually idiopathic
• neonatal septicemia
• omphalitis
• hepatocellular cancer
• umbilical vein catheterization for exchange transfusion

TREATMENT
• treat underlying condition
• possible shunt surgery

ICD-9-CM
452 portal vein thrombosis

 Postconcussion syndrome

DESCRIPTION Signs and symptoms that develop after concussion of the brain. Characteristics — amnesia, headache, dizziness, tinnitus, irritability, insomnia, difficulty in concentrating, sweating, heart palpitations. Usual course - acute; intermittent.

SYNONYMS
• posttraumatic brain syndrome

CAUSES
• mild head injury
• severe head injury

TREATMENT
• benzodiazepines

ICD-9-CM
310.2 postconcussion syndrome

 Postpoliomyelitis syndrome

DESCRIPTION A slow, progressive muscle weakness and deterioration of function in the previously affected muscles of an individual who had poliomyelitis at least 10 years earlier. The syndrome can appear 30 or more years after a partial or full recovery from the initial polio episode and is noninfectious. It usually involves those muscles most affected by the polio virus, but sometimes affects muscles that are fully recovered or never involved in the initial infection. Other symptoms include fatigue, muscle pain and fasciculations.

SYNONYMS
• polio, late effects
• postpoliomyelitis progressive muscular atrophy

CAUSES
• exact cause is unknown

TREATMENT
• physical and occupational therapy
• exercise, e.g., swimming
• consider changes in braces, medication or diet
• weight loss diet, if overweight
• respiratory support, if breathing is affected

ICD-9-CM
138 late effects of acute poliomyelitis

 Prader-Willi/Angelman syndrome

DESCRIPTION A congenital disorder of unknown etiology characterized by mental retardation, muscular hypotonia, obesity, short stature, hypogonadism and frequently developing insulin-resistant diabetes. Genetics - occasional small deletion of chromosome 15; sporadic; possible autosomal recessive. Usual course - progressive. When deletion is inherited from father the expression is Angelman's syndrome; when deletion is inherited from mother, the manifestations are Prader-Willi.

CAUSES
• hypothalamic dysfunction

TREATMENT
• dietary restrictions
• testosterone
• gastric bypass
• jaw wiring
• progesterone

ICD-9-CM
759.8 prader-willi syndrome

 Premature atrial contraction (PAC)

DESCRIPTION Premature, abnormal P waves. QRS complexes follow except in very early or blocked PAC. P wave may be buried in the preceding T wave or may be identified in the preceding T wave.

CAUSES
• congestive heart failure, coronary artery disease with ischemia, acute respiratory failure, chronic obstructive pulmonary disease, digitalis toxicity, aminophylline, adrenergic drugs, anxiety, caffeine

TREATMENT
• eliminate known causes

ICD-9-CM
427.61 premature atrial contraction

Premature ventricular contraction (PVC)

DESCRIPTION Irregular pulse. Ventricular beat occurs prematurely, followed by a compensatory pause after the premature ventricular contraction. QRS complex is wide and distorted. Most ominous when clustered, multifocal, with R wave on T pattern.

CAUSES
• multiple causes can include psychological stress, physiologic stress, drug toxicity (digitalis, aminophylline, tricyclic antidepressants, beta adrenergics (isoproterenol or dopamine)), caffeine, tobacco, electrolyte imbalances (especially hypokalemia)

TREATMENT
• lidocaine IV bolus and drip infusion
• procainamide IV if induced by digitalis toxicity
•stop digitalis. If caused by hypokalemia, give potassium chloride intravenous drip
• eliminate known causes

ICD-9-CM
427.69 premature ventricular contraction

 ## Primary lateral sclerosis

DESCRIPTION Degeneration of the lateral columns of the spinal cord. Characteristics — spastic paraplegia, rigidity of limbs, increased tendon reflexes, absence of nutritive and sensory disturbance. Usual course - chronic; slowly progressive.

CAUSES
• unknown
• existence as separate clinical entity questioned

TREATMENT
• none

ICD-9-CM
335.24 primary lateral sclerosis

 ## Proctalgia fugax

DESCRIPTION Abrupt, sharp or gripping-like pain in the anorectal area. The pain does not radiate. Often the pain wakes the individual in the night. Typically, relief occurs within seconds to minutes, although rare, the pain can be present for hours. The disorder is benign and there is no cure.

SYNONYMS
levator syndrome

CAUSES
• unknown; attributed to spasm of levator ani and coccygeal muscles, sometimes associated with stress or anxiety

TREATMENT
• reassuring patient of benign nature of disease is satisfactory in most cases
• warm baths
• periodic massage
• for severe pain, consider inhaled albuterol, oral clonidine, diltiazem

ICD-9-CM
564.6 anal spasm

 ## Progressive external ophthalmoplegia

DESCRIPTION Slowly progressive bilateral myopathy affecting the extraocular muscles. Characteristics — weakness of levators of the upper lids, ptosis, followed by total ocular paresis. Usual course - chronic; progressive.

SYNONYMS
• chronic dystrophic ophthalmoplegia

CAUSES
• unknown

TREATMENT
•none

ICD-9-CM
378.72 progressive external ophthalmoplegia

 ## Progressive hemiatrophy face

DESCRIPTION Atrophy of one half of the face which is usually progressive, but may eventually become stationary.

SYNONYMS
• Romberg's disease
• Parry-Romberg syndrome
• progressive hemifacial atrophy

CAUSES
• unknown
• possible lipodystrophy

TREATMENT
• plastic reconstructive surgery
• skin transplantation
• subcutaneous fat transplantation

ICD-9-CM
349.89 hemiatrophy, face, progressive.

 ## Progressive multifocal leukoencephalopathy

DESCRIPTION Serious, usually fatal viral disease. Characteristics — demyelination in white matter of the brain, but may be seen in the brain stem and cerebellum. It occurs secondary to lymphosarcoma and lymphatic myeloid leukemia. Usual course - progressive.

CAUSES
• latent papovavirus

TREATMENT
• cytosine arabinoside

ICD-9-CM
046.3 progressive multifocal leukoencephalopathy

 ## Prolactinoma

DESCRIPTION A pituitary adenoma which secretes prolactin, leading to increased serum levels of prolactin. Prolactinomas in women are presented with galactorrhea associated with amenorrhea. Though much less common for men, prolactinomas in men rarely produce galactorrhea and are later presented as larger, space-occupying tumors. Usual course - progressive.

SYNONYMS
• prolactin secreting pituitary adenoma
• PRL secreting pituitary adenoma

CAUSES
• prolactin-secreting pituitary microadenoma

TREATMENT
• transsphenoidal resection
• bromocriptine
• irradiation

ICD-9-CM
253.1 forbes-albright syndrome

 ## Pseudocyst pancreas

DESCRIPTION Unilocular cyst of the pancreas. Characteristics — tender mass in left upper quadrant, abdominal pain, weight loss, nausea, anorexia, jaundice. Usual course - acute; progressive.

CAUSES
• acute pancreatitis
• trauma
• pancreatic enzymes released into lesser omentum

TREATMENT
• needle aspiration
• internal drainage surgery
• external drainage

ICD-9-CM
577.2 cyst and pseudocyst of pancreas

 ## Pulmonary artery thrombosis

DESCRIPTION Blood clot in the pulmonary artery. Characteristics — dyspnea, weakness, chest pain, tachycardia, tachypnea.

CAUSES
• reduction in blood flow of pulmonary artery
• organization of previous embolism
• malignancy
• infection
• trauma
• intrinsic disease

TREATMENT
• anticoagulants

ICD-9-CM
415.1 pulmonary artery thrombosis

Pulmonary hypertension, secondary

DESCRIPTION Increased pressure in the pulmonary circulation above 30 millimeters of mercury systolic, and 12 millimeters of mercury diastolic, secondary to any of the listed causes.

CAUSES
• CHF, left ventricular failure, mitral stenosis, mitral regurgitation, myxoma, pulmonary embolism, interstitial fibrosis, sarcoidosis, asbestosis, radiation, alveolar hypoventilation, chronic obstructive pulmonary disease, chronic bronchitis, emphysema, ventricular septal defect, atrial septal defect, silicosis, anthrosilicosis, tuberculosis, SLE, scleroderma, dermatomyositis, connective tissue disorder, cystic fibrosis

TREATMENT
• corticosteroids, oxygen, cardiac catheterization, nitroprusside, hydralazine, diazoxid, isoproterenol, phentolamine, prazosin, verapamil, nifedipine, captopril

ICD-9-CM
416.8 secondary pulmonary hypertension

 ## Pulmonary infarction

DESCRIPTION Hemorrhagic consolidation of lung parenchyma resulting from thromboembolic pulmonary arterial occlusion. Usual course - acute.

CAUSES
• stasis, vein injury, hypercoagulable state, phlebitis, phlebothrombosis, thrombus, deep vein thrombosis, burn, surgery, oral contraceptives, trauma, hip fracture, immobilization, congestive heart failure, cardiomyopathy, subacute bacterial endocarditis, atrial myxoma, polycythemia rubra vera, sickle cell anemia, pancreatic carcinoma

TREATMENT
• anticoagulation
• heparin
• coumadin
• warfarin
• thrombolytic agent
• urokinase
• streptokinase
• embolectomy
• vena cava clip

ICD-9-CM
415.1 pulmonary embolism and infarction

Pulmonary interstitial fibrosis, idiopathic

DESCRIPTION Interstitial pneumonia, "nonspecific," or "usual." The term used when etiology leading to pulmonary fibrosis cannot be defined (about 50% of cases). Usual course - chronic; progressive.

SYNONYMS
• alveolocapillary block
• fibrosing alveolitis

CAUSES
• unknown
• loss of functional alveolarcapillary units
• inflammation

TREATMENT
• corticosteroids

ICD-9-CM
516.3 diffuse interstitial pulmonary fibrosis

 ## Pyogenic abscess liver

DESCRIPTION Bacterial abscess of the liver. Characteristics - fever, abdominal pain, anorexia, jaundice, hepatomegaly, elevated hemidiaphragm. Usual course - acute; relapsing.

CAUSES
• portal vein bacteremia
• systemic bacteremia
• ascending cholangitis
• direct extension
• trauma

TREATMENT
• aspiration
• antibiotics
• surgical drainage

ICD-9-CM
572.0 abscess of liver

 ## Pyrogenic shock

DESCRIPTION Shock associated with overwhelming infection, most commonly with gram-negative bacteria. Characteristics - fever, tachycardia, chills, myalgia, confusion, tachypnea, hypotension, nausea. Usual course - acute.

SYNONYMS
• septic shock
• endotoxic shock

CAUSES
• inadequate tissue perfusion following bacteremia
• escherichia coli
• klebsiella
• pseudomonas
• serratia
• neisseria meningitidis
• staphylococci; pneumococci; streptococci; bacteroides

TREATMENT
• respiratory support
• fluid replacement
• antibiotics
• vasoactive drugs

ICD-9-CM
785.59 septic shock

 ## Q fever

DESCRIPTION Acute, generally self-limited rickettsial infection. Characteristics — fever, chills, headache, myalgia, malaise, rash (rarely), pneumonitis, hepatitis, and endocarditis. No vector involved. Infection by inhalation of dust or aerosols derived from infected domestic animals. Usual course - abrupt; relapsing; chronic; usually mild. Endemic areas - Western USA; Australia; Africa; England; Mediterranean countries.

SYNONYMS
• Australian Q fever
• Balkan grippe
• nine mile fever
• hiberno-vernal bronchopneumonia
• Derrick-Burnet disease
• Query fever

CAUSES
• coxiella burnetii (rickettsia)
• aspiration of infected material
• contaminated raw milk ingestion
• infected animal conceptional product exposure

TREATMENT
• antibiotics

ICD-9-CM
083.0 Q fever

 ## Rat-bite fever, spirillary

DESCRIPTION Infection caused by a rat or mouse bite. Characteristics — wound heals promptly; inflammation recurs at bite site after 10 or more days, accompanied by relapsing fever and regional lymphadenitis; WBC elevated; myalgia, skin rash, chills, malaise, headache. Usual course - relapsing. Endemic areas - Asia; Europe; USA.

SYNONYMS
• sodoku

CAUSES
• spirillum minor-a spirochete
• rodent bite
• rodent scratch
• rodent-ingesting animal bite

TREATMENT
• antibiotics
• rapid bite cleaning

ICD-9-CM
026.9 rat-bite fever

 ## Rat-bite fever, streptobacillary

DESCRIPTION Bacterial infection caused by a rat or mouse bite, although occasionally associated with ingestion of contaminated milk or with the bite of a different rodent. Characteristics (10 or more days following the bite) — abrupt illness with chills, fever, vomiting, headache, arthralgia, backache, elevated WBC, morbilliform petechial skin rash. Usual course - relapsing. Endemic areas - Asia; Europe; USA.

CAUSES
• streptobacillus moniliformis
• rodent bite
• rodent scratch
• contaminated raw milk ingestion

TREATMENT
• antibiotics
• rapid bite cleansing

ICD-9-CM
026.9 rat-bite fever

 ## Relapsing fever

DESCRIPTION An acute infectious disease caused by arthropod-borne spirochetes. Clinically characterized by recurrent episodes of fever typically lasting three to five days, headache, arthralgia, myalgia, diarrhea, vomiting, coughing, eye and chest pain, splenomegaly. Two forms of the disease exist: louse-borne and tick-borne. Louse-borne relapsing fever occurs primarily in developing countries and is transmitted by body lice. Tick-borne relapsing fever is less severe and is caused by several species of Borrelia. It is transmitted by soft body ticks of the genus Ornithodoros.

SYNONYMS
• recurrent fever
• tick fever
• famine fever

CAUSES
• body lice
• body ticks

TREATMENT
• tetracyclines
• erythromycin
• penicillin

ICD-9-CM
087.9 fever

Renal artery stenosis

DESCRIPTION Occlusive disease of the renal arteries. This problem occurs in about 5% of patients with hypertension and is one form of hypertension that is surgically correctable. The disease is most often unilateral. Usual course - progressive.

CAUSES
• atherosclerosis
• fibromuscular dysplasia

TREATMENT
• surgery
• angioplasty
• antihypertensives

ICD-9-CM
440.1 renal artery stenosis

Renal infarction

DESCRIPTION Localized area of kidney necrosis caused by either renal arterial or venous occlusion. Characteristics - steady, aching, flank pain, fever, nausea, vomiting, hypertension, leukocytosis, proteinuria, microscopic hematuria. Renal imaging confirms the diagnosis. Usual course - acute.

CAUSES
• renal artery thrombosis
• renal emboli
• arteriosclerosis
• renal artery aneurysm
• fibrous dysplasia
• aortic dissection
• periarteritis nodosa
• vasculitis
• sickle cell disease
• scleroderma
• polycythemia
• trauma
• surgery
• cardiomegaly
• subacute bacterial endocarditis
• atrial myxoma
• rheumatic heart disease

TREATMENT
• surgery
• balloon angioplasty

ICD-9-CM
593.81 renal infarction

Renal vein thrombosis

DESCRIPTION Clotting within the renal vein. Characteristics — lumbar pain; dysuria; enlarged, tender kidney. Usual course - acute; chronic.

CAUSES
• abdominal operation
• CHF
• dehydration
• renal disease
• reduction in renal blood flow
• pregnancy
• constrictive pericarditis
• morbid obesity

TREATMENT
• anticoagulants
• corticosteroids

ICD-9-CM
453.3 embolism and thrombosis of renal vein

Reticulum cell sarcoma

DESCRIPTION Malignant histiocytic lymphoma made of a substance like embryonic connective tissue. Characteristics — fatigue, anorexia, weight loss, excessive sweating, fever, painless adenopathy, hepatosplenomegaly. Usual course - chronic; progressive; relapsing.

SYNONYMS
• reticulum cell lymphosarcoma
• diffuse histiocytic lymphoma
• reticulosarcoma

CAUSES
• unknown

TREATMENT
• chemotherapy
• radiotherapy
• surgery

ICD-9-CM
200.00 reticulosarcoma, nos

Retinal vein occlusion

DESCRIPTION One of the causes of sudden unilateral vision loss. Characteristics — extensive retinal hemorrhages; dilated, tortuous retinal veins. Usual course - acute.

SYNONYMS
• central retinal vein occlusion
• CRVO

TREATMENT
• panretinal photocoagulation

ICD-9-CM
362.35 central retinal vein occlusion

Retinoblastoma

DESCRIPTION Malignant congenital hereditary blastoma (autosomal dominant with high penetrance). Characteristics — appears in one or both eyes in children under 5 years of age, diagnosed initially by a bright white or yellow pupillary reflex. Usual course - progressive.

SYNONYMS
• glioma retina

CAUSES
• genetic

TREATMENT
• radiotherapy to preserve vision
• photocoagulation to preserve vision
• cryotherapy to preserve vision
• brachytherapy to preserve vision
• enucleation
• palliative radiotherapy for extraocular disease

ICD-9-CM
190.5 malignant neoplasm of the retina

Rhabdomyosarcoma

DESCRIPTION Highly malignant tumor of striated muscle. There are 3 forms - pleomorphic affecting predominantly the extremities of adults; alveolar form, occurring primarily in adolescents and young adults affecting muscles of extremities, trunk, and orbital region; embryonal form, occurring mainly in infants and children, affecting the head and neck, lower genitourinary tract, pelvis and extremities. Usual course - progressive.

SYNONYMS
• rhabdosarcoma

CAUSES
• fetal alcohol syndrome

TREATMENT
• surgical excision
• add radiotherapy in most cases
• group 2: add chemotherapy with vincristine plus dactinomycin
• group 3: add chemotherapy with vincristine plus dactinomycin
• combination chemotherapy for advanced disease

ICD-9-CM
171.9 malignant neoplasm of connective and soft tissue

Rheumatoid pneumoconiosis

DESCRIPTION Pneumoconiosis associated with rheumatoid arthritis. Characteristics — multiple spherical nodular lesions with clearly demarcated borders found throughout both lungs. Usual course: chronic; progressive.

SYNONYMS
• caplan syndrome
• rheumatoid lung with silicosis
• silicoarthritis

CAUSES
• unknown
• immune mechanism

TREATMENT
• manage complications

ICD-9-CM
714.81 caplan's syndrome

Rhinosporidiosis

DESCRIPTION Chronic, localized granulomatous infection of mucocutaneous tissues, especially the nose. Characteristics — nasal polyps, tumors, papillomas, or wart-like lesions. Other (rare) areas of infection include the conjunctiva, penis, anus, vagina, ears, pharynx, larynx. Usual course - progressive. Endemic areas - India; Sri-Lanka.

SYNONYMS
• rhinosporosis

CAUSES
• rhinosporidium seeberi

TREATMENT
• surgery

ICD-9-CM
117.0 rhinosporidiosis

Riboflavin deficiency

DESCRIPTION Deficiency of vitamin B2. Deficiency characteristics — cheilosis, photophobia, sore throat, glossitis, fissure tongue, seborrheic dermatitis. Usual course - acute; progressive.

SYNONYMS
• vitamin B2 deficiency
• ariboflavinosis

CAUSES
• inadequate dietary intake
• intestinal malabsorption

TREATMENT
• riboflavin administration

ICD-9-CM
266.0 ariboflavinosis

 Rickettsialpox

DESCRIPTION Mild, self-limited disease transmitted by a mite that is an ectoparasite of the house mouse. Characteristics — eschar-like primary skin lesion, generalize papulovesicular rash, headache, and backache. Usual course - acute; incubation period 10 days to 3 weeks after bite. Endemic areas - USA; Europe; Africa.

CAUSES
• Rickettsia akari
• bite from mite (vector) infected by rodent

TREATMENT
• tetracycline
• chloramphenicol

ICD-9-CM
083.2 rickettsialpox

 Ruptured chordae tendineae

DESCRIPTION Rupture of a tendinous chord that connects each cusp of atrioventricular valves to approximate papillary muscles in the heart ventricles. Characteristics include a dramatic wholosystolic apical murmur, precordial thrill, chest pain, dyspnea. Rupture of the chordae of the mitral valve is not uncommon. Usual course - acute; progressive.

CAUSES
• endocarditis
• trauma
• thoracic compression
• myxomatous perforation

TREATMENT
• diuretics
• surgical repair

ICD-9-CM
429.5 rupture of chordae tendineae

 Ruptured mitral papillary muscle

DESCRIPTION Rupture of conical muscular projections from walls of the cardiac ventricles, attached to cusps of the mitral arterioventricular valves by the chordae tendinae. Characteristics — pansystolic murmur, apical thrill, signs and symptoms of congestive heart failure. Usual course - acute; progressive.

SYNONYMS
• papillary muscle rupture

CAUSES
• myocardial infarction
• myocardial necrosis
• trauma

TREATMENT
• diuretics
• surgery

ICD-9-CM
429.6 rupture of papillary muscle

 Schatzki's ring

DESCRIPTION Ring-like narrowing of the distal esophagus at the squamo-columnar junction. It is probably congenital and measures 2-4 mm in the submucosa. Characteristics — dysphagia. X-ray with barium swallow confirms the diagnosis by displaying the annular constriction of the lower esophagus. Usual course - chronic; progressive.

SYNONYMS
• esophagogastric ring syndrome
• lower esophageal ring syndrome

CAUSES
• unknown

TREATMENT
• rubber dilatation of ring

ICD-9-CM
530.3 ; 750.3 Schatzki's ring

 Schistosomiasis haematobium

DESCRIPTION Parasitic disease caused by blood flukes of the genus Schistosoma haematobium. S. Haematobium causes symptoms in the genitourinary system or lower colon and rectum. Endemic in Africa, India, Middle East, Indian Ocean islands. Usual course - acute; chronic; intermittent; progressive.

SYNONYMS
• endemic hematuria
• urogenital schistosomiasis

CAUSES
• trematode Schistosoma haematobium
• fresh water snail reservoir

TREATMENT
• praziquantel
• metrifonate
• niridazole

ICD-9-CM
120.0 schistosomiasis due to Schistosoma haematobium

 Schistosomiasis japonica

DESCRIPTION Parasitic disease caused by blood flukes of Schistosoma japonica causing disturbances in the small intestine, colon, and rectum. Characteristics — may be asymptomatic, melena, diarrhea, hepatosplenomegaly. Endemic area - Africa, India, Middle East, Indian Ocean islands. Usual course - acute; chronic; intermittent; progressive.

SYNONYMS
• eastern schistosomiasis
• katayama disease
• yangtze river disease

CAUSES
• trematode Schistosoma japonica
• fresh water snail reservoir

TREATMENT
• praziquantel
• niridazole
• stibocaptate

ICD-9-CM
120.2 schistosomiasis due to Schistosoma japonicum

 Schistosomiasis mansoni

DESCRIPTION Parasitic disease caused by blood flukes of Schistosoma mansoni causing disturbances in the small intestine, colon, and rectum. Characteristics — diarrhea, weight loss, anorexia, melena, jaundice, hepatosplenomegaly. Endemic areas - Africa, South America, Caribbean, Middle East. May occur in Americans who lived in Puerto Rico. Usual course - acute; chronic; intermittent; progressive.

SYNONYMS
• intestinal bilharziasis
• schistosomal dysentery
• katayama fever
• Manson's schistosomiasis
• Schistosoma mansonii infection
• intestinal schistosomiasis

CAUSES
• trematode Schistosoma mansoni
• fresh water snail reservoir

TREATMENT
• praziquantel
• oxamniquine

ICD-9-CM
120.1 schistosomiasis due to Schistosoma mansoni

 Schistosomiasis of the liver, chronic

DESCRIPTION Parasitic disease caused by blood flukes of the genus Schistosoma that penetrate the skin and develop in the liver, causing fever, eosinophilia, urticaria, hepatosplenomegaly, lymphadenopathy, ascites, esophageal varices. Endemic areas - Africa, Asia, South America, Caribbean Islands.

SYNONYMS
• bilharziasis

CAUSES
• Schistosoma mansoni
• Schistosoma japonicum
• fresh water snails

TREATMENT
• oxamniquine
• praziquantel
• niridazole
• splenorenal anastomosis surgery

ICD-9-CM
120.9 schistosomiasis, unspecified

Schistosomiasis, cutaneous

DESCRIPTION Parasitic disease caused by blood flukes of the genus Schistosoma. Fresh and salt water mollusks are intermediate hosts. Characteristics — intense pruritus, stinging, macules, papules, and vesicles. Endemic areas - Hawaii, Florida, Great Lakes area. Usual course - acute; intermittent; relapsing.

SYNONYMS
• swimmer's itch
• clam digger's itch

CAUSES
• nonspecific Schistosome cercaria
• snail reservoir
• skin penetration
• abnormal host foreign body reaction

TREATMENT
• antipruritics
• antibiotics for secondary bacterial infections

ICD-9-CM
120.3 cutaneous schistosomiasis

Scleredema

DESCRIPTION Diffuse, symmetrical, wooden-like, non-pitting induration of the skin of face, head, shoulders, arms, thorax. Usually preceded by an infectious process. It occurs in association with diabetes mellitus. Resolves in 6 months to 2 years. Usual course - acute; chronic.

SYNONYMS
• scleredema adultorum of buschke

CAUSES
• unknown
• following streptococcal infection

TREATMENT
• self-limited
• unnecessary

ICD-9-CM
710.1 scleredema adultorum

Sclerosis of the brain

DESCRIPTION Familial form of leukoencephalopathy occurring in early life and running a slowly progressive course into adolescence or adulthood. Characteristics — nystagmus, ataxia, tremor, choreoathetotic movements, dyarthria, and mental deterioration.

SYNONYMS
• Pelizaeus-Merzbacher disease
• diffuse familial cerebral sclerosis
• aplasia axialis extracorticalis congenita

CAUSES
• genetic

TREATMENT
• supportive

ICD-9-CM
330.0 leukodystrophy

Scoliosis

DESCRIPTION A lateral curvature of the spine that may be found in the thoracic, lumbar, or thoracolumbar spinal segment. The curve may be convex to the right or to the left. Rotation of the vertebral column around its axis occurs and may cause rib cage deformity. May be associated with kyphosis (humpback) or lordosis (swayback). The most common type is idiopathic (80% of casses), usually begins about ages 8-10, is more common in girls than boys (4-5:1) and is classically asymptomatic.

CAUSES
• structural scoliosis
  ◊ idiopathic (may be transmitted as an autosomal dominant or multifactoral trait)
  ◊ congenital defects of the spine (hemivertebral or unilateral vertebral bridge)
  ◊ paralytic or musculoskeletal (due to polio, cerebral palsy, or muscular dystrophy)
• functional scoliosis
  ◊ poor posture
  ◊ uneven leg length

TREATMENT
• physical therapy and back exercises aimed at strengthening back muscles
• orthopedic back brace (sometimes worn for several years)
• if legs are of unequal length, a shoe lift for the shorter leg
• surgery to correct the deformity (severe cases only)

ICD-9-CM
737.30 scoliosis (and kyphoscoliosis), idiopathic
754.2 congenital musculoskeletal deformities of spine

Scurvy, infantile

DESCRIPTION Nutritional disease of children caused by ascorbic acid deficiency. Characteristics — weakness, anemia, spongy gums, mucocutaneous hemorrhages, brawny induration of calves and legs.

SYNONYMS
• vitamin C deficiency
• Barlow disease
• subperiosteal hematoma syndrome

CAUSES
• ascorbic acid deficiency

TREATMENT
• ascorbic acid
• fruit juice

ICD-9-CM
267 infantile scurvy

Seasonal affective disorder

DESCRIPTION Depression caused by dysfunction of circadian rhythms, that occurs most often in the winter months and is believed to be due to a decrease in exposure to full-spectrum light. In addition to feelings of sadness and anxiety, symptoms include hypersomnia, lethargy, carbohydrate craving and weight gain. Diagnosis usually requires a 2-3 year mood disturbance pattern, with the onset occurring in the autumn, and a remission in the spring. It occurs more commonly in women and among individuals living in the northern latitudes.

SYNONYMS
SAD

CAUSES
• exact cause is unknown; may be linked to amount of melatonin released by the pineal gland

TREATMENT
• phototherapy (light therapy) is preferential treatment
• MAO inhibitor or fluoxetine
• psychotherapy

ICD-9-CM
300.4 neurotic depression

Second degree AV block

DESCRIPTION Two subtypes:
• Type I or Wenckebach: P-R interval becomes progressively longer with each cycle until a non-conducted atrial beat occurs. After the dropped beat the P-R interval is shorter.
• Type II: Constant P-R intervals preceding a non-conducted atrial beat.
Ventricular rate is irregular. Atrial rhythm is regular.

SYNONYMS
• Mobitz type 1
• Wenckebach's period

CAUSES
• inferior wall myocardial infarction, digitalis toxicity, vagal stimulation

TREATMENT
• discontinue digitalis
• atropine if patient is symptomatic.

ICD-9-CM
426.13 second degree heart block

Selective IgA deficiency

DESCRIPTION The most common and mildest immunoglobulin deficiency (<15 mg/dL). IgA is the primary immunoglobulin in human saliva, nasal and bronchial fluids and intestinal secretions. It normally guards against bacterial and viral infections. The deficiency is lifelong and precautions need to be taken to prevent infections.

CAUSES
• autosomal dominant or recessive inheritance
• some drugs may cause transient IgA deficiency
• chromosome 18 abnormalities
• occurs in relatives patients with common variable immunodeficiency

TREATMENT
• no known cure
• treatment for associated diseases
• wear medical alerting identification

ICD-9-CM
279.01 selective IgA immunodeficiency

Sheehan's syndrome

DESCRIPTION Postpartum pituitary necrosis resulting form hypovolemia and shock in the immediate peri-partem period. Characteristics — endocrine deficiency syndromes due to loss of anterior lobe pituitary function. Usual course - progressive; acute.

SYNONYMS
• postpartum panhypopituitary syndrome
• postpartum hypopituitarism

CAUSES
• intrapartum hemorrhage
• postpartum hemorrhage
• postpartum infection
• peripheral vascular collapse
• vascular spasm
• DIC

TREATMENT
• hormone replacement therapy
• new pregnancy

ICD-9-CM
253.2 Sheehan's syndrome

Shigellosis

DESCRIPTION Acute infection of the bowel. Source of infection: excreta of infected individuals that may be indirectly spread by contaminated food. Incubation period - 1 to 4 days. Characteristics — sudden onset of fever, irritability, drowsiness, anorexia, nausea, vomiting, diarrhea, abdominal pain and distention. Stools show blood, pus and mucus.

CAUSES
• shigella ingestion

TREATMENT
• fluid replacement
• ampicillin
• tetracycline
• sulfamethoxazole-trimethoprim
• chloramphenicol

ICD-9-CM
004.9 shigellosis, unspecified

Short-bowel syndrome

DESCRIPTION A malabsorption syndrome resulting from massive resection of small bowel. Characteristics — diarrhea, steatorrhea, malnutrition. Usual course - chronic; progressive.

SYNONYMS
• massive bowel resection syndrome

CAUSES
• excessive resection of small bowel

TREATMENT
• parenteral nutrition
• low fat diet
• trace metal replacement
• mineral replacement
• vitamin replacement
• parenteral bile-salt sequestering agent
• H-2 receptor antagonist

ICD-9-CM
579.2 short bowel syndrome

Shoulder-hand syndrome

DESCRIPTION Clinical disorder of the upper extremity. Characteristics — pain and stiffness in the shoulder with puffy swelling and pain in the ipsilateral hand, sometimes occurring after myocardial infarction. Usual course - chronic; acute exacerbations.

SYNONYMS
• Steinbrocker syndrome
• reflex sympathetic dystrophy syndrome
• coronary-scapular syndrome
• postinfarction sclerodactylia

CAUSES
• reflex sympathetic stimulation
• cerebral vascular accident
• myocardial infarction
• upper extremity trauma

TREATMENT
• physical therapy
• analgesics
• oral steroids
• stellate ganglion block
• steroid injections

ICD-9-CM
337.9 shoulder-hand syndrome

Siderosis of the lung

DESCRIPTION Pneumoconiosis due to inhalation of iron particles. X-rays are abnormal, but there is no functional impairment and there are no symptoms. Usual course - chronic; acute; progressive.

SYNONYMS
• silver polisher lung
• welder lung

CAUSES
• inhalation of iron oxide dust

TREATMENT
• unnecessary

ICD-9-CM
503 siderosis of the lung

Silo filler disease

DESCRIPTION Pulmonary edema caused by nitrogen dioxide intoxication, which may take place among welders or silo fillers. Symptoms may not appear for 12 hours after exposure. Usual course - progressive; acute.

SYNONYMS
• nitrogen dioxide toxicity
• silage gas poisoning
• silo filler pneumoconiosis

CAUSES
• inhalation of nitrogen dioxide

TREATMENT
• bronchodilators
• mechanical ventilation
• supplemental oxygen

ICD-9-CM
506.9 silo fillers' disease

Silver poisoning

DESCRIPTION Permanent ashen-gray discoloration of the skin, conjunctiva, and internal organs resulting from long over-exposure to silver. Usual course - acute; chronic.

SYNONYMS
• argyria
• argyriasis

CAUSES
• absorption through skin
• inhalation of dust fumes
• accidental ingestion
• abuse of silver nose drops
• mining
• silver plating
• handling of metallic silver

TREATMENT
• emesis
• hydration
• gastric lavage
• activated charcoal

ICD-9-CM
985.8 argyria

Sinoatrial arrest or block

DESCRIPTION Unexpectedly long P-P interval interrupting normal sinus rhythm. Often terminated by a junctional escape beat or return to normal sinus rhythm. QRS complexes uniform, but irregular.

SYNONYMS
• Sinus arrest

CAUSES
• digitalis toxicity, quinidine toxicity, sick sinus syndrome

TREATMENT
• atropine, 0.5 mg intravenously
• Pacemaker for repeated episodes

ICD-9-CM
426.6 sinoatrial heart block

Sinus bradycardia

DESCRIPTION Rate of less than 60 beats per minute. A QRS complex follows each P wave.

CAUSES
• sick sinus syndrome, hypothyroidism, mechanical ventilation, inferior myocardial infarction, increased intracranial pressure, increased vagal tone (straining at stool), vomiting, intubation, treatment with beta-blockers and sympatholytic drugs

TREATMENT
• atropine, 0.5 mg every 5 minutes to total of 2.0 mg if needed
• temporary pacemaker if atropine fails

ICD-9-CM
427.89 other rhythm disorder

Sinus tachycardia

DESCRIPTION Cardiac rate greater than 100 beats per minute. May rarely increase to exceed 160 beats per minute. Every QRS complex follows a P wave.

CAUSES
• cardiac response to fever, anxiety, vigorous exercise, pain, dehydration, shock, left ventricular heart failure, cardiac tamponade, anemia, hyperthyroidism, hypovolemia, pulmonary embolus, myocardial infarction

TREATMENT
• treat the underlying cause

ICD-9-CM
427.89 other rhythm disorder

Smallpox

DESCRIPTION An acute infectious disease caused by pox virus. This disease is now extinct worldwide due to successful inoculation. Alastrim, a mild form of the disease is known as variola minor.

SYNONYMS
- variola
- variola major

CAUSES
- double-stranded DNA virus transmitted by inhalation
- rare family transmission

TREATMENT
- isolation, report to health department, meticulous fluid management, skin hygiene, antihistamines, antibiotics for secondary bacterial infections

ICD-9-CM
050.9 smallpox, nos

Somatoform disorders

DESCRIPTION A group of disorders in which there are physical symptoms for which no physical cause can be found. Included in this group are somatization disorder, conversion disorder, and body dysmorphic disorder. Hypochondriasis and chronic pain disorder (somatoform pain disorder) are also classified as somatoform disorders, but are covered in separate topics.
- Somatization disorder: multiple physical symptoms that recur over a period of several years with no medical basis. The patient has usually consulted numerous doctors for treatment and medications. This disorder was previous called hysteria. The symptoms often involve neurological problems (double vision), gynecological problems (painful menstruation) or gastrointestinal problems (abdominal pain).
- Conversion disorder: loss or change of a physical function (paralysis of an arm, blindness, seizures). The symptom is not intentionally produced or faked.
- Body dysmorphic disorder: preoccupation with an imagined defect in a normal-appearing person. The defect may be very minor, but the concern is blown out of proportion. The focus is often on skin wrinkles and blemishes, facial hair, shape of the nose, mouth or jaw.

CAUSES Exact cause is unknown

TREATMENT
- Psychotherapy
- Group therapy
- Family therapy

ICD-9-CM
306.9 unspecified psychophysiological malfunction

Sparganosis

DESCRIPTION Infection of animals, including fish and man, with a developmental stage of Diphyllobothrium. This stage has recently been referred to as a plerocercoid but the name sparganum has persisted. Therefore, infection of fish or other animals with the plerocercoid larvae is sparganosis. Fish-eating mammals, including man, are the final hosts. Usual course - chronic.

SYNONYMS
- larval diphyllobothriasis
- sparganosis (larval diphyllobothriasis)

CAUSES
- spirometra species
- larval diphyllobothrium ingestion from undercooked flesh
- animal flesh poultices

TREATMENT
- surgical excision only

ICD-9-CM
123.5 sparganosis

Spinal cord compression

DESCRIPTION Impingement on the spinal cord, usually by an extramedullary neoplasm. Characteristics — local back pain, hyperreflexia, Babinski's sign, weakness of lower extremities, sensory loss, loss of sphincter control. Back pain and weakness may last hours to days, but total loss of function control to the site of compression may take only minutes. Usual course - acute onset; chronic onset; often progressive primary disease.

CAUSES
- carcinoma of the lung
- breast carcinoma
- carcinoma of the prostate
- lymphoma
- neural malignancy
- herniated disk
- extradural abscess
- spinal tuberculosis
- rheumatoid arthritis
- cervical spondylosis

TREATMENT
- high dose corticosteroids
- radiotherapy
- surgery
- chemotherapy for primary tumor

ICD-9-CM
336.9 spinal cord compression, nos

Splenic agenesis syndrome

DESCRIPTION Congenital absence of the spleen, partial situs inversus viscerum accompanied by cardiac defects (right type atria, endocardial cushion defect). This is a familial disorder that is autosomal recessive with sporadic penetrance. Usual course - acute; chronic; progressive.

SYNONYMS
- Ivemark syndrome
- asplenia

CAUSES
- failure of normal asymmetry in morphogenesis

TREATMENT
- antibiotics
- cardiac surgery
- gastrointestinal surgery

ICD-9-CM
759.0 agenesis of the spleen

Squamous cell carcinoma, anterior tongue

DESCRIPTION Malignancy of the oral tongue that does not include the base of the tongue. Characteristics — located on lateral aspects of the undersurface of the tongue.

CAUSES
- unknown

TREATMENT
- surgery plus radiotherapy, depending on staging

ICD-9-CM
141.4 malignant neoplasm of anterior two-thirds of tongue

Squamous cell carcinoma, anus

DESCRIPTION These malignancies comprise 3-5% of rectal and anal cancers. Characteristics — fungating anal mass, tight sphincter, perineal pain and pressure. Usual course - insidious onset; surgical cure; progressive if untreated.

CAUSES
- condylomata
- rectal fistulae
- rectal fissures
- rectal abscesses
- leukoplakia of the anus
- irradiation

TREATMENT
- surgery
- radiotherapy

ICD-9-CM
154.3 malignant neoplasm of anus

Squamous cell carcinoma, bladder

DESCRIPTION Bladder malignancy frequently associated with parasitic infection or chronic mucosal irritation. Characteristics — highly infiltrative, poor prognosis, gross hematuria, dysuria. Usual course - progressive.

SYNONYMS
- epidermoid bladder carcinoma

CAUSES
- beta-naphthylamine
- 4-aminodiphenyl
- tobacco smoking
- chronic schistosoma haematobium infection
- aniline dye

TREATMENT
- endoscopic resection
- segmental bladder resection
- total cystectomy
- methotrexate
- cis-platin
- doxorubicin
- intravesical thiotepa
- preoperative radiotherapy
- supervoltage radiotherapy
- intracavitary radium
- interstitial implantations

ICD-9-CM
188.9 malignant neoplasm of the bladder

Squamous cell carcinoma, floor of the mouth

DESCRIPTION These account for 20,000 new cases of oral cancer each year. Appears most often as a red (erythroblastic) lesion at first appearing as an inflammatory lesion. Characteristics — lump in floor of the mouth; chronic, non-healing ulcer; foul breath odor; very few are indurated or raised. Usual course - progressive if not cured.

CAUSES
- tobacco
- alcohol
- poor oral hygiene
- epstein-barr virus
- chronic oral trauma
- plummer-vinson virus
- betel nut chewing

TREATMENT
- surgery plus radiotherapy depending on stage
- surgery plus radiotherapy depending on location

ICD-9-CM
144.9 malignant neoplasm of the floor of the mouth

Squamous cell
carcinoma, lung

DESCRIPTION   A type of bronchogenic carcinoma.
Characteristics — cough, hemoptysis, chest pain,
dyspnea, weight loss, fever. Usual course - usually
progressive.

SYNONYMS
• epidermoid carcinoma of the lung

CAUSES
• tobacco smoking
• radioisotopes
• asbestos
• halogen ethers
• polycyclic aromatic hydrocarbons
• tuberculosis
• nickel
• chromium
• inorganic arsenic
• iron ore
• printing inks
• other pollutants

TREATMENT
• surgery
• radiotherapy

ICD-9-CM
162.9 malignant neoplasm of the lung

 Squamous cell
carcinoma, nasopharynx

DESCRIPTION   Malignancy associated with tobacco
consumption and the Epstein-Barr virus. Characteristics —
nasal obstruction, epistaxis, tinnitus, facial pain, painless
upper neck mass, occipital and temporal headache. Usual
course - relapsing; early cure.

CAUSES
• nitrosamines
• Epstein Barr virus
• salted fish

TREATMENT
• high dose external beam radiotherapy
• surgical resection in selected patients

ICD-9-CM
147.9 malignant neoplasm of the nasopharynx

 Strabismus

DESCRIPTION   Deviation of one eye from parallelism
with the other

SYNONYMS
• Squint
• Cross eyes
• Heterotropia

CAUSES
• paralytic (nonconcomitant) strabismus - paralysis of one
or more ocular muscles. Nonparalytic (concomitant) -
unequal muscle tone.

TREATMENT
• treatment before age 6 years - complete eye exam;
corrective lenses or contact lenses; miotics; orthoptic
training; surgical restoration of muscle balance

ICD-9-CM
378.9 Unspecified disorder of eye movement

 Strongyloidiasis

DESCRIPTION   Infection with Strongyloides stercoralis
occurring widely in tropical and subtropical countries. Larvae
develop in the soil and penetrate the human skin on
contact. They travel to the lungs via the bloodstream and
thence to the trachea and esophagus and intestines. Usual
course - intermittent.

CAUSES
• parasitic infection caused by strongyloides stercorous
• penetration of the skin by larvae
• contaminated food ingestion
• autoinfection

TREATMENT
• thiabendazole

ICD-9-CM
127.2 strongyloidiasis

 Subacute combined
degeneration

DESCRIPTION   The neurologic manifestations of
pernicious anemia. Characteristics — peripheral
paresthesias, weakness, leg stiffness, unsteadiness,
lethargy, fatigue. Usual course - progressive.

SYNONYMS
• subacute combined degeneration of spinal cord
• combined system disease
• posterolateral sclerosis
• ataxic paraplegia
• neuroanemic syndrome
• funicular spinal disease
• Dana syndrome
• Putnam-Dana syndrome
• Lichtheim syndrome

CAUSES
• vitamin B12 deficiency
• pernicious anemia
• no intrinsic factor in gastric secretion

TREATMENT
• intramuscular cobalamin

ICD-9-CM
336.2 subacute combined degeneration of spinal cord in
diseases classified elsewhere

 Sulfur dioxide poisoning

DESCRIPTION   Irritant gas poisoning as an industrial
accident. Characteristics — cough, hemoptysis, wheezing,
retching, dyspnea, X-ray findings of diffuse mottled
infiltrates indicating pulmonary edema. Usual course -
acute; chronic; progressive; relapsing.

CAUSES
• cytotoxicity due to reactions between organic compounds
and nitrogen oxides
• oxidation to form sulfuric acid
• occupational exposure
• industrial cleaners

TREATMENT
• supportive
• oxygen
• bronchodilators
• eye dilution plus irrigation
• acid dilution
• analgesia
• corticosteroids
• dilute skin contact
• treat shock
• antibiotics

ICD-9-CM
987.3 poisoning, sulfur dioxide

 Sunburn

DESCRIPTION
• Characteristics - mild erythema with subsequent scaling,
pain, swelling, skin tenderness, blisters, fever, chills,
weakness, shock, secondary infections, miliaria-like
eruptions, exfoliation

CAUSES
• exposure to sunlight (or other ultraviolet light source)
following administration of phototoxicity-producing drugs
• overexposure to ultraviolet rays of UVB (2800 to 3200A);
danger increases proportionately to high altitude

TREATMENT
• prophylaxis with sunscreens rated 15 or better
• avoid additional exposure until wel
• use tap-water compresses
• avoid topical anesthetic lotions and ointments
• use oral corticosteroids for extensive, severe sunburn
(prednisone 10 mg qid for 4-6 days).

ICD-9-CM
692.71 Sunburn

 Superior sagittal sinus
thrombosis

DESCRIPTION   Blood clotting in the superior sagittal
sinus, a single venous sinus of the dura mater beginning in
front of the crista galli and extending backward in the
convex border of the falx cerebri. Characteristics — fever,
prostration, headache, obtundation, engorged scalp veins,
seizure, aphasia, hemiplegia. Usual course - acute.

SYNONYMS
• superior longitudinal sinus thrombosis

CAUSES
• infection
• extension from osteomyelitis
• dehydration
• trauma
• tumors

TREATMENT
• antimicrobials
• drainage
• surgery

ICD-9-CM
437.6 nonpyogenic thrombosis of intracranial venous sinus

 Syringomyelia

DESCRIPTION   Often associated with syringobulbia.
Fluid-filled cavity (syrinx) within the substance of the spinal
cord or brainstem.
• Characteristics - lack of sensation for noxious stimuli in
fingers (painless cut or burn). Capelike sensory defect over
shoulders and back. Spasticity and weakness of the lower
extremities. Muscular atrophy and fasciculations. Vertigo,
nystagmus

CAUSES
• congenital (50%), intramedullary tumors

TREATMENT
• surgical drainage of the syrinx; plugging obex in 4th
ventricle; section of spinal cord at filum terminale

ICD-9-CM
336.0 syringomyelia

Tabes dorsalis

DESCRIPTION Parenchymatous neurosyphilis in which there is slowly progressive degeneration of the posterior columns and roots and ganglia of the spinal cord. Occurs 15 to 20 years after initial syphilitic infection. Characteristics — lancinating lightning pains, urinary incontinence, ataxia, impaired position and vibratory sense, optic atrophy, hypotonia, hyporeflexia and trophic joint degeneration (Charcot's joints).

SYNONYMS
• tabetic neurosyphilis
• locomotor ataxia
• Duchenne's disease
• spinal cord syphilis

CAUSES
• treponema pallidum

TREATMENT
• penicillin, tetracycline, erythromycin
• anticonvulsants, carbamazepine, phenytoin
• surgery

ICD-9-CM
094.0 tabes dorsalis
094.89 other specified neurosyphilis

Takayasu syndrome

DESCRIPTION Pulseless disease. Progressive obliteration of the brachiocephalic trunk and the left subclavian and left common carotid arteries above their origin in the aortic arch. Characteristics — loss of pulse in both arms and carotids; symptoms associated with ischemia of the brain (synope, transient hemiplegia), eyes (transient blindness), face and arms. Usual course - progressive. Endemic areas - Orient.

SYNONYMS
• pulseless disease
• reverse coarctation
• Martorell syndrome
• brachiocephalic ischemia
• aortic arch syndrome

CAUSES
• unknown; autoimmune; hypersensitivity

TREATMENT
• corticosteroids
• surgery

ICD-9-CM
446.7 takayasu's disease

Tardive dyskinesia

DESCRIPTION A neurological syndrome characterized by involuntary and abnormal movements, usually involving bucco-oral muscles (but any muscle in the body can be affected). The movements include grimacing, sticking out the tongue, smacking and sucking of the lips, and sometimes, rapid movements of the arms and legs (chorea and athetosis). Tardive dyskinesia is associated with long-term use of neuroleptic drugs, usually appears late in the course of drug therapy and may persist indefinitely after discontinuation of the medication.

CAUSES
• up-regulation of dopamine receptors caused by long-term neuroleptic drug use (3 mos to years), prescribed for psychoses, also gastrointestinal and neurologic disorders

TREATMENT
• no effective treatment is available
• when possible, consider discontinuing the neuroleptic drug; some patients may prefer the movements to the possibility of relapse; also, discontinuance of the drug may not reverse tardive dyskinesia

ICD-9-CM
332.82 orofacial dyskinesia

Thallium poisoning

DESCRIPTION Poisoning due to ingestion of thallium compounds. Characteristics — vomiting, alopecia, neurologic and psychicsymptoms, (ataxia, restlessness, delirium, hallucinations, semicoma, blindness), liver and kidney damage. Thallium is commonly found in ant, rat, and roach poisons. Symptoms usually begin approximately 3 weeks after poisoning. Usual course - acute; progressive.

CAUSES
• thallium ingestion

TREATMENT
• gastric decontamination
• potassium ferric hexacyanoferrate
• skin decontamination
• forced diuresis
• hemoperfusion
• hemodialysis
• urine output maintenance
• supportive

ICD-9-CM
985.8 poisoning, thallium

Thrombocythemia (adult), idiopathic

DESCRIPTION Hemorrhagic thrombocythemia (one of the myeloproliferative syndromes). Characteristics — repeated spontaneous hemorrhages, either external or into the tissues and an extraordinary increase in the number of circulating platelets. Usual course - chronic; progressive.

SYNONYMS
• primary thrombocythemia
• essential thrombocythemia
• primary hemorrhagic thrombocythemia
• essential thrombocytosis
• primary thrombohemorrhagic thrombocytosis

CAUSES
• clonal megakaryocytic disorder

TREATMENT
• chemotherapy
• radiotherapy
• iron replacement
• plateletpheresis
• platelet anti-aggregating agents

ICD-9-CM
238.7 idiopathic thrombocythemia

Thymoma, malignant

DESCRIPTION Tumor derived from the epithelial or lymphoid elements of the thymus. Characteristics — cough, dyspnea, dysphagia, chest pain, weakness. Usual course - possibly acute; otherwise progressive.

CAUSES
• unknown

TREATMENT
• surgical thymectomy
• radiotherapy for invasive thymoma
• corticosteroids if radiotherapy fails
• chemotherapy for advanced disease

ICD-9-CM
164.0 malignant neoplasm of the thymus

Thyrotoxic heart disease

DESCRIPTION Heart disease associated with hyperthyroidism. Characteristics — atrial fibrillation, cardiac enlargement, congestive heart failure. Usual course - progressive; relapsing.

SYNONYMS
• hyperthyroid heart disease

CAUSES
• hyperthyroidism

TREATMENT
• treat underlying hyperthyroidism
• radioactive iodine
• surgery
• beta-adrenergic blockers

ICD-9-CM
242.9; 425.7 thyrotoxic heart failure

Thyrotoxic storm

DESCRIPTION Severe thyrotoxicosis accompanied by organ system decompensation. Characteristics — fever, severe tachycardia, dehydration, mental status abnormalities representing dysfunction of the cardiovascular and central nervous systems. Usual course - acute.

SYNONYMS
• thyrotoxicosis
• thyrotoxic crisis
• basedow crisis

CAUSES
• exacerbation of hyperthyroidism
• thyroid surgery
• infection
• trauma

TREATMENT
• fluids
• propylthiouracil
• iodine
• hydrocortisone
• external cooling
• beta-adrenergic blockers
• oxygen
• treat precipitating factors

ICD-9-CM
242.91 thyrotoxicosis without mention of goiter or other cause, with mention of thyrotoxic crisis or storm

Tinea barbae

DESCRIPTION Fungal infection involving the bearded area of the face and neck. Characteristics — kerion-like swellings and nodular swellings with marked crusting. Usual course - acute; chronic.

SYNONYMS
• tinea sycosis
• barber's itch
• beard ringworm

CAUSES
• fungal infection of coarse facial hair
• zoophilic dermatophytes

TREATMENT
• systemic antifungal agents
• systemic steroid added in severe inflammatory infections

ICD-9-CM
110.0 tinea barbae

Tinnitus

DESCRIPTION   A very common condition typified by the perception of sound in the absence of an acoustic stimulus. The sound may be of a buzzing, ringing, roaring, whistling or hissing quality or may involve more complex sounds that vary over time. It may be intermittent, continuous or pulsatile (synchronous with the heartbeat).

CAUSES
• damage to inner ear or cochlea
• middle ear infection or result from just about any ear disorder
• aneurysm's
• hardening of the arteries
• several medications

TREATMENT
• treat the underlying cause
• background music
• tinnitus masking device
• hearing aid for associated deafness

ICD-9-CM
388.3 tinnitus

Toluene poisoning

DESCRIPTION   A form of poisoning from toluene, a colorless liquid obtainable from coal tar. Toluene is an organic solvent used in rubber, plastic cements, paint removers, etc. Poisoning may result from inhalation or ingestion. Usual course - acute; chronic; progressive.

SYNONYMS
• toluol poisoning
• methylbenzene poisoning
• methylbenzol poisoning
• phenylmethane poisoning

CAUSES
• cytotoxicity

TREATMENT
• supportive; oxygen; bicarbonate
• CPR; gastric decontamination; skin decontamination; eye irrigation
• epinephrine contraindicated

ICD-9-CM
982.0 poisoning, toluene

Toxaphene poisoning

DESCRIPTION   Poisoning among agricultural workers using DDT. Characteristics — vomiting, paresthesias, malaise, course tremors, convulsions, pulmonary edema, ventricular fibrillation, respiratory failure. Usual course - acute; chronic; progressive.

SYNONYMS
• chlorinated camphene poisoning

CAUSES
• direct cytotoxicity
• diffuse neuronal excitation

TREATMENT
• gastric decontamination
• skin decontamination
• oxygen
• anticonvulsants
• avoid sympathomimetics
• supportive

ICD-9-CM
989.2 poisoning, toxaphene

Trachoma

DESCRIPTION   Chronic infectious disease of the conjunctiva and cornea. Characteristics — photophobia, pain, lacrimation. The organism is a bacterium, Chlamydia trachomatis. Usual course - acute; progressive. Endemic areas - Africa; Middle East; Asia; Central America.

SYNONYMS
• granular conjunctivitis
• Egyptian ophthalmia

CAUSES
• Chlamydia trachomatis
• transmission through birth canal

TREATMENT
• tetracyclines
• erythromycin
• sulfonamides

ICD-9-CM
076 trachoma
076.0 trachoma, initial stage
076.9 trachoma, unspecified

Transposition of the great vessels

DESCRIPTION   A congenital heart defect where the great arteries are reversed - the aorta arises from the right ventricle and the pulmonary artery from the left ventricle. This produces two noncommunicating circulatory systems (pulmonary and systemic. It often coexists with other congenital anomalies and affects boys 2 to 3 times more than females. Usual course - acute.

SYNONYMS
• complete dextrotransposition of the great arteries

CAUSES
• abnormal embryogenesis

TREATMENT
• balloon septostomy
• surgical redirection

ICD-9-CM
745.10 complete transposition of the great vessels

Trench fever

DESCRIPTION   Louse-borne disease occurring sporadically in Eastern Europe, Asia, North Africa and Mexico and producing multiple symptoms: fever, weakness, dizziness, severe leg and back pain.

SYNONYMS
• Wolhynia fever
• shin bone fever
• His-werner disease
• quintana fever

CAUSES
• Rochalimaea quintana transmitted by body lice

TREATMENT
• analgesics
• antipyretics
• delousing

ICD-9-CM
083.1 trench fever

Trichloroethylene poisoning

DESCRIPTION   Trichloroethylene is a widely used industrial solvent and formerly used as an inhalation anesthetic. Poisoning characteristics: dizziness, headache, delirium, vomiting, abdominal pain, jaundice, flush. Usual course - acute; chronic; progressive.

CAUSES
• decomposition to dichloroethylene
• decomposition to phosgene
• decomposition to carbon monoxide
• hepatotoxicity
• renal toxicity

TREATMENT
• supportive
• gastric decontamination
• remove contaminated clothing
• epinephrine contraindicated
• volume expanders
• diuretics for urine output maintenance

ICD-9-CM
982.3 poisoning, trichloroethylene

Trichostrongyliasis

DESCRIPTION   Infection by nematodes of the genus Trichostrongylus whose eggs are frequently mistaken for hookworms. Endemic areas - Middle East; Far East; Iran. Usually asymptomatic but may cause cramps and diarrhea. Usual course - acute.

SYNONYMS
• trichostrongyloidiasis

CAUSES
• trichostrongylus larvae ingestion

TREATMENT
• thiabendazole
• pyrantel pamoate

ICD-9-CM
127.6 trichostrongyliasis

Tricuspid atresia

DESCRIPTION   Absence of the orifice between the right atrium and ventricle. Circulation made possible by presence of an atrial septal defect, allowing blood to pass from the right to left atrium and then to the left ventricle and aorta. Intra-atrial communication due to anomalous embryonal development.
• Signs and symptoms include marked underdevelopment, severe cyanosis, clubbing of fingers, prominent jugular A wave, apical heave, pulmonic second sound absent, systolic murmur, enlarged liver, presystolic pulsation. EKG shows left axis deviation, left ventricular hypertrophy, tall P waves. Transposition of great vessels, patent foramen ovale and ventricular septal defect all may accompany tricuspid atresia.

CAUSES
• unknown

TREATMENT
• anticongestive therapy
• surgery to correct condition

ICD-9-CM
746.1 tricuspid valve atresia

Tricuspid regurgitation

DESCRIPTION Retrograde blood flow from the right ventricle to the right atrium due to inadequate apposition of the tricuspid valves. Characteristics — low output symptoms plus pulsations in the neck due to high jugular regurgitant waves from the transmitted right ventricular pressure. Usual course - acute; chronic.

SYNONYMS
• tricuspid valve insufficiency

CAUSES
• marked dilatation of right ventricle
• right ventricular failure
• rheumatic heart disease
• cor pulmonale
• congenital heart disease

TREATMENT
• treat underlying condition
• surgery
• tricuspid annuloplasty
• tricuspid valve replacement

ICD-9-CM
424.2 tricuspid valve insufficiency (nonrheumatic)

Tricuspid stenosis

DESCRIPTION Narrowing of the tricuspid orifice obstructing blood flow from the right atrium to the right ventricle. Characteristics — fatigue, enlarged liver, fluttering discomfort in the neck caused by giant A waves in the jugular pulse. Usual course - chronic; progressive.

SYNONYMS
• tricuspid valve stenosis

CAUSES
• rheumatic fever
• bacterial vegetations
• atrial thrombi
• tumors
• carcinoid heart disease
• fibroelastosis

TREATMENT
• sodium restriction
• digitalization
• diuretics
• surgery
• valvulotomy

ICD-9-CM
397.0 disease of tricuspid valve
424.2 tricuspid valve disorders, specified as nonrheumatic
746.1 tricuspid atresia and stenosis, congenital

Tropical eosinophilia

DESCRIPTION Subacute or chronic form of filariasis. Characteristics — episodic nocturnal wheezing and coughing, strikingly elevated eosinophilia and lung infiltrations. Usual course - chronic; progressive.

CAUSES
• adult wuchereria bancrofti worms
• adult brugia malayi worms

TREATMENT
• diethylcarbamazine

ICD-9-CM
518.3 tropical eosinophilia

Truncus arteriosus

DESCRIPTION Congenital anomaly in which there is a single arterial trunk arising from the heart, receiving blood from both ventricles and supplying blood to the coronary, pulmonary, and systemic circulations. Frequently co-exists with malformations of other organ systems.
• Characteristics - signs and symptoms begin during the first week of life and include poor development, minimal or absent cyanosis, marked hypertrophy of the heart, loud and clear second sound, harsh systolic murmur at the base and along the left sternal border, continuous bruit over the upper sternum, thrill with maximum intensity over base of the heart, dyspnea, wide pulse pressure.

CAUSES
• unknown

TREATMENT
• surgery
• anticongestive therapy

ICD-9-CM
745.0 truncus arteriosus

Trypanosomiasis, East African

DESCRIPTION Acute, severe, sometimes fatal form of African trypanosomiasis, transmitted by bites of tsetse flies. Usual course - acute; progressive; lethal within 1 year. Endemic areas - tropical East Africa.

SYNONYMS
• sleeping sickness
• Rhodesian sleeping sickness

CAUSES
• Trypanosoma brucei rhodesiense
• tsetse fly bites
• bushbuck antelope reservoir of infection

TREATMENT
• suramin prior to CNS involvement
• pentamidine prior to CNS involvement
• melarsoprol plus suramin pretreatment for CNS disease

ICD-9-CM
086.4 Rhodesian trypanosomiasis

Trypanosomiasis, West African

DESCRIPTION Chronic, less severe form of African trypanosomiasis. Disease persists for several months or years with central nervous system involvement late in its course. Usual course - chronic; intermittent; relapsing; progressive; delayed onset; successive bouts; intervening latent periods; may persist many years. Endemic areas - tropical West Africa; Central Africa.

SYNONYMS
• sleeping sickness
• Gambian sleeping sickness

CAUSES
• Trypanosoma brucei gambiense
• tsetse fly bites
• transplacental transmission
• human reservoir

TREATMENT
• suramin prior to CNS involvement
• pentamidine prior to CNS involvement
• melarsoprol plus suramin pretreatment for CNS disease

ICD-9-CM
086.3 Gambian trypanosomiasis

Tubular necrosis, acute

DESCRIPTION Acute renal tubular necrosis is a syndrome with multiple causes accounting for 70% of renal failure patients. Types include - stage 1: onset azotemia; stage 2: oliguria; stage 3: diuresis; stage 4: resolving diuresis
Usual course - acute; reversible;

SYNONYMS
• lower nephron nephrosis
• vasomotor nephropathy

CAUSES
• ischemia
• disseminated intravascular coagulation
• nephrotoxins
• trauma
• dehydration
• circulatory insufficiency

TREATMENT
• hemodialysis
• maintain renal perfusion
• maintain euvolemia
• diuretics
• vasopressors
• alkalinization

ICD-9-CM
584.5 acute renal failure with lesion of tubular necrosis

Uterine bleeding postmenopausal

DESCRIPTION Bleeding from female genital tract beginning one or more years following menopause. Characteristics - may occur from any part of the reproductive tract including uterus, cervix, vagina, vulva; bleeding may be heavy or light.

CAUSES
• Iatrogenic as a result of estrogen replacement therapy
• Infection, atrophy, tumors (benign or malignant), polyps, adnexal pathology. Endometrial carcinoma is the cause of 1/3 of all cases of postmenopausal bleeding.

TREATMENT
• D&C
• discontinue all exogenous estrogens, including creams, etc.
• definitive treatment depends on finding and treating underlying cause

ICD-9-CM
627.1 postclimacteric bleeding

Ventricular fibrillation

DESCRIPTION Ventricular rhythm rapid and chaotic. QRS complexes wide and irregular.

CAUSES
• myocardial infarction or ischemia, untreated ventricular tachycardia, electrolyte imbalances, digitalis or quinidine toxicity, electric shock, hypothermia

TREATMENT
• if pulse is absent, follow protocol using defibrillation, epinephrine, lidocaine, bretylium. Pronestyl, and sodium bicarbonate as indicated.

ICD-9-CM
427.41 ventricular fibrillation

Ventricular standstill

DESCRIPTION No QRS complexes. Symptoms include loss of consciousness. No peripheral pulses, blood pressure or respirations. Death.

SYNONYMS
• Asystole

CAUSES
• myocardial infarction or ischemia, untreated ventricular tachycardia, electrolyte imbalances, digitalis or quinidine toxicity, electric shock, hypothermia

TREATMENT
• follow protocol using epinephrine, defibrillation, lidocaine, bretylium. Pronestyl, and sodium bicarbonate as indicated.

ICD-9-CM
427.5 Asystole

 ## Ventricular tachycardia (VT)

DESCRIPTION Symptoms include chest pain, anxiety, palpitations, dyspnea, shock, coma, death. Ventricular rate usually regular at 140-220 beats per minute. QRS complexes are wide and bizarre.

CAUSES
• myocardial ischemia, infarction, or aneurysm, ventricular catheters, drug toxicity (digitalis or quinidine), hypokalemia, hypercalcemia, anxiety

TREATMENT
• lidocaine bolus if pulse is present. If pulse is absent, follow protocol using defibrillation, epinephrine, lidocaine, bretylium, Pronestyl, and sodium bicarbonate as indicated.

ICD-9-CM
427.1 ventricular tachycardia

 ## Vernal keratoconjunctivitis

DESCRIPTION Bilateral conjunctivitis associated with corneal epithelial changes. Most likely to occur in spring and fall in males aged 5-20.
• Characteristics - signs and symptoms include tearing; intense itching; redness of the conjunctiva; and a tenacious, mucoid discharge containing numerous eosinophils. Symptoms usually disappear during cold months.

CAUSES
• allergies (probably)

TREATMENT
• topical corticosteroid drops, (e.g., 0.1% dexamethasone drops q 2 h) with supplemental small oral doses if needed
• long-term maintenance treatment with 0.25 prednisolone acetate applied bid
• remember to check ocular pressure if steroids are needed for more than a few weeks

ICD-9-CM
372.13 vernal conjunctivitis

 ## Von Gierke's disease

DESCRIPTION An autosomal recessive glycogen storage disease, (Type Ia) Glucose-6-phosphatase deficiency affecting liver and kidneys. Characteristics — hepatomegaly, hypoglycemia, hyperuricaemia, xanthomas, bleeding, adiposity. Patients live into adulthood. May lead to symptomatic hypoglycemia. Patients needed added precautions when taking many drugs. Usual course - chronic; progressive.

SYNONYMS
• glucose-6-phosphatase deficiency type Ia
• hepatorenal glycogen storage disease

CAUSES
• genetic enzyme deficiency

TREATMENT
• frequent feeding
• allopurinol

ICD-9-CM
271.0 Von Gierke's disease

 ## Von Hippel-Lindau disease

DESCRIPTION One of the neurocutaneous syndromes (phakomatoses). 20% autosomal dominant chronic disease with variable expression. Characteristics - headache, loss of vision, unilateral ataxia, dizziness, retinal detachment, papilledema, macular star. Usual course - chronic.

SYNONYMS
• angioblastomatosis
• cerebelloretinal hemangioblastomatosis
• angiophakomatosis retinae et cerebelli

CAUSES
• genetic

TREATMENT
• surgery
• radiotherapy

ICD-9-CM
759.6 Von Hippel-Lindau disease

 ## Von Willebrand's disease

DESCRIPTION Group of hemorrhagic disorders in which the von Willebrand factor is either quantitatively or qualitatively abnormal. Usually inherited as an autosomal dominant trait though rare kindreds are autosomal recessive. Symptoms vary depending on severity and disease type but may include prolonged bleeding time, deficiency of factor VIII, and impaired platelet adhesion. Usual course - chronic.

SYNONYMS
• pseudohemophilia
• vascular hemophilia
• angiohemophilia

CAUSES
• no factor VIII associated proteins
• decreased factor VIII associated proteins activity

TREATMENT
• factor VIII replacement
• epsilon-aminocaproic acid
• DDAVP
• oral contraceptives to suppress menses

ICD-9-CM
286.4 von Willebrand's disease

 ## Waldenstrom's macroglobulinemia

DESCRIPTION Malignant neoplasm of cells with lymphocytic, plasmacytic or intermediate morphology which secrete an IgM M component. Usual course - slowly progressive; death 3-10 years. Genetics - slight increased familial incidence.

CAUSES
• IgM M-component secretion

TREATMENT
• chlorambucil
• plasmapheresis for hyperviscosity
• prednisone

ICD-9-CM
273.3 Waldenstrom's macroglobulinemia

 ## Werner's syndrome

DESCRIPTION Premature senility in an adult. Characteristics — early graying and some hair loss, cataracts, hyperkeratinization, and scleroderma-like changes in the skin of the lower extremities. Usual course - chronic.

SYNONYMS
• adult progeria
• progeria adultorum

CAUSES
• altered glycosaminoglycan turnover
• chromosomal instability

TREATMENT
• symptomatic

ICD-9-CM
259.8 Werner's disease or syndrome

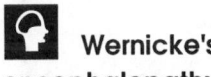 ## Wernicke's encephalopathy

DESCRIPTION Acute, subacute, or chronic neurological disorder. Characteristics — confusion, apathy, drowsiness, atoxic, nystagmus, ophthalmoplegia. Most commonly results from chronic alcohol abuse and accompanied by organic amnesia and other nutritional polyneuropathies. Usual course - acute; subacute; chronic.

SYNONYMS
• Wernicke syndrome
• Wernicke's disease
• Gayet-Wernicke syndrome

CAUSES
• thiamine deficiency

TREATMENT
• intravenous thiamine supplementation
• supportive measures

ICD-9-CM
265.1 Wernicke's encephalopathy

Neurofibromatosis

DESCRIPTION One of the neurocutaneous syndromes (phakomatoses). Clinical manifestation vary, but ususally include cafe-au-lait spots (more than 6 of over 1.5cm in diameter), neurofibromas (which degenerate into sarcomas in 10% of patients). Multiple associated congenital abnormalities have been described.

SYNONYMS
• von Recklinghausen disease

CAUSES
• congenital; autosomal dominant trait

TREATMENT
• Tumor excision as needed for pain or malignant transformation

ICD-9-CM
237.7 neurofibromatosis

 ## Sturge-Weber disease

DESCRIPTION One of the neurocutaneous syndromes (phakomatoses). Congenital capillary hemangiomas affect the skin of the face and neck, mucous membranes, meninges, and choroid. Anoxic injury to the cerebral cortex may occur resulting in seizure activity, mental retardation, and/or hemiparesis or hemianopsia.

SYNONYMS
• encephalotrigeminal angiomatosis

CAUSES
• congenital

TREATMENT
• anticonvulsants
• monitoring for glaucoma

ICD-9-CM
759.6 other hamartoses, NEC

 ## Whipple's disease

DESCRIPTION A malabsorption disorder. Characteristics — diarrhea, steatorrhea, skin pigmentation, arthralgia, arthritis, lymphadenopathy, and central nervous system lesions. Usual course - progressive; curative with treatment.

SYNONYMS
• lipophagic intestinal granulomatosis
• intestinal lipodystrophy
• secondary nontropical sprue

CAUSES
• probable bacterial infection

TREATMENT
• penicillin G
• ampicillin
• tetracycline
• corticosteroids

ICD-9-CM
040.2 Whipple's disease

 ## Wilson's disease

DESCRIPTION An inherited metabolic disorder characterized by excessive amounts of copper in the liver, brain, kidneys, and corneas. It can lead to tissue necrosis and fibrosis, which in turn can cause hepatic disease and neurologic changes. Without treament, it leads to fatal hepatic failure. Usual course - chronic.

SYNONYMS
• progressive lenticular degeneration
• Westphal-Struempell pseudosclerosis

CAUSES
• genetic

TREATMENT
• avoid copper-rich foods
• penicillamine, potassium sulfide, pyridoxine, zinc acetate as alternative to penicillamine

ICD-9-CM
275.1 Wilson's disease

 ## Wolff-Parkinson-White syndrome

DESCRIPTION A form of pre-excitation characterized by a short PR interval and long QRS interval with a delta wave associated with paroxysmal tachycardia (or atrial fibrillation). Usual course - intermittent.

SYNONYMS
• preexcitation syndrome
• anomalous atrioventricular excitation

CAUSES
• accessory atrioventricular pathway
• circus movement conduction due to AV reentrant tachycardia

TREATMENT
• vagal maneuvers
• antiarrhythmic agents
• cardioversion
• electrical pacing
• surgical ablation

ICD-9-CM
426.7 Wolff-Parkinson-White syndrome

 ## Yaws

DESCRIPTION Non-venereal, infectious, tropical disease usually affecting persons under the age of 15. Spread by direct contact. Characteristics — painless papule that grows into a papilloma. The papule heals, leaving a scar. Late manifestations: deforming lesions of bones, joints, and skin. Usual course - chronic; progressive. Endemic areas - tropical regions.

SYNONYMS
• frambesia
• buba
• pian

CAUSES
• skin contact
• treponema pertenue

TREATMENT
• penicillin

ICD-9-CM
102.9 yaws

 ## Yellow fever

DESCRIPTION An acute infectious disease primarily of the tropics, caused by a virus and transmitted to man by mosquitoes of the genus Aedes and Haemagogus. Usual course - acute. Endemic areas - Africa; South America.

CAUSES
• flavivirus
• mosquito bite
• Aedes aegypti

TREATMENT
• fluid replacement
• supportive therapy
• treatment for complications

ICD-9-CM
060.9 yellow fever

 ## Yersinia enterocolitica infection

DESCRIPTION Gram negative, facultatively anaerobic bacteria causing acute gastroenteritis and mesenteric lymphadenitis in children, and arthritis, septicemia, and erythema nodosum in adults. Transmitted through food, water, and person-to-person contact. Usual course - acute.

SYNONYMS
• yersinosis
• pasteurella pseudotuberculosis infection

CAUSES
• contaminated food ingestion

TREATMENT
• streptomycin
• gentamycin
• tetracycline
• chloramphenicol
• sulfamethoxazole-trimethoprim
• fluid replacement

ICD-9-CM
027.2 pasteurellosis

 ## Zygomycosis

DESCRIPTION Fungal infection typically seen in immunocompromised or debilitated patients. In healthy individuals, the organisms seldom cause infection. Several forms exist - gastrointestinal, rhinocerebral, disseminated mucormycosis, pulmonary, cutaneous, central nervous system. Prognosis is guarded.

SYNONYMS
• phycomycosis
• mucormycosis

CAUSES
• fungi of the class Zygomycetes

TREATMENT
• amphoterecin B
• surgical removal of necrotic tissue

ICD-9-CM
117.7 zygomycosis

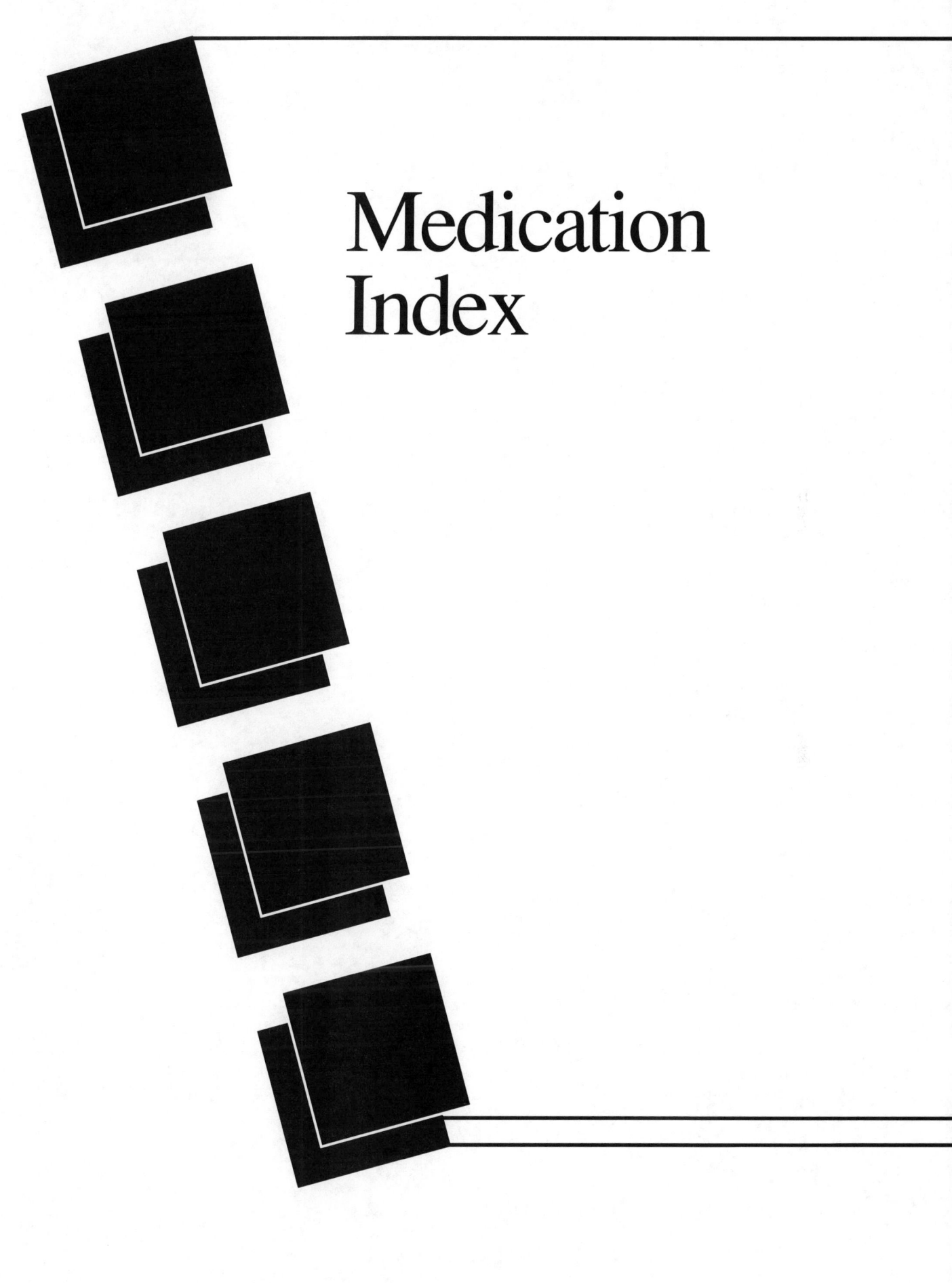

Medication
Index

Medication Index

acarbose
    Diabetes mellitus, non-insulin dependent (NIDDM)
    Hypoglycemia, diabetic
Accutane, see isotretinoin
acebutolol
    Hypertension, essential
acetaminophen
    Adenovirus infections
    Anemia, sickle cell
    Arthritis, osteo
    Blastomycosis
    Cervical spondylosis
    Costochondritis
    Cryptococcosis
    Fever of unknown origin (FUO)
    Herpangina
    Herpes zoster
    Influenza
    Mastalgia
    Measles, rubella
    Meningitis, viral
    Mononucleosis
    Mumps
    Osteonecrosis
    Pancreatitis
    Premenstrual syndrome (PMS)
    Roseola
    Scarlet fever
    Seizures, febrile
acetaminophen-butalbital
    Migraine
acetaminophen-butalbital-codeine
    Migraine
acetaminophen-codeine
    Anemia, sickle cell
    Epididymitis
    Meningitis, viral
    Renal calculi
acetazolamide
    Altitude illness
    Cryptococcosis
    Glaucoma, chronic open-angle
    Glaucoma, primary angle-closure
    Hypokalemic periodic paralysis
    Ocular chemical burns
    Pulmonary edema
    Retinitis pigmentosa
    Sleep apnea, obstructive
acetic acid
    Otitis externa
acetylcholine
    Primary pulmonary hypertension
acetylcysteine
    Acetaminophen poisoning
    Ocular chemical burns
Achromycin, see tetracycline
acrivastine
    Angioedema
    Urticaria
ACTH
    Dyshidrosis
    Gout
    Multiple sclerosis
Actigall, see ursodiol
Actinex, see masoprocol

actinomycin-D, see dactinomycin
Activase, see alteplase
activated charcoal
    Acetaminophen poisoning
    Salicylate poisoning
acyclovir
    Cervicitis
    Chickenpox
    Conjunctivitis
    Encephalitis, viral
    Erythema multiforme
    Herpes eye infections
    Herpes simplex
    Herpes zoster
    Herpes, genital
    Pneumonia, viral
    Proctitis
    Stevens-Johnson syndrome
Adapin, see doxepin
adenine arabinoside, see vidarabine
adenosine
    Primary pulmonary hypertension
adrenocorticotropic hormone, see ACTH
Adriamycin, see doxorubicin
Advil, see ibuprofen
AeroBid, see flunisolide
Afrin 12-Hour, see oxymetazoline
Afrin, see oxymetazoline
Afrinol, see pseudoephedrine
Albalon-A, see antazoline
albendazole
    Giardiasis
    Intestinal parasites
    Pinworms
    Pruritus ani
    Roundworms, intestinal
    Roundworms, tissue
    Tapeworm infestation
    Trichinosis
albumin
    Nephrotic syndrome
    Subdural hematoma
albuterol
    Anaphylaxis
    Asthma
    Bronchiectasis
    Chronic obstructive pulmonary disease & emphysema
    Cor pulmonale
    Near drowning
    Pneumonia, mycoplasma
    Respiratory syncytial virus (RSV) infection
alcohol-sulfur
    Acne rosacea
Aldactone, see spironolactone
alendronate
    Menopause
    Osteitis deformans
    Osteoporosis
Aleve, see naproxen
alfacalcidol
    Osteomalacia & rickets
Alkeran, see melphalan
all-trans-retinoic acid
    Leukemia
    Myelodysplastic syndromes (MDS)

Medication Index

Medication Index

Medication Index

Medication Index

Cardiac arrest
Diabetic ketoacidosis (DKA)
Salicylate poisoning
Bicillin LA, see penicillin, benzathine
bisacodyl
Constipation
Encopresis
bismuth subsalicylate
Diarrhea, acute
Peptic ulcer disease
bisoprolol
Hypertension, essential
bitolterol
Asthma
bleomycin
Bone tumor, primary malignant
Cervical malignancy
Hodgkin's disease
Kaposi's sarcoma
Pleural effusion
Testicular malignancies
Warts
Blocadren, see timolol
Bonine, see meclizine
boric acid
Vulvovaginitis, candidal
Botox, see botulinum toxin
botulinum toxin
Cerebral palsy
Stroke rehabilitation
Torticollis
Brethaire, see terbutaline
bretylium
Cardiac arrest
Hypothermia
British anti-Lewisite, see dimercaprol
bromocriptine
Amenorrhea
Brain injury, traumatic
Erectile dysfunction
Fertility problems
Fibrocystic breast disease
Galactorrhea
Hepatic encephalopathy
Hyperprolactinemia
Mastalgia
Parkinson's disease
Polycystic ovarian disease
Premenstrual syndrome (PMS)
brompheniramine
Rhinitis, allergic
budesonide
Laryngotracheobronchitis
Rhinitis, allergic
bumetanide
Hypertension, essential
Pulmonary edema
Buprenex, see buprenorphine
buprenorphine
Urolithiasis
bupropion
Depression
Post-traumatic stress disorder (PTSD)
Suicide
burrow's solution

Neurodermatitis
BuSpar, see buspirone
buspirone
Anxiety
Autism
Brain injury, traumatic
Dissociative disorders
Diverticular disease
Post-traumatic stress disorder (PTSD)
Premenstrual syndrome (PMS)
busulfan
Leukemia
Polycythemia vera
butoconazole
Onychomycosis
Vulvovaginitis, candidal
butorphanol
Migraine
C1-INH
Angioedema
C3F8, see perfluoropropane
cabergoline
Galactorrhea
Hyperprolactinemia
Cafergot, see ergotamine-caffeine
calamine lotion
Dermatitis, contact
Calan, see verapamil
Calcimar, see calcitonin
calcipotriene
Psoriasis
calcitonin
Hypercalcemia associated with malignancy
Osteitis deformans
Osteoporosis
calcitriol
Hypoparathyroidism
Osteomalacia & rickets
Vitamin deficiency
calcium
Endometriosis
Osteomalacia & rickets
Osteoporosis
Premenstrual syndrome (PMS)
calcium acetate
Renal failure, chronic
calcium carbonate
Glomerulonephritis, acute
calcium gluconate
Glomerulonephritis, acute
Hyperkalemia
Hypernatremia
Hypoparathyroidism
Otosclerosis (otospongiosis)
Rhabdomyolysis
calcium thioglycolate
Pseudofolliculitis barbae
cantharidin
Warts, plantar
Cantharone, see cantharidin
capsaicin
Arthritis, osteo
Bursitis
Herpes eye infections
Herpes zoster

Medication Index

Medication Index

Medication Index

Medication Index

Subphrenic abscess
Tetanus
Toxic shock syndrome
Toxoplasmosis
Tracheitis, bacterial
Vulvovaginitis, bacterial
Clinoril, see sulindac
clioquinol-hydrocortisone
    Dermatitis, diaper
clobetasol
    Dupuytren's contracture
    Neurodermatitis
    Psoriasis
    Vitiligo
clofazimine
    Leprosy
clofibrate
    Diabetes insipidus
    Hypertriglyceridemia
clomiphene
    Artificial insemination
    Fertility problems
    Polycystic ovarian disease
clomipramine
    Anxiety
    Autism
    Depression
    Dissociative disorders
    Hypochondriasis
    Obsessive compulsive disorder
    Post-traumatic stress disorder (PTSD)
    Premenstrual syndrome (PMS)
clonazepam
    Anxiety
    Causalgia syndrome
    Multiple sclerosis
    Porphyria
    Seizure disorders
    Trigeminal neuralgia
clonidine
    Alcoholism
    Attention deficit hyperactivity disorder
    Hypertension, essential
    Hypertensive emergencies
    Post-traumatic stress disorder (PTSD)
    Substance abuse
    Tourette's syndrome
clotrimazole
    Balanitis
    Candidiasis, mucocutaneous
    Corneal ulceration
    Dermatitis, diaper
    Glossitis
    Onychomycosis
    Pressure ulcer
    Tinea corporis
    Tinea cruris
    Tinea pedis
    Tinea versicolor
    Trichomoniasis
    Vulvovaginitis, candidal
    Vulvovaginitis, prepubescent
cloxacillin
    Furunculosis
    Paronychia

clozapine
    Parkinson's disease
    Schizophrenia
Clozaril, see clozapine
Co-trimoxazole, see trimethoprim-sulfamethoxazole
coal tar
    Dermatitis, atopic
    Dermatitis, seborrheic
    Dyshidrosis
    Pityriasis alba
    Psoriasis
cobalamin
    Vitamin deficiency
cocaine
    Epistaxis
cod liver oil
    Vitamin deficiency
codeine
    Altitude illness
    Arthritis, osteo
    Common cold
    Epstein-Barr virus infections
    Herpes zoster
    Mononucleosis
    Narcolepsy
    Sialadenitis
    Thyroiditis
Cogentin, see benztropine
Cognex, see tacrine
Colace, see docusate sodium
colchicine
    Amyloidosis
    Behçet's syndrome
    Gout
    Pericarditis
    Pseudogout (CPPD)
Colestid, see colestipol
colestipol
    Arteriosclerotic heart disease
    Hypercholesterolemia
colfosceril
    Respiratory distress syndrome, neonatal
collagenase
    Pressure ulcer
Colyte, see polyethylene glycol
Compazine, see prochlorperazine
Condylox, see podofilox
copolymer-1
    Multiple sclerosis
Cordarone, see amiodarone
Corgard, see nadolol
Cortenema, see hydrocortisone
corticosteroids
    Hepatitis, viral
Cortisporin, see neomycin-polymyxin B-hydrocortisone
cotrimoxazole
    Furunculosis
Coumadin, see warfarin
Creon, see pancreatic enzyme
Crixivan, see indinavir
cromoglycate
    Ulcerative colitis
cromolyn
    Asthma
cromolyn sodium

Medication Index

Medication Index

demecarium
   Glaucoma, chronic open-angle
demeclocycline
   Hyponatremia
   Inappropriate secretion of antidiuretic hormone
Demerol, see meperidine
Demser, see metyrosine
Denavir, see pencyclovir
Depakene, see valproic acid
Depakote, see divalproex
Depen, see penicillamine
Depo-Medrol, see methylprednisolone
Depo-Provera, see medroxyprogesterone
Desenex, see undecylenic acid
Desferal, see deferoxamine
desflurane
   Status epilepticus
desipramine
   Anorexia nervosa
   Brain injury, traumatic
   Bulimia nervosa
   Dementia
   Depression
   Enuresis
   Headache, tension
   Post-traumatic stress disorder (PTSD)
desmopressin
   Diabetes insipidus
   Enuresis
   Hemophilia
   Hypernatremia
   Urinary incontinence
Desogen, see desogestrel-ethinyl estradiol
desogestrel-ethinyl estradiol
   Contraception
desoximetasone
   Pruritus vulvae
Desyrel, see trazodone
dexamethasone
   Altitude illness
   Brain abscess
   Hirsutism
   Laryngotracheobronchitis
   Leukemia, acute lymphoblastic in adults (ALL)
   Meningitis, bacterial
   Meningococcemia
   Multiple myeloma
   Premature labor
   Reye's syndrome
   Uveitis
Dexedrine, see dextroamphetamine
dexfenfluramine
   Obesity
dextroamphetamine
   Attention deficit hyperactivity disorder
   Narcolepsy
dextromethorphan
   Common cold
DHE, see dihydroergotamine
Diabeta, see glyburide
Diabinese, see chlorpropamide
Diamox, see acetazolamide
diazepam
   Alcoholism
   Anxiety

   Bruxism
   Cerebral palsy
   Decompression sickness
   Eclampsia (toxemia of pregnancy)
   Insect bites & stings
   Labyrinthitis
   Lead poisoning
   Ménière's disease
   Multiple sclerosis
   Preeclampsia
   Status epilepticus
   Stroke rehabilitation
   Tetanus
   Torticollis
diazoxide
   Hypertensive emergencies
   Insulinoma
   Preeclampsia
Dibenzyline, see phenoxybenzamine
dibucaine
   Hemorrhoids
dichloroacetic acid
   Warts
   Warts, plantar
dichlorphenamide
   Glaucoma, chronic open-angle
diclofenac
   Cholecystitis
   Costochondritis
dicloxacillin
   Dermatitis, atopic
   Dermatitis, seborrheic
   Folliculitis
   Furunculosis
   Miliaria rubra
   Paronychia
   Vulvovaginitis, prepubescent
dicyclomine
   Irritable bowel syndrome
   Urinary incontinence
didanosine
   HIV infection & AIDS
Didronel, see etidronate
diethylcarbamazine
   Eosinophilic pneumonias
   Roundworms, tissue
diethylpropion
   Obesity
Diflucan, see fluconazole
Digibind, see digoxin Immune Fab
digoxin
   Atrial fibrillation
   Cardiomyopathy, end stage
   Complete atrioventricular (AV) canal
   Congestive heart failure
   Cor pulmonale
   Mitral stenosis
   Primary pulmonary hypertension
   Pulmonary edema
   Ventricular septal defect (VSD)
digoxin Immune Fab
   Digitalis toxicity
dihydroergotamine
   Headache, cluster
   Migraine

Medication Index

dihydrotachysterol, see vitamin D
diiodohydroxyquin
    Amebiasis
Dilantin, see phenytoin
diloxanide
    Amebiasis
    Intestinal parasites
diltiazem
    Angina
    Atrial fibrillation
    Cor pulmonale
    Hypertension, essential
    Idiopathic hypertrophic subaortic stenosis (IHSS)
    Primary pulmonary hypertension
    Raynaud's phenomenon
dimenhydrinate
    Hyperemesis gravidarum
    Ménière's disease
    Motion sickness
dimercaprol
    Lead poisoning
dimercaptosuccinic acid, see succimer
dinitrochlorobenzene
    Warts
dioctyl sodium sulfosuccinate, see docusate sodium
Dipentum, see olsalazine
diphenhydramine
    Anaphylaxis
    Angioedema
    Barotitis media
    Blastomycosis
    Cryptococcosis
    Dermatitis, contact
    Glossitis
    Herpangina
    Hyperemesis gravidarum
    Insect bites & stings
    Insomnia
    Ménière's disease
    Pemphigoid, bullous
    Pemphigus vulgaris
    Stomatitis
    Torticollis
    Transfusion reaction, hemolytic
    Urticaria
diphenidol
    Ménière's disease
diphenoxylate-atropine
    Diarrhea, acute
    Diarrhea, chronic
    Irritable bowel syndrome
    Ulcerative colitis
diphtheria antitoxin, equine
    Diphtheria
dipivefrin
    Glaucoma, chronic open-angle
dipyridamole
    Kawasaki syndrome
    Myeloproliferative disorders
    Scleroderma
    Transient ischemic attack (TIA)
disodium
    Milk-alkali syndrome
disodium etidronate
    Hypercalcemia associated with malignancy

disopyramide
    Atrial fibrillation
    Idiopathic hypertrophic subaortic stenosis (IHSS)
disulfiram
    Alcoholism
Ditropan, see oxybutynin
Diuril, see chlorothiazide
divalproex
    Dissociative disorders
    Hypochondriasis
    Seizure disorders
    Trigeminal neuralgia
DL-carnitine
    Diphtheria
DMSA, see succimer
DNase, see dornase alfa
DNCB, see dinitrochlorobenzene
dobutamine
    Cardiomyopathy, end stage
    Complete atrioventricular (AV) canal
    Congestive heart failure
    Pulmonary edema
    Respiratory distress syndrome, adult
    Shock, circulatory
    Ventricular septal defect (VSD)
docusate sodium
    Constipation
    Hearing loss
    Myocardial infarction
donepezil
    Alzheimer's disease
    Amyloidosis
    Dementia
Donnagel, see kaolin-pectin
Donnatal, see phenobarbital-hyoscyamine-atropine-hyoscine
dopamine
    Anaphylaxis
    Congestive heart failure
    Hepatorenal syndrome
    Insect bites & stings
    Shock, circulatory
    Status epilepticus
    Toxic shock syndrome
    Transfusion reaction, hemolytic
    Ventricular septal defect (VSD)
dornase alfa
    Cystic fibrosis
dorzolamide
    Glaucoma, chronic open-angle
    Glaucoma, primary angle-closure
doxazosin
    Aldosteronism, primary
    Hypertension, essential
    Pheochromocytoma
    Prostatic hyperplasia, benign (BPH)
doxepin
    Depression
    Dermatitis, stasis
    Neurodermatitis
    Post-traumatic stress disorder (PTSD)
    Urticaria
doxorubicin
    Bone tumor, primary malignant
    Gastric malignancy
    Hepatoma

Medication Index

Medication Index

Acne rosacea
Acne vulgaris
Animal bites
Bartonella infections
Blepharitis
Breast abscess
Bronchiolitis obliterans & organizing pneumonia
Cellulitis
Cervicitis
Cervicitis, ectropion & true erosion
Chancroid
Chlamydia pneumoniae
Chlamydial sexually transmitted diseases
Conjunctivitis
Dermatitis, atopic
Dermatitis, contact
Dermatitis, seborrheic
Diarrhea, acute
Diphtheria
Dyspepsia, functional
Erysipelas
Folliculitis
Furunculosis
Gingivitis
Glomerulonephritis, acute
Gonococcal infections
Hearing loss
Herpes eye infections
Hidradenitis suppurativa
Hordeolum (stye)
Impetigo
Laryngitis
Legionnaires' disease
Listeriosis
Lymphogranuloma venereum
Mitral stenosis
Nocardiosis
Paronychia
Pelvic inflammatory disease (PID)
Pertussis
Pharyngitis
Pneumonia, bacterial
Pneumonia, mycoplasma
Prostatitis
Pseudofolliculitis barbae
Psittacosis
Rape crisis syndrome
Scarlet fever
Sialadenitis
Syphilis
Typhus fevers
Urethritis
Vulvovaginitis, prepubescent
erythromycin-sulfisoxazole
    Otitis media
erythropoietin
    Renal failure, chronic
Eskalith, see lithium
Estar, see coal tar
Estrace, see estradiol
Estraderm, see estradiol
estradiol
    Anorexia nervosa
    Hyperparathyroidism
    Menopause

    Vulvovaginitis, estrogen deficient
estrogen
    Artificial insemination
    Hirsutism
estrogen, conjugated
    Amenorrhea
    Cervicitis, ectropion & true erosion
    Dysfunctional uterine bleeding (DUB)
    Menopause
    Menorrhagia
    Vulvovaginitis, estrogen deficient
    Vulvovaginitis, prepubescent
estropipate
    Menopause
ethacrynic acid
    Hypertension, essential
ethambutol
    Arthritis, infectious, granulomatous
    Tuberculosis
ethinyl estradiol
    Contraception
    Dysfunctional uterine bleeding (DUB)
ethionamide
    Leprosy
ethosuximide
    Seizure disorders
ethylestrenol
    Thrombophlebitis, superficial
etidronate
    Osteitis deformans
    Osteoporosis
etomidate
    Status epilepticus
etoposide
    Bone tumor, primary malignant
    Breast cancer
    Cervical malignancy
    Gastric malignancy
    Neuroblastoma
    Ovarian cancer
    Testicular malignancies
    Vaginal malignancy
etretinate
    Arthritis, psoriatic
    Cutaneous T cell lymphoma
    Dermatitis, exfoliative
    Lichen planus
    Lupus erythematosus, discoid
    Psoriasis
Eulexin, see flutamide
Eurax, see crotamiton
Ex-Lax, see phenolphthalein
Exelderm, see sulconazole
Exosurf, see colfosceril
factor IX
    Hemophilia
factor VIII
    Hemophilia
factor XIII
    Schönlein-Henoch purpura
famciclovir
    Chickenpox
    Cytomegalovirus inclusion disease
    Hepatitis, viral
    Herpes simplex

Medication Index

Herpes zoster
Herpes, genital
famotidine
    Burns
    Dysphagia
    Gastritis
    Gastroesophageal reflux disease
    Peptic ulcer disease
    Zollinger-Ellison syndrome
Famvir, see famciclovir
Fansidar, see sulfadoxine-pyrimethamine
felbamate
    Seizure disorders
Felbatol, see felbamate
Feldene, see piroxicam
felodipine
    Hypertension, essential
fenfluramine
    Autism
    Obesity
fenoprofen
    Headache, tension
ferriprotoporphyrin IX
    Porphyria
ferrous sulfate
    Iron deficiency anemia
fexofenadine
    Angioedema
    Barotitis media
    Rhinitis, allergic
    Urticaria
Fibercon, see polycarbophil
fibrinolysin-deoxyribonuclease
    Pressure ulcer
finasteride
    Prostatic hyperplasia, benign (BPH)
    Urinary incontinence
Fioricet, see acetaminophen-butalbital
Fiorinal #3, see acetaminophen-butalbital-codeine
Fiorinal #4, see acetaminophen-butalbital-codeine
fish oil
    Hypertriglyceridemia
Flagyl, see metronidazole
flavoxate
    Bladder injury
    Urinary incontinence
flecainide
    Atrial fibrillation
Fleet's, see sodium phosphate
Flexeril, see cyclobenzaprine
Floxin, see ofloxacin
fluconazole
    Candidiasis
    Candidiasis, mucocutaneous
    Coccidioidomycosis
    Cryptococcosis
    Histoplasmosis
    Onychomycosis
    Paronychia
    Sporotrichosis
    Tinea cruris
    Vulvovaginitis, candidal
flucytosine
    Arthritis, infectious, granulomatous
    Cryptococcosis

fludarabine
    Leukemia
fludrocortisone
    Addison's disease
    Carotid sinus syndrome
    Renal tubular acidosis (RTA)
Flumadine, see rimantadine
flumazenil
    Hepatic encephalopathy
flunisolide
    Chronic obstructive pulmonary disease & emphysema
    Rhinitis, allergic
fluocinonide
    Dermatitis, contact
fluorouracil
    Breast cancer
    Cervical dysplasia
    Cervical malignancy
    Condyloma acuminata
    Gastric malignancy
    Hepatoma
    Insulinoma
    Keratosis, actinic
    Ovarian cancer
    Vaginal malignancy
    Vulvar malignancy
    Warts
    Zollinger-Ellison syndrome
fluoxetine
    Anorexia nervosa
    Anxiety
    Autism
    Bulimia nervosa
    Dementia
    Depression
    Hypochondriasis
    Narcolepsy
    Obsessive compulsive disorder
    Post-traumatic stress disorder (PTSD)
    Premenstrual syndrome (PMS)
    Sleep apnea, obstructive
    Suicide
    Tourette's syndrome
fluphenazine
    Tourette's syndrome
flurazepam
    Fibromyalgia
    Insomnia
    Stroke rehabilitation
flurbiprofen
    Metatarsalgia
flutamide
    Hirsutism
    Prostatic cancer
    Prostatic hyperplasia, benign (BPH)
fluvastatin
    Arteriosclerotic heart disease
    Hypercholesterolemia
    Hypertriglyceridemia
fluvoxamine
    Bulimia nervosa
    Dementia
    Dissociative disorders
    Hypochondriasis
    Post-traumatic stress disorder (PTSD)

Medication Index

folic acid
  Anemia, sickle cell
  Fragile X syndrome
  Thalassemia
  Tropical sprue
folinic acid, see leucovorin
follicle-stimulating hormone
  Polycystic ovarian disease
Fortaz, see ceftazidime
Forvade, see cidofovir gel
Fosamax, see alendronate
foscarnet
  Herpes, genital
  Kaposi's sarcoma
  Pneumonia, viral
Foscavir, see foscarnet
fosinopril
  Hypertension, essential
fosphenytoin
  Status epilepticus
Fostril, see sulfur
framycetin
  Conjunctivitis
Fungizone, see amphotericin B
furazolidone
  Cholera
  Giardiasis
  Intestinal parasites
  Salmonella infection
  Typhoid fever
furosemide
  Ascites
  Asthma
  Cardiomyopathy, end stage
  Cirrhosis of the liver
  Complete atrioventricular (AV) canal
  Congestive heart failure
  Cor pulmonale
  Glomerulonephritis, acute
  Hyperparathyroidism
  Hypertension, essential
  Inappropriate secretion of antidiuretic hormone
  Milk-alkali syndrome
  Nephrotic syndrome
  Portal hypertension
  Pulmonary edema
  Renal failure, acute (ARF)
  Renal tubular acidosis (RTA)
  Subdural hematoma
  Transfusion reaction, hemolytic
Furoxone, see furazolidone
G-CSF, see granulocyte colony stimulating factor
gabapentin
  Porphyria
  Seizure disorders
gallium nitrate
  Hypercalcemia associated with malignancy
gamma globulin, see immune globulin, intravenous
gamma-hydroxybutyrate
  Narcolepsy
Gamulin Rh, see rho(D) immune globulin
ganciclovir
  Cytomegalovirus inclusion disease
  Kaposi's sarcoma
  Pneumonia, viral

Garamycin, see gentamicin
Gaviscon, see alumina-magnesium
gemfibrozil
  Arteriosclerotic heart disease
  Hypertriglyceridemia
gentamicin
  Anaerobic & necrotizing infections
  Appendicitis, acute
  Arthritis, infectious, bacterial
  Cellulitis
  Cellulitis, periorbital & orbital
  Cholecystitis
  Conjunctivitis
  Corneal ulceration
  Dermatitis, contact
  Diverticular disease
  Endocarditis, infective (part 2)
  Epididymitis
  Hearing loss
  Hordeolum (stye)
  Listeriosis
  Pelvic inflammatory disease (PID)
  Peritonitis, acute
  Pressure ulcer
  Prostatitis
  Puerperal infection
  Pyelonephritis
  Sepsis
  Subphrenic abscess
  Thrombophlebitis, superficial
  Tularemia
gentian violet
  Vulvovaginitis, candidal
glimepiride
  Diabetes mellitus, non-insulin dependent (NIDDM)
glipizide
  Diabetes mellitus, non-insulin dependent (NIDDM)
glucagon
  Anaphylaxis
  Hypoglycemia, diabetic
  Hypoglycemia, nondiabetic
  Insulinoma
Glucantime, see meglumine antimoniate
Glucotrol, see glipizide
glutaraldehyde
  Onychomycosis
Gly-Oxide, see carbamide peroxide
glyburide
  Diabetes mellitus, non-insulin dependent (NIDDM)
glycerin
  Glaucoma, primary angle-closure
glycolic acid
  Pseudofolliculitis barbae
glycopyrrolate
  Chronic obstructive pulmonary disease & emphysema
glypressin
  Portal hypertension
GM-CSF, see granulocyte-macrophage colony stimulating factor
gold
  Arthritis, juvenile rheumatoid (JRA)
  Arthritis, psoriatic
  Pemphigus vulgaris
GoLYTELY, see polyethylene glycol
goserelin
  Dysfunctional uterine bleeding (DUB)

Medication Index

Medication Index

Medication Index

Tendinitis
influenza vaccine
    Cystic fibrosis
    Influenza
INH, see isoniazid
insulin
    Diabetes mellitus, insulin-dependent (IDDM or Type I)
    Diabetic ketoacidosis (DKA)
    Hyperkalemia
    Rhabdomyolysis
interferon
    Chickenpox
    Cirrhosis of the liver
    Common cold
    Condyloma acuminata
    Cutaneous T cell lymphoma
    Idiopathic thrombocytopenic purpura (ITP)
    Kaposi's sarcoma
    Leukemia
    Macular degeneration, age-related (ARMD)
    Myelodysplastic syndromes (MDS)
    Myeloproliferative disorders
    Nephrotic syndrome
    Polycythemia vera
    Warts
    Zollinger-Ellison syndrome
interferon alfa-2a
    Hepatitis, viral
interferon alfa-2b
    Hepatitis, viral
interferon beta
    Multiple sclerosis
interferon gamma
    Leishmaniasis
interleukin-2
    Cutaneous T cell lymphoma
    Renal cell adenocarcinoma
interleukin-3
    Myelodysplastic syndromes (MDS)
Intron A, see interferon alfa-2b
Invirase, see saquinavir
iodide
    Arthritis, infectious, granulomatous
iodoquinol
    Amebiasis
    Balantidiasis
    Intestinal parasites
Iodotope I-131, see sodium iodine131
Iopidine, see apraclonidine
ipecac
    Acetaminophen poisoning
    Iron toxicity, acute
    Salicylate poisoning
ipodate sodium
    Hyperthyroidism
ipratropium
    Asthma
    Chronic obstructive pulmonary disease & emphysema
isoetharine
    Chronic obstructive pulmonary disease & emphysema
isoflurane
    Status epilepticus
isoflurophate
    Glaucoma, chronic open-angle
isometheptene - dichloralphenazone - acetaminophen

Headache, tension
    Migraine
isoniazid
    Amyloidosis
    Arthritis, infectious, granulomatous
    Silicosis
    Tuberculosis
isoproterenol
    Asthma
    Cardiac tamponade
    Primary pulmonary hypertension
    Stokes-Adams attacks
Isoptin, see verapamil
Isopto, see homatropine hydrobromide
isosorbide dinitrate
    Cardiomyopathy, end stage
    Complete atrioventricular (AV) canal
    Congestive heart failure
    Glaucoma, primary angle-closure
    Pulmonary edema
isotretinoin
    Acne rosacea
    Acne vulgaris
    Dermatitis, exfoliative
    Granuloma annulare
    Hidradenitis suppurativa
    Lichen planus
    Psoriasis
isoxsuprine
    Abortion, spontaneous
    Abruptio placentae
    Placenta previa
isradipine
    Hypertension, essential
    Migraine
itraconazole
    Aspergillosis
    Blastomycosis
    Histoplasmosis
    Onychomycosis
    Paronychia
    Sporotrichosis
    Tinea capitis
    Tinea corporis
    Tinea cruris
    Tinea pedis
ivermectin
    Roundworms, tissue
IVIG, see immune globulin, intravenous
kaolin-pectin
    Diarrhea, chronic
    Glossitis
Kaopectate, see attapulgite
Kapectolin, see kaolin-pectin
Kayexalate, see sodium polystyrene sulfonate
Keflex, see cephalexin
Keflin, see cephalothin
Kenalog in Orabase, see triamcinolone
Kenalog, see triamcinolone
ketamine
    Status epilepticus
ketoconazole
    Alopecia
    Arthritis, infectious, granulomatous
    Blastomycosis

Medication Index

Medication Index

liothyronine
  Thyroid malignant neoplasia
Lipitor, see atorvastatin
liposomal MTP-PE, see liposome-encapsulated muramyl tripeptide phosphatidylethanolamine
liposome-encapsulated muramyl tripeptide phosphatidylethanolamine
  Bone tumor, primary malignant
Liquimat, see alcohol-sulfur
liquor Carbonic Detergens
  Dermatitis, seborrheic
lisinopril
  Hypertension, essential
  Pulmonary edema
  Retinopathy, diabetic
  Ventricular septal defect (VSD)
lithium
  Brain injury, traumatic
  Bulimia nervosa
  Dissociative disorders
  Headache, cluster
  Hypochondriasis
  Inappropriate secretion of antidiuretic hormone
  Multiple sclerosis
  Suicide
Lo/Ovral, see norgestrel-ethinyl estradiol
Lomotil, see diphenoxylate-atropine
lomustine
  Renal cell adenocarcinoma
loperamide
  Diarrhea, acute
  Diarrhea, chronic
  Irritable bowel syndrome
  Ulcerative colitis
Lopid, see gemfibrozil
Lopressor, see metoprolol
Loprox, see ciclopirox
loratadine
  Angioedema
  Barotitis media
  Urticaria
lorazepam
  Alcoholism
  Anxiety
  Dementia
  Eclampsia (toxemia of pregnancy)
  Jet lag
  Myocardial infarction
  Neurodermatitis
  Schizophrenia
  Status epilepticus
  Suicide
losartan
  Hypertension, essential
Lotrimin, see clotrimazole
lovastatin
  Angina
  Arteriosclerotic heart disease
  Hypercholesterolemia
  Hypertriglyceridemia
Lovenox, see enoxaparin
Luminal, see phenobarbital
Lupron, see leuprolide
luteinizing hormone releasing hormone
  Uterine myomas

Luvox, see fluvoxamine
lymphokine-activated killer
  Renal cell adenocarcinoma
mafenide
  Burns
Magic Shave, see barium sulfide
magnesium
  Premenstrual syndrome (PMS)
magnesium citrate
  Constipation
magnesium hydroxide
  Peptic ulcer disease
magnesium salicylate
  Arthritis, osteo
magnesium sulfate
  Cardiac arrest
  Eclampsia (toxemia of pregnancy)
  Hypothermia
  Preeclampsia
  Premature labor
  Radiation sickness
malt soup extract
  Encopresis
Maltsupex, see malt soup extract
mannitol
  Brain injury, traumatic
  Burns
  Cryptococcosis
  Glaucoma, primary angle-closure
  Hypokalemic periodic paralysis
  Ocular chemical burns
  Renal failure, acute (ARF)
  Reye's syndrome
  Rhabdomyolysis
  Subdural hematoma
maprotiline
  Post-traumatic stress disorder (PTSD)
Marinol, see dronabinol
masoprocol
  Keratosis, actinic
Maxair, see pirbuterol
mazindol
  Obesity
mebendazole
  Intestinal parasites
  Pinworms
  Roundworms, intestinal
  Roundworms, tissue
  Trichinosis
mechlorethamine
  Cutaneous T cell lymphoma
  Hodgkin's disease
meclizine
  Hyperemesis gravidarum
  Labyrinthitis
  Ménière's disease
  Motion sickness
medroxyprogesterone
  Amenorrhea
  Breast cancer
  Contraception
  Dysfunctional uterine bleeding (DUB)
  Endometriosis
  Herpes eye infections
  Hirsutism

Medication Index

Menopause
Menorrhagia
Polycystic ovarian disease
Sleep apnea, obstructive
Uterine myomas
Vulvovaginitis, estrogen deficient
mefenamic acid
    Dysfunctional uterine bleeding (DUB)
    Menorrhagia
mefloquine
    Malaria
Mefoxin, see cefoxitin
Megace, see megestrol
megestrol
    Endometriosis
    Menorrhagia
    Uterine corpus malignancy
meglumine antimoniate
    Leishmaniasis
melatonin
    Insomnia
    Jet lag
Mellaril, see thioridazine
melphalan
    Amyloidosis
    Multiple myeloma
    Neuroblastoma
    Ovarian cancer
menotropins
    Artificial insemination
    Fertility problems
    Polycystic ovarian disease
meperidine
    Anemia, sickle cell
    Blastomycosis
    Diverticular disease
    Epstein-Barr virus infections
    Insect bites & stings
    Pancreatitis
    Peritonitis, acute
    Renal calculi
    Urolithiasis
Mepron, see atovaquone
mercaptopurine
    Crohn's disease
    Leukemia
    Leukemia, acute lymphoblastic in adults (ALL)
    Ulcerative colitis
mesalamine
    Crohn's disease
    Ulcerative colitis
mesna
    Bone tumor, primary malignant
    Cervical malignancy
    Neuroblastoma
    Ovarian cancer
    Testicular malignancies
mestranol
    Contraception
Metamucil, see psyllium
metaproterenol
    Chronic obstructive pulmonary disease & emphysema
    Cor pulmonale
    Near drowning
metaraminol

Priapism
metformin
    Diabetes mellitus, non-insulin dependent (NIDDM)
    Hirsutism
methadone
    Substance abuse
methazolamide
    Glaucoma, chronic open-angle
    Herpes eye infections
    Ocular chemical burns
methdilazine
    Rhinitis, allergic
Methergine, see methylergonovine
methimazole
    Hyperthyroidism
    Thyroiditis
methionine, see racemethionine
methocarbamol
    Bruxism
methotrexate
    Amyloidosis
    Arthritis, juvenile rheumatoid (JRA)
    Arthritis, psoriatic
    Arthritis, rheumatoid (RA)
    Asthma
    Behçet's syndrome
    Bone tumor, primary malignant
    Breast cancer
    Crohn's disease
    Cutaneous T cell lymphoma
    Dermatitis, exfoliative
    Ectopic pregnancy
    Gastric malignancy
    Leukemia
    Leukemia, acute lymphoblastic in adults (ALL)
    Pemphigus vulgaris
    Polymyositis/dermatomyositis
    Psoriasis
    Reiter's syndrome
    Sarcoidosis
    Systemic lupus erythematosus (SLE)
    Ulcerative colitis
    Wegener's granulomatosis
methoxsalen
    Vitiligo
methyl tert-butyl ether
    Cholelithiasis
methylcellulose
    Constipation
    Encopresis
methyldopa
    Aortic dissection
    Hypertension, essential
    Raynaud's phenomenon
methylergonovine
    Abortion, spontaneous
methylphenidate
    Attention deficit hyperactivity disorder
    Brain injury, traumatic
    Narcolepsy
methylprednisolone
    Anaphylaxis
    Asthma
    Cervical hyperextension injuries
    Cervical spine injury

Medication Index

Cervical spondylosis
Chronic obstructive pulmonary disease & emphysema
Lichen planus
Multiple sclerosis
Optic neuritis
Pseudogout (CPPD)
Tendinitis
methysergide
    Colorectal malignancy
    Headache, cluster
    Migraine
metipranolol
    Glaucoma, chronic open-angle
metoclopramide
    Bone tumor, primary malignant
    Breast cancer
    Cervical malignancy
    Dyspepsia, functional
    Dysphagia
    Esophageal tumors
    Gastric malignancy
    Gastroesophageal reflux disease
    Hiccups
    Migraine
    Neuroblastoma
    Ovarian cancer
    Testicular malignancies
    Uterine corpus malignancy
    Vaginal malignancy
metolazone
    Congestive heart failure
    Nephrotic syndrome
    Pulmonary edema
metoprolol
    Angina
    Atrial fibrillation
    Hypertension, essential
    Migraine
    Myocardial infarction
    Pheochromocytoma
Metrodin, see follicle-stimulating hormone
metronidazole
    Acne rosacea
    Amebiasis
    Anaerobic & necrotizing infections
    Appendicitis, acute
    Brain abscess
    Cellulitis
    Cervicitis
    Cervicitis, ectropion & true erosion
    Cholangitis
    Congenital megacolon
    Crohn's disease
    Diarrhea, acute
    Diverticular disease
    Gastritis
    Giardiasis
    Gonococcal infections
    Hepatic encephalopathy
    Intestinal parasites
    Lung abscess
    Pelvic inflammatory disease (PID)
    Peptic ulcer disease
    Peritonitis, acute
    Pseudomembranous colitis

    Puerperal infection
    Subphrenic abscess
    Trichomoniasis
    Urethritis
    Vulvovaginitis, bacterial
    Vulvovaginitis, prepubescent
metyrapone
    Cushing's disease and syndrome
metyrosine
    Pheochromocytoma
Mevacor, see lovastatin
Mezlin, see mezlocillin
mezlocillin
    Anaerobic & necrotizing infections
    Pneumonia, bacterial
    Puerperal infection
    Subphrenic abscess
MgSO4, see magnesium sulfate
Miacalcin Nasal Spray, see calcitonin
Miacalcin, see calcitonin
Micatin, see miconazole
miconazole
    Candidiasis, mucocutaneous
    Corneal ulceration
    Dermatitis, diaper
    Onychomycosis
    Pressure ulcer
    Tinea corporis
    Tinea cruris
    Tinea pedis
    Tinea versicolor
    Vulvovaginitis, candidal
    Vulvovaginitis, prepubescent
Micronase, see glyburide
Microsulfon, see sulfadiazine
micrurus fulvius antivenin
    Snake envenomations: Elapidae
Midamor, see amiloride
midazolam
    Status epilepticus
Midrin, see isometheptene - dichloralphenazone - acetaminophen
milk of magnesia
    Constipation
    Myocardial infarction
milrinone
    Cardiomyopathy, end stage
mineral oil
    Encopresis
    Rectal prolapse
Minipress, see prazosin
Minocin, see minocycline
minocycline
    Hidradenitis suppurativa
    Nocardiosis
minoxidil
    Alopecia
    Hypertension, essential
misoprostol
    Arthritis, osteo
    Arthritis, rheumatoid (RA)
    Gastritis
    Peptic ulcer disease
Mithracin, see plicamycin
mithramycin, see plicamycin

Medication Index

mitomycin
    Breast cancer
    Gastric malignancy
mitotane
    Cushing's disease and syndrome
Mitrolan, see polycarbophil
Modane, see phenolphthalein
mometasone
    Psoriasis
Monistat-Derm, see miconazole
Monistat, see miconazole
monopotassium phosphate
    Milk-alkali syndrome
morphine
    Anemia, sickle cell
    Brain injury, traumatic
    Burns
    Congestive heart failure
    Hip fracture
    Insect bites & stings
    Myocardial infarction
    Peritonitis, acute
    Pulmonary edema
    Renal calculi
    Urolithiasis
Motrin, see ibuprofen
Mucomyst, see acetylcysteine
mupirocin
    Dermatitis, diaper
    Folliculitis
    Furunculosis
    Impetigo
    Paronychia
    Pressure ulcer
Mustargen, see mechlorethamine
Mycelex, see clotrimazole
Mycostatin, see nystatin
Mylicon, see simethicone
Mysoline, see primidone
N-acetylcysteine, see acetylcysteine
n-Docosanol
    Herpes simplex
NAC, see acetylcysteine
nadolol
    Atrial fibrillation
    Headache, tension
    Hypertension, essential
    Migraine
    Pheochromocytoma
nafarelin
    Dysfunctional uterine bleeding (DUB)
    Dysmenorrhea
    Endometriosis
    Polycystic ovarian disease
nafcillin
    Anaerobic & necrotizing infections
    Arthritis, infectious, bacterial
    Brain abscess
    Cellulitis
    Cellulitis, periorbital & orbital
    Endocarditis, infective (part 2)
    Osteomyelitis
    Pneumonia, bacterial
    Thrombophlebitis, superficial
    Toxic shock syndrome

    Tracheitis, bacterial
naftifine
    Onychomycosis
    Tinea cruris
    Tinea pedis
Naftin, see naftifine
nalidixic acid
    Pyelonephritis
naloxone
    Cardiac arrest
    Cervical spine injury
    Hypothermia
    Status epilepticus
naltrexone
    Alcoholism
    Substance abuse
    Tourette's syndrome
naphazoline
    Conjunctivitis
Naprosyn, see naproxen
naproxen
    Ankylosing spondylitis
    Arthritis, juvenile rheumatoid (JRA)
    Carpal tunnel syndrome
    Costochondritis
    Dysfunctional uterine bleeding (DUB)
    Dysmenorrhea
    Epididymitis
    Erythema nodosum
    Fever of unknown origin (FUO)
    Headache, tension
    Low back pain
    Menorrhagia
    Metatarsalgia
    Reiter's syndrome
Narcan, see naloxone
Nardil, see phenelzine
Nasacort, see triamcinolone
Nasalcrom, see cromolyn sodium
Nasalide, see flunisolide
Navane, see thiothixene
Nebcin, see tobramycin
nedocromil
    Asthma
nefazodone
    Post-traumatic stress disorder (PTSD)
nelfinavir
    HIV infection & AIDS
Neo-Synephrine, see phenylephrine
Neoloid, see castor oil
neomycin
    Congenital megacolon
    Hepatic encephalopathy
    Hidradenitis suppurativa
    Portal hypertension
neomycin-polymyxin B-bacitracin
    Balanitis
    Conjunctivitis
    Pressure ulcer
neomycin-polymyxin B-hydrocortisone
    Hearing loss
    Mastoiditis
Neosporin, see neomycin-polymyxin B-bacitracin
neostigmine
    Myasthenia gravis

Medication Index

Neptazane, see methazolamide
netilmicin
    Pyelonephritis
Neurontin, see gabapentin
nevirapine
    HIV infection & AIDS
niacinamide
    Granuloma annulare
    Vitamin deficiency
nicardipine
    Hypertension, essential
    Stroke (Brain attack)
    Subarachnoid hemorrhage
niclosamide
    Intestinal parasites
    Tapeworm infestation
nicotinamide
    Diabetes mellitus, insulin-dependent (IDDM or Type I)
nicotinic acid
    Arteriosclerotic heart disease
    Hypercholesterolemia
    Hypertriglyceridemia
nifedipine
    Angina
    Causalgia syndrome
    Cor pulmonale
    Dysmenorrhea
    Dysphagia
    Eclampsia (toxemia of pregnancy)
    Frostbite
    Glomerulonephritis, acute
    Headache, cluster
    Hiccups
    Hypertension, essential
    Premature labor
    Primary pulmonary hypertension
    Raynaud's phenomenon
    Thromboangiitis obliterans (Buerger's disease)
Nilstat, see nystatin
nimodipine
    Cervical spine injury
    Headache, cluster
    Stroke (Brain attack)
    Subarachnoid hemorrhage
Nipride, see nitroprusside
nitrendipine
    Hypertension, essential
nitrogen mustard, see mechlorethamine
nitroglycerin
    Angina
    Congestive heart failure
    Hypertensive emergencies
    Pulmonary edema
    Raynaud's phenomenon
    Ventricular septal defect (VSD)
Nitropress, see nitroprusside
nitroprusside
    Aneurysm of the aorta
    Aortic dissection
    Hypertensive emergencies
    Pheochromocytoma
    Primary pulmonary hypertension
    Pulmonary edema
    Respiratory distress syndrome, adult
    Ventricular septal defect (VSD)

nitrous oxide
    Primary pulmonary hypertension
Nix, see permethrin
nizatidine
    Burns
    Dysphagia
    Gastritis
    Gastroesophageal reflux disease
    Peptic ulcer disease
Nizoral Shampoo, see ketoconazole
Nizoral, see ketoconazole
Noctec, see chloral hydrate
norepinephrine
    Shock, circulatory
norethindrone
    Menorrhagia
    Uterine myomas
norfloxacin
    Cirrhosis of the liver
    Conjunctivitis
    Epididymitis
    Rape crisis syndrome
    Salmonella infection
norgestrel-ethinyl estradiol
    Endometriosis
Normodyne, see labetalol
Noroxin, see norfloxacin
Norplant, see levonorgestrel
Norpramin, see desipramine
nortriptyline
    Dementia
    Depression
    Headache, tension
    Migraine
    Post-traumatic stress disorder (PTSD)
    Premenstrual syndrome (PMS)
Norvir, see ritonavir
NTG, see nitroglycerin
Nulytely, see polyethylene glycol
Nupercainal, see dibucaine
Nuprin, see ibuprofen
nystatin
    Balanitis
    Candidiasis, mucocutaneous
    Congenital megacolon
    Glossitis
    Laryngeal cancer
    Onychomycosis
    Stomatitis
    Vulvovaginitis, prepubescent
octreotide
    Diarrhea, chronic
    Dumping syndrome
    Insulinoma
    Portal hypertension
ofloxacin
    Bartonella infections
    Bronchitis, acute
    Brucellosis
    Cervicitis
    Cervicitis, ectropion & true erosion
    Chlamydial sexually transmitted diseases
    Epididymitis
    Folliculitis
    Gonococcal infections

Medication Index

Legionnaires' disease
Pelvic inflammatory disease (PID)
Salmonella infection
Urethritis
Ogen, see estropipate
olsalazine
Crohn's disease
Proctitis
omeprazole
Diarrhea, chronic
Dyspepsia, functional
Dysphagia
Gastritis
Gastroesophageal reflux disease
Peptic ulcer disease
Zollinger-Ellison syndrome
Oncovin, see vincristine
ondansetron
Bone tumor, primary malignant
Breast cancer
Bulimia nervosa
Cervical malignancy
Gastric malignancy
Hiccups
Neuroblastoma
Ovarian cancer
Testicular malignancies
Uterine corpus malignancy
Vaginal malignancy
Opticrom, see cromolyn sodium
Oragrafin, see ipodate sodium
Ornade, see phenylpropanolamine
Orthocept, see desogestrel-ethinyl estradiol
Ortholinum, see botulinum toxin
Orudis, see ketoprofen
Osteocalcin, see calcitonin
Ovral, see norgestrel-ethinyl estradiol
oxacillin
Blepharitis
Brain abscess
Cellulitis
Cellulitis, periorbital & orbital
Endocarditis, infective (part 2)
oxaprozin
Metatarsalgia
oxazepam
Anorexia nervosa
Myocardial infarction
oxiconazole
Onychomycosis
Tinea cruris
Tinea pedis
Oxistat, see oxiconazole
oxybutynin
Bladder injury
Multiple sclerosis
Urinary incontinence
oxycodone
Arthritis, osteo
oxycodone-acetaminophen
Epididymitis
Meningitis, viral
Pancreatitis
Renal calculi
Urolithiasis

oxymetazoline
Barotitis media
Common cold
oxytetracycline
Tropical sprue
oxytocin
Abortion, spontaneous
Abruptio placentae
paclitaxel
Breast cancer
Ovarian cancer
Pamelor, see nortriptyline
pamidronate
Hypercalcemia associated with malignancy
Osteitis deformans
Osteoporosis
Panafil, see papain
Pancrease MT, see pancreatic enzyme
pancreatic enzyme
Pancreatitis
pancuronium
Brain injury, traumatic
Tetanus
papain
Pressure ulcer
papaverine
Erectile dysfunction
paraldehyde
Seizures, febrile
Status epilepticus
Parlodel, see bromocriptine
paromomycin
Amebiasis
Giardiasis
paroxetine
Anxiety
Bulimia nervosa
Dementia
Depression
Post-traumatic stress disorder (PTSD)
Suicide
Pathocil, see dicloxacillin
Paxil, see paroxetine
PBZ, see tripelennamine
PCE, see erythromycin
Pediazole, see erythromycin-sulfisoxazole
PEG, see polyethylene glycol
pemoline
Attention deficit hyperactivity disorder
Narcolepsy
Pen Vee K, see penicillin V
Pen VK, see penicillin V
penbutolol
Hypertension, essential
pencyclovir
Herpes simplex
penicillamine
Arthritis, juvenile rheumatoid (JRA)
Arthritis, rheumatoid (RA)
Cirrhosis of the liver
Lead poisoning
Scleroderma
Urolithiasis
penicillin
Anemia, sickle cell

Medication Index

Medication Index

Medication Index

Medication Index

Proscar, see finasteride
prostacyclin
  Primary pulmonary hypertension
  Raynaud's phenomenon
prostaglandin E1, see alprostadil
protriptyline
  Depression
  Narcolepsy
  Post-traumatic stress disorder (PTSD)
  Sleep apnea, obstructive
Proventil, see albuterol
Provera, see medroxyprogesterone
Prozac, see fluoxetine
pseudoephedrine
  Barotitis media
  Common cold
  Rhinitis, allergic
  Urinary incontinence
PsoriGel, see coal tar
psyllium
  Anorexia nervosa
  Bulimia nervosa
  Constipation
  Encopresis
  Irritable bowel syndrome
PTU, see propylthiouracil
pyrantel pamoate
  Intestinal parasites
  Pinworms
  Roundworms, intestinal
pyrazinamide
  Arthritis, infectious, granulomatous
  Tuberculosis
pyrethrin
  Pediculosis
pyridostigmine
  Myasthenia gravis
pyridoxine
  Herpes gestationis
  Hyperemesis gravidarum
pyrimethamine
  Brain abscess
  Toxoplasmosis
PZA, see pyrazinamide
Questran, see cholestyramine
quinacrine
  Giardiasis
  Intestinal parasites
  Lupus erythematosus, discoid
quinagolide
  Galactorrhea
  Hyperprolactinemia
quinapril
  Hypertension, essential
quinidine
  Atrial fibrillation
  Malaria
quinine
  Malaria
rabies immune globulin, human
  Rabies
rabies vaccine adsorbed
  Rabies
rabies vaccine, human diploid cell
  Rabies

racemethionine
  Acetaminophen poisoning
raloxifene
  Osteoporosis
ramipril
  Hypertension, essential
ranitidine
  Burns
  Dysphagia
  Gastritis
  Gastroesophageal reflux disease
  Peptic ulcer disease
  Urticaria
  Zollinger-Ellison syndrome
ranitidine bismuth citrate
  Peptic ulcer disease
Redux, see dexfenfluramine
Refresh P.M., see carboxymethylcellulose
Refresh Plus, see hydroxypropyl methylcellulose
Regitine, see phentolamine
Reglan, see metoclopramide
Renova, see tretinoin
Rescriptor, see delaviridine
reserpine
  Aortic dissection
  Huntington's disease
  Hypertension, essential
  Raynaud's phenomenon
resorcinol-sulfur
  Acne rosacea
Resperidol, see resperidone
resperidone
  Alzheimer's disease
Restoril, see temazepam
Retin-A, see tretinoin
retinoic acid, see tretinoin
Retrovir, see zidovudine
ReVia, see naltrexone
Rezamid, see resorcinol-sulfur
RhIG, see rho(D) immune globulin
Rhinocort, see budesonide
rho(D) immune globulin
  Abortion, spontaneous
  Abruptio placentae
  Idiopathic thrombocytopenic purpura (ITP)
  Rh incompatibility
RhoGAM, see rho(D) immune globulin
ribavirin
  Bronchiolitis
  Hepatitis, viral
  Influenza
  Laryngotracheobronchitis
  Measles, rubeola
  Pneumonia, viral
  Respiratory syncytial virus (RSV) infection
riboflavin
  Vitamin deficiency
ricinoleic acid
  Constipation
Rid, see pyrethrin
RIF, see rifampin
Rifadin, see rifampin
rifampicin, see rifampin
rifampin
  Amyloidosis

Medication Index

Arthritis, infectious, granulomatous
Bartonella infections
Brucellosis
Endocarditis, infective (part 2)
Epididymitis
Furunculosis
Impetigo
Legionnaires' disease
Leprosy
Pneumonia, bacterial
Psittacosis
Silicosis
Tuberculosis
riluzole
    Amyotrophic lateral sclerosis
Rimactane, see rifampin
rimantadine
    Hepatitis, viral
    Influenza
    Pneumonia, viral
Risperdal, see risperidone
risperidone
    Autism
    Dissociative disorders
    Schizophrenia
Ritalin, see methylphenidate
ritodrine
    Abruptio placentae
    Placenta previa
    Premature labor
ritonavir
    HIV infection & AIDS
Rocephin, see ceftriaxone
Roferon-A, see interferon alfa-2a
Rogaine, see minoxidil
RSV immune globulin
    Respiratory syncytial virus (RSV) infection
RVA, see rabies vaccine adsorbed
saccharomyces bouldardii
    Pseudomembranous colitis
salicylic acid
    Psoriasis
    Warts
    Warts, plantar
salmeterol
    Asthma
    Chronic obstructive pulmonary disease & emphysema
salsalate
    Arthritis, osteo
    Low back pain
Sandostatin, see octreotide
Sansert, see methysergide
Santyl, see collagenase
saquinavir
    HIV infection & AIDS
Sarna, see hydrocortisone
Scabene, see lindane
scopolamine
    Herpes eye infections
    Labyrinthitis
    Ménière's disease
    Motion sickness
    Ocular chemical burns
    Uveitis
Sebulex, see sulphur-salicylic acid

secnidazole
    Amebiasis
    Diarrhea, acute
Seldane, see terfenadine
selegiline
    Alzheimer's disease
    Narcolepsy
    Parkinson's disease
selenium sulfide
    Tinea versicolor
Semprex, see acrivastine
senna
    Constipation
    Laxative abuse
Senokot, see senna
Septra, see trimethoprim-sulfamethoxazole
Serevent, see salmeterol
sertraline
    Anxiety
    Autism
    Brain injury, traumatic
    Bulimia nervosa
    Dementia
    Depression
    Obsessive compulsive disorder
    Post-traumatic stress disorder (PTSD)
    Premenstrual syndrome (PMS)
    Stroke rehabilitation
    Suicide
SF6, see sulfur hexafluoride
sigma-aminocaproic acid
    Anaphylaxis
silicone oil
    Retinal detachment
Silvadene, see silver sulfadiazine
silver nitrate
    Burns
    Molluscum contagiosum
    Onychomycosis
    Warts
silver sulfadiazine
    Burns
    Herpes zoster
    Pressure ulcer
simethicone
    Colic, infantile
    Irritable bowel syndrome
simvastatin
    Hypercholesterolemia
    Hypertriglyceridemia
Sinemet, see levodopa-carbidopa
Sinequan, see doxepin
Skelid, see tiludronate
SM, see streptomycin
SMX-TMP, see trimethoprim-sulfamethoxazole
sodium antimony gluconate
    Leishmaniasis
sodium bicarbonate
    Cardiac arrest
    Glossitis
    Hydronephrosis
    Hyperkalemia
    Hypernatremia
    Hypothermia
    Near drowning

Medication Index

Medication Index

Pseudogout (CPPD)
sulphur-salicylic acid
    Tinea versicolor
sumatriptan
    Headache, cluster
    Migraine
Suprax, see cefixime
Surgex, see calcium thioglycolate
Surmontil, see trimipramine
Survanta, see beractant
sutilains
    Pressure ulcer
Symmetrel, see amantadine
Synarel, see nafarelin
synthetic analogue, see octreotide
Synthroid, see levothyroxine
T3, see liothyronine
T4, see levothyroxine
Tacaryl, see methdilazine
tacrine
    Amyloidosis
    Dementia
tacrolimus
    Polymyositis/dermatomyositis
    Psoriasis
Tagamet, see cimetidine
talc
    Pneumothorax
Talwin, see pentazocine
tamoxifen
    Breast cancer
    Mastalgia
    Osteoporosis
tamsulosin
    Prostatic hyperplasia, benign (BPH)
TAO, see troleandomycin
Tapazole, see methimazole
Tavist, see clemastine
taxol
    Testicular malignancies
Taxol, see paclitaxel
TCA, see trichloroacetic acid
Tegison, see etretinate
Tegopen, see cloxacillin
Tegretol, see carbamazepine
teicoplanin
    Pseudomembranous colitis
temazepam
    Alzheimer's disease
    Dementia
    Fibromyalgia
    Insomnia
teniposide
    Neuroblastoma
Tenormin, see atenolol
Terazol, see terconazole
terazosin
    Aldosteronism, primary
    Hypertension, essential
    Pheochromocytoma
    Prostatic hyperplasia, benign (BPH)
terbinafine
    Onychomycosis
    Tinea capitis
    Tinea cruris

    Tinea pedis
terbutaline
    Abruptio placentae
    Asthma
    Chronic obstructive pulmonary disease & emphysema
    Placenta previa
    Premature labor
    Primary pulmonary hypertension
terconazole
    Vulvovaginitis, candidal
    Vulvovaginitis, prepubescent
terfenadine
    Angioedema
    Motion sickness
    Rhinitis, allergic
    Urticaria
terlipressin
    Portal hypertension
testosterone
    Pruritus vulvae
testosterone cypionate
    Erectile dysfunction
tetanus immune globulin, human
    Animal bites
    Tetanus
tetanus toxoid
    Animal bites
    Frostbite
    Tetanus
tetrabenazine
    Huntington's disease
tetracycline
    Acne rosacea
    Acne vulgaris
    Arthritis, infectious, granulomatous
    Balantidiasis
    Blepharitis
    Bronchiectasis
    Chlamydia pneumoniae
    Chlamydial sexually transmitted diseases
    Cholera
    Epididymitis
    Gastritis
    Hidradenitis suppurativa
    Intestinal parasites
    Lymphogranuloma venereum
    Malaria
    Pelvic inflammatory disease (PID)
    Peptic ulcer disease
    Plague
    Proctitis
    Prostatitis
    Pseudofolliculitis barbae
    Psittacosis
    Rape crisis syndrome
    Rocky Mountain spotted fever
    Syphilis
    Tropical sprue
    Typhus fevers
thalidomide
    Behçet's syndrome
    Leprosy
    Lupus erythematosus, discoid
    Macular degeneration, age-related (ARMD)
theophylline

Medication Index

Medication Index

Dermatitis, stasis
Dyshidrosis
Gingivitis
Glossitis
Granuloma annulare
Hidradenitis suppurativa
Keloids
Lichen planus
Lupus erythematosus, discoid
Neurodermatitis
Psoriasis
Rhinitis, allergic
triamterene
    Hypertension, essential
    Hypokalemic periodic paralysis
triazolam
    Dementia
    Fibromyalgia
    Insomnia
    Narcolepsy
trichloroacetic acid
    Condyloma acuminata
    Molluscum contagiosum
    Warts
    Warts, plantar
triethanolamine polypeptide oleate-condensate
    Hearing loss
trifluoperazine
    Schizophrenia
    Tourette's syndrome
trifluorothymidine
    Herpes eye infections
    Herpes simplex
trifluridine
    Conjunctivitis
trihexyphenidyl
    Parkinson's disease
trimethaphan
    Aortic dissection
    Hypertensive emergencies
trimethoprim
    Pneumonia, Pneumocystis carinii (PCP)
trimethoprim-sulfamethoxazole
    Arthritis, infectious, granulomatous
    Bronchiectasis
    Bronchitis, acute
    Brucellosis
    Cholera
    Cirrhosis of the liver
    Diarrhea, acute
    Epididymitis
    Intestinal parasites
    Legionnaires' disease
    Listeriosis
    Nocardiosis
    Otitis media
    Pneumonia, bacterial
    Pneumonia, Pneumocystis carinii (PCP)
    Prostatitis
    Pyelonephritis
    Radiation sickness
    Salmonella infection
    Sinusitis
    Typhoid fever
    Urinary tract infection in men

    Urinary tract infection in women
    Vulvovaginitis, prepubescent
    Wegener's granulomatosis
trimetrexate
    Pneumonia, Pneumocystis carinii (PCP)
trimipramine
    Depression
    Post-traumatic stress disorder (PTSD)
tripelennamine
    Rhinitis, allergic
trivalent A-B-E antitoxin
    Botulism
troglitazone
    Diabetes mellitus, non-insulin dependent (NIDDM)
troleandomycin
    Asthma
trypsin
    Pressure ulcer
Tums, see calcium carbonate
turosteride
    Prostatic hyperplasia, benign (BPH)
Tylenol #3, see acetaminophen-codeine
Tylenol, see acetaminophen
Tylox, see oxycodone-acetaminophen
U-100, see insulin
Ultram, see tramadol
Unasyn, see ampicillin-sulbactam
undecylenic acid
    Onychomycosis
    Tinea cruris
Unipen, see nafcillin
Urecholine, see bethanechol
Urispas, see flavoxate
Urocit-K, see potassium citrate
urokinase
    Arterial embolus & thrombosis
    Kawasaki syndrome
    Superior vena cava syndrome
    Thrombosis, deep vein (DVT)
ursodeoxycholic acid
    Cirrhosis of the liver
ursodeoxycholic acid, see ursodiol
ursodiol
    Cholecystitis
    Cholelithiasis
    Cirrhosis of the liver
valacyclovir
    Herpes simplex
    Herpes zoster
    Herpes, genital
Valium, see diazepam
valproic acid
    Causalgia syndrome
    Migraine
    Seizure disorders
    Seizures, febrile
    Status epilepticus
    Suicide
    Trigeminal neuralgia
Valtrex, see valacyclovir
Vancenase AQ, see beclomethasone
Vancocin, see vancomycin
vancomycin
    Brain abscess
    Cellulitis

Medication Index

Cellulitis, periorbital & orbital
Diarrhea, acute
Endocarditis, infective (part 2)
Epididymitis
Hepatic encephalopathy
Impetigo
Meningitis, bacterial
Osteomyelitis
Peritonitis, acute
Pneumonia, bacterial
Pseudomembranous colitis
Sepsis
Toxic shock syndrome
Vantin, see cefpodoxime
Vaponefrin, see epinephrine
Vaqta, see hepatitis A vaccine
varicella-zoster immune globulin
    Chickenpox
Vasocon-A, see antazoline
vasopressin
    Diverticular disease
    Portal hypertension
venlafaxine
    Depression
    Post-traumatic stress disorder (PTSD)
    Suicide
Ventolin, see albuterol
verapamil
    Angina
    Atrial fibrillation
    Headache, cluster
    Hypertension, essential
    Idiopathic hypertrophic subaortic stenosis (IHSS)
    Migraine
    Raynaud's phenomenon
Verelan, see verapamil
Vermox, see mebendazole
Verrusol, see cantharidin
Versed, see midazolam
Vibramycin, see doxycycline
Vicodin, see hydrocodone-acetaminophen
vidarabine
    Chickenpox
    Encephalitis, viral
    Herpes eye infections
    Herpes simplex
    Herpes zoster
    Herpes, genital
Videx, see didanosine
vinblastine
    Breast cancer
    Hodgkin's disease
    Idiopathic thrombocytopenic purpura (ITP)
    Kaposi's sarcoma
    Renal cell adenocarcinoma
vincristine
    Bone tumor, primary malignant
    Hodgkin's disease
    Idiopathic thrombocytopenic purpura (ITP)
    Kaposi's sarcoma
    Leukemia
    Leukemia, acute lymphoblastic in adults (ALL)
    Multiple myeloma
    Neuroblastoma
    Testicular malignancies

    Vaginal malignancy
    Wilms' tumor
Vioform-Hydrocortisone, see clioquinol-hydrocortisone
Vira-A, see vidarabine
Viracept, see nelfinavir
Viramune, see nevirapine
Virazole, see ribavirin
Viroptic, see trifluorothymidine
Vistaril, see hydroxyzine
vitamin A
    Fibrocystic breast disease
    Lacrimal disorders
    Measles, rubeola
    Retinitis pigmentosa
vitamin B-complex
    Glossitis
vitamin B12
    Anemia, pernicious
    Tropical sprue
vitamin B6
    Premenstrual syndrome (PMS)
    Vitamin deficiency
vitamin C
    Common cold
    Furunculosis
    Ocular chemical burns
    Pressure ulcer
    Vitamin deficiency
vitamin D
    Celiac disease
    Hypoparathyroidism
    Nephrotic syndrome
    Osteomalacia & rickets
    Osteoporosis
    Otosclerosis (otospongiosis)
    Renal failure, chronic
    Rhabdomyolysis
    Vitamin deficiency
vitamin E
    Alzheimer's disease
    Fibrocystic breast disease
    Glossitis
    Mastalgia
    Premenstrual syndrome (PMS)
    Vitamin deficiency
vitamin K
    Reye's syndrome
    Vitamin deficiency
Vivactil, see protriptyline
Voltaren, see diclofenac
Vontrol, see diphenidol
VP-16, see etoposide
VZIG, see varicella-zoster immune globulin
warfarin
    Atrial fibrillation
    Hip fracture
    Kawasaki syndrome
    Mitral stenosis
    Mitral valve prolapse
    Nephrotic syndrome
    Primary pulmonary hypertension
    Pulmonary embolism
    Thrombophlebitis, superficial
    Thrombosis, deep vein (DVT)
Wellbutrin, see bupropion

Medication Index

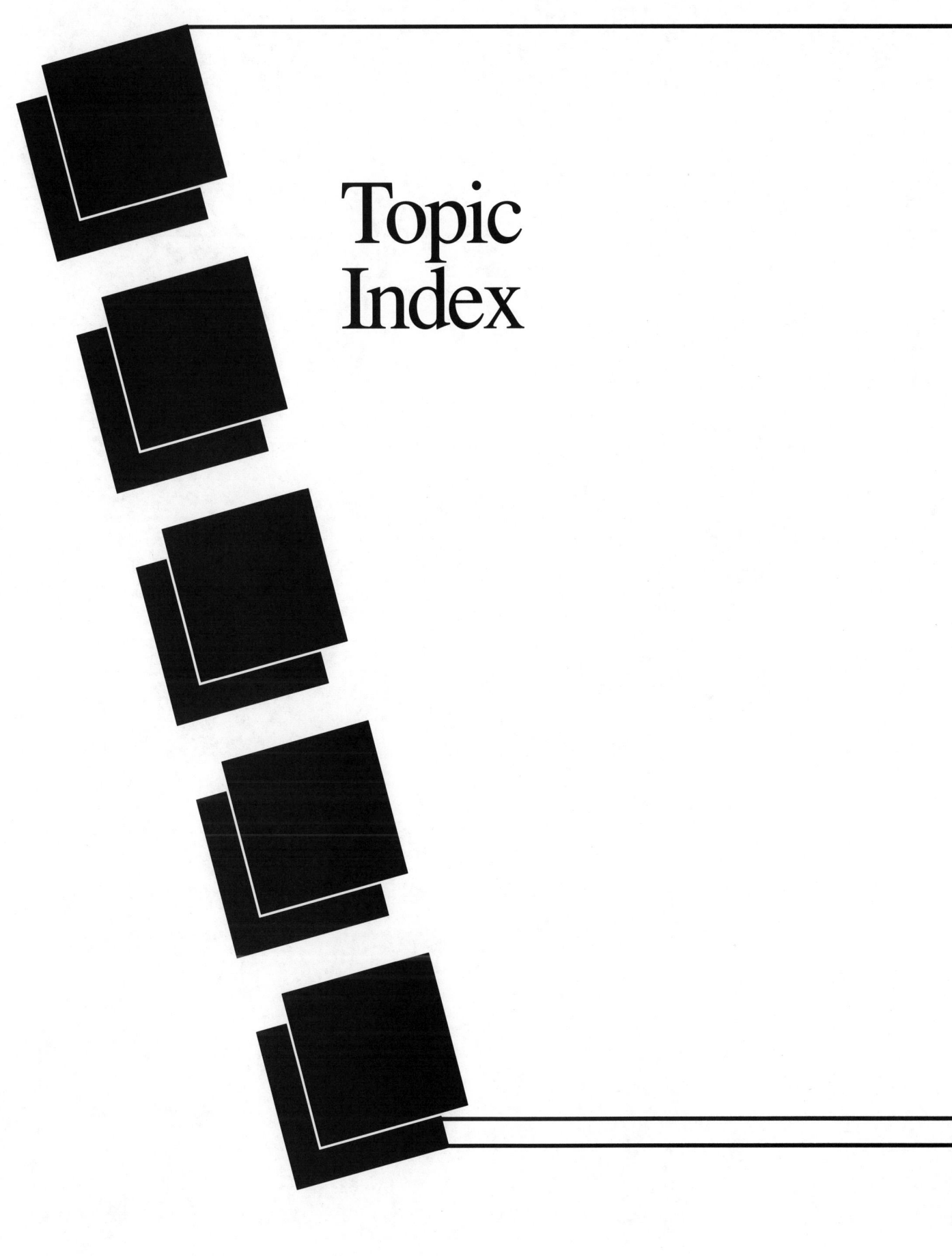

Topic
Index

Topic Index

Topic Index

Topic Index

Topic Index

Topic Index

Topic Index

Topic Index

Topic Index

Topic Index

Topic Index

Topic Index

Topic Index

Topic Index

Topic Index

Topic Index

Topic Index

Topic Index

Topic Index

Topic Index

Topic Index

Topic Index

Topic Index

Topic Index

Topic Index

Topic Index

Topic Index

Topic Index

Topic Index

Topic Index

chronic idiopathic 1203
cyclic 1203
malignant 1176
periodic 1203
nevus
fusco-caeruleus ophthalmo-maxillaris 1203
of ota 1203
newborn
Congenital anemia 382
Hemolytic disease 382
hyperbilirubinemia in the 1194
niacin deficiency disease 1205
NIDDM 310
Diabetes mellitus non-insulin dependent 310
Niemann-Pick disease 1203
nigricans, Acanthosis 1175
nil disease 1199
nine mile fever 1209
Nipple discharge 412
Nitrobenzene poisoning 1204
nitrobenzol toxicity 1204
nitrogen dioxide toxicity 1213
Nocardiosis 722
nocturnal
enuresis, Primary 362
hemoglobinuria, Paroxysmal 1205
upper airway occlusion 988
node syndrome, Mucocutaneous lymph 586
nodosa, Polyarteritis 828
nodosum, Erythema 380, 956
nodules, Milker's 1201
non-Hodgkin's, Lymphoma 1199
non-insulin dependent NIDDM, Diabetes mellitus 310
non-lipid reticuloendotheliosis 1198
Non-organic dyspepsia 342
Non-ulcer dyspepsia 342
Noncardiac pulmonary edema 916
nondiabetic, Hypoglycemia 534
Nonketotic diabetes mellitus 310
nonpuerperal galactorrhea 1190
Nonspecific vaginitis 1150
nonsuppurative pericarditis, Acute 788
nontropical sprue, secondary 1220
North American blastomycosis 128
Nosebleed 370
nuclear jaundice 1197
nutritional macrocytic anemia 1177

-O-

OAD Obstructive airways disease 232
Obesity 724
hypoventilation associated with extreme 1206
obliterans
Arteriosclerosis 1179
Buerger's disease, Thromboangiitis 1054
organizing pneumonia, Bronchiolitis 154
Obliterative bronchiolitis 154
Obsessive
compulsive disorder 726
compulsive neurosis 726
obstruction
Intestinal 572

Superior vena cava 1024
Urinary tract 504
Obstructive
airways disease, OAD 232
cardiomyopathy, Hypertrophic 552
lung disease, Chronic 232
nephropathy 504
pulmonary disease emphysema, Chronic 232
Sleep apnea 988
uropathy 504
occlusion
central retinal vein 1210
Coronary 708
Nocturnal upper airway 988
Retinal vein 1210
Occlusive
arterial disease 104
disease, Atherosclerotic 104
Ocular
chemical burns 728
injuries, Chemical 728
syndrome, Mucocutaneous 122
oculocraniosomatic neuromuscular disease 1196
oculodermal melanocytosis 1203
Oculosympathetic syndrome 498
Ohara's disease 1102
oil of mirbane toxicity 1204
Oliguric renal failure of cirrhosis 468
onset diabetes mellitus, Adult 310
Onychomycosis 730
open-angle, Glaucoma chronic 428
ophthalmia, Egyptian 1217
ophthalmicus, Herpes zoster 472
ophthalmo-maxillaris, nevus fusco-caeruleus 1203
ophthalmoplegia
chronic dystrophic 1208
hereditary external 1196
Progressive external 1208
ophthalmoplegia-plus 1196
Oppenheim-Urbach disease 1202
Optic
atrophy 732
neuritis 734
Oral
cavity neoplasms 736
Leukoplakia 620
rehydration 738
orbital, Cellulitis periorbital 190
organizing
pneumonia, Bronchiolitis obliterans 154
pneumonia, Cryptogenic 154
orgasm
in males, Inhibited 350
Inhibited female 978
origin FUO, Fever of unknown 392
Ornithosis 876
Osgood-Schlatter disease 740
Osler-Weber-Rendu disease 1194
Osteitis
deformans 742
fibrosa cystica 1177
osteo, Arthritis 84
osteoarthropathy, tabetic 1183
Osteoarthrosis 84
Osteochondritis

Topic Index

Topic Index

Topic Index

Topic Index

Topic Index

Topic Index

Topic Index

Topic Index

Topic Index

Topic Index

Topic Index

Topic Index

Topic Index

Topic Index